Part 3

HEART FAILURE

Part 4

RHYTHM AND CONDUCTION DISORDERS

Part 5

SYNCOPE, SUDDEN DEATH, AND CARDIOPULMONARY RESUSCITATION

Part 6

CORONARY HEART DISEASE

HURST'S
THE HEART

NOTICE

Medicine is an ever-changing science. As new research and clinical experience broaden our knowledge, changes in treatment and drug therapy are required. The authors and the publisher of this work have checked with sources believed to be reliable in their efforts to provide information that is complete and generally in accord with the standards accepted at the time of publication. However, in view of the possibility of human error or changes in medical sciences, neither the authors nor the publisher nor any other party who has been involved in the preparation or publication of this work warrants that the information contained herein is in every respect accurate or complete, and they disclaim all responsibility for any errors or omissions or for the results obtained from use of the information contained in this work. Readers are encouraged to confirm the information contained herein with other sources. For example and in particular, readers are advised to check the product information sheet included in the package of each drug they plan to administer to be certain that the information contained in this work is accurate and that changes have not been made in the recommended dose or in the contraindications for administration. This recommendation is of particular importance in connection with new or infrequently used drugs.

HURST'S THE HEART

VOLUME 2

TENTH EDITION

Editors

VALENTIN FUSTER M.D., Ph.D.
Director, The Zena and Michael A. Wiener Cardiovascular Institute
Richard Gorlin, M.D./Heart Research Foundation, Professor of Cardiology, Vice Chairman, Department of Medicine, The Mount Sinai School of Medicine
New York, New York

R. WAYNE ALEXANDER, M.D., PhD.
R. Bruce Logue Professor and Chair
Department of Medicine
Emory University School of Medicine
Atlanta, Georgia

ROBERT A. O'ROURKE, M.D.
Charles Conrad Brown Distinguished Professor in Cardiovascular Disease
University of Texas Health Science Center at San Antonio
San Antonio, Texas

Associate Editors

ROBERT ROBERTS, M.D.
Don W. Chapman Professor of Medicine and Chief of Cardiology
Professor of Cell Biology, Molecular Physiology and Biophysics, Director, Bugher Foundation Center for Molecular Biology in the Cardiovascular System
Baylor College of Medicine
Director, Specialized Center for Research in Heart Failure
Houston, Texas

SPENCER B. KING III, M.D.
J.B. and Dottie Fuqua Chair of Cardiology, The Fuqua Heart Center
Co-Director, Atlanta Cardiovascular Research Institute, Clinical Professor of Medicine
Atlanta, Georgia

HEIN J. J. WELLENS, M.D.
Professor and Chairman of the Department of Cardiology
Academic Hospital Maastricht
Maastricht, The Netherlands

McGRAW-HILL
Medical Publishing Division

New York St. Louis San Francisco Auckland Bogotá Caracas Lisbon London Madrid
Mexico City Milan Montreal New Delhi San Juan Singapore Sydney Tokyo Toronto

McGraw-Hill
A Division of The **McGraw-Hill** *Companies*

Hurst's
THE HEART
Tenth Edition

1234567890 DOWDOW 09876543210

ISBN 0-07-135694-0 (Single vol. ed.)
0-07-135693-2 (2-vol. set ed.)
0-07-135695-9 (Vol. 1)
0-07-135696-7 (Vol. 2)

This book was set in Times Roman by The PRD Group, Inc.
The editors were Darlene B. Cooke, Susan R. Noujaim, and Lester A. Sheinis.
The production supervisor was Richard C. Ruzycka.
The text designer was Marsha Cohen / Parallelogram Graphics.
The cover designer was Aimee Nordin.
The indexer was Irving Condé Tullar.
R. R. Donnelley and Sons Company was printer and binder.

This book is printed on acid-free paper.

Library of Congress Cataloging-in-Publication Data

Hurst's the heart / editors, Valentin Fuster ... [et al.].—10th ed.
p. ; cm.
Rev. ed. of: Hurst's the heart, arteries and veins. 9th ed. © 1998.
Includes bibliographical references and index.
ISBN 0-07-135694-0 (single vol.)—ISBN 0-07-135693-2 (2 vol. set)
1. Cardiovascular system—Diseases. 2. Heart—Diseases. I. Fuster, Valentin. II. Hurst's the heart, arteries and veins
[DNLM: 1. Cardiovascular Diseases. WG 100 H9662 2001]
RC667.H88 2001
616.1—dc21

00-061611

CONTENTS

Part 3

HEART FAILURE

Part 4

RHYTHM AND CONDUCTION DISORDERS

Part 5

SYNCOPE, SUDDEN DEATH, AND CARDIOPULMONARY RESUSCITATION

Part 6

CORONARY HEART DISEASE

Part 13

THE HEART, ANESTHESIA, AND SURGERY

Part 14

MISCELLANEOUS DISEASES AND CONDITIONS

Part 15

DISEASES OF THE GREAT VESSELS AND PERIPHERAL VESSELS

Part 16

COST-EFFECTIVE STRATEGIES, INSURANCE, AND LEGAL PROBLEMS

CONTRIBUTORS

Masood Akhtar, M.D.
Clinical Professor of Medicine
University of Wisconsin Medical School
Milwaukee Clinical Campus
Sinai Samaritan Medical Center
and St. Luke's Medical Center
Milwaukee Heart Institute
Milwaukee, Wisconsin
Chapter 26

R. Wayne Alexander, M.D., Ph.D.
R. Bruce Logue Professor and Chair
Department of Medicine
Emory University School of Medicine
Atlanta, Georgia
Chapters 6 and 42

Jeffrey L. Anderson, M.D.
Professor of Internal Medicine
Chief
Division of Cardiology
University of Utah School of Medicine
University of Utah Medical Center
Salt Lake City, Utah
Chapter 73

David S. Bach, M.D.
Associate Professor of Medicine
University of Michigan School of Medicine
University of Michigan
Ann Arbor, Michigan
Chapter 74

George L. Bakris, M.D.
Professor of Preventive Medicine and Internal Medicine
Vice-Chairman
Department of Preventive Medicine
Director
Hypertension Clinical Research Center
Rush-Presbyterian-St. Luke's Medical Center
Chicago, Illinois
Chapter 51

Ainat Beniaminovitz, M.D.
Assistant Professor of Medicine
Attending Physician
Columbia Presbyterian Medical Center
New York, New York
Chapter 69

Daniel S. Berman, M.D.
Professor of Medicine
University of California School of Medicine
Director, Nuclear Cardiology
Cedars Sinai Medical Center
Cedars-Sinai Medical Center
Los Angeles, California
Chapter 16

Gerald J. Berry, M.D.
Associate Professor of Pathology
Director of Cardiac Pathology
Stanford University School of Medicine
Stanford University Medical Center
Stanford, California
Chapter 22

Alan L. Bisno, M.D.
Professor and Vice-Chairman
Department of Medicine
University of Miami School of Medicine
Chief, Medical Service
VA Medical Center
Miami, Florida
Chapter 55

Henry R. Black, M.D.
Charles J. and Margaret Roberts Professor
Associate Dean for Research
Rush Medical College
Chair
Department of Preventive Medicine
Rush-Presbyterian-St. Luke's Medical Center
Chicago, Illinois
Chapter 51

Daniel G. Blanchard, M.D.
Associate Professor of Medicine
Director
Non-Invasive Cardiac Laboratories
University of California
San Diego Medical Center
UCSD Medical Center
San Diego, California
Chapter 13

Teresa J. Bohlmeyer, M.D.
Assistant Professor of Medicine
University of Colorado
Health Sciences Center
Division of Cardiology
UCHSC
Denver, Colorado
Chapter 66

Wendy M. Book, M.D.
Assistant Professor
Division of Cardiology
Emory University School of Medicine
Atlanta, Georgia
Chapter 71

Harisios Boudoulas, M.D., Ph.D.
Professor of Medicine and Pharmacy
Academician
Division of Cardiology
Ohio State University Medical Center
Director
Overstreet Teaching and Research Laboratory
Division of Cardiology
Ohio State University Medical Center
Columbus, Ohio
Chapter 32

Michael R. Bristow, M.D., Ph.D.
Professor of Medicine
Head
Division of Cardiology
Director
Temple Hoyne Buell Laboratories
Director
Heart Failure Program
Associate Director
Heart Transplant Program
University of Colorado Health Sciences Center
Denver, Colorado
Chapter 66

Bruce R. Brodie, M.D.
Clinical Professor of Medicine
Director
LeBauer Cardiovascular Research Foundation
University of North Carolina Teaching Service
The Moses H. Cone Memorial Hospital
Greensboro, North Carolina
Chapter 46

Christopher P. Cannon, M.D.
Assistant Professor of Medicine
Harvard Medical School
Associate Physician
Cardiovascular Division
Brigham and Women's Hospital
Associate Physical Cardiovascular Division
Brigham and Women's Hospital
Boston, Massachusetts
Chapter 44

Louis R. Caplan, M.D.
Professor of Neurology
Harvard Medical School
Chief
Cerebrovascular Disease
Beth Israel Deaconess Medical Center
Boston, Massachusetts
Chapter 89

Agustin Castellanos, M.D.
Director
Clinical Electrophysiology
Professor of Medicine
University of Miami—Jackson Memorial Hospital
Miami, Florida
Chapters 11, 24, 31

Simon Chakko, M.D.
Professor of Medicine
Department of Medicine
University of Miami School of Medicine
Chief
Cardiology Section
Veterans Affairs Medical Center
Chief
Cardiology Section
VA Medical Center
Miami, Florida
Chapter 55

Nisha Chandra-Strobos, M.D.
Professor and Director
Coronary Intensive Care Unit
Johns Hopkins Hospital
Division of Cardiology
Bayview Medical Center
Baltimore, Maryland
Chapter 34

Pamela Charney, M.D.
Professor of Clinical Medicine
Associate Professor of Clinical Obstetrics
& Gynecology and Women's Health
Director
General Internal Medicine
Women's Health Residency Track
Jacobi Medical Center—Adult Primary Care Pavilion
Bronx, New York
Chapter 87

Melvin D. Cheitlin, M.D.
Emeritus Professor of Medicine–UCSF
San Francisco General Hospital
San Francisco, California
Chapter 70

James T. T. Chen, M.D.
Professor of Radiology
Duke University Medical Center
Durham, North Carolina
Chapter 12

Michael B. Clark, M.D., F.A.C.C.
Chief Medical Director
Senior Vice President
Swiss RE Life & Health
Life Reassurance Corporation
Stamford, Connecticut
Chapter 95

Stephen D. Clements, Jr., M.D.
Professor of Medicine (Cardiology)
Emory University School of Medicine
Atlanta, Georgia
Chapter 49

Denton A. Cooley, M.D.
President and Surgeon-in-Chief
Texas Heart Institute
Surgeon-in-Chief
Texas Heart Institute
Houston, Texas
Chapter 77

Ralph B. D'Agostino, Sr., Ph.D.
Department of Mathematics
Boston University College of Arts and Sciences
Boston, Massachusetts
Chapter 1

Karina W. Davidson, Ph.D.
Assistant Research Professor
Mount Sinai School of Medicine
Integrative Behavioral Cardiology Program
The Zena and Michael A. Wiener Cardiovascular Institute
Mount Sinai Medical Center
New York, New York
Chapter 98

MICHAEL J. DAVIES, M.D.
Professor of Cardiovascular Pathology
St. George's Hospital Medical Center
London, England
Chapter 36

JOHN E. DEANFIELD, M.D.
Professor of Cardiology
Institute of Child Health
University College London
Consultant Cardiologist
Great Ormond Street Hospital for Children
London, United Kingdom
Chapter 64

ANTHONY N. DEMARIA, M.D.
Professor and Chief of Cardiology
University of California San Diego School of Medicine
UCSD Medical Center
San Diego, California
Chapter 13

REGIS DESILVA, M.D.
Associate Professor of Medicine
Harvard Medical School
Director of Medical Education
Cardiovascular Division
Beth Israel Deaconess Medical Center
Boston, Massachusetts
Chapter 29A

THOMAS F. DODSON, M.D.
Associate Professor of Surgery
Vice Chairman of Education
Program Director of General Surgery Residency Program
Emory University School of Medicine
Section of Vascular Surgery
The Emory Clinic
Atlanta, Georgia
Chapter 91

GERALD W. DORN III, M.D.
Professor of Medicine
Staff Cardiologist
University of Cincinnati Medical Center
Cincinnati, Ohio
Chapter 5

JOHN S. DOUGLAS, JR., M.D.
Professor of Medicine
Cardiology
Emory University School of Medicine
Director
Interventional Cardiology and Cardiac Catheterization Laboratories
Cardiac Cath Lab
Emory University Hospital
Atlanta, Georgia
Chapters 15, 40, 45

MARK DOYLE, M.D.
Associate Professor of Medicine
University of Alabama at Birmingham
Birmingham, Alabama
Chapter 18A

VICTOR J. DZAU, M.D.
Hersey Professor of the Theory and Practice of Physic (Medicine) and Chairman of Department of Medicine
Brigham and Women's Hospital
Boston, Massachusetts
Chapter 8

KIM A. EAGLE, M.D.
Albion Walter Henleh Professor of Internal Medicine
Chief
Division of Cardiology and Chief of Clinical Cardiology
Division of Cardiology
University of Michigan Medical Center
Ann Arbor, Michigan
Chapter 74

ROBERT H. ECKEL, M.D.
Professor of Medicine and of Physiology and Biophysics
University of Colorado Health Sciences Center
University of Colorado Health Sciences Center
Denver, Colorado
Chapter 83

WILLIAM D. EDWARDS, M.D.
Professor of Pathology
Mayo Graduate School of Medicine
Consultant in Pathology
Division of Anatomic Pathology
Mayo Clinic
Rochester, Minnesota
Chapter 2

WILLIAM J. ELLIOTT, M.D., Ph.D.
Professor of Preventive Medicine
Internal Medicine, and Pharmacology
Attending Physician
Rush University School of Medicine
Rush-Presbyterian-St. Luke's Medical Center
Chicago, Illinois
Chapter 51

DOMIEN ENGELEN, M.D.
Department of Cardiology
Academic Hospital Maastricht
Maastricht, The Netherlands
Chapter 43

MAURICE ENRIQUEZ-SARANO, M.D., F.A.C.C.
Associate Professor of Medicine
Consultant
Cardiovascular Diseases and Internal Medicine
Mayo Clinic
Rochester, Minnesota
Chapter 57

ERLING FALK, M.D., Ph.D.
Professor
Department of Cardiology Research
AARHUS University Hospital (Skejby)
Aarhus N, Denmark
Chapter 35

MICHAEL E. FARKOUH, M.D., F.R.C.P., M.Sc.
Assistant Professor of Medicine
Mount Sinai School of Medicine
Director
Telemetry Unit
Consultant
Mount Sinai Diabetes
Mount Sinai Medical Center
New York, New York
Chapter 78

ZAHI A. FAYAD, Ph.D.

Assistant Professor
Mount Sinai Medical School
Director
Cardiovascular MRI Research
Mount Sinai Medical Center
New York, New York
Chapter 18B

GERALD F. FLETCHER, M.D.

Professor of Medicine
Mayo Medical School
Jacksonville, Florida
Chapter 85

THOMAS R. FLIPSE, M.D.

Consultant
Cardiovascular Diseases
Mayo Clinic Jacksonville
Jacksonville, Florida
Chapter 85

THOMAS K. F. FOO, Ph.D.

Chief Scientist
Cardiovascular MRI
Development
Applied Science Laboratory
GE Medical Systems
Baltimore, Maryland
Chapter 18B

ROBERT H. FRANCH, M.D.

Professor of Medicine
Emory University School of Medicine
Atlanta, Georgia
Chapter 15

GARY S. FRANCIS, M.D.

Professor of Medicine
Director
Coronary Intensive Care Unit
George M. and Linda H. Kaufman
Center for Heart Failure
The Cleveland Clinic Foundation
Cleveland, Ohio
Chapter 20

O. HOWARD FRAZIER, M.D.

Chief
Cardiopulmonary Transplantation
Director
Surgery Research
Cullen Cardiovascular Research
Laboratories
Texas Heart Institute
Texas Medical Center
Houston, Texas
Chapter 77

MICHAEL D. FREED, M.D.

Associate Professor of Pediatrics
Harvard Medical School
Senior Associate in Cardiology
Children's Hospital
Boston, Massachusetts
Chapter 63

WILLIAM T. FRIEDEWALD, M.D.

Clinical Professor of Medicine and
Public Health
Columbia University School of
Medicine
Public Health Division of Epidemiology
Columbia-Presbyterian Medical Center
New York, New York
Chapter 95

WILLIAM H. FRISHMAN, M.D.

Professor of Medicine and
Pharmacology
Chairman
Department of Medicine
Director of Medicine
Westchester Medical Center
New York Medical College
Valhalla, New York
Department of Medicine
New York Medical College
Valhalla, New York
Chapters 21 and 81

VICTOR F. FROELICHER, M.D.

Professor of Medicine
Stanford University School of Medicine
Division of Cardiovascular Medicine
Director
ECG Exercise Lab
VA Medical Center
Palo Alto, California
Chapter 14

ROBERT L. FRYE, M.D.

Rose M. and Morris Eisenberg
Professor of Medicine
Mayo Clinic
Rochester, Minnesota
Chapter 57

VALENTIN FUSTER, M.D., Ph.D.

Director
The Zena and Michael A. Wiener
Cardiovascular Institute
Richard Gorlin, M.D./Heart Research
Foundation
Professor of Cardiology
Vice Chairman
Department of Medicine
The Mount Sinai School of Medicine
New York, New York
Chapters 18B, 35, 44, 78, 93

JOHN P. GASSLER, M.D.

Fellow
Cardiovascular Diseases
Cleveland Clinic Foundation
Cleveland, Ohio
Chapter 20

WILLIAM GERIN, M.D.

Associate Professor
The Zena and Michael A. Wiener
Cardiovascular Institute
The Mount Sinai School of Medicine
New York, New York
Chapter 98

GUIDO GERMANO, Ph.D.

Director
Nuclear Medicine Physics
Cedars-Sinai Medical Center
Associate Professor of Radiological
Science
University of California Los Angeles
School of Medicine
Los Angeles, California
Chapter 16

GARY GERSTENBLITH, M.D.

Professor of Medicine
The Johns Hopkins School of Medicine
Attending Physician
The Johns Hopkins Hospital
Director
Clinical Trials Cardiology Division
The John Hopkins Hospital
Baltimore, Maryland
Chapter 86

Edward M. Gilbert, M.D.
Associate Professor of Medicine
Director
Heart Failure Treatment Program
Division of Cardiology
University of Utah Health Sciences Center
Salt Lake City, Utah
Chapter 66

Anton P. M. Gorgels, M.D., Ph.D.
Department of Cardiology
Academic Hospital Maastricht
Maastricht, The Netherlands
Chapter 43

Kathy K. Griendling, M.D.
Professor of Medicine
Emory University School of Medicine
Emory University, Cardiology
Atlanta, Georgia
Chapter 6

Scott M. Grundy, M.D., Ph.D.
Professor of Internal Medicine
University of Texas
Southwestern Medical Center at Dallas
Director
Center for Human Nutrition
University of Texas, Southwestern Medical Center at Dallas
Dallas, Texas
Chapter 38

Gary L. Grunkemeier, M.D.
Director
Medical Data Research Center
Providence Health System
Portland, Oregon
Chapter 60

Robert J. Hall, M.D.
Director
Cardiac Education
St. Luke's Episcopal Hospital and Texas Heart Institute
Clinical Professor of Medicine
Baylor College of Medicine and University of Texas Medical School at Houston
St. Luke's Episcopal Hospital
Houston, Texas
Chapter 77

David G. Harrison, M.D.
Professor of Medicine
Emory University
Cardiology
Atlanta, Georgia
Chapter 6

Gerard Helft, M.D., Ph.D., A.C.C.A.
Research Fellow
Mount Sinai School of Medicine
The Zena and Michael A. Wiener Cardiovascular Institute
New York, New York
Chapter 18B

Brian D. Hoit, M.D.
Professor of Medicine
Case Western Reserve University
Co-director of Echocardiography
Attending Physician
University Hospitals of Cleveland
Cleveland, Ohio
Chapters 68 and 72

Larry H. Hollier, M.D., F.A.C.S., F.A.C.C., F.R.C.S. (Eng)
Julius Jacobson II, M.D.
Professor of Surgery
Chairman
Department of Surgery
Mount Sinai School of Medicine
Julius H, Jacobson II, M.D.
Professor of Vascular Surgery
Chairman
Department of Surgery
Mount Sinai Medical Center
New York, New York
Chapter 93

Carl C. Hug, Jr., M.D., Ph.D.
Attending Physician in Cardiothoracic Anesthesiology and Intensive Care
Emory University Hospital
Professor of Anesthesiology and Pharmacology
Emory University Hospital
Atlanta, Georgia
Chapter 49

Sharon A. Hunt, M.D.
Professor, Cardiovascular Medicine
Stanford University
Department of Cardiothoracic Surgery
Stanford, California
Chapter 22

Alberto Interian, Jr., M.D.
Professor of Medicine
Director
Electrophysiology Laboratory
Director
Electropathophysiology Laboratory
University of Miami School of Medicine
Division of Cardiology
Miami, Florida
Chapter 11

Mark E. Josephson, M.D.
Professor of Medicine
Harvard Medical School
Director
Harvard-Thorndike Electrophy
Beth Israel Deaconess Medical Center
Boston, Massachusetts
Chapter 33

William B. Kannel, M.D., M.P.H., F.A.C.C.
Professor of Medicine and Public Health
Boston University School of Medicine
Professor of Medicine and Public Health
Framingham Heart Study
Framingham, Massachusetts
Chapter 1

Samir R. Kapadia, M.D.
Acting Assistant Professor
University of Washington
Interventional Cardiologist
Puget Sound Health Care System
Seattle, Washington
Chapter 92

Joel A. Kaplan, M.D.

Dean
School of Medicine
Vice President for Health Affairs
University of Louisville School of Medicine
University of Louisville School of Medicine
Abell Administration Center
Louisville, Kentucky
Chapter 75

Marinka Kartalija, M.D.

Resident
Department of Internal Medicine
University of Utah School of Medicine
Salt Lake City, Utah
Chapter 73

Bradley B. Keller, M.D.

Chief
Division of Pediatric Cardiology
Director
Pediatric Cardiovascular Research Program
Jennifer Gill, Associate Professor of Pediatrics
Division of Pediatric Cardiology
University of Kentucky College of Medicine
Lexington, Kentucky
Chapter 9

Morton J. Kern, M.D.

Professor of Medicine
Director of Cardiac Catheterization Laboratory
St. Louis University Medical Center
St. Louis, Missouri
Chapter 15

Spencer B. King III, M.D.

Clinical Professor of Medicine
Emory University School of Medicine
J. B. and Dottie Fuqua Chair of Cardiology
The Fuqua Heart Center
Co-director
Atlanta Cardiovascular Research Institute
Atlanta, Georgia
Chapters 15 and 45

E. Martin Kloosterman, M.D.

Servicio de Electrofisiologia
Hospital Naval Pedro Mallo
Hospital Militar Cosme Argerich
Buenos Aires, Argentina
Chapter 24

Harlan Krumholz, M.D., M.Sc.

Associate Professor of Medicine
Cardiology
Yale University of Medicine
New Haven, Connecticut
Chapter 94

Edward G. Lakatta, M.D.

Adjunct Professor of Physiology
University of Maryland School of Medicine
Professor of Medicine
The Johns Hopkins School of Medicine
National Institute on Aging
Gerontology Research Center
Laboratory of Cardiovascular Science
Baltimore, Maryland
Chapter 86

Gaetano Antonio Lanza, M.D.

Assistant Professor
Catholic University of the Sacred Heart
Institute of Cardiology
Catholic University of the Sacred Heart
Rome, Italy
Chapter 37

Thierry H. LeJemtel, M.D.

Professor of Medicine
Albert Einstein College of Medicine
Bronx, New York
Chapter 21

Martin M. LeWinter, M.D.

Professor of Medicine
University of Vermont
Director
Cardiology Unit
University of Vermont
Fletcher Allen Health Care
MCHV Campus
Burlington, Vermont
Chapter 3

Richard P. Lewis, M.D.

Professor of Internal Medicine
Ohio State College of Medicine and Public Health
Columbus, Ohio
Chapter 32

Richard P. Lifton, M.D.

Chairman
Department of Genetics
Professor of Genetics
Internal Medicine and Molecular Biophysics and Biochemistry
Yale University School of Medicine
Associate Investigator
Howard Hughes Medical Institute
Yale University
New Haven, Connecticut
Chapter 7

Joseph Lindsay, Jr., M.D.

Director
Section of Cardiology
Washington Hospital Center
Professor of Medicine
The George Washington University
School of Health Care Sciences
Washington Hospital Center
Washington, District of Columbia
Chapter 88

Bernard Lown, M.D.

Professor of Cardiology (Emeritus)
Harvard School of Public Health
Senior Physician
Brigham and Women's Hospital
Brookline, Massachusetts
Chapter 29A

Bruce W. Lytle, M.D.

Surgeon
Department of Thoracic and Cardiovascular Surgery
The Cleveland Clinic Foundation
Cleveland, Ohio
Chapter 48

John J. Mahmarian, M.D.
Associate Professor of Medicine
Baylor College of Medicine
Assistant Director
Nuclear Cardiology Laboratory
The Methodist Hospital
Section of Cardiology
Baylor College of Medicine
Houston, Texas
Chapter 17

Joseph F. Malouf, M.D.
Associate Professor of Medicine
Cardiovascular Consultant
Mayo Clinic
Rochester, Minnesota
Chapter 2

Donna M. Mancini, M.D.
Associate Professor of Medicine
Medical Director
Cardiac Transplant
New York Presbyterian Hospital
New York, New York
Chapter 69

Michael L. Marin, M.D.
Henry Kaufmann Professor of
Vascular Surgery
Director of Endovascular Surgery
Mount Sinai Medical Center
New York, New York
Chapter 93

Roger R. Markwald, Ph.D.
Professor and Chairman
Department of Cell and Biology and
Anatomy
Medical University of South Carolina
Department of Cell Biology and
Anatomy
Charleston, South Carolina
Chapter 9

Barry J. Maron, M.D.
Director
Cardiovascular Research
Division, Minneapolis Heart Institute
Foundation
Minneapolis, Minnesota
Chapter 67

David J. Maron, M.D.
Assistant Professor of Medicine
Division of Cardiovascular Medicine
Director
Preventive Cardiology
Vanderbilt University Medical Center
Division of Cardiovascular Medicine
Nashville, Tennessee
Chapter 38

Attilio Maseri, M.D.
Professor of Cardiology
Director
Institute of Cardiology
Catholic University of the Sacred Heart
Institute of Cardiology
Rome, Italy
Chapter 37

Jay W. Mason, M.D.
Jack M. Gill Professor and Chairman
Department of Medicine
University of Kentucky
Lexington, Kentucky
Chapter 65

Hugh A. McAllister, Jr., M.D.
Chief
Department of Pathology
St. Luke's Episcopal Hospital
and Texas Heart Institute (Emeritus)
Clinical Professor of Pathology
Baylor College of Medicine
Adjunct Professor of Pathology
University of Texas Medical School
Houston, Texas
Chapter 77

John H. McAnulty, M.D.
Professor and Head of Cardiology
Oregon Health Sciences University
Portland, Oregon
Chapters 61 and 82

William M. McDonald, M.D.
Associate Professor
Department of Psychiatry and
Behavioral Sciences
Emory University School of Medicine
Fuqua Center for Late-Life Depression
Atlanta, Georgia
Chapter 80

James Metcalfe, M.D.
Professor of Medicine (Emeritus)
Oregon Health Sciences University
School of Medicine
Portland, Oregon
Chapter 82

Luisa Mestroni, M.D.
Associate Professor of Medicine
Director
Molecular Genetics
University of Colorado Cardiovascular
Institute
Director
Molecular Genetics
University of Colorado Cardiovascular
Institute
Fitzsimons Hospital
Aurora, Colorado
Chapter 66

William E. Mitch, M.D.
Director
Renal Division
Garland Herndon Professor of Medicine
Emory University School of Medicine
Emory University, Cardiology
Atlanta, Georgia
Chapter 84

Raul D. Mitrani, M.D.
Associate Professor of Medicine
Director
Arrhythmia and Pacemaker Center
University of Miami Medical Center–
Jackson Memorial Hospital
Miami, Florida
Chapter 31

Douglas C. Morris, M.D.
J. Willis Hurst, Professor and Vice
Chair
Department of Medicine
Emory University
Director
Emory Heart Center
Atlanta, Georgia
Chapter 49

Dominique L. Musselman, M.D.
Assistant Professor of Psychiatry
Psychiatry and Behavioral Sciences
Emory University School of Medicine
Atlanta, Georgia
Chapter 80

Robert J. Myerburg, M.D.
Director
Division of Cardiology
Professor of Medicine and Physiology
University of Miami School of Medicine
Division of Cardiology
Miami, Florida
Chapters 11, 24, 31

Elizabeth G. Nabel, M.D.
Scientific Director
Clinical Research Program
National Heart, Lung, and Blood Institute
National Institutes of Health
Bethesda, Maryland
Chapter 8

Ira S. Nash, M.D.
Associate Director
The Zena and Michael A. Wiener Cardiovascular Institute
Assistant Professor of Medicine
Mount Sinai School of Medicine
Mount Sinai Medical Center
New York, New York
Chapters 96 and 97

Steven D. Nelson, M.D.
Associate Professor of Medicine
Director
Cardiac Electrophysiology
Ohio State University Hospitals
Columbus, Ohio
Chapter 32

Charles B. Nemeroff, M.D., Ph.D.
Chair
Reunette W. Harris Professor and Chairman
Department of Psychiatry and Behavioral Sciences
Emory University School of Medicine
Atlanta, Georgia
Chapter 80

John H. Newman, M.D.
Chief of Medical Services
Elsa S. Harrigan Professor of Pulmonary Medicine
VAMC Nashville
Nashville, Tennessee
Chapter 54

Steve E. Nissen, M.D.
Professor of Medicine
Ohio State University
Vice-Chairman
Department of Cardiology
Cleveland Clinic Foundation
Cleveland, Ohio
Chapter 47

R. Joe Noble, M.D., F.A.C.C.
Clinical Professor of Medicine
Indiana University School of Medicine
Consulting Cardiologist
The Care Group
and St. Vincent's Hospital and Health Care Center
Northside Cardiology
Indianapolis, Indiana
Chapter 25

Peter A. O'Callaghan, M.D.
Clinical and Research Fellow in Cardiology
Department of Cardiological Sciences
St. Georges Hospital Medical School
London, England
Chapter 30

William W. O'Neill, M.D., F.A.C.C.
Director
Division of Cardiology
Co-Director
Beaumont Heart Center
William Beaumont Hospital
Royal Oak, Michigan
Chapter 46

Lionel H. Opie, M.D., D.Phil, F.R.C.P.
Professor of Medicine
Co-Director
Cape Heart Centre
University of Cape Town Medical School
Cape Town, South Africa
Chapter 81

Robert A. O'Rourke, M.D.
Charles Conrad Brown, Distinguished Professor in Cardiovascular Disease
University of Texas Health Science Center
San Antonio, Texas
Chapters 10, 40, 58

George Osol, Ph.D.
Professor and Director of Research
Department of Obstetrics and Gynecology
University of Vermont College of Medicine
Burlington, Vermont
Chapter 3

Eegen C. Palma, M.D., F.A.C.C.
Assistant Professor of Medicine
Albert Einstein College of Medicine
Electrophysiologist
Montefiore Medical Center
Division of Cardiology
Bronx, New York
Chapter 28

Stephen O. Pastan, M.D.
Associate Professor of Medicine
Emory University School of Medicine
Atlanta, Georgia
Chapter 84

Thomas A. Pearson, M.D., M.P.H., Ph.D.
Albert D. Kaiser Professor and Chair
Community and Preventive Medicine
Professor of Medicine
University of Rochester School of Medicine and Dentistry Attending Physician
Department of Medicine
Director
Preventive Cardiology Clinic
Co-Director
Stony Heart Program
University of Rochester Medical Center
Rochester, New York
Chapter 38

Thomas G. Pickering, M.D., D.Phil
Professor of Medicine
Director
Integrative and Behavioral Cardiology Program
The Zena and Michael Wiener Cardiovascular Institute
Mount Sinai Medical Center
New York, New York
Chapter 98

Duane S. Pinto, M.D.
Cardiology Fellow
Clinical Instructor in Medicine
Beth Israel Deaconess Medical Center
Divison of Cardiology
Boston, Massachusetts
Chapter 33

Gerald M. Pohost, M.D.
Mary Gertrude Waters Professor of Cardiovascular Medicine
Professor of Medicine and Radiology
University of Alabama
Birmingham, Alabama
Chapter 18A

Paul Poirier, M.D., F.R.C.P.C.
Associate Professor of Medicine
Laval University School of Medicine
Director
Cardiac Rehabilitation Program
Quebec Heart Institute
Laval Hospital
Quebec, Canada
Chapter 83

Michael Poon, M.D.
Assistant Professor of Medicine (Cardiology)
Director of the Mount Sinai Pulmonary Hypertension Program
Medical Director of the Joseph H. Hazen Ambulatory Cardiac Care Center
Mount Sinai Medical Center
New York, New York
Chapter 93

Craig M. Pratt, M.D.
Director
Coronary Care Unit
Professor of Medicine
Baylor College of Medicine
The Methodist Hospital
Houston, Texas
Chapter 42

Eric N. Prystowsky, M.D.
Director
Clinical Electrophysiology Laboratory
St. Vincent Hospital
Indianapolis, Indiana
Consulting Professor of Medicine
Duke University Medical Center
Durham, North Carolina
Northside Cardiology, PC
Indianapolis, Indiana
Chapter 25

Shahbudin H. Rahimtoola, M.D.
George C. Griffith Professor of Cardiology
Division of Cardiology
LAC + USC Medical Center
Los Angeles, California
Chapters 56, 57, 60, 61

Elliot J. Rayfield, M.D.
Clinical Professor of Medicine
Mount Sinai School of Medicine
Attending Physician
Mount Sinai Hospital
New York, New York
Chapter 78

David L. Reich, M.D.
Vice Chair for Academic Affairs
Co-Director of Cardiothoracic Anesthesia
Professor of Anesthesiology
Mount Sinai Medical School
Department of Anesthesiology
New York, New York
Chapter 75

Paul M. Ridker, M.D., M.P.H.
Associate Professor of Medicine
Harvard Medical School
Director
Center for Cardiovascular Disease Prevention
Birgham and Women's Hospital
Harvard Medical School
Boston, Massachusetts
Chapter 38

Stefano Rigattieri, M.D.
Resident in Cardiology
Catholic University of the Sacred Heart
Institute of Cardiology
Rome, Italy
Chapter 37

William C. Roberts, M.D.
Medical Director
Baylor Cardiovascular Institute
Clinical Professor of Medicine
Hahnemann Medical School
Philadelphia, Pennsylvania
Baylor Cardiovascular Institute
Baylor University Medical Center
Dallas, Texas
Chapter 76

Robert Roberts, M.D.
Don W. Chapman Professor of Medicine
Chief of Cardiology
Professor of Cell Biology
Director of Bugher Foundation Center for Molecular Biology
Baylor College of Medicine
Houston, Texas
Chapters 4, 7, 9, 42, 62

Luz-Maria Rodriguez, M.D.

Associate Professor of Cardiology
University of Maastricht
Staff Physician
Cardiology
University Hospital Maastricht
The Netherlands
Maastricht, The Netherlands
Chapter 29

Thom W. Rooke, M.D.

Professor of Medicine
Mayo Clinic
Rochester, Minnesota
Chapter 90

Lewis J. Rubin, M.D.

Professor of Medicine
Director of Pulmonary Critical Care Medicine
University of California San Diego
Director
Division of Pulmonary/Critical Care Medicine
UCSD Medical Center
La Jolla, California
Chapter 52

Jeremy N. Ruskin, M.D.

Director
Cardiac Arrhythmia Service
Massachusetts General Hospital
Associate Professor of Medicine
Harvard Medical School
Boston, Massachusetts
Chapter 30

Thomas J. Ryan, M.D.

Professor of Medicine
Boston University School of Medicine
Senior Consultant
and Emeritus Chief of Cardiology
Boston, Massachusetts
Chapter 42

Merle A. Sande, M.D.

Professor and Chairman
Department of Medicine
Clarence M. and Ruth N. Birrer
Presidential Endowed Chair in Internal Medicine
University of Utah School of Medicine
Salt Lake City, Utah
Chapter 73

Tommaso Sanna, M.D.

Consultant
Catholic University of the Sacred Heart
Institute of Cardiology
Rome, Italy
Chapter 37

Stephen F. Schaal, M.D.

Professor of Medicine
Ohio State University
College of Medicine and Public Health
Columbus, Ohio
Chapter 32

Hartzell V. Schaff, M.D.

Stuart W. Harrington
Professor of Surgery
Division of Cardiology
Mayo Clinic
Rochester, Minnesota
Chapter 57

Melvin M. Scheinman, M.D.

Professor of Medicine
University of California San Francisco
Medical Center
San Francisco, California
Chapter 28

Heinrich R. Schelbert, M.D., Ph.D.

Professor of Pharmacology and Radiological Sciences
Chief
Nuclear Medicine Services
Department of Molecular and Medical Pharmacology
UCLA School of Medicine
Los Angeles, California
Chapter 19

Robert C. Schlant, M.D.

Professor of Medicine (Cardiology)
Emory University School of Medicine
Atlanta, Georgia
Chapter 40

John S. Schroeder, M.D.

Professor of Medicine
Stanford University School of Medicine
Stanford, California
Chapter 22

Steven P. Schulman, M.D.

Associate Professor of Medicine
Director of CCU
The Johns Hopkins University School of Medicine
Baltimore, Maryland
Chapter 86

Robert J. Schwartz, Ph.D.

Professor of Cell Biology
Baylor College of Medicine
Houston, Texas
Chapter 9

James B. Seward, M.D.

Professor of Medicine & Pediatrics
Director
Echocardiography Laboratory
Consultant in Cardiovascular Diseases
Mayo Clinic
Rochester, Minnesota
Chapter 2

James Shaver, M.D.

Professor of Cardiovascular Disease
University of Texas Health Science Center
San Antonio, Texas
Chapter 10

Leslee J. Shaw, M.D.

Associate Professor of Medicine and Health Policy and Management
Director
Technology Evaluation Center
Emory University
Rowland School of Public Health
Atlanta, Georgia
Chapter 16

Halit Silbershatz, Ph.D.

Associate Director of Biometrics
Pfizer Pharmaceuticals, Inc.
New York, New York
Chapter 1

Mark Silverman, M.D.

Professor of Cardiovascular Disease
University of Texas Health Service Center
San Antonio, Texas
Chapter 10

ROBERT B. SMITH III, M.D.
John E. Skandalakis, Professor of Surgery
Emory University School of Medicine
Medical Director
Emory University Hospital
Chief
Vascular Surgery
Atlanta, Georgia
Chapter 91

ANDREW L. SMITH, M.D.
Assistant Professor
Division of Cardiology
Emory University School of Medicine
Medical Director
Heart Failure and Transplant Programs
Emory Health Care
Atlanta, Georgia
Chapter 71

EDMUND H. SONNENBLICK, M.D.
Professor of Medicine
Albert Einstein College of Medicine
Bronx, New York
Chapters 20 and 21

ALBERT STARR, M.D.
Professor of Surgery
Oregon Health Sciences University
Director
Heart Institute
Providence St. Vincent Medical Center
Starr Wood Cardiac Group
Portland, Oregon
Chapter 60

PANAGIOTIS N. SYMBAS, M.D.
Professor of Cardiothoracic Surgery
Emory University
Director of Cardiothoracic Surgery
Grady Hospital
Atlanta, Georgia
Chapter 79

A. JAMIL TAJIK, M.D.
Thomas J. Watson, Jr., Professor of Medicine and Pediatrics
Chair
Division of Cardiovascular Diseases
Consultant
Division of Cardiovascular Diseases
Mayo Clinic
Rochester, Minnesota
Chapter 2

VICTOR F. TAPSON, M.D., F.C.C.P.
Associate Professor
Division of Pulmonary and Critical Care
Director
Lung Transplant Program
Duke University Medical Center
Durham, North Carolina
Chapter 53

THOMAS J. THOM, B.A.
Epidemiology and Biometry Program
Division of Heart and Vascular Diseases
National Heart, Lung, and Blood Institutes
Bethesda, Maryland
Chapter 1

CARL TIMMERMANS, M.D.
Associate Professor of Cardiology
University of Maastricht
Staff Physician
Cardiology
University Hospital Maastricht
Maastricht, The Netherlands
Chapter 29

JEFFREY A. TOWBIN, M.D.
Professor of Pediatrics (Cardiology) and Molecular and Human Genetics
Associate Chief
Pediatrics Director
Heart Failure and Transplant Program
Texas Children's Hospital Foundation
Chair
Pediatric Molecular Cardiac Research
Molecular and Human Genetics
Baylor College of Medicine
Houston, Texas
Chapter 62

KENT VELAND, M.D.
Professor Emeritus
Department of OB/GYN
Stanford University School of Medicine
Stanford, California
Chapter 82

ALBERT L. WALDO, M.D.
The Walter H. Pritchard Professor of Cardiology and Professor of Medicine
Case Western Reserve University
Cleveland, Ohio
Director
Cardiac Electrophysiology Program
Division of Cardiology
University Hospitals of Cleveland
Cleveland, Ohio
Chapter 23

BRUCE F. WALLER, M.D.
Clinical Professor of Medicine and Pathology
Indiana University School of Medicine
Director
Cardiovascular Pathology Registry
St. Vincent Hospital
Cardiologist
The Care Group
Medical Director
The Care Group Laboratory
Indianapolis, Indiana
Chapter 39

RICHARD A. WALSH, M.D.
John H. Hord Professor
and Chairman of the Department of Medicine
Case Western Reserve University
Physician-in-Chief
University Hospitals of Cleveland
Cleveland, Ohio
Chapter 5

CAROLE A. WARNES, M.D., M.R.C.P., F.A.C.C.
Professor of Medicine
Mayo Medical School
Consultant Division of Cardiovascular Diseases
Internal Medicine
Pediatric Cardiology
and Adult Congenital Heart Disease Clinic
Mayo Clinic
Rochester, Minnesota
Chapter 64

DAVID D. WATERS, M.D.
Professor of Medicine
University of California, San Francisco
Division of Cardiology
San Francisco General Hospital
San Francisco, California
Chapter 41

WILLIAM S. WEINTRAUB, M.D.
Professor of Medicine
Cardiology
Director
Emory Center for Outcomes Research (ECOR)
Emory University
Division of Cardiology
Atlanta, Georgia
Chapter 94

MYRON L. WEISFELDT, M.D.
Chairman
Department of Medicine
Samuel Bard Professor of Medicine
Columbia University College of Physicians and Surgeons
Columbia Presbyterian Medical Center
New York, New York
Chapter 34

HEIN J. J. WELLENS, M.D.
Professor of Cardiology
University of Maastricht
Chairman
Department of Cardiology
University Hospital Maastricht
Maastricht, The Netherlands
Chapters 29 and 43

NANETTE K. WENGER, M.D.
Professor of Medicine (Cardiology)
Emory University School of Medicine
Consultant
Emory Heart and Vascular Center
Chief of Cardiology
Grady Memorial Hospital
Emory University School of Medicine
Atlanta, Georgia
Chapter 50

PAUL WENNBERG, M.D.
Instructo of Medicine
Senior Associate Consultant
Cardiovascular Division
Mayo Clinic
Rochester, Minnesota
Chapter 90

ANDY WESSELS, Ph.D.
Professor
Medical University of South Carolina
Medical University of South Carolina
Chapter 9

SUSAN WILANSKY, M.D.
Medical Director
Non-Invasive Cardiac Imaging
St. Luke's Episcopal Hospital/Texas Heart Institute
St. Luke's Episcopal Hospital
Houston, Texas
Chapter 77

ANDREW L. WITT, Ph.D.
Professor and Associate Chairman
Department of Pharmacology
College of Physicians and Surgeons
Columbia University
New York, New York
Chapter 23

RAYMOND L. WOOSLEY, M.D., Ph.D.
Professor and Chairman
Department of Pharmacology
Georgetown University Medical Center
Washington, District of Columbia
Chapter 27

STEPHEN G. WORTHLEY, M.B.B.S., F.R.A.C.P.
Research Fellow
Mount Sinai School of Medicine
The Zena and Michael A. Wiener Cardiovascular Institute
New York, New York
Chapter 18B

SANJAY S. YADAV, M.D.
Director, Carotid Intervention
Staff Cardiologist
Vascular Medicine
The Cleveland Clinic Foundation
Cleveland, Ohio
Chapter 92

PREFACE

In 1966 the first edition of Hurst's *The Heart* was published after more than five years of planning by Dr. J. Willis Hurst and his colleagues at Emory University. This was the first textbook on cardiovascular disease to be multiauthored and comprehensive with expert discussions on the basic science of cardiovascular diseases and the diagnosis and treatment of specific disorders involving the heart arteries, and veins.

Contributing authors were carefully chosen and the various chapters of the textbook were meticulously reviewed by the editors to provide completeness without overlap. This 1966 text was extensively referenced and the index of the book was written by the contributing authors and editors themselves. The first edition of *The Heart* was designed as a reference source for its readers as well as providing clinically relevant material for use in the diagnosis and treatment of cardiovascular disease in the 1960s.

The tenth edition of *The Heart* is considerably different from the previous nine editions. It approaches the entire discipline of cardiovascular disease, from basic science through clinical disease states, with all chapters written by most prominent experts in the field. Thus, from the description of the latest advances in molecular cardiology, including the promising cardiovascular applications of the human genome project, the book approaches in depth all the recent major advances in clinical cardiology, including the description of the most up-to-date practice guidelines.

Sixteen new chapters have been added and about 60 percent of the chapters have been radically modified. Specifically new, and we believe unique, aspects of this tenth edition of *The Heart* are the following:

1. Within the basic section of the book there are three new chapters devoted to molecular, cellular, and vessel wall biology;
2. also, in the basic section there are three new chapters devoted to the human genome, molecular development and embriology, and genetic therapy;
3. as a practical new understanding of the anatomy of *The Heart*, the group at the Mayo Clinic has written an outstanding chapter based on clinical imaging;
4. in the section devoted to diagnostic modalities, there are four new superb chapters on computed tomography of the heart, magnetic resonance imaging of the heart, magnetic resonance imaging of the vascular systsem, and cardiac positron emission tomography;
5. two timely new clinincal chapters; diabetes in cardiovascular disease and cardiac disease in women;
6. a new aspect of this tenth edition is a chapter on practice guidelines in cardiovascular disease, which we expect will be very practical for the daily approach to the patient and as a teaching tool for residents and fellows;
7. finally, there is a new and unique chapter on extended cardiovascular medicine, which, we predict, outlines a strong trend toward the future.

From the moment that the outstanding group of authors accepted to participate in this tenth edition of *The Heart* to the moment of the book appearing on the shelves has only taken fifteen months. This is an absolute record for a textbook of this size and complexity. Such an approach represents the highest tribute and acknowledgment to our authors for their extraordinary and timely contribution.

We thank J. Willis Hurst, M.D., editor of the first seven editions, for his constant and enthusiastic encouragement, as well as Robert C. Schlant, M.D., who contributions to the first nine editions of *The Heart* have been responsible for the foundation of this tenth edition. Importantly, this edition would not have been possible without the many extensive contributions and personal sacrifices of two individuals at McGraw-Hill, Darlene B. Cooke and Susan R. Noujaim. We would also like to thank Lester A. Sheinis and Richard C. Ruzycka for their efforts in getting the book produced on time.

Finally we wish to acknowledge the support of our families and the many sacrifices they have made to make this volume possible. Our wives remain our greatest support and strength; Maria Fuster, Jane W. Alexander, Suzann O'Rourke, Donna Roberts, Gail King, and Inez Wellens.

HURST'S
THE HEART

C H A P T E R 47

CORONARY INTRAVASCULAR ULTRASOUND IMAGING

Steven E. Nissen

Although angiography continues to serve as the primary imaging modality used to assess the anatomy of coronary artery disease, intravascular ultrasound has matured into an important alternative method for examination of the coronaries during diagnostic or interventional catheterization.[1-8] Studies comparing angiography and intravascular ultrasound have demonstrated important differences in quantitative and qualitative findings.[7-11] Unlike angiography, which portrays the vessel as a silhouette of the lumen, intravascular ultrasound provides tomographic images that portray not only the lumen but also the deeper intramural structures within the vessel wall. The ability of ultrasound to penetrate and image soft tissue enables direct visualization of the atheroma, providing insights into the pathophysiology of coronary disease not obtainable by any other technique. Accordingly, intraluminal ultrasound imaging is now commonly utilized to confirm, refute, or supplement angiographic data in patients with coronary disease.[8]

RATIONALE FOR INTRAVASCULAR ULTRASOUND

Limitations of Angiography

Visual interpretation of angiograms exhibits significant observer variability, and necropsy examination is often discordant with the apparent angiographic severity of lesions.[12-18] In comparison to postmortem evaluation, angiography often significantly underestimates the extent of atherosclerosis.[13,18] Angiographic assessment of lesion severity is strikingly discordant with measurements of the physiologic effects of stenoses.[19] Angiography depicts coronary anatomy from a planar two-dimensional silhouette of the contrast-filled lumen. However, coronary lesions are often complex, with markedly distorted or eccentric luminal shapes, and mechanical interventions (other than stenting) exaggerate luminal eccentricity by fracturing or dissecting the atheroma.[9,20,21] The angiographic appearance of the postintervention vessel often reveals an enlarged but "hazy" lumen. This indistinct, broadened angiographic silhouette may overestimate actual vessel diameter and misrepresent the gain in lumen size.[21]

The traditional method for characterizing angiographic lesion severity depends upon visual or computer measurements of the percentage stenosis. This process requires comparison of luminal dimensions within both the lesion and an adjacent, uninvolved "normal" reference segment. However, necropsy studies demonstrate that coronary disease is frequently diffuse and contains no truly normal reference segment.[18] In the presence of diffuse disease, calculation of percent stenosis will predictably underestimate disease severity. Diffuse, concentric, and symmetrical disease affecting the entire vessel may result in the angiographic appearance of a small but normal artery.[21] Angiography is also confounded by the phenomenon of coronary "remodeling," observed histologically as the outward displacement of the external vessel wall in segments with atherosclerosis.[22] This adventitial enlargement attenuates lumen encroachment, thereby concealing the presence of the atheroma on angiography. Although such lesions do not restrict blood flow, clinical studies have demonstrated that these minimal, nonobstructive lesions represent an important cause of acute coronary syndromes.[23] Angiographically unrecognized disease virtually always underlies an ergonovine-positive response in symptomatic patients with a "normal" coronary angiogram.[24]

Theoretical Advantages of Ultrasound

Intravascular ultrasound has several unique properties of theoretical value in the detection and quantitation of coronary disease.[25,26] The cross-sectional perspective of ultrasound permits visualization of the full 360-degree circumference of the vessel wall. Accordingly, measurement of lumen area can be determined by planimetry independent of the radiographic projection or magnification.[7,21,25,26] The tomographic perspective of ultrasound enables evaluation of vessels difficult to assess by angiographic techniques, including diffusely diseased segments and bifurcation or ostial lesions. The ability to directly image the atheroma represents a truly unique capability not possible using any other commonly available imaging modality.

IMAGING TECHNOLOGY

Catheter Design

Intracoronary ultrasound equipment consists of two major components: a catheter incorporating a miniaturized transducer and a console containing the electronics necessary to reconstruct the image. High frequencies (20 to 50 MHz) are employed, resulting in excellent theoretical resolution (axially <100 μm and laterally <250 μm). Two dissimilar technical approaches to transducer design exist: mechanically rotated devices and multielement electronic arrays[1–5] (Fig. 47-1). Each design has yielded small intravascular devices suitable for coronary imaging, typically ranging in size from 2.6 to 3.5 Fr (diameter of 0.86 to 1.17 mm). To facilitate subselective coronary cannulation and catheter exchanges, ultrasound catheters provide a lumen for a movable guidewire. Most systems generate images at a temporal frequency of 30 frames per second for recording on videotape.

Limitations and Artifacts

Intravascular ultrasound devices generate artifacts that may adversely affect image quality, alter interpretation, or reduce quantitative accuracy.[27] Ring-down artifact arises from acoustic oscillations in the piezoelectric transducer, resulting in high-amplitude signals that preclude imaging close to the transducer surface. Accordingly, the "acoustic" size of catheters is slightly larger than their physical size. Since the minimum size of current devices is approximately 0.9 mm, some severe stenoses cannot be imaged prior to intervention. Geometric distortion can result from imaging in an oblique plane (not perpendicular to the long axis of the vessel), resulting in an elliptical rather than circular imaging plane.[28]

Mechanical, but not electronic, transducers may exhibit cyclical oscillations in rotational speed, resulting in an artifact known as nonuniform rotational distortion (NURD).[27] This artifact arises from mechanical friction within the catheter drive shaft during the portions of its rotational cycle. This speed variation produces readily visible distortion often observed as circumferential stretching of a portion of the image with compression of the contralateral vessel wall. NURD is most evident when the drive shaft is bent into a small radius of curvature by a tortuous vessel. Improvements in the mechanical precision of ultrasound devices have reduced the impact of the artifact, but it still remains troublesome during some examinations.

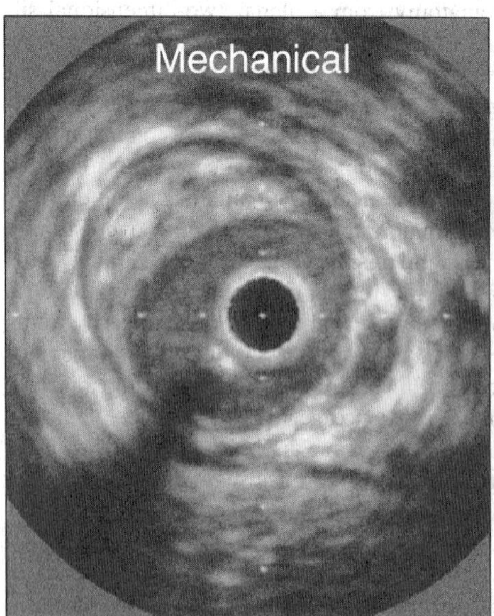

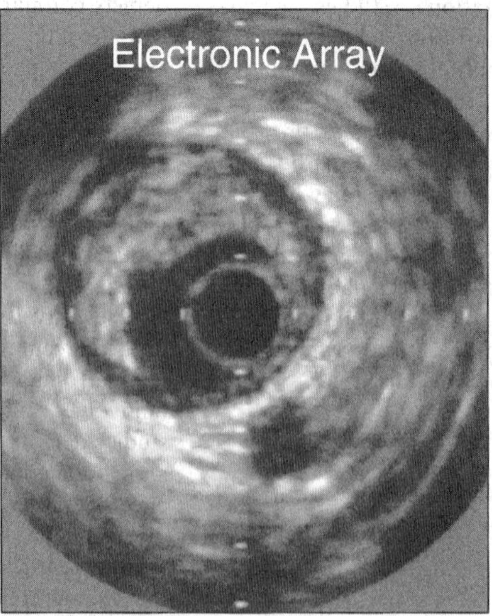

FIGURE 47-1 Mechanical and electronic array of intravascular ultrasound images. In the left panel, an intravascular ultrasound image produced using a mechanical type of catheter is illustrated. In the right panel, a similar plaque in a different patient illustrates an image acquired using a multiple-element electronic array.

CORONARY IMAGING

Examination Technique

Standard interventional techniques for intracoronary catheter delivery are used for intraluminal ultrasound examination. Intravenous heparin [to maintain activated clotting time (ACT) >200 to 250 s] and intracoronary nitroglycerin (100 to 300 μg) are routinely administered, although there are no controlled studies documenting the necessity for anticoagulation. Using a 7- or 8-Fr guiding catheter, the operator advances a steerable guidewire to subselectively cannulate the vessel. A stable guiding catheter position with good support is desirable, since current ultrasound catheters have less trackability and a larger profile than modern balloon angioplasty catheters. The operator carefully advances or retracts the imaging catheter over the wire to examine the vessel in real time, recording images on videotape for subsequent quantitative or qualitative analysis.

Some centers use a motorized pullback device to withdraw the catheter at a constant speed (between 0.25 and 1 mm/s, most frequently 0.5 mm/s). However, a single pullback, even when controlled by a precise motor, may be insufficient for a complete diagnostic ultrasound examination. Accordingly, motorized pullback is most often used to "survey" the coronary prior to more prolonged and thorough examination of sites of interest. Side branches, visualized with both angiography and ultrasound, are often used as landmarks to facilitate interpretation. Some practitioners advocate use of a uniform format, electronically rotating the ultrasound image so that branches appear in a standardized orientation. For example, imaging of the left anterior descending is often performed with the septal branches at 6 o'clock and the left circumflex appearing at about 9 o'clock.

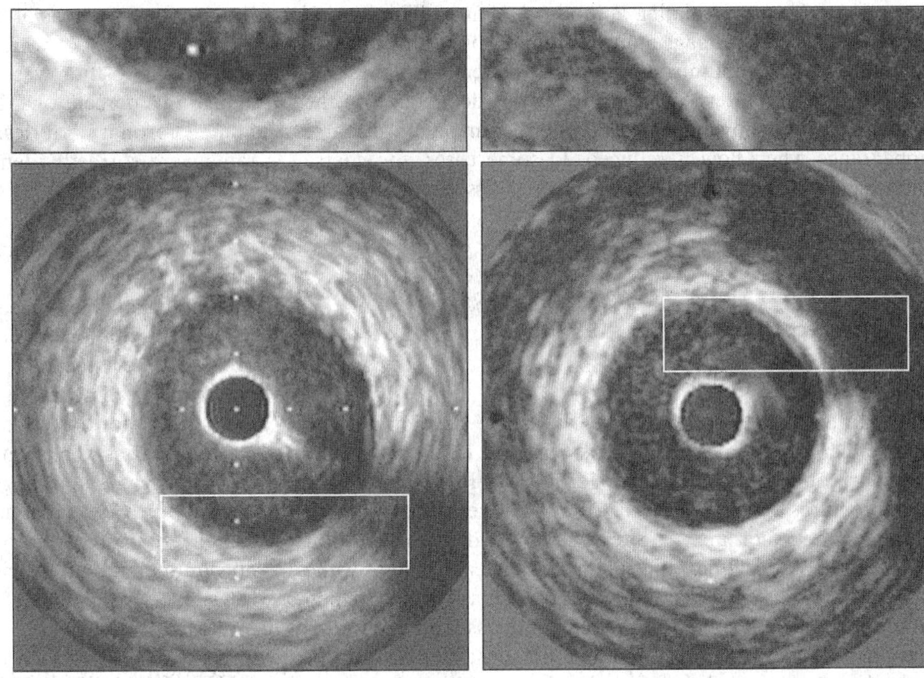

FIGURE 47-2 Two variants of normal coronary anatomy by intravascular ultrasound. In both images, a magnified view of the area contained within the rectangle is shown at the top. In the left panel, there is a monolayered artery; in the right panel, the artery has a trilaminar structure.

Safety of Coronary Ultrasound

Although intravascular ultrasound requires intracoronary instrumentation, studies have demonstrated few serious untoward effects.[29-31] The most frequently encountered complication is focal coronary spasm, which usually responds rapidly to intracoronary nitroglycerin. Data from European centers reported a 1.1 percent complication rate in 718 ultrasound examinations.[30] Another report from 28 centers (2207 studies) documented spasm in 2.9 percent and major complications such as occlusion or dissection judged to have a "certain relation" to instrumentation in 0.4 percent.[29] In both studies, complications (spasm, vessel dissection, or guidewire entrapment) occurred in patients undergoing angioplasty rather than diagnostic imaging.[44] In 170 cardiac transplant recipients (240 studies), there was no morbidity, but spasm occurred in 20 patients (8.3 percent) despite pretreatment with nitroglycerin.[31] Any intracoronary instrumentation carries the potential risk of intimal injury or vessel dissection. Accordingly, most laboratories limit credentialing for this procedure to personnel with interventional training.

Normal Coronary Anatomy

Studies performed either in vivo or using excised, pressure-distended vessels have characterized the appearance of normal coronaries by intravascular ultrasound.[32-36] Important determinants of vessel wall appearance include both the normal arterial structure and the inherent properties of ultrasound. An ultrasound reflection occurs at a tissue boundary whenever there is an abrupt change in acoustic impedance. Normally, two strong acoustic interfaces are visualized by ultrasound—the leading edge of the intima (at the interface between the blood-filled lumen and the endothelium) and the outer border of the media (at the junction of media and external elastic membrane). Underlying the trailing edge of the intima, a middle sonolucent layer is usually evident, which is composed principally of the tunica media. The echodense intima and adventitia with a sonolucent medial layer often give the wall a trilaminar appearance. However, this pattern is not a universal finding; in 30 to 50 percent of normal segments, a thin intimal layer reflects ultrasound poorly, which results in a monolayer appearance[35] (Fig. 47-2).

In a necropsy study, the ultrasound-derived intimal thickness in segments with three layers was significantly greater than for monolayered sites (0.24 ± 0.1 versus 0.11 ± 0.06 mm, $p <$ 0.001). The mean age in the three-layered group was greater, 42.8 ± 9.8 versus 27.1 ± 8.5 years ($p < 0.001$).[37] Other studies demonstrate that a trilaminar appearance is dependent not only on the age but also on the histologic characteristics of the vessel. A three-layered appearance is consistently observed if an internal elastic membrane state is present.[38] However, if an internal elastic membrane is absent, a trilaminar appearance is observed only when the collagen content of the media is low. In older "normal" subjects, intimal thickening usually results in a pattern of two distinct echogenic layers sandwiching a sonolucent intermediate layer. In nearly all cases, the deepest arterial layers exhibit a characteristic "onionskin" pattern, representing the adventitia and periadventitial tissues with an indistinct outer vessel border.

In both normal and abnormal arteries, the lumen exhibits faint, finely textured, swirling echoes that arise from acoustic reflections from circulating blood elements. This blood "speckle" may assist image interpretation by providing a means to confirm the communication between dissection planes and the lumen. The pattern of blood speckle is dependent on the velocity of flow, showing increased intensity and a more coarse appearance when flow is reduced. In some cases, the coarse blood speckle can mimic the appearance of tissue, complicating image interpretation.

CHARACTERIZATION OF ATHEROSCLEROSIS

Atheroma Composition

The subtle changes that occur early in the development of atherosclerosis, such as fatty streaks, are not visible using current ultrasound devices. Atherosclerotic arteries exhibit a variety of features that reflect the distribution, severity, and composition of the atheroma.[32-34] Sites with limited disease exhibit generalized or focal thickening of the intimal leading edge, while advanced lesions appear as large echogenic masses encroaching upon the lumen. A comparative study of ultrasound and histology in 1100 fresh necropsy sections demonstrated that lipid-laden lesions are usually hypoechoic.[32] Soft, low-intensity echoes most often represent fibromuscular lesions and very bright echoes are observed within dense fibrous or calcified tissues (Fig. 47-3). In highly echogenic plaques, foci of calcification are recognized by attenuation of ultrasound penetration, which obscures deeper layers, a phenomenon known as "acoustic shadowing." In lipid-laden or fibromuscular lesions, a prominent echogenic overlying fibrous "cap" may be observed.

The echogenicity of the plaque components is dependent not only on the acoustic properties of tissue but also on the acquisition settings (gain, compression, etc.). Accordingly, most classification schemes compare the echogenicity of the plaque to the surrounding adventitia to correct for differences in ultrasound technique. However, in plaques containing a zone of reduced echogenicity, it is not possible to determine whether these represent areas of lipid deposition, thrombus, or necrotic degeneration, all of which can appear as zones of low density. Plaque composition was accurately predicted by ultrasound imaging in 96 percent of 112 quadrants from 21 freshly explanted human coronary arteries.[29] Fibrous and calcified plaque quadrants were correctly identified in almost all incidences (100 of 103, or 97 percent), but only 7 of 9 quadrants (78 percent) with predominantly lipid deposits were correctly identified.

Accordingly, some caution is warranted in the intravascular ultrasound classification of atheroma composition. Although currently available devices produce detailed views of the vessel wall, interpretation employs visual inspection of acoustic reflections to determine morphology. Different histologic features may exhibit comparable acoustic properties, and methods do not yet exist for objective or automated classification of atheromatous lesions. Thus, intravascular ultrasound can delineate the thickness and echogenicity of vessel wall structures but does not provide actual histology. Despite these limitations, the classification of coronary plaques into the categories of soft, fibromuscular, and calcified has important clinical implications.

Detection of Calcification

Ultrasound imaging has shown superiority over fluoroscopy or angiography in the detection of coronary calcification. In a series of 110 patients undergoing intervention, target lesion calcification was detected by ultrasound and fluoroscopy in 84 and 50 patients, respectively (76 versus 14 percent, $p < 0.001$).[39] Another retrospective study analyzed calcification by angiography and ultrasound in 183 interventional patients.[40] Assessment by the two techniques was concordant in 92 and discordant in 91 cases. Calcification was detected in 138 patients by ultrasound and 63 by fluoroscopy, showing a sensitivity and specificity for angiography of 46 and 82 percent, respectively. When calcium was detected angiographically, calcification by ultrasound often subtended >90 degrees and was superficial to the lumen in location. If no calcification could be visualized on the angiogram, the chance of detecting a large superficial arc of calcium by ultrasound was low (12 percent).

Ultrasound calcification is a major determinant of the arterial response to intervention, portending a greater risk of dissection following balloon angioplasty, less tissue retrieval with directional atherectomy, and greater benefit with the use of rotational atherectomy.[41,42] Because of the importance of calcium in the selection of interventional devices, most classification schemes quantify calcification, usually by measuring the circumferential angle subtended by calcified plaque.[39] Commonly, the axial length of the calcified portion of the lesion is also reported and the depth of calcification assessed, described as superficial when the calcium re-

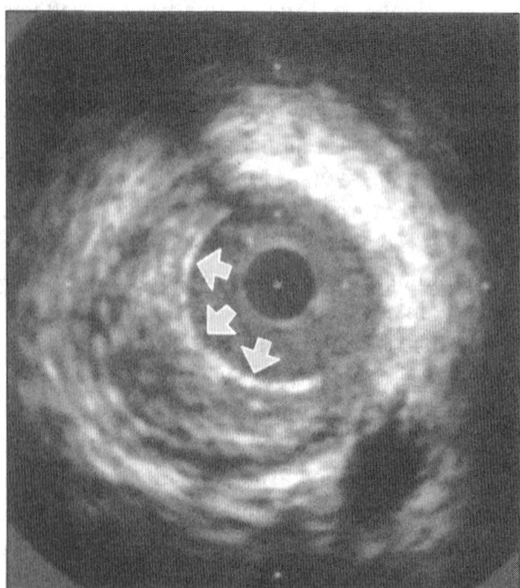

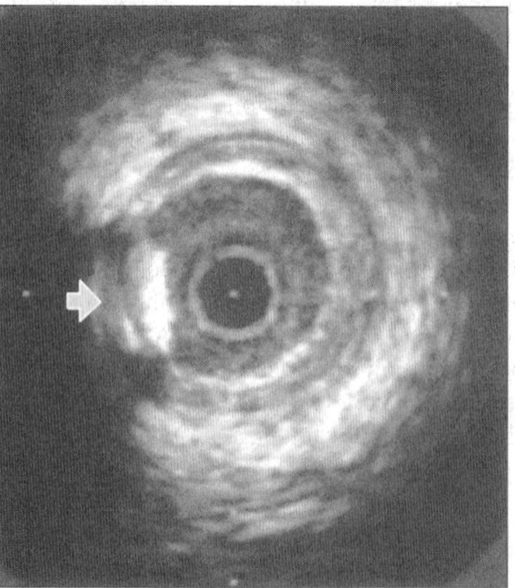

FIGURE 47-3 Atheroma morphology by intravascular ultrasound. In the left panel, a large, "soft," lipid-laden atheroma with a thin fibrous cap is shown (*arrows*). It is eccentric, involving only about 50 percent of the vessel wall. In the right panel, a circumferential atheroma with an area of focal calcification is evident (*arrow*).

mains in contact with the luminal surface and deep if no portion of the calcium deposit is superficial.

Arterial Remodeling

This term refers to a change in arterial dimensions associated with the development of atherosclerosis. In a necropsy study of 136 human left main coronary arteries, Glagov et al. originally described focal arterial enlargement at atherosclerotic sites, reporting a positive correlation between external elastic membrane (EEM) area and the area occupied by atheroma ($r = 0.44$, $p < 0.001$).[22] At sites with area stenosis less than 40 percent, the increase in arterial size "overcompensated" for the plaque deposition, leading to an increase in absolute lumen area. With more advanced lesions (area stenosis >40 percent), the degree of arterial enlargement or remodeling was blunted, resulting in a smaller lumen area. The authors hypothesized that this phenomenon represented a compensatory mechanism to preserve lumen size.

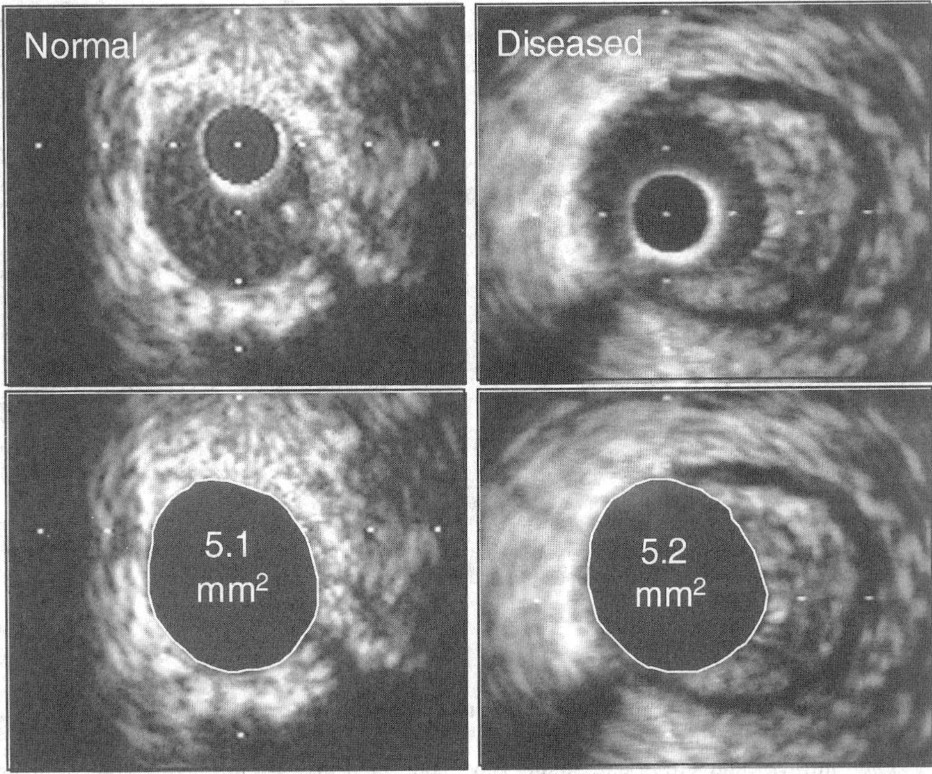

FIGURE 47-4 Example of coronary remodeling. In the left upper panel, a normal segment of the circumflex coronary is illustrated. In the right upper panel, an atherosclerotic segment of the coronary a few millimeters proximal to the normal segment is shown. In the bottom two panels, measurements taken at each of the sites show very similar cross-sectional areas. The preservation of lumen area results in a coronary angiogram that is normal despite the presence of a large atherosclerotic plaque in the involved segment.

The findings of Glagov et al. were later confirmed in vivo by intravascular ultrasound imaging[43,44] (Fig. 47-4). In 80 ultrasound cross sections obtained from 44 patients undergoing coronary interventions, EEM area correlated closely with plaque area ($r = 0.79$, $p = 0.0001$). In this study, lumen area increased with early atherosclerosis, confirming the phenomenon of overcompensation in early stages of the disease. With more advanced atherosclerosis, there was a correlation between increasing area stenosis and decreasing lumen area ($r = 0.58$, $p = 0.0001$).[43] Compensatory enlargement has also been demonstrated by ultrasound in superficial femoral arteries; however, there was no difference between lesions less than and greater than 40 percent stenosis.[45]

In recent years, ultrasound studies have demonstrated a new dimension to arterial remodeling: negative remodeling.[46,47] At diseased sites, the EEM area may actually be reduced in size, contributing to luminal narrowing rather than compensating for it. In 51 femoral arteries, EEM area was smaller at lesions than adjacent reference sites, with a negative correlation between stenosis severity and EEM area reduction ($r = 0.62$ by histology and 0.66 by ultrasound, $p < 0.001$ for both).[46] "Inadequate" remodeling, defined as an EEM area within the lesion less than 78 percent of a proximal reference site, has also been described in the coronaries of patients with stable angina.[47] Although 91 of 603 lesions (15 percent) fit this definition, there was a highly variable response among lesions within the same patient. However, when remodeling is defined in this fashion, there is an assumption that the reference EEM area represents the original vessel size, which may not be correct, since angiographic reference sites are invariably diseased according to ultrasound.

Although the exact mechanisms of compensatory or negative remodeling remain unclear, these phenomena have important clinical implications. Compensatory remodeling represents an important factor in the underestimation of the severity of atherosclerosis by angiography. Remodeling may influence the estimation of the vessel size during coronary interventions. Recently, negative remodeling has been implicated in restenosis following debulking and balloon angioplasty.[48]

Unstable Plaque and Thrombi

An emerging application of intracoronary ultrasound is the characterization of the atheroma associated with acute coronary syndromes (Fig. 47-5). The typical angiographic appearance of a ruptured plaque is a stenosis with an eccentric or ulcerated lumen, often with overhanging edges (Ambrose type II lesion).[49-54] However, retrospective reviews of angiograms of patients performed before an episode of unstable angina usually reveal minimal disease within the culprit lesion segment.[51] These studies highlight the inability of angiography to identify "rupture-prone" lesions. Histologic examination of unstable plaques after rupture usually reveals a lipid-laden plaque with a thin fibrous cap.[49] Based on these observations, it has been postu-

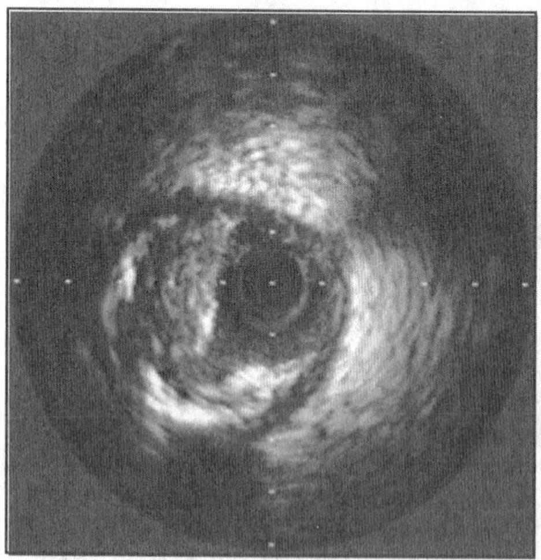
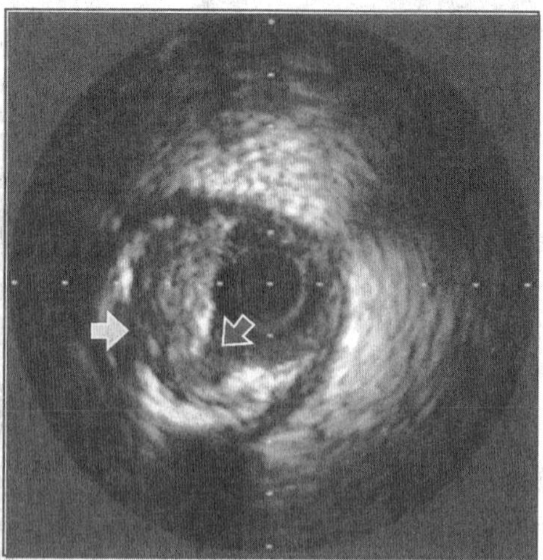

FIGURE 47-5 Ruptured coronary plaque. In these two identical images, the anatomy of a ruptured coronary plaque is illustrated. There is a large lipid core with a fracture of the fibrous cap (*right panel, arrow*). This image was obtained a few days after hospitalization of this patient for a unstable coronary syndrome.

lated that the size of the lipid pool and the thickness of the fibrous cap are more important than severity of stenosis in predicting plaque rupture.[52]

Some intravascular ultrasound studies have confirmed the presence of an echolucent atheroma within culprit lesions in patients with acute coronary syndromes. In a small study of 22 stable and 43 unstable angina patients, type II eccentric lesions were detected on the angiograms in 18 percent of stable and 40 percent of unstable angina patients. Echolucent plaques were more frequently observed in patients with unstable than in those with stable angina syndromes (74 versus 41 percent, $p < 0.01$).[11] Recent and intriguing intravascular ultrasound studies have examined the relationship between remodeling and the type of clinical presentation. The culprit lesions in 76 patients with acute coronary syndromes were compared with lesions in 40 patients with stable angina. In the unstable patients, both EEM and plaque areas were significantly larger than the corresponding measurements in the stable patients ($p = 0.02$ for both). Positive remodeling was more prevalent in the unstable group (51 versus 18 percent, $p = 0.002$) and negative remodeling more prevalent in the stable group (58 versus 33 percent, $p = 0.002$).[55]

The formation of intraluminal thrombi at a ruptured or fissured plaque is considered to be the hallmark of acute coronary syndromes.[56] Angiographic criteria for diagnosis of a coronary thrombus, the presence of haziness, an intraluminal filling defect, and/or irregular lumen contour are not sensitive.[54] Small observational studies have attempted to differentiate the ultrasound appearance of thrombus, defined as hypoechoic material projecting into the lumen with a slight synchronous pulsation and a distinct acoustic interface, from more echogenic plaque[57,58] (Fig. 47-6). However, in vitro studies have revealed limitations in the reliability of intravascular ultrasound diagnosis of thrombi (sensitivity of 57 percent and specificity of 91 percent), considerably inferior to angioscopy (sensitivity and specificity of 100 percent).[56] Radiofrequency analysis of ultrasound signals has shown some promise in differentiating between thrombus and plaque, although the clinical application is not yet feasible.[59,60]

DIAGNOSTIC CLINICAL APPLICATIONS

Quantitative Luminal Measurements

A broad spectrum of therapeutic decisions hinge upon assessment of coronary luminal dimensions. Accordingly, in diagnostic and interventional practice, quantitation of vascular dimensions represents an important clinical application of intravascular ultrasound. Several studies have compared luminal measurements by intravascular ultrasound and quantitative angiography.[6,7] For vessels without atherosclerosis, most studies document a close correlation between angiographic and ultrasonic coronary dimensions, although a few studies suggest slightly larger measurements by ultrasound.[7] However, in patients with atherosclerotic arteries, most investigators report only a moderate correlation between ultrasonic and angiographic dimensions, with the greatest disparities in vessel segments with a noncircular lumen shape.[5,7,10] This reduced correlation is probably explained by the irregular, noncircular cross-sectional profile of diseased vessels, which cannot be adequately measured using angiography.[10]

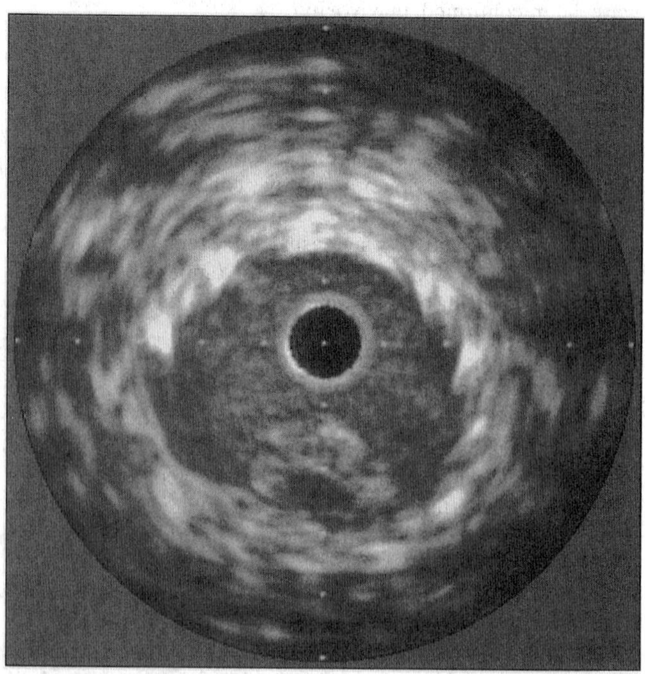

FIGURE 47-6 Thrombus within a coronary stent. In this intravascular ultrasound image, a stent is well visualized. There is a globular mass projecting into the lumen at 6 o'clock; it probably represents a large thrombus.

Quantitation of Atherosclerosis

Analysis of intravascular ultrasound images permits quantitative measurements of the extent and severity of coronary atherosclerosis[26] (Fig. 47-7). However, the inherent properties of ultrasound require utilization of different anatomic landmarks than those serving classic histology. In all ultrasound imaging, reflections at the leading edge of any interface are located precisely at the boundary where acoustic impedance abruptly changes. However, the position of the trailing edge of any anatomic structure is determined by multiple nonanatomic factors, including ultrasound beam properties, particularly the wavelength (frequency). Thus, leading-edge measurements accurately describe the location of a boundary, whereas trailing-edge measurements are unreliable. As previously noted, strong reflections are generally produced at two locations, the leading edge of the intima and the border between the media and the external elastic membrane. The position of the trailing edge of the intima is not accurately localized in intravascular ultrasound images. Accordingly, quantitative measurements must calculate the atheroma's cross-sectional area by subtracting the area bounded by the intimal leading edge from the area enclosed by the external elastic membrane. This approach results in a slight overestimation of atheroma volume (in comparison to histology) by including the area of the media within the calculation.

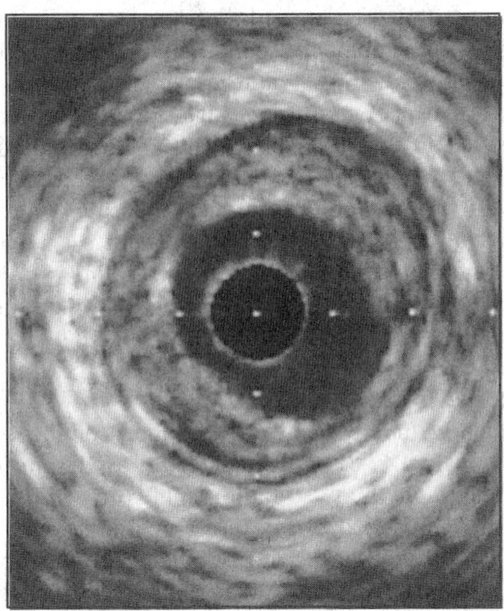

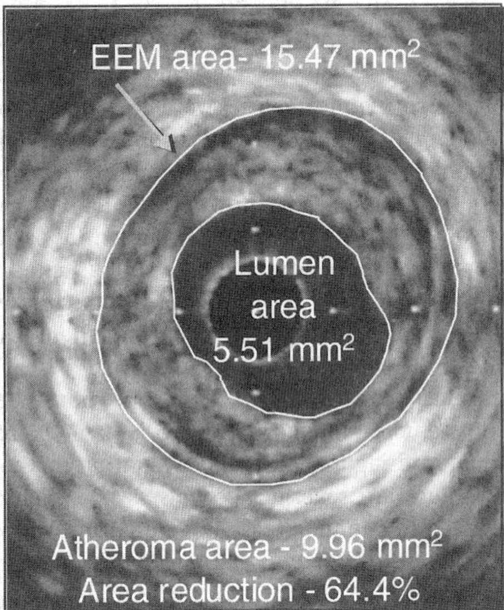

FIGURE 47-7 Boundaries for intravascular ultrasound measurements. In these two identical images, an atherscle-rotic plaque is well visualized. The right panel illustrates the planimetry typically employed to measure the extent of the atherosclerotic disease. Both the lumen and external elastic membrane (EEM) are measured. The atheroma area represents the difference between the EEM and the lumen areas. The area reduction is calculated as the atheroma area divided by the EEM area multiplied by 100.

NORMAL INTIMAL THICKNESS

The threshold for abnormal intimal thickness by intravascular ultrasound is controversial, particularly since the categorical classification of a continuous variable, intimal thickness, as normal and abnormal is inherently arbitrary. In various histologic and ultrasound studies, normal intimal thickness ranges between 0.10 and 0.35 mm and the normal medial thickness ranges from 0.15 to 0.25 mm. In a necropsy study, normal intimal thickness not including media was age-dependent, averaging 0.21 mm in 21- to 25-year-olds, 0.22 mm in 26- to 30-year-olds, and 0.25 mm in 36- to 40-year-olds.[37] In a comparative study, intravascular ultrasound measurements of the intima plus media averaged 20 percent greater than histological measurements.[61,62] Considering the histologic and ultrasound data, most clinical studies have defined the ultrasound measurement threshold for coronary disease as an intimal thickness ≥0.5 mm.[63-67] Currently, there is no well-defined threshold for normal values for other measures, like intimal cross-sectional area.

The tomographic orientation of intravascular ultrasound represents an additional problem in quantifying atherosclerosis. Since each image contains information from only a thin "slice" of the vessel, global measures of atheroma burden require the integration of multiple cross sections. One successful approach to this conundrum employs a motorized device to steadily and progressively withdraw the ultrasound catheter through the interrogated vessel, typically at 0.5 to 1.0 mm/s. Since motor speed is kept constant, the operator can obtain a series of cross sections separated by a constant, recurring time interval; these are individually measured and then summated to approximate total atheroma burden using Simpson's rule. A second approach to atheroma quantitation employs three-dimensional (3D) reconstruction of the vessel from the two-dimensional ultrasound tomograms.[68] Unfortunately 3D methods are exceedingly complex, have many unresolved confounding variables, and remain largely unvalidated.

Atheroma Distribution

The circumferential distribution of the atheroma varies from nearly symmetrical plaques to very eccentric lesions in which the entire atheroma is located on one side of the artery. Assessed by ultrasound, the majority of plaques are eccentric, with a maximum atheroma thickness more than twice the minimum plaque thickness.[69] Studies have demonstrated a poor correlation between the apparent circumferential pattern by angiography and the actual plaque distribution revealed by ultrasound examination.[69] Such studies demonstrate the inaccuracy inherent in determining plaque distribution from the projected two-dimensional silhouette of the lumen (angiography). This observation has important implications for guidance of coronary interventions, particularly techniques for selective plaque removal, such as directional atherectomy.

Angiographically Unrecognized Disease

In patients undergoing angiography for clinically suspected coronary artery disease, no angiographic evidence of narrowing is present in 10 to 15 percent of cases. In these patients, intravascular ultrasound commonly detects atherosclerosis at angiographically normal sites.[21,25,26,70,71] Using intravascular ultrasound, atherosclerotic abnormalities were documented in 21 of 44 patients (48 percent) with suspected coronary artery disease and normal coronary angiograms.[70] Combining ultrasound and functional assessment (coronary flow reserve and endothelium-mediated vasodilator response), only 36 percent of patients in this cohort were completely normal. Other studies demonstrate that, if any luminal irregularity is present by angiography, ultrasound will usually demonstrate atherosclerosis at nearly all other examined sites.[21] The prevalence of atherosclerosis at angiographically normal sites confirms the finding, previously reported from necropsy studies, that coronary involvement is frequently underestimated using angiographic evaluation methods[12,13] (Fig. 47-8).

There are several mechanisms by which angiography may underestimate the presence, extent, or severity of atherosclerosis.[21] First, to detect focal narrowing, angiography relies upon comparison of the interrogated site to an adjacent uninvolved segment. However, the involved vessel is often reduced in caliber along its entire length, containing no truly normal segment for comparison. The angiographer may erroneously conclude that the vessel is simply "small in caliber." Overlapping structures and mechanical limits in x-ray positioning may prevent the angiographer from obtaining optimal radiographic projections (orthogonal to the lesion). Accordingly, eccentric plaques that occupy only a portion of the vessel circumference represent an important source of false-negative angiography. At atherosclerotic sites, compensatory enlargement of the vessel wall overlying the plaque often preserves lumen diameter, resulting in false-negative angiography because the lumen size in the involved segment is identical to that of adjacent, uninvolved segments. Finally, radiographic foreshortening can conceal short "napkin-ring" lesions.

For each of these mechanisms of false-negative angiography, intravascular ultrasound has been employed to confirm the presence and estimate the extent of atherosclerosis.[21] However, the long-term clinical implications of angiographically unrecognized atherosclerosis remain uncertain since no outcomes-based research has demonstrated a worse prognosis for patients with atherosclerosis detected only by ultrasound. However, several investigators have demonstrated that plaques with minimal to moderate angiographic narrowing are the most likely lead to acute coronary syndromes. Accordingly, the presence of angiographically occult coronary disease may have prognostic significance. Studies are currently under way to determine the value of ultrasound in predicting the clinical outcome in patients with angiographically unrecognized coronary disease.

Lesions of Uncertain Severity

Angiographers commonly encounter lesions that elude accurate characterization despite thorough examination using multiple radiographic projections. Difficult-to-assess sites include ostial or bifurcation lesions and moderate stenoses (angiographic severity ranging from 40 to 75 percent) in patients whose symptomatic status is difficult to evaluate. For ambiguous lesions, ultrasound provides a tomographic perspective, independent of the radiographic projection, that may permit quantification of the lesion. In two prospective series, intracoronary ultrasound changed the management strategy in approximately 20 percent of the examinations performed immediately prior to coronary intervention.[72,73] In both studies, however, operator selection of patients for ultrasound examination may have resulted in an overestimation of the true impact of ultrasound imaging on clinical decision making.

Angiographic assessment of left main coronary artery (LMCA) obstruction represents a particularly vexing clinical problem.[14] Radiographic contrast in the aortic cusp can obscure the ostium, and "streaming" of contrast from the injection vortex can result in a false impression of luminal narrowing. The LMCA is often short in length, leaving no normal "reference" segment. The bifurcation or trifurcation of the LMCA into daughter branches may produce vessel overlap, thereby concealing a stenosis. Intravascular ultrasound is commonly used to quantify LMCA lesions when angiographic interpretation is uncertain.[74] The technique for examination consists of subselective placement of the ultrasound transducer in the circumflex or anterior descending, followed by slow pullback to the aorta with the guiding catheter disengaged. There is no consensus regarding the threshold for critical LMCA obstruction. However, an area stenosis >50 percent or an absolute area <9 mm^2 has been proposed as a threshold.[74]

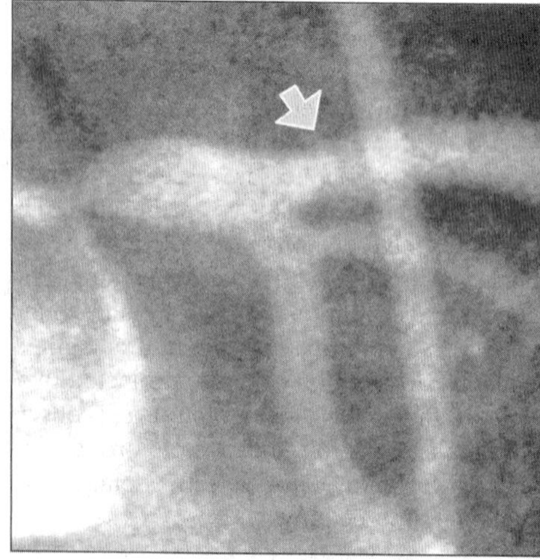
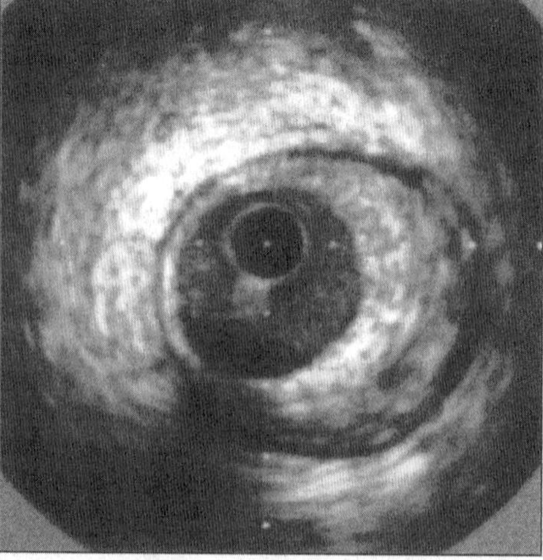

FIGURE 47-8 Underestimation of coronary atherosclerosis by angiography. In the angiogram in the left panel, a relatively minor lesion of the left anterior descending coronary is illustrated (*arrow*). In the right panel, this lesion is depicted by intravascular ultrasound and consists of a large eccentric atherosclerotic plaque that appears much more extensive than would be suspected from the angiogram.

Cardiac Allograft Disease

Transplant coronary artery disease is the leading cause of death beyond the first year after cardiac transplantation, with a reported incidence of 15 to 20 percent per year.[75] Although most transplant centers perform arteriograms annually for screening, these surveillance studies often fail to detect atherosclerosis prior to a clinical event.[76,77] Necropsy studies have demonstrated that angiography systematically underestimates coronary atherosclerosis in transplant recipients.[77] Patients may have diffuse vessel involvement that, for reasons already enumerated, conceals the atherosclerosis from the angiographer. Many active transplant centers now routinely perform intravascular ultrasound at the time of annual catheterization in all recipients. Investigations using ultrasound to detect transplant vasculopathy report a very high incidence of abnormal intimal thickening in 80 percent of patients at 1 year and in more than 92 percent studied 4 or more years after transplantation.[65–67,79–83]

Recent studies have revealed two pathways to transplant-associated atherosclerosis. Some patients receive atherosclerotic plaques transmitted via the donor heart, while others develop an immune-mediated vasculopathy.[67,81] Despite a young donor age, lesions of conventional atherosclerosis are frequently present in donor hearts. At a mean donor age of only 32 years, atherosclerosis, defined as a maximal intimal thickness ≥0.5 mm, was evident in 56 percent of patients.[67] Multivariate analysis demonstrated donor age ($p = 0.0001$) and male donor gender ($p = 0.0006$) to be important predictors of atherosclerosis. Ultrasound imaging was a necessity for accurate detection of donor lesions, since the sensitivity of angiography was only 43 percent. The natural history of donor lesions after transplantation is largely unknown. Since angiography is relatively insensitive, ultrasound remains the most important method used to study the early atherosclerotic lesion. In the first year after transplantation, progression occurred in 42 percent of patients.[82]

INTERVENTIONAL CLINICAL APPLICATIONS

Preinterventional Imaging

Several studies have demonstrated that ultrasound imaging of interventional target lesions may influence the approach to therapy. In one study (313 lesions), the intended revascularization strategy before ultrasound imaging was compared with the treatment actually performed.[42] In 40 percent of cases, the intended strategy was altered based on the ultrasound findings, most often ultrasound assessment of lesion composition or eccentricity (26 percent). Although there was a relatively close correlation between angiographic and ultrasonic lumen diameter ($r = 0.83$), a disagreement between the two methods was cited as the reason for altering the procedure in 13 percent of lesions. In another small, nonrandomized study ($n = 56$) of ultrasound guidance of balloon angioplasty or directional atherectomy, operators reclassified lesion characteristics after ultrasound in 68 percent of patients and the therapeutic approach was modified in 48 percent. Ultrasound measurements revealed a smaller lumen diameter than expected from angiography, leading to balloon upsizing in 34 percent of angioplasty cases.[84]

Several studies have purported to show benefits of ultrasound imaging prior to implantation of coronary stents.[85,86] The preliminary results of one prospective study identified vessel calcification as one of the predictors of "inadequate" stent expansion.[85] For ostial lesions, ultrasound imaging is sometimes used to determine whether the lesion involves the "true" ostium or spares the most proximal few millimeters, which may assist optimal stent positioning. When stents are used to treat dissections, ultrasound may reveal involvement of a longer segment than can be appreciated by angiography. This may be particularly relevant in "bailout" stenting for threatened abrupt closure, where it may be preferred to cover the full length of the dissection.[86] Despite promising data, reports on preinterventional imaging must be interpreted with caution. There are no prospective, controlled trials demonstrating a superior outcome using an ultrasound-guided approach. Study patients were not randomized, allowing for bias in selection of more complex cases for ultrasound guidance, which would likely emphasize the contributions of imaging. Furthermore, cases in which the operators were unable to advance the ultrasound catheter through the lesion were systematically excluded.

Imaging during Specific Interventions

BALLOON ANGIOPLASTY

Ultrasound guidance of balloon sizing has been proposed as a means to improve procedural result and late clinical outcome for percutaneous transluminal coronary angioplasty (PTCA).[87] In a study of 104 lesions, ultrasound was performed after obtaining a "satisfactory" angiographic result and revealed remodeling at the lesion or extensive plaque within the reference segment in 73 percent of the cases. In this subset, the balloon-to-artery ratio was increased from 1.12 ± 0.15 to 1.30 ± 0.17 ($p < 0.0001$) and the resulting angiographic minimal lumen diameter increased from 1.95 ± 0.5 to 2.21 ± 0.5 mm. Ultrasound lumen area improved from 3.16 ± 1.0 to 4.52 ± 1.1 mm^2 ($p > 0.0001$). Following ultrasound-guided balloon upsizing, the incidence of angiographic dissection was not increased (37 versus 40 percent, $p = 0.67$). However, the study was too small to demonstrate any effect upon intermediate or long-term clinical restenosis rates.

Intravascular ultrasound studies have evaluated the mechanisms of luminal enlargement following balloon angioplasty. Prior necropsy studies in patients who expired shortly after balloon angioplasty have described plaque fracture or disruption as the most common mechanism of dilatation.[20] Most ultrasound studies have confirmed that dissection is the most important mechanism of luminal enlargement, occurring in 40 to 80 percent of patients.[9,41,88–92] Identification of dissection or fracture is based on the visualization of blood flow in the newly created lumen, sometimes aided by injection of saline or iodinated contrast to opacify the lumen via microbubbles. Wall disruptions can be further defined by measuring the circumferential extent, length, and/or maximal depth of the dissection. One small study reported that calcified lesions had a higher incidence of dissection (67 versus 25 percent, $p = 0.03$) with a trend toward restenosis in lesions with no dissection.[41] Following iliac artery angioplasty, ultrasound evidence of dissection was noted in all 40 cases, accounting for 72 percent of the total lumen gain.[89]

Several alternative mechanisms for luminal enlargement not discernible by angiography have been identified using ultrasound, including arterial wall stretching and plaque compression, or "axial redistribution."[93–95] The contribution of vessel stretch to lumen gain following balloon angioplasty has been validated in experimental and clinical investigations. A peripheral angioplasty study reported that plaque area was reduced by 33 percent, accounting for only 20 percent of lumen gain.[89]

However, studies using automatic pullback devices have shown that "compression" actually represents redistribution of plaque along the long axis of the vessel.[95] The prognostic significance of different mechanisms of luminal enlargement remains under investigation.

DIRECTIONAL ATHERECTOMY

Directional coronary atherectomy (DCA) is currently performed relatively uncommonly. DCA devices incorporate a rotating circular blade to remove atherosclerotic plaque from the luminal surface. This process requires the inflation of a balloon within the housing of the cutter, leading to invagination of the plaque into the open window on the cutting surface.[96] Because angiographic and/or ultrasound calcification is a well-documented predictor of failure of directional atherectomy, ultrasound imaging has been advocated for guidance of atherectomy, particularly for preintervention lesion selection.[97,98] Ultrasound imaging can differentiate between superficial calcium, which predicts poor tissue retrieval, and deep calcium, which does not appear detrimental to favorable results. In 70 atherectomy patients, lesion calcification was detected by ultrasound in 63 percent, compared with 22 percent by angiography. Ultrasound-detected calcification resulted in reduced lumen gain and a smaller final lumen area.[97]

The additional spatial perspective provided by ultrasound may assist in the orientation of atherectomy cuts. However, successful application is complex because precise orientation of the ultrasound image remains difficult, relying primarily upon anatomic features such as side branches to orient the image. Repeated ultrasound examinations are sometimes performed between passes of the DCA device to determine the extent of plaque removal and the need for additional cuts. Ultrasound studies before and after directional atherectomy confirm that plaque removal is the primary mechanism of luminal enlargement[91,97] (Fig. 47-9). In 25 treated lesions, plaque reduction accounted for 78 percent of total lumen gain. Plaque area was reduced from 14.3 ± 0.8 to 10.5 ± 0.7 mm^2, whereas EEM area increased only slightly, from 16.7 ± 0.8 to 17.5 ± 0.8 mm^2, $p < 0.02$. Ultrasound studies show that despite a successful angiographic result, 40 to 60 percent of the target site is still occupied by atheroma.

Some investigators have proposed that achieving a larger lumen after atherectomy using ultrasound guidance would result in a lower restenosis rate. This hypothesis was tested in a multicenter registry (the Optimal Atherectomy Restenosis Study, or OARS) in which residual stenosis was reduced from 64 to 7 percent with ultrasound guidance.[98] The angiographic restenosis rate at 6 months was 28.9 percent and the 1-year target lesion revascularization rate was 17.8 percent. In the CAVEAT trial, DCA failed to reduce late events as compared with PTCA with or without ultrasound guidance.[99] Moreover, most atherectomy trials were performed without adjuvant therapy with GPIIb/IIIa inhibitors. It remains untested whether a larger postprocedure lumen and lower restenosis rate can be achieved using ultrasound guidance without a concomitant increase in complications.

ROTATIONAL ABLATION

Rotational ablation employs a high-speed (up to 200,000 rpm) diamond-coated burr to debulk atheroma. Theoretically, this device minimizes injury to the normal arterial wall by "differential cutting," in which normal elastic tissue is deflected away from the burr while relatively inelastic atheroma is not displaced and is therefore abraded by rotation of the burr. Clinical indications for rotational ablation include calcified segments or lesions that resist balloon dilatation. Rotational ablation is also sometimes used in long lesions, ostial lesions, and in-stent restenosis.[100-104] Demonstration of a heavily calcified vessel by angiography or ultrasound is often cited by operators as an indication for rotational ablation. However, there is a poor correlation between ultrasound and fluoroscopy in assessing the presence or extent of calcification. Accordingly, ultrasound is sometimes employed prior to rotational ablation to confirm or refute the presence of calcification. Vessels revascularized using rotational ablation are often diffusely diseased, and the "normal" dimension can be difficult to determine by angiography. Therefore, ultrasound is sometimes used to size the vessel and determine the largest burr that can be safely employed.

Intravascular ultrasound studies have confirmed the principle of selective plaque removal or differential cutting. In 48 lesions treated with rotational ablation, atheroma area decreased from 15.7 ± 4 to 13.0 ± 5 mm^2 and the arc of calcium decreased slightly from 227 ± 107 to 209 ± 107 degrees, $p < 0.05$.[104] Vessel expansion or dissection was noted in a minority of cases and did not contribute significantly to lumen gain. The residual narrowing of the cross-sectional area measured by ultrasound averaged 74 percent. Following rotational ablation, the residual lumen is usually round or ellipsoid and may have a 15 to 20

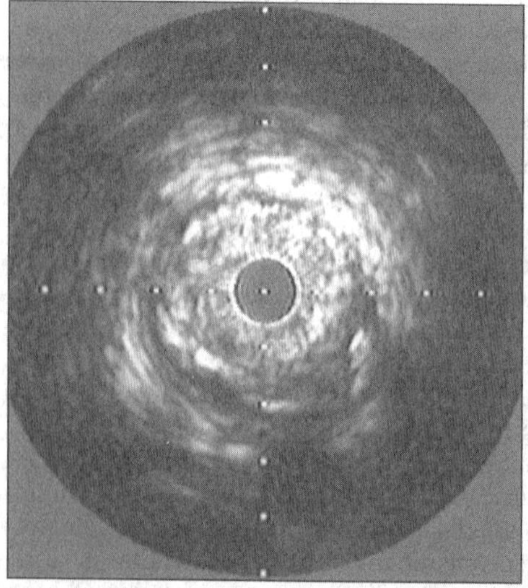

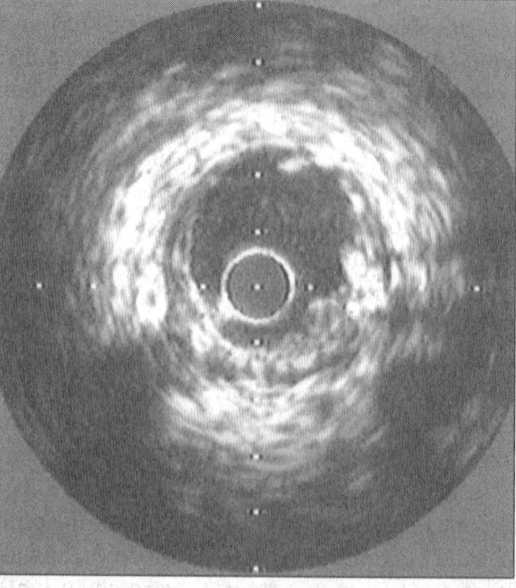

FIGURE 47-9 Directional coronary atherectomy. In the left panel, an intravascular ultrasound prior to atherectomy is shown. In the right panel, following directional atherectomy, extensive plaque removal is evident with a slightly irregular surface produced by the cutting action of the atherectomy device.

percent greater area than the largest burr used, presumably due to lateral movement of the burr during the procedure.

Luminal Measurements Postintervention

A poor correlation has been reported for comparisons of ultrasound and angiography in assessment of residual stenosis following balloon angioplasty, with measurements that are usually smaller by ultrasound than by angiography.[9,41,88–92] Two factors probably influence the overly optimistic tendency of angiographic imaging.[21] At the reference site, angiography tends to underestimate the diameter of the normal "reference" vessel because of the frequent presence of unrecognized atherosclerosis. At the target site, angiography tends to overestimate the actual gain in luminal diameter because contrast material penetrates into complex cracks and fissures produced by the intervention, giving the appearance of an enlarged lumen. To calculate a postprocedure percent diameter stenosis, the diameter at the target site (an overestimate) is divided by the reference diameter (an underestimate), resulting in a more favorable impression of the actual gain in luminal dimensions. Quantitative angiography showing a residual stenosis of 10 to 15 percent is commonly associated with a 60 to 80 percent atheroma burden.

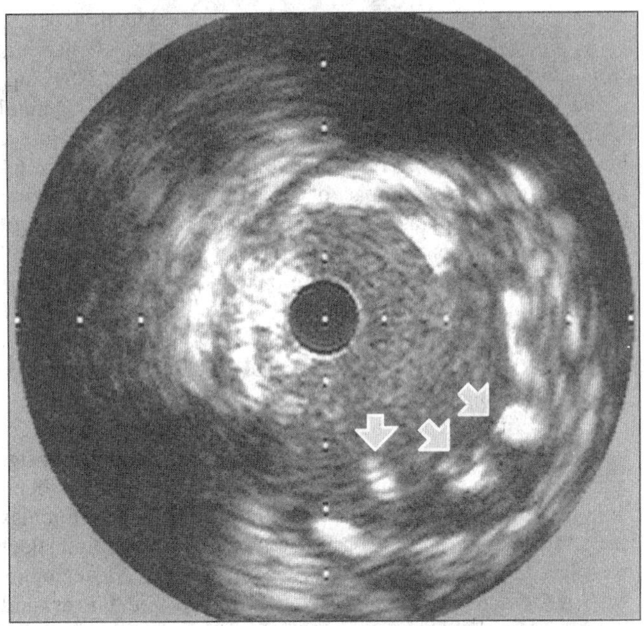

FIGURE 47-10 Underdeployed coronary stent. In this example, intravascular ultrasound images show several stent struts (*arrows*) that are not in full contact with the underlying vessel wall. This process is referred to as incomplete stent apposition.

Coronary Stent Deployment

INITIAL STUDIES OF ULTRASOUND GUIDANCE

The use of stents in percutaneous revascularization has increased exponentially over the last few years. Intravascular ultrasound imaging has played a pivotal role in understanding and optimizing the benefits of stent therapy.[105–107] In initial trials leading to FDA approval, articulated slotted-tube stents were deployed using moderate balloon pressures (6 to 10 atm).[108,109] To reduce subacute thrombosis, patients received aggressive anticoagulation with both antiplatelet and antithrombotic agents, including warfarin, for 3 to 6 months. Initial studies demonstrated a reduction in the restenosis rate compared with balloon angioplasty but reported a high incidence of hemorrhagic complications and longer hospital stays. A pioneering report detailing the intravascular ultrasound experience of Colombo et al. in Milan, Italy, significantly altered the understanding of optimal stent deployment and prevention of subacute thrombosis.[107] Ultrasound examination revealed a mean residual stenosis of 51 percent following angiographically guided stent deployment, with frequent incomplete stent apposition (Fig. 47-10).

Because stents are porous structures, angiographic contrast can flow outside of a partially deployed stent, resulting in the angiographic appearance of full deployment, despite the presence of incomplete apposition. In the Milan study, the operators performed additional balloon inflations at higher pressures (typically 18 to 20 atm) or used a larger balloon (or both), reducing final ultrasound residual stenosis to 34 percent and reporting a subacute thrombosis rate of only 0.3 percent with the use of no systemic antithrombotic agents (antiplatelet therapy only). It is now widely accepted that high-pressure deployment of the stents dramatically reduces the incidence of subacute thrombosis and obviates the need for acute and chronic administration of antithrombotic agents.[110,111] Subsequently, routine high-pressure deployment without ultrasound imaging became the standard of therapy.

ROUTINE VERSUS NONROUTINE ULTRASOUND

Following the widespread acceptance of high-pressure postdilatation with antiplatelet rather than anticoagulation regimens, the further benefit of ultrasound imaging has been debated.[86,110–114] Some investigators have suggested that despite routine use of high-pressure postdilatation, ultrasound-guided therapy can improve procedural results.[86,114] In a retrospective analysis of 315 lesions treated by high-pressure stenting, ultrasound was defined as "beneficial" if imaging resulted in further interventions that increased stent area by >25 percent or identified other lesions that required treatment.[115] Prior to ultrasound, the mean inflation pressure was 14.7 ± 3.2 atm, but only 47 percent of stents were considered "optimally" deployed. Additional ultrasound-triggered inflations improved in-stent lumen area by more than 25 percent in 83 lesions (26 percent of patients), and additional procedures were performed in lesions identified by ultrasound in 51 (16 percent). Final in-stent area improved from 6.9 ± 2.2 to 8.0 ± 1.93 mm² ($p < 0.001$). Procedural results were "improved" in 39 percent of the cases following ultrasound imaging.[115] It is now generally accepted that after high-pressure coronary stenting, ultrasound imaging results in additional procedures in approximately 20 to 40 percent of cases.

Since in-stent restenosis is predominantly determined by the degree of intimal hyperplasia, a larger lumen can theoretically accommodate more tissue growth without flow-limiting obstruction.[116] However, it remains uncertain whether ultrasound-guided "optimal" expansion translates into better clinical outcome. A randomized trial in 164 patients of ultrasound-guided stenting demonstrated a 6.3 percent absolute reduction in restenosis rate, which was not statistically significant because the study was powered to detect a 50 percent reduction of the restenosis rate.[117] A nonrandomized substudy of 538 patients from the Stent Anticoagulation Regimen Study (STARS) compared the outcome of ultrasound and angiographically guided stenting. The ultrasound arm achieved a significantly larger lumen area and a 39 percent relative reduction in clinical restenosis.[118] However, the impact of the more aggressive dilatation on restenosis rates has not been adequately examined by prospective trials. It remains conceivable that increased vessel wall injury from a larger high-pressure balloon will yield less favorable long-term results.

ULTRASOUND IMAGING OF PERISTENT SEGMENTS

Ultrasound imaging of "reference" segments following stenting may be useful in identifying reference segment disease or dissections that require additional interventions. The presence of significant peristent flow-limiting lesions or dissections has been linked to higher likelihood of stent thrombosis.[119] These findings are often angiographically occult or appear as areas of indistinct vessel border "haziness." In 201 stent patients, 31 segments with peristent angiographic haziness were detected. Ultrasound imaging revealed an angiographically inapparent obstructive lesion in 15, a peristent wall injury in 14, and mild intimal thickening in the remaining 2 segments.[120] The extent of neointimal hyperplasia at the stent margins has been linked to preexisting reference-segment disease.[121] In stenting as a "bailout" for dissection, intravascular ultrasound is more sensitive in detecting the extent of dissection, often revealing a greater true length than is evident from angiography, which may be helpful in guiding vessel salvage.

OPTIMAL PROCEDURAL GOALS OF ULTRASOUND GUIDED STENTING

Although ultrasound guidance of stenting has been practiced for several years, there is no consensus regarding optimal procedural end points. Colombo initially recommended achieving ≥60 percent of the average proximal and distal reference areas but later altered the definition to ≥100 percent of the distal reference lumen area.[105–107] Other definitions of optimal expansion include ≥90 percent of the distal reference area, ≥80 percent or ≥90 percent of the average reference area, a "lumen symmetry index" >0.7, and/or full coverage of reference-segment disease or dissections.[122,123] In most clinical trials, procedural end points are not achieved in the majority of cases. In the Optimal Stent Implantation Trial, the target of >90 percent of the average reference or >100 percent of the smaller reference area were not achieved in half the patients at an inflation pressure of 15 atm and only 60 percent of patients at 18 atm.[122] In the Angiography Versus Intravascular Ultrasound Directed Stent Placement (AVID) trial, the target end point of ≥90 percent of the distal reference area was not achieved in >70 percent of 225 patients.[124]

Recent reports have questioned the clinical relevance of using the stent-to-reference ratios as target for ultrasound-guided stenting. In 165 patients, target vessel revascularization was predicted by final in-stent lumen area (OR 1.4, 95 percent CI 1.1–1.9) and not the ratio of stent-to-reference area (OR 1.1, 95 percent CI 0.85–1.6).[112] Repeat revascularization was required in 30 percent of patients with a minimum in-stent lumen area <5 mm^2 but only 3 percent of cases with an area exceeding 9 mm^2. In another large cohort undergoing ultrasound-guided stenting, restenosis was inversely related to the minimum in-stent area.[125] An area of 9 mm^2 was achieved in 23 percent, but the incidence of restenosis in this subgroup was only 8 percent, compared with 29 percent in the remaining patients, $p < 0.0001$. Thus, commonly employed ultrasound end points based upon a predefined stent-to-reference ratio are both difficult to achieve and correlate weakly with clinical outcome.[125–127] Ultrasound studies have demonstrated that the degree of in-stent neointimal hyperplasia is independent of final lumen size, which may explain the higher restenosis rates in smaller vessels and poorly expanded stents.[116] If acute lumen gain is not adequate to accommodate subsequent tissue proliferation, there is significant late loss and restenosis.

Intravascular Ultrasound and Restenosis

A more complete understanding of restenosis has evolved from serial ultrasound measurements of plaque and lumen areas following balloon angioplasty and directional atherectomy.[128,129] In some studies, serial ultrasound examinations have shown that a late reduction in total vessel area (chronic negative remodeling) is an important mechanism of restenosis after interventional procedures.[129] These observations suggest that mechanical interventions to prevent chronic recoil (such as stenting) may be more important in preventing restenosis than interventions designed to prevent intimal hyperplasia. If further validated, this concept may explain the lower restenosis rate observed in randomized multicenter studies comparing balloon angioplasty and stent implantation.[108,109]

In 212 native coronary lesions in 209 patients following intervention, the ultrasound cross-sectional area with the smallest lumen area at late follow-up was compared with the matching site obtained immediately following the intervention.[129] At follow-up examination, there was a significant decrease in EEM area and an increase in plaque area ($p < 0.0001$ for both) that combined to reduce lumen area. More than 70 percent of lumen loss was attributable to the decrease in EEM area, whereas the neointimal area accounted for only 23 percent of the decrease in lumen area. The change in lumen area correlated more strongly with the change in EEM area ($r = 0.75$, $p < 0.0001$) than with the change in plaque area ($r = 0.28$, $p < 0.0001$). At lesions that demonstrated an increase in EEM area at follow-up (47 percent), there was no change or an actual gain in lumen area and a reduction in angiographic restenosis (26 versus 62 percent for lesions with a decrease in EEM area at follow-up, $p < 0.0001$).

Other investigators have suggested a bidirectional remodeling response following percutaneous coronary interventions: early adaptive enlargement and late shrinkage of the vessel. In a unique study, 61 lesions in 57 patients who underwent balloon angioplasty or atherectomy were examined by intravascular ultrasound in a serial manner—before and immediately after the intervention and after 24 h, 1 month, and 6 months.[48] The lumen area significantly improved during the first month following the intervention but significantly decreased at 6 months. Simultaneously, the EEM area increased in the first month but later decreased at 6 months. However, plaque area steadily increased from immediately postintervention to the 6-month follow-up. Thus the changes in lumen size closely tracked the changes in EEM area ($r = 0.72$, $p = 0.0001$). Although the increase in plaque area correlated with lumen loss, the correlation was not as strong ($r = 0.34$, $p = 0.0008$). The lumen gain observed during the first month was solely due to the compensatory vessel enlargement, whereas the late lumen loss was mostly caused by vessel shrinkage but also by progressive neointimal hyperplasia.

Investigations employing quantitative angiography have demonstrated that late lumen loss is significantly greater with stents than with balloon angioplasty. This, however, is offset by the much larger acute lumen gain, such that the net gain at follow-up is significantly greater with stenting.[108,109] Intravascular ultrasound has been employed to examine the mechanism of stent restenosis. Unlike the restenotic response to other percutaneous devices, which is a mixture of arterial remodeling and neointimal growth, stent restenosis is almost exclusively due to the neointimal proliferation.[129] In a serial study using intravascular ultrasound of stented coronary segments, there was no significant change in the area bound by stent struts, indicating that stents can withstand and resist the arterial remodeling process.[130] In some cases, restenosis develops at the margins of the stent. Predictors of stent restenosis have been identified by multivariate analysis, including the smaller reference vessel and lumen size, the larger plaque burden at the reference segments, and the smaller achieved in-stent lumen area at the stent margins.[121]

FUTURE DIRECTIONS

The technology and clinical role for intravascular ultrasound examination of the coronaries continues to evolve. Technological advances in intravascular imaging are anticipated, including further reductions in the size of imaging catheters and higher-frequency ultrasound catheters, yielding significantly better spatial resolution.[131,132] Although high-frequency probes enable better axial and lateral resolution, there are significant trade-offs in moving beyond the current 30-MHz frequency. For example, penetration is likely to be impaired in comparison with more conventional devices, and greater backscatter from blood cells at high frequencies may interfere with discrimination of the interface between lumen and vessel wall. However, if catheter miniaturization continues, a shorter wavelength will be important in preserving near-field image quality. It remains apparent that the physical limits of intravascular imaging technology have not been reached. Accordingly, further improvements in the performance of these devices are anticipated.

Analysis of backscattered ultrasound signals has been used by several investigators to perform "tissue characterization" of coronary plaques. Intrinsic characteristics of the backscattered ultrasound signals—including the amplitude distribution, frequency response, and power spectrum of the signal—convey specific information about tissue types.[133] Soft plaque consists of an amorphous collection of lipid substances, fibrosis, cholesterol clefts, and a variable amount of collagen and elastin. Thrombus, on the other hand, consists of a fairly organized layering of fibrous strands packed with a dense collection of red blood cells. The ability of computer-based analysis of the unprocessed radiofrequency backscatter to differentiate the histologic layers of the normal vessel wall remains investigational.

Three-dimensional reconstruction of intravascular ultrasound has been proposed as a means to facilitate understanding of the spatial relationship between the structures within different tomographic cross sections.[134] Despite the promise of these methods, many unresolved problems remain. The algorithms applied for 3D reconstruction do not consider the presence of curvatures of the vessel and assume that the catheter passes in a straight line through the center of consecutive cross sections. The systolic expansion of the coronary vessel and the movements of the catheter within the vessel during the cardiac cycle also generate artifacts. Accordingly, the reconstructed images should not be considered faithful representations of the vessel and should not be used for volumetric plaque determination. Simultaneous digitization of biplane fluoroscopic tracking of the radiopaque transducer and catheter tip has the potential to overcome some of these limitations, but is practical only for small-scale research purposes.[135]

SUMMARY

The equipment, technique, and applications for intravascular ultrasound imaging continue to evolve, finding increasingly common usage in clinical practice and research. The insights provided by the unique ability of intravascular ultrasound to directly image coronary plaques have contributed greatly to our understanding of the nature of atherosclerosis and the effects of interventional devices.

References

1. Bom N, Lancee CT, Van Egmond FC. An ultrasonic intracardiac scanner. *Ultrasonics* 1972; 10:72–76.
2. Yock PG, Johnson EL, Linker DT. Intravascular ultrasound: Development and clinical potential. *Am J Cardiac Imaging* 1988; 2:185–193.
3. Roelandt JR, Bom NY, Serruys PW. Intravascular high-resolution real-time, two-dimensional echocardiography. *Int J Cardiac Imaging* 1989; 4:63–67.
4. Hodgson JM, Graham SP, Savakus AD, et al. Clinical percutaneous imaging of coronary anatomy using an over-the-wire ultrasound catheter system. *Int J Cardiac Imaging* 1989; 4:187–193.
5. Nissen SE, Grines CL, Gurley JC, et al. Application of a new phased-array ultrasound imaging catheter in the assessment of vascular dimensions: In vivo comparison to cineangiography. *Circulation* 1990; 81:660–666.
6. Tobis JM, Mallery J, Mahon D, et al. Intravascular ultrasound imaging of human coronary arteries in vivo. *Circulation* 1991; 83:913–926.
7. Nissen SE, Gurley JC, Grines CL, et al. Intravascular ultrasound assessment of lumen size and wall morphology in normal subjects and patients with coronary artery disease. *Circulation* 1991; 84:1087–1099.
8. Nissen SE, Di Mario C, Tuzcu EM. Intravascular ultrasound, angioscopy, doppler, and pressure measurement. In: *Topol Cardiovascular Medicine*. Philadelphia: Lippincott-Raven Publishers; 1997.
9. Tobis JM, Mallery JA, Gessert J, et al. Intravascular ultrasound cross-sectional arterial imaging before and after balloon angioplasty in vitro. *Circulation* 1989; 80:873–882.
10. Topol EJ, Nissen SE. Our preoccupation with coronary luminology: The dissociation between clinical and angiographic findings in ischemic heart disease. *Circulation* 1995; 92:2333–2342.
11. Hodgson JM, Reddy KG, Suneja R, et al. Intracoronary ultrasound imaging: Correlation of plaque morphology with angiography, clinical syndrome and procedural results in patients undergoing coronary angioplasty. *J Am Coll Cardiol* 1993; 21:35–44.
12. Arnett EN, Isner JM, Redwood CR, et al. Coronary artery narrowing in coronary heart disease: Comparison of cineangiographic and necropsy findings. *Ann Intern Med* 1979; 91:350–356.

13. Grodin CM, Dydra I, Pastgernac A, et al. Discrepancies between cineangiographic and post-mortem findings in patients with coronary artery disease and recent myocardial revascularization. *Circulation* 1974; 49:703–709.
14. Isner JM, Kishel J, Kent KM. Accuracy of angiographic determination of left main coronary arterial narrowing. *Circulation* 1981; 63:1056–1061.
15. Vlodaver Z, Frech R, van Tassel RA, Edwards JE. Correlation of the antemortem coronary angiogram and the postmortem specimen. *Circulation* 1973; 47:162–168.
16. Zir LM, Miller SW, Dinsmore RE, et al. Interobserver variability in coronary angiography. *Circulation* 1976; 53:627–632.
17. Galbraith JE, Murphy ML, Desoyza N. Coronary angiogram interpretation: Interobserver variability. *JAMA* 1981; 240:2053–2059.
18. Roberts WC, Jones AA. Quantitation of coronary arterial narrowing at necropsy in sudden coronary death. *Am J Cardiol* 1979; 44:39–44.
19. White CW, Wright CB, Doty DB, et al. Does visual interpretation of the coronary arteriogram predict the physiologic importance of a coronary stenosis? *N Engl J Med* 1984; 310:819–824.
20. Waller BF. "Crackers, breakers, stretchers, drillers, scrapers, shavers, burners, welders, and melters": The future treatment of atherosclerotic coronary artery disease? A clinical-morphologic assessment. *J Am Coll Cardiol* 1989; 13:969–987.
21. Topol EJ, Nissen SE. Our preoccupation with coronary luminology: The dissociation between clinical and angiographic findings in ischemic heart disease. *Circulation* 1995; 92:2333–2342.
22. Glagov S, Weisenberg E, Zarins CK, et al. Compensatory enlargement of human coronary arteries. *N Engl J Med* 1987; 316:1371–1375.
23. Little WC, Constantinescu M, Applegate RJ, et al. Can arteriography predict the site of a subsequent myocardial infarction in patients with mild-to-moderate coronary artery disease? *Circulation* 1988; 78:1157–1166.
24. Yamagishi M, Miyatake K, Tamai J, et al. Detection of atherosclerosis at the site of focal vasospasm in angiographically normal or minimally narrowed coronary segments by intravascular ultrasound. *J Am Coll Cardiol* 1994; 23:352–357.
25. Nissen SE, Gurley JC. Application of intravascular ultrasound to detection and quantitation of coronary atherosclerosis. *Int J Cardiac Imaging* 1991; 6:165–177.
26. Nissen SE, DeFranco A, Tuzcu EM. Detection and quantification of atherosclerosis: The emerging role for intravascular ultrasound. In: Fuster V, ed., *Syndromes of Atherosclerosis: Correlations of Clinical Imaging and Pathology*. Armonk, NY; Futura; 1996:291.
27. TenHoff H, Korbijn A, Smit ThH, et al. Image artifacts in mechanically driven ultrasound catheters. *Int J Cardiac Imaging* 1989; 4:195–199.
28. Di Mario C, Madretsma S, Linker D, et al. The angle of incidence of the ultrasonic beam: A critical factor for the image quality in intravascular ultrasonography. *Am Heart J* 1993; 125: 442–448.
29. Hausmann D, Erbel R, Alibelli-Chemarin MJ, et al. The safety of intracoronary ultrasound: A multicenter survey of 2207 examinations. *Circulation* 1995; 91:623–630.
30. Batkoff BW, Linker DT. Safety of intracoronary ultrasound: Data from a multicenter European registry. *Cathet Cardiovasc Diagn* 1996; 38:238–241.
31. Pinto FJ, St Goar FG, Gao SZ, et al. Immediate and one-year safety of intracoronary ultrasonic imaging: Evaluation with serial quantitative angiography. *Circulation* 1993; 88:1709–1714.
32. Gussenhoven EJ, Essed CE, Lancee CT, et al. Arterial wall characteristics determined by intravascular ultrasound imaging: An in vitro study. *J Am Coll Cardiol* 1989; 4:947–952.
33. Potkin BN, Bartorelli AL, Gessert JM, et al. Coronary artery imaging with intravascular high-frequency ultrasound. *Circulation* 1990; 81:1575–1585.
34. Nishimura RA, Edwards WD, Warnes CA, et al. Intravascular ultrasound imaging: In vitro validation and pathologic correlation. *J Am Coll Cardiol* 1990; 16:145–154.
35. Fitzgerald PJ, St Goar FG, Connolly AJ, et al. Intravascular ultrasound imaging of coronary arteries: Are three layers the norm? *Circulation* 1992; 86:154–158.
36. St Goar FG, Pinto FJ, Alderman EL, et al. Intravascular ultrasound imaging of angiographically normal coronary arteries: An in vivo comparison with quantitative angiography. *J Am Coll Cardiol* 1991; 18:952–958.
37. Velican D, Velican C. Comparative study on age-related changes and atherosclerotic involvement of the coronary arteries of male and female subjects up to 40 years of age. *Atherosclerosis* 1981; 38:39–50.
38. Maheswaran B, Leung CY, Gutfinger DE, et al. Intravascular ultrasound appearance of normal and mildly diseased coronary arteries: Correlation with histologic specimens. *Am Heart J* 1995; 130:976–986.
39. Mintz GS, Popma JJ, Pichard AD, et al. Patterns of calcification in coronary artery disease: A statistical analysis of intravascular ultrasound and coronary angiography in 1,155 lesions. *Circulation* 1995; 91:1959–1965.
40. Tuzcu EM, Berkalp B, DeFranco AC, et al. The dilemma of diagnosing coronary calcification: Angiography versus intravascular ultrasound. *J Am Coll Cardiol* 1996; 27:832–838.
41. Honye J, Mahon DJ, Jain A, et al. Morphological effects of coronary balloon angioplasty in vivo assessed by intravascular ultrasound imaging. *Circulation* 1992; 85:1012–1025.
42. Mintz GS, Pichard AD, Kovach JA, et al. Impact of preintervention intravascular ultrasound imaging on transcatheter treatment strategies in coronary artery disease. *Am J Cardiol* 1994; 73:423–430.
43. Hermiller JB, Tenaglia AN, Kisslo KB, et al. In vivo validation of compensatory enlargement of atherosclerotic coronary arteries. *Am J Cardiol* 1993; 71:665–668.
44. Ge J, Erbel R., Zamorano J, et al. Coronary artery remodeling in atherosclerotic disease: An intravascular ultrasonic study in vivo. *Coron Artery Dis* 1993; 4:981–986.
45. Losordo DW, Rosenfield K, Kaufman J, et al. Focal compensatory enlargement of human arteries in response to progressive atherosclerosis: In vivo documentation using intravascular ultrasound. *Circulation* 1994; 89:2570–2577.
46. Pasterkamp G, Wensing PJ, Post MJ, et al. Paradoxical arterial wall shrinkage may contribute to luminal narrowing of human atherosclerotic femoral arteries. *Circulation* 1995; 91:1444–1449.
47. Mintz GS, Kent KM, Pichard AD, et al. Contribution of inadequate arterial remodeling to the development of focal coronary artery stenoses: An intravascular ultrasound study. *Circulation* 1997; 95:1791–1798.
48. Kimura T, Kaburagi S, Tamura T, et al. Remodeling of human coronary arteries undergoing coronary angioplasty or atherectomy. *Circulation* 1997; 96:475–483.
49. Richardson PD, Davies MJ, Born GV. Influence of plaque configuration and stress distribution on fissuring of coronary atherosclerotic plaques. *Lancet* 1989; 2:941–944.
50. Kalbfleisch SJ, McGillem MJ, Simon SB, et al. Automated quantitation of indexes of coronary lesion complexity: Comparison between patients with stable and unstable angina. *Circulation* 1990; 82:439–447.
51. Ambrose JA, Winters SL, Arora RR, et al. Angiographic evolution of coronary artery morphology in unstable angina. *J Am Coll Cardiol* 1986; 7:472–478.
52. Loree HM, Kamm RD, Stringfellow RG, Lee RT. Effects of fibrous cap thickness on peak circumferential stress in model atherosclerotic vessels. *Circ Res* 1992; 71:850–858.

53. Levin DC, Fallon JT. Significance of the angiographic morphology of localized coronary stenoses: Histopathologic correlations. *Circulation* 1982; 66:316–320.
54. Ambrose JA, Winters SL, Stern A, et al. Angiographic morphology and the pathogenesis of unstable angina pectoris. *J Am Coll Cardiol* 1985; 5:609–616.
55. Shoenhagen P, Ziada KM, Kapadia SR, et al. Extent and direction of arterial remodeling in stable versus unstable coronary syndromes: An intravascular ultrasound study. *Circulation* 2000; 101:598–603.
56. Siegel RJ, Ariani M, Fishbein MC, et al. Histopathologic validation of angioscopy and intravascular ultrasound. *Circulation* 1991; 84:109–117.
57. Kearney P, Erbel R, Rupprecht HJ, et al. Differences in the morphology of unstable and stable coronary lesions and their impact on the mechanisms of angioplasty: An in vivo study with intravascular ultrasound. *Eur Heart J* 1996; 17:721–730.
58. Bocksch W, Schartl M, Beckmann S, et al. Intravascular ultrasound imaging in patients with acute myocardial infarction. *Eur Heart J* 1995; 16(suppl J):46–52.
59. Bridal SL, Fornes P, Bruneval P, Berger G. Parametric (integrated backscatter and attenuation) images constructed using backscattered radio frequency signals (25–56 MHz) from human aortae in vitro. *Ultrasound Med Biol* 1997; 23:215–229.
60. Hiro T, Leung CY, Karimi H, et al. Angle dependence of intravascular ultrasound imaging and its feasibility in tissue characterization of human atherosclerotic tissue. *Am Heart J* 1999; 137:476–481.
61. Wong M, Edelstein J, Wollman J, Bond MG. Ultrasonic-pathological comparison of the human arterial wall: Verification of intima-media thickness. *Arterioscler Thromb* 1993; 13:482–486.
62. Potkin BN, Bartorelli AL, Gessert JM, et al. Coronary artery imaging with intravascular high-frequency ultrasound. *Circulation* 1990; 81:1575–1585.
63. Tuzcu EM, Hobbs H, Rincon G, et al. Occult and frequent transmission of atherosclerosis coronary disease with cardiac transplantation. *Circulation* 1995; 91:1706–1713.
64. Mehra MR, Ventura HO, Stapleton DD, Smart FW. The prognostic significance of intimal proliferation in cardiac allograft vasculopathy: A paradigm shift (review). *J Heart Lung Transplant* 1995; 14:6 Pt. 2, S207–S211.
65. Escobar A, Ventura HO, Stapleton DD, et al. Cardiac allograft vasculopathy assessed by intravascular ultrasonography and nonimmunologic risk factors. *Am J Cardiol* 1994; 74: 1042–1046.
66. Rickenbacher PR, Pinto FJ, Chenzbraun A, et al. Incidence and severity of transplant coronary artery disease early and up to 15 years after transplantation as detected by intravascular ultrasound. *J Am Coll Cardiol* 1995; 25:171–177.
67. Tuzcu EM. DeFranco AC, Goormastic M, et al. Dichotomous pattern of coronary atherosclerosis 1 to 9 years after transplantation: Insights from systematic intravascular ultrasound imaging. *J Am Coll Cardiol* 1996; 27:839–846.
68. Gil R, von Birgelen C, Prati F, et al. Usefulness of three-dimensional reconstruction for interpretation and quantitative analysis of intracoronary ultrasound during stent deployment. *Am J Cardiol* 1996; 77:761–764.
69. Mintz GS, Popma JJ, Pichard AD, et al. Limitations of angiography in the assessment of plaque distribution in coronary artery disease: A systematic study of target lesion eccentricity in 1446 lesions. *Circulation* 1996; 93:924–931.
70. Erbel R, Ge J, Bockisch A, et al. Value of intracoronary ultrasound and Doppler in the differentiation of angiographically normal coronary arteries: A prospective study in patients with angina pectoris. *Eur Heart J* 1996; 17:880–889.
71. Mintz GS, Painter JA, Pichard AD, et al. Atherosclerosis in angiographically "normal" coronary artery reference segments: An intravascular ultrasound study with clinical correlations. *J Am Coll Cardiol* 1995; 25:1479–1485.
72. Lee DY, Eigler N, Luo H, et al. Effect of intracoronary ultrasound imaging on clinical decision making. *Am Heart J* 1995; 129:1084–1093.
73. Mintz GS, Pichard AD, Kovach JA, et al. Impact of preintervention intravascular ultrasound imaging on transcatheter treatment strategies in coronary artery disease. *Am J Cardiol* 1994; 73:423–430.
74. Hermiller JB, Buller CE, Tenaglia AN, et al. Unrecognized left main coronary artery disease in patients undergoing interventional procedures. *Am J Cardiol* 1993; 71:173–176.
75. Uretsky BF, Kormos RL, Zerbe TR, et al. Cardiac events after heart transplantation: Incidence and predictive value of coronary arteriography. *J Heart Transplant* 1992; 11:S45–S50.
76. O'Neill BJ, Pflugfelder PW, Single NR, et al. Frequency of angiographic detection and quantitative assessment of coronary arterial disease one and three years after cardiac transplantation. *Am J Cardiol* 1989; 63:1221–1226.
77. Dressler FA, Miller LW. Necropsy versus angiography: How accurate is angiography? *J Heart Lung Transplant* 1992; 11(part2):S56–S59.
78. Johnson DE, Alderman EL, Schroeder JS, et al. Transplant coronary artery disease: Histopathological correlations with angiographic morphology. *J Am Coll Cardiol* 1991; 17:449–457.
79. Yeung AC, Davis SF, Hauptman PJ, et al. Incidence and progression of transplant coronary artery disease over 1 year: Results of a multicenter trial with use of intravascular ultrasound. Multicenter Intravascular Ultrasound Transplant Study Group. *J Heart Lung Transplant* 1995; 14:6, S215–S220.
80. Kerber S, Rahmel A, Heinemann-Vechtel O, et al. Angiographic, intravascular ultrasound and functional findings early after orthotopic heart transplantation. *Int J Cardiol* 1995; 49:119–129.
81. St Goar FG, Pinto FJ, Alderman EL, et al. Detection of coronary atherosclerosis in young adult hearts using intravascular ultrasound. *Circulation* 1992; 86:756–763.
82. Kapadia SR, Nissen SE, Ziada KM, et al. Development of transplant vasculopathy and progression of donor-transmitted atherosclerosis: A comparison by serial intravascular ultrasound imaging. *Circulation* 1998; 98:2672–2678.
83. Kapadia SR, Crowe TD, Ziada KM, et al. Natural history of donor transmitted atherosclerosis in transplant patients: Serial intravascular ultrasound study. *J Am Coll Cardiol* 1998; 31:856–862.
84. Impact of intravascular ultrasound on device selection and endpoint assessment of interventions: Phase I of the GUIDE trial (abstr). *J Am Coll Cardiol* 1993; 21:134A.
85. Hoffmann R, Mintz GS, Popma JJ, et al. Treatment of calcified coronary lesions with Palmaz-Schatz stents: An intravascular ultrasound study. *Eur Heart J* 1998; 19:1224–1231.
86. Russo RJ. Ultrasound-guided stent placement. *Cardiol Clin* 1997; 15:49–61.
87. Stone GW, Hodgson JM, St Goar FG, et al. Improved procedural results of coronary angioplasty with intravascular ultrasound-guided balloon sizing: The CLOUT pilot trial: Clinical Outcomes with Ultrasound Trial (CLOUT) investigators. *Circulation* 1997; 95:2044–2052.
88. Gil R, Di Mario C, Prati F, et al. Influence of plaque composition on mechanisms of percutaneous transluminal coronary balloon angioplasty assessed by ultrasound imaging. *Am Heart J* 1996; 131:591–597.
89. Losordo DW, Rosenfield K, Pieczek A, et al. How does angioplasty work? Serial analysis of human iliac arteries using intravascular ultrasound. *Circulation* 1992; 86:1845–1858.
90. Potkin BN, Keren G, Mintz GS, et al. Arterial responses to balloon coronary angioplasty: An intravascular ultrasound study. *J Am Coll Cardiol* 1992; 20:942–951.

91. Braden GA, Herrington DM, Downes TR, et al. Qualitative and quantitative contrasts in the mechanisms of lumen enlargement by coronary balloon angioplasty and directional coronary atherectomy. *J Am Coll Cardiol* 1994; 23:40–48.
92. van der Lugt A, Gussenhoven EJ, Stijnen T, et al. Comparison of intravascular ultrasonic findings after coronary balloon angioplasty evaluated in vitro with histology. *Am J Cardiol* 1995; 76:661–666.
93. Mintz GS, Pichard AD, Kent KM, et al. Axial plaque redistribution as a mechanism of percutaneous transluminal coronary angioplasty. *Am J Cardiol* 1996; 77:427–430.
94. Botas J, Clark DA, Pinto F, et al. Balloon angioplasty results in increased segmental coronary distensibility: A likely mechanism of percutaneous transluminal coronary angioplasty. *J Am Coll Cardiol* 1994; 23:1043–1052.
95. Mintz GS, Pichard AD, Kent KM, et al. Axial plaque redistribution as a mechanism of percutaneous transluminal coronary angioplasty. *Am J Cardiol* 1996; 77:427–430.
96. Simpson JB, Selmon MR, Robertson GC, et al.Transluminal atherectomy for occlusive peripheral vascular disease. *Am J Cardiol* 1988; 61:96G–101G.
97. Matar FA, Mintz GS, Pinnow E, et al. Multivariate predictors of intravascular ultrasound end points after directional coronary atherectomy. *J Am Coll Cardiol* 1995; 25:318–324.
98. Simonton CA, Leon MB. Baim DS, et al. "Optimal" directional coronary atherectomy: Final results of the Optimal Atherectomy Restenosis Study (OARS). *Circulation* 1998; 97:332–339.
99. Topol EJ, Leya F, Pinkerton CA, et al., on behalf of the CAVEAT Study Group. A comparison of coronary angioplasty with directional atherectomy in patients with coronary artery disease. *N Engl J Med* 1993; 329:221–227.
100. MacIsaac AI, Bass TA, Buchbinder M, et al. High speed rotational atherectomy: Outcome in calcified and noncalcified coronary artery lesions. *J Am Coll Cardiol* 1995; 26:731–736.
101. De Franco AC, Nissen SE, Tuzcu EM, Whitlow PL. Incremental value of intravascular ultrasound during rotational coronary atherectomy. *Cathet Cardiovasc Diagn* 1996; (suppl. 3): 23–33.
102. Sharma SK, Duvvuri S, Dangas G, et al. Rotational atherectomy for in-stent restenosis: Acute and long-term results of the first 100 cases. *J Am Coll Cardiol* 1998; 32:1358–1365.
103. Schiele F, Meneveau N, Vuillemenot A, et al. Treatment of in-stent restenosis with high speed rotational atherectomy and IVUS guidance in small 3.0 mm vessels. *Cathet Cardiovasc Diagn* 1998; 44:77–82.
104. Kovach JA, Mintz GS, Pichard AD, et al. Sequential intravascular ultrasound characterization of the mechanisms of rotational atherectomy and adjunct balloon angioplasty. *J Am Coll Cardiol* 1993; 22:1024–1032.
105. Nakamura S, Colombo A, Galglione S, et al. Intracoronary ultrasound observations during stent implantation. *Circulation* 1994; 89:2026–2034.
106. Goldberg SL, Colombo A, Nakamura S, et al. Benefit of intracoronary ultrasound in the deployment of Palmaz-Schatz stents. *J Am Coll Cardiol* 1994; 24:996–1003.
107. Colombo A, Hall P, Nakamura S, et al. Intracoronary stenting without anticoagulation accomplished with intravascular ultrasound guidance. *Circulation* 1995; 91:1676–1688.
108. Serruys PW, de Jaegere P, Kiemeneij F, et al., on behalf of the Benestent Study Group. A comparison of balloon-expandable-stent implantation with balloon angioplasty in patients with coronary artery disease. *N Engl J Med* 1994; 331:489–495.
109. Fischman DL, Leon MB, Baim DS, et al. A randomized comparison of coronary-stent placement and balloon angioplasty in the treatment of coronary artery disease. *N Engl J Med* 1994; 331:496–501.
110. Morice MC, Breton C, Bunouf P, et al. Coronary stenting without anticoagulation, without intravascular ultrasound: Results of the French registry. *Circulation* 1995; 92(suppl I):I-796.
111. Sandardas MA, McEniery PT, Aroney CN, Bett JHN. Elective implantation of intracoronary stents without intravascular ultrasound guidance or subsequent warfarin. *Cathet Cardiovasc Diagn* 1996; 37:355–359.
112. Goods CM, Al-Shaibi KF, Yadav SS, et al. Utilization of the coronary balloon-expandable coil stent without anticoagulation or intravascular ultrasound. *Circulation* 1996; 93:1803–1808.
113. Karrillon GJ, Morice MC, Benveniste E, et al. Intracoronary stent implantation without ultrasound guidance and with replacement of conventional anticoagulation by antiplatelet therapy. 30-day clinical outcome of the French Multicenter Registry. *Circulation* 1996; 94:1519–1527.
114. Prati F, Gil R, Di Mario C, et al. Is quantitative angiography sufficient to guide stent implantation? A comparison with three-dimensional reconstruction of intracoronary ultrasound images. *G Ital Cardiol* 1997; 27:328–336.
115. Allen KM, Undemir C, Shaknovich A, et al. Is there need for intravascular ultrasound after high pressure dilatation of Palmaz-Schatz stents (abstr). *J Am Coll Cardiol* 1996; 27:138A.
116. Hoffmann R, Mintz GS, Pichard AD, et al. Intimal hyperplasia thickness at follow-up is independent of stent size: A serial intravascular ultrasound study. *Am J Cardiol* 1998; 82:1168–1172.
117. Schiele F, Meneveau N, Vuillemenot A, et al. Impact of intravascular ultrasound guidance in stent deployment on 6-month restenosis rate: A multicenter, randomized study comparing two strategies—with and without intravascular ultrasound guidance. RESIST Study Group (REStenosis after Ivus guided STenting). *J Am Coll Cardiol* 1998; 32:320–328.
118. Fitzgerald PJ, Hayase M, Mintz GS, et al. CRUISE: Can routine intravascular ultrasound influence stent expansion? Analysis of outcomes. *J Am Coll Cardiol* 1998; 31:396A.
119. Schuhlen H, Hadamitzky M, Walter H, et al. Major benefit from antiplatelet therapy for patients at high risk for adverse cardiac events after coronary Palmaz-Schatz stent placement: Analysis of a prospective risk stratification protocol in the Intracoronary Stenting and Antithrombotic Regimen (ISAR) trial. *Circulation* 1997; 95:2015–2021.
120. Ziada KM, Tuzcu EM, De Franco AC, et al. Intravascular ultrasound assessment of the prevalence and causes of angiographic "haziness" following high-pressure coronary stenting. *Am J Cardiol* 1997; 80:116–121.
121. Hoffmann R, Mintz GS, Kent KM, et al. Serial intravascular ultrasound predictors of restenosis at the margins of Palmaz-Schatz stents. *Am J Cardiol* 1997; 79:951–953.
122. de Jaegere P, Mudra H, Figulla H, et al. Intravascular ultrasound-guided optimized stent deployment: Immediate and 6 months clinical and angiographic results from the Multicenter Ultrasound Stenting in Coronaries Study (MUSIC Study). *Eur Heart J* 1998; 19:1214–1223.
123. Stone GW, St Goar F, Fitzgerald P, et al. The Optimal Stent Implantation Trial: Final core lab angiographic and ultrasound analysis (abstr). *J Am Coll Cardiol* 1997; 29:369A.
124. Russo RJ, Nicosia A, Teirstein PS, Investigators AVID. Angiography versus intravascular ultrasound-directed stent placement. *J Am Coll Cardiol* 1997; 29:369A.
125. Kasaoka S, Tobis JM, Akiyama T, et al. Angiographic and intravascular ultrasound predictors of in-stent restenosis. *J Am Coll Cardiol* 1998; 32:1630–1635.
126. Ziada KM, Tuzcu EM, De Franco AC, et al. Absolute, not relative, post-stent lumen area is a better predictor of clinical events (abstr). *Circulation* 1996; 94:I-453.
127. Moussa I, Di Mario C, Moses J, et al. The predictive value of different intravascular ultrasound criteria for restenosis after coronary stenting (abstr). *J Am Coll Cardiol* 1997; 29:60A.
128. Mintz GS, Popma JJ, Pichard AD, et al. Intravascular ultrasound

predictors of restenosis after percutaneous transcatheter coronary revascularization. *J Am Coll Cardiol* 1996; 27:1678–1687.
129. Mintz GS, Popma JJ, Pichard AD, et al. Arterial remodeling after coronary angioplasty: A serial intravascular ultrasound study. *Circulation* 1996; 94:35–43.
130. Painter JA, Mintz GS, Wong SC, et al. Serial intravascular ultrasound studies fail to show evidence of chronic Palmaz-Schatz stent recoil. *Am J Cardiol* 1995; 75:398–400.
131. Lockwood GR, Ryan LK, Foster FS. A 45 to 55 MHz needle-based ultrasound system for invasive imaging. *Ultrason Imaging* 1993; 15:1–13.
132. Foster FS, Knapik DA, Machado JC, et al. High-frequency intra-coronary ultrasound imaging. *Semin Intervent Cardiol* 1997; 2:33–41.
133. Linker DT, Kleven A, Gronningsaether A, et al. Tissue characterization with intra-arterial ultrasound: Special promise and problems. *Int J Cardiol Imaging* 1991; 6:255–263.
134. von Birgelen C, de Vrey EA, Mintz GS, et al. ECG-gated three-dimensional intravascular ultrasound: Feasibility and reproducibility of the automated analysis of coronary lumen and atherosclerotic plaque dimensions in humans. *Circulation* 1997; 96:2944–2952.
135. Evans JL, Ng KH, Wiet SG, et al. Accurate three-dimensional reconstruction of intravascular ultrasound data: Spatially correct three-dimensional reconstructions. *Circulation* 1996; 93:567–576.

C H A P T E R 48

CORONARY BYPASS SURGERY

Bruce W. Lytle

Coronary bypass surgery as a planned consistent approach for the treatment of patients with angiographically documented coronary atherosclerosis was begun by Sones, Favaloro, and colleagues in 1967. Many previous schemes for surgical myocardial revascularization, direct and indirect, had been attempted, including pericardial pouderage, mammary artery implantation (Vineberg operation), coronary endarterectomy, and "blind" bypass grafting without the angiographic definition of coronary lesions.[1,2] The concept behind the concerted effort undertaken by cardiologists and cardiac surgeons at The Cleveland Clinic Foundation in 1967 was that the symptoms and clinical events associated with coronary artery disease (CAD) were related to stenotic coronary artery lesions that could be specifically identified by coronary angiography, and if those lesions could be treated with bypass grafting, unfavorable symptoms and events would be less common. Experience has shown that concept to be correct but also has shown that atherosclerosis is a progressive disease.

In the early years of coronary bypass grafting, the vast majority of grafts were reversed segments of saphenous vein anastomosed to the aorta and to the coronary arteries distal to coronary stenoses (Fig. 48-1*A*). It was rapidly obvious that effective bypass surgery relieved symptoms of angina, and during the decade 1970–1980, the practice of coronary artery surgery exploded. Improvements in instrumentation, technology, and surgical training were rapid, and by 1980, bypass surgery had evolved into a microsurgical procedure usually performed with optical assistance at many hundreds of medical centers around the world.

EARLY RANDOMIZED TRIALS OF BYPASS SURGERY VERSUS MEDICAL TREATMENT

During the 1970s, multiple investigations were initiated to examine the long-term outcomes of patients receiving initial bypass grafting compared with those treated initially with medical management. The most influential were multicenter, randomized trials of patients with chronic stable angina: the Veteran's Administration study of patients with chronic stable angina (VA study),[3] the European Coronary Surgery Study (ECSS),[4] and the Coronary Artery Surgery Study (CASS).[5,6] These trials randomized patients with angiographically documented coronary stenoses to either initial medical management or initial treatment with bypass surgery, and their primary emphasis was survival. In the two largest trials (ECSS and CASS), severely symptomatic patients were excluded from randomization, and in all these trials, patients who experienced the onset or persistence of severe symptoms were allowed to change from medical to surgical treatment, a phenomenon called *crossover*. Analyses of outcomes were performed on an "intention to treat" basis. That is, patients who were randomized to the medical treatment group but who later decided to have surgery were still considered part of the medically treated group, and patients randomized to surgery who did not actually receive surgery were still considered part of the surgically treated group.

All these trials showed there were some patient subsets that experienced a higher survival rate if they received initial surgical management rather than initial medical treatment, although those subsets varied among the trials. Not surprisingly, the patients who benefited the most from surgery in terms of survival were patients at the highest risk of death without operation. Individual trials noted improved survival rates for patients with significant left main stenosis, three-vessel disease with abnormal left ventricular (LV) function, and two- or three-vessel disease with a more than 75 percent stenosis in the proximal left anterior descending (LAD) coronary artery. The clinical descriptors of an abnormal baseline electrocardiogram (ECG) or a strongly positive exercise test helped to define patient subsets with improved survival rates with surgery. Recently, a metaanalysis that included the three major trials and some smaller ones

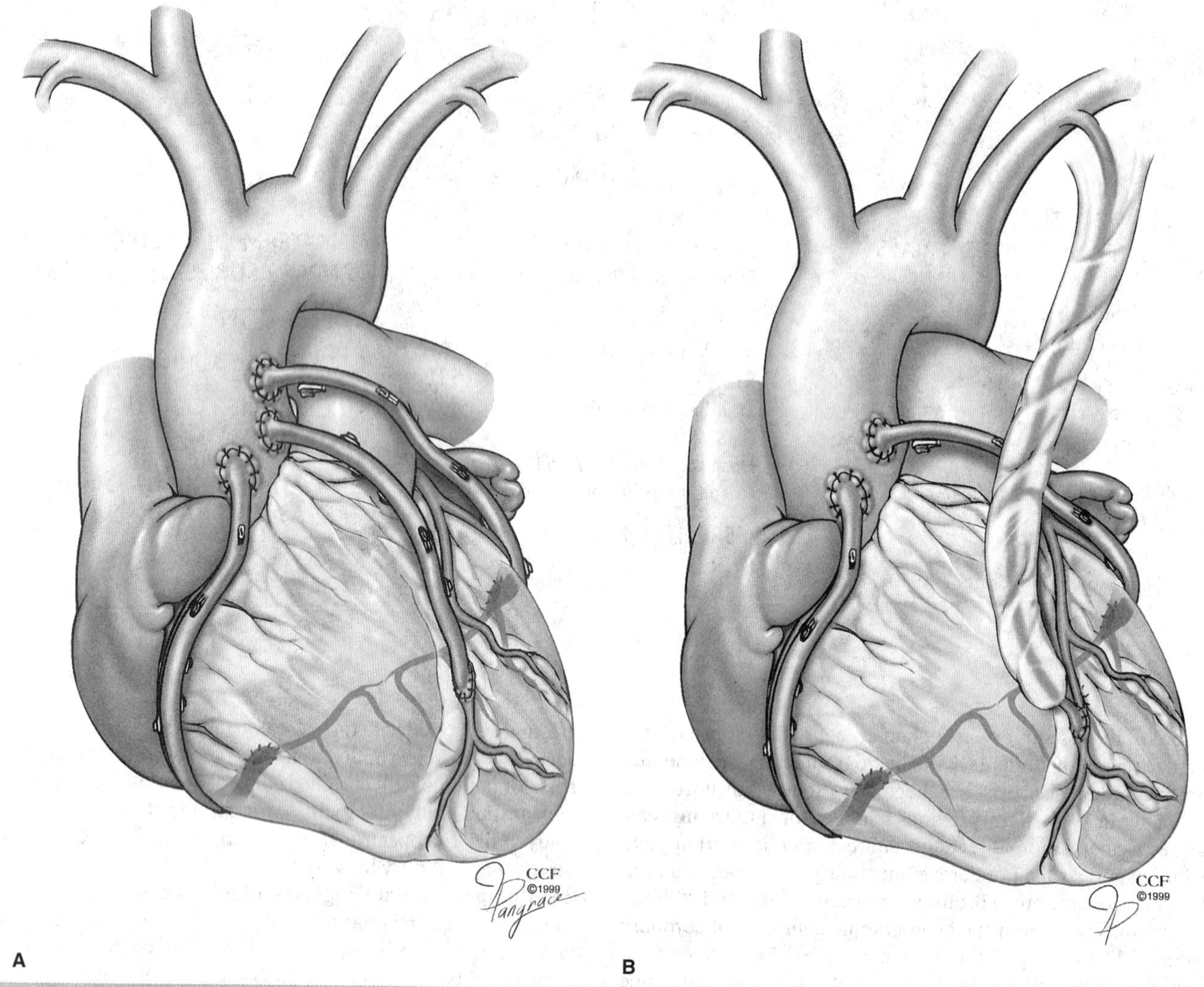

FIGURE 48-1 *A*. Most early coronary bypass operations involved only aorta to coronary saphenous vein grafts. *B*. The use of a left ITA to LAD artery graft improves clinical outcomes, and combining this strategy with vein grafts to other coronary arteries has become the standard bypass operation.

confirmed the observations of the individual trials but also seemed to show a significant survival benefit for patients with triple-, double-, or even single-vessel disease that included a proximal LAD stenosis regardless of whether they had normal or abnormal LV function. For patients without a proximal LAD stenosis, surgery improved the survival rate for only patients with left main stenosis or triple-vessel disease. In addition, the surgically treated patients had fewer symptoms at 5 postoperative years and took fewer antianginal medications.

The degree of benefit achieved with initial bypass surgery diminished with time both in terms of survival and with regard to symptom status.[8] There were multiple reasons for this. First, the status of the surgically treated patients deteriorated based on late graft failure and the progression of native vessel atherosclerosis. Very few patients in these early trials received internal thoracic artery (ITA) grafts or were treated with platelet inhibitors or lipid-lowering agents, strategies we now know significantly improved long-term outcomes after surgery. Second, the status of the "medically treated" patients actually improved slightly because a large proportion of those patients "crossed over" and underwent bypass surgery, although they were still analyzed as part of the medically treated group. In the three major studies, 40 to 44 percent of the total medically treated patient population had undergone bypass surgery by 10 postoperative years, including 65 percent of patients with left main disease and 48 percent of patients with three-vessel disease.[7] Finally, when all-cause mortality is the end point, any two survival curves eventually will meet at zero.

Randomized clinical trials as described earlier have the advantage that they lessen the influence of bias in the selection of treatment once patients are entered into the study, but they have the disadvantage that bias may be exerted at the point of inclusion into the trial. In all these trials, a minority of patients presenting for evaluation met the criteria for entry into the trial, and of those who met the criteria for entry, a minority actually were randomized. In the case of CASS, however, patients who were not randomized were followed prospectively in a registry, and that registry has produced observational studies that continue to provide useful information.

Among the important conclusions from the CASS Registry are that asymptomatic patients with 50 percent or more of left main stenosis and patients with left main equivalent (70 percent or more stenosis of the proximal LAD and circumflex vessels) have improved survival with surgery.[9,10] For severely symptomatic patients, bypass surgery improved the survival rates of those with three-vessel disease regardless of whether they had normal or abnormal LV function, even if those patients did not have severe proximal coronary artery stenoses.[11] Also, surgically treated patients who were completely revascularized fared better than incompletely revascularized patients, particularly if they had abnormal LV function.[12]

Outcomes for patients with unstable angina based on either progressive symptoms or rest angina with electrocardiographic changes were tested in the Veterans Administration Cooperative Study. Patients with rest angina and abnormal LV function had greatly improved survival with initial surgery. Patients with progressive angina did not appear to have a worse survival rate if they were treated initially with medical therapy, but 19 percent of this group crossed over to surgery within 30 days of randomization, and by 96 months, 45 percent had crossed over to surgery.[13]

Although these trials were undertaken relatively early in the history of coronary bypass surgery and today we can expect lower operative mortality rates and improved long-term outcomes after operation based on the use of arterial grafts, platelet inhibitors, and lipid-lowering agents, the observations from these studies provide the fundamental basis for the development of indications for bypass surgery even today.[2,14]

EVOLUTION OF THE OPERATION AND PATIENT POPULATION

In the early years of bypass surgery, surgical candidates usually were relatively young, had limited coronary artery disease, good LV function, and few comorbid conditions. The operation was almost always performed through a median sternotomy with the use of cardiopulmonary bypass. To achieve a surgical field and allow operations to be done on a still heart, either cold fibrillation or intermittent ischemic arrest was a common strategy. The operation involved bypass grafts of reversed segments of greater saphenous vein from the aorta to the distal coronary arteries (see Fig. 48-1*A*). In a small number of centers, the left ITA was used as a bypass graft, usually as a graft to the LAD artery (see Fig. 48-1*B*), but this strategy was not common.

Throughout the 1970s and 1980s, operations for bypass surgery became progressively safer for multiple reasons. Surgeons became better trained, and surgical experience increased. Optical assistance became routine, and microsurgical instrumentation improved. Cardiac anesthesia developed as a subspecialty, and postoperative care protocols became more routinized. Intraoperative myocardial protection improved with the use of cardioplegia, a strategy whereby a combination of cardiac standstill and effective myocardial protection was achieved by injecting cardioplegic solution (usually containing high potassium concentrations) into the coronary circulation. The use of this strategy allowed extensive coronary reconstructions to be achieved consistent with effective myocardial protection and made surgical treatment of extensive and severe coronary atherosclerosis possible with safety.

In addition, the population of patients undergoing bypass surgery changed to an older population with more extensive coronary stenoses, a higher incidence of left main stenoses, abnormal LV function, and more frequent comorbid conditions. Table 48-1 shows the changes in preoperative descriptors for patients undergoing primary coronary surgery at The Cleveland Clinic Foundation for selected years from 1967 to 1996, and Table 48-2 shows similar changes between 1980 and 1990 in a countrywide population as recorded by the Society of Thoracic Surgeons National Database.[15] The bypass surgery population changed for multiple reasons. Improved technology and experience made it possible to operate on more complex and sicker patients with reasonable risk. Also, the randomized trials demonstrated that the patients who have the most to gain from surgery were patients with left main or multivessel disease and abnormal LV function. Furthermore, the U.S. population has been aging, and older patients have high expectations for their activity level. Finally, in the early 1980s, the advent of percutaneous anatomic treatments for coronary stenoses (i.e., PCTA) provided an alternative treatment for patients with limited coro-

TABLE 48-1 Preoperative Clinical Characteristics for the First 1000 Patients per Year Undergoing Elective Primary Isolated Coronary Bypass Grafting (The Cleveland Clinic Foundation)

Clinical Variable	1967–1970	1973	1976	1979	1982	1985	1988	1990	1994	1996
Age (yr, median)	50	53	55	56	59	62	64	65	64	65
Men (%)	85	89	89	88	84	80	78	76	75	71
Severe angina (T)	19	21	24	20	17	23	26	34	30	34
Diabetes (%)	7	7	6	7	9	13	19	24	24	27
Age ≥70 yr (%)	0.2	0.5	3	4	10	17	26	32	28	34
Single-vessel disease* (%)	56	17	15	10	8	5	3	5	9	9
Double-vessel disease* (%)	31	33	28	28	25	25	19	25	29	26
Triple-vessel disease* (%)	13	50	57	62	67	71	78	70	60	63
Left main coronary stenosis (≥50%) (%)	9	8	12	12	13	13	16	17	19	19
Left ventricular asynergy (%)	41	41	45	54	55	56	57	51	48	39

The terms *single, double-*, and *triple-vessel disease* refer to the number of the three main coronary vessels (left anterior descending, circumflex, and right coronary arteries) that have stenoses ≥50%.

TABLE 48-2 Comparison of Patient Characteristics 1980 to 1990, The Society of Thoracic Surgery Database*

Characteristic	1980	1990	*P* Value
Age (y)	58.5 ± 9.11	64.1 ± 10.2	<0.001
EF	0.62 ± 0.15	0.51 ± 0.14	<0.001
Female	17.04	26.98	<0.005
Diabetes mellitus	11.73	22.8	<0.005
MI <21 days before CABG	0.34	12.47	<0.005
Cardiogenic shock	0.51	1.61	<0.010
Unstable angina	28.51	47.84	<0.005
Left main disease	6.93	11.7	<0.005
Reoperation	1.88	7.01	<0.005
Nonelective operation	4.11	18.22	<0.005

*Values are shown as percentages except for age and EF, which are shown as mean ± standard deviation.

ABBREVIATIONS: CABG = coronary artery bypass grafting; EF = ejection fraction; IABP = intraaortic balloon pump; MI = myocardial infarction.

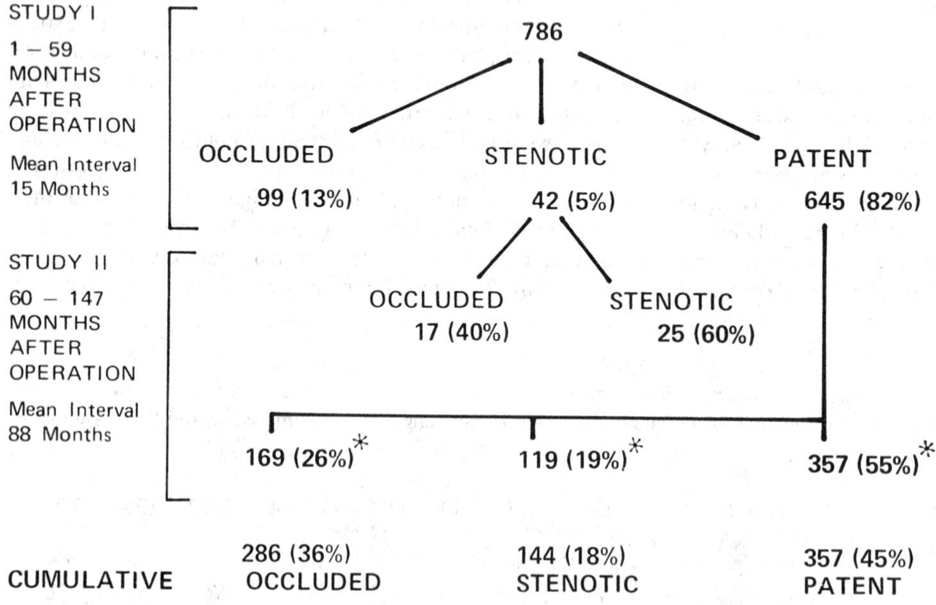

FIGURE 48-2 Data from serial postoperative angiography of saphenous vein to coronary artery grafts. Any graft narrowing was considered a stenosis. Percentages not marked with an asterisk refer to the total number of grafts (786). Percentages marked with an asterisk refer to grafts originally patent. Treatment with postoperative platelet inhibitors and lipid-lowering agents was not used for these patients. (Used with permission from Lytle BW, Loop FD, Cosgrove DM, et al. Long-term (5 to 12 years) serial studies of internal mammary artery and saphenous vein coronary bypass grafts. *J Thorac Cardiovasc Surg* 1985; 89:250.)

nary lesions, removing many of those patients from the surgical population.

TYPES OF BYPASS GRAFTS AND THEIR OUTCOMES

Saphenous Vein Grafts

The most important technical change in coronary surgery has been in the types of grafts that are used. By 1980, angiographic studies at multiple centers had shown that early vein graft patency rates were favorable (80–90 percent within the first postoperative year). Early patency rates were influenced by surgical technique, gender (men experienced better patency rates), the coronary artery grafted (LAD artery patency rates were better than circumflex and right coronary artery rates), the size of the vessel grafted, and the indications for repeat study (routine studies demonstrating better patency rates than studies performed because of symptoms). Coronary risk factors did not appear to influence early patency rates.[1,16–20] However, sequential studies of patent vein grafts demonstrated substantial late attrition. Fitzgibbon et al.[17] studied 590 vein grafts that were patent at 1 postoperative year and found that when studied late (>5 years after operation) 30 percent of patent grafts had become occluded, and 76 percent had angiographic evidence of pathologic changes. Fitzgibbon et al.[17] and Bourassa et al.[16] found a 2.1 percent yearly rate of occlusion of vein grafts up to 5 years after operation, but Bourassa et al.[20] noted a 5.3 percent yearly occlusion rate between 6 and 11 years after operation. Data from sequential The Cleveland Clinic Foundation studies (Fig. 48-2) showed that of vein grafts patent without stenosis 1 to 5 years after operation, only 55 percent remained angiographically perfect 6 to 12 years after surgery.[19] In addition, the attrition rate of patent grafts was not related to the coronary vessel grafted but was related to coronary risk factors such as diabetes and hyperlipidemia.[18,19]

The pathologic changes found in stenotic or occluded vein grafts are different at different postoperative intervals.[21-25] Grafts occluded within 1 or 2 months of surgery exhibit thrombosis, often associated with endothelial disruption. Grafts examined more than a few months after surgery consistently exhibit a hypercellular, proliferative hyperplasia involving the intima—intimal fibroplasia. Intimal fibroplasia is a concentric lesion that evolves into a more fibrotic lesion. It may cause fixed stenoses and may be associated with occlusion but usually is not. However, it appears to be the substrate for the development of vein graft atherosclerosis (VGA), the process that leads to many late graft stenoses or occlusions.

VGA is different from native coronary atherosclerosis. Native coronary artery atherosclerosis is a proximal, eccentric, and intermittent lesion that usually is covered by a fibrous cap. VGA is distributed throughout the length of vein grafts, it is circumferential, it is not encapsulated, and it is extremely friable. With time, the early circumferential lesion often progresses to eccentric lesions causing severe stenoses (Fig. 48-3). Because of its friability and nonencapsulated nature, VGA is a dangerous lesion. Embolization of atherosclerotic debris is a major risk during percutaneous interventions on vein grafts and during reoperations, and it is probable that spontaneous embolization may occur.[20,26] VGA usually is not recognized before 2 to 3 years after operation and does not appear to cause much graft attrition before 5 postoperative years. However, grafts that become occluded more than 5 years after operation usually exhibit thrombosis superimposed on VGA, and the increased rate of graft attrition seen more than 5 years after operation appears to be due in large part to VGA.

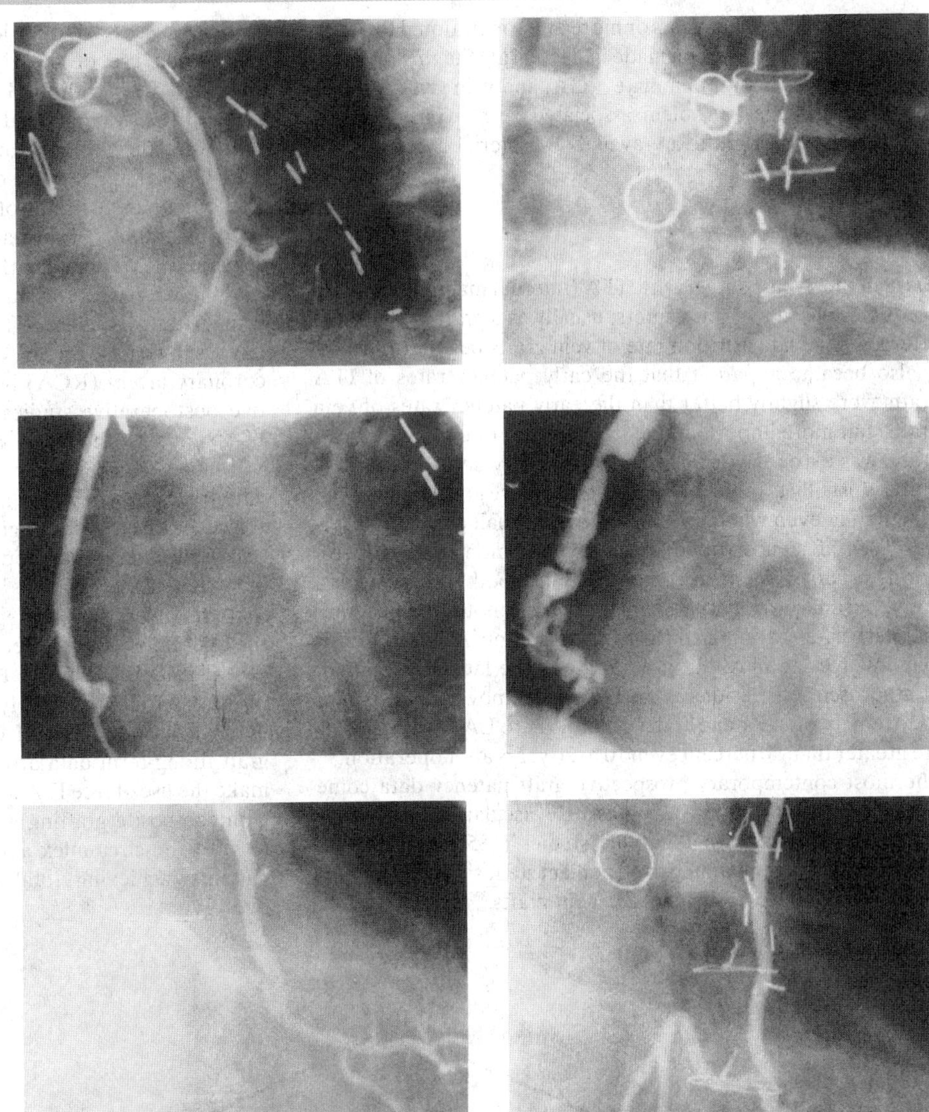

FIGURE 48-3 Angiographic anatomy 1 year after operation (*left*) showing patent vein grafts to the LAD artery and RCA and an ITA graft to the circumflex artery. Seven years later, the LAD artery vein graft is occluded, the RCA graft exhibits diffuse irregular stenoses characteristic of VGA, and the ITA graft is unchanged. (Used with permission from Lytle BW, Loop FD, Cosgrove DM, et al. Long-term (5 to 12 years) serial studies of internal mammary artery and saphenous vein coronary bypass grafts. *Thoracic Cardiovasc Surg* 1985; 89:250.)

Since the early studies of vein grafts cited earlier, substantial progress has been made in the prevention of vein graft attrition. First, multiple randomized, prospective trials have shown that the perioperative and long-term treatment of patients who received vein grafts with platelet inhibitors have significantly decreased the occlusion rate of saphenous vein grafts at 1 year after operation to 6 to 11 percent.[27,28] Second, lipid-lowering trials using a cholesterol-niacin combination or using an aggressive regimen of Pravastatin to lower low-density lipoprotein cholesterol levels have been shown to decrease the progression of angiographic lesions in vein grafts, including a decrease in the rate of occlusion 5 to 15 years after operation.[29,30] Importantly, a clinical trial (CARE trial) of 1091 patients who survived a myocardial infarction (MI), had average cholesterol levels, and underwent bypass surgery showed that treatment with Pravastatin decreased the risk of death and nonfatal MI over a 5-year follow-up.[31] Thus multiple studies appear to show that outcomes for patients receiving vein grafts today can be expected to be better than those noted in studies from the 1970s. Furthermore, some vein grafts provide very long-term benefit. For patients studied 16 to 20 years after operation Lawrie et al.[32] noted 46 percent vein graft patency and Fitzgibbon et al.[20] noted a 50 percent patency rate 15 years or more after operation. However, although progress has been made in decreasing the *rate* of VGA, these strategies do not eliminate VGA, and vein graft attrition remains the biggest problem associated with bypass surgery. Fortunately, other grafts are available—arterial bypass grafts.

ITA Grafts

Early in the bypass surgery era, ITA (internal mammary artery) grafts were used in a few centers, usually as a graft to the LAD artery. As the late attrition rate of vein grafts began to surface, it also became apparent that the early patency rates of ITA grafts were slightly better than the early patency rates of vein grafts, but more important, the late attrition rate of patent ITA grafts was extremely low[1,19] (Fig. 48-4). Early occlusion of ITA grafts is usually technically related, since these grafts can remain functioning even when used to graft very small coronary arteries. ITA graft stenosis or occlusion beyond 6 months after operation is usually related to competition in blood flow through a native coronary artery that is not severely stenotic and becomes manifest as a "string sign" or diffuse spasm. Atherosclerosis may involve the ITA, but it is rare, and the late development of atherosclerotic lesions in an ITA graft known to be patent is extremely rare. Patency rates of left ITA to LAD artery grafts are greater than 90 percent even 10 to 20 years after operation.[1,19] The most contemporary prospective graft patency data come from the Bypass Surgery Angioplasty Revascularization Investigation (BARI) trial angiographic studies (135 patients) that documented 1-year patency (<50 percent stenosis) of 98 percent for ITA grafts and 87 percent for vein grafts.[33]

The success of the left ITA to LAD artery graft has led to the use of the right ITA as a bypass graft, usually simultaneously with the left ITA (bilateral ITA grafting). The right ITA has been used as an in situ graft and as a "free" graft with the proximal anastomosis constructed either to the left ITA (Fig. 48-5*A*) or to the aorta (see Fig. 48-5*B*). Although patency rates of ITA grafts have been highest when used to graft the LAD artery–diagonal system, Dion et al.[34] restudied 135 pedicled ITA to circumflex artery grafts 13 months after operation and noted a 95 percent patency rate. Longer-term studies of ITA to circumflex artery grafts also have showed favorable outcomes.[1] ITA grafts to the right coronary artery (RCA) have been less frequent and prospective postoperative studies are rare, but long-term patency of ITA grafts to the RCA is possible.

Studies of aorta to coronary ITA grafts have tended to show patency rates not quite as good as those of pedicled grafts. However, these types of grafts can exhibit 20-year patency, and once they are patent, they appear to remain free from graft atherosclerosis.[1,34]

A relatively new strategy is composite arterial grafting with the right ITA used as a free graft anastomosed to the left ITA[35,36] (see Fig. 48-4*B*). This strategy allows more flexibility in the use of the right ITA, and early data show patency rates of 91 to 95 percent within a year of operation for this type of free ITA graft. Long-term data are not available, but this strategy may make the use of free ITA grafts more effective. Once experience with composite grafting is gained, the right ITA may be used to graft the circumflex and right coronary systems in selected patients, achieving total arterial revascularization with the two ITAs.

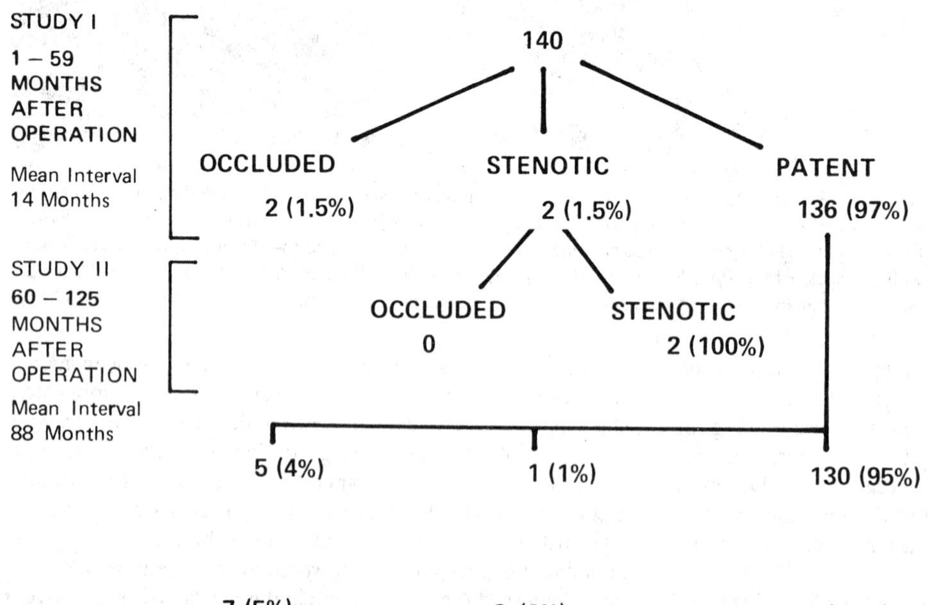

FIGURE 48-4 Data from serial postoperative angiography of ITA to coronary artery grafts. Percentages not marked with an asterisk refer to the total number of grafts (140). Percentages marked with an asterisk refer to grafts originally patent. (Used with permission from Lytle BW, Loop FD, Cosgrove DM, et al. Long-term (5 to 12 years) serial studies of internal mammary artery and saphenous vein coronary bypass grafts. *J Thorac Cardiovasc Surg* 1985; 89:252.)

Clinical Impact of ITA Grafts

The high and stable patency rate of the left ITA to LAD artery graft also produces improved clinical outcomes. No large randomized studies have compared ITA and vein grafts, but in a large observational study published in 1986, Loop et al.[37] showed that patients who received a left ITA to LAD artery graft (with or without vein grafts to the circumflex and RCA branches) had better 10-year survival rates when compared with patients who received only vein grafts (Fig. 48-6). This observation was true for patients with single-, double-, or triple-vessel disease. In addition, the ITA graft patients underwent fewer reoperations (4 versus 8 percent) and had fewer cardiac-related hospitalizations. Data from CASS have extended the observed benefits of ITA grafting to 15 to 18 years after operation.[38]

Logic seems to dictate that if one ITA graft is good, two ITA

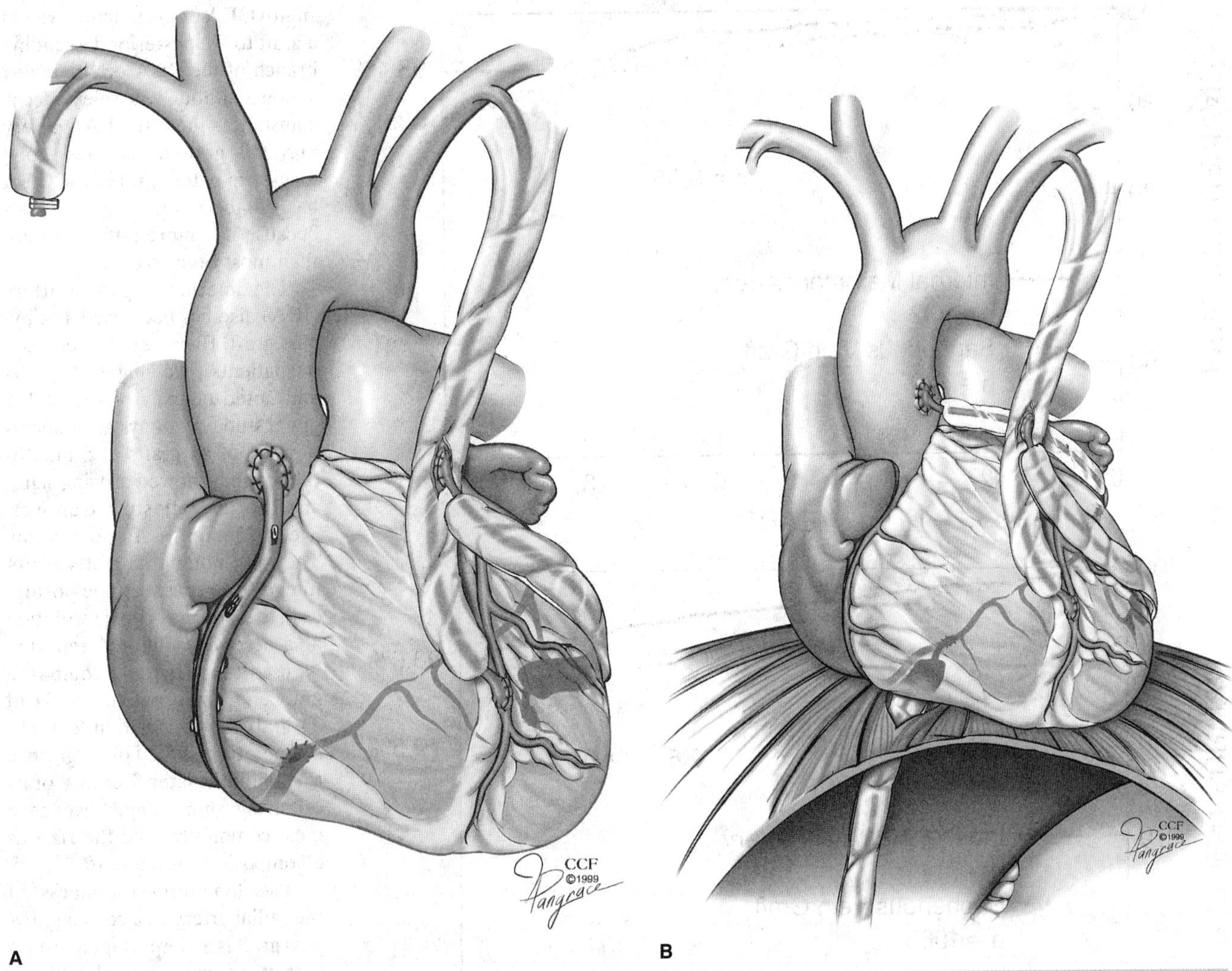

FIGURE 48-5 *A*. Bilateral ITA grafting with the right ITA used as a composite (from left ITA) graft to the circumflex coronary artery and a vein graft to the RCA. *B*. Total arterial revascularization with an aorta to coronary right ITA to circumflex graft, the radial artery used as a composite graft from the left ITA to diagonal coronary artery, the left ITA used as a graft to the anterior descending coronary artery, and an in situ GEA graft to the RCA.

grafts may improve outcomes further. However, the strategy of bilateral ITA grafting has not become widespread. Bilateral ITA grafting makes the bypass operation more difficult, some studies have shown an increase in the risk of wound complications, and the outcomes for patients receiving a single ITA to LAD artery graft are very good, particularly over the first postoperative decade. Furthermore, because of the importance of the LAD coronary artery in many patients, improved results may be difficult to show if LAD artery revascularization is secure. And indeed, a number of retrospective studies have shown either no benefit or relatively little incremental benefit of bilateral ITA grafting over single ITA grafting. These studies involved either small patient numbers or relatively short follow-up intervals. Recently, we retrospectively reviewed a large series of patients receiving single or bilateral ITA grafts and found an improved 12-year survival rate for the patients receiving bilateral ITA grafts, as well as a decreased risk of reoperation or percutaneous intervention over that same time frame[39] (Fig. 48-7). Another recent study that confirmed these observations also involves relatively large patient numbers.[40] It is probable that the incremental benefit of bilateral ITA grafting over single ITA grafting may be less than the benefit of a left ITA to LAD artery graft over only vein grafts. Nonetheless, it does appear that bilateral ITA grafting does offer incremental benefit.

Other Arterial Bypass Grafts

The gastroepiploic artery (GEA) was used for Vineberg-type myocardial implantation prior to the bypass grafting era, and its use as a coronary bypass graft was begun by Suma and Pym in 1986. Suma reported a 94 percent (253 of 268) patency rate within 2 months of operation and 47 of 50 GEA grafts (94 percent) patent at 2 to 5 postoperative years.[41] In situ GEA grafts have had better patency rates than free grafts. When late attrition has occurred, it has appeared to be related to native coronary artery competitive flow. Anecdotal angiographic studies have documented the patency of GEA grafts 9 to 10 years after operation and have not shown evidence of the occurrence of graft atherosclerosis. The GEA is prone to spasm, and intraluminal vasodilators have been used by many of its proponents.

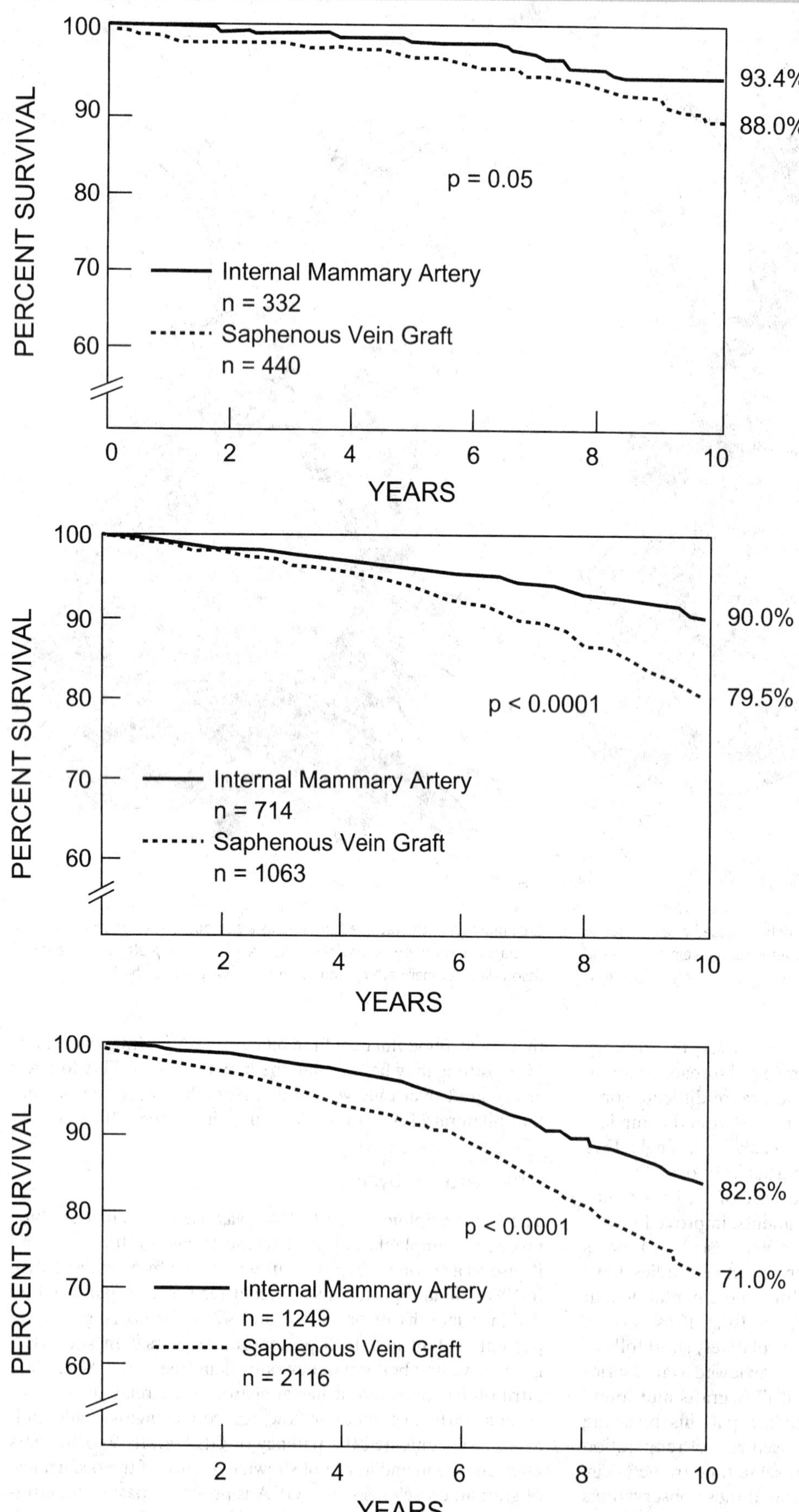

In situ GEA grafts function well as a graft to the posterior descending branch of the RCA or circumflex system, although in selected circumstances the distal LAD artery may be grafted. Despite good long-term patency rates, the GEA has not become a popular graft because it is more difficult to use than most other conduits.

The inferior epigastric artery (IEA) also has been used as a bypass graft. Buche et al.[42] reported on patients receiving IEA grafts and noted patency of 132 of 135 grafts studied 11 days after operation, 44 of 48 grafts at 8 months (although 8 showed a string sign), and 25 of 29 grafts studied an average of 25 months after operation. They also noted that grafts exhibiting diffuse spasm at one postoperative study may show resolution at a second. Califiore[36] reported on use of the IEA as a composite graft and noted patency in 34 of 34 grafts studied within 2 weeks of operation and 20 of 21 grafts 6 to 14 months later. Because of its relatively short length, we have most commonly used the IEA as a composite arterial graft.

The long-term usefulness of the radial artery as a coronary bypass graft is an important question that is as yet incompletely answered. The radial artery is a long graft that is easily procured and has very favorable size and handling characteristics. However, it is a thicker, more muscular artery than the ITA, and when it was used by Carpentier[44] and others[43] in the early 1970s, patency rates were not favorable. Recently, its use has been revisited along with the use of calcium-channel

FIGURE 48-6 Survival for patients with an ITA to LAD artery graft with and without vein grafts to other coronary vessels compared with survival for patients with only vein grafts. An ITA to LAD artery graft was associated with significantly better survival for patients with single- (*top*), double- (*middle*), or triple-vessel (*bottom*) disease. (Used with permission from Loop FD, Lytle BW, Cosgrove DM, et al. Influence of the internal-mammary-artery graft on 10-year survival and other cardiac events. *N Engl J Med* 1986; 314:106.)

blocking agents to prevent postoperative spasm, and Broadman et al.[45] and Acar et al.[46] have reported early (<6 months) patency rates of greater than 90 percent. Acar et al.[46] reported 75 radial grafts studied within 2 weeks of operation with 1 occluded graft and 4 with spasm. At 1 year, 61 grafts were restudied, with 4 occluded and 2 stenotic. At 4 to 7 years after operation, 50 patients underwent repeat study, and of 64 radial artery grafts, 10 were occluded, 1 had a string sign, and 53 (83 percent) looked perfect. In the same patients, 91 percent of left ITA grafts were patent. Possati et al.[47] performed serial studies after radial artery grafting and documented an 87 percent perfect patency at 5 postoperative years, compared with 98 percent left ITA patency and 69 percent vein graft patency in the same patients. Early diffuse radial artery graft abnormalities in 7 patients disappeared by the 5-year angiogram.[47] At this point the jury is still out on radial artery grafts. They are not as reliable in terms of patency as left ITA grafts are but may be superior to vein grafts over the long term if they are resistant to late graft atherosclerosis.

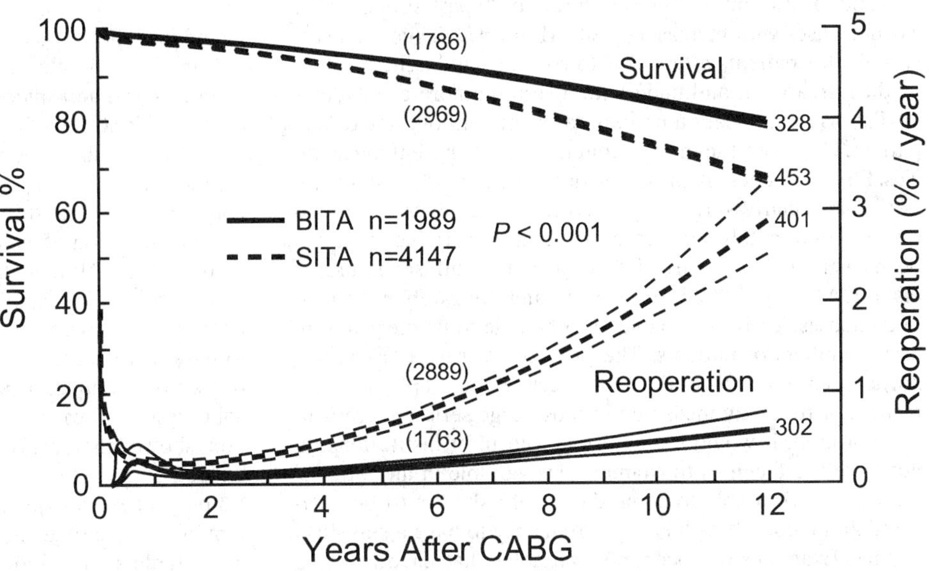

FIGURE 48-7 Comparison of survival and reoperation hazard function curves in propensity-matched patients receiving bilateral ITA grafts (BITA) and single ITA grafts (SITA) with or without additional vein grafts. CABG, coronary artery bypass grafting. (Used with permission from Lytle BW, Blackstone EH, Loop FD, et al. Two internal thoracic artery grafts are better than one. *J Thorac Cardiovasc Surg* 1999; 117:855–872.)

Total arterial revascularization is an appealing concept, but its clinical importance is not yet certain. For some patients, total arterial revascularization can be achieved solely with the use of ITA grafts, but for many others, other arterial grafts are needed. Bergsma et al.[48] reported on a group of 256 selected patients with triple-vessel disease revascularized with two ITA grafts and a GEA graft. These relatively good-risk patients experienced an expected good survival rate, but it was also noted that over a mean follow-up period of 51 months, 85.7 percent experienced no angina, an impressive figure. Much longer-term follow-up is needed. Realistically, it is unlikely that most coronary surgeons will use GEA grafts routinely, but if the long-term patency rates of radial artery grafts are superior to vein grafts, total arterial revascularization will become common.

CURRENT OPERATIVE STRATEGIES AND RISKS

Standard Operative Strategies

Currently, most operations for primary isolated coronary revascularization are still performed through a median sternotomy with the aid of cardiopulmonary bypass. Aortic occlusion and cold potassium-based cardioplegia (delivered antegrade through the aortic root or retrograde through a catheter in the coronary sinus) are used to achieve an immobile surgical field consistent with intraoperative myocardial protection. Standard revascularization techniques involve the use of an in situ left ITA to graft the coronary artery, and in most centers, vein grafts are then employed to graft the other vessels.

Hospital Mortality

Overall hospital mortality rates for primary bypass surgery vary between 1 and 4 percent. Mortality rates in the voluntary countrywide Society of Thoracic Surgeons Database ranged from 3.46 to 3.78 percent (including reoperations) from 1990 to 1994.[49] The unadjusted mortality rate for patients undergoing primary operations in New York State (a compulsory registry with subsequent public disclosure) from 1993 to 1995 was 1.9 percent,[50] and single-institution reviews have noted overall mortality rates of 1 percent or less for elective patients.[1] Multiple database analyses have been devoted to the identification of variables that can be used to predict in-hospital outcomes and adjust for patient selection. A recent review of the seven largest data sets available in the literature found that 7 variables were predictive of in-hospital death in all data sets: acuteness of operation, age, prior cardiac surgery, gender, LV ejection fraction, left main coronary artery percent stenosis, and number of coronary systems with more than 70 percent stenosis.[51] Acuteness of operation, age, and previous surgery had the greatest predictive value. Also identified were 13 variables that added some predictive value to the core variables: percutaneous transluminal angioplasty (PCTA) during the same admission, MI less than 1 week prior to operation, angina, ventricular arrhythmia, congestive heart failure, mitral regurgitation, diabetes, cerebral vascular disease, peripheral vascular disease, chronic obstructive pulmonary disease (COPD), and serum creatinine.

In the spectrum of clinical settings ranging from stable angina, to unstable angina with electrocardiographic changes, to recent subendocardial infarction, to recent Q-wave MI, and to cardiogenic shock, there has been an increased operative risk associated with increasing degrees of ischemia and decreasing degrees of LV function. Modern methods of myocardial protection have diminished the impact of unstable angina. However, operations for postinfarction ischemia and shock still generate substantial risk, and the mortality rate of bypass surgery after MI decreases with increasing post-MI interval. Thus the usual strategy for patients after MI is to control acute ischemia with medical treatment and undertake operation more electively.

The risk-stratification process has value for both doctor and patient. However, the process contains some inherent inaccuracies. First, variables are measured differently in different institutions, particularly variables related to the acuteness of operation. Second, databases record and analyze variables that can be measured. Some variables, such as the diffuse nature of distal CAD, are difficult to measure and are rarely contained in databases. Third, a variable must be able to be measured in large numbers of patients. The presence of severe ascending aortic atherosclerosis as defined by echocardiography is a risk factor not routinely measured in most large series. Were it to be measured, it would be important, but most institutions do not have the facilities to examine this variable in all patients. Fourth, for a variable to be predictive of risk, it must be measured and recorded with enough frequency to have a statistical impact. Examples of uncommon variables that have a strong impact on operative mortality include hepatic cirrhosis, congenital clotting disorders, severe protamine allergies, and previous mediastinal radiation therapy.

Coronary bypass surgery is a very scrutinized treatment. Overall mortality rates tend to be maintained in a narrow range in part because that scrutiny engenders careful patient selection if overall mortality rates begin to rise. Burack et al.[52] studied the New York State Department of Health Cardiac Surgery Reporting System (CSRS) and found evidence that high-risk patients were being denied bypass surgery. Certainly, not all institutions should perform all operations, and it probably is of benefit for high-risk patients to undergo surgery in selected institutions. However, in a milieu of medical economics where patient mobility may be limited, care must be exerted such that high-risk patients are not denied potentially lifesaving operations.

One operation-related variable that has been associated with decreased in-hospital risk is the use of ITA grafts. At one time there was concern that ITA use would increase risk. However, multiple retrospective studies from different data sets and during different surgical periods have shown that use of the ITA graft is associated with a decrease in hospital mortality rather than an increase.[53,54]

One advantage of identifying characteristics that predict high risk is that patients who are at extremely low risk also may be identified. For example, during the years 1995–1998, the STS Database recorded 25,776 patients who underwent a primary elective bypass operation, had a LV ejection fraction of greater than 50 percent, and did not have peripheral vascular disease, carotid disease, renal failure, a prior MI, or an intraaortic balloon pump. For these good-risk patients, 98 deaths occurred for a 0.38 percent mortality rate.[55]

Hospital Morbidity

PERIOPERATIVE MI

Since the early years of bypass surgery, improved strategies for myocardial protection have evolved, and significant perioperative MI has become less frequent. Today most surgeons employ aortic occlusion combined with some type of cardioplegia injected into the cardiac vascular system to produce a still heart. Originally, cardioplegic solutions were asanguineous, cold, high in potassium, and injected into the aortic root. Modifications of this basic strategy have included addition of blood, addition of metabolic substrates, warming some or all of the cardioplegic solution, and delivery of cardioplegia retrograde through the coronary sinus into the cardiac venous system.

The definition of what constitutes a perioperative MI varies among studies but with the use of cardioplegia, the risk of hemodynamically significant perioperative MI in elective patients is very low, and it has become difficult in such patients to show incremental benefit of any of the cardioplegia modifications. For example, a trial of warm blood cardioplegia versus cold crystalloid cardioplegia in primary elective bypass operations showed that rates of MI (1.4 versus 0.8 percent), intraaortic balloon pump use (1.4 versus 2.0 percent), and death (1.0 versus 1.6 percent) were equivalent.[56] For patients undergoing operation in the face of acute ischemia based either on failed PCTA or unstable angina, blood cardioplegia does appear to provide incremental benefit.[57,58] Retrograde delivery through the coronary sinus and coronary venous system provides more effective delivery during reoperations, in the setting of acute coronary ischemia, or if the aortic valve is insufficient.[59]

For the period of time needed to complete even extensive coronary revascularization operations using standard techniques, the metabolic environment created by these cardioplegic strategies appears to be sufficient for protection. Significant perioperative MI, when it occurs, appears to be based on anatomic causes, acute coronary occlusion, graft failure, or incomplete revascularization.

NEUROLOGIC COMPLICATIONS

Adverse neurologic events after coronary bypass surgery may negatively affect overall outcomes, and at a period in time where myocardial protection has diminished the impact of perioperative MI, the perioperative risk of cerebral complications is still under intense investigation. A recent multicenter study authored by Roach et al.[60] separated postoperative neurologic abnormalities into focal strokes (type I) and diffuse encephalopathies (type II). In this study, the total number of adverse outcomes was 6.1 percent, divided between type I (3.1 percent) and type II (3.0 percent). Advanced age and hypertension predicted an increased risk for both types of deficits.

Focal strokes (type I) appear to have multiple causes, including carotid or intracranial vascular disease, embolic phenomena based on interventricular or atrial thrombi or postoperative atrial fibrillation, and atheroembolization from the aorta, probably the most common cause. In fact, in the study by Roach et al.,[60] the greatest predictor of a type I deficit was proximal aortic atherosclerosis as noted by the surgeon. Hartman et al.[61] have associated the risk of stroke with the severity of aortic atherosclerosis as defined by transesophageal echocardiography, and Blauth et al.[62] associated the presence of ascending aortic atherosclerosis with evidence of atherosclerotic emboli to multiple organ systems. There are multiple techniques available to diminish the impact of aortic atherosclerosis, including alternative arterial cannulation sites, single aortic cross-clamping, circulatory arrest and aortic replacement, and surgery without cardiopulmonary bypass. Which strategy will produce the best outcomes will vary according to the particular pathology involved, but the most important point is recognition by the surgeon of the existence of the problem. Other predictors of type I deficit have included a history of stroke, diabetes, unstable angina, peripheral vascular disease, and a total carotid occlusion.

Variables that were predictive of type II deficits in the Roach et al. study included a history of alcohol abuse, atrial fibrillation, prior coronary artery bypass grafting (CABG), peripheral vascular disease, and congestive heart failure. The anatomic basis of type II deficits is not known, but many authors have noted some evidence of gaseous or particulate embolization associated with cardiopulmonary bypass. Strategies designed to minimize microembolization associated with cardiopulmonary bypass includes the use of membrane oxygenators, arterial filters, alpha-stat extracorporeal circulation acid-base management, and avoidance of cerebral hyperthermia. Another appealing concept is the performance of bypass surgery without the use of cardiopulmonary bypass, and logic would seem to dictate that this strategy would decrease the incidence of both types of neurologic complications. This issue is currently being intensively investigated.

The presence of carotid stenoses, symptomatic or asymptomatic, in a patient undergoing bypass surgery creates both a short- and a long-term risk of stroke. Studies of patients over age 65 with carotid Duplex scans have defined the predictors of 80 percent or more carotid stenoses as female gender, peripheral vascular disease, previous transient ischemic attack (TIA) or stroke, smoking history, and left main stenoses.[63] The majority of patients aged 65 or older had one of these characteristics, and it may be logical to screen all patients in that age group undergoing bypass surgery. Regardless of age, patients with a previous stroke, TIA, or carotid bruit should undergo Duplex screening, and any patients evidencing symptoms characteristic of vertebrobasilar insufficiency should have further studies.

The patient with simultaneous carotid and coronary disease is at higher risk than the patient with only CAD regardless of which therapeutic approach is used. Staged operations with carotid endarterectomy performed first has been shown to be safe but has been applied in very selected patients with less severe CAD. Patients undergoing bypass surgery in the face of a severe uncorrected carotid stenosis are at increased risk of stroke, and patients with bilateral stenoses are at a greatly increased risk of stroke.[64,65] Many experienced centers recommend combined carotid endarterectomy and coronary surgery for patients with carotid stenoses who are undergoing primary bypass operations, although even with this approach stroke and mortality rates are slightly worse than those for patients with isolated CAD.[66]

WOUND COMPLICATIONS

Deep sternal wound complications represent a serious adverse outcome and occur in 0.5 to 4 percent of cases depending on patient selection. Obesity and diabetes have been implicated in multiple studies as factors increasing the risk of sternal complications. There is some evidence that aggressive treatment of blood glucose levels with intravenous insulin may decrease the risk of infection in diabetic patients. No studies have shown that the use of a single ITA graft increases the risk of sternal wound complications, but some authors have implicated bilateral ITA grafting, particularly for diabetic patients.[67] Dissection of the ITA as a skeletonized artery rather than as a pedicle may leave collateral circulation to the sternum intact and diminish the impact of ITA use.

DIFFERENTLY INVASIVE BYPASS SURGERY

New concepts in how bypass surgery is being performed are now under exploration: operations done through small incisions (minimally invasive bypass surgery) and operations performed without the use of cardiopulmonary bypass (beating-heart or off-pump surgery). Stimuli for these changes include the maturation of small incision or endoscopic technology for the performance of thoracic and general surgery and the desire to decrease incision-related and cardiopulmonary bypass–related morbidity (and perhaps mortality) related to coronary surgery.

Small-incision and beating-heart concepts have been combined in an operation during which a small left anterior thoracotomy is used to prepare a left ITA graft that is then anastomosed to the LAD coronary artery under direct vision (MIDCAB or LAST operation) (Fig. 48-8). Endoscopic technologies sometimes have been used for the ITA preparation but usually not for creation of the anastomosis. Early studies showed that this approach was possible but also noted an increased risk of ITA graft failure associated with this strategy. However, with increased surgical experience, results clearly have improved.[68,69] Because the left ITA-LAD operation using standard techniques (median sternotomy and cardiopulmonary bypass) is extremely safe and produces excellent 20-year outcomes, the only major risks of bypass surgery that are likely to be diminished with the MIDCAB approach are wound complications. However, it is the hope that this less invasive approach may have cosmetic,

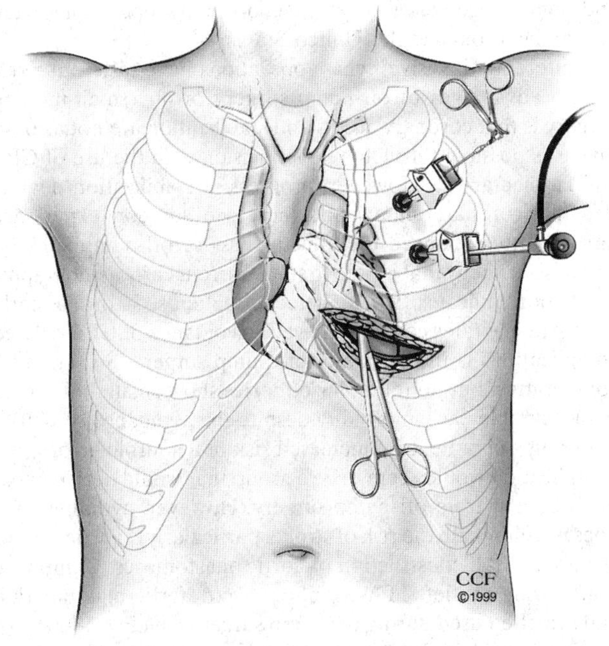

FIGURE 48-8 A small left anterior thoracotomy may be used to construct a limited anastomosis without the use of CPB, or with the use of percutaneous CPB, more vessels are accessible through this small incision. Endoscopic preparation of the left ITA graft may be employed.

hospital stay, time loss from work, and cost advantages. The disadvantage of a limited-access, off-pump operation is that a limited number of coronary vessels can be grafted through any one incision. To approach this issue, three directions are being pursued: small-incision surgery with cardiopulmonary bypass (CPB), large-incision surgery without CPB, and robotics surgery.

A percutaneous CPB system has been developed that involves femoral arterial and venous cannulation and percutaneous cannulas that allow balloon occlusion of the ascending aorta and the delivery of antegrade and retrograde cardioplegia. This approach allows aortic occlusion, cardiac arrest, and decompression, making the coronary vessels more accessible through a small left thoracotomy. The disadvantages of this approach are that coronary exposure may not be ideal, the right ITA and GEA arteries are difficult to use as grafts, the patient undergoes the risks of CPB, and the patient is exposed to vascular-related risks of catheter placement such as aortic dissection and atherosclerotic embolization. Industry sources appear to show that an early increased risk of aortic dissection has lessened with experience and that the risks of death and stroke are not obviously out of line.[70] The possible benefits of this approach are a decrease in wound complications and a faster return to full activity. In carefully selected patients, these goals seem achievable.

A more common differently invasive strategy is to use a median sternotomy incision to improve coronary artery access but avoid the use of CPB, bypass surgery being performed on the beating heart. Beating-heart surgery was employed in the early years of bypass surgery, and although poor angiographic outcomes led to its decline, it never disappeared completely. Many surgeons continued to perform small numbers of off-pump operations for patients at particularly high risk for CPB, and some large series of elective off-pump operations were accumulated outside the United States.[71,72]

Differently invasive bypass operations have different risks. The disadvantages of off-pump surgery or any small-incision surgery is that coronary access and stabilization are not as optimal as is possible through a large incision with the use of CPB and cardiac arrest. However, progress in stabilization devices and intracoronary shunts and increased surgeon experience have greatly enhanced the effectiveness of off-pump surgery, and it is a strategy that is here to stay. Current early angiographic evaluation indicates that for selected patients, favorable early graft patency rates can be achieved. Avoidance of CPB-related complications is the upside of off-pump surgery. So far, large comparative, but nonrandomized series show small differences in measurable early morbidity despite the avoidance of CPB.[73] Subgroups of patients at increased risk of a neurologic or renal complication would seem to be a group that would derive maximum benefit from off-pump surgery. However, avoiding CPB does not eliminate the risk of stroke, particularly if aortic clamps are used in the construction of aortic anastomoses. Composite grafts using the left ITA as inflow avoid aortic manipulation and are often used during off-pump surgery (see Fig. 48-5*A*, *B*).

The use of robotics-type visualization and manipulative technology is in its infancy but offers the possibility of expanding the extent of operations that can be performed through small incisions with or without CPB. The development of effective anastomotic stapling devices will greatly expand the possibilities for robotics bypass surgery.

LONG-TERM OUTCOMES AFTER BYPASS SURGERY

Late survival after bypass surgery is related to the patient's cardiac status at the time of operation, the bypass operation, progression of atherosclerosis, noncardiac comorbidity, and fate. Recent follow-up of 8221 surgical patients from the CASS Registry documented overall survival of 96, 90, 74, 56, and 45 percent at 1, 5, 10, 15, and 18 postoperative years, respectively.[74] These figures are inferior to those for the age-sex-matched U.S. population. Noted in other follow-up studies is that 55 percent of deaths over the first postoperative decade were cardiac in nature.[75]

Age is a major determinant of survival. In the CASS review, very young and very elderly patients had a decreased survival rate. The lack of ITA grafting in the CASS population almost certainly had a detrimental effect on the survival of young patients, but no studies of patients 40 years of age or under have ever shown survival rates equivalent to age-matched controls. However, elderly patients, while having a diminished survival when compared with younger patients, actually have survival rates better than those for age-matched controls, an effect that begins to be observed around age 60.[74]

LV function is the cardiac-related variable most closely related to long-term survival. In addition, left main stenosis, a proximal LAD artery stenosis, and the number of significantly stenotic coronary arteries all have influenced survival in most studies. The late survival of patients treated medically is dramatically influenced by these cardiac variables, but bypass surgery at least partially ameliorates their impact.[74] In our study analyzing the impact of arterial revascularization, a proximal LAD artery stenosis had no effect on late survival, and left main disease and the number of systems diseased had minor influence.[39] In no long-term study has bypass surgery completely obliterated the impact of abnormal LV function on late survival.

Risk factors for atherosclerosis also decrease late survival, most particularly cigarette smoking, hypercholesterolemia, hypertension, and diabetes. Smoking decreases the survival rate, and stopping smoking returns the patient to a nonsmoker's prognosis.[76] High elevations in total cholesterol are related to a decreased survival in some studies,[77] and there is suggestive evidence that pharmacologic treatment may improve the survival rate for these patients. Diabetes severe enough to require treatment is associated with a decreased late survival rate, but it is not yet clear whether or not glycemic control will improve the late survival rate of surgically treated patients. However, it has been shown that close control of diabetes does improve long-term outcomes for medically treated patients, and logic would dictate the importance of this approach despite bypass surgery.

As discussed previously, the surgical strategies of the left ITA-LAD artery graft and bilateral ITA grafting incrementally improve the late survival.

The impact of incomplete revascularization on long-term outcome is of increasing importance with the emergence of PCTA and minimally invasive bypass operations, strategies that may involve less complete revascularization than can be achieved with standard bypass surgical techniques. Definitions of what *incomplete revascularization* is have varied, and it is difficult to separate incomplete revascularization as a surgical strategy from incomplete revascularization as a marker of bad coronary and noncoronary atherosclerosis. Retrospective multivariate analyses of The Cleveland Clinic Foundation data identified incomplete revascularization as a risk factor for late death, but not a strong one.[77] A CASS Registry study by Bell et al.[12] noted a strong negative effect of incomplete revascularization on the late survival of patients with abnormal LV function who underwent bypass surgery, and Jones and Weintraub[78] observed a negative effect on patients with normal LV function.

Incomplete revascularization as a surgical strategy was examined in a study by Tasdemir et al.[72] that reviewed patients having off-pump bypass surgery. In this study, incomplete revascularization (usually of the circumflex system) was sometimes accepted in order to be able to perform bypass surgery without CPB. Failure to revascularize the circumflex system was a risk factor for early death and cardiac events, but late follow-up was not available.

REOPERATION

Atherosclerosis is a progressive disease, and some patients eventually will undergo repeat bypass surgery. A study reviewing patients undergoing primary bypass surgery in the 1970s noted a cumulative incidence of reoperation of 2.7, 11.4, and 17.3 percent at 5, 10, and 12 years after bypass, respectively.[79] Young age, normal LV function, single- or double-vessel disease, severe symptoms, incomplete revascularization, and not having an ITA graft were all factors increasing the likelihood of a reoperation. Today, the availability of PCTA, use of arterial grafts, and possibly risk factor control will diminish the rate of reoperation. However, recurrent ischemic syndromes will develop in some patients with previous surgery, and reoperation will sometimes be required.

Patients who are candidates for reoperation are different from those having primary surgery. Today, the typical candidate for reoperation underwent primary surgery more than 10 years ago, had triple-vessel disease at that time, and needs reoperation at least in part because of graft failure. The atherosclerotic process is advanced, and such patients have a high incidence of noncardiac atherosclerosis. Their cardiac atherosclerosis is severe, and they have a higher prevalence of aortic atherosclerosis, left main stenosis, severe distal CAD, and abnormal LV function than patients undergoing primary surgery. They usually have the unique characteristics of having their myocardial blood supply dependent on ITA grafts, being at risk for injury, or having atherosclerotic vein grafts that create the possibility of coronary atheroembolism. In addition, few data are available that help to define the indications for reoperation, particularly for patients who are not severely symptomatic. None of the randomized trials included patients with previous bypass surgery, and since their myocardium is usually jeopardized at least in part by vascular pathology different from native coronary artery atherosclerosis, generalization from the randomized studies is unwise.

To examine outcomes for patients with prior surgery who developed recurrent ischemic syndromes, we performed two retrospective, nonrandomized studies of patients who underwent repeat angiography after primary bypass surgery. The first involved patients who did not undergo prompt reoperation and compared outcomes with patients with vein graft stenoses with patients without vein graft stenoses.[80] This study showed that late (≥5 years) stenoses in vein grafts are more dangerous lesions than are native coronary lesions. For example, patients 5 years or more after operation with a 50 percent or greater stenosis in the LAD artery vein graft had survival of 70 and 50 percent 2 and 5 years after angiography compared with survival rates of 97 and 70 percent for patients whose LAD coronary artery was jeopardized by a 50 percent or greater native vessel stenosis.

The second study involved patients with stenotic vein grafts and compared outcomes for those who underwent repeat surgery with those who were treated without initial reoperation.[81] Treatment was not randomized, and the patients who underwent repeat surgery were more symptomatic. Patients with late (≥5 years) stenoses in vein grafts had better survival rates with surgery, and the patients who particularly benefited were those with an atherosclerotic vein graft to the LAD coronary artery. The patients with a 50 percent or greater LAD artery graft stenosis had immediate and obvious benefit, but even those with a 20 to 50 percent stenosis had an improved survival rate with surgery when followed for 5 years (Fig. 48-9). Patients with late stenoses in non-LAD artery grafts also appeared to have improved late survival unless they had a patent ITA to LAD artery graft. Patients with early vein graft stenoses did not have an improved late survival rate with surgery, although patients who underwent reoperation had fewer symptoms at late follow-up.

All studies that have examined large numbers of patients undergoing reoperation have noted an increased in-hospital risk when compared with patients undergoing primary surgery. The STS National Database noted an overall risk of 7.14 percent for reoperations from 1980 to 1990,[15] and The Cleveland Clinic Foundation studies have documented a risk of 3 to 4 percent for a first reoperation from 1967 through the present.[82–84]

The increased risk of reoperation is related in large part to an increased risk of perioperative MI. Graft injury, atherosclerotic embolization from vein grafts or the aorta, incomplete revascularization due to diffuse disease or lack of bypass conduit, and technical difficulty with severely atherosclerotic coronary vessels are anatomic causes of perioperative MI that are either unique to reoperation or more common in that setting. The use of retrograde cardioplegia has been of major benefit in the management of atherosclerotic vein grafts and patent ITA grafts, but avoiding perioperative MI during reoperation still represents a challenge.

In the reoperative setting, emergency operation produces a large increase in risk. Definitions of *emergency* vary among studies, but the lesson is the same. For example, in the STS National Database, primary operation had a risk of 2.24 percent for elective operation versus 5.7 percent for emergencies, whereas elective reoperations had a 5.33 percent risk compared with 12.69 percent for emergencies.[15] Left main stenosis, advanced age, congestive heart failure, female gender, and numbers of stenotic vein grafts have been other factors associated with increased risk.

In general, the long-term outcomes after reoperation are slightly inferior to those after primary surgery. Loop et al.[83] noted a 69 percent 10-year survival for 2429 hospital survivors of a first reoperation. LV function was the variable having the strongest impact on survival. Reoperations tend to achieve less perfect revascularization than primary procedures, and by 5 to 6 postoperative years, about 50 percent of reoperative patients have some angina, although in few patients is it severe.[82]

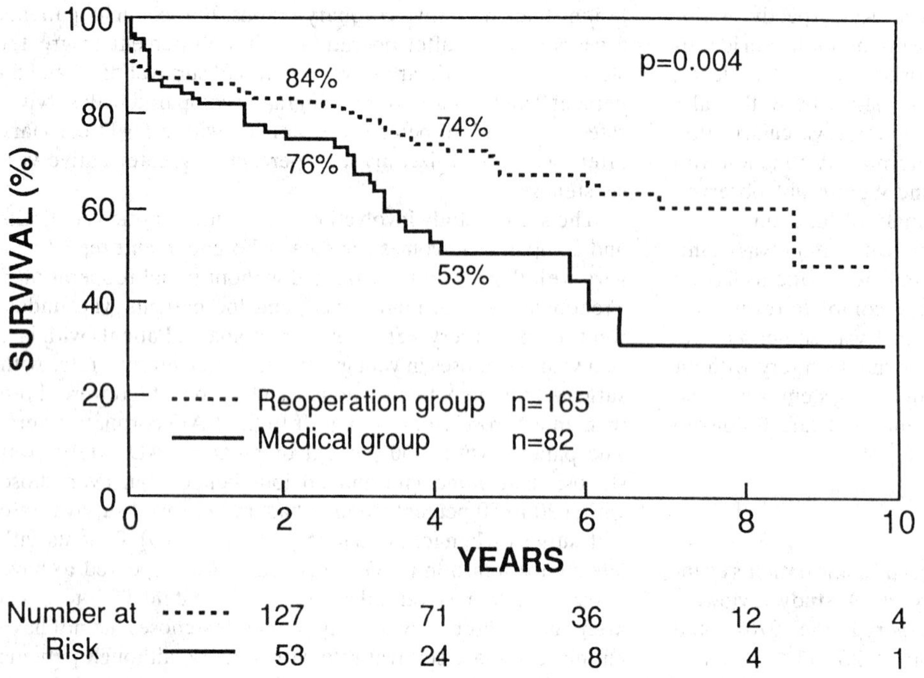

FIGURE 48-9 Patients with late (>5 years after operation) stenoses in venous grafts to the LAD coronary artery have better survival with reoperation than with medical treatment. (Used with permission from Lytle BW, Loop FD, Taylor PC, et al. The effect of coronary reoperation on the survival of patients with stenoses in saphenous vein bypass grafts to coronary arteries. *J Thorac Cardiovasc Surg* 1993; 605-14.)

PCTA VERSUS CABG

The advent of PCTA brought another invasive treatment for coronary atherosclerosis into the arena. Observational studies have identified many of the benefits (low procedure-related morbidity, early return to full activity, feasibility of multiple procedures) and disadvantages (not feasible for many patients, incomplete revascularization, restenosis, acute coronary occlusion) of PCTA. To compare PCTA and surgery for selected patient subgroups, multiple randomized trials have been undertaken.

A three-armed trial [The Medicine, Angioplasty or Surgery Study (MASS)] randomized 214 patients with severe (>80 percent) proximal LAD artery stenoses to medical treatment, PCTA, or bypass surgery (CABG).[85] During a 5-year follow-up, the primary end points of MI, death, and refractory angina occurred for 6 CABG patients, 29 PCTA patients, and 17 medically treated patients ($p = 0.001$). Considering repeat revascularization, death, and MI as events, event-free survival at 5 years was 98.6 percent after CABG, 93.9 percent after PCTA, and 88.9 percent for medically treated patients. The percentage of patients free of angina were CABG, 72.7 percent; PCTA, 64.7 percent; and medically treated, 25.8 percent. There was no difference, however, among the groups in the likelihood of death.

Multiple randomized, prospective trials have compared PCTA versus CABG for the treatment of multivessel CAD. The design of these trials has been to test the question of whether or not an initial strategy of PCTA compromises patient survival. The multicenter Bypass Angioplasty Revascularization Investigation (BARI) trial is the largest such trial (1792 patients randomized in 18 centers), and the single-center Emory Angioplasty Surgery Trial (EAST) is the other U.S. study.[86,87] Included in these trials were patients with stable or unstable angina who were good angiographic candidates for PCTA.

Of the spectrum of patients with coronary atherosclerosis who are considered for revascularization, a minority were included in these trials. Patients with left main stenosis of 50 percent or more were purposely excluded. In the BARI trial, more than half the patients who were potentially randomizable were excluded because of anatomy unfavorable for PCTA, and of the patients judged suitable, only half were randomized. A majority of BARI patients had two-vessel disease (59 percent) and normal LV function, and a minority (37 percent) had a proximal LAD artery lesion. Thus the BARI trial (and EAST patients had similar baseline characteristics) included very few patients who had been shown to have improved survival with CABG in the medicine versus surgery trials of the 1970s. In particular, the PCTA versus CABG trials are underpowered to detect a difference in survival for patients with multivessel disease and abnormal LV function because very few of such patients were randomized.

At approximately a 5-year follow-up interval, overall survival rates have been equivalent for the PCTA and CABG groups in both BARI and EAST. In the BARI trial, the subgroup of patients with treated diabetes had much worse survival with PCTA (Fig. 48-10). The survival advantage of the CABG group was present only if an ITA graft was used. Nondiabetic patients had equivalent survival.[88]

There were large differences between the PCTA and CABG groups in the need for repeat revascularization. Repeat revascularization was required in 54 percent of PCTA patients in both BARI and EAST versus 8 percent in the BARI CABG group and 13 percent in the EAST CABG group. There were smaller differences in symptom status and the need to take antianginal medications in favor of CABG. Detailed discussion of the limitation of these trials and the limitations in the conclusions that can be drawn from these trials have been described in detail by American College of Cardiology/American Heart Association task forces.[2,14] However, among the limitations of these trials in terms of current recommendations for the treatment of a broad spectrum of patients with multivessel CAD are the following: (1) The benefit of PCTA for high-risk patients (those subsets for whom surgery prolongs survival) has not been established because of the small number of such patients included in these randomized trials. (2) Only good angiographic candidates for PCTA were included, and the results of these trials cannot be extended to patients with more marginal suitability for PCTA. (3) Few PCTA patients received intracoronary stents. (4) Few surgical patients had extensive arterial revascularization. (5) None of the protocols included lipid-lowering therapy.

Observational studies have the disadvantage of bias in treatment selection but may have an advantage of being more inclusive. A recent large study from the New York State Cardiac Procedure Registries detailed a 3-year outcome of 29,646 CABG patients and 29,930 PCTA patients.[50] This study found a survival advantage for CABG for all patients with a proximal LAD artery lesion regardless of whether they had single-, double-, or triple-vessel disease.

Comparative trials of PCTA and CABG have involved patients with stable or unstable angina but not "beat the clock" treatment of acute MI. Currently, thrombolysis, PCTA, or both are the strategies employed for the vast majority of patients with acute MI.

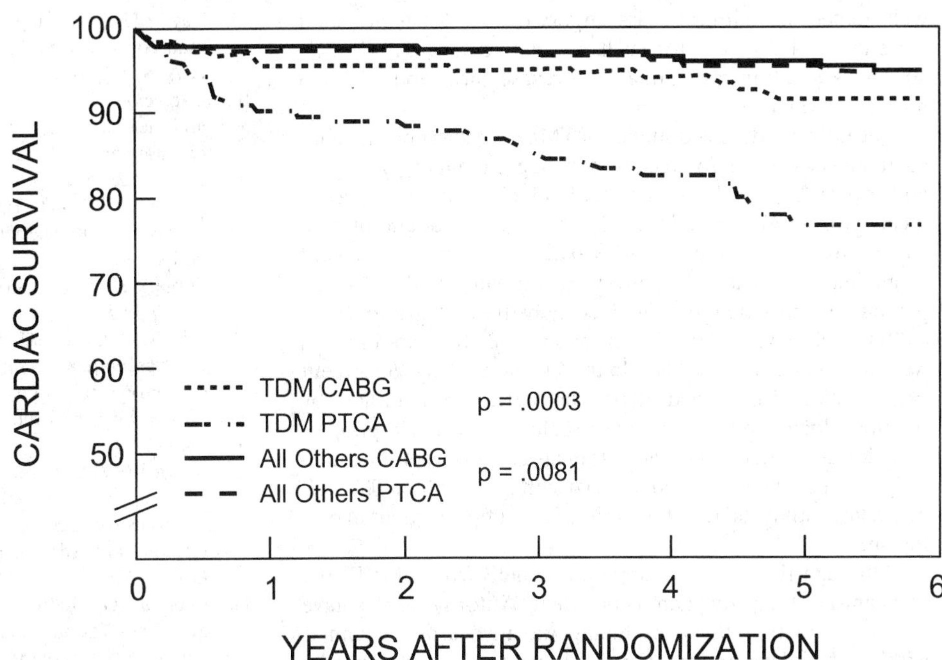

FIGURE 48-10 BARI trial patients with treated diabetes had worse survival following PCTA than following CABG ($p = 0.003$). Patients without diabetes had equivalent survival. (Used with permission from BARI Investigators. Influence of diabetes on 5-year mortality and morbidity in a randomized trial comparing CABG and PTCA in patients with multivessel disease. *Circulation* 1997; 96:1761–1769.)

There are no randomized studies of PCTA versus CABG for patients with previous bypass surgery. The percutaneous treatment of VGA usually has not been effective. Despite the use of stents, there is a high rate of restenosis and cardiac events.[89] Furthermore, it appears that these cardiac events are often serious ones, MI and/or death. Pathologies that are not based on VGA may be treated effectively with PCTA, including graft anastomotic stenoses, early vein graft stenoses, and native vessel stenoses. Patients with large amounts of myocardium jeopardized by atherosclerotic vein grafts usually should be treated with reoperation. However, generalizations are difficult for these complex patients, and therapeutic decisions are best made by interventional cardiologists, cardiac surgeons, and clinical cardiologists working in concert.

INDICATIONS FOR BYPASS SURGERY

In the individual case, recommendations concerning bypass surgery may be influenced by comorbid conditions that greatly increase operative risk or that limit the patient's ultimate life span. However, some generalizations can be made.[2,14] Patients with 50 percent or greater left main stenosis or multivessel disease with a proximal LAD artery stenosis and abnormal LV function should have a recommendation of surgery regardless of their symptom status. Individual randomized trials and meta-analyses have shown clearly a survival benefit for these patients, and there is no evidence that PCTA is safe in these subgroups.

Diabetic patients with multilesion, multivessel disease including a proximal LAD artery lesion should have surgery regardless of LV function and symptom status. Survival is better with CABG than with medical treatment, and PCTA is clearly not an equivalent intervention in terms of survival.

Patients with multivessel disease that include a proximal LAD artery lesion and demonstrable ischemia should have a recommendation for revascularization. If these patients are nondiabetic with normal LV function and are good angiographic candidates for PCTA, it appears that PCTA does not compromise 5-year survival, and the options of PCTA and CABG should be discussed with the patient.

For patients with single-vessel disease based on a proximal LAD artery lesion, survival appears equivalent with medical therapy, PCTA, and CABG, and all options are reasonable, although CABG patients have had fewer events and symptoms over 5 years.

For other subsets of patients with multivessel disease, surgery may be a reasonable choice for the treatment of symptoms in the face of demonstrable ischemia. The choice between PCTA and CABG for these patients should be based on coronary vascular anatomy and patient preference.

For patients with previous bypass surgery and a significant ($\geq$50 percent) late stenosis in a vein graft to the LAD coronary artery, surgery should be recommended regardless of symptoms. For patients in other anatomic subgroups, the risk-benefit situation is complex. Usually reoperation is undertaken to treat severe symptoms and/or large areas of ischemic jeopardy.

TRANSMYOCARDIAL LASER REVASCULARIZATION

The concept of achieving myocardial revascularization by the creation of channels in the myocardium to allow perfusion of blood directly from the LV cavity to coronary sinusoids has been investigated since the 1950s. Early experiments involved mechanically created channels, but more recently, lasers of various wavelengths have been used. The increasing population of patients with severe distal native vessel atherosclerosis (usually occurring years after previous bypass surgery) who may not be well treated with either bypass surgery or PCTA has provided impetus to the search for such alternative revascularization strategies, and transmyocardial laser revascularization (TMLR) may be of value.

Recently, randomized studies of TMLR versus medical management have been conducted involving patients with angina and severe CAD judged untreatable by conventional invasive means. Both CO_2 and holmium lasers were tested, and in both studies, over 70 percent of TMLR patients noted improvement in angina at 1 year postoperatively compared with 13 to 32 percent improvement in the medically treated group ($p < 0.001$).[90,91] Survivals of the TMLR and medically treated groups were the same in both studies. In the CO_2 laser study, 20 percent of patients had improved myocardial perfusion as judged by pharmacologic stress testing with thallium-201 single-photon-emission computed tomography (versus 27 percent of the medically treated group with worse perfusion; $p = 0.002$). The holmium laser study did not show a significant improvement in perfusion.

Although there is some apparent benefit from TMLR, the mechanism of improvement is not clear. Autopsy studies have noted granulation tissue occluding the myocardial channels within a few days of operation, and angina relief may not be immediate. Denervation and microcollateral stimulation have been suggested as possible mechanisms of angina relief. TMLR appears to have a role in revascularization but currently does not appear to produce the degree or the consistency of improved myocardial perfusion that can be achieved when bypass surgery or PCTA is possible. The indications for TMLR are still in evolution.

References

1. Lytle BW, Cosgrove DM. Coronary artery bypass surgery. In: Wells SA, ed. *Current Problems in Surgery*. St. Louis: Mosby–Year Book; 1992; 29:733–807.
2. Eagle KA, Guyton RA, Davidoff R, et al. ACC/AHA guidelines for coronary artery bypass graft surgery: Executive summary and recommendations: A report of the American College of Cardiology/American Heart Association Task Force on Practice Guidelines (Committee to Revise the 1991 Guidelines for Coronary Artery Bypass Graft Surgery). *J Am Coll Cardiol* 1999; 34:1262–1346.
3. Peduzzi P. Eighteen-year follow-up in the Veterans Affairs Cooperative Study of coronary artery bypass surgery for stable angina: The VA Coronary Artery Bypass Surgery Cooperative Study Group. *Circulation* 1992; 86:121–130.
4. Varnauskas E and The European Coronary Surgery Study Group. Twelve-year follow-up of survival in the randomized European Coronary Surgery Study. *N Engl J Med* 1988; 319:332–337.
5. Passamani E, Davis KB, Gillespie MJ, et al. A randomized trial of coronary artery bypass surgery: Survival of patients with a low ejection fraction. *N Engl J Med* 1985; 312:1665–1671.
6. Alderman EL, Bourassi MG, Cohen LS, et al. Ten-year follow-up of survival and myocardial infarction in the randomized Coronary Artery Surgery Study. *Circulation* 1990; 82:1629–1646.
7. Yusuf S, Zucker D, Peduzzi P, et al. Effect of coronary artery bypass graft surgery on survival: Overview of 10-year results from randomised trials by the Coronary Artery Bypass Graft Surgery Trialists Collaboration. *Lancet* 1994; 344:563–570.
8. Rogers WJ, Coggin CJ, Gersh BJ, et al. Ten-year follow-up of quality of life in patients randomized to receive medical therapy or coronary artery bypass graft surgery: The Coronary Artery Surgery Study (CASS). *Circulation* 1990; 82:1647–1658.
9. Taylor HA, Deumite NJ, Chaitman BR, et al. Asymptomatic left main coronary artery disease in the Coronary Artery Surgery Study (CASS) registry. *Circulation* 1989; 79:1171–1179.
10. Caracciolo EA, Davis KB, Sopko G, et al. Comparison of surgical and medical group survival in patients with left main equivalent coronary artery disease: Long-term CASS experience. *Circulation* 1995; 91:2335–2344.
11. Myers WO, Schaff HV, Gersh BJ, et al. Improved survival of surgically treated patients with triple vessel coronary artery disease and severe angina pectoris: A report from the Coronary Artery Surgery Study (CASS) registry. *J Thorac Cardiovasc Surg* 1989; 97:487–495.
12. Bell MA, Gersh BJ, Schaff HV, et al. Effect of completeness of revascularization on long-term outcome of patients undergoing coronary artery bypass surgery: A report from the Coronary Artery Surgery Study (CASS) Registry. *Circulation* 1992; 86: 446–457.
13. Sharma GV, Deupree RH, Khuri SF, et al. Coronary bypass surgery improves survival in high-risk unstable angina: Results of a Veterans Administration Cooperative study with an 8-year follow-up. Veterans Administration Unstable Angina Cooperative Study Group. *Circulation* 1991; 84(suppl III):III-260–III-267.
14. Gibbons RJ, Chatterjee K, Daley J, et al. ACC/AHA/ACP-ASIM guidelines for the management of patients with chronic stable angina: A report of the American College of Cardiology/American Heart Association Task Force on Practice Guidelines (Committee on Management of Patients with Chronic Stable Angina). *J Am Coll Cardiol* 1999; 33:2092–2197.
15. Edwards FH, Clark RE, Schwartz M. Coronary artery bypass grafting: The Society of Thoracic Surgeons National Database experience. *Ann Thorac Surg* 1994; 57:12–19.
16. Bourassa MG, Campeau L, Lesperance J. Changes in grafts and coronary arteries after coronary bypass surgery. *Cardiovasc Clin* 1991; 21:83–100.
17. Fitzgibbon GM, Leach AJ, Kafka HP, et al. Coronary bypass graft fate: Long-term angiographic study. *J Am Coll Cardiol* 1991; 17:1075.
18. Campeau L, Enjalbert M, Lesperance M, et al. The relation of risk factors to the development of atherosclerosis in saphenous vein bypass grafts and the progression of disease in the native circulation. *N Engl J Med* 1984; 311:1329–1332.
19. Lytle BW, Loop FD, Cosgrove DM, et al. Long-term (5 to 12 years) serial studies of internal mammary artery and saphenous vein coronary bypass grafts. *J Thorac Cardiovasc Surg* 1985; 89:248–258.
20. Fitzgibbon GM, Kafka HP, Leach AJ, et al. Coronary bypass graft fate and patient outcome: angiographic follow-up of 5065 grafts related to survival and reoperation in 1388 patients during 25 years. *J Am Coll Cardiol* 1996; 28:616–626.
21. Vlodaver Z, Edward JE. Pathologic changes in aortic-coronary arterial saphenous vein grafts. *Circulation* 1971; 44:719–728.
22. Ratliff NB, Myles JL. Rapidly progressive atherosclerosis in aortocoronary saphenous vein grafts: Possible immuno-mediated disease. *Arch Pathol Lab Med* 1989; 113:772–776.
23. Fitzmaurice M, Ratliff NB. Immunoglobulin deposition in atherosclerotic aortocoronary saphenous vein grafts. *Arch Pathol Lab Med* 1990; 114:388–393.
24. Barboriak JJ, Pintar K, Korns ME. Atherosclerosis in aortocoronary vein grafts. *Lancet* 1974; 2:611–614.
25. Neitzel GF, Barboriak JJ, Pintar K, et al. Atherosclerosis in aortocoronary bypass grafts: Morphologic study and risk factor analysis 6 to 12 years after surgery. *Arteriosclerosis* 1986; 6:594–600.
26. Keon WJ, Heggtveit HA, Leduc J. Perioperative myocardial infarctions caused by atheroembolization. *J Thorac Cardiovasc Surg* 1982; 84:849–855.
27. Gavaghan TP, Gebski V, Baron DW. Immediate postoperative aspirin improves vein graft patency early and late after coronary

artery bypass graft surgery: A placebo-controlled, randomized study. *Circulation* 1991; 83:1526–1533.

28. Goldman S, Copeland J, Moritz T, et al. Starting aspirin therapy after operation: Effects on early graft patency. *Circulation* 1991; 84:520–526.
29. The Post Coronary Artery Bypass Graft Trial Investigators. The effect of aggressive lowering of low-density lipoprotein cholesterol levels and low-dose anticoagulation on obstructive changes in saphenous-vein coronary-artery bypass grafts. *N Engl J Med* 1997; 336:153–162.
30. Blankenhorn DH, Nessim SA, Johnson RL, et al. Beneficial effects of combined colestipol-niacin therapy on coronary atherosclerosis and coronary venous bypass grafts. *JAMA* 1987; 257: 3233–3240.
31. Flaker GC, Warnica JW, Sacks FM. et al. Pravastatin prevents clinical events in revascularized patients with average cholesterol concentrations: Cholesterol and Recurrent Events (CARE) investigators. *J Am Coll Cardiol* 1999; 34:106–112.
32. Lawrie GM, Morris GC Jr., Earle N. Long-term results of coronary bypass surgery: Analysis of 1698 patients followed 15 to 20 years. *Ann Surg* 1991; 213:377–385.
33. Whitlow PL, Dimas AP, Bashore TM, et al. Relationship of extent of revascularization with angina at one year in the Bypass Angioplasty Revascularization Investigation (BARI). *J Am Coll Cardiol* 1999; 34:1750–1759.
34. Dion R, Etienne PY, Verhelst R, et al. Bilateral mammary grafting: Clinical, functional, and angiographic assessment in 400 consecutive cases. *Eur J Cardiothorac Surg* 1993; 7:287–294.
35. Tector AJ, Amundsen S, Schmahl TM, et al. Total revascularization with T grafts. *Ann Thorac Surg* 1994; 57:33–39.
36. Califiore AM, DiGiammarco G, Lucimi N, et al. Composite arterial conduits for a wide arterial myocardial revascularization. *Ann Thorac Surg* 1994; 58:185–190.
37. Loop FD, Lytle BW, Cosgrove DM, et al. Influence of the internal-mammary artery graft on 10-year survival and other cardiac events. *N Engl J Med* 1986; 314:1–6.
38. Cameron A, Davis KB, Green G, et al. Coronary bypass surgery with internal-thoracic-artery grafts: Effects on survival over a 15-year period. *N Engl J Med* 1996; 334:216–219.
39. Lytle BW, Blackstone EH, Loop FD, et al. Two internal thoracic artery grafts are better than one. *J Thorac Cardiovasc Surg* 1999; 117:855–872.
40. Buxton BF, Komeda M, Fuller JA, Gordon I. Bilateral internal thoracic artery grafting may improve outcome of coronary artery surgery: Risk-adjusted survival. *Circulation* 1998; 98:III-1–III-6.
41. Suma H, Amano A, Horii T, et al. Gastroepiploic artery graft in 400 patients. *Eur J Cardiothorac Surg* 1996; 10:6–11.
42. Buche M, Schroeder E, Gurne O, et al. Coronary artery bypass grafting with the inferior epigastric artery: Midterm clinical and angiographic results. *J Thorac Cardiovasc Surg* 1995; 109:553–560.
43. Fisk RL, Brooks CH, Callaghan JC, et al. Experience with the radial artery for coronary artery bypass. *Ann Thorac Surg* 1976; 21:513–518.
44. Carpentier A. Selection of coronary bypass: Anatomic, physiological and angiographic consideration of vein and mannary artery bypass. *J Thorac Cardiovasc Surg* 1975; 70:414–431.
45. Brodman RF, Frame R, Camacho M, et al. Routine use of unilateral and bilateral radial arteries for coronary bypass graft surgery. *J Am Coll Cardiol* 1996; 28:959–963.
46. Acar C, Ramsheyi A, Pagny J. et al. The radial artery for coronary artery bypass grafting: Clinical and angiographic results at five years. *J Thorac Cardiovasc Surg* 1998; 116:981–989.
47. Possati G, Gardino M, Alessandrini F, et al. Mid-term clinical and angiographic results of radial artery grafts used for myocardial revascularization. *J Thorac Cardiovasc Surg* 1998; 116:1015–1021.
48. Bergsma TM, Grandjean JG, Voors AA, et al. Low recurrence of angina pectoris after coronary artery bypass graft surgery with bilateral internal thoracic and right gastroepiploic arteries. *Circulation* 1998; 97:2402–2405.
49. Edwards FH, Grover FL, Shroyer AL, et al. The Society of Thoracic Surgeons National Cardiac Surgery Database: Current risk assessment. *Ann Thorac Surg* 1977; 63:903–908.
50. Hannan EL, Racz MJ, McCallister BD, et al. A comparison of three-year survival after coronary artery bypass graft surgery and percutaneous transluminal coronary angioplasty. *J Am Coll Cardiol* 1999; 33:63–72.
51. Jones RH, Hannan EL, Hammermeister KE, et al. Identification of preoperative variables needed for risk adjustment of short-term mortality after coronary bypass graft surgery: The Working Group Panel on the Cooperative CABG Database Project. *J Am Coll Cardiol* 1996; 28:1478–1487.
52. Burack JH, Impellizzai P, Homel P, et al. Public reporting of surgical mortality: A survey of New York State cardiothoracic surgeons. *Ann Thorac Surg* 1999; 68:1195–1202.
53. Cosgrove DM, Loop FD, Lytle BW, et al. Does internal mammary artery grafting increase surgical risk? *Circulation* 1985; 72(suppl 2):170–174.
54. Grover FL, Johnson RR, Marshall G, et al. Impact of mammary grafts on coronary bypass operation mortality and morbidity. *Ann Thorac Surg* 1994; 57:559–569.
55. Edwards FH for STS Database. Personal communication, 1999.
56. Martin TD, Craver JM, Gott JP, et al. Prospective, randomized trial of retrograde warm blood cardioplegia: Myocardial benefit and neurologic threat. *Ann Thorac Surg* 1994; 57:298–302.
57. Bottner RK, Wallace RB, Visner MS, et al. Reduction of myocardial infarction after emergency coronary artery bypass grafting for failed coronary angioplasty with use of a normothermic perfusion cardioplegia protocol. *J Thorac Cardiovasc Surg* 1971; 101:1069–1075.
58. Christakis GT, Fremes SE, Weisel RD, et al. Reducing the risk of urgent revascularization for unstable angina: A randomized clinical trial. *J Vasc Surg* 1986; 3:764–772.
59. Buckberg GD. Strategies and logic of cardioplegic delivery to prevent, avoid and reverse ischemic and reperfusion damage. *J Thorac Cardiovasc Surg* 1987; 93:127–139.
60. Roach GW, Kanchuger M, Mangano CM, et al. Adverse cerebral outcomes after coronary bypass surgery: Multicenter study of Perioperative Ischemia Research Group and the Ischemia Research and Education Foundation investigators. *N Engl J Med* 1996; 335:1857–1863.
61. Hartman GS, Yao FS, Bruefach M III. Severity of aortic atheromatous disease diagnosed by transesophageal echocardiography predicts stroke and other outcomes associated with coronary artery surgery: A prospective study. *Anesth Analg* 1996; 83:701–708.
62. Blauth CI, Cosgrove DM, Webb BW, et al. Atheroembolism from the ascending aorta: An emerging problem in cardiac surgery. *J Thorac Cardiovasc Surg* 1992; 103:1104–1112.
63. Berens ES, Kouchoukos NT, Murphy SF, Wareing TH. Preoperative carotid artery screening in elderly patients undergoing cardiac surgery. *J Vasc Surg* 1992; 15:313–321.
64. Salasidis GC, Latter DA, Steinmetz OK, et al. Carotid artery duplex scanning in preoperative assessment for coronary artery revascularization: The association between peripheral vascular disease, carotid artery stenosis and stroke. *J Vasc Surg* 1995; 21:154–160.
65. Hertzer NR, Loop FD, Beven EG, et al. Surgical strategy for simultaneous coronary and carotid disease: A study including prospective randomization. *J Vasc Surg* 1989; 9:455–463.
66. Akins CW, Moncure AC, Daggett WM, et al. Safety and efficacy of concomitant carotid and coronary artery operations. *Ann Thorac Surg* 1995; 60:311–317.
67. Loop FD, Lytle BW, Cosgrove DM, et al. Sternal wound complications after isolated coronary bypass grafting: Early and late mortal-

ity, morbidity and cost of care. *Ann Thorac Surg* 1990; 49:179–187.

68. Possati G, Gandino M, Alessandrini F, et al. Systematic clinical and angiographic follow-up of patients undergoing minimally invasive coronary artery bypass. *J Thorac Cardiovasc Surg* 1998; 115: 785–790.
69. Calafiore AM, Teodori G, DiGiammao G, et al. Minimally invasive coronary artery surgery: The LAST operation. *Semin Thorac Cardiovasc Surg* 1997; 9:305–311.
70. Galloway AC, Shemin R, Glower DD et al. First report of the Port-Access International Registry. *Ann Thorac Surg* 1999; 67:51–58.
71. Buffolo E, deAndrade CS, Branco JN, et al. Coronary artery bypass grafting without cardiopulmonary bypass. *Ann Thorac Surg* 1996; 61:63–66.
72. Tasdemir O, Vural KM, Karagoz H, et al. Coronary artery bypass grafting on the beating heart without the use of extracorporeal circulation: Review of 2052 cases. *J Thorac Cardiovasc Surg* 1998; 116:68–73.
73. Iaco AL, Contini M, Teodori G, et al. Off or on bypass: What is the safety threshold? *Ann Thorac Surg* 1999; 68:1486–1489.
74. Myers WO, Blackstone EH, Davis K, et al. CASS Registry. Long term surgical survival. *J Am Coll Cardiol* 1999; 33:488–498.
75. Kirklin JW, et al. ACC/AHA Task Force Report: Guidelines and indications for coronary artery bypass surgery. *J Am Coll Cardiol* 1991; 17:543.
76. Cavender JB, Rogers WJ, Fisher LD, et al. Effects of smoking on survival and morbidity in patients randomized to medical or surgical therapy in the Coronary Artery Surgery Study (CASS): 10-year follow-up. *J Am Coll Cardiol* 1992; 20:287–294.
77. Cosgrove DM, Loop FD, Lytle BW, et al. Determinants of 10-year survival after primary myocardial revascularization. *Ann Surg* 1985; 202:480–490.
78. Jones EL, Weintraub WS. The importance of completeness of revascularization during long-term follow-up after coronary artery operation. *J Thorac Cardiovasc Surg* 1996; 112:227–237.
79. Cosgrove DM, Loop FD, Lytle BW, et al. Predictors of reoperation after myocardial revascularization. *J Thorac Cardiovasc Surg* 1986; 92:811–821.
80. Lytle BW, Loop FD, Taylor PC, et al. Vein graft disease: The clinical impact of stenoses in saphenous vein grafts to coronary arteries. *J Thorac Cardiovasc Surg* 1992; 103:831–840.
81. Lytle BW, Loop FD, Taylor PC, et al. The effect of coronary reoperation on the survival of patients with stenoses in saphenous vein to coronary bypass grafts. *J Thorac Cardiovasc Surg* 1993; 105:605–614.
82. Lytle BW, Loop FD, Cosgrove DM, et al. Fifteen hundred coronary reoperations: Results and determinants of early and late survival. *J Thorac Cardiovasc Surg* 1987; 93:847–859.
83. Loop FD, Lytle BW, Cosgrove DM, et al. Reoperation for coronary atherosclerosis: Changing practice in 2509 consecutive patients. *Ann Surg* 1990; 212:378–386.
84. Lytle BW, McElroy D, McCarthy PM, et al. Influence of arterial coronary bypass grafts on the mortality in coronary reoperations. *J Thorac Cardiovasc Surg* 1994; 107:675–683.
85. Hueb WA, Sowes PR, deOliveira SA, et al. Five-year follow-up of the Medicine, Angioplasty, or Surgery Study (MASS): A prospective, randomized trial of medical therapy. Balloon angioplasty or bypass surgery for single proximal left anterior descending coronary artery stenosis. *Circulation* 1999; 100(supp II):II-107–II-113.
86. Bypass Angioplasty Revascularization Investigation (BARI). Comparison of coronary bypass surgery with angioplasty in patients with multivessel disease. *N Engl J Med* 1996; 335: 217–225.
87. King SB, Lembo NJ, Weintraub WS, et al. A randomized trial comparing coronary angioplasty with coronary bypass surgery: Emory Angioplasty versus Surgery Trial (EAST). *N Engl J Med* 1994; 331:1044–1050.
88. BARI Investigators. Influence of diabetes on 5-year mortality and morbidity in a randomized trial comparing CABG and PTCA in patients with multivessel disease. *Circulation* 1997; 96:1761–1769.
89. Savage MP, Douglas JS Jr., Fischman DL, et al. Stent placement compared with balloon angioplasty for obstructed coronary bypass grafts. Saphenous Vein De Novo Trial Investigators. *N Engl J Med* 1997; 337:740–747.
90. Frazier OH, March RJ, Horvath KA, et al. Transmyocardial revascularization with a carbon dioxide laser in patients with end-stage coronary artery disease. *N Engl J Med* 1999; 341:1021–1028.
91. Allen KB, Dowling RD, Fudge TL, et al. Comparison of transmyocardial revascularization with medical therapy in patients with refractory angina. *N Engl J Med* 1999; 341:1029–1036.

CHAPTER 49

MANAGEMENT OF THE PATIENT AFTER CARDIAC SURGERY

Douglas C. Morris / Stephen D. Clements, Jr. / Carl C. Hug, Jr.

The initial management of the patient following cardiac surgery is primarily focused in specialized intensive care units. The unique pathophysiologic alterations associated with hypothermia and cardiopulmonary bypass (CPB)[1] mandated that a specialized environment, including intensive monitoring and offering sophisticated electrophysiologic, hemodynamic, and mechanical intervention supervised by specially trained critical care nurses, be available. While CPB is no longer universally applied in cardiac surgery, the multiple management problems posed by cardiac patients as a consequence of their preoperative status, effects of residual anesthetic drugs, success of the operative procedure, and intraoperative complications continue to demand specialized treatment. When direct coronary artery bypass grafting is done without CPB, the primary concerns are bleeding (residual heparin, surgical hemostasis), hypothermia, myocardial ischemia, and injury. The use of CPB accentuates these concerns and adds those of a generalized inflammatory response.

ROLE OF VASCULAR CANNULAE, LIFE SUPPORT, AND MONITORING IN THE IMMEDIATE POSTOPERATIVE PERIOD

On arrival in the ICU, the patient is still under the effects of anesthesia and hypothermia, often receiving one or more drugs affecting the systemic circulation, and, in most cases, mechanically ventilated. The patient typically arrives from the operating room with the necessary apparatus for monitoring the following parameters: heart rate and rhythm; arterial, central venous, pulmonary artery, and pulmonary artery occlusion pressures (PAOP); cardiac output; urinary output; mediastinal drainage; body temperature; and arterial oxygen saturation (SpO_2) and end-tidal carbon dioxide tension ($ETCO_2$). Immediately upon arrival in the ICU, reliable monitoring of the previously mentioned variables should be instituted. Once the patient is satisfactorily connected to the bedside monitors and ventilator, all the hemodynamic measurements should be recorded, the patient's level of consciousness and comfort should be assessed, a portable supine chest x-ray should be acquired, and a 12-lead electrocardiogram obtained.

Most of the apparatus attached to the patient upon arrival in the ICU serves a dual purpose. A pulmonary artery catheter not only allows monitoring of pulmonary artery pressures but can also be used to estimate the filling pressure of the left ventricle, cardiac output, and body core temperature. The peripheral arterial cannula provides a continuous pulse-wave tracing of systemic blood pressure and ready access to arterial blood sampling for laboratory analysis. *Regular periodic assessments of arterial blood gases, especially after a major change in ventilator settings, are essential unless continuous $ETCO_2$ and SpO_2 by pulse oximetry are being monitored.* $ETCO_2$ and SpO_2 are reliable in guiding the weaning of mechanical ventilation and tracheal extubation. Monitoring of these parameters has been used very effectively in "fast-track" protocols. Assessment of volume loss is based on chest and mediastinal tube drainage plus urine output. The endotracheal tube secured in the correct position with an appropriately inflated cuff is essential for positive-pressure ventilation of the lungs. Confirmation of bilateral breath sounds and absence of tracheal air leak versus cuff inflation should be made upon arrival in the ICU and after suctioning secretions from the oropharynx. The endotracheal tube's position should be ascertained on the initial chest x-ray. The endotracheal tube also allows for suctioning of bronchial secretions and reduces (but does not eliminate) the risk of oropharyngeal and gastric reflux secretions entering the trachea and bronchi. The endotracheal tube can often be removed the evening of surgery if the patient is conscious, is able to protect the airway, has good ventilatory mechanics and muscle strength, and is able to take on the work of breathing. Most patients can have the pulmonary artery catheter removed within 12 to 24 h if cardiovascular drug therapy is at minimum levels. The peripheral arterial cannula can be removed once cardiovascular function is satisfactory and the need for blood sampling is at a routine daily level. The urinary catheter is usually removed when the patient is ambulatory unless there is a vigorous diuresis or an increased risk of urinary retention. Chest tubes are generally removed when the total drainage is less than 100 mL per tube over 8 h.

The primary factor that differentiates cardiac surgery from other forms of surgery is CPB. With such improvements in extracorporeal technology as membrane oxygenation, arterial blood filtration, and blood sparing techniques, the noncardiac complications have been significantly reduced. Major improvements in myocardial protection technology coupled with changes in anesthetic and CPB techniques now frequently allow extubation within several hours of surgery.[2] Intraoperative management has now evolved to the point of minimizing the need for cardiopulmonary support after surgery, thereby allowing the patient to recover satisfactory vital function more rapidly than before. As a consequence, mechanical ventilation and other measures can be discontinued much earlier, and the patient can be safely and comfortably transferred from the ICU within the first 6 to 24 h, a process that has been termed *fast-tracking*.[3]

Individuals undergoing "off pump" procedures also have the potential for rapid recovery and early extubation and removal of catheters and chest tubes, and can be sitting up in the chair the next morning ready for transfer.

Fast-tracking describes efforts to minimize the duration of the patient's stay in the ICU or postanesthesia care unit and to allow the early, safe transfer of the cardiac surgical patient to a so-called step-down level of monitored care. Early extubation and transfer should require that the patient's status is characterized as follows: awake or easily aroused, neurologically intact, cooperative, and comfortable; stable, satisfactory hemodynamics; normothermia; satisfactory spontaneous ventilation; normal coagulation with minimal chest tube drainage; satisfactory urine output, electrolyte, and acid-base balance.[4]

EARLY POSTOPERATIVE MANAGEMENT

Pathophysiologic Consequences of Cardiopulmonary Bypass

The basic pathophysiology during the early postoperative period revolves around the following variables: transient left ventricular dysfunction, capillary leak, warming from hypothermia, mediastinal bleeding, and emergence from anesthesia.

The likely presence of left ventricular dysfunction during the first 24 h postoperatively with a gradual recovery to preoperative levels is suggested by studies based upon hemodynamic data, nuclear scanning, and metabolic techniques. While improvements in surgical techniques, cardioplegia delivery, and other myocardial protection measures achieved in the past decade would have been expected to lessen this complication, the reported prevalence of early ventricular dysfunction (90 percent) did not change between 1979 and 1990.[5] This transient myocardial depression has been attributed by some authors to inadequate myocardial protection or the effects of cold cardioplegia,[6,7] but the bulk of the evidence incriminates the inflammatory state induced by CPB as the primary causative factor.[1]

The inflammatory state induced by CPB involves platelet-endothelial cell interactions and vasospastic responses that result in low-flow states in the coronary circulation.[8] The inflammatory reaction causes vascular endothelial adhesion molecules to attract inflammatory cells that subsequently adhere to the vascular endothelium. These inflammatory cells mediate much of the subsequent injury by the release of oxygen radicals or proteolytic enzymes.[9] This release of oxygen-free radicals in response to reperfusion injury is now generally accepted as the explanation for the transient postoperative ventricular dysfunction.[10–12] Depressed myocardial function seems to be unrelated to CPB time, number of coronary artery grafts, preoperative medications, or postoperative core temperature. Ventricular function is generally depressed by 2 h and is at its worse at 4 to 5 h after CPB. Significant recovery of function usually occurs by 8 to 10 h, and full recovery is reached by 24 to 48 h.[13] Systemic vascular resistance, while not rising immediately after surgery, increases as ventricular function worsens. This rise in systemic vascular resistance is likely secondary to reduced ventricular function and the need to maintain systemic blood pressure and, per se, is not a major causative factor of depressed cardiac contractility. The confounding effect of vasopressor drugs used in an attempt to increase systemic blood pressure must be recognized.

The inflammation-mediated production of oxygen-free radicals and release of proteolytic enzymes by neutrophils also damages the endothelial cells. The "gatekeeper" function of the endothelium is disturbed and capillary permeability increases, resulting in edema.[9] The capillary leak syndrome may last from a few hours up to 1 to 2 days, depending to a large degree on the duration of CPB. When the capillary leak ceases and interstitial edema fluid is mobilized, intravascular volume overload is a threat. At this time, diuretics are beneficial to eliminate excessive fluid.

Hypothermia predisposes the patient to cardiac dysrhythmias, increases systemic vascular resistance, precipitates shivering (which increases O_2 consumption and CO_2 production), and impairs coagulation.[13] Hypothermia with the patient's core temperature below 35°C frequently recurs after rewarming to 37°C (98.6°F) at the end of CPB. This fall in core temperature reflects the loss of heat from the surgical field after CPB, exposure of the patient to ambient temperature, and incomplete rewarming of peripheral tissues, especially fat and muscle. If the patient is hypothermic upon arrival in the ICU, monitoring the temperature of noncore body sites such as a finger or toe can assure complete assessment of rewarming. Hypothermia causes peripheral vasoconstriction and contributes to the hypertension frequently seen after cardiac surgery. Furthermore, hypothermia causes a decrease in cardiac output by producing bradycardia along with the increase in vascular resistance. As the patient is rewarmed, large increases in O_2 consumption, and CO_2 production can occur, with a consequent increase in demand on cardiovascular and pulmonary functions.[14]

Hypercarbia will cause catecholamine release, tachycardia, and pulmonary hypertension. If the patient cannot increase the cardiac output and O_2 delivery, venous hemoglobin desaturation and metabolic acidosis will result. Most believe that the patient should be passively rewarmed by warm air (e.g., Bear Hugger) and that shivering should be eliminated by the administration of meperidine (25 to 50 mg) and muscle relaxants.[15] As body temperature increases, the vasoconstriction and hypertension associated with hypothermia are replaced by vasodilatation, tachycardia, and hypotension. Volume loading during the rewarming process helps reduce the rapid swings in blood pressure. Vasopressors (e.g., norepinephrine) may be required to maintain an adequate systemic blood pressure.

The commonly reported prevalence of severe postoperative bleeding (more than 10 U of blood transfused) following cardiac surgery is between 3 and 5 percent. In some hospitals, 25 percent of all blood products are dedicated to cardiac surgery.[16] While approximately one-half of the patients who undergo reoperation for excessive bleeding exhibit incomplete surgical hemostasis, the remainder bleed because of various acquired hemostatic defects, most often related to acquired platelet dysfunction.[17] The factors that predispose to bleeding following CPB are residual heparin effect, platelet dysfunction (which may be intensified by preoperative drug therapy, e.g., aspirin and $GPII_bIII_a$ inhibitors), clotting-factor depletion, inadequate surgical hemostasis, hypothermia, and postoperative hypertension. CPB decreases both platelet count and function. Hemodilution causes platelet counts to fall rapidly to about 50 percent of preoperative values. Within minutes after instituting CPB, the bleeding time is prolonged and platelet aggregation is impaired. The bleeding time usually normalizes by 2 to 4 h after CPB. The platelet count usually requires several days to return to normal levels. While the exact mechanism responsible for the transient platelet dysfunction remains undefined, it appears to be related to contact of platelets with the synthetic surfaces of the extracorporeal oxygenator and to hypothermia. Reductions in the plasma concentrations of coagulation factors II, V, VII, IX, X, and XIII due to hemodilution occur during CPB, but these coagulation factors remain well above levels considered adequate for hemostasis and generally normalize within the first 12 h after surgery. Moreover, while bleeding after CPB is often attributed to excessive fibrinolysis, the decrease in both plasminogen and fibrinogen levels during CPB is due to hemodilution and not consumption.[17] Upon returning from the operating room after exploration for bleeding, a common report is that no localized site of bleeding occurred and only diffuse oozing was found. Less frequently, a specific site such as an internal mammary pedicle will be identified.

MANAGEMENT OF COMMON POSTOPERATIVE SYNDROMES

Vasoconstriction with Hypertension and Borderline Cardiac Output

Increased arteriolar resistance as a consequence of hypothermia and increased levels of circulating catecholamines, plasma renin, or angiotensin II is present in most postoperative cardiac patients. The usual criterion for pharmacologic lowering of blood pressure in postoperative patients is a mean arterial blood pressure 10 percent above the upper level of normal (>90 mmHg). Patients with a friable aorta or friable suture lines might be subjected to a lower mean arterial pressure to prevent dehiscence. The mean arterial blood pressure is monitored because it is most reflective of systemic vascular resistance. As the hypothermic patient is rewarmed, a short-acting vasodilator (nitroprusside, nitroglycerin, or nicardipine) can be infused intravenously to maintain mean arterial pressure at 80 to 90 mmHg. Intravascular volume should be maintained at a relatively high level (PAOP of 14 to 16 mmHg) in anticipation of vasodilation upon rewarming and to enhance cardiac output and peripheral perfusion. If the cardiac index is marginal (2.0 to 2.2 L/min/m^2), an inotropic drug should be administered in addition to the vasodilator.

Vasodilatation and Hypotension

This condition, which generally appears during rewarming, is most effectively prevented and best treated by fluid administration. The specific volume expander selected should be based upon a determination of the predominant factor leading to the hypovolemia. If the predominant factor is a capillary leak syndrome with generalized edema, the use of colloids could aggravate the situation as the oncotic elements pass into the interstitium and exacerbate tissue edema. If vasodilatation with increased venous capacitance is the major problem, colloids will provide longer-lasting augmentation of intravascular volume. Hetastarch (administered in 250- to 500-mL increments) provides sustained volume expansion equal to 5 percent albumin, at a significant reduction in cost. It does, however, have a tendency to increase bleeding. If fluid administration has increased PAOP appropriately (e.g., 14 to 16 mmHg for a normal ventricle or 18 to 22 mmHg for a noncompliant ventricle) and systemic blood pressure remains marginal, vasopressor or inotropic drugs should be administered. Generally, a PAOP above 15 mmHg in the postoperative period is of little benefit due to a "flattening" of the diastolic function curve, which accompanies the decline in systolic function.[18] An inotropic vasopressor should be infused if more than 1 or 2 L of fluid have been administered and the PAOP is not rising. In some patients after cardiac surgery, fluid administration produces a substantial increase in left ventricular end-diastolic volume without changing PAOP. Whether this is due to an open pericardium with overdistension of the left ventricle or some other factor is unclear.[19] If the blood pressure is marginal and the cardiac index is over 2.0 L/min/m^2, norepinephrine or dopamine is the preferable agent. If the cardiac index is less than 2.0 L/min/m^2, an inotropic agent should be administered initially.

Normal Ventricular Systolic Function and Low Cardiac Output

This set of circumstances is often noted in small women with systemic hypertension and in patients undergoing aortic valve replacement for aortic stenosis. The likely explanation is diastolic dysfunction. The problem should be managed by volume expansion with the intent to elevate PAOP to levels as high as 20 to 25 mmHg if necessary. Sinus rhythm and atrioventricular synchrony are essential and, if not present, should be restored.

In the absence of other reasons for diastolic dysfunction, the possibility of cardiac compression from clots in the mediastinum and pericardial space should be considered. If volume expansion does not lead to hemodynamic improvement, transesophageal echocardiography (TEE) should be used to establish or exclude the presence of clots or other causes of low output. If the information derived from TEE does not permit explanation and/or resolution of the problem, the patient should return to the operating room for exploration.

A rather characteristic presentation of cardiac compression is the patient who initially has significant mediastinal bleeding that ceases rather abruptly. The patient then becomes hypotensive, with high PAOP and central venous pressure and progressively increasing inotropic drug requirements. Cardiac compression from clots in the pericardial space should be suspected and, if time allows, confirmed by TEE. Rapid clinical deterioration demands immediate exploration of the pericardial space.

APPROACH TO POSTOPERATIVE CARDIOVASCULAR PROBLEMS

Low Cardiac Output Syndrome

Satisfactory cardiac performance following cardiac surgery is usually indicated by a cardiac index greater than 2.2, L/min/m^2 with a heart rate below 100 beats per minute. Marginal cardiac function is present with a cardiac index between 2.0 and 2.2 L/min/m^2. A cardiac index below 2.0 L/min/m^2 is unacceptably low, and therapeutic intervention is indicated. Clinical signs of the adequacy or inadequacy of organ perfusion must be incorporated into any assessment of cardiac performance.

ASSESSMENT

The most common causes of low cardiac output postoperatively are related to a decreased left ventricular preload. The decreased preload, in turn, can likely be attributed to hypovolemia (due to bleeding or to vasodilatation as a consequence of warming or of drugs), cardiac tamponade, or right ventricular dysfunction. Alternative explanations for low cardiac output include decreased contractility due to a preexisting low ejection fraction or to intra- or postoperative ischemia or infarction. Perioperative myocardial ischemia or infarction is usually due to poor intraoperative myocardial protection, incomplete myocardial revascularization, coronary artery spasm, coronary embolism of atherosclerotic debris or air, prolonged systemic hypotension, or severe acute anemia. Tachy- or bradyarrhythmias decrease cardiac output by reducing ventricular preload (e.g., decreased diastolic filling time, loss of atrial contraction or atrioventricular synchrony) or by reducing the number of effective ventricular contractions per minute. Substantial increases in systemic vascular resistance (i.e., vasoconstriction) impede ventricular ejection and lower cardiac output. Vasodilatation from sepsis or anaphylaxis resulting in systemic hypotension could lead to reduced coronary blood flow and myocardial ischemia. Sepsis (an unlikely occurrence in the immediate postoperative period) is also associated with the production of myocardial depressant factors. Anemia may result in reduced blood viscosity (a major determinant of total peripheral resistance) leading to hypotension and decreased oxygen delivery to the heart. The hypotension in anemia, however, is most often due to changes in effective blood volume rather than to the changes in viscosity.

ETIOLOGY AND MANAGEMENT

The multiple variables constantly monitored usually provide sufficient clues as to the cause of low cardiac output. If there is no obvious noncardiac cause such as anaphylaxis or anaphylactoid reaction, acidosis, severe anemia, or marked alterations in body temperature, then the first step is to optimize the preload (PAOP of 15 to 18 mmHg). The next step is to optimize the heart rate by either cardiac pacing or antiarrhythmic drugs. Postoperative myocardial performance is usually best at a rate of 90 to 100 beats per minute. If these measures prove unsuccessful, pharmacologic intervention with inotropic agents, vasodilators, vasopressors, or a combination of these drugs must be considered. The selection of drugs should be based upon the balance of their effects on heart rate, contractility, ventricular preload, and systemic vasculature resistance (Table 49-1). The presence of elevated left- and right-sided filling pressures, a recent cessation of mediastinal drainage, and progressively increasing inotropic drug-dosage requirements suggests tamponade, which should be relieved emergently. TEE has been very helpful in clarifying these situations. The final therapeutic step, if the preceding measures have proved inadequate, is the use of aortic counterpulsation (i.e., intraaortic balloon pump) or another type of cardiac assist device.

TABLE 49-1 Medications Used in Low Cardiac Output Syndrome

Medication	Hemodynamic Properties	Dosage Range
Dopamine	Low dose—dopaminergic effect Moderate dose—inotropic effect High dose—vasopressor effect	2–20 μg/kg/min
Dobutamine	Positive inotropic agent	2–20 μg/kg/min
Epinephrine	Positive inotropic agent	1–4 μg/min
Amrinone	Positive inotropic agent	10–15 μg/kg/min
Isoproterenol	Potent inotropic agent Pronounced chronotropic effect	0.5–10 μg/min
Norepinephrine	Potent vasopressor effect; inotropic effect	1–100 μg/min
Phenylephrine	Potent vasopressor agent	10–500 μg/min

Hypertension

MANAGEMENT

A variety of medications are available for control of hypertension, and the drug selected should depend on the hemodynamic status of the patient, the cardiovascular effects of the drug, and the patient's other medical problems. Systemic hypertension in the presence of a high left ventricular filling pressure and marginal cardiac output is most appropriately treated by an arterial vasodilator. Nitroprusside relaxes vascular smooth muscle in arterial resistance vessels (both systemic and pulmonary) and in venous capacitance vessels. The potential exists with nitroprusside for dilation of the coronary resistance vessels and production of a coronary steal syndrome by shunting blood away from any ischemic areas. The advantages of the drug are its very rapid onset and the rapid dissipation of its effects. The risks with this agent are rapid and excessive hypotension and the potential for either acute cyanide toxicity or thiocyanate toxicity with prolonged use.[19]

Nitroglycerin is primarily a venous dilator, although it produces varying degrees of arterial vasodilatation, especially at high doses. Its major role in treating systemic hypertension is in the patient with high filling pressures and active myocardial ischemia.[20] Nicardipine is a potent systemic and coronary vasodilator without the risk of coronary steal, and it has no significant effect on the venous system. It can, therefore, effectively control postoperative hypertension without reducing the filling pressures or causing a coronary steal. While its onset of action is rapid (1 to 2 min), its elimination half-life is about 40 min. Unlike some calcium channel blockers, this agent lacks a negative inotropic effect and has no effect on atrioventricular conduction.[21] Hydralazine is a direct arterial vasodilator, which is usually administered in intermittent intravenous or intramuscular doses. Hydralazine-induced arterial vasodilation may produce a compensatory tachycardia. This drug is frequently resorted to in patients who are hemodynamically stable but remain hypertensive several days after surgery and cannot yet take or absorb oral medications.

When the hypertension is associated with a normal cardiac output and a relatively rapid sinus heart rate or a propensity toward dysrhythmias, a drug with negative inotropic and chronotropic properties is desirable. Esmolol is a cardioselective, ultrashort-acting beta blocker, which also produces a rapid and titratable control of the blood pressure accompanied by a decrease in heart rate. The drug is usually tolerated satisfactorily by patients with a history of bronchospasm because of its relatively high selectivity for $beta_1$-type adrenergic receptors. It is not ideal for patients with impaired cardiac contractility, particularly in the presence of elevated filling pressures.[22] Diltiazem is an arterial vasodilator that has a mild negative inotropic effect and a more potent negative chronotropic effect. Verapamil is a less potent vasodilator but with more potent negative inotropic, chronotropic, and dromotropic effects. It can be administered intravenously by either boluses or continuous infusion. Labetalol has both alpha- and beta-blocking properties as well as a direct vasodilatory effect. Its predominant effect is as a beta blocker, especially in the intravenous form. The angiotensin-converting enzyme inhibitor enalaprilat, which is the active form of enalapril, can be administered intermittently by the intravenous route. This agent is usually reserved for the patient who is hemodynamically stable with either a normal or reduced cardiac output but with hypertension expected to persist (Table 49-2).

Arrhythmias

GENERAL CONSIDERATIONS AND SINUS TACHYCARDIA

The most common rhythm disturbance immediately after cardiac surgery is sinus tachycardia. This condition is appropriately treated by searching for and correcting the underlying cause (pain, anxiety, low cardiac output, anemia, fever, or beta-blocker withdrawal). The second most common arrhythmia is ventricular ectopy. Again, an underlying cause such as myocardial ischemia, hypokalemia, hypomagnesemia, hypoxia, or administration of sympathomimetic drugs must be sought and corrected if possible. It is also important to review the patient's preoperative record to determine if the patient had preexisting ectopy. Patients with chronic ventricular ectopy frequently have their ectopy exaggerated postoperatively.[23] In the presence of active myocardial ischemia, pharmacologic suppression is advisable for complex ventricular ectopy. In the first 12 h after coronary bypass surgery, myocardial ischemia must be suspected and is difficult to exclude; accordingly, the preceding policy for ectopy suppression should be adhered to with the possible exception of those with known chronic ectopy. Lidocaine is the drug of choice in most instances. The loading dose of lidocaine is approximately 3 mg per kilogram of ideal body weight given over 20 min. One approach is to give an initial bolus of 75 mg, following by 50 mg every 5 min to a total dose of 225 mg. An alternative is to give a priming dose of 75 mg, followed by a loading infusion of 150 mg over 20 min. The usual initial maintenance infusion is 1.5 to 2.5 mg/min. If the arrhythmia is uncontrolled, one can give another bolus of 25 to 50 mg and increase the infusion rate. The chances of toxicity rise signifi-

TABLE 49-2 Intravenous Antihypertensive Agents

Drug	Peak Effect	Duration	Dosage
Nitroprusside	Immediate	2–5 min	0.3–1.0 μg/kg/min
Nitroglycerine	Immediate	2–5 min	5–100 μg/min infusion
Nicardipine	5–60 min	20–40 min	2.5 mg over 5 min; may repeat times 4 at 10-min intervals; infusion 2–15 mg/h
Esmolol	2–5 min	8–10 min	1-min loading infusion of 0.25–0.5 mg/kg; sustained infusion of 50–200 μg/kg/min
Enalaprilat	15–30 min	6 h or more	0.625–1.25 mg slowly over 5 min every 6 h
Hydralazine	15–20 min	3–4 h	5- to 10-mg bolus may be repeated every 15 min; up to total of 40 mg
Diltiazem	3–30 min	3 h	20- to 25-mg bolus may repeat; infusion of 10–20 mg/h
Verapamil	2–3 min	20–40 min	5- to 10-mg bolus; may repeat in 10 min; infusion of 3–25 mg/h
Labetalol	5–15 min	2–6 h	20-mg bolus over 2 min; then 40- to 80-mg boluses every 15 min until effect achieved (to total dose of 300 mg)

cantly at infusion rates above 4 mg/min, especially in individuals greater than 65 years of age. If the ectopy does not respond to lidocaine, the option is to not use an antiarrhythmic agent unless ventricular tachycardia occurs *or* to use intravenous amiodarone. Pacing the heart at a faster rate may prove successful in suppressing the ectopy.

VENTRICULAR TACHYCARDIA AND FIBRILLATION

After cardiac surgery, a few patients develop sustained ventricular tachycardia (either monomorphic or polymorphic) or ventricular fibrillation. These profound rhythm disturbances may develop in the absence of evidence of acute myocardial ischemia or infarction or electrolyte imbalance. In most cases the patients have had previous myocardial infarction and have undergone "complete" revascularization, including regions likely to be nonviable. Reperfusion of these areas that probably include viable as well as nonviable myofibrils embedded in the healed infarct may lead to altered dispersion of repolarization. These changes support development of reentry arrhythmias.[23] The ventricular tachycardia in these patients uncommonly responds to lidocaine and usually requires amiodarone. In some instances, a combination of amiodarone and a beta blocker is required. In a rare circumstance, aortic counterpulsation has seemed to be of benefit.

Every encounter with a wide complex tachycardia requires careful consideration as to the possibility of supraventricular tachycardia with aberrant conduction. In the presence of atrial fibrillation with a rapid ventricular response, right bundle branch aberrant conduction often mimics ventricular tachycardia. Care must be given to avoid lidocaine in these situations, because it may result in an even more rapid ventricular rate.

Wide complex tachyarrhythmias in the range of 250 to 300 beats per minute should suggest the presence of an anomalous conduction pathway. The mechanism of this arrhythmia usually involves atrial flutter, with one-to-one conduction or atrial fibrillation with a very fast ventricular response involving an anomalous pathway. Once this is recognized, procainamide becomes the drug of choice, since it does have favorable therapeutic effects on the bypass track tissue. Lidocaine and verapamil should be avoided if the presence of an anomalous pathway is suspected (see also Chap. 24).

SUPRAVENTRICULAR ARRHYTHMIAS

The most common supraventricular dysrhythmias, with the exception of sinus tachycardia, are atrial fibrillation and atrial flutter. These rhythm disturbances occur in 10 to 30 percent of patients following cardiac surgery. The predominant predisposing factor in the development of atrial fibrillation is the patient's age. The prevalence of atrial fibrillation in postoperative cardiac patients <40 years of age is as low as 3.7 percent, while the prevalence is at least 28 percent in patients >70 years. Atrial fibrillation is most likely to appear on the second postoperative day. Within 1 to 3 days, 80 percent of these patients will return to sinus rhythm with only digoxin or beta-blocker therapy.[24–26] The prophylactic use of beta blockers has a protective effect against the development of atrial fibrillation or flutter. This beneficial effect has been demonstrated with any one of several beta blockers, administered in low or high doses and started preoperatively or postoperatively. Neither digoxin nor verapamil has demonstrated effective prophylaxis against atrial fibrillation or flutter.[27]

Preoperative oral administration of amiodarone also reduces the prevalence of postoperative atrial fibrillation.[28] The major limitation to the widespread application of this prophylactic approach is the apparent need for a 7-day preoperative treatment period. An accelerated loading regimen over 1 to 2 days may be effective, but is unproved.[29]

Intravenous infusions of either esmolol or diltiazem can be used to control the ventricular rate with atrial fibrillation or flutter. Esmolol is given as a 1-min loading infusion of 0.25 to 0.5 mg/kg, followed by a sustained infusion of 50 to 200 μg/kg/min. Diltiazem is administered as a bolus of 20 to 25 mg (which may be repeated), followed by an infusion of 10 to 15 mg/h.

Atrial epicardial pacing wires provide the means of atrial pacing to convert some cases of atrial flutter to sinus rhythm.[25] Short bursts (15 to 30 s) of atrial pacing at rates of 300 to 600 per minute may be effective in converting atrial flutter. Approximately 10 percent of patients with atrial fibrillation require electrical cardioversion to restore sinus rhythm. If hemodynamic compromise is present and aggravated by a supraventricular tachyarrhythmia, cardioversion should be used immediately rather than later.

Intravenous ibutilide (1 mg infused over 10 min to be repeated once if necessary) is the most effective pharmacologic means of converting recent-onset atrial flutter. The drug is much less effective (in the range of 30 to 50 percent) for conversion of recent-onset atrial fibrillation. The disadvantage of ibutilide is the propensity for causing torsades de pointes in 2 to 4 percent of patients.[29]

CONDUCTION DEFECTS

The prevalence of intraventricular conduction abnormalities after coronary bypass surgery is reported to be from 1 to 45 percent, with approximately 10 percent being the most commonly reported frequency. The most common conduction defect is right bundle branch block, which may be due to selective sensitivity of the right bundle to the effects of hypothermia and the extracorporeal circulation process. Only about 5 percent of the patients are left with a permanent conduction abnormality, and the prognosis for these patients is no worse than it is for comparable patients with no conduction defect.[30,31] The development of high-degree (second- or third-degree) atrioventricular block is an indication for temporary pacing via epicardial pacing wires. Atrioventricular block is not as common as either bundle branch block or fascicular block, but it does occur, especially after aortic valve surgery.

Respiratory Management

EXPECTED RESPIRATORY CHANGES AFTER CARDIAC SURGERY

Pulmonary problems are the most significant cause of morbidity following cardiac surgery. The pain associated with sternotomy and, especially, with thoracotomy has a deleterious effect on the patient's willingness to breathe deeply and cough. Pain caused by the presence of chest tubes may also interfere with normal respiratory function. Phrenic nerve damage can result in diaphragmatic dysfunction. More commonly, the diaphragm is passively displaced cephalad by abdominal contents (gastrointestinal intraluminal air and fluid and edematous bowel) in the anesthetized, paralyzed patient supported by mechanical ventilation. Elevated left side of the heart filling pressures may cause alveolar edema and, in some patients, increased capillary permeability may exist. Insertion of an oro- or nasogastric tube by the anesthesiologist while the patient is under general anesthesia is recommended.

Atelectasis is the most common pulmonary complication, occurring in about 70 percent of patients following cardiac surgery with CPB.[32] During CPB, the lungs are not perfused and are usually allowed to collapse. Once the lungs are reexpanded, a variable amount of atelectasis remains. While the atelectasis might be microscopic, intermediate degrees (subsegmental and segmental) are common. The preponderance of atelectasis occurs in the left lower lobe because of its compression during cardiac surgery, the tendency to suction more thoroughly the right mainstem bronchus during blind naso-orotracheal suctioning, and the frequent surgical practice of opening the left pleural space to facilitate dissection of the left internal mammary artery. Evidence for a depletion of surfactant after cardiopulmonary bypass is lacking.[33]

After thoracotomy, both lung and chest wall compliance decrease significantly. The maximum decrease occurs at approximately 3 days, but the decrease persists to a lesser degree 6 or more days after sternotomy. Alterations in chest wall mechanics lead to a decrease in the forced expiratory volume (FEV_1) and the functional residual capacity (FRC). The changes in the FEV_1 may persist for 6 weeks. In addition to these changes in flows and volumes, reduced inspiratory strength and uncoordinated rib cage expansion occur. These changes result in an increase in respiratory rate and a decrease in tidal volume, a decrease in respiratory efficiency, and an increase in oxygen cost of breathing. The atelectasis and decrease in lung volume result in ventilation:perfusion mismatch and shunting. The clinical manifestation is a decrease in arterial PO_2 and hemoglobin saturation.[33]

There is little evidence of a significant increase in lung water after routine CPB. When increased capillary permeability exists, it is usually related to elevated cardiac filling pressures.[33]

BASIC CONCEPTS OF OXYGENATION AND ALVEOLAR VENTILATION

The goals of mechanical ventilation are the maintenance of satisfactory arterial oxygenation and CO_2 removal. Direct measurement of PaO_2 is generally used to assess the overall adequacy of blood oxygenation, while pulse oximetry (SpO_2) is used to monitor peripheral arterial hemoglobin saturation on a continuous basis. An $SpO_2 > 90$ percent is considered to be acceptable, but it may be associated with a marginal PaO_2. The oxygen-hemoglobin dissociation curve portrays this relationship (Fig. 49-1). The shoulder of this sigmoid curve lies at a PaO_2 of approximately 65 mmHg. A PaO_2 below this level will result in a precipitous fall in the oxygen saturation of hemoglobin. With hypothermia or with profound respiratory alkalosis, the curve will shift to the left, resulting in more avid binding of oxygen to hemoglobin and less release of oxygen to the tissues. The patient will likely be receiving 100 percent oxygen during transfer from the operating room to the ICU or postanesthesia care unit. The FIO_2 should be gradually decreased to 0.4 as tolerated to minimize adsorption atelectasis and pulmonary O_2 toxicity. Mechanical ventilation is also used to maintain alveolar ventilation, which regulates the arterial blood CO_2 tension

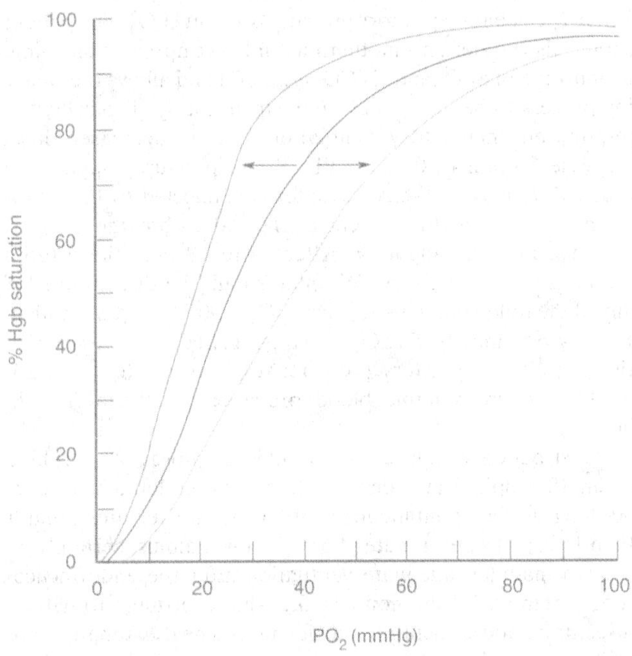

FIGURE 49-1 Oxygen-hemoglobin dissociation curve. The curve depicts the saturation of hemoglobin at increasing levels of PaO_2. A shift of the curve to the left increases the affinity of hemoglobin for oxygen and a shift to the right decreases the affinity.

($PaCO_2$). Alveolar ventilation is regulated by controlling the tidal volume and the respiratory rate. Generally, the ventilator should maintain an exhaled minute ventilation of 6 to 8 L/min. Decreasing the tidal volume below 8 to 10 mL/kg may result in alveolar hypoventilation and atelectasis. Mild hypocarbia ($PaCO_2$ of 30 to 35 mmHg) is satisfactory immediately after surgery, but more profound respiratory alkalosis should be avoided because it leads to hypokalemia and a leftward shift of the oxygen-hemoglobin dissociation curve (decreased oxygen release to the tissues). Hypocarbia is best corrected by reducing the ventilator rate.

Hypercarbia in the immediate postoperative period usually indicates that minute ventilation is inadequate. The problem can be rectified primarily by increasing the ventilator rate; in some cases it is appropriate to increase the tidal volume as well. Later, as the patient is weaned from the ventilator, hypercarbia may reflect opioid analgesia (a necessary side effect of satisfactory analgesia) or compensatory hypoventilation in response to a metabolic alkalosis, most likely due to excessive diuresis. Acetazolamide (Diamox), 250 to 500 mg intravenously every 6 h, is beneficial in correcting a primary metabolic alkalosis. Severe hypercarbia should raise a concern about mechanical problems such as ventilator malfunction, endotracheal tube malposition, or a pneumothorax.[5] Occasionally, hypoxemia and even hypotension may develop in the mechanically ventilated patient due to a tension pneumothorax or hemothorax. If the latter are suspected, assessment of breath sounds and a chest x-ray are indicated for confirmation.

VENTILATORY WEANING AND EXTUBATION

Ventilatory support should be reduced as tolerated when the cardiovascular system has become stable and the arterial oxygen tension is satisfactory [$PaO_2 > 70$ mmHg, with FIO_2 of 0.5 and

PEEP (peak end-expiratory pressure) of 5 cm H_2O]. The patient should also be alert, normothermic, and have no active bleeding. Monitoring of SpO_2 and $ETCO_2$ is helpful and allows the weaning process to be done safely and expeditiously. Typically, the intermittent mandatory ventilation rate is decreased in a stepwise fashion to 0. Then PEEP and pressure support are reduced. Finally, a T-piece adapter is connected to the endotracheal tube and the patient is allowed to breathe oxygen-enriched air spontaneously. After 30 to 60 min, the arterial blood gases are analyzed. Weaning should be discontinued if any of the following signs appear: $SpO_2 < 90$; $PaO_2 < 60$ mmHg; $ETCO_2 > 50$ mmHg; $PaCO_2 > 55$ mmHg; pH < 7.30; 10-mmHg rise in pulmonary artery pressure; respiratory rate > 30; 20-mmHg rise in systemic blood pressure; or 20-beat rise in heart rate.[5]

Most patients require low to moderate doses of morphine or another opioid in order to tolerate the endotracheal tube. As long as the spontaneous ventilatory rate remains greater than 15 breaths per minute, the patient will almost certainly be able to maintain adequate ventilation after the endotracheal tube is removed. Common mistakes that contribute to patient discomfort and difficulty in achieving tracheal extubation are (1) trying to sedate the patient with benzodiazepines only, which have no antitussive effect and (2) avoiding opioids for fear of respiratory depression.

BRONCHOSPASM

Severe bronchospasm during CPB is an unusual event, but it can occur. A few patients cannot have their chest cavity closed at the end of surgery because of hyperinflated lungs. The most likely cause of this fulminant bronchospasm is activation of human C5a anaphylatoxin by the extracorporeal circulation. Other likely causes of bronchospasm in the postoperative period are cardiogenic pulmonary edema; simple exacerbation of preexisting bronchospastic disease triggered by instrumentation, secretions, or cold anesthetic gas; beta-adrenergic blockers in susceptible individuals; and allergic reaction to protamine.[32]

The initial therapy of bronchospasm in the postoperative patient, once a diagnosis of heart failure is excluded, should be inhaled $beta_2$-agonists (terbutaline, metaproterenol, albuterol) and/or inhaled cholinergic agents (ipratropium bromide or glycopyrrolate). In the inhaled form these rather potent bronchodilators have minimal cardiovascular effects. In addition to their bronchodilator effect, these agents may augment mucociliary transport and aid in clearing secretions. A combination of $beta_2$-agonists and cholinergic agents should be tried in the patient refractory to a single agent. Even more refractory bronchospasm requires either a short course of systemic steroids or intravenous aminophylline. In addition to being a bronchodilator, aminophylline is a mild diuretic, increases the central nervous system respiratory drive, improves respiratory muscle function, and may decrease pulmonary artery pressure. It is, however, arrhythmogenic and chronotropic.

Postoperative Oliguria and Renal Insufficiency

ETIOLOGY

The use of radiocontrast agents in the days immediately preceding cardiac surgery may embarrass renal function, as manifested by a rise in blood urea nitrogen and serum creatinine values. Following CPB, there is a substantial incidence of postoperative renal dysfunction (up to 30 percent) but a relatively low incidence of severe renal impairment requiring dialysis (1 to 5 percent). Renal blood flow and glomerular filtration rate are reduced by 25 to 75 percent during bypass, with partial but not complete recovery in the first day after CPB. This reduction in renal function is attributed to renal artery vasoconstriction, hypothermia, and loss of pulsatile perfusion during CPB. Angiotensin II levels are higher with nonpulsatile flow as compared to pulsatile flow. While renal dysfunction cannot be consistently related to the systemic blood pressure and pump flow rate during nonpulsatile bypass, there is a definite relation between the incidence of postbypass renal dysfunction and the duration of CPB. In addition to the duration of CPB, the risk of developing postbypass renal failure seems to be a function of the patient's underlying renal function (also affected by age) and the perioperative circulatory status. The histologic changes that accompany renal impairment after cardiopulmonary bypass are characteristic of tubular necrosis. The tubular cells seem to be the most susceptible to acute reductions in renal perfusion.[33]

MANAGEMENT

There are three agents (so-called renoprotective drugs) that might be used during CPB to prevent an ischemic insult to the kidneys. Mannitol used in the CPB priming fluid may moderate ischemic insult, probably by volume expansion and hemodilution. It also initiates an osmotic diuresis, which prevents tubular obstruction and may serve as a free radical scavenger. Furosemide appears to improve renal blood flow when given during bypass. So-called renal dose dopamine (1 to 2.5 μg/kg/min based on ideal body weight) may maintain renal blood flow and urine output. Once renal failure has developed, none of these drugs is likely to offer any beneficial effect. A megadose of furosemide (200 to 300 mg) may be tried, but if there is no diuretic response, it should not be repeated. Similarly, a single dose of mannitol (12.5 to 25 mg) either with or without furosemide could be tried but not repeated if there is no effect. Whenever possible, it is advisable to avoid potentially nephrotoxic agents in the early postoperative period. Examples of such include radiologic contrast agents, aminoglycoside antibiotics, and angiotensin-converting enzyme inhibitors.

Postoperative Gastrointestinal Dysfunction

GASTROINTESTINAL CONSEQUENCES OF CARDIOPULMONARY BYPASS

The gastrointestinal consequences of CPB appear to be minimal. Reviews of the subject report a 1 percent prevalence.[32,33] Most patients eat within 24 to 48 h after an uncomplicated elective procedure. The limited investigations of the gastrointestinal tract after cardiac surgery have found a slight decrease in hepatic and pancreatic blood flow during cooling and rewarming on bypass and a decrease in gastric pH.[32,34] Transient elevations in liver function tests and hyperamylasemia may occur after cardiac surgery, and the risk factors include long CPB time, multiple transfusions, and multiple valve replacements. Appearance of jaundice portends a poor prognosis.[35] Severe gastrointestinal complications are usually ischemic in nature and are often associated with a low-output syndrome.[32] The use of opioids as part of general anesthesia and postoperative pain management contributes to gastrointestinal dysfunction (cramping, ileus, and constipation) and to postoperative nausea and vomiting. The nausea and vomiting can be minimized by use of a naso- or orogastric tube to maintain gastric decompression intraoperatively and early in the postoperative period, with the additional benefit of improving thoracoabdominal compliance to positive-pressure ventilation.

Postoperative Metabolic Disorders

POTASSIUM IMBALANCE

There are multiple factors that can produce large and rapid shifts in the serum potassium levels during and after CPB. These factors include the following: (1) high-potassium cardioplegia solution used during surgery; (2) renal dysfunction with associated oliguria and decreased clearance of potassium; (3) low cardiac output states accompanied by oliguria and acidosis; (4) hemolyzed red blood cells' release of potassium; (5) potassium lost by diuresis; and (6) diabetes mellitus interference with cellular uptake of potassium, unless insulin is infused intra- and postoperatively. The principal detrimental effects of these potassium shifts is on the electrical activity of the heart. The electrocardiographic signs of hyperkalemia and hypokalemia are described in Chap. 11. The electrocardiographic changes of hyperkalemia do not necessarily appear in the classic progressive manner; they are more related to the rate of rise in serum potassium rather than to the absolute serum concentration. The therapy of severe hyperkalemia should include counteracting the toxic cardiac effects of the elevated potassium with intravenous calcium gluconate or calcium chloride and lowering the serum level of potassium with sodium bicarbonate and/or administration of regular insulin and glucose. Hypokalemia does not usually become clinically evident until the serum potassium concentration is $<$2.5 meq/L, and at these levels it can be associated with severe ventricular tachyarrhythmias. Another consequence of potassium depletion is metabolic alkalosis as the hydrogen ions replace potassium ions within the cells. Hypokalemia is treated with the intravenous administration of KCl at a rate of no more than 10 to 15 meq/h. The serum potassium rises approximately 0.1 meq/L for each 2 meq of KCl administered. Large doses of KCl should be administered by a central venous catheter because of the caustic effect of potassium on peripheral veins.

HYPOMAGNESEMIA

Hypomagnesemia is common following cardiac surgery using CPB. Magnesium mimics potassium in its effects on the electrical activity of the heart. The cause of the hypomagnesemia is unknown, but it is probably multifactorial. Many patients will be hypomagnesemic preoperatively due to the use of loop diuretics, thiazides, digoxin, or alcohol and to the effects of type I diabetes mellitus. Magnesium is usually lost in the urine during CPB. Patients with postoperative hypomagnesemia develop atrial and ventricular dysrhythmias more frequently and require more prolonged mechanical ventilatory support than do patients with normal magnesium levels.[36] Magnesium administration also seems to improve stroke volume and cardiac index in the early postoperative period.[37] Magnesium can be administered as magnesium sulfate (2 g in 100-mL solution) to raise serum levels to 2 meq/L.

HYPERGLYCEMIA

During CPB there is a rise in blood glucose levels. The elevation is modest during hypothermia and becomes more marked during rewarming. This rise in glucose is due in part to increased glucose mobilization related to dramatic increases in cortisol, catecholamine, and growth hormone levels during CPB. Also, there is an apparent failure of insulin secretion, particularly during hypothermia, probably related to inhibition of the insulin secretory response by the elevated catecholamines. This blunting of the insulin response persists for the first 24 h after surgery. These changes are exaggerated in the diabetic patient.[38] Insulin requirements are likely to be 7 times greater than the preoperative requirements during the first 4 h postoperatively. Furthermore, such insulin resistance is exacerbated by catecholamines, diuretics, and blood transfusions.[39] These multiple factors make the diabetic patient susceptible to hyperosmolar, hyperglycemia, nonketotic diabetic coma.[40]

Postoperative Fever

Fever is a common occurrence in the postoperative patient. It is generally a consequence of pleuropericarditis, atelectasis, or phlebitis. Since 70 percent of patients have atelectasis after cardiac surgery, it is the most likely etiology of postoperative fever.[32] A reasonable assumption in a patient with a core temperature $<$38°C (100.4°F) and no evidence of phlebitis or presence of a pericardial or pleural rub is that the source of the fever is atelectasis. The appropriate therapeutic approach is to encourage intensified efforts at incentive spirometry and coughing. Any fever $>$38.5°C (101.3°F) warrants blood, sputum, and urine cultures. A white blood cell count (total and differential) and a chest x-ray should also be obtained.

Sternal wound infections occur in 0.4 to 5 percent of patients after sternotomy.[41–43] Multiple factors have been identified as increasing the risk of developing sternal wound infection. These include pneumonia, prolonged mechanical ventilation (especially with tracheostomy), emergency operations, postoperative hemorrhage with mediastinal hematoma, early reexploration, obesity, diabetes mellitus, and use of bilateral internal mammary grafts. While some studies have not found a higher prevalence of sternal wound infections with bilateral mammary grafts, the bulk of the evidence argues to the contrary. Perhaps some of the conflicting results can be explained by the fact that different degrees of devascularization of the sternum occur, depending on the particular technique used to harvest the internal mammary artery. The greatest risk for sternal infection seems to be in diabetic patients who receive bilateral internal mammary grafts.[43] Debate continues as to whether the most appropriate initial treatment is debridement and closure or open packing and subsequent plastic surgical closure with a muscle flap.

Approximately 1 percent of patients who have had coronary artery bypass surgery experience leg wound infections that necessitate extra care. Leg infections seem to occur more frequently in obese women, especially if the thigh veins are harvested.[44]

Neurologic and Neurophysiologic Dysfunction

MECHANISM

The mechanisms thought to account for most cerebral injury during cardiac surgery are macroembolization of air, debris from aortic atheroma, or left ventricular thrombus; microembolization of aggregates of granulocytes, platelets, and fibrin; and cerebral hypoperfusion. Death or disabling stroke occurs in about 2 percent of patients, with another 3 percent experiencing transient or minor functional disability secondary to cerebral infarction.[45] Focal neurologic deficits resulting from intraoperative events are usually noted within the first 24 to 48 h after surgery.

ENCEPHALOPATHY AND DELIRIUM

Alteration of mental status (encephalopathy and delirium) will be seen in approximately 30 percent of patients after cardiopulmonary bypass.[45] While the appearance of these encephalopathic symptoms likely reflects cerebral injury, other causes must be excluded, including drugs, sepsis, fever, hypoxemia, ethanol withdrawal, renal failure, and hyperosmolar state. Postoperative encephalopathic changes, varying from mild confusion and disorientation to protracted somnolence or agitation and hallucinations, may appear at any time during the hospital stay.[46] In fact, some physicians will not accept a diagnosis of postcardiotomy delirium unless the delirium develops following a lucid interval of 2 to 5 days after surgery. Studies of this condition have not identified any consistent risk factors, but advancing age, duration of CPB, and sleep deprivation have been frequently associated. The prevalence of this condition has remained rather constant since the early days of cardiac surgery involving CPB, but there has been a shift in the clinical presentation. Currently, the condition seems to present with disorientation rather than with hallucinations, paranoid ideation, and agitation noted earlier.[46] Recognition of this entity is important because the family can be assured that the patient's mental status is likely to recover. Agitation and acute psychosis in these patients usually respond to intravenous haloperidol, 2 to 10 mg, repeated as needed to produce adequate sedation.

BRACHIAL PLEXOPATHY AND ULNAR NERVE DYSFUNCTION

Another serious neurologic complication of cardiac surgery is brachial plexopathy. This neurologic dysfunction, involving C8 and T1, usually results from mechanical trauma secondary to sternal retraction but may be due to penetration by a posterior fractured segment of the first rib or injury during internal jugular cannulation. There is no specific therapy for this condition, and recovery can take as long as 6 months, with a few cases being permanent.[47] Ulnar nerve dysfunction may result from malpositioning of the upper extremities during surgery, which results in pressure being exerted on the ulnar nerve at the elbow.

References

1. Cameron D. Initiation of white cell activation during cardiopulmonary bypass: Cytokines and receptors. *J Cardiovasc Pharmacol* 1996; 27(suppl 1):S1–S5.
2. Chong JL, Pillai R, Fisher A, et al. Cardiac surgery, moving away from intensive care. *Br Heart J* 1992; 68:430–433.
3. Aps C. Fast-tracking in cardiac surgery. *Br J Hosp Med* 1995; 54:139–142.
4. Jindosi A, Aps C, Neville E, et al. Postoperative cardiac surgical care: An alternative approach. *Br Heart J* 1993; 69:59–64.
5. Bojar RM. *Manual of Perioperative Care in Cardiac and Thoracic Surgery*, 2d ed. Boston: Blackwell Scientific; 1994.
6. Levy JH, Salemenpera MT, Bailey JM, Ramsey JG. Postoperative circulatory control. In: Kaplan JA, ed. *Cardiac Anesthesia*, 3d ed. Philadelphia: Saunders; 1993:1168–1193.
7. Swanson DK, Myerowitz PD. Effect of reperfusion temperature and pressure on the functional and metabolic recovery of preserved hearts. *J Thorac Cardiovasc Surg* 1983; 86:242–251.
8. Gold JP, Roberts AJ, Hoover EL, et al. Effects of prolonged aortic cross clamping with potassium cardioplegia on myocardial contractility in man. *Surg Forum* 1979; 30:252–254.
9. Spiess BD. Ischemia—a coagulation problem? *J Cardiovasc Pharmacol* 1996; 27(suppl 1):S38–S41.
10. Verrier E. The microvascular cell and ischemia-reperfusion injury. *J Cardiovasc Pharmacol* 1996; 27(suppl 1):S26–S30.
11. Bolli R. Oxygen derived free radicals and postischemic myocardial dysfunction. *J Am Coll Cardiol* 1988; 12:239–249.
12. Przyklenk K, Kloner RA. "Reperfusion injury" by oxygen derived free radicals? *Circ Res* 1989; 64:86–96.
13. Breisblatt WM, Stein KI, Wolfe CJ, et al. Acute myocardial dysfunction and recovery: A common occurrence after coronary bypass surgery. *J Am Coll Cardiol* 1990; 15:1261–1269.
14. Donati F, Maille JG, Blain R, et al. End-tidal carbon dioxide tension and temperature changes after coronary artery bypass surgery. *Can Anaesth Soc J* 1985; 32:272–277.
15. Ralley FE, Wynando JE, Rams JG, et al. The effects of shivering on oxygen consumption and carbon dioxide production in patients rewarming from hypothermic cardiopulmonary bypass. *Can J Anaesth* 1988; 35:332–337.
16. Woodman RC, Harker LA. Bleeding complications associated with cardiopulmonary bypass. *Blood* 1990; 76:1680–1697.
17. Harker L, Malpass TW, Branson HE, et al. Mechanism of abnormal bleeding in patients undergoing cardiopulmonary bypass: Acquired transient platelet dysfunction associated with selective alpha-granule release. *Blood* 1980; 56:824–834.
18. Ellis RJ, Mangano DT, Van Dyke DC. Relationship of wedge pressure to end diastolic volume in patients undergoing myocardial revascularization. *J Thorac Cardiovasc Surg* 1979; 78:605–613.
19. Palmer RF, Lasseter KC. Drug therapy: Sodium nitroprusside. *N Engl J Med* 1975; 292:294–297.
20. Flaherty JT, Magee PA, Gardner TL, et al. Comparison of intravenous nitroglycerin and sodium nitroprusside for treatment of acute hypertension developing after coronary bypass surgery. *Circulation* 1982; 65:1072–1077.
21. Lambert CR, Hill JA, Feldman RL, et al. Effects of nicardipine on exercise- and pacing-induced myocardial ischemia in angina pectoris. *Am J Cardiol* 1987; 60:471–476.
22. Gray RJ, Bateman TM, Czer LS, et al. Comparison of esmolol and nitroprusside for acute postcardiac surgical hypertension. *Am J Cardiol* 1987; 59:887–891.
23. Topol EJ, Lerman BB, Baughman KL, et al. De novo refractory ventricular tachyarrhythmias after coronary revascularization. *Am J Cardiol* 1986; 57:57–59.
24. Leith JW, Thomson D, Baird DK, Harris PJ. The importance of age as a predictor of atrial fibrillation and flutter after coronary artery bypass grafting. *J Thorac Cardiovasc Surg* 1990; 100:338–342.
25. Hashimoto K, Ilstrup DM, Schaff HV. Influence of clinical and hemodynamic variables on risk of supraventricular tachycardia after coronary artery bypass. *J Thorac Cardiovasc Surg* 1991; 101:56–65.
26. Fuller JA, Adams GG, Buxton B. Atrial fibrillation after coronary artery bypass grafting. Is it a disorder of the elderly? *J Thorac Cardiovasc Surg* 1989; 97:821–825.
27. Andrews TC, Reimold SC, Berlin JA, Antman EM. Prevention of supraventricular arrhythmias after coronary artery bypass surgery. A meta-analysis of randomized controlled trials. *Circulation* 1991; 84(suppl III):III-236–III-244.
28. Baerman JM, Kirsch MM, de Buitleir M, et al. Natural history

and determinates of conduction defects following coronary artery bypass surgery. *Ann Thorac Surg* 1987; 44:150–153.

29. Tuzcu EM, Emre A, Goormastic M, Loop FD. Incidence and prognostic significance of intraventricular conduction abnormalities after coronary bypass surgery. *J Am Coll Cardiol* 1990; 16:607–610.
30. Sladden RN, Berkowitz DE. Cardiopulmonary bypass and the lung. In: Gravlee GP, Davis RF, Utley IR, eds. *Cardiopulmonary Bypass*. Baltimore: Williams & Wilkins; 1993:468–487.
31. Ramsey J. The respiratory, renal and hepatic systems: Effects of cardiac surgery and cardiopulmonary bypass. In: Mora CT, ed. *Cardiopulmonary Bypass*. New York: Springer; 1995:147–168.
32. Hanks JB, Curtis SE, Hanks BB, et al. Gastrointestinal complications after cardiopulmonary bypass. *Surgery* 1982; 92:394–400.
33. Welling RE, Rath R, Albers JE, Glaser RS. Gastrointestinal complications after cardiac surgery. *Arch Surg* 1986; 121:1178–1180.
34. Mori A, Watanabe K, Onoe M, et al. Regional blood flow in the liver, pancreas, and kidney during pulsatile and nonpulsatile perfusion under profound hypothermia. *Jpn Circ J* 1988; 52: 219–227.
35. Collins JD, Bassendine MF, Ferner R, et al. Incidence and prognostic importance of jaundice after cardiopulmonary bypass surgery. *Lancet* 1983; 1:1119–1123.
36. Aglio LS, Stanford GG, Maddi R, et al. Hypomagnesemia is common following cardiac surgery. *J Cardiothorac Anesth* 1991; 5:201–208.
37. England MR, Gordon G, Salem M, Chernow B. Magnesium administration and dysrhythmias after cardiac surgery: A placebo-controlled, double-blind, randomized trial. *JAMA* 1993; 269:2369–2370.
38. Frater RW, Oka Y, Kadish A, et al. Diabetes and coronary artery surgery. *Mt Sinai J Med* 1982; 49:237–240.
39. Elliott MJ, Gill GV, Home PD, et al. A comparison of two regimens for the management of diabetes during open-heart surgery. *Anesthesiology* 1984; 60:364–368.
40. Seki S. Clinical features of hyperglycemia, nonketotic diabetic coma associated with cardiac operations. *J Thorac Cardiovasc Surg* 1986; 91:8678–8687.
41. Ulicny KS, Hiradzka SF. The risk factors of median sternotomy infection: A current review. *J Cardiac Surg* 1991; 6:338–351.
42. Hazelrigg SR, Wellons HA, Schneider JA, Kolm P. Wound complications after median sternotomy: Relationship to internal mammary grafting. *J Thorac Cardiovasc Surg* 1989; 98:1096–1099.
43. Grossi EA, Esposito R, Harris LJ, et al. Sternal wound infections and use of internal mammary artery grafts. *J Thorac Cardiovasc Surg* 1991; 102:342–347.
44. De Laria GA, Hunter JA, Goldin MD, et al. Leg wound complications associated with coronary revascularization. *J Thorac Cardiovasc Surg* 1981; 81:403–407.
45. Breuer AC, Furlan AJ, Hanson MR, et al. Central nervous system complications of coronary artery bypass graft surgery: Prospective analysis of 421 patients. *Stroke* 1983; 14:82–87.
46. Smith LW, Dimsdale JE. Postcardiotomy delirium: Conclusions after 25 years? *Am J Psychiatry* 1989; 146:452–458.
47. Shaw PJ, Bates D, Cartlidge NE, et al. Early neurological complications of coronary artery bypass surgery. *Br Med J* 1985; 91:1384–1387.

CHAPTER 50

REHABILITATION OF THE PATIENT WITH CORONARY HEART DISEASE

Nanette K. Wenger

Cardiac rehabilitation, an essential component of the long-term comprehensive management strategy for coronary patients, includes an individualized regimen of physical activity and health education and counseling appropriate for the individual patient's needs and specific cardiac problem.[1] *Cardiac rehabilitation* is described by the American College of Cardiology as "those exercise and counseling services which reduce symptoms or improve cardiac function"[2] and by the U.S. Public Health Service as "comprehensive, long-term programs involving medical evaluation, prescribed exercise, cardiac risk factor modification, education, and counseling." Initially, these services were recommended for patients following myocardial infarction (MI); subsequently, they were applied after coronary artery bypass graft (CABG) surgery or for patients with chronic stable angina pectoris. More recently, the U.S. Health Care Financing Administration concluded[3] that heart transplant patients and patients who had undergone percutaneous transluminal coronary angioplasty (PTCA) could benefit from prescribed cardiac rehabilitation. The Clinical Practice Guideline *Cardiac Rehabilitation*[4] documented the benefits of rehabilitative services for patients with heart failure and left ventricular (LV) systolic dysfunction and recommended their application.

The current short hospital stay for uncomplicated MI necessitates early ambulation and an accelerated educational regimen, with deferral of most teaching and counseling to the outpatient setting. Early discharge from the hospital is characteristic for patients after successful myocardial reperfusion by coronary thrombolysis or acute primary angioplasty. Patients recovering from CABG surgery typically undergo rapid ambulation, have a short hospital stay, and constitute an increasing percentage of patients referred for cardiac rehabilitation.[5] Such patients without prior MI characteristically have good ventricular function and favorable survival and are at low risk for proximate coronary events. Many require protracted guidance for coronary risk reduction; early counseling appears to aid in averting physiologic and psychological disability. Most patients following successful PTCA have brief hospital stays, good functional status, and early resumption of employment and other activities.[6,7] Patients with stable angina without recent MI constitute almost one-fourth of the total coronary population but are undeserved in terms of rehabilitative care. They are frequently not referred for formal rehabilitative services, often due to lack of insurance reimbursement. This population often has substantial loss of productivity and reduction in the quality of life and requires comprehensive medical management, with needs that may exceed those of patients after uncomplicated MI. With the aging of the U.S. population, coronary rehabilitative care is now provided to many elderly patients,[8,9] as well as to many patients with severe and complicated coronary illness. There is increasing contemporary emphasis on education and counseling as additional cornerstones of rehabilitative care, using the behavioral approach to assist patients in coronary risk reduction and other cardiovascular health-related goals[10–12]; on psychosocial assessment and interventions; and on occupational assessment and vocational counseling.

Each year almost 1 million survivors of MI are candidates for cardiac rehabilitation services in the United States, in addition to more than 7 million patients with stable angina pectoris and patients following revascularization with CABG surgery (367,000 patients in 1996, 44 percent under age 65) or PTCA and other transcatheter interventional procedures (482,000 in 1996, 51 percent younger than age 65). Of these several million patients with coronary heart disease for whom benefits can be anticipated from cardiac rehabilitation, only 11 to 20 percent participated in formal rehabilitation programs.[4,13] Among patients with acute MI enrolled in the Global Utilization of Streptokinase and tPA for Occluded Coronary Arteries (GUSTO) trial, 38 percent of U.S. patients and 32 percent of Canadian patients attended cardiac rehabilitation programs.[14] A U.S. national survey of 500 cardiac rehabilitation programs highlighted the underrepresentation of women, nonwhites, and those older than age 65.[15] Heart failure is the most common discharge diagnosis for hospitalized Medicare patients in the United States and the fourth most common discharge diagnosis for all hospitalized patients. Although coronary heart disease (CHD) is not etiologic in all these patients, it is a substantial contributor to heart failure. Application of cardiac rehabilitation services to patients with heart failure (as well as after cardiac transplantation) has gained increasing acceptance as its benefits and safety have been documented. An estimated 4.7 million patients with heart failure are potential candidates for cardiac rehabilitation.[4]

Nonetheless, this component of cardiac care is underutilized despite its efficacy and cost-effectiveness.[16,17]

EXERCISE TRAINING

Although no single randomized trial of exercise training demonstrated a reduction in mortality and morbidity in patients following MI, in part owing to inadequate sample size and/or duration of follow-up, to high dropout rates, etc., favorable trends occurred in several. Metaanalysis[16,18] of pooled data from large prospective, randomized exercise trials suggest as much as a 25 percent survival advantage for exercising subjects at 3-year follow-up following MI. This benefit cannot be attributed solely to exercise training, since many studies included coronary risk reduction as well as exercise. The reduction in mortality approaches that resulting from pharmacologic management of patients following MI with beta-blocking drugs and of patients with LV systolic dysfunction with angiotensin-converting enzyme (ACE) inhibitor therapy. The reduction in cardiovascular mortality was 26 percent in multifactorial randomized trials of cardiac rehabilitation as compared with 15 percent in trials that involved solely exercise training. There is no evidence that cardiac rehabilitation exercise training changes the rates of nonfatal reinfarction.[4,11]

The evidence-based Clinical Practice Guideline *Cardiac Rehabilitation* of the U.S. Department of Health and Human Services[4] highlights the beneficial effect of cardiac rehabilitation exercise training on exercise tolerance as one of the most clearly established favorable outcomes for coronary patients with angina pectoris, MI, CABG surgery, and PTCA and for patients with compensated heart failure or a decreased LV ejection fraction. This approach particularly benefits patients with decreased exercise tolerance.[19] Improved exercise tolerance was evident for both women and men and also occurred in elderly patients. The most consistent benefit resulted from exercise training at least three times weekly for 12 or more weeks' duration. The duration of aerobic exercise sessions varied from 20 to 40 min, at an intensity approximating 70 to 85 percent of the baseline exercise test heart rate. Improvement in exercise tolerance occurred with lower-intensity exercise as well.[20–22] Maintenance of exercise training is required to sustain improvement in exercise tolerance.

No significant increase in cardiovascular complications or other serious adverse outcomes was reported in any randomized, controlled trial of exercise training in coronary patients. These randomized, controlled trials involved 3932 patients following MI, 745 patients with catheterization-documented coronary disease, 215 patients following CABG surgery, and 139 following PTCA. No deterioration in measures of exercise tolerance was reported in any patients undergoing exercise training, nor did any controlled study document significantly greater improvement in exercise tolerance in control patient groups compared with exercising patients.

The improvement in functional capacity with exercise training, averaging 20 percent after recovery from MI, is associated with a reduction in activity-related symptoms: angina, dyspnea, fatigue, and at times claudication. Exercise training results in (1) an improvement in oxygen transport, evident as an increase in maximal cardiac output and oxygen consumption, (2) a reduction in heart rate, systolic blood pressure, and thereby myocardial oxygen requirement at rest and at submaximal work levels, and (3) and more rapid return to normal of the exercise heart rate.

The improvement in functional capacity and decrease in activity-related symptoms following usual moderate-intensity exercise training appear to be related primarily to peripheral adaptations. These include an increase in oxygen extraction and use by trained skeletal muscle, with a decrease in myocardial oxygen demand and requirement for coronary blood flow at submaximal exercise. The redistribution of cardiac output, decrease in systemic vascular resistance, and autonomic nervous system adaptations (particularly lowering of the heart rate) result in a decreased rate-pressure product at submaximal levels of exertion. High-intensity, long-term endurance exercise may effect cardiac (central) adaptations, possibly including improved ventricular contractility and increased maximal stroke volume in selected coronary patients[23]; such intensive exercise training is feasible for only a small subset of coronary patients. There is no evidence that exercise training as a sole intervention alters the angiographic characteristics of coronary lesions, increases coronary blood flow or myocardial oxygen supply, or stimulates the formation of a coronary collateral circulation in humans. No consistent improvement in cardiac hemodynamic measurements or ventricular systolic function has resulted from exercise training.[24,25] Exercise training, however, may improve skeletal muscle functioning in patients with heart failure.[26] Exercise training can decrease evidence of myocardial ischemia, as measured by exercise electrocardiogram (ECG) testing, ambulatory ECG recording, and radionuclide perfusion imaging.[27,28] In several randomized clinical trials, apparently spontaneous improvement in resting ejection fraction after MI occurred in both exercising and control populations, rendering suspect the improvements in ejection fraction described in observational studies of exercise training. There were no consistent changes in ventricular arrhythmia related to exercise rehabilitation.

Clinical benefits of exercise training include a decrease in the symptoms of angina pectoris in patients with coronary disease[27] and the symptoms of heart failure in patients with LV systolic dysfunction.[29,30] The improvement in electrocardiographic and nuclear cardiology measures of myocardial ischemia provides objective support for the symptomatic improvement.

Exercise training of patients with LV systolic dysfunction provided added symptomatic improvement to that achieved by appropriate medication.[30]

The decrease in symptoms and improvement in functional status that result from exercise training can enable a return to remunerative employment as well as to leisure and recreational activities.[31] For more impaired coronary patients, including many elderly ones, even a modest increase in functional capacity can help maintain independence.[8,9,32–35]

Guidelines for Prescriptive Exercise Training[36]

Individualized medically prescribed physical activity is the hallmark of rehabilitative exercise training. Standards and guidelines have been promulgated by a number of professional organizations.[2,37–43] The prescriptive components of exercise training include its "dosage," determined by the intensity, frequency, and duration of exercise; the types of exercise; and the rate of progression of exercise intensity. Coronary patients should not exercise at a level higher than that documented to produce an appropriate cardiovascular response during testing. The predischarge (or early posthospitalization) exercise test, typically performed for risk stratification, can serve as the basis for initial exercise recommendations. It is inappropriate to use age-predicted target heart rates for coronary patients; disease, therapies, and prior levels of training or fitness may influence the heart rate response to exercise.

Prescription of target heart rate range is based on the results of exercise testing. Although in prior years patients were advised to exercise to a target heart rate range between 70 and 85 percent of the highest level safely achieved at exercise testing,[44] exercise intensities in the 50 to 70 percent heart rate range have produced comparable improvement in functional capacity and endurance and may provide greater safety because of the lower risk of cardiovascular complications with unsupervised exercise.[21,22,45] These lower rates are less likely to produce discomfort that may deter long-term exercise adherence. The documented efficacy of lower-intensity exercise training to improve aerobic capacity has increased both its applicability and acceptance.[1,21,22] Particularly for unfit patients or those with lower exercise capacities, the increased comfort of lower-intensity exercise may encourage adherence, although increased duration of training may be required. Comparable favorable effects on quality of life occurred with low- and high-intensity exercise.[46] An alternative method for calculating target heart rate involves 70 to 85 percent of the difference between peak exercise test heart rate and resting heart rate, added to resting rate. This method may be advantageous in patients whose heart rate is attenuated by beta-blocking or other drugs.

The basic design of an exercise session involves an initial 5 to 10 min of warm-up exercise, i.e., stretching and range-of-motion activities that enable musculoskeletal and circulatory readiness for exercise. This is followed by a 20- to 40-min endurance component that initially involves walk-run sequences or exercise on a stationary bicycle or treadmill; for these activities, skill is a minimal component of the intensity of work demand.

When space for exercise is limited, "station" training may be preferable, with participants serially using bicycle ergometry, arm ergometry, rowing machines, and treadmills. When more space is available, gymnasium-type programs can accommodate larger numbers of patients for walk-jog activities and floor exercises; some facilities have indoor or outdoor tracks. A final 5- to 10-min cool-down period entails a gradual decrease in intensity that allows the heart rate to slow and averts postexercise hypotension. Three exercise sessions weekly appear adequate, and a greater frequency does not significantly improve aerobic capacity. Aerobic games, as a recreational component, add variety to an exercise program and improve adherence; they also provide upper body exercise. Because the oxygen cost of these activities varies with each patient's skills and competitiveness, they should be limited early in exercise training.

As the level of training increases, recreational activities in which skill often influences the intensity of work may add variety to the exercise regimen. Enjoyable, effective endurance activities include rope skipping, bicycling, skating, swimming, rowing, and aerobic dancing; both rope-skipping and swimming (for unskilled swimmers) impose higher workloads and should be undertaken carefully.

Characteristics of Aerobic (Dynamic) and Strength (Isometric) Exercise Training

Aerobic (dynamic) exercise, rhythmic repetitive movements of large muscle groups, traditionally is prescribed for coronary patients. The physiologic response, an increase in heart rate, parallels the intensity of activity, and an increase in stroke volume occurs in young and middle-aged patients. In most elderly patients, the increase in heart rate predominates, with little increase in stroke volume. Systolic blood pressure increases progressively with exercise intensity, with maintenance of or slight decrease in diastolic blood pressure and widening of the pulse pressure.

By contrast, with strength (isometric) training, the increase in heart rate is modest, and the increase in cardiac output is slight. There is a substantial increase in systolic blood pressure with high-intensity isometric activity, particularly in unfit individuals; this may provoke angina, ventricular dysfunction, and/or arrhythmias and is the basis for limiting isometric activity in coronary patients with a low exercise capacity. Once a reasonable aerobic capacity is achieved, combined aerobic and strength training exercises in coronary patients may produce substantial training effects and improve muscle strength,[47] with resulting improvement in endurance and the ability to return to active occupational and recreational lifestyles.[48] Studies document the effectiveness of mild to moderate resistive exercise training in selected patients with coronary heart disease.[49–52] The absence of signs or symptoms of myocardial ischemia, abnormal hemodynamic changes, and cardiovascular complications suggests that resistance exercise training is safe for coronary patients who have previously participated in aerobic exercise training. A major change in contemporary exercise programs is the inclusion of strength training for appropriately selected coronary patients. Most reported studies have involved small numbers of low-risk male patients, 70 years or younger, with minimal functional aerobic impairment and with normal or near-normal LV function. The extent to which the safety and effectiveness of resistance training demonstrated by these studies can be extrapolated to other populations of coronary patients (e.g., women, older patients of both genders with low aerobic fitness, or patients at moderate to high cardiovascular risk) is not known.[4]

Arm versus Leg Exercise Training

Because exercise training is predominantly muscle-specific, both arm and leg exercises should be included in exercise rehabilitation.[53] The heart rate and blood pressure responses to leg work decrease following leg training, with only modest improvement in the response to arm work. Following arm training, the most prominent decreases in heart rate and blood pressure response occur with arm work. In one study, improvement in exercise response of the untrained limb was only 50 to 75 percent of the trained limb, suggesting that about half the increase in trained-limb performance is due to a generalized training effect; the remainder reflects predominantly improved oxygen extraction by trained skeletal muscle.

Since walk-run sequences or exercise on a stationary bicycle or treadmill train primarily leg muscles, supplementary arm exercise training is accomplished by selected repetitive calisthenics, shoulder wheels, rowing machines, and arm ergometers. When data from leg exercise testing are used to prescribe arm exercise, a reduction of about 10 beats per minute in target heart rate range is appropriate. The workload for arm training is about half that for leg training.[53] Since most occupational and recreational activities entail both arm and leg work (and often predominantly arm work), arm exercise training should be included in rehabilitative exercise.

The Effect of Cardiovascular Drugs on Exercise Training

Exercise training can occur in patients receiving antianginal drugs, which may lessen symptoms and improve the ability to exercise.[54] Although beta-blocking drugs decrease the heart rate and blood pressure response to exercise, they do not attenuate the improvement in physical work capacity that results from exercise training. Exercise testing undertaken to prescribe exercise should be performed with patients receiving medications that are planned for their training.

The Role of Exercise Testing in Coronary Rehabilitation

Graded exercise testing, using either a treadmill or a bicycle protocol, is safely performed within the initial weeks following MI.[55] Most centers currently test patients to a sign- or symptom-limited end point because heart rate limits are often inaccurate as a result of antianginal therapy effects on heart rate. Treadmill testing typically entails serial 3-min stages of walking, beginning at slow speed, initially on the level, and then at increasing speed and elevations; comparable test protocols are available for a bicycle ergometer (see Chap. 14). Arm testing may be undertaken in patients with claudication or musculoskeletal problems that make leg testing not feasible.[56]

The results of predischarge exercise tests, performed with or without radionuclide studies, contribute independent prognostic information for risk stratification.[55] High-risk patients are characterized by having a low exercise capacity [peak workload below 4 to 6 metabolic equivalents (METs)]; the occurrence of angina, ischemic ST-segment abnormalities, and/or exercise-induced hypotension at low levels of exercise; and the development of ventricular arrhythmias at low levels of exercise. Radionuclide evidence of myocardial ischemia or LV dysfunction with exercise also indicates an adverse prognosis. Predischarge exercise testing also identifies low-risk patients with a favorable prognosis who do not require additional diagnostic testing, are well-suited for accelerated rehabilitation, and for whom early discharge home and prompt resumption of preinfarction activities, including return to work, can be recommended.[55,57] The exercise test can help define safe levels of activity and guide the surveillance necessary during exercise rehabilitation. This permits simple, effective, accelerated, and less costly rehabilitation for low-risk coronary patients, reserving financial and personnel resources for high-risk patients who may derive substantial benefit from supervised exercise training. Satisfactory performance of an exercise test, coupled with explanation of its relationship to activities to be undertaken at home, may lessen the common fear of postinfarction patients that physical activity may result in reinfarction or death.[58] Such counseling also has been associated with an early return to work.[31]

Safety of Rehabilitative Exercise Training

The Clinical Practice Guideline *Cardiac Rehabilitation*[4] highlights the safety of cardiac rehabilitation exercise training in that randomized, controlled trials involving over 4500 coronary patients showed no increase in morbidity or mortality. A questionnaire survey of 142 U.S. cardiac rehabilitation programs, involving patients participating in exercise rehabilitation between 1980 and 1984, reported a low rate of nonfatal MI of 1 per 294,000 patient-hours and a cardiac mortality rate of 1 per 784,000 patient-hours.[59] Twenty-one episodes of cardiac arrest occurred, with successful resuscitation of 17 patients. A 1978 report[44] also described a low rate of fatal cardiac events during or immediately following exercise training: 1 per 116,400 patient-hours of participation. Definitive information is not available regarding the effect of levels of supervision and of ECG monitoring of exercise training on safety.

IMPLEMENTATION OF CARDIAC REHABILITATIVE CARE

Inpatient, or Hospital, Phase

The major components of rehabilitative care for patients hospitalized for a coronary event include progressive resumption of physical activity (early ambulation) and education and counseling of both patient and family (see also Chap. 42).

EARLY AMBULATION

Early ambulation is designed to limit the detrimental effects of deconditioning: reduced physical work capacity and maximal oxygen uptake; orthostatic intolerance, characterized by orthostatic hypotension and tachycardia (due both to hypovolemia and to a lessened cardiovascular reflex response); increase in blood viscosity owing to a decrease in plasma volume disproportionate to the decrease in red blood cell mass; and decrease in pulmonary ventilation. The decrease in muscle mass and muscular contractile strength renders muscular contraction inefficient, with more oxygen required for comparable work.

Guidelines[60] for physical activity in the coronary or surgical intensive care unit are for initial low-intensity exercise (1–2 METs), with gradual progression in work demand; supervision of progressive ambulation permits detection of inappropriate responses. Patients are encouraged to feed themselves, perform personal care, use a bedside commode, and sit in a bedside chair. Cardiac work is less in the seated than in the supine position. Sitting in a chair two or three times daily limits the hypovolemia of immobilization and resulting orthostatic hypotension. Exposure to gravitational stress, rather than physical activity intensity, appears to be the determinant in limiting hypovolemia, cardiac underfilling, and deterioration of oxygen transport capacity with effort intolerance.[61] Patients perform selected arm and leg exercises designed to maintain muscle tone and increase flexibility and joint mobility. Incentive spirometry is important for postoperative patients.

Disproportionate responses[60] to low-level activity include chest discomfort, dyspnea, or palpitations; a heart rate in excess of 100 beats per minute or lower than 50 beats per minute; ST-segment displacement on the electrocardiographic monitor; appearance of arrhythmias; or a decrease of more than 10 to 15 mmHg in systolic blood pressure. Although the latter usually indicates ischemic ventricular dysfunction, the vasodilator effect of nitrate, calcium channel blocking drugs, or ACE inhibitor therapy also must be considered. A systolic blood pressure response during low-level activity of more than 180 mmHg or a diastolic pressure response of more than 110 mmHg is an indication for antihypertensive therapy. Appropriate responses to ambulation indicate that the patient can progress to higher-intensity activity; disproportionate responses require activity restriction and clinical reassessment for unrecognized cardiac ischemia or ventricular dysfunction.

The major prescriptive hospital activity is walking, with stepwise increases in pace and distance. Patients who must climb steps at home should practice this in the hospital. Most household tasks require a work intensity of 2 to 3 METs. Electrocardiographic telemetry monitoring during ambulation is indicated for selected patients, e.g., those with serious ventricular arrhythmias or asymptomatic myocardial ischemia. A protocol for early ambulation and concomitant educational activities for patients with MI is applicable, with minor modifications, to postoperative coronary patients (Table 50-1).

Neither early ambulation nor early hospital discharge adversely affects the short- or long-term morbidity or mortality of appropriately selected coronary patients.[60,62] Benefits include prevention of deconditioning, decrease in pulmonary atelectasis and thromboembolic complications, lessened anxiety and depression, and an enhanced sense of well-being, related to improved functional status. Improved functional status of patients at hospital discharge has been associated with an earlier and more complete return to work.

EDUCATION AND COUNSELING OF HOSPITALIZED PATIENTS AND THEIR FAMILIES[63]

The current abbreviated hospital stay limits the ability of health professionals to address the informational and learning needs of the patient, spouse, and family; to assist them through recovery; and to prepare them adequately for convalescence. Answering the questions or concerns of patients in a coronary or surgical intensive care unit (or during the preprocedure phase for elective coronary angioplasty or bypass surgery) can provide reassurance. Education includes a brief explanation of the medical or surgical problem(s), tests anticipated in subsequent days, and familiarization with procedures and equipment; this information helps patients adjust to a situation perceived as life-threatening. The temporary nature of most restrictions should be emphasized, citing that improved coronary status with recovery lessens the intensity of surveillance and care.

During the remainder of the hospitalization, providing more information and planning for discharge are appropriate. Increased knowledge can lessen anxiety and improve adherence to recommendations. Patients should be instructed about medications—the purpose, dosage, desired effects, and potential adverse responses of each. Many patients have not taken medications prior to a coronary event and may be unfamiliar with the problems of taking medications. Patients and family members should be taught the appropriate response to new or recurrent symptoms and how to gain access to emergency medical care.

Outpatient, or Ambulatory, Phase

About 70 percent of contemporary survivors of MI are younger than 70 years of age[10] and many patients following successful myocardial revascularization procedures are at low risk for proximate coronary events. Exercise rehabilitation for most low-risk coronary patients, particularly following myocardial revascularization, begins shortly after discharge from the hospital; these patients usually progress rapidly in increasing their intensity and duration of exercise, often without supervision. Coronary patients who are elderly; those with significant comorbidity, myocardial ischemia, heart failure, or serious arrhythmias; those with complications of MI or CABG surgery; or those with severe angina may require exercise surveillance of variable duration.[2,37,39,55] Outpatient exercise rehabilitation is best described by the characteristics of the exercise training and the requirements, duration, and complexity of surveillance, based on the patient's clinical and risk factor status, rather than by traditional phases of earlier years that typically had fixed durations and composition. This is concordant with responding to an individual patient's needs for exercise training rather than requiring a patient to conform to program phases or requirements.

THERAPEUTIC EXERCISE TRAINING

Therapeutic exercise training typically lasts for 8 to 12 weeks. Initial home exercise may involve progressive walking and walk-jog sequences or serial increases in the intensity and duration of use of a stationary bicycle. Videotapes may help guide and pace home exercise and are available for varying intensities of exercise training. Home-based exercise rehabilitation optimally includes planned communication and management by rehabilitation nurses and other specially trained personnel.[10,11]

In the early years of outpatient exercise rehabilitation, few patients had continuous ECG monitoring because ECG telemetry was not widely available. In subsequent years, complication rates were described as being lower in exercise programs with continuous ECG monitoring.[44] It remains unknown, however, whether ECG monitoring, closer medical supervision, and/or differences in exercise intensity were the safety determinants. More recently, continuous ECG monitoring has not been shown to provide added safety for low-risk patients during supervised exercise[59]; as a result, ECG monitoring is currently recommended only for high-risk patients and other selected patients with problems in exercising,[1,2,4,39] although some recommend more extensive ECG monitoring. Often, ECG monitoring is

TABLE 50-1 Inpatient Rehabilitation: Five-Step Myocardial Infarction Program (Revised 1996: Grady Memorial Hospital/Emory University School of Medicine)

Step	Date	M.D. Initials	Nurse/ Exer Specialist Notes	Supervised Exercise	CCU/Step Down Unit Activity	Educational Activity
				CCU		
1	——			Active and passive ROM all extremities in bed Teach patient ankle plantar and dorsiflexion—repeat hourly when awake	Partial self-care Feed self Dangle legs on side of bed Use bedside commode Sit in chair 15 min, 1–2 times/day	Orientation to CCU Personal emergencies, social service aid as needed Bedside teaching (CCU staff)
2	——			Active ROM all extremities, sitting on side of bed or bedside chair	Sit in chair 15–30 min, 2–3 times/day Complete self-care	Orientation to rehabilitation team, program Smoking cessation Educational literature if requested Planning transfer from CCU
				STEP DOWN UNIT		
3	——			Warm-up exercises, 2–2.5 METs: Stretching ROM Calisthenics Walk in hall 50–75 ft and back at slow pace	Sit in chair ad lib Walk in room Walk to class with supervision Out of bed as tolerated	Normal cardiac anatomy and function Development of atherosclerosis What happens when myocardial infarction occurs Coronary risk factors and their control Diet
4	——			Teach pulse counting, Borg Scale ROM and calisthenics, 3 METs Practice walking few stair-steps Walk 300–500 ft bid Instruct on home exercise	Tepid shower or tub bath, with supervision Walk in corridor prn	Heart attack management: Medications Exercise Surgery Response to symptoms Family, community adjustments on return home Work simplification techniques (as needed)
5	——			Continue above activities Check pulse counting Walk up flight of steps Walk 500 ft bid Continue home exercise instruction; present information regarding outpatient exercise program	Continue all previous activities Predischarge exercise test (as appropriate)	Discharge planning Medications, diet, activity Return appointments Schedules tests Return to work Community resources Educational literature Medication cards

NOTE: 1 foot = 0.30 meter.

SOURCE: Reprinted with permission of Grady Memorial Hospital/Emory University School of Medicine.

undertaken solely owing to its requirement for insurance reimbursement rather than based on medical need. Many patients in supervised exercise programs without continuous ECG monitoring or patients exercising independently can be taught either to check their heart rate response intermittently to ensure that it remains in the prescribed target heart rate range or to estimate exercise intensity by the rating of perceived exertion, as described by Borg.[64] In supervised settings, heart rate response can be documented by intermittent use of defibrillator paddles as ECG leads. A technique of value in maintaining appropriate exercise intensity in unsupervised settings is the "talk test," wherein patients exercise only to the level that permits continued conversation with an exercising companion, a level generally below the anaerobic threshold at which respiratory rate accelerates.

High-risk coronary patients may require supervised and often ECG-monitored exercise. These patients are characterized by having a markedly reduced exercise capacity, severely depressed ventricular function, complex ventricular arrhythmias, exercise-induced angina, ischemia, or hypotension at low exercise intensities, and/or the inability to self-monitor exercise heart rate. Because of their increased risk for adverse events, exercise training should occur, at least initially, in a medically supervised and probably ECG-monitored setting.[65] Because exercise-related cardiac complications may be increased not only in proximity to an acute coronary event, the need and duration of ECG surveillance of exercise for these high-risk patients remain uncertain. The uniform success of resuscitation with supervised exercise, despite the rarity of its application, suggests that exercise supervision may be beneficial for selected patients.[59]

Although recent studies document the efficacy of home-based exercise training and risk reduction guided by a specialized cardiac nurse manager, data are not available as to the efficacy of long-term risk reduction or long-term compliance with unsupervised exercise in the absence of management and supervision strategies. Several studies showed that all training regimens appeared to increase functional capacity more rapidly than occurred spontaneously.[11,29,30,47] Supervision of exercise may not entail an "all or nothing" approach; intermittent supervision may be feasible in a community facility, there may be periodic telephone transmission of the exercise ECG of patients who exercise at home, patients may use inexpensive heart rate monitors during home exercise, or a combination of these techniques may be used. It is not known whether any of these approaches improves adherence to exercise or exercise safety; several studies of independent exercise showed a lack of coronary risk reduction.

The Clinical Practice Guideline *Cardiac Rehabilitation*[4] highlights alternative approaches to the delivery of cardiac rehabilitation services, other than traditional supervised group interventions, as effective and safe for carefully selected clinically stable patients. Transtelephonic and other means of monitoring and surveillance of patients can extend cardiac rehabilitation beyond the setting of supervised, structured, group-based rehabilitation. The feasibility, safety, and efficacy of these alternative strategies for exercise rehabilitation must be assessed in more diverse populations of patients with stable coronary heart disease, particularly elderly patients, those with ventricular dysfunction, and other patients of higher risk status.

MAINTENANCE EXERCISE TRAINING

Once patients attain their initial exercise goals, maintenance training can be undertaken or continued in community recreational facilities or at home. Because lifetime regular physical activity is necessary to maintain physical fitness, patients must achieve reasonable independence in exercising and remain involved in an exercise regimen that is social, enjoyable, convenient, and appropriate. Most coronary patients with prior exercise restrictions who can safely attain a 7- to 8-MET level of performance can safely progress to unsupervised exercise. Patients leaving supervised exercise programs may require counseling regarding the selection and initiation of long-term exercise in the community or at home.

EDUCATION AND COUNSELING OF AMBULATORY CORONARY PATIENTS[36]

The behavioral approach to coronary risk reduction encourages and enables coronary patients to manage their illness, adopt and maintain healthy lifestyles, and improve adherence to medications and other recommended regimens.[66,67] Metaanalysis of 28 controlled trials of patient education showed that "education programs have demonstrated a measurable impact on blood pressure, mortality, exercise, [and] diet" and that other parameters are positively affected, although less consistently.[68] A combination of education, counseling, and behavioral intervention strategies seems most effective in promoting health, reducing risk, and favorably altering lifestyle.[4,10,66] Whether the same interventions are equally effective for men and women and across the life span remains unanswered because few studies have enrolled patients over 70 years of age or included women.

Patients with diagnosed coronary disease are at the highest risk for disability and death and thus constitute patients for whom untreated risk factors are most damaging.[69] Cardiac rehabilitation services provide an integrating structure for the multiple risk-reduction components of secondary prevention.

There is no evidence that the performance of CABG surgery per se encourages favorable modification of coronary risk status postoperatively.[70,71] Postoperative recurrence of coronary symptoms or deterioration of function following saphenous vein CABG surgery relates predominantly to progression of the underlying atherosclerosis both in the graft vessels and in the native circulation. Control of hypertension, diabetes, hyperlipidemia, and obesity and cessation of cigarette smoking,[72,73] with adoption of a physically active lifestyle, even at advanced age, may slow progression or induce regression of atherosclerosis and decrease the occurrence of subsequent coronary events.

Community resources that may be helpful in rehabilitation should be identified: counseling and guidance services, home-care agencies, vocational rehabilitation facilities and services for job training and placement, services for financial aid, outpatient coronary rehabilitation programs, and postcoronary groups or clubs. Participation in community heart clubs or educational groups may further facilitate rehabilitation; coronary risk reduction and other skills learned and practiced in these settings may encourage health-related behaviors and aid in reinforcing maintenance of these changes. Acquisition of knowledge appears to affect favorably both behaviors involving implementing recommendations for care and coping behaviors.[63]

CORONARY POPULATIONS WITH SPECIAL REHABILITATION NEEDS

Elderly Coronary Patients

Elderly patients constitute a high percentage of those with MI, CABG surgery, and PTCA and other transcatheter revascularization procedures. Complications of MI and myocardial revascularization are more frequent in the elderly, with prolongation of both immobilization and hospitalization predisposing to deconditioning; early ambulation can limit functional deterioration and decrease depression. In both medical and surgical coronary intensive care settings, the major educational strategy involves concise and repeated explanations, reassurance, and time and place orientation to help avert confusion and delirium. Teaching energy-conserving techniques for self-care and performance of household tasks helps maintain independent living, an outcome valued by elderly patients. Modification of conventional coronary risk factors is feasible and warranted, given the greater prevalence and severity of coronary disease at elderly age.

Elderly patients are also at high risk of disability following a coronary event. Recent trials of exercise rehabilitation have begun to include patients over 65 years of age and to evaluate outcomes in the elderly coronary population specifically. Although few studies and no randomized, controlled trials have addressed the efficacy and safety of exercise training and multifactorial rehabilitation in the elderly, the available studies provide important new information for clinical practice.

Elderly coronary patients in posthospital exercise regimens have exercise trainability comparable with that of younger patients participating in similar exercise rehabilitation,[35,74] with elderly women and men showing comparable improvement. One report found that exercise testing before hospital discharge was feasible in about half of patients aged 70 years or older with MI, enabling accurate risk stratification and exercise prescription.[75] No complications or adverse outcomes of exercise training in elderly patients were described in any cardiac rehabilitation study. Nonetheless, rates of entry referral to and participation in exercise rehabilitation were substantially lower among elderly than among younger patients,[9,33] and older women were even less likely to be referred than were older men.[34] Elderly patients are less fit after a coronary event, in part because of decreased fitness prior to the event. Adherence to exercise training was high (90 percent) in the reported studies,[35] and significant reduction in coronary risk factors occurred in elderly patients who participated in multifactorial cardiac rehabilitation.[9]

For elderly patients who exercise independently, emphasis should be placed on the importance of warm-up and cool-down activities because of the delayed return of the exercise heart rate to normal at elderly age. Walking provides an adequate training stimulus for many elderly patients because it constitutes a significant percentage of the decreased aerobic capacity of aging.[76] Running, jumping, and other high-impact activities should be limited to avoid musculoskeletal complications. Walking, bicycle ergometry, and/or walking in a pool in shallow water can favorably modify the decreased joint mobility of aging; enhance neuromuscular coordination, balance, and stability and thereby lessen propensity for falls; and improve endurance. Elderly individuals who exercise independently should be cautioned to decrease their exercise intensity in hot and humid environments.

Coronary Patients with Heart Failure

Impairment of exercise capacity with heart failure appears in part due to inadequate nutritive blood flow to skeletal muscle; factors other than lack of increase in cardiac output with exercise seem important, including the ability to decrease peripheral vascular resistance and possibly the adequacy of right ventricular function (see also Chap. 20). Patients with heart failure and normal cardiac output responses to exercise frequently improve their functional capacity with exercise training, whereas those with severe hemodynamic dysfunction with exercise often do not.[77] A combination of LV systolic dysfunction and residual myocardial ischemia may limit trainability. The ventricular ejection fraction predicts poorly both exercise capacity and the potential for improvement of exercise performance with training; some patients with substantial ventricular dysfunction have a normal exercise capacity and no symptoms or impairment of lifestyle.[78]

Most studies of exercise training of patients with heart failure and moderate to severe LV systolic dysfunction do not demonstrate deterioration in LV volume, wall thickness, or function.[79,80] Randomized, controlled clinical trial data of exercise training in postinfarction patients with an ejection fraction less than 40 percent showed that long-term home-based exercise may attenuate the unfavorable remodeling response and even improve ventricular function over time.[79] Peripheral (skeletal muscle) adaptations appear to mediate the improvement in exercise tolerance; exercise training can substantially correct the impaired oxidative capacity of skeletal muscle in chronic heart failure.[81] Exercise training also may improve peripheral artery endothelial function in patients with chronic heart failure.[82] Exercise training can augment both the symptomatic and functional benefits of ACE inhibitor therapy.[30] Even small improvements in symptomatic status and functional capacity can exert a substantial favorable impact on quality of life. Improved clinical outcomes are also described.[83] In both the supervised and at-home settings, low- to moderate-intensity exercise regimens provide benefit, although adverse events may occur in this high-risk patient group.[4]

Although the initial exercise training programs of patients with ventricular systolic dysfunction were predominantly supervised, typically with continuous ECG monitoring, other studies have described moderate-intensity, unsupervised exercise as safe and effective.[84,85] The optimal duration of exercise supervision and the duration and need for ECG monitoring of these patients remain uncertain but should be guided by clinical evidence of exercise-related ischemia and/or arrhythmia.[29] In a study of 105 ambulatory cardiac transplant candidates, nonsupervised prescribed walking at a target heart rate range close to baseline exercise test-determined anaerobic threshold produced significant improvement in peak maximal oxygen consumption and peak exercise tolerance in 38 of 68 clinically stable patients without adverse effects. After an average of 6 months of such exercise, 31 of these 38 patients improved sufficiently to be removed from the transplant list, with improvement persisting to 2 years.[86]

Additional important components of rehabilitative care for patients with significant activity limitations include teaching work simplification, particularly the pacing of daily living activities; working in a seated rather than a standing position; and taking frequent rest periods between activities.

Patients with Implanted Pacemakers and Cardioverter-Defibrillators

Exercise prescription is determined by the characteristics of the implanted pacemaker. Because most patients likely to exercise currently receive rate-responsive pacemakers, exercise testing can ascertain the appropriateness of the sensor response to the exercise intensity,[87] and reprogramming can be undertaken as needed.

The exercise target heart rate range for patients with implanted cardioverter-defibrillators should be set at 20 to 30 beats per minute below the threshold rate of the device to fire. This also enables appropriate work-related activities.[88] Coparticipants in the exercise setting must be reassured that they cannot be harmed by physical contact with a patient whose cardioverter-defibrillator discharges.

PSYCHOLOGICAL ASPECTS OF CORONARY REHABILITATION[36]

The importance of psychosocial variables in the prognosis of patients with established coronary disease has received increasing attention during the past decade. Although the type A behavior pattern previously received emphasis, currently the hostility component of type A behavior is regarded as its most adverse feature. High levels of anger and hostility appear associated with increased cardiac morbidity and mortality.[89,90]

Other major psychological problems in coronary patients involve anxiety, depression, denial, and dependence.[91] Denial of presenting symptoms may limit or delay access to care, often with adverse outcomes. "Appropriate" denial, characterized by confidence in a favorable outcome, often an effective coping strategy of patients with a coronary event, is associated with a favorable prognosis. Anxiety, which is often the initial psychological manifestation at hospitalization, is related to a fear of dying and may progress to depression as patients contemplate their potential inability to resume former family, occupational, and community roles. Anxiety and depression, the most common psychological complications of infarction, contribute to the failure to make satisfactory life adjustments, to return to work, to return to sexual function, and to engage in social activities subsequent to hospital discharge. Depression is reported to precede MI in 30 to 50 percent of patients. Depression is associated with increased morbidity and mortality following MI and CABG surgery[92,93]; patients with depression were five times more likely to die during the initial 6 months following MI than nondepressed patients.[94] Depression may be associated with social isolation, which may serve as an independent risk factor. The 6-month mortality of patients living alone was double that of patients living with others (16 versus 8 percent), and follow-up study of patients with angiographically documented coronary disease showed a 50 percent 5-year mortality rate among those most socially isolated, compared with 17 percent among those without these characteristics. The impact of social isolation on prognosis appeared independent of ventricular ejection fraction and other physiologic prognostic factors. Interventions against depression and social isolation following MI are currently being evaluated.

Many patients with successful physical recovery following MI or myocardial revascularization often have residual psychological impairment.[91] Two major strategies that appear to limit this complication are education and counseling and the initiation of a physical activity regimen. Many patients remain psychologically disabled because, inappropriately, they perceive an excessive severity of infarction and vulnerability to sudden death; safe resumption of physical activity provides reassurance and restores self-confidence.[58] In randomized exercise trials, exercising patients returned to sexual activity, to work, and to a near-normal lifestyle more rapidly and had greater improvements in work capacity, income, and job responsibility.[95] Both physical and psychosocial benefits occurred even with low-intensity exercise, particularly among older and sicker coronary patients. Despite the paucity of controlled studies, consistent moderate psychosocial benefit appears to result from combinations of structured exercise, education, and counseling.[63,96] Although the contribution of peer support in a group program has not been ascertained, it may be helpful given the predictive power of social isolation for coronary mortality.[97]

VOCATIONAL ASPECTS OF CORONARY REHABILITATION[36]

A major goal of rehabilitative care for nonelderly patients recovered from MI or myocardial revascularization is resumption of gainful employment, a change in occupation if needed, and the resulting economic and psychological benefits. In the 1980s, about 80 percent of patients who recovered from uncomplicated MI and who were younger than 65 years of age and employed at the time of infarction returned to work within 2 to 3 months, typically resuming former jobs.[98] Despite this favorable early return to work, subsequent cessation of employment was high, with as much as a 20 percent decrement in continued employment between 6 months and 1 year. Comparable data are not available for patients with complications of MI or residual functional impairment, although their return to work is estimated at 25 to 33 percent.

These data contrast markedly with work resumption following CABG surgery. Despite a substantial decrease in symptoms, improvement in functional capacity, and reported enhancement of life quality and participation in leisure activities, return to work following coronary bypass surgery has been much less favorable than anticipated.[99,100] No difference in 10-year employment status was described between patients randomized to medical and surgical treatment in the Coronary Artery Surgery Study (CASS).[101] Return to work following PTCA is comparable with that following CABG surgery, although PTCA patients are reported to return to work more promptly.[100] Other reports described lack of confidence in the ability to return to work following PTCA, even when patients were physically able to do so.[102]

Most studies of the return to work have involved predominantly or exclusively men; recent examination of working women with coronary disease showed them to have a longer convalescence and even lesser return to work; whether this is a gender issue or reflects older age or greater occurrence of depression among women warrants study.[103]

For patients younger than 65 years of age following MI or myocardial revascularization, the indirect health care costs of disability, including lessened productivity, loss of income, welfare payments, and unemployment insurance costs, must be considered when the cost-effectiveness of rehabilitation is determined.[57,104–106] Coronary heart disease is the leading problem in the United States for which adults receive premature disability benefits under the Social Security system; almost one-fourth of men and women receiving Social Security disability allowances have permanent disability due to coronary disease. Following both MI and myocardial revascularization, symptomatic and functional improvement correlates poorly with the return to work and resumption of preillness lifestyle, with psychosocial status appearing as a more important determinant.[99] Since only about 15 percent of the U.S. labor force currently performs manual labor and this percentage decreases with older age, the severity of angina or heart failure in coronary patients only rarely precludes or delays return to work. Many nonmedical factors negatively influence resumption of employment: older age, adequate nonwork income, anxiety or depression, activity-induced symptoms, lower social class and less education, jobs involving high-level physical activity (more common among blue-collar workers), and perception of the coronary illness as job-related. Patients who fail to resume employment within 6 months after a coronary event are unlikely ever to do so.[107]

Among the medical reasons for failure to return to work are unwarranted medical restrictions or, even more commonly, lack of professional assurance of the safety of so doing.[107] Exercise testing performed for risk stratification also can be used for work evaluation; it permits a relatively precise assessment of function that may help allay the apprehensions of the patient,[58] family,[108] physician, and employer about the capability and safety of return to work.[109] One randomized, controlled trial of occupational work assessment in a health maintenance organization population early following MI, identifying low-risk patients and counseling them about the appropriateness of prompt return to work, effected a 32 percent reduction in the duration of convalescence.[31] Extrapolation of exercise test data to job requirements should include an analysis of the job to be performed and differences in temperature, environment, intellectual demands, relation to meals, travel requirements, and emotional stress, among others. Nonetheless, patients without evidence of ischemia or arrhythmia during a symptom-limited standard exercise test typically are free of these problems when occupational static and dynamic work are combined.[110] Arm ergometry may be preferable for occupational assessment of patients who perform predominantly arm work.[53]

Furthermore, since most occupational work is intermittent, with brief periods of strenuous activity and longer intervals of low-level activity or rest, occupational myocardial work demand is lower than for the same level of steady-state exercise; cardiac output, blood pressure, and oxygen uptake do not approach steady state until about 2 min after the onset of work, explaining the tolerance of patients with modest cardiac impairment and limitation of cardiac output for significant workloads of short duration, when adequate rest periods are interspersed. Recommendations for full-time work should be for work levels approximating 30 percent of measured physical work capacity. Guidelines are available to assist physicians in assessing and establishing the employment of patients with coronary heart disease.[111]

Other nonmedical considerations also influence postinfarction or postrevascularization employment, particularly the financial, social, disability, and compensation benefits of not returning to work. Although appropriate physician and employer attitudes may facilitate reemployment, the viewpoint of the patient appears the major determinant. In a number of studies, the patient's preoperative perception about ability to return to work appeared to be the most important determinant.

Benefits to employers of cardiac rehabilitative care for their employees include earlier return to work, less disability, less absenteeism, reduced financial expenditures for sickness and disability payments, reduced training costs for replacement of personnel, and greater productivity.[1] Employers thus should encourage coronary rehabilitative care as a component of their managed care plans.

References

1. Report of the WHO Expert Committee, Wenger NK, Expert Committee Chairman. *Rehabilitation after Cardiovascular Diseases, with Special Emphasis on Developing Countries.* WHO Tech. Rep. Series No. 831, Geneva: World Health Organization; 1993.
2. American College of Cardiology. Position report on cardiac rehabilitation: Recommendations of the American College of Cardiology on cardiovascular rehabilitation. *J Am Coll Cardiol* 1986; 7:451.
3. Agency for Health Care Policy and Research. *Cardiac Rehabilitation Programs.* Health Technology Assessment Report No. 3, DHHS Publication No. AHCPR 92-0015. Rockville, MD: U.S. Department of Health and Human Services, Public Health Service, Agency for Health Care Policy and Research; December 1991.
4. Wenger NK, Froelicher ES, Smith LK, et al. *Cardiac Rehabilitation.* Clinical Practice Guideline No. 17, AHCPR Publication No. 96-0672. Rockville, MD: U.S. Department of Health and Human Services, Public Health Service, Agency for Health Care Policy and Research and the National Heart, Lung, and Blood Institute; October 1995.
5. Ben-Ari E, Kellermann JJ, Fishman EZ, et al. Benefits of long-term physical training in patients after coronary artery bypass grafting: A 58-month follow-up and comparison with a nontrained group. *J Cardiopulm Rehabil* 1986; 6:165.
6. Raft D, McKee DC, Popio KA, et al. Life adaptation after percutaneous transluminal coronary angioplasty and coronary artery bypass grafting. *Am J Cardiol* 1985; 56:395.
7. Ben-Ari E, Rothbaum DA, Linnemeir TJ, et al. Benefits of a monitored rehabilitation program versus physician care after emergency percutaneous transluminal coronary angioplasty: Follow-up of risk factors and rate of stenosis. *J Cardiopulm Rehabil* 1989; 7:281.
8. Ades PA, Waldmann ML, Gillespie C. A controlled trial of exercise training in older patients. *J Gerontol* 1995; 50A:M7.
9. Lavie CJ, Milani RV, Littman AB. Benefits of cardiac rehabilitation and exercise training in secondary coronary prevention in the elderly. *J Am Coll Cardiol* 1993; 22:678.
10. DeBusk RF, Houston Miller N, Superko HR, et al. A case-management system for coronary risk factor modification after acute myocardial infarction. *Ann Intern Med* 1994; 120:721.
11. Haskell WL, Alderman EL, Fair JM, et al. Effects of intensive multiple risk factor reduction on coronary atherosclerosis and

clinical cardiac events in men and women with coronary artery disease. The Stanford Coronary Risk Intervention Project (SCRIP). *Circulation* 1994; 89:975.
12. Schuler G, Hambrecht R, Schlierf G, et al. Regular physical exercise and low-fat diet: Effects on progression of coronary artery disease. *Circulation* 1992; 86:1.
13. Leon AS, Certo C, Comoss P, et al. Scientific evidence of the value of cardiac rehabilitation services with emphasis on patients following myocardial infarction: I. Exercise conditioning component (position paper). *J Cardiopulm Rehabil* 1990; 10:79.
14. Mark DB, Naylor CD, Hlatky MA, et al. Use of medical resources and quality of life after acute myocardial infarction in Canada and the United States. *N Engl J Med* 1994; 331:1130.
15. Thomas RJ, Houston Miller N, Lamendola C, et al. National survey on gender differences in cardiac rehabilitation programs: Patient characteristics and enrollment patterns. *J Cardiopulm Rehabil* 1996; 16:402.
16. O'Connor GT, Buring JE, Yusuf S, et al. An overview of randomized trials of rehabilitation with exercise after myocardial infarction. *Circulation* 1989; 80:234.
17. Oldridge N, Furlong W, Feeny D, et al. Economic evaluation of cardiac rehabilitation soon after acute myocardial infarction. *Am J Cardiol* 1993; 72:154.
18. Oldridge NB, Guyatt GH, Fischer ME, et al. Cardiac rehabilitation after myocardial infarction: Combined experience of randomized clinical trials. *JAMA* 1988; 260:945.
19. Balady GJ, Jette D, Scheer J, et al, and the Massachusetts Association of Cardiovascular and Pulmonary Rehabilitation Database Co-Investigators. Changes in exercise capacity following cardiac rehabilitation in patients stratified according to age and gender: Results of the Massachusetts Association of Cardiovascular and Pulmonary Rehabilitation Multicenter Database. *J Cardiopulm Rehabil* 1996; 16:38.
20. Rechnitzer PA, Cunningham DA, Andrew GM, et al. Relation of exercise to the recurrence rate of myocardial infarction in men: Ontario Exercise-Heart Collaborative Study. *Am J Cardiol* 1983; 51:65.
21. Blumenthal JA, Rejeski WJ, Walsh-Riddle M, et al. Comparison of high and low-intensity exercise training early after acute myocardial infarction. *Am J Cardiol* 1988; 61:26.
22. Goble AJ, Hare DL, Macdonald PS, et al. Effect of early programmes of high and low intensity exercise on physical performance after transmural acute myocardial infarction. *Br Heart J* 1991; 65:126.
23. Ehsani AA, Biello DR, Schultz J, et al. Improvement of left ventricular contractile function by exercise training in patients with coronary artery disease. *Circulation* 1986; 74:350.
24. Kennedy CC, Spiekerman RE, Lindsay MI Jr, et al. One-year graduated exercise program for men with angina pectoris: Evaluation by physiologic studies and coronary arteriography. *Mayo Clin Proc* 1976; 51:231.
25. Hung J, Gordon EP, Houston N, et al. Changes in rest and exercise myocardial perfusion and left ventricular function 3 to 26 weeks after clinically uncomplicated acute myocardial infarction: Effects of exercise training. *Am J Cardiol* 1984; 54:943.
26. Sullivan MJ, Higginbotham MB, Cobb FR. Exercise training in patients with severe left ventricular dysfunction: Hemodynamic and metabolic effects. *Circulation* 1988; 78:506.
27. Todd IC, Ballantyne D. Effect of exercise training on the total ischaemic burden: An assessment by 24-hour ambulatory electrocardiographic monitoring. *Br Heart J* 1992; 68:560.
28. Sebrechts CP, Klein JL, Ahnve S, et al. Myocardial perfusion changes following 1 year of exercise training assessed by thallium-201 circumferential count profiles. *Am Heart J* 1986; 112:1217.
29. Coats AJS, Adamopoulos S, Meyer TE, et al. Effects of physical training in chronic heart failure. *Lancet* 1990; 335:63.
30. Meyer TE, Casadei B, Coats AJS, et al. Angiotensin-converting enzyme inhibition and physical training in heart failure. *J Intern Med* 1991; 230:407.
31. Dennis C, Houston-Miller N, Schwartz RG, et al. Early return to work after uncomplicated myocardial infarction: Results of a randomized trial. *JAMA* 1988; 260:214.
32. Ades PA, Grunvald MH. Cardiopulmonary exercise testing before and after conditioning in older coronary patients. *Am Heart J* 1990; 120:585.
33. Ades PA, Hanson JS, Gunther PGS, et al. Exercise conditioning in the elderly coronary patient. *J Am Geriatr Soc* 1987; 35:121.
34. Ades PA, Waldman ML, Polk DM, et al. Referral patterns and exercise response in the rehabilitation of female coronary patients aged ≥62 years. *Am J Cardiol* 1992; 69:1422.
35. Williams MA, Maresh CM, Esterbrooks DJ, et al. Early exercise training in patients older than age 65 years compared with that in younger patients after acute myocardial infarction or coronary artery bypass grafting. *Am J Cardiol* 1985; 55:263.
36. Wenger NK, Smith LK, Froelicher ES, et al, eds. *Cardiac Rehabilitation: A Guide to Practice in the 21st Century.* New York: Marcel Dekker; 1999.
37. Balady GJ, Fletcher BJ, Froelicher ES, et al. Cardiac rehabilitation programs: A statement for healthcare professionals from the American Heart Association. *Circulation* 1994; 90:1602.
38. American College of Sports Medicine Position Stand. Exercise for patients with coronary artery disease. *Med Sci Sports Exerc* 1994; 26:i.
39. Health and Public Policy Committee, American College of Physicians. Cardiac rehabilitation services. *Ann Intern Med* 1988; 109:671.
40. American Association of Cardiovascular and Pulmonary Rehabilitation. *Guidelines for Cardiac Rehabilitation Programs.* Champaign, IL: Human Kinetics; 1991.
41. Wenger NK, Balady GJ, Cohn LH, et al. Ad Hoc Task Force on Cardiac Rehabilitation: Cardiac rehabilitation services following PTCA and valvular surgery. Guidelines for use. *Cardiology* 1990; 19:4.
42. Wenger NK, Haskell WL, Kanter K, et al. Ad Hoc Task Force on Cardiac Rehabilitation: Cardiac rehabilitation services after cardiac transplantation. Guidelines for use. *Cardiology* 1991; 20:4.
43. NIH Consensus Development Panel on Physical Activity and Cardiovascular Health. Physical activity and cardiovascular health. *JAMA* 1996; 276:241.
44. Haskell WL. Cardiovascular complications during exercise training of cardiac patients. *Circulation* 1978; 57:920.
45. DeBusk RF, Haskell WL, Miller NH, et al. Medically directed at-home rehabilitation soon after uncomplicated acute myocardial infarction: A new model for patient care. *Am J Cardiol* 1985; 55:251.
46. Worcester MC, Hare DL, Oliver RG, et al. Early programmes of high and low intensity exercise and quality of life after acute myocardial infarction. *B Med J* 1993; 307:1244.
47. Kelemen MH, Stewart KJ, Gillian RE, et al. Circuit weight training in cardiac patients. *J Am Coll Cardiol* 1986; 7:38.
48. Franklin BA, Bonzheim K, Gordon S, et al. Resistance training in cardiac rehabilitation. *J Cardiopulm Rehabil* 1991; 11:99.
49. Kelemen MH. Resistive training safety and assessment guidelines for cardiac and coronary prone patients. *Med Sci Sports Exerc* 1989; 21:675.
50. Sparling PB, Cantwell JD, Dolan CM, et al. Strength training in a cardiac rehabilitation program: A six-month follow-up. *Arch Phys Med Rehabil* 1990; 71:148.
51. Stewart KJ, Mason M, Keleman MH. Three-year participation in circuit weight training improves muscular strength and self-efficacy in cardiac patients. *J Cardiopulm Rehabil* 1988; 8:292.
52. Wilke NA, Sheldahl LM, Levandoski SG, et al. Transfer effect of upper extremity training to weight carrying in men with ischemic heart disease. *J Cardiopulm Rehabil* 1991; 11:365.

53. Franklin BA. Exercise testing, training and arm ergometry. *Sports Med* 1985; 2:100.
54. Wenger NK. Ischemic heart disease: Exercise training, selected aspects of pharmacologic therapy, and drug-exercise interactions. *Emory J Med* 1989; 3:253.
55. Ryan TJ, Antman EM, Brooks NH, et al. 1999 Update: ACC/AHA guidelines for the management of patients with acute myocardial infarction. A report of the American College of Cardiology/American Heart Association Task Force on Practice Guidelines (Committee on Management of Acute Myocardial Infarction). *J Am Coll Cardiol* 1999; 34:890; Executive Summary and Recommendations. *Circulation* 1999; 100:1016.
56. Balady GJ, Weiner DA, Rose L, et al. Physiologic responses to arm ergometry exercise relative to age and gender. *J Am Coll Cardiol* 1990; 16:130.
57. Picard MH, Dennis C, Schwartz RG, et al. Cost-benefit analysis of early return to work after uncomplicated acute myocardial infarction. *Am J Cardiol* 1989; 63:1308.
58. Ewart CK, Taylor CB, Reese LB, et al. Effects of early postmyocardial infarction exercise testing on self-perception and subsequent physical activity. *Am J Cardiol* 1983; 51:1076.
59. Van Camp SP, Peterson RA. Cardiovascular complications of outpatient cardiac rehabilitation programs. *JAMA* 1986; 256:1160.
60. Wenger NK. In-hospital exercise rehabilitation after myocardial infarction and myocardial revascularization: Physiologic basis, methodology, and results. In: Wenger NK, Hellerstein H, eds. *Rehabilitation of the Coronary Patient,* 3d ed. New York: Churchill-Livingstone; 1992:351.
61. Hung J, Goldwater D, Convertino VA, et al. Mechanisms for decreased exercise capacity after bed rest in normal middle-aged men. *Am J Cardiol* 1983; 51:344.
62. Rowe MH, Jelinek MV, Liddell N, et al. Effect of rapid mobilization on ejection fractions and ventricular volumes after acute myocardial infarction. *Am J Cardiol* 1989; 63:1037.
63. Maeland JG, Havik OE. The effects of an in-hospital educational programme for myocardial infarction patients. *Scand J Rehabil Med* 1987; 19:57.
64. Borg GA. Psychophysical bases of perceived exertion. *Med Sci Sports Exerc* 1982; 14:377.
65. Williams RS, Miller H, Koisch FP Jr, et al. Guidelines for unsupervised exercise in patients with ischemic heart disease. *J Cardiac Rehabil* 1981; 1:213.
66. Blumenthal JA, Levenson RM. Behavioral approaches to secondary prevention of coronary heart disease. *Circulation* 1987; 76(suppl I):I-130.
67. Ornish D, Brown SE, Scherwitz LW, et al. Can lifestyle changes reverse coronary heart disease? The Lifestyle Heart Trial. *Lancet* 1990; 336:129.
68. Mullen PD, Mains DA, Velez R. A meta-analysis of controlled trials of cardiac patient education. *Patient Educ Couns* 1992; 19:143.
69. Fuster V, Pearson TA. 27th Bethesda Conference: Matching the intensity of risk factor management with the hazard for coronary disease events. *J Am Coll Cardiol* 1996; 27:957.
70. CASS Principal Investigators and Their Associates. Coronary Artery Surgery Study (CASS): A randomized trial of coronary artery bypass surgery. Quality of life in patients randomly assigned to treatment groups. *Circulation* 1993; 68:951.
71. Leaman DM, Brower RW, Meester GT. Coronary artery bypass surgery: A stimulus to modify existing risk factors? *Chest* 1982; 81:16.
72. Kottke TE, Battista RN, DeFriese GH, et al. Attributes of successful smoking cessation interventions in medical practice: A meta-analysis of 39 controlled trials. *JAMA* 1988; 259:2883.
73. Fiore MC, Smith SS, Jorenby DE, et al. The effectiveness of the nicotine patch for smoking cessation: A meta-analysis. *JAMA* 1994; 271:1940.
74. Shephard RJ. The scientific basis of exercise prescribing for the very old. *J Am Geriatr Soc* 1990; 38:62.
75. Saunamaki KI. Early post-myocardial infarction exercise testing in subjects 70 years or more of age: Functional and prognostic evaluation. *Eur Heart J* 1984; 5(suppl E):93.
76. Bruce RA, Larson EB, Stratton J. Physical fitness, functional aerobic capacity, aging, and responses to physical training or bypass surgery in coronary patients. *J Cardiopulm Rehabil* 1989; 9:24.
77. Wilson JR, Groves J, Rayos G. Circulatory status and response to cardiac rehabilitation in patients with heart failure. *Circulation* 1996; 94:1567.
78. Litchfield RL, Kerber RE, Benge JW, et al. Normal exercise capacity in patients with severe left ventricular dysfunction: Compensatory mechanisms. *Circulation* 1982; 66:129.
79. Giannuzzi P, Temporelli PL, Corrà U, et al., for the ELVD Study Group. Attenuation of unfavorable remodeling by exercise training in postinfarction patients with left ventricular dysfunction: Results of the Exercise in Left Ventricular Dysfunction (ELVD) Trial. *Circulation* 1997; 96:1790.
80. Dubach P, Myers J, Dziekan G, et al. Effect of exercise training on myocardial remodeling in patients with reduced left ventricular function after myocardial infarction: Application of magnetic resonance imaging. *Circulation* 1997; 95:2060.
81. Adamopoulos S, Coats AJS, Brunotte F, et al. Physical training improves skeletal muscle metabolism in patients with chronic heart failure. *J Am Coll Cardiol* 1993; 21:1101.
82. Hornig B, Maier V, Drexler H. Physical training improves endothelial function in patients with chronic heart failure. *Circulation* 1996; 93:210.
83. Belardinelli R, Georgiou D, Cianci G, et al. Randomized, controlled trail of long-term moderate exercise training in chronic heart failure: Effects on functional capacity, quality of life, and clinical outcome. *Circulation* 1999; 99:1173.
84. Squires RW, Lavie CJ, Brandt TR, et al. Cardiac rehabilitation in patients with severe ischemic left ventricular dysfunction. *Mayo Clin Proc* 1987; 62:997.
85. Williams RS. Exercise training of patients with ventricular dysfunction and heart failure. In: Wenger NK, ed. *Exercise and the Heart,* 2d ed. Philadelphia: Davis; 1985:219.
86. Stevenson LW, Steimle E, Fonarow G, et al. Improvement in exercise capacity of candidates awaiting heart transplantation. *J Am Coll Cardiol* 1995; 25:163.
87. Tamarisk NK. Enhancing activity levels of patients with permanent cardiac pacemakers. *Heart Lung* 1988; 17:698.
88. Kalbfleisch KR, Lehmann MH, Steinman RT, et al. Reemployment following implantation of the automatic cardioverter defibrillator. *Am J Cardiol* 1989; 64:199.
89. Williams RB Jr, Barefoot JC, Haney TL, et al. Type A behavior and angiographically documented coronary atherosclerosis in a sample of 2289 patients. *Psychosom Med* 1988; 50:139.
90. Helmers KF, Krantz DS, Howell RH, et al. Hostility and myocardial ischemia in coronary artery disease patients: Evaluation by gender and ischemic index. *Psychosom Med* 1993; 55:29.
91. Razin AM. Psychosocial intervention in coronary artery disease: A review. *Psychosom Med* 1982; 44:363.
92. Schleifer SL, Macari-Hinson MM, Coyle DA, et al. The nature and course of depression following myocardial infarction. *Arch Intern Med* 1989; 149:1785.
93. Frasure-Smith N, Lesperance F, Talajic M. Depression and 18-month prognosis after myocardial infarction. *Circulation* 1995; 91:999.
94. Frasure-Smith N, Lesperance F, Talajic M. Depression following myocardial infarction: Impact on 6-month survival. *JAMA* 1993; 270:1819.

95. Stern MJ, Cleary P. National Exercise and Heart Disease Project: Psychosocial changes observed during a low-level exercise program. *Arch Intern Med* 1981; 141:1463.
96. Maeland JG, Havlik OE. Psychological predictors for return to work after a myocardial infarction. *J Psychosom Res* 1987; 31:471.
97. Orth-Gomer K, Unden A-L, Edwards M-E. Social isolation and mortality in ischemic heart disease: A 10-year follow-up study of 150 middle-aged men. *Acta Med Scand* 1988; 224:205.
98. Wenger NK, Hellerstein HK, Blackburn H, et al. Physician practice in the management of patients with uncomplicated myocardial infarction: Changes in the past decade. *Circulation* 1982; 65:421.
99. Walter PJ, ed. *Return to Work after Coronary Artery Bypass Surgery: Psychosocial and Economic Aspects.* Berlin: Springer-Verlag; 1985.
100. Russell RO Jr, Abi-Mansour P, Wenger NK. Return to work after coronary bypass surgery and percutaneous transluminal angioplasty: Issues and potential solutions. *Cardiology* 1986; 73:306.
101. Rogers WJ, Coggin CJ, Gersh BJ, et al, for the CASS Investigators. Ten-year follow-up of quality of life in patients randomized to receive medical therapy or coronary artery bypass graft surgery. The Coronary Artery Surgery Study (CASS). *Circulation* 1990; 82:1647.
102. Fitzgerald ST, Becker DM, Celentano DD, et al. Return to work after percutaneous transluminal coronary angioplasty. *Am J Cardiol* 1989; 64:1108.
103. Walling A, Tremblay GJ, Jobin J, et al. Evaluating the rehabilitation potential of a large population of post-myocardial infarction patients: Adverse prognosis for women. *J Cardiopulm Rehabil* 1988; 8:99.
104. Ades PA, Huang D, Weaver SO. Cardiac rehabilitation participation predicts lower rehospitalization costs. *Am Heart J* 1992; 123:916.
105. Levin LA, Perk J, Hedback B. Cardiac rehabilitation: A cost analysis. *J Intern Med* 1991; 230:427.
106. Oldridge N, Furlong W, Feeny D, et al. Economic evaluation of cardiac rehabilitation soon after acute myocardial infarction. *Am J Cardiol* 1993; 72:154.
107. Almeida D, Bradford JM, Wenger NK, et al. Return to work after coronary bypass surgery. *Circulation* 1983; 68(suppl II):II-205.
108. Taylor CB, Bandura A, Ewart CK, et al. Exercise testing to enhance wives' confidence in their husbands' cardiac capability soon after clinically uncomplicated acute myocardial infarction. *Am J Cardiol* 1995; 55:635.
109. Hellerstein HK. Vocational aspects of rehabilitation: Work evaluation.In: Wenger NK, Hellerstein HK, eds. *Rehabilitation of the Coronary Patient,* 3d ed. New York: Churchill-Livingstone; 1992:523.
110. Hung J, McKillip J, Savin W, et al. Comparison of cardiovascular response to combined static-dynamic effort, postprandial dynamic effort and dynamic effort alone in patients with chronic ischemic heart disease. *Circulation* 1982; 65:1411.
111. 20th Bethesda Conference. Insurability and employability of the patient with ischemic heart disease, October 3–4, 1988. *J Am Coll Cardiol* 1989; 14:1003.

P A R T S E V E N

SYSTEMIC ARTERIAL HYPERTENSION

CHAPTER 51

HYPERTENSION: EPIDEMIOLOGY, PATHOPHYSIOLOGY, DIAGNOSIS, AND TREATMENT

Henry R. Black / George L. Bakris / William J. Elliott

INTRODUCTION

Hypertension is the most common disease-specific reason for which Americans visit a physician. It is currently among the leading causes of morbidity and mortality in the world and is expected to have an even greater impact on the health of the public as more of the world becomes developed.[1] In addition to the morbidity and mortality directly attributable to hypertension, high blood pressure (BP) is a powerful risk factor (a condition or characteristic of an individual or a population) that in this case increases the likelihood that an individual or population will develop a wide variety of cardiovascular (CV) diseases (Table 51-1).[2–5] Hypertension even has been associated with an increased risk of certain cancers.[6–8] Some authors have failed to appreciate this relationship when attributing certain cancers to particular antihypertensive treatments.[9]

All health care providers routinely encounter patients whose BP is elevated. In patients with definite hypertension (see below), the paramount consideration is the choice of treatment, but in an increasing number of individuals, lowering BP may be beneficial even if definite hypertension cannot be diagnosed. In the next decade, it is expected that more and more patients will become candidates for antihypertensive therapy, especially as trials demonstrate the benefits of treatment and pharmacologic approaches become safer and more effective. Furthermore, many citizens, perhaps of the majority of those over 40 years of age, who do not yet meet the criteria for pharmacologic treatment for hypertension will benefit from lifestyle modification, a presumably safe and cost-effective public health approach to reducing BP. Many of the lifestyle habits that lower BP or slow the rate of rise of BP probably should be incorporated into everyone's lifestyle very early.

This chapter reviews the risks imparted by elevated BP, discusses the pathophysiology of hypertension, and analyzes currently available and recommended tools to measure BP and evaluate patients with hypertension. Treatment both with and without drugs is discussed in light of the explosion of information furnished by clinical trials and the newer approaches to lowering BP created by an enhanced understanding of the mechanisms responsible for raising it. The techniques of molecular biology and the contribution of genetics to hypertension have dramatically increased physicians' appreciation of the complexity of the problem.

Hypertension is a disorder of circulatory regulation. The now-classic mosaic theory of the etiology of hypertension, which first was proposed in 1949 by Page, can be endorsed even more

TABLE 51-1 Risks Associated with Hypertension

Cerebrovascular disease	Renal insufficiency
Coronary artery disease	Peripheral vascular disease
Heart failure	Premature mortality

enthusiastically in light of current knowledge.[10] No longer can one expect a simple explanation of why BP is elevated in an individual patient or expect that a single approach to therapy will be successful in the majority of those who are treated.

However, with all the progress that has been made in identifying the risks associated with elevated BP and all the efforts to develop ways to lower BP and prove that they work, the situation in the United States leaves much to be accomplished.[11,12] Only 27.4 percent of hypertensive Americans ages 18 to 74 in the period 1991 to 1994 had a BP of <140/90 mmHg, the current goal.[11] The data are still worse for those ≥75 years of age, and the goal may well be too high in some subpopulations of hypertensives, particularly those with diabetes mellitus (DM) and/or renal disease with proteinuria. The record in the rest of the world is much worse.[13–17] Although the United States does better than other countries, much still needs to be done here and elsewhere. One must understand hypertension better to give optimal care to the 1.2 billion hypertensives estimated to be living by the year 2010. Physicians must strive to prevent as much of the enormous morbidity and premature mortality that one can predict will result.

DEFINITION

Blood pressure is a continuous variable, and whatever number is used to define hypertension will be arbitrary. In the past several decades, the levels at which definite hypertension is defined as beginning have changed from >160/95 mmHg to >140/90 mmHg. Although there is still some disagreement, most authorities now agree on several important principles:

TABLE 51-2 Threshold Values for "Normal" versus "Abnormal" BP (in mmHg)

Source	Office Readings	Home Readings	ABPM Readings
JNC VI	140/90		
Ohasama	140/90	137/84	
French	140/90	127/83	
ASH	140/90	135/85	135/85
Staessen	140/90		133/82

SOURCE: Adapted from JNC VI: The sixth report on the Joint National Committee on Prevention, Detection, Evaluation, and Treatment of High Blood Pressure (JNC VI). *Arch Intern Med* 1997; 157:2413–2443. Ohasama: Tsuji I, Imai Y, Nagai K, et al. Proposal of reference values for home blood pressure measurement: Prognostic criteria based on a prospective observation of the general population in Ohasama, Japan. *Am J Hypertens* 1997; 10:409–418. French Society of Hypertension: De Gaudemaris R, Chau NP, Maillion JM. Home blood pressure variability, comparison with office readings and proposal for reference values: Groupe de la Mesure, French Society of Hypertension. *J Hypertens* 1994; 12:831–838. ASH: Pickering T. Recommendations for use of home (self) and ambulatory blood pressure monitoring: American Society of Hypertension Ad Hoc Panel. *Am J Hypertens* 1996; 9:1–11. Staessen: Staessen JA, O'Brien ET, Atkins N, Amery AK. Short report: Ambulatory blood pressure in normotensive compared with hypertensive subjects: The Ad-Hoc Working Group. *J Hypertens* 1993; 11:1289–1297.

- Hypertension should be defined by both systolic and diastolic BP levels.
- Simply defining and consequently categorizing individuals as hypertensive or not only on the basis of their BP levels neglects the value of using the presence or absence of other risk factors, comorbidity, and target organ damage (TOD) to assess prognosis and ultimately to guide therapy. Thus, the Sixth Joint National Committee on Prevention, Detection, Evaluation and Treatment of High Blood Pressure (JNC VI), the World Health Organization/International Society of Hypertension (WHO/ISH), and the British Hypertension Society (BHS) use a more comprehensive system to define hypertension[11,18,19] (Table 51-2). These definitions are based on properly measured office readings (see below). The definitions of hypertension for home and ambulatory measurements are different. Blood pressure >135/85 mmHg for 24-h ambulatory monitoring or home monitoring is the usual level considered to be where hypertension starts.[20,21] Although home or ambulatory measurements are useful, it is not appropriate routinely to use those values to diagnose most individuals. Office readings remain the standard. In certain situations, especially when an individual claims to have multiple "normal" readings outside the physician's office (see below), it may be reasonable to rely more on out-of-office measurements.
- The treatment approach to individuals with elevated BP should not focus simply on the BP level, which assesses the relative risk that is imparted by that BP, but also on the remainder of the CV risk profile, which estimates the absolute risk of events that an individual with that particular BP and risk profile will face. In the JNC VI classification and stratification of hypertension, for example, the stages (optimal to normal to high normal through stages 1 to 3) represent increasing relative risk as BP rises, while risk group A-C denotes increasing absolute risk as other risk factors and TOD are superimposed on the level of BP[11] (Table 51-3).

It is not of major significance whether hypertensives are classified as being in a stage as recommended by JNC VI or a class per WHO/ISH.[11,18] What is important is that one base the evaluation and care of hypertensive patients on more than the BP number. Black and Yi have suggested that reimbursement for care of a hypertensive patient be based on the stage and risk group into which that patient falls, but to date such a system has not been implemented.[22]

EPIDEMIOLOGY AND RISK

Physicians generally do not concern themselves with reducing BP when it is elevated because of the specific clinical problems they can attribute to that elevation. Instead, hypertension is treated because of the increased risk of mortality and CV disease that results from having an elevated BP (Table 51-1).

These risks have been well documented in numerous epidemiologic studies, beginning with the Framingham Heart Study and many others in the 1950s and 1960s and extending to the present.[23–29] More recently, meta-analyses of pooled data have confirmed the robust, continuous relationship between BP level

TABLE 51-3 JNC VI Stratification of Cardiovascular Risk and Links to Initial Treatment Strategy

		Risk Group		
		A	B	C
	No. of Risk Factors	0	1 (not DM[a])	≥2 (or DM)
	Target organ damage	Absent	Absent	Present
	Cardiovascular disease	Absent	Absent	Present
BP stage				
High normal (130–139/85–89)		LM[b] only	LM only	LM plus drug therapy
Stage 1 (140–159/90–99)		LM for 12 months	LM for 6 months	LM plus drug therapy
Stage 2 (160–179/100–109)		LM plus drug therapy	LM plus drug therapy	LM plus drug therapy
Stage 3 (≥180/≥110)		LM plus drug therapy	LM plus drug therapy	LM plus drug therapy

[a]DM = diabetes mellitus.
[b]LM = lifestyle modifications.

and cerebrovascular disease and coronary artery disease (CAD) in both western and eastern populations.[30,31] In addition, BP is directly related to left ventricular hypertrophy (LVH) and heart failure (HF), peripheral vascular disease (PVD), carotid atherosclerosis, renal disease, and "subclinical disease."[4,5,32,33] Kannel and colleagues in the Framingham Heart Study have documented the fact that CV risk factors tend to cluster in hypertensives.[34] Hypertensives are more likely to have dyslipidemias, especially elevated serum triglycerides and low levels of high-density lipoprotein cholesterol (HDL-C), and type 2 DM. The common denominator may be insulin resistance, perhaps as a result of the frequent association of hypertension and obesity.[35]

In the last several years, it has become increasingly clear that the risks attributed to hypertension are much more strongly related to the level of systolic BP than to diastolic BP, especially in those over age 50 or 60 years.[36,37] The observation that systolic BP predicts events and TOD better than diastolic BP was persuasively argued in the early 1970s, but it took until 1993, in the Fifth Report of the Joint National Committee on the Detection, Evaluation and Treatment of Hypertension, before systolic BP was given even equal weight to diastolic BP in classification systems.[36,38]

Some have argued that one should not measure diastolic BP other than perhaps to calculate pulse pressure (PP).[39,40] Pulse pressure, the difference between systolic and diastolic BP, is an even better predictor of risk than is systolic BP in most of the epidemiologic studies done to date.[41–46] A wide PP, unless it is a result of aortic insufficiency or an arteriovenous malformation, is a simple clinical indicator of stiffer and less compliant large central arteries and significant arterial damage. Franklin and colleagues, again using data from the Framingham Heart Study cohort, showed that at all levels of systolic BP (even as low as 110 to 130 mmHg), risk is less with higher diastolic BPs.[46] More recent analyses by this group have suggested that these findings may be relevant only in those over age 60, and so it is not appropriate to ignore those with elevated diastolic BP level if their systolic readings are not above normal. The classification systems cited above have been careful not to include PP either in defining the risks of hypertension or in recommending treatment. A recently published position paper from the National High Blood Pressure Education Program has cautioned physicians not to rely on PP measurements until more support is gathered for this position.[47]

With the exception of hypertensive encephalopathy, it has long been felt that few, if any, clinical symptoms can be attributed to increased BP levels. This may have to be reevaluated, however, as newer and very well tolerated drugs are developed and as improved methods of assessing subtle symptoms are perfected. Clinical trials with angiotensin receptor blockers (ARBs), for example, consistently show that the members of the actively treated group have fewer adverse reactions than do those given placebo.[48,49] Furthermore, in the Treatment of Mild Hypertension Study (TOMHS) and the Hypertension Optimum Treatment (HOT) trial, the group with the lowest BP had the fewest complaints.[50,51] These trials utilized a wide variety of drugs to reduce BP and clearly showed not only that lowering BP is safe but that hypertensives treated to lower levels feel better. Hypertension may not be the asymptomatic condition it has long been thought to be.

ECONOMICS

Cost considerations are playing an increasingly important role in the pharmacologic management of hypertension in the United States, and they have always been a major consideration in the rest of the world. No regimen, no matter how carefully and appropriately selected, will be effective if the patient cannot afford it. Moreover, if antihypertensive agents do not appear on the national formulary or the formulary of the insurance company from which a patient gets medication, the cost will not be covered and the patient may not be willing or able to purchase them. Generic preparations are available for every class of antihypertensive agent except ARBs, and these generic preparations tend to be the least expensive options for initial therapy. In general, branded calcium antagonists (CAs) are the most expensive, with ARBs and angiotensin-converting enzyme inhibitors (ACE-Is) the next most expensive drugs. For many of the fixed-dose combinations now available, the cost is less than what would be paid for the individual components if they were purchased separately. It is also customary for fixed-dose combinations that include a thiazide diuretic to cost no more than does the nondiuretic component alone.

A careful analysis of the economics of hypertension treatment has to include more than what is spent on drugs, patient visits, or laboratory tests.[52,53] For many affected (and especially high-risk) patients, the extremely expensive complications of under- and/or untreated hypertension far outweigh the inconvenience and costs associated with effective treatment.[53] Current estimates are that in the United States in the year 2000, hypertension will cost approximately $37.2 billion.[54] Nearly half this total is spent on indirect costs (death benefits for the families of those who die from untreated hypertension, disability payments for stroke survivors, time away from work, and transportation costs, to name a few) and payments to hospitals and nursing homes.[54] Both of these expenses could be reduced if hypertension treatment were more effective in controlling BP and reducing the risk of the clinical sequelae of hypertension, including myocardial infarction (MI), HF, stroke, and end-stage renal disease (ESRD).[55]

PATHOPHYSIOLOGY

Hypertension is a disorder of BP regulation and results from a multitude of causes. Control of BP involves a complex interaction among the kidneys, the central nervous system (CNS) and peripheral nervous system (PNS), and the vascular endothelium thoughout the body as well as a variety of the other organs, such as the adrenal and pituitary glands. The heart is the organ that responds to many of the changes mediated by these systems. It also secretes hormones locally and systemically that interact with substances produced elsewhere and help regulate BP levels. In those genetically predisposed to develop hypertension, an imbalance occurs among the various systems that modulate the level of BP. The sympathetic nervous system (SNS), the renin-angiotensin-aldosterone (RAA) system, vasopressin (VP), nitric oxide (NO), and a host of vasoactive peptides, including endothelin, adrenomedullin, and others produced by the heart and a host of different cells (endothelial and vascular smooth cells, for example), modulate the responses of these systems and help maintain BP over a range commensurate with optimum physical and mental activity. Additionally, these systems affect the ability of the kidney to handle sodium (Na^+) and volume, which Guyton and colleagues feel is the primary controller of BP.[56]

Sympathetic Nervous System and Renal Sodium Handling

Guyton and colleagues noted that while the SNS and the RAA system are important for short-term changes in BP, ultimately it is the kidney that is responsible for long-term blood volume and BP control.[56] High-pressure baroreceptors in the carotid sinus and aortic arch respond to acute elevations in systemic BP by causing a reflex vagal bradycardia that is mediated though the parasympathetic system and inhibition of sympathetic output from the CNS. Low-pressure cardiopulmonary receptors in the atria and ventricles likewise respond to increases in atrial filling by increasing heart rate (HR) through inhibition of the cardiac SNS, increasing atrial natriuretic peptide (ANP) release, and inhibiting VP release.[57–59] These reflexes are largely controlled centrally, particularly in the nucleus tractus solitarii of the dorsal medulla. This vasomotor center also receives input from the limbic system and hypothalamus in response to emotional or psychological stress.

The consequences of SNS stimulation are peripheral vasoconstriction, an increase in HR, release of norepinephrine from the adrenals, and a resultant rise in systemic BP. The increase in SNS activity also plays a role in mediating local vascular hypertrophy and stiffness. Renal efferent sympathetics also are activated and cause internal vasoconstriction with a fall in renal blood flow and an increase in renal vascular resistance.[60] The renal SNS also directly stimulates Na^+ reabsorption and renin release from the juxtaglomerular apparatus.[60–62] Thus, the SNS and CNS have effects on renal handling of Na^+.

Hyperactivity of the SNS has been described in patients with essential hypertension, particularly in the young and those with "high-normal" BP (130 to 139/80 to 89 mmHg).[63,64] Elevated plasma norepinephrine levels with increased HR and cardiac indexes have been described in people with newly diagnosed hypertension.[64] These individuals frequently show exaggerated BP responses to emotional (mental arthimetic) and physical stressors such as ice-water immersion. Additionally, a subset of these patients exhibit elevated plasma renin levels that may reflect beta-adrenergic stimulation of renin secretion.

A defect in baroreceptor sensitivity has been postulated to be responsible for abnormal responsiveness of the SNS and thus may contribute to the increase in BP and HR variability noted in some hypertensive patients.[65] SNS activity also is increased in certain high-risk groups with hypertension, including African-Americans, those with obesity, those with insulin resistance, and those who ingest or inhale certain agents, such as nicotine, alcohol, cyclosporine, and cocaine.[66–68] A very small subset of patients may have hypertension caused by compression of the lateral medulla by cranial nerves and/or vessels.[60] This results in increased SNS activity. Selective decompression of these nerves may ameliorate the hypertension in rare instances. Activation of the CNS/SNS also may result from renal afferent sympathetics from the kidney in hypertensive patients. In experimental models of hypertension, renal sympathectomy resulted in a reduction in BP.[60,64]

The influence of the SNS on Na^+ handling in the kidney also has been examined in detail.[69] Several studies have linked SNS hyperactivity with greater than normal increases in BP in response to a given Na^+ load.[70–73] Indeed, Dahl and Heine were the first to show that hypertension can be transferred from a hypertensive Dahl salt-sensitive rat to a nonhypertensive Dahl salt-resistant rat by transplantation of the kidney.[70] Patients with essential hypertension and associated renal failure have been cured of the underlying hypertension by renal transplantation from a normotensive donor.[74]

Most authorities believe that the mechanism by which the kidney causes hypertension is impairment in the excretion of Na^+.[60,61,71,75–78] This impairment may be related to genetic changes in various Na^+ exchangers in the proximal and distal tubules that result in altered responses to stimulation by the SNS and the RAA system. Epidemiologic studies have linked the relative Na^+ content in the diet with the prevalence of hypertension in various populations, although the value of dietary Na^+ restriction in reducing BP remains controversial (see below).[79,80] Interventional studies with Na^+ restriction and/or loading have revealed that the BP responses in many hypertensive patients are "salt-sensitive": Their BP rises with a salt load.[81,82] In addition, several studies have shown that salt loading of patients with essential hypertension results in a net total body Na^+ accumulation. Three genetic diseases associated with hypertension in childhood (Liddle's syndrome, the syndrome of apparent mineralocorticoid excess, and glucocorticoid-remediable aldosteronism) all are associated with increased reabsorption of Na^+ by the kidney.[83]

A genetically mediated defect in the ability of the kidney to excrete Na^+ does not readily explain certain observations:

- Young hypertensive subjects appear to excrete Na^+ normally or supernormally.
- Individuals with high-normal BP may have a low blood volume.
- As many as 40 percent of people with hypertension do not show a change in BP with Na^+ loading ("salt resistance").
- With aging, salt sensitivity increases both in frequency and in degree such that by age 70, the majority of hypertensive patients are salt-sensitive.

In fact, it has been argued from meta-analyses that salt restriction is not important either in normotensives or in patients with hypertension under age 40.[84,85] All these findings are consistent with the possibility that the defect in Na^+ excretion in hypertensive patients is acquired rather than genetically determined. It should be kept in mind, however, that abnormal Na^+ handling is a mechanism that contributes to elevating BP in many but probably not all patients with hypertension.

The Renin-Angiotensin-Aldosterone System

The RAA system is one of the most important physiologic mediators that regulate blood volume and BP. Plasma angiotensinogen, which is released primarily from the liver, is acted on by renin from the kidney to generate angiotensin I, which is further degraded in the presence of angiotensin-converting enzyme to angiotensin II (AII). In addition to the systemic RAA system, there is now evidence that a local RAA system is present in blood vessels, the heart, the kidney, and elsewhere, where it may mediate local effects (such as tissue remodeling) independent of circulating renin or angiotensinogen levels.

Most of the actions of AII are mediated by the AT_1 receptor and include stimulating vascular smooth muscle contraction and hypertrophy, increasing cardiac contractility, stimulating the SNS in the CNS and PNS, increasing NO production, causing aldosterone and VP release, and increasing thirst (Table 51-4).[86] Within the kidney, stimulation of the AT_1 receptor by AII also causes renal vasoconstriction (especially of the efferent arteriole and vasa rectae), a fall in renal blood flow, and an increase in renal vascular resistance.[87] Angiotensin II also increases Na^+ reabsorption both by increasing aldosterone release and through direct effects on the proximal tubule. Additionally, AII increases the sensitivity of the tubuloglomerular (TG) feedback response.

Angiotensin subtype 2 (AT_2) receptors also are stimulated by angiotensin II. These receptors produce virtually opposite actions in some experimental systems and are clearly active during fetal development (Table 51-4). Their role in healthy adults and even in those with cardiac or vascular damage is still uncertain.

The role of the RAA system in essential hypertension is complex. Whereas plasma renin activity (PRA) is elevated in 20 percent of hypertensive patients, PRA is either normal (50 percent) or low (30 percent) in the majority. However, in many patients with normal plasma renin levels, PRA may be inappropriately high in relation to total body Na^+. This has been suggested by the observation that Na^+ depletion accentuates and Na^+ infusion blunts changes in PRA levels in patients with hypertension. Additional evidence to support this concept comes from the observation that BP in these patients frequently is reduced after the use of ACE-Is or ARBs.[88]

Sealey and colleagues have suggested that the reason for widely varying PRA levels may be nephron heterogeneity within individual kidneys, in which there are some ischemic nephrons that make excess renin and other hyperfiltering nephrons in which renin secretion is suppressed.[89] They postulated that the increased renin release from the ischemic nephrons enters the circulation and then leads to AII generation, which causes inappropriate vasoconstriction and Na^+ reabsorption in the other hyperfiltering nephrons. This results in Na^+ retention and the development of hypertension.

Unfortunately, this is only part of the explanation, since PRA is relatively low in African-Americans and the elderly, two populations with a high prevalence of hypertension and a high rate of complications from hypertension. Low PRA, however, does not necessarily mean that the RAA is not active, since tissue effects and local actions are not necessarily evident from PRA alone.

TABLE 51-4 Characteristics and Functions of AT_1 and AT_2 Receptors

AT_1 Receptors
Always expressed
Mediate vasoconstriction
Mediate growth
Smooth muscle proliferation
Stimulate connective tissue deposit in media
Facilitate low-density lipoprotein cholesterol transport to media
Inhibit endothelial function
Mediate renal tubular sodium reabsorption
AT_2 Receptors
Increased expression during stress or injury
Mediate vasodilatation
Inhibit growth (antiproliferation)
Decreased renal absorption of sodium

Vasopressin

While VP has been clearly shown *not* to play a role in the genesis of essential hypertension, it does play an important role in the maintenance of established hypertension, especially in African-Americans.[90] In African-Americans, studies have shown that selective inhibition of V_1A receptors reduces systolic BP by an additional 8 to 12 mmHg in the presence of a high-salt diet (suppression of the RAA system) and clonidine (suppression of SNS).[91,92] Interestingly, this is not observed in whites. In light of the interaction between arginine vasopressin (AVP), AII, and endothelin on cellular growth and vascular responsiveness, it appears that AVP may have a potentiating effect on one of these other hormones.[93]

Endothelin

Endothelin is known to be the most potent vasoconstrictor in humans.[94] Comparative studies with AII have demonstrated not only that the endothelin family of hormones has cellular actions similar to those of AII but that the two hormones work in concert to potentiate each other's vascular and cellular effects.[95] Given this, however, the specific role of endothelin in the etiology of essential hypertension is minimal.[96] It plays a far more important role in cyclosporine-induced hypertension and decreased renal function as well as in maintaining BP in people with HF.[97]

Endothelin is the major mechanism by which cyclosporine constricts the afferent arteriole of the kidney and reduces renal function. Calcium antagonists and endothelin receptor blockade prevent this reduction. Additionally, endothelin A receptors have been shown to play a major role in contributing to the maintenance of elevated renal perfusion pressure in patients with HF.[98]

Nitric Oxide

Nitric oxide is the vasodilator produced by the endothelium in response to vasoconstrictor hormones, and so the contribution of NO to the maintenance of normal BP is vitally important.[99,100] Defects in NO release or synthesis that are induced by atherosclerosis or that are genetically programmed are a major determinant in predisposing individuals to the development of atherosclerosis and hypertension.[101] NO serves as a major counterbalancing factor that maintains BP within the range necessary to maintain organ perfusion but avoid injury. It counterbalances vasoconstrictive hormones, cytokines such as AII, platelet-derived growth factor (PDGF), tumor necrosis factor-alpha, and other hormones that stimulate its release. Transgenic animal models that do not have the ability to synthesize NO have very high BP and die of CV causes earlier than do animals that can produce NO.

Additionally, NO plays a major role in the genesis of hypertension in people who are insulin-resistant. The underlying mechanisms and the factors that may govern the interaction between insulin and NO have been studied extensively in healthy people and insulin-resistant subjects. It appears that a genetic and/or acquired defect of NO synthesis could represent a central defect that triggers many of the metabolic, vascular, and sympathetic abnormalities characteristic of insulin-resistant states, all of which may predispose to CV.[102]

Ion Transport Abnormalities

A number of dietary factors affect the SNS, the CNS, and the RAA system in those genetically predisposed to develop hypertension. These dietary factors, such as high Na^+ intake and low potassium (K^+), Ca^{2+}, and/or magnesium (Mg^{2+}) intake, may produce, worsen, or attenuate changes in BP. Substantial evidence from animal models of hypertension as well as diabetic and nondiabetic hypertensive individuals supports an association between the hypertension and changes in intracellular pH as well as electrolyte composition.[103–121] These observations have led to various hypotheses regarding the importance of one ion relative to others.

Numerous investigators have documented increases in cytosolic free Na^+ concentrations in cells of hypertensive or diabetic patients compared with age- and sex-matched normotensive or nondiabetic controls.[103–105] These increases result from altered activity of the Na^+/H^+ antiporter and the Na^+/Li^+ countertransporter. These increases in intracellular Na^+ are highly correlated with the presence of an elevated diastolic BP.

The relationship between intracellular Mg^{2+} and BP is less clearly defined. Data from experimental models of hypertension as well as from patients with hypertension demonstrate an inverse relation between intracellular Mg^{2+} concentration and BP elevation.[106,107] The primary mechanism responsible for this relative reduction in intracellular Mg^{2+} relates to Na^+-dependent Mg^{2+} efflux through the plasmalemma membrane.[112]

Increases in the intracellular Ca^{2+} concentration are seen commonly in obese and essential hypertensive subjects.[105,110] Like Na^+, these changes reflect altered membrane ion transport activity. Early clinical studies demonstrated that oral Ca^{2+} ingestion reduces BP, but the results from clinical trials do not consistently show a reduction in BP after Ca^{2+} supplementation.[120,121]

Increased K^+ intake is well known to have effects on BP control through multiple mechanisms, including opening K^+ channels in the vasculature, altering sympathetic neuronal output, and increasing vasodilatory prostaglandins.[122–125] This is exemplified by the fact that hypokalemia in patients will blunt reductions in blood pressure by antihypertensive medication, perhaps because it results in the closure of K^+ channels.

Potassium also plays a role in modulating vascular responsiveness in salt-sensitive individuals. In a recent clinical study, increasing dietary K^+ for 3 weeks in 16 predefined salt-sensitive subjects and 42 salt-resistant subjects resulted in the conversion of all salt-sensitive subjects from nocturnal nondipping to dipping status[126] (see below). These results suggest that a positive relationship between dietary K^+ intake and BP modulation can exist even when daytime BP is unchanged by a high-K^+ diet.[126]

Taken together, these data suggest that both univalent and divalent cations affect vascular responses to stimuli such as those mediated by the RAA and the SNS. Changes in vascular responses are linked to altered function of membrane ion transporters (Na^+/H^+ antiporter, Na^+/K^+/ATPase, Mg^{2+}/Na^+ exchanger, Ca^{2+}/H^+ exchanger, Ca^{2+} ATPase, and others). Both the Na^+/K^+/ATPase and the Ca^{2+}/ATPase pumps are important in maintaining the Ca^{2+} homeostasis of the cell.

Extracellular Volume Homeostasis

Whereas an acute infusion of saline administered to animals with experimentally induced hypertension will initially raise blood volume and cardiac output, the increase in cardiac output is transient and is replaced by a rise in systemic vascular resistance (SVR).[71,72]

There are several potential mechanisms for this observation. First, the normal response to a salt load is inhibition of the SNS. However, it is known that in salt-sensitive patients, the SNS is not inhibited and even may be activated with a salt load.[127,128] A possible explanation is that in the setting of renal dysfunction or intrarenal ischemia, salt loading triggers an intense tuboglomerular feedback signal that activates the renal afferent SNS. This renal response subsequently triggers a CNS response. Indeed, there is evidence that renal afferent nerves activate CNS sympathetic activity in both experimental hypertension and chronic renal disease.

Second, parabiotic experiments have suggested there may be circulating factors in salt-loaded animals with hypertension that are responsible for some of the increase in SVR. One class of factors is circulating $Na^+/K^+/ATPase$ inhibitors, which have been documented in some patients with essential hypertension.[129–131] These substances, one of which is ouabain, are digitalis-like and adrenally derived. Blaustein has suggested that these substances, which presumably are secreted in an attempt to facilitate Na^+ excretion, may have the adverse consequence of increasing intracellular Na^+ and thus facilitating Na^+-Ca^{2+} exchange in vascular smooth muscle cells. This would lead to a rise in intracellular Ca^{2+} and stimulate vascular smooth muscle contraction, vasoconstriction, and a rise in SVR.[110]

A third mechanism is the loss of a vasodepressor substance. There is good evidence that a lipid-like vasodepressor factor termed adrenomedullin is expressed in some of the interstitial cells in the renal medulla and the juxtamedullary region. Release of this factor into the circulation appears to depend on medullary blood flow and can be inhibited if activation of renal SNS or inhibition of NO reduces blood flow.[60] Thus, one might expect to see lower circulating levels of this substance in the setting of tubulointerstitial (TI) injury and intrarenal ischemia.

Fourth, the increase in pressure associated with a saline load could cause increased tension in the peripheral vasculature, leading to microvascular rarefaction (which has been observed in the forearms and nail beds of patients with essential hypertension) that could raise the SVR. An increased pressure load on the vessels also could result in compensatory vascular hypertrophy mediated by local growth factors and the local RAA system. Indeed, there is evidence that AII, PDGF, and basic fibroblast growth factor are involved in these processes.

Mechanisms of Na^+ Retention in Essential Hypertension

A rise in systemic BP normally is associated with brisk natriuresis. This is thought to be due to a transient rise in pressure in the peritubular capillaries in the juxtamedullary region, with a subsequent increase in interstitial pressure and a backflow of Na^+ through the paracellular space of the proximal tubule. Numerous studies have confirmed that most patients with essential hypertension have a defect in the pressure natriuresis curve, in which higher systemic pressures are required to excrete a Na^+ load.[132,133]

A second mechanism for decreased Na^+ excretion is an enhancement of TG feedback. Tubuloglomerular feedback is a reflex vasoconstriction that occurs with chloride delivery to the macula densa, and the vasoconstrictive response will reduce glomerular filtration and Na^+ excretion. TG feedback can be enhanced in the setting of increased local vasoconstrictors such as AII and adenosine or by a reduction in local vasodilators such as NO. TG feedback appears to be enhanced in models of experimental hypertension.[132,134]

Finally, alterations in intrarenal vasoactive mediators may be involved in the impairment of Na^+ excretion in patients with hypertension. In both experimental and human hypertension, there may be low levels of renal vasodilators, such as prostaglandins, dopamine, and NO as well as elevated levels of renal vasoconstrictors such as AII and adenosine and increased activity of the renal SNS. In addition to their effects of enhancing TG feedback, alterations in the levels of these agents could contribute to net Na^+ reabsorption because of their direct effects on tubular Na^+ transport.

Some studies have shown that TI injury can be induced in rats with either catecholamine (phenylephrine) or AII infusion and that subsequently these animals will develop hypertension when placed on a high-salt diet.[134] Evaluation of these biopsies demonstrated focal areas of peritubular capillary rarefaction. This also has been observed in kidney biopsies of patients with essential hypertension. The loss of peritubular capillaries could help explain the impairment of pressure natriuresis. The ischemia related to the vasoconstriction and capillary loss could lead to alterations in the various vasoactive mediators. Indeed, there is some evidence that NO levels fall and adenosine levels rise with TI injury and ischemia, and this could contribute to the enhanced TG feedback that has been observed.[135,136]

While this pathway links a hyperactive SNS or RAA system with TI injury and salt-dependent hypertension, it is likely that TI injury induced in other ways could result in salt-sensitive hypertension. Indeed, it is of interest that TI disease is associated with reflux nephropathy, chronic pyelonephritis, DM, cyclosporine, radiation, lead and analgesic nephropathy, hypercalcemia/nephrocalcinosis, and gout, all of which are strongly associated with hypertension. In addition, it is noteworthy that many high-risk groups associated with salt-dependent essential hypertension, such as aged persons, obese persons, and African-Americans, have a high prevalence of TI disease.

Insulin Resistance

Insulin resistance is a metabolic disorder that is manifested by a reduction in peripheral skeletal muscle utilization of glucose.[35] To fully understand the contribution of insulin resistance to the genesis of hypertension, one has to evaluate the effects of insulin resistance and hyperinsulinemia on factors that contribute to BP elevation. High levels of insulin cause sodium retention and other vascular effects, such as cellular proliferation and matrix expansion.[137] In the presence of hyperinsulinemia, neurohumoral factors such as AII, endothelin, and VP also potentiate proliferation of endothelial and vascular smooth muscle cells.[138] Lastly, the effect of insulin on various growth factors contributes to the development of vascular injury through its potentiation of the atherosclerotic process.[139] These factors in a person genetically predisposed to develop nephropathy can potentiate injury to the vasculature and end organs.

It should be noted, however, that not all subjects with insulin resistance have all the associated components of insulin resistance syndrome or syndrome X, i.e., lipid abnormalities, hyperuricemia, type 2 DM, glucose intolerance, hypertension, microalbuminuria, left ventricular hypertrophy, salt sensitivity, and obesity, among others. Studies in the normotensive offspring of hypertensive nondiabetic parents demonstrate the presence of insulin resistance.[140,141] This is also true for nondiabetic first-degree relatives of patients with type 2 DM.[142] Thus, a genetic predisposition seems to be needed to develop this syndrome.

TABLE 51-5 Candidate Genes Associated with Hypertension and Cardiovascular Risk

- Monogenic forms
  - Glucocorticoid-remediable aldosteronism
  - Liddle's syndrome
- Polygenic forms that affect
  - Angiotensinogen gene
  - Na^+-Li^+ countertransport
  - Epithelial amiloride-sensitive sodium channel
  - Nitric oxide generation
  - Alpha-adducin
  - G_3 beta subunit (intracellular signal transduction)
  - Insertion/deletion of ACE gene

Genetic Factors

Commonly accepted candidate genes associated with the genesis of hypertension are summarized in Table 51-5. Insulin resistance is clearly associated with hypertension. A possible genetic link between the presence of insulin resistance and the development of hypertension has been proposed.[143–146] Recent studies also have identified insulin resistance in the normotensive offspring of parents with essential hypertension. Saad and coworkers evaluated the association between insulin resistance and the propensity to develop hypertension in different racial groups.[147] Those investigators examined Pima Indians, whites, and blacks who were normotensive and nondiabetic. They noted that Pima Indians had higher fasting plasma insulin concentrations than did whites or blacks and lower whole body glucose disposal. They also noted a strong correlation between fasting plasma insulin concentrations and the rate of glucose disposal in whites but not in Pima Indians or blacks. Thus, the development of hypertension does not necessarily correlate with the presence of either hyperinsulinemia or insulin resistance in certain racial groups.

Work by various investigators to isolate a "hypertensive gene" or group of genes has been ongoing for many years. Abnormalities in the angiotensinogen gene identified by Caufield and coworkers provide evidence to link mutations in the angiotensinogen gene to the pathogenesis of essential hypertension.[148] A study of 179 hypertensive sibpairs from 69 type 2 diabetic kindreds showed that specific changes in the linkage of the angiotensinogen gene were highly correlated with the presence of hypertension.[149]

The delineation of a gene profile that will predict who will develop hypertension is near. A number of federally funded studies to gather sib pairs and families to identify candidate genes that predispose individuals to the development of hypertension are under way. Data from these studies may lead to the identification of such genes within the next 5 to 10 years. Thus, until these genetic profiles are delineated, it will be necessary to rely on the data garnered from epidemiologic studies to identify subjects at risk for the development of hypertension and CV events.

These are several clear examples of genetic influences in hypertension.

GLUCOCORTICOID-REMEDIABLE ALDOSTERONISM

This is an inherited autosomal dominant disorder that mimics an aldosterone-producing adenoma.[150] An important clinical clue to diagnosing this disease is the age at onset of hypertension. Patients with glucocorticoid-remediable aldosteronism (GRA) typically are diagnosed with high BP as children, whereas patients with other mineralocorticoid excess states, such as aldosterone-producing adenomas (APA) and idiopathic adrenal hyperplasia, usually are diagnosed in the third through sixth decades of life. A strong family history of hypertension is the rule, often associated with early death of affected family members from cerebrovascular accidents, as is seen characteristically in some GRA families.

In GRA, the RAA system is suppressed and aldosterone secretion is regulated solely by ACTH. As a result, plasma aldosterone levels usually decline during the course of an upright posture study, similar to what is seen in patients with APA.[151–153] The administration of exogenous ACTH to patients with GRA is associated with aldosterone hyperresponsiveness compared with normal subjects.[153] Moreover, in contrast to normal subjects in whom continuous ACTH administration is associated with a rise and a subsequent fall in aldosterone to basal levels over days, patients with GRA exhibit an exuberant aldosterone response that is sustained as long as ACTH is infused.

GRA is caused by a genetic mutation that results in a hybrid or chimeric gene product fusing nucleotide sequences of the 11-hydroxylase and aldosterone synthase genes.[154,155] Characterization of this chimeric gene indicates that it arose from unequal crossing between 11-hydroxylase and aldosterone synthase genes.[155] These two genes are located in close proximity on human chromosome 8, are 95 percent homologous in nucleotide sequence, and have an identical intron-exon structure. The structure of the duplicated gene contains the 5′ regulatory sequences that confer the ACTH responsiveness of 11-hydroxylase fused to more distal coding sequences of the aldosterone synthase gene.[153,154] Therefore, this hybrid gene is expected to be regulated by ACTH and have aldosterone synthase activity. This hybrid gene allows ectopic expression of aldosterone synthase activity in the ACTH-regulated zona fasciculata, which normally produces cortisol.[156,157] This abnormal gene duplication can be detected readily by southern blotting, allowing for direct genetic screening for this disorder with a small blood sample.

GLUCOCORTICOID RESISTANCE

The structure, growth, and secretory activity of the adrenal cortical zona fasciculata are regulated largely by ACTH. Only cortisol can inhibit ACTH release. An increase in ACTH release raises the levels of cortisol, which then inhibits the release of ACTH. This continuous inhibitory feedback effect of cortisol on ACTH release is interrupted in patients with glucocorticoid resistance. In this disorder, although cortisol levels are exceedingly high, ACTH release is not inhibited, leading to uninhibited ACTH secretion, which in turn stimulates the adrenal cortex to produce 11-deoxycorticosterone (DOC).[157] If sufficient DOC is secreted, salt and water retention ensue, precipitating hypertension and hypokalemia. Animal studies indicate that the mechanism for this may in part be related to changes in hippocampal steroid receptor building.[158]

Animal studies also indicate that an expressional downregulation of endothelial cell nitric oxide synthase (NOS III) may contribute to the hypertension caused by glucocorticoids. Ingestion of dexamethasone by telemetrically instrumented rats increased BP progressively over 7 days. Plasma oxidation products of NO decreased to 40 percent, and the expression of endothelial NOS III was found to be downregulated in the aorta and several other tissues in glucocorticoid-treated rats. Dexamethasone treatment significantly attenuated the relaxation to the endothelium-dependent vasodilator acetylcholine but not to the endothelium-independent vasodilator S-nitroso-*N*-acetyl-D,L-penicillamine. Additionally, incubation of human umbilical vein endothelial cells or bovine aortic endothelial cells with several glucocorticoids reduced NOS III mRNA and protein expression to 60 to 70 percent of control, an effect that was prevented by the glucocorticoid receptor antagonist mifepristone.[159]

LIDDLE'S SYNDROME

Liddle's syndrome is an autosomal dominant disorder that mimics the signs and symptoms of mineralocorticoid excess.[160] The fault appears to lie with continuously avid Na^+ channels in the distal nephron, resulting in excessive salt absorption and K^+ wasting (despite negligible aldosterone production) and severe hypertension.[161,162] A prominent feature is premature death from stroke or HF. The clinical manifestations can be corrected by triamterene and amiloride but not by spironolactone. Triamterene and amiloride directly block the Na^+ channel, whereas spironolactone inhibits Na^+ absorption by binding the aldosterone receptor.

The cellular defect associated with this syndrome is located on the apical portion of the tubule where the epithelial Na^+ channel (EnaC) located on the apical membrane plays a critical role in Na^+ absorption. Mutations in this channel cause diseases of Na^+ homeostasis, including a genetic form of hypertension (Liddle's syndrome inhibits cAMP-mediated stimulation of EnaC). Thus, the apical Na^+ channels and transepithelial Na^+ current are inhibited. Experimental data indicate that cAMP-mediated translocation of EnaC to the cell surface is defective in patients with Liddle's syndrome.[163]

DIAGNOSIS OF HYPERTENSION

Estimation of the pressure generated by the heart during its normal contractile cycle has been measured for more than 100 years. The value of such readings in predicting prognosis was recognized in the early 1930s by insurance companies, which probably have the best data correlating causal BP measurements and the risk of future disability and death.[164] Since the second half of the 1800s, palpation of the pulse and appreciation of the contour and pressure within a peripheral artery were skills learned only through extensive experience. Such subjective observations were supplanted by objective (albeit indirect) measurements after the introduction of the Riva-Rocci sphygmomanometer in the late nineteenth century.[165,166] This instrument was refined by Janeway and Korotkoff, who characterized the sounds heard when using a stethoscope placed over the compressed artery in 1906.[167–169] Even today, the terminology introduced by Korotkoff is still used: Systolic BP is recognized when clear and repetitive tapping sounds are heard; diastolic BP is recorded when the sounds disappear. Exceptions to these general rules are still recognized among patients who have audible sounds even down to zero mmHg and in obstetric patients: In both situations, the "muffling" of the sounds (Korotkoff phase IV) is recorded either in addition to the phase V measurement or as the diastolic BP, respectively.[170]

Techniques of Measuring Blood Pressure

The proper technique for accurate BP measurement typically is taught very early during medical training but then seldom is followed.[171–173] Many expert panels have made recommendations regarding the methodology of BP measurement, that frequently do not agree in all details, but several general principles can be extracted[174–177]:

TABLE 51-6 Blood Pressure Cuff Names and Sizes

Cuff	Width, cm	Length, cm
Newborn	2.5–4.0	5.0–9.0
Infant	4.0–6.0	11.5–18.0
Child	7.5–9.0	17.0–19.0
Normal adult	11.5–13.0	22.0–26.0
Large adult	14.0–15.0	30.5–33.0
Thigh	18.0–19.0	36.0–38.0

- There are six sizes of commonly available BP cuffs (Table 51-6). Using a smaller than recommended cuff on a larger arm typically results in an overestimation of casual BP. In obese or muscular persons, the large adult-size cuff is required for all those with an arm circumference at the mid-humerus over 38 cm. In very large individuals, a "thigh" cuff is often necessary.[178]
- In accurately measuring BP, the deflation rate of the column of mercury should be 2 to 3 mmHg/s. The lower rate of deflation should be used for persons with HRs less than 72 beats per minute (bpm); the more rapid deflation is appropriate only for those with resting tachycardia. If the precision of measurement is to be at least 2 mmHg, the observer should have the opportunity to hear at least one Korotkoff sound at each 2-mmHg gradation of the mercury column. Thus, the proper deflation rate depends on the HR of the subject and is unlikely to be more than 3 mmHg/s if a precise BP measurement is desired.
- It is unusual for a single BP measurement to be an accurate indicator of future CV risk; multiple measurements made on different occasions are more likely to be helpful in deciding whether a particular person ought to have his or her BP lowered. Although it is traditional to average the second and third of a series of BP measurements in a single position (e.g., supine, seated, or standing) and record this as the "average BP" at a given visit, recent "quality care guidelines" mandate instead the recording of individual BP measurements, with the lowest on a given date being the one of greatest interest to auditors. For these reasons, it is quickly becoming "standard practice" to record individual readings and is especially important to measure BP in several positions (including standing), since the auditors record only the lowest BP reading (in any position) as the "BP taken at that visit."[179] The BP readings of many physicians participating in managed care audits are being judged as a "quality of care" indicator, and recording the largest number of BP measurements in several positions offers the greatest opportunity to have at least one which is deemed "acceptable."[179]
- Most of the long-term data on hypertension and its treatment were derived from "casual" measurements made with a mercury sphygmomanometer and stethoscope in a health care provider's office. Physicians and patients often are more interested and impressed by BP readings taken in other settings (e.g., home monitors or ambulatory BP monitoring devices, both of which are discussed further below), but the great

majority of data linking BP measurements to adverse clinical sequelae (including MI, stroke, and death) were made in the traditional fashion in the physician's office, and for now, office readings taken by a trained professional should be the BP used for diagnosing and treating hypertensives in all but a few special situations.

Blood pressure is subject to a large degree of intrinsic variability. Several steps can be taken to minimize this variability, including the following:

- Taking multiple measurements, especially when the pulse is irregular (e.g., atrial fibrillation). This is necessary because ventricular filling pressures vary considerably as a result of variability of diastolic filling time.[180] Blood pressure variability is especially pronounced in older persons with primarily or exclusively systolic BP evaluations.
- Centering the bladder of the cuff over the brachial artery with its lower edge within 2.5 cm of the antecubital fossa. This leaves enough space so that the stethoscope head can be applied inferiorly without touching the cuff (and generating background noise).
- Having the subject rest silently and comfortably (with back support if seated) for at least 5 min before the measurement.
- Abstaining from drinking caffeine or alcohol-containing beverages or tobacco use within 30 min before a BP measurement.
- Questioning the subject regarding the most recent meal or evacuation of bowels or bladder. Distended abdominal viscera not only are painful but routinely cause elevations in BP, presumably related to anxiety and pain. Older persons typically have a lower BP postprandially; thus, it is often necessary to inquire about and record when the last meal was eaten.
- Assuring that the arm is supported at the level of the heart. Both muscular work (of tensed muscles around the elbow) and hydrostatic pressure caused by a "dangling arm" increase the pressure necessary to obliterate the pulse and lead to overestimates of systolic BP.
- Listening over the brachial artery by using the bell of the stethoscope with minimal pressure exerted on the skin. At the conclusion of the BP measurement, there should be no lasting indentations in the area where the head of the stethoscope was placed. Otherwise the systolic BP is likely to be overestimated and the diastolic BP to be underestimated because too great a pressure was exerted directly over the artery.
- The "peak inflation level" of the mercury column should be determined by using palpation of the radial artery before the stethoscope is applied. For all subsequent BP measurements, the cuff typically should be inflated 20 mmHg higher than the pressure at which the palpable pulse at the radial artery disappears. Important prognostic information may be missed if the "auscultatory gap" is not detected; this risk is minimized by determining the peak inflation level by palpation before the stethoscope is applied.[181]
- Although mercury columns traditionally have been used in the measurement of BP, environmental concerns associated with elemental mercury are increasing. In Sweden and many other countries, elemental mercury is forbidden in the workplace. Nonetheless, sphygmomanometers used in the measurement of BP should be calibrated frequently and routinely against such standards (typically every 6 months) to assure accuracy.
- Attempting to avoid "terminal digit preference." Traditionally, BP measurements have been made to the nearest 2 mmHg (the typical markings on a mercury sphygmomanometer). Theoretically, in a large collection of systolic and diastolic BP measurements, there should be an equal number of readings ending in 0, 2, 4, 6, or 8 mmHg. It is often instructive to compare the actual distribution of terminal digits with the 20 percent expected for each one. This typically reveals a preference for 0 (in inpatient medical services, where BP readings are typically precise to ±10 mmHg) or 8 (for outpatients in a managed care organization being graded on how many people are <140/90 mmHg).
- Measurements of BP in both arms typically are obtained at the initial visit, and the arm with the higher BP is used thereafter if the difference is greater than 10/5 mmHg. In such situations, there is often concern about coarctation of the aorta or Takayasu's arteritis or moyamoya disease, but seldom is this seen on ultrasonography or other confirmatory testing. Blood pressure measurement in a leg should be commonplace in all young hypertensives at the first visit and may be useful in older people as a peripheral indicator of aortic insufficiency ("Hill's sign").
- Assuring that the equipment used to measure BP is in good working order. Many sphygmomanometers (even in hospitals) are in poor repair and should be cleaned, calibrated, and fitted with nonleaking tubing and properly sized cuffs. The interest in BP measurements recently demonstrated by agencies that certify health systems for quality has improved the chance that any given patient will be hospitalized in a bed with properly maintained BP-measuring equipment.

Home Blood Pressure Measurements

The technology for obtaining accurate and reproducible BP measurements outside the traditional medical environment has improved greatly in the last 20 years. Many types of machines now exist (Table 51-7) that are convenient, inexpensive, and relatively accurate. Even persons with hearing difficulties, problems with hand-eye coordination, and other disabilities can operate semiautomatic devices with digital readouts and printers to estimate BP. Some authorities feel that such devices should be provided to every person with elevated BP, but others are concerned about overinterpretation of the data, which generally have not been used commonly in clinical decision making in clinical trials and should not be used routinely in practice to make diagnostic or therapeutic decisions.

Home BP readings are typically lower (by an average of 12/7 mmHg) than measurements taken in the traditional medical environment, even in normotensive subjects.[21] Home readings tend to be better correlated with both the extent of TOD and the risk of future mortality than are readings taken in the physician's office.[182] Home readings can be helpful in evaluating symptoms suggestive of hypotension, especially if the symptoms are intermittent or infrequent. During treatment, reliable home readings can lower costs by substituting for multiple visits to health care providers.[183] Persons who routinely measure BP at home probably have a better prognosis than do those who do not because of both selection bias (they tend to be more interested in their BP than are those who refuse to purchase and use a home BP machine) and social support (when a friend or

TABLE 51-7 Advantages and Disadvantages of Methods of BP Measurement Available to Patients in the Outpatient Setting

Attribute	Anaeroid with Stethoscope	Oscillometric with Stethoscope	Oscillometric with Digital Readout
Coordination necessary	Yes	Yes	Less so
Affected by presbyacusis	Yes	Yes	No
Affected by presbyopia	Yes	Less so	Less so
Widely available	Yes	Less so	Increasingly
Inexpensive	Yes	Less so	Increasingly
Good-quality results	Yes, with effort	Yes, with effort	Yes
Increases patients' interest in managing BP	Yes	Yes	Yes
Battery-powered	No	Yes	Yes
Affected by impaired grip strength	Yes	No	No
Independently validated by prospective studies	No	No	No

spouse becomes involved in measurement and overseeing pill-taking and appointment-keeping behaviors).

Home BP readings should be interpreted cautiously, carefully, and conservatively.[184] There are no data from long-term clinical studies that based all treatment decisions solely on home readings, but several preliminary reports show benefit from supplementing office BP measurements with home readings.[185,186] Several studies have shown that prognosis is better predicted by home readings than by one or two "casual" BP measurements.[187–189] Many of the factors that contribute to BP variability are more difficult to control in the home environment, including intrinsic circadian variation, food and alcohol ingestion, exercise, and stress. The possibility that home BP measurements will become an obsession is also a disadvantage. If home readings are to be taken, most authorities recommend that the instrument be calibrated against a mercury sphygmomanometer by using a Y-tube and that the technique of the measurer be checked. Home readings can be a useful adjunct to information obtained in the physician's office, especially when the two are widely disparate. One long-term study showed that people with much lower home BP readings (compared with those in the physician's office) suffer fewer major CV events than do people who have elevated readings both in the office and at home.[187,190] The authors recommend that patients who are interested in and capable of measuring their BP at home do it at a fixed time of the day and record all the readings obtained. The physician then can review them during the office visit and strive to educate the patients about the difficulties of interpretation of the readings.

Ambulatory Blood Pressure Monitoring

Extensive research has led to a better definition of the role of automatic recorders that measure BP frequently over a 24-h period during a person's usual daily activities (including sleep). Despite the acquisition and dissemination of excellent data, however, the use of these devices by practitioners in the United States has been extremely limited, mostly because of a lack of reimbursement by third-party payers. As a research tool, however, the advantages and disadvantages of ambulatory blood pressure monitoring (ABPM) have been well documented (Table 51-8), normal values have been defined (Table 51-2), and multiple publications correlating abnormal patterns of ABPM with adverse outcomes have appeared.[191,192] Several expert panels have defined the special situations in which ABPM is particularly useful (Table 51-9).

Several varieties of ABPM devices are currently available. In the United States, those which measure BP indirectly (i.e., without arterial cannulation) use either an auscultatory or an oscillometric technique. The former type uses a microphone placed over the artery to detect Korotkoff sounds in the traditional fashion. The latter measures biophysical oscillations of the brachial artery, which are compared (using a standardized algorithm) with those observed with a mercury sphygmomanometer: Systolic BP is determined directly from the threshold oscillation, mean arterial pressure is estimated, and diastolic

TABLE 51-8 Advantages and Disadvantages of Ambulatory Blood Pressure Monitoring

ADVANTAGES

- Many BP and pulse measurements during 24-h period
- Measures diurnal variation (including during sleep)
- Measures BP and pulse during daily activities
- Can identify "white coat" hypertension
- No "alerting response"
- No placebo effect
- Better correlation with target organ damage than other methods

DISADVANTAGES

- Cost
- Limited availability of equipment
- Disruption of daily activities from noise/discomfort (e.g., sleep quality, flaccid arm during measurement)
- Limited "normative" data
- Limited guidelines (or consensus) for interpretation of data in individuals
- Few long-term prospective studies demonstrating utility compared with traditional (and much less expensive) BP measurements

SOURCE: Adapted from Elliott WJ, Black HR. Special situations and special considerations. In: Hollenberg NK, ed. *Hypertension: Mechanism and Treatment.* Volume 1 of Braunwald EB, ed. *Atlas of Heart Disease.* Philadelphia: Current Medicine; 1995:12-1.

TABLE 51-9 Situations in Which ABPM is Useful

"High-normal" blood pressure without target organ damage
Office or "white coat" hypertension
Refractory hypertension
Episodic hypertension
Symptoms consistent with hypotension associated with antihypertensive medication
Hypertension with autonomic dysfunction
Nocturnal hypertension
Evaluation of efficacy of antihypertensive drugs in clinical research

SOURCE: Adapted from the National High Blood Pressure Education Program's Working Group Report on Ambulatory Blood Pressure Monitoring. *Arch Intern Med* 1990; 150:2270–2280.

BP is calculated. Both types of monitors are small (<450 g), simple to apply and use, accurate, relatively quiet and tolerable, and powered by two to four small batteries. Data from 80 to 120 measurements of BP and pulse typically are stored in a small microprocessor and then downloaded into a desktop computer, which then edits the readings and prints the report.

None of the currently available ABPM devices is completely without problems. Devices that rely on direct measurements require 24 h of arterial cannulation, which is potentially dangerous, and rarely are used even for research. Indirect measurements of BP using auscultatory techniques can be confused by ambient noise levels even if R-wave gating is used (this requires the electrocardiographic leads to be attached to the chest). Oscillometric techniques require that the subject keep the arm straight and flaccid during the measurement and can be completely confused if the subject has a tremor. The interpretation of ABPM readings may be enhanced by a diary of the subject's activities, but such diaries are not always completed.

ABPM makes it possible to measure BP routinely during sleep and has reawakened interest in the circadian variation of HR and BP. Most normotensives and perhaps 80 percent of hypertensives have at least a 10 percent drop in BP during sleep compared with the daytime average. Although there may be some important demographic confounders (blacks and the elderly have less prominent "dips"[193,194]), several prospective studies have shown an increased risk of CV events among those with a "nondipping" BP or pulse pattern.[195–197] However, there is concern, based on several Japanese studies, that elderly persons with more than a 20 percent difference between nighttime and daytime average BPs ("excessive dippers") may suffer unrecognized ischemia in "watershed areas" (of the brain and other organs) during sleep if their BP declines below the autoregulatory threshold.[198]

During the last 15 years, research has demonstrated an important correlation between ABPM readings and the prevalence and extent of TOD in hypertensives. Compared with "casual" BP measurements (obtained in the health care provider's office), ABPM measurements clearly are a better predictor of LVH, cardiac function, and overall scores summing optic, carotid, cardiac, renal, and peripheral vascular damage resulting from elevated BP.[199–201] Ambulatory BP monitoring also may be useful in identifying the small minority of typically unrecognized patients [61 of 234 (26 percent) in New York City] with "white coat normotension" who have normal BP readings in the physician's office but elevated ABPM readings with LVH and carotid wall thickening similar to that usually seen in sustained hypertensives.[202]

Perhaps the most important data demonstrating the value of ABPM have come from recent end-point studies of CV events (death, MI, stroke). In the first published study of outcomes in central Italy, ABPM was the best predictor of future CV events; "nondipper hypertensives" had approximately three times the risk of hypertensives whose BP was ≥10 percent lower at night compared to daytime ("dippers").[195] A population-based study involving 1572 men and women of ABPM versus casual and home BPs has been ongoing since 1987 in Ohasama, Japan.[188] After an average of approximately 5 years of follow-up, there was no significant relationship between one casual BP measurement and future CV mortality. However, there was a highly significantly increased risk of CV death in the quintile with the highest ABPM, and the lowest risk was found in those in the lowest quintile of ABPM.[189] The value of ABPM in refractory hypertension was demonstrated in a study of 86 hypertensive people taking on average three antihypertensive medications daily.[203] Follow-up data were collected approximately 4 years after an ABPM was performed; the patients having ABPM results in the lowest tertile had significantly lower rates of CV complications: 2.2 versus 9.5 versus 13.5 events per 100 patient-years. These data suggest that ABPM may be helpful in sorting out which patients with elevated office BP measurements who already are taking multiple antihypertensive medications ought to have intensified treatment and which ones can be spared the additional expense and risk. A subsidy of the Systolic Hypertension in Europe (Syst-EUR) trial involved 808 patients who had ABPM in addition to the usual clinic BP measurements before randomization to placebo or active treatment.[197] In the group randomized to placebo, ABPM was clearly a better predictor of future CV events than was the office BP measurement. Active treatment reduced the difference in prognosis among ambulatory and office measurements. Furthermore, the risk of a CV event was much higher in patients who did not display a nocturnal decline in BP. These data suggest (but do not prove) that the poor prognosis seen with nondipping hypertension can be mitigated by active antihypertensive treatment.

White Coat Hypertension

Since the advent of technology that allows accurate BP measurement outside the health care provider's office, it has been estimated by many but not all reports that 10 to 20 percent of American hypertensives have substantially lower BP measurements in other settings.[204] The name *white coat hypertension* has been given to the situation in which BP measurements outside the health care setting are considerably lower than those in it even though the "white coat" itself is unlikely to be the only factor that increases BP. Careful studies originally done in Italy and later corroborated in other countries show that BP rises in response to an approaching physician who is not previously known to the subject. This apparently does not happen if the subject is approached by a nurse even if she or he is wearing a white coat.

The clinical consequences and prognostic significance of white coat hypertension have been hotly debated in the medical literature for some years. One school of thought suggests that if a person has an acute rise in BP caused by stress related to an approaching physician, similar elevations in BP are likely whenever a stressful stimulus is encountered. Thus, some of the literature supports the concept that the white coat response is merely a precursor to "more substantial and more sustained hypertension."[205] This point of view is buttressed by the realization that in several clinical and population-based studies, white coat hypertension also is found in people with a greater prevalence of subclinical risk factors for CV, including LVH, a family history of hypertension and heart disease, hypertriglyceridemia, elevated fasting insulin levels, and lower HDL-C levels.[205–208]

A second school of thought, based on more careful and conservative definitions of the white coat effect, proposes that some individuals consistently show a similar and marked elevation in BP in response to the health care environment. Using somewhat more stringent criteria than the studies cited above, several long-term studies have shown a greatly reduced risk of either TOD or major CV sequelae among people with lower BPs measured either at home or by 24-h BP monitoring compared with measurements taken in the same person in the physician's office.[187,190,195] Whether the future risk of such individuals for CV events is similar (or even identical) to that of completely normotensive people is open to question. A third group has claimed that white coat hypertension simply represents regression to the mean in those with considerable BP variability.[204]

The best approach to the treatment of white coat hypertension is unresolved. Clearly, such individuals would benefit from lifestyle modification, which presumably would reduce the probability of progression to sustained hypertension. Completely abstaining from antihypertensive medication in "white coat hypertensives" appears unwise. Verdecchia and colleagues have published data indicating that in the long term, the risk of future CV events did not differ between white coat and sustained hypertensives when both were treated with antihypertensive medications.[209] Whether intensive treatment with continuous antihypertensive medication is warranted for only temporary increases in BP is debatable. Clearly, the treatment and repeated ABPM sessions required to monitor therapy would not be very cost-effective. The cost-effectiveness of ABPM to diagnose and monitor people with white coat hypertension has been estimated by several groups, primarily because 10 to 20 percent of hypertensives might be spared the cost of treatment and close follow-up.[210–212] One ABPM session annually has been set as the upper limit of what most American health plans could afford.[213] Several authoritative groups have recommended that ABPM be used sparingly in the general antihypertensive population but may be more widely used in managed care, veterans' hospitals, and other situations where minimal incremental direct costs are involved.[213,214]

EVALUATION OF THE HYPERTENSIVE PATIENT

Six key issues must be addressed during the initial office evaluation of a person with elevated BP readings:

- Documenting an accurate diagnosis of hypertension (see above)
- Defining the presence or absence of TOD related to hypertension
- Screening for other CV risk factors that often accompany hypertension
- Stratifying risk for CVD (according to risk Group A, B, or C in JNC VI)[11]
- Assessing whether the person is likely to have an identifiable cause of hypertension (secondary hypertension) and should have further diagnostic testing to confirm or exclude the diagnosis
- Obtaining data that may be helpful in the initial choice and subsequent choice of therapy

There are many diagnostic possibilities for explaining a single set of elevated BP readings (Tables 51-10 and 51-11). Aside from those who take one of several types of drugs known to elevate BP, many persons with only one elevated BP reading will have their BP decline and return to the normal range. This is the reason for recommending multiple encounters (at least two or three) before a diagnosis of hypertension is firmly established.

Routine Evaluation in All Hypertensive Patients

The recommendations of JNC VI and other national and international expert panels limit the number of and the expense related to initial tests for the routine evaluation of a hypertensive patient[11,18,19] (Table 51-12). Those which are used in assessing the presence or absence of TOD include physical examination, blood urea nitrogen (BUN)/creatinine, electrolytes, urinalysis, and an electrocardiogram (ECG). Assessing the number of CV risk factors can be accomplished with the medical history, chemistry panel [glucose, total cholesterol (TC), triglycerides], and urinalysis. The JNC VI suggests stratifying patients' risk for CV into three risk groups (Table 51-3). Other national expert panels have even more elaborate systems for linking the assessment of CV risk and the intensity of antihypertensive treatment.[19,215]

Several elements of the evaluation of a hypertensive patient warrant further comment. The physical examination needs to be "directed" toward looking for clues that might indicate an identifiable secondary cause of hypertension such as an abdominal or flank bruit, which would be a sign of visceral atherosclerosis or perhaps renal artery fibromuscular disease, or an abdominal or flank mass that might be a pheochromocytoma or a polycystic kidney.

Proper examination of the optic fundus often is neglected even though it is a valuable tool for evaluating hypertensive patients. In the years before effective antihypertensive drug therapy became available, the most important predictor of future CV mortality and morbidity was not the level of BP but in the appearance of TOD in the optic fundi.[216] Although the prognosis of hypertensive patients has improved greatly since that time, the appreciation of hypertension-related changes in the optic fundus is still important in the assessment of both the severity and the duration of elevated BP. The optic fundus is the only site in the entire body where blood vessels can be examined directly. Very few patients with a recent onset of hypertension have Keith-Wagener-Barker (KWB) grade III or IV fundi (Table 51-13).

Arteriosclerosis can be directly recognized, and the severity and duration of previous hypertension can be estimated through the appreciation of abnormalities of the retinal arteries.[217] The

TABLE 51-10 Causes of Hypertension

I. Systolic and diastolic hypertension
  A. Primary, essential or idiopathic
  B. Secondary
    1. Renal
      a. Renal parenchymal disease
        (1) Acute glomerulonephritis
        (2) Chronic nephritis
        (3) Polycystic disease
        (4) Diabetic nephropathy
        (5) Hydronephrosis
      b. Renovascular
        (1) Renal artery stenosis
        (2) Intrarenal vaculitis
      c. Renin-producing tumors
      d. Renoprival
      e. Primary sodium retention (Liddle's syndrome, Gordon's syndrome)
    2. Endocrine
      a. Acromegaly
      b. Hypothyroidism
      c. Hyperthyroidism
      d. Hypercalcemia (hyperparathyroidism)
      e. Adrenal
        (1) Cortical
          (a) Cushing's syndrome
          (b) Primary aldosteronism
          (c) Congenital adrenal hyperplasia
          (d) Apparent mineralocorticoid excess (licorice)
        (2) Medullary: pheochromocytoma
      f. Extraadrenal chromaffin tumors
      g. Carcinoid
      h. Exogenous hormones
        (1) Estrogen
        (2) Glucocorticoids
        (3) Mineralocorticoids
        (4) Sympathomimetics
        (5) Tyramine-containing foods and monoamine oxidase inhibitors
    3. Coarctation of the aorta
    4. Pregnancy-induced hypertension
    5. Neurologic disorders
      a. Increased intracranial pressure
        (1) Brain tumor
        (2) Encephalitis
        (3) Respiratory acidosis
      b. Sleep apnea
      c. Quadriplegia
      d. Acute porphyria
      e. Familial dysautonomia
      f. Lead poisoning
      g. Guillain-Barré syndrome
    6. Acute stress, including surgery
      a. Psychogenic hyperventilation
      b. Hypoglycemia
      c. Burns
      d. Pancreatitis
      e. Alcohol withdrawal
      f. Sickle cell crisis
      g. After resuscitation
      h. Postoperative
    7. Increased intravascular volume
    8. Alcohol and drug use
II. Systolic hypertension
  A. Increased cardiac output
    1. Aortic valvular insufficiency
    2. Arteriovenous fistula, patent ductus arteriosus
    3. Thyrotoxicosis
    4. Paget's disease of bone
    5. Beriberi
    6. Hyperkinetic circulation
  B. Rigidity of aorta
III. Iatrogenic hypertension (see Table 51-11)

SOURCE: Kaplan NM. Systemic hypertension: Mechanisms and diagnosis. In: Braunwald E, ed. *Heart Disease,* 5th ed. Philadelphia: Saunders; 1997:807.

TABLE 51-11 Drugs Known to Elevate Blood Pressure

Nonsteroidal anti-inflammatory drugs
Sympathomimetic amines (e.g., phenylpropanolamines)
Estrogen and estrogen analogs (e.g., oral contraceptive pills and hormone replacement therapy)
Methylxanthines (e.g., theophylline, caffeine, theobromine)
Cyclosporine
Erythropoietin
Cocaine
Nicotine
Phencyclidine ("angel dust")
"Herbal ecstasy" (and other ephedra-containing substances)
Withdrawal from certain drugs (e.g., beta blockers, alpha agonists, opioids, ethanol, calcium antagonists)

TABLE 51-12 Routine Tests Recommended by JNC VI for the Initial Evaluation of a Hypertensive Patient

Serum chemistry (glucose, potassium, creatinine)
Urinalysis
Electrocardiogram

TABLE 51-13 Keith-Wagener-Barker Classification of Optic Fundi

Grade	Characteristic Finding
I	Arterial tortuosity, localized arterial spasm or narrowing (relative to neighboring vein), "silver wiring"
II	Extensive or generalized arteriolar narrowing, resulting in arteriovenous crossing changes ("arterial nicking")
III	Hemorrhages or exudates
IV	Papilledema

normal yellowish-white color of the retinal arteries gradually changes to a reddish-brown tone ("copper wire"), and the ratio of artery/vein diameters is reduced from the normal 2:3 to less than 1:3. Over time, the column of blood within the artery gradually diminishes and the artery is reduced to a whitish thread ("silver wire") despite a persistent (albeit reduced) flow of blood. "AV nicking" is perhaps the most easily recognized ocular abnormality in hypertension. When the thickened artery containing blood at elevated pressure compresses a low-pressure, thin-walled vein within the shared adventitial sheath, the vein disappears from view. Hypertension is therefore both epidemiologically and pathophysiologically a risk factor for retinal vein occlusion, although this is not a common occurrence.[218,219] When arterial blood flow is reduced sufficiently to cause infarction of underlying retinal tissue, round to oval white patches with fluffy borders are formed ("cytoid bodies" or "cotton-wool spots"). When there is breakdown in the blood-retinal barrier (caused by a ruptured aneurysm, neovascularization—typically in diabetics—or "blowout" hemorrhages resulting from hypertension), intraretinal "flame-shaped" hemorrhages can be recognized on direct ophthalmoscopy. The leakage of plasma into the macular space often causes an acute reduction in vision and leaves behind the "macular star figure" for years thereafter. Grade IV retinopathy (papilledema), which is the hallmark of either retinal vein occlusion or a hypertensive emergency, usually is caused by ischemia in the optic nerve circulation resulting from increased intraocular or intracranial pressure and diminished axoplasmic flow in the optic nerve fibers. In some cases, particularly when BP is not exceedingly high and there is no other evidence of acute TOD from a hypertensive emergency, another cause should be sought. Papilledema without other evidence of hypertensive retinopathy generally is due to another etiology.

The impact of controlling hypertension on ophthalmic end points (e.g., vision loss, retinal hemorrhages, and laser photocoagulation procedures) has not received much attention in the general medical literature. There are nonetheless several reports of reduced risk of these end points in several clinical trials that assessed their incidence prospectively, particularly among diabetic hypertensives.[220-222]

Cardiac Evaluation

One of the most important elements of the physical examination of hypertensive patients is the cardiac examination. An atrial (S_4) gallop is an extremely common finding and may be a vital clue to the presence of hypertensive heart disease.

A key part of the laboratory evaluation is directed at determining whether LVH is present. The ECG is currently recommended by nearly all authorities as part of the initial evaluation of persons with hypertension. Not only is the ECG useful in documenting previously undetected MI, myocardial ischemia, and/or cardiac rhythm disturbances, it is the least expensive and possibly the most cost-effective way to diagnose and/or exclude LVH. Although several studies have suggested that compared with echocardiography, computed axial tomography (CAT), or magnetic resonance imaging (MRI) of the heart, the ECG is perhaps only 10 to 50 percent sensitive (depending on which criteria are used) and at best 80 percent specific, the expense of these more accurate methods of screening for LVH limits their use.[223-225] A "limited echocardiogram" that accurately calculates left ventricular (LV) size at a very affordable price and also provides information about ventricular geometry has been recommended by several authorities but has not been commonly endorsed by third-party or other payers.[226]

The prognostic significance of LVH among hypertensive patients is well established. Left ventricular hypertrophy often is thought of as the "hemoglobin A_{1c} of BP," since it is an objective measure of both the severity and the duration of elevations in BP. In the Framingham Heart Study, ECG evidence of LVH was associated with an approximately threefold increase in the incidence of CV events.[227] Echocardiographically detected LVH appears to predict an even greater incremental increase in the risk of future CV events, although the geometry of the ventricle also may play a role.[228,229] Hypertension typically is associated with concentric hypertrophy of the ventricle, perhaps as a result of concentric remodeling, which in one series carried a fourfold increased risk of cardiac morbidity and mortality (compared with nonhypertrophied hearts).[230] Eccentric hypertrophy, which is seen in response to exercise in athletes, imparted only a twofold increased risk of events in the same series.[229] In several reports from various locales, in both univariate and multivariate models, LVH was the most powerful of any of the traditional CV risk factors in predicting not only death or MI but also stroke, HF, and other CV end points.[228,229,231,232] Although research studies including thousands of people have demonstrated the importance of echocardiographically determined measurements of LV mass, there is concern that the intrinsic variability of a single echocardiogram is sufficiently high (perhaps 10 to 15 percent) that serial determinations in a usual hypertensive individual are unlikely to be cost-effective. The exception may be a person with stage 1 hypertension, in whom the presence of this form of LVH would lead to a reclassification of the patient and indicate the need for antihypertensive drug therapy earlier than it might have been given if the clinician had thought the patient was free of TOD.

LVH is associated both epidemiologically and pathophysiologically with intimal hyperplasia of the epicardial coronary arteries, increased coronary vascular resistance, increased severity and frequency of ventricular dysrhythmias, decreased flow reserve, and reduced diastolic relaxation. At the extreme, diastolic dysfunction and restrictive cardiomyopathy result clinically in "flash pulmonary edema" despite a normal ejection fraction. Although this phenomenon is not well understood, some feel that hypertension plays the major role in the pathogenesis of this syndrome, which has been identified in up to 40 percent of patients presenting to the hospital with HF.[233] The important prognostic role of LVH was demonstrated and separated from possible subclinical coronary disease in a consecutive series of 785 patients who had cardiac catheterization.[234] After

4 years of follow-up in patients with echocardiographically documented LVH, the risk of dying was increased twofold if there was coronary artery disease (CAD) but more than fourfold if CAD was not present.[234] Echocardiographically defined LVH was the most powerful risk factor for death.

The most contentious aspect of LVH is the importance of its reversal and how to achieve it. While early data from several centers indicate a better prognosis among patients with echocardiographically determined LVH whose LV mass index is reduced (typically by pharmacologic treatment of hypertension) compared with those whose index increases over time, the large therapeutic trials directed primarily at this question are still ongoing. There are major controversies, supported by separate meta-analyses with differing conclusions, about whether certain classes of antihypertensive drug therapy are more effective at quickly reducing LV mass, but these changes have not been correlated with a reduced risk of CV events in large numbers of patients.[235–237] Most studies agree that LVH is unlikely to regress without reducing BP; most authorities therefore recommend spending resources on achieving BP control rather than on serial echocardiograms to see if the LV mass index is returning toward normal.

Renal Evaluation

Current recommendations for the evaluation of renal function include just a measure of BUN and serum creatinine and a dipstick to detect heavy proteinuria. A more extensive search for microalbuminuria (MA), as defined by the presence of albumin in the urine above the normal range of less than 30 mg/day but below the detectable range with the conventional dipstick methodology, i.e., 300 mg/day, is also warranted.[238] Data from several pioneering studies done over the last two decades have demonstrated that MA is not only a predictor of diabetic complications but also a powerful independent risk factor for CV disease.[238–240] Moreover, MA predicts the development of ischemic CV events related to the development of atherosclerosis. Numerous clinical studies in persons with either type 1 or type 2 DM as well as those with renal disease have demonstrated higher CV mortality in those with MA.[239–244]

The prevalence of MA in patients with type 2 DM is about 20 percent (range, 12 to 36 percent) and affects about 30 percent of people with type 2 DM older than 55 years of age.[242–244] The prevalence of MA ranges from 5 to 40 percent among nondiabetic persons with essential hypertension.[244] The reason for this high variability in MA prevalence among those with essential hypertension relates to both the duration of BP control and associated lipid abnormalities, especially low-density lipoprotein cholesterol (LDL-C) levels.[245] A second related predictor is the duration of hypertension.[246] In this way, MA may be a marker of BP control, since BP control with all agents, except dihydropyridine CA and central or peripheral sympathetic blockers, reduces albuminuria.[247] Subsequent chronic renal failure occurs at a rate of 1 percent per annum in those with type 2 DM; the risk for those with type 1 DM approaches 75 percent after 10 years, while for those with essential hypertension, it is less than 1 percent over 5 years.[247,248]

Some studies have shown that the amount of MA present in a person is proportional to the severity of systolic, diastolic, and mean BP elevation as measured by either clinic or 24-h ambulatory BP monitoring.[249,250] This observation has been corroborated by the results of a clinical study of 211 untreated men with MA and essential hypertension.[251] This study agreed with the findings of previous investigators and showed that patients with MA had higher BP levels.[249] Another Italian population study with 1567 participants revealed an 18-mmHg higher systolic BP in the group of nondiabetic people with MA.[252] Lastly, circadian abnormalities of BP seen in nondippers (see above), who are known to be at higher risk for CV, also have a higher prevalence of MA.[253,254]

The exact pathophysiology of how MA contributes to or accelerates the atherosclerotic process is uncertain. The current understanding, however, suggests that MA is an indicator of increased vascular permeability and, hence, altered barrier function of the endothelium.[249,250,252–255] People with MA have an elevated transcapillary escape rate of albumin regardless of whether they have preexisting DM. Moreover, it has been argued that when albumin leaks into the interstitial space, cellular injury occurs secondary to free radicals and cytokine production enhanced by the presence of albumin. More recently, some authors have suggested that MA is another element of the metabolic components of syndrome X[256–258] (see above).

Simply using a conventional dipstick that can detect only higher levels of urinary protein (>300 mg/24 h) means that the clinician will miss the opportunity to characterize a patients' prognosis more precisely at the initial visit. Dipsticks that detect MA are available and inexpensive. Perhaps all hypertensives with "trace" proteinuria (generally 300 to 500 mg/day) when measured by conventional dipsticks should have a spot urine measurement of the albumin/creatinine ratio.[238] Routine assessment of MA in diabetic patients is well advised, but in hypertensives without DM, its value is still debatable. In part, this is due to the relatively low prevalence of MA in the nondiabetic population and the uncertainty of the significance of its modification in these groups.

Studies found that subjects with MA and type 2 DM have approximated total mortality of 8 percent and CV mortality of 4 percent annually. These values are up to four times higher than those of patients without MA.[258] Similar increases in CV mortality also are present in people with MA and without diabetes. In several series, the CV event rate in nondiabetic people with MA and hypertensives was twofold to fourfold higher than it was in those without MA.[259]

In several studies, people with MA had larger LV mass and higher degrees of LVH.[260–262] This has been documented by both ECG and echocardiographic criteria. However, this finding was not consistent in other populations that were relatively young (age between 18 and 45) and had stage 1 hypertension. This association of MA with LVH may be related to a higher BP load.

Evaluation of the Vasculature

One of the hallmarks of the hypertensive circulation is decreased vascular compliance. Acutely, elevated BP affects the elastic behavior of both large and small arteries such that the muscular layers of the arterial wall are unable to relax as quickly and transmit pressure waves as easily and reproducibly as they can when BP is lower. This is a passive and reversible phenomenon that typically lasts minutes to hours. Over a prolonged period, however, there is a gradual infiltration of the internal elastic lamina of blood vessels with thinned, split, and frayed elastic fibers and a laying down of new intercellular matrix; in extreme cases, medial necrosis is found within the arterial wall. This process, which is attributed to aging, hypertension, or a combination of the two, often is described as "arteriosclerosis," since it leads to chronic and generally irreversible stiffening of the arterial tree.[263]

There are several methods of assessing arterial compliance (Table 51-14), but most are invasive, expensive, or not widely used in clinical medicine.[264] Several new methods for calculating total arterial compliance are based on pulse contour analysis but have not been tested in large population-based studies to prove their value in estimating CV risk.[265,266] Blacher and associates showed in 710 subjects from the Framingham Heart Study that pulse wave velocity is higher in subjects with known atherosclerotic CV.[267] Whether this measure will be used routinely to evaluate hypertensives remains to be seen.

Pseudohypertension is the name given to the rare circumstance in which BP measurements by the usual indirect sphygmomanometry are much higher than direct intraarterial measurements; these differences usually are attributed to very "stiff" and calcified arteries that are nearly impossible to compress with the bladder in the usual BP cuff. The "Osler maneuver" (palpating the walls of the brachial artery when blood flow has been interrupted by inflating the cuff higher than systolic pressure) has been recommended as a simple measure to diagnose this condition, but several reports have found it less sensitive and specific than was reported initially, and the authors do not recommend using it.[268] Because making the diagnosis of pseudohypertension requires a potentially dangerous and expensive intraarterial measurement (and perhaps an infusion of an intravenous antihypertensive agent to "calibrate" the difference between indirect and direct BP measurements), few clinicians routinely check for and diagnose pseudohypertension.

The benefits of lowering BP in older patients with "stiff" arteries, however, are well established. Three clinical trials specifically in isolated systolic hypertension [systolic blood pressure (SBP) ≥160 mmHg with diastolic blood pressure (DBP) <90 or <95 mmHg] proved that older individuals with BP elevations only in systolic BP (a typical finding in patients with reduced vascular compliance) have a reduced risk of CV events with pharmacologic treatment.[269–271] Whether arterial compliance should be measured as a predictor of CV risk and measured serially over time is controversial; perhaps it would not be as cost-effective as serial BP determinations during treatment.

Other Evaluation

Other blood tests such as PRA and serum insulin or newly appreciated markers of CV risk such as C-reactive protein have been abandoned for routine or even specialized evaluation or have not been proved to be sensitive or specific enough to warrant inclusion in the evaluation of all hypertensive patients.[272]

Evaluation for Identifiable Causes of Hypertension

There are many identifiable causes of hypertension (secondary hypertension). In patients with some of these causes, the elevation of BP can be eliminated with specific treatment such as angioplasty or surgery therapy or by removing the agent that caused the hypertension. By far the most common identifiable cause is chronic renal failure. Although chronic renal disease almost never can be cured, the hypertension associated with it often can be controlled with adequate dialysis without the use of drugs. Renal artery stenosis, pheochromocytoma, and primary aldosteronism, however, are potentially curable. These conditions are encountered commonly enough that the clinician seeing a hypertensive patient must have a high index of suspicion in the appropriate clinical setting and should order the specialized tests necessary to screen for and confirm the diagnosis. Other etiologies, such as specific enzyme deficiencies, coarctation of the aorta, and Ask-Upmark kidney, are distinctly rare. This section will cover only the most common etiologies listed in Table 51-10. If a secondary cause of hypertension is suspected, a referral to a hypertension specialist may be appropriate.[11,19]

RENOVASCULAR HYPERTENSION

Patients with this form of secondary hypertension often have stage 3 hypertension and considerable TOD and are at risk of losing renal function. At least 90 percent of cases of renovascular hypertension now are due to renal artery atherosclerosis, with only 10 percent being due to fibromuscular dysplasia or unusual causes.[273,274] Atherosclerotic renal artery stenosis is a disease

TABLE 51-14 Methods for Determining Arterial Compliance

	Measured in	Invasive?	Drawbacks
Direct methods			
Angiography	Aorta	Yes	Expensive
Echocardiography	Aorta	No	Expensive
Echo tracking	Peripheral arteries	No	Not widely available
Intravascular ultrasound	Peripheral arteries	Yes	Expensive
Venous occlusion plethysmography	Peripheral arteries	No	Time- and operator-intensive
Indirect methods			
Stroke volume/pulse pressure ratio	Total arterial compliance	No	Reproducibility questionable
Pulse wave velocity	Segmental arteries	No	Limited to large arteries
Fourier pulse analysis	Peripheral arteries	No	Reproducibility questionable
Total compliance	Total arterial compliance	No	Expensive
Pulse contour analysis	Total arterial compliance	No	Time- and operator-intensive

TABLE 51-15 Testing for Renovascular Hypertension: Clinical Index of Suspicion as a Guide to Selecting Patients for Workup

Low (should not be tested)
- Stage 1 or 2 hypertension in the absence of clinical clues

Moderate (noninvasive test recommended)
- Stage 3 hypertension
- Hypertension refractory to standard therapy
- Abrupt onset of sustained stages 2–3 hypertension at age <20 years
- Hypertension with a suggestive abdominal bruit (long, high-pitched, and localized to the region of the renal artery)
- Stages 2–3 hypertension (diastolic BP exceeding 105 mmHg) in a smoker, a patient with evidence of occlusive vascular disease (cerebrovascular, coronary, peripheral, vascular), or a patient with unexplained but stable elevation of serum creatinine

High (may consider proceeding directly to arteriography)
- Stage 3 hypertension with either progressive renal insufficiency or refractoriness to aggressive treatment, particularly in a patient who has been a smoker or has other evidence of occlusive arterial disease
- Accelerated or malignant hypertension (grade III or IV retinopathy)
- Hypertension with recent elevation of serum creatinine, either unexplained or reversibly induced by an angiotensin-converting enzyme inhibitor
- Moderate to severe hypertension with incidentally detected ansymmetry of renal size

SOURCE: Modified from Mann SL, Pickering TG. Detection of renovascular hypertension: State of the art: 1992. *Ann Intern Med* 1992; 117:845.

of older individuals. Characteristically, these patients develop hypertension after age 50 or have a history of hypertension that had been relatively easy to control and became refractory. A large proportion of these patients have evidence of vascular disease elsewhere (carotids, coronaries, and peripheral circulation, in particular), and the majority are cigarette smokers, often heavy smokers.[275] Although it is more common in whites, blacks also can develop atherosclerotic renovascular hypertension.[276,277] Fibromuscular dysplasia tends to affect young white women in whom BP tends to rise abruptly to stage 3 during the third decade of life. Abdominal or frank bruits are heard commonly, and renal function is usually normal when the diagnosis is entertained.

Laboratory Testing The objective of laboratory testing in patients suspected of having renovascular hypertension is not only to verify that arterial lesions are present but also to determine that the lesion that is discovered is in fact the cause of the patient's hypertension.[273] The clinical situations in which renovascular disease should be suspected are listed in Table 51-15.

The tests used to confirm the clinical suspicion that a patient has renovascular hypertension are biochemical or depend on a variety of imaging techniques (Table 51-16).

Biochemical Measurement of serum K^+ (which, if low, may indicate hyperaldosteronism) or PRA (which, if high, may confirm activation of the RAA system) plays no role in the further case finding for renovascular hypertension because the sensitivity and specificity are too low.[278] Even measuring the PRA after captopril (the so-called captopril test) has a sensitivity of only 60 to 70 percent, although better results have been obtained in some series.[278] Measuring the concentration and activity of renin simultaneously from each renal vein and computing the renal vein renin ratio was a very popular approach at one time, but the sensitivity and specificity for detection of renovascular hypertension with this test are both approximately 75 percent, unacceptably low for an invasive procedure that requires special expertise and sophisticated measurements.[278] This ratio may still be useful to help prove that an anatomic lesion is also the cause of a patient's hypertension but should not be used as a screening tool.

Imaging Rapid-sequence intravenous pyelography and standard renal scanning were the earliest noninvasive imaging studies used for diagnosing renovascular hypertension.[278] Even though in expert hands each has reasonable sensitivity (65 to 70 percent for scanning and 75 percent for pyelography), neither has a place in the diagnostic approach any longer. Renal duplex ultrasound has the advantage of being noninvasive and widely available. In some laboratories, the sensitivity of this test approaches 90 to 95 percent.[279] However, the presence of abdominal gas or fat may make it difficult to visualize the renal arteries, and the test is very operator-dependent. In specialized centers with special expertise and in selected patients, it may be a useful test. In most settings, however, little is gained by using this technique. Magnetic resonance angiography with gadolinium is a new approach to visualization of the renal arteries that is becoming widely available and is noninvasive.[280] However, until the quality of the images improves and the cost becomes lower, this technique is not likely to replace angiography when visualization of the renal arteries is felt to be necessary.

The two imaging modalities currently favored are isotopic renography with labeled dethylenetriamine pentaacetic acid (DTPA) (a measure of glomerular filtration) of MAG-3 (a

TABLE 51-16 Detection of Renovascular Hypertension

Biochemical
- Serum K^+
- PRA
- Renal vein renin activity
- Split renal function tests

Imaging
- Rapid-sequence intravenous pyelography
- Renography
- Captopril or enalaprilat renography
- Intraarterial digital substraction angiography
- Standard angiography
- Duplex renal ultrasound
- Magnetic resonance angiography

measure of renal blood flow) with captopril and intraarterial digital subtraction angiography.[273] Isotopic renography with captopril is a minimally invasive test that detects a discrepancy between perfusion and function of the kidneys. The overall sensitivity and specificity are 90 percent when done carefully, especially in patients whose prior probability of having renovascular hypertension is judged to be high.[273,278] Only ACE-Is and ARBs need to be stopped before the test is performed, and adverse reactions from the single dose of captopril are rare. Isotopic renography with captopril also provides functional information. If the time to peak activity is initially normal and becomes abnormal after captopril ("captopril-induced changes"), the likelihood of cure or improvement after revascularization is high.[273]

Intraarterial digital subtraction angiography has become the invasive procedure of choice to demonstrate definitively the renal artery anatomy and determine whether an arterial lesion is present. Although an arterial puncture is required, the needle used is small and the dye load is modest. In addition, the type of lesion (ostial, nonostial, or branch) can be determined. In some centers, percutaneous renal angioplasty is done at the same time if it is felt to be indicated. The authors are not in favor of doing revascularization unless evidence has been obtained (a positive captopril renogram with captopril-induced changes or a renal vein renin ratio >1.5) that the lesion is functionally significant. The presence of anatomic renal artery stenosis does not mean that the lesion is responsible for the elevation in BP (functional renal artery stenosis).[273]

When considering whether to proceed with these studies, the clinician must consider how the data will be used. In a number of hypertensive patients with renovascular hypertension, BP is controlled adequately with medical therapy. If the risk of surgery or angioplasty is viewed as unacceptably high or if the patient will not consent to having a revascularization procedure if a remediable lesion is discovered, any specific further evaluation may not be appropriate.

PHEOCHROMOCYTOMA

Patients with pheochromocytoma are almost always symptomatic on presentation.[281] These patients usually have a characteristic cluster of complaints that occur in paroxysms or "spells." The description of the spell tends to be typical and is usually the same in each patient. The spells may occur many times a day or may be separated by weeks or months.[282] Often there is a characteristic trigger (change in position, certain foods, trauma, pain, or drugs) that if present should greatly increase the clinician's index of suspicion of pheochromocytoma. Hypertension is not usually paroxysmal, as has often been stated, with some BP readings elevated and some normal. Most measurements are in fact in the hypertensive range, although wide variability is the rule. The three most common symptoms of pheochromocytoma are headache, diaphoresis, and palpitations[282] (Table 51-17). Many other symptoms, particularly anxiety, weakness, and tremulousness, are also quite common. The pattern of symptoms can provide guidance about the predominant hormone secreted by the tumor. When norepinephrine is the primary hormone produced, pallor is usually the symptom. Flushing is more likely if substantial amounts of epinephrine are produced.

Laboratory Testing for Pheochromocytoma Whereas it is possible and sometimes desirable to manage hypertensive patients with renovascular hypertension or mineralocorticoid-excess states with medical therapy, it is almost always imperative to remove a pheochromocytoma. As with renovascular hypertension, once the clinical presentation suggests that a pheochromocytoma may be the cause of a patient's hypertension, a variety of tests are available to confirm the diagnosis (Table 51-18). If a pheochromocytoma is suspected, the next step is to obtain biochemical confirmation of an increase in catecholamine production. The authors prefer to measure 24-h urinary excretion of total catecholamines (norepinephrine, epinephrine, or dopamine) or their metabolites (vanillylmandelic acid or metanephrine).[282] In some laboratories, 24-h urinary metanephrines are the most sensitive and specific in the diagnosis (both approximately 85 percent and 90 percent), but when done precisely, there is little to choose in regard to which should be measured. When the two or three of these compounds are quantitated and several samples are analyzed, both the sensitivity and the

TABLE 51-17 Symptoms and Signs of Pheochromocytoma

Symptoms[a]	Frequency, %
Headaches	40–96
Diaphoresis	40–74
Palpitations	45–70
Pallor	40–45
Nervousness and/or anxiety	22–43
Tremulousness	29–31
Signs[b]	**Frequency, %**
Hypertension	>90
Sustained	50–60
Intermittent	2–50
Paroxysms	50
Weight loss (hypermetabolic state)	80
Funduscopic changes	50–70
Orthostatic hypotension	40–70

[a]Infrequent symptoms: flushing, Raynaud's phenomenon, nausea, seizures, dizziness, dyspnea, and abdominal, chest, or arm pain.
[b]Infrequent signs: acrocyanosis, bradycardia, fever, and glucose intolerance.

TABLE 51-18 Diagnostic Tests for Pheochromocytoma

- Biochemical
  - Urinary free catecholamines
  - Urinary vanilylmandelic acid
  - Urinary metanephrines
  - Plasma catecholamines (or metanephrines)
  - Clonidine suppression test
- Imaging studies
  - Computed axial tomography
  - Magnetic resonance imaging
  - ^{131}I-meta-iodobenzylguanidine
  - Abdominal ultrasound
  - Adrenal vein or vena caval drainage
  - Angiography

specificity of the tests improve. Attention must be paid to the conditions under which the sample is collected, and urinary creatinine also should be measured to verify that the collection represents the 24-h excretion. To reduce the number of false-positive results, the patient should be in a nonstressful situation when the sample is obtained.

In the authors' view, only when the urinary assays are borderline can the measurement of plasma catecholamines be useful. If plasma catecholamines (norepinephrine plus epinephrine) levels exceed 2000 pg/mL in the basal state, the presence of a pheochromocytoma is highly likely. If the levels are less than 1000 pg/mL, the diagnosis is very unlikely, whereas in patients with plasma catecholamine levels between 1000 and 2000 pg/mL, the clonidine suppression test may be useful.[283] If plasma catecholamine levels do not suppress after the administration of 0.3 mg of oral clonidine in an appropriately prepared and monitored patient, a further aggressive search for a pheochromocytoma is warranted.

The choice of which initial imaging procedure to obtain is also somewhat controversial. CT scanning is a highly sensitive imaging modality that will locate nearly all pheochromocytomas, especially those in the adrenal gland or the abdomen. MRI has the advantage of not requiring contrast material (which is sometimes necessary with CT scanning) and is also helpful in localizing nonadrenal or nonabdominal pheochromocytomas. Enhancement of the T2-weighted images happens virtually only with pheochromocytomas and adrenal carcinomas, helping distinguish adrenal masses that are not biochemically active (so-called incidentalomas) from metabolically active or malignant tumors.

The use of I-meta-iodobenzylguanidine scanning has been particularly helpful when a pheochromocytoma is suspected but is not clearly located with CT or MRI. This radiopharmaceutical is a guanethidine analog that is concentrated in pheochromocytomas and other neural crest tumors.[284] Using total-body scanning helps localize the tumor if the initial CT or MRI scans are negative or equivocal. The sensitivity of this test exceeds 90 percent, but it is not uniformly available.

PRIMARY ALDOSTERONISM

In a hypertensive patient receiving no treatment who demonstrates significant hypokalemia (serum K^+ ≤3.2 meq/L) with renal K^+ wasting (24-h urinary K^+ >30 meq), PRA below 1 ng/mL, and elevated plasma or urinary aldosterone values, the diagnosis is unequivocal. Often, however, the diagnosis is not obvious because the values are not as definitive; in such cases, multiple measurements are needed during salt loading.

The single best test in people with normal renal function for identifying patients with primary aldosteronism is the measurement of 24-h urinary aldosterone excretion during salt loading[285,286] (Table 51-19). An excretion rate of >14 μg of aldosterone in 24 h after 3 days of salt loading (greater than 200 meq/day) distinguishes most patients with primary aldosteronism from those with essential hypertension. Only 7 percent of patients with primary aldosteronism have values that fall within the range for essential hypertension. In contrast, a substantial number (about 39 percent) of patients with primary aldosteronism have plasma aldosterone values that fall within the range for essential hypertension.[287] The findings of hypokalemia and suppressed PRA provide corroborative evidence, but the absence of either or both does not preclude the diagnosis.

TABLE 51-19 Diagnostic Studies for Mineralocorticoid Excess States

Biochemical
Serum potassium
Plasma renin activity
Plasma aldosterone
Plasma aldosterone/renin ratio
24-h urinary aldosterone excretion
Plasma 18-hydroxycorticosterone
Plasma 18-oxocortisol
Plasma 18-hydroxycortisol
Adrenal vein sampling for aldosterone
Imaging studies
Abdominal ultrasound
Computed axial tomography
Iodocholesterol scanning
Adrenal venography

A substantial number of patients with primary aldosteronism, however, do not present with hypokalemia; serum K^+ concentration is normal in 7 to 38 percent of reported cases.[288,289] In addition, 10 to 12 percent of patients with proven tumors may not have hypokalemia during short-term salt loading. Plasma renin activity <1 ng/mL per hour or one that fails to rise above 2 ng/mL per hour after salt and water depletion and upright posture has been used as an additional test to exclude primary aldosteronism.[288] However, a significant number (about 35 percent) of patients with the disease have values that rise >2 ng/mL per hour when appropriately stimulated.[286] In addition, about 40 percent of subjects with essential hypertension have suppressed PRA, and 15 to 20 percent of these patients have values <2 ng/mL per hour under conditions of stimulation.

The plasma aldosterone/renin ratio has been used to define the appropriateness of PRA for the circulating concentrations of aldosterone.[286] It is assumed that the volume expansion associated with excessive aldosterone production inhibits the synthesis of renin without affecting the autonomous production of aldosterone. Both tests are subject to the same limitations: First, there is inherent variability of plasma levels of aldosterone even in the presence of a tumor, and this translates into variability in the absolute value of the ratio; second, the use of drugs that result in marked and prolonged stimulation of renin long after their discontinuation may alter the ratio.

The most common cause of primary aldosteronism is an aldosterone-producing adenoma (70 to 80 percent of all proven cases). Approximately 20 to 30 percent of cases are caused by hyperplasia of the zona glomerulosa layer of the adrenal cortex (bilateral adrenal hyperplasia). Some reports suggest the occurrence of a syndrome intermediate between adenoma and hyperplasia.[288] The distinction between these two processes is important because surgical intervention is likely to be curative in the majority of adenomas and fails to reduce BP in patients with bilateral adrenal hyperplasia.

An adenoma is likely in the presence of spontaneous hypokalemia <3.0 meq/L, plasma 18-hydroxycorticosterone values >100 ng/dL, and an anomalous postural decrease in plasma aldosterone concentration.[289,290] In addition, adenomas are largely unresponsive to changes in sodium balance and appear to be exquisitely sensitive to ACTH, unlike hyperplasias, which are more sensitive to angiotensin II infusions.[290] Plasma 18-hydroxycorticosterone values <100 ng/dL, a postural increase in aldosterone, or both, are findings usually associated with hyperplasia, but they do not completely rule out the presence of an adenoma.[291]

An adrenal CT scan should be considered the initial step in tumor localization. It is noninvasive, and all adenomas ≥1.5 cm in diameter can be located accurately. Only 60 percent of nodules measuring between 1 and 1.4 cm in diameter are detected by CT scanning. Nodules <1 cm in diameter are very difficult, if not impossible, to demonstrate. The overall sensitivity of localizing adenomas by high-resolution CT scanning exceeds 90 percent.[292] Adrenal venous aldosterone levels should be measured when the biochemical findings are highly suggestive of an adenoma, but the adrenal CT scan is ambiguous.[293]

Medical therapy is indicated in patients with adrenal hyperplasia, patients with adenoma who are poor surgical risks, and patients with bilateral adrenal adenomas that may require bilateral adrenalectomy. Total bilateral adrenalectomy has no place in the management of primary aldosteronism.

The long-standing experience has been that the hypertension associated with primary aldosteronism is salt- and water-dependent and is best treated with sustained salt and water depletion.[294] The usual doses of diuretic agents are hydrochlorothiazide 25 to 50 mg/day or furosemide 80 to 160 mg/day in combination with either spironolactone 100 to 200 mg/day or amiloride 10 to 20 mg/day. These combinations usually result in prompt correction of hypokalemia and normalization of BP within 2 to 4 weeks.

In the majority of these patients, surgical excision of an aldosterone-producing adenoma leads to normotension as well as reversal of the biochemical defects. One year postoperatively, about 70 percent of patients are normotensive, but 5 years postoperatively, only 53 percent remain normotensive. The restoration of normal K^+ homeostasis is permanent. Patients undergoing surgery should receive drug treatment for a least 8 to 10 weeks both to decrease BP and to correct metabolic abnormalities. These patients have a significant K^+ deficiency that must be corrected preoperatively because hypokalemia increases the risk of cardiac arrhythmias during anesthesia.

After the removal of an aldosterone-producing adenoma, selective hypoaldosteronism usually occurs even in patients whose PRA had been stimulated with chronic diuretic therapy. Potassium supplementation therefore should be given cautiously, and serum K^+ values should be monitored closely. Sufficient residual mineralocorticoid activity often is left to prevent excessive renal retention of K^+ provided that Na^+ intake is adequate. Abnormalities in aldosterone production can persist for as long as 3 months after tumor removal.

OTHER FORMS OF IDENTIFIABLE SECONDARY HYPERTENSION

In addition to these three most common and potentially curable forms of identifiable secondary hypertension, there are a vast number of rare conditions in which the cause of the hypertension cannot be found (Table 51-10). These include enzyme deficiencies such as 17-β-hydroxylase deficiency and 17-α-hydroxylase deficiency, other congenital disorders such as the Ask-Upmark kidney, trauma such as the Page kidney, urologic causes such as hydronephrosis, endocrine abnormalities such as Cushing's syndrome and Cushing's disease, and even infectious etiologies such as renal tuberculosis.[274] Although the practicing clinician may never encounter a patient with any of these disorders, it is incumbent on him or her to know that these unusual conditions may present with hypertension and that the elevated BP may be the first clue to the diagnosis. Two causes of identifiable hypertension are not rare, and all clinicians will see patients with iatrogenic hypertension and those with sleep apnea (Table 51-11). Any of the drugs or other substances listed in the table should be stopped before one concludes that a patient has hypertension. The relation of sleep apnea to hypertension and obesity has long been recognized.[295,296] The typical clinical presentation of sleep apnea (daytime drowsiness, snoring) in an obese hypertensive should alert the clinician to this disorder.

TREATMENT OF HYPERTENSION

Patients with JNC VI stage 2 or 3 hypertension (SBP ≥160 mmHg or DBP ≥100 mmHg) and those in risk group C (those with DM and those with clinical CV) should receive drug therapy once their hypertension has been diagnosed and confirmed.[11] Furthermore, the length of time the clinician should rely on lifestyle modifications before starting drug therapy has been clarified in JNC VI and is based on risk estimates, not just on the level of BP (Table 51-3). Those with stage 1 hypertension (SBP 140 to 159 mmHg and/or DBP 90 to 99 mmHg) who have no other risk factors or end-organ damage (so-called risk group A) can be treated only with lifestyle modification for up to 1 year even if goal BP is not reached before drug therapy should be considered necessary. Since male sex and age over 60 years are considered risk factors, only women under 60 years of age are in group A.

Patients with stage 1 hypertension who are in risk group B (other CV risk factors but no TOD or DM) should receive pharmacologic therapy after only a 6-month trial of lifestyle modification unless goal BP is achieved without drugs. Those in risk group C [TOD, clinical cardiovascular disease (CVD), and/or DM) should be treated with pharmacologic agents and lifestyle modification even if they have high-normal BP (SBP 130 to 139 mmHg and/or DBP 85 to 89 mmHg).

Lifestyle Modification

The JNC VI recommended weight loss for obese hypertensive patients, modification of dietary Na^+ intake to ≤100 mmol/day, and modification of alcohol intake to no more than two drinks per day.[11] It also recommended an increase in physical activity for all patients with hypertension who have no specific condition that would make such a recommendation not applicable or safe. However, for many of the authors' patients these suggestions are not practicable or already are being implemented. For such patients, drug therapy may be indicated even sooner in group A and group B hypertensive patients.

There is little doubt that lifestyle factors such as diet, exercise, and stress can affect BP. There is a strong positive correlation between the level of body weight and body mass index (weight/height) and the level of BP.[297] The relationship of dietary Na^+ and BP is equally clear, especially at low and modest intakes of Na^+ and in those deemed to be salt-sensitive. Other nutrients, such as K^+, the omega-3 fatty acids present in fish oil, and possibly Ca^{2+} and Mg^{2+}, are inversely related to BP level. Sedentary individuals who do little, if any, aerobic exercise usually have higher BPs than do appropriately matched controls even when one controls for other confounding variables.[298] The relationship of stress to BP is somewhat less clear. Physical or mental stress will raise BP temporarily, but the relationship of chronic anxiety and stress has been more difficult to demonstrate.

The appreciation of these relationships has naturally led to numerous attempts to lower BP by modifying lifestyle (Table 51-20). The most important trial that evaluated the benefits of lifestyle modification, including weight loss, was the Trial of Hypertension Prevention (TOHP-1).[299] This study was large ($n = 2182$) and randomized and compared the benefits of weight loss, Na^+ reduction, or stress reduction to usual care and also compared K^+ supplements at 60 meq/day or Ca^{2+} at 1.0 g/day or Mg^{2+} at 15 mmol/day or fish oil at 3.0 g of omega-3 fatty acid to placebos. The weight loss, Na^+ reduction, and stress management were given to 308, 327, and 240 participants, respectively, for 18 months. The group assigned to supplementation (Mg^{2+}, Ca^{2+}, or placebo) then was rerandomized to fish oil, K^+, or placebo. In addition, 589 participants received usual care, giving this trial the ability to judge the efficacy of these treatments more objectively than any prior studies could. The nutritional treatments were delivered by trained nutritionists using group and individual sessions to maximize the adherence to the regimen and presumably its efficacy. The long period of treatment and observation in TOHP-1 also provided important information about the "natural history" of the efficacy of these therapies. TOHP-1 showed that weight loss was the most effective lifestyle modification, reducing BP by 2.9/2.3 mmHg in association with an average weight loss of 3.9 kg. Sodium reduction was the only other therapeutic modality that reduced BP a significant amount (1.7/0.9 mmHg) with a reduction of 44 meq/day of Na^+. All the other arms of the study (K^+, Ca^{2+}, Mg^{2+}, fish oil supplements, and stress management) failed to demonstrate any reduction in BP compared with placebo or usual care. Whereas there were physiologic markers that indicated that the nutritional approaches and weight loss did at least partially achieve their objectives, the stress management techniques used were not effective. Perhaps successful stress management might lower BP.

TABLE 51-20 Lifestyle Modifications That Lower Blood Pressure

PRIMARY LIFESTYLE MODIFICATIONS

1. Reduction of body weight (5-kg threshold; 10 kg reduces BP ~10/8 mmHg)
2. Reduction in dietary salt consumption (target 100 mmol/day; can lower BP ~12/10 mmHg, but individual responses vary)
3. Increase physical activity to 30–45 min, four times a week (can lower BP 8/4 mmHg and often helps control weight)
4. Increased consumption of fruits and vegetables (at least 4 servings/day; can lower BP ~6/3 mmHg and often helps reduce salt consumption)
5. Moderation of alcohol consumption (target 10–20 g ethanol for women, 20–30 g for men; can lower BP up to 8/4 mmHg in those who have more than 5 drinks/day)
6. Stress management (randomized clinical trials outside the workplace have been unconvincing, but many psychologists still recommend the approach despite a lack of detailed protocols that uniformly lower BP)

OTHER LIFESTYLE MODIFICATIONS THAT ARE ROUTINELY RECOMMENDED

1. Tobacco avoidance (lowers cardiovascular risk independently of any effect on BP)
2. Fish consumption (improves lipid profiles and cardiovascular risk more than expected if BP effect alone is operative)
3. Increasing dietary fiber (improves lipid profiles and cancer risk independently of effect on BP)

LIFESTYLE MODIFICATIONS THAT ARE NOT ROUTINELY RECOMMENDED

1. Biofeedback
2. Dietary calcium supplementation
3. Dietary magnesium supplementation
4. Micronutrient supplements

SOURCE: Whelton PK, Appel LJ, Espeland MA, et al., for the TONE Collaborative Research Group. Sodium restriction and weight loss in the treatment of hypertension in older persons: A randomized controlled trial of nonpharmacologic interventions in the Elderly (TONE). *JAMA* 1998; 279:839–846. Appel LJ, Moore TJ, Obarzanek E, et al. A clinical trial of the effects of dietary patterns on blood pressure. *N Engl J Med* 1997; 336:1117–1124. Bao DG, Mori TA, Burke V, et al. Effects of dietary fish and weight reduction on ambulatory blood pressure in overweight hypertensives. *Hypertension* 1998; 32:710–717. Arakawa K. Antihypertensive mechanism of exercise. *J Hypertens* 1993; 11:223–229. Beilin LJ. Stress, coping, lifestyle and hypertension: A paradigm for research, prevention and non-pharmacological management of hypertension. *Clin Exp Hypertens* 1997; 19:739–752.

TOMHS also evaluated the long-term benefit of lifestyle modification.[300] This study compared five classes of antihypertensives (diuretics, CAs, ACE-Is, alpha blockers, and beta blockers) to placebo in middle-aged subjects with minimal elevations of BP (average BP of 140/91 mmHg when the study started) and superimposed these pharmacologic treatments on a comprehensive lifestyle regimen that included weight loss, Na^+ restriction, alcohol reduction, and exercise. A subgroup of the cohort got lifestyle modification with placebo. In TOMHS, the nutritional advice and the exercise program were presented to the participants and monitored by certified nutritionists and trained exercise physiologists. The subjects were seen frequently in group and individual sessions. The group given placebo reduced BP from 140/91 to 132/82 mmHg (a reduction of 9.1/8.6 mmHg) and sustained that level for the 4.4 years of study follow-up, even though the reduction of the Na^+ intake, amount of weight loss, and the increase in exercise did not reach study goals. Perhaps the most important finding in TOMHS was the statistically significantly fewer number of CV events ($p < .03$), in the group given pharmacologic treatment plus lifestyle modification. These patients achieved an average BP of 125/79 mmHg, a reduction of 16/12 mmHg. Even though the lifestyle modification was successful and sustained, the group given drugs had statistically significantly fewer CV events ($p < .03$), probably because their BP was lower.

The inevitable conclusion from this trial is that even successful lifestyle modification that brings BP to the current goals does not reduce morbidity and probably mortality as well as does the combination of drugs and lifestyle adjustments that brings BP down even further. The fact that the value of BP reduction in preventing CV complications with pharmacologic agents could be demonstrated in a group at such low risk calls into question the current emphasis on delaying treatment with drugs even in low-risk individuals while the patient and provider try to get BP to goal without them. In a subsequent paper, Grimm and colleagues also showed that quality of life, as assessed by a very extensive questionnaire delivered on multiple occasions during TOMHS, showed that subjects felt best in all the ways studied when their BP was lowest.[50] This result was seen whether they were on active pharmacologic treatment with lifestyle modification or on lifestyle modification alone. These data lead the authors to believe that physicians should strive to get the maximum BP reduction that can be achieved safely and do so by combining treatments and not restrict their approach to one modality or the other.

More recent studies have combined the two most successful lifestyle modifications (weight loss and Na^+ restriction) in prospective, randomized, and well-controlled long-term trials. The Trials of Hypertension Prevention-2 (TOHP-2) studied the value of weight loss and Na^+ restriction in a 2 × 2 factorial design against usual care.[301] The group assigned to both Na^+ reduction and weight loss did the best at 6 months [BP fell 4.0/2.8 mmHg (usual care subtracted)], while those receiving a single modality did not experience as much of a BP reduction (3.7/2.7 mmHg for the weight loss only group, 2.9/1.6 mmHg for the Na^+ reduction only group, also usual care subtracted). The disturbing finding here was that most of this reduction was gone by the 3-year follow-up, with the combined treatment having reduced BP by only 1.1/0.6 mmHg at that time. This finding highlights another difficulty with lifestyle modification: the high recidivism rate seen in virtually all long-term studies. While adherence to a drug regimen is notoriously poor, adherence to lifestyle modification is, if anything, even worse. As in TOHP-1, the regimen was delivered by highly trained nutritionists in group and individual sessions and is consequently not an inexpensive way to reduce BP.

The second long-term, randomized, and well-controlled study directly assessing the value of lifestyle modification was the Trial of Nonpharmacologic Interventions in the Elderly (TONE).[302] This study also evaluated the efficacy of weight loss and Na^+ reduction, but in a different population and with a somewhat different objective. Only hypertensives 60 to 80 years of age were enrolled, and all already were on single-drug pharmacologic treatment. The objective of TONE was to see whether the imposition of a formal lifestyle approach, again taught by highly trained professionals, would allow hypertensives to go off their medications. The results were equally disappointing. After 30 months, when the study ended, 44 percent of the actively treated subjects were able to stay off antihypertensives (they did not have a CV event or have BP rise to levels that were considered too high not to be given drugs: >150/90 mmHg) compared with 38 percent of those not getting active lifestyle modification. While this was statistically significant ($p < .001$), it means that 56 percent of successfully treated hypertensives needed to resume drug therapy even when given the best possible lifestyle regimen available administered by experts.

The value of alcohol reduction also has been addressed by a recently published clinical trial (PATHSI).[303] This study took 641 patients at seven Department of Veterans Affairs clinics who were actively employed and completely functional but had at least six alcoholic drinks per day. The subjects reduced their alcohol intake nearly 20 percent once they entered into the study and before their randomization to intensive counseling or usual care was done. Those in the intensive counseling group were seen frequently and were able to reduce their average alcohol consumption to 2.0 drinks per day, which was significantly better than the usual care group (3.3 drinks per day). In spite of this, BP and events were not different at the end of this 2-year trial.

Appel and associates showed in the Dietary Approaches to Stop Hypertension (DASH) trial that a diet rich in fruit and vegetables lowered BP by 2.8/1.1 mmHg more than did the control diet.[304] The fruit and vegetable diet was designed to contain K^+ and Mg^{2+} at the 75th percentile of the usual American diet, while the control diet was at the 25th percentile. A "combination" diet that also contained foods rich in Ca^{2+} and was lower in total and saturated fat content lowered BP by 5.5/3.0 mmHg more than did the control diet. In the hypertensive subjects in DASH (n = 133 of 459), the BP reduction was impressive (11.4/5.5 mmHg). Although this study was short (only 8 weeks) and may not be generalizable to the population since it was carried out in four centers with special expertise, this approach offers great promise for using nutritional management to prevent hypertension in individuals with high-normal BP. The DASH diet provides high amounts of K^+, Mg^{2+}, and Ca^{2+} in the food eaten, not as supplements, and also limits the dietary fat and saturated fat intake in a diet only modestly low in Na^+ (3000 mg/24 h). Further studies done over longer periods in a less highly selected cohort will be needed to verify these results and determine whether the DASH diet will be a valuable therapeutic tool for the general population.

While treatment modalities such as K^+, Ca^{2+}, and/or Mg^{2+} supplements, fish oil, and garlic have advocates, careful and objective assessment of the data leads one to the conclusion that lifestyle modification should be primarily adjunctive to drug therapy in hypertensives, especially now that so many well-tolerated agents have been developed and it has been proved that lowering BP with drugs reduces morbidity and mortality.[305–309] No study of lifestyle modification in hypertensives has demonstrated that life is prolonged or CV events prevented.

The recommendations for lifestyle modification from JNC VI and other guideline committees also include smoking cessation.[11] The reason for the inclusion of this recommendation was to improve CV health rather than because of a proven direct relationship between smoking and hypertension. A direct relationship between smoking and BP, in fact, had not been demonstrated in epidemiologic studies, and often the opposite (BP lower in smokers) was observed.[310] It is now clear, however, that cigarette smoking increases BP and HR transiently (for about 15 min) and that the rise in both is gone by 30 min. The mechanism is the increase in catecholamine secretion induced by smoking. Since the authors recommend that office readings be taken no sooner than 30 min after smoking and caffeine ingestion (another substance that transiently raises BP), one may well miss the elevation of BP caused by smoking if it is measured when the patient has not smoked. Indeed, ABPM studies have shown that smokers have significantly higher BP on days when they smoke compared with days when they do not.[311] The recommendation not to smoke is clearly appropriate, and it is worthwhile not only because of enhanced CV health but also because smoking induces a rise in BP.

The lack of proof of efficacy or effectiveness when using lifestyle modification to treat or even prevent hypertension does not mean that physicians should abandon their efforts to encourage patients to lose weight; restrict their Na^+ intake; eat generous amounts of K^+, Mg^{2+}, Ca^{2+}, and fish; exercise regularly; drink only moderately if they wish to; stop smoking; and reduce stress. What one needs to realize is that the most important thing is to lower BP, perhaps to the lowest tolerable level, and to do so safely and without excessive personal or societal cost. The tension between advocates of lifestyle modification and those who consider it at best no more than an adjunct is not useful. The recommendations for modifying lifestyle are still very appropriate for the general population. If adopted, they will prevent or delay the virtually inevitable rise in BP that occurs with age and many hypertensives will be able to reduce BP further than might be achieved with drugs alone. Lifestyle modification is the primary public heath approach to trying to reduce the prevalence of hypertension and the average BP in the society. If successful, such modification is likely to save more lives and prevent more MIs, strokes, and episodes of HF than can be prevented by using drugs in those who are already hypertensive.

PHARMACOLOGIC THERAPY

The primary goal of BP reduction is to achieve the recommended goal BP by using the least intrusive means possible.[11] *Intrusive* has several interpretations: economic, office visits, adverse effects, and convenience. The choice of the drug with which to begin therapy is probably the most important decision the clinician must make when treating hypertensive patients. Approximately half the patients physicians treat will respond to the first choice and can tolerate most rational options. If physicians choose wisely, the first choice will be successful in getting BP to goal, and that will be the drug on which the patient remains for what is usually an indefinite period of therapy. Since the remainder will need additional treatment, the choice of the first drug must be done with an eye toward what can be added to achieve that goal.

Classification of Antihypertensive Agents

Antihypertensive agents can be classified in a number of ways. Some are effective parentally and are indicated only for a hypertensive crisis, and others (the overwhelming majority) are used orally for chronic therapy. Antihypertensive agents are further classified by pharmacologic class and alleged primary mechanism of action (Table 51-21). There are more than 80 effective antihypertensive drugs and 40 fixed-dose combinations from which to choose. This provides physicians with many options but can make the choice seem more perplexing than it should be. All the drugs that are available lower BP safely and, in appropriate doses, essentially to the same degree. Some classes are more likely than others to reduce BP to goal with monotherapy and with acceptable tolerability. Those agents are appropriate choices for initial treatment.

Surrogate versus Clinical End Points

Physicians are no longer willing simply to look at the degree of BP reduction when making a choice of antihypertensive therapy. Clinical end points are the events that physicians are trying to prevent in treating hypertension. So-called surrogate (or intermediate) end points are factors that may contribute to clinical end points and can be affected favorably or unfavorably by treatment. Blood pressure reduction is a surrogate or intermediate end point, since the reason for treating hypertension is to reduce the morbidity and mortality associated with elevated BP, not simply to lower BP. Physicians now expect and demand proof that the selection made will prevent hypertension-related clinical end points. Data from large and prospective clinical trials that are designed to evaluate the ability of a drug to reduce hypertension-related CV events as well as or better than an otherwise reasonably alternative drug are the reliable means to use in choosing from among the otherwise bewildering number of options.

Before 1997, only diuretics and beta blockers had been shown to reduce the morbidity and mortality in clinical trials in hypertension. Dihydropyridine (DHP), CAs, and ACE-Is were added to the list after the Syst-EUR trial was completed.[270] This trial used the DHP CA nitrendipine, followed by enalapril and hydrochlorothiazide, if needed, to get BP to goal. It was only in 1999, when the Captopril Prevention Project (CAPPP) was published, that the ability of an ACE-I to reduce morbidity and mortality in a trial that enrolled subjects because they were hypertensive was demonstrated.[312] That project showed that a regimen starting with the ACE-I captopril achieved the same overall benefit in reducing morbidity and mortality as did one that began with diuretics or beta blockers (so-called conventional therapy).[312] Certain interesting findings need further study. For example, the group randomized to conventional therapy had statistically significantly fewer strokes, and the group given the ACE-I had a lower incidence of new DM and better outcomes in those with known type 2 DM. A more recent active comparison study, the second Swedish Trial of Hypertension in Older Persons (STOP-2), again confirmed that both ACE-Is and DHP CA reduce morbidity and mortality as well as but clearly not better than do diuretics and beta blockers.[313] In STOP-2, conventional treatment was not better than newer agents at preventing strokes, and the ACE-I group did not have less incident DM. This trial failed to confirm the intriguing findings from CAPPP.

Numerous studies have shown the value of ACE-Is in saving the lives of patients with HF, in those with an MI, and in those with type 1 DM with nephropathy and proteinuria.[314–317] Many of the subjects in these trials had hypertension but were enrolled in the studies because they had these other conditions, and so one needs to be cautious about whether these data can be extrapolated to hypertensives who do not have these complications. A major new trial, the Heart Outcome Prevention Evaluation (HOPE) trial, was published in 2000.[318] This trial demonstrated that treatment with the ACE-I ramapril significantly reduced CV events compared with placebo in participants with multiple CV risk factors who had an average BP of 138/78 mmHg.[318] However, HOPE did not have an active comparator, and the group on ramapril did have a modestly lower BP (3/2 mmHg). Although the investigators claimed that this small difference in BP could not explain most of the benefit of ramapril, it is still possible that it was the reduction in BP rather than the ACE-I that was responsible for the dramatic reduction in events.

In the next few years, approximately 30 more events trials will be completed.[319] Table 51-22 lists some of the more important trials in progress. When some or all of these trials are published, it should be known with some degree of certainty whether lowering BP is all that matters or whether a particular drug or class of drugs should be selected because it or they prevent hypertension-related events more effectively. The largest of these trials (42,448 subjects), the Antihypertensive and Lipid Lowering Trial to Prevent Heart Attack (ALLHAT), is due to be completed in 2003.[320] ALLHAT compares diuretics to DHP CAs, ACE-Is, and alpha blockers. Acute MI in the primary end point. In February 2000, the alpha-blocker arm of the ALLHAT trial was stopped because of a 25 percent higher CV mortality and twofold increase in HF when doxazosin was compared to chlorthalidone.[321] The primary end point was not different between the two groups. Here too, there was a difference in BP control. The chlorthalidone group had a 3/0 mmHg lower BP almost from the start compared with those getting doxazosin. Thus, the question of the degree BP reduction versus how one chooses to achieve it remains open.

It is of great interest that the participants receiving the alpha blocker had lower TC, triglycerides, and serum glucose and higher serum K^+ than did those on the diuretic.[321] If metabolic surrogate end points are important, all these changes would predict that alpha-blocker-treated subjects should have fewer events than do those on chlorthalidone. The opposite was the case. Another trial, the Controlled ONset Verapamil INvestigation of Cardiovascular Endpoints (CONVINCE), will be completed in 2002.[322] This study compares a nondihydropyridine CA (verapamil) to diuretics/beta blockers in 16,600 older hypertensives. This trial will indicate whether this class of CA will prevent mortality and morbidity as well as or better than conventional therapy does. It also will evaluate the importance of circadian variation in BP since the verapamil preparation used is designed to be given at night and released in concert with the morning rise in BP (see below). Event trials of ARBs in older high-risk hypertensives [Valsartan Amlodipine Long Term Use Evaluation (VALUE)] in hypertensives with ECG LVH (the Losartan Intervention for End Point Reduction–LIFE), and in those with diuretic nephropathy are in progress and will be finished in the next few years.[319,323]

Individualizing Therapy

In view of the many effective options available, the physician must pay very close attention to each patient's needs and plan his or her regimen accordingly. Each patient must be treated as an individual, not as a member of a population, and so the drug chosen must be compatible with that individual patient's preferences, lifestyle, and job requirements. Whatever is selected, it must be affordable. No amount of therapeutic wisdom will be effective if the patient does not have the funds to purchase the physician's choice.

Goal of Therapy

One must strive to reduce SBP to below 140 mmHg and to reduce DBP to below 90 mmHg, the goal currently articulated by several guidelines committees.[11,18,19] In diabetic patients, the recommended goal is lower (SBP <130 mmHg and DBP <85 mmHg). JNC VI recommended these more stringent goals for those with DM without proof from a clinical trial to support this aggressive approach. The subsequent publication of the HOT study and the United Kingdom Diabetes Prevention Study (UKDPS) provided the solid evidence that was needed to support this recommendation.[324,325] In patients with renal disease and at least 1 g of proteinuria per day, JNC VI recommended an even lower goal (SBP <125 mmHg and DBP <75 mmHg). This too was not an "evidence-based" recommendation but was based on the expectation that a still lower BP would be helpful in preventing morbidity and mortality in this population of hypertensives.[326] The African-American Study of Kidney Disease (AASK) will provide definitive evidence for or against this very stringent goal.[327] Whether this more aggressive goal should be extended to other subpopulations, such as those with prevalent CVD, remains to be proved.

One of the perceived limitations to achieving this lower level of BP control was the fear that lowering BP too far might be harmful, the concept of the "J" curve. Several investigators had pointed out that subjects treated to diastolic BP level below 85 mmHg had higher rates of MI than did those whose on-treatment diastolic BP was between 85 and 90 mmHg.[328,329] However, an increased risk for those with low diastolic BP is also evident in populations and in the placebo groups of several trials.[330,331] Furthermore, the Systolic Hypertension in the Elderly Program (SHEP) treated individuals down to an average diastolic BP of 67 mmHg and prevented MIs compared with those with an average of 71 mmHg.[269] Definite proof that aggressive treatment is not harmful has come from the HOT and UKPDS trials.[324,325] These studies showed no increase in the incidence of CV events in the groups randomized to the lowest levels of BP control, but HOT could not show that those treated to the lowest goal necessarily did the best. Both demonstrated reduced risk in hypertensives with DM and did not support the contention that hypertensives with known CAD would be at risk if treated aggressively. Both support the more aggressive BP treatment goals now recommended by guidelines committees (Table 51-23).

While the benefits of this level of aggressive therapy have not been proved conclusively, clinical trial results suggest that more events would be prevented with these treatment goals than with higher levels, with little if any harm to the patient. Another aspect, that of cost, was addressed in an analysis by Elliott and colleagues.[332] They compared the putative cost/effectiveness ratio of treating to a goal of [140/90 mmHg (JNC V) compared with 130/85 mmHg (JNC VI)] in hypertensives with type 2 DM.[11,38] Their theoretical analysis suggested that the

TABLE 51-21 Pharmacologic Properties of Commonly Used Antihypertensive Agents

Drug	Dose, mg/day	Doses per Day	Mechanisms of Action	Special Considerations
Diuretics				
Thiazides and related drugs	12.5–25	1	Decreased body sodium and extracellular fluid volume	More effective antihypertensive agents than loop diuretics unless serum creatinine is ≥2.0 mL/min or creatinine clearance is ≤50 mL/min
Hydrochlorothiazide				
Loop diuretics				
Furosemide	20–320	2	Inhibit $2Cl^{-}Na^{+}$ pump	Effective even in patients with advanced renal or congestive heart failure
Bumetanide	0.5–5	2	Ascending loop of Henle	
Ethacrynic acid	25–100	2		
Torsemide	5–20	1		
Fixed-dose diuretics (potassium-sparing)			Increase K^{+} reabsorption	Weak diuretics
Hydrochlorothiazide/amiloride				
HCTZ/triamterene				
Spironolactone	25–100	2–3	Aldosterone antagonist	May cause hyperkalemia in patients with serum creatinine >2.5 mg/dL, particularly when combined with ACE inhibitors, K^{+} supplements, or NSAIDs
Triamterene	50–100	2		
Adrenergic inhibitors				
Beta blockers				
Cardioselective			Inhibit $beta_1$ receptors, decrease CO	In higher doses, also inhibit $beta_2$ receptors
Atenolol	25–100	1	Increase SVR, decrease plasma renin activity (PRA)	
Metoprolol	50–200	1–2		
Noncardioselective			Inhibit $beta_1$ and $beta_2$ receptors	More likely to cause metabolic side effects
Nadolol	20–240	1		
Propranolol	40–240	1–2		
Timolol	20–40	2		
With intrinsic sympathomimetic activity (ISA)				
Acebutolol	200–1200	2	Partial agonist activity on beta-adrenergic receptors	No clear advantage except for less bradycardia and metabolic side effects than other beta blockers
Pindolol	10–60	2		
Antiadrenergic agents				
Centrally acting				
α-Methyldopa	250–1500	2	Stimulate $alpha_2$-adrenergic receptors in the brainstem, resulting in inhibition of efferent sympathetic activity; decrease SVR	Sudden withdrawal may result in hypertensive crisis
Clonidine	0.1–0.6	2		
Clonidine TTS	0.1–0.3	Once a week		
Guanfacine	1–3	1		
Peripherally acting				
Guanethidine	10–100	1	Inhibit norepinephrine release from sympathetic nerve terminals Decrease SVR	Frequently cause orthostatic hypotension and sexual dysfunction

Reserpine	0.05–0.25	1	Depletion of norepinephrine	Causes frequent neurologic symptoms; $alpha_1$-receptor blockers
Doxazosin	2–16	1	Inhibit $alpha_1$-adrenergic receptors.	First-dose effect; postural hypotension; useful for prostatic hypertrophy
Prazosin	2–20	1–2	Decrease SVR; CO same or increases	
Terazosin	1–20	1		
Alpha/beta blockers				
Labetalol	200–800	2–3	Blocks alpha- and beta-adrenergic receptors (7:1 beta:alpha blockade)	Same as beta blockers
Carvedilol	3.75–25	2	Blocks alpha- and beta-adrenergic receptors (3:1 beta:alpha blockade)	Same as beta blockers
ACE inhibitors				
Benazepril	10–40	1–2	Block conversion of angiotensin I to angiotensin II; decrease aldosterone; may increase bradykinin and vasodilatory prostaglandins; decrease SVR; no change in CO	When added to diuretics, may cause hypotension; may cause hyperkalemia in patients with renal failure, those with hypoaldosteronism, those receiving K-sparing diuretics or NSAIDs
Captopril	12.5–100	2–3		
Cilazapril	2.5–5	1–2		
Enalapril	2.5–40	1–2		
Fosinopril	10–40	1		
Lisinopril	5–40	1		
Perindopril	1–16	1–2		Can cause acute renal failure in patients with bilateral renal artery stenosis, renal artery stenosis of a solitary kidney, creatinine >3 mg/dL, or severe heart failure
Quinapril	5–80	1–2		
Ramipril	1.25–20	1		
Spirapril	12.5–50	1–2		
Trandolapril	1–4	1		
Calcium antagonists			Blocks entry of calcium into smooth muscle cells, resulting in vasodilation; decreases SVR; blunts increases in exercise heart rate	
Diltiazem	90–360	3–4		
Diltiazem CD	180–360	1		
Verapamil	80–480	2–3		May cause heart block, particularly when combined with beta blocker
Verapamil SR	120–480	1–2		
Verapamil-Covera HS	180–240	1 (at bedtime)		
Dihydropyridines				
Amlodipine	2.5–10	1	Same as diltiazem and verapamil	More potent vasodilators than diltiazem and verapamil; may cause dizziness, headache, tachycardia, flushing, edema
Felodipine	5–20	1	Do not blunt increase in exerise heart rate	
Isradipine	2.5–10	2		
Nicardipine	60–120	3		
Nifedipine	30–120	3		
Nifedipine (GITS)	30–120	1		
Nisoldipine	10–10	1–2		
Direct vasodilators				
Hydralazine	50–200	2–4	Direct relaxation of smooth muscle cells, causing arteriolar vasodilation secondary to opening $[K^+]$ channels	Limited efficacy if given alone due to fluid retention and reflex vasodilation; should be combined with a diuretic and a beta blocker to prevent edema and tachycardia
Minoxidil	2.5–80	1		

TABLE 51-21 Pharmacologic Properties of Commonly Used Antihypertensive Agents (*Continued*)

Combination Drugs for Hypertension	
Drug	Trade Name
Beta-adrenergic blockers and diuretics	
Atenolol 50 or 100 mg and chlorthalidone 25 mg	Tenoretic
Bisoprolol fumarate 2.5, 5, or 10 mg, and hydrochlorothiazide 6.25 mg	Ziac[a]
Metoprolol tartrate 50 or 100 mg and hydrochlorothiazide 25 or 50 mg	Lopressor HCT
Nadolol 40 or 80 mg and bendroflumethiazide 5 mg	Corzide
Propranolol hydrochloride 40 or 80 mg and hydrochlorothiazide 25 mg	Inderide
Propranolol hydrochloride (extended release) 80, 120, or 160 mg and hydrochlorothiazide 50 mg	Inderide LA
Timolol maleate 10 mg and hydrochlorothiazide 25 mg	Timolide
ACE inhibitors and diuretics	
Benazepril hydrochloride 5, 10, or 20 mg, and hydrochlorothiazide 6.25, 12.5, or 25 mg	Lotensin HCT
Captopril 25 or 50 mg and hydrochlorothiazide 15 or 25 mg	Capozide[a]
Enalapril maleate 5 or 10 mg and hydrochlorothiazide 12.5 or 25 mg	Vaseretic
Lisinopril 10 or 20 mg and hydrochlorothiazide 12.5 or 25 mg	Prinzide, Zestoretic
Angiotensin II receptor antagonists and diuretics	
Losartan potassium 50 mg and hydrochlorothiazide 12.5 mg	Hyzaar
Calcium antagonists and ACE inhibitors	
Amlodipine besylate 2.5 or 5 mg and benazepril hydrochloride 10 or 20 mg	Lotrel
Diltiazem hydrochloride 180 mg and enalapril maleate 5 mg	Teczem
Verapamil hydrochloride (extended release) 180 or 240 mg and trandolapril 1, 2, or 4 mg	Tarka
Felodipine 5 mg and enalapril maleate 5 mg	Lexxel
Other combinations	
Triamterene 37.5, 50, or 75 mg, and hydrochlorothiazide 25 or 50 mg	Dyazide, Maxide
Spironolactone 25 or 50 mg and hydrochlorothiazide 25 or 50 mg	Aldactazide
Amiloride hydrochloride 5 mg and hydrochlorothiazide 50 mg	Moduretic
Guanethidine monosulfate 10 mg and hydrochlorothiazide 25 mg	Esimil
Hydralazine hydrochloride 25, 50, or 100 mg, and hydrochlorothiazide 25 or 50 mg	Apresazide
Methyldopa 250 or 500 mg and hydrochlorothiazide 15, 25, 30, or 50 mg	Aldoril
Reserpine 0.125 mg and hydrochlorothiazide 25 or 50 mg	Hydropres
Reserpine 0.10 mg, hydralazine hydrochloride 25 mg, and hydrochlorothiazide 15 mg	Ser-Ap-Es
Clonidine hydrochloride 0.1, 0.2, or 0.3 mg, and chlorthalidone 15 mg	Combipres
Methyldopa 250 mg and chlorothiazide 150 or 250 mg	Aldochlor
Reserpine 0.125 or 0.25 mg and chlorthalidone 25 or 50 mg	Demi-Regroton
Reserpine 0.125 or 0.25 mg and chlorothiazide 250 or 500 mg	Diupres
Prazosin hydrochloride 1, 2, or 5 mg, and polythiazide 0.5 mg	Minizide

[a]Approved first-line medications.

TABLE 51-22 Long-Term Outcome–Based Clinical Trials of Antihypertensive Agents in Progress

Acronym (Name)	First-Line Agent	Comparator	Patients	Comments
ALLHAT (Antihypertensive and Lipid Lowering Prevention of Heart Attack Trial)	Amlodipine, Doxazosin, Lisinopril	Chlorthalidone	42,448 in 625 centers in United States and Canada	Doxazosin arm stopped prematurely; 6-year follow-up planned
ANBP-2 (Australian National Blood Pressure Trial No. 2)	ACE inhibitor	Diuretic	6000 65–84-year-old Australians	5-year follow-up planned
ASCOT (Anglo-Scandinavian Cardiac Outcomes Trial)	Calcium antagonist or ACE inhibitor	Diuretic or beta blocker	18,000 residents of Scandinavia or United Kingdom	5-year follow-up planned
CONVINCE (Controlled-Onset Verapamil Investigation of Cardiovascular Endpoints)	COER-verapamil	HCTZ or atenolol	16,602 in 661 centers worldwide	5-year follow-up planned
ELSA (European Lacidipine Study of Atherosclerosis)	Lacidipine	Beta blocker	2251 European patients with known atherosclerosis	4-year follow-up planned
HYVET (Hypertension in the Very Elderly Trial)	ACE inhibitor (± diuretic)	Placebo	2100 patients >80 years old	5-year follow-up planned
INSIGHT (International Nifedipine GITS Study Intervention as a Goal in Hypertension Treatment)	Nifedipine GITS	HCTZ plus amiloride	6592 patients in nine European countries	3-year minimum follow-up planned
LIFE (Losartan Intervention for Endpoint Reduction)	Losartan	Atenolol	9194 patients in >300 centers worldwide	ECG LVH only; 4-year follow-up planned
NICS-EH (National Intervention Cooperative Study in Elderly Hypertensives)	Calcium antagonist	Diuretic	1000 Japanese >60 years old	5 year follow-up planned
NORDIL (Nordic Diltiazem Study)	Diltiazem	Diuretic or beta blocker	11,000 patients in 480 centers in Sweden and Norway	5-year follow-up planned
SHELL (Systolic Hypertension in the Elderly Long-Term Lacidipine Trial)	Lacidipine	Diuretic	4800 Europeans with isolated systolic hypertension	Compares 3.5-year incidence of cardiovascular morbidity/mortality
VALUE (Valsartan Amlodipine Long-Term Utilization Evaluation)	Valsartan (±HCTZ)	Amlodipine (±HCTZ)	14,400 patients in 1000 centers in 31 countries	6 years follow-up, 1450 primary end points expected

aggressive approach would save money. Even though more drugs would be needed, the reduction in both direct costs (hospitalization for the greater number of events that would occur in those with higher BP) and indirect costs (lost work) would more than balance the money spent for additional antihypertensives, any costs related to adverse reactions, and the extra visits to providers necessary to get BP to the lower goal.

TABLE 51-23 Goal Blood Pressure

General population without diabetes or renal disease	<140/90 mmHg
Diabetes	<130/85 mmHg
Renal disease with >1 g proteinuria	<125/75 mmHg
Isolated systolic hypertension	<140 mmHg

Factors to Consider in Choosing an Initial Antihypertensive Agent

There are 10 factors that should always be considered when initial therapy is chosen and other drugs are added (if additional agents are needed to reduce BP to goal) (Table 51-24).

EFFICACY

JNC VI made the distinction between surrogate and clinical end points when it provided guidelines for selecting treatment that were based on efficacy, defined as the reduction of morbid-

TABLE 51-24 Factors in the Choice of Agents for Antihypertensive Therapy

1. Efficacy
2. Comorbidity and other risk factors
3. Safety (adverse reactions and side effects)
4. Demographic considerations
5. Special situations
6. Dose schedule (dosage and chronotherapy)
7. Drug interactions
8. Adherence
9. Mechanism of action of drug and pathophysiology of patient's hypertension
10. Cost

ity and mortality. Now four classes of drugs (thiazide diuretics, beta blockers, long-acting DHP CAs, and ACE-Is) have been shown to reduce CV end points when used as the initial therapy for hypertension in appropriately designed and implemented clinical trials. Other agents, such as peripheral sympatholytics (reserpine and guanethidine), centrally acting alpha agonists (alpha-methyldopa), and vasodilators (hydralazine), also have been used in clinical trials as the second, third, or even fourth agent to be added to get BP under control. None is an option for initial therapy because they are relatively poorly tolerated compared with the agents that are recommended as initial therapy or need to be taken together with diuretics to lower BP effectively in the long term. Other drugs, such as alpha/beta blockers and ARBs, that are effective as monotherapy and are well tolerated, have not yet been shown to reduce clinical end points. Alpha blockers are valuable as adjunctive therapy, but the early data from ALLHAT have shown that this class should not be used as the initial treatment for hypertension unless symptomatic relief of benign prostatic hypertrophy (BPH) is needed.[321] Many would now recommend that a man with hypertension and BPH get another drug along with the alpha blocker as part of an antihypertensive regimen.

COMORBIDITY AND OTHER RISK FACTORS

JNC VI has recognized two other factors that may alter the correct choice of initial treatment in an individual hypertensive patient:

- Data from events trials that were conducted in subjects with other conditions (e.g., type 1 DM, acute MI, HF, and after HOPE, those considered to be at high risk for CV events) but in which many subjects with hypertension were enrolled. These trials were the basis for the JNC VI designation of a "compelling" indication (Table 51-25)
- Individual patients may have certain comorbid conditions for which a specific agent may be appropriate even though no trial has been completed in which that agent has been compared to drugs for which clinical trial data are currently available. This was the basis of the JNC VI recommendation for a drug to be indicated or contraindicated as a "specific" indication even though randomized clinical trials might not be available to support that decision (Table 51-26). A "specific" indication tries to codify clinical judgment, or that which any reasonable clinician would do to care for all the health needs of his or her patients. For the most part, these

TABLE 51-25 Considerations in Individualizing Antihypertensive Drug Therapy

Indication[a]	Drug Therapy
DM (type 1) with proteinuria	ACE-I
HF (systolic)	ACE-I, diuretics, beta blockers, aldosterone receptor blockers
Isolated systolic hypertension (older patients)	Diuretics (preferred), DHP CAs
MI	Beta blockers (non-ISA), ACE-Is (systolic dysfunction)

[a]Compelling indications unless contraindicated.
SOURCE: Modified from JNC VI.

recommendations do not add classes of drugs to the list of those which are favored because of a reduction in clinical end points but instead alter the choice of which class should be selected for initial therapy. Good examples are osteoporosis and thiazide diuretics and angina pectoris and beta blockers.

The factors that influence the specific indications are generally the presence of other risk factors and active clinical problems. These conditions may and often should alter the initial and subsequent choice of antihypertensive therapy in an individual patient. An appreciation of the fact that the drugs prescribed to reduce BP can improve or adversely affect other clinical conditions is the basis for the JNC VI recommendation that although diuretics and beta blockers should be used when a patient has "uncomplicated" hypertension, the presence of these comorbid conditions clearly affects that decision.

This approach was also used by the BHS.[19] In those guidelines, similar language to that in JNC VI was used, but the BHS considered the presence of some of these comorbid conditions to be a compelling reason rather than a specific one to choose a particular class of drugs even though a trial had not been completed proving the value of those agents in patients with these conditions. The lessons from the Evaluation of Losartan in the Elderly II trial (ELITE II), which failed to show any advantage of an ARB over an ACE-I (see below), and ALLHAT are that it is best to demand and wait for evidence that an agent prevents events before recommending to clinicians that they should feel "compelled" to prescribe that class.

Dyslipidemias Hypertensive patients who have lipid abnormalities (which may be present in as many as 50 percent of those treated for hypertension) probably should not be treated with drugs that worsen their particular dyslipidemia. Although it has not been proved that the changes in serum lipids caused by certain classes of antihypertensive agents are harmful, it is certainly reasonable to choose an equally effective drug that is lipid-neutral or one that may improve the lipid profile.[333] In large doses (>25 mg/day), thiazide diuretics and related compounds such as chlorthalidone raise TC and LDL-C 5 to 10 percent at least transiently and may lower HDL-C 2 to 4 percent. Serum triglycerides are increased 15 to 30 percent.[334] With the

TABLE 51-26 Drugs That May Have Favorable or Unfavorable Effects on Comorbid Conditions

Condition	Drugs
Favorable	
Angina	Beta blockers, Ca^{2+} antagonists
Atrial tachycardia and fibrillation	Beta blockers, CA nondihydropyridines
Cyclosporine-induced hypertension	Ca^{2+} antagonists (caution with the dose of cyclosporine)
DM (types 1 and 2) with proteinuria	ACE-Is (preferred), CAs (nondihydropyridines), low-dose diuretics
HF	ACE-Is, losartan, K^+-sparing agents, beta-blockers
Liver disease	Beta blockers
Peripheral vascular disease	Alpha-blockers, CAs
Pregnancy	Labetalol hydrochloride, methyldopa
DM (type 2)	ACE-Is
Dyslipidemia	Alpha blockers
Essential tremor	Beta blockers
Hyperthyroidism	Beta blockers
Migraine	Beta blockers (noncardioselective), Ca^{2+} antagonists (nondihydropyridine)
MI	Beta blockers (cardioselective)
Osteoporosis	Thiazide diuretics
Preoperative hypertension	Beta blockade
Prostatism (benign prostatic hyperplasia)	Alpha blockers
Renal insufficiency (caution in renovascular disease)	ACE-Is, ARBs, K^+-sparing agents for hypertension and creatinine >3 mg/dL
Unfavorable	
Bronchospastic disease	Beta blockers
Depression	Beta blockers, central alpha agonists, reserpine
DM (types 1 and 2)	Beta blockers, high-dose diuretics
Dyslipidemia	Beta blockers (non-ISA), diuretics (high-dose)
Gout	Diuretics
Second- or third-degree heart block	Beta blockers, Ca^{2+} antagonists (nondihydropyridine)
Renal insufficiency, renovascular disease	ACE-Is, ARBs

doses that are currently recommended (using up to but no more than 25 mg of hydrochlorothiazide), there is little if any alterations in these parameters. The beta blockers that do not have intrinsic sympathomimetic activity lower HDL-C even more (10 percent) and also raise triglycerides (approximately 20 percent) without affecting TC or LDL.[335] Beta blockers that do have intrinsic sympathomimetic activity and alpha/beta blockers are lipid-neutral.

Conversely, one could choose to add to therapy using a peripheral alpha blocker in patients with dyslipidemias who are already being treated with agents known to reduce CV events, such as beta blockers, ACE-Is, and diuretics.[333,336] These drugs reduce TC and LDL cholesterol approximately 8 to 10 percent, triglycerides 15 percent, and HDL-C 10 to 15 percent. The ALLHAT results mentioned above call into question the wisdom of this approach.[321] ACE-Is do not affect serum lipids, and in some studies benefits similar to those seen with alpha blockers have been observed. ARBs and CAs are lipid-neutral.[334,335]

Other sympatholytics do not affect the lipid profile, and direct vasodilators (e.g., hydralazine) raise HDL-C and lower triglycerides and TG even when used in combination with thiazide diuretics.

Glucose and Insulin and Diabetes Mellitus Antihypertensive drugs may affect glucose metabolism and worsen or improve insulin sensitivity.[333] The magnitude and direction of the drug-induced changes seen in glucose and insulin are very similar to what occurs with lipids. Peripheral alpha blockers and some ACE-Is (captopril, enalapril, trandolapril, and perindopril) may improve insulin sensitivity.[337] Not only do some ACE-Is improve insulin sensitivity, all have been shown to reduce urinary protein excretion, which may contribute to the renal benefit seen in patients with DM. Both moderate- to high-dose thiazides and beta blockers worsen insulin sensitivity and occasionally precipitate glucose intolerance. Beta blockers increase the risk of developing clinical DM by up to 25 percent.[338] In spite of these metabolic changes, in SHEP, treatment with low-dose chlorthalidone (plus atenolol or reserpine in some volunteers) reduced clinical events in the diabetic subgroup even more than it did in nondiabetics.[339] In the HOPE trial and in CAPPP, incident diabetes was prevented.[312,318] These findings, if confirmed by ALLHAT (STOP-2 did not demonstrate that ACE-Is prevented new DM), indicate that patients at high risk of becoming diabetic (the obese and those with glucose intolerance or other components of syndrome X) also might benefit from treatment with ramapril or an ACE-I.

Hypertensives with Diabetes Mellitus The combination of hypertension and DM confers much more risk for CV events and renal failure than does either one alone. Angiotensin-converting enzyme inhibitors, diuretics, and beta blockers have been shown consistently to reduce CV and renal risk. There are very few data on other classes of antihypertensive agents, although there are some preliminary studies with ARBs and CAs. JNC VI recommended that clinicians should feel "compelled" to give hypertensive patients with type 1 DM an ACE-I only because the only randomized clinical trial that has clearly demonstrated the utility of ACE-Is in reducing clinical events was done in a group of type 1 diabetic patients with hypertension.[316] Although no large, long-term events trials have been completed that have proved the special value of ACE-Is in patients with type 2 DM, many feel that the benefit shown for type I diabetic patients also can be assumed to occur for type 2 diabetic patients, and so ACE-Is were recommended by JNC VI as a specific indication.[11] Others argue that if BP control is achieved, it does not matter what drug or drugs are used. In UKPDS, the group that received the ACE inhibitor captopril did no better than did the group that received atenolol. This lends some support to the argument that BP control, not how it is accomplished, is the key factor in reducing events in type 2 diabetic patients.[325]

Although some experts have raised concern about the safety of DHP CAs in type 2 diabetic patients, the Syst-EUR study, in which these drugs were the initial therapy, demonstrated that the benefit accrued was greater in diabetic patients than it was in other patients.[340] Just as with SHEP, the results of a properly done clinical trial disproved surrogate end-point-based hypotheses from other sources of data such as observational studies, case-control studies, and meta-analyses of smaller trials.

Trials of CV mortality involving nondihydropyridine CAs in high-risk hypertensive patients have not been completed. However, nondihydropyridine CAs have been shown to reduce CV mortality after an MI and slow the progression of diabetic nephropathy.[341,342] Moreover, their use in combination with ACE-Is lowers urinary protein excretion, and unlike DHP CAs, they have additive effects to reduce proteinuria independent of BP reduction.[343,344] This combination appears to be particularly useful in diabetic patients with nephropathy and proteinuria.

From the available data, it would appear that in people with DM, the most important factor in reducing mortality and preserving renal function is reducing BP to goal (Table 51-23).

Left Ventricular Hypertrophy and Heart Failure Left ventricular hypertrophy results from chronic elevations in arterial pressure that cause cardiac myocyte hypertrophy and remodeling of the coronary resistance vessels. This leads to perivascular fibrosis of the intramyocardial arteries and arterioles. Over time, these changes in the myocardium contribute to the development of ventricular wall stiffness and diastolic dysfunction.[345]

Left ventricular hypertrophy is a robust independent risk factor for CV and premature mortality.[227] It is especially common in the elderly, particularly in elderly women, and often is associated with diastolic dysfunction. It appears that all antihypertensive agents that are recommended for initial therapy reduce LV mass. Data from meta-analyses have suggested that agents that block the RAA system reduce LV mass better than do other antihypertensive agents.[235] However, TOMHS and the Veterans Administration (VA) study of monotherapy found that there was no difference among antihypertensive agents in their ability to regress LVH.[236,237] Moreover, in TOMHS, nutritional hygienic measures such as weight loss, reduced Na^+ and alcohol intake, and exercise were effective by themselves in regressing LV mass. Perhaps the most important factor responsible for LV mass regression is the prolonged reduction of systolic BP.

Heart Failure Hypertension has been identified as a major risk factor for the subsequent development of HF, the onset of which typically occurs many years later.[346] For many un- or undertreated hypertensives, LVH is an important intermediate step, resulting in "hypertensive heart disease" with impaired LV filling and increased ventricular stiffness. This type of HF (which has been seen in up to 40 percent of hospitalized patients with an antecedent history of hypertension) is commonly called diastolic dysfunction.[233] The more common type of "systolic dysfunction" associated with a reduced LV ejection fraction most often is due to previous MI (for which hypertension is also an important risk factor). In a meta-analysis of clinical trials in hypertension, there was a 42 percent reduction in HF incidence among hypertensives randomized to either a low-dose diuretic or a beta blocker.[342]

Distinguishing between the two subtypes of HF is most easily done by quantitation of the LV ejection fraction.[347] The results dictate the therapy. Patients with low ejection fractions ("systolic HF") improve both BP and long-term prognosis with ACE-Is and diuretics, to which are sometimes added beta blockers, spironolactone, and/or other drugs.[314,347–349] The role of ARBs is controversial unless cough or other adverse effects preclude an ACE-I. In the first (but small) direct comparison of captopril and losartan [Evaluation of Losartan In The Elderly (ELITE)], there was a survival benefit (a tertiary hypothesis) attributed to the ARBs, which the larger study (ELITE II), with exactly the same protocol, did not confirm.[350] If cough or other adverse effects of an ACE-I preclude its use, an ARB becomes the rational choice. Ongoing research may define the benefit of using both an ACE-I and an ARB simultaneously in patients with systolic HF. The role of DHP CAs and other direct-acting vasodilators (e.g., hydralazine in combination with isosorbide dinitrate) remains controversial.[351] Most authorities recommend these drugs as second- or third-line therapy (after maximum doses of ACE-Is and/or ARBs) if BP is still elevated. Recently, in the Randomized Aldactone Evaluation Study (RALES) trial, spironolactone, an aldosterone antagonist, in doses that do not lower BP reduced morbidity and mortality in patients with HF, most of whom were already taking ACE-Is, aspirin, and diuretics.[349] Many of these patients were also on beta blockers.

Treatment of hypertension with diastolic dysfunction and HF has not been as well studied, but most authorities recommend using drugs that reduce HR, increase diastolic filling time, and allow the heart muscle to relax more fully: beta blockers or nondihydropyridine CAs.[352,353] Although these options make physiologic sense, no randomized clinical trials have had outcomes that demonstrate their long-term efficacy.[352]

Valvular Disease The coexistence of hypertension and valvular heart disease is, for most affected patients, simply an occurrence of two common conditions in the same person. There are few syndromes or scenarios in which the two are pathophysiologically connected, but there are some circumstances in which their coexistence has clinical importance, especially in regard to choosing antihypertensive drug therapy.

A murmur of aortic sclerosis is found in approximately 21 to 26 percent of adults over 65 years of age. Recent data from the CV Health Study showed that 29 percent of the 5621 subjects age 65 and over had this valvular abnormality detected on echocardiography; it was found much more commonly among hypertensives and those with LVH.[354] Perhaps most important, its presence was associated with a 50 percent increased risk of CV events over an average of 5 years of follow-up. After adjustment for risk factor differences at baseline (e.g., hypertension), only one of four studied end points retained statistical significance. Calcific aortic stenosis is about 10 times less common but often must be evaluated more extensively, usually with an echocardiogram. Aortic insufficiency in hypertensives is found almost exclusively in patients with isolated systolic hypertension and is most easily recognized by the murmur and several peripheral signs.[355] Unloading the LV with arteriolar vasodilators has long been recommended on a pathophysiologic basis and has been shown in a long-term trial against digoxin to prolong the time until valvular replacement surgery was required.[356] Although nifedipine was used in the study, it is likely that any vasodilator would be more effective than a weakly positive inotropic agent.

Mitral valvular disease is less common than it was in past decades, primarily because of efforts to treat streptococcal pharyngitis. Mitral stenosis is still seen occasionally in citizens of developing countries but is not commonly associated with systemic hypertension. Since digoxin typically is used to control the ventricular rate in atrial fibrillation, antihypertensive drugs that interfere with the excretion of digoxin should be used cautiously. Mitral insufficiency is also less common than it was in the past, but there are few problems specific to this disease that affect hypertension and its therapy.

The right-sided cardiac valves seldom need be considered in the treatment of patients with systemic hypertension. In patients with primary (or secondary) pulmonary hypertension (which can be treated with the usual antihypertensive drugs, although with less success), the status of the right-sided heart valves takes on increased significance.[357] Occasionally, insufficiency of the tricuspid valve is the major diagnostic clue to carcinoid heart disease (associated with weight loss drugs but rarely associated with hypertension).[358]

Microalbuminuria MA is a predictor of CV and renal death in patients with DM.[359–361] The class of antihypertensive medications known to have the most potent effects on reducing MA is the ACE-Is.[317,359–363] These agents reduce albuminuria by reducing intraglomerular pressure as well as decreasing glomerular size selectivity and partially restoring membrane charge.[362,363] The effects of different classes of antihypertensive agents on MA as well as related metabolic parameters are summarized in Table 51-27.

TABLE 51-27 Effects of Drugs on Microalbuminuria and Proteinuria

Decrease levels
ACE inhibitors
Angiotensin receptor blockers
Alpha/beta blockers
Nondihydropyridine CAs
Beta blockers
Diuretics
Increase levels
Short-acting dihydropyridine CAs
Minoxidil
No effect
Dihydropyridine CAs (long acting)
Alpha blockers
Central alpha agonists (clonidine, methyldopa)

Both ACE-Is and nondihydropyridine CAs reduce albuminuria and together have additive antialbuminuric effects, in part independently of further reductions in BP.[359,364,365]

The ACE-Is and ARBs are the antihypertensive agents that most consistently reduce proteinuria in response to their BP-lowering effect. Moreover, in the absence of hypertension, these agents prevent the increase of MA to proteinuria and in many cases normalize protein excretion in patients with MA.[366] Nondihydropyridine CAs (diltiazem and verapamil) also have some utility in reducing urinary protein excretion in hypertensive patients with kidney disease.[364] In two studies, these drugs had antiproteinuric effects similar to those of ACE-Is in hypertensive diabetic patients with chronic renal disease and heavy proteinuria.[367,368] Some studies have shown that a high Na^+ intake blunts the antiproteinuric and antihypertensive effects of an ACE-I.[369,370] Increasing dietary salt despite not affecting BP appears to abolish the antiproteinuric effect of the nondihydropyridine CA diltiazem, and so attention should be paid to Na^+ intake in patients with MA/or proteinuria.[368,369] Since there are so many more data, including events data, about ACE-I than about any other agents, including ARBs, ACE-Is should be the first-line treatment of hypertension in DM and should be included in all antihypertensive regimens in such patients if tolerated.

Renal Dysfunction Any agent or group of agents that adequately lowers BP to levels <130/85 mmHg will slow the progression of nephropathy. Aggressive BP reduction (<125/75 mmHg) is needed to maximally slow the progression of renal disease, especially among patients with elevated serum creatinine. Aggressive BP reduction (<125/75 mmHg) is needed to maximally slow the progression of renal disease, especially among patients with an elevated serum creatinine ≥1.4 mg/dL.[11] ACE-Is will slow the progression of diabetic and nondiabetic nephropathy, assuming BP reduction to levels below 140/90 mmHg.

In spite of the evidence from many long-term clinical trials, there is a general hesitancy among clinicians to use ACE-Is in such patients. This stems from a rise in serum creatinine that predictably occurs when the drug is given. It is common to see increases in serum creatinine of up to 25 percent above baseline within 2 to 3 months of ACE-inhibitor initiation. An analysis of long-term clinical trials has confirmed that this reduction in renal function plateaus within a month.[371] In a study from Scandinavia, ACE-Is were discontinued after an average follow-up of 6 years of therapy. The glomerular filtration rate (GFR) returned to levels not significantly different from baseline even though within the first 4 months after ACE-I initiation there was a clear initial reduction in GFR by an average of 8 to 10 percent below baseline.[372] This return to baseline GFR has not been reported with any other class of antihypertensive agent studied and suggests that ACE-Is prevented the expected deterioration of renal function over time. If the serum creatinine continues to rise, especially after 1 month of therapy, evaluation for renal artery stenosis may be indicated.

There are also concerns about hyperkalemia. This should be worrisome only if the serum K^+ rises ≥0.5 meq/L.

The role of ARBs in the treatment of nephropathy and reducing CV events has not been settled. All animal studies and one completed clinical trial in patients with HF suggest that these agents are as good as ACE-Is in slowing the progression of renal disease and reducing proteinuria and CV events.[360,365] Whether ARBs are better than ACE-Is or even equivalent remains to be proved. Two ongoing clinical trials in subjects with diabetic nephropathy are scheduled to be completed by 2002 and will answer the question definitively.[319]

Thus, while any class of antihypertensive agent may be used to achieve this new recommended lower level of BP to preserve renal function, certain principles should be kept in mind.

- BP will never be controlled adequately in patients with significant renal insufficiency (serum creatinine >1.8 mg/dL) without the use of a diuretic (usually a loop diuretic).
- Long-acting loop diuretics are preferred, or if furosemide is used, it needs to be given twice a day.
- Various combinations of medications will be needed to achieve BP reduction. One of these drugs should contain an ACE-I. If side effects are noted with the ACE-I, an ARB may be substituted to ensure renal protection and BP reduction.

Since CV is the most common cause of death in people with renal disease, beta blockers clearly also have a role in therapy. These agents do not have synergistic or additive effects on BP in the presence of agents such as clonidine.[373]

Coronary Artery Disease Since hypertension is a major risk factor for CAD, it is not surprising that a large number of patients have both conditions. It is unlikely on ethical grounds that a placebo-controlled trial will be done with any single antihypertensive drug in such patients. The presence of CAD in a patient with hypertension is likely to influence both the choice of drugs used to treat the patient and the BP goal to be achieved. Because both beta blockers and CAs are effective antihypertensive agents with major antianginal efficacy, they are often the preferred agents for initial treatment, especially in the common setting of unstable angina pectoris.[374] A recent meta-analysis suggested that the former are more effective, although the latter are more commonly used.[375] The recent HOPE trial showed a large survival benefit for high-risk hypertensives (most of whom had known CAD) treated with ramapril.[318] None of the volunteers in HOPE had known HF at enrollment in which this degree of benefit would have been expected. This has been interpreted by some as evidence in favor of this class of medication or even for this specific agent for all hypertensive patients with CAD.

The issue of how low to reduce BP in the setting of CAD is controversial. The concept of the J-shaped curve has been supported by data in patients with coronary disease, mostly using beta blockers.[328] Diastolic pressures less than 82 mmHg were associated with a higher risk of coronary events, and the rationale proposed was that since coronary artery filling occurs during diastole, reducing perfusion pressure during this time might increase coronary ischemia. These and other data led to the HOT study, in which 18,790 hypertensive patients without known coronary disease were randomized to one of three diastolic BP goals: ≤90, ≤85, and ≤80 mmHg.[324] After 3.8 years, there were no significant differences in major CV events across the groups, suggesting that there is no increase in risk from lowering diastolic BPs below 80 mmHg. It is unlikely that a similar study in patients with CAD will be done, but some still recommend caution in lowering BP below 85 mmHg in patients with angina and/or known CAD. JNC VI indicates that "BP should be lowered to the usual target range (<140/90 mmHg), and even lower BP is desirable if angina persists."[11] The World Health Organization/International Society of Hypertension's Collaborative Trialists' Group is collecting patient-specific outcome data and eventually may have sufficient power from the clinical trials in this registry for a post hoc analysis comparing levels of achieved BP control among 270,000 hypertensives with or without CAD.[319] Even after such data become available, it probably will be advisable to use beta blockers, CAs, and perhaps nitrates for hypertensive patients with CAD to achieve a slightly lower than usual BP target and to recommend aspirin and intensive treatment of dyslipidemias. Appropriate precautions must be taken for hypertensives also using sildenafil citrate (Viagra). To date, no antihypertensives seem to confer any increased risks when used with this agent, but all nitrate-containing preparations are contraindicated.

After Stroke Although hypertension is perhaps the most powerful risk factor for acute stroke and "clinically evident cerebrovascular disease is an indication for antihypertensive treatment," optimal BP management depends on the nature, cause, and chronology of the neurologic symptoms.[376] In the immediate setting of acute ischemic stroke, there is controversy about the optimal level of acceptable BP. Appropriate concern has been expressed about possible reduction in blood flow to "watershed" areas of the brain that are already poorly perfused if BP is reduced pharmacologically.[377] Many neurologists have observed acute worsening of cerebrovascular function and evolving neurologic deficits when BP has been reduced "too much" or "too quickly." Most physicians therefore are uncomfortable reducing BP to <180/100 mmHg. Many do not institute treatment until mean arterial pressure is >130 mmHg (e.g., BP >200/100 mmHg), except in the setting of concomitant hemorrhagic transformation or another hypertensive emergency (e.g., aortic dissection, MI, renal failure with bleeding).[378] This level of BP is at least supported by the exclusion criterion from the National Institutes of Health (NIH)-sponsored rt-PA for acute stroke trial; patients with BP >185/110 mmHg were prohibited from getting the thrombolytic agent and were instead suggested to receive antihypertensive therapy.[379] The optimal drug therapy for acute stroke-related hypertension is also ill defined, but most authorities prefer intravenously administered, short-acting agents because they can be discontinued quickly if a patient's neurologic condition deteriorates acutely.[378]

SAFETY (ADVERSE REACTIONS AND SIDE EFFECTS)

The two primary types of adverse reactions and side effects that occur with antihypertensive therapy are clinical and biochemical (Table 51-21). Clinical side effects are directly evident to the patient and are perceived by the patient or the clinician to be related to the drug. The appearance of these adverse reactions requires that the drug be stopped, the dose be reduced, or the patient be willing to remain on therapy until he or she becomes able to tolerate the side effect or until it disappears. The drugs recommended for initial therapy generally cause fewer clinical side effects than do other drugs at doses that lower BP.[11,18,19]

Biochemical side effects may lead to clinically evident adverse reactions (e.g., hypokalemia from thiazide diuretics causing muscle weakness, palpitations, nocturia, or polyuria), but usually the biochemical problems that occur with antihypertensive agents are more troublesome to the clinician than they are to the patient.

The importance of biochemical side effects is usually not that they result in clinically evident problems but the danger that these drug-related permutations of lipids, glucose, or insulin may aggravate other risk factors and accelerate the clinical impact of dyslipidemias, glucose intolerance, or insulin resistance. Whether the minor and often short-term effects on triglycerides, HDL-C, or TG that result from therapy with thiazides or beta blockers are responsible for an increase in ischemic heart disease remains to be proved. It is of great interest that in ALLHAT the biochemical profile of the group receiving the alpha blocker seemed favorable (lower triglycerides, TG, and glucose and higher K^+) compared with the group on chlorthalidone, yet the diuretic prevented CV events more successfully.[321] The remaining treatment arms of ALLHAT (DHP CA and ACE-I versus diuretic) should definitely delineate the role of these metabolic changes.

At the doses that are now recommended, these changes and the electrolyte disturbances noted with thiazides are modest, although it is still possible that at high doses, thiazides could reduce serum K^+ sufficiently to increase the rate of sudden cardiac death. Whether the increases in insulin resistance that are seen with thiazide diuretics and beta blockers and the hypokalemia that is seen with thiazide diuretics have precipitated DM sooner or in patients who would not otherwise have become diabetic also remains to be proved. Although it is not certain that these metabolic adverse reactions are clinically relevant, it may be prudent to select another option for patients with DM or a dyslipidemia so long as BP is reduced to goal. Certain types of dual therapy also may ameliorate biochemical adverse reactions. Angiotensin-converting enzyme inhibitors and ARBs and thiazides, when given together, produce few, if any, of the metabolic abnormalities associated with thiazides alone.[380] Several fixed-dose combinations or these classes of drugs are available and may be appropriate as initial therapy[11] (Table 51-21).

The incidence of clinical side effects tends to rise with increasing doses with all classes of drugs, with the exception of ACE-Is and ARBs. Patients who develop an adverse reaction on a high dose of a drug or on a dose they previously tolerated do not necessarily need to have that drug discontinued. Instead, the dose can be lowered and another antihypertensive can be added to reduce BP to goal. The primary problems with ACE-Is are cough and angioedema, both of which tend to be idiosyncratic and occur with all representatives of that class of agents. Reducing the dose or changing to a different ACE-I is rarely helpful. Angiotensin-converting enzyme inhibitors should be increased to the maximum recommended dose before therapy is abandoned or another agent is added unless a low-dose fixed-dose combination is felt to be more appropriate. Angiotensin II receptor blockers as a class appear to be the best tolerated of all currently available antihypertensive agents.[381] Although some experts feel that they should be reserved for initial therapy only in patients who have developed a cough with ACE-Is, they are also an excellent option for patients who have no complaints when treatment is started and patients in whom a drug that primarily blocks the RAA system appears to be a good option. When VALUE and LIFE are completed, it will be known whether ARBs are as good a choice as the other four classes of antihypertensives available.

DEMOGRAPHIC CONSIDERATIONS

Blacks and Other Ethnic Minorities Some classes of antihypertensive agents reduce BP more or less effectively in certain ethnic groups. Thiazide diuretics, for example, are more effective in blacks than in whites, whereas ACE-Is, ARBs, and beta blockers are more effective at lower doses in whites. Many blacks respond to agents that block the RAA system, but they often need higher doses than do whites or Asians.[382] Studies in African-Americans have demonstrated that starting with higher doses of an ACE-I makes this class quite efficacious in lowering BP in this population.[383] Therefore, if a black hypertensive patient would benefit from the special properties that these drugs may have in type 1 diabetic patients or in HF, for example, they definitely should be used even if additional agents will be needed to get BP to goal. Peripheral alpha blockers, alpha/beta blockers, and CAs are equally effective in all types of hypertensive patients in all ethnic groups. In general, the response rates to antihypertensive agents in Hispanics is intermediate between that seen in whites and that seen in blacks, while east Asians, though not necessarily south Asians (patients from the Indian subcontinent), often need lower doses than do whites.

The Elderly All classes of antihypertensive agents lower BP effectively in older persons, although the doses needed to reach goal are often lower than the doses necessary in young and middle-aged hypertensive patients.[384,385] Certain drugs and certain classes of drugs, however, should be avoided or used with caution in older hypertensives. These include agents, such as peripheral alpha blockers, that can exacerbate the postural fall in BP seen more frequently in older individuals with baroreceptor dysfunction; nondihydropyridine CAs and beta blockers that may aggravate subtle or subclinical conduction defects or precipitate systolic dysfunction and HF; and verapamil, which may not be well tolerated in some older persons already bothered by constipation. Cough from an ACE-I may be more common in older women. Diuretics and dihydropyridine DHP CAs have both been shown to reduce morbidity and mortality in older persons with stage 2 or 3 isolated systolic hypertension, making them excellent choices in such patients.[269–271] What is often forgotten in regard to many classes is that the benefits of effective treatment are more evident in older hypertensives who are at higher risk than are younger hypertensives.[385] Therapy should not be withheld for fear of toxicity or lack of efficacy in the elderly.

Children The diagnosis and treatment of hypertension in children are different from those in adults, primarily because of the limited experience with antihypertensive drug therapy in children and the low risk of CV events in younger individuals.[386,387] Most pediatricians are very comfortable measuring and monitoring BP in their patients, but few nonnephrologists commit the expected 1 percent of their patients to drug therapy. Because of a higher incidence of secondary hypertension than there is in adults, most hypertensive children have at least an evaluation of the kidneys and urinary tract before beginning treatment.[387]

The diagnosis of hypertension in pediatric patients is truly population-based, since the 5 percent of children with the highest BP are diagnosed with "significant hypertension" and the highest 1 percent are deemed eligible for pharmacologic treat-

TABLE 51-28 Antihypertensive Drugs Frequently Used in Children

Drug	Initial Dose	Usual Maximum Dose
Intravenously administered		
Sodium nitroprusside	0.5 μg/kg/min	8 μg/kg/min
Labetalol	1 mg/kg/h	3 mg/kg/h
Orally administered		
Hydrochlorothiazide	1 mg/kg/day	2–3 mg/kg/day
Furosemide	1 mg/kg/day	12 mg/kg/day
Bumetanide	0.02–0.05 mg/kg/day	0.3 mg/kg/day
Propranolol	1 mg/kg/day	8 mg/kg/day
Atenolol	1 mg/kg/day	8 mg/kg/day
Captopril (for neonates)	0.03 mg/kg/day	2 mg/kg/day
Captopril (for children)	1.5 mg/kg/day	6 mg/kg/day
Enalapril	0.15 mg/kg/day	40 mg/day
Nifedipine (extended release)	0.25 mg/kg/day	3 mg/kg/day
Prazosin	0.05–0.1 mg/kg/day	0.5 mg/kg/day
Minoxidil	0.1–0.2 mg/kg/day	1 mg/kg/day

SOURCE: Adapted from Sinaiko AR. Current concepts: Hypertension in children. *N Engl J Med* 1996; 335:1968–1973.

ment.[387] The diagnostic cutoffs for hypertension in youth are age- and weight-dependent, and "growth charts" for plotting the progress of a child's BP against age often are completed by pediatricians for height, weight, and, more recently, BP. More frequent measurements and attention to BP are warranted when a child's BP exceeds the 90th percentile. Treatment of hypertension in children begins with lifestyle modifications, since they are likely to be beneficial as a child grows into adolescence and adulthood.[386,387] Because few registration studies of antihypertensive drugs include children (owing to informed consent complexities and risk management issues), there are limited data on the benefits of specific drugs in hypertensive children. Although the recommended treatment algorithm is based on time-tested drug use in adults, there is a growing awareness of the possibility of long-term adverse effects with diuretics and especially beta blockers (which make exercise more difficult and may lead to weight gain) and a growing use of both ACE-Is and CAs. Antihypertensive drugs that are used frequently in children are shown in Table 51-28; the doses typically are based on the body weight of the child.

SPECIAL SITUATIONS

Pregnancy Hypertension is found in about 10 percent of pregnancies and is the major cause of perinatal morbidity and mortality in most developed countries. Because of the unique patient population, hypertension in pregnancy has a special definition, four specific types, and a treatment algorithm that recognizes the need to assess outcomes in both mother and baby. Since most pregnancies are managed by obstetricians, most of the authoritative pronouncements about this condition have been advanced by expert panels drawn from that discipline.[388,389] In the United States, hypertension in pregnancy is defined as either BP >140/90 mmHg on two measurements at least 4 h apart or a diastolic BP >110 mmHg at any time during pregnancy or up to 6 weeks postpartum.[389]

The classification of hypertension in pregnancy typically requires some knowledge of BP status before conception. If there was preexisting hypertension, the patient is said to have "chronic hypertension," which can be diagnosed before 20 weeks' gestation and persists at least 42 days postpartum. Preeclampsia is hypertension appearing after 20 weeks' gestation, associated with proteinuria (at least 300 mg per 24-h collection or 2+ on a random dipstick), which typically resolves within 42 days after delivery. Hypertension with superimposed preeclampsia is a combination of the two. The term *Hypertension unclassified* typically is used only when none of the above criteria are met and the BP status before conception or during the first trimester is unknown.

There has been a great effort to elaborate both the cause and the effective treatment for preeclampsia, but neither has been identified. A large number of demographic, genetic, laboratory parameters, and other factors have been associated with a higher risk of preeclampsia, but none has been accepted as the underlying "cause" (Table 51-29). Even more interesting are recent clinical trials that attempted to prevent preeclampsia with low-dose aspirin or Ca^{2+} supplementation.[390,391] Despite a great deal of evidence in smaller studies, typically in high-risk women, the large NIH-sponsored megatrials have been unsuccessful in showing benefit from these inexpensive preventive measures. In addition, since aspirin tends to delay parturition and increase the likelihood of bleeding, few obstetricians routinely recommend it.

Treatment of elevated BP during pregnancy traditionally has begun with bed rest, followed by methyldopa as the primary drug, based on its long history of efficacy and lack of adverse

TABLE 51-29 Factors Associated with Altered Risk of Preeclampsia

- Genetic markers
  - Angiotensinogen gene polymorphism
  - Tumor necrosis factor–alpha gene polymorphism
  - Mitochondrial transfer RNA gene mutation
- Congenital thrombophelias
  - Resistance to activated protein C (factor V Leiden, perhaps the most common form of hereditary prothrombotic disorder)
  - Mutation in gene for prothrombin factor II
  - Hyperhomocysteinemia (mutation C677T)
  - Protein S deficiency
  - Antiphospholipid antibody syndrome
  - Protein C and antithrombin deficiencies

SOURCE: Adapted from Shear R, Leduc L, Rey E, Moutquin J-M. Hypertension in pregnancy: New recommendations for management. *Curr Hypertens Reports* 1999; 1:529–539.

effects on babies. For severe hypertension (BP >160 or 169/109 mmHg) in outpatients that is not controlled with these measures to a diastolic BP between 90 and 100 mmHg, hydralazine, labetalol, and nifedipine routinely are added in succession.[392,393] Angiotensin-converting enzyme inhibitors and ARBs are contraindicated because of renal abnormalities in the fetus, and diuretics typically are avoided because of the risk for oligohydramnios. For intrapartum management, until delivery can be achieved, intravenous Mg^{2+} sulfate has been a mainstay for the prevention of progression of preeclampsia to seizures and other more serious complications.

Hypertension during pregnancy also carries prognostic significance for future health problems as the woman ages. Sixty percent of women with early-onset preeclampsia have abnormalities on renal biopsy and a higher risk of persistent hypertension after delivery. Women who develop hypertension during pregnancy not only are at higher risk for hypertension later in life but also have a roughly twofold increase in the risk of death from CAD.

Hypertensive Emergencies and Urgencies Although great strides have been made in the treatment of hypertension since the First Report of the Joint National Committee on Detection, Evaluation, and Treatment of High Blood Pressure in 1977, some patients still present to physicians' offices and emergency departments with hypertensive crises.[393] Fortunately, there now are excellent medications available for both acute, in-hospital treatment and outpatient management; these improvements have led to a decrease in the 1-year mortality rate after a hypertensive emergency from 80 percent (1928) to 50 percent (1955) to only 10 percent (Fig. 51-1).

The primary pathophysiologic abnormality in patients who experience hypertensive crises is the alteration of autoregulation in certain vascular beds (especially cerebral and renal), which often is followed by frank arteritis and ischemia in vital organs.[394] Autoregulation is the ability of blood vessels to dilate or constrict to maintain normal organ perfusion. Normal arteries from normotensive individuals can maintain flow over a wide range of mean arterial pressures, usually 60 to 150 mmHg. Chronic elevations of BP cause compensatory functional and structural changes in the arterial circulation and shift the autoregulatory curve to the right; this allows hypertensive patients to maintain normal perfusion and avoid excessive blood flow at higher BP levels.[395] When BP increases above the autoregulatory range, tissue damage occurs. An understanding of autoregulation is also important for therapy, since the sudden lowering of BP into a range that would otherwise be considered normal may reduce BP below the autoregulatory capacity of the hypertensive circulation and lead to inadequate tissue perfusion (Fig. 51-2). In the later stages of a hypertensive crisis, pathologists can demonstrate cerebral edema and both acute and chronic inflammation of the medium and small arteries and arterioles, often associated with necrosis.

Hypertensive crises occur in a variety of clinical settings. The most common is a chronic and often untreated patient with stage 3 essential hypertension (i.e., usual BP ≥ 180/110) whose BP rises above the autoregulatory range, triggering the pathophysiologic sequence outlined above. Identical crises can occur, however, any time there is an acute or rapid rise in BP in a normotensive or minimally hypertensive individual, such as a child or a woman during pregnancy. Hypertensive crises can most easily be recognized by the association of an extremely

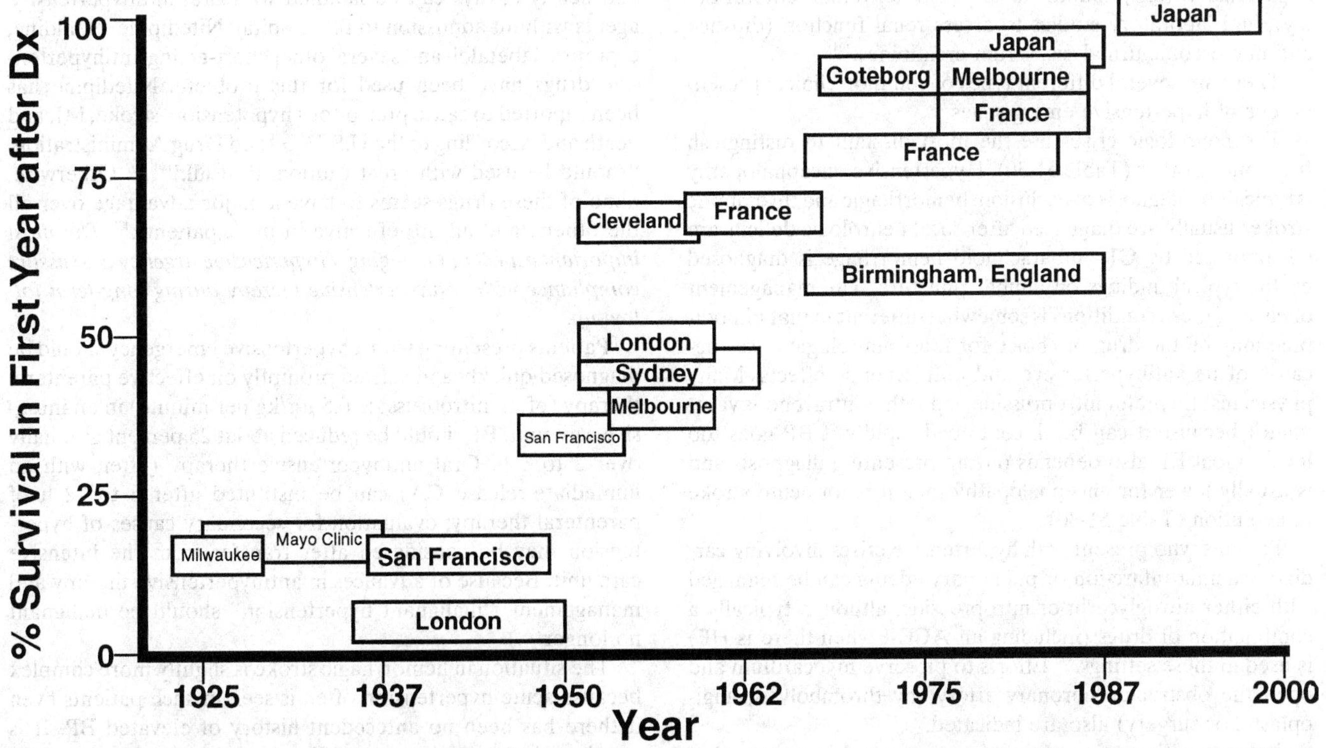

FIGURE 51-1 Improvement in 1-year survival from 1925 to 1999 among patients presenting with a hypertensive emergency. (From Elliott WJ. Hypertensive emergencies. In: Hollenberg SM, Kelly RF, eds. *Critical Care Clinics on Acute Cardiac Care.* New York: Saunders; in press.)

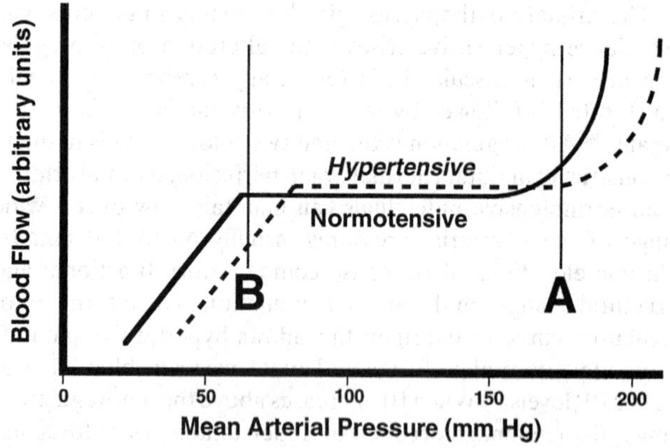

FIGURE 51-2 Blood pressure versus flow relationships in normotensive (*dark curve*) and hypertensive (*dotted curve*) persons, based on cerebral blood flow data of Strandgaard et al.[395] Chronically hypertensive persons can autoregulate their blood flow within the normal range despite higher blood pressures (e.g., vertical line "B"). Lowering BP in the setting of a hypertensive emergency to what might be considered "normal" (in a normotensive person, e.g., vertical line A) probably will put BP below the autoregulatory threshold and may compromise local circulation.

elevated BP with physical examination or laboratory findings that indicate acute TOD. The actual levels of BP are of little import.

The initial evaluation of a severely hypertensive patient includes a thorough inspection of the optic fundi (looking for acute hemorrhages, exudates, or papilledema); a mental status assessment; a careful cardiac, pulmonary, and neurologic examination; a quick search for clues that might indicate secondary hypertension (e.g., abdominal bruit, striae, radial-femoral delay); and laboratory studies to assess renal function (dipstick and microscopic urinalysis, serum creatinine).[394]

There are several different types of common clinical presentations of hypertensive emergencies.

The neurologic crises are the most difficult to distinguish from one another (Table 51-30). Hypertensive encephalopathy is typically a diagnosis of exclusion; hemorrhagic and thrombotic strokes usually are diagnosed after focal neurologic deficits are corroborated by CT. Subarachnoid hemorrhage is diagnosed by the typical findings on lumbar puncture. The management of each of these conditions is somewhat different in that nimodipine may be the drug of choice for most neurologic crises because of its antihypertensive and anti-ischemic effects. Many physicians still prefer nitroprusside or another intravenous vasodilator because it can be discontinued rapidly if BP goes too low.[396] Goal BP also depends on the presenting diagnosis and is usually lower for encephalopathy than it is for acute stroke in evolution (Table 51-30).

Patients who present with hypertensive crises involving cardiac ischemia/infarction or pulmonary edema can be managed with either nitroglycerin or nitroprusside, although typically a combination of drugs (including an ACE-I when there is HF) is used in these settings.[396] Efforts to preserve myocardium and open the obstructed coronary artery (by thrombolysis, angioplasty, or surgery) also are indicated.

Patients with aortic dissection are managed in a somewhat different fashion.[397] A beta blocker is added to the intravenous vasodilator, and the goal BP is much lower: Typically 120 mmHg systolic is recommended, but 100 mmHg systolic may be even better. Pharmacologic therapy is only a temporary adjunct to definitive surgical therapy, which should be planned with dispatch, although long-term medical therapy may be more appropriate in some patients.[398]

Hypertensive crises involving the kidney commonly are followed by a further deterioration in renal function even when BP is lowered properly. Some physicians prefer fenoldopam to nicardipine or nitroprusside in this setting because of its lack of toxic metabolites and specific renal vasodilating effects.[396,399,400] Blood pressure should be reduced about 10 percent during the first hour and a further 10 to 15 percent during the next 1 to 3 h. The need for acute dialysis often is precipitated by BP reduction, but many patients are able to avoid dialysis in the long term if BP is carefully and well controlled during follow-up.

Hypertensive crises resulting from catecholamine excess states [pheochromocytoma, monoamine oxidase (MAO) inhibitor crisis, cocaine intoxication, etc.] are best managed with an intravenous alpha blocker (phentolamine), with the beta blocker added later, if necessary. Many patients with severe hypertension caused by sudden withdrawal of antihypertensive agents (e.g., clonidine) are easily managed by reinstituting such therapy.

Hypertensive crises during pregnancy must be managed in a more careful and conservative manner because of the presence of the fetus. Magnesium sulfate, methyldopa, and hydralazine are the drugs of choice, with oral labetalol and nifedipine being drugs of second choice in the United States. Delivery of the infant often assists in the management of hypertension in pregnancy and often is hastened by the obstetrician under these conditions.

Hypertensive urgencies are situations in which acute TOD is not present; they require somewhat less aggressive management and nearly always can be handled with oral antihypertensive agents without admission to the hospital. Nifedipine, clonidine, captopril, labetalol, and several other short-acting antihypertensive drugs have been used for this problem. Nifedipine has been reported to cause precipitous hypotension, stroke, MI, and death and, according to the U.S. Food and Drug Administration, "should be used with great caution, if at all."[401,402] Otherwise, none of these drugs seems to have a major advantage over all the others, and all are effective in most patients.[403] *The most important aspect of managing a hypertensive urgency is to assure compliance with antihypertensive therapy during long-term follow-up.*

Patients presenting with a hypertensive emergency should be diagnosed quickly and started promptly on effective parenteral therapy (often nitroprusside 0.5 μg/kg per minute) in an intensive care unit. BP should be reduced about 25 percent gradually over 2 to 3 h. Oral antihypertensive therapy (often with an immediate-release CA) can be instituted after 6 to 12 h of parenteral therapy; evaluation for secondary causes of hypertension may be considered after transfer from the intensive care unit. Because of advances in antihypertensive therapy and management, "malignant hypertension" should be malignant no longer.

The situation in hemorrhagic stroke is slightly more complex because acute hypertension often is seen in such patients even if there has been no antecedent history of elevated BP. It is not clear if acute BP lowering will reduce or increase the complication rates (from worsened cerebral ischemia in other areas or making a zone surrounding the hemorrhage ischemic). As a result, it is recommended not to treat hypertension beyond a

TABLE 51-30 Types of Hypertension Crises with Suggested Drug Therapy and BP Targets

Type of Crisis	Drug of Choice	BP Target
Neurologic		
Hypertensive encephalopathy	Nitroprusside[a]	25% reduction in mean arterial pressure over 2–3 h
Intracranial hemorrhage or acute stroke in evolution	Nitroprusside[a] (controversial)	0–25% reduction in mean arterial pressure over 6–12 h (controversial)
Acute head injury/trauma	Nitroprusside[a]	0–25% reduction in mean arterial pressure over 2–3 h (controversial)
Subarachnoid hemorrhage	Nimodipine	Up to 25% reduction in mean arterial pressure in previously hypertensive patients, 130–160 systolic in normotensive patients
Cardiac		
Ischemia/infarction	Nitroglycerin or nicardipine	Reduction in ischemia
Heart failure	Nitroprusside[a] or nitroglycerin	Improvement in failure (typically 10–15% decrease in BP)
Aortic dissection	Beta blocker plus nitroprusside[a]	120 mmHg systolic in 30 min (if possible)
Renal		
Hematuria or acute renal impairment	Fenoldopam	0–25% reduction in mean arterial pressure over 1–12 h
Catecholamine excess states		
Pheochromocytoma	Phentolamine	To control paroxysms
Drug withdrawal	Drug withdrawn	Typically only one dose necessary
Pregnancy-related eclampsia	$MgSO_4$, methyldopa, hydralazine	Typically <90 mmHg diastolic but often lower

[a]Some physicians prefer an intravenous infusion or either fenoldopam or nicardipine, neither of which has potentially toxic metabolites, to nitroprusside. Recent studies have shown improvements in renal function during therapy with the former compared to nitroprusside.

SOURCE: Updated from Elliott WJ, Black HR. Hypertension crises. In: Parillo JE, Bone RC, eds. *Clinical Care Medicine: Principles of Diagnosis and Management.* Philadelphia: Mosby Year Book; 1990:565.

mean arterial pressure of >130 mmHg, and even then it is controlled rather more slowly into an intermediate range (e.g., 160/100 mmHg). Some have claimed that previously hypertensive patients with acute intracerebral hemorrhage should be managed even less aggressively.

Appropriate BP reduction in the setting of acute subarachnoid hemorrhage is even more controversial.[379] Even associating higher BP levels with higher rates of rebleeding has been difficult. If BP lowering is desired (e.g., if mean arterial pressure is >130 mmHg), a short-acting intravenous drug (e.g., nitroprusside) typically is recommended, since it can be discontinued quickly and the patient can be given fluids to restore the previous BP level if the neurologic status worsens.

DOSE SCHEDULE (DOSAGE AND CHRONOTHERAPY)

It is clear that BP needs to be controlled for 24 h. Preparations that are active once a day are easier for patients to remember to take, but adherence to treatment may not be substantially worse if twice-a-day preparations are used. In fact, patients may be better protected if they fail to remember to take one dose of a twice-a-day medication and be uncovered for 12 hours than if they skip a once-a-day pill and are unprotected for a considerably longer period.

In addition to "controlling BP" over 24 h, regimens should pay some attention to the circadian rhythm of BP and HR. Many of the sequelae of hypertension have a strong circadian variation, with a peak incidence in the early morning. Recent meta-analyses have quantitated the excess risk of heart attack during the period from 6 A.M. to noon at 40 percent, sudden cardiac death at 29 percent, and stroke at 49 percent compared with what would be expected if these events happened evenly or randomly throughout the day.[404,405] Since most patients administer antihypertensive agents in the morning, most authorities recommend long-acting drugs that should cover the early-morning period, when blood pressure, pulse, and cardiovascular risk are highest. Although many of the currently used medications have short intrinsic elimination half-lives, pharmaceutical technology has made available several methods of making sustained-release compounds from short-acting drugs.[406,407]

Recently, a chronobiological approach to antihypertensive therapy has become available.[407] This is currently available only for two preparations of verapamil.[408] These drug-delivery systems release active drug for 18 to 20 h, beginning between 2 A.M. and 4 A.M., leaving the patient with no active drug in the circulation from about 10 P.M. to 2 A.M. The rationale for this approach is that BP falls normally at night coincident with the usual circadian rhythm and active drug might cause excessive lowering of BP during the middle of the night.[409] These sustained-release preparations provide adequate active drug as the BP rises before awakening and during the peak time of CV events (the period between 6 A.M. and noon). The same matching of drug delivery to BP is not achieved by giving "homeostatically" designed drugs (i.e., all the others) at night. Such agents were designed for morning use, and giving them at night causes the risk of lowering BP too far during sleep.[198]

The putative advantage of such a system is that it would not excessively lower BP during sleep (when BP is typically at its nadir anyway) and would deliver an agent that is both hypotensive and HR-lowering at the time of day when BP, HR, and CV risk are nearly maximal.[198] The long-term consequences of this strategy are being tested in the CONVINCE trial with 16,602 subjects; conclusions may be available in 2002.[322]

DRUG INTERACTIONS

The selection of the initial agent to treat hypertension must be done with the understanding that many hypertensive patients may not reach goal BP on that agent alone and will therefore need additional antihypertensive therapy. Furthermore, many hypertensive patients need to take medications for other conditions, and so the problem of drug–drug interactions is particularly pertinent.

Certain combinations of antihypertensive agents are particularly effective, such as thiazide diuretics with beta blockers, ACE-Is, or ARBs.[380] Combinations of ACE-Is with CAs (both DHP and non-DHP) are also effective. Moreover, combinations of the two subtypes of CAs are synergistic with regard to BP reduction.[409] Dihydropyridine CAs and beta blockers are also very effective combinations. Nondihydropyridine CAs and beta blockers should not be used because of the risk of excessive bradycardia and conduction defects. Thiazide diuretics are also effective with all other antihypertensive drugs, including CAs, and always should be included in a triple-drug regimen. Little is known about the efficacy of combining alpha blockers with central and peripheral sympatholytics or with ACE-Is or ARBs.

Recently, a series of low-dose fixed-dose combinations have been introduced that have fewer clinical side effects than occur when the components are used as monotherapy (Table 51-21). The best example is the combination of a DHP CA with an ACE-I. These fixed-dose combinations have a significantly lower incidence of edema than that seen when a DHP CA is given alone.[380] The incidence of cough, however, is not lessened when these drugs are combined. The appeal of a low-dose fixed-dose combination is that BP can be reduced further with fewer adverse reactions with two drugs at lower doses than might occur when one or the other component is pushed to the full dose. The added advantage is that the patient needs to take fewer pills to get BP to goal and so adherence to the regimen tends to improve (see below).

Most commonly used antihypertensives do not have any serious drug–drug interactions with anticoagulants, platelet inhibitors, or antibiotics. Nondihydropyridine CAs, beta blockers, and possibly telmisartan (an ARB) must be used with care in patients who are taking digitalis preparations.[381] Nonsteroidal anti-inflammatory agents may raise BP and interfere with the activity of all antihypertensive agents because of their Na^+-retaining properties.[410]

ADHERENCE

Fewer than 50 percent of patients continue taking the initially prescribed antihypertensive drug therapy for a year.[411,412] The proportion who properly adhere to therapy improves only modestly when the drugs and medical care are provided free of charge. Recent estimates indicate that about 10 percent of the overall expenditures on hypertension in the United States are wasted because of nonadherence to medical advice and antihypertensive drug therapy.[413] Patients who do not follow the advice of their physicians and do not take their medications correctly have an *infinite* cost/benefit ratio because they incur all the cost associated with the therapy but derive *none* of the benefits of treatment.

TABLE 51-31 Strategies to Improve Medication Adherence

- Educate patient regarding proper use of medications
- Improve patient's social support network (e.g., spouse or caretaker)
- Increase patient's autonomy and involvement in decision making (when appropriate)
- Remove barriers to compliance with pill taking
- Integrate into activities of daily living (e.g., brushing teeth)
- Avoid large ("horse") pills
- Avoid bad-tasting formulations (e.g., lactulose, quinine)
- Simplify the therapeutic regimen
  - Minimize number of pills
  - Minimize frequency of pill taking
  - Minimize inconvenience of pill taking
- Provide positive attitude and positive reinforcement about achieving therapeutic goals
- Maintain continuity of care with same practitioner
- Use well-tolerated antihypertensive drug therapy individualized for each patient

Assessing adherence with antihypertensive medications is generally difficult, but several simple measures often are recommended.[11,38,414] Some medications induce physical signs that are absent in those who have not recently taken them, e.g., bradycardia with beta blockers, orthostatic BP change with alpha blockers, and an increase in serum urate with diuretics. A telephone call to the patient's pharmacy generally will reveal how many times the prescribed medications have been refilled during the last year.[415] Several interventions have been advocated to improve adherence with medications (Table 51-31).

There is concern, however, that administering long-acting drugs will lower blood pressure to a relatively constant degree during the day and night. This may lead to hypoperfusion of vital organs during the night that will not be symptomatic.[408]

MECHANISM OF ACTION OF THE DRUG AND PATHOPHYSIOLOGY OF THE PATIENT'S HYPERTENSION

Some have felt that physicians could be much more successful in treating hypertensive patients if they could base therapy on the reason why the patient is hypertensive (the pathophysiologic abnormality responsible for the patient's hypertension) and match that information to the mechanism of action of antihypertensive drugs. If physicans truly could know precisely why an individual was hypertensive and easily and safely obtain such information, treating hypertension would be not be complicated. If it really were known exactly how drugs work, those decisions would be much simpler. This approach, while intellectually appealing, has problems.

The first difficulty is that attempts to profile patients either biochemically using PRA, for example, or hemodynamically by measuring cardiac output and peripheral vascular resistance are too expensive and potentially invasive to do in everyone. In addition, these methods are not precise enough to provide the kind of necessarily definitive information needed to predict the response to therapy in a particular patient. Furthermore, trying to base therapy on the presumed pathophysiology in an individual or group of individuals would be expected to have is also imprecise. This approach runs the risk of denying certain patients the potential benefits of certain classes of drugs. Although it is true that blacks and older persons tend on the average to have low or suppressed PRA, many do not. Also, many patients with a low PRA will respond to drugs, such as ACE-Is or ARBs, that are less effective on the average in hypertensives with this renin profile. In the VA trial of monotherapy, selecting initial treatment on the basis of PRA was less effective than simply using age and ethnicity (thiazide diuretics and CAs for older patients and blacks and ACE-Is and beta blockers for whites and in those less than 60 years of age).[382] However, neither method correctly predicted a good response in more than 63 percent of the patients.

The second issue that complicates this approach is that many, if not all, drugs have more complex mechanisms of action than they were originally thought to have and work well in patient subgroups in whom they were supposed to be ineffective. For example, thiazide diuretics not only reduce plasma volume but also are vasodilators after 4 weeks of therapy. It should not have been surprising that these agents are effective and very well tolerated in older persons even though many of those patients tend to have a modestly decreased plasma volume compared with younger hypertensives. Although it is true that ACE-Is usually suppress the endocrine RAA system, the antihypertensive effect is still evident even when plasma AII concentration returns to pretreatment levels. This is good evidence that there is a tissue site of action for these drugs or that other mechanisms, perhaps the stimulation of bradykinin or NO, participate in how ACE-Is lower BP and that the initial formulation of their mechanism of action was incomplete. This also explains why some patients with low PRA (a measure of the activity of the *endocrine* RAA system) respond well to these agents or to ARBs, which suppress the RAA system at the angiotensin AT_1 receptor in tissues throughout the body. Calcium antagonists were presumed to work best in older hypertensives and in those with suppressed PRA, but these agents are equally effective in all subgroups of hypertensives.[237]

Perhaps the major flaw in the reasoning that drugs can be used to "probe" the pathophysiologic abnormality causing a patient's hypertension is the concept that there is one overriding abnormality responsible for that patient's elevated BP. In all likelihood, more than one, if not many, of the systems that control BP, many of which are discussed in this chapter, are dysfunctional simultaneously and single or combinations of pharmacologic agents that reduce BP do so by correcting more than one abnormality.[10]

The choice of initial therapy therefore should be based primarily on evidence from clinical trials that document a reduction in CV events and/or renal disease progression. However, despite the fact that one cannot precisely determine the mechanism or mechanisms of action of drugs and that it is impossible to elucidate precisely why a particular patient is hypertensive, the empirical approach to treating hypertension dramatically reduced the rate of stroke and CAD after physicians began to treat hypertension aggressively. This approach, though far from perfect, has paid dividends.

COST

The economics of hypertension and its therapy are complex, but the simple fact is that if a person cannot afford to pay for the drug chosen by the health care provider, the completed prescription will do little good in the long term.[52,53] Many pharmacists and businesspeople associated with health care believe that the agent with the lowest purchase price is the best, but this oversimplification omits the costs of extra visits to health care providers, laboratory testing, and adverse drug experiences that result in emergency room visits or hospitalization.[415] Such global evaluations of the economics of hypertension and its therapy are rare. It is possible for a more expensive but better-tolerated drug (e.g., an ARB) to actually be less expensive in the long term than another agent that produces many side effects, some of which must be evaluated by laboratory testing, physician visits, and even hospitalization. There is also the possibility that some of the newer (and currently more expensive) agents are more effective in lowering BP and reducing cardiovascular events (which currently account for 82 percent of expenditures related to hypertension in the United States) than are some of the older agents; this alone may be sufficient to make them more cost-effective than the time-tested agents.

Generically available drugs are usually less expensive to purchase than their branded counterparts and are strongly favored in most managed care pharmacy plans by both mandates to physicians and lower copayments by patients.[416] Some organized health care plans insist that the first month of antihypertensive therapy always involve a low-dose thiazide diuretic because of its proven efficacy and low cost. Although JNC VI "favored" low-dose diuretics and beta blockers for uncomplicated hypertension, it did, for the first time, suggest that hypertensives with another "compelling condition" would benefit even more from other classes of antihypertensive agents. There are now more data to suggest that in the long term it matters more what BP level is achieved during treatment than which agent is chosen initially to begin the lowering.

Many authorities are concerned that achieving the new, lower target BPs for diabetic and renally impaired hypertensives will cost more, as it will require more visits to health care providers and more antihypertensive medications. These increases in short-term expenditures are likely, however, to be offset by a lower future incidence of expensive outcomes, including heart attack, stroke, ESRD, and HF, at least for diabetic patients over age 60 in the United States.[332]

Many proposals for reducing the high cost of antihypertensive therapy have been advanced. JNC VI has suggested withholding drug therapy for 6 to 12 months from those at low risk (risk groups A and B) with stage 1 hypertension and giving it instead to patients in risk group C with BP ≥130/85 mmHg.[11] In stage 2 to 3 hypertension, wider use of combination drug tablets has been advocated, as these tablets typically cost much less than two separate prescriptions for the same doses of individual agents. Some formularies and pharmacy benefits managers prefer agents that have all doses priced identically, with the theory that a pill splitter can then be used to divide one tablet into two or more days' treatment. Aggressive health care plans have implemented strategies that prohibit the use of more expensive medications (e.g., ARBs) unless two physicians independently ascribe an adverse effect to a less expensive drug (e.g., an ACE-I), and others require three separate ACE-Is to be administered sequentially before an ARB can be dispensed.

Until a universal pharmacy benefits program is instituted, there are likely to be wide variations in the pricing and cost of antihypertensive agents. Although it is difficult for physicians to stay abreast of fluctuations in these costs, it is important that all health care providers attempt to provide tolerable antihypertensive medications at the lowest possible cost for the benefit of the patient, the health plan, and the national budget.

SUMMARY AND RECOMMENDATIONS

Although there are numerous options and many sources of error, the successful pharmacologic treatment of a hypertensive patient need not be too complicated, although it also should not be oversimplified. Once the diagnosis has been established and the routine evaluation and any more complex tests believed to be necessary have been completed, lifestyle modification should begin. Lifestyle modification should be given time to work unless the patient is in a group for which drug therapy is indicated (together with lifestyle modifications at the initiation of treatment). Drug therapy is indicated in all hypertensive patients if goal BP is not reached with lifestyle modification alone.

The following steps are recommended for choosing a regimen and then altering it until the goal is reached:

- Deal first with cost. If the patient is unable to afford any but the least expensive drugs or cannot pay for the one that is selected, price becomes the primary issue.
- Ascertain whether other risk factors or comorbidity is present. Avoid drugs that may worsen these factors or conditions and choose the ones that may tend to improve them.
- Find out what clinical adverse reactions the patient would find the most troublesome and avoid agents that are more likely to cause or exacerbate these problems. Some patients are not concerned by certain side effects that are very troublesome for others.
- Consider demographic issues and select the class of drug with a higher probability of success if options are available.
- Start with the lowest effective dose and plan to see the patient within 2 to 4 weeks unless the severity of the patient's hypertension or another problem warrants an earlier visit. Carry out appropriate biochemical monitoring when necessary. In some patients, start with a fixed-dose combination when it appears appropriate.
- Increase the dose if goal BP has not been reached or if there has been only a minimal response. Do not increase the first dose or any dose prematurely. Give each dose adequate time to be fully effective. If intolerable side effects occur and are likely to be drug-related or if there has been no response, only then switch to another appropriate agent for monotherapy.
- Continue the process of dose titration and monitoring until the maximum recommended dose has been reached. Stopping before the full dose has been reached leads to a situation in which the patient is treated with multiple agents at subtherapeutic doses when only one or two drugs are necessary.
- If the drug of first choice fails to reduce BP to goal, add a second agent that has a different mechanism of action and is known to have additive antihypertensive effects to the first-choice agent. A fixed-dose combination that combines two drugs in the desired doses also could be used at this time.
- Titrate the second drug to the full dose, as was done for the first drug, and continue appropriate monitoring. If the two-drug combination fails, consider a specific cause for the patient's refractory hypertension, and if none is evident, add a third drug, being sure that a diuretic is part of the regimen. Consider a referral to a hypertension specialist.
- Plan to see a patient who is at goal at least once every 3 months to be sure that BP control is sustained.
- Reinforce the need for adherence to the regimen and always question each patient carefully about adverse reactions. Although some patients will not reach goal with this approach even with the many effective treatment options that are available, most will come under control or close to it. Patients who do this can anticipate substantial long-term benefit with an extended life expectancy and a much reduced risk of stroke, ischemic heart disease, HF, and probably renal failure and dementia.

CONCLUSION

Although treating high BP can be costly and at times seem unrewarding, the benefits to individual patients and to society make the effort worthwhile. Physicians must be careful not to become apathetic about hypertension. The problem has not been solved and will not be solved until all hypertensive patients are able to avail themselves of what has been among the most successful examples of preventive medicine.

References

1. Murray CJ, Lope AD. Evidence-based health policy—lessons from the Global Burden of Disease Study. *Science* 1996; 274(5288):740–743.
2. Kannel WB. Blood pressure as a cardiovascular risk factor: Prevention and treatment. *JAMA* 1996; 275:1571–1576.
3. MacMahon S, Rodgers A. The epidemiological association between blood pressure and stroke: Implications for primary and secondary prevention. *Hypertens Res* 1994; 17(suppl I):S23–S32.
4. Klag MJ, Whelton PK, Randall BL, et al. Blood pressure and end-stage renal disease in men. *N Engl J Med* 1996; 334:13–18.
5. Criqui MH, Langer RD, Fronek A, et al. Large vessel and isolated small vessel peripheral arterial disease. In: Fowkes FCR, ed. *Epidemiology of Peripheral Vascular Disease.* Ireland: Springer-Verlag; 1991:85.
6. Xie L, Wu K, Xu N, et al. Hypertension is associated with a high risk of cancer. *J Hum Hypertens* 1999; 13(5):295–301.
7. Rosengren A, Himmelmann A, Wihelmsen L, et al. Hypertension and long-term cancer incidence and mortality among Swedish men. *J Hypertens* 1998; 16(7):933–940.
8. Hamet P. Cancer and hypertension: A potential for crosswalk? *J Hypertens* 1997; 15(12 part 2):1573–1577.
9. Grossman E, Messerli FH, Goldbourt U. Does diuretic therapy increase the risk of renal cell carcinoma? *Am J Cardiol* 1999; 83(7):1090–1093.
10. Page IH. The mosaic theory. In: Page IH, ed. *Hypertension Mechanisms.* Orlando, FL: Grune & Stratton; 1987:910.
11. The Sixth Report of the Joint National Committee on Prevention, Detection, Evaluation, and Treatment of High Blood Pressure (JNC VI). *Arch Intern Med* 1997; 157:2413–2446.
12. Berlowitz DR, Ash AS, Hickey EC, et al. Inadequate management of blood pressure in a hypertensive population. *N Engl J Med* 1998; 339(27):1957–1963.

13. Colhoun HM, Dong W, Poulter NR. Blood pressure screening, management, and control in England: Results from the health survey for England 1994. *J Hypertens* 1998; 16:747–752.
14. De Backer G, Myny K, De Henauw S, et al. Prevalence, awareness, treatment and control of arterial hypertension in an elderly population in Belgium. *J Hum Hypertens* 1998; 12:701–706.
15. Stergiou GS, Thomopoulou GC, Skeva I, Moutokalakis TD. Prevalence, awareness, treatment, and control of hypertension in Greece: The Didima study. *Am J Hypertens* 1999; 12:959–965.
16. Joffres MR, Ghardirian P, Fondor JG, et al. Awareness, treatment, and control of hypertension in Canada. *Am J Hypertens* 1997; 10:1097–1102.
17. Zanchetti A. Antihypertensive therapy: Pride and prejudice. *J Hypertens* 1995; 13:1522–1528.
18. 1999 World Health Organization–International Society of Hypertension Guidelines for the Management of Hypertension: Guidelines Subcommittee. *J Hypertens* 1999; 17(2):151–183.
19. Ramsay LE, Williams B, Johnston GD, et al. British Hypertension Society guidelines for hypertension management 1999: Summary. *BMJ* 1999; 319:630–635.
20. Pickering T. Recommendations for use of home (self) and ambulatory blood pressure monitoring: American Society of Hypertension Ad Hoc Panel. *Am J Hypertens* 1996; 9:1–11.
21. Tsuji I, Imai Y, Nagai K, et al. Proposal of reference values for home blood pressure measurement: Prognostic criteria based on a prospective observation of the general population in Ohasama, Japan. *Am J Hypertens* 1997; 10:409–418.
22. Black HR, Yi JY. A new classification for hypertension based on relative and absolute risk with implications for treatment and reimbursement. *Hypertension* 1996; 28:719–724.
23. Kannel WB. Blood pressure as a cardiovascular risk factor: Prevention and treatment. *JAMA* 1996; 275(20):1571–1576.
24. Van den Hoogen PCW, Feskens EJM, Nagelkerke NJD, et al., for the Seven Countries Study Research Group. The relation between blood pressure and mortality due to coronary heart disease among men in different parts of the world. *N Engl J Med* 2000; 342:1–8.
25. Cholesterol, diastolic blood pressure, and stroke: 13,000 strokes in 450,000 people in 45 prospective cohorts: Prospective studies collaboration. *Lancet* 1995; 346(8991–8992):1647–1653.
26. MacMahon S, Peto R, Cutler J, et al. Blood pressure, stroke, and coronary heart disease: I. Prolonged differences in blood pressure: Prospective observational studies corrected for the regression dilution bias. *Lancet* 1990; 335(8692):756–774.
27. Stamler J, Stamler R, Neaton JD. Blood pressure, systolic and diastolic, and cardiovascular risks: US population data. *Arch Intern Med* 1993; 153:598–615.
28. Psaty BM, Furberg CD, Kuller LH, et al. Isolated systolic hypertension and subclinical CVD in the elderly: Initial findings from the Cardiovascular Health Study. *JAMA* 1992; 268:1287–1291.
29. Lee ML, Rosner BA, Weiss ST. Relationship of blood pressure to cardiovascular death: The effects of pulse pressure in the elderly. *Ann Epidemiol* 1999; 9:101–107.
30. Collins R, Peto R, MacMahon S, et al. Blood pressure, stroke, and coronary heart disease: II. Short-term reductions in blood pressure: Overview of randomized drug trials in their epidemiologic context. *Lancet* 1990; 335:827–838.
31. Blood pressure, cholesterol, and stroke in eastern Asia: Eastern Stroke and Coronary Heart Disease Collaborative Research Group. *Lancet* 1998; 352(9143):1801–1807.
32. Kannel WB, Gordon T, Castelli WP, Margolis JR. Electrocardiographic left ventricular hypertrophy and risk of coronary heart disease: The Framingham Study. *Ann Intern Med* 1970; 72: 813–822.
33. Kuller LH, Shemanski L, Psaty BM, et al. Subclinical disease as an independent risk factor for cardiovascular disease. *Circulation* 1995; 92:720–726.
34. Kannel WB. Risk stratification in hypertension: New insights from the Framingham Study. *Am J Hypertens* 2000; 13:3S–10S.
35. Ferrannini E, Natali A, Capaldo B, et al. Insulin resistance, hyperinsulinemia, and blood pressure. *Hypertension* 1997; 30:1144–1149.
36. Kannel WB, Gordon T, Schwartz MJ. Systolic versus diastolic blood pressure and risk of coronary heart disease: The Framingham Study. *Am J Cardiol* 1971; 27:335–346.
37. Black HR, Kuller LH, O'Rourke MF, et al. The first report of the Systolic and Pulse Pressure (SYPP) Working Group on systolic and pulse pressure. *J Hypertens* 1999; 17(suppl 5):S3–S14.
38. Joint National Committee on Detection, Evaluation, and Treatment of High Blood Pressure. The Fifth Report of the Joint National Committee on Detection, Evaluation, and Treatment of High Blood Pressure (JNC V). *Arch Intern Med* 1993; 153:154–183.
39. Fisher CM. The ascendancy of diastolic blood pressure over systolic. *Lancet* 1985; 2:1349–1350.
40. Black HR. The paradigm has shifted, to systolic blood pressure. *Hypertension* 1999; 34:386–387.
41. Madhavan S, Ooi WL, Cohen J, Alderman MH. Relation of pulse pressure and blood pressure reduction to the incidence of myocardial infarction. *Hypertension* 1994; 23:395–401.
42. Pannier B, Brunel P, el Aroussy WE, et al. Pulse pressure and echocardiographic findings in essential hypertension. *J Hypertens* 1989; 7:127–132.
43. Verdecchia P, Schillaci G, Borgioni C, et al. Ambulatory pulse pressure: A potent predictor of total cardiovascular risk in hypertension. *Hypertension* 1998; 32:983–988.
44. Benetos A, Safar M, Rudnichi A, et al. Pulse pressure: A predictor of long-term cardiovascular mortality in a French male population. *Hypertension* 1997; 30:1410–1415.
45. Benetos A, Rudnichi A, Safar M, Guise L. Pulse pressure and cardiovascular mortality in normotensive and hypertensive subjects. *Hypertension* 1998; 32:560–564.
46. Franklin SS, Khan SA, Wong ND, et al. Is pulse pressure useful in predicting risk for coronary heart disease? The Framingham Heart Study. *Circulation* 1999; 100:354–360.
47. Izzo JL, Levy D, Black HR. Clinical advisory statement: Importance of systolic blood pressure in older Americans. *Hypertension* 2000; 35:1021–1024.
48. Messerli FH, Weber MA, Brunner HR. Angiotensin II receptor inhibition: A new therapeutic principle. *Arch Intern Med* 1996; 156:1957–1965.
49. Bauer JH, Reams GP. The angiotensin II type 1 receptor antagonist: A new class of antihypertensive drugs. *Arch Intern Med* 1995; 155:1361–1368.
50. Grimm RH, Grandits GA, Cutler JA, et al., for the TOMHS Research Group. Relationships of quality of life measures to long-term lifestyle and drug treatment in the Treatment of Mild Hypertension Study. (TOMHS) *Arch Intern Med* 1997; 157: 638–648.
51. Wiklund I, Halling K, Ryden-Bergsten T, Fletcher A. Does lowering the blood pressure improve the mood? Quality-of-life results from the Hypertension Optimal Treatment (HOT) study. *Blood Pressure* 1997; 6(6):357–364.
52. Stason WB. Economic impact of blood pressure. In: Black HR, Izzo JL Jr, eds. *Hypertension Primer*, 2d ed. Dallas, TX: American Heart Association; 1999:286.
53. Elliott WJ. Economic considerations in the management of hypertension. In: Black HR, Izzo JL Jr, eds. *Hypertension Primer,* 2d ed. Dallas, TX: American Heart Association; 1999:289.
54. *American Heart Association's Heart & Stroke Facts. Statistical Supplement.* Dallas, TX: American Heart Association; 2000:24.
55. Elliott WJ. The current inadequate control of hypertension: How

can we do better? In: Kaplan NM, ed. *Hypertension Therapy Annual.* London: Martin Dunitz; 2000:1.

56. Guyton AC, Coleman TG, Cowley AW, et al. Arterial pressure regulation: Overriding dominance of the kidneys. *Am J Med* 1972; 52:584–594.
57. Morimoto S, Sasaki S, Itoh H, et al. Sympathetic activation and contribution of genetic factors in hypertension with neurovascular compression of the rostral ventrolateral medulla. *J Hypertens* 1999; 17(11):1577–1582.
58. Laitinen T, Hartikainen J, Niskanen L, et al. Sympathovagal balance is major determinant of short-term blood pressure variability in healthy subjects. *Am J Physiol* 1999; 276(4 part 2): H1245–H1252.
59. Adamopoulos S, Rosano GM, Ponikowski P, et al. Impaired baroreflex sensitivity and sympathovagal balance in syndrome X. *Am J Cardiol* 1998; 82(7):862–868.
60. DiBona GF, Kopp UC. Neural control of renal function. *Physiol Rev* 1997; 77:76–97.
61. Kurokawa K. Kidney, salt and hypertension: How and why. *Kidney Int* 1996; 49(suppl 55):S46–S51.
62. Muirhead EE. Renal vasodepressor mechanisms: The medullipin system. *J Hypertens* 1993; 5:S53–S58.
63. Julius S, Schork MA. Predictors of hypertension. *Ann NY Acad Sci* 1978; 304:38–58.
64. Julius S, Valentini M. Continuing on J. P. Henry's path: Studies of physiology and pathophysiology of cardiopulmonary receptors in humans. *Acta Physiol Scand Suppl* 1997; 640:122–124.
65. Narkiewicz K, Pesek CA, Kato M, et al. Baroreflex control of sympathetic nerve activity and heart rate in obstructive sleep apnea. *Hypertension* 1998; 32(6):1039–1043.
66. Ryuzaki M, Stahl LK, Lyson T, et al. Sympathoexcitatory response to cyclosporin A and baroreflex resetting. *Hypertension* 1997; 29(2):576–582.
67. Ligtenberg G, Blankestijn PJ, Oey PL, et al. Reduction of sympathetic hyperactivity by enalapril in patients with chronic renal failure. *N Engl J Med* 1999; 340(17):1321–1328.
68. Watanabe K, Sekiya M, Tsuruoka T, et al. Relationship between insulin resistance and cardiac sympathetic nervous function in essential hypertension. *J Hypertens* 1999; 17(8):1161–1168.
69. Yuasa S, Li X, Hitomi H, et al. Sodium sensitivity and sympathetic nervous system in hypertension induced by long-term nitric oxide blockade in rats. *Clin Exp Pharmacol Physiol* 2000; 27(1–2): 18–24.
70. Dahl LK, Heine M, Primary role of renal homografts in setting chronic blood pressure levels in rats. *Circ Res* 1975; 36:692–696.
71. Muntzel M, Drueke T. A comprehensive review of the salt and blood pressure relationship. *Am J Hypertens* 1992; 5:1s–42s.
72. Luft FC, Rankin LI, Bloch R, et al. Cardiovascular and humoral responses to extremes of sodium intake in normal black and white men. *Circulation* 1979; 60:697–706.
73. Folkow B, Ely DL. Cardiovascular and sympathetic effects of 240-fold salt intake variations—studies in rats with implications to man. *Acta Physiol Scand* 1989; 136:89–96.
74. Rettig R, Schmitt B, Pelzl B, Speck T. The kidney and primary hypertension: Contributions from renal transplantation studies in animals and humans. *J Hypertens* 1993; 11(9):883–891.
75. Weir MR. Impact of salt intake on blood pressure and proteinuria in diabetes: Importance of the renin-angiotensin system. *Miner Electrolyte Metab* 1998; 24(6):438–445.
76. Sever PS, Poulter NR. A hypothesis for the pathogenesis of essential hypertension: The initiating factors. *J Hypertens* 1989; 7(suppl 1):9s–12s.
77. Joseph JG, Prior IAM, Salmond CE, Stanley D. Elevation of systolic and diastolic blood pressure associated with migration: The Tokelau Island Migrant Study. *J Chronic Dis* 1983; 36: 507–516.
78. Weinberger M, Fineberg N. Sodium and volume sensitivity of blood pressure: Age and pressure change over time. *Hypertension* 1991; 18:67–71.
79. Sanchez RA, Gimenez MI, Migliorini M, et al. Erythrocyte sodium-lithium countertransport in non-modulating offspring and essential hypertensive individuals: Response to enalapril. *Hypertension* 1997; 30(1 part 1):99–105.
80. Aviv A. Recent advances in cellular Ca^{++} homeostasis: Implications to altered regulations of cellular Ca^{++} and Na^{+}-H^{+} exchange in essential hypertension. *Curr Opin Cardiol* 1996; 11(5):477–482.
81. Cappuccio FP, Markandu ND, Carney C, et al. Double-blind randomized trial of modest salt restriction in older people. *Lancet* 1997; 350(9081):850–854.
82. Wedler G, Brier M, Wiersbitsky M, et al. Sodium kinetics in salt-sensitive and salt-resistant normotensive and hypertensive subjects. *J Hypertens* 1992; 10:663–669.
83. Lifton R. Molecular genetics of human blood pressure variation. *Science* 1996; 272:676–680.
84. Alam S, Johnson AG. A meta-analysis of randomized controlled trials (RCT) among healthy normotensive and essential hypertensive elderly patients to determine the effect of high salt (NaCl) diet of blood pressure. *J Hum Hypertens* 1999; 13(6):367–374.
85. He J, Whelton PK, Appel LJ, et al. Long-term effects of weight loss and dietary sodium reduction on incidence of hypertension. *Hypertension* 2000; 35(2):544–549.
86. Timmermans PB. Angiotensin II receptor antagonists: An emerging new class of cardiovascular therapeutics. *Hypertens Res* 1999; 22(2):147–153.
87. Myers BD, Deen WM, Brenner BM. Effects of norepinephrine and angiotensin II on the determinants of glomerular ultrafiltration and proximal tubule fluid reabsorption in the rat. *Circ Res* 1975; 25:663–673.
88. Weber MA. Angiotensin II receptor antagonist in the treatment of hypertension. *Cardiol Rev* 1997; 5:72–80.
89. Sealey JE, Blumenfeld JD, Bell GM, et al. On the renal basis for essential hypertension: Nephron heterogeneity with discordant renin secretion and sodium excretion causing a hypertensive vasoconstriction-volume relationship. *J Hypertens* 1988; 6(10): 763–777.
90. Thibonnier M, Kilani A, Rahman M, et al. Effects of the nonpeptide V(1) vasopressin receptor antagonist SR49059 in hypertensive patients. *Hypertension* 1999; 34(6):1293–1300.
91. Bakris GL, Kusmirek SL, Smith AC, et al. Calcium antagonism abolishes the antipressor action of vasopressin (V1) receptor antagonism. *Am J Hypertens* 1997; 10(10 part 1):1153–1158.
92. Bakris G, Bursztyn M, Gavras I, et al. Role of vasopressin in essential hypertension: Racial differences. *J Hypertens* 1997; 15(5):545–550.
93. Bakris GL, Re RN. Endothelin modulates angiotensin II-induced mitogenesis of human mesangial cells. *Am J Physiol* 1993; 264(6 part 2):F937–F942.
94. Yanagisawa M, Kurihara H, Kimura S, et al. A novel potent vasoconstrictor peptide produced by vascular endothelial cells. *Nature* 1988; 332(6163):411–415.
95. Gardener SM, March JE, Kemp PA, Bennett T. Cardiovascular responses to angiotensins I and II in normotensive and hypertensive rats: Effects of NO synthase inhibition or ET receptor antagonism. *Br J Pharmacol* 1999; 128(8):1795–1803.
96. Krum H, Viskoper RJ, Lacourciere Y, et al. The effect of an endothelin-receptor antagonist, bosentan, on blood pressure in patients with essential hypertension: Bosentan Hypertension Investigators. *N Engl J Med* 1998; 338(12):784–790.
97. Taler SJ, Textor SC, Canzanello VJ, Schwartz L. Cyclosporin-induced hypertension: Incidence, pathogenesis and management. *Drug Saf* 1999; 20(5):437–449.
98. Moe GW, Albermaz A, Naik GO, et al. Beneficial effects of long-

term selective endothelin type A receptor blockade in canine experimental heart failure. *Cardiovasc Res* 1998; 39(3):571–579.

99. Higashi Y, Oshima T, Ozono R, et al. Effect of L-arginine infusion on systemic and renal hemodynamics in hypertensive patients. *Am J Hypertens* 1999; 12(1 part 1):8–15.
100. Cardillo C, Panza JA. Impaired endothelial regulation of vascular tone in patients with systemic arterial hypertension. *Vasc Med* 1998; 3(2):138–144.
101. Vogel RA. Cholesterol lowering and endothelial function. *Am J Med* 1999; 107(5):479–487.
102. Sartori C, Scherrer U. Insulin, nitric oxide and the sympathetic nervous system: At the crossroads of metabolic and cardiovascular regulation. *J Hypertens* 1999; 17(11):1517–1525.
103. Canessa M, Spalvins A, Adragna N, Falkner B. Red cell sodium cotransport and countransport in normotensive and hypertensive blacks. *Hypertension* 1984; 6:344–351.
104. Garay RP, Dagher G, Permollet MG, et al. Inherited defect in Na^+-K^+ cotransport system in erythrocytes from essential hypertensive patients. *Nature* 1980; 284:281–283.
105. Hilton PJ. Cellular sodium transport in essential hypertension. *N Engl J Med* 1986; 314:22–29.
106. Resnick LM. Ionic basis of hypertension, insulin resistance, vascular disease and related disorders. *Am J Hypertens* 1993; 6:123S–134S.
107. Resnick L, Gupta R, Sosa R, et al. Intracellular pH in human and experimental hypertension. *Proc Natl Acad Sci USA* 1987; 84:7663–7667.
108. Batlle DC, Sharma AM, Alsheikha MW, et al. Renal acid excretion and intracellular pH in salt sensitive genetic hypertension. *J Clin Invest* 1993; 91:2178–2184.
109. Tepel M, Bauer S, Husseini S, et al. Increased cytosolic free sodium in platlets from type 2 diabetic patients is associated with hypertension. *J Endocrinol* 1993; 138:565–572.
110. Draznin B. Cytosolic calcium and insulin resistance. *Am J Kidney Dis* 1993; 21(suppl 3):32–38.
111. Andronico G, Mangano MT, Piazza G, et al. Cellular cation exchange in arterial hypertension: Effects of insulin resistance. *J Hypertens* 1993; 11(suppl 5):S274–S275.
112. Picado MJ, de la Sierra A, Aguilera MT, et al. Increased activity of the Mg^{++}/Na^+ exchanger in red blood cells from essential hypertensive patients. *Hypertension* 1994; 23(6 part 2):987–991.
113. Ng LL, Dudley C, Bomford J, Hawley D. Leukocyte intracellular pH and Na^+/H^+ antiport activity in human hypertension. *J Hypertens* 1989; 7:471–475.
114. Resnick LM, Barbagallo M, Gupta RK, Laragh JH. Ionic basis of hypertension in diabetes mellitus: Role of hyperglycemia. *Am J Hypertens* 1993; 6(5 part 1):413–417.
115. Papageorgiou P, Morgan KP. Intracellular free Ca^{2+} is elevated in hypertrophic aortic muscle from hypertensive rats. *Am J Physiol* 1991; 29:H507–H515.
116. Ruiz-Palomo F, Toledo T. Primary Na^+/H^+ exchanger dysfunction: A possible explanation for insulin resistance syndrome. *Med Hypotheses* 1993; 41:186–189.
117. Williams B, Howard RL. Glucose-induced changes in Na^+/H^+ antiport activity and gene expression in cultured vascular smooth muscle cells: Role of protein kinase C. *J Clin Invest* 1994; 93:2623–2631.
118. Ng LL, Davies JE. Abnormalities in Na^+/H^+ antiporter activity in diabetic nephropathy. *J Am Soc Nephrol* 1992; 3(suppl 4): S50–S55.
119. Aviv A. Cytosolic Ca^{2+}, Na^+/H^+ antiport, protein kinase C trio in essential hypertension. *Am J Hypertens* 1994; 7:205–212.
120. McCarron DA, Reusser ME. Finding consensus in the dietary calcium-blood pressure debate. *J Am Coll Nutr* 1999; 18(suppl 5):398S–405S.
121. Kotchen TA, McCarron DA. Dietary electrolytes and blood pressure: A statement for healthcare professionals from the American Heart Association Nutrition Committee. *Circulation* 1998; 98(6):613–617.
122. Ishimitsu T, Tobian L. High potassium diets reduce endothelial permeability in stroke-prone spontaneously hypertensive rats. *Clin Exp Pharmacol Physiol* 1996; 23(3):241–245.
123. Tobian L. Dietary sodium chloride and potassium have effects on the pathophysiology of hypertension in humans and animals. *Am J Clin Nutr* 1997; 65(suppl 2):606S–611S.
124. Ishimitsu T, Tobian L, Uehara Y, et al. Effect of high potassium diets on the vascular and renal prostaglandin system in stroke-prone spontaneously hypertensive rats. *Prostaglandins Leukot Essent Fatty Acids* 1995; 53(4):255–260.
125. Fujimoto S, Ikegami Y, Isaka M, et al. K(+) channel blockers and cytochrome P450 inhibitors on acetylcholine-induced, endothelium-dependent relaxation in rabbit mesenteric artery. *Eur J Pharmacol* 1999; 384(1):7–15.
126. Wilson DK, Sica DA, Miller SB. Effects of potassium on blood pressure in salt-sensitive and salt-resistant black adolescents. *Hypertension* 1999; 34(2):181–186.
127. Campese VM. Salt-sensitive hypertension: Renal and cardiovascular implications. *Nutr Metab Cardiovasc Dis* 1999; 9(3): 143–156.
128. Luft FC, Grim CE, Higgins JT, Weinberger MH. Differences in response to sodium administration in normotensive white and black subjects. *J Lab Clin Med* 1977; 90:555–562.
129. Blaustein MP, Hamlyn JM. Role of a natriuretic factor in essential hypertension: A hypothesis. *Ann Intern Med* 1983; 98:785–792.
130. McCarron DA, Morris CD, Henry HJ, Stanton JL. Blood pressure and nutrient intake in the United States. *Science* 1984; 224:1392–1398.
131. De Wardener HE, MacGregor GA. The relation of a circulating sodium transport inhibitor (the natriuretic hormone?) to hypertension. *Medicine (Baltimore)* 1983; 62:310–326.
132. Guyton AC, Langston JB, Navar G. Theory for renal autoregulation by feedback at the juxtaglomerular apparatus. *Circ Res* 1964; 14/15(suppl I):1187–1197.
133. Campese VM, Parise M, Karubian F, Bigazzi R. Abnormal renal hemodynamics in black salt sensitive patients with hypertension. *Hypertension* 1991; 18:805–821.
134. Johnson RJ, Schreiner GF. Hypothesis: The role of acquired tubulointerstitial disease in the pathogenesis of salt-dependent hypertension. *Kidney Int* 1997; 52:1169–1179.
135. Zou AP, Nithipatikom K, Li PL, Cowley AW Jr. Role of renal medullary adenosine in the control of blood flow and sodium excretion. *Am J Physiol* 1999; 276(3 part 2):R790–R798.
136. Szentivanyi M Jr, Zou AP, Maeda CY, et al. Increase in renal medullary nitric oxide synthase activity protects from norepinephrine-induced hypertension. *Hypertension* 2000; 35(1 part 2): 418–423.
137. Stehouwer CDA, Lambert J, Donker AJM, Van Hinsbergh VWM. Endothelial dysfunction and pathogenesis of diabetic angiopathy. *Cardiovasc Res* 1997; 34:55–68.
138. Bakris GL, Walsh MF, Sowers JR. Endothelium/mesangium interactions: Role of insulin-like growth factors. In: Sowers JR, ed. *Endocrinology of the Vasculature.* Totowa, NJ: Humana Press; 1996:341.
139. Sowers JR, Sowers PS, Peuler JD. Role of insulin resistance and hyperinsulinemia in the development of hypertension and atherosclerosis. *J Lab Clin Med* 1994; 123:647–652.
140. Forsblom CM, Eriksson JG, Ekstrand AV, et al. Insulin resistance and abnormal albumin excretion in non-diabetic first-degree relatives of patients with NIDDM. *Diabetologia* 1995; 38:363–369.
141. Andersen UB, Dige-Petersen H, Frandsen EK, et al. Basal insulin-level oscillations in normotensive individuals with genetic predisposition to essential hypertension exhibit an irregular pattern. *J Hypertens* 1997; 15(10):1167–1173.
142. Forsblom CM, Eriksson JG, Ekstrand AV, et al. Insulin resistance

and abnormal albumin excretion in non-diabetic first-degree relatives of patients with NIDDM. *Diabetologia* 1995; 38:363–369.
143. Kurtz TW, Spence MA. Genetics of essential hypertension. *Am J Med* 1993; 94:77–84.
144. Dowse GK, Collins VR, Alberti KG, et al. Insulin and blood pressure levels are not independently related in Maritians of Asian Indian, Creole or Chinese origin: The Maritius noncommunicable disease study group. *J Hypertens* 1993; 11:297–307.
145. Charles MA, Pettitt DJ, Hanson RL, et al. Familial and metabolic factors related to blood pressure in Pima Indian children. *Am J Epidemiol* 1994; 140:123–131.
146. Ferrannini E, Guzzigoli G, Bonadonna R, et al. Insulin resistance in essential hypertension. *N Engl J Med* 1987; 317:350–357.
147. Saad MF, Lillioja S, Nyomba BL, et al. Racial differences in the relation between blood pressure and insulin resistance. *N Engl J Med* 1991; 324(11):733–739.
148. Caufield M, Lavender P, Farrall M, et al. Linkage of the angiotensinogen gene to essential hypertension. *N Engl J Med* 1994; 330:1629–1633.
149. Lesage S, Velho G, Vionnet N, et al. Genetic studies of the renin-angiotensin system in arterial hypertension associated with non-insulin-dependent diabetes mellitus. *J Hypertens* 1997; 15(6): 601–606.
150. Bravo EL, Tarazi RC, Dustan HP, et al. The changing clinical spectrum of primary aldosteronism. *Am J Med* 1983; 74:641–652.
151. Bravo EL, Dustan HP, Tarazi RC, et al. Clinical implications of primary aldosteronism with resistant hypertension. *Hypertension* 1988; 11(suppl I):1–207.
152. Ganguly A, Grim CE, Weinberger MH. Anomalous postural response in glucocorticoid-suppressible hyperaldosteronism. *N Engl J Med* 1981; 305:991–993.
153. Ganguly A, Weinberger MH, Guthrie GP, et al. Adrenal steroid response to ACTH in glucocorticoid-suppressible hyperaldosteronism. *Hypertension* 1984; 6:563–567.
154. Lifton RP, Dluhy RG, Powers M, et al. A chimeric 11-hydroxylase/aldosterone synthase gene causes glucocorticoid-remediable aldosteronism and human hypertension. *Nature* 1992; 355:262–265.
155. Lifton RP, Dluhy RG, Powers M, et al. Hereditary hypertension caused by chimeric gene duplications and ectopic expression of aldosterone synthase. *Nat Genet* 1992; 2:66–74.
156. Pascoe L, Curnow KM, Slutsker L, et al. Glucocorticoid-suppressible hyperaldosteronism results from hybrid genes created by unequal crossovers between CYP11B1 and CYP11B2. *Proc Natl Acad Sci USA* 1992; 89:8327–8331.
157. Woodland E, Tunny TJ, Hamlet SM, et al. Hypertension corrected and aldosterone responsiveness to renin-angiotensin restored by long-term dexamethasone in glucocorticoid-suppressible hyperaldosteronism. *Clin Exp Pharmacol Physiol* 1985; 12:245–248.
158. Hastings NB, Orchinik M, Aubourg MV, McEven BS. Pharmacological characterization of central and peripheral type I and type II adrenal steroid receptors in the prairie vole, a glucocorticoid-resistant rodent. *Endocrinology* 1999; 140(10):4459–4469.
159. Wallerath T, Witte K, Schafer SC, et al. Down-regulation of the expression of endothelial NO synthase is likely to continue to glucocorticol-mediated hypertension. *Proc Natl Acad Sci USA* 1999; 96(23):13,357–13,362.
160. Kondo K, Saruta T, Saito I, et al. Benign deoxycorticosterone producing adrenal tumor. *JAMA* 1976; 236:1042.
161. Liddle GW, Bledsoe T, Coppage WS. A familial renal disorder simulating primary aldosteronism but with negligible aldosterone secretion. *Trans Assoc Am Phys* 1963; 76:199.
162. Botero-Velez M, Curtiss JJ, Warnock DG. Liddle's syndrome revisited: A disorder of sodium reabsorption in the distal tubule. *N Eng J Med* 1994; 300:178.
163. Kellenberger S, Gautschi I, Rossier BC, Schild L. Mutations causing Liddle syndrome reduce sodium-dependent downregulation of the epithelial sodium channel in the Xenopus oocyte expression system. *J Clin Invest* 1998; 101:2741–2750.
164. Gubner RS. Systolic hypertension: A pathogenetic entity: Significance and therapeutic considerations. *Am J Cardiol* 1962; 9:773–776.
165. Brown WC, O'Brien ET, Semple PF. The sphygmomanometer of Riva Rocci 1896–1996. *J Hum Hypertens* 1996; 10:723–724.
166. Mancia G. Scipione Riva-Rocci. *Clin Cardiol* 1997; 20:503–504.
167. Janeway TC. A clinical study of hypertensive cardiovascular disease. *Arch Intern Med* 1913; 12:752–786.
168. Laher M, O'Brien E. In search of Korotkoff. *BMJ* 1982; 285:1796–1798.
169. Segall HN. How Korotkoff, the surgeon, discovered the auscultatory method of measuring arterial pressure. *Ann Intern Med* 1975; 83:561–562.
170. Franx A, Evers IM, van der Pant KA, et al. The fourth sound of Korotkoff in pregnancy: A myth. *Eur J Obstet Gynecol Reprod Biol* 1998; 76:53–59.
171. Bailey RH, Bauer JH. A review of common errors in the indirect measurement of blood pressure. *Arch Intern Med* 1993; 153:2741–2748.
172. Villegas I, Arias IC, Botero A, Escobar A. Evaluation of the technique used by health-care workers for taking blood pressure. *Hypertension* 1995; 26:1204–1206.
173. Practice imperfect [editorial]. *Lancet* 1991; 337:1195–1196.
174. Abbott D, Campbell N, Carruthers-Czyzewski P, et al. Guidelines for measurement of blood pressure, follow-up and lifestyle counseling: Canadian Coalition for High Blood Pressure Prevention and Control. *Can J Public Health* 1994; 85(suppl 2):S29–S43.
175. Cooper KM. Measuring blood pressure: The right way. *Nursing* 1992; 22:75.
176. Frohlich ED, Grim C, Labarthe DR, et al. Recommendations for Human Blood Pressure Determination by Sphygmomanometers: Report of a Special Task Force Appointed by the Steering Committee, American Heart Association. *Hypertension* 1988; 11:210A–222A.
177. Baker RH, Ende J. Confounders of auscultatory blood pressure measurement. *J Gen Intern Med* 1995; 10:223–231.
178. Stolt M, Sjonell G, Astrom H, et al. Improved accuracy of indirect blood pressure measurement in patients with obese arms. *Am J Hypertens* 1993; 6:66–71.
179. National Committee for Quality Assurance (NCQA). *HEDIS 3.0, Vol. 1* Washington, DC: NCQA; 1997.
180. Stewart MJ, Gough K, Padfield PL. The accuracy of automated blood pressure measuring devices in patients with controlled atrial fibrillation. *J Hypertens* 1995; 13:297–300.
181. Cavallini MC, Roman MJ, Blank SG, et al. Association of the auscultatory gap with vascular disease in hypertensive patients. *Ann Intern Med* 1996; 124:877–883.
182. Ohkubo T, Imai Y, Tsuji I, et al. Home blood pressure measurement has a stronger predictive power for mortality than does screening blood pressure measurement: A population-based observation in Ohasama, Japan. *J Hypertens* 1998; 16:971–975.
183. Soghikian K, Casper SM, Fireman BH, et al. Home blood pressure monitoring: Effect on use of medical services and medical costs. *Med Care* 1992; 30:855–865.
184. Appel LJ, Stason WB. Ambulatory blood pressure monitoring and blood pressure self-measurement in the diagnosis and management of hypertension. *Ann Intern Med* 1993; 118:867–882.
185. Gerin W, Pickering TG, Holland JK, Alter R. Telephone-linked home blood pressure monitoring may improve management [abstract]. *Am J Hypertens* 1999; 12:163.
186. Mengden T, Beltran B, Weisser B, et al. Long-term control of blood pressure guided by daily self-measurement is superior to usual office-based care [abstract]. *J Hypertens* 1999; 17 (suppl 3):30.

187. Perloff D, Sokolow M, Cowan R. The prognostic value of ambulatory blood pressures. *JAMA* 1983; 249:2792–2798.
188. Imai Y, Ohkubo T, Tsuji I, et al. Prognostic value of ambulatory and home blood pressure measurements in comparison to screening blood pressure measurements: A pilot study in Ohasama. *Blood Press Monit* 1996; 1(suppl 2):51–58.
189. Ohkubo T, Imai Y, Tsuji I, et al. Prediction of mortality by ambulatory blood pressure monitoring versus screening blood pressure measurements: A pilot study in Ohasama. *J Hypertens* 1997; 15:357–364.
190. Perloff D, Sokolow M, Cowan RM, Juster RP. Prognostic value of ambulatory blood pressure measurements: Further analyses. *J Hypertens* 1989; 7(suppl 3):S3–S10.
191. Staessen JA, O'Brien ET, Atkins N, Amery AK. Short report: Ambulatory blood pressure in normotensive compared with hypertensive subjects: The Ad-Hoc Working Group. *J Hypertens* 1993; 11:1289–1297.
192. Rasmussen SL, Torp-Pedersen C, Borch-Johnsen K, Ibsen H. Normal values for ambulatory blood pressure and differences between casual blood pressure and ambulatory blood pressure: Results from a Danish population survey. *J Hypertens* 1998; 16:1415–1424.
193. Gretler DD, Fumo MT, Nelson KS, Murphy MB. Ethnic differences in circadian hemodynamic profile. *Am J Hypertens* 1994; 7:7–14.
194. Staessen JA, Bieniaszewski L, O'Brien E, et al. Nocturnal blood pressure fall on ambulatory monitoring in a large international database. *Hypertension* 1997; 29:30–39.
195. Verdecchia P, Porcellati C, Schillaci G, et al. Ambulatory blood pressure: An independent predictor of prognosis in essential hypertension. *Hypertension* 1994; 24:793–801.
196. Verdecchia P, Schillaci G, Borgioni C, et al. Adverse prognostic value of a blunted circadian rhythm of heart rate in essential hypertension. *J Hypertens* 1998; 16:1335–1343.
197. Staessen JA, Thijs L, Fagard R, et al. Predicting cardiovascular risk using conventional vs. ambulatory blood pressure in older patients with systolic hypertension. *JAMA* 1999; 282:589–596.
198. Elliott WJ. Circadian variation in blood pressure: Implications for elderly patients. *Am J Hypertens* 1999; 12:43S–49S.
199. Kleinert HD, Harshfield GA, Pickering TG, et al. What is the value of home blood pressure measurement in patients with mild hypertension? *Hypertension* 1984; 6:574–578.
200. White WB, Schulman P, McCabe EM, Day HM. Average daily blood pressure, not office pressure, determines cardiac function in patients with hypertension. *JAMA* 1989; 261:873–877.
201. Palatini P, Penzo M, Ricioppa A, et al. Clinical relevance of nighttime blood pressure and of daytime blood pressure variability. *Arch Intern Med* 1992; 152:1855–1860.
202. Liu JE, Roman MJ, Pini R, et al. Cardiac and arterial target organ damage in adults with elevated ambulatory and normal office blood pressure. *Ann Intern Med* 1999; 131:564–572.
203. Redon J, Campos C, Narciso ML, et al. Prognostic value of ambulatory blood pressure monitoring in refractory hypertension: A prospective study. *Hypertension* 1998; 31:712–718.
204. Pearce KA, Grimm RH Jr, Rao S, et al. Population-derived comparisons of ambulatory and office blood pressures: Implications for the determination of usual blood pressure and the concept of white coat hypertension. *Arch Intern Med* 1992; 152: 750–756.
205. Weber MA, Neutel JM, Smith DHG, Graettinger WF. Diagnosis of mild hypertension by ambulatory blood pressure monitoring. *Circulation* 1994; 90:2291–2298.
206. Muscholl MW, Hense HW, Brockel U, et al. Changes in left ventricular structure and function in patients with white coat hypertension: Cross sectional survey. *BMJ* 1998; 317:565–570.
207. Owens PE, Lyons SP, Rodriguez SA, O'Brien ET. Is elevation of clinic blood pressure in patients with white coat hypertension who have normal ambulatory blood pressure associated with target organ changes? *J Hum Hypertens* 1998; 12:743–748.
208. Julius S, Jamerson K, Mejia A, et al. The association of borderline hypertension with target organ changes and higher coronary risk: The Tecumseh Blood Pressure Study. *JAMA* 1990; 264:354–358.
209. Verdecchia P, Schillaci G, Borgioni C, et al. Prognostic significance of the white coat effect. *Hypertension* 1997; 29:1218–1224.
210. Krakoff LR, Schechter C, Fahs M, Andre M. Ambulatory blood pressure monitoring: Is it cost-effective? *J Hypertens* 1991; 9(suppl):S28–S30.
211. Krakoff LR. Ambulatory blood pressure monitoring can improve cost-effective management of hypertension. *Am J Hypertens* 1993; 6(suppl):220S–224S.
212. Yarows SA, Khoury S, Sowers JR. Cost effectiveness of 24-hour ambulatory blood pressure monitoring in evaluation and treatment of essential hypertension. *Am J Hypertens* 1994; 7:464–468.
213. Appel LJ, Stason WB. Ambulatory blood pressure monitoring and blood pressure self-measurement in the diagnosis and management of hypertension. *Ann Intern Med* 1993; 118:867–882.
214. Sheps SG, Clement DL, Pickering TG, et al. Ambulatory blood pressure monitoring: Hypertensive Diseases Committee, American College of Cardiology position statement. *J Am Coll Cardiol* 1994; 23:1511–1513.
215. Jackson R, Barham P, Bills J, et al. Management of raised blood pressure in New Zealand: A discussion document. *BMJ* 1993; 307:107–110.
216. Keith NM, Wagener HP, Barker NW. Some different types of essential hypertension: Their course and prognosis. *Am J Med Sci* 1939; 197:332–343.
217. Tso MOM, Jampol LM. Pathophysiology of hypertensive retinopathy. *Ophthalmology* 1982; 89:1132–1145.
218. The Eye Disease Case-Control Study Group. Risk factors for branch retinal vein occlusion. *Am J Ophthalmol* 1993; 116: 286–296.
219. The Eye Disease Case-Control Study Group. Risk factors for central retinal vein occlusion. *Arch Ophthalmol* 1996; 114: 545–554.
220. Macular Photocoagulation Study Group. Laser photocoagulation for justrafoveal choroidal neovascularization: Five-year results from randomized clinical trials. *Arch Ophthalmol* 1994; 112: 500–509.
221. Knowler WC, Bennett PH, Ballintine EJ. Increased incidence of retinopathy in diabetics with elevated blood pressure: A six-year follow-up study in Pima Indians. *N Engl J Med* 1980; 302:645–650.
222. Turner R, Holman R, Stratton I, et al., for the United Kingdom Prospective Diabetes Study Group. Tight blood pressure control and risk of macrovascular and microvascular complications in type 2 diabetes: UKPDS 38. *BMJ* 1998; 317:707–713.
223. Levy D, Labib SB, Anderson KM, et al. Determinants of sensitivity and specificity of electrocardiographic criteria for left ventricular hypertrophy. *Circulation* 1990; 81:815–820.
224. Molloy TJ, Okin PM, Devereux RB, Kligfield P. Electrocardiographic detection of left ventricular hypertrophy by the simple QRS-voltage duration product. *J Am Coll Cardiol* 1992; 20:1180–1186.
225. Okin PM, Roman MJ, Devereux RB, Kligfield P. Electrocardiographic identification of increased left ventricular mass by simple voltage duration products. *J Am Coll Cardiol* 1995; 25:417–423.
226. Black HR, Weltin G, Jaffe CC. The limited echocardiogram: A modification of standard echocardiography for use in the routine evaluation of patients with systemic hypertension. *Am J Cardiol* 1991; 67:1027–1030.
227. Levy D, Salomon MS, D'Agostino RB, et al. Prognostic implications of baseline electrocardiographic features and their serial changes in subjects with left ventricular hypertrophy. *Circulation* 1994; 90:1786–1793.

228. Levy D, Garrison RJ, Savage DD, et al. Prognostic implications of echocardiographically determined left ventricular mass in the Framingham Heart Study. *N Engl J Med* 1990; 322:1561–1566.
229. Koren MJ, Devereux RB, Casale PN, et al. Relation of left ventricular mass and geometry to morbidity and mortality in uncomplicated essential hypertension. *Ann Intern Med* 1991; 114: 345–352.
230. Devereux RB, de Simone G, Ganau A, et al. Left ventricular hypertrophy and hypertension. *Clin Exp Hypertens* 1993; 15: 1025–1032.
231. Bikkina M, Levy D, Evans JC, et al. Left ventricular mass and risk of stroke in an elderly cohort: The Framingham Heart Study. *JAMA* 1994; 272:33–36.
232. Verdecchia P, Schillaci G, Borgioni C, et al. Prognostic significance of serial changes in left ventricular mass in essential hypertension. *Circulation* 1998; 97:48–54.
233. Soufer R, Wohlgelernter D, Vita NA, et al. Intact systolic ventricular function in clinical congestive heart failure. *Am J Cardiol* 1985; 55:1032–1036.
234. Liao Y, Cooper RS, McGee DL, et al. The relative effects of left ventricular hypertrophy, coronary artery disease, and ventricular dysfunction on survival among black adults. *JAMA* 1995; 273:1592–1597.
235. Dahlöf B, Pennert K, Hansson L. Reversal of left ventricular hypertrophy in hypertensive patients: A metaanalysis of 109 treatment studies. *Am J Hypertens* 1992; 5:95–110.
236. Liebson PR, Grandits GA, Dianzumba S, et al, for the Treatment of Hypertension Study Research Group. Comparison of five antihypertensive monotherapies and placebo for change in left ventricular mass in patients receiving nutritional hygienic therapy in the Treatment of Mild Hypertension Study (TOMHS). *Circulation* 1995; 91:698–706.
237. Gottdiener JS, Reda DJ, Massie BM, et al, for the VA Cooperative Study Group on Antihypertensive Agents. Effect of single-drug therapy on reduction of left ventricular mass in mild to moderate hypertension: Comparison of six antihypertensive agents; The Department of Veterans Affairs Cooperative Study Group on Antihypertensive Agents. *Circulation* 1997; 95:2007–2014.
238. Keane WF, Eknoyan G. Proteinuria, albuminuria, risk, assessment, detection, elimination (PARADE): A position paper of the National Kidney Foundation. *Am J Kidney Dis* 1999; 33(5):1004–1010.
239. Yudkin JS, Forest RD, Jackson CA. Microalbuminuria as predictor of vascular disease in non-diabetic subjects: Islington Diabetes Survey. *Lancet* 1988; 2:530–533.
240. Borch-Johnsen K, Feldt-Rasmussen B, Strandgaard S, et al. Urinary albumin excretion: An independent predictor of ischemic heart disease. *Arterioscler Thromb Vasc Biol* 1999; 19(8):1992–1997.
241. Mogensen CE. Microalbuminuria predicts clinical proteinuria and early mortality in maturity-onset diabetes. *N Engl J Med* 1984; 310:356–360.
242. Stepheson JM, Kenny S, Stevens LK, et al, and the WHO Multinational Study Group. Proteinuria and mortality in diabetes: The WHO multinational study of vascular disease in diabetes. *Diabetes Med* 1995; 12:149–155.
243. Gosling P. Microalbuminuria and cardiovascular risk: A word of caution. *J Hum Hypertens* 1998; 12:211–213.
244. Dinneen SF, Gerstein HC. The association of microalbuminuria and mortality in non-insulin-dependent diabetes mellitus: A systemic overview of the literature. *Arch Intern Med* 1997; 157: 1413–1418.
245. Bakris GL, Randall O, Rahman M, et al, for the AASK Study Group. Associations between cardiovascular risk factors and glomerular filtration rate at baseline in the African American Study of Kidney Disease (AASK) trial (abstract). *J Am Soc Nephrol* 1998; 9:139.
246. Mimran A, Ribstein J, Du Cailar G, Halimi JM. Albuminuria in normals and essential hypertension. *J Diabet Complications* 1994; 8:150–156.
247. Tarif N, Bakris GL. Preservation of renal function: The spectrum of effects by calcium channel blockers. *Nephrol Dial Transplant* 1997; 12:2244–2250.
248. Pontremoli R. Microalbuminuria in essential hypertension—its relation to cardiovascular risk factors. *Nephrol Dial Transplant* 1996; 11:2113–2134.
249. Bigazzi R, Bianchi S. Microalbuminuria as a marker of cardiovascular and renal disease in essential hypertension. *Nephrol Dial Transplant* 1995; 10(suppl 6):10–14.
250. Pontremoli R, Sofia A, Ravera M, et al. Prevalence and clinical correlates of microalbuminuria in essential hypertension: The MAGIC study. *Hypertension* 1997; 30:1135–1143.
251. Pedrinelli R, Dell'Omo G, Penno G, et al. Microalbuminuria and pulse pressure in hypertensive and atherosclerotic men. *Hypertension* 2000; 35(1 part 1):48–54.
252. Cirillo M, Senigalliese L, Laurenzi M, et al. Microalbuminuria in nondiabetic adults: Relation of blood pressure, body mass index, plasma cholesterol levels, and smoking: The Gubbio Population Study. *Arch Intern Med* 1998; 158:1933–1939.
253. Bianchi S, Bigazzi R, Baldari G, et al. Diurnal variations of blood pressure and microalbuminuria in essential hypertension. *Am J Hypertens* 1994; 7:23–29.
254. Redon J, Liao Y, Lozano JV, et al. Ambulatory blood pressure and microalbuminuria in essential hypertension: Role of circadian variability. *J Hypertens* 1994; 12:947–953.
255. Jensen JS. Renal and systemic transvascular albumin leakage in severe atherosclerosis. *Arterioscler Thromb Vasc Biol* 1995; 15:1324–1329.
256. Alzaid AA. Microalbuminuria in patients with type 2 diabetes: An overview. *Diabetes Care* 1996; 19:79–89.
257. Stehouwer CDA, Lambet J, Donker AJM, van Hinsberg VWM. Endothelial dysfunction and pathogenesis of diabetic angiopathy. *Cardiovasc Res* 1997; 34:55–68.
258. Gosling P. Microalbuminuria: A marker of systemic disease. *Br J Hosp Med* 1995; 54:285–290.
259. Agewall S, Wikstrand J, Ljungman S, Fagerberg B. Usefulness of microalbuminuria in predicting cardiovascular mortality in treated hypertensive men with and without diabetes mellitus. *Am J Cardiol* 1997; 80:164–169.
260. Cerasola G, Cottone S, D'lgnoto G, et al. Microalbuminuria as a predictor of cardiovascular damage in essential hypertension. *J Hypertens* 1989; 7:S332–S333.
261. Pedrinelli R, Di Bello V, Catapano G, et al. Microalbuminuria is a marker of left ventricular hypertrophy but not hyperinsulinemia in non-diabetic atherosclerotic patients. *Arterioscler Thromb* 1993; 12:947–953.
262. Palatini P, Graniero GR, Mormino P, et al. Prevalence and clinical correlates of microalbuminuria in stage I hypertension: Results from the Hypertension and Ambulatory Recording Venetian Study (HARVES). *Am J Hypertens* 1996; 9:334–341.
263. Virmani R, Avolio AP, Mergner WJ, et al. Effect of aging on aortic morphology in populations with high and low prevalence of hypertension and atherosclerosis: Comparison between Occidental and Chinese communities. *Am J Pathol* 1991; 139:1119–1129.
264. Glasser SP, Arnett DK, McVeigh GE, et al. Vascular compliance and cardiovascular disease: A risk factor or marker? *Am J Hypertens* 1997; 10:1175–1189.
265. Simon A, Megnien JL, Levenson J. Detection of preclinical atherosclerosis may optimize the management of hypertension. *Am J Hypertens* 1997; 10:813–824.
266. Kelly R, Hayward C, Avolio A, O'Rourke M. Noninvasive deter-

mination of age-related changes in the human arterial pulse. *Circulation* 1989; 80:1652–1659.
267. Blacher J, Asmar R, Djane S, London GM. Aortic pulse wave velocity as a marker of cardiovascular risk in hypertensive patients. *Hypertension* 1999; 33(5):1111–1117.
268. Messerli FH, Ventura HO, Amodeo C. Osler's maneuver and pseudohypertension. *N Engl J Med* 1985; 312:1548–1551.
269. The SHEP Cooperative Study Group. Prevention of stroke by antihypertensive drug treatment in older persons with isolated systolic hypertension. *JAMA* 1991; 265:3255–3264.
270. Staessen JA, Fagard R, Thijs L, et al, for the Systolic Hypertension in Europe (Syst-EUR) Trial Investigators. Morbidity and mortality in the placebo-controlled European Trial on Isolated Systolic Hypertension in the Elderly. *Lancet* 1997; 360:757–764.
271. Liu L, Wang J, Gong L, et al, for the Systolic Hypertension in China (Syst-China) Collaborative Group. Comparison of active treatment and placebo in older Chinese patients with isolated systolic hypertension. *J Hypertens* 1998; 16:1823–1829.
272. Ridker PM, Glynn RJ, Hennekens CH. C-reative protein adds to the predictive value of total and HDL-cholesterol in determining risk of first myocardial infarction. *Circulation* 1998; 97:2007–2011.
273. Setaro JF, Saddler MC, Chen CC, et al. Simplified captopril renography in diagnosis and treatment of renal artery stenosis. *Hypertension* 1991; 18:289–298.
274. Stair DC, Rios WA, Black HR. Atypical causes of curable renovascular hypertension: A review. *Prog Cardiovasc Dis* 1990; 33(3)185–210.
275. Black HR, Cooper KA. Cigarette smoking and atherosclerotic renal artery stenosis. *J Clin Hypertens* 1986; 2(4):322–330.
276. Emovon OE, Klotman PE, Dunnick NR, et al. Renovascular hypertension in blacks. *Am J Hypertens* 1996; 9(1):18–23.
277. Setaro JF, Chen CC, Hoffer PB, Black HR. Captopril renography in the diagnosis of renal artery stenosis and the prediction of improvement with revascularization. *Am J Hypertens* 1991; 4(12 part 2):698S–705S.
278. Mann SL, Pickering TG. Detection of renovascular hypertension: State of the art: 1992. *Ann Intern Med* 1992; 117:845.
279. Helenon O, Melki P, Correas JM, et al. Renovascular disease: Doppler ultrasound. *Semin Ultrasound CT MR* 1997; 18(2): 136–146.
280. Leung DA, Hoffman U, Pfammatter T, et al. Magnetic resonance angiography versus duplex sonography for diagnosing renovascular disease. *Hypertension* 1999; 33(2):726–731.
281. Yi J, Bakris GL. Pheochromocytoma. In: Conn RB, Borer WZ, Snyder JW, eds. *Current Diagnosis 9*. New York: Saunders; 1997:794.
282. Stein PP, Black HR. A simplified diagnostic approach to pheochromocytoma: A review of the literature and report of one institution's experience. *Medicine* (*Baltimore*) 1991; 70:46–66.
283. Bravo EL. Evolving concepts in the pathophysiology, diagnosis, and treatment of pheochromocytoma. *Endocr Rev* 1994; 15: 356–368.
284. Jalil N, Pattou FN, Combemale F, et al. Effectiveness and limits of preoperative imaging studies for the localization of pheochromocytomas and paragangliomas: A review of 282 cases: French Association of Surgery (AFC), The French Association of Endocrine Surgeons (AFCE). *Eur J Surg* 1998; 164(1):23–28.
285. Ferriss JB, Beevers DG, Brown JJ, et al. Clinical, biochemical, and pathological features of low renin ("primary") hyperaldosteronism. *Am Heart J* 1978; 95:375–381.
286. Lins PW, Adamson U. Plasma aldosterone-plasma renin activity ratio: A simple test to identify patients with primary aldosteronism. *Acta Endocrinol* (*Copenh*) 1986; 113:564.
287. Ganguly A. Primary aldosteronism. *N Engl J Med* 1998; 339(25):1828–1834.
288. Biglieri EG, Irony I, Kater Cl. Identification and implications of new types of mineralocorticoid hypertension. *J Steroid Biochem* 1989; 32:199.
289. Biglieri EG, Schambelan M. The significance of elevated levels of plasma 18-hydroxycorticosterone in patients with primary aldosteronism. *J Clin Endocrinol Metab* 1979; 49:87.
290. Ganguly A, Melada GA, Luetscher JA, et al. Control of plasma aldosterone in primary aldosteronism: Distinction between adenoma and hyperplasia. *J Clin Endocrinol Metab* 1973; 37:765.
291. Fraser R, Beretta-Piccoli C, Brown JJ, et al. Response of aldosterone and 18-hydroxycorticosterone to angiotensin II in normal subjects and patients with essential hypertension: Conn's syndrome and non-tumorous hyperaldosteronism. *Hypertension* 1991; 3(suppl I):87.
292. Geisinger MA, Zelch MA, Bravo EL, et al. Primary hyperaldosteronism: Comparison of CT, adrenal venography, and venous sampling. *AJR* 1983; 141:299.
293. Melby JC, Spark RF, Dale S, et al. Diagnosis and localization of aldosterone-producing adenomas by adrenal vein catheterization. *N Engl J Med* 1967; 277:1050.
294. Bravo EL, Dustan HP, Tarazi RC. Spironolactone as a nonspecific treatment for primary aldosteronism. *Circulation* 1973; 48:491.
295. Stradling JR, Crosby JH. Relation between systemic hypertension and sleep hypoxaemia or snoring: Analysis in 748 men drawn from general practice. *BMJ* 1990; 300:75–78.
296. Nieto FJ, Young TB, Lind BK, et al. Association of sleep-disordered breathing, sleep apnea, and hypertension in a large community-based study. *JAMA* 2000; 283:1829–1836.
297. Ledoux M, Lambert J, Reeder BA, Depres JP. Correlation between cardiovascular disease risk factors and simple anthropometic measures: Canadian Heart Health Surveys Research Group. *Can Med Assoc J* 1997; 157(suppl 1):S46–S53.
298. Fagard RH. Physical fitness, and blood pressure. *J Hypertens* 1993; 11(suppl 5):S47–S52.
299. The Trials of Hypertension Prevention Collaborative Research Group. The effects of nonpharmacologic interventions on blood pressure of persons with high normal levels: Results of the Trials of Hypertension Prevention, phase I [published erratum appears in *JAMA* 1992; 267:2330]. *JAMA* 1992; 267:1213–1220.
300. Neaton JD, Grimm RH, Prineas RJ, et al. Treatment of mild hypertension study: Final results. *JAMA* 1993; 270:713–724.
301. The Trials of Hypertension Prevention Collaborative Research Group. Effects of weight loss and sodium reduction intervention on blood pressure and hypertension incidence in overweight people with high-normal blood pressure: The Trials of Hypertension Prevention, phase II. *Arch Intern Med* 1997; 157:657–667.
302. Whelton PK, Appel LJ, Espeland MA, et al., for the TONE Collaborative Research Group. Sodium restriction and weight loss in the treatment of hypertension in older persons: A randomized controlled trial of nonpharmacologic interventions in the Elderly (TONE). *JAMA* 1998; 279:839–846.
303. Cushman WC, Cutler JA, Hanna E, et al., for the PATHS Group. The Prevention and Treatment of Hypertension Study (PATHS): Effects of an alcohol treatment program on blood pressure. *Arch Intern Med* 1998; 152:1197–1207.
304. Appel LJ, Moore TJ, Obarzanek E, et al. A clinical trial of the effects of dietary patterns on blood pressure. *N Engl J Med* 1997; 336:1117–1124.
305. Whelton PK, He J, Cutler JA, et al. Effects of oral potassium on blood pressure: Meta-analysis of randomized controlled clinical trials. *JAMA* 1997; 277:1624–1632.
306. Sacks FM, Brown LE, Appel L, et al. Combinations of potassium, calcium, and magnesium supplements in hypertension. *Hypertension* 1995; 26:950–956.
307. Sacks FM, Willett WC, Smith A, et al. Effect of blood pressure of potassium, calcium, and magnesium in women with low habital intake. *Hypertension* 1998; 31:131–138.

308. Morris MC, Sacks FM, Rosner B. Does fish oil lower blood pressure: A meta-analysis of controlled trials. *Circulation* 1993; 88:523–533.
309. Issacsohn JL, Moser M, Stein EA, et al. Garlic powder and plasma lipids and lipoproteins: A multicenter, randomized, placebo-controlled trial. *Arch Intern Med* 1998; 158(11):1189–1194.
310. Minami J, Ishimitus T, Matsouka H. Effects of smoking cessation on blood pressure and heart and heart rate variability in habitual smokers. *Hypertension* 1999; 33(1 part 2):586–590.
311. Bolinder G, de Faire U. Ambulatory 24 hour blood pressure monitoring in healthy, middle-aged smokeless tobacco users, smokers, and nontobacco users. *Am J Hypertens* 1998; 11(10):1153–1163.
312. Hansson L, Lindholm LH, Niskanen L, et al. Effect of angiotensin-converting-enzyme inhibition compared with conventional therapy on cardiovascular morbidity and mortality in hypertension: The Captopril Prevention Project (CAPPP) randomised trial. *Lancet* 1999; 353(9153):611–616.
313. Hansson L, Lindholm LH, Ekborn T, et al. Randomised trial of old and new antihypertensive drugs in elderly patients: Cardiovascular mortality and morbidity. The Swedish Trial in Old Patients with Hypertension-2 study. *Lancet* 1999; 354(9192):1751–1756.
314. Garg R, Yusuf S, for the Collaborative Group on ACE Inhibitor Trials. Overview of randomized trials of angiotensin-converting enzyme inhibitors on mortality and morbidity in patients with heart failure. *JAMA* 1995; 273:1450–1456.
315. Pfeffer MA, Braunwald E, Moyé LA, et al, for the SAVE investigators. Effect of captopril on mortality and morbidity in patients with left ventricular dysfunction after myocardial infarction: Results of the Survival and Ventricular Enlargement Trials. *N Engl J Med* 1992; 327:669–677.
316. Lewis EJ, Hunsicker LG, Bain RP, Rohde RD, for the Collaborative Study Group. The effect of angiotensin-converting-enzyme inhibition on diabetic nephropathy. *N Engl J Med* 1993; 329:1456–1462.
317. Maschio G, Alberti D, Janin G, et al, for the Angiotensin-Converting-Enzyme Inhibition in Progressive Renal Insufficiency Study Group. Effect of the angiotensin-converting-enzyme inhibitor benazepril on the progression of chronic renal insufficiency. *N Engl J Med* 1996; 334:939–945.
318. Yusuf S, Sleight P, Pogue J, et al. Effects of an angiotensin-converting-enzyme inhibitor, ramipril, on death from cardiovascular causes, myocardial infarction, and stroke in high-risk patients: The Heart Outcomes Prevention Evaluation (HOPE) study investigators. *N Engl J Med* 2000; 342:145–153.
319. 1999 World Health Organization–International Society of Hypertension Guidelines for the management of hypertension: Guidelines Subcommittee. *J Hypertens* 1999; 17(2):151–183.
320. Davis BR, Cutler JA, Gordon DJ, et al. Rationale and design for the antihypertensive and lipid lowering treatment to prevent heart attack trial (ALLHAT). *Am J Hypertens* 1996; 9:342–360.
321. The ALLHAT Officers and Coordinators for the ALLHAT Collaborative Research Group. Major cardiovascular events in hypertensive patients randomized to doxazosin vs. chlorthalidone: The Antihypertensive and Lipid-Lowering Treatment to Prevent Heart Attack Trial (ALLHAT). *JAMA* 2000; 283:1967–1975.
322. Black HR, Elliott WJ, Neaton JD, et al. Rationale and design for the Controlled ONset Verapamil INvestigation of Cardiovascular Endpoints (CONVINCE) trial. *Controlled Clin Trials* 1998; 19(4):370–390.
323. Dahlof B, Devereux RB, Julius S, et al. Characteristics of 9194 patients with left ventricular hypertrophy: The LIFE study: Losartan Intervention For Endpoint Reduction in Hypertension. *Hypertension* 1998; 32(6):989–997.
324. Hansson L, Zandretti A, Carruthers SG, et al. Effects of intensive blood pressure lowering and low-dose aspirin in patients with hypertension: Principal results of the Hypertension Optimal Treatment (HOT) randomised trial: The HOT Study Group. *Lancet* 1998; 351:1755–1762.
325. Tight blood pressure control and risk of macrovascular and microvascular complications in type 2 diabetes: UKPDS 38: UK Prospective Diabetes Study Group. *BMJ* 1998; 317:703–713.
326. Lazarus JM, Bourgoignie JJ, Buckalew VM, et al. Achievement and safety of a low blood pressure goal in chronic renal disease: The Modification of Diet in Renal Disease Study Group. *Hypertension* 1997; 29:641–650.
327. Wright JS Jr, Kusek JW, Toto RD, et al. Design and baseline characteristics of participants in the African-American Study of Kidney Disease and Hypertension Pilot Study for the AASK pilot study investigators. *Controlled Clin Trials* 1996; 17:3S–16S.
328. Cruickshank JM, Thorpe JM, Zacharias FJ. Benefits and potential harm of lowering high blood pressure. *Lancet* 1987; 1:581–584.
329. Farnett L, Murlow CD, Linn WD, et al. The J curve phenomenon and the treatment of hypertension: Is there a point beyond which pressure reduction is dangerous? *JAMA* 1991; 265:489–495.
330. D'Agostino RB, Belanger AJ, Kannel WB, Cruickshank JM. Relation of low diastolic blood pressure to coronary heart disease death in presence of myocardial infarction: The Framingham Study. *BMJ* 1991; 303(6799):385–389.
331. Fletcher AE, Bulpitt CJ. How far should blood pressure be lowered? *N Engl J Med* 1992; 326:251–254.
332. Elliott WJ, Weir DR, Black HR. Cost-effectiveness of lowering treatment goal of JNC VI for diabetic hypertensives. *Arch Intern Med* 2000; 160:1277–1283.
333. Black HR. Metabolic considerations in the choice of therapy for the hypertensive patient. *Am Heart J* 1991; 121:707–715.
334. Kasiske BL, Ma JZ, Kalil R, Louis TA. Effects of antihypertensive therapy on serum lipids. *Ann Intern Med* 1995; 122:133–141.
335. Grimm RH, Flack JM, Grandits GA, et al, for the TOMHS Research Group. Long term effects on plasma lipids of diet and drugs to treat hypertension. *JAMA* 1996; 275:1549–1556.
336. Jones DW, Sands CD. Effects of doxazosin and hydrochlorothiazide on lipid levels in Korean patients with essential hypertension. *J Cardiovasc Pharmacol* 1993; 22(3):431–437.
337. Elisaf MS, Theodorou J, Pappas H, et al. Effectiveness and metabolic effects of perindopril and diuretics combination in primary hypertension. *J Hum Hypertens* 1999; 13(11):787–791.
338. Gress TW, Nieto FJ, Shahar E, et al, for the Atherosclerosis Risk in Communities Study. Hypertension and antihypertensive therapy and the risk factors for the type 2 diabetes mellitus. *N Engl J Med* 2000; 342:905–912.
339. Curb JD, Pressel SL, Cutler J, et al. Effect of diuretic-based antihypertensive treatment on cardiovascular disease risk in older diabetics with isolated systolic hypertension *JAMA* 1996; 276(23):1886–1892.
340. Tuomilehto J, Rastenyte D, Birkenhager WH, et al. Effects of calcium-channel blockade in older patients with diabetes and systolic hypertension: Systolic Hypertension in Europe Trial Investigators (Syst-Eur). *N Engl J Med* 1999; 340(9):677–684.
341. Yusuf S, Held P, Furberg C. Update of effects of calcium channel antagonists in myocardial infarction or angina in light of the second Danish Verapamil infarction trial (DAVIT-II) and other recent studies. *J Am Col Cardiol* 1991; 67:1295–1297.
342. Psaty BM, Smith NL, Siscovick DS, et al. Health outcomes associated with antihypertensive therapies used as first-line agents: A systematic review and meta-analysis. *JAMA* 1997; 277:739–745.
343. Bakris GL, Weir MR, DeQuattro V, McMahon FG. Effects of an ACE inhibitor/calcium antagonist combination on proteinuria in diabetic nephropathy. *Kidney Int* 1998; 54:1283–1289.
344. Bakris GL, Griffin KA, Picken MM, Bidani AK. Combined effects of an angiotensin converting enzyme inhibitor and a calcium antagonist on renal injury. *J Hypertens* 1997; 15:1181–1185.
345. Weber KT, Sun Y, Guarda E. Structural remodeling in hyperten-

sive heart disease and the role of hormones. *Hypertension* 1994; 23(part 2):869–877.
346. Douglas PS. Diastolic dysfunction: Old dog, new tricks [editorial]. *Am Heart J* 1999; 37:777–778.
347. Konstam MA, Dracup K, Baker DW, et al. Heart Failure: Evaluation and Care of Patients with Left Ventricular Systolic Dysfunction: Clinical Practice Guideline. No. 11. (AHCPR Publication #94-0612). Rockville, MD: Agency for Healthcare Policy and Research; 1994.
348. Hjalmarson A, Goldstein S, Faberberg B, et al. Effects of controlled-release metoprolol on total mortality, hospitalizations, and well-being in patients with heart failure: The Metoprolol CR/XL Randomized Intervention Trial in Congestive Heart Failure (MERIT-HF). *JAMA* 2000; 283:1295–1302.
349. Pitt B, Zannad F, Remme WJ, et al, for the Randomized Aldactone Evaluation Study (RALES) investigators. The effect of spironolactone on morbidity and mortality in patients with severe heart failure. *N Engl J Med* 1999; 341:709–717.
350. Pitt B, for the ELITE investigators. Results of the Evaluation of Losartan In The Elderly (ELITE) Trial. *Lancet* 1997; 349:757–762.
351. Packer MA, for the PRAISE Study Group. Final results of the Prospective Randomized Amlodipine Ischemia and Survival Evaluation Study. *N Engl J Med* 1996; 335:1107–1111.
352. Williams JF, Bristow MR, Fowler MB, et al. Guidelines for the evaluation and management of heart failure: Report of the American College of Cardiology/American Heart Association Task Force on Practice Guidelines (Committee on Evaluation and Management of Heart Failure). *J Am Coll Cardiol* 1995; 26:1376–1398.
353. Setaro JF, Zaret BL, Schulman DS, et al. Usefulness of verapamil for congestive heart failure associated with abnormal left ventricular diastolic filling and normal left ventricular systolic performance. *Am J Cardiol* 1990; 66:981–986.
354. Otto CM, Lind BK, Kitzman DW, et al. Association of aortic-valve sclerosis with cardiovascular mortality and morbidity in the elderly. *N Engl J Med* 1999; 341:142–147.
355. Sapira JD. Quincke, de Musset, Duroziez and Hill: Some aortic regurgitations. *South Med J* 1981; 74:459–467.
356. Scognamiglio R, Rahimtoola SH, Fasoli G, et al. Nifedipine in asymptomatic patients with severe aortic regurgitation and normal left ventricular function. *N Engl J Med* 1994; 331:689–694.
357. Rich S, Kaufmann E, Levy PS. The effect of high doses of calcium-channel blockers on survival in primary pulmonary hypertension. *N Engl J Med* 1992; 327:76–81.
358. Khan MA, Herzog CA, St. Peter JV, et al. The prevalence of cardiac valvular insufficiency assessed by transthoracic echocardiography in obese patients treated with appetite-suppressant drugs. *N Engl J Med* 1999; 339:713–718.
359. Remuzzi G, Ruggenenti P, Benigni A. Understanding the nature of renal disease progression. *Kidney Int* 1997; 51:2–15.
360. Tarif N, Bakris GL. Renal components of the hypertensive syndrome. *J Cardiovas Risk* 1997; 4(4):271–278.
361. The GISEN group. Randomized placebo-controlled trial of effect of ramipril on decline in glomerular filtration rate and risk of terminal renal failure in proteinuric, non-diabetic nephropathy. *Lancet* 1997; 349:1857–1863.
362. Benigni A, Remuzzi G. Glomerular protein trafficking and progression of renal disease to terminal uremia. *Semin Nephrol* 1996; 16(3):151–159.
363. Brown S, Walton C, Crawford P, Bakris GL. Comparative renal hemodynamic effects of an ACE inhibitor or calcium antagonist on progression of diabetic nephropathy in the dog. *Kidney Int* 1993; 43:1210–1218.
364. Kloke HJ, Branten AJ, Huysmans FT, Wetzels JF. Antihypertensive treatment of patients with proteinuric renal diseases: Risks or benefits of calcium channel blockers? *Kidney Int* 1998; 53(6):1559–1573.
365. Tarif N, Bakris GL. Angiotensin II receptor blockade and progression of renal disease in nondiabetic patients. *Kidney Int* 1997; 52(suppl 63):S-67–S-70.
366. Ravid M, Brosh D, Levi Z, et al. Use of enalapril to attenuate decline in renal function in normotensive, normoalbuminuric patients with type 2 diabetes mellitus: A randomized, controlled trial. *Ann Intern Med* 1998; 128(12 part 1):982–988.
367. Abbott K, Smith AC, Bakris GL. Effects of dihydropyridine calcium antagonists on albuminuria in diabetic subjects. *J Clin Pharmacol* 1996; 36:274–279.
368. Bakris GL, Smith AC. Effects of sodium intake on albumin excretion in patients with diabetic nephropathy treated with long-acting calcium antagonists. *Ann Intern Med* 1996; 125(3):201–203.
369. Bakris GL, Weir MR. Salt intake and reductions in arterial pressure and proteinuria: Is there a direct link? *Am J Hypertens* 1996; 9:200S–206S.
370. Heeg JE, de Jong PE, van der Hem GK, de Zeeuw D. Efficacy and variability of the antiproteinuric effect of ACE inhibition by lisinopril. *Kidney Int* 1989; 36(2):272–279.
371. Bakris GL, Weir MR. ACE inhibitor associated elevations in serum creatinine: Is this a cause for concern? *Arch Intern Med* 2000; 160:685–693.
372. Parving HH, Rossing P, Hommel E, Smidt UM. Angiotensin-converting enzyme inhibition in diabetic nephropathy: Ten years' experience. *Am J Kidney Dis* 1995; 26(1):99–107.
373. The National Kidney Foundation Hypertension and Diabetes Executive Committee Working Group. Treatment of hypertension in adults with diabetes to preserve renal function: A position paper. *Am J Kidney Dis,* in press.
374. Yeghiazarians Y, Braunstein JB, Askari A, Stone PH. Medical progress: Unstable angina pectoris. *N Engl J Med* 2000; 342:101–114.
375. Heidenreich PA, McDonald KM, Hastie T, et al. Meta-analysis of trials comparing beta-blockers, calcium antagonists, and nitrates for stable angina. *JAMA* 1999; 281:1927–1936.
376. Powers WJ. Acute hypertension after stroke: The scientific basis for treatment decisions. *Neurology* 1994; 43:461–467.
377. Adams HP, Brott TG, Crowell RM, et al. Guidelines for the management of patients with acute ischemic stroke: A statement for healthcare professionals from a special writing group of the Stroke Council, American Heart Association. *Stroke* 1994; 25:1901–1914.
378. The National Institute of Neurological Disorders and Stroke rt-PA Stroke Study Group. Tissue plasminogen activator for acute ischemic stroke. *N Engl J Med* 1995; 333:1581–1587.
379. Mayberg MR, Batjer HH, Dacey R, et al. Guidelines for the management of aneurysmal subarachnoid hemorrhage: A statement for healthcare professionals from a special writing group of the Stroke Council, American Heart Association. *Circulation* 1994; 90:2592–2605.
380. Epstein M, Bakris GL. Newer approaches to antihypertensive therapy: Use fixed dose combination therapy. *Arch Intern Med* 1996; 156:1969–1978.
381. Bakris GL, Weber MA, Black HR, Weir MR. Clinical efficacy and safety profiles of AT1 receptor antagonists. *Cardiovasc Rev Reports* 1999; 20:77–100.
382. Preston RA, Materson BJ, Reda DJ, et al, for the Department of Veterans Affairs Cooperative Study Group on Antihypertensive Agents. Age-race subgroup compared to renin profile as predictors of blood pressure response to antihypertensive therapy in 1031 patients: Results of the VA cooperative study. *JAMA* 1998; 280(13):1168–1172.
383. Weir MR, Gray JM, Paster R, Saunders E. Differing mechanisms of action of angiotensin-converting enzyme inhibition in black

and white hypertensive patients: The Trandolapril Multicenter Study Group. *Hypertension* 1995; 26(1):124–130.

384. National High Blood Pressure Education Program Working Group. National High Blood Pressure Education Program Working Group Report on Hypertension in the Elderly. *Hypertension* 1994; 23:275–285.
385. Lever AF, Ramsay LE. Treatment of hypertension in the elderly. *J Hypertens* 1995; 13:571–579.
386. Update on the Task Force Report (1987) on High Blood Pressure in Children and Adolescents: A Working Group Report from the National High Blood Pressure Education Program: National High Blood Pressure Education Program Working Group on Hypertension Control in Children and Adolescents. *Pediatrics* 1996; 98:649–658.
387. Sinaiko AR. Current concepts: Hypertension in children. *N Engl J Med* 1996; 335:1968–1973.
388. National High Blood Pressure Education Program Working Group on Hypertension in Pregnancy. Report of the National High Blood Pressure Education Program Working Group on Hypertension in Pregnancy. *Am J Obstet Gynecol* 1990; 163:1689–1712.
389. Helewa ME, Burrows RF, Smith J, et al. Report of the Canadian Hypertension Society Consensus Conference: Definition, evaluation, and classification of hypertensive disorders in pregnancy. *Can Med Assoc J* 1997; 157:715–725.
390. Caritis S, Sibai B, Hauth J, et al. Low-dose aspirin to prevent preeclampsia in women at high risk. *N Engl J Med* 1998; 338:701–705.
391. Levine RJ, Hauth JC, Curet LB, et al. Trial of calcium to prevent preeclampsia. *N Engl J Med* 1997; 337:69–76.
392. Kaplan NM. Management of hypertensive emergencies. *Lancet* 1994; 344:1335–1338.
393. Gifford RW Jr. Management of hypertensive crises. *JAMA* 1991; 266:829–835.
394. Elliott WJ, Black HR. Hypertensive emergencies and aortic dissection. *Curr Ther Crit Care Med* 1997; 185–191.
395. Strandgaard S, Paulson OR. Hypertensive disease and the cerebral circulation. In: Laragh JH, Brenner BM, eds. *Hypertension: Pharphysiology, Diagnosis, and Management*, Vol 1. New York: Raven Press; 1990:399.
396. Cohn JN, Burke LP. Nitroprusside. *Ann Intern Med* 1979; 91:752–757.
397. Dmowski AT, Carey MJ. Aortic dissection. *Am J Emerg Med* 1999; 17:372–375.
398. Chen K, Varon J, Wenker OC, et al. Acute thoracic aortic dissection: The basics. *J Emerg Med* 1997; 15:859–867.
399. Post JB IV, Frishman WH. Fenoldopam: A new dopamine agonist for the treatment of hypertensive urgencies and emergencies. *J Clin Pharmacol* 1998; 38:2–13.
400. Wallin JD, Fletcher E, Ram CV, et al. Intravenous nicardipine for the treatment of severe hypertension. *Arch Intern Med* 1989; 149:2662–2669.
401. Grossman E, Messerli FH, Grodzicki T, et al. Should a moratorium be placed on sublingual nifedipine capsules given for hypertensive emergencies and pseudoemergencies? *JAMA* 1996; 276:1328–1331.
402. Stason WB, Schmid CH, Niedzwiecki D, et al. Safety of nifedipine in patients with hypertension: A meta-analysis. *Hypertension* 1997; 30:7–14.
403. Grossman E, Ironi AN, Messerli FH. Comparative tolerability profile of hypertensive crises treatments. *Drug Saf* 1998; 19: 99–122.
404. Cohen MC, Rohtla KM, Lavery CE, et al. Meta-analysis of the morning excess of acute myocardial infarction and sudden cardiac death. *Circulation* 1997; 79:1512–1515.
405. Elliott WJ. Circadian variation in the timing of stroke onset: A meta-analysis. *Stroke* 1998; 29:992–996.
406. Elliott WJ, Prisant LM. Drug delivery systems for antihypertensive agents. *Blood Pressure Monit* 1997; 2:53–60.
407. Smolensky MH, Portaluppi F. Chronopharmacology and chronotherapy of cardiovascular medications: Relevance to prevention and treatment of coronary heart disease. *Am Heart J* 1999; 137(4 part 2):S14–S24.
408. White WB, Black HR, Elliott W, et al. Comparison of effects of controlled onset extended release verapamil at bedtime and nifedipine gastrointestinal therapeutic system on arising on early morning blood pressure, heart rate, and the heart rate–blood pressure product. *Am J Cardiol* 1998; 81:424–431.
409. Saseen JJ, Carter BL, Brown TE, et al. Comparison of nifedipine alone and with diltiazem or verapamil in hypertension. *Hypertension* 1996; 28(1):109–114.
410. Matersson HRB, Pope JE, Anderson JJ, Felson DT. A meta-analysis of the effects of nonsteroidal anti-inflammatory drugs on blood pressure. *Arch Intern Med* 1993; 153(4): 477–484.
411. Jones JK, Gorkin L, Lian JF, et al. Discontinuation of and changes in treatment after start of new courses of antihypertensive drugs: A study of a United Kingdom population. *BMJ* 1995; 311:293–296.
412. Bloom BS. Continuation of initial antihypertensive medication after one year of therapy. *Clin Ther* 1998; 20:671–681.
413. Levine M. Costs associated with noncompliance. In: Leenen, FHH, ed. *Patient Compliance and the Long-Term Management of Hypertension.* Montréal: STA Communications; 1996:21.
414. Elliott WJ. Compliance Strategies. In: Alderman MH, Mitch WE, eds. *Current Opinion in Nephrology and Hypertension,* Vol 3. Philadelphia: Current Science; 1994:271.
415. Hilleman DE, Mohiuddin SM, Lucas BD Jr, et al. Cost-minimization analysis of initial antihypertensive therapy in patients with mild-to-moderate essential diastolic hypertension. *Clin Ther* 1994; 16:88–102.
416. Drugs for Hypertension. *The Medical Letter on Drugs & Therapeutics.* 1999; 41:23–28.

PART EIGHT

PULMONARY HYPERTENSION AND PULMONARY DISEASE

CHAPTER 52

PULMONARY HYPERTENSION

Lewis J. Rubin

Pulmonary hypertension is a hemodynamic abnormality common to a variety of conditions that is characterized by increased right ventricular (RV) afterload and work. The clinical manifestations, natural history, and reversibility of pulmonary hypertension depend heavily on the nature of the pulmonary vascular lesions and the etiology and severity of the hemodynamic disorder. For example, subacute or chronic hypoxia predominantly causes increased muscularization of the small muscular pulmonary arteries and arterioles while leaving the intima relatively intact. Relief of the hypoxia improves or occasionally reverses the process with little or no pathologic residue.[1,2] In contrast, the lesions of systemic sclerosis (scleroderma), which tend to be confined to the intima of the small pulmonary arteries and arterioles, are usually progressive and irreversible. In contrast to scleroderma and chronic hypoxia, which spare the pulmonary capillary bed, the pulmonary capillaries are the primary site of involvement in pulmonary capillary hemangiomatosis.[3] Because of its large capacity, its great distensibility, its low resistance to blood flow, and the modest amounts of smooth muscle in the small arteries and arterioles, the pulmonary circulation is not predisposed to become hypertensive. When total cross-sectional area is decreased, such as by destruction or obliteration of lung tissue or occlusive lesions in the resistance vessels, pulmonary arterial pressures increase. The degree of pulmonary hypertension that develops is a function of the amount of the pulmonary vascular tree that has been eliminated. Pulmonary hypertension is usually secondary to cardiac or pulmonary disease. Although primary pulmonary hypertension (PPH) is uncommon, it has attracted considerable attention as a distinctive clinical entity in which intrinsic pulmonary vascular disease is free of the complicating features of secondary pulmonary hypertension contributed by diseases of the heart and/or lungs. Mild or even moderate pulmonary hypertension can exist for a lifetime without becoming evident clinically. For example, native residents at high altitude, in whom mild to moderate pulmonary hypertension is a natural result of sustained exposure to hypoxia, can function normally. When pulmonary hypertension does become manifest clinically, the symptoms tend to be nonspecific (Table 52-1).

DEFINITIONS

Pulmonary *arterial* hypertension can be either acute or chronic. The acute form is usually a result of either pulmonary embolism (see Chap. 53) or the adult respiratory distress syndrome. This chapter deals with *chronic* pulmonary arterial hypertension.

Pulmonary *venous* hypertension usually is encountered clinically as a consequence of left ventricular (LV) failure or mitral valvular disease. Occasionally, it may occur in the course of fibrosing mediastinitis. Only rarely is the entity known as pulmonary veno-occlusive disease (PVOD) encountered. Even though pulmonary hypertension may be confined, at the outset, to the pulmonary veins (e.g., in acute mitral insufficiency), sooner or later pulmonary arterial hypertension supervenes. The hallmarks of pulmonary venous hypertension are pulmonary congestion and edema. For practical purposes, pulmonary venous hypertension is said to exist when pulmonary venous (or left atrial) pressure rises above 15 mmHg.

Cor pulmonale signifies the presence of pulmonary hypertension in the setting of chronic respiratory disease.[4] The degree of pulmonary hypertension that develops in patients with chronic lung disease tends to be less severe than in connective tissue diseases, chronic thromboembolic disease, or primary pulmonary hypertension. Pulmonary hypertension may be severe, however, in some patients with interstitial lung disease.

TABLE 52-1 Symptoms of Primary Pulmonary Hypertension

Dyspnea	Palpitations
Fatigue	Orthopnea
Dizziness	Cough
Syncope	Hoarseness
Chest pain	

NORMAL PULMONARY CIRCULATION

Structure

Immediately before birth, pulmonary and systemic arterial blood pressures are about equal and on the order of 70/40 mmHg, with a mean of 50 mmHg. Immediately after birth, with closure of the ductus arteriosus and initiation of ventilation, pulmonary arterial pressure falls rapidly to about one-half of systemic levels. Thereafter, pulmonary arterial pressures gradually decrease over several weeks to reach adult levels[5] (see also Chap. 70).

In some neonates, the normal pulmonary hypertension of the fetus fails to recede normally, generally due to either a developmental anomaly or a relentless increase in pulmonary vascular tone. In such infants, the persistent pulmonary hypertension and RV failure may become life-threatening. Surgical intervention or temporizing measures, such as the use of inhaled nitric oxide (NO) or extracorporeal membrane oxygenation (ECMO), may be useful in reversing the pulmonary vascular abnormalities.[6]

In the normal adult at sea level, the small muscular arteries and arterioles in the lungs are thin-walled and contain very little smooth muscle. In contrast, in the fetus or the adult who has lived under hypoxic conditions (e.g., native residents at high altitude), the media of the arterioles are thickened, and the muscle extends distally into precapillary vessels that are ordinarily devoid of muscle; i.e., the precapillary vessels undergo "remodeling."[7]

Endothelium and Endothelium–Smooth Muscle Interactions

In addition to its role as a semipermeable barrier between blood and interstitium, the endothelium serves a wide array of biologically important functions, the net effect of which is the processing of blood flowing through the lungs. Among these functions are the synthesis, uptake, storage, release, and metabolism of vasoactive substances; transduction of blood-borne signals; modulation of coagulation and thrombolysis; regulation of cell proliferation; engagement in the local inflammatory and proliferative reactions to injury; involvement in immune reactions; and angiogenesis (see also Chap. 4). Some of the enzymes involved in these processes, such as the angiotensin-converting enzyme, are found on the surface of endothelial cells; others, such as 5′-nucleotidase, are found within the cell.[8] Hence it is appropriate to regard endothelium as an organ with diverse metabolic and endocrine functions, one that is unique because of its strategic location as a continuous, monolayered lining of blood vessels throughout the body. It is also important to bear in mind that the lungs contain the largest expanse of endothelium in the body.

The cells that comprise the monolayered endothelial lining communicate not only with each other by anatomic junctions and bridges but also with the underlying smooth muscle by way of biologically active substances.[9] This interaction participates in regulating normal vasomotor tone as well as in response to the administration of vasoactive substances. It is not difficult to imagine that damage to the lining cells, proliferation of the intima, or hypertrophy of the smooth muscle will upset the normal interplay.

Hemodynamics

For the adult pulmonary circulation, the definition of *normal* depends on the altitude. The normal pulmonary hemodynamics of adults residing at sea level and above sea level are compared in Table 52-2. At *sea level,* a cardiac output of 5 to 6 L/min is associated with a pulmonary arterial pressure of about 20/12 mmHg, with a mean of about 15 mmHg. At an altitude of 15,000 ft, the same level of blood flow is associated with somewhat higher pressures (see Table 52-2). Pulmonary arterial pressures also tend to increase somewhat with age.

A pressure drop of only 5 to 10 mmHg between the pulmonary artery and left atrium accompanies the cardiac output of 5 to 6 L/min (see Table 52-2). Determination of pulmonary vascular resistance, calculated as the ratio of the difference in mean pressure at the two ends of the pulmonary vascular bed (pulmonary arterial pressure minus left atrial pressure divided by the cardiac output; see Table 52-2), has proved to be a practical clinical tool for assessing the hemodynamic state of the pulmonary circulation and for distinguishing between active and passive changes in the pulmonary resistance vessels (e.g., the effect of administering a vasodilator agent to a patient with pulmonary hypertension). In practice, since the left atrium may not be readily accessible, pulmonary wedge pressure generally is substituted for left atrial pressure.

Another approach to defining certain characteristics and the behavior of the pulmonary arterial tree, i.e., elastic properties and geometry, is the calculation of pulmonary arterial input

TABLE 52-2 Values for Normal Pulmonary Circulation at Sea Level and Altitude

	Sea Level	Altitude (~15,000 ft)
Pulmonary arterial pressure (P_{PA}), mmHg	20/12, 15	38/14, 25
Cardiac output (Q), L/min	6.0	6.0
Left atrial pressure (P_{LA}), mmHg	5.0	5.0
Pulmonary vascular resistance (PVR),[a] (mmHg/L)/min (R units)	1.7	3.3

[a] $PVR = \frac{P_{PA} - P_{LA}}{Q} = \frac{15 - 5}{6} = 1.67$ R units. To convert T units to CGS units (dynes·s/cm^5), multiply R units by 80.

impedance. This approach has more physiologic than clinical value. It takes into account the pulsatile nature of pulmonary arterial pressures and flow. Like vascular resistance, it is defined as a ratio. But instead of a ratio involving *mean* pressures and blood flow, the ratio is of the amplitudes of pulsatile pressure to oscillatory flow near the beginning of the pulmonary artery at a particular frequency. Values for the ratio are obtained by resolving mathematically the pulsatile pressure and flow curves into their sinusoidal components.

Although calculated pulmonary vascular resistance has proved useful in assessing the state of the normal and abnormal pulmonary circulation, and even though a change in calculated resistance often can be helpful in deciding whether pulmonary vasoconstriction or vasodilatation has occurred, translation of a calculated ratio into vasomotor activity has to be made with caution.[4] For example, changes in calculated pulmonary vascular resistance are not readily interpretable when a vasodilator agent evokes multiple hemodynamic changes simultaneously (e.g., simultaneous changes in pulmonary vascular pressures and blood flow). Also, a clinical shortcut, such as the substitution in the numerator of the pulmonary arterial pressure for the pressure *drop* between the pulmonary artery and left atrium, may be useful empirically but deprives the calculation of any physiologic meaning. Finally, the clinical significance of a value calculated for pulmonary vascular resistance depends heavily on the implications of the hemodynamic changes on the work of the right ventricle. For example, the same decrease in calculated pulmonary vascular resistance brought about by two different pulmonary vasodilators may affect the work of the right ventricle differently: Should one agent elicit a *decrease* in pulmonary arterial pressure along with an *increase* in cardiac output (an ideal response), it is more apt to be of long-term benefit than another agent that, while increasing the cardiac output, fails to decrease the pulmonary arterial pressure.

In the normal lung, a considerable increase in cardiac output, i.e., two to three times that at rest, generally increases pulmonary arterial pressure by only a few millimeters of mercury. On the other hand, in pulmonary hypertensive states, in which the distensibility and extent of the pulmonary vascular bed have been restricted by disease, pulmonary arterial pressure increases along with even small increments in pulmonary blood flow. Changes in pulmonary blood volume are much more subtle than changes in blood pressure or flow in their hemodynamic effects; they are also much more difficult to quantify. Clinical clues can be helpful in recognizing that the pulmonary blood volume has increased. Often a fullness of the pulmonary vascular pattern on the chest radiograph along with evidences of interstitial edema suggests that pulmonary blood volume has increased acutely. In chronic mitral stenosis or LV failure, the pulmonary blood volume is not only increased but is also redistributed toward the apices of the lungs, i.e., "cephalization."

Autonomic innervation of the pulmonary vascular tree plays much less of a role in modulating vasomotor tone than do local stimuli, particularly hypoxia. Indeed, hypoxia can exert its pulmonary pressor effect in the isolated lung, i.e., one that is devoid of external innervation. The mechanism by which hypoxia exerts its local pressor effect is not fully characterized but appears to involve altered smooth muscle cell membrane ion channel activity.[2] Acidosis potentiates the hypoxic pressor effect. Hypercapnia also exerts a pulmonary pressor effect, presumably by way of the local acidosis that it generates, but it is less powerful than hypoxia as a pulmonary vasoconstrictor agent.

PULMONARY HYPERTENSION: GENERAL FEATURES

Clinical Manifestations

Pulmonary hypertension is a final common hemodynamic consequence of multiple etiologies and diverse mechanisms. As noted earlier, most cases of pulmonary hypertension are secondary (Table 52-3). Among the underlying causes of pulmonary hypertension are mechanical compression and distortion of the resistance vessels of the lungs (e.g., by diffuse pulmonary fibrosis), hypoxic vasoconstriction (e.g., in severe obstructive airways or diffuse parenchymal diseases), intravascular obstruction (e.g., thromboemboli or tumor emboli), and combinations of mechanical and vasoconstrictive influences. The significance of pulmonary hypertension, however, is that if it is uncontrolled, it leads to RV failure. Once pulmonary arterial pressures reach systemic levels, RV failure becomes inevitable.

Special Studies

The "gold standard" for the diagnosis of pulmonary hypertension is right-sided heart catheterization. This technique enables the direct determination of right atrial and ventricular pressures, pulmonary arterial pressure, pulmonary wedge pressure (as an approximation of pulmonary venous pressure), pulmonary blood flow (cardiac output), and the responses of these parameters to interventions (vasodilators, oxygen, exercise). From the measurements and samples obtained during cardiac catheterization, pulmonary vascular resistance can be calculated (see Table 52-2). As a rule, noninvasive methods are less reliable and less informative.

CHEST RADIOGRAPHY

The findings on the chest radiograph depend on the duration of the pulmonary hypertension and the etiology. The characteristic findings of pulmonary hypertension are enlargement of the pulmonary trunk and hilar vessels in association with attenuation (pruning) of the peripheral pulmonary arterial tree (Fig. 52-1). Right-sided heart enlargement can be best detected radiographically on the lateral view as fullness in the retrosternal airspace. In secondary pulmonary hypertension, changes in the lungs (e.g., hyperinflation, fibrosis) and in the position of the heart and diaphragm often mask the radiologic changes of pulmonary hypertension. Contrast angiography has a role in the workup for pulmonary hypertension when chronic thromboembolic disease, which may be treated surgically, is suspected.[8]

THE ELECTROCARDIOGRAM

The electrocardiogram (ECG) can disclose hypertrophy of the right ventricle and is more reliable in respiratory disorders that do not involve the parenchyma of the lungs (e.g., alveolar hypoventilation and sleep apnea) than in obstructive airways disease or parenchymal lung disease.

ECHOCARDIOGRAPHY

The amount of reliable information obtained by Doppler and two-dimensional echocardiography depends greatly on the com-

TABLE 52-3 Nomenclature and Classification of Pulmonary Hypertension

DIAGNOSTIC CLASSIFICATION

1. Pulmonary arterial hypertension
    1.1 Primary pulmonary hypertension
        (a) Sporadic
        (b) Familial
    1.2 Related to
        (a) Collagen-vascular disease
        (b) Congenital systemic to pulmonary shunts
        (c) Portal hypertension
        (d) HIV infection
        (e) Drugs/toxins
            (1) Anorexigens
            (2) Other
        (f) Persistent pulmonary hypertension of the newborn
        (g) Other
2. Pulmonary venous hypertension
    2.1 Left-side atrial or ventricular heart disease
    2.2 Left-side valvular heart disease
    2.3 Extrinsic compression of central pulmonary veins
        (a) Fibrosing mediastinitis
        (b) Adenopathy/tumors
    2.4 Pulmonary veno-occlusive disease
    2.5 Other
3. Pulmonary hypertension associated with disorders of the respiratory system and/or hypoxemia
    3.1 Chronic obstructive pulmonary disease
    3.2 Interstitial lung disease
    3.3 Sleep-disordered breathing
    3.4 Alveolar hypoventilatory disorders
    3.5 Chronic exposure to high altitude
    3.6 Neonatal lung disease
    3.7 Alveolar-capillary dysplasia
    3.8 Other
4. Pulmonary hypertension due to chronic thrombotic and/or embolic disease
    4.1 Thromboembolic obstruction of proximal pulmonary arteries
    4.2 Obstruction of distal pulmonary arteries
        (a) Pulmonary embolism (thrombus, tumor, ova and/or parasites, foreign material)
        (b) In-situ thrombosis
        (c) Sickle cell disease
5. Pulmonary hypertension due to disorders directly affecting the pulmonary vasculature
    5.1 Inflammatory
        (a) Schistosomiasis
        (b) Sarcoidosis
        (c) Other
    5.2 Pulmonary capillary hemangiomatosis

mitment of individual clinics to standardizing and perfecting these noninvasive techniques. In general, echocardiographic techniques have proved useful in providing a measure of RV thickness as an index of RV hypertension. In some clinics, reliable estimates of the level of pulmonary hypertension have been obtained by determining regurgitant flows across the tricuspid and pulmonic valves using continuous-wave Doppler echocardiography.[9] In patients in whom the pulmonic valve has been visualized, its behavior during the cardiac cycle also has been used to estimate the level of pulmonary arterial pressure. Probably one of the more rewarding applications of echocardiography has been as an alternative to repeated cardiac catheterization in tracing the course of the disease and in assessing the effects of therapeutic interventions (e.g., pulmonary vasodilators) in some patients (see also Chap. 13).

LUNG SCANS

Ventilation-perfusion scans are of most value in the diagnosis and exclusion of pulmonary thromboembolic disease (see below).

RADIONUCLIDE STUDIES

The response of the RV ejection fraction to exercise is assessed in some clinics using radionuclide angiography. Scintigraphy using thallium-201 also has been useful in detecting hypertrophy of the right ventricle due to pulmonary hypertension (see also Chap. 16).

LUNG BIOPSY

The sampling of lung tissue by open thoracotomy or thoracoscopy occasionally is helpful in identifying the etiology of the pulmonary hypertension, e.g., in the setting of suspected pulmonary vasculitis. However, the procedure carries substantial risk in these hemodynamically compromised individuals. Attempts to predict responsiveness to vasodilators on the basis of lung biopsy have met with limited success.[10]

SECONDARY PULMONARY HYPERTENSION

Cardiac and/or respiratory diseases are the most common causes of secondary pulmonary hypertension. Pulmonary thromboembolic disease ranks third. Cardiac disease leads to pulmonary hypertension by increasing pulmonary blood flow (e.g., large left-to-right shunts) or by increasing pulmonary venous pressure (e.g., LV failure). Almost invariably, secondary influences such as intimal proliferation in the pulmonary resistance vessels add a component of obstructive pulmonary vascular disease.[11] In respiratory disease, the predominant mechanism for the pulmonary hypertension is an increase in resistance to pulmonary blood flow arising from perivascular parenchymal changes coupled with pulmonary vasoconstriction due to hypoxia. In pulmonary thromboembolic disease, clots in various stages of organization and affecting pulmonary vessels of different size increase resistance to blood flow.[11]

Cardiac Disease

The mechanisms of pulmonary hypertension usually are quite different in acquired disorders of the left side of the heart than in those of congenital heart disease.

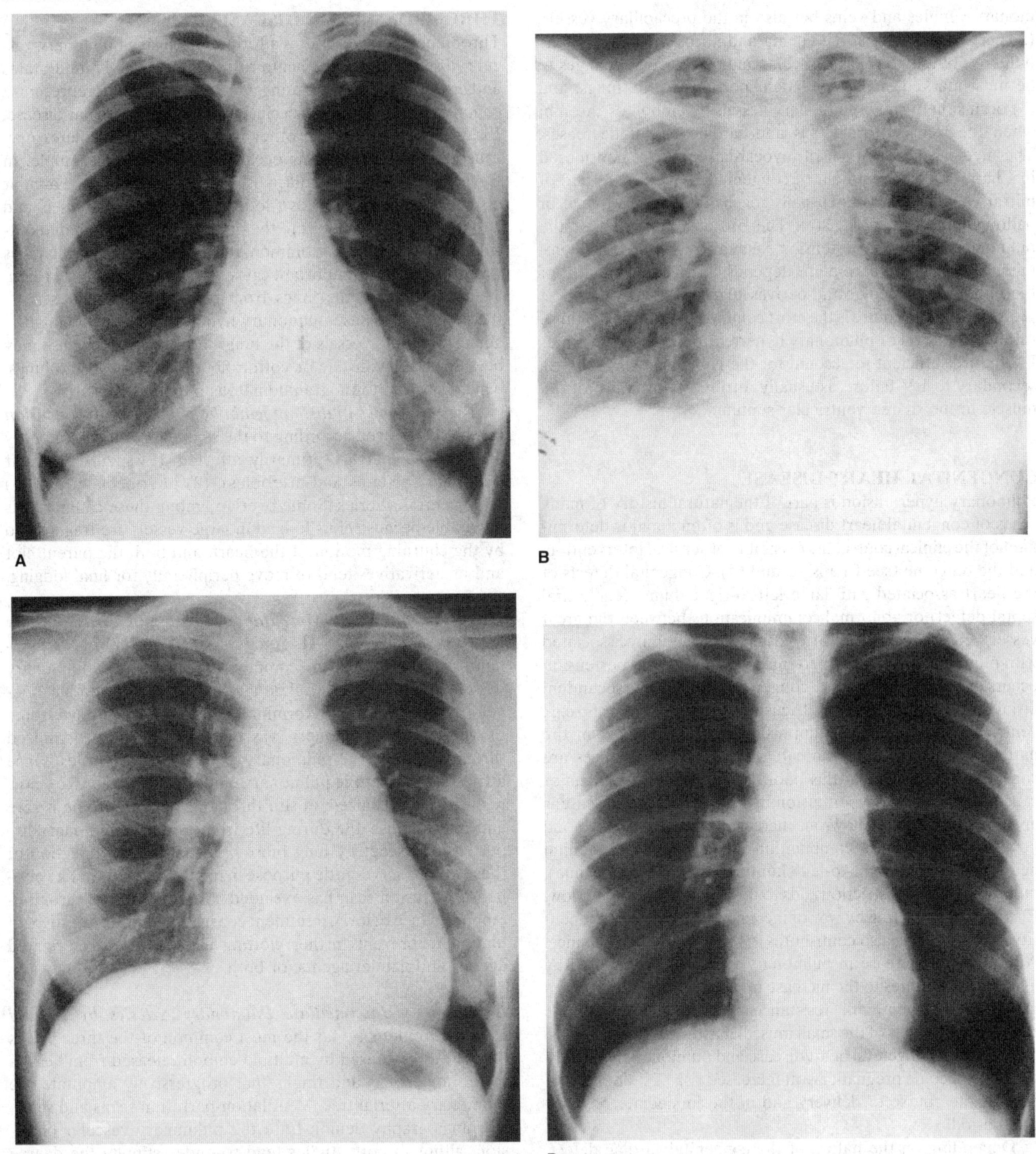

FIGURE 52-1 Cardiac silhouette in four patients with severe pulmonary hypertension on admission to the hospital: *A,B.* Primary pulmonary hypertension showing different stages in the evolution of right-sided heart failure. *C.* Widespread pulmonary fibrosis. *D.* Systemic lupus erythematosus proven by lung biopsy. This radiograph is indistinguishable from that of primary pulmonary hypertension.

ACQUIRED DISORDERS OF THE LEFT SIDE OF THE HEART

LV failure is the most common cause of pulmonary hypertension. Among the various etiologies, myocardial disorders and lesions of the mitral and aortic valves predominate. Both categories of lesions lead to an increase in pulmonary venous pressure that, in turn, evokes an increase in pulmonary arterial pressure. Presumably, the increase in pulmonary arterial pressure is reflex in origin. In time, three types of morphologic changes supervene: (1) occlusive intimal and medial changes not only in pulmonary venules and veins but also in the precapillary vessels, (2) perivascular interstitial edema and fibrosis that, under the influence of gravity, cause vascular and perivascular changes to be most marked in the dependent portions of the lungs, and (3) occlusion of small pulmonary vessels by emboli or thrombi when the right ventricle fails and cardiac output decreases. The medical management of myocardial failure is considered in Chap. 21. The treatment of congenital heart disease and of mitral valvular disease is usually mechanical (e.g., surgical or balloon mitral valvuloplasty). The prospect for relief of the pulmonary venous hypertension, such as by mitral valve commissurotomy or replacement, depends on the reversibility of the pulmonary vascular and perivascular lesions.

Although LV failure is the most common cause of RV failure, rarely is the level of pulmonary hypertension that accompanies LV failure sufficient to account for the RV failure. RV failure, secondary to LV failure, is usually attributed to failure of the muscle in the shared ventricular septum.

CONGENITAL HEART DISEASE

Pulmonary hypertension is part of the natural history of many types of congenital heart disease and is often a major determinant of the clinical course, the feasibility of surgical intervention, and the outcome (see Chaps. 63 and 64). Congenital defects of the heart associated with large left-to-right shunts (e.g., atrial septal defect) or abnormal communications between the great vessels (e.g., patent ductus arteriosus) are commonly associated with pulmonary arterial hypertension. Pulmonary hypertension occurs in both "pretricuspid" congenital defects (e.g., secundum atrial septal defect) and "posttricuspid" congenital defects (e.g., ventricular septal defect). Important differences exist in the natural history of these two categories. Their differences are considered elsewhere in this book (see Chap. 70). The major cause of pulmonary hypertension in congenital heart disease is an increase in blood flow, an increase in resistance to blood flow, or most often, a combination of the two. In congenital heart disease with right-to-left shunting (systemic hypoxemia), pulmonary vasoconstriction adds to the resistance to blood flow. Erythrocytosis, acting by way of increased viscosity and propensity to thrombosis, also contributes to the increase in resistance. Although the increase in pulmonary vascular tone elicited by hypoxia contributes to the increase in pulmonary vascular resistance, the predominant resistance is offered by anatomic changes in the walls of the small muscular arteries and arterioles. Patients with congenital heart disease and pulmonary hypertension who become pregnant are at increased risk of sudden death both in the course of delivery and in the immediate postpartum period.

Depending on the nature of the congenital cardiac defect, vasodilators sometimes are helpful in diminishing heightened pulmonary vasomotor tone. Caution is required in administering such agents to patients with congenital heart disease because of the potential to increase right-to-left shunting by reducing systemic vascular resistance to a greater degree than its pulmonary counterpart. Phlebotomy, with replacement of fluid (e.g., plasma or albumin), is helpful in congenital cyanotic heart disease in which severe hypoxemia has evoked a large increase in red cell mass. Once again, caution is required to avoid depletion of iron stores and to avoid reduction in the circulating blood volume.

THROMBOEMBOLIC DISEASE

Thromboembolic disease is a form of occlusive pulmonary vascular disease. It may be acute or chronic. In the United States and Europe, clots originating in peripheral veins represent a common cause of chronic occlusive pulmonary vascular disease. Elsewhere in the world, other intravascular particulates may cause pulmonary vascular occlusive disease. For example, in Egypt, where schistosomiasis is endemic, pulmonary vascular disease stemming from ova lodged in pulmonary vessels and hypersensitivity reactions to the organism (usually situated outside the lungs) is not uncommon. In some parts of Asia, filariasis is reputed to be an important cause of pulmonary hypertension. Tumor emboli to the lungs from extrapulmonary sites (e.g., the breast) can cause pulmonary hypertension by invading the adjacent minute vessels of the lungs. Intravenous drug use may be associated with talc or cotton fiber embolism to the lungs, which can result in a granulomatous pulmonary arteritis.

The *syndromes of thromboembolic pulmonary hypertension* can be categorized according to the segments of the pulmonary arterial tree that are primarily affected: (1) small (muscular pulmonary arteries and arterioles), (2) intermediate, and (3) large central arteries. Some overlap among these categories is inevitable because clots lodged in large vessels are fragmented by the churning motion of the heart, and both the parent clot and its derivatives tend to move peripherally for final lodging.

Occlusion of Small Muscular Arteries and Arterioles by Organized Thrombi At autopsy, small thrombi, predominantly recent in origin, are commonplace in the small pulmonary vessels of patients with pulmonary hypertension who have developed heart failure preterminally. In contrast is the syndrome of widespread pulmonary vascular occlusion by organized thrombi in the small pulmonary arteries and arterioles. Once attributed to multiple pulmonary emboli, these lesions are now regarded as organized, in situ thrombi.[12] The syndrome is rare and indistinguishable during life from primary pulmonary hypertension except by lung biopsy. Histologic identification of these lesions serves little purpose in management. After a ventilation-perfusion scan has excluded chronic proximal thromboembolism (see below), treatment consists of long-term anticoagulation to prevent further clotting using warfarin or related agents, antiplatelet agents, or both.

Occlusion of Intermediate Pulmonary Arteries by Emboli This syndrome is by far the most common of the three.[12] It is thought to be caused by multiple emboli released from vessels in the upper legs and thighs that progressively amputate the pulmonary arterial tree. Ventilation-perfusion scans and selective angiography demonstrate the pulmonary vascular occlusion, although both studies tend to underestimate the degree of obstruction compared with direct inspection of the vascular tree at surgery or postmortem (see Chap. 53). The major therapeutic concern in these patients is to exclude chronic proximal pulmonary thromboembolism (see below) and to prevent recurrent thromboemboli. Treatment involves the use of anticoagulants of the warfarin type and antiplatelet agents.

Chronic Proximal Pulmonary Thromboembolism In some patients who have survived large to massive pulmonary emboli, resolution fails to occur, and the clots become organized and incorporated into the walls of the major pulmonary arteries,

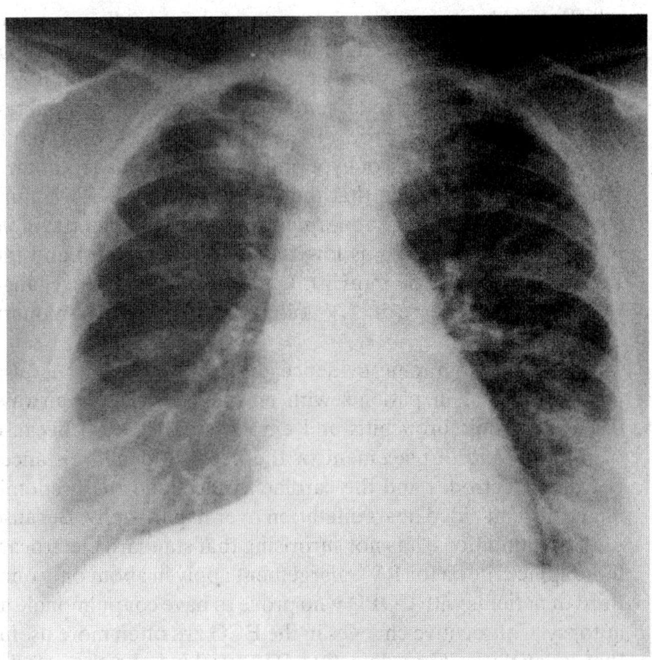

A

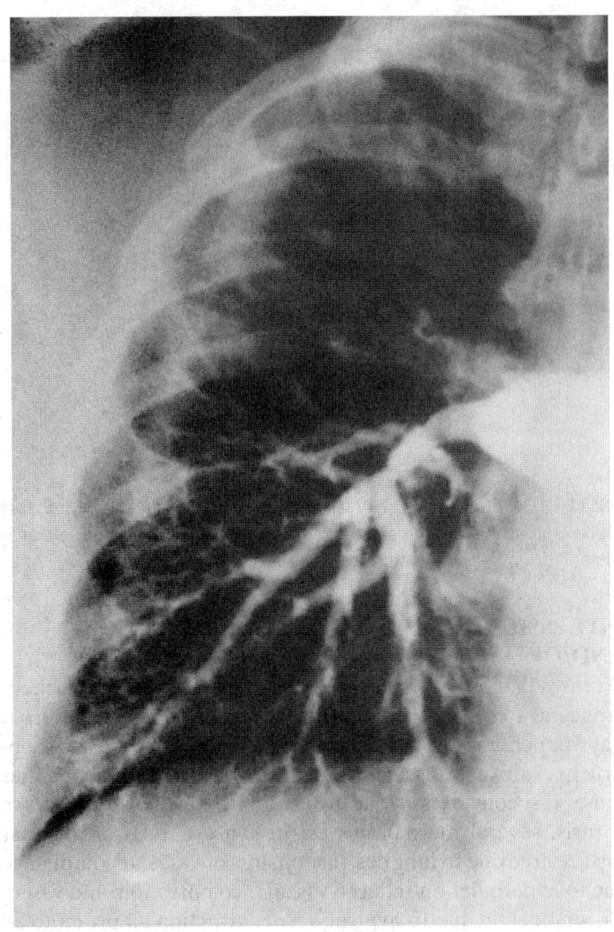

B

FIGURE 52-2 Pulmonary hypertension due to organized clot in central pulmonary arteries. Dramatic relief after pulmonary thromboendarterectomy. *A*. Chest radiograph. The right upper lobe is strikingly hypoperfused, and the vasculature on the left is quite prominent, reflecting redirection of the pulmonary blood flow to open vessels. *B*. Angiogram. The flow to the right upper lung is interrupted by the large central clot.

leading to pulmonary hypertension (Fig. 52-2). Overwhelming the capacity of the local fibrinolytic mechanisms also allows the clot to propagate, to obstruct large segments of the pulmonary vascular bed, and to decrease the compliance of the central pulmonary vessels. By the time the diagnosis is made, the obstructing lesions in the central pulmonary arteries have become an integral part of the vascular wall through the processes of endothelialization and recanalization.[12]

The importance of recognizing *proximal* pulmonary thromboembolism as a cause of pulmonary hypertension is the possibility of relieving the pulmonary hypertension by surgical intervention, i.e., by pulmonary thromboendarterectomy. Ventilation-perfusion lung scanning is the critical diagnostic test. As a rule, patients with proximal pulmonary thromboembolism show two or more segmental perfusion defects. If the perfusion defects are segmental or larger, selective pulmonary angiography is called for to define the location, extent, and number of pulmonary vascular occlusions.[13,14] Cardiac catheterization for selective pulmonary angiography also enables hemodynamic assessment. Fiberoptic angioscopy, helical computed tomographic scanning, and magnetic resonance imaging may be helpful in defining the lesions of proximal thromboembolic pulmonary hypertension[15] (see also Chap. 53).

Surgery is advocated for patients with pulmonary hypertension who have persistent clot in lobar or more proximal pulmonary arteries after at least 6 months of anticoagulation. Thromboendarterectomy is done via a median sternotomy using deep hypothermic cardiopulmonary bypass with intermittent periods of circulatory arrest. Postoperatively, hemodynamic improvement is usually quite dramatic.[8,14] Reperfusion pulmonary edema can be a severe complication immediately after the obstruction has been relieved. In experienced hands, mortality is on the order of 5 percent. After the operation, patients are placed on lifelong anticoagulants. A filter is usually placed in the inferior vena cava to further prevent recurrence.

Respiratory Diseases and Disorders

In addition to intrinsic pulmonary diseases, disturbances in respiratory muscle function or in the control of breathing also can lead to pulmonary hypertension. Among the intrinsic lung diseases are those affecting the airways (e.g., chronic bronchitis) as well as those affecting the parenchyma (i.e., emphysema, pulmonary fibrosis). Among the ventilatory disorders are the syndromes of alveolar hypoventilation due to respiratory muscle weakness and sleep-disordered breathing.

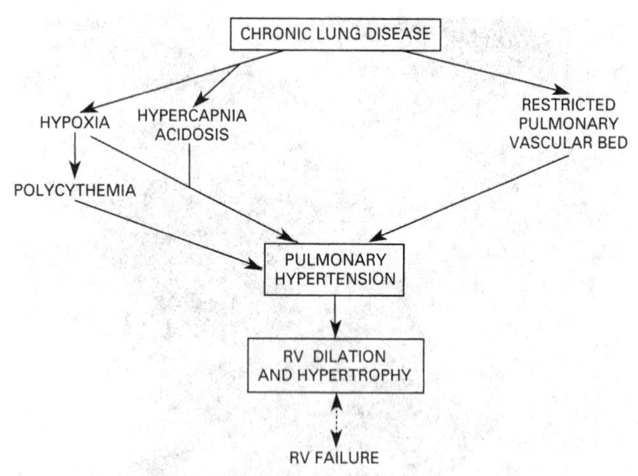

FIGURE 52-3 The evolution of RV failure in chronic obstructive airways disease (chronic bronchitis and emphysema; COPD). The factors on the left arise primarily from the bronchitis; those on the right from emphysema.

INTRINSIC DISEASES OF THE LUNGS AND/OR AIRWAYS

Diseases that affect the parenchyma of the lungs or the tracheobronchial tree can elicit pulmonary hypertension in different ways depending on the underlying disease (Fig. 52-3). In obstructive airways disease, ventilation-perfusion abnormalities cause vasoconstriction due to arterial hypoxemia. In diffuse fibrosis, several mechanisms act in concert: Loss of vascular surface area due to lung destruction, loss of vascular compliance due to hyperinflation-induced vascular compression, and vascular remodeling due to hypoxic vasoconstriction all promote an increased pulmonary vascular resistance.

INTERSTITIAL FIBROSIS

Pulmonary sarcoidosis, asbestosis, and idiopathic and radiation-induced fibrosis are common causes of widespread pulmonary fibrosis that culminates in cor pulmonale. Dyspnea and tachypnea generally dominate the clinical picture of interstitial fibrosis; cough is rarely prominent. As a rule, severe pulmonary hypertension occurs toward the end of the illness, when hypoxemia and hypercapnia are present at rest (see Fig. 52-1). RV failure is a common sequel.

Systemically administered vasodilators have no proven place in dealing with the pulmonary hypertension associated with interstitial fibrosis and may worsen intrapulmonary gas exchange. Recent experience with inhaled vasodilators, such as the prostacyclin analogue iloprost, is encouraging and suggests the possibility of producing selective pulmonary vasodilator and/or antiproliferative effects in this population.[16] Oxygen therapy, particularly during daily activity or sleep, can be important in attenuating the hypoxic pulmonary pressor response. Glucocorticoids and other potent immunosuppressive agents are the mainstay of therapy and often effect some symptomatic relief. The advent of lung transplantation has widened greatly the therapeutic horizons for dealing with widespread interstitial fibrosis.

CHRONIC OBSTRUCTIVE AIRWAYS DISEASE

Chronic bronchitis and emphysema [chronic obstructive pulmonary disease (COPD)] are the most common causes of cor pulmonale in patients with intrinsic pulmonary disease.[17,18] Cystic fibrosis is an example of a mixed airways and parenchymal lung disease in which pulmonary hypertension plays a significant role in outcome.

Cor pulmonale is encountered in two different settings: *acutely* in the setting of decompensation, which is often due to an acute respiratory infection, and *chronically* when progressive lung disease and worsening gas exchange lead to unremitting vascular remodeling.

The "gold standard" for diagnosing pulmonary hypertension in patients with COPD is right-sided heart catheterization. Noninvasive studies, such as echocardiography, have proved useful in some centers.[19,20] RV enlargement, the cardinal sign of pulmonary hypertension, can be difficult to discern in obstructive airways disease because of hyperinflation and cardiac rotation.[21] Once suspicion is raised that the clinical picture of RV failure stems from gas exchange abnormalities, an arterial blood sample will confirm that the P_{O_2} is low ($P_{O_2} < 40$–50 mmHg) and the P_{CO_2} is high ($P_{CO_2} > 50$ mmHg). Derangement in gas exchange to this degree is rare in LV failure unless overt pulmonary edema is present.

Electrocardiographic evidence of RV hypertrophy is also often equivocal in patients with chronic obstructive airways disease (chronic bronchitis and emphysema, COPD) because of rotation and displacement of the heart, widened distances between electrodes and the cardiac surface, and the predominance of right-sided heart dilatation over hypertrophy. Because of these limitations, it is not surprising that standard electrocardiographic criteria for RV enlargement apply in about only one-third of patients with COPD who prove to have cor pulmonale at autopsy. Consecutive changes in the ECG are often more useful than a single ECG in detecting RV overload. As the arterial P_{O_2} drops to abnormal levels (e.g., <60–70 mmHg while awake), T waves tend to become inverted, biphasic, or flat in the right precordial leads (V_1 to V_3); the mean electrical axis of the QRS shifts 30° or more to the right of the patient's usual axis; ST segments become depressed in leads II, III, and aV_F; and right bundle-branch block (incomplete or complete) often appears. These changes tend to reverse as arterial oxygenation improves (see also Chap. 11).

In the patient with COPD with acute cor pulmonale precipitated by a bout of bronchitis or pneumonia, the goal of therapy is to maintain tolerable levels of arterial oxygenation while waiting for the upper respiratory infection to subside. Supplemental oxygen, such as 28% oxygen delivered by a Venturi mask, generally suffices to relieve arterial hypoxemia and to restore pulmonary arterial pressures to normal. Considerable improvement also may be accomplished even in the individual who has chronic pulmonary hypertension by sustained (>18 h/day) breathing of oxygen-enriched air.

Once the right ventricle has failed, inotropic agents should be used cautiously because of the threat of arrhythmias posed by arterial hypoxemia and respiratory acidosis. Moreover, after adequate oxygenation has been achieved, the need for digitalis and diuretics often decreases because the hemodynamic burden on the right ventricle decreases. Even though acute cor pulmonale is largely reversible, each bout appears to leave behind a slightly higher level of pulmonary hypertension after recovery.[17]

Arterial blood gas composition is the therapeutic compass to the control of pulmonary hypertension in COPD. The degree of hypoxia may be underestimated by blood sampling while the patient is awake and at rest, since hypoxemia is more marked during sleep and with physical activity. Determinations of the oxygen saturation during sleep or with ambulation using pulse oximetry are helpful in optimally prescribing supplemental oxygen.

Ensuring the return of arterial oxygenation toward normal is much more vital than is the administration of inotropic agents.[22] When respiratory infection has triggered the episode of pulmonary hypertension, a vital strategy for achieving a lasting improvement in arterial oxygenation is the administration of an appropriate antibiotic. While awaiting the salutary effects of antibiotic therapy, attention is paid to hydration, to postural drainage, and to adequate alveolar ventilation.

Phlebotomy, once popular because of the prospect that increased blood viscosity contributes importantly to the pulmonary hypertension, has fallen into disuse. Polycythemia is rarely severe enough to be a serious problem in cor pulmonale associated with bronchitis and emphysema, and when its is present, it is usually indicative of inadequate relief of hypoxemia with optimal use of supplemental oxygen.

Vasodilators recently have been tried in various types of secondary pulmonary hypertension, including that due to COPD.[23] The agents tried are the same as those outlined for *primary* pulmonary hypertension. They run the risk of aggravating arterial hypoxemia by exaggerating ventilation-perfusion abnormalities. Unfortunately, the efficacy of vasodilator agents in secondary pulmonary hypertension has proved to be far less impressive or predictable than in primary pulmonary hypertension. To date, the safest and most effective approach to pulmonary vasodilatation in obstructive lung disease with arterial hypoxemia is the use of supplemental oxygen.[23]

CONNECTIVE TISSUE DISEASES

Pulmonary vascular disease is an important component of certain connective tissue diseases. Among these, the more common are systemic lupus erythematosus (SLE), the scleroderma spectrum of diseases, and dermatomyositis.[24] The lesions may take the form of interstitial inflammation and fibrosis, obliterative disease, or vasculitis, either singly or in combination. Although pulmonary hypertension can complicate many connective tissue diseases, it has been documented most often in SLE and progressive systemic sclerosis (scleroderma) and its variant syndromes. The possibility has been raised that primary pulmonary hypertension is an inflammatory, or autoimmune, disease. This prospect has gained support from the occasional instances in which the lesions are confined to the pulmonary arterial tree without interstitial involvement and similarities in the histologic appearance of the vascular lesions. The high frequency of both collagen-vascular disease and primary pulmonary hypertension in women and the occurrence of Raynaud's phenomenon in up to 20 percent of patients with primary pulmonary hypertension has been used as additional evidence.[25] Finally, there is a high incidence of positive serologic tests for antibodies (ANA, anti-Ku), particularly in women with primary pulmonary hypertension. With respect to the pathogenesis of the two disorders, the idea has been raised that both the Raynaud's phenomenon and an increase in pulmonary vascular tone represent a widespread vasoconstrictive pulmonary-systemic disorder. However, this hypothesis has not gained universal support.

The lungs and pleura are frequently involved in SLE, with a reported frequency of up to 70 percent. Patients with pulmonary hypertension and SLE are predominantly women; most of these patients also exhibit Raynaud's phenomenon.

The histopathologic lesions in these patients resemble those of primary pulmonary hypertension. Pulmonary hypertension in these patients may originate in microthrombi secondary to the hypercoagulable state caused by lupus anticoagulant or anticardiolipin antibodies in the blood. Less likely is the hypothesis of generalized vasoconstriction noted earlier. Unfortunately, treatment of pulmonary hypertension associated with SLE using either anticoagulants or pulmonary vasodilators has had only modest success. This poor outcome contrasts with the results obtained in patients with active pulmonary vasculitis, who may either improve or stabilize their vascular disease with immunosuppressive agents.

In progressive systemic sclerosis (scleroderma) and its variants, such as the CREST syndrome (*c*alcinosis, *R*aynaud's syndrome, *e*sophageal involvement, *s*clerodactyly, and *t*elangiectasia) and in overlap syndromes (e.g., mixed connective tissue disease), the incidence of pulmonary vascular disease is high. In these patients, pulmonary hypertension is the cause of considerable morbidity and mortality. In a prospective study involving cardiac catheterization of patients with progressive systemic sclerosis or the CREST syndrome variant, pulmonary hypertension, either as an isolated finding or in association with pulmonary parenchymal or cardiac disease, was found in up to one-third of patients with progressive systemic sclerosis and in up to one-half of patients with the CREST syndrome.[26] The pulmonary vascular disease may be independent of pulmonary or other visceral disease. As in the case of SLE, the pathology of these lesions is often indistinguishable from that of primary pulmonary hypertension. Vasodilator therapy has not proved to be highly effective; however, continuous intravenous epoprostenol recently has been shown to improve hemodynamics and exercise tolerance.[27]

ALVEOLAR HYPOVENTILATION IN PATIENTS WITH NORMAL LUNGS

In patients who hypoventilate despite normal lungs (alveolar hypoventilation), the primary pathogenetic mechanism is alveolar hypoxia potentiated by respiratory acidosis.[28] These abnormal alveolar and arterial blood gases play the same role in eliciting pulmonary hypertension in patients with alveolar hypoventilation as in those in whom the abnormal alveolar and blood gases are the result of ventilation-perfusion abnormalities. In individuals with normal lungs, the alveolar hypoventilation generally originates from an inadequate ventilatory drive (e.g., after encephalitis), covert obstruction of the upper airways (e.g., in the sleep apnea syndromes), an ineffective chest bellows (e.g., after poliomyelitis or polymyositis), or lungs entrapped by neoplasm or fibrosis (e.g., in trapped lung caused by asbestosis).

Regardless of etiology, whether pulmonary hypertension will occur in patients with alveolar hypoventilation and normal lungs depends on the whether there is sufficient alveolar and arterial hypoxia to raise pulmonary arterial pressures considerably. In the sleep apnea syndromes, severe arterial hypoxemia and pulmonary hypertension that develop initially only during sleep may become self-perpetuating and carry over into wakefulness, although this only occurs in those with severe disturbances in respiration during sleep.[29]

For the patient with alveolar hypoventilation with combined respiratory and cardiac (right ventricular) failure, the highest therapeutic priority is to improve oxygenation. Assisted ventilation, particularly during sleep, may be particularly helpful in improving oxygenation and reducing hypercapnia (e.g., continuous positive airway pressure) breathing. Pharmacologic therapy is rarely needed for patients with alveolar hypoventilation because of the efficiency of assisted ventilation coupled with oxygen therapy in promoting pulmonary vasodilatation.

PRIMARY (UNEXPLAINED) PULMONARY HYPERTENSION

Definition

PPH is a disorder intrinsic to the pulmonary vascular bed that is characterized by sustained elevations in pulmonary artery pressure and vascular resistance that generally lead to RV failure and death.[25] The diagnosis of PPH requires the exclusion on clinical grounds of other conditions that can result in pulmonary artery hypertension[30] (see Table 52-3). PPH is a rare disease, with an incidence of 1 to 2 per million.[31] Its prevalence is about 0.1 to 0.2 percent of all patients who come to autopsy.

The clinical diagnosis of PPH rests on three different types of evidence: (1) clinical, radiographic, and electrocardiographic manifestations of pulmonary hypertension, (2) hemodynamic features consisting of abnormally high pulmonary arterial pressures and pulmonary vascular resistance in association with normal left-sided filling pressures and a normal or low cardiac output, and (3) exclusion of the causes of secondary pulmonary hypertension.

SPECIAL TYPES

Certain associations of PPH have attracted interest because of their prospects for shedding light on some etiologies. These include so-called anorexigen-induced pulmonary hypertension, familial pulmonary hypertension, human immunodeficiency virus (HIV) infection–associated pulmonary hypertension, and portal-pulmonary hypertension.[30–33] In each of these, the clinical findings and the histologic appearance of the lungs at autopsy are identical to those which characterize the sporadic form of PPH. This diversity in associations underscores the likelihood that so-called PPH is the final common expression of heterogeneous etiologies.

General Features

After puberty, females predominate, those between 10 and 40 years of age being most often affected. Before puberty, no sex difference is discernible. The textbook picture of a patient with PPH is that of a young woman in the prime of life who develops one or more of the symptoms in Table 52-1 without discernible cause. Sex and age are sometimes useful in distinguishing clinically between the likelihood of PPH and pulmonary thromboembolic disease. The latter generally favors men, particularly in their later years.[25]

As a rule, median survival of patients can be predicted on the basis of the New York Heart Association functional classification: 6 months for class IV, 2½ years for class III, and 6 years for classes I and II. Unless interrupted by sudden death, which occurs in approximately 15 percent of patients, the usual downhill course terminates in intractable RV failure.[34]

Etiology

The common denominator in the pathogenesis of PPH appears to be injury to the layers of the vascular wall of the small muscular pulmonary arteries and arterioles.[35] In response to injury, the intima of these vessels proliferates so that the endothelium changes from a single flat layer to a piled-up projection that narrows the caliber of the vascular lumen. Along with intimal proliferation, the media of the affected vessels hypertrophy.[36]

The primary site of injury in PPH remains uncertain. Recent studies have implicated an intrinsic defect in ion channel function and calcium homeostasis in vascular smooth muscle,[37] whereas others have shown that endothelial function is disturbed, leading to altered production or handling of a variety of endothelial-derived vasoactive substances.[35] These abnormalities, coupled with altered platelet-endothelial interactions that predispose to intravascular thrombosis, lead to an inexorable course of enhanced vascular reactivity, proliferation and remodeling, and progressive obliterative vasculopathy. Diverse etiologies seem to be capable of eliciting PPH[38] (Table 52-4). For example, ingestion of the anorexigens fenfluramine and its isomer dexfenfluramine has been demonstrated to markedly increase the risk of PPH,[31] ingestion of toxic oil elicited an outbreak of pulmonary hypertension in Spain,[39] and HIV infection, even in the absence of the acquired immune deficiency syndrome, also has been implicated.[32]

For a long while, virtually all reports of PPH dealt with sporadic cases. An epidemic in Europe between 1967 and 1970 that was linked to the use of Aminorex, an anorectic agent, raised the prospect of hereditary predisposition, since only 1 in 1000 who took the drug developed pulmonary hypertension. More recently, the fenfluramines have been associated with both severe pulmonary hypertension and valvular heart disease.[31,40] The recent toxic oil epidemic in Spain has reinforced

TABLE 52-4 Suggested Mechanisms for Primary Pulmonary Hypertension

Proposed Mechanism	Evidence
Early/sustained vasoconstriction kinetics	Altered smooth muscle cell calcium Endothelial dysfunction
Genetic predisposition identified	Familial disease with gene locus ?Susceptibility with exposures, e.g., anorexigens, HIV, portal hypertension
Pulmonary thrombosis/embolism arteries/arterioles	Widespread occlusion of ?Altered endothelial-platelet interaction
Autoimmune disease	Raynaud's phenomenon and antinuclear antibodies common, female gender predilection

the concept of individual susceptibility to pulmonary vasotoxic agents.[39]

In recent years, an increasing number of patients have been identified in whom PPH is genetically linked.[41] In these individuals, the hereditary pattern is that of autosomal dominance with incomplete penetrance. The locus of the familial gene recently has been localized to the long arm of chromosome 2.[42] One major insight provided by the families with PPH is the diversity of pulmonary vascular lesions in members of the same family.[41]

Pathology

The evolution of PPH depends on progressive attenuation of the pulmonary arterial tree, which gradually increases pulmonary vascular resistance to the point of eliciting RV strain and failure. The seat of the disease is in the small pulmonary arteries (between 40 and 100 mm in diameter) and arterioles. The obliterative lesions can affect one or more layers of these vessels. In some instances, medial hypertrophy predominates; in others, it is the intima that proliferates. In addition, evidence of inflammation also may be present[36] (Fig. 52-4).

Histologic examination of the lung identifies a constellation of pulmonary precapillary lesions that are consistent with the clinical diagnosis of PPH, i.e., plexiform lesions, angiomatoid lesions, concentric intimal fibrosis, and necrotizing arteritis. The pathologist is often hard-pressed to distinguish between organized clots in small vessels that initiate the pulmonary hypertension and those which result from the obliterative pulmonary vascular disease. Recent clots in small pulmonary arteries and arterioles are common at autopsy in patients with PPH, particularly when the right ventricle has failed and cardiac output falls. Although similar clots may not have initiated the pulmonary hypertension process in PPH, it seems reasonable that more often they are complicating features that aggravate and exaggerate pulmonary vascular obstruction.

Pathophysiology

The hemodynamic hallmarks of PPH in the resting patient were indicated earlier: a combination of a high pulmonary arterial pressure, a normal or low cardiac output, and a normal left atrial (pulmonary wedge) pressure. As a result of this hemodynamic pattern, calculated pulmonary vascular resistance is high, generally leading to the logical conclusion that the resistance vessels, i.e., the small muscular arteries and arterioles, are the predominant sites of vascular obstruction. During exercise, as cardiac output increases, pulmonary arterial pressures increase further; the increments in pressure in the pulmonary hypertensive circuit are much more striking than in the normotensive pulmonary circulation owing to the inability to dilate existing vasculature or recruit unused vessels to accommodate the rise in pulmonary blood flow.

Pulmonary vasodilators are currently administered acutely for testing the responsiveness of the pulmonary circulation.[30] Among these, inhaled NO and intravenous prostacyclin have become the "gold standards." Several clinical and hemodynamic changes are sought as desirable end points: (1) improvement in exercise tolerance and in the quality of life; the increase in physical capacity, attributable to an increase in cardiac output, in turn improves oxygen delivery to peripheral organs and tissues; (2) a decrease in the level of pulmonary arterial hypertension, with evidence of regression of RV hypertrophy or dilatation, or both; (3) a decrease in calculated pulmonary vascular resistance; optimally, this decrease should entail an increase in cardiac output (with minimal increase in heart rate) accompanied by a decrease in pulmonary arterial pressure; and (4) since pulmonary vasodilators are also systemic vasodilators, pulmonary vasodilatation has to be effected without evoking undue systemic hypotension and tachycardia.

The combination of right-sided heart catheterization and vasodilator testing is particularly useful not only for defining the hemodynamic state of the patient but also in providing a hemodynamic baseline for future invasive and noninvasive studies, such as serial echocardiograms.

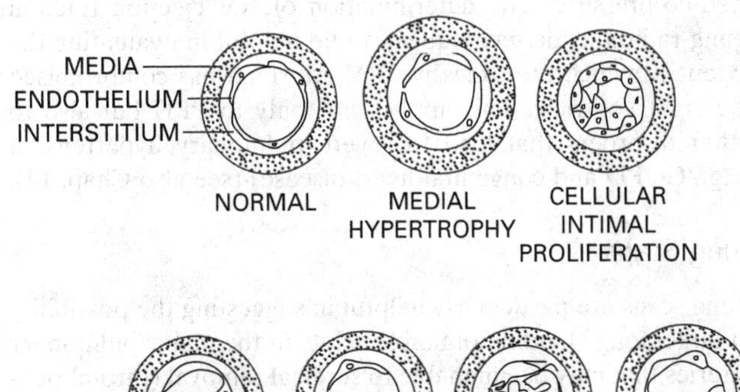

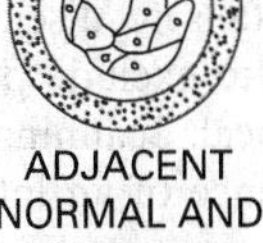

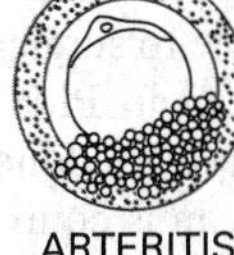

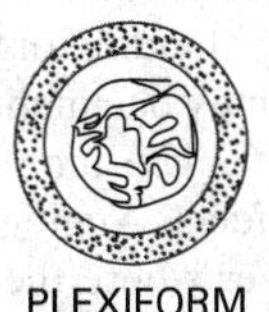

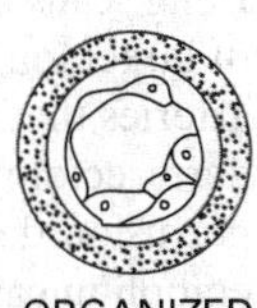

FIGURE 52-4 Vascular lesions in primary pulmonary hypertension. The plexiform lesion, once believed to be the histologic hallmark of primary pulmonary hypertension, has emerged as only one feature of a constellation of lesions.

Clinical Picture

In its early stages, the disease is difficult to recognize. In the sporadic case, the first clue is often an abnormal chest radiograph (see Fig. 52-1) or ECG indicative of RV hypertrophy (Fig. 52-5). Both are late manifestations. The existence of RV enlargement is generally confirmed by echocardiography. By the time these changes appear, however, pulmonary hypertension is moderate to severe. Initial complaints, particularly easy fatigability and dyspnea, tend to be discounted, i.e., attributed to being "out of shape," except when the index of suspicion is high, e.g., with a history of ingestion of anorectic agents or of familial pulmonary hypertension (see Table 52-1).

When the disease is advanced, the activities of daily life are progressively circumscribed by increasing nonspecific discomfort. Dyspnea, particularly during physical activity, becomes incapacitating. Some patients develop an angina type of chest pain along with breathlessness. Other common symptoms are weakness, fatigue, and exertional or postexertional syncope (see Table 52-1). Infrequently, an enlarged pulmonary artery causes hoarseness because of compression of the left recurrent laryngeal nerve. In time, right-sided heart failure develops.

Patients with severe pulmonary hypertension seem prone to sudden death. Death has occurred unexpectedly during normal activities, cardiac catheterization, and surgical procedures and after the administration of barbiturates or anesthetic agents.

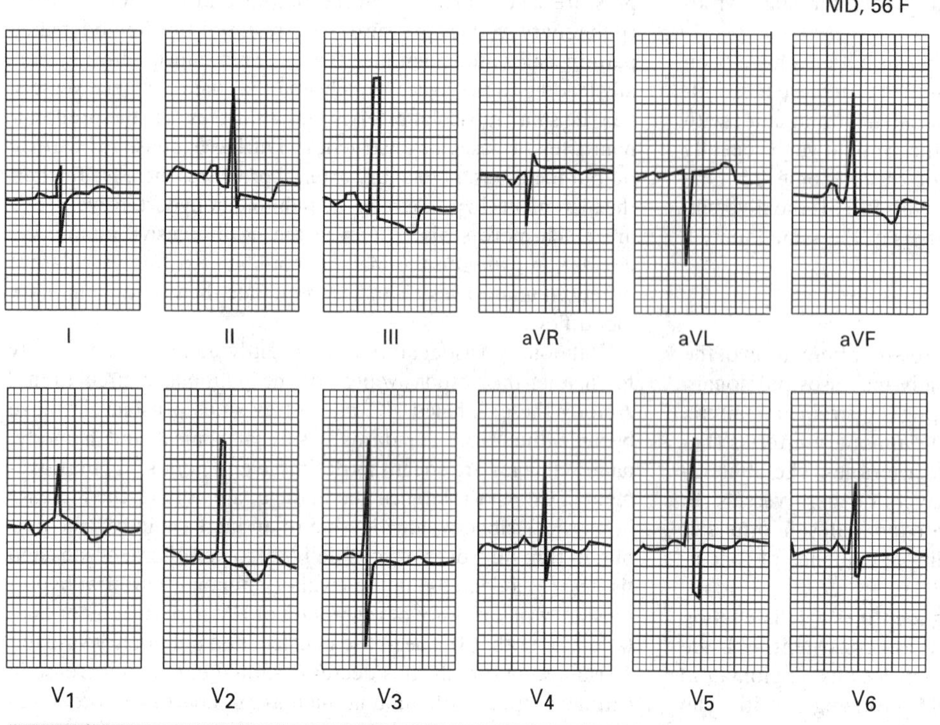

FIGURE 52-5 ECGs in patients with primary pulmonary hypertension and cor pulmonale.

The mechanisms for sudden death are not clear and may include arrhythmias or acute pulmonary thromboembolism. In a few instances, severe bradycardia and atrioventricular (AV) dissociation have preceded cardiac arrest.

It was noted earlier that as far as clinical manifestations and physical examination are concerned, PPH has an advantage over secondary pulmonary hypertension in that its manifestations are not obscured by those of underlying cardiac or respiratory disease. On physical examination, the jugular venous pulse usually shows a prominent *a* wave. RV hypertrophy causes a heave along the left sternal border, and a distinct systolic impulse is palpable over the region of the main pulmonary artery (see Chap. 10). The pulmonic component of the second sound is markedly accentuated, the second heart sound is narrowly split, and an ejection click is heard in the pulmonic area. Often a fourth heart sound emanating from the hypertrophied right ventricle is heard at the lower left sternal border. The murmur of tricuspid regurgitation is best heard along the sternal border with the patient in the supine position and can be accentuated with inspiration. In some patients, a midsystolic murmur is audible at the pulmonic area; as pulmonary arterial pressures approximate systemic arterial levels, the murmur of pulmonary valvular regurgitation often appears (see also Chap. 10).

The onset of RV failure is accompanied by jugular venous distention and a gallop (S_3); inspiration intensifies the gallop. The liver becomes enlarged and tender, and hepatojugular reflux can be elicited. Hydrothorax and ascites are seen as RV failure progresses.

Special Studies

Direct determination of pulmonary circulatory pressures by right-sided heart catheterization is the only way to definitively establish the diagnosis of pulmonary hypertension; however, other studies that are less direct can strongly suggest that it is present. Since the diagnosis of "primary" is one of exclusion, a number of tests are undertaken, usually in the hope of identifying a more treatable disease than PPH.[38]

CHEST RADIOGRAPHY AND ELECTROCARDIOGRAPHY

In the early stages, the chest radiograph is generally normal. Later it shows cardiac enlargement in association with enlargement of the pulmonary trunk, while the peripheral pulmonary arterial branches are attenuated; the lung fields appear oligemic (see Fig. 52-1). Although fullness of the central pulmonary arterial trunks and peripheral "pruning" are distinctive, appearances vary somewhat from patient to patient in accord with the level and pace of the pulmonary hypertension and the age of the patient. Radiographic evidence of RV enlargement usually becomes overt only late in the course of the pulmonary hypertension. The ECG almost always shows right axis deviation, RV hypertrophy, and, usually, right atrial enlargement (see Chap. 11).

THE ECHOCARDIOGRAM

Two-dimensional echocardiography confirms the enlargement and hypertrophy of the right atrium and ventricle, tricuspid regurgitation, and pulmonic valvular regurgitation. At the same time, LV structure and function are normal. The magnitude of the velocity of the tricuspid regurgitant jet using Doppler techniques can provide a noninvasive estimate of RV peak systolic pressure. The determination of RV ejection fraction using radionuclide techniques can be helpful in evaluating the extent to which the excessive RV afterload has compromised the right ventricle. This applies not only to PPH but also to other disorders that lead to severe pulmonary hypertension (e.g., COPD and congenital heart disease) (see also Chap. 14).

Lung Scans

Lung scans are particularly helpful in suggesting the possibility of large, long-standing organized clots in the major pulmonary arteries that may be amenable to surgical removal (thromboendarterectomy). The lung scan in PPH fails to disclose major perfusion defects. Angiography is done to exclude pulmonary emboli in cases where the scan is equivocal. Scanning over the brain or kidneys may disclose the presence of an intracardiac or intrapulmonary right-to-left shunt.

RIGHT-SIDED HEART CATHETERIZATION

Cardiac catheterization is invaluable in quantifying the hemodynamic abnormalities, in excluding cardiac causes of pulmonary arterial hypertension, and in assessing the hemodynamic responses of the heart and pulmonary circulation to vasodilator agents.[4]

Diagnosis

The diagnosis of PPH rests on two pillars: (1) the detection of pulmonary hypertension and (2) the exclusion of known causes of high pulmonary arterial pressure. The history is of utmost importance. Before categorizing pulmonary hypertension as "primary" or "unexplained," due regard must be paid to the exclusion of known etiologies (see Table 52-3), particularly thromboembolic disease and connective tissue disorders. Account also should be taken of the likelihood of familial disease. Pulmonary function tests are useful in excluding diffuse pulmonary disorders, particularly interstitial fibrosis and granuloma. Serologic testing can point the way to covert connective tissue disorders. Abnormal liver function tests can signal the coexistence of portal and pulmonary hypertension. The value of cardiac catheterization in eliminating acquired or congenital heart disease was indicated earlier. Unfortunately, by the time pulmonary hypertension complicating heart disease is recognized, the anatomic lesions often are too far advanced for the obliterative pulmonary vascular disease to be reversible. One notable exception is the dramatic improvement that often follows surgical removal of organized clots from the walls of major pulmonary arteries.

Treatment

For the past few decades, treatment of PPH has repeatedly turned to the use of vasodilators in the hope that an increase in pulmonary vascular tone contributed importantly to the high pulmonary arterial pressures. Although the bulk of the pulmonary vascular obstruction was clearly anatomic, vasodilators offered the prospect not only of decreasing pulmonary arterial pressures somewhat, and therefore the hemodynamic burden on the right ventricle, but also of prompting reversibility of the anatomic lesions, such as muscular hypertrophy, that resulted simply from the high pulmonary arterial pressures. Unfortunately, the use of vasodilators, which could affect the systemic as well as the pulmonary circulation and which often were accompanied by undesirable side effects, led to progressive disenchantment with one agent after another.

The situation has changed considerably during the past decade. The introduction of acute vasodilator testing for responsiveness helped to confirm the idea that in about one-third of patients, heightened pulmonary vasomotor tone helped to sustain the pulmonary hypertension. An optimal "responder" to acute testing manifested an increase in cardiac output along with a decrease in pulmonary arterial pressure and in pulmonary vascular resistance without affecting systemic arterial pressure unduly. Improvement in exercise tolerance accompanied the increase in cardiac output. Another landmark was the introduction of calcium channel blocking agents that could be taken orally, and in general, those who were highly responsive during acute testing could be maintained at lower pulmonary arterial pressures by these agents. A third insight was that even patients who failed to satisfy the criteria for a good hemodynamic response to acute vasodilator testing might respond to continuous infusion of epoprostenol. Indeed, a substantial number of such patients have been treated in this way for years, and even more have used continuous intravenous epoprostenol as a transition to transplantation of the lung or lungs or of heart and lungs. During this evolution, heart-lung and then lung transplantation became increasingly feasible and available, although the donor supply is still a limiting factor.

As a result of these advances, a patient with PPH has several therapeutic options, ranging from oral calcium channel blocking agents to continuous infusion of prostacyclin to lung transplantation. However, none of these modalities is free of complications. The oral calcium channel blocking agents generally have to be administered in large doses that are often accompanied by undesirable side effects.[43] The continuous infusion of a vasodilator, such as prostacyclin, runs the risks not only of a permanently placed intravenous catheter but also of drug-related side effects that can preclude dose increases.[44,45] Transplantation offers the substitution of immunosuppression and its attendant risk of infection as a better option than chronic cor pulmonale and RV failure.[46] Despite the limitations of each of these therapeutic modalities, together they provide a graduated therapeutic approach that has provided, at each stage, a better quality of life for many individuals with PPH. Moreover, they have prompted the search for agents that can be used in place of prostacyclin, which, until now, has required intravenous infusion; prostacyclin analogues that are delivered subcutaneously and by aerosol are currently under investigation. Other novel approaches include chronic ambulatory NO, which can be administered by inhalation.

VASODILATOR AGENTS

Various agents have been tried over the years as pulmonary vasodilators. These include α-adrenergic antagonists, β-adrenergic agonists, diazoxide, hydralazine, nitrates, and angiotensin-converting enzyme inhibitors. In general, these have not withstood the test of time. Experience has taught that untoward reactions can occur with any pulmonary vasodilator, even when low doses are used. Three categories of agents continue to hold promise, however: calcium channel blocking agents, arachidonic acid metabolites, and NO.

DRUGS THAT BLOCK CALCIUM TRANSPORT

The designation *calcium channel blocker* refers to a heterogeneous group of agents of different structural, pharmacologic, and electrophysiologic properties. The agents in this category currently receiving the most clinical attention as potential pulmonary vasodilators are nifedipine and diltiazem. Of the two, nifedipine is the more popular. Verapamil generally is not used because of its undesirable negative inotropic effect.

Nifedipine Note that this use is not listed in the manufacturer's directive. Nifedipine is a synthetic agent that is unrelated to other vasoactive or cardiotonic drugs. It is a potent systemic vasodilator that is used for the treatment of coronary vasospasm. Although it has significant direct negative inotropic effects, these are usually not prominent clinically because of the reflex sympathetic stimulation of the heart; it does not possess antiarrhythmic properties. It is now the preferred agent for therapy of patients who manifest acute vasoreactivity when tested with short-acting agents under hemodynamic monitoring.

Sustained-release preparations are used, with the dosage generally titrated to the maximal tolerable level based on avoiding untoward systemic effects, i.e., hypotension, headache, dizziness, and flushing. Considerable caution is necessary in administering the higher dosages, however, because side effects can occur precipitously and be life-threatening. In one study, 64 patients with PPH were treated acutely with high doses of calcium channel blockers. Seventeen patients responded to treatment with nifedipine (13 patients) or diltiazem (4 patients) and were alive after 5 years.[46]

In experienced centers, the trial of nifedipine or diltiazem orally is preceded by use of testing of acute vasoreactivity using one or more of three agents: (1) inhaled NO, in concentrations of 10 to 40 ppm for 5 to 10 min, (2) prostacyclin (PGI_2, Epoprostenol, Flolan), administered intravenously in increasing doses (starting dose of 1–2 ng/kg/min followed by successive increments every 15 min of 2 ng/kg/min until a maximal dose of 12 ng/kg/min is reached or until side effects preclude further increases), and (3) adenosine (50–200 ng/kg/min). Only patients who manifest significant reductions in pulmonary vascular resistance (usually >20–30 percent), resulting from a fall in pulmonary artery pressure without systemic hypotension and accompanied by an unchanged or increased cardiac output, are considered candidates for chronic therapy with oral calcium channel antagonists.

Arachidonic Acid Metabolites Epoprostenol (Flolan, prostacyclin, PGI_2), a metabolite of arachidonic acid, and its analogues continue to be a major focus of attention as treatments for a variety of forms of pulmonary hypertension. The pulmonary endothelium elaborates prostacyclin into the bloodstream, where it has a short biologic half-life, i.e., 2 to 3 min. In principle, it is attractive for the treatment of pulmonary hypertension on several accounts: (1) it is a pulmonary vasodilator, (2) it inhibits platelet aggregation, and (3) it inhibits proliferation of vascular smooth muscle. Unfortunately, it suffers the disadvantage of requiring continuous intravenous infusion, which is currently being done using portable pumps.[44,45] Analogues that can be given orally, subcutaneously, or by the inhaled route are under investigation. Success in long-term management recently has been reported using aerosolized iloprost, a stable prostacyclin analogue.[16,47] Currently, its most effective use is for long-term management in patients with severe (NYHA classes III or IV) primary pulmonary hypertension who are unresponsive to or are not candidates for therapy with calcium channel blockers.[44,45,48]

Nitric Oxide NO is synthesized in endothelial cells from one of the guanidine nitrogens of L-arginine by the enzyme NO synthase. It has proved to be the endothelial-derived relaxing factor that contributes to the low initial tone of the pulmonary circulation. It has the advantage of other vasodilators of selectively relaxing pulmonary vessels without affecting systemic arterial pressure. It is currently being used as a test of vasoreactivity in a wide variety of pulmonary hypertensive states including PPH and also has been used to control pulmonary hypertension in the syndrome of persistent pulmonary hypertension in the newborn.[49,50,51]

Anticoagulants Since 1984, when Fuster et al.[52] in a nonrandomized clinical trial showed that long-term survival was improved in patients with PPH by anticoagulant therapy (warfarin in low doses), the use of anticoagulants has been incorporated into the therapeutic regimen in patients with PPH. This practice is supported by the high incidence of antemortem clots found at autopsy in the small pulmonary arteries and arterioles of patients with PPH. Moreover, in a recent trial that separated "responders" from "nonresponders" to calcium channel blockers, survival was significantly better in those given warfarin than in those who were not anticoagulated.[43] The advent of RV failure increases the propensity for clotting in the pulmonary circulation. The usual goal of anticoagulation is to achieve and maintain an INR of 2 to 2.5.[53]

ATRIAL SEPTOSTOMY

Blade-balloon atrial septostomy has been performed in patients with severe RV pressure and volume overload refractory to maximal medical therapy.[54] The goal of this approach is to decompress the overloaded right heart and improve systemic output of the underfilled left ventricle. Improvements in exercise function and signs of severe right-sided heart dysfunction such as syncope and ascites have been observed. Since the creation of an interatrial communication will result in an increased venous admixture, worsening hypoxemia is an expected outcome. The size of the septostomy that is created should be monitored carefully to achieve the ideal balance of optimizing systemic oxygen transport and reducing right-sided heart filling pressures without overfilling a noncompliant left ventricle or producing extreme degrees of venous admixture.

LUNG TRANSPLANTATION

Only one-third of patients with PPH are responsive to long-term oral vasodilator therapy. Of the remainder, approximately 65 to 75 percent maintain sustained clinical improvement with long-term continuous intravenous therapy using prostacyclin. When pulmonary hypertensive disease has progressed, or threatens to progress, to the stage of RV failure, the physician and patient are left with few therapeutic options other than lung transplantation. Lung transplantation is currently being done at specialized centers and is almost invariably handicapped by a shortage of donor lungs, which can lead to long delays. Single- or double-lung transplantation has largely replaced heart-lung transplantation. Often, hemodynamic improvement is dramatic,[55] but transplantation for PPH poses not only a considerable surgical risk but also the prospect of opportunistic infections that accompanies lifelong immunosuppression.[56] Rejection phenomena, notably bronchiolitis obliterans, are the major limiting factor to prolonged survival. The median survival after lung transplantation is approximately 3 years.[46] Recurrence of PPH after transplantation has not been reported.

Prognosis

The diagnosis of PPH carries with it a poor prognosis unless medical or surgical therapy succeeds in decreasing pulmonary vascular resistance. Although death usually occurs within a few years after the onset of symptoms, instances of long-term survival do occur. Although sudden death accounts for 10 to 15 percent of all PPH-related deaths, the prognosis is largely determined by the severity of pulmonary hypertension and right-sided heart dysfunction.[34]

PULMONARY VENO-OCCLUSIVE DISEASE AND PULMONARY CAPILLARY HEMANGIOMATOSIS

These are the least common of all types of unexplained pulmonary hypertension. Not infrequently, the patient is thought to have primary pulmonary hypertension until manifestations inconsistent with pulmonary precapillary disease, such as pulmonary congestion and edema or severe hypoxemia, redirect attention to the vascular bed distal to the arterioles, i.e., the capillaries, pulmonary small veins, and venules. The pathogenetic mechanism of POVD is unknown but may begin as an inflammatory-thrombotic process in the small pulmonary veins and venules and ends in fibrous obliteration of the venous and venular lumens. Presumably as a secondary phenomenon, the distal pulmonary arterial tree also develops obstructive lesions that are generally proliferative ("reactive") rather than inflammatory in nature; the intervening capillary bed is generally normal. The pulmonary veno-occlusive lesions have been attributed to an inflammatory response to vascular injury, followed by thrombosis and scarring. Among the postulated etiologies (based on exceedingly sparse evidence) are viral illness, chemotherapy, toxins, autoimmune disease, and mediastinal fibrosis.[36]

Both POVD and capillary hemangiomatosis can be familial. When the pulmonary hypertension is suspected of originating distal to the pulmonary capillary bed, mitral valve disease, myocardial dysfunction, or even left atrial myxoma has a greater likelihood of being the cause than does POVD.

Clinical Picture

Predominantly children and young adults are affected, but the age has ranged from infancy to 48 years. Clinical suspicion of this disorder generally arises when a patient with congested and edematous lungs proves to have a normal mitral valve and left ventricle.

The cardinal signs are dyspnea and fatigue on exertion in conjunction with evidence of pulmonary hypertension; the pulmonary venous rather than pulmonary arterial etiology is suggested by radiologic evidence of postcapillary pulmonary hypertension without evidence of involvement of the left side of the heart (Fig. 52-6*A*). Pleural effusions are common. Cyanosis, syncope, hemoptysis, and finger clubbing have been inconsistent findings. Moderate to severe hypoxemia, due to intrapulmonary shunting through the abnormal capillary network, is a hallmark of capillary hemangiomatosis. Rarely, systemic embolization may occur.

Hemodynamics

Cardiac catheterization discloses a high pulmonary arterial pressure with a normal pulmonary wedge (and LV end-diastolic) pressure. The low wedge pressure has been attributed to discontinuities and channels of high resistance between the pulmonary capillaries and the pulmonary and bronchial venous channels so that wedging interrupts all sources of flow distal to the area blocked by the catheter.[30] When epoprostenol is administered to a patient with POVD, an acute pulmonary edema pattern may ensue, resulting from increasing pulmonary blood flow in the face of downstream vascular obstruction.[48,57] Although not universally present, this response is virtually diagnostic of POVD. Patients with capillary hemangiomatosis may experience worsening hypoxemia with epoprostenol, attributable to increased shunting through the low-resistance capillary meshwork.

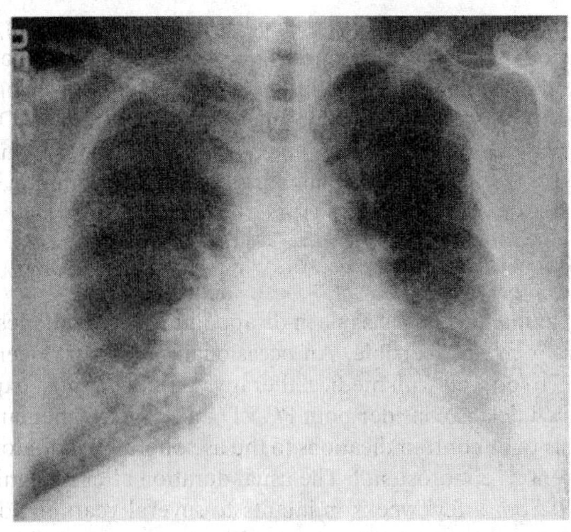
A

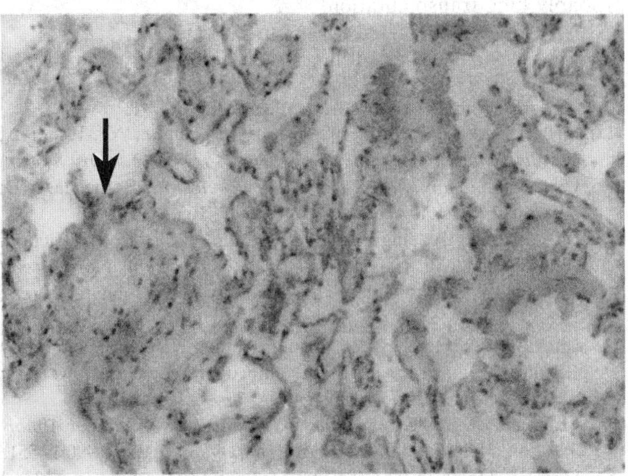
B

FIGURE 52-6 POVD proven by open lung biopsy. *A*. Chest radiography. Pulmonary interstitial edema is marked at both bases. *B*. Lung biopsy. In addition to obliterative pulmonary venular disease, the pulmonary arterioles (*arrow*) showed intimal proliferation and medical hypertrophy. (Courtesy of Dr. G. G. Pietra.)

Pathology

Few lung biopsies have been done during life. At autopsy, both lungs are involved. The lungs are the seat of congestion, edema, and focal fibrosis, which may become extensive. The venous lesions may be more marked in one region than in another. Although the small pulmonary arteries as well as the small pulmonary veins are affected, the lesions are different (see Fig. 52-6*B*). Most striking are the morphologic changes in the pulmonary veins and venules, which are narrowed or occluded by intimal proliferation and fibrosis; up to 95 percent of the veins and venules may be affected in this way, but complete occlusion is uncommon. Bronchial veins and bronchopulmonary anastomoses share in the occlusive process. Hypertrophy in the walls of the pulmonary arteries may be quite striking. POVD, to varying degrees, also may coexist with capillary hemangiomatosis. Thrombi in the pulmonary arteries are common.[36]

Treatment

Medical management has been disappointing, since the lesions generally are irreversible. An occasional patient has been reported to do well with medical therapy,[58] although most experienced clinicians consider both POVD and capillary hemangiomatosis to be contraindications to the use of oral vasodilators or intravenous epoprostenol. The usual duration after recognition ranges from a few weeks in infants to several years in adults, with 7 years being the maximum. The treatment of choice is probably lung transplantation.

References

1. Fishman AP. Pulmonary circulation. In: Fishman AP, Fisher A, eds. *The Handbook of Physiology*, Sec 3: *The Respiratory System*, vol I: *Circulation and Nonrespiratory Functions*. Bethesda, MD: American Physiological Society; 1985:93–165.
2. Fishman AP. The enigma of hypoxic pulmonary vasoconstriction. In: Fishman AP, ed. *The Pulmonary Circulation: Normal and Abnormal*. Philadelphia: University of Pennsylvania Press; 1990:109–130.
3. Eltorky MA, Headley AS, Winer-Muram H, et al. Pulmonary capillary hemangiomatosis: A clinicopathologic review. *Ann Thorac Surg* 1994; 57:772–776.
4. Fishman AP, ed. *The Pulmonary Circulation: Normal and Abnormal*. Philadelphia: University of Pennsylvania Press; 1990:1–551.
5. Harris P, Heath D. The structure of the normal pulmonary blood vessels after infancy. In: Harris P, Heath D, eds. *The Human Circulation: Its Form and Function in Health and Disease*. Edinburgh: Churchill-Livingstone; 1986:30–47.
6. Kinsella JP, Abman SH. Recent developments in the pathophysiology and treatment of persistent pulmonary hypertension of the newborn. *J Pediatr* 1995; 126:853–864.
7. Reid LM. Vascular remodeling. In: Fishman AP, ed. *The Pulmonary Circulation: Normal and Abnormal*. Philadelphia: University of Pennsylvania Press; 1990:259–282.
8. Moser KM, Auger WR, Fedullo PF. Chronic major vessel thromboembolic pulmonary hypertension. *Circulation* 1990; 81:1735–1743.
9. Beard JT II, Bryd BF III. Saline contrast enhancement of trivial Doppler tricuspid regurgitation signals for estimating pulmonary arterial pressure. *Am J Cardiol* 1988; 62:486–488.
10. Palevsky HI, Schloo BL, Pietra GG, et al. Primary pulmonary hypertension: Vascular structure, morphometry, and responsiveness to vasodilator agents. *Circulation* 1989; 80:1207–1221.
11. Edwards WD. The pathology of secondary pulmonary hypertension. In: Fishman AP, ed. *The Pulmonary Circulation: Normal and Abnormal*. Philadelphia: University of Pennsylvania Press; 1990:329–342.
12. Fedullo PF, Auger WR, Channick RN, et al. Chronic thromboembolic pulmonary hypertension. *Clin Chest Med* 1995; 16:353–374.
13. Ryan KL, Fedullo PF, Davis GB, et al. Perfusion scans underestimate the severity of angiographic and hemodynamic compromise in chronic thromboembolic pulmonary hypertension. *Chest* 1988; 93:1180–1185.
14. Jamieson SW, Auger WR, Fedullo PF, et al. Experience and results with 150 pulmonary thromboendarterectomy operations over a 29-month period. *J Thorac Cardiovasc Surg* 1993; 106:116–127.
15. Ricou F, Nicod PH, Moser KM, Peterson KL. Catheter-based intravascular ultrasound imaging of chronic thromboembolic pulmonary disease. *Am J Cardiol* 1991; 67:749–752.
16. Olschewski H, Ardeschir H, Walmrath D, et al. Inhaled prostacyclin and iloprost in severe pulmonary hypertension secondary to lung fibrosis. *Am J Respir Crit Care Med* 1999; 160:600–603.
17. Weitzenblum E, Oswald M, Mirhom R, et al. Evolution of pulmonary haemodynamics in COPD patients under long-term oxygen therapy. *Eur Respir J* 1989; 2(suppl 7):669S–673S.
18. Fishman AP. A century of primary pulmonary hypertension. In: Rubin LJ, Rich S, eds. *Primary Pulmonary Hypertension*. New York: Marcel Dekker; 1997:1–18.
19. Matthay RA, Shub C. Imaging techniques for assessing pulmonary artery hypertension and right ventricular performance with special reference to COPD. *J Thorac Imag* 1990; 5:47–67.
20. Tramarin R, Torbicki A, Marchandise B, et al. Doppler echocardiographic evaluation of pulmonary artery pressure in chronic obstructive pulmonary disease: A European multicentre study. *Eur Heart J* 1991; 12:103–111.
21. Maeda S, Katsura H, Chida K, et al. Lack of correlation between P pulmonale and right atrial overload in chronic obstructive airways disease. *Br Heart J* 1991; 65:132–136.
22. Weitzenblum E, Sautegeau A, Ehrhart M, et al. Long-term oxygen therapy can reverse the progression of pulmonary hypertension in patients with chronic obstructive pulmonary disease. *Am Rev Respir Dis* 1985; 131:493–498.
23. Brown G. Pharmacologic treatment of primary and secondary pulmonary hypertension. *Pharmacotherapy* 1991; 11:137–156.
24. Yousem SA. The pulmonary pathologic manifestations of the CREST syndrome. *Hum Pathol* 1990; 21:467–474.
25. Rich S, Dantzker DR, Ayres SM, et al. Primary pulmonary hypertension: A national prospective study. *Ann Intern Med* 1987; 107:216–223.
26. Shuck JW, Oetgen WJ, Tesar JT. Pulmonary vascular response during Raynaud's phenomenon in progressive systemic sclerosis. *Am J Med* 1985; 78:221–227.
27. Badesch D, Brundage B, Tapson V, et al. Continuous intravenous epoprostenol for pulmonary hypertension due to scleroderma: Spectrum of disease. *Ann Intern Med* 2000; 132:425–434.
28. Fishman AP. Pulmonary hypertension and cor pulmonale. In: Fishman AP, ed. *Pulmonary Diseases and Disorders*, 2d ed. New York: McGraw-Hill; 1988:999–1048.
29. Chaouat AE, Weitzenblum E, Krieger J, et al. Pulmonary hemodynamics in the obstructive sleep apnea syndrome: Results in 220 consecutive patients. *Chest* 1996; 109:380–386.
30. Rubin LJ. Primary pulmonary hypertension. *N Eng J Med* 1997; 336:111–117.
31. Abenhaim L, Moride Y, Brenot F, et al. Appetite-suppressant drugs and the risk of primary pulmonary hypertension. *N Engl J Med* 1996; 335:609–616.
32. Speich R, Jenni R, Opravil M, et al. Primary pulmonary hypertension in HIV infection. *Chest* 1991; 100:1268–1271.
33. Kuo PC, Plotkin JS, Rubin LJ. Distinctive clinical features of portopulmonary hypertension. *Chest* 1997; 112:980–986.
34. D'Alonzo GE, Barst RJ, Ayres SM, et al. Survival in patients with primary pulmonary hypertension. *Ann Intern Med* 1991; 115:343–349.
35. Voelkel NF, Tuder RM, Weir EK. Pathophysiology of primary pulmonary hypertension: In Rubin LJ, Rich S, eds. *Primary Pulmonary Hypertension*. New York: Marcel Dekker; 1997:83–133.
36. Pietra G. Pathology of primary pulmonary hypertension. In: Rubin LJ, Rich S, eds. *Primary Pulmonary Hypertension*. New York: Marcel Dekker, 1997:19–62.
37. Yuan JXJ, Aldinger AM, Juhaszova M, et al. Dysfunctional voltage-gated K^+ channels in pulmonary artery smooth muscle cells

of patients with primary pulmonary hypertension. *Circulation* 1998; 98:1400–1406.
38. Gaine SP, Rubin LJ. Primary pulmonary hypertension. *Lancet* 1998; 353:719–725.
39. Lopez-Sendon J, Sanchez MAG, De Juan MJM, Coma-Canella I. Pulmonary hypertension in the toxic oil syndrome. In: Fishman AP, ed. *The Pulmonary Circulation: Normal and Abnormal*. Philadelphia: University of Pennsylvania Press; 1990:385–396.
40. Connolly HD, Crary JL, McGoon MD, et al. Valvular heart disease associated with fenfluramine-phentermine. *N Engl J Med* 1997; 337:581–588.
41. Loyd J, Newman J. Familial primary pulmonary hypertension: Clinical patterns. *Am Rev Respir Dis* 1984; 129:194–197.
42. Nichols W, Koller D, Slovis B, et al. Localization of the gene for familial primary pulmonary hypertension to chromosome 2q31-32. *Nature Gen* 1997; 15:277–280.
43. Rich S, Kaufmann E, Levy PS. The effect of high doses of calcium-channel blockers on survival in primary pulmonary hypertension. *N Engl J Med* 1992; 327:76–81.
44. Barst RJ, Rubin LJ, McGoon MD, et al. Survival in primary pulmonary hypertension with long-term continuous intravenous prostacyclin. *Ann Intern Med* 1994; 121:409–415.
45. Rubin LJ, Mendoza J, Hood M, et al. Treatment of primary pulmonary hypertension with continuous intravenous prostacyclin (epoprostenol). *Ann Intern Med* 1991; 112:485–591.
46. Arcasoy SM, Kohoff RM. Lung transplantation. *N Engl J Med* 1999; 340:1081–1091.
47. Olschewski H, Walmrath D, Schermuly R, et al. Aerosolized prostacyclin and iloprost in severe pulmonary hypertension. *Ann Intern Med* 1996; 124:820–824.
48. Barst RJ, Rubin LJ, Long WA, et al. A comparison of continuous intravenous epoprostenol (prostacyclin) with conventional therapy for primary pulmnary hypertension. *N Engl J Med* 1996; 334:296–302.
49. Sitbon O, Brenot F, Denjean A, et al. Inhalednitric oxide as a screening vasodilator agent in primary pulmonary hypertension: A dose-response study and comparison with prostacyclin. *Am J Respir Crit Care Med* 1995; 151:384–389.
50. Lunn RJ. Inhaled nitric oxide therapy. *Mayo Clin Proc* 1995; 70:247–255.
51. Pepke-Zaba J, Higenbottam T, Dinh-Xuan AT, et al. Inhaled nitric oxide as a cause of selective pulmonary vasodilation in pulmonary hypertension. *Lancet* 1991; 338:1173–1174.
52. Fuster V, Steele PM, Edwards WD, et al. Primary pulmonary hypertension: Natural history and the importance of thrombosis. *Circulation* 1984; 70:580–585.
53. Medical management. In: Rubin LJ, Rich S, eds. *Primary Pulmonary Hypertension*. New York: Marcel Dekker; 1996:271–286.
54. Kerstein D, Levy PS, Hsu DT, et al. Blade balloon atrial septostomy in patients with severe primary pulmonary hypertension. *Circulation* 1995; 91:2028–2035.
55. Pasque MK, Kaiser LR, Dresler CM, et al. Single lung transplantation for pulmonary hypertension. *J Thorac Cardiovasc Surg* 1992; 103:475–481.
56. Katayama Y, Cremona G, Wallwork J, Higenbottam T. Transplantation for primary pulmonary hypertension. In: Rubin LJ, Rich S, eds. *Primary Pulmonary Hypertension*. New York: Marcel Dekker; 1996:287–304.
57. Davis LL, deBoisblanc BP, Glynn CE, et al. Effect of prostacyclin on microvascular pressures in a patient with pulmonary veno-occlusive disease. *Chest* 1995; 108:1754–1756.
58. Palevsky HI, Pietra GG, Fishman AP. Pulmonary veno-occlusive disease and its response to vasodilator agents. *Am Rev Respir Dis* 1990; 142:426–429.

C H A P T E R 53

PULMONARY EMBOLISM

Victor F. Tapson

Approximately 100,000 patients in the United States die each year directly due to acute pulmonary embolism (PE), with another 100,000 deaths occurring in patients with concomitant disease in whom PE contributes significantly to the demise of the patient.[1,2] A substantial number of patients die from PE prior to being diagnosed. Many of these deaths appear to be preventable. Autopsy studies have repeatedly documented the high frequency with which PE has gone unsuspected and undetected.[3] Despite advances in diagnostic technology and therapeutic approaches, PE remains underdiagnosed and prophylaxis continues to be dramatically underutilized. Pulmonary embolism nearly always results from deep venous thrombosis (DVT) of the proximal deep veins of the legs, that is, including the popliteal veins, and their vicinity, although axillary and subclavian vein thrombi may also embolize. Venous thromboembolism (VTE) represents the clinical spectrum of DVT and PE and occurs extraordinarily commonly in hospitalized patients, particularly after major surgery.

Because DVT and PE are so commonly clinically unsuspected, considerable diagnostic and therapeutic delays result and substantial morbidity and mortality are the ultimate consequence. The risk factors for DVT are discussed below, followed by the pathophysiology of acute PE. Because of the potential overlap with regard to the diagnostic approach to suspected DVT and PE, these are discussed in the same section. The principles of management of DVT and PE are addressed. Finally, the less common entity of chronic thromboembolic pulmonary hypertension is reviewed.

ACUTE DEEP VENOUS THROMBOSIS: RISK FACTORS AND PATHOGENESIS

Virchow proposed that the pathogenesis of DVT was based upon several potential initiating events, including stasis, venous injury, and hypercoagulability. Risk factors for DVT are based upon these processes (Table 53-1). Thrombosis may develop within the lumen of any vein as well as in the right side of the heart. Extensive investigation has been undertaken of the veins of the lower extremities, since most significant PE originate from this location. Although thrombi may form at any point along the vein wall, most originate in valve pockets. The veins of the calf are the most common site of origin, with subsequent extension of the clot prior to embolization.[4] If the clot does propagate, it usually remains attached at its base and floats in the vein more proximally. Eventually, it may expand to fill the vessel entirely, with both retrograde and further proximal extension. If embolization does not occur, the thrombosis can partially or completely resolve via three mechanisms, which include recanalization, organization, and lysis. Fatal PE is the most feared complication of DVT. Chronic thrombophlebitis with recurrent pain and swelling can be incapacitating. Fre-

TABLE 53-1 Risk Factors for Venous Thromboembolism

- Acquired factors
  - Age greater than 40
  - Prior history of venous thromboembolism
  - Prior major surgical procedure
  - Trauma
  - Hip fracture
  - Immobilization/paralysis
  - Venous stasis
  - Varicose veins
  - Congestive heart failure
  - Myocardial infarction
  - Obesity
  - Pregnancy/postpartum period
  - Oral contraceptive therapy
  - Cerebrovascular accident
  - Malignancy
  - Severe thrombocythemia
  - Paroxysmal nocturnal hemoglobinuria
  - Antiphospholipid antibody syndrome (including lupus anticoagulant)
- Inherited factors
  - Antithrombin III deficiency
  - Factor V Leiden (activated protein C resistance)
  - Prothrombin gene (G20210A) defect
  - Protein C deficiency
  - Protein S deficiency
  - Dysfibrinogenemia
  - Disorders of plasminogen
  - Hyperhomocysteinemia

quently more than one risk factor for venous thrombosis is present and knowledge of these risk factors provides the rationale for both prophylaxis and clinical suspicion.

Acquired Risk Factors

Most venous thrombi arise in venous valves, where blood flow tends to stagnate. The increased frequency of thrombosis with advanced age and immobilization further emphasizes the importance of stasis in thrombogenesis. Immobility, regardless of the cause, discourages venous return and contributes to stasis. Acute paraplegia significantly increases the risk of DVT (particularly in the paralyzed limb), and the period of highest risk appears to be the first 2 weeks after the onset of the paralysis.[5] Prolonged bed rest or long automobile or airplane trips may be the only obvious risk factors in patients developing thromboemboli. Obesity also appears to increase the risk of VTE. Information extrapolated from the Prospective Investigation of Pulmonary Embolism Diagnosis (PIOPED) suggests that the relationship of obesity and VTE are not entirely understood and that further clarification would be useful.[6] Although obesity is commonly believed to be a significant risk, it is likely that immobility and stasis are contributing factors. Age appears to increase mortality due to PE,[7] and it appears that PE is suspected less commonly prior to death in the elderly patient.[8] The risk of VTE is particularly high in those of the elderly with concomitant cardiac disease or cancer.

Antecedent pulmonary thromboembolism forecasts an appreciable risk of recurrence in the hospitalized patient. Surgical patients with a previous history of VTE who do not receive prophylaxis develop postoperative DVT in more than 50 percent of cases.[9] Surgery itself significantly enhances the risk. Even surgery patients without significant additional risk factors develop venography-proven DVT in nearly 20 percent of cases if neither pharmacologic nor mechanical prophylaxis is applied.[10] Prophylactic anticoagulation is initiated either prior to surgery or shortly thereafter to prevent the development of intraoperative and early postoperative thrombosis. Total hip and total knee replacement patients not receiving prophylaxis develop DVT in more than 50 percent of cases.[11] These orthopedic settings have been comprehensively investigated, prompted by the increasing use of low-molecular-weight heparin (LMWH). Spinal or pelvic surgery place patients at particularly high risk for VTE.

Trauma, particularly of the lower extremities and pelvis, heightens the risk of DVT. Pulmonary embolism has been identified at autopsy in as many as 60 percent of patients with lower extremity fractures,[12] and mortality has been attributed to PE in as many as 50 percent of patients dying after hip fracture.[13] The incidence of VTE increases with time after the traumatic event. Autopsy-confirmed PE in patients surviving for less than 24 h after trauma has been demonstrated in 3.3 percent, increasing to 5.5 percent in those surviving up to 7 days. Pulmonary emboli occurred in 18.6 percent of those surviving for a longer period.[14] Venous catheters (particularly in the jugular, subclavian, or femoral veins) traumatize veins as well as serving as potential nidi for thrombosis. Associated cancer or immobility is often present in these individuals. Symptomatic PE can originate from catheter-induced (or non-catheter-induced) upper extremity thrombi, although this appears much less commonly than when the leg or pelvic veins are the source. Upper extremity (axillary-subclavian) thrombosis may also occur due to the effort-induced syndrome described by Paget-Schroetter.[15]

Recent epidemiologic analyses as well as autopsy data suggest that patients with cardiac and malignant disease are particularly predisposed to VTE.[7,16] Although myocardial infarction without anticoagulation has been associated with a significant incidence of DVT, more recent therapeutic strategies have had a beneficial impact.[17] Several of the large, multicenter, placebo-controlled acute myocardial infarction trials have indicated that the use of thrombolytic therapy has reduced the incidence of VTE.[18,19]

Malignancies clearly augment the risk of VTE, although the precise pathogenesis of thromboembolism in cancer is not well understood.[16] It is clear, however, that numerous mechanisms—including intrinsic tumor procoagulant activity and extrinsic factors such as chemotherapeutic agents and indwelling access catheters—contribute to this process. The thrombophilic tendency associated with cancer is often amplified by weakness and reduced ambulation with venous stasis. A recent analysis, based upon data from the PIOPED trial, revealed that of 399 patients with PE, 73 (18.3 percent) had cancer.[7] Pancreatic, lung, gastric, genitourinary tract, and breast malignancies are associated with a particularly high risk of DVT and PE. It appears that about half of all cancer patients and about 90 percent of those with metastases exhibit abnormalities of one or more coagulation parameter. The most common abnormalities include elevation of clotting factor levels (fibrinogen, factors

V, VIII, IX, and XI), fibrinogen and fibrin degradation products, and thrombocytosis.[16]

Most tumor cells produce both tissue factor and cancer procoagulant.[16,20] Tissue factor appears to be the primary coagulant factor implicated in promoting fibrin deposition and is expressed in situ as well as in isolated cells of numerous cancers.[21] Tumor cell expression of tissue factor also promotes metastatic dissemination.[21] Cancer procoagulant is a cysteine protease that activates factor X. Mucin, a glycoprotein produced by certain tumors, possesses a sialic acid moiety that may nonenzymatically cleave factor X to Xa. Plasminogen activator inhibitor type 1 (PAI-1) is secreted by numerous tumor cells and inhibits plasmin generation, augmenting the thrombophilic state as well as possibly also promoting tumor metastasis dissemination.[21] Other procoagulant properties of tumor cells include expression of cytokines such as IL-1β and tumor necrosis factor alpha (TNF-α), which, in turn, regulate expression of procoagulants and mediate interactions between tumor cells, platelets, leukocytes, and endothelial cells. Thrombin, certain cytokines, and growth factors such as vascular endothelial growth factor (VEGF) can stimulate endothelial cells to synthesize tissue factor, further potentiating a procoagulant surface and leading to fibrin deposition on vessel walls. Activated protein C inhibitor may contribute to a prothrombotic state, as it can inhibit both fibrinolysis and the protein C anticoagulant pathway.[21]

Chemotherapy, with resulting neutropenia and sepsis, often necessitates hospitalization and bed rest, which contributes further to the high risk of VTE. Following the administration of various chemotherapeutic agents, changes in the levels of coagulation factors, suppression of anticoagulant and fibrinolytic activity, and direct endothelial damage have been documented clinically and experimentally.[22] Hormonal therapy, particularly tamoxifen in breast cancer adjuvant therapy, is also associated with an increased risk of thromboembolism, particularly when combined with chemotherapy. The thrombophilic state induced by chemotherapeutic agents has recently been reviewed.[22] Further comprehensive research will more clearly elucidate the mechanisms underlying thrombophilia in cancer patients. In spite of the clear association, there is no convincing evidence that an aggressive search for cancer is warranted in patients presenting with apparently idiopathic DVT.[23]

Pregnancy and the postpartum period are the most common settings in which women under age 40 acquire thromboembolic disease. Venous thrombosis develops in these settings five times more often than in age-matched women not on oral contraceptives.[24] Although DVT appears to be more common in the third-trimester and postpartum than prior to delivery, the risk is clearly considerable throughout pregnancy.[24] Cesarean section further augments the risk. Oral contraceptives are associated with the development of VTE, although the precise risk has been controversial.[25] The risk increases with third-generation agents (agents containing desogestrel or gestodene as the progestogen component).[26,27] Results from a clinical trial evaluating hormonal replacement therapy indicated that such therapy increased the incidence of VTE in women 45 to 64 years of age. A yearly total of 16.5 cases of VTE per 100,000 women may be attributed to hormonal replacement therapy.[28] The risk of VTE also appears to be highest during the first year of exposure to hormonal replacement.[29] It has not been clearly established that previous use increases the risk.[30] Although such therapy is associated with obvious benefits, physicians must consider other potential risk factors for VTE before prescribing hormonal replacement therapy.

Other disease states and clinical settings enhance the risk of VTE. Most intensive care unit patients can be considered at risk for VTE because of their multiple risk factors, including significant underlying disease, immobility, and venous injury due to trauma or central venous catheters. These patients should receive some form of DVT prophylaxis and a high index of suspicion for VTE should be maintained in appropriate clinical circumstances.

Inherited Risk Factors

Inherited thrombophilias result in variable degrees of VTE risk. Individuals with, for example, antithrombin III or factor V Leiden deficiency without significant superimposed risk factors such as surgery or immobilization often do not suffer from VTE until an additional risk factor develops. The factor V Leiden mutation is a common genetic polymorphism associated with activated protein C resistance and appears to be present in approximately 4 to 6 percent of the general population.[31] The relative risk of a first idiopathic venous thrombosis among men heterozygous for the mutation has been shown to be three- to sevenfold higher than that of those not affected.[31] Another thrombophilic mutation has been identified in the 3′ untranslated region of the prothrombin gene (substitution of A for G at position 20210), and this mutant allele is present in 2 percent of the general population.[32] This prothrombin gene defect increases the risk of DVT by a factor of 2.7 to 3.8.[32–33] It appears that carriers of both factor V Leiden and the prothrombin G20210A defect have an increased risk of recurrent DVT after a first episode and are candidates for lifelong anticoagulation.[34] There has been increasing interest in the potential role of homocysteine in VTE. In vitro, homocysteine has potentially thrombogenic effects, including injury to vascular endothelium and antagonism of the synthesis and function of nitric oxide.[35] Coexisting hyperhomocysteinemia has been shown to increase the risk for thrombosis in patients with factor V Leiden.[36] However, the thermolabile methylenetetrahydrofolate reductase gene variant is not independently associated with thrombosis, emphasizing that the precise role of homocysteine in venous thrombosis is unclear. Thus, interactions between the genetic factors (defects in enzymes) that control homocysteine metabolism and nutritional factors (folate, vitamin B_6, and vitamin B_{12} deficiencies) that affect homocysteine metabolism appear to warrant additional investigation with regard to VTE. It would appear certain that additional inherited thrombophilic disorders will be identified that may explain some of the "idiopathic" cases.

ACUTE PULMONARY EMBOLISM: PATHOPHYSIOLOGY

Gas-Exchange Abnormalities

The effect of PE on oxygenation and hemodynamics depends upon the extent of obstruction of the pulmonary vascular bed and the severity of underlying cardiopulmonary disease. Hypoxemia develops in the preponderance of patients with PE and has been attributed to various mechanisms. When no previous cardiopulmonary disease is present, lung regions with low ventilation/perfusion ratios and shunting due to perfusion of atelectatic areas appear to be the predominant mechanisms of hypoxemia. Hypoxemia leads to an increase in sympathetic tone with systemic vasoconstriction and may actually increase venous return with augmentation of stroke volume, at least initially, if there is no significant underlying cardiac or pulmonary pathology already present.

Hemodynamic Alterations

Massive emboli can cause profound hemodynamic compromise. In the setting of massive emboli, cardiac output is diminished but may be initially sustained as the mean right atrial pressure increases. The increased pulmonary vascular resistance impedes right ventricular outflow with a reduction in left ventricular preload. When no underlying cardiopulmonary disease is present, occlusion of 25 to 30 percent of the vascular bed by emboli results in a rise in pulmonary artery pressure (PAP). As the extent of vascular obstruction increases, hypoxemia worsens, stimulating vasoconstriction and a further rise in PAP. Greater than 50 percent obstruction of the pulmonary arterial bed is generally present before there is substantial elevation of the mean pulmonary artery pressure. When the extent of embolic occlusion approaches 75 percent, the right ventricle must generate a systolic pressure in excess of 50 mmHg and a mean PAP of greater than 40 mmHg to preserve pulmonary perfusion.[37] Although a hypertrophied right ventricle (in an otherwise normal patient) may theoretically be capable of achieving pressures this high, a normal right ventricle is unable to and will fail.[37] In reality, individuals with significant underlying cardiopulmonary disease and superimposed PE are more inclined to develop a more profound deterioration in cardiac output than normal individuals with PE, whether or not right ventricular hypertrophy is present. Furthermore, a depressed cardiac output in the absence of an elevated right atrial pressure suggests that the PE is superimposed upon preexisting cardiac disease. Right ventricular failure develops more frequently in the setting of PE when the patient has underlying coronary artery disease.[38] Aggressive hemodynamic support may sustain some patients with massive embolism at least temporarily, even when the right ventricle is dilated and hypocontractile, but any further increment in embolic burden may be fatal.

DIAGNOSIS OF DEEP VENOUS THROMBOSIS AND PULMONARY EMBOLISM

Venous thromboembolism represents the spectrum of one disease. Most clinically significant PE arise from the prior development of DVT in the lower extremities, with subsequent embolization to the lungs. Patients may present with symptoms of either DVT, PE, or both. At the present time, the diagnostic strategy involves recognition of certain symptoms and signs of DVT and/or PE and usually involves an imaging study directed at either the legs or the lungs, depending upon the presentation. Ventilation/perfusion ($\dot{V}/\dot{Q}$) scanning has been the diagnostic cornerstone for patients with suspected PE for decades. However, the contrast-enhanced computed tomography (CT) scan is being used increasingly as experience and technology improve. The diagnostic approach to acute DVT and PE has recently been exhaustively reviewed and presented as clinical practice guidelines by the American Thoracic Society.[39]

Lower extremity ultrasound is the most common leg study utilized, and the $\dot{V}/\dot{Q}$ scan still appears to be the most frequently utilized lung imaging study. It is important to realize that an increasingly common diagnostic strategy in patients presenting with suspected PE but with a nondiagnostic lung imaging study is to perform a lower extremity study in hopes of proving that DVT is present.

History and Physical Examination

The clinical diagnosis of both DVT and PE, based upon the history and physical examination, are insensitive and nonspecific. Patients with lower extremity DVT may be asymptomatic or may have erythema, warmth, pain, swelling, and/or tenderness. These findings are not specific for DVT but suggest the need for further evaluation. The differential diagnosis of DVT includes cellulitis, edema from other causes, musculoskeletal pain, or trauma (some of these may be concomitant and may or may not be related). Pulmonary embolism must always be considered when unexplained dyspnea is present. Dyspnea as well as pleuritic chest pain and hemoptysis are common in PE but are nonspecific. Coughing may be present, and while sometimes caused by PE, it more commonly occurs with bronchitis or pneumonia. It is far less common than shortness of breath. Anxiety, light-headedness, and syncope are all symptoms that may be caused by PE but may also be due to a number of other entities that result in hypoxemia or hypotension. Tachypnea and tachycardia are the most common signs of PE but are also nonspecific. Syncope or sudden hypotension should suggest the possibility of massive PE. The cardiac and pulmonary physical examinations are both nonspecific. A pleural rub or accentuated pulmonic component of the second heart sound may suggest PE but can also be explained by other disorders. In spite of the limitations of the history and physical examination for DVT and PE, the index of clinical suspicion becomes a more useful parameter when considered in conjunction with additional studies and $\dot{V}/\dot{Q}$ scanning.[40] Dyspnea, tachypnea, clear lung fields, and hypoxemia may often be attributed to a flare of chronic obstructive disease or asthma when underlying PE is present. Thus, diagnostic efforts aimed at possible VTE should still be considered despite alternative explanations if risk factors and the clinical setting are suggestive.

Laboratory Testing

Routine laboratory testing is not useful in proving or refuting the presence of DVT or PE but may be helpful in confirming or excluding alternative or concomitant diagnoses. For example, leukocytosis and pulmonary infiltrates may suggest pneumonia, and worsening hypercapnia in a patient with known chronic obstructive lung disease may suggest a flare of the underlying lung disease. It is important to realize, however, that acute PE can develop in the setting of other cardiopulmonary disorders that do not exclude the possibility of concomitant PE.

D-DIMER TESTING

The D-dimer is a specific derivative of cross-linked fibrin. Measurement of circulating plasma D-dimer has been comprehensively evaluated as a diagnostic test for acute VTE, both independently and together with other diagnostic measures. A normal enzyme-linked immunosorbent assay (ELISA) appears to be sensitive in excluding PE. When the D-dimer level is 500 μg/L or greater, the sensitivity and specificity for PE have been shown to be 98 and 39 percent, respectively.[41] The sensitivity of the plasma D-dimer appears to remain high up to 1 week after presentation. In another prospective analysis, 96 percent of 79 patients with high-probability $\dot{V}/\dot{Q}$ scans had an elevated D-dimer concentration.[42] Thus, increased levels of cross-linked fibrin degradation products are an indirect but suggestive marker of intravascular thrombosis in addition to indicating fibrinolysis. Although the sensitivity of the D-dimer appears high, the specificity is not high enough to be diagnostic. Patients with both suspected and proven DVT and PE often have underlying disease states that also cause the D-dimer to be elevated.

When clinical studies comparing D-dimer with the results of other diagnostic tests for VTE are reviewed, there appear to be appreciable differences in assay performance, heterogeneity among the patient population, and inconsistent use of definitive diagnostic criteria for venous thromboembolism.[43,44] The number of available D-dimer assays, including rapid bedside assays, is increasing. It appears that results of clinical studies utilizing one manufacturer's D-dimer assay cannot be extrapolated to another study using another manufacturer's assay. No single assay has been established as superior to all the others. The ELISA assays are sensitive but cannot be performed rapidly. The latex tests, while rapid, have not been proven to be sufficiently sensitive. A rapid, quantitative, immunoturbidimetric technique has been evaluated that recognizes the D-dimer epitope by using antibody-coated latex particles.[45] In at least one study, the degree of abnormality of this D-dimer test appeared to correlate with the extent of the DVT, with proximal thrombosis producing higher D-dimer levels.[45] In addition, patients presenting immediately after the onset of symptoms were found to have higher D-dimer levels than patients examined after a few days. Thus, certain quantitative D-dimer tests may prove to offer additional information regarding the acuity and extent of thromboembolic disease. Future studies of D-dimer techniques should be rigorous with regard to the definitive presence or absence of DVT and/or PE as well as addressing issues such as duration of symptoms, presence of comorbid disease, and extent of thrombosis.

Recently, both DVT and PE management studies have been performed, with therapeutic decisions based, to some extent, upon D-dimer results. When a bedside whole-blood agglutination D-dimer assay and impedance plethysmography were both negative in patients with suspected DVT and anticoagulation was withheld, the negative predictive value was 98.5 percent (95 percent confidence interval, 96.3–99.6) based upon 3 months of follow-up.[46] For the D-dimer test alone, the negative predictive value was 97.2 percent. A diagnostic protocol including an assessment of clinical probability, $\dot{V}/\dot{Q}$ scan, ELISA plasma D-dimer, and lower extremity ultrasound (US) was utilized in 308 consecutive patients presenting to the emergency room with suspected PE.[47] Of these patients, 106 (34 percent) had diagnostic $\dot{V}/\dot{Q}$ scans (high probability in 63 and normal in 43). The noninvasive evaluation was diagnostic in 125 patients (62 percent). In 48 patients, PE was ruled out by a nondiagnostic lung scan together with low clinical probability. In 53 cases, it was ruled out by a quantitative D-dimer of less than 500 μg/L. Only 77 of the 202 patients with nondiagnostic $\dot{V}/\dot{Q}$ scans required pulmonary angiography. At 6 months follow-up, only 2 of the 199 patients in whom the diagnostic protocol had ruled out PE had a VTE event. Using the same cutoff value for the quantitative D-dimer, these investigators subsequently reported that of 198 patients with suspected PE and a D-dimer <500 μg/L, 196 were free of PE, one had PE, and one was lost to follow-up.[48] Thus, the negative predictive value of the D-dimer was approximately 196 of 198 (99 percent). Although these data represent the work of only one group of investigators, they are promising. Rapid bedside assays are becoming more available and additional outcome studies will help to clarify their role. At present, plasma D-dimer measurements should be interpreted with caution and in the context of other diagnostic tests.

ARTERIAL BLOOD GAS ANALYSIS

Hypoxemia, while not universal, is extremely common in acute PE. Some patients, particularly young individuals without underlying cardiopulmonary disease may have a normal Pa_{O_2}. In a retrospective study of hospitalized patients with PE, the Pa_{O_2} was greater than 80 mmHg in 29 percent of patients less than 40 years old, compared with 3 percent in the older group.[49] However, the alveolar-arterial (A-a) difference was elevated in all patients. Thus, as age increases, it becomes even less likely that a patient with PE will have a normal room air Pa_{O_2}. In the PIOPED, a subset of patients suspected of PE without a history or evidence of underlying cardiac or pulmonary disease was evaluated, and the Pa_{O_2} and A-a difference values were compared.[50] Patients with and without PE could not be distinguished based upon either of these values. However, the A-a difference was elevated by more than 20 mmHg in 76 of 88 (86 percent) patients with PE. The diagnosis of acute PE cannot be excluded based upon a normal Pa_{O_2}, and although the A-a difference is usually elevated, it may very rarely be normal in patients without preexisting cardiopulmonary disease. An important tenet should be that unexplained hypoxemia, particularly in the setting of risk factors for DVT, should suggest the possibility of PE.

Electrocardiography

Electrocardiography (ECG) cannot be relied upon to rule in or rule out PE, though ECG proof of a clear alternative diagnosis, such as myocardial infarction, is useful when PE is among the possible diagnoses. The potential coexistence of PE together with another process must, however, be a consideration. ECG findings in acute PE are generally nonspecific and include T-wave changes, ST-segment abnormalities, and left- or right-axis deviation. The changes that do occur are likely caused by right ventricular dilation. The "classic" S1Q3T3 pattern described by McGinn and White[51] in 1935 in seven patients with acute cor pulmonale secondary to PE was subsequently demonstrated to be present in about 10 percent of PE cases.[52] In patients without underlying cardiac or pulmonary disease from the Urokinase Pulmonary Embolism Trial (UPET), electrocardiographic abnormalities were documented in 87 percent of patients with proven PE.[53] These findings were not specific for PE, however. In this clinical trial, 26 percent of patients with massive or submassive PE and 32 percent of those with massive PE had manifestations of acute cor pulmonale, such as the S1 Q3 T3 pattern, right bundle-branch block, P-wave pulmonale, or right axis deviation. Such changes are thus seen in a minority of patients. The low frequency of specific ECG changes associated with PE was confirmed in the PIOPED study.[50] It has been recently suggested that the anterior subepicardial ischemic pattern is the most frequent ECG sign of massive PE.[54]

Chest Radiography

The chest radiograph is abnormal in the majority of patients with PE, but the findings are nonspecific. Atelectasis, pulmonary infiltrates, pleural effusion, and mild elevation of a hemidiaphragm may be present.[50] Classic radiographic evidence of pulmonary infarction (Hampton's hump) or decreased vascularity (Westermark's sign) are suggestive but uncommon. A normal chest radiograph in the presence of significant dyspnea and hypoxemia without evidence of bronchospasm or anatomic cardiac shunt is strongly suggestive of PE. In most situations, however, the chest radiograph cannot be used to definitively diagnose or exclude PE. Although exclusion of other processes such as pneumonia, congestive heart failure, pneumothorax, or rib fracture (which may cause symptoms similar to acute PE) is important, PE often coexists with other underlying lung diseases.

Imaging Studies for Pulmonary Embolism

VENTILATION/PERFUSION SCANNING

Ventilation/perfusion scanning has been the pivotal diagnostic test for approaching suspected PE for many years. However, even in patients in whom PE is ultimately proven, the $\dot{V}/\dot{Q}$ scan is most commonly nondiagnostic. Certain $\dot{V}/\dot{Q}$ scan readings are of substantial utility, however. Normal and high-probability scans are considered diagnostic. A normal perfusion scan excludes the diagnosis of PE with enough certainty that further diagnostic testing is unnecessary. Matching areas of decreased ventilation and perfusion in the presence of a normal chest radiograph suggests a process other than PE. However, low- or intermediate-probability (nondiagnostic) scans are commonly found with PE, and particularly when clinical suspicion is high, additional testing is necessary. In the PIOPED study, the utility of $\dot{V}/\dot{Q}$ scanning combined with clinical assessment of patients with suspected PE was prospectively evaluated.[40] Patients with PE had scans that were of high, intermediate, or low probability, but so did most individuals without PE. Although the specificity of high-probability scans was 97 percent, the sensitivity was only 41 percent. Of interest, 33 percent of patients with intermediate-probability scans and 12 percent of patients with low-probability scans were diagnosed definitively with PE by pulmonary arteriography. When the clinical suspicion of PE was considered very high, the positive predictive value of high-probability scans for PE was 96 percent. More interestingly, in those with high clinical suspicion and intermediate- and low-probability scans, it was 66 and 40 percent, respectively. Thus, further diagnostic testing for PE should be performed even when the lung scan is of low or intermediate probability if the clinical setting suggests PE. Although the $\dot{V}/\dot{Q}$ scan may sometimes be diagnostic of PE or exclude the possibility with sufficient certainty, it is often nondiagnostic. The latter fact emphasizes the need to further improve our diagnostic resources.

PULMONARY ARTERIOGRAPHY

Pulmonary arteriography is the established "gold standard" diagnostic technique for the diagnosis of PE. It is a very sensitive and specific test. However, for smaller (subsegmental) emboli, it appears less accurate. Two referee readers from the PIOPED agreed on the presence or absence of subsegmental emboli in only 66 percent of cases.[55] In another study, using selective pulmonary arteriography, there was excellent agreement on main, lobar, and segmental emboli but only 13 percent agreement on subsegmental emboli.[56] The significance of such emboli is unclear, however, and may depend upon the presence of underlying cardiopulmonary disease, the extent of concurrent DVT, and the continued presence or absence of risk factors for DVT. Arteriography is safe in most instances. Complications related to this technique among 1111 patients suspected of PE in the PIOPED study included death in 0.5 percent and major nonfatal complications in 1 percent.[55] An increasingly utilized alternative to pulmonary arteriography is to perform lower extremity studies when the $\dot{V}/\dot{Q}$ scan is nondiagnostic; if DVT is discovered, the therapeutic approach is generally the same as if an arteriogram were positive for PE. If serial lower extremity testing is negative, the chances of significant PE or morbidity from a subsequent event appears unlikely.[57] However, the ease with which serial testing can be performed is variable, and arteriography is often the best alternative when the leg test is negative, since the sensitivity of ultrasound for DVT is substantially lower in patients with asymptomatic DVT. Lower extremity testing is being increasingly utilized in patients with nondiagnostic lung scans and in stable patients; this appears to be appropriate.[39] Pulmonary arteriography has also been performed at the bedside utilizing a Swan-Ganz catheter.[58] However, accurate interpretation of arteriography, particularly in the case of submassive emboli, is crucial.

ECHOCARDIOGRAPHY

Echocardiography is not usually used for approaching the patient with suspected PE, although it may suggest its presence in some clinical settings, and it has been suggested as a potential means by which to determine the need for thrombolytic therapy.[59] Echocardiography can often be performed more rapidly than either $\dot{V}/\dot{Q}$ scanning or pulmonary arteriography and may suggest hemodynamically significant PE.[60] Studies of patients with documented PE have revealed that more than 80 percent of patients have imaging or Doppler abnormalities of right-ventricular size or function that may suggest acute PE.[60,61] However, patients who are acutely ill with suspected PE often have underlying cardiac or pulmonary disorders such as chronic obstructive lung disease, and neither right-ventricular dilation nor hypokinesis can be reliably used even as indirect evidence of PE in these settings. Intravascular ultrasound imaging has been utilized in both the experimental and clinical setting to image large emboli.[62–64] This technique can be performed at the bedside. Although the technique may be less sensitive and specific and more time-consuming in the setting of smaller emboli, further investigation may be warranted.

COMPUTED TOMOGRAPHY

Contrast-enhanced spiral (helical) CT scanning has been increasingly investigated and utilized in patients with clinically suspected acute and chronic PE. This technique involves continuous movement of the patient through the scanner with concurrent scanning by a constantly rotating gantry and detector system.[65] A helix of projecting data is obtained. Continuous volume acquisitions can be obtained during a single breath, and with newer scanners, breath-holding may be less important. Rapid scans can be obtained, facilitating imaging in critically ill patients. Limitations of helical CT scanning in early clinical studies included poor visualization of horizontally oriented vessels in the right middle lobe and lingula because of volume averaging.[66] The peripheral areas of the upper and lower lobes may be inadequately scanned and the presence of intersegmental lymph nodes may result in false-positive studies. Multiplanar reconstructions in coronal, sagittal, or oblique planes aid in distinguishing lymph nodes from emboli (see also Chap. 17).

Computed tomography scanning may reveal emboli in the main, lobar or segmental pulmonary arteries with >90 percent sensitivity and specificity.[66–69] Accurate results have been reported for large PE.[70,71] However, for subsegmental emboli, the sensitivity and specificity appear to be lower. The incidence of isolated subsegmental emboli appears to be approximately 6 to 30 percent, with the former figure likely being more representative.[55,72] Of note, even with the gold standard diagnostic test (arteriography), two referee readers from the PIOPED agreed on the presence or absence of subsegmental emboli in only 66 percent of cases.[55] Another study, using selective pulmonary arteriography, indicated excellent agreement on main, lobar, and segmental emboli but only 13 percent agreement on subsegmental emboli.[56] Thus, this apparent limitation with spiral CT scanning is also a concern with angiography. The incorporation of CT scanning into diagnostic algorithms for PE is being endorsed increasingly.[73] However, no prospective multicenter randomized clinical trials large enough to unequivocally prove the sensitivity and specificity of contrast-enhanced CT scanning in patients with suspected PE have been performed. Most have been single-center trials of moderate size. The value of CT for large emboli appears clear, however.

Sensitivity and specificity data from several large studies evaluating helical CT scanning for acute PE are shown in Table 53-2. Contrast-enhanced electron-beam CT also appears useful in diagnosing acute PE.[69,74] In one comparison with pulmonary angiography, only 8 of 720 vascular zones (1.1 percent) were considered inadequately visualized with electron-beam CT. As with spiral CT, three-dimensional reconstruction techniques can be applied to the pulmonary vessels to better define vessels located within the plane that has been sectioned. Another important advantage of these CT techniques over the $\dot{V}/\dot{Q}$ scan is the concomitant ability to define nonvascular structures such as airway, parenchymal, and pleural abnormalities, lymphadenopathy, and cardiac and pericardial disease. Prospective randomized clinical trials comparing these techniques with the standard diagnostic approach to PE will help to determine their precise role. It appears that CT scanning is being increasingly utilized.

TABLE 53-2 Sensitivity and Specificity for Contrast-Enhanced CT Scanning for Acute Pulmonary Embolism

References	Number of Patients	Sensitivity (%)	Specificity (%)
Spiral CT			
Remy-Jardin[66]	72	90	86
Remy-Jardin[67]	42	100	96
Goodman[68]	20	86[a]	92[a]
		63[b]	89[b]
van Rossum[70]	124	97	98
van Rossum[71]	45	95	97
Sostman[77]	28	73	97
Electron-beam CT			
Teigen[69]	60	65	97
Teigen[74]	25	95	80

[a]Main, lobar and segmental emboli.
[b]All emboli including peripheral.

MAGNETIC RESONANCE IMAGING

Magnetic resonance imaging (MRI) is also being utilized to evaluate clinically suspected PE at some centers.[75,76] One clinical trial compared MRI with spiral CT: the average sensitivity of CT for five observers was 75 percent and of MRI 46 percent.[77] The average specificity of CT was 89 percent, compared with 90 percent for MRI. Sensitivity and specificity values for expert readers were higher, however. Spiral CT may be somewhat more useful than MRI for detecting PE at the present time, but MRI has several attractive advantages, including excellent sensitivity and specificity for the diagnosis of DVT. As in the case of CT scanning, the diagnosis of entities other than PE using MRI is a major advantage over the $\dot{V}/\dot{Q}$ scan.

Diagnostic algorithms for patients presenting with suspected DVT and PE have been recommended in the American Thoracic Society Consensus Statement and allow for a certain degree of flexibility with regard to specific diagnostic modalities utilized.[39]

Imaging Studies for Deep Venous Thrombosis

A number of diagnostic techniques can be utilized to evaluate the patient with suspected DVT. Compression US is the most common technique used in the United States and in many other areas of the world. Impedance plethysmography is used at some centers, and a number of important clinical trials have been performed utilizing this technique. MRI appears to have some important advantages, but it has not generally been used as a first-line test. Venography remains the gold standard, but has been necessary less often at many centers in view of the accuracy of US. Each diagnostic technique has advantages and limitations. Although diagnostic algorithms may be suggested for suspected DVT, these are institution-specific, depending upon resources and available expertise with certain techniques. Newer diagnostic testing modalities, such as scanning with technetium 99m–labeled glycopeptide IIb/IIIa receptor antagonists, appear promising but will not be discussed.[78]

CONTRAST VENOGRAPHY

Although contrast venography remains the gold standard for the diagnosis of DVT, it has been less commonly used since the advent of US. Venography should be performed whenever noninvasive testing is nondiagnostic or impossible to perform. It is an invasive procedure that may result in superficial phlebitis or hypersensitivity reactions, but it is generally safe and accurate.

IMPEDANCE PLETHYSMOGRAPHY

Impedance plethysmography has been carefully studied in patients presenting with suspected acute DVT. It has proven reliable for the detection of proximal DVT (including that occurring in and above the popliteal vein). Preliminary studies suggested greater than 90 percent sensitivity and 97 percent specificity for DVT involving the proximal lower extremity, although less than 30 percent of isolated calf vein thromboses were detected.[79,80] Although this modality is sometimes portable, it does require access to the calf and thigh for electrode and cuff placement. The specificity of IPG is affected by disorders that obstruct venous outflow, such as tumor or hematoma. Plaster casts or external fixation of extremities limits the utility of this technique. Some investigators have emphasized the potential limitations of IPG.[81] Among the limitations of the technique are its inability to detect asymptomatic/nonobstructive proximal DVT, or calf DVT and its lack of utility for diagnoses other than DVT.[39] It is used much less commonly than compression US.

ULTRASONOGRAPHY

Compression US with venous imaging is a portable, accurate, and widely available diagnostic technique for proximal lower extremity DVT. Combined with a Doppler reading, this technique is referred to as *duplex ultrasonography*. Ultrasound technology has been further sophisticated by the development of color duplex instrumentation that display Doppler frequency shifts as color superimposed on the gray-scale image. The color duplex images display both mean blood flow *velocity,* expressed as a change in hue or saturation, and *direction* of blood flow, displayed as red or blue. US imaging techniques can also identify or suggest the presence of pathology other than DVT—for example, Baker's cysts, hematomas, lymphadenopathy, arterial aneurysms, superficial thrombophlebitis, and abscesses may be suggested or diagnosed.[82] The sensitivity and specificity of US for symptomatic proximal DVT has been well above 90 percent in most recent clinical trials.[83,84] There are limitations, including insensitivity for asymptomatic DVT (less than 50 percent), operator dependence, the inability to accurately distinguish acute from chronic DVT in symptomatic patients, and insensitivity for calf vein thrombosis.[85–87] Compared with other technology, it is relatively inexpensive and is the preferred diagnostic modality for the straightforward case of symptomatic suspected proximal DVT.

MAGNETIC RESONANCE IMAGING

Magnetic resonance imaging (MRI) has clear advantages as a diagnostic test for suspected DVT and appears to be an accurate noninvasive alternative to venography.[88] A major feature of this technique is excellent resolution of the inferior vena cava and pelvic veins.[89,90] Preliminary experience with MRI suggests that it is at least as accurate as contrast venography or US imaging and more sensitive than US for pelvic vein thrombosis.[88–90] Simultaneous bilateral lower extremity imaging can be accomplished, and MRI appears to accurately distinguish acute from chronic DVT. This technique appears to be useful in distinguishing other entities such as cellulitis or a Baker's cyst from acute DVT. As with many other diagnostic techniques, its utility depends to a certain degree on the experience on the part of the reader. There is the additional advantage of evaluating a patient for the entire spectrum of VTE in one imaging session by scanning the legs and pelvis as well as the lungs. MRI is used by some medical centers when the initial diagnostic test (usually US) is nondiagnostic (see also Chap. 18).

PREVENTION OF DEEP VENOUS THROMBOSIS

Background

Prophylaxis for DVT is effective.[91] A substantial reduction in the incidence of DVT can be accomplished when individuals at risk receive appropriate preventive care, as such measures appear to be grossly underutilized. A review of the use of prophylaxis for DVT in 16 Massachusetts hospitals revealed that such therapy was administered to only 44 precent of high-risk patients in teaching hospitals and only 19 percent in nonteaching hospitals.[92] The frequency of prophylaxis ranged from 9 to 56 percent among hospitals. Another retrospective analysis revealed that only 97 of 250 patients (39 percent) at *very high risk* for DVT received any form of prophylaxis and that of these 97, only 64 (66 percent) received appropriate care.[93] Prophylaxis can be pharmacologic (anticoagulation) or nonpharmacologic. Low-molecular-weight heparin (LMWH) products have been increasingly utilized in clinical practice for both prevention and treatment of established VTE. Extensive literature is now available supporting the use of these preparations for DVT prevention. The LMWH preparations are advantageous in that they produce a more predictable dose response and are administered subcutaneously only once or twice daily (without monitoring) depending on the preparation (see "Management of Established Venous Thromboembolism," below).[94] Early ambulation whenever possible is always recommended in postoperative patients.

General Medical Patients

Patients are stratified according to DVT risk, and certain prophylactic measures are more appropriate for some patients than for others. Generally, low-dose anticoagulation with standard, unfractionated heparin or LMWH is indicated in medical or surgical patients deemed at risk for DVT. When standard heparin is used for prophylaxis in general medical patients, 5000 U delivered subcutaneously every 8 to 12 h is generally adequate. LMWHs have also been studied in general medical patients. In a large double-blind, randomized clinical study comparing two different doses of subcutaneous LMWH (enoxaparin) delivered once daily to acutely ill medical patients, the higher dose (40 mg) proved more effective than the lower dose (20 mg).[95] The incidence of DVT was 5.5 percent in the former group and 14.9 percent in the latter.

When prophylactic anticoagulation is contraindicated, mechanical devices (intermittent pneumatic compression) are utilized. Anticoagulation together with pneumatic compression is appropriate in patients deemed at exceptionally high risk or with multiple risk factors for DVT.

General Surgical Patients

In general surgery patients, a number of prophylactic strategies have been employed. An overview of the results of randomized trials in surgical patients demonstrated the substantial benefit of DVT prophylaxis.[91] In this review of more than 70 randomized trials involving 16,000 patients, it was demonstrated that perioperative use of subcutaneous heparin could prevent about half of all PE and about two-thirds of all DVT. In a large meta-analysis, the value of prophylaxis to reduce the incidence of DVT was confirmed; it was also suggested that intermittent pneumatic compression plus the use of gradient compression stockings may result in the lowest incidence of postoperative DVT.[96] Other combined treatments were associated with lower rates than heparin alone and appear appropriate in patients at exceptionally high risk. For those patients undergoing minor operations who are less than 40 years old and have no additional risk factors for DVT, no prophylaxis other than early ambulation is recommended. Older patients undergoing major operations without additional risk factors should receive either standard, unfractionated heparin, LMWH, or intermittent pneumatic compression. When additional risk factors are present in the latter group, standard heparin every 8 h or LMWH should be administered. Enoxaparin has been FDA-approved for prophylaxis in patients undergoing elective abdominal surgery (40 mg subcutaneously once daily). A second preparation, dalteparin, has also been approved in the United States for once-daily use as prophylaxis for elective abdominal surgery.

Other High-Risk Patients

Certain orthopedic populations at particularly high risk for acute DVT have been carefully studied with well-designed randomized clinical trials, which led to the approval of enoxaparin by the FDA for prophylaxis against DVT in patients undergoing elective total hip or knee replacement. The approved dosing regimens are 30 mg subcutaneously twice daily initiated within 12 to 24 h after surgery, and 40 mg once daily initiated preoperatively. The duration of prophylaxis depends upon whether the patient is ambulatory and upon additional risk factors. At least one large randomized, placebo-controlled clinical trial suggested a lower incidence of DVT with more prolonged (1 month) outpatient prophylaxis in this patient population.[97] LMWHs have also been evaluated in trauma patients at risk for DVT and have proven efficacious in this patient population.[98] Intermittent pneumatic compression should be utilized if anticoagulation prophylaxis is contraindicated.

A number of LMWH preparations are currently being investigated. It is important to realize that these preparations are not identical and the results of clinical trials with one agent cannot be extrapolated to another. Detailed recommendations for DVT prophylaxis are published and updated every 2 to 3 years (American College of Chest Physicians Consensus).[99]

MANAGEMENT OF ESTABLISHED VENOUS THROMBOEMBOLISM

Assuring adequate oxygenation and hemodynamic support for PE is of paramount importance. Such supportive measures for massive PE are discussed further on in this chapter (see "Hemodynamic Management of Massive Pulmonary Embolism," below). Pain control and elevation of the leg are recommended for DVT, particularly severe, symptomatic acute iliofemoral DVT. Certain recommendations, such as bed rest in patients with established DVT, have not been well substantiated, but this measure should be instituted when significant symptoms are present. The major focus for effective therapy of VTE involves anticoagulation.

Anticoagulation

When DVT or PE is diagnosed or strongly suspected, anticoagulation therapy should be initiated immediately unless contraindications exist. The diagnosis must be confirmed if anticoagulation is to be continued.

STANDARD, UNFRACTIONATED HEPARIN

Standard heparin has been the time-honored parenteral anticoagulant based upon its prompt antithrombotic effect in preventing thrombus growth. The major anticoagulant effect of heparin is accounted for by a unique pentasaccharide with a high-affinity binding sequence to antithrombin III, which is present on only one-third of heparin molecules.[100] The interaction of heparin with antithrombin III markedly accelerates its ability to inactivate thrombin, factor Xa, and factor IXa. Heparin also catalyzes the inactivation of thrombin by a second plasma cofactor, heparin cofactor II. Heparin does not directly dissolve thrombus, but it allows the fibrinolytic system to act unopposed and more readily reduces the size of the thromboembolic burden.[100] Although thrombus growth can be prevented, early recurrence can develop even during therapeutic anticoagulation.

When intravenous standard, unfractionated heparin is instituted, the activated partial thromboplastin time (APTT) should be aggressively followed at 6-h intervals until it is consistently in the therapeutic range of 1.5 to 2.0 times control values.[101] This range corresponds to a heparin level of 0.2 to 0.4 U/mL as measured by protamine sulfate titration. Heparin can be administered by several protocols, but a weight-based approach has been shown to substantially enhance the chances of attaining the therapeutic range quickly. Heparin can be administered as an intravenous bolus of 5000 U followed by a maintenance dose of at least 30,000 to 40,000 U every 24 h by continuous infusion.[102] The lower dose is administered if the patient is considered at high risk for bleeding. This aggressive approach decreases the risk of subtherapeutic anticoagulation and, although supratherapeutic levels are sometimes achieved initially, bleeding complications do not appear to be increased.[102] More recent data continue to support aggressive heparin dosing. An alternative regimen consisting of a bolus of 80 U/kg followed by 18 U/kg/h has been recommended.[103,104] Subsequent adjusting of the heparin dose should also be weight-based (Table 53-3). This approach was recommended by the recent American College of Chest Physicians (ACCP) Consensus Conference on Antithrombotic Therapy.[104] Warfarin therapy may be initiated as soon as the APTT is therapeutic and heparin should be maintained until a therapeutic International Normalized Ratio (INR) of 2.0 to 3.0 has been overlapped with a therapeutic APTT for 2 consecutive days. This initial anticoagulation approach applies to both acute DVT and PE. Although proximal lower extremity thrombus is more likely to result in PE, calf thrombi should still be treated aggressively with anticoagulation or followed with noninvasive testing over 10 to 14 days for extension into the popliteal vein.[105,106] The spectrum of upper extremity venous thrombosis is variable and includes patients with peripherally and centrally placed intravenous catheters as

TABLE 53-3 Nomogram for Heparin Therapy in Acute Venous Thromboembolism

The initial heparin dose is 80 U/kg bolus, then 18 U/kg/h.
Subsequent dose modifications, based on APTT as follows:

APTT		
(Sec)	(Times Control)	Heparin Dose Adjustment
<35	<1.2	80 U/kg bolus, then increase by 4 U/kg/h
35 to 45	1.2 to 1.5	40 U/kg bolus, then increase by 2 U/kg/h
46 to 70	1.5 to 2.3	No change
71 to 90	2.3 to 3	Decrease infusion rate by 2 U/kg/h
>90	>3	Hold infusion 1 h, then decrease rate by 3 U/kg/h

SOURCE: American College of Chest Physicians Guidelines[104] and Raschke et al.[103]

well as those with underlying malignancy. Symptomatic patients with documented upper extremity DVT should be anticoagulated.[107] Prophylacticanticoagulation in patients with long-term indwelling catheters should also be instituted.[104,108]

LOW-MOLECULAR-WEIGHT HEPARIN

Mechanisms of Action and Pharmacology Low-molecular-weight heparin is being utilized increasingly for acute venous thromboembolism. These agents differ in a number of respects from standard, unfractionated heparin. Standard heparin consists of lengthy glycosaminoglycan polymers that are heterogenous in size, with a mean molecular weight of approximately 15,000 Da. LMWHs, also glycosaminoglycans, are prepared by chemical or enzymatic depolymerization and are approximately one-third of the size of unfractionated heparin. These LMWH fractions are also diverse, with a mean molecular weight of 4000 to 5000 Da. The difference in size between unfractionated heparin and LMWH results in an altered anticoagulant profile.[109] Only one-third of the LMWH molecules contain the pentasaccharide required for antithrombin III binding. Maximal inhibition of thrombin requires the binding of heparin to both antithrombin III and the activated enzyme. In contrast, the accelerated inactivation of factor Xa by the heparin/antithrombin III combination requires only the binding of unfractionated heparin to antithrombin III and does not require the formation of the ternary complex. Heparin molecules smaller than 18 saccharide units are unable to bind thrombin and antithrombin III simultaneously, precluding maximal acceleration of the inactivation of thrombin by antithrombin III. These smaller LMWH molecules do, however, retain their ability to catalyze the inhibition of factor Xa by antithrombin III. For this reason, LMWH fractions appear to have relatively more anti-Xa than antithrombin activity and significantly less effect upon the APTT. While the ratio of anti-Xa to antithrombin of heparin is 1:1, the LMWH preparations have significantly higher ratios. In addition, other anticoagulant properties such as stimulation of tissue factor pathway–inhibitor release appear to be responsible for the effect of these agents, suggesting more reason for variability among them.[109] While the different preparation methods result in products with similar molecular profiles, structural variations remain, which impart significant differences in their biologic actions. Chemical modifications of various portions of the molecules, charge density, and the degree of desulfation all affect the characteristics of the final product. Because of these differences, antithrombin III activity, the effects on tissue-factor-pathway inhibitor, platelet factor 4, and heparin cofactor II would be expected to be different for the different preparations. Other potential dissimilarities between heparin and LMWH and between the individual LMWH preparations include differences in stimulation of the release of tissue plasminogen activator and prostacyclin. A major advantage of these preparations over unfractionated heparin is substantially enhanced bioavailability. This has been shown to differ for different LMWH preparations as well. Each of the LMWH compounds should be considered a distinct agent and they should not, at the present time, be considered interchangeable. Important characteristics and advantages of the LMWH preparations are shown in Tables 53-4 and 53-5.

Clinical Trials and Indications Numerous clinical trials have strongly suggested the efficacy and safety of LMWH for treatment of established acute proximal DVT, using recurrent symptomatic VTE as the primary outcome measure.[110–116] Treatment with LMWH is more convenient for the patient and for the nursing staff for several reasons. A continuous intravenous line is not required, as these agents can be administered once or twice per day subcutaneously at therapeutic doses. In most cases monitoring of the APTT is not required. Patients can be monitored by measuring levels of factor X, and certain patient populations, such as significantly obese individuals or those with renal insufficiency, are probably best managed with such monitoring. There has not been com-

TABLE 53-4 A Comparison of Low-Molecular-Weight Heparin with Unfractionated Heparin

Characteristic	UFH[a]	LMWH[b]
Mean molecular weight	12,000–15,000	4000–6000
Protein binding	Substantial	Minimal
Anti-Xa activity	Substantial	Substantial
Anti-IIa activity	Substantial	Minimal
Platelet inhibition	Substantial	Minimal
Vascular permeability	Moderate	None
Microvascular permeability	Substantial	Minimal
Elimination (predominant)	Hepatic/macrophages	Renal

[a]Unfractionated heparin.
[b]Low-molecular-weight heparin.

TABLE 53-5 Potential Advantages of Low-Molecular-Weight Heparins over Unfractionated Heparin

Efficacy: Comparable or superior[a]
Safety: Comparable or superior[b]
Bioavailability: Superior
Subcutaneous administration
Once or twice daily dosing
No laboratory monitoring[c]
Less phlebotomy
Earlier ambulation
Home therapy in certain patient subsets

[a]Based upon objectively documented recurrence rates in clinical trials.
[b]Based upon rates of major and minor bleeding in clinical trials.
[c]In certain patient populations (significant obesity, renal insufficiency), monitoring has been suggested.

plete agreement on the approach to these individuals. Outpatient therapy for stable patients with DVT is increasing significantly. In two large, randomized (Canadian and European) trials, therapy with LMWH (enoxaparin and fraxiparine, respectively) was compared with that using standard weight-based unfractionated heparin.[110,111] The LMWH patients were treated entirely as outpatients or continued at home after a brief hospitalization. The outpatient LMWH regimens proved safe and effective. Three meta-analyses examined the use of LMWH compared with unfractionated heparin in the initial treatment of acute proximal DVT.[117–119] Although there was overlap among the clinical trials included in the analyses, they have helped to confirm the efficacy and safety of LMWH for the treatment of established DVT. At the present time, only one LMWH (enoxaparin) is FDA-approved for use in the United States for treatment of established DVT in the outpatient setting or for DVT (with or without PE) in the inpatient setting. Unlike the regimen for prophylaxis, in which a fixed dose of enoxaparin is utilized, a weight-based dosing regimen is employed for treatment of established VTE. For outpatient therapy, the recommended dose of enoxaparin is 30 mg subcutaneously every 12 h, while for inpatient treatment both 30 mg every 12 h and 40 mg once daily have been studied and FDA-approved. In addition to being more convenient, the LMWH preparations appear to be cost-effective, particularly when outpatient therapy is utilized.[120] Some of the different LMWH products and their prophylaxis and treatment regimens are listed in Table 53-6. The appropriate steps in instituting anticoagulation with enoxaparin for established VTE, including outpatient therapy, are shown in Table 53-7.

LONG-TERM THERAPY FOR DEEP VENOUS THROMBOSIS AND PULMONARY EMBOLISM

Documented proximal DVT or PE should be treated for 3 months with oral warfarin, keeping the INR at 2.0 to 3.0. Individuals unable to take warfarin can be treated with long-term subcutaneous heparin or LMWH. More prolonged therapy is indicated when significant risk factors persist. Furthermore, patients in whom no clear risk factors exist (idiopathic VTE) appear to benefit from more prolonged anticoagulation.[121] In a double-blind study, patients completing 3 months of anticoagulation for a first episode of idiopathic VTE were randomized to receive either warfarin (INR 2.0 to 3.0) or placebo for an additional 24 months, and there was a substantial reduction in recurrences in the warfarin group without a statistically significant increase in bleeding.[121] Both short- and long-term anticoagulation guidelines are outlined in the ACCP Consensus Conference guidelines.[104]

OTHER ANTICOAGULANTS

Newer anticoagulants are being explored. Heparin works indirectly, requiring antithrombin III as a cofactor, and its effects vary considerably between patients. Hirudin is a direct thrombin inhibitor that has several advantages over heparin, including efficacy against fibrin clot–bound thrombin. It does not require any cofactors and is not inactivated by platelet factor 4 or plasma proteins. This drug, derived from the saliva of the medicinal leach (*Hirudo medicinalis*), appears promising. Data from several clinical myocardial infarction trials suggested that hirudin is at least as safe as heparin.[122,123] Recombinant hirudin has been examined for prophylaxis of DVT in patients receiving total hip replacement and resulted in a low rate of proximal DVT.[124] As with heparin, these direct thrombin inhibitors have very narrow therapeutic indices. Other direct thrombin inhibitors and substances such as selective factor Xa inhibitors and tissue factor pathway inhibitor (TFPI) merit further investigation in the treatment of acute VTE.[125–130]

TABLE 53-6 Doses of Low-Molecular-Weight for Prevention and Treatment of Venous Thromboembolism

LMWH	Prevention	Treatment
Enoxaparin	30 mg q12h or 40 mg qd	1 mg/kg bid, 1.5 mg/kg qd[a]
Dalteparin	2500 to 5000 Xa U qd	200 Xa U/kg qd
Tinzaparin	75 Xa U/kg qd	175 Xa U/kg qd
Nadroparin	41 to 62 U/kg qd	<50 kg 4100 Xa U q12h
		50 to 75 kg 6150 Xa U q12h
		>70 kg 9200 Xa U q12h
Reviparin	4200 Xa U qd	35 to 45 kg 3500 Xa U q12h
		46 to 60 kg 4200 Xa U q12h
		>60 kg 6300 Xa U q12h
Ardeparin	50 Xa U/kg q 12h	Not evaluated

[a]Enoxaparin is the only LMWH approved for use in the United States for established DVT. It is indicated in patients who present with DVT (with or without concomitant PE). A dose of either 1.5 mg/kg or 1 mg/kg q12h has proven effective for inpatients with DVT +/− PE. Outpatient studies have been with 1 mg/kg q12h. It would appear highly likely that the once-daily dose would be adequate for outpatients, particularly since these patients tend to be stable and *may* have smaller thrombotic burdens.

TABLE 53-7 Initiating Low-Molecular-Weight Heparin for Established Deep Venous Thrombosis

Establish diagnosis of DVT[a] (with or without pulmonary embolism)
Be certain that no contraindications to anticoagulation exist
If diagnosis is strongly *suspected* but not yet proven and the patient is at low bleeding risk, initiate therapy (be certain that proof of thrombosis is established as quickly as possible)
If *outpatient therapy* is being considered, be certain patient is appropriate (medically stable, no massive DVT, pulmonary embolism absent, compliant, ability to self-administer LMWH[b] or have family or home health access for this)
Outpatient program established (patient must know who to contact, where/when to follow up)
Regimen
- Enoxaparin initiated administered subcutaneously[c,d]
- Warfarin initiated at 5 to 10 mg qd on day 1
- The INR[e] checked and goal is 2.0 to 3.0
- The APTT is not monitored (consider checking platelet count at day 3 to 5)
- Enoxaparin continued for at least 5 days or until the INR is therapeutic for 2 consecutive days

[a]Deep venous thrombosis.
[b]Low-molecular-weight heparin.
[c]This is the only FDA-approved LMWH for treatment of established DVT with or without pulmonary embolism.
[d]1 mg/kg q12h is the FDA-approved dose for inpatient or outpatient therapy, while 1.5 mg/kg qd is approved for inpatient use.
[e]International Normalized Ratio.

COMPLICATIONS OF ANTICOAGULATION

Complications of heparin include bleeding and heparin-induced thrombocytopenia (HIT). The rates of major bleeding in recent trials using standard heparin by continuous infusion or high-dose subcutaneous injection have been less than 5 percent.[104] Heparin-induced thrombocytopenia typically develops 5 or more days after the initiation of heparin therapy, and occurs in 5 to 10 percent of patients.[131–133] If a patient is placed on heparin for VTE and the platelet count progressively decreases to 100,000/mm^3 or less, heparin therapy should be discontinued. Although the risk of HIT appears to be lower with LMWH, it is important for clinicians to realize that HIT can occur with the use of either form of heparin.[134] Over the past decade, there have been many important advances in the pathogenesis, diagnosis, and treatment of HIT, which represents one of the most common immune-mediated adverse drug reactions.[135] This entity is caused by heparin-dependent IgG antibodies that recognize complexes of heparin and platelet factor 4, leading to activation of platelets via platelet Fc gamma IIa receptors. Formation of procoagulant, platelet-derived microparticles, and, possibly, activation of endothelium generate thrombin in vivo. The generation of thrombin helps to account for the strong association between HIT and thrombosis, including the recently recognized syndrome of warfarin-induced venous limb gangrene. This syndrome develops during warfarin treatment of HIT and deep venous thrombosis when acquired protein-C deficiency leads to the inability to regulate thrombin generation in the microvasculature. The diagnosis of HIT can be made confidently when one or more typical clinical events (most frequently, thrombocytopenia with or without thrombosis) occur in a patient with detectable HIT antibodies. The pivotal role of thrombin generation in this syndrome provides a rationale for the use of anticoagulants that reduce thrombin generation (danaparoid) or inhibit thrombin (lepirudin).

Vena Cava Interruption

In patients with established VTE in whom heparin therapy cannot be continued, inferior vena cava (IVC) filter placement can be undertaken to prevent lower extremity thrombi from embolizing to the lungs. These devices have been widely used for nearly two decades. The essential indications for filter placement include contraindications to anticoagulation, recurrent embolism while on adequate therapy, and significant bleeding complications during anticoagulation.[136] Filters are sometimes placed in the setting of massive PE when it is believed that any further emboli might be lethal.[136] A number of filter devices exist, but the Greenfield filter design has been most widely used. These devices can be inserted via the jugular or femoral vein and are effective. Complications are unusual.[137] Possible mechanisms of IVC filter failure include filter migration; improper filter positioning, allowing thrombi to bypass the filter; and formation of thrombosis proximal to the filter or on the proximal tip of the filter with subsequent embolization. Rare complications include clinically significant perforation of the IVC, migration to the heart, and displacement of the filter during insertion. Rarely, these devices may erode into the wall of the IVC. Occasionally, IVC obstruction due to thrombosis at the filter site may occur. Deaths due to filter placement are extraordinarily uncommon. Anticoagulation is generally continued when a filter is placed unless it is contraindicated. Temporary filters have been placed in individuals deemed at extremely high risk for DVT yet unable to receive anticoagulant prophylaxis, such as certain trauma patients.[138]

Thrombolytic Therapy

Acceleration of clot lysis in PE using thrombolytic therapy was first documented several decades ago.[139–141] The prospective, multicenter, randomized UPET evaluated 160 patients with arteriographically proven PE.[53] Thrombolysis was accelerated in patients receiving urokinase compared with those on heparin when pulmonary arteriograms and lung perfusion scans were examined 24 h after treatment. Subsequently, the difference between the two groups diminished and by day 5 the improvement in each group was similar. There were no differences in the frequency of recurrent PE or mortality rate within 2 weeks of treatment. The lack of reduction in mortality may have been explained by the fact that only 7 percent of the patients in the clinical trial were classified as having massive PE with shock. The second phase of this clinical trial also documented the efficacy of streptokinase administered over 24 h.

Both urokinase and streptokinase were approved for use in pulmonary embolism. In 1980, the National Institutes of Health issued consensus guidelines for PE thrombolysis and recommended thrombolytic therapy for patients with obstruction of blood flow to a lobe or multiple pulmonary segments and for patients with hemodynamic compromise regardless of the size of the PE.[142] Recombinant tissue plasminogen activator (t-PA) was subsequently approved for use for the treatment of PE and is administered as a 100-mg intravenous infusion delivered over 2 h.[143] Even shorter infusion durations have been evaluated, and future clinical trials may lead to wider acceptance of these regimens. At present, the above t-PA regimen is the most rapidly administered protocol that is currently approved for use.

At the present time, the clearest indication for the use of thrombolytic therapy is in patients with hemodynamic instability (hypotension) when there are no concomitant contraindications.[144,145] Patients with severely compromised oxygenation should also be considered.[144] Stable patients with a significant embolic load are individualized, often receiving treatment in the absence of absolute or relative contraindications. For example, a strong case for thrombolytic therapy can be made when the embolic load visualized on the imaging study is extensive (defect involving the equivalent of half of the pulmonary vascular bed) or with echocardiographic evidence of right ventricular dysfunction without clear hemodynamic instability.[146,147] Another setting in which thrombolytic therapy may be considered is when extensive DVT accompanies a submassive PE. No clinical studies have been undertaken to support this indication. Perhaps future trials will clarify more controversial guidelines.

The recommendations for use of thrombolytic therapy in PE have been carefully reviewed.[146] Potential indications are presented in Table 53-8. Approved regimens for the treatment of PE are presented in Table 53-9. Coagulation assays are not necessary during thrombolysis, since the approved regimens are administered as fixed doses. Heparin should be withheld until the thrombolytic infusion is completed. The APTT is then determined and heparin is initiated without a loading dose if this value is less than twice the upper limit of normal. If the APTT exceeds this value, the test is repeated every 4 h until it is safe to proceed with heparin. The method of delivery of thrombolytic agents has also been investigated. Although a number of investigators have employed standard or low-dose intrapulmonary arterial thrombolytic infusions in order to deliver a high concentration of drug in close proximity to the clot,[148,149] intravenous therapy appears adequate in most settings.[150] More direct techniques, such as catheter-directed administration of intraembolic thrombolytic therapy are discussed below.

TABLE 53-8 Thrombolytic Therapy in Venous Thromboembolism: Potential Indications[a]

- Hypotension related to PE[b]
- Severe hypoxemia
- Lobar or greater perfusion defect[c]
- Right ventricular dysfunction associated with PE
- Extensive deep vein thrombosis

[a]All indications require careful review of contraindications to thrombolytic therapy.
[b]This indication is widely accepted.
[c]This indication was supported by NIH guidelines in 1980.[142] However, administration of thrombolytic therapy based upon a lobar defect alone *in the absence of other indications* is not widely practiced.

TABLE 53-9 Thrombolytic Therapy for Acute Pulmonary Embolism: Approved Regimens

- Streptokinase: 250,000 U IV (loading dose over 30 min); then 100,000 U/h for 24 h[a]
- Urokinase: 2000 U/lb IV (loading dose over 10 min); then 2000 U/lb/h for 12 to 24 h
- Tissue-type plasminogen activator: 100 mg IV over 2 h

[a]Streptokinase administered over 24 to 72 h at this loading dose and rate has also been approved for use in patients with extensive DVT.

The use of thrombolytic therapy for DVT without PE is more controversial. A comprehensive review of the literature suggests that use of streptokinase may be associated with a reduction in postphlebitic syndrome when used for acute DVT, although bleeding is increased with thrombolytic therapy.[151] Future studies may clarify the role of thrombolytic therapy for DVT. It is reasonable to consider systemic thrombolytic therapy in patients with proximal occlusive DVT associated with significant swelling and symptoms when there are no absolute or relative contraindications.

The major complication resulting from thrombolytic therapy is bleeding. These agents are not fibrin-specific and any clot, whether pathologic or protective, is subject to lysis. Although hemorrhagic complications in the UPET were relatively high, further experience with thrombolytic therapy has suggested that adverse effects are reduced when venous cut-downs and unnecessary arterial phlebotomy are avoided.[152] Thus, when thrombolytic therapy is administered, invasive procedures should be minimized. The most devastating complication associated with this treatment is the development of intracranial hemorrhage.[153] Clinical trials have suggested that this occurs in significantly less than 1 percent of patients. Contraindications to systemic thrombolytic therapy in VTE are listed in Table 53-10. Bleeding related to thrombolytic therapy requires immediate management. Bleeding from vascular puncture sites should be addressed with manual compression followed by a pressure dressing. Intracranial bleeding requires immediate discontinuation of thrombolytics or anticoagulants, and emergent neurologic and neurosurgical consultation should be obtained. A noncontrasted brain CT scan should be performed. Retroperitoneal hemorrhage may develop from a vascular puncture above the inguinal ligament and may be life-threatening. Severe or refractory bleeding should be addressed with transfusion of 10 U of cryoprecipitate and 2 U of fresh frozen plasma, and heparin

TABLE 53-10 Thrombolytic Therapy for Acute Pulmonary Embolism: Contraindications

Absolute
- Intracranial tumor or hemorrhagic stroke
- Previous head trauma or cranial surgery
- Active or recent gastrointestinal/internal bleeding

Relative
- Thrombocytopenia or coagulopathy
- Uncontrolled severe hypertension
- Cardiopulmonary resuscitation
- Surgery or biopsy within the previous 10 days

can be reversed with protamine. A comprehensive review of thrombolytic therapy for acute VTE has been published.[154]

Catheter-Directed Techniques

The intravenous route has been the primary method of delivery, but local thrombolytic therapy has been utilized in massive PE. Intrapulmonary arterial delivery of thrombolytic agents by bolus or prolonged infusion with or without concomitant heparin has been utilized for massive PE (see "Thrombolytic Therapy," above).[148,149] These studies have generally been small and uncontrolled. Although intrapulmonary arterial delivery of thrombolytic agents appears to offer no advantage over the intravenous route,[150] *intraembolic* thrombolytic infusions may offer advantages over merely infusing the agents into the pulmonary artery. Such techniques have been applied in both animal models of PE and in patients, with enhanced thrombolysis.[155,156] Lower than conventional doses of t-PA or urokinase are delivered via a catheter imbedded directly within massive emboli over 10 to 20 min.[155,156] Combining thrombolytic therapy via direct delivery (at low doses) with the possible mechanical benefits of direct intraembolic infusion could prove advantageous over the intravenous route, particularly in the setting of contraindications to thrombolytic therapy. Larger randomized studies would be needed to demonstrate the efficacy, potential advantages, and safety of such techniques. The implementation of these techniques, as well as the catheter-directed administration of intraembolic thrombolytic therapy described above, depend upon the experience of the medical team involved. Transvenous embolectomy without thrombolysis, via a suction-catheter device, has been proven quite effective by some[157,158] but is not widely performed. In an experience spanning 7 years, one group successfully extracted emboli in 11 of 18 patients with massive PE utilizing this technique; 13 survived their hospital stay while 5 died.[158]

Catheter-directed techniques have been successfully employed in the setting of acute iliofemoral DVT utilizing urokinase doses ranging from 1.4 to 16 million U delivered over an average of 30 h.[159,160] Results from a national registry of patients with iliofemoral thrombosis treated with local, catheter-directed therapy indicates that this approach is frequently successful.[160] Randomized trials may be appropriate.

Surgical Embolectomy

Pulmonary embolectomy may be performed in the setting of acute massive PE. The advent of thrombolytic therapy has reduced the number of potential candidates, but contraindications to these agents are relatively common. Although many patients die from PE before surgical embolectomy can be performed, some deteriorate hours after the initial episode, suggesting that surgery may occasionally be appropriate. In one case series of 71 embolectomies performed for acute PE using cardiopulmonary bypass, hospital mortality was 29 percent.[161] However, the mortality in those patients who had not sustained a cardiac arrest preoperatively was only 11 percent.

Hemodynamic Management of Massive Pulmonary Embolism

Massive PE should always be a consideration in the setting of the sudden onset of hypotension or extreme hypoxemia. Electromechanical dissociation or sudden cardiac arrest should always make massive PE suspect. If the patient is stable enough, lung imaging (generally $\dot{V}/\dot{Q}$ scan or spiral CT scan) should be performed when possible. Echocardiography may support the diagnosis of massive PE and may also suggest that aggressive intervention including thrombolytic therapy be considered.[146,147] When massive PE associated with hypotension and/or severe hypoxemia is suspected, supportive treatment is immediately initiated. Intravenous saline can be rapidly infused, but caution is recommended because right ventricular function is often markedly compromised. Dopamine or norepinephrine appear to be the favored choices of vasoactive therapy in massive PE and should be administered if the blood pressure is not rapidly restored.[162] Death from massive PE results from right ventricular failure, and dobutamine has been recommended by some as a means by which to augment right ventricular output.[163,164] A vasopressor such as norepinephrine combined with dobutamine might offer optimal results, and further exploration of such combined therapy would prove enlightening. Oxygen therapy is administered and thrombolytic therapy should be administered if hypotension is present and there are no contraindications. Intubation and mechanical ventilation are instituted as needed to support respiratory failure. Surgical embolectomy may be indicated, particularly if thrombolytic therapy cannot be administered.

CHRONIC THROMBOEMBOLIC PULMONARY HYPERTENSION

In the majority of cases of acute PE, the patient either dies or completely recovers; however, a substantial residual thromboembolic burden occasionally remains and/or continues to form.[165,166] In these patients, the clot becomes organized and adherent and is not amenable to thrombolysis. If the obstruction becomes extensive, pulmonary hypertension develops. At least 50 percent of patients who develop chronic thromboembolic pulmonary hypertension have no documented history of DVT or PE, and this feature greatly impedes the diagnosis. Most patients have no identifiable coagulopathy. Dyspnea with exertion and fatigue are the most common complaints. The nonspecific nature of these findings may substantially delay the correct diagnosis. The physical examination generally reveals a right ventricular heave, a loud P_2, a right ventricular S_3, and tricuspid regurgitation consistent with pulmonary hypertension. In 20 percent of patients, one or more murmurs may be auscultated over the lung fields.

The chest radiograph usually reveals right ventricular enlargement and enlarged main pulmonary arteries. ECG changes are consistent with pulmonary hypertension. Arterial blood gases generally reveal hypoxemia with a widened A-a difference, although some patients may only demonstrate exercise-induced hypoxemia. Echocardiography documents pulmonary hypertension and enlargement of the right ventricle. Chest CT scanning is prudent and may reveal other rare causes of pulmonary hypertension, such as mediastinal fibrosis, and may, in fact, demonstrate evidence of chronic thrombi. With chronic thromboembolic pulmonary hypertension, the $\dot{V}/\dot{Q}$ scan nearly always indicates a high probability of PE, but occasionally it is less impressive. Right heart catheterization and pulmonary arteriography are performed, both to establish the diagnosis with certainty and to determine operability. Pulmonary angioscopy has frequently proven complementary to arteriography in assessing these patients.

Although anticoagulation should be instituted and IVC filters are recommended in patients with chronic thromboembolic pulmonary hypertension, the only means by which to alleviate symptoms and affect survival is with surgery. The University of California at San Diego has been a leading center for the evaluation and surgical therapy of these patients. Pulmonary thromboendarterectomy is performed via median sternotomy on cardiopulmonary bypass, and the overall mortality, which has continued to improve, is now less than 5 percent. Lung transplantation can sometimes be performed in patients in whom thrombi are too distal to extract.

SUMMARY

Venous thromboembolism represents a spectrum consisting of DVT and PE. It is a common cause of death, particularly in hospitalized patients with significant risk factors, and is frequently not diagnosed until autopsy. The history and physical examination for both DVT and PE consist of suggestive but generally very nonspecific findings. These findings, particularly in the setting of risk factors for VTE, are important in raising the level of suspicion for VTE, leading to diagnostic testing. Preventive measures in patients at risk are crucial. Anticoagulation represents appropriate therapy for most patients with VTE. Low-molecular-weight heparins are being used increasingly in established VTE as well as for prophylaxis. Thrombolytic therapy should be considered in massive PE in the absence of contraindications, and guidelines for the use of these agents is evolving. Placement of a filter in the inferior vena cava is indicated when anticoagulation is contraindicated. Newer agents such as direct thrombin inhibitors are being explored. Future clinical trials will help to clarify the roles of both the newer diagnostic modalities and therapeutic strategies.

References

1. Anderson FA, Wheeler HB. Venous thromboembolism: Risk factors and prophylaxis. *Clin Chest Med* 1995; 16:235–251.
2. Dalen JE, Alpert JS. Natural history of pulmonary embolism. *Prog Cardiovasc Dis* 1975; 17:257–270.
3. Lindblad B, Eriksson A, Bergquist D. Autopsy-verified pulmonary embolism in a surgical department: Analysis of the period from 1951 to 1988. *Br J Surg* 1991; 78:849–852.
4. Cotton LT, Clark C. Anatomical localization of venous thrombosis. *Ann R Coll Surg Engl* 1965; 36:214–224.
5. Lamb GC, Tomski MH, Kaufman J, et al. Is chronic spinal cord injury associated with increased risk of venous thromboembolism? *J Am Paraplegia Soc* 1993; 16:153–156.
6. Layish DT, DeLong DM, Tapson VF. Relationship between obesity and pulmonary embolism: A review of the PIOPED data. *Chest* 1996; 110:53S.
7. Carson JL, Kelley MA, Duffy A, et al. The clinical course of pulmonary embolism. *N Engl J Med* 1992; 326:1240–1245.
8. Goldhaber SZ, Hennekens CH, Evans DA, et al. Factors associated with correct antemortem diagnosis of major pulmonary embolism. *Am J Med* 1982; 73:822–826.
9. Kakkar VV, Howe CT, Nicolaides AN, et al. Deep vein thrombosis of the legs: Is there a "high risk" group? *Am J Surg* 1970; 120:527–530.
10. Clagett GP, Reisch JS. Prevention of venous thromboembolism in general surgical patients: Results of a meta-analysis. *Ann Surg* 1988; 208:227–240.
11. Clagett GP, Anderson FA Jr, Geerts W, et al. Prevention of venous thromboembolism. *Chest* 1998; 114:531S–560S.
12. Fisher M, Michele A, McCann W. Thrombophlebitis and pulmonary infarction associated with fractured hip. *Clin Res* 1963; 11:407.
13. Fitts, WT Jr, Lehr HB, Bitner RL, et al. An analysis of 950 fatal injuries. *Surgery* 1964; 56:663–668.
14. Coon WW. Risk factors in pulmonary embolism. *Surg Gynecol Obstet* 1976; 143:385–390.
15. Haire WD. Arm vein thrombosis. *Clin Chest Med* 1995; 16:341.
16. Falanga A, Rickles FR. Pathophysiology of the thrombophilic state in the cancer patient. *Semin Thromb Hemostas* 1999; 25:173–182.
17. Handley AJ, Emerson PA, Fleming PR. Heparin in the prevention of deep vein thrombosis after myocardial infarction. *BMJ* 1972; 2:436–438.
18. Gruppo Italiano per lo Studio della Streptochinasi nell'Infarto Miocardico (GISSI). Effectiveness of intravenous thrombolytic treatment in acute myocardial infarction. *Lancet* 1986; 1:397–402.
19. ISIS-2 Collaborative Group. Randomized trial of IV streptokinase, oral aspirin, both or neither among 17,187 cases of suspected acute myocardial infarction. *Lancet* 1988; 2:349–360.
20. Rickles FR, Levine MN, Edwards RL. Hemostatic alterations in cancer patients. *Cancer Met Rev* 1992; 11:291–311.
21. Carroll VA, Binder BR. The role of the plasminogen activation system in cancer. *Semin Thromb Hemostas* 1999; 25:183–198.
22. Lee AYY, Levine MN. The thrombophilic state induced by therapeutic agents in the cancer patient. *Semin Thromb Hemostas* 1999; 25:137–146.
23. Sorensen HT, Mellemkjaer L, Steffensen FH, et al. The risk of a diagnosis of cancer after primary deep venous thrombosis or pulmonary embolism. *N Engl J Med* 1993; 38:1169–1173.
24. Toglia MR, Weg JG. Current concepts: Venous thromboembolism during pregnancy. *N Engl J Med* 1996; 335:108–114.
25. Stadel BV. Oral contraceptives and cardiovascular disease. *N Engl J Med* 1981; 305:672–677.
26. Weiss N. Third-generation oral contraceptives: How risky? *Lancet* 1995; 346:1570.
27. World Health Organization Collaborative Study of Cardiovascular Disease and Steroid Hormone Contraception. Venous thromboembolic disease and combined oral contraceptives: Results of international multicentre case-control study. *Lancet* 1995; 346: 1575–1582.
28. Daly E, Vessey MP, Hawkins MM, et al. Risk of venous thromboembolism in users of hormone replacement therapy. *Lancet* 1996; 348:977–980.
29. Jick H, Derby LE, Wald MyersM, et al. Risk of hospital admission for idiopathic venous thromboembolism among users of postmenopausal estrogens. *Lancet* 1996; 348:981–983.
30. Grodstein F, Stampfer MJ, Goldhaber SZ, et al. Prospective study of exogenous hormones and risk of pulmonary embolism in women. *Lancet* 1996; 348:983–987.
31. Ridker PM, Hennekens CH, Lindpainter K, et al. Mutation in the gene coding for coagulation factor V and the risk of myocardial infarction, stroke, and venous thrombosis in apparently healthy men. *N Engl J Med* 1995; 332:912.
32. Poort SR, Rosendaal FR, Reitsma PH, et al. A common genetic variation in the 3′-untranslated region of the prothrombin gene is associated with elevated plasma prothrombin levels and an increase in venous thrombosis. *Blood* 1996; 88:3698–3703.
33. Hillarp A, Zoller B, Svensson PJ, Dahlback B. The 20210A of the prothrombin gene is a common risk factor among Swedish outpatients with verified deep venous thrombosis. *Thromb Haemostas* 1997; 78:990–992.
34. DeStefano V, Martinelli I, Mannucci PM, et al. The risk of recur-

rent deep venous thrombosis among heterozygous carriers of both factor V Leiden and the G20210A prothrombin mutation. *N Engl J Med* 1999; 341:801–806.
35. D'Angelo A, Selhub J. Homocysteine and thrombotic disease. *Blood* 1997; 90:1–11.
36. Ridker PM, Hennekens CH, Selhub J, et al. Interrelation of hyperhomocysteinemia, factor V Leiden, and risk of future venous thromboembolism. *Circulation* 1997; 95:1777–1782.
37. Benotti JR, Dalen JE. The natural history of pulmonary embolism. *Clin Chest Med* 1984; 5:403.
38. McIntyre KM, Sasahara AA. The ratio of pulmonary artery pressure to pulmonary vascular obstruction. *Chest* 1977; 71:692.
39. Tapson VF, Carroll BA, Davidson BL, et al. The Diagnostic Approach to Acute Venous Thromboembolism. American Thoracic Society Consensus Statement and Clinical Practice Guidelines. *Am J Resp Crit Care Med* 1999; 160:1043–1066.
40. The PIOPED Investigators. Value of the ventilation/perfusion scan in acute pulmonary embolism: Results of the prospective investigation of pulmonary embolism diagnosis. *JAMA* 1990; 263:2753–2759.
41. Bounameaux H, Cirafici P, DeMoerloose P, et al. Measurement of D-dimer in plasma as diagnostic aid in suspected pulmonary embolism. *Lancet* 1991; 337:196.
42. Rowbotham BJ, Egerton-Vernon J, Whitaker AN, et al. Plasma cross-linked fibrin degradation products in pulmonary embolism. *Thorax* 1990; 45:684–687.
43. Becker DM, Philbrick JT, Bachhuber TL, Humphries JE. D-dimer testing and acute venous thromboembolism: A shortcut to accurate diagnosis? *Arch Intern Med* 1996; 156:939–946.
44. Moser KM. Diagnosing pulmonary embolism: D-dimer needs rigorous evaluation. *BMJ* 1994; 309:1525–1526.
45. Knecht MF, Heinrich F. Clinical evaluation of an immunoturbidimetric D-dimer assay in the diagnostic procedure of deep vein thrombosis and pulmonary embolism. *Thromb Res* 1997; 88: 413–417.
46. Ginsberg JS, Kearon C, Douketis J, et al. The use of D-dimer testing and impedance plethysmographic examination in patients with clinical indications of deep venous thrombosis. *Arch Intern Med* 1997; 157:1077–1081.
47. Perrier A, Bounameaux H, Morabia A, et al. Diagnosis of pulmonary embolism by a decision analysis-based strategy including clinical probability, D-dimer levels, and ultrasonography: A management study. *Arch Intern Med* 1996; 156:531–536.
48. Perrier A, Desmarais S, Goehring C, et al. D-dimer testing for suspected pulmonary embolism in outpatients. *Am J Respir Crit Care Med* 1997; 156:492–496.
49. Green RM, Meyer TJ, Dunn M, Glassroth J. Pulmonary embolism in younger adults. *Chest* 1992; 101:1507–1511.
50. Stein PD, Terrin ML, Hales CA, et al. Clinical, laboratory, roentgenographic, and electrocardiographic findings in patients with acute pulmonary embolism and no pre-existing cardiac or pulmonary disease. *Chest* 1991; 100:598–603.
51. McGinn S, White PD. Acute cor pulmonale resulting from pulmonary embolism. *JAMA* 1935; 104:1473–1480.
52. Sokolow M, Katz LN, Muscovitz AN. The electrocardiogram in acute pulmonary embolism. *Am Heart J* 1940; 19:166–184.
53. The Urokinase Pulmonary Embolism Trial; A national cooperative study. *Circulation* 1973; 47(suppl. II):1–108.
54. Ferrari E, Imbert A, Chevalier T, et al. The ECG in pulmonary embolism. Predictive value of negative T waves in precordial leads: 80 case reports. *Chest* 1997; 111:537–543.
55. Stein PD, Athanasoulis C, Alavi A, et al. Complications and validity of pulmonary angiography in acute pulmonary embolism. *Circulation* 1992; 85:462–468.
56. Quinn MF, Lundell CJ, Klotz TA, et al. Reliability of selective pulmonary arteriography in the diagnosis of acute pulmonary embolism. *AJR* 1987; 149:469–471.
57. Hull RD, Raskob G, Ginsberg JS, et al. A noninvasive strategy for the treatment of patients with suspected pulmonary embolism. *Arch Intern Med* 1994; 154:289–297.
58. Rosengarten PL, Tuxen DV, Weeks AM. Whole lung pulmonary angiography in the intensive care unit with two portable chest x-rays. *Crit Care Med* 1990; 18:459–460.
59. Nass N, McConnell MV, Goldhaber SZ, et al. Recovery of regional right ventricular function after thrombolysis for pulmonary embolism. *Am J Cardiol* 1999; 83:804–806.
60. Come PC. Echocardiographic evaluation of pulmonary embolism and its response to therapeutic interventions. *Chest* 1992; 101: 151S–162S.
61. Kasper W, Meinertz T, Kersting F, et al. Echocardiography in assessing acute pulmonary hypertension due to pulmonary embolism. *Am J Cardiol* 1980; 45:567–572.
62. Tapson VF, Davidson CJ, Gurbel PA, et al. Rapid and accurate diagnosis of pulmonary emboli in a canine model using intravascular ultrasound imaging. *Chest* 1991; 100:1410–1413.
63. Tapson VF, Davidson CJ, Kisslo KB, et al. Rapid visualization of massive pulmonary emboli utilizing intravascular ultrasound. *Chest* 1994; 105:888–890.
64. Ricou F, Nicod PH, Moser KM, Peterson KL. Catheter-based intravascular ultrasound imaging of chronic thromboembolic pulmonary disease. *Am J Cardiol* 1991; 67:749–752.
65. Remy-Jardin M, Remy J. Spiral CT angiography of the pulmonary circulation. *Radiology* 1999; 212:615–636.
66. Remy-Jardin M, Remy J, Wattinne L, Giraud F. Central pulmonary thromboembolism: Diagnosis with spiral volumetric CT with the single-breath-hold technique: Comparison with pulmonary angiography. *Radiology* 1992; 185:381–387.
67. Remy-Jardin M, Remy J, Deschildre F, et al. Diagnosis of pulmonary embolism with spiral CT: Comparison with pulmonary angiography and scintigraphy. *Radiology* 1996; 200:699–706.
68. Goodman LR, Curtin JJ, Mewissen MW, et al. Detection of pulmonary embolism in patients with unresolved clinical and scintigraphic diagnosis: Helical CT versus angiography. *AJR* 1995; 164:1369–1374.
69. Teigen CL, Maus TP, Sheedy PF, et al. Pulmonary embolism: Diagnosis with contrast-enhanced electron-beam CT and comparison with pulmonary angiography. *Radiology* 1995; 194: 313–319.
70. van Rossum AB, Pattynama PM, Treurniat FE, et al. Spiral CT angiography for detection of pulmonary embolism: Validation in 124 patients. *Radiology* 1995; 197(P):303.
71. van Rossum AB, Treurniat FE, Kieft GJ, et al. Role of spiral volumetric computed tomographic scanning in the assessment of patients with clinical suspicion of pulmonary embolism and an abnormal ventilation perfusion scan. *Thorax* 1996; 51:23–28.
72. Oser RF, Zuckerman DA, Gutirrez FR, Brink JA. Anatomic distribution of pulmonary embolism at pulmonary arteriography: Implications for spiral and electron-beam CT. *Radiology* 1996; 199:31–35.
73. Goodman LR, Lipchik RJ. Diagnosis of acute pulmonary embolism: Time for a new approach. *Radiology* 1996; 199:25–27.
74. Teigen CL, Maus TP, Sheedy PF, et al. Pulmonary embolism: Diagnosis with electron-beam CT. *Radiology* 1993; 188:839–845.
75. Meaney JFM, Weg JG, Chenevert TL, et al. Diagnosis of pulmonary embolism with magnetic resonance angiography. *N Engl J Med* 1997; 336:1422–1427.
76. Tapson VF. Pulmonary embolism—New diagnostic approaches. *N Engl J Med* 1997; 336:1449–1451.
77. Sostman HD, Layish DT, Tapson VF, et al. Prospective comparison of helical CT and MR imaging in clinically suspected acute pulmonary embolism. *JMRI* 1996; 6:275.
78. Mousa SA, Bozarth JM, Edwards S, et al. Novel technetium-99m–labeled platelet GPIIb/IIIa receptor antagonists as poten-

tial imaging agents for venous and arterial thrombosis. *Coron Artery Dis* 1998; 9:131–141.
79. Hull R, Hirsh J, Powers P. Impedance plethysmography: The relationship between venous filling and sensitivity and specificity for proximal vein thrombosis. *Circulation* 1978; 58:898–902.
80. Hull R, van Aken WG, Hirsh J, et al. Impedance plethysmography using the occlusive cuff technique in the diagnosis of venous thrombosis. *Circulation* 1976; 53:696–700.
81. Anderson DR, Lensing AWA, Wells PS, et al. Limitations of impedance plethysmography in the diagnosis of clinically suspected deep-vein thrombosis. *Ann Intern Med* 1993; 118:25–30.
82. Borgstede JP, Clagett GE. Types, frequency, and significance of alternative diagnoses found during duplex Doppler venous examinations of the lower extremities. *J Ultrasound Med* 1992; 11:85–89.
83. Lensing AW, Levi MM, Buller HR, et al. Diagnosis of deep-vein thrombosis using an objective Doppler method. *Ann Intern Med* 1990; 113:9–13.
84. White R, McGahan JP, Daschbach MM, Hartling MM. Diagnosis of deep-vein thrombosis using duplex ultrasound. *Ann Intern Med* 1989; 111:297–304.
85. Cronan JJ, Leen V. Recurrent deep venous thrombosis: Limitations of ultrasound. *Radiology* 1989; 170:739–742.
86. Killewich LA, Bedford GR, Beach KW, Strandness DE. Diagnosis of deep venous thrombosis: A prospective study comparing duplex scanning to contrast venography. *Circulation* 1989; 79: 810–814.
87. Davidson BL, Elliott CG, Lensing AWA. Low accuracy of color Doppler ultrasound in the detection of proximal leg vein thrombosis in asymptomatic high-risk patients. *Ann Intern Med* 1992; 117:735–738.
88. Evans AJ, Tapson VF, Sostman HD, et al. The diagnosis of deep venous thrombosis: A prospective comparison of venography and magnetic resonance imaging. *Chest* 1992; 102:120S.
89. Witty LA, Tapson VF, Evans AJ, et al. MRI versus ultrasound: A radiologic and clinical evaluation of DVT. *Am Rev Respir Dis* 1993; 147:A998.
90. Burke B, Sostman HD, Carroll BA, Witty LA. The diagnostic approach to deep venous thrombosis: Which technique? *Clin Chest Med* 1995; 16:253–268.
91. Collins R, Scrimgeour A, Yusuf S, Peto R. Reduction in fatal pulmonary embolism and venous thrombosis by perioperative administration of subcutaneous heparin. *N Engl J Med* 1988; 318:1162–1173.
92. Anderson FA Jr, Brownell W, Goldberg RJ, et al. Physician practices in the prevention of venous thromboembolism. *Ann Intern Med* 1991; 115:591–595.
93. Bratzler DW, Raskob GE, Murray CK, et al. Underuse of venous thromboembolism prophylaxis for general surgery patients: Physician practices in the community hospital setting. *Arch Intern Med* 1998; 158:1909–1912.
94. Tapson VF, Hull R. Management of venous thromboembolic disease: The impact of low-molecular-weight heparin. *Clin Chest Med* 1995; 16:281–294.
95. Samama MM, Cohen AT, Darmon JY, et al. A comparison of enoxaparin with placebo for the prevention of venous thromboembolism in acutely ill medical patients. *N Engl J Med* 1999; 341:793–800.
96. Colditz GA, Tuden RL, Oster G. Rates of venous thrombosis after general surgery: Combined results of randomised clinical trials. *Lancet* 1986; 2:143.
97. Bergqvist D, Benoni G, Bjorgello XX, et al. Low-molecular-weight heparin (enoxaparin) as prophylaxis against venous thromboembolism after total hip replacement. *N Engl J Med* 1996; 335:696–700.
98. Geerts WH, Jay RM, Code KI, et al. A comparison of low-dose heparin with low-molecular-weight heparin as prophylaxis against venous thromboembolism after major trauma. *N Engl J Med* 1996; 335:701–707.
99. Clagett GP, Anderson FA Jr, Geerts WH, et al. Prevention of venous thromboembolism. *Chest* 1998; 114(suppl):531S–560S.
100. Hirsh J, Warkentin TE, Raschke R, et al. Heparin and low-molecular-weight heparin. Mechanisms of action, pharmacokinetics, dosing considerations, monitoring, efficacy, and safety. *Chest* 1998; 114:489S–510S.
101. Hull RD, Raskob GE, Hirsh J, et al. Continuous intravenous heparin compared with intermittent subcutaneous heparin in the initial treatment of proximal vein thrombosis. *N Engl J Med* 1986; 315:1109–1114.
102. Hull R, Raskob G, Rosenbloom D, et al. Optimal therapeutic level of heparin therapy in patients with venous thrombosis. *Arch Intern Med* 1992; 152:1589–1595.
103. Raschke RA, Reilly BM, Guidry JR, et al. The weight-based heparin dosing nomogram compared with a "standard care" nomogram. *Ann Intern Med* 1993; 119:874.
104. Hyers TM, Agnelli G, Hull RD, et al. Antithrombotic therapy for venous thromboembolic disease. *Chest* 1998; 114:561S–578S.
105. Lagerstedt CI, Olsson C-G, Fagher BO, Oqvist BW. Need for long-term anticoagulant treatment in symptomatic calf-vein thrombosis. *Lancet* 1985; 2:515–518.
106. Moser KM et al. Is embolic risk conditioned by location of deep venous thrombosis? *Ann Intern Med* 1981; 94:439–444.
107. Prandoni P, Polistena P, Bernardi E, et al. Upper extremity deep vein thrombosis. *Arch Intern Med* 1997; 157:57–62.
108. Randolph AG, Cook DJ, Gonzalez CA, et al. Benefit of heparin in central venous and pulmonary artery catheters: A meta-analysis of randomized controlled trials. *Chest* 1998; 113:165–171.
109. Nader HB, Walenga JM, Berkowitz SD, et al. Preclinical differentiation of low molecular weight heparins. *Semin Thromb Hemost* 1999; 25(suppl 3):63–72.
110. Levine M, Gent M, Hirsh J, et al. A comparison of low molecular-weight-heparin administered primarily at home with unfractionated heparin administered in the hospital for proximal deep vein thrombosis. *N Engl J Med* 1996; 334:677–681.
111. Koopman MM, Prandoni P, Piovella F, et al. Low molecular-weight-heparin versus heparin for proximal deep vein thrombosis. *N Engl J Med* 1996; 334:682–687.
112. A Collaborative European Multicentre Study. A randomized trial of subcutaneous low-molecular-weight heparin (CY216) compared with intravenous unfractionated heparin in the treatment of deep vein thrombosis. *Thromb Haemostas* 1991; 65:251–256.
113. Hull RD, Raskob GE, Pineo GF, et al. Subcutaneous low molecular-weight heparin compared with continuous intravenous heparin in the treatment of proximal-vein thrombosis. *N Engl J Med* 1992; 326:975–983.
114. Prandoni P, Lensing AWA, Buller HR, et al. Comparison of subcutaneous low-molecular-weight heparin with intravenous standard heparin in proximal deep vein thrombosis. *Lancet* 1992; 339:441–445.
115. Simonneau G, Charbonnier B, Decousus H, et al. Subcutaneous low-molecular-weight heparin compared with continuous intravenous unfractionated heparin in the treatment of proximal deep vein thrombosis. *Arch Intern Med* 1993; 153:1541–1546.
116. Lindmarker P, Holmstrom M, Granqvist S, et al. Fragmin once daily subcutaneously in a fixed dose compared with continuous intravenous unfractionated heparin in the treatment of deep venous thrombosis. *Thromb Haemostas* 1993; 69:648.
117. Siragusa S, Cosmi B, Piovella F, et al. Low-molecular-weight heparins and unfractionated heparin in the treatment of patients with acute venous thromboembolism: Results of a meta-analysis. *Am J Med* 1996; 100:269–270.
118. Lensing AWA, Prins MH, Davidson BL, Hirsh J. Treatment of deep venous thrombosis with low-molecular-weight heparins: A meta-analysis. *Arch Intern Med* 1995; 155:601–607.

119. Leizorovicz A, Simonneau G, Decousus H, Boissel JP. Comparison of efficacy and safety of low molecular weight heparins and unfractionated heparin in initial treatment of deep venous thrombosis. *BMJ* 1994; 309:299–304.
120. O'Brien B, Levine M, Willan A, et al. Economic evaluation of outpatient treatment with low-molecular-weight heparin for proximal vein thrombosis. *Arch Intern Med* 1999; 159:2298–2304.
121. Kearon C, Gent M, Hirsh J, et al. A comparison of three months of anticoagulation with extended anticoagulation for a first episode of idiopathic venous thromboembolism. *N Engl J Med* 1999; 340:901–907.
122. The Global Use of Strategies to Open Occluded Coronary Arteries (GUSTO) IIB Investigators. A comparison of recombinant hirudin with heparin for the treatment of acute coronary syndromes. *N Engl J Med* 1996; 335:775–782.
123. Antman EM for the TIMI 9B Investigators. Hirudin in acute myocardial infarction: Thrombolysis and thrombin inhibition in MI (TIMI) 9B trial. *Circulation* 1996; 94:911–921.
124. Eriksson BI, Wille-Jorgensen P, Kalebo P, et al. A comparison of recombinant hirudin with a low-molecular-weight heparin to prevent thromboembolic complications after total hip replacement. *N Engl J Med* 1997; 337:1329–1335.
125. Gustafsson D, Elg M, Lenfors S, et al. Effects of inogatran, a new low molecular weight thrombin inhibitor, in rat models of venous and arterial thrombosis, thrombolysis and bleeding time. *Blood Coagul Fibrinolysis* 1996; 7:69–79.
126. Roux S, Tschopp T, Baumgartner HR. Effects of napsagatran, a new synthetic thrombin inhibitor and of heparin in a canine model of coronary artery thrombosis: Comparison with a ex vivo annular perfusion chamber model. *J Pharmacol Exp Ther* 1996; 277:71–78.
127. Valjii K, Arun K, Bookstein JJ. Use of a direct thrombin inhibitor (argatroban) during pulse-spray thrombolysis in experimental thrombosis. *J Vasc Intervent Radiol* 1995; 6:91–95.
128. Nicolini FA, Lee P, Malycky JL, et al. Selective inhibition of factor Xa during thrombolytic therapy markedly improves coronary artery patency in a canine model of coronary thrombosis. *Blood Coagul Fibrinolysis* 1996; 7:39–48.
129. Abildgaard U. Relative roles of tissue factor pathway inhibitor and antithrombin in the control of thrombogenesis. *Blood Coagul Fibrinolysis* 1995; 6(suppl 1):S45–S49.
130. Pineo GF, Hull RD. Thrombin inhibitors as anticoagulant agents. *Curr Opin Hematol* 1999; 6:298–303.
131. Kelton JG, Sheridan D, Santos A, et al. Heparin-associated thrombocytopenia: Laboratory studies. *Blood* 1988; 79:925–930.
132. Amiral J, Bridey F, Dreyfus M, et al. Platelet factor 4 complexed to heparin is the target for antibodies generated in heparin-induced thrombocytopenia. *Thromb Haemost* 1992; 68:95–96.
133. Visentin GP, Ford SE, Scott JP, Aster RH. Antibodies from patients with heparin-induced thrombocytopenia/thrombosis are specific for platelet factor 4 complexed with heparin or bound to endothelial cells. *J Clin Invest* 1994; 93:81–88.
134. Warkentin TE, Levine MN, Hirsh J, et al. Heparin-induced thrombocytopenia in patients treated with low-molecular-weight heparin or unfractionated heparin. *N Engl J Med* 1995; 332:1330–1335.
135. Warkentin TE. Heparin-induced thrombocytopenia: A ten-year retrospective. *Annu Rev Med* 1999; 50:129–147.
136. Greenfield LJ. Vena caval interruption and pulmonary embolectomy. *Clin Chest Med* 1984; 5:495–505.
137. Becker DM, Philbrick JT, Selby JB. Inferior vena cava filters: Indications, safety, effectiveness. *Arch Intern Med* 1992; 152: 1985–1994.
138. Hughes GC, Smith TP, Eachempati SR, et al. The use of a temporary vena caval interruption device in high-risk trauma patients unable to receive standard venous thromboembolism prophylaxis. *J Trauma* 1999; 46:246–249.
139. Johnson AJ, McCarthy WR. The lysis of artificially induced intravascular clots in man by intravenous infusion of streptokinase. *J Clin Invest* 1959; 38:1627–1643.
140. Miller GAH, Gibson RV, Sutton GC. Treatment of pulmonary embolism with streptokinase. *BMJ* 1969; 1:812–815.
141. Sasahara AA, Cannilla JE, Belks JJ, et al. Urokinase therapy in clinical pulmonary embolism. *N Engl J Med* 1969; 277:1168–1173.
142. NIH: Symposium: Thrombolytic therapy in thrombosis: A National Institutes of Health Consensus Development Conference. *Ann Intern Med* 1980; 93:141–143.
143. Goldhaber SZ, Kessler CM, Heit J, et al. A randomized controlled trial of recombinant tissue plasminogen activator versus urokinase in the treatment of acute pulmonary embolism. *Lancet* 1988; 2:293–298.
144. Witty LA, Steinfeld AD, Tapson VF. Thrombolytic therapy in acute pulmonary embolism: Physician attitudes. *Arch Intern Med* 1994; 154:1601–1604.
145. Goldhaber SZ. Evolving concepts in thrombolytic therapy for pulmonary embolism. *Chest* 1992; 101(suppl):183S–185S.
146. Goldhaber SZ, Haire WD, Feldstein ML, et al. Alteplase versus heparin in acute pulmonary embolism: Randomized trial assessing right ventricular function and pulmonary perfusion. *Lancet* 1993; 341:507–510.
147. Nass N, McConnell MV, Goldhaber SZ, et al. Recovery of regional right ventricular function after thrombolysis for pulmonary embolism. *Am J Cardiol* 1999; 83:804–806.
148. Leeper KV Jr, Popovich J Jr, Lesser BA, et al. Treatment of massive acute pulmonary embolism. The use of low doses of intrapulmonary arterial streptokinase combined with full doses of systemic heparin. *Chest* 1988; 93:234–240.
149. The UKEP study. Multicentre clinical trial on two local regimens of urokinase in massive pulmonary embolism. *Eur Heart J* 1987; 8:2–10.
150. Verstraete M, Miller GAH, Bounameaux H, et al. Intravenous and intrapulmonary recombinant tissue-type plasminogen activator in the treatment of acute massive pulmonary embolism. *Circulation* 1988; 77:353–360.
151. Rogers LQ, Lutcher CL. Streptokinase therapy for deep vein thrombosis: A comprehensive review of the literature. *Am J Med* 1990; 88:389–395.
152. Sane DC, Califf RM, Topol EJ, et al. Bleeding during thrombolytic therapy for acute myocardial infarction: Mechanisms and management. *Ann Intern Med* 1989; 111:1010–1022.
153. Gore JM. Prevention of severe neurologic events in the thrombolytic era. *Chest* 1992; 101:124S–130S.
154. Dalen JE, Alpert JS, Hirsh J. Thrombolytic therapy for pulmonary embolism. Is it safe? Is it effective? *Arch Intern Med* 1997; 157:2550–2556.
155. Tapson VF, Gurbel PA, Royster R, et al. Pharmacomechanical thrombolysis of experimental pulmonary emboli: Rapid low-dose intraembolic therapy. *Chest* 1994; 106:1558–1562.
156. Tapson VF, Davidson CJ, Bauman R, et al. Rapid thrombolysis of massive pulmonary emboli without systemic fibrinogenolysis: Intra-embolic infusion of thrombolytic therapy. *Am Rev Respir Dis* 1992; 145:A719.
157. Greenfield LJ, Kimmell GO, McCurdy WC. Transvenous removal of pulmonary emboli by vacuum-cup catheter technique. *J Surg Res* 1969; 9:347–352.
158. Timsit JF, Reynaud P, Meyer G, Sors H. Pulmonary embolectomy by catheter device in massive PE. *Chest* 1991; 100:655–658.
159. Semba CP, Dake MD. Iliofemoral deep venous thrombosis: Aggressive therapy with catheter-directed thrombolysis. *Radiology* 1994; 191:487–494.
160. Mewissen MW, Seabrook GR, Meissner MH, et al. Catheter-directed thrombolysis for lower extremity deep venous thrombosis: Report of a national multicenter registry. *Radiology* 1999; 211:39–49.

161. Gray HH, Morgan JM, Paneth M, Miller GAH. Pulmonary embolectomy: Indications and results. *Br Heart J* 1987; 57:572.
162. Tapson VF, Witty LA. Massive pulmonary embolism: Diagnostic and therapeutic strategies. *Clin Chest Med* 1996; 16:329.
163. Jardin F, Genevray B, Brun-ney D, Margairaz A. Dobutamine: a hemodynamic evaluation in pulmonary embolism shock. *Crit Care Med* 1985; 13:1009–1012.
164. Manier G, Castaing Y. Influence of cardiac output on oxygen exchange in acute pulmonary embolism. *Am Rev Respir Dis* 1992; 145:130–136.
165. Shure D. Chronic thromboembolic pulmonary hypertension: Diagnosis and treatment. *Semin Respir Crit Care Med* 1996; 17:7.
166. Fedullo PF, Auger WR, Channick RN, et al. Chronic thromboembolic pulmonary hypertension. *Clin Chest Med* 1995; 16: 353–374.

CHAPTER 54

CHRONIC COR PULMONALE

John H. Newman

DEFINITION

Cor pulmonale is a term that describes the pathologic effects of lung dysfunction on the right side of the heart. Pulmonary hypertension is the link between lung dysfunction and the heart in cor pulmonale. Cor pulmonale occurs as a late manifestation of many diseases of the lung, but the common thread in each case is increased right ventricular afterload. Cor pulmonale can be an elusive clinical diagnosis because pulmonary hypertension can exist without clinical manifestations and because clinical signs, such as dyspnea, may be shared with the underlying disease. Acute pulmonary hypertension leads to acute dilatation of the right ventricle; chronic pulmonary hypertension leads to ventricular hypertrophy followed by dilatation. The presence of overt right-sided heart failure is not essential to make the diagnosis of cor pulmonale, but right-sided heart failure is a common consequence. The clinical manifestations of cor pulmonale relate to alterations in cardiac output, salt and water homeostasis, and in most cases, gas exchange in the lung. Right-sided heart dysfunction secondary to left-sided heart failure, valvular dysfunction, or congenital heart disease is excluded in the definition of cor pulmonale.[1] Pulmonary venous obstruction is a cause of cor pulmonale; pulmonary venoocclusive disease is usually considered in the spectrum of primary pulmonary hypertension.

As a concept, cor pulmonale was introduced over 200 years ago, but the exact origin of the term is uncertain.[2] Osler[3] commented in the first edition of his textbook that "hypertrophy of the right ventricle . . . results from increased resistance in the pulmonary circulation, as in cirrhosis of the lung and emphysema." McGinn and White[4] apparently were the first to use the term *acute cor pulmonale* in the discussion of a case of acute, massive thromboembolism in 1935. William Harvey's discussion of the relationship of the lung and right side of the heart in *De Motu Cordis*[5] showed remarkable insight into the limitations of the right ventricle.

INCIDENCE, ETIOLOGIES, AND PATHOLOGY

Emphysema and chronic bronchitis cause over 50 percent of cases of cor pulmonale in the United States. The prevalence of cor pulmonale is difficult to determine because cor pulmonale does not occur in all cases of chronic lung disease and because routine physical examination and laboratory tests are relatively insensitive to the presence of pulmonary hypertension. The prevalence of chronic obstructive lung disease in the United States is about 15 million, directly resulting in approximately 70,000 deaths per year and contributing to about 160,000 other deaths.[6] It has been estimated that cor pulmonale accounts for 5 to 10 percent of organic heart disease. Cor pulmonale was present in 20 to 30 percent of admissions for heart failure in one study.[7] It is likely that cor pulmonale is a complication in a high percentage of cases. Gazes[8] found that 9.2 percent of cases of heart disease that came to autopsy had right heart abnormalities.

Chronic cor pulmonale occurs most frequently in adult male smokers, although the incidence in women is increasing as heavy smoking in females becomes more prevalent. A list of all diseases that may lead to cor pulmonale would be extensive and is not included in this chapter, but the major types of disease processes are listed in Table 54-1. Two important causes of cor pulmonale, thromboembolism and primary pulmonary hypertension, are discussed in Chaps. 52 and 53.

Chronic Obstructive Pulmonary Disease

Chronic obstructive pulmonary disease (COPD) causes cor pulmonale through several interrelated mechanisms, including hypoventilation, hypoxemia from ventilation-perfusion ($\dot{V}/\dot{Q}$) mismatch, and reduction of perfused surface area.[9,10] Patients with more prominent hypoxemia and alveolar hypoventilation develop erythrocytosis, edema, and early onset of cor pulmonale ("blue bloaters").[10] Patients in whom dyspnea on exertion is

TABLE 54-1 Etiologies of Chronic Cor Pulmonale by Mechanism of Pulmonary Hypertension

I. Hypoxic vasoconstriction
   A. Chronic bronchitis and emphysema, cystic fibrosis
   B. Chronic hypoventilation
      1. Obesity
      2. Sleep apnea
      3. Neuromuscular disease
      4. Chest wall dysfunction
   C. High-altitude dwelling and chronic mountain sickness (Monge's disease)
II. Occlusion of the pulmonary vascular bed
   A. Pulmonary thromboembolism, parasitic ova, tumor emboli
   B. Primary pulmonary hypertension
   C. Pulmonary venocclusive disease/pulmonary capillary hemangioma
   D. Sickle cell disease/sickle crisis/marrow embolism
   E. Fibrosing mediastinitis, mediastinal tumor
   F. Pulmonary angiitis from systemic disease
      1. Collagen vascular diseases
      2. Drug-induced lung disease
      3. Necrotizing and granulomatous arteritis
III. Parenchymal disease with loss of vascular surface area
   A. Bullous emphysema, $alpha_1$ antiproteinase deficiency, hyperinflation
   B. Diffuse bronchiectasis, cystic fibrosis
   C. Diffuse interstitial disease
      1. Pneumoconiosis
      2. Sarcoid, idiopathic pulmonary fibrosis, histiocytosis X
      3. Tuberculosis, chronic fungal infection
      4. Adult respiratory distress syndrome
      5. Collagen vascular disease (autoimmune lung disease)
      6. Hypersensitivity pneumonitis

the most prominent symptom have less hypoventilation and less hypoxemia at rest and therefore develop cor pulmonale later ("pink puffers"). Some of the differences between blue bloaters and pink puffers may relate to ventilatory drives; patients with low drives may be more likely to fit the blue-bloater category, whereas pink puffers strive to maintain normal arterial pH and gas tensions.[12] Another hypothesis is that blue bloaters have more inflammatory bronchitis and that pink puffers suffer more from pure emphysema.[10] *Physical examination* in advanced COPD shows an increase in the thoracic diameter, flattened diaphragms, hyperresonance to percussion, decreased breath sounds with expiratory wheezes, distant heart sounds, distended neck veins during expiration, and a palpable liver. Liver enlargement and leg edema are manifestations of fluid retention, and right-sided heart failure and may or may not be present. The *chest roentgenogram* may show characteristic changes of emphysema such as hyperlucent lungs, bullae, increased anteroposterior (AP) diameter, and flattened diaphragms. In some cases, increased bronchovascular markings and air bronchograms suggest the presence of thickened or inflamed airways. On the other hand, the chest roentgenogram may not show characteristic findings or be indicative of the severity of the physiologic impairment. Pulmonary function tests show an increased residual volume and total lung capacity, decreased forced vital capacity (FVC), and markedly decreased expiratory flow rates (FEV_1, FEF_{25-75}). Arterial blood studies at rest can be normal when disease is mild but in severe disease show decreased P_{O_2}, increased P_{CO_2}, and decreased pH. With cor pulmonale, P_{O_2} is likely to be below 55 mmHg. Desaturation increases with exercise and frequently during sleep. The $\dot{V}/\dot{Q}$ inequality and alveolar hypoventilation both contribute to the hypoxemia. A P_{CO_2} above 45 mmHg at rest defines net alveolar hypoventilation. Asthma is a form of COPD that rarely, if ever, leads to chronic cor pulmonale, probably because asthma is usually a disease of intermittent airways obstruction.

Cor pulmonale in COPD is related to the severity of lung dysfunction, and pulmonary hypertension is a manifestation of advanced disease. Exercise limitation in COPD is usually due to limitation of ventilatory capacity, not cardiac reserve, although sedentary patients develop deconditioning, which reduces exercise performance. No single test of lung function—such as spirometry, lung volumes, carbon monoxide diffusing capacity (DL_{CO}), blood gas tension, or radiography—is highly predictive of cor pulmonale because abnormalities such as reduced surface area and hypoxic vasoconstriction add independently to pulmonary artery pressure.[10]

Diffuse Interstitial Lung Disease

These patients have dyspnea, tachypnea, exercise intolerance, and occasionally clubbing of the digits. Basilar crackles are heard frequently on auscultation of the chest and may persist throughout inspiration. The *chest roentgenogram* shows diffuse reticular, reticulonodular, or fibrotic lesions, but the appearance does not always correlate well with physiologic impairment. In some disease presentations, such as desquamative interstitial pneumonitis, there may be an alveolar filling pattern with air bronchograms. A lung biopsy frequently is required to identify the basic pathologic process, and even then the exact etiology may not always be determined. Transbronchial biopsy can be diagnostic in some interstitial diseases such as sarcoidosis, and bronchoalveolar lavage may point to a diagnosis in many cases.[13] *Pulmonary function tests* show a restrictive process with reduced lung volumes, decreased compliance, and decreased diffusing capacity without airway obstruction. The vital capacity is reduced, and the forced expiratory volume in 1 s (FEV_1) as a percentage of FVC is usually at least 80 percent. At first, P_{O_2} decreases during exercise but is kept at normal levels at rest by hyperventilation. As the disease becomes more severe, P_{O_2} is low at rest. The course and prognosis of interstitial lung disease depend on the specific etiology, and there is wide variation among and within diseases.[13]

The presence of cor pulmonale in interstitial lung disease implies extensive lung dysfunction, perhaps with vascular involvement (as in systemic lupus erythematosus), and cor pulmonale may not occur even in end-stage disease. Treatment of idiopathic pulmonary fibrosis frequently is unsatisfactory despite the use of high-dose corticosteroids and either cyclophosphamide or azathiopirine. Recent trials using interferon-alpha with corticosteroids show promise of improved efficacy.[14]

Hypoventilation Syndromes

Some disorders (i.e., kyphoscoliosis) may impair or restrict mechanisms of ventilation, causing general alveolar hypoventilation and alveolar hypoxia.[15] Extreme obesity may be associated with hypoventilation, cyanosis, polycythemia, and somnolence (without intrinsic lung disease), often called the *pickwickian syndrome*.[16] Patients with daytime somnolence, morning headaches, and personality disturbances have been found to have periodic apnea during sleep associated with sleep deprivation, loud snoring, hypoxemia, and hypercapnia caused by upper airway obstruction (i.e., by the tongue, enlarged tonsils, or collapse of pharyngeal walls). Brainstem abnormalities such as Arnold-Chiari malformation also may cause respiratory center depression and primary hypoventilation. Neuromuscular diseases such as postpolio syndrome and chronic Guillain-Barré syndrome may present with cor pulmonale and right-sided heart failure.[17] Diagnosis of hypoventilation is confirmed by blood gas analysis, a depressed ventilatory response to inhaled CO_2, tests of pulmonary hypoventilation, or sleep studies. It has become apparent that disordered ventilation during sleep is a major component of many hypoventilation syndromes.[18] In all cases of hypoventilation, the main stimulus for pulmonary hypertension is hypoxic vasoconstriction, a response of the pulmonary arterioles to alveolar hypoxia. The respiratory acidosis that may accompany hypoventilation augments the vasoconstrictor response to hypoxia. Noninvasive assisted nocturnal ventilation with continuous positive airway pressure (CPAP), with or without added O_2 is the most efficacious therapy in most patients with nocturnal hypoventilation.[17]

Pulmonary Vascular Disease

Chronic cor pulmonale is a consequence of several diseases that involve the pulmonary vessels. Primary pulmonary hypertension and recurrent (or unresolved) pulmonary emboli are described in detail in Chaps. 59 and 60. Sickle cell disease, from SS or SC hemoglobinopathy, can cause cor pulmonale after multiple episodes of pulmonary infarction from focal pulmonary sickling, fat embolism, or thromboembolism.[18,19] Pulmonary venoocclusive disease is a rare disease of the pulmonary veins that presents with pulmonary hypertension and variable pulmonary infiltrates. It occasionally occurs in human immune deficiency virus (HIV) infection and after bone marrow transplantation.[20]

Cirrhosis of the liver is usually associated with pulmonary vasodilatation, but occasionally a disorder clinically and pathologically identical to primary pulmonary hypertension emerges.[21] HIV infection is a new cause of pulmonary vascular disease resembling primary pulmonary hypertension.[22] Collagen-vascular disease can cause cor pulmonale by primary vasculitis as well as by diffuse interstitial fibrosis. Systemic sclerosis, systemic lupus erythematosus (SLE), and rheumatoid arthritis (RA) are the collagen-vascular diseases that most commonly cause pulmonary arteritis. Patients with SLE and RA frequently present with primary interstitial lung disease. Occasionally, the presentation is that of cor pulmonale without interstitial disease but with primary pulmonary arteritis.[23] Cor pulmonale is not reported as a feature of Goodpasture's syndrome or idiopathic pulmonary hemosiderosis. Historically, dietary pulmonary hypertension has occurred as a result of the use of Aminorex in Europe, contaminated canola oil in Spain, and in eosinophilia myalgia syndrome in the United States related to contaminated tryptophan.[24] The new anorectic drug dexfenfluramine has caused pulmonary hypertension in France and recently has been banned in the United States by the Food and Drug Administration (FDA) because of its association with primary pulmonary hypertension and perhaps valvular dysfunction.[25]

PATHOPHYSIOLOGY

Increased pulmonary vascular resistance (PVR) and pulmonary hypertension are central mechanisms in all cases of cor pulmonale.[10] Physiologic mechanisms of pulmonary arterial pressure are shown in Table 54-2. These variables can be described in part by Poiseuille's law. Fortunately, most pulmonary diseases and disorders do not produce enough pulmonary hypertension to cause cor pulmonale.

Normal Pulmonary Circulation

The primary function of this unique high-flow, low-pressure, low-resistance system is to provide blood for gas exchange, and it is ideally structured for this function. It receives and transmits the entire cardiac output at low hydrostatic pressures primarily because of three characteristics: (1) the pulmonary arteries are thin-walled with little resting muscular tone, (2) there is negligible vasomotor control by the autonomic nervous system at rest in the adult, and (3) many small arterioles and alveolar capillaries produce a high surface area that can be recruited when needed to expand the pulmonary vascular bed, resulting in a decreased PVR. Normal mean pulmonary artery pressure (PAP) is about 12 to 17 mmHg; PAP above 20 mmHg at rest

TABLE 54-2 Genesis of Pulmonary Vascular Pressure: Poiseuille's Law

$$\text{Ppa} = \text{CO}\left(\frac{8}{\pi} \times n \times \frac{1}{N} \times \frac{1}{r^4}\right) + \text{Pla}$$

Flow = cardiac output (usually ↑ elevated in COPD; if PRV is fixed. ↑ CO will ↑ PAP).

$\frac{8}{\pi}$ = numerical constant related to tubular structure of vessels.

n = blood viscosity (increased in polycythemia vera, secondary erythrocytosis, and cryoglobulinemia).

N = number of perfused vessels of a particular radius. N is decreased in any occlusive or destructive disease (see Table 61-1). N for pulmonary capillaries is >200 million.

$\frac{1}{r^4}$ = radius of a vessel is a critical determinant of flow (r is decreased by vasoconstriction, luminal obstruction, or hyperinflation. A change in r from 1 to 2 units changes resistance 16-fold).

Pla = left atrial pressure. Passive pulmonary hypertension can result from left atrial pressure elevation due to either LV or valvular disease.

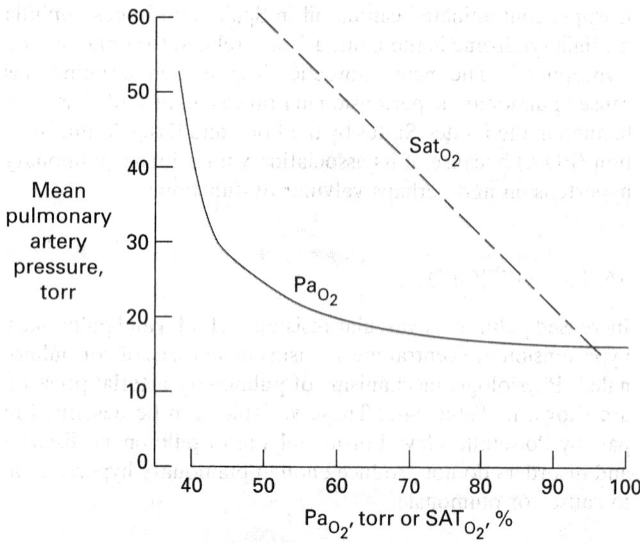

FIGURE 54-1 Pulmonary arterial pressure as a function of Pa_{O_2} or oxyhemoglobin saturation in humans. Pulmonary arterial pressure rises sharply as Pa_{O_2} decreases below 55 mmHg. (Redrawn from Reeves JT, Grover RF. High altitude pulmonary hypertension and pulmonary edema. *Prog Cardiol* 1975; 4:105, and from Burrows B. Anaerobic infections of the lung and pleural space. *Am Rev Respir Dis* 1974; 110:64, with permission.)

suggests pulmonary hypertension. Flow of blood from the main pulmonary artery (PA) through the pulmonary capillaries to the left atrium is accomplished by a pressure drop of only 5 to 9 mmHg, compared with an arterial-to-venous gradient of 90 mmHg in the systemic circuit. Thus normal PVR is 10- to 20-fold less than systemic vascular resistance.

Pulmonary Hypertension

The effective cross-sectional area of the pulmonary vascular bed must be reduced by 25 to 50 percent before any change in PAP can be detected at rest. Exercise causes increased PAP because of increased pulmonary blood flow in the normal bed, and exercise will dramatically raise PAP if the vascular bed is reduced. Obliterative vascular diseases increase PVR by vascular luminal occlusion, whereas diffuse interstitial diseases act primarily by compression and obliteration of small vessels. Hyperinflation in COPD increases PVR partly by compressing intraalveolar vessels, reducing the cross-sectional area of the bed. It is now well established, however, that arteriolar constriction resulting from alveolar hypoxia is the predominant cause of pulmonary hypertension in chronic airways diseases.[1,10,26,27]

PULMONARY ARTERIOLAR CONSTRICTION

The most important cause of pulmonary vasoconstriction is alveolar hypoxia. The mechanism of hypoxic pulmonary vasoconstriction is unknown. It is thought to be due either to mediator release from some unknown effector cell or a direct action of hypoxia on pulmonary vascular smooth muscle K channels.[28,29] The degree of hypoxic vasoconstriction depends primarily on the alveolar P_{O_2}, and when alveolar P_{O_2} is less than 55 mmHg, PAP rises sharply (Fig. 54-1). When PAP is greater than 40 mmHg due to hypoxia, arterial oxygen saturation is very likely less than 75 percent.[26] There is large individual variability in the hypoxic pressor response, and hypoxic vasoconstriction is enhanced by acidosis and blunted by alkalosis. Acidosis also has a mild direct pressor effect on the pulmonary circulation.[28] Extensive investigations into the mechanism of hypoxic vasoconstriction have shown that many local and circulating mediators of pulmonary vascular tone are capable of modulating the hypoxic pressor response but that no single mediator yet discovered is solely or predominantly responsible[28] (Table 54-3).

Hypoxic vasoconstriction in a region of lung where ventilation is diminished probably serves to maximize net arterial oxygenation by diverting blood from the hypoxic region to better-ventilated areas. Because the pulmonary vascular bed is capable of significant recruitment, localized hypoxic vasoconstriction does not cause pulmonary hypertension. Generalized hypoxia causes generalized hypoxic vasoconstriction and the development of pulmonary hypertension (Fig. 54-2). In COPD, the first episodes of alveolar hypoxia may occur during sleep, and it gradually becomes more prevalent thereafter.[30] Any cause of alveolar hypoventilation (see Table 54-1) can result in chronic cor pulmonale through the mechanism of hypoxic pulmonary vasoconstriction, including entities as different as diffuse emphysema and kyphoscoliosis[9,15] (see also Chap. 59).

OTHER CONTRIBUTIONS TO PULMONARY HYPERTENSION

Increases in cardiac output and blood volume or direct effects of acidosis and/or hypoxia on the myocardium may contribute to pulmonary hypertension. Increased blood flow such as occurs with exercise engenders an increased PAP, and in such a situation, the effects of hypoxia and acidosis also will be exaggerated.[26] Sustained or repetitive severe hypoxemia causes secondary erythrocytosis. Blood viscosity increases rapidly after the hematocrit exceeds about 55 percent, raising PVR and also decreasing cerebral function. If left ventricular failure (LVF) is superimposed on an already reduced pulmonary vascular bed, pulmonary hypertension will be augmented by elevated downstream left atrial pressure. Once established, pulmonary hypertension may be self-perpetuating. A sustained increase in PAP in patients with diffuse lung disease causes muscular hypertrophy in the walls of small arteries, with extension of muscle toward alveolar vessels, further increasing PVR and

TABLE 54-3 Endogenous Pulmonary Vasomotor Tone

Dilator	Constrictor
Beta-adrenergic	Alpha-adrenergic agonists
Histamine H_2	Histamine H_1
Prostacyclin (PGI_2), PGE_1	PGE_2, PGF_{1a}, Thromboxane A_2PGD_2
Acetylcholine*	Serotonin
Oxygen	Hypoxia
Bradykinin	Angiotensin II
Vasoactive intestinal polypeptide	Platelet activating factor
	Endothelin
Nitric oxide	Leukotriene C_4/D_4
Atrial natriuretic peptide	Vasopressin
Adenosine	

*The response of the pulmonary vascular bed is tone-dependent. When the pulmonary circulation is preconstricted, acetylcholine is a vasodilator through the release of endothelium-derived NO.

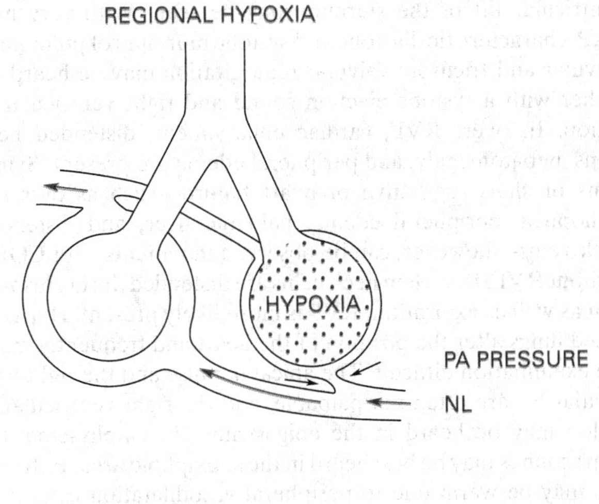

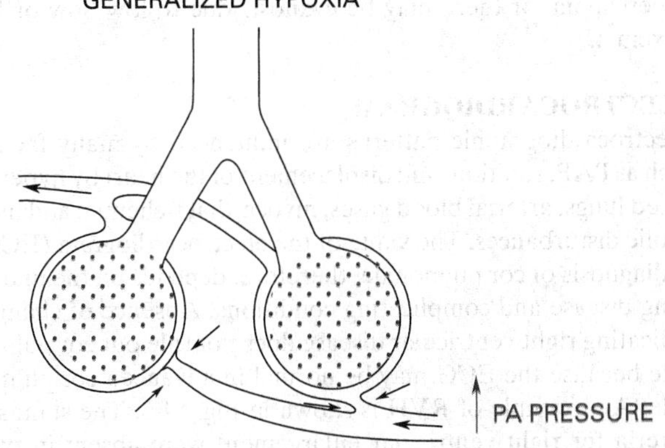

FIGURE 54-2 Hypoxic pulmonary vasoconstriction maximizes arterial oxygenation by diverting blood away from areas of regional hypoxia toward better-ventilated zones. Generalized hypoxia causes generalized hypoxic vasoconstriction and results in pulmonary hypertension. (From Newman JH. Pulmonary vascular reactivity in primary pulmonary edema. *Semin Respir Med* 1983; 4:299; reproduced with permission of the publisher. Courtesy of J. V. Weil.)

PAP. Chronic hypoxia alone results in muscularization of pulmonary arterioles and exaggerated increases in PAP with stimuli.[26,31]

Right Ventricular Response to Pulmonary Hypertension

The right ventricle is thin-walled and eccentric and better able to handle an increase in volume load than to meet an increased pressure load.[10] The primary cause of right ventricular strain and failure (RVF), therefore, is a chronic pressure load (afterload). Small increases in PAP may result in large increases in right ventricular work. Pulmonary hypertension at rest indicates a high baseline resistance, and small changes in blood flow will cause large increases in PAP.

Response of the right ventricle to pulmonary hypertension depends on the acuteness and severity of the pressure load. Acute cor pulmonale (see Chaps. 59 and 60) occurs after a sudden and severe stimulus (i.e., massive pulmonary emboli) with ventricular dilatation and failure but without hypertrophy. Acute cor pulmonale may develop within minutes to hours. Chronic cor pulmonale, however, is associated with a more slowly evolving and slowly progressive hypertension,[33] and the response involves increased protein synthesis and right ventricular hypertrophy (RVH).[34] The severity of the hypertension, the rapidity with which it becomes severe, and the possible eventual onset of RVF are influenced by factors that intercede intermittently, such as (1) *alterations in ventilatory function,* causing alveolar pressure changes with effects on chamber function, (2) *alterations in gas exchange,* with more or less severe hypoxemia, hypercapnia, and acidosis, and (3) *alterations in volume load,* as influenced by exercise, heart rate, polycythemia, or renal retention of salt and water associated with cor pulmonale. At some stage, the myocardium is unable to function at the high-pressure load, dilates, and fails. RVF may occur relatively early in some patients with chronic bronchitis and emphysema because of sustained hypoxemia and hypercarbia, but it occurs later in patients with diffuse interstitial lung disease because the degree of RVH helps to maintain blood flow even when PAP is high.[33] Extreme pulmonary hypertension and RVH can occur in normal persons living at high altitude (>10,000 ft, or 3033 m) with no evidence for heart failure.[34] Thus the right ventricle can develop into an efficient high-pressure pump over time and sustain normal function for months to years.

Left Ventricular Function in Cor Pulmonale

Dysfunction of the left ventricle occurs in some patients with cor pulmonale, but the evidence available indicates that cor pulmonale per se does not cause disease of the left side of the heart. The likelihood in most cases is that left-sided heart dysfunction coexisting with cor pulmonale results from other known causes, such as coronary ischemia or systemic hypertension. Left ventricular failure is a serious complication in cor pulmonale because the increase in left atrial pressure and in lung water further impairs lung function, increases the work of breathing, increases PAP, impairs gas exchange, and may induce respiratory failure. When underlying disease of the left ventricle is present, the direct effects of hypoxia, hypercapnia, and acidosis arising from primary lung disease may precipitate left ventricular failure.[10,35,36]

Several lines of evidence point to mechanical effects of lung dysfunction and right ventricular dilatation on performance of the left ventricle.[36,37] Wide swings in transpulmonary pressure in obstructive lung disease can reduce left ventricular filling and increase left ventricular afterload.[38] Hypertrophy and elevated end-diastolic pressure of the right ventricle in cor pulmonale can reduce left ventricular compliance and impair left ventricular filling through effects on the shared ventricular septum.[39] Despite these effects, most patients with chronic cor pulmonale demonstrate normal resting cardiac output, normal pulmonary artery wedge pressure, and normal resting left ventricular ejection fraction.[40] The majority of patients with abnormal left ventricular ejection fraction in either compensated or decompensated chronic lung disease probably have demonstrable coronary artery disease.

Edema Formation and Cor Pulmonale

Peripheral edema occurs in some cases of chronic cor pulmonale. The mechanism of edema formation is poorly understood but is probably related to increased systemic venous pressure, hypercarbia, and hypoxemia.[10,41] The presence of pulmonary hypertension per se does not appear to be sufficient to cause fluid retention until right atrial pressure becomes elevated. Decreased clearance of aldosterone from the passively congested liver contributes to salt retention but is likely not an initiating event. Plasma volume is increased, however, in chronic cor pulmonale.[10]

Hypercarbia stimulates plasma renin activity, and hypercarbic, edematous patients with COPD have increased plasma levels of aldosterone and antidiuretic hormone.[42,43] This pattern occurs despite oxygen therapy in these patients. Thus not only increased salt retention but also impaired water excretion contributes to edema in chronic hypercapnia. Atrial natriuretic peptide is elevated in cor pulmonale in response to elevated right atrial pressure and perhaps acidosis.[10] Severe hypoxemia is associated with reduced renal blood flow and glomerular filtration rate and a decrease in urine sodium excretion.[10] Other mechanisms of edema formation are increased systemic capillary hydrostatic pressure, related to increased venous pressure and blood volume; and perhaps inappropriate release of arginine vasopressin.[10] Many mechanisms appear to be operating to produce edema in chronic cor pulmonale, several of which are related to the primary pulmonary dysfunction, especially in COPD. The exact mechanisms and sequence of events leading to edema are difficult to determine in any specific case. Pulmonary edema and pleural effusion are not seen as a consequence of chronic cor pulmonale.

CLINICAL MANIFESTATIONS OF COR PULMONALE

Symptoms

Clinical manifestations of cor pulmonale are often obscured by the signs and symptoms of underlying disease and therefore are closely related to the pulmonary disease or disorder. It is necessary first to recognize the type and severity of lung disease and then to look for cor pulmonale.

There is no history that is specific for cor pulmonale. Episodes of leg edema, atypical chest pain, dyspnea on exertion, exercise-induced peripheral cyanosis, prior respiratory failure, and excessive daytime somnolence are all historical clues suggesting the presence of cor pulmonale. Chest pain may be due to strain or distortion of the chest wall (musculoskeletal) or may be related to right ventricular ischemia. Cough and complaints of easy fatigability are common. Some patients with nocturnal hypoventilation and sleep apnea may present with personality changes, mild systemic hypertension, and headache. Shortness of breath is nearly a universal symptom in cor pulmonale. The degree of activity that leads to dyspnea should be quantified because patients reduce activities to avoid dyspnea. Thus the naive question of whether a patient is short of breath may lead to a negative reply because the patient is less and less active. Abdominal pain may result from liver and bowel congestion if RVF is present.

Physical Examination

The earliest signs are those associated with long-standing pulmonary hypertension. The most sensitive sign for pulmonary hypertension is an accentuated pulmonary component of S_2, which also may be palpable in the pulmonic area, and right ventricular lift of the sternum may be seen. With very high PAP, characteristic diastolic and systolic murmurs of pulmonary valvular and tricuspid valvular regurgitation may be heard together with a systolic ejection sound and right ventricular S_3 gallop. In overt RVF, cardiac enlargement, distended neck veins, hepatomegaly, and peripheral edema are present. Symptoms or signs suggestive of heart failure—such as dyspnea, orthopnea, peripheral edema, palpable liver, and distended neck veins—however, can be observed in patients with COPD without RVF. But when neck veins are distended during inspiration as well as expiration, RVF is more likely present. Hyperinflated lungs alter the position of the heart and frequently make the examination difficult. The apical impulse and the right ventricular lift are often not palpable, and the right ventricular S_3 gallop may be heard in the epigastrium. In emphysema, the heart sounds may be best heard in the subxiphoid area. Extremities may be warm due to peripheral vasodilatation caused by hypercapnia, or there may be cyanosis due to low flow or hypoxemia.

ELECTROCARDIOGRAM

Electrocardiographic patterns are influenced by many factors such as PAP, rotation, and displacement of the heart by hyperinflated lungs, arterial blood gases, myocardial ischemia, and metabolic disturbances. The value of the electrocardiogram (ECG) in diagnosis of cor pulmonale, therefore, depends on the underlying disease and complicating conditions. Absence of changes indicating right ventricular disease does not rule out cor pulmonale because the ECG may be normal in advanced cor pulmonale. An example of RVH is shown in Fig. 54-3. The standard criteria for right ventricular enlargement were absent in two-thirds of patients with COPD who had RVH on postmortem examination.[1] It has been suggested that when classic RVH changes are absent, diagnosis should be based on the combination of rS in V_5 to V_6, RAD, qR in aV_R, and P pulmonale.[44] Tall peaked P waves in leads II and aV_F may reflect positional changes rather than right atrial enlargement. Right bundle-branch block occurs in about 15 percent of patients. A pattern of S_1, Q_3, and T_3 carries reasonable sensitivity and specificity for cor pulmonale in COPD.[45] Arrhythmias are infrequent in uncomplicated cor pulmonale, but when present, they are mostly supraventricular and may reflect blood gas abnormalities, hypokalemia, or excess of drugs such as digitalis, theophylline, and beta agonists. Multifocal atrial tachycardia is associated with decompensated COPD and is best treated by attention to the underlying disease rather than by antiarrhythmic drugs. Ventricular arrhythmias, when they occur, are associated with a high mortality.

CHEST ROENTGENOGRAM

The radiographic findings of pulmonary hypertension in patients with normal lung parenchyma (such as in primary pulmonary hypertension) are well described[46,47] (Fig. 54-4). Most diseases that cause cor pulmonale have grossly abnormal chest roentgenograms, and the radiologic diagnosis of pulmonary hypertension in these diseases is more difficult. Right ventricular enlargement may be difficult to detect in the vertical heart of emphysema, and comparison with previous films may be helpful. In the most obvious cases of cor pulmonale, there is right ventricular and PA enlargement, but pulmonary hypertension precedes right ventricular dilatation. One indicator of pulmonary hypertension is measurement of the dimensions of the right and left PAs. Enlargement is considered to exist if the diameter of the right descending PA is greater than 16 mm and the left descending PA is greater than 18 mm.[48] These findings occurred in 43 of 46 patients with known pulmonary hypertension, but the true sensitivity and specificity of these measurements are not known.

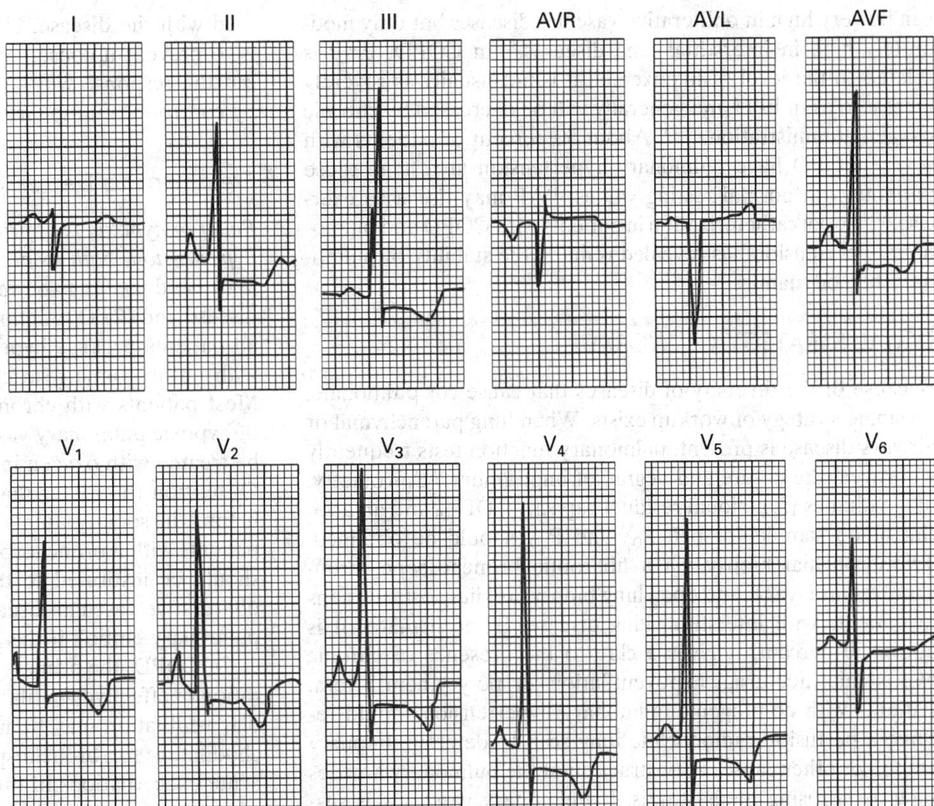

FIGURE 54-3 Electrocardiogram in a patient with cor pulmonale. The mean QRS axis is +120°. The tall, peaked P waves indicate right atrial enlargement. The tall R waves in leads V_1 to V_3 and deep S wave in V_6 and the associated T-wave changes indicate RVH. (From Voelkel NF, Reeves JT. Primary pulmonary hypertension. In: Moser KM, ed. *Pulmonary Vascular Diseases*. New York: Marcel Dekker; 1979; reproduced with permission of the publisher and the author. Courtesy of J. R. Pryor.)

ECHOCARDIOGRAM

Advances in echocardiography make this a useful test where cor pulmonale is suspected.[49] The standard M mode reliably detects right ventricular dilatation and is best able to display the anteriormost right ventricular wall near the interventricular septum. Two-dimensional echocardiography allows improved visualization of right ventricular chamber size and wall thickness, as well as changes in the interventricular septum resulting from RVH.[49,50] Because the right ventricle is asymmetric, measurement of right ventricular volume is difficult even with two-dimensional views. Right ventricular pressure overload usually is detected by hypertrophy of the anterior right ventricular wall and by dilatation of the chamber. Hypertrophy of the septum can be found, and paradoxical septal encroachment into the left ventricular chamber can be seen in severe cor pulmonale.[53] Right ventricular volume overload, as in atrial septal defect, causes dilatation as the predominant finding, often in association with abnormal ventricular septal motion.[51]

Echo-Doppler techniques have become the noninvasive standard to detect pulmonary hypertension and to measure cardiac output. These techniques are relatively accurate when PAP is above 30 mmHg, but they may not detect milder but pathologic pulmonary hypertension.[52–53] Echo Doppler is useful for longitudinal follow-up of pharmacologic treatment of pulmonary hypertension and cor pulmonale.

RIGHT-SIDED HEART CATHETERIZATION

Right-sided catheterization is the only technique available for the direct measurement of PAP, PA wedge pressure, and cardiac output. It is occasionally important in differentiating cor pulmonale from left ventricular dysfunction when the clinical presentation is confusing. This is especially true in patients with primary pulmonary hypertension (PPH) or unresolved pulmonary emboli, where airway function may appear normal, or with restrictive cardiomyopathy (see Chap. 75). In cor pulmonale, PA diastolic pressure is usually significantly higher than wedge pressure, unlike LVF or mitral stenosis, where the diastolic–wedge pressure gradient is smaller in most patients. Mean PAP

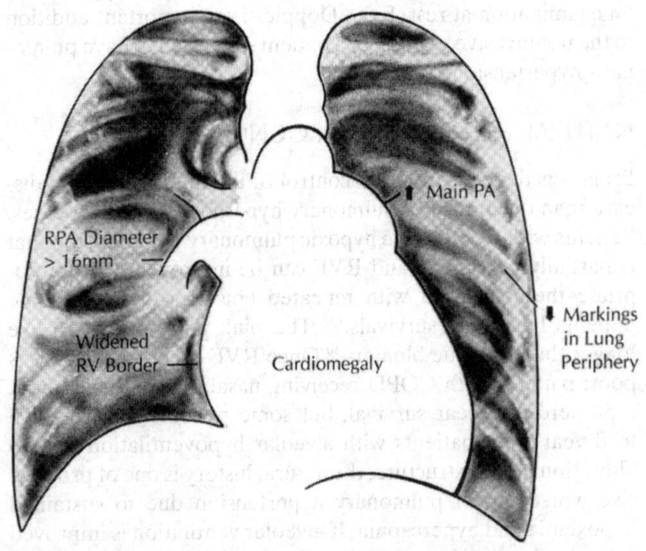

FIGURE 54-4 Classic features of the chest radiograph in severe pulmonary hypertension. The enlarged pulmonary arteries can be mistaken for hilar adenopathy, and the large main pulmonary artery obscures the aortic arch. Right descending PA diameter greater than 16 mm suggests severe pulmonary hypertension.

can be very high in obliterative vascular diseases but only moderately high in interstitial lung diseases.[36] In COPD, PAP is related to the level of hypoxemia; it is not usually as severely increased as in PPH and generally will be decreased by chronic oxygen administration.[26,54,55] About 50 percent of patients with severe COPD have pulmonary hypertension at rest; in those patients with normal resting values, PAP may rise with exercise.[10,54] Serial catheterization in patients with COPD and pulmonary hypertension has revealed remarkable stability of pulmonary hemodynamics.[56]

USUAL STRATEGY OF WORKUP

Because of the diversity of diseases that cause cor pulmonale, no single strategy of workup exists. When lung parenchymal or airways disease is present, pulmonary function tests frequently will reveal the nature and degree of impairment.[57] Spirometry, lung volumes (functional residual capacity), DL_{CO}, and an arterial blood sample for pH, P_{O_2}, and P_{CO_2} should be obtained. Transbronchial biopsy via a fiberoptic bronchoscope, bronchoalveolar lavage, and open lung biopsy are diagnostic options in patients with interstitial lung disease. If the hematocrit is above 50 percent, it gives a clue to the presence of chronic hypoxemia, nocturnal hypoventilation, or polycythemia vera. Patients with cryptogenic pulmonary hypertension should receive a perfusion radionuclide lung scan to detect pulmonary emboli or other causes of obstruction of the pulmonary arteries such as fibrosing mediastinitis. If pulmonary vasculitis is suspected, serum can be screened for the presence of antinuclear antibody, hepatitis B surface antigen, rheumatoid factor, and cryoglobulins. Factor V_{Leiden} is likely to be a frequent abnormality in thrombotic pulmonary hypertension,[58] and the antiphospholipid antibody syndrome may cause cor pulmonale.[59]

Polysomnography should be performed in patients with cor pulmonale and any sign or symptoms of sleep apnea. Exercise tests occasionally will reveal desaturation or ventilatory limitations that denote significant lung dysfunction not appreciated on examination at rest. Echo Doppler is an important addition to the noninvasive workup of a patient suspected to have pulmonary hypertension.

NATURAL HISTORY AND PROGNOSIS

Prognosis depends more on control of the underlying lung disease than on control of pulmonary hypertension in most cases. Patients with COPD have hypoxic pulmonary hypertension that is partially reversible, and RVF can be improved with appropriate therapy. Even with repeated episodes of RVF, some patients have long survivals.[1,10] The pink puffers tend to live longer than the blue bloaters.[10] Once RVF occurs, prognosis is poor; patients with COPD receiving nasal oxygen have about a 50 percent 2-year survival, but some patients survive for 5 to 8 years.[27] In patients with alveolar hypoventilation but no alteration in lung structure, the natural history is one of progressive worsening of pulmonary hypertension due to sustained hypoxemia and hypercapnia. If alveolar ventilation is improved prior to the development of nonreversible changes in vessel walls, the prognosis is good.

MEDICAL TREATMENT

The underlying lung disease is the focus of therapy and is the best way to reduce the right ventricular pressure work associated with the disease. If RVF has not appeared, a major goal is to prevent its onset. When it appears, it should be treated, but the response will be poor unless cardiac work is reduced by control of pulmonary hypertension.

Treatment to Decrease Pulmonary Hypertension

Relief of hypoxia is of prime importance in reducing pulmonary hypertension, both to prevent and to treat cor pulmonale. This may be done in two ways: (1) treatment of the underlying disease and (2) O_2 administration.[55] Neither will lower PAP in all patients because hypertension is often intractable in those with an anatomic restriction of the pulmonary vascular bed. Most patients with chronic cor pulmonale have a component of hypoxic pulmonary vasoconstriction, and all patients should be treated with oxygen in amounts adequate to restore arterial O_2 tension to greater than 60 mmHg. Corticosteroids may be helpful in some patients with interstitial lung disease and in patients with a bronchospastic component of COPD. Measures should be instituted to treat the systemic disease with which obliterative vascular disease is associated or to prevent further pulmonary emboli if this is the problem.

In COPD, the primary focus is relief of hypoxemia by restoration of effective ventilation or by O_2 administration. Net alveolar ventilation may be improved by therapy, including bronchodilators for bronchospasm, antibiotics to prevent or treat acute exacerbations of bronchitis, bronchial toilet for removal of secretions, and avoidance of airway irritants such as tobacco smoke. Nocturnal aspiration of gastric fluid is now known to be a common cause of exacerbation of chronic lung disease. Tranquilizers, sedatives, and narcotics should be avoided in unstable patients and patients with hypoventilation. Correction of hypoxia and acidosis may produce a striking reduction in PAP. In diseases that alter lung function but not structure, effective alveolar ventilation must be restored by treatment of the underlying disease or by use of mechanical ventilation. Short-term ventilatory stimulants may be useful in some cases of decreased ventilatory drives, although nasal CPAP has become the first choice in most cases of sleep apnea.[10]

Adequate oxygenation may prevent the onset of heart failure, both acutely and over a long period of time. Any patient with cor pulmonale and RVF should be given sufficient O_2 to restore P_{O_2} to levels above 60 mmHg, but it should be given cautiously when P_{CO_2} is high and the threat of respiratory acidosis is present. Oxygen therapy is usually well tolerated in patients with stable lung disease but not in patients with acute acidosis or respiratory muscle fatigue. When low-flow nasal O_2 causes significant increases in P_{CO_2}, mechanical ventilation may be required to relieve hypoxia. Studies have shown conclusively that home oxygen therapy, nocturnal or continuous, is beneficial in keeping patients with severe COPD functioning better for longer periods of time; it may be effective both in treating cor pulmonale and in postponing its onset.[27,55] Continuous 24 h/day oxygen therapy is the desired goal in most patients, because desaturation occurs during both sleep and physical activity.

Treatment of Heart Failure

Cor pulmonale is heart disease, and while treatment of the lung disease and relief of hypoxia are necessary to reduce cardiac work, general principles of management of heart failure apply. Diuretics and phlebotomy can be appropriate measures for treatment of RVF. Pulmonary vasodilators are efficacious in some patients with primary pulmonary hypertension but are of unproven value in cor pulmonale from COPD.[61]

Beneficial effects of digitalis are not as obvious as in LVF, and arrhythmias caused by digitalis may occur at relatively low serum levels in patients with hypoxia and acidosis. Susceptibility to digitalis intoxication is enhanced in pulmonary disease.[62] Its use in cor pulmonale therefore has been controversial. Nevertheless, studies have shown that *digitalis improves right ventricular function in cor pulmonale, and it is an appropriate drug for treatment of RVF when given cautiously and at carefully controlled dosage levels*.[63] It should not be used during the acute phases of respiratory insufficiency when there are large fluctuations in levels of hypoxemia and acidosis but is reserved for the time when the patient is stabilized. Heart rate in this setting cannot be used as a guide for the level of digitalization. It is also reasonable to question whether or not patients with cor pulmonale who continue to have overt RVF after relief of hypoxemia in intensive therapy for the underlying lung disease will benefit from the use of digitalis. Digitalis is appropriate if there is known or suspected concurrent left ventricular systolic dysfunction.

Vasodilator therapy to reduce right ventricular afterload has been recognized as a potential treatment strategy for several years. Vasodilator therapy has the disadvantage of being secondary therapy that is not aimed at the primary lung dysfunction. Vasodilator use has not become widespread because of small observed reductions in pulmonary hypertension and occasional worsening of gas exchange.[61]

Diuretics are effective in the treatment of RVF, and indications for their use are the same as in other forms of heart disease. Pulmonary function is improved by diuretics in patients with COPD who have hypervolemia.[64] The effects of diuretics should be monitored carefully by measurement of arterial P_{O_2}, P_{CO_2}, and pH because acid-base abnormalities are often present in cor pulmonale. Contraction alkalosis can be a problem in hypercarbic patients with a large buffer base who have had vigorous diuresis.

When the hematocrit is above 55 to 60 percent, phlebotomy may reduce PAP and PVR and possibly improve right ventricular function.[65] The phlebotomy should be in small volumes (200–300 mL) and done cautiously.

SURGICAL TREATMENT

There is no surgical treatment for most diseases that cause chronic cor pulmonale. Pulmonary embolectomy is extremely efficacious for unresolved pulmonary emboli causing chronic thrombotic pulmonary hypertension (see Chap. 60). Adenoidectomy in children with chronic airways obstruction and uvulopalatopharyngeoplasty in selected patients with sleep apnea can relieve cor pulmonale related to hypoventilation. Single-lung, double-lung, and heart-lung transplantations are all used for salvage in the terminal phase of several diseases complicated by cor pulmonale.[66] *The diseases most commonly treated by lung transplantation are primary pulmonary hypertension, emphysema, idiopathic pulmonary fibrosis, and cystic fibrosis.* Two-year survival for single- and double-lung transplant has risen to 60 percent, still lower than the approximately 80 percent for heart transplant alone. One interesting finding is that the right ventricle can recover function after lung transplant even after the chronic stress of severe pulmonary hypertension. Volume-reduction surgery for selected patients with emphysema improves ventilatory function and gas exchange, and the long-term benefit of this approach is under study.[67]

References

1. Palevsky HI, Fishman AP. Chronic cor pulmonale. *JAMA* 1990; 263:2347–2354.
2. Richards DW. The right heart and the lung with some observations on teleology: The J. Burns Amberson Lecture. *Am Rev Respir Dis* 1966; 94:691–702.
3. Osler W. *The Principles and Practice of Medicine*. New York: Appleton; 1892:628–640.
4. McGinn S, White PD. Acute cor pulmonale resulting from pulmonary embolism, its clinical recognition. *JAMA* 1935; 104:1473–1480.
5. Harvey W. *Exercitatio de Motu Cordis et Sanguinis in Animalibus*. Francofurti: Guilielem Fitzeri; 1628 (Leake CD, transl). Springfield, IL: Charles C Thomas; 1928.
6. Standards for the diagnosis and care of patients with chronic obstructive pulmonary disease: ATS statement. *Am J Respir Crit Care Med* 1995; 152(55):S77–S120.
7. A report of the Surgeon General. *Chronic Obstructive Lung Disease: The Health Consequences of Smoking*. Rockville, MD: U.S. Department of Health and Human Services; 1984:189.
8. Gazes PC. *Clinical Cardiology: A Bedside Approach*. Philadelphia: Lea & Febiger; 1990:301–320.
9. Thurlbeck WM. Pathophysiology of chronic obstructive pulmonary disease. *Clin Chest Med* 1990; 11:389–403.
10. MacNee W. Pathophysiology of cor pulmonale in chronic obstructive pulmonary disease. State of the art. *Am J Pulm Crit Care Med* 1994; 150(4):833–892, 1158–1163.
11. Jamal K, Fleetham JA, Thurlbeck WM. Cor pulmonale: Correlation with central airway lesions, peripheral airway lesions, emphysema and control of breathing. *Am Rev Respir Dis* 1990; 141:1172–1177.
12. Mountain R, Zwillich C, Weil J. Hypoventilation in obstructive lung disease. *N Engl J Med* 1978; 298:521–525.
13. Schwarz MI, King TE Jr, eds. *Interstitial Lung Diseases*. St Louis: Mosby–Year Book; 1998.
14. Ziesche R, Hofbauer E, Wittman K, et al. A preliminary study of long-term IF gamma 1-b and low dose prednisolone in pulmonary fibrosis. *N Engl J Med* 1999; 341:1264–1270.
15. Bergofsky EH. Respiratory failure in disorders of the thoracic cage. *Am Rev Respir Dis* 1979; 119:643–669.
16. Burwell CS, Robin ED, Whaley RD, Bickelmann AG. Extreme obesity associated with alveolar hypoventilation—A Pickwickian syndrome. *Am J Med* 1956; 21:811–818.
17. Strohl KP, Rogers RM. Obstructive sleep apnea. *N Engl J Med* 1996; 334:99–104.
18. Gerry JL, Buckley BH, Hutchins GM. Clinicopathologic analysis of cardiac dysfunction in 52 patients with sickle cell anemia. *Am J Cardiol* 1978; 42:211–216.
19. Weil JV, Castro O, Malik AB, et al. Pathogenesis of lung disease in sickle hemoglobinopathies. *Am Rev Respir Dis* 1993; 148:249–256.
20. Swenson SJ, Tashjian JH, Myers JL, et al. Pulmonary veno-occlusive disease: CT findings in eight patients. *AJR* 1996; 167:937–940.
21. Lange PA, Stoller JK. The hepatopulmonary syndrome. *Ann Intern Med* 1995; 122:521–529.
22. Coplan N, Shinony R, Ioachim H. Primary pulmonary hypertension associated with human immunodeficiency viral infection. *Am J Med* 1990; 89:96–99.
23. Winslow TM, Ossipov MA, Fazio GP, et al. Five year follow-up of the prevalence and progression of pulmonary hypertension in systemic lupus erythematosus. *Am Heart J* 1995; 129:510–515.
24. Brenot F, Simonneau G. Risk factors for primary pulmonary hypertension. In: Rubin LJ, Rich S, eds. *Primary Pulmonary Hyper-*

tension, Vol 99: *Lung Biology in Health and Disease*. New York: Marcel Dekker; 1997:131–147.
25. Mark EJ, Patalas ED, Chang HT, et al. Fatal pulmonary hypertension associated with short term use of fenfluramine and phentermine. *N Engl J Med* 1997; 337:602–606.
26. Burrows B. Arterial oxygenation and pulmonary hemodynamics in patients with chronic airways obstruction. *Am Rev Respir Dis* 1974; 110(suppl):64–70.
27. Nocturnal Oxygen Therapy Trial Group. Continuous or nocturnal oxygen therapy in hypoxemic chronic obstructive lung disease: A clinical trial. *Ann Intern Med* 1980; 93:391–398.
28. Voelkel N. Mechanisms of hypoxic pulmonary vasoconstriction. *Am Rev Respir Dis* 1986; 133:1186.
29. Michelakis ED, Archer SL, Weir EK. Acute hypoxic pulmonary vasoconstriction: A model of O_2 sensing. *Physiol Res* 1995; 44:361–367.
30. Douglas NJ, Flenley DC. Breathing during sleep in patients with obstructive lung disease. *Am Rev Respir Dis* 1990; 141:1065–1070.
31. Enson Y. Pulmonary heart disease: Relation of pulmonary hypertension to abnormal lung structure and function. *Bull NY Acad Med* 1977; 53:551–566.
32. Meerson FX. *The Failing Heart: Adaptation and Maladaptation*. New York: Raven Press; 1983:51.
33. Enson Y, Thomas HM, Bosken CH, et al. Pulmonary hypertension in interstitial lung disease: Relation of vascular resistance to abnormal lung structure. *Trans Assoc Am Phys* 1975; 88:248–255.
34. Grover RF. Pulmonary circulation in animals and man in high altitude. *Ann NY Acad Sci* 1965; 127:632–639.
35. Fishman AP. The left ventricle in chronic bronchitis and emphysema. *N Engl J Med* 1971; 285:402–404.
36. Murphy ML, Adamson J, Hutcheson F. Left ventricular hypertrophy in patients with chronic bronchitis and emphysema. *Ann Intern Med* 1974; 81:307–313.
37. Matthay RA, Berger HO. Cardiovascular function in cor pulmonale. *Clin Chest Med* 1983; 4:269–295.
38. Buda AJ, Pinsky MR, Ingels NB, et al. Effect of intrathoracic pressure on left ventricular performance. *N Engl J Med* 1979; 301:453–459.
39. Bermis CE, Sehur JR, Borkenhagen D, et al. Influence of right ventricular filling pressure on left ventricular pressure and dimension. *Circ Res* 1974; 34:498–504.
40. Santamore WB, Dell-Italia LJ. Ventricular interdependence: Significant left ventricular contributions to right ventricular systolic function. *Prog Cardiovasc Dis* 1998; 40:289–308.
41. Bichet D, Schrier RS. Cardiac failure, liver disease and nephrotic syndrome. In: Schrier JR, Gottschalk C, eds. *Diseases of the Kidney*. Boston: Little, Brown; 1993:2453–2491.
42. Farber MO, Roberts LR, Weinberger MH, et al. Abnormalities of sodium and H_2O handling in chronic obstructive lung disease. *Arch Intern Med* 1982; 142:1326–1330.
43. Stewart AG, Waterhouse JC, Billings CG, et al. Effects of ACE inhibition on sodium excretion in patients with hypoxemic COPD. *Thorax* 1994; 49:995–998.
44. Lehtonen J, Sutinen S, Ikaheimo P, Paako P. Electrocardiographic criteria for the diagnosis of right ventricular hypertrophy verified at autopsy. *Chest* 1988; 93:839–842.
45. Murphy ML, Hutcheson F. The electrocardiographic diagnosis of right ventricular hypertrophy in chronic obstructive pulmonary disease. *Chest* 1974; 65:622–627.
46. Moore CB, Kraus WL, Dork DS. The relationship between pulmonary arterial pressure and roentgenographic appearance in mitral stenosis. *Am Heart J* 1959; 58:576–581.
47. Chang CH. The normal roentgenographic measurement of the right descending pulmonary artery in 1,085 cases. *AJR* 1962; 87:929–935.
48. Matthay RA, Schwarz MI, Ellis JH. Pulmonary artery hypertension in chronic obstructive pulmonary disease: Chest radiographic assessment. *Invest Radiol* 1981; 16:95–100.
49. Cacho A, Prokash R, Sarne R, Kaushik VS. Usefulness of two-dimensional echocardiography in diagnosing right ventricular hypertrophy. *Chest* 1983; 84:154–157.
50. Hagan A, DeMaria A. Diseases of the right heart. In: *Clinical Applications of Two Dimensional Echocardiography*. Boston: Little, Brown; 1985:270.
51. Louie EK, Rich S, Levitshy S, Brundage BH. Doppler echocardiographic demonstration of the differential effects of RV pressure and volume overload on LV geometry and filling. *J Am Coll Cardiol* 1992; 19:84–91.
52. Kitabatake A, Michitoshi I, Asao M, et al. Noninvasive evaluation of pulmonary hypertension by a pulsed Doppler technique. *Circulation* 1983; 68:302–309.
53. Schiller N. Pulmonary artery pressure estimation by Doppler and two-dimensional echocardiography. *Cardiol Clin* 1990; 8:277–287.
54. Kawakami Y, Kishi F, Yamamoto H, et al. Relation of oxygen delivery, mixed venous oxygenation and pulmonary hemodynamics to prognosis in COPD. *N Engl J Med* 1983; 308:1045–1049.
55. Tarpy SP, Edlli BR. Long-term oxygen therapy. *N Engl J Med* 1995; 333:710–715.
56. Weitzenblum E, Loiseau A, Hirth C, et al. Course of pulmonary hemodynamics in patients with chronic obstructive pulmonary disease. *Chest* 1979; 75:656–662.
57. Crapo RO. Pulmonary function testing. *N Engl J Med* 1994; 331:25–31.
58. Ridker P, Hennekens CH, Lindpaintner K, et al. Mutation in the gene coding for coagulation factor V and the risk of infarction, stroke, and venous thrombosis in apparently healthy men. *N Engl J Med* 1995; 332:912–917.
59. Asherson RA, Khamashta MA, Ordi-Ros, et al. The primary antiphospholipid syndrome: Major clinical and serological features. *Medicine* 1989; 68:366–374.
60. Kryger MH. Management of obstructive sleep apnea. *Clin Chest Med* 1992; 13:481–492.
61. Wiedemann H, Matthay R. Cor pulmonale in chronic obstructive pulmonary disease circulatory pathophysiology and management. *Clin Chest Med* 1990; 11:523–545.
62. Green LH, Smith TW. The use of digitalis in patients with pulmonary disease. *Ann Intern Med* 1977; 87:459–465.
63. Smith DE, Bissett JK, Phillips JR, et al. Improved right ventricular systolic time intervals after digitalis in patients with cor pulmonale and chronic obstructive pulmonary disease. *Am J Cardiol* 1978; 41:1299–1304.
64. Gertz I, Hedenstierna G, Wester PO. Improvement in pulmonary function with diuretic therapy in the hypervolemic and polycythemic patient with chronic obstructive pulmonary disease. *Chest* 1979; 75:146–151.
65. Weisse AB, Moschos CB, Frank MJ, et al. Hemodynamic effects of staged hematocrit reduction in patients with stable cor pulmonale and severely elevated hematocrit levels. *Am J Med* 1975; 58:92–98.
66. Patterson GA, Cooper JD. Lung transplantation. *Chest Surg Clin North Am* 1995; 3:1.
67. Cooper JD, Trulock EP, Triantafillon AN, et al. Bilateral pneumectomy (volume reduction) for chronic obstructive pulmonary disease. *J Thorac Cardiovasc Surg* 1995; 109:106–116.

P A R T N I N E

Valvular Heart Disease

C H A P T E R 55

ACUTE RHEUMATIC FEVER

Simon Chakko / Alan L. Bisno

DEFINITION

Rheumatic fever is an inflammatory disease that occurs as a delayed nonsuppurative sequel to group A streptococcal infection of the pharynx. It involves the heart, joints, central nervous system, skin, and subcutaneous tissues with varying frequency. Its clinical manifestations include migratory polyarthritis, fever, carditis, and, less frequently, Sydenham's chorea, subcutaneous nodules, and erythema marginatum. Rheumatic fever is a clinical syndrome for which no specific diagnostic test exists. No symptom, sign, or laboratory test result is pathognomonic, although several combinations of them are diagnostic. Its importance relates to involvement of the heart, which, though rarely fatal during the acute stage, may lead to rheumatic valvular disease, a chronic and progressive condition that causes cardiac disability or death many years after the initial event.

ETIOLOGY

Antecedent infection of the upper respiratory tract with the group A streptococcus is necessary for the development of rheumatic fever. Cutaneous streptococcal infection may lead to acute glomerulonephritis but has never been demonstrated to cause rheumatic fever. The evidence establishing the group A streptococcus as the etiologic agent of rheumatic fever is only indirect, because the organism cannot be recovered from the lesions and there is no experimental animal model. Nevertheless, the evidence from clinical, immunologic and epidemiologic studies is overwhelming.

At least one-third of patients deny previous sore throat, and cultures of the pharynx are often negative for group A streptococci at the onset of rheumatic fever. However, an antibody response to streptococcal extracellular products can be demonstrated in almost all cases,[1] and the attack rate of acute rheumatic fever is strongly correlated with the magnitude of the antibody response.[2]

A clear sequential relationship between outbreaks of streptococcal pharyngitis or scarlet fever and rheumatic fever has been demonstrated in epidemiologic studies of military recruit camps, and such outbreaks can be eradicated when streptococcal infection is controlled by chemotherapy.[3] Prompt and effective penicillin therapy of streptococcal pharyngitis prevents the initial attack of rheumatic fever (so-called primary prevention),[4] and continuous chemoprophylaxis against streptococcal infection (secondary prophylaxis) prevents its recurrences.[5]

EPIDEMIOLOGY

Rheumatic fever is a major health problem in the developing countries of Asia, Africa, the Middle East, and Latin America. It is difficult for physicians trained in North America to comprehend the magnitude of the problem. A World Health Organization survey conducted between 1986 and 1990 estimated the prevalence of rheumatic fever and chronic rheumatic heart disease per 1000 schoolchildren to be 12.6 in Zambia, 10.2 in Sudan, and 7.9 in Bolivia.[6] Hospital statistics from many developing countries reveal that 10 to 35 percent of all cardiac admissions are for rheumatic fever and rheumatic heart disease.[6,7] It has been estimated that there are at least 50,000 cases of rheumatic fever annually in India and more than 1 million people with rheumatic heart disease.[7] Exceedingly high attack rates have been reported among aboriginal populations in New Zealand and Australia.[8]

Acute rheumatic fever is most common among children in the 5- to 15-year age group. There is no clear-cut sex predilection, although there is a female preponderance in rheumatic mitral stenosis and in Sydenham's chorea. The attack rate of acute rheumatic fever following untreated exudative tonsillitis varies, depending upon the epidemiologic circumstances and the rheumatogenic potential of prevalent streptococcal strains. This rate has been reported to approximate 3 percent during epidemics in military recruit camps[9] but only 0.4 percent after endemically occurring infections in untreated children in civilian populations.[10] Acute rheumatic fever is more likely to occur after those streptococcal infections judged to be more severe by clinical and immunologic criteria (i.e., exudative tonsillopharyngitis, vigorous rises in serum titers of antistreptolysin O, and prolonged convalescent streptococcal throat carriage). Nevertheless, approximately one-third of the cases occur after asymptomatic streptococcal infections. A striking feature of the epidemiology of acute rheumatic fever is the propensity of patients who have suffered an initial attack to experience recurrences of the disease following group A streptococcal infections.

Strains of group A streptococci vary in their propensity to elicit acute rheumatic fever. Although the precise factor or factors that confer this property are unknown, highly rheumatogenic strains share certain biological characteristics. Only a limited number of the more than 90 streptococcal M-protein types have been strongly and repetitively associated with rheumatic fever.[11] These strains are often heavily encapsulated, a feature manifest by the formation of mucoid colonies on blood-agar plates. Their M-protein molecules share a particular surface-exposed antigenic domain against which rheumatic fever patients mount a strong immunoglobulin G response.[12] These characteristics were established, however, by study of rheumatic fever cases and outbreaks in the United States and Great Britain; they remain to be validated for cases occurring in third-world countries or among aboriginal populations.

The twentieth century witnessed a dramatic decline in the incidence of rheumatic fever and rheumatic heart disease in the industrialized nations.[13] The incidence of rheumatic fever and the prevalence of rheumatic heart disease are now very low in North America and western Europe. Rates fewer than 2 per 100,000 schoolchildren have been reported from several areas in the United States. The disease is very rare in affluent suburban populations[14] but persists among disadvantaged families dwelling in the crowded inner cities.[14,15] The higher incidence rates reported among blacks than among whites appear to be due to socioeconomic rather than genetic factors.

The reasons for the recent decline in the incidence of rheumatic fever in developed countries are multifactorial. One of the factors was likely an improvement in living standards, including a decrease in household crowding. Crowding favors interpersonal spread of group A streptococci and probably enhances streptococcal virulence by human passage. Although the diminution was well under way prior to the introduction of penicillin, this highly effective antimicrobial may have contributed to the decline in initial attacks of rheumatic fever and clearly contributed to a decrease in mortality by preventing repetitive attacks in patients compliant with programs of secondary prophylaxis.

There is no evidence of a decline in the frequency of streptococcal pharyngitis concomitant with the dramatic decline in rheumatic fever incidence. This strongly suggests that there have been changes in the rheumatogenicity of streptococcal strains currently prevalent in civilian populations of North America and western Europe. This concept was further validated by the isolation of strains manifesting the above-mentioned rheumatogenic phenotypic characteristics during a resurgence of rheumatic fever that occurred in certain American communities toward the end of the century (see below).

In the mid-1980s, after decades of decline, outbreaks of rheumatic fever occurred in numerous cities and in two military recruit camps in the United States.[13,16] Strains of group A streptococci recovered from patients with acute rheumatic fever and their families and those found in community and training camp surveys were generally high-mucoid and often belonged to well-established rheumatogenic serotypes (serotypes 3 and 18). A survey of hospitals conducted by the American Heart Association indicated that the reported outbreaks were focal and not nationwide.[17] The largest epidemic occurred in Salt Lake City, Utah, and the surrounding intermountain area,[18] where over 500 cases were diagnosed between 1985 and 1999.

Surprisingly, the epidemiologic features of several of the civilian outbreaks—including the largest one in Salt Lake City—differed from the traditional patterns described above in that the victims were predominantly white middle-class children living in the suburbs. Only one-third of the children with rheumatic fever in Salt Lake City had a sore throat of sufficient severity that the parents considered taking them to a physician.[19] Most such outbreaks appear to have subsided during the 1990s, but that in Salt Lake City is continuing as of this writing.

PATHOGENESIS

The exact mechanism by which the group A streptococcus causes rheumatic fever remains unexplained. Possibilities include (1) toxic effects of streptococcal products, particularly streptolysins S or O, which are capable of inducing tissue injury; (2) a serum sickness–like reaction; and (3) autoimmune phenomena induced by the similarity or identity of certain streptococcal antigens to wide variety of human tissue antigens.[20] Although no mechanism has been unequivocally proven, autoimmunity or, more precisely, molecular mimicry appears to be most likely.[21] There are shared epitopes between cardiac myosin and streptococcal M protein that lead to cross-reactive humoral and T-cell immunity against group A streptococci and the heart.[22] Epitopes of streptococcal M protein also share antigenic determinants with heart valves, sarcolemmal membrane proteins, synovium, and articular cartilage.[23] Circulating antibodies that react with neurons of the caudate and subthalamic nuclei and with group A streptococcal cell membranes have been found in many children with Sydenham's chorea.[24] Injection of streptococcal mucopeptide-polysaccharide cell wall complex can induce chronic nodular lesions in the dermal connective tissue in experimental animals.[25] These cross-reactive and toxic phenomena could explain many of the clinical manifestations of rheumatic fever, but, in the absence of a credible animal model of the disease, there is no direct proof that they do so.

During active rheumatic carditis both the number of helper (CD4) lymphocytes and the ratio of CD4 to CD8 cells are increased in the heart valves, and the production of interleukin-1 and interleukin-2 is reportedly increased.[26,27] Scarring and collagen deposition in the valves and destruction of myocytes may result.

The fact that, even in severe epidemics of exudative pharyngitis, rheumatic fever affects only a small proportion of infected persons, coupled with the known familial aggregation of rheumatic fever cases, has long suggested the possibility of a genetic predisposition to rheumatic attacks. Studies of the distribution of class 1 HLA antigens in rheumatics versus controls have been inconclusive. A statistically significant association has been reported between certain of the class II HLA antigens (HLA-DR2 in blacks[28] and HLA-DR4 in whites[29]) and rheumatic fever. An intriguing potential link between the genetic constitution of the human host and susceptibility to rheumatic fever is the identification of certain alloantigens that are expressed in a higher proportion of circulating B lymphocytes of rheumatic subjects and their family members than in those of patients with poststreptococcal glomerulonephritis or normal controls.[30]

PATHOLOGY

Acute rheumatic fever is characterized by exudative and proliferative inflammatory lesions of the connective tissue, most notably of the heart, joints, and subcutaneous tissue. When carditis ensues, all layers of the heart are involved. Pericarditis is common and fibrinous pericarditis is occasionally present. The pericardial inflammation usually resolves over time with no clinically significant sequelae, and tamponade is rare. In fatal cases, myocardial involvement leads to globular enlargement involving all four chambers of the heart. In the myocardium, initially there is fragmentation of collagen fibers, lymphocytic infiltration, and fibrinoid degeneration. This is followed by the appearance of myocardial Aschoff nodules, which are considered pathognomonic of acute rheumatic fever. The Aschoff nodule consists of an area of central necrosis surrounded by lymphocytes, plasma cells, and large mononuclear and giant multinucleate cells. Many of these cells have an elongated nucleus with a clear area just within the nuclear membrane ("owl-eyed nucleus"). These cells are called *Anitschkow myocytes*, although histochemical studies suggest that they are of macrophage-histiocyte origin.[31] Aschoff nodules may also be found in endomyocardial biopsy specimens obtained from patients with acute rheumatic carditis.[32]

Endocardial involvement is responsible for chronic rheumatic valvulitis.[33] Small fibrinous, verrucous vegetations, 1 to 2 mm in diameter, are seen on the atrial surface at sites of valve coaptation and on the chordae tendineae. Even when no vegetations are present, there is edema and inflammation of the valve leaflets. A thickened and fibrotic patch (MacCallum's patch) may be found in the posterior left atrial wall. It is believed to be the effect of the mitral regurgitant jet impinging on the left atrial wall.[33] Healing of the valvulitis leads to granulation and fibrosis of the leaflets and fusion of the chordae. Valvular stenosis or incompetence may result. The mitral valve is involved most frequently, followed by the aortic valve. Tricuspid and pulmonic valves are usually spared.

CLINICAL MANIFESTATIONS

Rheumatic fever may involve different organ systems such as heart, joints, skin, and central nervous system. The clinical picture depends upon the systems involved, and the manifestations may appear singly or in various combinations (Table 55-1). Five clinical features (carditis, polyarthritis, chorea, subcutaneous nodules, and erythema marginatum) are so characteristic of the disease that they are classified as major manifestations according to the Jones criteria (Table 55-2).[34] Additional findings such as fever, arthralgia, heart block, and acute-phase reactants in the blood (i.e., elevation of erythrocyte sedimentation rate and serum concentration of C-reactive protein) are commonly present in acute rheumatic fever but are nonspecific in nature and are therefore classified as minor manifestations.

The latent period from the onset of streptococcal sore throat to the onset of initial and recurrent attacks of rheumatic fever varies between 1 and 5 weeks with a median of 19 days. The mode of onset is quite variable. An abrupt onset with fever and toxicity is common in patients in whom acute polyarthritis is the presenting complaint. The onset may be insidious or even subclinical when mild carditis is the initial manifestation. Most attacks begin with polyarthritis, and occasionally this may be preceded by abdominal pain and fleeting signs of peritoneal inflammation, which may be misdiagnosed as acute appendicitis.

TABLE 55-1 Clinical Manifestations of Acute Rheumatic Fever

General
- High fever, lassitude, prostration, tachycardia

Cardiac
- Cardiomegaly, congestive heart failure
- Acute pericarditis, pericardial effusion
- Apical pansystolic murmur (mitral regurgitation)
- Apical middiastolic murmur (Carey Coombs)
- Basal diastolic (aortic regurgitation)

Dermatologic
- Subcutaneous nodules
- Erythema marginatum

Rheumatologic
- Arthralgia
- Migratory polyarthritis

Neurologic
- Sydenham's chorea

TABLE 55-2 Guidelines for the Diagnosis of the Initial Attack of Rheumatic Fever (Jones criteria, updated in 1992)[a]

Major Manifestations	Minor Manifestations	Supporting Evidence for Antecedent Group A Streptococcal Infection
Carditis	Clinical findings	Positive throat culture or rapid streptococcal antigen test
Polyarthritis	Arthralgia	
Chorea	Fever	
Erythema marginatum	Laboratory findings	Elevated or rising streptococcal antibody titer
Subcutaneous nodules	Elevated acute phase reactants	
	Erthrocyte sedimentation rate	
	C-reactive protein	
	Prolonged P-R interval	

[a]If supported by evidence of preceding group A streptococcal infection, the presence of two major manifestations or one major and two minor manifestations indicates a high probability of acute rheumatic fever.

SOURCE: From Dajani et al.[34] Reproduced by permission of *JAMA* 1992; 268:2069–2073, copyrighted 1992, American Medical Association.

Overall, arthritis occurs in approximately 75 percent of first attacks, carditis in 40 to 50 percent, chorea in 15 percent, and subcutaneous nodules and erythema marginatum in less than 10 percent.[35] These figures may vary widely, however.

Carditis

Carditis is the only manifestation of acute rheumatic fever that has the potential to cause long-term disability and death. Severe mitral regurgitation (or, possibly, severe myocarditis) may precipitate intractable heart failure and may be fatal during the acute phase of the disease. Fortunately, this complication is quite rare. Carditis, if present, usually appears within the first 3 weeks of the illness. The cardiac involvement is frequently mild or even asymptomatic, but occasionally the course can be fulminant. The diagnosis of carditis requires the presence of one of the following four manifestations: (1) organic cardiac murmurs not previously present, (2) cardiomegaly, (3) pericarditis, (4) congestive heart failure.

Valvulitis is associated with characteristic murmurs that are almost always present unless they are obscured by a loud pericardial friction rub, a large pericardial effusion, or low cardiac output. Mitral regurgitation leads to a blowing holosystolic murmur best heard at the apex and radiating to the axilla and occasionally to the base of the heart or the back. Hemodynamic and surgical pathologic studies conducted in South African patients suggest that mitral annular dilatation is usually the initial abnormality and predisposes to lengthening or rupture of the chordae tendineae and prolapse of the anterior leaflet.[36,37] Increased flow across the mitral valve in the presence of valvulitis may produce a middiastolic murmur (Carey Coombs murmur) that follows an S_3 gallop. This murmur is always accompanied by a systolic murmur of mitral regurgitation. It is not diagnostic of rheumatic fever because other conditions that lead to increased flow across the mitral valve can cause a similar murmur, and in children an S_3 gallop can be physiologic. The Carey Coombs murmur can be differentiated from the diastolic rumble of mitral stenosis by the absence of an opening snap, presystolic accentuation, and loud first sound. A high-pitched decrescendo basal diastolic murmur of aortic regurgitation may also be heard. It is best heard along the left sternal border, over the aortic area, in expiration with the patient leaning forward (see also Chap. 57).

Myocarditis in the absence of valvulitis is not likely to be rheumatic in origin. Tachycardia is common. S_3, S_4, or summation gallops may be audible. Cardiomegaly may be noted on the chest roentgenogram or echocardiogram. In acute congestive heart failure, rapid distention of the hepatic capsule may lead to right-upper-quadrant discomfort and tenderness. Congestive heart failure is usually caused by left ventricular volume overload associated with severe mitral or aortic regurgitation.

In the presence of pericarditis, a pericardial friction rub or muffled heart sounds due to a large effusion may be noted. The presence of effusion should be confirmed by echocardiography. Large effusions leading to tamponade are rare. Pericarditis in the absence of valvular involvement is rarely due to acute rheumatic fever, and other causes should be sought.[34]

Polyarthritis

Arthritis is the most frequent major manifestation of rheumatic fever.[38] Any joint may be affected, but involvement of larger joints such as knees, ankles, elbows, and wrists is more common. The spine is only rarely affected. Several joints are involved in quick succession, and each for a brief period of time, resulting in the typical picture of migratory polyarthritis accompanied by signs and symptoms of an acute febrile illness. A striking feature of rheumatic arthritis is its dramatic response to salicylate therapy. Thus, the typical migratory polyarthritis pattern may not be present if effective anti-inflammatory therapy is administered early in the course of the disease.

The synovial fluid contains numerous white blood cells with a marked preponderance of polymorphonuclear leukocytes. Bacterial cultures are sterile. Inflammation of any one joint subsides spontaneously within a week and the entire bout of polyathritis rarely lasts more than 4 weeks. Resolution is complete with no residual joint damage. A possible exception is the so-called Jaccoud deformity of the metacarpophalangeal joints. This is a periarticular fibrosis and not a true synovitis, and its relation to rheumatic fever is unclear.[39]

Subcutaneous Nodules

These nodules are seen in only 1 to 21 percent of patients with rheumatic fever.[38] They are most often associated with carditis and rarely appear as an isolated manifestation of rheumatic fever. They are round, firm, painless, freely movable subcutaneous lesions varying in size from 0.5 to 2.0 cm. They occur in crops and are usually found over bony surfaces and over tendons such as elbows, knees, and wrists, the occiput and vertebrae (Fig. 55-1). They last for a week or two and disappear spontaneously. Similar nodules also occur in rheumatoid arthritis and systemic lupus erythematosus.

Erythema Marginatum

This rash is usually found on the trunk and proximal parts of the extremities, with the face being spared. It begins as an

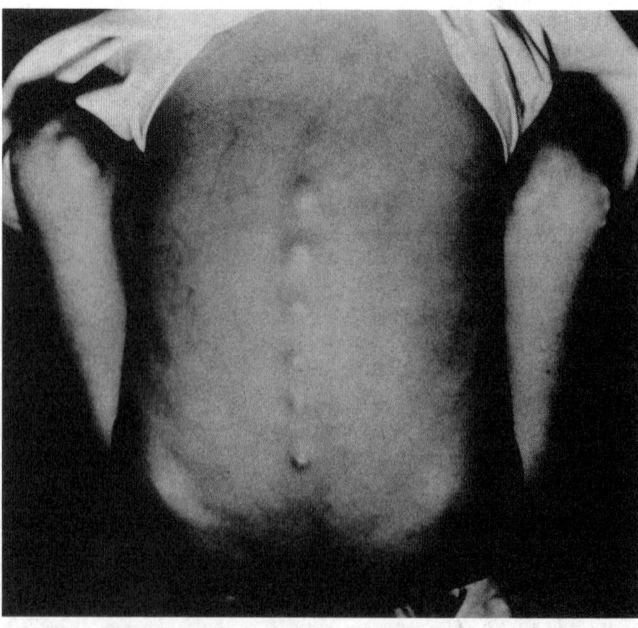

FIGURE 55-1 Subcutaneous nodules on the spine and elbows. (Courtesy of Dr. Benedict F. Massell.)

erythematous macule or papule that extends outward while skin in the center returns to normal. Lesions may merge and form serpiginous patterns. They are never pruritic or indurated, blanch on pressure, and are not influenced by anti-inflammatory therapy. The rash is evanescent, migrating from place to place and leaving no residual scarring. Individual lesions may appear and disappear in minutes to hours. Erythema marginatum has also been reported in sepsis, drug reactions, and glomerulonephritis.

Sydenham's Chorea (St. Vitus Dance)

This neurologic disorder often occurs in isolation, either unaccompanied by other major manifestations of rheumatic fever or after a latent period of several months, at a time when all other manifestations of rheumatic fever have subsided. It is characterized by rapid, purposeless, involuntary movements, most noticable in the extremities and face. The arms and legs flail about in erratic, jerky, uncoordinated movements. The speech is usually slurred and jerky. The involuntary movements disappear during sleep and may be suppressed by sedation. The patient is unable to sustain a tetanic muscular contraction. Emotional lability is characteristic of Sydenham's chorea and may often precede other neurologic manifestations. The duration of the chorea is variable, and its severity may wax and wane. Most patients recover in 6 months. Long-term sequelae such as convulsions, learning disabilities, and behavior problems are rare but have been reported in a small number of patients. Experience with brain imaging is limited but isolated case reports suggest that magnetic resonance imaging or computed tomographic scans may reveal abnormalities in the caudate nuclei, putamen, and substantia nigra.[40]

Rarely, chorea may be due to other conditions that affect the basal ganglia, including collagen vascular, endocrine, neoplastic, genetic, metabolic, and infectious disorders.[41] Perhaps the most frequent differential diagnostic consideration is systemic lupus erythematosus. The relationship of chorea occurring during pregnancy (chorea gravidarum) to acute rheumatic fever remains unclear.

Minor Manifestations

Minor manifestations of rheumatic fever include fever, arthralgia, and laboratory evidences of inflammation (Table 55-2). Fever usually ranges from 38.4 to 40°C and rarely lasts for more than 3 to 4 weeks. Arthralgia is pain in one or more joints without objective evidence of inflammation. In diagnosing rheumatic fever using the Jones criteria, arthralgia should not be considered a minor manifestation when arthritis is present.

Other Clinical Features

Abdominal pain in rheumatic fever is the result of peritoneal inflammation and may be confused with acute appendicitis or sickle cell crisis. Because it occurs at the onset of the illness, other manifestations of rheumatic fever may not yet be present. Epistaxis has been reported as a manifestation of rheumatic fever, but it is not clear to what extent it may be attributable to the large doses of aspirin administered for treatment of the disease. Tachycardia may be out of proportion to fever and persists during sleep.

LABORATORY FINDINGS

A mild to moderate normochromic normocytic anemia and leukocytosis with an increased proportion of polymorphonuclear leukocytes are common. Elevated serum levels of C-reactive protein and an increased erythrocyte sedimentation rate are almost always present, indicating acute inflammation. An exception is "pure" chorea, which may appear after these markers of inflammation have returned to normal.

Throat cultures are usually negative for group A streptococci by the time rheumatic fever appears. Streptococcal antibody tests provide evidence for antecedent streptococcal infection and include antistreptolysin O (ASO), anti-DNAse B, and antihyaluronidase. These antibodies reach peak titer at about the time of onset of acute rheumatic fever. The ASO is elevated in 80 percent or more of patients with rheumatic fever. A battery of these three tests will establish the presence of immunologically significant infection with group A streptococcus in 95 percent of patients.[42] The normal ranges for these titers vary depending upon the test used, patient's age, and geographic locale. ASO titers greater than 200 Todd units per milliliter in adults and 320 Todd units in children are generally considered elevated. In patients seen early during the course of rheumatic fever, rising antibody titers may be seen. An elevated streptococcal antibody titer is not diagnostic of rheumatic fever, but the diagnosis is very unlikely if all three tests (ASO, anti-DNAse B, and antihyaluronidase) are negative (see section on "Diagnosis" below (or exceptions).

Electrocardiogram

Persistent sinus tachycardia that does not resolve during sleep is common in the presence of carditis.[43] Sinus bradycardia and sinus arrhythmia may be present in some patients and can be abolished by the administration of atropine. Prolongation of the PR interval is a common abnormality. In various studies, the incidence varied from 10 to 84 percent.[43] A recent study of the resurgence of rheumatic fever[18] described the electrocardiographic findings in 232 patients. Alterations in atrioventricular conduction were noted in 74 patients (32 percent). Of these, 66 had a prolonged PR interval, 4 had transient episodes of AV block, and 4 had transient episodes of AV dissociation.

Some investigators have suggested that the AV conduction delay is a manifestation of carditis.[43] However, the response to atropine and the lack of correlation with clinical carditis suggests that this is a nonspecific finding.[34] Transient complete heart block that causes Stokes-Adams attacks has been described. Bundle-branch blocks are rare. Atrial flutter and fibrillation have been described in the presence of carditis. Low QRS voltage may be noted if a large pericardial effusion is present.

Echocardiogram

Few studies have used echocardiography to evaluate and follow up patients with rheumatic carditis.[44] During the resurgence of rheumatic fever in Salt Lake City, two-dimensional and Doppler echocardiograms were performed in children with rheumatic fever.[18] During the acute phase of rheumatic carditis, echocardiographic evidence of mitral regurgitation ws often found even when a murmur was not audible ("silent mitral regurgitation").

Valvular thickening and the presence of nodular lesions on the body and tips of the mitral leaflet have been described.[45] These are most likely echocardiographic equivalents of rheumatic verrucae. The key features of rheumatic mitral valvulitis were annular dilation and elongation of the chordae to the anterior leaflet, resulting in mitral regurgitation with a posterolaterally directed jet.[18] In an echocardiographic study of 73 patients with active rheumatic carditis and mitral regurgitation, it was noted that 90 percent of patients had elongated mitral valve chordae, 94 percent had prolapse of the anterior leaflet of the mitral valve, and 96 percent had annular dilation.[46] The resulting mitral regurgitant jet was directed toward the posterolateral wall of the left atrium. The site where this jet strikes the posterior left atrial wall corresponds with the site of endocardial thickening described at autopsy as MacCallum's patch. Rheumatic carditis can be differentiated from the common mitral valve prolapse syndrome because only the coapting portion of the anterior mitral leaflet prolapses and there is no billowing of the medial portion of the leaflet.

In the past congestive heart failure seen in acute rheumatic fever was attributed to myocarditis. Recent echocardiographic studies have shown that patients with rheumatic fever and congestive heart failure have preserved left ventricular systolic function and severe mitral regurgitation.[45,47] Thus the etiology of heart failure appears to be acute mitral regurgitation and not myocarditis.[19,44] Although these findings are interesting, experience is limited, and it is not yet clear the extent to which echocardiography has incremental diagnostic value when added to the clinical findings in the diagnosis of carditis or in ascertaining the likelihood of development of chronic rheumatic heart disease.

Endomyocardial Biopsy

Rheumatic fever is basically a clinical syndrome for which no specific diagnostic test exists. However, the presence of Aschoff nodules on histologic specimens obtained at surgery and autopsy can be considered diagnostic of rheumatic fever. Percutaneous transvenous myocardial biopsy is now feasible and may be useful in the diagnosis.[48] Aschoff nodules and interstitial mononuclear infiltrates with or without myocyte necrosis have been described in the myocardial biopsy specimens of four patients with acute rheumatic fever.[49–52] To determine the role of myocardial biopsy in the diagnosis of rheumatic carditis, a prospective study was performed in 54 patients.[32] Among 11 patients with definite clinical rheumatic carditis, 3 (27 percent) had Aschoff nodules in the biopsy specimen; the remainder had evidence of myocarditis, but the abnormalities were not diagnostic of rheumatic carditis. Among patients with suspected rheumatic carditis, myocardial specimens were diagnostic only in a minority of cases. The investigators concluded that the role of myocardial biopsy in the diagnosis of rheumatic fever was limited.

DIAGNOSIS

The diagnostic criteria for acute rheumatic fever were originally proposed by T. Duckett Jones 1944 and have been later modified and updated by the American Heart Association (Table 55-2).[34] Based on their diagnostic importance, clinical and laboratory findings are divided into major and minor manifestations. If supported by evidence of a preceding group A streptococcal infection, the presence of two major manifestations, or of one major and two minor manifestations indicates a high probability of acute rheumatic fever. Supporting evidence of a previous group A streptococcal infection is a prerequisite for fulfilling the criteria.

There are some circumstances in which the diagnosis of rheumatic fever can be made without strictly adhering to the Jones criteria. Chorea may not occur until several months after the antecedent streptococcal pharyngeal infection. Isolated carditis that does not provoke congestive failure may not be recognized during the acute phase of illness yet may persist for months. In these situations, markers of inflammation may no longer be present and antistreptococcal antibody titers may have returned to normal by the time the illness comes to light. Moreover, in patients with previous rheumatic fever or established rheumatic heart disease, recurrences are common and a presumptive diagnosis of a recurrence may be made in the presence of a single major or several minor manifestations.[34]

Overdiagnosis must be avoided. Following well-documented group A streptococcal pharyngitis, vague signs and symptoms and nonspecific laboratory abnormalities may appear. Discomfort in the extremities, borderline temperature elevation, increased intensity of functional murmurs, tachycardia, elevated erythrocyte sedimentation rate, and prolonged PR interval may occur in the absence of major manifestations. These patients do not develop rheumatic heart disease on follow-up.[34] Thus the diagnosis of rheumatic fever should not be made in the absence of major manifestations. There is no evidence that temporarily withholding salicylates or corticosteriods has any adverse effect on the long-term prognosis. Thus premature administration of these drugs before the symptoms become distinct should be avoided.

Because acute rheumatic fever can have such diverse manifestations (acute polyarthritis, congestive heart failure, chorea, or combinations of these) and because there is no specific diagnostic test for the disease, the differential diagnostic possibilities in an individual case may be quite broad. Among the diseases that need most frequently to be differentiated are rheumatoid arthritis, juvenile rheumatoid arthritis, systemic lupus erythematosus, serum sickness, sickle cell crisis or cardiopathy, rubella arthritis, septic arthritis (especially gonococcal arthritis in adolescent patients), Lyme disease, infective endocarditis, viral myocarditis, and early stages of Henoch-Schönlein purpura. Less frequent differential diagnostic considerations include gout, sarcoidosis, Hodgkin's disease, and leukemia. Choreiform movements have been described in patients with systemic lupus erythematosus, neoplasms involving the basal ganglia, Legionnaire's disease, hypoparathyroidism, antiphospholipid syndrome, Wilson's disease, and Huntington's disease. Chorea is also seen occasionally in women taking oral contraceptives, and during pregnancy ("chorea gravidarum").

In areas of low rheumatic fever incidence, the Jones criteria are perhaps most useful in excluding the diagnosis. The specificity of the criteria is most problematic when the diagnosis is based upon acute polyarthritis as a single major manifestation plus laboratory findings indicative of acute inflammation. In such cases, there must be clear-cut supporting laboratory evidence of recent streptococcal infection and alternative diagnoses must be carefully ruled out.

TREATMENT

Antibiotics neither modify the course of the disease nor prevent the development of rheumatic carditis. Nevertheless, a course of antibiotics to eradicate group A streptococci remaining in the pharynx and tonsils is usually given. Penicillin G benzathine (1.2 million units intramuscularly as a single injection) is the treatment of choice for patients who are not allergic to penicillin. Erythromycin is prescribed for the penicillin-allergic patient. An oral cephalosporin is an acceptable alternative if the penicillin allergy is not of the immediate type. Following this, continuous prophylactic therapy is given to prevent streptococcal pharyngitis (see below).

Anti-inflammatory drugs provide dramatic clinical improvement but are not curative and do not prevent development of rheumatic heart disease.[53] Aspirin is very effective in reducing fever, toxicity, and inflammation of the joints. It is given as tolerated in a dosage of 90 to 100 mg/kg/day in children and 6 to 8 g/day in adults in divided doses every 4 h. A serum salicylate level of 20 to 25 mg/dL is adequate. Adverse effects include salicylism and gastrointestinal bleeding. The precise dose of aspirin is determined by the severity of symptoms, clinical response, salicylate levels, and tolerance to the drug. After 2 weeks of therapy, a reduced dose of aspirin may be used for another 6 weeks.

Corticosteroids are used in patients with carditis manifest by heart failure and in patients who do not tolerate aspirin or whose symptoms do not respond well to this drug. Prednisone 40 to 60 mg a day in divided doses is given for 2 to 3 weeks and the dosage is gradually reduced over the following 3 weeks. In some patients symptoms of rheumatic fever may reappear when the anti-inflammatory therapy, especially steroids, is stopped. Continuing aspirin therapy for 1 month after steroids are discontinued can prevent this. Although the use of nonsteroidal anti-inflammatory drugs seems reasonable in patients who cannot tolerate salicylates and who do not require corticosteroids, there is a paucity of data on the use of these agents in acute rheumatic fever. Thus, their role in management remains to be defined.

Congestive heart failure is managed in the conventional manner. Digoxin should be used cautiously in the presence of myocarditis. After the acute attack subsides, the level of physical activity is determined by the cardiac status. Patients without residual cardiac disease do not require restriction of physical activity. In the rare instances in which patients with acute rheumatic fever develop intractable heart failure, mitral valve repair or replacement may be life-saving (see also Chap. 57).

TABLE 55-3 Secondary Prevention of Rheumatic Fever (Prevention of Recurrent Attacks)

Agent	Dose	Mode
Benzathine penicillin G	1 200 000 U every 4 weeks[a]	Intramuscular
	or	
Penicillin V	250 mg twice daily	Oral
	or	
Sulfadiazine	0.5 g once daily for patients ≤27 kg (60 lb)	Oral
	1.0 g once daily for patients >27 kg (60 lb)	
For individuals allergic to penicillin and sulfadiazine		
Erythromycin	250 mg twice daily	Oral

[a]In high-risk situations, administration every 3 weeks is justified and recommended.
SOURCE: From Dajani et al.[55] Reproduced by permission of *Pediatrics* 1995; 96:758–764.

PROGNOSIS

Manifestations of chronic rheumatic heart disease include mitral and aortic insufficiency or stenosis, congestive heart failure, and atrial fibrillation. The ultimate cardiac prognosis of an individual rheumatic fever attack is rather directly related to the severity of cardiac involvement during the acute phase provided that the patient is protected from recurrent attacks (see below). In the United Kingdom—United States Collaborative Study,[54] only 6 percent of the patients with no carditis or only questionable carditis during their attack of acute rheumatic fever were found to have heart murmurs when reexamined 10 years later. Heart disease was present at follow-up in 30 percent of the patients initially found to have only apical systolic murmurs, in 40 percent of those with basal diastolic murmurs during the acute phase, and in 68 percent of those who initially suffered from congestive heart failure, pericarditis, or both. Some patients with "pure" chorea may later develop rheumatic heart disease, even though carditis was not recognized during the

TABLE 55-4 Duration of Secondary Rheumatic Fever Prophylaxis

Category	Duration
Rheumatic fever with carditis and residual heart disease (persistent valvular disease[a])	At least 10 years since last episode and at least until age 40 years, sometimes lifelong prophylaxis
Rheumatic fever with carditis but no residual heart disease (no valvular disease[a])	10 years or well into adulthood, whichever is longer
Rheumatic fever without carditis	5 years or until age 21 years, whichever is longer

[a]Clinical or echocardiographic evidence.
SOURCE: From Dajani et al.[55] Reproduced by permission of *Pediatrics* 1995; 96:758–764.

initial attack. In such cases, however, it may be that the initial findings of carditis were no longer prominent by the time that chorea (which often occurs after a long latent period) manifested itself.

Prevention

The risk of developing rheumatic fever following a symptomatic or asymptomatic streptococcal infection is much higher in patients who have experienced a previous attack than in nonrheumatic individuals. In some studies the recurrence rate following immunologically confirmed streptococcal upper respiratory infection has been as high as 16 percent.[2] In patients with rheumatic heart disease, recurrent attacks lead to progressive damage. Although patients who did not suffer carditis initially are less prone to develop it in the event of a recurrence, exceptions do occur. It is therefore crucial that rheumatic fever patients be protected optimally from streptococcal infections. This is accomplished by continuous antimicrobial prophylaxis.[55]

The recommended prophylactic regimens are shown in Table 55-3. The optimal duration of antibiotic prophylaxis remains controversial. The risk of acute rheumatic fever declines with age and the number of years since previous attack. The recommendations of the American Heart Association for the duration of secondary prophylaxis are given in Table 55-4. The decision to discontinue rheumatic fever prophylaxis must be individualized on the basis of risk of recurrence and the probable consequence of a recurrence. It should be noted that health care workers, individuals who have contact with schoolchildren, military recruits, and residents of areas with a high incidence of rheumatic fever are at increased risk for streptococcal infection. This fact should be taken into account when considering discontinuation of prophylaxis.

References

1. Stollerman GH. The epidemiology of primary and secondary rheumatic fever. In: Uhr JW, ed. *The Streptococcus, Rheumatic Fever and Glomerulonephritis*. Baltimore: Williams & Wilkins; 1964: 311–337.
2. Taranta A, Wood HF, Feinstein AR, et al. Rheumatic fever in children and adolescents. A long-term epidemiologic study of subsequent prophylaxis, streptococcal infections, and clinical sequelae. IV. Relation of the rheumatic fever recurrence rate per streptococcal infection to the titers of streptococcal antibodies. *Ann Intern Med* 1964; 60(suppl 5):47–57.
3. Frank PF, Stollerman GH, Miller LF. Protection of a military population from rheumatic fever. *JAMA* 1965; 193:755–783.
4. Wannamaker LW, Rammelkamp CH Jr, Denny FW, et al. Prophylaxis of acute rheumatic fever by treatment of preceding streptococcal infection with various amounts of depot penicillin. *Am J Med* 1951; 10:673–695.
5. Wood HF, Feinstein AR, Taranta A, et al. Rheumatic fever in children and adolescents. A long-term epidemiologic study of subsequent prophylaxis, streptococcal infections, and clinical sequelae: III. Comparative effectiveness of three prophylaxis regimens in preventing streptococcal infections and rheumatic recurrences. *Ann Intern Med* 1964; 60(suppl 5):31–46.
6. World Health Organization. WHO programme for the prevention of rheumatic fever/rheumatic heart disease in 16 developing countries: Report from phase I (1986–90). *Bull WHO* 1992; 70:213–218.
7. Vijaykumar M, Narula J, Reddy KS, Kaplan EL. Incidence of rheumatic fever and prevalence of rheumatic fever disease in India. *Int J Cardiol* 1994; 43:221–228.
8. Carapetis JR, Wolff DR, Currie BJ. Acute rheumatic fever and rheumatic heart disease in the top end of Australia's Northern Territory. *Med J Aust* 1996; 164:146–149.
9. Rammelkamp CH, Denny FW, Wannamaker LW. Studies on the epidemiology of rheumatic fever in the armed services. In: Thomas L, ed. *Rheumatic Fever*. Minneapolis: University of Minnesota Press; 1952:72–89.
10. Siegel AC, Johnson EE, Stollerman GH. Controlled studies of streptococcal pharyngitis in a pediatric population: I. Factors related to the attack rate of rheumatic fever. *N Engl J Med* 1961; 265:559–566.
11. Bisno AL. The concept of rheumatogenic and non-rheumatogenic group A streptococci. In: Read SE, Zabriskie JB, eds. *Streptococcal Diseases and the Immune Response*. New York: Academic Press; 1980:789–803.
12. Bessen DE, Veasy LG, Hill HR, et al. Serologic evidence for a class I group A streptococcal infection among rheumatic fever patients. *J Infect Dis* 1995; 172:1608–1611.
13. Bisno AL. Group A streptococcal infections and acute rheumatic fever. *N Engl J Med* 1991; 325:783–793.
14. Land MA, Bisno AL. Acute rheumatic fever: A vanishing disease in suburbia. *JAMA* 1983; 249:895–898.
15. Ferguson GW, Shultz JM, Bisno AL. Epidemiology of acute rheumatic fever in a multi-ethnic, multi-racial U.S. urban community: The Miami-Dade experience. *J Infect Dis* 1991; 164:720–725.
16. Wallace MR, Garst PD, Papadimos TJ, Oldfield EC. The return of acute rheumatic fever in young adults. *JAMA* 1989; 262:2557–2561.
17. Taubert KA, Rowley AH, Shulman ST. Seven-year national survey of Kawasaki disease and acute rheumatic fever. *Pediatr Infect Dis J* 1994; 13:704–708.
18. Veasy LG, Tani LY, Hill HR. Persistence of acute rheumatic fever in the intermountain area of the United States. *J Pediatr* 1994; 124:9–16.
19. Veasy LG. Lessons learned from the resurgence of rheumatic fever in the United States. In: Narula J, Virmani R, Reddy KS, Tandon R, eds. *Rheumatic Fever*. Washington, DC: Armed Forces Institute of Pathology; 1999:69–78.
20. Stollerman GH. Rheumatogenic streptococci and autoimmunity. *Clin Immunol Immunopathol* 1991; 61:131–142.
21. Zabriskie JB. Rheumatic fever: A model for the pathological consequences of microbial-host mimicry. *Clin Exp Rheumatol* 1986; 4:65–73.
22. Cunningham M. Molecular mimicry between group A streptococci and myosin in the pathogenesis of acute rheumatic fever. In: Narula J, Virmani R, Reddy KS, Tandon R, eds. *Rheumatic Fever*. Washington, DC: Armed Forces Institute of Pathology; 1999:135–165.
23. Baird RW, Bronze MS, Kraus W, et al. Epitopes of group A streptococcal M protein shared with antigens of articular cartilage and synovium. *J Immunol* 1991; 146:3132–3137.
24. Husby G, van de Rijn I, Zabriskie JB, et al. Antibodies reacting with cytoplasm of subthalamic and caudate nuclei neurons in chorea and rheumatic fever. *J Exp Med* 1976; 144:1094–1110.
25. Schwab JH, Cromartie WJ. Immunological studies on a C polysaccharide complex of group A streptococci having a direct toxic effect on connective tissue. *J Exp Med* 1960; 111:295–307.
26. Morris K, Mohan C, Wahi PL, et al. Increase in activated T cells and reduction in suppressor/cytotoxic T cells in acute rheumatic fever and active heart disease: A longitudinal study. *J Infect Dis* 1993; 167:979–983.
27. Morris K, Mohan C, Wahi PL, et al. Enhancement of IL-1, IL-2 production and IL-2 receptor generation in patients with acute rheumatic fever and active rheumatic heart disease: A prospective study. *Clin Exp Immunol* 1993; 91:429–436.
28. Ayoub EM, Barrett DJ, Maclaren NK, Krischer JP. Association

of class II human histocompatibility leukocyte antigens with rheumatic fever. *J Clin Invest* 1986; 77:2019–2026.
29. Anastasiou-Nana MI, Anderson JL, Carlquist JF, Nanas JN. HLA-DR typing and lymphocyte subset evaluation in rheumatic heart disease: A search for immune response factors. *Am Heart J* 1986; 112:992–997.
30. Khanna AK, Buskirk DR, Williams RC Jr, et al. Presence of a non-HLA B cell antigen in rheumatic fever patients and their families as defined by a monoclonal antibody. *J Clin Invest* 1989; 83:1710–1716.
31. Chopra P, Wanniang J, Kumar AS. Immunochemical and histochemical profile of Aschoff bodies in rheumatic carditis in excised left atrial appendages: An immunoperoxidase study in fresh and paraffin-embedded tissue. *Int J Cardiol* 1992; 34:199–207.
32. Narula J, Chopra P, Talwar KK, et al. Does endomyocardial biopsy aid in the diagnosis of active rheumatic carditis? *Circulation* 1993; 88(part 1):2198–2205.
33. Virmani R, Farb A, Burke AP, Narula J. Pathology of acute rheumatic carditis. In: Narula J, Virmani R, Reddy KS, Tandon R, eds. *Rheumatic Fever*. Washington, DC: Armed Forces Institute of Pathology; 1999:217–234.
34. Dajani AS, Ayoub E, Bierman FZ, et al. Guidelines for the diagnosis of rheumatic fever: Jones criteria, updated 1992. *JAMA* 1992; 268:2069–2073.
35. Sanyal SK, Thapar MK, Ahmed SH, et al. The initial attack of acute rheumatic fever during childhood in North India: A prospective study of the clinical profile. *Circulation* 1974; 49:7–12.
36. Barlow JB. Aspects of active rheumatic carditis. *Aust N Z J Med* 1992; 22:592–600.
37. Marcus RH, Sareli P, Pocock WA, Barlow JB. The spectrum of severe rheumatic mitral valve disease in a developing country: Correlations among clinical presentation, surgical pathologic findings, and hemodynamic sequelae. *Ann Intern Med* 1994; 120:177–183.
38. Bisno AL. Noncardiac manifestations of rheumatic fever. In: Narula J, Virmani R, Reddy KS, Tandon R, eds. *Rheumatic Fever*. Washington, DC: Armed Forces Institute of Pathology; 1999:245–256.
39. Stollerman GH. *Rheumatic Fever and Streptococcal Infection*. New York: Grune & Stratton; 1975:147–180.
40. Heye N, Jergas M, Hotzinger H, et al. Sydenham chorea: Clinical, EEG, MRI and SPECT findings in the early stage of the disease. *J Neurol* 1993; 240:121–123.
41. Swedo SE. Sydenham's chorea: A model for childhood autoimmune neuropsychiatric disorders. *JAMA* 1994; 272:1788–1791.
42. Stollerman GH, Lewis AJ, Schultz I, Taranta A. Relationship of immune response to group A streptococci to the course of acute, chronic and recurrent rheumatic fever. *Am J Med* 1956; 20:163–169.
43. Krishnan SC, Kushwaha SS, Josephson ME. Electrocardiographic abnormalities and arrhythmias in patients with acute rheumatic fever. In: Narula J, Virmani R, Reddy KS, Tandon R, eds. *Rheumatic Fever*. Washington, DC: Armed Forces Institute of Pathology; 1999:287–298.
44. Minich LL, Tani LY, Veasy LG. Role of echocardiography in the diagnosis and follow-up evaluation of rheumatic fever. In: Narula N, Virmani R, Reddy KS, Tandon R, eds. *Rheumatic Fever*. Washington, DC: Armed Forces Institute of Pathology; 1999:307–318.
45. Vasan RS, Shrivastava S, Vijayakumar M, et al. Echocardiographic evaluation of patients with acute rheumatic fever and rheumatic carditis. *Circulation* 1996; 94:73–82.
46. Marcus RH, Sareli P, Pocock WA, et al. Functional anatomy of severe mitral regurgitation in active rheumatic carditis. *Am J Cardiol* 1989; 63:577–584.
47. Essop MR, Wisenbaugh T, Sareli P. Evidence against a myocardiac factor as the cause of left ventricular dilation in active rheumatic carditis. *J Am Coll Cardiol* 1993; 22:826–829.
48. Narula J, Narula N, Southern JF, Chopra P. Endomyocardial biopsy for the diagnosis of rheumatic carditis. In: Narula J, Virmani R, Reddy KS, Tandon R, eds. *Rheumatic Fever*. Washington, DC: Armed Forces Institute of Pathology; 1999:319–328.
49. Echigo S, Kamiya T, Baba K, et al. A case of congestive cardiomyopathy with histological findings suggesting rheumatic carditis by endomyocardial biopsy. *Jpn Circ J* 1980; 44:823–826.
50. Ursell PC, Alballa A, Fenoglio JJ Jr. Diagnosis of acute rheumatic carditis by endomyocardial biopsy. *Hum Pathol* 1982; 13:677–679.
51. Marboe CC, Knowles DMII, Weiss MB, Fenoglio JJ Jr. Monoclonal antibody identification of mononuclear cells in endomyocardial biopsy specimens from a patient with rheumatic carditis. *Hum Pathol* 1985; 16:332–338.
52. Byck PL, Listinsky CM, Cooper TB, Papapeitro SE. Acute congestive heart failure in a 55-year-old man. Rheumatic carditis diagnosed by endomyocardial biopsy. *Arch Pathol Lab Med* 1990; 114:526–527.
53. Thatai D, Turi ZG. Current guidelines for the treatment of patients with rheumatic fever. *Drugs* 1999; 57:545–555.
54. United Kingdom and United States Joint Report on Rheumatic Heart Disease. The natural history of rheumatic fever and rheumatic heart disease: Ten-year report of a cooperative clinical trial of ACTH, cortisone and aspirin. *Circulation* 1965; 32:457–476.
55. Dajani A, Taubert K, Ferrieri P, et al. Treatment of acute streptococcal pharyngitis and prevention of rheumatic fever: A statement for health professionals. Committee on Rheumatic Fever, Endocarditis, and Kawasaki Disease of the Council on Cardiovascular Disease in the Young, the American Heart Association. *Pediatrics* 1995; 96:758–764.

CHAPTER 56

AORTIC VALVE DISEASE

Shahbudin H. Rahimtoola

The assessment and management of patients with valvular heart disease has undergone many changes in the past four decades. The incidence of acute rheumatic fever has declined, and as a result rheumatic heart disease is not the most important cause of valve disease in the developed countries. Prolapse of the mitral valve and congenital aortic valve disease are now the most common valvular lesions. Valve surgery has been the major therapeutic advance in treating patients with severe valve disease; in fact, most patients with severe valve disease are now considered candidates for surgery. Echocardiography/Doppler ultrasound has a very important role in the diagnosis and follow-up of these patients. Cardiac catheterization/angiography remains an extremely important diagnostic procedure that is needed in almost all patients being considered for interventional therapy. Catheter balloon valvuloplasty is a useful technique for the treatment of some stenotic cardiac valves.

AORTIC VALVE STENOSIS

Aortic stenosis (AS) is obstruction to outflow of blood flow from the left ventricle to the aorta. The obstruction may be at the valve, above the valve (supravalvular), or below the valve (subvalvular).[1] Supravalvular AS is a congenital lesion. Subvalvular AS results either from a discrete fibromuscular obstruction, which is a congenital lesion, or from a muscular obstruction (hypertrophic cardiomyopathy).

Etiology

The most common causes of AS are congenital,[2,3] rheumatic, and calcific (degenerative) (Table 56-1). Calcific AS is seen in patients 35 years of age or older and is the result of calcification of a congenital or rheumatic valve or of a normal valve that has undergone "degenerative" changes.[4] Recent data suggest that degenerative/calcific AS may represent an immune reaction to antigens present in the valve[5] and is related to atherosclerosis.[6]

Rare causes of AS include obstructive, infective vegetations that are usually large, e.g., those seen in fungal endocarditis. Atherosclerotic AS is seen most frequently in patients with severe hypercholesterolemia and is observed in children and young adults with homozygous type II hyperlipoproteinemia.[7,8] Paget's disease of the bone,[9] end-stage renal disease,[10,11] systemic lupus erythematosus, rheumatoid involvement, ochronosis,[12] and irradiation are other rare causes of AS.

At the present time, calcific AS in the older patient is the most common valve lesion requiring valve replacement.[4,13] Among patients under the age of 70, congenital bicuspid valve accounted for one-half of the surgical cases; degenerative changes were the cause in 18 percent.[4] In contrast, in those aged 70 or older, degenerative changes accounted for almost one-half of the surgical cases and a congenital bicuspid valve for approximately one-quarter of the cases (Fig. 56-1).

Pathology

In congenital AS, the valve may be unicuspid, bicuspid, or tricuspid, depending on the patient's age.[14] In patients under the age of 15 years, over 80 percent of stenotic valves are either unicuspid or bicuspid and 15 to 20 percent are tricuspid. In patients aged 15 to 65 years, 60 percent are bicuspid, 10 percent are unicuspid, and 25 to 30 percent are tricuspid. In patients 65 years of age or over, 90 percent of the valves are tricuspid and 10 percent are bicuspid. Unicuspid valves produce severe obstruction in infancy and are the most frequent malformation found in fatal valvular AS in children under the age of 1 year.[2] Congenital bicuspid valves can produce severe obstruction to left ventricular (LV) outflow after the first few years of life.[3] The valvular abnormality produces turbulent flow, which traumatizes the leaflets and eventually leads to fibrosis, rigidity, and calcification of the valve. In a congenitally abnormal tricuspid aortic valve, the cusps are of unequal size and have some degree of commissural fusion; the third cusp may be diminutive. Eventually, the abnormal structure leads to changes similar to those seen in a bicuspid valve, and significant LV outflow obstruction often results. In calcific AS (so called "degenerative") early

TABLE 56-1 Etiology of Aortic Valve Stenosis

I. Congenital
II. Acquired
  A. Rheumatic
  B. Calcific (degenerative/autoimmune)
  C. Rare causes
    1. Obstructive infective vegetations
    2. Homozygous type II hyperlipoproteinemia
    3. Paget's disease of bone
    4. Systemic lupus erythematosus
    5. Rheumatoid involvement
    6. Ochronosis (alkaptonuria)
    7. Irradiation

changes show chronic inflammatory cell infiltrate (macrophages and T lymphocytes), lipid in lesion and in adjacent fibrosa and thickening of fibrosa with collagen and elastin.[6] These patients also have a higher incidence of risk factors for coronary atherosclerosis.[15]

Rheumatic AS results from adhesions and fusion of the commissures and cusps. The leaflets and the valve ring become vascularized, which leads to retraction and stiffening of the cusps. Calcification occurs, and the aortic valve orifice is reduced to a small triangular or round opening, which is frequently regurgitant as well as stenotic. Importantly, the heart exhibits other evidence of rheumatic heart disease—namely, involvement of the mitral valve and presence of Aschoff's nodules in the myocardium.

Rheumatoid AS is extremely rare and results from nodular thickening of the valve leaflets and the involvement of the proximal part of the aorta. In severe forms of hypercholesterolemia, lipid deposits occur not only in the aortic wall but also in the aortic valve and occasionally produce AS.

The LV is concentrically hypertrophied.[16] The hypertrophied cardiac muscle cells are increased in size, with their transverse diameters ranging from 15 to 70 μm (normal, 10 to 15 μm). There is an increase of connective tissue,[17–19] and a variable amount of fibrous tissue (collagen fibrils) in the interstitial tissue. Usually, the cardiac muscle cells do not degenerate in patients with AS. Myocardial ultrastructural changes[20] may account for the LV systolic dysfunction that occurs late in the disease; such changes include unusually large nuclei, loss of myofibrils, accumulation of mitochondria, large cytoplasmic areas devoid of contractile material, and proliferation of fibroblasts and collagen fibers in the interstitial space.

Subclinical calcific emboli are commonly found in calcific AS if diligently sought at autopsy.

Pathophysiology

With reduction in the *aortic valve area* (AVA), energy is dissipated during the transport of blood from the LV to the aorta. The AVA has to be reduced by about 50 percent of normal before a measurable gradient can be demonstrated in humans.[21] When a pressure gradient develops between the left ventricle and the ascending aorta, LV pressure rises; aortic pressure remains within the normal range until end-stage heart failure occurs. The relationship of the AVA to cardiac output and pressure gradient is discussed in Chap. 57. As LV pressure rises, ventricular wall stress increases, which leads to impaired LV function. The heart normalizes wall stress by becoming hypertrophic. Since AS develops slowly, hypertrophy develops in proportion to increased intraventricular pressure, and myocardial stress remains normal.[22] *Thus, the major compensatory mechanism by which the heart copes with LV outflow obstruction is ventricular hypertrophy.* LV mass in patients with severe AS undergoing valve replacement averages 229 g/m^2 (normal, 105 g/m^2);[22] at autopsy, left ventricles weighing as much as 1000 g have been reported. LV volume, however, is within the normal range,[22] and so there is a considerable thickening of the LV wall.

The diastolic properties of the LV are affected in AS.[23–27] This diastolic abnormality results from a combination of impaired myocardial relaxation with altered chamber compliance because the hypertrophied LV per se offers increased resistance to filling, and from increased myocardial stiffness because of structural alterations.[27] As a result, LV end-diastolic pressure is elevated, but this is not necessarily a measure of LV failure. Powerful atrial contraction produces the required LV filling and results in an elevated LV end-diastolic pressure (atrial booster pump function).[28,29] The necessary LV filling and fiber length to achieve an adequate stroke volume are achieved by atrial systole, which occupies only a small part of the cardiac cycle. Therefore there is a transient increase in left atrial pressure due to the large *a* wave, but mean left atrial pressure remains in the normal range or is only minimally increased (Fig. 56-2).

Left atrial contraction is therefore of considerable benefit to these patients.

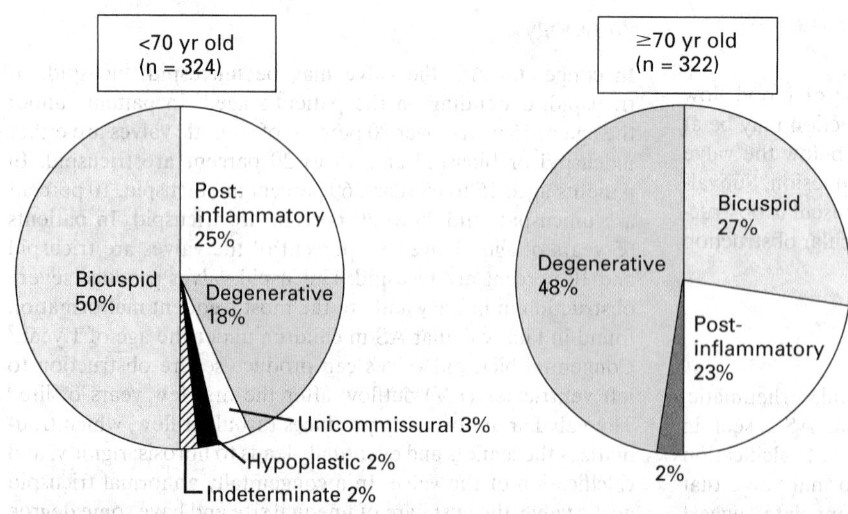

FIGURE 56-1 Etiology of aortic stenosis in patients under the age of 70 years (*left panel*); congenital bicuspid valve accounted for one-half of the surgical cases. In those aged 70 or older (*right panel*), "degenerative" changes accounted for almost one-half of the surgical cases. (From Passik et al.,[4] with permission.)

Loss of effective atrial contraction, either because of atrial fibrillation or because of an inappropriately timed atrial contraction [e.g., that associated with first-degree heart block or with atrioventricular (AV) dissociation], results in elevations of mean left atrial pressure, reduction of cardiac output, or both and may precipitate clinical heart failure with pulmonary congestion.

Patients with severe LV hypertrophy may exhibit LV diastolic dysfunction, which may produce the syndrome of clinical heart failure (paroxysmal nocturnal dyspnea, orthopnea, and even pulmonary edema) even if LV systolic pump function is normal. In patients 60 years of age or older, a higher percentage of women (41 percent) than men (14 percent) have "excessive" hypertrophy, that is, greater amounts of hypertrophy in spite of similar degrees of severity of AS.[30] They have "supernormal" LV systolic pump function (high LV ejection fraction) and a small, thick-walled chamber with lower end-systolic wall stress (Table 56-2).

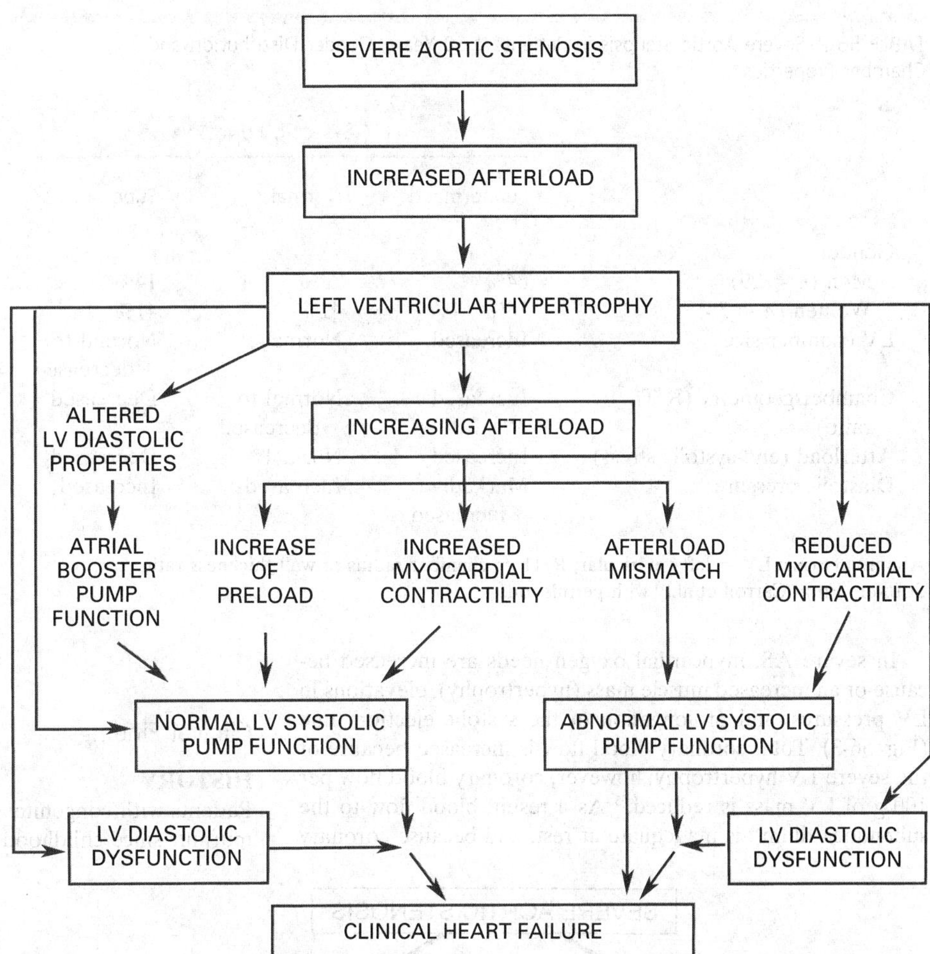

FIGURE 56-2 Illustration of some aspects of the pathophysiology in severe aortic stenosis (see text). The heart responds to AS by hypertrophy, and LV systolic pump function remains normal. LV hypertrophy may alter the LV diastolic properties. As a result, LV end-diastolic pressure is elevated; but powerful atrial contraction produces the required LV filling and fiber length (atrial booster pump function).

As LV afterload continues to increase, the LV uses two additional compensatory mechanisms, namely, increase of preload and increase of myocardial contractility. Both of these help maintain normal LV systolic pump function.

When the limit of the preload reserve has been reached (afterload mismatch) or myocardial contractility is reduced, LV systolic pump function becomes abnormal.

Clinical heart failure is usually a result of abnormal LV systolic pump function; diastolic dysfunction may also be present in some patients. Clinical heart failure in those with normal LV systolic pump function is a result of LV diastolic dysfunction. (Copyright © by S. H. Rahimtoola, M.B., F.R.C.P., M.A.C.P., M.A.C.C. See Ref. 93.)

LV systolic pump function is determined by myocardial (muscle) function and by a combination of LV afterload and preload. Thus, impaired LV systolic pump function (as measured by ejection fraction) may be the result of afterload-preload mismatch,[31] impaired myocardial function, or both. LV systolic pump function is normal in most patients with severe AS. When the LV hypertrophy alone is not adequate to overcome the outflow obstruction, the left ventricle uses the Frank-Starling mechanism (preload reserve) to maintain systolic pump function. When the preload reserve is no longer adequate, a reduction of LV systolic pump function occurs (Fig. 56-2). In AS, major use of the preload reserve is not a good compensatory mechanism. Even small increases in LV volume may result in major increases in LV end-diastolic pressure because the LV is on the very steep portion of its diastolic pressure-volume curve, and the corresponding increase in mean left atrial pressure produces pulmonary edema. Thus, clinical heart failure may be a result of either LV diastolic dysfunction in the presence of normal LV systolic function or impaired myocardial function producing LV systolic dysfunction, with or without associated LV diastolic dysfunction. Eventually, pulmonary artery, right ventricular, and right atrial pressures are elevated. Peripheral edema results from increases in systemic venous pressure and salt and water retention.

In most patients with AS, cardiac output is in the normal range and initially increases normally with exercise. Later, as the severity of AS increases progressively, the cardiac output remains within the normal range at rest, but, on exercise, it no longer increases in proportion to the amount of exercise undertaken or does not increase at all (fixed cardiac output). With the development of heart failure, there is a reduction in the resting cardiac output and a tachycardia. As a result, stroke volume may be so lowered that it results in a small gradient across the LV outflow tract in spite of severe AS. As the patient's age increases, there is a progressive decrease of cardiac output with exercise and a progressive increase of LV end-diastolic pressure at equal levels of AVA. This may be related only to LV diastolic dysfunction and is most marked in the older patient.[32]

TABLE 56-2 Severe Aortic Stenosis in Patients ≥60 Years, Gender Distribution and Chamber Properties

	LV SYSTOLIC FUNCTION		
	Subnormal	Normal	Supernormal
Gender			
Men (n = 29)	64%	22%	14%
Women (n = 34)	18%	41%	41%
LV chamber size	Increased	Normal	Normal to decreased
Chamber geometry (R/Th ratio)	Increased	Normal to decreased	Decreased
Afterload (end-systolic stress)	Increased	Normal	Decreased
Diastolic pressure	Markedly increased	Increased	Increased

ABBREVIATIONS: LV = left ventricular; R/Th = chamber radius to wall thickness ratio.
SOURCE: From Carroll et al.,[30] with permission.

In severe AS, myocardial oxygen needs are increased because of an increased muscle mass (hypertrophy), elevations in LV pressures, and prolongation of the systolic ejection time (Fig. 56-3). Total coronary blood flow is increased because of the severe LV hypertrophy; however, coronary blood flow per 100 g of LV mass is reduced.[33] As a result, blood flow to the subendocardium[34] is inadequate at rest; and because coronary vasodilator reserve is reduced,[35] myocardial blood flow is also reduced further, relative to need, on exercise. Coronary blood flow is reduced because of a reduced coronary perfusion pressure (the elevated LV end-diastolic pressure lowers the diastolic aortic-LV pressure gradient) and also because the hypertrophied myocardium compresses the coronary arteries as they traverse the myocardium to supply blood to the subendocardium (systolic "milking" of intramural arteries). As a result, patients may have classic angina pectoris even in the absence of *coronary artery disease* (CAD). Associated obstructive CAD from atherosclerosis further increases the imbalance between myocardial oxygen needs and supply (Fig. 56-2).

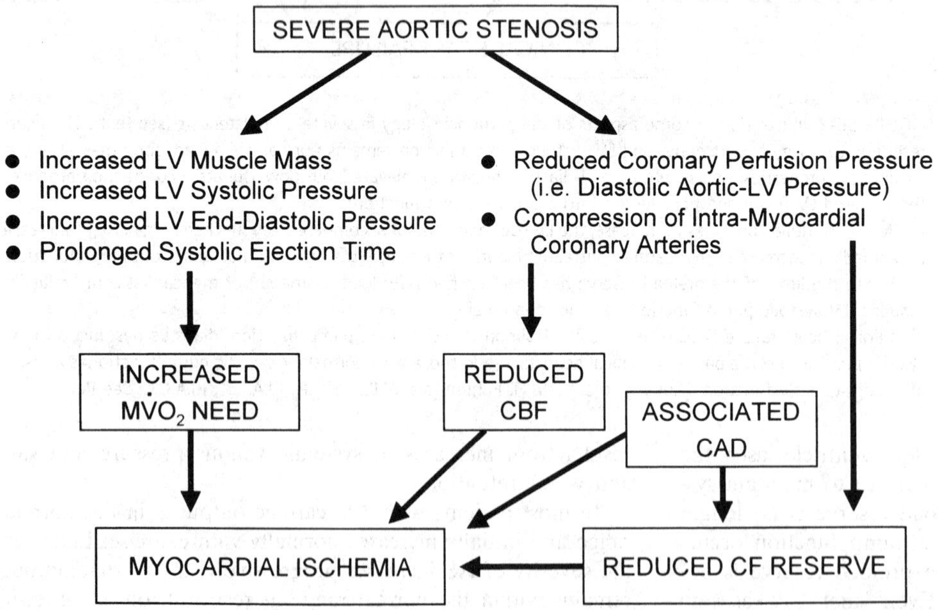

Clinical Findings

HISTORY

Patients with congenital valve stenosis may give a history of a murmur since childhood or infancy; those with rheumatic stenosis may have a history of rheumatic fever. Most patients with valvular AS, including some with severe valve stenosis, are asymptomatic. The symptoms of AS are angina pectoris, syncope, exertional presyncope, dyspnea (on exertion, orthopnea, paroxysmal nocturnal dyspnea, pulmonary edema), and the symptoms of heart failure. Once symptoms occur in a patient with severe AS, the life span of the patient is very short without surgical treatment. Sudden cardiac death is stated to occur in 5 percent of patients with AS. It occurs only in those with severe valve stenosis, most of whom have had some cardiac symptoms before the fatal episode. Typical angina pectoris occurs with or without associated CAD and results from an imbalance between myocardial oxygen needs and supply (Fig. 56-3).

Syncope is the result of reduced cerebral perfusion. Syncope occurring on effort is caused by either systemic vasodilatation in the presence of a fixed or inadequate cardiac output, an arrhythmia, or both.[36-38] Syncope at rest

FIGURE 56-3 In severe aortic stenosis, myocardial oxygen needs are increased because of increased muscle mass (hypertrophy), increases in LV pressures, and prolongation of the systolic ejection time. Total coronary blood flow is increased; however, coronary blood flow per 100 g of LV mass is reduced because of a reduction in diastolic aortic-LV pressure gradient and "systolic milking" of the coronary arteries in the hypertrophied LV as they traverse the myocardium from the epicardium to endocardium to supply the subendocardial myocardial region. Thus, these patients may have myocardial ischemia, particularly in the subendocardial region. Coronary vasodilator reserve, i.e., the ability of the coronary blood flow to increase with vasodilatation, is also significantly reduced, and thus the myocardial ischemia can be markedly exacerbated on effort. Associated obstructive coronary artery disease can be expected to further exacerbate the myocardial ischemia. (Copyright © by S. H. Rahimtoola, M.B., F.R.C.P., M.A.C.P., M.A.C.C. See Ref. 93.)

is usually due to a transient ventricular tachyarrhythmia, from which the patient recovers spontaneously. Other possible causes of syncope include transient atrial fibrillation or transient AV block, during which the ventricle is deprived of the powerful atrial booster pump function and/or the ventricular rate is slow.

Dyspnea on exertion, orthopnea, paroxysmal nocturnal dyspnea, and pulmonary edema result from varying degrees of pulmonary venous hypertension. Systemic venous congestion with enlargement of the liver and peripheral edema result from increased systemic venous pressure and salt and water retention. There is an increased incidence of gastrointestinal arteriovenous malformations.[39,40] As a result, these patients are susceptible to gastrointestinal hemorrhage and anemia. Calcific systemic embolism may occur.[41,42]

PHYSICAL FINDINGS

There is a spectrum of physical findings in patients with AS, depending on the severity of the stenosis, stroke volume, LV function, and the rigidity and calcification of the valve (Table 56-3). The arterial pulse rises slowly, taking a longer time than normal to reach peak pressure, and the peak is reduced (*parvus et tardus*);[43] the pulse pressure may be narrowed. The anacrotic notch on the upstroke is best appreciated in the carotid arteries. The more severe the valve stenosis, the lower the anacrotic notch on the arterial pulse. A systolic thrill may be felt in the carotid arteries. The jugular venous pulse is normal unless the patient is in heart failure. In the absence of heart failure, the heart size is normal. The cardiac impulse is heaving and sustained in character, and there may be a palpable fourth heart sound (S_4). An aortic systolic thrill is often present at the base of the heart. In 80 to 90 percent of adult patients with severe AS, there is an S_4 gallop sound, a midsystolic ejection murmur that peaks late in systole, and a single second heart sound (S_2) because A_2 and P_2 are superimposed or A_2 is absent or soft. There is often a faint early diastolic murmur of minimal aortic regurgitation. In the young patient with valvular AS, a systolic ejection sound (systolic ejection click) initiates the systolic murmur but later tends to disappear as AS becomes severe. The S_2 may be paradoxically split due to late A_2, and there may be no early diastolic murmur. In many patients, particularly the elderly, the systolic ejection murmur is atypical, may be soft, is described as a seagull sound (or musical, or cooing), and may be heard only at the apex of the heart (Gallavardin phenomenon). In the presence of heart failure, the jugular venous pressure is often increased, the left ventricle is dilated, a third heart sound is present, and the systolic murmur may be very soft or absent. Thus, the clinical features on physical examination may resemble those of heart failure from a variety of causes, such as dilated cardiomyopathy, rather than AS (see also Chap. 10).

Severe valvular AS is common in patients 60 years of age or older.[13,44] The clinical features in many of these patients tend to be somewhat different from those typical of younger patients.[44] Systemic hypertension is common, being present in about 20 percent of the patients, half of whom have moderate or severe systolic and diastolic hypertension. A fifth of the patients first present in congestive heart failure. The male: female ratio is 2:1. Because of thickening of the arterial wall and its associated lack of dispensability, the arterial pulse rises normally or even rapidly, and the pulse pressure is wide. The S_2 is either absent or single. As noted above, the murmur may be high-pitched and musical and may radiate from the base to the apex or may be heard best at the apex, mimicking mitral regurgitation.

CHEST X-RAY

The characteristic finding is a normal-sized heart with a dilated proximal ascending aorta (poststenotic dilation). Calcium in the aortic valve can be seen on the lateral film but is better appreciated by fluoroscopy with image intensification. In the current era, calcification is most easily recognized on two-

TABLE 56-3 Physical Examination of Patients with Varying Severity of Aortic Valve Stenosis

	Mild	Moderate	Severe + Normal LV Function	Severe + LV Dysfunction	Severe + Heart Failure[a]
Arterial pulse	Normal	Slowly rising	*Parvus et tardus*	*Parvus et tardus*	Small volume
Jugular venous pulse	Normal	Normal	Normal	Normal	±
Carotid thrill	±	±	±	±	±
Cardiac impulse	Normal	Heaving	Heaving, sustained palpable *a* wave	Heaving	Heaving or reduced
Precordial thrill	±	±	Usually ++	±	–
Auscultation					
S_4	–	±	++	+	–
S_3	–	–	–	±	+
ESS	+	±	–	–	–
Peak of ESM	Early systole	Mid-systole	Late systole	Late to mid-systole, soft	Mid-systole, soft or absent
S_2	Normal	Normal or single	Single or paradoxical	Single	Single

[a]There may be signs of mitral and tricuspid regurgitation and of pulmonary hypertension.

ABBREVIATIONS: S_4 = fourth heart sounds (presystolic gallop); S_3 = third heart sound (diastolic gallop); ESS = ejection systolic sound; ESM = ejection systolic murmur; S_2 = second heart sound.

dimensional echocardiography. Calcium in the aortic valve is the hallmark of AS in adults 40 to 45 years of age.[45,46] In patients aged 45 years or above, the diagnosis of severe AS is doubtful if there is no calcium in the aortic valve. The presence of calcium, however, does not necessarily mean that the valve is stenotic or that the AS is severe. In patients with heart failure, the cardiac size is increased because of dilatation of the left ventricle and left atrium; the lung fields show pulmonary edema and pulmonary venous congestion with redistribution of blood flow. In the presence of heart failure, the right ventricle and the right atrium may be dilated.

ELECTROCARDIOGRAM

The *electrocardiogram* (ECG) in severe AS shows LV hypertrophy with or without secondary ST-T-wave changes. It is important to recognize, however, that in about 10 to 15 percent of patients with severe AS, LV hypertrophy cannot be appreciated on the ECG. In fact, the ECG may be entirely normal in some of these patients. The P-wave abnormality (P = 0.12 s) of left atrial enlargement and/or hypertrophy and/or conduction delay is present in over 80 percent.[47] The ECG may show left bundle branch block, right bundle branch block with left or right axis deviation, or, occasionally, isolated right bundle branch block.[48–50] In some patients, the conduction abnormality results from aortic valve calcification extending into the specialized conducting tissue, which may even produce heart block. The patients are usually in sinus rhythm. The presence of atrial fibrillation indicates the presence of either associated mitral valve disease, CAD, or heart failure secondary to aortic valve disease. Atrial fibrillation is relatively common in the elderly with calcific AS, probably because of the increased presence of associated diseases.

Laboratory Investigations

ECHOCARDIOGRAPHY/DOPPLER ULTRASOUND

Echocardiography/Doppler (echo/Doppler) ultrasound (Chap. 13) is an extremely important and useful noninvasive test. On the echocardiogram, the aortic valve leaflets normally are barely visible in systole, and the normal range of aortic valve opening is 1.6 to 2.6 cm. In the presence of a bicuspid aortic valve, eccentric valve leaflets may be seen. The aortic valve leaflets may appear to be thickened as a result of calcification and/or fibrosis; however, the older patient without valve stenosis may also have thickened cusps. The aortic valve may have a reduced opening, but this also occurs in other conditions in which the cardiac output is reduced. The LV hypertrophy often results in thickening of both the interventricular septum and the posterior LV wall. The LV cavity size is normal. All these abnormalities are better appreciated on two-dimensional echocardiography. When LV systolic function is impaired, the left ventricle and left atrium are dilated and the percentage of dimensional shortening is reduced.

In many patients, the severity of AS is incorrectly estimated by M-mode or two-dimensional echocardiography. Neither is a completely reliable technique for assessing the severity of AS. The presence of normal movement of thin aortic leaflets on the echocardiogram, however, is strong evidence against severe AS in adults.

Echo/Doppler, when properly applied, is extremely useful for estimating the valve gradient and AVA noninvasively.[50–56] When compared with results obtained at cardiac catheterization, the standard error of the estimate of mean gradient in the best laboratories is 10 mmHg.[57] Thus, the mean gradient by Doppler can be expected to be within ±20 mmHg (95 percent confidence level) of that obtained at catheterization.[57] Similarly, the AVA will be within ±0.3 cm^2 of that obtained at cardiac catheterization.[57] A recent study of 156 patients compared AVA obtained by cardiac catheterization with that obtained by Doppler ultrasound.[58] Of 125 patients with AVA 0.8 cm^2 at cardiac catheterization, in 36 (29 percent) Doppler-estimated AVA was ≥0.9 cm^2. In all 7 patients with AVA >1.0 cm^2 by cardiac catheterization, Doppler-estimated AVA was 1.0 cm^2; the findings in these 7 patients must be interpreted cautiously because they were likely to be a highly selected subgroup. Guidelines for assessing severity of AS based on Doppler-obtained gradients are shown in Table 56-4. In a study of 636 patients studied by cardiac catheterization, no single aortic valve gradient was found to be both sensitive and specific for severe AS. A mean gradient of ≥50 mmHg or a peak gradient ≥60 mmHg were "specific" with a 90 percent or more positive predictive value. It was not possible to find a lower limit with 90 percent negative predictive value.[59] Thus, a mean gradient of <50 mmHg is compatible with mild, moderate, or severe AS.

TABLE 56-4 Suggested Conservative Guidelines for Relating Severity of Aortic Stenosis to Doppler Gradients in Adults with Normal Cardiac Output and Normal Average Heart Rate

Peak Gradient, mmHg	Mean Gradient, mmHg	Severe AS
≥80	≥70	Highly likely
60–79	50–69	Probable
<60	<50	Uncertain

SOURCE: From Rahimtoola,[57] with permission.

Transesophageal echo/Doppler ultrasound is very useful in defining the aortic valve abnormality and in assessing its severity when an adequate examination cannot be obtained with the transthoracic technique.

CARDIAC CATHETERIZATION/ANGIOGRAPHY

Cardiac catheterization remains the standard technique to assess the severity of AS "accurately." This is done by measuring simultaneous LV and ascending aortic pressures and measuring

TABLE 56-5 A Suggested Grading of the Degree of Aortic Stenosis

Aortic Stenosis	AVA, cm^2	AVA Index, cm^2/m^2
Mild	>1.5	>0.9
Moderate	>1.0–1.5	>0.6–0.9
Severe[a]	≤0.8–1.0	≤0.4–0.6

[a]Patients with AVAs that are at borderline values between the moderate and severe grades (0.9–1.1 cm^2; 0.55–0.65 cm^2/m^2) should be considered individually.
ABBREVIATIONS: AVA = aortic valve area.
SOURCE: From Rahimtoola,[57] with permission.

TABLE 56-6 Aortic Valve Disease: Indications for Coronary Arteriography

Patients ≥35 years
Patients <35 years:
- Left ventricular dysfunction
- Symptoms or signs suggesting CAD
- Two or more risk factors for premature CAD (excluding gender)

ABBREVIATIONS: CAD = coronary artery disease.
SOURCE: From Rahimtoola,[57] with permission.

cardiac output by either the Fick principle or the indicator dilution technique. The AVA can be calculated (see Chap. 15). It is important to calculate AVA.[59] AS can be considered to be severe when the valve area is 1.0 cm^2 or less or the AVA index is 0.6 cm^2 per square meter or less (Table 56-5).[57] The state of LV systolic pump function can be quantitated by measuring LV end-diastolic and end-systolic volumes and ejection fraction. *It must be recognized that ejection fraction may underestimate myocardial function in the presence of the increased afterload of severe AS.*

The presence of CAD and its site and severity can be estimated only by selective coronary angiography, which should be performed in all patients 35 years of age or older being considered for valve surgery and in those <35 years if they have LV systolic dysfunction, symptoms or signs suggesting CAD, or two or more risk factors for premature CAD (excluding gender) (Table 56-6). The incidence of associated CAD will vary considerably depending on the prevalence of CAD in the population.[57,60] It was reported to be 50 percent in patients with AS and 20 percent in patients with aortic regurgitation.[57] In general, in persons 50 years of age or older, it is about 50 percent (Table 56-7).[44,61-63]

TABLE 56-7 Isolated Aortic Valve Replacement: Incidence of Associated Coronary Artery Disease

	VA Co-op Study[a]	Mayo Clinic[b]	MGH[c] (80–89 years)
Total number of patients	643	618	64
Patients with coronary artery disease	312	321	37
%	49%	52%	58%
1 VD	17%	22%	27%
2 VD	17%	14%	19%
3 VD	15%	17%	13%
Additional LMCAD	—	5%	3%

[a]Sethi GK et al.[61]
[b]Mullany CJ et al.[62]
[c]Levinson JR et al.[63]
ABBREVIATIONS: LMCAD = left main coronary artery disease; MGH = Massachusetts General Hospital; VA = Veterans Administration; VD = vessel disease.

GATED BLOOD POOL RADIONUCLIDE SCANS

Gated blood pool radionuclide scans provide information on ventricular function similar to that provided by two-dimensional echocardiography and LV cineangiography. These studies are of particular value in the occasional patient in whom LV cineangiography is unsuccessful and echocardiographic studies are suboptimal.

EXERCISE TESTS

It is usually recommended that exercise tests of any kind not be undertaken in patients with severe AS unless there is a specific reason for such studies. Exercise tests in these patients may precipitate ventricular tachyarrhythmias and ventricular fibrillation. If there is doubt about the severity of AS and concern that the patient's symptoms may not be caused by AS, it is usually wise to document the absence of severe AS before performing an exercise test. Occasionally, in a patient with severe AS who denies all symptoms, a closely monitored exercise test by experienced and skilled physician(s) may be needed to assess exercise capacity but should usually *only* be undertaken after exclusion of associated significantly obstructive CAD.

AMBULATORY ECG RECORDING

Ambulatory ECG recordings may be needed in an occasional patient suspected of having an arrhythmia[64,65] or painless ischemia. Occasionally, patients with mild or moderate AS who are symptomatic may be suspected of having an arrhythmia or painless ischemia as a cause of the symptoms. At times, in asymptomatic patients with severe AS, one may need to determine if the patient has painless ischemia (see also Chap. 25).

PROVOCATIVE DIAGNOSTIC TEST

In an occasional patient, the severity of the AS may be in doubt because of a small stroke volume and small mean aortic valve gradient. The AS may be severe or mild to moderate, and the calculated AVA may be very small because of severe stenosis or because the small stroke volume only opens the valve to a limited extent; thus, the AVA will be determined to be small even on echo/Doppler ultrasound. Infusion of an inotropic agent such as dobutamine, which results in increases of stroke volume and heart rate, usually helps one to make a correct diagnosis. In these circumstances, it is important to measure cardiac output and LV and aortic pressures simultaneously and meticulously, both before and during dobutamine infusion. Whether the AS is mild or severe the gradient increases with dobutamine infusion; however, in mild AS the AVA increases significantly; but in severe AS the AVA does not increase or increases minimally (approximately 10 percent).

Clinical Decision Making

There are a number of steps involved in clinical decision making in patients with valvular heart disease (Table 56-8).[57] The first is a complete clinical evaluation, which includes history, physical examination, ECG, and chest x-ray. Next, disease of all cardiac valves, ventricular function, and hemodynamic effects as well as CAD, other cardiovascular disease, and disease of other organs should be diagnosed and the severity assessed. Before proceeding to additional testing, it is important to list the question(s) to be answered and to be reasonably certain that these

TABLE 56-8 Steps in Clinical Decision Making in Patients with Valvular Heart Disease

1. Perform a complete clinical evaluation
   - History
   - Physical examination
   - Electrocardiogram
   - Chest x-ray film
2. Diagnose and assess severity of disease
   - All valves
   - Ventricular function
   - Hemodynamic effects
   - Coronary artery disease
   - Other cardiovascular disease
   - Effects on other body organs
   - Other organ diseases
3. List questions that need answering
4. Be reasonably certain these questions need to be answered
5. Perform test(s) most likely to provide these answers in one's own institution with the following criteria:
   - Reliability
   - Accuracy
   - Lowest risk to patients
   - Reasonable (or lowest) cost
6. Review results of test(s)
7. Make an overall assessment of patient
8. Make recommendations regarding management

SOURCE: From Rahimtoola,[57] with permission.

questions need to be answered. The test(s) that are most likely to provide these answers *in the clinician's own institution* should then be performed, with the following criteria being kept in mind: reliability, accuracy, lowest risk to patient, and reasonable (lowest) cost. The results of the test(s) should be reviewed as they become available, and an overall evaluation/assessment of the patient and, finally, recommendations regarding management should be made.

In a prospective, blinded study of consecutive patients with valvular heart disease, the sensitivity and specificity of diagnosis of AS and the accuracy of assessment of severity of AS were determined (Table 56-9).[66] This study revealed the following important points: (1) Clinical evaluation was sensitive, highly specific, and reasonably accurate in diagnosing AS and was very accurate in assessing its severity when AS was moderate or severe. This emphasizes the importance of a thorough clinical evaluation of the patient. (2) Echo/Doppler ultrasound improved the accuracy of this assessment to a certain extent. (3) The reason clinical evaluation and echo/Doppler do not have a 100 percent specificity is the inability in an occasional patient to distinguish mild AS from turbulence across a normal or slightly diseased aortic valve. (4) Both clinical evaluation and echo/Doppler ultrasound are excellent in diagnosing the AS as being at least moderate or severe. (5) An important difficulty in diagnosis by clinical evaluation and by echo/Doppler is in not being able to separate accurately all patients with moderate AS from those with severe AS.

TABLE 56-9 Clinical Decision Making Utilizing Clinical Evaluation and Echo/Doppler in Patients with Aortic Stenosis

	After Clinical Evaluation, %	After Echo/Doppler, %
Diagnosis of AS		
Sensitivity	78	100
Specificity	92	92
Accuracy of diagnosis		
All levels of severity	48	65
Moderate or severe AS	100	100

SOURCE: From Kotlewski et al.,[66] with permission.

Natural History and Prognosis

Valvular AS is frequently a progressive disease, the severity increasing over time.[67–71] The factors that control this progression and the time it takes for severe outflow obstruction to develop are unknown; however, it appears that in the older patient, AS may progress at about twice the rate that it does in the younger patient.[72] In a study of 142 patients with "mild" stenosis (catheterization-proven AVA >1.5 cm^2),[73] the rate of progression to severe stenosis was 8 percent in 10 years, 22 percent in 20 years, and 38 percent in 25 years. At 25 years, 38 percent still had mild AS (Table 56-10). The duration of the asymptomatic period after the development of severe AS is also unknown; some recent data suggest that it may be less than 2 years. The outcome of the asymptomatic patient with severe AS is not known. In the study of 123 asymptomatic patients aged 63 ± 16 years, the actuarial probability of death or aortic valve surgery was 7 ± 5 percent at 1 year, 38 ± 8 percent at 3 years, and 74 ± 10 percent at 5 years.[74] The event rate at 2 years for peak aortic jet velocity by Doppler ultrasound of >4 m/s was 79 ± 18 percent, for 3 to 4 m/s was 66 ± 13 percent, and for <3 m/s was 16 ± 16 percent. However, the limitations of gradients and of aortic peak velocity obtained by Doppler ultrasound should be kept in mind.[75] The overwhelming majority of adults with severe AS who are seen by cardiologists have symptoms.

Severe disease in adults is lethal, particularly if the patient is symptomatic, with a prognosis that is worse than for many forms of neoplastic disease.[57] The 3-year mortality is approximately 36 to 52 percent, the 5-year mortality is about 52 to 80 percent, and the 10-year mortality is 80 to 90 percent.[57] A recent study of elderly patients (average age 77 years) showed 1-year and 3-year mortalities were 44 and 75 percent, respectively.[76] With the onset of severe symptoms (angina, syncope, or heart

TABLE 56-10 Natural History of Mild[a] Aortic Stenosis (n = 142)

	10 Years	20 Years	25 Years
Mild	88%	63%	38%
Moderate	4%	15%	25%
Severe	8%	22%	38%

[a]Mild stenosis is defined here as an aortic valve area >1.5 cm^2.
SOURCE: From Horstkotte and Loogen,[73] with permission.

TABLE 56-11 Average Survival of Symptomatic Patients with Severe AS

	Autopsy Data,[a] Years	Post Cardiac Catheterization,[b] Months
Overall	3	23
Angina	5	45
Syncope	3	27
Heart failure	<2	11

[a]From Ross and Braunwald.[77]
[b]From Horstkotte and Loogen.[73]

failure), the average life expectancy is 2 to 3 years (Table 56-11).[73,77] Almost all patients with heart failure are dead in 1 to 2 years.[73,77] A combination of symptoms is much more ominous, a sign of a greatly reduced survival. Sudden death, like syncope, occurs in the presence of severe AS. Its exact incidence is difficult to determine but may be about 5 percent.[77] Most but not all of these patients have had some cardiac symptoms before the fatal episode; at times, the only symptom has been exertional presyncope. Patients with aortic valve "sclerosis" have an approximately 50 percent increase in cardiovascular mortality and myocardial infarction.[78] This incidence is lower than in patients with AS, and aortic sclerosis appears to be a marker for vascular atherosclerosis.

Management

All patients with AS need antibiotic prophylaxis against infective endocarditis (see Chap. 73). Those in whom the valve lesion is of rheumatic origin need additional prophylaxis against recurrence of rheumatic fever. Patients with mild or moderate stenosis rarely have symptoms or complications and do not need any specific medical therapy (Table 56-12). In mild stenosis, the patient should be encouraged to lead a normal life. Those with moderate AS should avoid moderate to severe physical exertion and competitive sports. In patients with mild or moderate AS, if atrial fibrillation should occur, it should be reverted rapidly to sinus rhythm. In severe AS, reversion to sinus rhythm often becomes a matter of some urgency.

Operation should be advised for the symptomatic patient who has severe AS. In young patients, if the valve is pliable and mobile, simple commissurotomy or valve repair may be feasible; the operative mortality is <1 percent.[79] It will relieve outflow obstruction to a major degree. In such patients, catheter balloon valvuloplasty is the procedure of choice in experienced and skilled centers. Both of these are palliative procedures that postpone valve replacement for many years. Older patients and even young patients with calcified, rigid valves need valve replacement. The natural history of symptomatic patients with severe AS is dismal, i.e., a 10-year mortality of 80 to 90 percent, but there is good outcome after surgery, particularly in patients without any comorbid cardiac and noncardiac conditions. Given the unknown natural history of the asymptomatic patient with severe AS, which may not be benign,[57] it is reasonable to recommend surgery even to the asymptomatic patient. There is, however, no consensus about valve replacement in the truly asymptomatic patient. Clearly, if the patient has LV dysfunction, then valve replacement should be performed. Some recommend

TABLE 56-12 Medical Treatment of Patients with Aortic Valve Stenosis

- I. Antibiotic prophylaxis
  - A. Infective endocarditis (Chap. 82)
  - B. Recurrent rheumatic carditis (Chap. 62)
- II. Restriction of activities
  - A. Severe exercise
  - B. Competitive sports
- III. Arrhythmias
  - A. Prevent and/or control
  - B. Restore sinus rhythm, if possible
- IV. Cardiac medications (only if essential)
  - A. Avoid negative inotropic and proarrhythmic agents if possible
  - B. Diuretics—use cautiously
  - C. Arteriolar and venodilators—use cautiously
- V. Follow-up of asymptomatic patients
  - A. Mild AS: Every 2–5 years
  - B. Moderate AS: Every 6–12 months
  - C. Develop symptoms: Immediate

SOURCE: Copyright S. H. Rahimtoola, M.B., F.R.C.P., M.A.C.P., M.A.C.C. See Ref. 93.

TABLE 56-13 Severe Aortic Valve Stenosis: Indications for Surgery

- I. All symptomatic patients
  - A. LV function normal: as soon as possible
  - B. LV dysfunction: urgent
  - C. Heart failure: emergent
- II. Asymptomatic patients
  - A. Patients undergoing surgery for CAD, aorta, other valves
  - B. Associated significantly obstructed CAD
  - C. LV dysfunction
  - D. Progressive decline of LVEF
  - E. Marked or excessive LVH:
    1. ≥11–12 mm in smaller people, e.g., women
    2. ≥13–14 mm in larger people, e.g., men
  - F. Patients aged ≥60–65 years
  - G. "Very" severe AS ≤0.7 cm²; 0.4 cm²/m²
  - H. Others:
    1. Abnormal response to exercise
       a. Hypotension/no or minimal increase of BP
       b. Ischemia
       c. LV dysfunction
       d. Arrhythmias
    2. Arrhythmias
       a. Ventricular/Atrial tachyarrhythmias
       b. A-V block >1° AVB

ABBREVIATIONS: LV = left ventricular; AVA = aortic valve area; CAD = Coronary artery disease.
SOURCE: Copyright © by Shahbudin H. Rahimtoola, M.B., F.R.C.P., M.A.C.P., M.A.C.C. See Ref. 93.

TABLE 56-14 Aortic Valve Replacement (AVR) Operative Mortality and Late Survival: Effect of Coronary Bypass Surgery (CBS)

	1982–1983	1967–1976					
	Operative Mortality, %	Operative Mortality, %	All Patients, %	1 VD, %	2 VD, %	3 VD, %	LMCAD, %
AVR + no CAD	1.4	4.5	63	—	—	—	—
AVR + CAD + CBS	4.0	6.3	49	38	28	34	11
AVR + CAD + no CBS	9.4	10.3	36	65	22	13	1

ABBREVIATIONS: CAD = coronary artery disease, VD = vessel disease, LMCAD = left main coronary artery disease.
SOURCE: From Mullany et al.,[62] with permission.

valve replacement in all asymptomatic patients with severe AS, while others would recommend it in those with AVA $\leq$0.7 cm^2 and in selected patients with AVA of 0.76 to 1.0 cm^2 (Table 56-13).

The operative mortality of valve replacement is about 5 percent or less (see Chap. 61).[57,61,62] In patients without associated CAD, heart failure, or other comorbid factors, it may be 1 to 2 percent in centers with experienced and skilled staff.[62] Patients with associated CAD should have coronary bypass surgery at the same time as valve surgery because it results in a lower operative and late mortality (Table 56-14). The operative mortality in octogenarians or older is much higher: up to 6 percent for isolated aortic valve replacement and up to 10 percent for those undergoing aortic valve replacement and associated coronary bypass surgery.

In severe AS, valve replacement results in an improvement of survival (Fig. 56-4),[73,80] even in those with normal preoperative LV function. LV function remains normal postoperatively if perioperative myocardial damage has not occurred.[22,57,81,82] LV hypertrophy regresses toward normal;[22,57,81,82] after 2 years, the regression continues at a slower rate for up to 8 to 10 years after valve replacement.[82] In those with excessive LV hypertrophy preoperatively,[30] the hypertrophy may regress slowly or not at all. These patients may have persistent severe LV diastolic dysfunction, which may be a difficult clinical problem both in the early postoperative period and after hospital discharge. Their clinical picture subsequently resembles that of patients with hypertrophic cardiomyopathy without outflow obstruction, and they may have to be treated as such. Surviving patients are functionally improved. After aortic valve replacement, the 10-year survival is 60 percent or better and the 15-year survival is 45 percent or better.[83] Approximately one-half of the late deaths are not related to the prosthesis but to associated cardiac abnormalities and other comorbid conditions.[83] Thus, the late survival will vary in different subgroups of patients. The older patients ($\geq$65 years) have a relative 10-year survival (actual survival compared to an age- and gender-matched person in the population) after valve replacement that is significantly better than that of those who are younger (<65 years)—94 percent versus 81 percent (Fig. 56-5).[84]

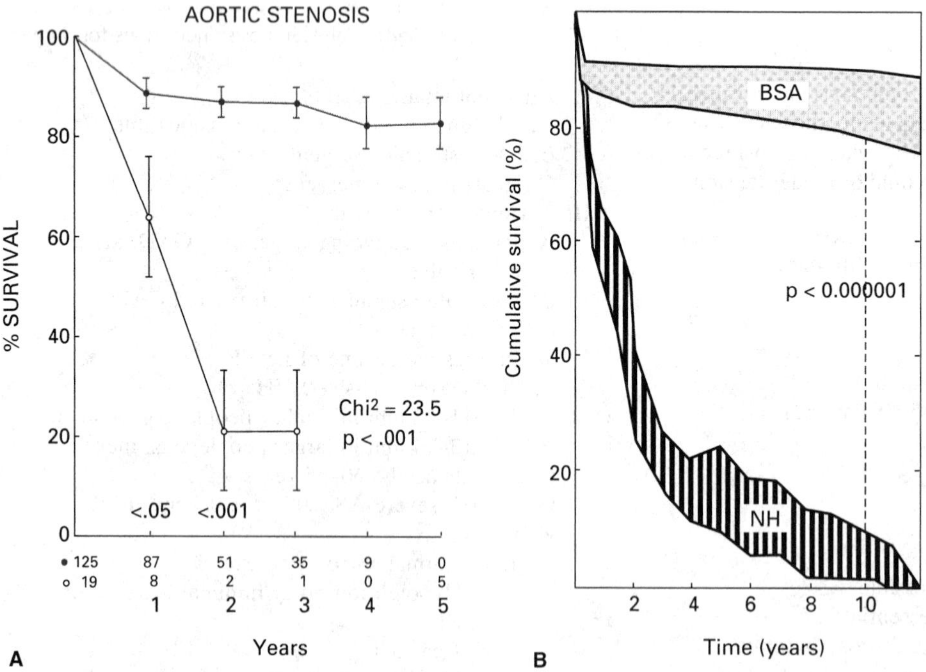

FIGURE 56-4 There are no prospective randomized trials of aortic valve replacement in severe aortic stenosis, and there are unlikely to be any in the near future. Two studies have compared the results of aortic valve replacement with medical treatment during the same time period in symptomatic patients with normal LV systolic pump function. *Panel A.* Patients who had valve replacement (*closed circles*) had a much better survival than those treated medically (*open circles*). (From Schwarz et al.,[80] with permission.)

Panel B. Patients who were treated with valve replacement (BSA) had a better survival than those treated medically (NH). (From Horstkotte and Loogen,[73] with permission.)

These differences in survival between those treated medically and surgically are so large that there is a great deal of confidence that aortic valve replacement significantly improves the survival of those with severe AS.

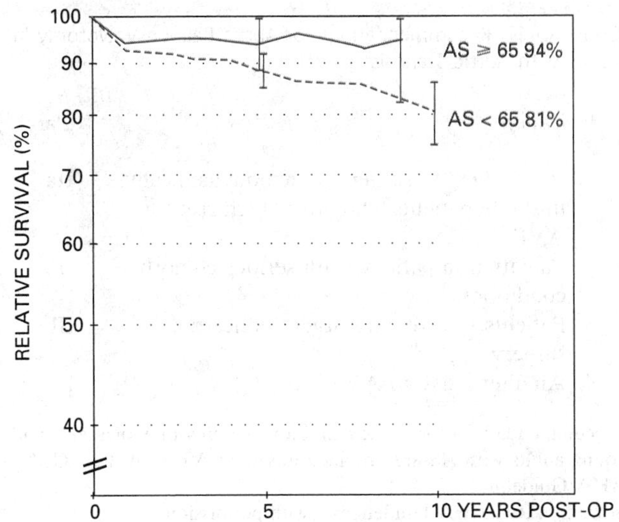

FIGURE 56-5 Data from the Karolinska Institute in Sweden provided an interesting perspective on the long-term survival after valve replacement in patients aged ≥65 years. They examined the relative survival, i.e., compared the survival of the patient who had undergone aortic valve replacement with another age- and sex-matched person in the same population. Patients under the age of 65 had a relative survival of 81 percent, significantly lower than 100 percent. On the other hand, patients aged ≥65 years who underwent valve replacement had a relative survival of 94 percent at the end of 10 years—not significantly different from 100 percent. These data indicate that (1) survival following valve replacement for AS in patients aged ≥65 years is identical to an age- and sex-matched individual in the population who does not have AS and (2) the late relative survival of patients aged 65 years or greater is much better than that of patients under the age of 65. (From Lindblom et al.,[84] with permission.)

Patients who present with heart failure should be hospitalized and treated with digitalis, diuretics, and *angiotensin-converting enzyme* (ACE) inhibitors and should undergo surgery as soon as possible. ACE inhibitors should be used extremely cautiously if at all. The patient must be monitored and hypotension avoided; a "significant" fall in blood pressure is an indication to discontinue or reduce the dose of ACE inhibitor. If heart failure does not respond satisfactorily and rapidly to medical therapy, surgery becomes a matter of considerable urgency.[85] Catheter balloon valvuloplasty can be an important bridge procedure in selected critically ill patients.[85] It usually improves the patients' hemodynamics and makes them better candidates for valve replacement. Valve replacement in patients with AS and heart failure can be performed at an operative mortality of 10 percent or less.[86] Although this is higher than in patients not in heart failure, the risk is justified because late survival in those who survive the operation is excellent and is far superior to that which can be expected with medical therapy; the 7-year survival of patients who survive operation is 84 percent.[87] The survival is lower in those with associated CAD.[86] The impaired LV function improves in all such patients provided that there has been no perioperative myocardial damage; it becomes normal in two-thirds of the patients (Fig. 56-6).[88] In some patients the improvement is less marked.[86] This is more likely in those with longer duration of preoperative LV dysfunction and in those with associated CAD. In addition, the operative survivors are functionally much improved. LV hypertrophy and dilatation (if present preoperatively) regress toward normal. Despite the

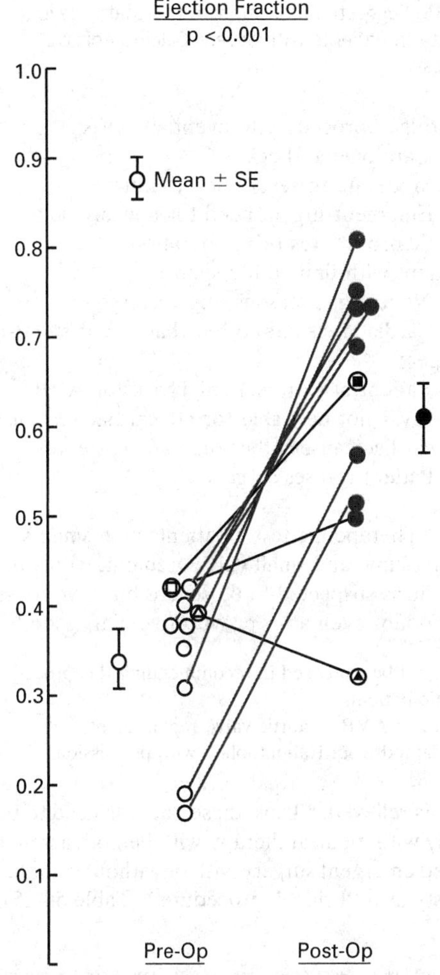

FIGURE 56-6 Examination of changes in LV ejection fraction in each individual patient. In those who had aortic stenosis with LV systolic dysfunction and clinical heart failure, the LV ejection fraction after aortic valve replacement increased from 0.34 to 0.63. All but one patient showed an improvement in LV ejection fraction; the only patient who showed a deterioration in ejection fraction suffered a perioperative myocardial infarction and had complete heart block, and the only patient who showed only a small increase in ejection fraction had had a myocardial infarct prior to valve replacement. Note that ejection fraction normalized in two-thirds of the patients, and in the two patients with the lowest ejection fraction (0.18 and 0.19), the ejection fraction normalized in both.

These data indicate that there is probably no lower limit of ejection fraction at which time these patients become inoperable. This also indicates that the lower the ejection fraction, the more urgent the need for valve replacement. (From Smith et al.,[88] with permission.)

excellent results of valve replacements in patients with severe AS who are in heart failure, it is important to recognize that surgery should *not* be delayed until heart failure develops.

In the data bases of older patients who underwent catheter balloon valvuloplasty, 6 percent of the patients were in cardiogenic shock.[89,90] The hospital mortality in such patients was very high, almost 50 percent. After hospital discharge, the subsequent mortality is also very high if the patients have not had

TABLE 56-15 Suggested Indications for Catheter Balloon Valvuloplasty in Patients with Severe Calcific Aortic Valve Stenosis[a]

I. "Bridge" procedure to eventual AVR
   A. Cardiogenic shock
   B. Moderate to severe heart failure
   C. Emergent/urgent need for noncardiac therapeutic procedures (e.g., operation)
II. Patient with limited life span
   A. Noncardiac reasons (e.g., carcinoma)
   B. Cardiac reason(s) other than aortic stenosis
III. Others
   A. Patient at extremely high risk for AVR
   B. AVR not desirable for noncardiac reasons or cardiac causes other than aortic stenosis
   C. Patient refuses surgery
IV. Rare
   A. "Therapeutic test": patients with small stroke volume and small valve gradient, with valve stenosis suspected to be severe but severity in doubt even after provocative diagnostic tests

[a]Caution should be exercised in recommending this procedure in asymptomatic patients.
ABBREVIATIONS: AVR = aortic valve replacement.
SOURCE: Adapted from Rahimtoola,[85] with permission.

their stenosis relieved.[90] Thus, these patients need to be treated aggressively with medical therapy with hemodynamic monitoring and need emergent surgery with or without catheter balloon valvuloplasty as a "bridge" procedure[85] (Table 56-15).

TABLE 56-16 Recommendations for Aortic Valve Replacement in Aortic Stenosis

Indication	Class
1. Symptomatic patients with severe AS	I
2. Patients with severe AS undergoing coronary artery bypass surgery	I
3. Patients with severe AS undergoing surgery on the aorta or other heart valves	I
4. Patients with moderate AS undergoing coronary artery bypass surgery or surgery on the aorta or other heart valves (see sections III.F.6., III.F.7., and VIII.D. of the ACC/AHA Guidelines)	IIa
5. Asymptomatic patients with severe AS and	
• LV systolic dysfunction	IIa
• Abnormal response to exercise (e.g., hypotension)	IIa
• Ventricular tachycardia	IIb
• Marked or excessive LV hypertrophy (≥15 mm)	IIb
• Valve area <0.6 cm^2	IIb
6. Prevention of sudden death in asymptomatic patients with none of the findings listed under indication 5	III

SOURCE: ACC/AHA Guidelines,[91] with permission.

TABLE 56-17 Recommendations for Aortic Balloon Valvotomy in Adults with Aortic Stenosis[a]

Indication	Class
1. A "bridge" to surgery in hemodynamically unstable patients who are at high risk for AVR	IIa
2. Palliation in patients with serious comorbid conditions	IIb
3. Patients who require urgent noncardiac surgery	IIb
4. An alternative to AVR	III

[a]Recommendations for aortic balloon valvotomy in adolescents and young adults with AS are provided in section VI.A. of the ACC/AHA Guidelines.
SOURCE: ACC/AHA Guidelines,[91] with permission.

The role of catheter balloon valvuloplasty in the older patient has now been clarified.[57,85] In calcific AS after catheter balloon valvuloplasty, the average increase in AVA is 0.3 cm^2 and the final AVA usually averages 0.8 cm^2; thus, many patients continue to have severe AS.[57,85,89] The 30-day, 1-year, and 3-year mortalities average 14, 35, and 71 percent, respectively, in the older patient (average age 78 ± 9 years) with calcific AS,[89] a mortality rate that may be similar to the natural history of this lesion. This technique is indicated[85] as a bridge procedure in those who need emergent noncardiac surgery and in those who are in heart failure (or in cardiogenic shock), who have an expected limited short life span when operative risks are considered to be prohibitively high, and who refuse surgery. When performed as a bridge procedure, valve surgery should not be unduly delayed. On rare occasions, it may be considered as a therapeutic test in patients in whom AS is suspected to be severe but the severity of the AS is in doubt after all standard tests have been performed (Table 56-15), including provocative diagnostic tests to assess mean aortic gradient, stroke volume, and AVA before and after infusion of dobutamine. Catheter balloon valvuloplasty is the procedure of choice in young patients who have pliable, noncalcified valves with commissural fusion (see Chap. 63).

The recommendations of the American College of Cardiology/American Heart Association (ACC/AHA) Practice Guidelines are shown in Tables 56-16 and 56-17.[91] Guidelines *are not* and *should not* be the law. Application of these guidelines to clinical practice should be based on the following principles: (1) classes I and III applies to all patients in these classes unless there is a specific clinical circumstance not to do so; (2) class II applies to patients in this class depending on the clinical conditions of the patients and the skill and experience at the individual medical center.

ACUTE AORTIC REGURGITATION

Etiology

The two most common causes of acute *aortic regurgitation* (AR) are infective endocarditis and prosthetic valve dysfunction.[92] Other causes include dissection of the aorta, systemic hypertension, and trauma.[93,94] AR associated with dissection of the aorta indicates that the dissection involves the ascending aorta down to the aortic valve annulus/root. AR associated with systemic hypertension is usually mild and transient; it is associated with severe elevation of aortic pressure, and, when the systemic hypertension is controlled, the AR usually disappears unless permanent changes have occurred in the aortic valve annulus/root or valve leaflets.

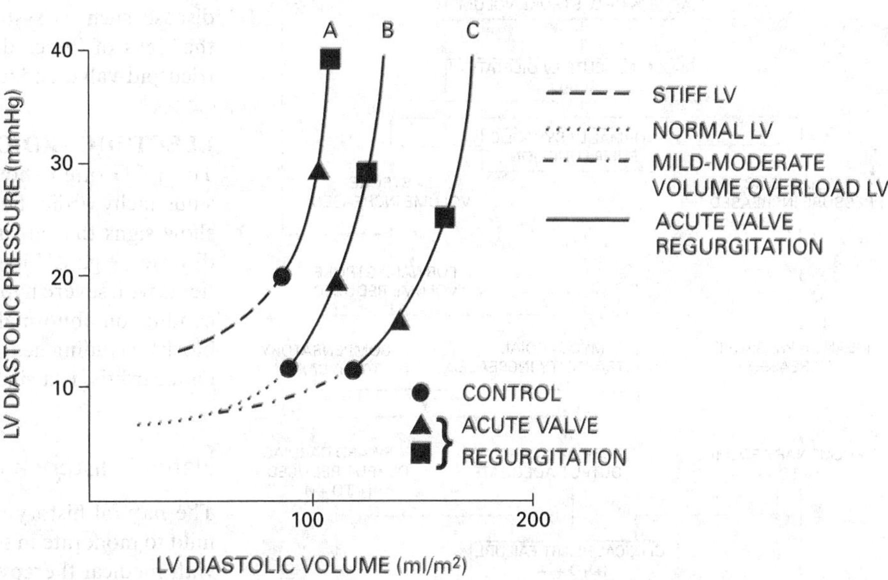

FIGURE 56-7 The left ventricular (LV) diastolic pressure-volume (P-V) relationship in acute valve regurgitation. The volume overload of acute AR produces a rapid increase of LV diastolic pressure in a patient with normal LV diastolic P-V prior to the acute AR (*curve B*). The LV diastolic pressure will rise more or less precipitously as a result of the volume overload of acute AR, depending on whether the LV is already stiff (*curve A*) or is somewhat dilated from a previous volume overload (*curve C*). (From Rahimtoola,[98] with permission.)

Pathophysiology

The LV diastolic pressure-volume relationship plays a very important role in the pathophysiology of acute valve regurgitation (Fig. 56-7).[95,96] Two features should be considered:[92] (1) The ability of the left ventricle to dilate acutely is limited; as a result, the volume overload of acute AR produces a rapid increase of LV diastolic pressure (curve B in Fig. 56-7). (2) The LV diastolic pressure-volume relationship before the onset of acute AR. If the left ventricle is already stiff or less compliant than normal from an associated lesion (e.g., AS or systemic hypertension), the LV diastolic pressure will rise more precipitously as a result of the volume overload of acute AR (curve A) than if the LV were normal (curve B). On the other hand, if the left ventricle is somewhat dilated from a previous lesion, for example, mild AR (curve C), initially the LV pressure will rise more gradually with acute AR but may subsequently rise to the same high levels as that seen with a normal or stiff LV.

Acute AR that is mild produces little or no hemodynamic abnormality, for example, when associated with systemic hypertension. Increasing severity of regurgitation produces greater degrees of hemodynamic abnormalities, and severe AR often produces the clinical picture of "heart failure."

Acute AR that is severe results in a large volume of regurgitant blood; therefore, the volume of blood in the LV in diastole is increased. In an acute situation, the LV end-diastolic volume can only increase mildly (no more than 20 to 30 percent) and the LV diastolic pressure-volume relationships are particularly important. The LV systolic pump function is initially normal (Fig. 56-8). The increased LV diastolic pressure results in increases in mean left atrial and pulmonary venous pressures and produces varying degrees of pulmonary edema.[97] The normal LV systolic pump function in the presence of LV dilatation results in an increase of LV stroke volume. A large percentage of the LV stroke volume is returned to the LV in diastole, however; as a result, the forward stroke volume is reduced. The LV uses two mechanisms: an increase of myocardial contractility and, importantly, a compensatory tachycardia to maintain an adequate forward cardiac output. As a result, the forward cardiac output may be appropriate initially. If the compensatory mechanisms are inadequate, however, forward cardiac output is reduced. Pulmonary edema, with or without an adequate cardiac output, produces the picture of clinical heart failure.[97] Subsequently, LV systolic pump function may become abnormal; when that occurs, the pulmonary edema is further increased and the forward cardiac output is further reduced, leading to more severe manifestations of clinical heart failure.

Clinical Findings

HISTORY, PHYSICAL FINDINGS

The clinical presentations of patients with acute AR are those relating to preexisting disorders that have caused the acute AR. For example, patients may have peripheral signs of infective endocarditis, a history of trauma, or severe chest pain of aortic dissection. The other clinical presentations are those related to the AR itself. If the AR is mild, the patient is usually asymptomatic. In the symptomatic patient, the symptoms are those of heart failure.

On physical examination, the symptomatic patient with acute severe AR usually has a tachycardia. The arterial pulse shows an increased rate of rise of pressure. Systolic pressure is usually normal unless there is very severe heart failure; however, the diastolic pressure is in the normal range or may be decreased. The pulse pressure is usually normal. Thus, although the classic peripheral signs of chronic, severe AR are often absent, an important diagnostic clue is the rapid rate of rise of arterial pressure. The usual clinical signs of heart failure may be present. On examination of the precordium, the LV impulse is normal or slightly displaced to the left; it is usually hyperkinetic unless LV systolic dysfunction is present. The first heart sound is soft, and the second heart sound is often single and is soft. If pulmonary hypertension is present, P_2 is loud and there is a loud S_3

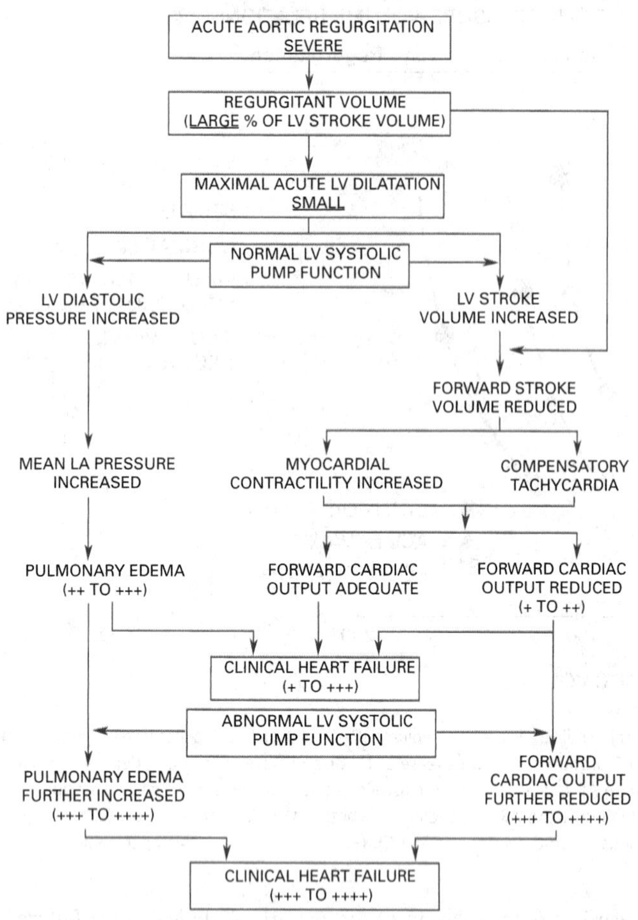

FIGURE 56-8 Pathophysiology of acute severe aortic regurgitation. Acute AR that is severe results in a large volume of regurgitant blood; therefore, the volume of blood in the left ventricle in diastole is increased. In an acute situation, the LV end-diastolic volume can only increase mildly (no more than 20 to 30 percent) and the LV diastolic pressure-volume relationships are particularly important (see Fig. 56-1). The subsequent findings are dependent on LV systolic pump function, LV diastolic pressure-volume relationship, myocardial contractile state, and compensatory tachycardia (see text for details). (Copyright © by S. H. Rahimtoola, M.B., F.R.C.P., M.A.C.P., M.A.C.C. See Ref. 93.)

gallop sound, but an S_4 gallop sound is absent. The clinical sine qua non of AR is the AR murmur, an early or immediate, blowing, decrescendo diastolic murmur beginning after A_2 that is best heard with the diaphragm of the stethoscope. Having the patient sit up and lean forward with the breath held in expiration facilitates the audibility of the murmur in difficult cases. The murmur may be short and soft if the ascending aortic pressure equalizes with LV pressure in early or middiastole. An Austin Flint murmur, if present, occurs in middiastole (see also Chap. 10).

An important clinical picture in intravenous drug abusers[92] includes: (1) a peripheral arterial pulse that has a rapid rate of rise and fall, even though the pulse pressure is small; (2) the telltale signs of intravenous drug abuse; (3) sinus tachycardia; and (4) "normal" heart size with pulmonary edema on chest x-ray.

CHEST X-RAY

The chest x-ray shows a "normal" heart size with pulmonary edema; however, some enlargement of all cardiac chambers and the main pulmonary artery may be present. The aorta is not dilated unless aortic annular/root disease or dissection of the aorta is the cause of the acute AR. The aorta may also be dilated in the older patient and/or in those with an associated disease such as systemic hypertension. The lungs may show the signs of infected pulmonary emboli if there is associated tricuspid valve endocarditis.

ELECTROCARDIOGRAM

The ECG often shows nonspecific ST-T-wave changes and a sinus tachycardia; however, it may be normal. The ECG may show signs that are usually found in the associated causative disorder, e.g., LV hypertrophy with ST-T-wave changes in patients with severe hypertension. The ECG may show a variety of conduction abnormalities (atrioventricular and bundle branch block) including heart block, which, in the presence of infective endocarditis, is a sign of paravalvular/myocardial abscess.

Natural History and Prognosis

The natural history of this condition is variable. If the AR is mild to moderate in severity, these patients are likely to do well with medical therapy. Eventually, the changes of chronic AR will be seen. In patients with severe AR, the natural history depends on whether or not they have heart failure.[98] If heart failure is present, which is common, the prognosis is very poor without valve surgery unless the heart failure can be very easily controlled with medical therapy.

Management

DIAGNOSIS OF AORTIC REGURGITATION

In most instances, the diagnosis can be made by clinical evaluation, which includes the history, physical examination, electrocardiography, and chest x-ray. The diagnosis by physical examination in an acutely ill patient who is in extremis may be difficult.

Transthoracic echo/Doppler ultrasound is an important and valuable noninvasive procedure that should be used in every instance. It will demonstrate the AR and its severity and will provide useful information about the size and function of the left ventricle and other valvular and cardiac abnormalities. If the transthoracic method is not adequate, for example, in the very ill patient, then the transesophageal method should be used (see Chap. 13).

Echocardiography shows the diastolic flutter of the anterior leaflet of the mitral valve. In addition, the echocardiogram may show vegetations on the aortic valve, prolapse of an aortic valve leaflet into the left ventricle in diastole, and premature mitral valve closure. The mitral valve may be seen to open for only a short time because the stroke volume is limited. Occasionally, the aortic valve leaflets have been totally destroyed, and none are seen on the echocardiogram. Doppler ultrasound can easily demonstrate the AR and provides an estimate of its severity.

Cardiac catheterization and angiography, including coronary arteriography, show the abnormal physiology described, and aortography shows gross AR. These modalities may be needed to make the diagnosis and are usually indicated before surgical intervention. Coronary arteriography is indicated in the appropriate patient (see above). In the extremely ill patient, there is often a need for clinical judgment with regard to the tests that are essential.

Other tests (cine-computed tomography, including fast cine-computed tomography, radionuclide gated blood scan, or ambulatory ECG) may be needed in very special conditions.

DIAGNOSIS OF THE ETIOLOGY OF ACUTE AORTIC REGURGITATION

The diagnosis of the etiology is usually made during the clinical evaluation by finding the usual clinical characteristics of the underlying lesion. Additional laboratory tests will be needed to confirm the diagnosis—for example, blood cultures in those with suspected infective endocarditis.

Echo/Doppler ultrasound (transthoracic and transesophageal) examination is also extremely valuable in diagnosing the underlying lesion. Its widespread availability and comparative ease of use, especially in the very acutely ill patient, make it the noninvasive procedure of choice. The availability of biplane and omniplane transesophageal probes further enhances its value as a diagnostic tool.

Magnetic resonance imaging (MRI) has a very high specificity for the diagnosis of dissection of the aorta[99,100] and, if available, should be used in all hemodynamically stable patients if the diagnosis has not already been made. The availability of biplane or omniplane transesophageal echocardiography markedly improves the specificity and diagnostic accuracy of transesophageal echocardiography. Angiography is also an effective and time-honored method of diagnosing dissection of the aorta.

In summary, clinical evaluation is available in all institutions; echo/Doppler ultrasound is available in almost all institutions. The use of the other tests depends on the availability of equipment and the skill and experience of personnel using the equipment for this purpose at each institution.

BEDSIDE HEMODYNAMIC MONITORING

In acute disorders affecting the left ventricle, there may be a phase lag between the rise in pulmonary venous pressure and the appearance of pulmonary edema on the chest x-ray film. As a result, the reliability of the chest x-ray in demonstrating the presence and severity of elevated left atrial pressure initially is less than satisfactory in the acutely ill patient.[101] If the assessment of left atrial pressure is made by physical examination and chest x-ray, a significant number of errors may be made in these patients with an acute cardiac problem. Therapeutic decisions based on incorrect assessments may result in significant problems; for example, inappropriate diuresis may result in a fall of cardiac output, or inappropriate volume loading may result in a further increase in left atrial pressure. Furthermore, the optimization of filling pressures and cardiac output may not be made accurately in acute heart failure without measuring their actual values. Thus, use of a balloon flotation catheter for bedside hemodynamic monitoring is required in most if not almost all acutely ill patients with acute AR.

TREATMENT

Treatment of the heart failure is directed toward reducing pulmonary venous pressure and increasing cardiac output. In all patients, treatment is also directed toward correcting or controlling the etiologic disease/disorder and/or the altered pathophysiologic state (Table 56-18).[92,98]

Vasodilators (intravenous nitroprusside for an acute, severe condition) are useful and important in the management of these patients.[102] Vasodilators will produce a reduction of left atrial v wave and mean left atrial pressure. They produce a reduction in LV end-diastolic and end-systolic volumes and an increase in LV ejection fraction. The regurgitant fraction and regurgitant volume are reduced; as a result, the forward stroke volume and cardiac output are increased.[102] Digitalis therapy is of significant benefit in the management of heart failure. The combination of various agents (vasodilators, diuretics, and digitalis) tends to produce the maximum benefit in an individual patient; intravenous nitroprusside is often necessary in the acutely ill patient.

TABLE 56-18 Treatment of Heart Failure in Acute Valve Regurgitation

I. Correct or control altered pathophysiologic state
   A. Reduce pulmonary venous pressure
      1. Diuresis
      2. Vasodilation
      3. Control heart rate and maintain sinus rhythm (digitalis, cardioversion, antiarrhythmics)
   B. Increase cardiac output
      1. Reduction of valve regurgitation (vasodilators)
      2. Inotropic stimulation (digitalis, dobutamine)
   C. Improve left ventricular systolic dysfunction
      1. Reduce pulmonary venous pressure
      2. Increase cardiac output
      3. ACE inhibitors
II. Correct or control underlying disease or disorder
   A. Antibiotics for infective endocarditis
   B. Pharmacologic therapy for systemic hypertension
   C. Surgery for valve regurgitation in infective endocarditis, prosthetic valve dysfunction, dissection of the aorta, trauma

SOURCE: From Rahimtoola,[92] with permission.

Surgical therapy (valve replacement/valve repair or appropriate surgery for dissection of the aorta) is the cornerstone of the most definitive therapy currently available for heart failure in these patients. The management of the patient with heart failure or suspected heart failure is outlined in Fig. 56-9.[98] If the valve regurgitation is due to *dissection of the aorta,* the need for cardiac surgery is an emergency, even if the regurgitation is mild or moderate, because AR indicates involvement of the ascending aorta down to the region of the aortic valve annulus/root (see also Chap. 88). The outcome of the patient with heart failure due to infective endocarditis is very poor with medical therapy but is improved with valve replacement.[103] The indications for surgery in *infective endocarditis* are listed in Table 56-19.[81] Infective endocarditis due to special organisms (e.g., fungi) can only rarely be controlled by pharmacologic therapy alone, and surgery is almost always needed. In these and some other conditions, valve surgery may be needed even if the AR is only mild or moderate. It must be recognized, however, that in 90 to 95 percent of patients needing surgery for endocarditis, the indication for valve surgery is heart failure. When the heart failure is a result of *prosthetic valve dysfunction* or *trauma,* the need for surgery can be an emergency, an urgent situation, or

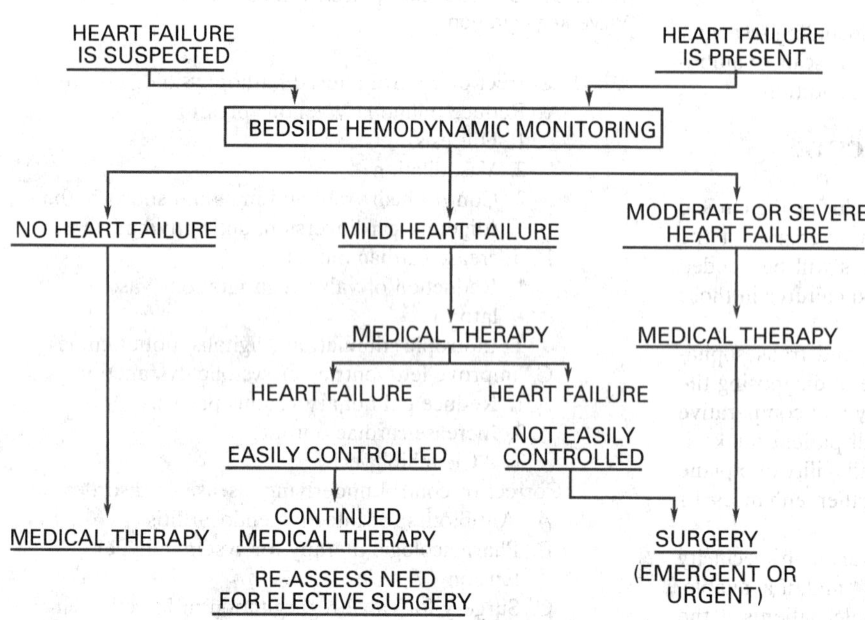

FIGURE 56-9 Role of bedside hemodynamic monitoring in acute aortic regurgitation. All patients with acute AR probably should have this procedure. If the AR is mild and there are no significant hemodynamic abnormalities, then the balloon flotation catheter can be withdrawn. On the other hand, if the AR is moderate to severe and there are significant hemodynamic abnormalities, then the balloon flotation catheter is left in place to guide therapy in the management of these acutely ill patients. If the hemodynamic abnormalities are mild, the patient is treated medically. If these abnormalities are easily controlled, medical therapy is continued and periodic reassessments are made to assess the need for elective surgery. If the hemodynamic abnormalities are not easily corrected or the hemodynamic abnormalities initially are moderate/severe, then surgery is undertaken either emergently or urgently. (From Rahimtoola,[98] with permission.)

an elective procedure. Prosthetic valves are inherently stenotic. When regurgitation is superimposed, it produces a pressure plus volume overload on the left ventricle that the ventricle may not handle very well acutely. Furthermore, valve regurgitation may be a sign of bioprosthetic valve degeneration or prosthetic endocarditis; in both conditions, prosthetic valve replacement is usually needed even if the valve regurgitation is mild to moderate. Trauma may result in AR from damage to valve leaflets or aortic annulus/root or from dissection of the aorta. If trauma produces dissection of the aorta and AR, the need for surgery may be an emergent one.

In some instances, the heart failure can be controlled completely with pharmacologic therapy, and the left ventricle and left atrium are able to dilate and adapt to the volume overload; in such instances, surgical therapy may be delayed, perhaps for a considerable period of time.

TABLE 56-19 Indications for Surgery in Infective Endocarditis

- Congestive heart failure
- Infection
  - Uncontrolled by antibiotic therapy
  - Fungal
  - Usually with staphylococcal infection of aortic or mitral valves
  - *Serratia*
  - Usually with gram-negative bacillary infection
- Recurrent septic systemic emboli despite adequate antibiotic therapy
- Perivalvular and myocardial abscesses
- Structural damage to valve in association with other catastrophes (e.g., ruptured sinus of Valsalva)
- Very large mobile vegetation

SOURCE: From Rahimtoola,[81] with permission.

CHRONIC AORTIC REGURGITATION

Etiology

In North America, the most common cause of chronic, isolated severe AR is aortic root/annular dilatation that is presumably the result of medial disease. Other common causes include a congenital (bicuspid) valve, previous infective endocarditis, and rheumatic disease.[93,94] Chronic AR also occurs in association with a variety of other diseases (Table 56-20). Between 40 and 60 percent of the surgically removed valves from patients with isolated severe regurgitation are classified as idiopathic. Half of these (or 20 to 30 percent of all the valves removed) show histologic criteria of myxomatous degeneration.[104]

Pathology

During systole the aortic root/annulus expands by an increase of 14 to 16 percent of the diameter (twice the radius).[105] This

TABLE 56-20 Etiology of Chronic Aortic Valve Regurgitation

- Aortic root dilatation
- Congenital bicuspid valve
- Previous infective endocarditis
- Rheumatic
- In association with other diseases
  - Congenital lesions, e.g., supravalvular or discrete subvalvular AS, ventricular septal defect, and aneurysm of the sinus of Valsalva
  - Connective tissue disease, e.g., Marfan syndrome, osteogenesis imperfecta, and Ehlers-Danlos syndrome
  - Autoimmune diseases, e.g., ankylosing spondylitis, rheumatoid arthritis, and systemic lupus erythematosus
  - Various forms of aortitis and arteritis, e.g., giant-cell arteritis and Takayasu's disease
  - Syphilis

causes the commissural attachments to spread apart, initiating the opening of the valves. These movements are continued during LV systole, which produces the forward motion of the blood. The length of the free edge of the cusps equals the diameter of the aortic root/annulus, or roughly one-third of the perimeter. Therefore, dilatation of the aortic root/annulus, if it is not accompanied by an enlargement of the cusps, results in AR.[104]

Depending on the cause, the valve cusps may show thickening, shortening, commissural lesions, or calcification (Fig. 56-10).[106] Regardless of the cause, the LV is dilated and hypertrophied; some of the largest ventricles have been described in association with chronic severe AR. Little pockets may be seen in the LV outflow tract. These are pouches out of the endocardial lining formed by the regurgitant jet(s) striking the left ventricle.

The myocardium is hypertrophied, with replication of sarcomeres in series, elongation of fibers, and wall thickening. The wall is not as thickened as in patients with AS. Ultrastructural changes in the myocardial cells are similar to those seen in AS; an important difference, however, is the frequent presence of degenerated cardiac muscle cells in patients with severe AR. Cardiac muscle cells with mild degeneration show focal myofibrillar lysis, with preferential loss of thick myofilament and focal proliferation of tubules of the sarcoplasmic reticulum. Moderately degenerated muscle cells show a marked decrease

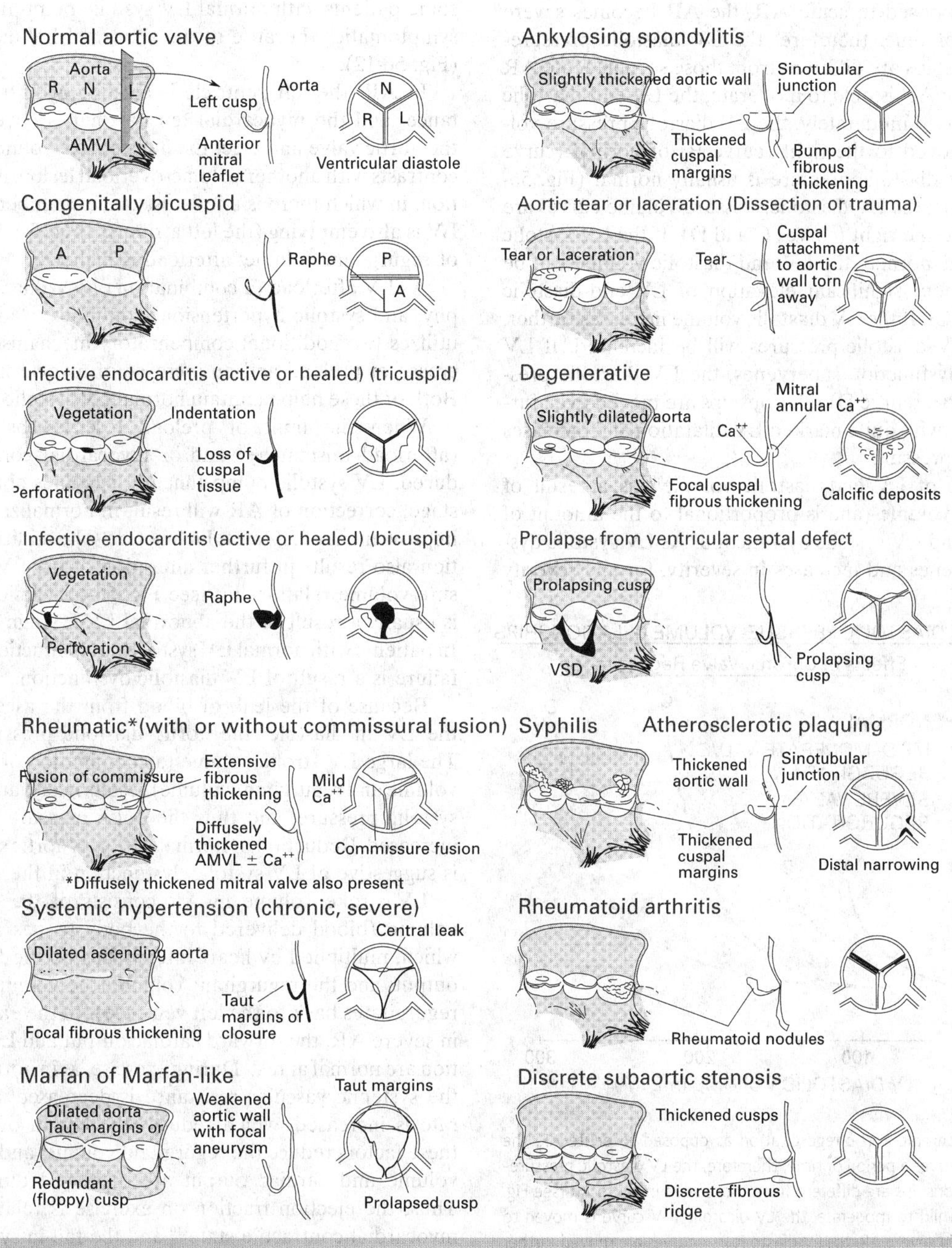

FIGURE 56-10 Pathologic findings in aortic regurgitation depending on the etiology of the AR. (From Waller,[106] with permission.)

in the number of myofibrils and T tubules and proliferation of sarcoplasmic reticulum, mitochondria, or both. Severely degenerated muscle cells usually are present in areas of marked fibrosis; they are often atrophic, have thickened basement membranes, and have lost their intercellular connections. These degenerated cardiac muscle cells may represent the ultrastructural basis for impaired LV function, which is seen more commonly in severe AR than in severe AS.

In patients with rheumatoid arthritis and ankylosing spondylitis, nodules on the outer surface of the anterior leaflet of the mitral valve have been described.

Pathophysiology

In chronic as opposed to acute AR, the AR becomes severe over a period of time; therefore, the LV diastolic pressure-volume relationships are different from those seen in acute AR (Fig. 56-7). If the AR is mild to moderate, the LV end-diastolic volume is increased moderately, the LV diastolic pressure-volume curve is moved to the right (curve B) of normal (curve A), and the LV diastolic pressure is usually normal (Fig. 56-11). In severe AR, the LV diastolic pressure-volume curves are moved further to the right (curves C and D). If the LV systolic pump function is normal, the LV end-diastolic volume can be quite large without significant elevation of LV end-diastolic pressure (curve C). If the LV diastolic volume increases further, however, the LV diastolic pressures will be increased. If LV systolic pump dysfunction supervenes, the LV diastolic pressure-volume curve (curve D) relationships are moved even further to the right, with quite marked LV dilatation and increases in LV diastolic pressure.

The increase of LV end-diastolic volume[107] is a result of the regurgitant volume (and is proportional to the amount of regurgitation) and LV systolic dysfunction. As LV systolic dysfunction supervenes and increases in severity, for any severity of regurgitant volume the LV end-diastolic volume increases further in an attempt to maintain LV stroke volume.

Severe chronic AR results in a large regurgitant volume (a large percentage of LV stroke volume). The left ventricle responds by dilating (average LV end-diastolic volume in patients undergoing surgery was 205 mL/m^2);[22] the dilatation is proportional to the amount of the regurgitant volume. The subsequent large LV stroke volume produces LV systolic hypertension. Both of these increase LV wall stress (afterload), which can result in an impairment of LV function. The heart responds by becoming hypertrophied (average LV mass in patients undergoing valve surgery was 222 g/m^2),[22] and LV systolic pump function remains normal. There is also an alteration of the LV diastolic pressure-volume relationship (Fig. 63-11). As a result, some patients with normal LV systolic pump function become symptomatic[108] because of the abnormal LV diastolic function (Fig. 56-12).

In AR, the left ventricle is ejecting against systemic resistance, and the myocardial tension that is developed to open the aortic valve and eject the huge stroke volume is great. This contrasts with another volume-overload lesion, mitral regurgitation, in which there is a low-resistance chamber into which the LV is also emptying (the left atrium). Thus, for the same degree of regurgitant volume, afterload is higher in AR.

As LV afterload (a combination of LV dilatation, hypertrophy, and systolic hypertension) continues to increase, the LV utilizes two additional compensatory mechanisms, namely, increase of preload and an increase of myocardial contractility. Both of these help maintain normal LV systolic pump function.

When the limit of preload reserve has been reached (afterload mismatch)[31] and/or myocardial contractility is reduced, LV systolic pump function becomes abnormal. At this stage, correction of AR will result in normalization or marked improvement of LV systolic function. The additional LV dilatation also results in further alteration of the LV diastolic pressure-volume relationship (see Fig. 56-6). Clinical heart failure is usually a result of the abnormal LV systolic pump function. In patients with normal LV systolic pump function, clinical heart failure is a result of LV diastolic dysfunction.

Because of the leak of blood from the ascending aorta to the LV in diastole, the aortic diastolic pressure is reduced. The large LV stroke volume (a combination of forward stroke volume and regurgitant volume) results in elevation of the aortic systolic pressure, and thus the pulse pressure is considerably increased. Reduction or normalization of aortic systolic pressure is suggestive of LV systolic dysfunction in these patients.

LV stroke volume in AR consists of the forward stroke volume (blood delivered to the body tissues and the heart), which, multiplied by heart rate, makes up the forward cardiac output, and the regurgitant volume (the volume of blood that regurgitates back to the left ventricle). In the early stages, even in severe AR, the forward cardiac output and LV ejection fraction are normal at rest. During exercise, as in normal individuals, the systemic vascular resistance is decreased[109] and the heart rate is increased, which reduces the length of diastole. Both these factors reduce the regurgitant volume, and forward stroke volume and cardiac output are increased during exercise.[109] Thus, the ejection fraction on exercise is related to both the myocardial contractile state[110] and the fall in systemic vascular resistance.[109] Accordingly, a decline in ejection fraction on exercise cannot be used as a specific marker of LV function in these

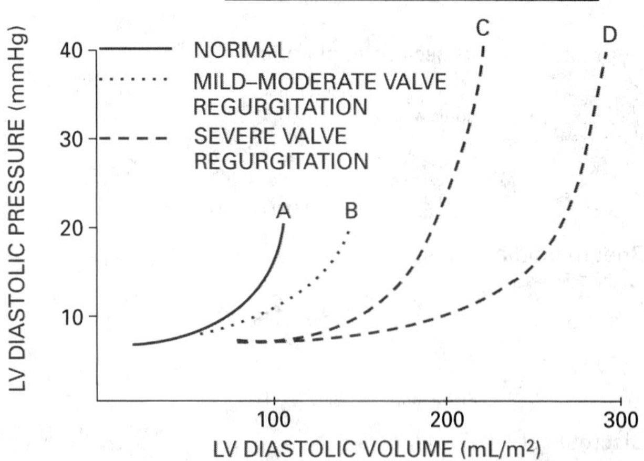

FIGURE 56-11 In chronic aortic regurgitation as opposed to acute AR, the AR becomes severe over a period of time; therefore, the LV diastolic pressure-volume (P-V) relationships are different from those seen in acute AR (see Fig. 56-7). If the AR is mild to moderate, the LV diastolic P-V curve is moved to the right (*curve B*). In severe AR, the LV diastolic P-V curves are moved further to the right, depending on whether the LV systolic pump function is normal (*curve C*) or abnormal (*curve D*). (From Rahimtoola,[98] with permission.)

patients unless the change in systemic vascular resistance has also been measured. A fall of normal resting ejection fraction to less than 0.50 on exercise, however, has been shown to correlate with reduced total body oxygen consumption[103] and increased left atrial pressure during exercise.[109,111] Further impairment of LV function produces demonstrable abnormalities at rest; there is a further increase in LV end-diastolic volume, which helps to maintain forward stroke volume. The resting LV ejection fraction is reduced, and mean left atrial pressure begins to increase. Even at this stage, the forward cardiac output may be maintained in the normal range. The increases in left atrial pressure may produce various grades of pulmonary edema. Finally, in the state of severe heart failure, the ejection fraction may be low, LV end-diastolic volume is large, and LV end-diastolic pressure is greatly increased and is associated with increases in left atrial, pulmonary, right ventricular, and right atrial pressures. Forward cardiac output is no longer normal. An increase in systemic venous pressure in association with salt and water retention produces engorgement of systemic organs (e.g., the liver) as well as peripheral edema.

In severe AR, myocardial oxygen needs are increased because of increases in LV diastolic and systolic volumes, LV muscle mass (hypertrophy), and LV pressures as well as by prolongation of systolic ejection time. Total coronary blood flow is increased. Coronary reserve, the ability of the coronary blood flow to increase with vasodilatation, however, is significantly reduced,[112–114] probably because of a reduced diastolic aortic-LV pressure gradient and compression of intramyocardial coronary arteries (systolic "milking" of intramural arteries). Therefore, myocardial ischemia is often present on stress in these patients.[112–114] Some patients with severe AR may complain of angina pectoris on effort even in the absence of epicardial CAD. Associated obstructive CAD can be expected to exacerbate further the myocardial ischemia (see Fig. 56-13).

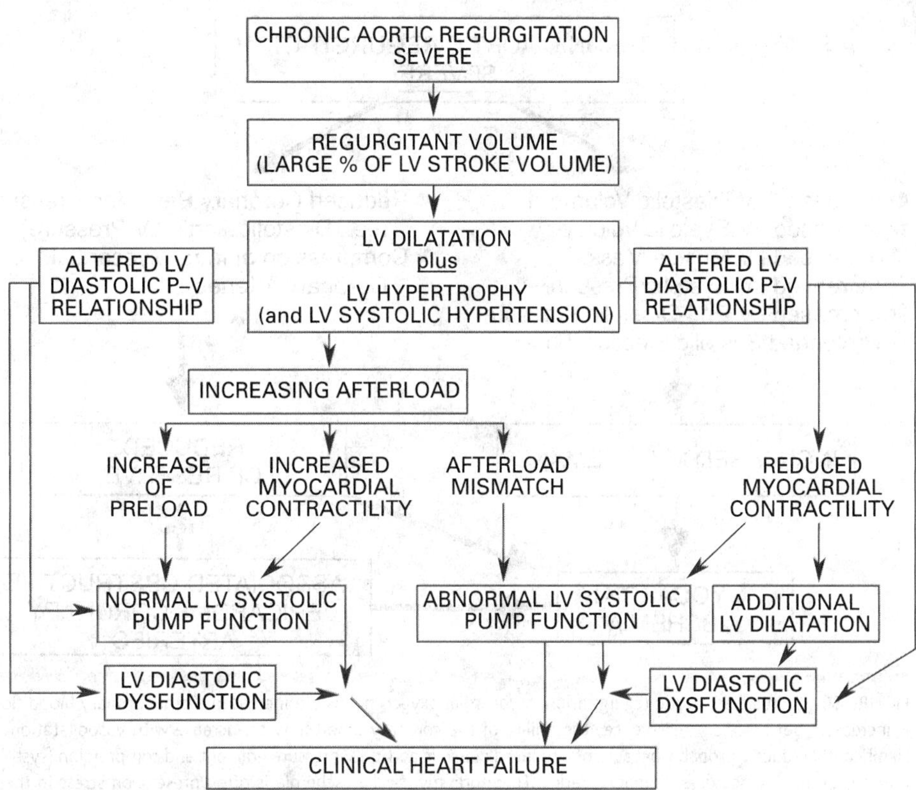

FIGURE 56-12 Severe chronic aortic regurgitation results in a large regurgitant volume (a large percentage of LV stroke volume). The left ventricle responds by dilating; the subsequent large LV stroke volume results in the production of LV systolic hypertension. There is an alteration of the LV diastolic pressure-volume (P-V) relationship. However, some patients with normal LV systolic pump function become symptomatic because of the abnormal LV diastolic function. As LV afterload (a result of LV dilatation, hypertrophy, and systolic hypertension) continues to increase, the LV utilizes two additional compensatory mechanisms, i.e., increase of preload and an increase of myocardial contractility. Both of these help maintain normal LV systolic pump function.

When the limit of preload reserve has been reached (afterload mismatch) and/or myocardial contractility is reduced, LV systolic pump function becomes abnormal. The additional LV dilatation also results in further alteration of the LV diastolic P-V relationship.

Clinical heart failure is usually a result of the abnormal LV systolic pump function; diastolic dysfunction may also be present in some patients. Clinical heart failure in those with normal LV systolic pump function is a result of LV diastolic dysfunction. (Copyright © by S. H. Rahimtoola, M.B., F.R.C.P., M.A.C.P., M.A.C.C. See Ref. 93.)

Clinical Features

HISTORY

Patients with mild to moderate AR usually do not have symptoms that can be attributed to the heart. Even patients with severe AR may be asymptomatic. They may complain of pounding of the head or palpitations, which result from their awareness of the beating of a dilated left ventricle that undergoes a large volume change in systole, during either sinus beats or postectopic beats. The main symptoms of severe AR result from elevated pulmonary venous pressures and include dyspnea on exertion, orthopnea, and paroxysmal nocturnal dyspnea. When congestive heart failure occurs, patients complain of fatigue and weakness. Angina pectoris occurs in 20 percent of such patients and may be present even if the coronary arteries are normal. Angina associated with syphilitic AR may be due to associated ostial stenosis of the coronary arteries. In such patients, angina often occurs at rest and is difficult to control.

PHYSICAL EXAMINATION

A variety of interesting but not very useful clinical signs may be present in patients with chronic severe AR. These include *de Musset's sign* (bobbing of the head with each heartbeat), *Traube's sign* (pistol-shot sound heard over the femoral artery), *Duroziez's sign* (systolic murmur over the femoral artery when

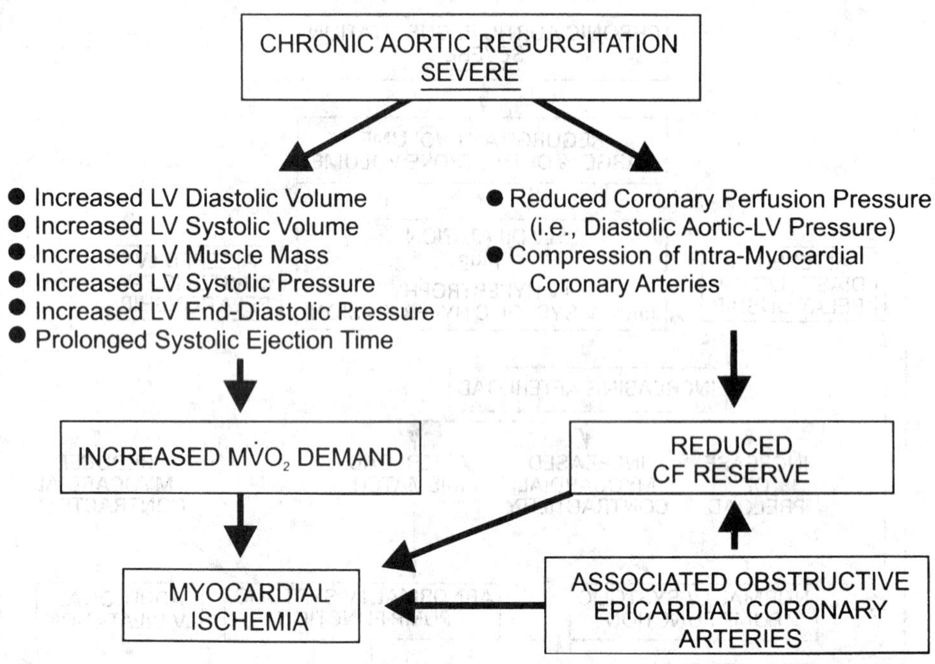

FIGURE 56-13 In severe aortic regurgitation, myocardial oxygen needs are increased. Total coronary blood flow is increased, but coronary reserve, i.e., the ability of the coronary blood flow to increase with vasodilatation, is significantly reduced, probably because of a reduced diastolic aortic-LV pressure gradient and compression (systolic milking) of intramyocardial coronary arteries. Therefore, myocardial ischemia is often present on stress in these patients. Associated obstructive coronary artery disease can be expected to further exacerbate the myocardial ischemia. (Copyright © by S. H. Rahimtoola, M.B., F.R.C.P., M.A.C.P., M.A.C.C. See Ref. 93.)

it is compressed proximally and diastolic murmur when it is compressed distally), and *Quincke's pulse* (capillary pulsations that can be detected by pressing a glass slide on the patient's lip or transmitting a light through the patient's fingertips).

The arterial pulse is very characteristic and consists of an abrupt distention with a rapid rise and a quick collapse *(Corrigan's pulse)*. The arterial pulse may be bisferiens, a double impulse during systole. The systolic arterial pressure is increased (in severe AR it averages 145 to 160 mmHg), the diastolic pressure is reduced (in severe AR it averages 45 to 60 mmHg), and the Korotkoff's sounds persist down to 0 mmHg. Even in such instances, however, the recorded intraarterial pressure rarely falls below 30 mmHg. The vasoconstriction that occurs in the presence of heart failure may result in some elevation of the arterial diastolic pressure and should not be interpreted as an improvement in severity of AR. Similarly, LV systolic dysfunction can produce a fall of systolic blood pressure that should not be considered to be an improvement of the AR. The fall of systolic pressure along with elevation of diastolic pressures tends to normalize the pulse pressure. The jugular venous pressure is normal except in heart failure and in those rare instances in which the greatly dilated ascending aorta obstructs the superior vena cava.

On inspection, the chest may rock and the cardiac impulse may be visible. The cardiac impulse is hyperdynamic (Table 56-21). There may be a systolic thrill at the base of the heart, over the carotids, and in the suprasternal notch. This results from a large LV stroke volume across a diseased aortic valve. A diastolic thrill signifies severe AR. The first heart sound is usually soft because the mitral valve leaflets are close to each other at the onset of systole, or there may be premature valve closure. This is exaggerated if the PR interval is prolonged. The S_2 is usually single because the aortic valve does not close properly[115] or because the LV ejection time is prolonged and the P_2 may not be heard. Often, a systolic ejection murmur, which is sometimes very loud, is present. The clinical sine qua non of AR is an early or immediate, blowing, decrescendo diastolic murmur beginning after A_2. It is best heard with the diaphragm of the stethoscope at the left sternal border or, in difficult instances, by having the patient sit up and lean forward and by auscultating in held respiration at the end of a deep expiration. In severe AR, the murmur may be holodiastolic. When it is soft, its intensity can be increased by having the patient perform isometric exercise, for example, a handgrip, which increases aortic diastolic pressure. At times, this murmur is better heard along the right sternal border, which should draw attention to the possibility that the cause of the AR is aortic root/annular disease (see also Chap. 10). Classically, rupture of the sinus of Valsalva into the right heart chambers produces a continuous murmur.

In many patients with severe AR, an Austin Flint murmur[116] (see Chap. 10) is present in presystole and/or mid-diastole. Two inferences can be drawn from the presence of an Austin Flint murmur: (1) it signifies that the AR is severe and (2) it requires that associated mitral stenosis be excluded. The most helpful sign at the bedside is the response of the murmur to the inhalation of amyl nitrite. The vasodilatation produced by amyl nitrite increases forward flow, reduces the regurgitant volume, and results in the Austin Flint murmur becoming much softer or disappearing. On the other hand, the increased cardiac output and the tachycardia accentuate or increase the murmur of mitral stenosis. Alternatively, echocardiography can easily demonstrate the presence of organic mitral stenosis.

With severe LV dilatation and/or LV systolic dysfunction, secondary mitral regurgitation may be present with the characteristic holosystolic murmur. Heart failure may be associated with pulmonary congestion/edema, pulmonary hypertension, right ventricular enlargement, tricuspid regurgitation, elevated jugular venous pressure, hepatomegaly, and peripheral edema (see Chap. 20).

CHEST X-RAY

The LV is increased in size, and this can be appreciated on the chest x-ray by an increase in the cardiothoracic ratio. Since the upper limit of normal of the cardiothoracic ratio is 0.49, many patients with increased LV size have an enlarged ventricular volume and may still have a cardiothoracic ratio within the normal range. A better noninvasive quantification of LV size

TABLE 56-21 Physical Examination of Patients with Varying Severity of Chronic Aortic Valve Regurgitation

	Mild	Moderate	Severe	Severe + LV Systolic Dysfunction	Severe + Heart Failure + LV Systolic Dysfunction
Arterial pulse	Normal	Corrigan's + to + +	Corrigan's + + +	Corrigan's + +	Corrigan's +
Arterial pressure					
Systolic	Normal	Increased + to + +	Increased + + +	Increased + +	Normal/+
Diastolic	Normal	Decreased + to + +	Decreased + + + to + + + +	Decreased + + to + + +	Decreased +
Pulse pressure	Often normal	Increased + to + +	Increased + + + to + + + +	Increased + + to + + +	Increased +
Cardiac impulse	Often normal	Hyperdynamic	Very hyperdynamic visible ± chest may rock	Hyperdynamic	May be hypodynamic
Precordial thrill:					
Systolic	−	±	±	±	−
Diastolic	−	−	±	±	−
Auscultation:					
S_4	−	−	−	−	−
S_1	Normal	Often soft	Soft	Soft	Soft
S_2	Normal	Normal or single	Often single	Often single	Often single
S_3	−	+	+ + to + + +	+ + +	+ + +
ESM	±	+	+ to + +	+ to + +	+
AoDM	+	+ +	+ + + to + + + +	+ + to + + +	+ to + +
Austin Flint murmur	−	−	±	−	−

ABBREVIATIONS: S_1 and S_2 = first and second heart sounds; S_3 = third heart sound (diastolic gallop); S_4 = fourth heart sound (presystolic gallop); ESM = ejection systolic murmur; AoDM = aortic diastolic murmur; − absent; + + + + most prominent; ± present or absent.

can be obtained by echocardiography. The ascending aorta is dilated throughout, and there may be calcium in the aortic valve. With increased filling pressures in the later stages, there might be evidence of an enlarged left atrium and an increased left atrial and pulmonary venous pressure, which are manifested in the pulmonary vascular shadows by a redistribution of blood flow, pulmonary congestion, and pulmonary edema. In the presence of heart failure, enlargement of the right atrium and superior vena cava may be appreciated. Calcification that is limited to the ascending aorta is strongly suggestive of luetic aortitis.

ELECTROCARDIOGRAM

The ECG shows LV hypertrophy with or without associated secondary ST-T-wave changes. In a small percentage of patients, ECG evidence of LV hypertrophy is absent in spite of severe AR. Conduction abnormalities, such as atrioventricular block or left or right bundle branch block with or without axis deviation, may be present. The PR interval may be prolonged,[117] particularly in patients with ankylosing spondylitis. The rhythm is usually sinus. The presence of atrial fibrillation should make one suspect the presence of associated mitral valve disease or heart failure.

ECHOCARDIOGRAPHY

The sign of AR on echocardiography is diastolic fluttering of the anterior leaflet of the mitral valve. Echocardiography is of particular value for excluding the presence of associated mitral stenosis in patients with an Austin Flint diastolic murmur. LV dimensions are increased, and if ventricular function is normal, the percentage of dimensional shortening is normal. Because of the increase in LV dimensions caused by volume overload, there is separation between the open anterior leaflet of the mitral valve and the endocardial surface of the interventricular septum (septal–E point separation), but this does not necessarily indicate impaired LV function when AR is present. In AR, as in other volume-overload lesions, the response in mild volume overload is an elongation of the heart. Since M-mode echocardiography takes a pencil look at the short axis of the heart, LV dimensions by M-mode echocardiography may appear to be normal. In such patients, two-dimensional echocardiography is much superior to the M-mode technique for assessing LV volumes and systolic function. A dilated ascending aorta can be detected on echocardiography, as can an enlarged left atrium. Aortic valve vegetations suggest infective endocarditis. Some other conditions can easily be detected by echocardiography, for example, prolapse of the aortic leaflet into the left ventricle in diastole. Doppler ultrasound is useful for diagnosing and assessing the severity of AR. There is a significant incidence of false-positive mild regurgitation. There is also an overlap between the various grades of severity of assessment of AR by Doppler when compared to angiography. Transesophageal echocardiography is a useful technique when transthoracic echocardiogram is unsatisfactory and in certain instances for identifying the anatomy of the valve leaflets and aortic root/

annulus; it is essential to evaluate if the valve is suitable for repair. Echo/Doppler ultrasound is also very useful for assessing disease of other valves.

CARDIAC CATHETERIZATION/ANGIOGRAPHY

Cardiac catheterization allows the measurement of intracardiac and intravascular pressures and cardiac output, both at rest and during exercise, and can demonstrate the changes described under "Pathophysiology," above. In addition, other valvular disease—for example, mitral stenosis, aortic stenosis, and mitral regurgitation—can be excluded. LV angiography demonstrates enlarged LV volumes and allows the calculation of LV volumes and LV ejection fraction. Angiography performed with injection of contrast medium in the ascending aorta demonstrates AR and allows a semiquantitative assessment of the degree of AR. In addition, the angiogram demonstrates the dimensions of the aortic root and the state of the ascending aorta. The indications for selective coronary angiography are the same as for aortic stenosis (see Table 56-6).

GATED BLOOD POOL RADIONUCLIDE SCANS

Gated blood pool radionuclide scans also allow the measurement of LV volumes and ejection fraction. In addition, with this technique, it is possible to quantify the amount of AR. These scans, however, assess regurgitation present at both the aortic and mitral valves. Thus, if both valves are incompetent, the total amount of regurgitation present at both valves will be measured. This technique also allows measurement of LV ejection fraction on exercise and on serial studies.

TREADMILL EXERCISE TEST

A treadmill exercise test provides an objective assessment of the degree of functional impairment and documentation of arrhythmias related to exertion. In some patients, however, the exercise test may remain normal despite deterioration of LV function.

AMBULATORY ECG RECORDING

Ambulatory ECG recording may be needed in an occasional patient suspected of having an arrhythmia.

MAGNETIC RESONANCE IMAGING

MRI can demonstrate AR but is rarely needed clinically.

Clinical Decision Making

Please see the equivalent section under "Aortic Valve Stenosis," above. The sensitivity, specificity, and accuracy of diagnosis of chronic AR are shown in (Table 56-22).[66] The following should be noted: (1) The sensitivity, specificity, and accuracy of diagnosing AR after clinical evaluation are good but not quite as good as in AS; (2) echo/Doppler ultrasound improves these criteria to a greater extent than in AS; (3) the difficulties lie in accurately distinguishing patients with mild AR from normal individuals and those with moderate AR and in distinguishing between moderate AR and severe AR; and (4) both clinical evaluation and echo/Doppler ultrasound are excellent in diagnosing the AR as being moderate or severe.

TABLE 56-22 Clinical Decision Making Utilizing Clinical Evaluation versus Echo/Doppler in Patients with Aortic Regurgitation

	After Clinical Evaluation, %	After Echo/Doppler, %
Diagnosis of AR		
Sensitivity	66	79
Specificity	76	74
Accuracy of diagnosis		
All levels of severity	43	57
Moderate or severe AR	91	100

SOURCE: From Kotlewski et al.,[66] with permission.

Natural History and Prognosis

Patients with mild AR that does not progress should have a normal life expectancy. Their major risk is the development of infective endocarditis and further valve destruction. Patients with moderate AR, if their disease does not progress, would be expected to have a life expectancy that is reasonably close to the normal range. The disease does progress, however, and mortality at the end of 10 years appears to be about 15 percent.

Patients with severe AR are known to have a long asymptomatic period before the condition is discovered. In asymptomatic patients with normal LV function at rest, symptoms and/or LV dysfunction (and/or sudden death) develop at the rate of about 3 to 6 percent per year. The predictor of development of symptoms is LV systolic dysfunction at rest.[118–122] In patients with normal LV systolic function at rest (Table 56-23), the predictors of development of LV systolic dysfunction and/or symptoms are an increased LV size (LV dimension at end-diastole of ≥70 mm and at end-systole of ≥50 mm,[119–121] and LV end-diastolic volume index of ≥150 mL/m^2),[123] and abnormal LV ejection fraction on exercise of <0.50.[111] In smaller people, for example, in women,[122] these values are too large and have to be corrected for body size. The corrected dimensions for end diastole and end systole are 35 mm/m^2 and 25 mm/m^2, respectively. Sudden death in asymptomatic patients appears to occur only in those with a massively dilated left ventricle (LV end-diastolic dimension of ≥80 mm).[119] It is likely that LV dysfunction first appears on exercise and later also at rest; eventually, heart failure ensues.

TABLE 56-23 Chronic Severe Aortic Regurgitation: Asymptomatic + Normal LV Function at Rest

		Likelihood of Symptoms or LV Dysfunction or Death, % per Year
LV end-diastolic dimension	≥70 mm	10
	<70 mm	2
LV end-systolic dimension	≥50 mm	19
	40–49 mm	6
	<40 mm	0

SOURCE: From Bonow et al.,[119] with permission.

Severe symptoms, however, may occur even when LV systolic pump function is normal at rest (see "Pathophysiology," above). The 5-year mortality of symptomatic patients with severe AR is about 25 percent, and the 10-year mortality averages 50 percent.[118] Once symptoms occur in patients with AR, it is likely that the rate of deterioration will be rapid. Most patients with angina are dead within 4 years.[124] The 2- to 3-year mortality of those with heart failure is 50 to 70 percent. In a recent study, the mortality was 4.7 percent per year, in the symptomatic patient it was 9.4 percent per year[125] and in the asymptomatic patient 2.8 percent, which was not significantly different from age- and gender-matched individuals in the population. In the symptomatic patient, those in the New York Heart Association (NYHA) classes III and IV had an annual mortality of 24.6 percent per year, while in the class II patient it was 6.3 percent per year. In asymptomatic patients, those with LV ejection fraction <0.55, the annual mortality was 5.8 percent per year, and in those with LV end-systolic dimension ≥25 mm/m², it was 7.8 percent per year.[125]

Management

All patients with AR need antibiotic prophylaxis to prevent infective endocarditis. Patients with AR of a rheumatic origin need antibiotic prophylaxis to prevent recurrences of rheumatic carditis. Patients with syphilitic AR need a course of antibiotics to treat syphilis.

Patients with mild AR need no specific therapy (Table 56-24). They do not need to restrict their activities and can lead a normal life. Patients with moderate AR also usually need no specific therapy. These patients, however, should avoid heavy physical exertion, competitive sports, and isometric exercise.

The value of long-term vasodilators to produce an improvement in LV size and function has been evaluated in two placebo-controlled randomized trials. In the hydralazine trial,[126] 36 percent of the patients were in NYHA functional class II, and patients had moderate to severe AR. Hydralazine produced modest reduction of LV end-diastolic volume and a small increase in ejection fraction at the end of 2 years; however, because of side effects, long-term compliance was poor,[126] which probably accounted for the extremely modest beneficial effects.[127] In asymptomatic patients with severe AR,[128] a calcium channel blocking agent, long-acting nifedipine, produced significant reductions in blood pressure and LV end-diastolic volume and mass and major increases in LV ejection fraction at the end of 1 year. Almost all patients completed the trial. Recently, a prospective randomized trial in *asymptomatic* patients with *normal LV systolic* function[120] showed that at the end of 6 years, 34 ± 6 percent of patients treated with digoxin developed LV systolic dysfunction and/or symptoms and thus needed valve replacement, compared to 15 ± 3 percent of patients treated with long-acting nifedipine ($p < .001$) (Fig. 56-14); 90 percent (23 of 26) of those who needed valve replacement had developed LV systolic dysfunction with or without symptoms; only 3 had become symptomatic without developing LV systolic dysfunction. Accordingly, all asymptomatic patients with severe AR and normal LV systolic function should be treated with a vasodilator (calcium antagonists long-acting nifedipine) unless there is a contraindication to its use.

The role of nifedipine in patients with moderate AR has not been studied. In view of its beneficial effects in severe AR, long-acting nifedipine could be used in selected patients with moderate AR if there are no contraindications to its use. An acute study showed that nifedipine was superior to an ACE inhibitor,[129] and a 6-month trial showed that the results with captopril were similar to placebo.[130] One study with quinapril involved 10 patients, many of whom had moderate AR.[131] In another study with enalapril, most patients had mild to moderate AR and many had severe systemic hypertension.[132] Moreover, there are no published data to show that ACE inhibitor therapy reduces the need for valve surgery. In brief, ACE inhibitors are not of proven benefit in asymptomatic patients with AR and with normal LV systolic function.

Symptomatic patients with severe AR need medical and surgical treatment. Medical treatment (Table 56-24) consists of the administration of digitalis, diuretics, and vasodilators. Digitalis acts by increasing myocardial contractility, often reducing LV end-diastolic volume while increasing the LV ejection fraction and also the cardiac output if it is reduced in the resting state. Digitalis is clearly indicated in patients with symptoms.

TABLE 56-24 Medical Treatment of Patients with Aortic Regurgitation

I. Antibiotic prophylaxis
 A. Infective endocarditis
 B. Recurrent rheumatic carditis
II. Restriction of activities (moderate/severe AR)
 A. Severe exercise
 B. Competitive sports
III. Arrhythmias
 A. Prevent and/or control
 B. Restore sinus rhythm, if possible
IV. Cardiac medications
 A. Asymptomatic, normal LV function
  1. Mild AR: None
  2. Moderate AR: ? Nifedipine long-acting
  3. Severe AR: Nifedipine long-acting
 B. Severe AR symptomatic (while waiting for surgery)
  1. Normal LV function: Nifedipine long-acting
  2. LV dysfunction: Digitalis; ACE inhibitors; Hydralazine ± nitrates, if needed; Diuretics, if needed; Dobutamine, if needed
 C. Severe AR + heart failure:
  Digitalis, diuretics, ACE inhibitors
  Hydralazine + nitrates
  IV nitroprusside, if IV therapy needed
  Dobutamine, if needed
V. Follow-up of asymptomatic patient
 A. Mild AR: Every 2–5 years
 B. Moderate AR: Every 1–2 years
 C. Severe AR: Every 6–12 months
 D. Develop symptoms: Early or immediate

SOURCE: Copyright © by S. H. Rahimtoola, M.B., F.R.C.P., M.A.C.P., M.A.C.C. See Ref. 93.

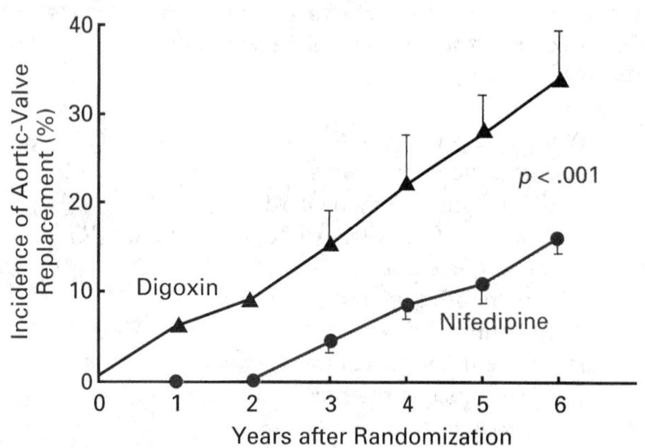

FIGURE 56-14 The role of long-term nifedipine therapy in asymptomatic patients with severe AR and normal LV systolic pump function was evaluated in 143 asymptomatic patients in a prospective randomized trial. By actuarial analysis, at 6 years, 34 ± 6 percent of patients in the digoxin group underwent valve replacement, versus 15 ± 3 percent of those in the nifedipine group, $p < .001$.

This randomized trial demonstrates that long-term vasodilator therapy with nifedipine reduces and/or delays the need for aortic valve replacement in asymptomatic patients with severe AR and normal LV systolic pump function. (From Scognamiglio et al.,[120] with permission.)

The need for and benefits of this therapy in asymptomatic patients have not been well documented. Diuretics are of value when the left atrial pressure is elevated and in the presence of heart failure.

Vasodilators are either arterial, venous, or both. Vasodilators act by reducing the peripheral arterial resistance, which favors forward cardiac output and reduces regurgitant volume; initially, the total LV stroke volume remains unchanged. If the left atrial pressure is elevated and LV ejection fraction reduced, vasodilators frequently result in an improvement in both.

Long-term hydralazine therapy in symptomatic patients results in significant benefit in only 20 to 35 percent of patients.[57] Those who are likely to benefit cannot be predicted. Vasodilators are indicated in patients who refuse surgery or are not operative candidates for any reason.

Vasodilators are also indicated for short-term therapy in patients awaiting valve replacement to optimize their hemodynamics (reduce filling pressures and increase cardiac output) and thus reduce their operative risks. If LV systolic function is normal, they can be given long-acting nifedipine. If they have abnormal LV systolic function, they should be treated with digitalis and ACE inhibitors; diuretics and hydralazine, with or without nitrates, can be used if needed. Small doses of hydralazine (50 mg) are without therapeutic effect in AR, and larger doses (≥100 mg) need to be given only twice daily;[133] the twice-daily regimen reduces the incidence of side effects. Hydralazine should be started in small doses and gradually increased, depending on patient tolerance of the drug.

Vasodilators are of considerable short-term benefit in patients in functional classes III and IV or heart failure. All such patients need digitalis, diuretics, and ACE inhibitors. In patients in functional class IV with heart failure, vasodilators should ideally be started after the institution of bedside hemodynamic monitoring—that is, measurement of pulmonary artery wedge pressure and cardiac output with the use of balloon flotation catheters. Hemodynamic monitoring accurately identifies patients who need the therapy, since clinical judgments can be wrong. It establishes whether arterial dilators alone will suffice or whether additional venodilators are needed. Finally, it provides information on the optimum dosage of vasodilator therapy. After the initial hemodynamic measurements are made, arterial dilators are given in progressively increasing dosage until an optimum effect on cardiac output has been obtained. If cardiac output does not show any further increase but left atrial pressure is still very high, additional venodilator therapy should be given. If the patient is very ill or the hemodynamic abnormalities are marked, intravenous therapy (e.g., sodium nitroprusside) is the vasodilator of first choice. In this situation, intravenous vasodilator therapy should be used only with bedside hemodynamic monitoring. Inotropic agents, such as dobutamine, may be needed to improve LV function and increase cardiac output. Low-dose dopamine may be of value to increase urinary output.

Patients with severe chronic AR need valve surgery. The correct timing of surgical therapy is now better defined but is not fully clarified. Valve replacement should be performed before irreversible LV dysfunction occurs. The major problem, however, is identifying the precise point at which LV dysfunction will occur. Here, two major difficulties are encountered: (1) patients may already have impaired LV systolic pump function at rest when they first present or at the time of the first symptom and (2) patients with severe symptoms may have normal LV systolic pump function. Patients may be in NYHA functional class III (symptoms with less than ordinary activity), with a normal LV ejection fraction,[108] or they may be in functional class I (asymptomatic), with a reduced LV ejection fraction.[108] A reduced LV ejection fraction demonstrated by two-dimensional echocardiography and/or radionuclide ventriculography is the best noninvasive indicator of depressed LV systolic function.

Decisions about surgery in AR should be based on the clinical functional class and on the LV ejection fraction at rest (Table 56-25).[134] Patients with chronic severe AR who are symptomatic (NYHA functional classes II to IV) need valve replacement. Although there may be some disagreement about recommending valve replacement to patients with normal ejection fraction who are in functional class II, we currently would do so. The benefit from valve replacement has been demonstrated even when the LV ejection fraction is 0.25 or less.[135] As opposed to AS, in which there is no lower level of ejection fraction that indicates inoperability, it is likely that some patients with AR and a very low ejection fraction become inoperable. This level has not been precisely defined but may be about 0.15 or less. There is a need to individualize the need for valve replacement in those with very severe LV systolic dysfunction at rest, in those with very severe LV dilatation (LV end-diastolic volume index ≥300 mL/m^2),[136] and in those with a small regurgitant volume, with a ratio of regurgitant volume to end-diastolic volume of 0.14[137] (Table 56-25). Recent data indicate that patients with severe AR, LV end-diastolic dimension on echocardiography of ≥80 mm, and mild to moderate reduction of LV ejection fraction (mean 0.43) can obtain benefit from valve replacement.[138] Postoperatively, they are symptomatically improved, LV ejection fraction increases, and LV size is reduced; the 5- and 10-year survivals are 87 and 71 percent, respectively.

Although the issue is controversial in some countries, we believe that patients who are in NYHA functional class I

TABLE 56-25 Chronic Severe Aortic Regurgitation: Indications for Surgery[a]

- I. Symptomatic patients
  - A. LV function normal: As soon as possible
  - B. LV dysfunction: Urgent
  - C. Heart failure: Emergent
  - D. Individualize if:
    1. Very severe LV dysfunction (LVEF ≤0.20)
    2. Severe LV dilatation (LVEDD ≥80 mm with severe LV dysfunction; LVEDVI ≥300 ml/m²)
    3. Small RgV (RgV/EDV ≤0.14)
- II. Asymptomatic patients
  - A. LV systolic dysfunction (LVEF ≤0.50–0.54)
  - B. Normal LV systolic function
    1. Associated cardiovascular diseases requiring surgery
       - a. CAD
       - b. Other valve disease
       - c. Ascending aortic aneurysm
    2. Large LV
       LVEDD ≥70–75 mm; 35–38 mm/m²
       LVESD ≥50–55 mm; 25–27 mm/m²
       LVEDVI ≥150 ml/m²
       PLUS PA wedge on exercise ≥20–22 mmHg
    3. Progressive changes in LV size and function
       Increase of LVEDD and/or LVESD
       Decrease of LVEF

[a]Valve replacement/valve repair.
ABBREVIATIONS: CAD = coronary artery disease; EF = ejection fraction; EDD = end-diastolic dimension; EDVI = end-diastolic volume index; RgV = regurgitant volume; EDV = end-diastolic volume; PAW = pulmonary artery wedge.
SOURCE: Copyright © by S. H. Rahimtoola, M.B., F.R.C.P., M.A.C.P., M.A.C.C. See Ref. 93.

(asymptomatic) and have a reduced ejection fraction at rest should be offered aortic valve replacement. If the ejection fraction is normal at rest, one should consider valve replacement in NYHA functional class I patients if they have severe obstructive CAD and/or need surgery for other valve disease (Table 56-25). It is suggested that patients undergo an exercise test during right heart catheterization if the left ventricle is large (LV end-diastolic volume ≥150 mL/m², LV internal dimension on M-mode echocardiography of ≥70 mm at end diastole and ≥50 mm at end systole) and/or the LV ejection fraction shows a new, persistent reduction to 0.54 to 0.60; if the patients have reduced exercise capacity on treadmill testing; or if ambulatory ECG monitoring demonstrates ventricular tachyarrhythmias. Valve replacement is recommended if the pulmonary artery wedge pressure during exercise ≥20 to 24 mmHg. Patients with associated significant CAD should have coronary bypass surgery performed at the time of valvular surgery (see "Aortic Valve Stenosis," above, and Table 56-14).

Aortic valve replacement, with or without associated coronary bypass surgery for obstructive CAD, can be performed at many surgical centers with an operative mortality of 5 percent or less (see Chap. 66). In those without associated CAD or reduced LV systolic function, the operative mortality may be

TABLE 56-26 Recommendations for Aortic Valve Replacement in Chronic Severe Aortic Regurgitation

Indication	Class
1. Patients with NYHA functional Class III or IV symptoms and preserved LV systolic function, defined as normal ejection fraction at rest (ejection fraction ≥0.50)	I
2. Patients with NYHA functional class II symptoms and preserved LV systolic function (ejection fraction ≥0.50 at rest) but with progressive LV dilatation or declining ejection fraction at rest on serial studies or declining effort tolerance on exercise testing	I
3. Patients with Canadian Heart Association functional Class II or greater angina with or without CAD	I
4. Asymptomatic or symptomatic patients with mild to moderate LV dysfunction at rest (ejection fraction 0.25 to 0.49)	I
5. Patients undergoing coronary artery bypass surgery or surgery on the aorta or other heart valves	I
6. Patients with NYHA functional Class II symptoms and preserved LV systolic function (ejection fraction ≥0.50 at rest) with stable LV size and systolic function on serial studies and stable exercise tolerance	IIa
7. Asymptomatic patients with normal LV systolic function (ejection fraction >0.50) but with severe LV dilatation (end-diastolic dimension >75 mm or end-systolic dimension >55 mm)[a]	IIa
8. Patients with severe LV dysfunction (ejection fraction <0.25)	IIb
9. Asymptomatic patients with normal systolic function at rest (ejection fraction >0.50) and progressive LV dilatation when the degree of dilatation is moderately severe (end-diastolic dimension 70 to 75 mm, end-systolic dimension 50 to 55 mm)	IIb
10. Asymptomatic patients with normal systolic function at rest (ejection fraction >0.50) but with decline in ejection fraction during	
• Exercise radionuclide angiography	IIb
• Stress echocardiography	III
11. Asymptomatic patients with normal systolic function at rest (ejection fraction >0.50) and LV dilatation when degree of dilatation is not severe (end-diastolic dimension <70 mm, end-systolic dimension <50 mm)	III

[a]Consider lower threshold values for patients of small stature of either gender. Clinical judgment is required.
SOURCE: ACC/AHA Guidelines,[91] with permission.

in the range of 1 to 2 percent. If aortic valve replacement is successful and uncomplicated, LV volume and hypertrophy regress but do not return to normal; the beneficial effects on LV size, volume, and mass continue to be seen up to 5 years after surgery.[82,139,140] Impaired LV systolic pump function improves postoperatively in 50 percent or more of patients;[135] this improvement is more likely to occur if LV dysfunction has been present preoperatively for 12 months or less, and in this subgroup LV ejection fraction usually normalizes.[140] Even if LV systolic pump function does not improve, there is a reduction in end-diastolic volume and hypertrophy;[125] from a cardiac point of view, this is advantageous to the patient. The 5-year survival of patients undergoing aortic valve replacement in severe AR is 85 percent (this figure includes operative and late cardiac deaths).[134] The 5-year survival of patients with LV ejection fraction ≥0.45 is 87 percent, versus 54 percent in patients with an ejection fraction <0.45.[134] Late survival after valve replacement for chronic severe AR is best predicted by variables indicative of LV systolic pump function. Both the operative mortality and late survival are dependent on cardiac and LV function and associated noncardiac comorbid factors (see "Aortic Valve Stenosis," above, and Chap. 66).

Indeed, in general, the major factors influencing outcome in patients with valvular heart disease are: LV dysfunction and its magnitude, duration of LV dysfunction, degree of LV dilatation, greater NYHA functional class, older age, associated CAD, and comorbid conditions.

New techniques of aortic valve repair are being developed and evaluated, and early results are encouraging in selected subgroups.[105,141,142] It is possible that selected patients may eventually need to have valve repair rather than valve replacement for AR.

The recommendations of the ACC/AHA Practice Guidelines are shown in Table 56-26.[91] Guidelines are *not* and should *not* be the Law. Application of such guidelines to clinical practice should be based on the following principles: (1) classes I and III applies to all patients in these classes unless there is a specific clinical circumstance not to do so; (2) class II applies to patients in this class depending on the clinical conditions of the patients and the skill and experience at the individual medical center.

References

1. Roberts WC. Valvular, subvalvular and supravalvular aortic stenosis: Morphologic features. *Cardiovasc Clin* 1973; 5:97.
2. Moller JH, Nakib A, Elliott RS, Edwards JE. Symptomatic congenital aortic stenosis in the first year of life. *J Pediatr* 1966; 69:728–734.
3. Braunwald E, Goldblatt A, Aygen MM, et al. Congenital aortic stenosis: I. Clinical and hemodynamic findings in 100 patients. II. Surgical treatment and the results of operation. *Circulation* 1963; 27:426–462.
4. Passik CS, Ackerman DM, Pluth JR, Edwards WD. Temporal changes in the causes of aortic stenosis: A surgical pathological study of 646 cases. *Mayo Clin Proc* 1987; 62:119–123.
5. Olsson N, Dalsgaaro C-J, Haegerstrand A, et al. Accumulation of T lymphocytes and expression of interleukin-2 receptors in nonrheumatic stenotic aortic valves. *J Am Coll Cardiol* 1994; 23:1162–1170.
6. Otto CM, Knusisto J, Reichenbach D, et al. Characterization of the early lesion of "degenerative" valvular aortic stenosis: Historical and immunohistochemical studies. *Circulation* 1994; 90:844–853.
7. Narang NK, Andrew AMR, Chaudhury HR, Gaba BS. Aortic stenosis due to familial hypercholesterolemic xanthomatosis: A case report with brief review of literature. *Indian Heart J* 1978; 30:189–192.
8. Deutscher S, Rockette HE, Krishnaswami V. Diabetes and hypercholesterolemia among patients with calcific aortic stenosis. *J Chronic Dis* 1984; 37:407–415.
9. Strickberger SA, Schulman SP, Hutchins GM. Association of Paget's disease of bone with calcific aortic valve disease. *Am J Med* 1987; 82:953–956.
10. Maher ER, Pazianas M, Curtis JR. Calcific aortic stenosis: A complication of chronic uraemia. *Nephron* 1987; 47:119–122.
11. Maher ER, Young G, Smyth-Walsh B, et al. Aortic and mitral valve calcification in patients with end-stage renal disease. *Lancet* 1987; 2:875–877.
12. Dereymaeker L, Van Parijs G, Bayart M, et al. Ochronosis and alkaptonuria: Report of a new case with calcified aortic valve stenosis. *Acta Cardiol* 1990; 45:87–92.
13. Selzer A. Changing aspects of the natural history of valvular aortic stenosis. *N Engl J Med* 1987; 31:91–98.
14. Roberts WC. The structural basis of abnormal cardiac function: A look at coronary, hypertensive, valvular, idiopathic myocardial, and pericardial heart disease. In: Levine JJ, ed. *Clinical Cardiovascular Physiology*. New York: Grune & Stratton; 1976.
15. Stewart BF, Siscovick P, Lind B, et al. Clinical factors associated with calcific aortic valve disease. *J Am Coll Cardiol* 1997; 29: 630–634.
16. Kennedy JW, Twiss RD, Blackmon JR, Dodge HT. Quantitative angiography: III. Relationships of left ventricular pressure, volume, and mass in aortic valve disease. *Circulation* 1968; 38:838–845.
17. Bertrand ME, LaBlanche JM, Tilmant PY, et al. Coronary sinus blood flow at rest and during isometric exercise in patients with aortic valve disease: Mechanism of angina pectoris in presence of normal coronary arteries. *Am J Cardiol* 1981; 47:199–205.
18. Bonow RO. Left ventricular structure and function in aortic valve disease. *Circulation* 1989; 79:966–969.
19. Krayenbuehl HP, Hess OM, Monrad ES, et al. Left ventricular myocardial structure in aortic valve disease before, intermediate, and later after aortic valve replacement. *Circulation* 1989; 79:744–755.
20. Schwarz F, Flameng W, Schaper J, et al. Myocardial structure and function in patients with aortic valve disease and their relation to postoperative results. *Am J Cardiol* 1978; 41:661–669.
21. Tobin JR Jr, Rahimtoola SH, Blundell PE, Swan HJC. Percentage of left ventricular stroke work loss: A simple hemodynamic concept for estimation of severity in valvular aortic stenosis. *Circulation* 1967; 35:868–879.
22. Pantely G, Morton MJ, Rahimtoola SH. Effects of successful, uncomplicated valve replacement on ventricular hypertrophy, volume, and performance in aortic stenosis and aortic incompetence. *J Thorac Cardiovasc Surg* 1978; 75:383–391.
23. Hess OM, Ritter M, Schneider J, et al. Diastolic stiffness and myocardial structure in aortic valve disease before and after replacement. *Circulation* 1984; 69:855–865.
24. Murakami T, Hess O, Gage JE, et al. Diastolic filling dynamics in patients with aortic stenosis. *Circulation* 1986; 73:1162–1174.
25. Dineen E, Brent BN. Aortic valve stenosis: Comparison of patients to those without chronic congestive heart failure. *Am J Cardiol* 1986; 57:419–422.
26. Fifer MA, Borow KM, Colan SD, Lorell BH. Early diastolic left ventricular function in children and adults with aortic stenosis. *J Am Coll Cardiol* 1985; 5:1147–1154.
27. Hess OM, Villari B, Krayenbuehl HP. Diastolic dysfunction in aortic stenosis. *Circulation* 1993; 87(suppl IV):73–76.

28. Braunwald E, Frahm CJ. Studies on the Starling's law of the heart. IV: Observations on the hemodynamic functions of the left atrium in man. *Circulation* 1961; 24:633–642.
29. Stott DK, Marpole DGF, Bristow JD, et al. The role of left atrial transport in aortic and mitral stenosis. *Circulation* 1970; 41:1031–1041.
30. Carroll JD, Carroll EP, Feldman T, et al. Sex-associated differences in left ventricular function in aortic stenosis of the elderly. *Circulation* 1992; 86:1099–1107.
31. Ross J Jr. Afterload mismatch and preload reserve: A conceptual framework for the analysis of ventricular function. *Prog Cardiovasc Dis* 1976; 18:255–264.
32. Bache RJ, Wang Y, Jorgensen CR. Hemodynamic effects of exercise in isolated valvular aortic stenosis. *Circulation* 1971; 44:1003.
33. Johnson LL, Sciacca RR, Ellis K, et al. Reduced left ventricular myocardial blood flow per unit mass in aortic stenosis. *Circulation* 1978; 57:582–590.
34. Vinten-Johansen J, Weiss HR. Oxygen consumption in subepicardial and subendocardial regions of the canine left ventricle—The effect of experimental acute valvular aortic stenosis. *Circ Res* 1980; 46:139–145.
35. Marcus ML, Doty DB, Horatzka LF, et al. Decreased coronary reserve: A mechanism for angina pectoris in patients with aortic stenosis and normal coronary arteries. *N Engl J Med* 1982; 307:1362–1366.
36. Grech ED, Ramsdale DR. Exertional syncope in aortic stenosis: Evidence to support inappropriate left ventricular baroreceptor response. *Am Heart J* 1991; 121:603–606.
37. Schwartz LS, Goldfischer J, Sprague GJ, Schwartz SP. Syncope and sudden death in aortic stenosis. *Am J Cardiol* 1969; 23:647–658.
38. Kulbertus HE. Ventricular arrhythmias, syncope and sudden death in aortic stenosis. *Eur Heart J* 1988; 9(suppl E):51–52.
39. Shoenfeld Y, Eldar M, Bedazovsky B, et al. Aortic stenosis associated with gastrointestinal bleeding: A survey of 612 patients. *AmHeart J* 1980; 100:179–182.
40. Love JW. The syndrome of calcific aortic stenosis and gastrointestinal bleeding: Resolution following aortic valve replacement. *J Thorac Cardiovasc Surg* 1982; 83:779–783.
41. Pleet AB, Massey EW, Vengrow ME. TIA, stroke, and the bicuspid aortic valve. *Neurology* 1981; 31:1540–1542.
42. Brockmeier LB, Adolph RJ, Gustin BW, et al. Calcium emboli to the retinal artery in calcific aortic stenosis. *Am Heart J* 1981; 101:32–37.
43. Wood P. Aortic stenosis. *Am J Cardiol* 1958; 1:553–571.
44. Murphy ES, Lawson RM, Starr A, Rahimtoola SH. Severe aortic stenosis in the elderly: State of left ventricular function and result of valve replacement on ten-year survival. *Circulation* 1981; 64(suppl II):184–188.
45. Szamosi A, Wassberg B. Radiologic detection of aortic stenosis. *Acta Radiol Diagn* 1983; 24:201.
46. Siegel RJ, Maurer G, Navatpumin T, Shah PK. Accurate noninvasive assessment of critical aortic valve stenosis in the elderly (abstr). *J Am Coll Cardiol* 1983; 1:639.
47. Gooch AS, Calatayud JB, Rogers PA, Garman PA. Analysis of the P wave in severe aortic stenosis. *Dis Chest* 1966; 49:459–463.
48. Thompson R, Mitchell A, Ahmed M, et al. Conduction defects in aortic valve disease. *Am Heart J* 1979; 98:3–10.
49. Nair CK, Aronow WS, Stokke K, et al. Cardiac conduction defects in patients older than 60 years with aortic stenosis and without mitral annular calcium. *Am J Cardiol* 1984; 53:169–172.
50. Rosenbaum M, Elizari M, Lazari J. *Los Hemibloques*. Buenos Aires: Paidos; 1968:363.
51. Galan A, Zoghbi WA, Quiñones MA. Determination of severity of valvular aortic stenosis by Doppler echocardiography and relation of findings to clinical outcome and agreement with hemodynamic measurements determined at cardiac catheterization. *Am J Cardiol* 1991; 67:1007–1012.
52. Agatston AS, Chengot M, Rao A, et al. Doppler diagnosis of valvular aortic stenosis in patients over 60 years of age. *Am J Cardiol* 1985; 56:106–109.
53. Skjaerpe T, Hegrenaes L, Hatle L. Noninvasive estimation of valve area in patients with aortic stenosis by Doppler ultrasound and two-dimensional echocardiography. *Circulation* 1985; 72:810–815.
54. Yeager M, Yock PG, Popp RL. Comparison of Doppler-derived pressure gradient to that determined at cardiac catheterization in adults with aortic valve stenosis: Implications for management. *Am J Cardiol* 1986; 57:644–648.
55. Currie PJ, Seward JB, Reeder GS, et al. Continuous-wave Doppler echocardiographic assessment of severity of calcific aortic stenosis: A simultaneous Doppler-catheter correlative study in 100 adult patients. *Circulation* 1985; 71:1162–1169.
56. Oh JK, Taliercio CP, Holmes DR Jr, et al. Prediction of the severity of aortic stenosis by Doppler aortic valve area determination: Prospective Doppler-catheterization in 100 patients. *J Am Coll Cardiol* 1988; 11:1227–1234.
57. Rahimtoola SH. Perspective on valvular heart disease: Update II. In: Knoebel S, ed. *An Era in Cardiovascular Medicine*. New York: Elsevier; 1991:45–70.
58. Roger VL, Tajik AJ, Reeder GS, et al. Effect of Doppler echocardiography on utilization of hemodynamic cardiac catheterization in the preoperative evaluation of aortic stenosis. *Mayo Clin Proc* 1996; 71:141–149.
59. Griffith MJ, Carey C, Coltart DJ, et al. Inaccuracies of using aortic valve gradients alone to grade severity of aortic stenosis. *Br Heart J* 1989; 62:372–378.
60. Enriquez-Sarano M, Klodas E, Garratt KN, et al. Secular trends in coronary atherosclerosis—Analysis in patients with valve regurgitation. *N Engl J Med* 1996; 335:316–322.
61. Sethi GK, Miller DC, Sonchek J, et al. Clinical, hemodynamic and angiographic predictors of operative mortality in patients undergoing single valve replacement. *J Thorac Cardiovasc Surg* 1987; 93:884–887.
62. Mullany CJ, Elveback ER, Frye RL, et al. Coronary artery disease and its management: Influence on survival in patients undergoing aortic valve replacement. *J Am Coll Cardiol* 1987; 10:66–72.
63. Levinson JR, Akins CW, Buckley MJ, et al. Octogenarians with aortic stenosis: Outcome after aortic valve replacement. *Circulation* 1989; 80(suppl I):49–56.
64. Klein RC. Ventricular arrhythmias in aortic valve disease: Analysis of 102 patients. *Am J Cardiol* 1984; 53:1079–1083.
65. von Olshausen K, Schwarz F, Apfelbach J, et al. Determinants of the incidence and severity of ventricular arrhythmias in aortic valve disease. *Am J Cardiol* 1983; 51:1103–1109.
66. Kotlewski A, Kawanishi DT, McKay CR, et al. The relative value of clinical examination, echocardiography with Doppler and cardiac catheterization with angiography in the evaluation of aortic valve disease. In: Bodnar E, ed. *Surgery for Heart Valve Disease*. London: ICR; 1990:66–72.
67. Jonasson R, Jonsson B, Nordlander R, et al. Rate of progression of severity of valvular aortic stenosis. *Acta Med Scand* 1983; 213:51–54.
68. Nestico PF, DePace NL, Kimbiris D, et al. Progression of isolated aortic stenosis: Analysis of 29 patients having more than one cardiac catheterization. *Am J Cardiol* 1983; 52:1054–1058.
69. Hoagland PM, Cook EF, Wynne J, Goldman L. Value of noninvasive testing in adults with suspected aortic stenosis. *Am J Med* 1986; 80:1041–1050.
70. Cohen LS, Friedman WF, Braunwald E. Natural history of mild congenital aortic stenosis elucidated by serial hemodynamic studies. *Am J Cardiol* 1972; 30:1–5.
71. Cheitlin MD, Gertz EW, Brundage BH, et al. Rate of progression

of severity of valvular aortic stenosis in the adult. *Am Heart J* 1979; 98:689–700.

72. Wagner S, Selzer A. Patterns of progression of aortic stenosis: A longitudinal hemodynamic study. *Circulation* 1982; 65:709–712.
73. Horstkotte D, Loogen F. The natural history of aortic valve stenosis. *Eur Heart J* 1988; 9(suppl E):57–64.
74. Otto CM, Burwash JG, Legget ME, et al. Prospective study of asymptomatic valvular aortic stenosis: Clinical, echocardiographic, and exercise predictors of outcome. *Circulation* 1997; 95:2262–2270.
75. Rahimtoola SH. Prophylactic valve replacement for mild aortic valve disease at time of surgery for other cardiovascular disease? . . . NO. *J Am Coll Cardiol* 1999; 33:2009–2015.
76. Holmes DR Jr, Nishimura RA, Reeder GS. In-hospital mortality after balloon valvuloplasty: Frequency and associated factors. *J Am Coll Cardiol* 1991; 17:189–192.
77. Ross J Jr, Braunwald E. Aortic stenosis. *Circulation* 1968; 36(suppl IV):61–67.
78. Otto CM, Lind BK, Kitzman DW, et al. Association of aortic valve sclerosis with cardiovascular mortality and morbidity in the elderly. *N Engl J Med* 1999; 341:142–147.
79. Kirklin JW, Barratt-Boyes BG. Congenital valvular aortic stenosis. In: *Cardiac Surgery*. New York: Wiley; 1986:972–988.
80. Schwarz F, Banmann P, Manthey J, et al. The effect of aortic valve replacement on survival. *Circulation* 1982; 66:1105–1110.
81. Rahimtoola SH. Valvular heart disease: A perspective. *J Am Coll Cardiol* 1983; 1:199–215.
82. Monrad ES, Hess OM, Murakami T, et al. Time course of regression of left ventricular hypertrophy after aortic valve replacement. *Circulation* 1988; 77:1345–1355.
83. Hammermeister KL, Sethi GK, Henderson WG, et al. A comparison of outcomes in men 11 years after heart-valve replacement with a mechanical valve or bioprosthesis. *N Engl J Med* 1993; 328:1289–1296.
84. Lindblom D, Lindblom U, Qvist J, Lundström H. Long-term relative survival rates after heart valve replacement. *J Am Coll Cardiol* 1990; 15:566–573.
85. Rahimtoola SH. Catheter balloon valvuloplasty for severe calcific aortic stenosis: A limited role. *J Am Coll Cardiol* 1994; 23:1076–1078.
86. Connolly HM, Oh JK, Orszulak TA, et al. Aortic valve replacement for aortic stenosis with severe left ventricular dysfunction: Prognostic indicators. *Circulation* 1997; 95:2395–2400.
87. Rahimtoola SH, Starr A. Valvular surgery. In: Braunwald E, Mock M, Watson J, eds. *Congestive Heart Failure: Current Research and Clinical Applications*. Orlando, FL: Grune & Stratton; 1982:89–93.
88. Smith N, McAnulty JH, Rahimtoola SH. Severe aortic stenosis with impaired left ventricular function and clinical heart failure: Results of valve replacement. *Circulation* 1978; 58:255–264.
89. Otto CM, Mickel MC, Kennedy JW, et al. Three-year outcome after balloon aortic valvuloplasty: Insights into prognosis of valvular aortic stenosis. *Circulation* 1994; 89:642–650.
90. Moreno PR, Jang I-K, Newell JB, et al. The role of percutaneous aortic balloon valvuloplasty in patients with cardiogenic shock and critical aortic stenosis. *J Am Coll Cardiol* 1994; 23:1071–1075.
91. Bonow RO, Carabello B, de Leon AC Jr, et al. ACC/AHA guidelines for the management of patients with valvular heart disease: A report of the American College of Cardiology/American Heart Association Task Force on Practice Guidelines (Committee on Management of Patients with Valvular Heart Disease). *J Am Coll Cardiol* 1998; 32:1486–1588.
92. Rahimtoola SH. Recognition and management of acute aortic regurgitation. *Heart Dis Stroke* 1993; 2:217–221.
93. Braunwald E. Valvular heart disease. In: Braunwald E, ed. *Heart Disease*, 4th ed. Philadelphia: Saunders; 1992:1007–1077.
94. Rahimtoola SH. Valvular heart disease. In: Stein J, ed. (O'Rourke RA, Cardiology Section ed). *Internal Medicine*, 4th ed. St. Louis: Mosby–Year Book; 1994:202–234.
95. Belenkie I, Rademaker A. Acute and chronic changes after aortic valve damage in the intact dog. *Am J Physiol* 1981; 241:H95–H103.
96. Welch GH Jr, Braunwald E, Sarnoff SJ. Hemodynamic effects of quantitatively varied experimental aortic regurgitation. *Circ Res* 1957; 5:546–551.
97. Rahimtoola SH. Aortic regurgitation. In: Rahimtoola SH, ed. *Atlas of Heart Diseases: Valvular Heart Disease*. Vol XI. Philadelphia: Current Medicine; 1997:7.1–7.26.
98. Rahimtoola SH. Management of heart failure in valve regurgitation. *Clin Cardiol* 1992; 15(suppl I):22–27.
99. Nienaber CA, von Kodolitsch Y, Nicholas V, et al. The diagnosis of thoracic aortic dissection by noninvasive imaging procedures. *N Engl J Med* 1993; 328:1–9.
100. Cigarroa JE, Isselbacher EM, De Sanctis RW, Eagle KA. Diagnostic imaging in the evaluation of suspected aortic dissection: Old standards and new directions. *N Engl J Med* 1993; 328:35–43.
101. Kostuk W, Barr JW, Simon AL, Ross J Jr. Correlations between the chest film and hemodynamics in acute myocardial infarction. *Circulation* 1973; 48:624–632.
102. Chatterjee K, Parmley WW, Swan HJC, et al. Beneficial effects of vasodilator agents in severe mitral regurgitation due to dysfunction of subvalvular apparatus. *Circulation* 1973; 48:684–690.
103. Richardson JV, Karp RB, Kirklin JW, Dismukes WE. Treatment of infective endocarditis: A 10-year comparative analysis. *Circulation* 1978; 58:589–597.
104. Tonnemacher D, Reid CL, Kawanishi DT, et al. Frequency of myxomatous degeneration of the aortic valve as a cause of isolated aortic regurgitation severe enough to warrant aortic valve replacement. *Am J Cardiol* 1987; 60:1194–1196.
105. Antunes M. Repair for acquired valvular heart disease. In: Rahimtoola SH, ed. *Atlas of Heart Diseases: Valvular Heart Disease*. Vol XI. Philadelphia: Current Medicine; 1997:12.1–12.23.
106. Waller BF. Rheumatic and nonrheumatic conditions producing valvular heart disease. In: Frankl WS, Brest AN, eds. *Cardiovascular Clinics—Valvular Heart Disease: Comprehensive Evaluation and Management*. Philadelphia: Davis; 1986:30–31.
107. Miller GAH, Kirklin JW, Swan HJC. Myocardial function and left ventricular volumes in acquired valvular insufficiency. *Circulation* 1965; 31:374–384.
108. Karaian CH, Greenberg BH, Rahimtoola SH. The relationship between functional class and cardiac performance in patients with chronic aortic insufficiency. *Chest* 1985; 88:553–557.
109. Kawanishi DT, McKay CR, Chandraratna PAN, et al. Cardiovascular response to dynamic exercise in patients with chronic symptomatic mild-to-moderate and severe aortic regurgitation. *Circulation* 1986; 73:62–72.
110. Shen WF, Roubin GS, Choong CY-P, et al. Evaluation of relationship between myocardial contractile state and left ventricular function in patients with aortic regurgitation. *Circulation* 1985; 71:31–38.
111. Boucher CA, Wilson RA, Kanarek DJ, et al. Exercise testing in asymptomatic or minimally symptomatic aortic regurgitation: Relationship of left ventricular ejection fraction to left ventricular filling pressure during exercise. *Circulation* 1983; 67:1091–1100.
112. Falsetti HL, Carroll RJ, Cramer JA. Total and regional myocardial blood flow in aortic regurgitation. *Am Heart J* 1979; 97:485–493.
113. Uhl GS, Boucher CA, Oliveros RA, Murgo JP. Exercise-induced myocardial oxygen supply-demand imbalance in asymptomatic or mildly symptomatic aortic regurgitation. *Chest* 1981; 80:686–691.
114. Nittenburg A, Foult JM, Antony I, et al. Coronary flow and resistance reserve in patients with chronic aortic regurgitation, angina pectoris, and normal coronary arteries. *J Am Coll Cardiol* 1988; 11:478–486.

115. Sabbah HN, Khaja F, Anbe DT, Stein PD. The aortic closure sound in pure aortic insufficiency. *Circulation* 1977; 56:859–863.
116. Schaefer RA, McAnulty JH, Starr A, Rahimtoola SH. Diastolic murmurs in the presence of Starr-Edwards mitral prosthesis: With emphasis on the genesis of the Austin Flint murmur. *Circulation* 1975; 51:402–409.
117. Roberts WC, Day PJ. Electrocardiographic observations in clinically isolated, pure, and chronic, severe aortic regurgitation: Analysis of 30 necropsy patients aged 19 to 65 years. *Am J Cardiol* 1985; 55:431–438.
118. Rapaport E. Natural history of aortic and mitral valve disease. *Am J Cardiol* 1975; 35:221–227.
119. Bonow RO, Lakatos E, Maron BJ, Epstein SE. Serial long-term assessment of the natural history of asymptomatic patients with chronic aortic regurgitation and normal left ventricular systolic function. *Circulation* 1991; 84:1625–1635.
120. Scognamiglio R, Rahimtoola SH, Fasoli G, et al. Nifedipine in asymptomatic patients with severe aortic regurgitation and normal left ventricular function. *N Engl J Med* 1994; 331:689–695.
121. Tornos MP, Olona M, Permanyer-Miralda G, et al. Clinical outcome of severe asymptomatic chronic aortic regurgitation: A long-term prospective follow-up study. *Am Heart J* 1995; 130:333–339.
122. Klodas E, Enrique-Sarano M, Tajik AJ, Mullany CJ, et al. Surgery for aortic regurgitation in women: Contrasting indications and outcomes compared with men. *Circulation* 1996; 94:2472–2478.
123. Siemienczuk D, Greenberg B, Morris C, et al. Chronic aortic insufficiency: Factors associated with progression to aortic valve replacement. *Ann Intern Med* 1989; 110:587–592.
124. McKay CR, Rahimtoola SH. Natural history of aortic regurgitation. In: Gaasch WH, Levine HJ, eds. *Chronic Aortic Regurgitation*. Boston: Kluwer Academic; 1980:1–17.
125. Dujardin KS, Enriquez-Sarano M, Schaff HV, et al. Mortality and morbidilty of aortic regurgitation in clinical practice: A long-term follow-up study. *Circulation* 1999; 99:1851–1857.
126. Greenberg B, Massie B, Bristow JD, et al. Long-term vasodilator therapy of chronic aortic insufficiency: A randomized double-blinded, placebo-controlled clinical trial. *Circulation* 1988; 78:92–103.
127. Rahimtoola SH. Vasodilator therapy in chronic severe aortic regurgitation. *J Am Coll Cardiol* 1990; 16:430–432.
128. Scognamiglio R, Rasoli G, Ponchia A, Dalla-Volta S. Long-term nifedipine unloading therapy in asymptomatic patients with chronic severe aortic regurgitation. *J Am Coll Cardiol* 1990; 16:424–429.
129. Rothlisberger C, Sareli P, Wisenbaugh T. Comparison of single-dose nifedipine and captopril for chronic severe aortic regurgitation. *Am J Cardiol* 1993; 72:799–804.
130. Wisenbaugh T, Sinovich V, Dullabh A, Sareli P. Six month pilot study of captopril for mildly symptomatic, severe isolated mitral and isolated aortic regurgitation. *J Heart Valve Dis* 1994; 3:197–204.
131. Schon HR, Dorn R, Barthel P, Schömig A. Effects of 12 months quinapril therapy in asymptomatic patients with chronic aortic regurgitation. *J Heart Valve Dis* 1994; 3:500–509.
132. Lin M, Chian H-T, Lin S-L, et al. Vasodilator therapy in chronic asymptomatic aortic regurgitation: Enalapril versus hydralazine. *J Am Coll Cardiol* 1994; 24:1046–1053.
133. McKay CR, Nanna M, Kawanishi DT, et al. Importance of internal controls, statistical methods, and side effects in acute vasodilator trials: A study of hydralazine kinetics in patients with aortic regurgitation. *Circulation* 1985; 72:865–872.
134. Greves J, Rahimtoola SH, McAnulty JH, et al. Preoperative criteria predictive of late survival following valve replacement for severe aortic regurgitation. *Am Heart J* 1981; 101:300–308.
135. Clark DG, McAnulty JH, Rahimtoola SH. Valve replacement in aortic insufficiency with left ventricular dysfunction. *Circulation* 1980; 61:411–421.
136. Taniguchi K, Nakano S, Hirose H, et al. Preoperative left ventricular function: Minimal requirement for successful late results of valve replacement for aortic regurgitation. *J Am Coll Cardiol* 1987; 10:510–518.
137. Levine HJ, Gaasch WH. Ratio of regurgitant volume to end-diastolic volume: A major determinant of ventricular response to surgical correction of chronic volume overload. *Am J Cardiol* 1983; 52:406–410.
138. Klodas E, Enriquez-Sarano M, Tajik AJ, et al. Aortic regurgitation complicated by extreme left ventricular dilation: Long-term outcome after surgical correction. *J Am Coll Cardiol* 1996; 27:670–677.
139. Gaasch WH, Carroll JD, Levine HJ, Criscitiello MG. Chronic aortic regurgitation: Prognostic value of left ventricular end-systolic dimension and end-diastolic radius/thickness ratio. *J Am Coll Cardiol* 1983; 1:775–782.
140. Bonow RO, Dodd JT, Maron BJ, et al. Long-term serial changes in left ventricular function and reversal of ventricular dilatation after valve replacement for chronic aortic regurgitation. *Circulation* 1988; 78:1108–1120.
141. Cosgrove DM, Rosenkranz ER, Hendren WG, et al. Valvuloplasty for aortic insufficiency. *J Thorac Cardiovasc Surg* 1991; 102:571–577.
142. Duran C, Kumar N, Gometza B, Al Halees Z. Indications and limitations of aortic valve reconstruction. *Ann Thorac Surg* 1991; 52:447–454.

CHAPTER 57

MITRAL VALVE DISEASE*

Shahbudin H. Rahimtoola / Maurice Enriquez-Sarano / Hartzell V. Schaff / Robert L. Frye

MITRAL STENOSIS

Etiology

Mitral stenosis (MS), an obstruction to blood flow between the left atrium (LA) and the left ventricle (LV), is caused by abnormal mitral valve function. In virtually all adult patients, the cause of MS is previous rheumatic carditis.[1] About 60 percent of patients with rheumatic mitral valve disease do not give a history of rheumatic fever or chorea, and about 50 percent of patients with acute rheumatic carditis do not eventually have clinical valvular heart disease.[2] Other causes of MS are all uncommon or rare and are listed in Table 57-1.[2–10] Congenital MS is uncommon. It is usually caused by a "parachute" deformity of the valve, in which shortened chordae tendineae insert in a large, single papillary muscle. MS, usually rheumatic, in association with atrial septal defect is called *Lutembacher's syndrome*. A rare cause of MS is massive mitral valve annular calcification. This process occurs most frequently in elderly patients and produces MS by limiting leaflet motion. When stenosis is present, it is usually mild in degree. Other causes of obstruction to LA outflow include a LA myxoma, massive LA ball thrombus, and cor triatriatum, in which a congenital membrane is present in the LA.

Pathology

Acute rheumatic carditis is a pancarditis involving the pericardium, myocardium, and endocardium. In temperate climates and developed countries, there is usually a long interval (averaging 10 to 20 years) between an episode of rheumatic carditis and the clinical presentation of symptomatic MS. In tropical and subtropical climates and in less developed countries, the latent period is often shorter, and MS may occur during childhood or adolescence (see Chap. 55).

The pathologic hallmark of rheumatic carditis is an Aschoff's nodule. The most common lesion of acute rheumatic endocarditis is mitral valvulitis. In this condition the mitral valve has vegetations along the line of closure and the chordae tendineae. Mitral regurgitation (MR) may be present during the acute episode of rheumatic carditis.

MS is usually the result of repeated episodes of carditis alternating with healing and is characterized by the deposition of fibrous tissue. MS may result from fusion of the commissures, cusps, or chordae, or a combination of these.[9,10] Ultimately, the deformed valve is subject to nonspecific fibrosis and calcification. Lesions along the line of closure result in fusion of the commissures and contracture and thickening of the valve leaflets. The chordal lesions are manifest as shortening and fusion of these structures. The combination of commissural fusion, valve leaflet contracture, and fusion of the chordae tendineae results in a narrow, funnel-shaped orifice, which restricts the flow of blood from the LA to the LV. The rapidity with which patients become symptomatic may depend on the number and severity of repeated bouts of rheumatic valvulitis. Frequently, the rheumatic episodes are not clinically apparent.

In pure MS, the LV is usually normal, but there may be evidence of previous carditis with deposition of fibrous tissue. The LA is enlarged and hypertrophied as a consequence of LA hypertension. Mural thrombi are often found in the LA, particularly if atrial fibrillation has been present. Calcification of the mitral valve frequently also involves the mitral annulus.

Pathophysiology

The pathophysiologic features of MS all result from obstruction of the flow of blood between the LA and the LV. With reduction in valve area, energy is lost to friction during the transport of blood from the LA to the LV. Accordingly, a pressure gradient is present across the stenotic valve. The relationship between valve area, cardiac output, flow period, and average diastolic gradient between the LA and the LV is defined by the formula of Gorlin and Gorlin (Chap. 15).

It is readily apparent that maintaining cardiac output when

* Mitral stenosis section written by Dr. Rahimtoola. Mitral regurgitation section written by Drs. Enriquez-Sarano, Schaff, and Frye.

TABLE 57-1 Causes of Mitral Stenosis

	Involved Structure(s)			
Cause	Leaflet	Chordae	Commissures	Other
Rheumatic fever	+	+	+	
Congenital	+	+		Single papillary muscle
Active infective endocarditis	+			Vegetation
Neoplasm				Mass, pulmonary vein obstruction
Massive annular calcification	+	0	0	Rigid annulus
Systemic lupus erythematosus	+	+	+	Verrucous vegetations may extend into papillary muscles
Carcinoid				Atrial septal defect or lung tumor in order to affect left heart
Methysergide therapy	+	+		Serotonin agonist/antagonist
Hunter-Hurler syndromes				Mucopolysaccharide deposits
Fabry's disease				Aramide trihexoxide deposits
Whipple's disease				PAS-positive macrophage deposits
Rheumatoid arthritis	+	+	+	PAS-positive plasma cell infiltrate

SOURCE: From Kawanishi DT, Rahimtoola SH. Mitral stenosis. In: Rahimtoola SH, ed. *Valvular Heart Disease. II.* St. Louis: Mosby; 1996:8.1–8.24.

the valve area is small requires a large gradient and thus an elevated LA pressure. Similarly, an increased demand for cardiac output (CO), such as occurs during exercise or pregnancy, results in an increase in gradient and high LA pressures. More subtle is the effect of the length of the diastolic flow period on the relationship between CO and gradient. The time available for diastole is that part of the cardiac cycle occupied by isovolumic contraction and relaxation or by ejection. As the heart rate increases, the total amount of time spent during systole increases despite a reduction in the systolic time per beat.[11,12] *Thus, time available for diastole decreases as the heart rate increases.* Because blood can flow through the mitral valve only during diastole, the flow rate is inversely proportional to the duration of the flow period at a constant stroke volume. Of course, a higher flow rate results in a greater loss of energy to friction and requires a larger gradient and higher LA pressures. It is important to remember that the gradient from LA to LV is a function per beat, not per minute. Thus, the gradient is dependent on the stroke volume and the diastolic filling time as well as the LV diastolic pressure.

The pressure gradient between the LA and the LV, which increases markedly with increased heart rate or CO, is responsible for LA hypertension. The LA gradually enlarges and hypertrophies. Pulmonary venous pressure rises with LA pressure increase and is passively associated with an increase in pulmonary arterial (PA) pressure (Fig. 57-1). In up to 20 percent of patients, the pulmonary vascular resistance is also elevated,[13] which further increases PA pressure. PA hypertension results in *right ventricular* (RV) hypertrophy and RV enlargement. The changes in RV function eventually result in *right atrial* (RA) hypertension and enlargement and systemic venous congestion; frequently, tricuspid regurgitation also occurs. In a small percentage of patients, there may be regional or global LV systolic dysfunction, the cause or causes of which are not fully understood.[14–18]

Pulmonary venous hypertension alters lung function in several ways. Distribution of blood flow in the lung is altered, with a relative increase in flow to the upper lobes and therefore in physiologic dead space. Pulmonary compliance generally decreases with increasing pulmonary capillary pressure, increasing the work of breathing, particularly during exercise. Chronic changes in the pulmonary capillaries and pulmonary arteries include fibrosis and thickening. These changes protect the lungs from the transudation of fluid into the alveoli (alveolar pulmonary edema). Indeed, it is not uncommon to find patients with severe MS whose resting PA wedge pressure (indirect LA pressure) exceeds 25 to 30 mmHg. Capillary and alveolar thickening, which help protect against pulmonary edema, further add to the abnormalities of ventilation and perfusion. Pulmonary vascular changes cause an elevated pulmonary vascular resistance.

In some patients with high pulmonary vascular resistance and RV dysfunction, CO may be low. The body maintains oxygen consumption by extracting more oxygen from the arterial blood, and the mixed venous oxygen content falls. The hemoglobin-O_2 dissociation curve is shifted to the right, facilitating the unloading of oxygen from hemoglobin to the tissues. The reduced CO may result in a *surprisingly small gradient* across the mitral valve despite severe stenosis. Although pulmonary congestion may be less striking in these patients, the CO does not increase normally with exercise, and, typically, the patients are severely limited by fatigue.

Long-standing MS with severe PA hypertension and resultant RV dysfunction may be accompanied by chronic systemic venous hypertension. Tricuspid regurgitation is frequently present, even in the absence of intrinsic disease of this valve. Functional pulmonic regurgitation may also be present. Dependent edema formation and visceral congestion directly reflect elevated systemic venous pressure and salt and water retention. Chronic passive congestion in the liver leads to central lobular necrosis and eventually to cardiac cirrhosis.

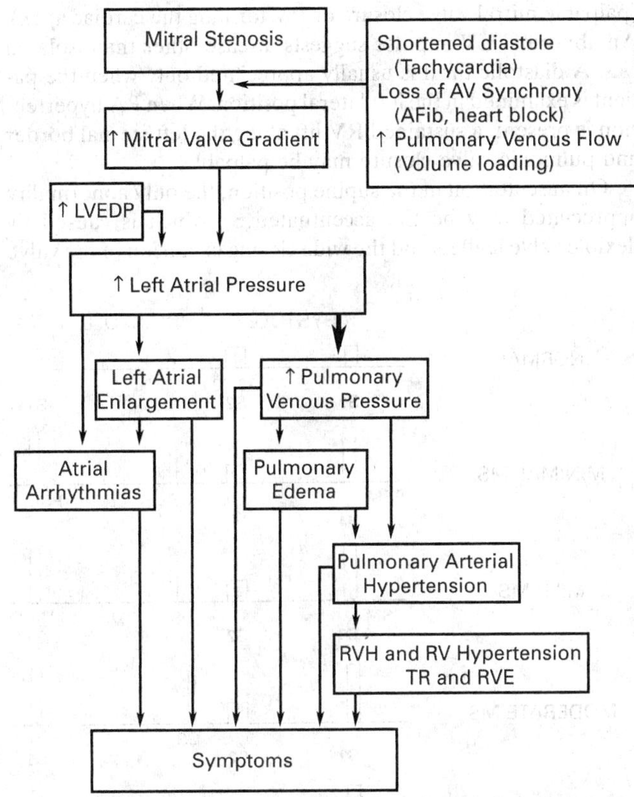

FIGURE 57-1 Pathophysiology of mitral stenosis. Mitral stenosis results in a diastolic pressure gradient from the LA to the LV. The actual gradient is dependent on the mitral valve area and the mitral valve *flow per diastolic second*. As a result, there is an elevation of LA pressure and therefore also of pulmonary venous pressure. Physiologic and pathologic changes—such as tachycardia and atrial fibrillation (which shorten diastole and may also result in loss of effective atrial contraction) or pregnancy, volume loading, and left-to-right shunts (at ventricular and aortopulmonary levels), which increase pulmonary venous flow—will increase the mitral valve gradient as well as LA and pulmonary venous pressures. An increased LV diastolic pressure will also result in further increase of LA pressure. An elevated LA pressure has several important effects; these include enlargement of the left atrium, atrial arrhythmias, and an increase of pulmonary venous pressure. Pulmonary venous hypertension may result in pulmonary edema and pulmonary arterial hypertension. PA hypertension and RV ventricular hypertension results in RV hypertrophy and may result in tricuspid regurgitation and RV enlargement. All of these changes contribute to producing symptoms. In addition, a fixed or even reduced cardiac output will also contribute to the symptomatic state of the patient. [Copyright by S. H. Rahimtoola. M.B., F.R.C.P., M.A.C.P., M.A.C.C. (Ref. 10).]

Clinical Findings

HISTORY

An asymptomatic interval is usually present between the initiating event of acute rheumatic fever and the presentation of symptomatic MS (averaging 10 to 20 years).[13,19] During this interval, the patient feels well (Table 57-2). Initially, there is little or no gradient at rest, but with increased cardiac output, LA pressure rises and exertional dyspnea develops. As mitral valve obstruction increases, dyspnea occurs at lower work levels. The progression of disability is so subtle and so protracted that patients may adapt by circumscribing their lifestyles. It becomes

TABLE 57-2 Symptoms Associated with Mitral Stenosis

On exertion
Dyspnea, wheezing, cough
Fatigue
Diminished activity/or pace of activity
Palpitations
Feeling faint, presyncope, syncope
At rest
Cough, wheezing
Paroxysmal nocturnal dyspnea
Orthopnea
Hemoptysis
Hoarseness (Ortner's syndrome)
From complications of MS

SOURCE: Copyright S. H. Rahimtoola, M.B., F.R.C.P, M.A.C.P., M.A.C.C. (Ref. 10).

imperative, then, to document what activities the patient can perform without symptoms and at what activity level symptoms begin; failure to do this often results in an underestimation of disability.

As obstruction progresses, the patients note orthopnea and paroxysmal nocturnal dyspnea that apparently results from redistribution of blood to the thorax on assuming the supine position. With severe MS and elevated pulmonary vascular resistance, fatigue rather than dyspnea may be the predominant symptom. Dependent edema, nausea, anorexia, and right-upper-quadrant pain reflect systemic venous congestion resulting from elevated systemic venous pressure and salt and water retention.

Palpitations are a frequent complaint in patients with MS and may represent frequent premature atrial contractions or paroxysmal atrial fibrillation/flutter. Of patients with severe symptomatic MS, 50 percent or more have chronic atrial fibrillation. Paroxysmal atrial fibrillation may produce pulmonary edema in some patients with MS. The acute increase in LA pressure that produces pulmonary edema results both from a decrease in the diastolic flow period caused by increased heart rate and from a loss of atrial transport function.

Systemic embolism, a frequent complication of MS, may result in stroke, occlusion of extremity arterial supply, occlusion of the aortic bifurcation, and visceral or myocardial infarction. Atrial fibrillation, increasing age of the patient, increasing LA size, and a previous history of embolism are associated with an increased incidence of systemic embolism[13] (Table 57-3).

Hemoptysis may result from a variety of causes. It is usually due to increased pulmonary venous pressure. Sputum may be blood-stained with paroxysmal nocturnal dyspnea, pink frothy sputum may result from rupture of alveolar capillaries associated with acute pulmonary edema or from pulmonary infarction due to pulmonary embolism, or hemoptysis may be severe and profuse (pulmonary apoplexy). The latter results from rupture of thin-walled, dilated bronchial veins, and although usually not fatal, it may be life-threatening because of aspiration pneumonia or massive hemorrhage. The edematous bronchial mucosa is more likely to be associated with chronic bronchitis, especially in cold and wet climates; it can also result in blood-stained sputum.

TABLE 57-3 Complications of Mitral Stenosis

Arrhythmias
- Atrial flutter/fibrillation

Embolism
- Systemic-cerebral, coronary, abnormal, peripheral, pulmonary

Acute pulmonary edema
Pulmonary arterial hypertension
Right ventricular hypertrophy/dilatation
Tricuspid regurgitation
Clinical heart failure
Left ventricular dysfunction
Chest pain/angina
Infective endocarditis

SOURCE: Copyright by S. H. Rahimtoola, M.B., F.R.C.P., M.A.C.P., M.A.C.C. (Ref. 10).

Exertional chest pain, typical of angina pectoris, may be present in some patients with severe MS but normal coronary arteries. Severe PA hypertension has been postulated as a cause. Infective endocarditis is an uncommon complication of pure MS.

Progression of symptoms in MS is generally slow but relentless. Thus, a sudden change in symptoms rarely reflects a change in valve obstruction. Rather, there is usually a noncardiac precipitating event or paroxysmal atrial fibrillation. Fever, pregnancy, hyperthyroidism, and noncardiac surgery, all of which increase CO, can precipitate decompensation in patients with moderate to severe MS.

PHYSICAL FINDINGS

During the latent, presymptomatic interval, incidental physical findings may be normal or may provide evidence of mild MS. Frequently, the only characteristic finding noted at rest will be a loud S_1 and a presystolic murmur. A short diastolic decrescendo rumble may be heard only with exercise. In patients with symptomatic stenosis, the findings are more obvious, and careful physical examination usually leads to the correct diagnosis (Chap. 10).

The general appearance of the patient in MS is usually normal. The MS facies, characterized by malar flush (pinkish-purple patches on the cheeks),[13] is uncommon and is caused by peripheral cyanosis, which is usually associated with a low CO, systemic vasoconstriction, and severe PA hypertension. Tachypnea may be present if LA pressure is high. The arterial pulse is normal except for irregularity in atrial fibrillation and is of low volume when CO is reduced. All peripheral pulses should be carefully examined because of the frequency of systemic embolism. The jugular venous pressure may be normal or may show evidence of elevated RA pressure. A prominent *a* wave is a result of RV hypertension/hypertrophy or of associated tricuspid stenosis. A prominent *v* wave is caused by tricuspid regurgitation. Atrial fibrillation produces an irregular venous pulse with absent *a* waves. The chest findings may be normal or may reveal signs of pulmonary congestion with rales or pleural fluid (dullness and absent breath sounds). Marked LA enlargement may produce egophony at the tip of the left scapula.

The precordium is usually unremarkable on inspection. On palpation, the apical impulse should feel normal or is tapping (palpable mitral valve closure or RV forming the cardiac apex). An abnormal LV impulse suggests disease other than isolated MS. A diastolic thrill is usually appreciated only when the patient is examined in the left lateral position. When PA hypertension is present, a sustained RV lift along the left sternal border and pulmonic valve closure may be palpable.

On auscultation in the supine position, the only abnormality appreciated may be the accentuated S_1, which is caused by flexible valve leaflets and the wide closing excursion of the valve

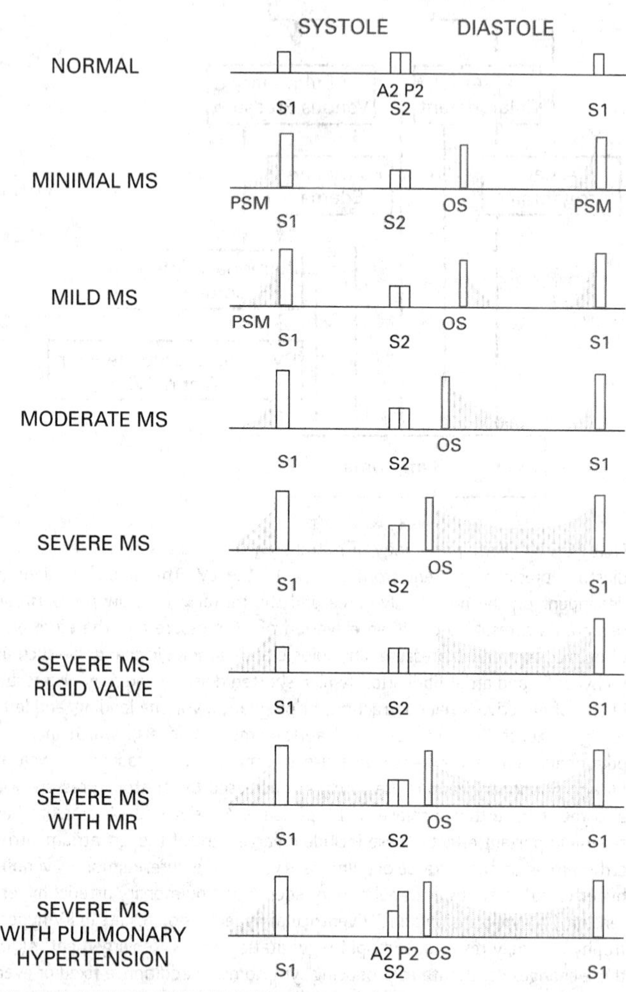

FIGURE 57-2 Auscultatory signs of MS in patients in sinus rhythm are illustrated. These include a presystolic murmur, loud first heart sound (S_1), an opening snap (OS), and a middiastolic murmur (low-pitched, decrescendo diastolic rumble, rumbling murmur). These signs may be accentuated or at times may be heard only by placing the patient in the left lateral decubitus position. Importantly, these signs are helpful in assessing the severity of the MS; as the MS becomes more severe, the S_2-OS interval is shortened and the length of the middiastolic rumble is increased. In mild OS, the S_2-OS interval is long and the diastolic murmur is short. In moderate MS, the S_2-OS interval is shorter, and although the diastolic murmur is longer at rest, there is usually a gap between the end of the murmur and the onset of the presystolic murmur. In severe MS, the S_2-OS interval is short (usually 0.04 to 0.06 s) and the diastolic murmur is a full-length murmur. With PA hypertension, P_2 is increased in intensity. In the presence of a rigid mitral valve (with or without calcification), S_2 is soft and the OS is usually not heard. A holosystolic murmur of mitral regurgitation may be present. (Adapted and modified from Kawanishi DT, Rahimtoola SH. Mitral stenosis. In: Rahimtoola SH, ed. *Valvular Heart Disease II*. St. Louis: Mosby; 1996:8.1–8.24. Copyright by S. H. Rahimtoola, M.B., F.R.C.P., M.A.C.P., M.A.C.C.)

leaflets[20] (see also Chap. 10). Failure to examine the patient in the left lateral position accounts for most of the missed diagnoses of symptomatic MS. The diastolic rumble is heard best with the bell of the stethoscope applied at the apical impulse. Nevertheless, the murmur may be localized, and the region around the apical impulse also should be auscultated. The *opening snap* (OS) occurs when the movement of the domed mitral valve into the LV is suddenly stopped.[20] It is heard best with the diaphragm and is often most easily appreciated midway between the apex and the left sternal border. In this intermediate region, the S_1, the pulmonary component of the second heart sound (P_2), and the OS can be identified. The auscultatory signs of MS in sinus rhythm and in atrial fibrillation are illustrated in Figs. 57-2 and 57-3.

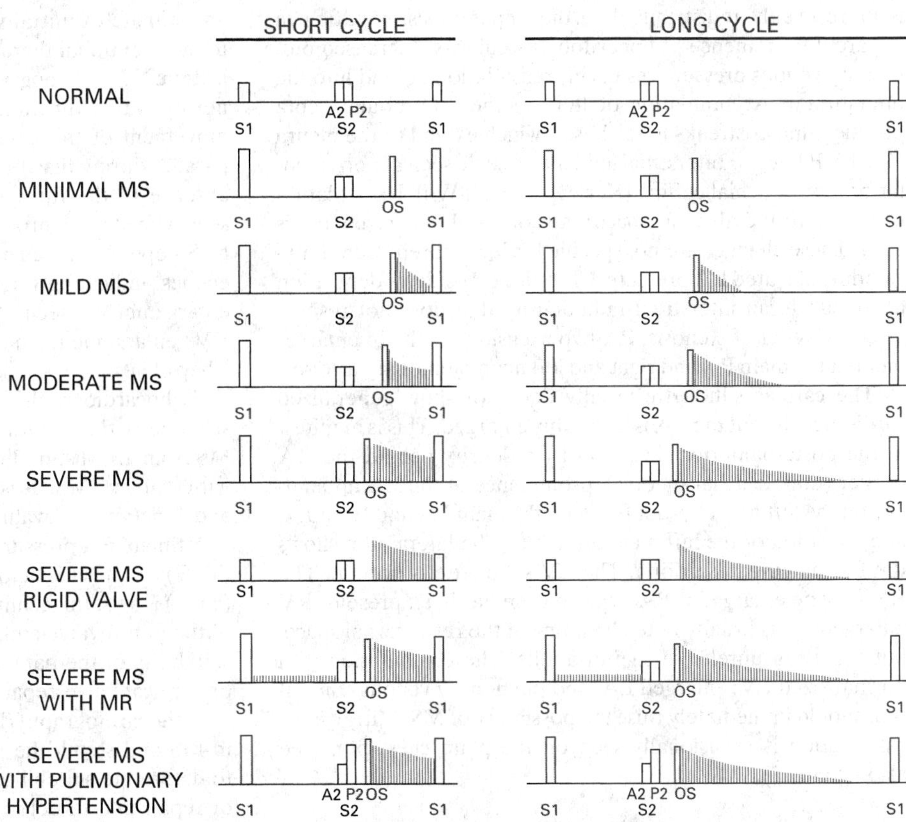

FIGURE 57-3 Auscultatory signs of MS in atrial fibrillation are illustrated. The presystolic murmur is absent. The loud S_1 and the OS are still heard. In the short cycles, the duration of diastole is short and the middiastolic rumble occupies the whole of diastole (*left panel*). In the long cycles (*right panel*), the length of middiastolic murmur is related to the severity of MS. As the MS becomes more severe, the length of this murmur is increased. In atrial fibrillation, with a slow ventricular response and very long R-R intervals, the middiastolic rumble may not occupy the whole diastolic period and the presystolic murmur is usually absent. Thus, one may get the impression that the MS is moderate rather than severe. Increasing the heart rate—for example, with brief physical exertion—may produce more characteristic auscultatory findings. Alternatively, when the ventricular rate in atrial fibrillation is rapid or in short cycles, the auscultatory findings may suggest a more severe degree of MS than is really the case (*left panel*). (Adapted and modified from Kawanishi DT, Rahimtoola SH. Mitral stenosis. In: Rahimtoola SH, ed. *Valvular Heart Disease. II*. St. Louis: Mosby; 1996:8.1–8.24. Copyright 1996 by S. H. Rahimtoola, M.B., F.R.C.P., M.A.C.P., M.A.C.C.)

The OS occurs after the LV pressure falls below LA pressure in early diastole. When LA pressure is high, as in severe MS, the snap occurs earlier in diastole (Fig. 57-2). The converse is true with mild MS. The interval between A_2 and the OS varies from 40 to 120 ms. Although the OS is present in most cases of MS, it is absent in patients with stiff, fibrotic, or calcified leaflets. Thus, absence of the OS in severe MS suggests that mitral valve replacement rather than commissurotomy may be necessary.

The low-pitched diastolic rumble follows the OS and is best heard with the bell of the stethoscope. In some patients with low cardiac output or mild MS, brief exercise, such as situps or walking, is adequate to increase flow and bring out the murmur. The murmur is low-pitched, rumbling, and decrescendo. In general, the more severe the MS, the longer the murmur (Fig. 57-2). Presystolic accentuation of the murmur occurs in sinus rhythm and has been reported even in atrial fibrillation. In the latter situation, a brief "presystolic" accentuation is due to narrowing of the mitral orifice produced by ventricular systole before the final, completeclosure of the mitral valve and the mitral component of S_1. A diastolic rumble is not diagnostic of MS and may be heard with increased flow across a normal mitral valve—for example, in ventricular septal defect with a large left-to-right shunt.

The two most important auscultatory signs of severe MS are a short A_2-OS interval (usually 40 to 60 ms) and a full-length diastolic rumble. The A_2-OS interval may be longer if there is associated moderate/severe aortic regurgitation, and the OS may be absent when the mitral valve is rigid. The diastolic murmur may not be full-length in severe MS if the stroke volume is low and there is no tachycardia.

Systolic murmurs also may be heard in association with the murmur of MS. A blowing, holosystolic murmur at the apex suggests associated MR; whereas a systolic blowing murmur heard best at the lower left sternal border that increases with inspiration usually signifies tricuspid regurgitation. The Graham Steell murmur is a high-pitched diastolic decrescendo murmur of pulmonic regurgitation caused by severe PA hypertension. In most patients with MS, such a murmur usually indicates AR instead. In general, a left-sided S_3 is not compatible with severe MS with the possible exception of concomitant severe AR and/or significant LV systolic dysfunction. If an S_3 and a rumble are present, MR is usually the predominant lesion (see also Chap. 10).

ROENTGENOGRAM

The posteroanterior and lateral chest films are often so typical that experienced clinicians can make the tentative diagnosis from them. The thoracic cage is normal. The lung fields show evidence of elevated pulmonary venous pressure. Blood flow is more evenly redistributed to the upper lobes, resulting in apparent prominence of upper-lobe vascularity. Increased pulmonary venous pressure results in transudation of fluid into the interstitium. Accumulation of fluid in the interlobular septa produces linear streaks in the bases, which extend to the pleura (Kerley B lines).[21] Interstitial fluid may also be seen as perivascular or peribronchial cuffing (Kerley A lines). With transudation of fluid into the alveolar spaces, alveolar pulmonary edema is seen. These changes are not specific for MS but represent long-standing elevated LA pressure. Chronic hemosiderin deposition can result in an interstitial radiodensity that does not resolve after the relief of stenosis. PA hypertension results in enlargement of the main PA and right and left main pulmonary arteries.

The cardiac silhouette usually does not show generalized cardiomegaly, but the LA is invariably enlarged. This is manifest in the posteroanterior chest film by a density behind the RA border (double atrial shadow), prominence of the LA appendage on the left heart border between the main PA and LV apex, and elevation of the left main bronchus. The lateral film shows the LA bulging posteriorly. The LV silhouette is normal. The RV may be enlarged if PA hypertension has been present. RV enlargement is usually noted by filling of the retrosternal space, but this is an unreliable sign in adults. The combination of a normal-sized LV, enlarged LA, and pulmonary venous congestion should immediately raise the possibility of MS. Mitral valve calcification is occasionally seen on the plain chest film (see also Chap. 12).

ELECTROCARDIOGRAM

The *electrocardiogram* (ECG) is not usually as helpful as the chest x-ray. Patients in sinus rhythm may have a widened P wave caused by interatrial conduction delay and/or prolonged LA depolarization. Classically, the P wave is broad and notched in lead II and biphasic in lead V_1; it measures 0.12 s or more. Atrial fibrillation is common. LV hypertrophy is almost never present unless there are associated lesions. RV hypertrophy may be present if PA hypertension is marked (see also Chap. 11).

CLINICAL INDICATIONS OF SEVERE MITRAL STENOSIS

Some clinical features make it virtually certain that MS is severe. These include (1) moderate to severe PA hypertension as indicated by clinical and ECG evidence of RV hypertrophy or PA hypertension or both and/or (2) moderate to severe elevation of LA pressure as indicated by orthopnea, a short P_2-OS interval, a diastolic rumble that occupies the whole length of a long diastolic interval in patients with atrial fibrillation, and pulmonary edema on the chest x-ray. In both these clinical circumstances, one must be certain that there is no other cause for elevated LA pressure and that LA hypertension is not caused mainly by a correctable transient elevation of LV diastolic pressure.

Laboratory Tests

ECHOCARDIOGRAPHY/DOPPLER ULTRASOUND

Echocardiography/Doppler ultrasound has proved to be both sensitive and specific for MS when adequate studies are done (Chap. 13).[22–25] False-positive and false-negative results are uncommon. M-mode and two-dimensional echocardiography do not reliably predict the severity of MS. Doppler studies provide an estimate of mitral valve area that is within ± 0.4 cm^2 (prior to interventional therapy) of that obtained by cardiac catheterization.[26] The echographic findings of MS reflect the loss of normal valve function. The fusion of commissures results in movement of the anterior and posterior leaflets anteriorly in parallel during diastole. In patients in sinus rhythm, there is an absence of the further opening of the valve that is normally seen with atrial contraction. Other findings include decreased E-to-F slope, decreased mitral valve leaflet excursion, and multiple echoes, indicating thickening or calcification of the valve. LA enlargement is seen. Abnormal pulmonary valve motion and RV enlargement may signify PA hypertension (see also Chap. 13).

Echocardiography is of great value in patients with equivocal signs, in patients with gross PA hypertension, to differentiate MS from an Austin Flint murmur of AR, and in the rare patient with "silent" MS. It is used to assess LV, RV, and atrial size and function; to evaluate the aortic and tricuspid valves; and to estimate PA pressure. When transthoracic echocardiography (TTE) is unsatisfactory, transesophageal echocardiography (TEE) is a useful technique to assess LA thrombus, the anatomy of the mitral valve and subvalvular apparatus, and to assess the suitability of the patient for catheter balloon commissurotomy or surgical valve repair.

Echocardiography/Doppler ultrasound is a most useful test in MS and should be performed in all patients. It is essential to determine suitability of the valve for commissurotomy and/or repair and to determine the likely result.

CARDIAC CATHETERIZATION/ANGIOGRAPHY

In most patients with disabling symptoms from presumed MS, right and left heart catheterization should be performed as part of a preoperative assessment. Simultaneous measurement of cardiac output and the gradient between the LA and the LV and calculation of valve area remain the "gold standard" for assessing the severity of MS (Chap. 15). LV angiography assesses the competence of the mitral valve, an important determinant of operability for mitral commissurotomy. Quantification of LV function provides a useful prognostic indicator of operative and late survival and of the expected functional result. Aortic valve function should be evaluated in all patients. Selective supraventricular aortography should be performed in all patients unless there is a contraindication. Tricuspid valve function can be assessed when there is a question of coexisting lesions. In certain circumstances—for example, in a patient with suspected severe MS who has a small gradient and mildly elevated LA pressure—dynamic exercise in the catheterization laboratory with measurement of mitral valve gradient, CO and LA and PA pressures can be extremely useful. Another example is a patient with significant symptoms in whom the findings at rest suggest moderate (or even mild) MS. Selective coronary arteriography establishes the site, severity, and extent of coronary artery disease and should be performed in patients with angina, in those with LV dysfunction, in those with risk factors for coronary artery disease, and in those 35 years of age or older who are being considered for interventional therapy.

OTHER INVESTIGATIONS

In most clinical situations, other investigations are not needed. Occasionally, a treadmill exercise test to evaluate functional capacity may be very useful clinically—for example, when a patient denies symptoms in spite of severe hemodynamic abnormalities.

Clinical Decision Making

The reader is referred to the section on aortic stenosis in Chap. 57. In a prospective blinded study of consecutive patients with valvular heart disease, the sensitivity and specificity of diagnosis of MS by clinical evaluation was 86 and 87 percent, respectively. The accuracy of diagnosis of MS for moderate to severe stenosis was 92 percent by clinical evaluation and 97 percent by echocardiography/Doppler ultrasound.[27] This emphasizes the importance of a thorough clinical evaluation. The principal difficulty with both clinical evaluation and echocardiography/Doppler ultrasound is being able to accurately separate in all instances mild from moderate MS and moderate from severe MS.

Natural History and Prognosis

The population presenting with MS is changing because of the sharp decline in the incidence of acute rheumatic fever in the past 40 years (see also Chap. 55). Native-born American citizens with symptomatic MS are presenting at an older age. Young adults in the third and fourth decades with symptomatic MS are more likely to come from low socioeconomic backgrounds and from the inner city or to be immigrants, particularly from Latin America, the Middle East, Africa, or Asia. Therefore, the latent period between acute rheumatic fever and symptomatic MS is variable and appears to be related to the presence of repeated streptococcal infection. Women with MS outnumber men by almost two to one. The most important feature of the asymptomatic interval is the susceptibility to repeated bouts of both rheumatic valvulitis and streptococcal infection. The mechanism for the progression from no symptoms to mild to severe symptoms is progressive stenosis of the mitral valve.

With the onset of exertional dyspnea and fatigue, the valve area is usually reduced to one-half to one-third its normal size. Further small reductions in valve area markedly obstruct flow and result in symptoms with minimal exertion. The interval from initial mild symptoms to disabling symptoms may be 10 years. During this time, the patient is at some risk of death (see below). Permanent injury may result from atrial fibrillation with rapid ventricular rate, resulting in pulmonary edema, and from systemic embolus. Unfortunately, it is not possible to predict who is at risk of embolism. When late functional class II or functional class III symptoms are present, the valve area is usually 1.0 cm^2 or less (in an occasional patient the valve area is 1.2 or 1.3 cm^2), and both rest and exercise hemodynamics are deranged.[2] Further small reductions in valve area result in symptoms at rest.

The 10-year survival of patients with MS who are asymptomatic is approximately 84 percent and that of those who are mildly symptomatic is 34 to 42 percent (Fig. 57-4).[28–30] The 10-year survival of patients who are moderately or severely symptomatic and who do not have therapy is 40 percent or less, and the survival at 20 years is less than 10 percent.[28–30] Patients in the New York Heart Association functional class IV have a very poor survival without treatment[28]: 42 percent at 1 year and 10 percent or less at 5 years. All are dead by 10 years (Fig. 57-5).

Management

MS can be prevented through two approaches (Table 57-4). First, all streptococcal infections should be diagnosed rapidly and correctly treated (Chap. 55). This prevents most initial episodes of acute rheumatic fever. Second, all patients with known previous acute rheumatic fever/rheumatic carditis with or without obvious valve disease should receive appropriate antibiotic prophylaxis against recurrent streptococcal infection (Chap. 55).

Although the incidence of infective endocarditis is low in isolated MS, all patients exposed to bacteremia should receive appropriate prophylaxis against infective endocarditis (Chap. 73). Family and vocational planning should be considered. Women with this disease should consider bearing children before symptoms occur, since pregnancy is usually well tolerated with mild MS. Occupations that require strenuous exertion in middle age and later should probably be avoided if possible. In patients with moderate or severe MS, activities such as strenuous exercise and competitive sports should be restricted.[9]

When patients reach the symptomatic threshold, medical treatment may be of some benefit. Digitalis offers no improvement for the patient with normal sinus rhythm and normal LV function. When atrial fibrillation is present, however, digitalis plays a critical role in controlling ventricular rate. In selected patients, beta-adrenergic blocking agents, diltiazem, or amiodarone may be added if digoxin alone is not satisfactory in controlling ventricular rate at rest or on exercise. Beta-adrenergic blocking agents should be used with great caution or not at all in patients with impaired LV function, associated significant aortic stenosis, or other associated severe valvular disease. Digoxin and diltiazem or digoxin and low-dose amiodarone are probably the two best combined regimens. Diuretics reduce pulmonary congestion and peripheral edema and allow most patients freedom from severe salt restriction. For the patient with mild symptoms, maintenance of sinus rhythm is desirable. Cardioversion of atrial fibrillation and maintenance of sinus rhythm using antiarrhythmic therapy with either digitalis and quinidine or digitalis and amiodarone should be offered to these patients. In patients who need interventional therapy, cardioversion is usually performed after completion of the procedure. Anticoagulation with warfarin is usually begun about 3 weeks in advance of cardioversion and for 4 weeks after the procedure.[31] Patients with chronic atrial fibrillation and those with a previous history of embolism should receive anticoagulation with warfarin (International Normalized Ratio, or INR, of 2 to 3) unless there is a specific contraindication.

There are no randomized trials of surgery versus medical therapy. Roy and Gopinath's study[29] showed that in comparable patients, surgical commissurotomy was associated with a better survival than medical therapy in patients with class II symptoms as well as in those with class III and IV symptoms (Fig. 57-6).

Unless there is a contraindication, surgery should be recommended to an MS patient with functional class III or IV symptoms (Table 57-5). For younger patients with a pliable, noncalcified valve and without important mitral regurgitation, this means valve repair. The hemodynamic results of surgical commissurotomy are excellent.[9,32,33] Because of the low morbidity and mortality of mitral commissurotomy/valve repair,[9,32–34] surgery is also offered to those patients when functional class II symptoms are present. The results of successful commissurot-

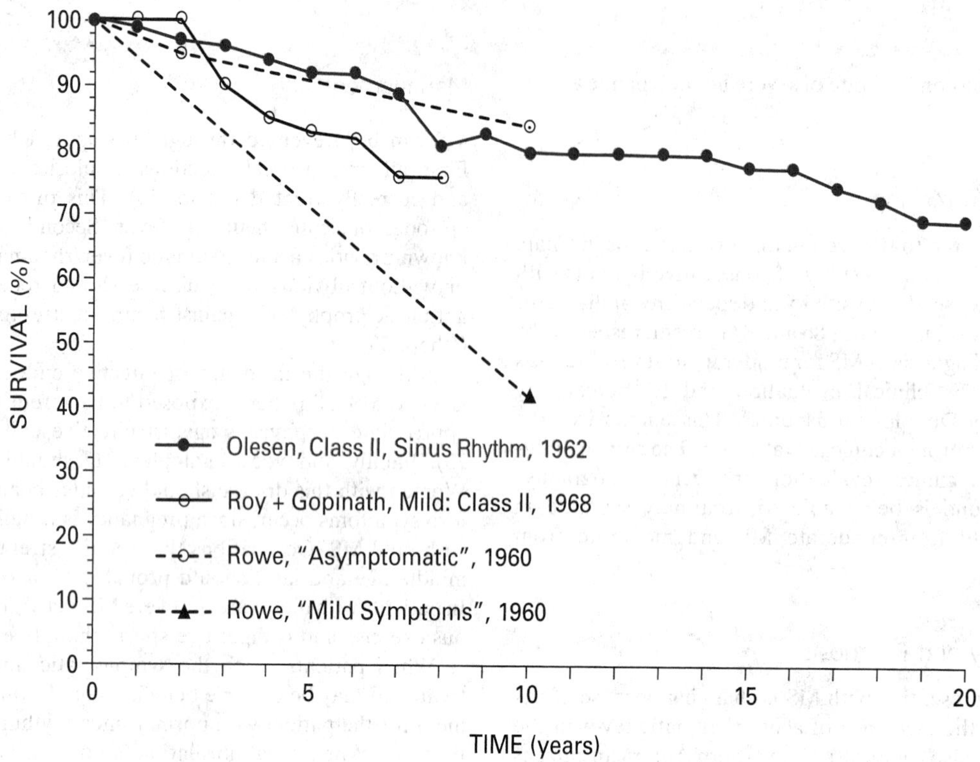

FIGURE 57-4 This figure depicts the survival of patients with MS who initially where asymptomatic or had mild symptoms and were treated medically. In the 1960 study of Rowe and coworkers[30] (*dashed lines*), 52 percent of 250 patients with "auscultatory MS" who presented between 1925 and 1947 were asymptomatic; their 10-year survival was 84 percent. The lower dashed line represents the survival in the 42 percent of patients who had mild symptoms on clinical presentation; their 10-year survival was 42 percent.[30] The data of Olesen, 1962[27] (*upper solid curve connecting solid symbols*), show the survival in the 21 percent of 271 symptomatic MS patients who had class II symptoms. Their 10- and 20-year survival was 34 and 14 percent, respectively. The data of Roy and Gopinath, 1968[29] (*lower solid curve connecting open symbols*), also show the survival in patients with class II symptoms. (From Kawanishi DT, Rahimtoola SH. Mitral stenosis. In: Rahimtoola SH, ed. *Valvular Heart Disease. II.* St. Louis: Mosby; 1996:8.1–8.24.)

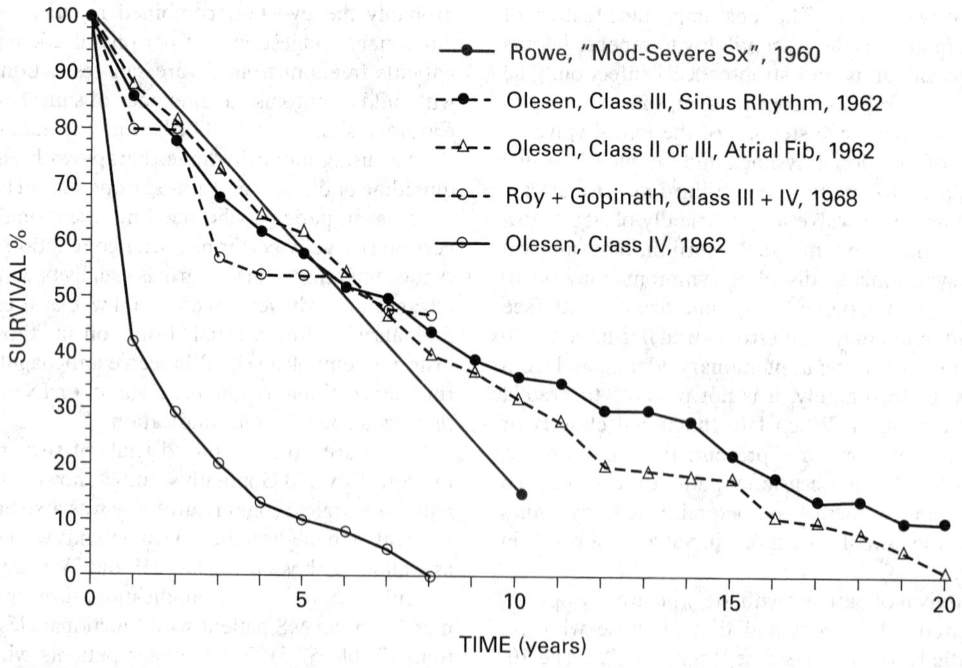

FIGURE 57-5 Survival of patients with MS and moderate or advanced (severe) symptoms is shown. Patients who were in NYHA functional class IV (Olesen, class IV, 1962)[28] had a 42 percent 1-year survival and all patients had died within 8 years. The other four survival curves are of patients who were in functional classes II to IV, and their survival curves are similar, with 5-, 10-, and 15-year approximate survivals of 60, 40, and 20 percent, respectively; at 20 years, less than 10 percent of the patients were still alive.[28-30] Thus, the survival in this group of patients with more advanced symptoms is much worse than that of patients who were initially asymptomatic or minimally symptomatic (see Fig. 57-4). (From Kawanishi DT, Rahimtoola SH. Mitral stenosis. In: Rahimtoola SH, ed. *Valvular Heart Disease. II.* St. Louis: Mosby; 1996:8.1–8.24.)

TABLE 57-4 Medical Treatment of Mitral Stenosis

Prevention
- Primary
  - Treatment of streptococcal group A infection
- Secondary (antibiotic prophylaxis)
  - Recurrent rheumatic fever
  - Infective endocarditis

Restrict activities (moderate/severe MS)
- Severe exercise
- Competitive sports

Arrhythmias
- Prevent and/or control
- Restore sinus rhythm if possible

Cardiac medications
- Use only if essential
- Diuretics—use cautiously
- Anticoagulants for systemic/pulmonary emboli
- Elevated pulmonary venous pressure—diuretics
- Heart failure—digitalis, diuretics, ACE inhibitors

Follow-up of asymptomatic patients

Mild MS	Every 2–5 years
Moderate MS	Every 1–2 years
Severe MS	Every 6–12 months if interventional therapy not performed
Development of symptoms	Early or "immediate"

SOURCE: Copyright by S. H. Rahimtoola, M.B., F.R.C.P., M.A.C.P., M.A.C.C. (Ref. 10).

TABLE 57-5 Indications for Interventional Therapy for Severe Mitral Stenosis

- All severely symptomatic patients (functional classes III and IV)
- All mildly symptomatic patients (functional class II)[a,b]
- Asymptomatic patients[a,b]
  - Pulmonary artery hypertension
  - Episodic pulmonary edema
  - Atrial fibrillation (persistent or repeated episodes)
  - Thromboembolism (systemic/pulmonary)
  - Severe mitral stenosis (valve suitable for CBC/surgical valve repair)

[a]Catheter balloon commissurotomy (CBC)/surgery.
[b]Individualize depending on patient characteristics; suitability of patient for CBC/surgical valve repair versus valve replacement, skill and experience of interventional team.
SOURCE: Copyright by S. H. Rahimtoola, M.B., F.R.C.P., M.A.C.P., M.A.C.C. (Ref. 10).

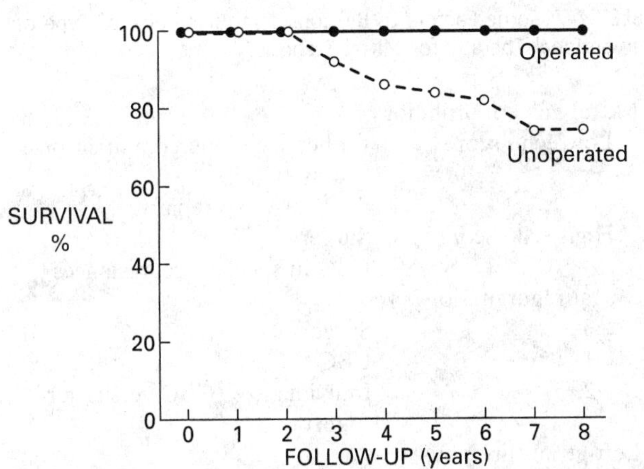

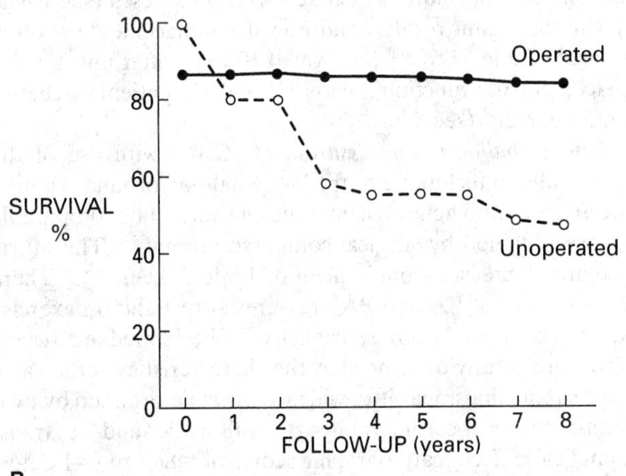

FIGURE 57-6 Comparison of survival of patients with class II symptoms (*left panel*) and class III and IV symptoms due to MS (*right panel*).[29] Survival of patients treated medically (unoperated) is indicated by the broken line and with surgical closed mitral commissurotomy (operated) by the solid line. In patients treated by surgical commissurotomy, there were no operative or late deaths in those with mild symptoms and no late deaths in those with class III and IV symptoms. There is a clear improvement in survival in operated patients. The 5-year mortality with medical treatment alone in those with class III and IV symptoms approaches 50 percent (also see Fig. 57-5); with surgery, there is no appreciable mortality following recovery from the procedure. [From Roy SB, Gopinath N. Mitral stenosis. *Circulation* 1968; 38(suppl v):68–76.]

TABLE 57-6 Mitral Stenosis: Results of Mitral Valve Replacement in 33 Patients

	Mitral Stenosis	
	Pre-MVR[a]	Post-MVR
LV end-diastolic pressure, mmHg	11 ± 5	12 ± 6
Mean PA wedge pressure, mmHg	36 ± 15	28 ± 14[b]
Mean systolic PA pressure, mmHg	54 ± 24	42 ± 22[c]
Cardiac index, $L/min/m^2$	2.1 ± 1.5	2.3 ± 0.6
LV EDVI, mL/m^2	79 ± 18	72 ± 24
LV ESVI, mL/m^2	41 ± 13	39 ± 21
LVEF	0.48 ± 0.10	0.47 ± 0.14
Mitral regurgitant volume, mL	—	—
Regurgitant volume/end-diastolic volume	—	—
Mitral valve gradient, mmHg	15 ± 7	8 ± 3[b]
Mitral valve area, cm^2	1.2 ± 0.4	1.8 ± 0.6[b]

[a]MVR = mitral valve replacement.
[b]$p < .001$.
[c]$p < .01$ comparing before and after mitral valve replacement artery.
SOURCE: Crawford MH et al.[36]

omy are excellent; in experienced and skilled centers, surgical mortality is less that 1 percent. Late mortality at 10 years is less than 5 percent, the thromboembolism rate is 2 percent per year or less, and the reoperation rate ranges from 0.5 to 4.5 percent per year. The return of symptoms after commissurotomy/valve repair is usually the result of an incomplete operation, other valvular lesions, refusion of mitral commissures, or deterioration of myocardial function. In less developed countries, excellent results have been reported in a very high percentage of young patients for up to 25 years.[35]

For the older patient with a stiff or calcified valve or when moderate mitral regurgitation is present, mitral valve replacement is usually performed. Valve replacement carries a higher operative mortality than does commissurotomy (up to 5 percent) and the morbidity associated with prostheses (see Chap. 60). Hemodynamic results of mitral valve replacement are often not ideal (Table 57-6).[36,37] Survival at 10 years after mitral valve replacement for functional class III and IV patients is better than 60 percent (see Chap. 60).

Catheter balloon commissurotomy (CBC) with use of the double balloon technique or the Inoue balloon produces immediate and 3-month hemodynamic and clinical results comparable to those obtained by surgical commissurotomy.[38–41] The mitral valve area increases from a mean of 1.0 to 2.0 cm^2.[26,32,38] There are reductions of LA and PA pressures at rest and on exercise and an increase of exercise capacity.[39] The immediate results of CBC are greatly influenced by the characteristics of the valve and its supporting apparatus, which are best determined by two-dimensional echocardiography (transthoracic and/or transesophageal).[22] Echocardiographic scores of ≤8 or of 0–1 determined by the two different methods provide a clue to the best immediate results. Repeat CBC or mitral valve replacement is needed in 20 percent of patients within 5 to 7 years. Late survival is poorer in those in whom functional class IV, higher echocardiographic score, higher LV end-diastolic pressure, or higher PA systolic pressure is present prior to the CBC.[42–47] In one study, the 7-year survival was 95 ± 1 percent and the event-free survival was 65 ± 6 percent.[47] The 7-year event-free survival ranged from 13 to 90 percent in various subgroups. The 7-year event-free survival was best predicted by the post-CBC mitral valve area (≥1.5 cm^2) and PA wedge pressure (18 mmHg); the 7-year event-free survival was 90 ± 6 percent.[47] In the appropriate patient and in centers with skilled and experienced staff, CBC is the procedure of first choice for relief of severe MS. Factors to be taken into account choosing between surgery and CBC in an individual patient are shown in Table 57-7.

The recommendations of the ACC/AHA Practice Guidelines are shown in Tables 57-8, 57-9, and 57-10.[48] Guidelines are *not* and should *not* be the law. Application of guidelines to clinical practice should be based on the following principles: (1) classes I and III apply to all patients in these classes unless there is a specific clinical circumstance contradicting this and (2) class II applies to patients in this class depending on the clinical condition of the patient and the skill and experience at the individual medical center.

NORMAL MITRAL STRUCTURE AND FUNCTION

The mitral valve is a complex structure formed by four elements[49,50]:

1. The annulus is asymmetrical, with a fixed portion (corresponding to the anterior leaflet) shared with the aortic

TABLE 57-7 Some Factors to Be Considered in Choice of Type of Interventional Therapy for Mitral Stenosis[a]

Mitral valve morphology	
Low echo score:	Catheter balloon commissurotomy (CBC)
	Surgical valve repair
High echo score:	Surgery
	CBC in special circumstances
Mitral regurgitation	
≥3+:	Surgery
≤1+:	CBC
2+:	Individualize (CBC versus surgery)
Left atrial thrombus	
Surgery	
CBC in special circumstances	
Need for other cardiac surgery	
Surgery	
CBC in special circumstances	

[a]In centers with skilled and experienced interventional teams.
SOURCE: Copyright by S. H. Rahimtoola. M.B., F.R.C.P., M.A.C.P., M.A.C.C. (Ref. 10).

TABLE 57-8 Recommendations for Percutaneous Mitral Balloon Valvotomy

Indication	Class
1. Symptomatic patients (NYHA functional class II, III, or IV), moderate or severe MS (mitral valve area ≤1.5 cm^2),[a] and valve morphology favorable for percutaneous balloon valvotomy in the absence of left atrial thrombus or moderate to severe MR	I
2. Asymptomatic patients with moderate or severe MS (mitral valve area ≤1.5 cm^2)[a] and valve morphology favorable for percutaneous balloon valvotomy who have pulmonary hypertension (pulmonary artery systolic pressure >50 mmHg at rest or 60 mmHg with exercise) in the absence of left atrial thrombus or moderate to severe MR	IIa
3. Patients with NYHA functional class III–IV symptoms, moderate or severe MS (mitral valve area ≤1.5 cm^2),[a] and a nonpliable calcified valve who are at high risk for surgery in the absence of left atrial thrombus or moderate to severe MR	IIa
4. Asymptomatic patients, moderate or severe MS (mitral valve area ≤1.5 cm^2)[a] and valve morphology favorable for percutaneous balloon valvotomy who have new onset of atrial fibrillation in the absence of left atrial thrombus or moderate to severe MR	IIb
5. Patients in NYHA functional class III–IV, moderate or severe MS (MVA ≤1.5 cm^2), and a nonpliable calcified valve who are low-risk candidates for surgery	IIb
6. Patients with mild MS	III

[a]The committee recognizes that there may be variability in the measurement of mitral valve area and that the mean transmitral gradient, pulmonary artery wedge pressure, and pulmonary artery pressure at rest or during exercise should also be taken into consideration.
SOURCE: ACC/AHA Guidelines,[48] with permission.

TABLE 57-9 Recommendations for Mitral Valve Repair for Mitral Stenosis

Indication	Class
1. Patients with NYHA functional class III–IV symptoms, moderate or severe MS (mitral valve area ≤1.5 cm^2),[a] and valve morphology favorable for repair if percutaneous mitral balloon valvotomy is not available	I
2. Patients with NYHA functional class III–IV symptoms, moderate or severe MS (mitral valve area ≤1.5 cm^2),[a] and valve morphology favorable for repair if a left atrial thrombus is present despite anticoagulation	I
3. Patients with NYHA functional class III–IV symptoms, moderate or severe MS (mitral valve area ≤1.5 cm^2),[a] and a nonpliable or calcified valve with the decision to proceed with either repair or replacement made at the time of the operation	I
4. Patients in NYHA functional class I, moderate or severe MS (mitral valve area ≤1.5 cm^2),[a] and valve morphology favorable for repair who have had recurrent episodes of embolic events on adequate anticoagulation	IIb
5. Patients with NYHA functional class I–IV symptoms and mild MS	III

[a]The committee recognizes that there may be a variability in the measurement of mitral valve area and that the mean transmitral gradient, pulmonary artery wedge pressure, and pulmonary artery pressure at rest or during exercise should also be considered.
SOURCE: ACC/AHA Guidelines,[48] with permission.

TABLE 57-10 Recommendations for Mitral Valve Replacement for Mitral Stenosis

Indication	Class
1. Patients with moderate or severe MS (mitral valve area ≤1.5 cm^2)[a] and NYHA functional class III–IV symptoms who are not considered candidates for percutaneous balloon valvotomy or mitral valve repair	I
2. Patients with severe MS (mitral valve area ≤1 cm^2)[a] and severe pulmonary hypertension (pulmonary artery systolic pressure >60 to 80 mmHg) with NYHA functional class I–II symptoms who are not considered candidates for percutaneous balloon valvotomy or mitral valve repair	IIa

[a]The committee recognizes that there may be a variability in the measurement of mitral valve area and that the mean transmitral gradient, pulmonary artery wedge pressure, and pulmonary artery pressure should also be considered.
SOURCE: ACC/AHA Guidelines,[48] with permission.

annulus and a dynamic portion (corresponding to the posterior leaflet) that represents most of the circumference of the annulus.

2. The two leaflets are asymmetrical; the anterior has the greater length of tissue but occupies a smaller portion of the circumference of the annulus than the posterior.
3. The chordae join each papillary muscle to the corresponding commissure and the adjoining halves of both leaflets and maintain the two leaflets in a position allowing coaptation.
4. The two papillary muscles and the adjacent wall attach the mitral apparatus to the LV.

Mitral competence during systole is normally ensured, first, by a large area of coaptation between leaflets allowing high friction resistance to abnormal valve movement and, second, by the systolic position to the anterior leaflet parallel to the direction of blood flow. The mechanism of MR frequently combines abnormal function of more than one anatomic element, which fact underlines the complexity of conservative surgery for restoration of normal mitral function.

MITRAL REGURGITATION

Mitral regurgitation (MR) is characterized by an abnormal reversed blood flow from the left ventricle (LV) to the left atrium (LA). The etiologic profile of MR is now dominated by degenerative and ischemic causes in developed countries. The development of noninvasive assessment with transesophageal echocardiography, color-flow imaging and Doppler methods of quantitation of regurgitation has transformed diagnostic approaches. With improved understanding of the impact of LV dysfunction on outcome, and most importantly with major advances in conservative surgery, the management of MR has become far more proactive.

Etiology and Mechanism (Table 57-11)

MR is often referred to as *organic* if there is an intrinsic valve disease or *functional* if the valve is structurally normal but leaks due to an extravalvular abnormality. Ischemic MR may be organic (ruptured papillary muscle) or functional (LV dysfunction). Nonischemic MR may be organic (e.g., rheumatic) or functional (e.g., cardiomyopathy).

RHEUMATIC DISEASE

Rheumatic MR is rarely pure, and in most cases is associated with stenosis and fusion of the commissures (Fig. 57-7, Plate 86). Severe rheumatic MR requiring surgical correction is still frequent in developing countries but is now rare in developed countries.[51] The underlying lesion is retractile fibrosis of leaflets and chordae, causing loss of coaptation. The secondary dilatation of the mitral annulus tends to further decrease the contract between leaflets. Elongated or ruptured chordae are infrequent.

DEGENERATIVE MITRAL REGURGITATION

These causes are often associated with valve prolapse, an abnormal movement of the leaflets into the LA during systole due to inadequate chordal support (elongation or rupture) and excessive valvular tissue. In western countries, mitral prolapse represents the most frequent causes leading to surgery for severe MR.[51] Degenerative MR can be separated in three categories:

- The mitral valve prolapse syndrome, characterized by diffuse myxomatous infiltration, discussed in detail in Chap. 58 (Fig. 57-8, Plate 87).
- The degenerative "primary" ruptured chordae, which involves the posterior more often than the anterior leaflet and occurs more often in men than in women. There is usually no excessive tissue, but enlargement of the annulus may occur as in any MR. The involved leaflet may present with a myxomatous infiltration,[52] but the other leaflet usually remains normal. Calcification of the mitral annulus or systemic hypertension may precede the occurrence of the ruptured chordae. Isolated ruptured cord may occasionally be due to blunt thoracic trauma and endocarditis (secondary forms).
- Degenerative MR without prolapse, which is usually mild and due to valve sclerosis or isolated annular calcification; here regurgitation is secondary to deformation of the valves of annulus (Fig. 57-9, Plate 88).

INFECTIVE ENDOCARDITIS

Infective endocarditis accounts for about 5 percent of cases of severe MR. Vegetations may produce mild MR by interposition between leaflets. Severe endocarditic MR is usually related to ruptured chordae and less frequently to destruction of mitral tissue involving either the leaflet's edges or a perforation (Fig. 57-10, Plate 89).

ISCHEMIC AND FUNCTIONAL MITRAL REGURGITATION

Ischemic and functional MR—i.e., due to LV wall dysfunction secondary to ischemia, scarring, aneurysm, cardiomyopathy, or myocarditis—have in common the same mechanism: the coaptation of intrinsically normal leaflets is incomplete. Rupture of

TABLE 57-11 Mitral Regurgitation: Mechanisms

Etiology	Mechanism	Echocardiographic Appearance
Rheumatic	Retraction	Thickened chordae/ leaflets
Lupus erythematosus	Thickening	Normal or restricted motion
Anticardiolipin syndrome		
Carcinoid		
Ergot lesions		
Postradiation		
Degenerative	Prolapsed leaflets	Prolapsing/flail leaflets
Marfan syndrome	Ruptured chords	Redundant tissue
Ehlers-Danlos syndrome		Ruptured chords
Traumatic MR		
Ischemic (infarction)	Ruptured papillary muscle	Flail leaflet
Myocardial disease	Dilatation of annulus	Normal leaflets
Ischemic (chronic)	Traction anterior leaflet	Reduced motion of leaflets
Cardiomyopathies		
Infiltrative disease	Thickened leaflet	Thickened leaflets
Hypereosinophilic syndrome	Loss of coaptation	Reduced motion
Endomyocardial fibrosis		
Hurler's disease		
Endocarditis	Destructive lesions	Perforations
		Flail leaflets
Congenital	Cleft leaflet	Cleft leaflet
	Transposed valve	Tricuspid valve

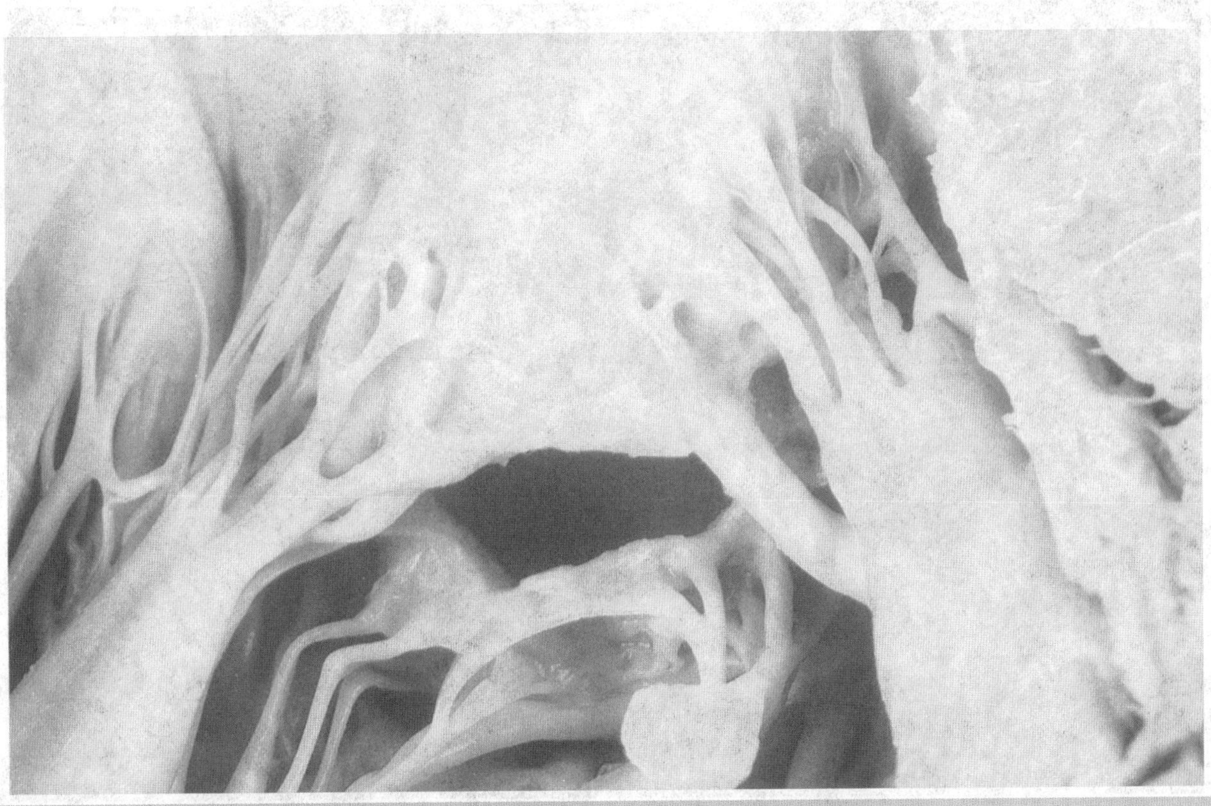

FIGURE 57-7 (Plate 86) Anatomic example of rheumatic MR. Note the thickening of the leaflet and chordae and the retraction of the mitral tissue. (Courtesy of Dr. W. D. Edwards.)

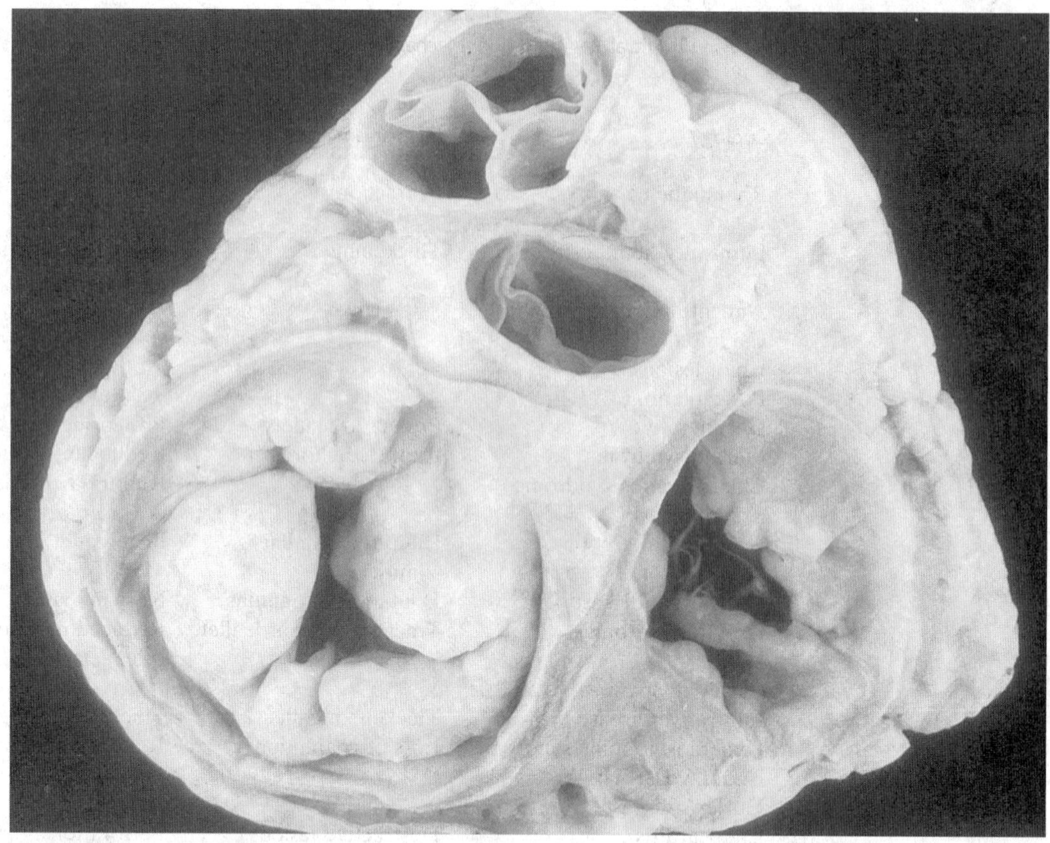

FIGURE 57-8 (Plate 87) Anatomic example of MR due to mitral valve prolapse seen from the atrial view (the mitral orifice is on the left of picture). Note the redundancy of the leaflets with excess tissue. (Courtesy of Dr. W. D. Edwards.)

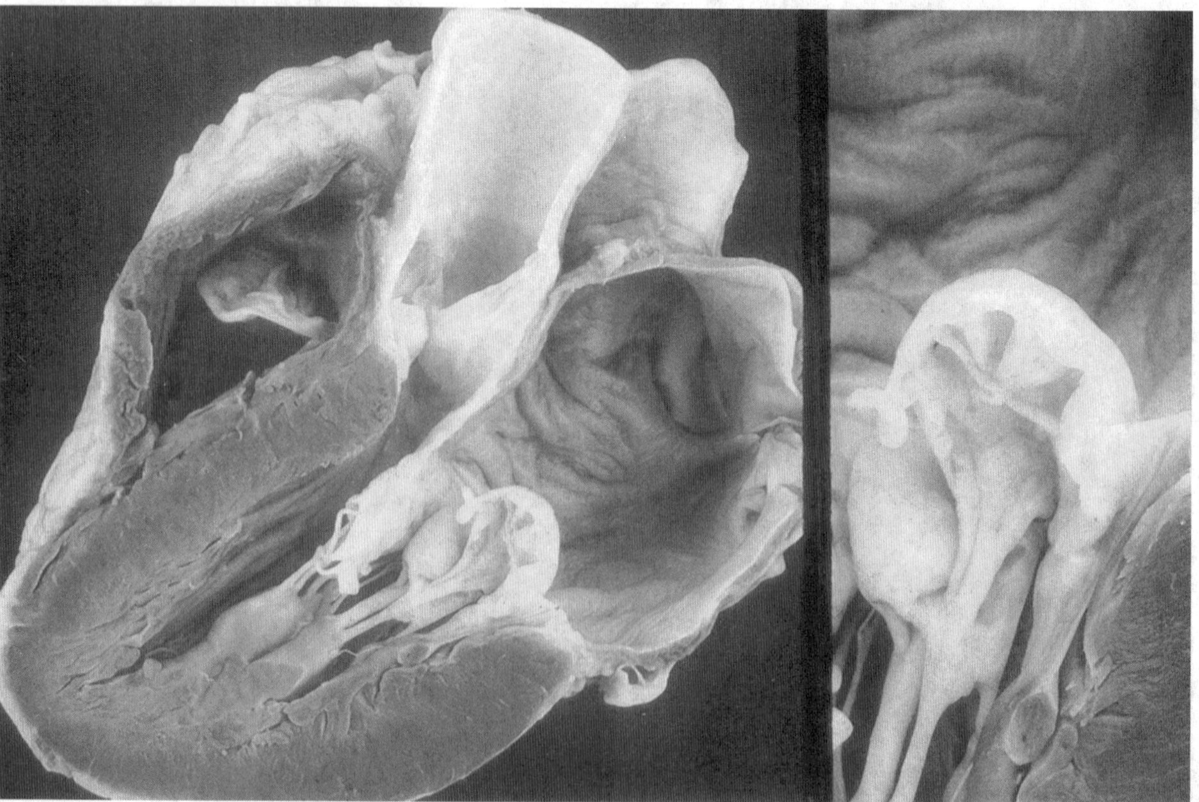

FIGURE 57-9 (Plate 88) Anatomic example of a flail posterior leaflet with ruptured chord. On the right of the picture, closeup view of the ruptured chord. Otherwise the left atrium is enlarged and the valvular tissue normal. (Courtesy of Dr. W. D. Edwards.)

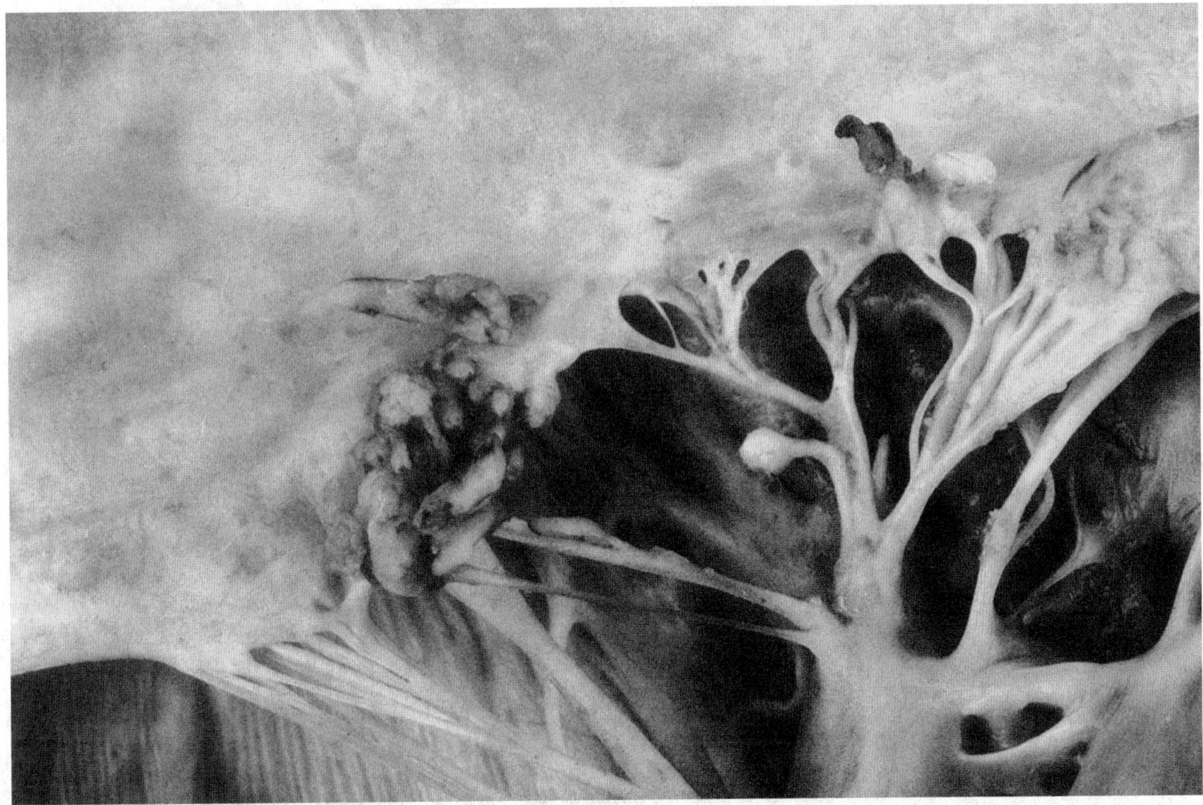

FIGURE 57-10 (Plate 89) Anatomic example of MR due to endocarditis. Note the vegetations of the anterior leaflet and the ruptured chords. (Courtesy of Dr. W. D. Edwards.)

papillary muscle produces MR because of the flail leaflet and involves in 80 percent of cases the posteromedial papillary muscle and is most often associated with infarction of the adjacent ventricular wall.[53] It is the rarest form of heart rupture and of ischemic MR. Complete rupture is rapidly fatal without surgery, and partial or single-head rupture of the papillary muscle more often allows emergency surgery[53] (Fig. 57-11, Plate 90).

OTHER CAUSES OF MITRAL REGURGITATION

MR is observed very frequently with color-flow imaging, even in patients without cardiac disease. However, clinically significant MR may be found in (1) *connective tissue disorder,* Marfan syndrome, Ehlers-Danlos syndrome, pseudoxanthum elasticum, osteogenesis imperfecta, Hurler's disease, systemic lupus erythematosus, and anticardiolipin syndrome; (2) penetrating or nonpenetrating *cardiac trauma;* (3) *myocardial disease*—hypertrophic cardiomyopathy or sarcoidosis; (4) *endocardial lesions* due to hypereosinophilic syndrome, endocardial fibroelastosis, carcinoid tumors, ergot toxicity, radiation toxicity, diet or drug toxicity[54]; (5) *congenital* lesions such as cleft mitral valve isolated or associated with persistent atrioventricular canal, corrected transposition with or without Ebstein's abnormality of the left atrioventricular valve, and (6) *cardiac tumors.*

Pathophysiology

The abnormal coaptation of the mitral leaflets creates a *regurgitant orifice* during systole. The systolic pressure gradient between the LV and LA is the driving force of the regurgitant flow, which results in a *regurgitant volume.* This regurgitant volume represents a percentage of the total ejection of the LV and may be expressed as the *regurgitant fraction.* The regurgitant volume creates a volume overload by entering the LA in systole and the LV in diastole, modifying LV loading and function.

CHRONOLOGY OF REGURGITATION

The pressure gradient between the LV and atrium begins with mitral closure (simultaneous to S_1) and persists after closure of the aortic valve (S_2) until the mitral valve opens.[55] Thus, timing of regurgitant flow is determined by that of the regurgitant orifice and is most often holosystolic. Various dynamic changes in the regurgitant orifice can be observed depending on its cause.[56] With small regurgitant orifices, the regurgitant orifice declines with the ventricular volume tending to limit regurgitation to early systole.[55] Conversely, in valve prolapse, the regurgitant orifice appears or increases late in systole and variations of regurgitant flow throughout systole are the complex results of combined effects of changes of regurgitant orifice and gradient.[56,57]

DEGREE AND CONSEQUENCES OF REGURGITATION

The degree of volume overload depends on three factors, the area of the regurgitant orifice,[58] the regurgitant gradient, and the regurgitant duration. The volume overload is usually less severe in mitral than in aortic regurgitation, despite a usually

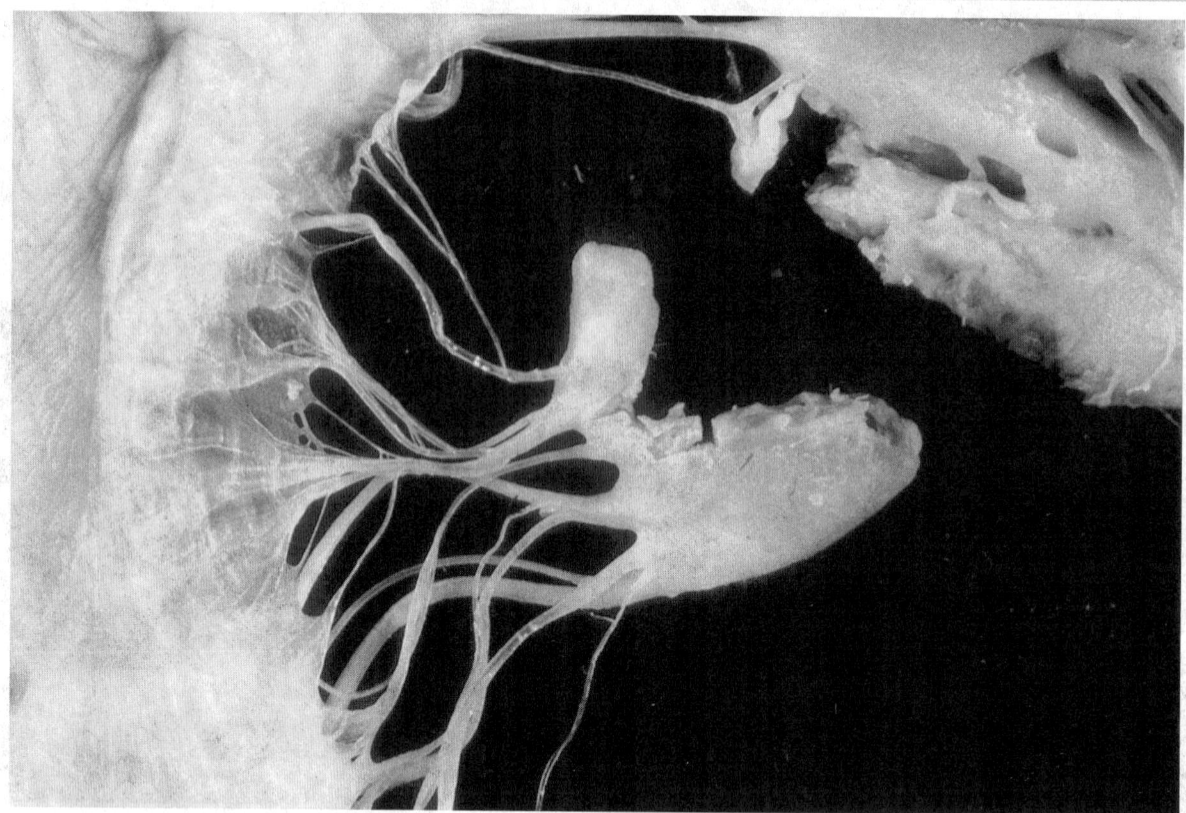

FIGURE 57-11 (Plate 90) Anatomic example of a ruptured posterior papillary muscle. Note the normal valvular tissue otherwise. (Courtesy of Dr. W. D. Edwards.)

larger regurgitant gradient and orifice.[58] Such differences are related to a shorter duration of MR during the cardiac cycle in mitral than in aortic regurgitation.[58]

The degree of MR is not fixed and may vary with interventions. Vasodilators may be beneficial,[59] but the change in regurgitant orifice area rather than that of ventriculoatrial gradient is the main mechanism of this effect. In functional[60] and organic MR,[61] the regurgitant orifice increases with increased afterload or ventricular volume and decreases with decreased afterload or improved contractility, but it is not influenced by changes in heart rate.[61]

The regurgitant energy produced by the LV translates into two components: the kinetic energy (regurgitant volume) and the potential energy (elevation of atrial pressure). The typical left atrial pressure change is the V wave,[62] which nevertheless, is not specific for MR. The height of the V wave and more generally left atrial pressure is mainly determined by left atrial compliance.[62] In acute MR, the LA is less compliant than in chronic MR and the MR produces a marked increase in LA pressure. The atrial V wave, in turn, decreases the ventriculoatrial gradient and, thus, for any effective regurgitant orifice,[58] tends to limit the regurgitant volume. When MR becomes chronic, the LA dilates, the V wave is less prominent, and it does not limit the regurgitant volume; the LA pressure may be normal even with severe MR.[63] At that stage, usually the cardiac output is decreased but the pulmonary pressures are often normal. Pulmonary hypertension in MR is poorly understood and mostly observed in elderly patients.

LEFT VENTRICULAR FUNCTION

With MR the LV is dilated, but less so than in aortic regurgitation of comparable degree.[64] LV end-diastolic volume and wall stress are increased,[64] and the ventricle's shape becomes spherical. End-systolic volume is increased in chronic MR but end-systolic wall stress is usually normal.[65] The myocardial mass is increased proportionately to LV dilatation.[66]

LV function is difficult to characterize because of the changes in preload and afterload. It has been suggested that normalization of ejection fraction (EF) to the preload would provide an appropriate assessment of LV function. Afterload is more difficult to assess because the MR may decrease the instantaneous impedance to ejection, but the measure of afterload provided by end-systolic wall stress is within the normal range.[65] However the usual inverse correlation between end-systolic wall stress and EF is also observed in MR.[67] Complex indices using the afterload—such as the end systolic wall stress,[68] or maximum elastance,[65] normalized to the LV volume—have been proposed and may be sensitive to subtle changes in function.

LV dysfunction is a frequent and dismal complication of MR.[69,70] The mechanism of LV hypertrophy is a reduction in protein degradation, but the mechanisms leading to interstitial fibrosis and LV dysfunction remain mysterious. Experimentally, LV dysfunction is not due to changes in coronary blood flow. The changes in myofiber contractility parallel those in LV function[71] and are associated with reduced myofiber content,[72] but the cause of the myofiber dysfunction and the explanation of its high incidence have not been clarified.

During diastole, LV relaxation is prolonged but chamber stiffness is reduced.[73] Age and decreased systolic function[73] are associated with increased chamber stiffness. The significance of the diastolic abnormalities is unclear.

ISCHEMIC AND FUNCTIONAL MITRAL REGURGITATION

The pathophysiology of ruptured papillary muscles is poorly known. In chronic ischemic or functional MR, the primary disease involves the LV, which is often contracting poorly. However, MR may be determined more by localized LV deformation than by the systolic function. The apical and inferior traction on papillary muscles leads to leaflet tethering and tenting and subsequently to MR.[74,75] In ischemic or functional as opposed to organic (due to primary valvular disease) MR, the regurgitant volume is usually small,[76] and the LV and atrial dilatation is in excess to the degree of MR.[58] Nevertheless, MR is associated with elevated left atrial pressure[58] and poor outcome[77]; it is also a marker of sensitivity to vasodilators.

HORMONAL ACTIVATION

In organic MR, natriuretic peptides are elevated in experimental[78] and clinical[79] studies. The main determinant of elevation of atrial natriuretic peptide is the elevation of atrial pressures.[79] In our experience, brain natriuretic peptide is more a marker of LV remodeling than of altered hemodynamics. The value of natriuretic peptide levels as markers of hemodynamics, LV function, and prognosis is not established yet.

The activation of the renin-angiotensin system is not fully understood. In dogs with organic MR, systemic activation of the renin-angiotensin system is rare,[80] but tissue levels of angiotensin II are markedly elevated.[81,82] The role of angiotensin in the development of hypertrophy and fibrosis are not fully clarified.

Clinical Presentation

The sex distribution has changed in parallel to the changes in etiology of MR. With the decrease in rheumatic heart disease, severe MR is now predominantly seen in males (65 to 75 percent). The prevalence of MR increases with age[83]; therefore, patients with severe MR most often present in the sixth decade of life.[84]

The clinical presentation—including symptoms, physical findings, electrocardiographic and radiographic change—is determined by the degree, rapidity of development, and cause of MR and by LA and LV function and compliance.

SYMPTOMS

Patients with mild MR usually have no symptoms. Severe MR is diagnosed most often because of the murmur when no or minimal symptoms are present.[84] Fatigue and mild dyspnea on exertion are the most usual symptoms and are rapidly improved by rest. The administration of diuretics and progressive self-limitation of physical activity may prevent the occurrence of more severe symptoms. Severe dyspnea on exertion or, more rarely, paroxysmal nocturnal dyspnea, frank pulmonary edema, or even hemoptysis may be observed later in the course of the disease. Such severe symptoms may be triggered by a new onset of atrial fibrillation, or increase in degree of MR, the occurrence of endocarditis or ruptured chordae, or a change in LV compliance or function.

With severe MR of *acute onset,* symptoms are usually more dramatic—pulmonary edema or congestive heart failure—but will progressively subside with administration of diuretic and increased LA compliance. A syndrome of sudden onset of atypical chest pain and dyspnea may occur with abrupt chordal rupture. Rupture of papillary muscle usually has a dramatic presentation, with cardiogenic shock or a severe pulmonary edema. Pulmonary edema may also be observed in transient severe papillary muscle dysfunction.

Sudden death as the initial presentation of MR is rare.[85]

PHYSICAL EXAMINATION

Blood pressure is usually normal. Carotid upstroke is brisk.

Cardiac palpation may show laterally displaced, diffuse, and brief apical impulse with enlarged LV. An apical thrill is characteristic of severe MR. The left sternal border lift is observed with right ventricular dilatation and may be difficult to distinguish from the left atrial lift due to the dilated, expansive LA, which is more substernal and lower.

S_1 is included in the murmur and is usually normal but may be increased in rheumatic disease. S_2 is usually normal but may be paradoxically split if the LV ejection time is markedly shortened. The presence of a third heart sound (S_3) is directly related to the volume of the regurgitation in patients with organic MR.[86] It is often associated with an early diastolic rumble due to the increased mitral flow in diastole even without mitral stenosis (Chap. 10). The S_3 and diastolic rumble are low-pitched sounds and may be difficult to detect without careful auscultation in the left lateral decubitus position. The S_3 increases with expiration. In ischemic-functional MR, S_3 corresponds more often to restrictive LV filling. An atrial gallop (S_4) is heard mainly in MR of recent onset and in ischemic/functional MR in sinus rhythm. Midsystolic clicks are markers of valve prolapse (Chaps. 10 and 11).

The hallmark of MR is the systolic murmur, most often holosystolic, including first and second heart sounds. If an opening snap or S_3 is mistakenly interpreted as S_2, the murmur may appear midsystolic. Only a careful examination beginning at the base of the heart to identify the second heart sound and progressing toward the apex will allow clear recognition of the nature of the murmur. The murmur is of the blowing type but may be harsh, especially in valve prolapse. The maximum intensity is usually at the apex, and it may radiate to the axilla in rheumatic or anterior leaflet prolapse, affecting primarily the anterior leaflet. In posterior leaflet prolapse, the jet is usually superiorly and medially directed and the murmur radiates towards the base of the heart.[87] The murmur may be heard in the back, in the neck, and sometimes on the skull. In the cases where the murmur radiates to the base, it may be difficult to distinguish from the murmur of aortic stenosis or obstructive cardiomyopathy, and pharmacologic maneuvers showing that the murmur decreases with amyl nitrite and increases with methoxamine strongly suggest MR. Murmur intensity does not increase with postextrasystolic beats and usually parallels the degree of MR,[88] but in myocardial infarction severe MR may be totally silent[89] (see Chap. 10).

Murmurs of shorter duration usually correspond to mild MR; they may be mid or late systolic in mitral valve prolapse or early systolic in functional MR.

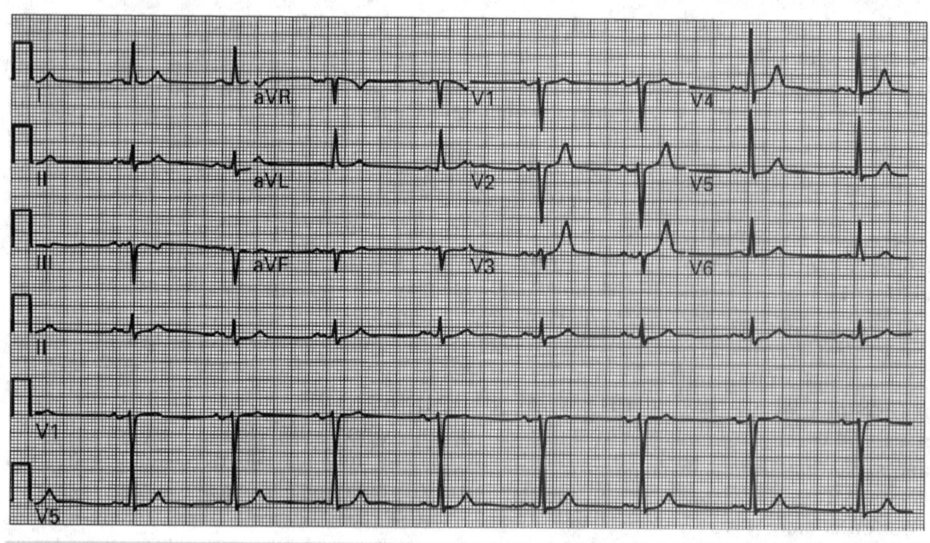

FIGURE 57-12 Electrocardiogram of a patient with severe MR. Note LA enlargement, as indicated by notched p waves (lead I and rhythm strip lead II).

ELECTROCARDIOGRAM

The most frequent feature of MR is atrial fibrillation which was found in approximately 50 to 60 percent of earlier series and is now present in approximately 50 percent of surgically corrected MR.[90] Patients in sinus rhythm may present with signs of left atrial enlargement (Fig. 57-12). LV hypertrophy is more rarely seen and may be associated with secondary ST-T abnormalities.[91] Right ventricular hypertrophy is uncommon. The electrocardiogram, especially in acute MR, may be entirely normal. In ischemic MR, Q waves in the inferior leads or left bundle-branch block is often noted.

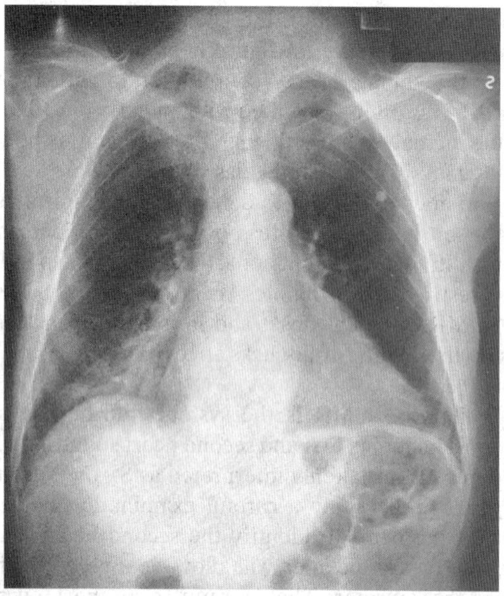

FIGURE 57-13 Chest roentgenogram of a patient with severe MR. Note the cardiomegaly and enlargement of the LA body and appendage.

CHEST ROENTGENOGRAM

Cardiomegaly may be present in chronic MR or in ischemic/functional MR (Fig. 57-13). LA body and appendage dilatation is frequent but giant LA is rare and is usually seen in severe mixed valve disease. Although valvular calcifications are rare, annular calcification seen as a C-shaped density below the posterior leaflet is frequent. Because LA pressure is frequently normal even with severe MR, signs of pulmonary hypertension or pulmonary edema are rarely observed.

CLINICAL SYNDROMES

The clinical presentation of patients with MR can be schematically separated in four syndromes, summarized in Table 57-12.

Laboratory Tests

DOPPLER ECHOCARDIOGRAPHY

Doppler echocardiography has an important role in the assessment of MR using two-dimensional echocardiography with directed M-mode measurements, color-flow imaging, pulsed and continuous-wave Doppler, and transesophageal echocardiography (TEE). Quantitative measurements of flow and detailed hemodynamic assessment should be routinely performed. The goals of Doppler echocardiography are (1) to assess the mor-

TABLE 57-12 Mitral Regurgitation: Clinical Presentations

	MVP Syndrome	Chronic MR	Acute MR	Ischemic/Functional MR
Symptoms	Chest pain	Fatigue	Pulmonary edema	CHF
Physical examination	Midsystolic click, murmur	Loud murmur S_3	Loud murmur S_4	Soft murmur S_3, S_4
Electrocardiogram	ST-T changes	Atrial fibrillation	Normal	Q waves, left bundle-branch block
Chest x-ray	Pectus excavatum	Cardiomegaly	Normal heart size, pulmonary edema	Cardiomegaly, pulmonary edema

phology of the mitral valve (etiology and mechanism), (2) to assess the degree of MR, and (3) to assess ventricular and atrial function (see also Chap. 13).

Morphology The features of the most common causes are indicated below.

Rheumatic MR is characterized by thickening of the leaflets and chordae. The posterior leaflet has reduced mobility whereas the anterior leaflet may be doming if commissural fusion is associated. A valvular prolapse is usually not present unless a ruptured chordae or active rheumatic carditis are present. Similar lesions are observed in lupus or anticardiolipin syndrome, in which transesophageal echocardiography may also show small vegetations.

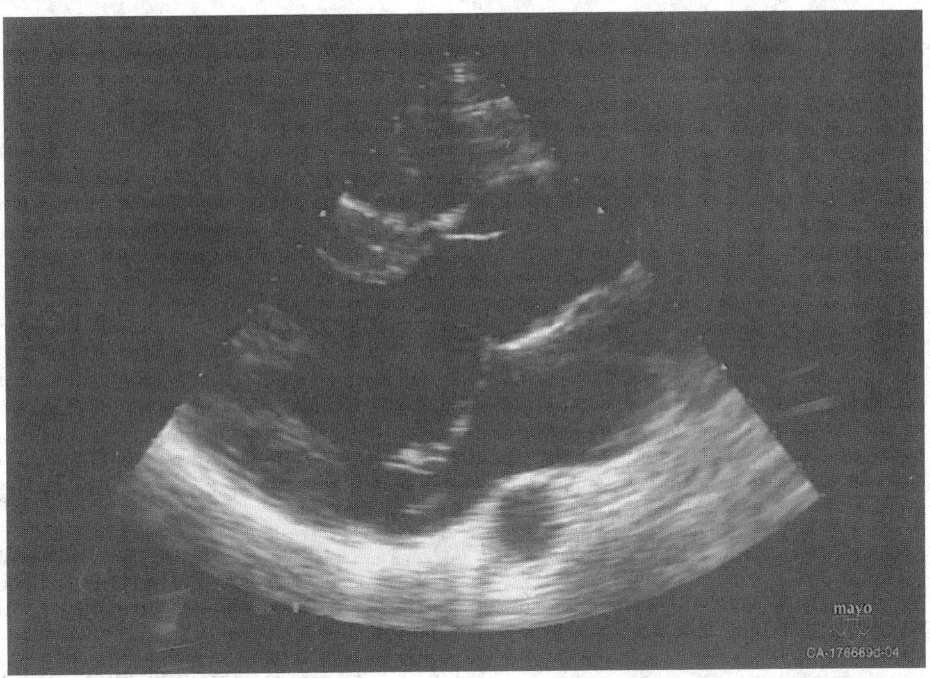

FIGURE 57-14 Echocardiogram of a bileaflet mitral valve prolapse seen from the parasternal long-axis view.

In *degenerative MR,* prolapse is observed with the passage of valvular tissue beyond the annulus plane in the long-axis view (Fig. 57-14). Some features are important:

- Myxomatous changes with diffusely thickened leaflets and excessive valvular tissue
- Localization of the leaflet involved (most often the posterior) confirmed by the initial direction of the jet
- The presence of mitral annular calcification, which may represent a limitation for conservative surgery if extensive and severe
- Flail segments appearing as complete eversion of the segment with or without the small floating echo of ruptured chordae[92] (Fig. 57-15)

The usual mechanism in endocarditic MR, flail leaflets, is relatively easy to diagnose.[92] Perforations are more difficult to diagnose. Mitral annular abscesses are rare and are best detected by TEE. Vegetations can be seen on leaflets or on ruptured chords with superior sensitivity by TEE.[93]

In ischemic/functional MR, the finding of a dilated annulus[94,95] is nonspecific[76] and annular descent is reduced. The features of ischemic heart disease may be observed as regional wall motion abnormalities.[94] The leaflet tissue is normal. The mitral tenting due to the abnormal traction by the principal chordae on the anterior leaflet reduces the area of coaptation of the two leaflets and therefore allows for a central jet of MR.[94,95]

With papillary muscle rupture,[53] MR is due to the flail leaflet. The diagnosis is based on visualization of a small mass of muscle attached to chordae and floating freely during the cardiac cycle.

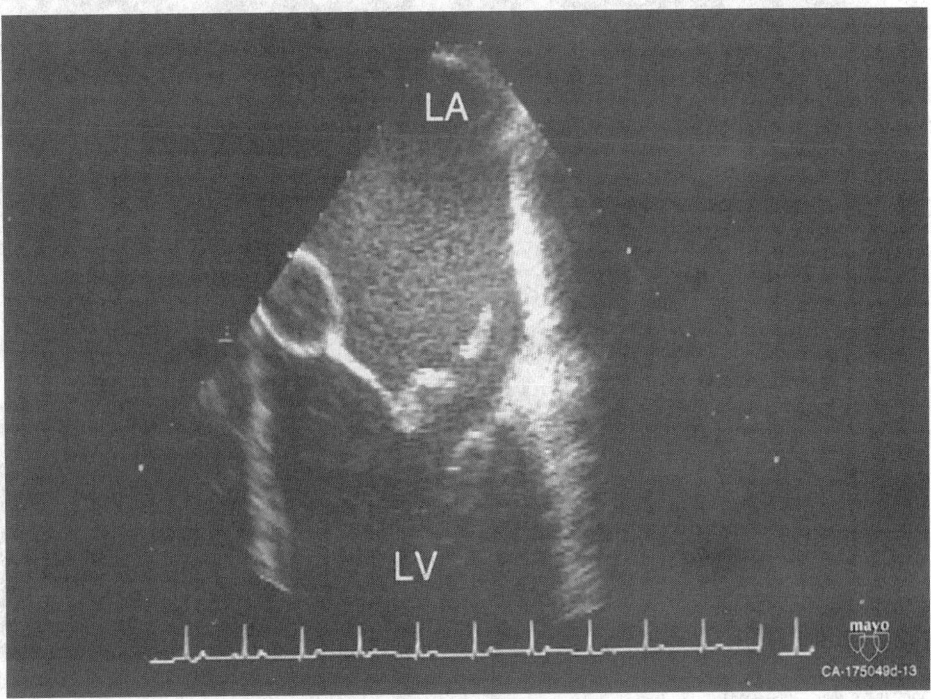

FIGURE 57-15 Transesophageal echocardiography (*horizontal plane*) of a flail anterior leaflet. The ruptured chord is seen at the tip of the anterior leaflet.

TABLE 57-13 Assessment of Severity of Mitral Regurgitation

Clinical		
Systolic thrill		
Murmur intensity		
S_3		
Diastolic rumble		
Laboratory		
Qualitative		
Large jet ≥8 cm² (echo-Doppler)		
Pulmonary vein reversal (Doppler, angiography)		
Dense contrast in LA (angiography)		
Quantitative		
	Criteria:	Regurgitant volume ≥60 mL
		Regurgitant fraction ≥50%
		Effective regurgitant orifice ≥40 mm²
	Method:	Doppler echocardiography
		Quantitative Doppler
		Quantitative 2D echo
		Amplitude weighted mean velocity
		Proximal isovelocity surface area (PISA)
		Radionuclide angiography
		Quantitative LV angiography

Assessment of Severity of Regurgitation (Table 57-13)

SEMIQUANTITATIVE METHODS COLOR-FLOW IMAGING JET ANALYSIS The origin and direction of the jet is related to etiology. Jet length and ratio of jet to left atrial area (or more simply jet area)[96] have been suggested as good indices of MR severity. Small jets consistently correspond to mild MR.[76] However, color-flow imaging has significant limitations, intrinsically related to the nature of regurgitant jets (Chap. 13). The extent of a jet is determined by its momentum and thus as much by regurgitant velocity as by regurgitant flow. Also, jets are constrained by the LA and expand more in large LAs.[76] The eccentric jets of valve prolapse[97] impinge on the LA wall and tend to underestimate MR[76] (Fig. 57-16, Plate 91). Central jets of functional MR expand markedly in the enlarged LA, and this tends to overestimate MR[76] (Fig. 57-17, Plate 92). TEE usually shows larger jets but does not suppress these limitations of color-flow imaging (Chap. 13).

VENA CONTRACTA MEASUREMENT The vena contracta is the region of the regurgitant flow immediately below the flow convergence through the regurgitant orifice.[98] Therefore, direct measurement of vena contracta width provides an index of the regurgitant orifice area. The vena contracta width appears superior to jet measurements and can be obtained either through transesophageal[98] or transthoracic echocardiography.[99]

The *pulmonary venous velocity profile* is useful to assess the degree of MR.[100] Systolic reversal in pulmonary veins is a strong argument for severe MR but is related not only to MR severity but also to jet direction and LA pressure.[101] Consequently, pul-

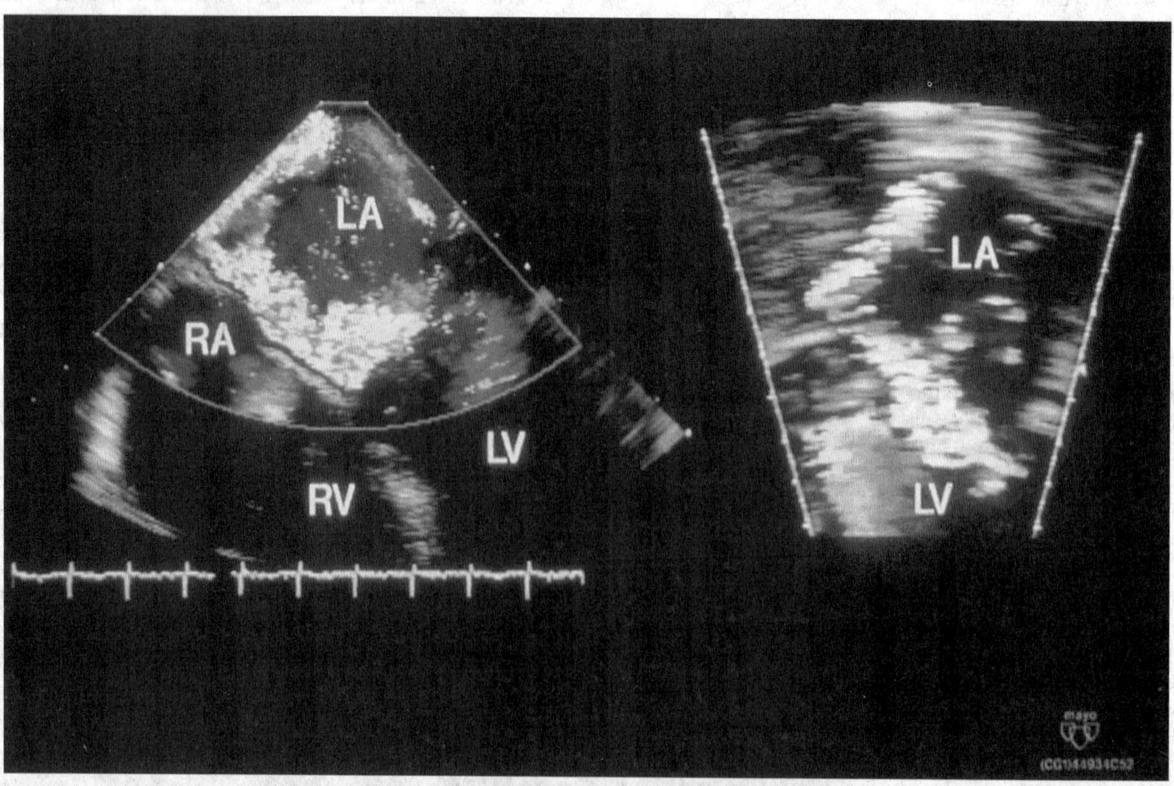

FIGURE 57-16 (Plate 91) Color-flow imaging of an eccentric jet (flail posterior leaflet). *Left:* Transesophageal (*horizontal plane*) echocardiography. *Right:* Transthoracic echocardiography. Note that with both modalities the jet is thinned, impinging on the atrial wall and tending to underestimate this severe regurgitation.

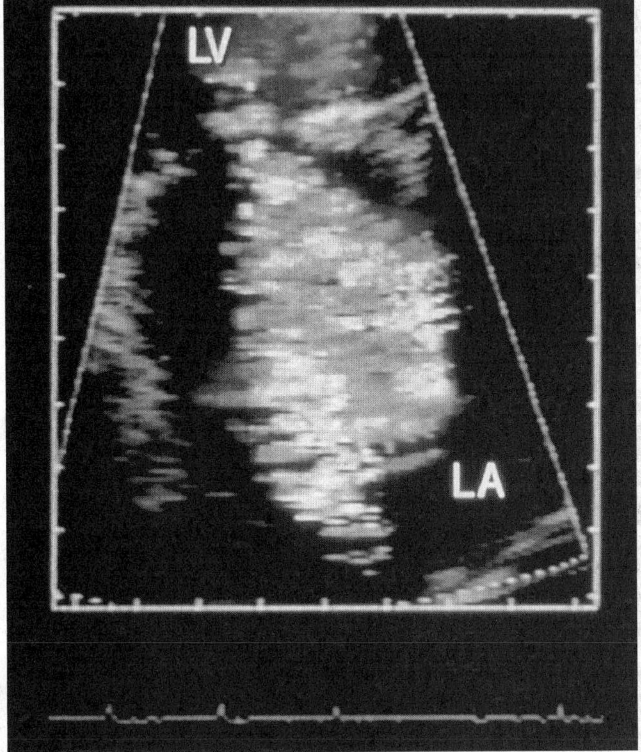

FIGURE 57-17 (Plate 92) Color flow imaging of a central jet of a functional mitral regurgitation by transthoracic echocardiography. Note that the jet is free, expands in the left atrium, and tends to overestimate this moderate regurgitation.

monary venous reversal may be absent or asymmetric in severe MR[101] (Fig. 57-18).

QUANTITATIVE METHODS *The goal* of quantitative methods is to measure the volume overload expressed as the regurgitant volume (difference between the total and forward stroke volume) or fraction (proportion of LV ejection volume regurgitated in the LA). The lesion's severity is expressed as the effective regurgitant orifice (ERO) area and calculated as follows[58,102]: ERO = regurgitant flow/regurgitant velocity or ERO = regurgitant volume/regurgitant TVI, where the TVI is the time velocity integral of the regurgitant jet.

The *practical* quantitation of MR can be performed using various methods:

- *Quantitative Doppler* is based on the calculation of the mitral and aortic stroke volumes using pulsed-wave Doppler.[103] The principle is simple and applicable in most cases, but the measurement of the mitral stroke volume is technically demanding, with a significant learning phase.[103]
- *Quantitative two-dimensional echocardiography* is of similar principle but is based on measurement of LV volumes for total stroke volume calculation.[104]
- The *proximal isovelocity surface area* (PISA) method, conversely, directly measures regurgitant flow by analyzing the flow convergence proximal to the regurgitant orifice (Fig. 57-19, Plate 93) and is based on the principle of conservation of mass. Because color-flow mapping allows precise determination of velocity in the flow-convergence region, the regurgitant flow can be calculated. Using regurgitant flow and velocity, regurgitant orifice and volume can be calculated.[102] This method is simple and accurate if the assumptions are respected. (See also Chap. 13.)

Assessment of Left Ventricular and Atrial Function The technique of guided M-mode diameters is used for assessment of LV size, mass, and wall stress.[90,105,106] LV volumes can be reliably measured by two-dimensional echocardiography. The EF can be calculated or estimated. M-mode diameter or volume can assess the LA size by two-dimensional echocardiography.

RADIONUCLIDE STUDIES

Radionuclide angiography can be used to estimate the LV end-diastolic and end-systolic volume as well as the right and LV EF. The detection of exercise-induced LV dysfunction is frequent. However the significance of such measurement on the long-term prognosis has not been analyzed in large series of patients. A comparison of the counts measured over the RV and LV allows the calculation of the regurgitant fraction.

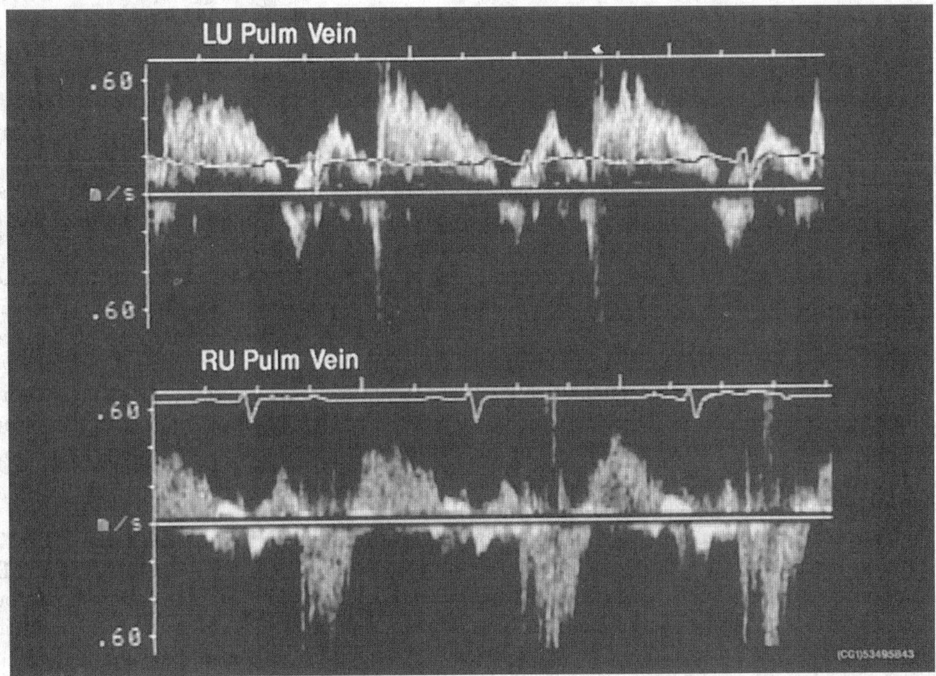

FIGURE 57-18 Pulmonary venous flow of a patient with MR due to a flail posterior leaflet (by transesophageal echocardiography). Note that the flow is asymmetrical, with preserved systolic flow in the left upper pulmonary vein and systolic reversal in the right upper pulmonary vein.

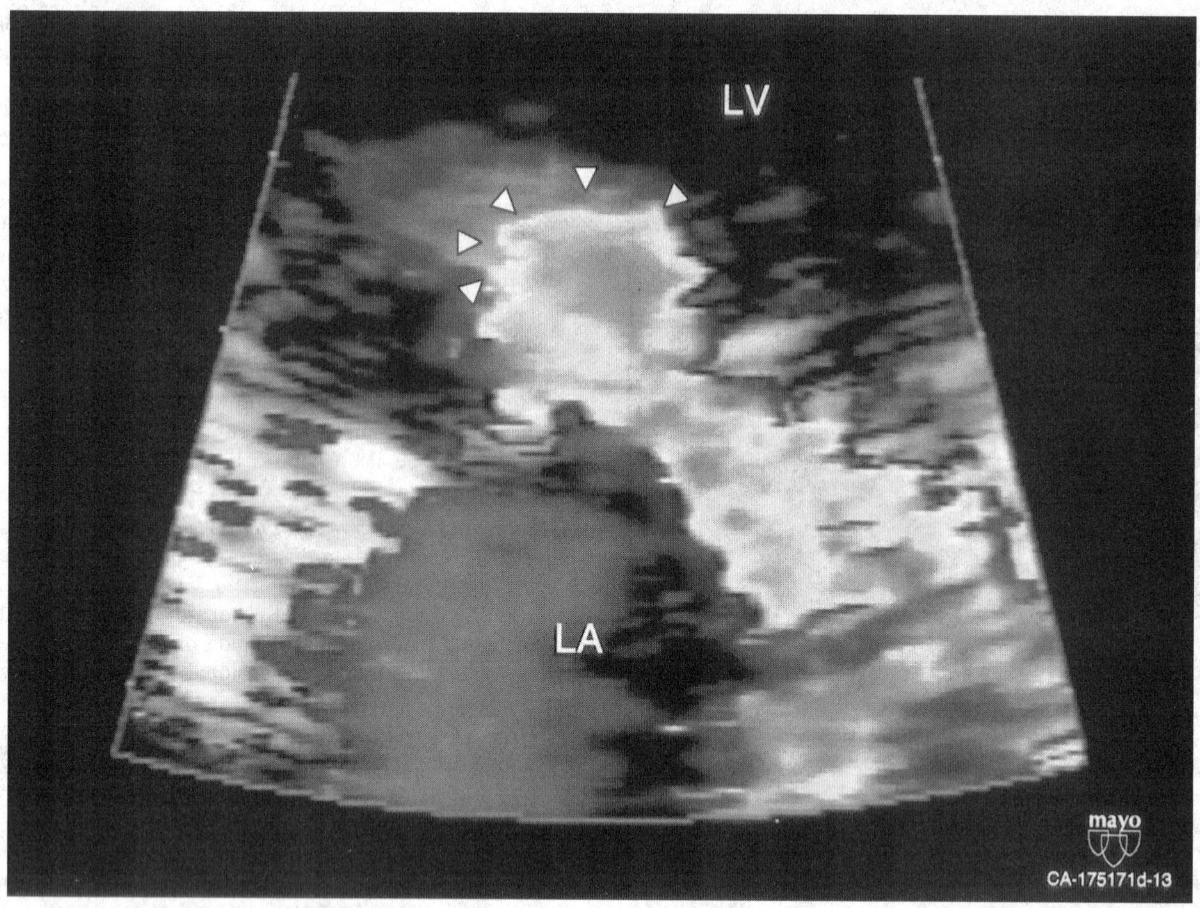

FIGURE 57-19 (Plate 93) Color flow imaging of the proximal flow convergence of a mitral regurgitation due to a flail posterior leaflet (by transthoracic echocardiography). The downward baseline shift of the color-flow scale enlarges the size of the flow convergence, which is easily measurable.

CARDIAC CATHETERIZATION

Cardiac catheterization is utilized to assess hemodynamic status, the severity of MR, LV function, and coronary anatomy.

The major hemodynamic consequences of MR are reduction of cardiac output and elevation of pulmonary artery wedge pressure. Marked pulmonary hypertension is rarely present. The large V wave of the pulmonary wedge pressure is more frequent in acute than in chronic MR but can be observed in other disease such as ventricular septal defect or heart failure with reduced left atrial compliance without MR (Fig. 57-20).

The assessment of MR degree can be obtained by LV selective angiography and can be qualitatively graded in three or four grades on the basis of the degree and persistence of opacification of the LA.[107] Although time-honored, this method has limitations, like all qualitative methods.[108] Quantitation of MR can be obtained by comparing the angiographic stroke volume to the forward stroke volume, calculated by the Fick or thermodilution methods,[109] to calculate the regurgitant volume and fraction. The angiographic stroke volume usually overestimates the true stroke volume and corrections have been used to minimize the overestimation of the regurgitant volume. Subtraction of two stroke volumes introduces a potentially high range of error, which cannot be verified by combined methods or by repeating the measurements; therefore this method is rarely utilized.

The assessment of LV function can be performed using quantitative angiography. LV volumes correlate strongly to the regurgitant volume, duration and etiology of MR, and LV function. The most frequently utilized indices of LV function are end-systolic volume and EF, which are useful prognostic indices.[70,110] High-fidelity pressure recording with LV angiography allows calculation of more complex indices of LV distensibility in diastole[73] and of wall stress, maximum LV elastance, and LV systolic stiffness. The additional value of these complex measurements has been investigated in small groups of patients and remains to be defined in larger populations.

Selective coronary angiography allows definition of coronary anatomy. Obstructive coronary atherosclerosis continues to be frequent even in the absence of angina,[111] and coronary angiography is ordinarily performed in patients more than 40 to 50 years of age.

STRATEGY OF UTILIZATION OF LABORATORY TESTING

Not all the tests should be performed in all patients[112] (Fig. 57-21). Because transthoracic Doppler echocardiography confirms the diagnosis and degree of MR and of associated valvular diseases and provides a unique assessment of mitral lesions, it is performed in most cases for the initial diagnostic assessment, for follow-up, and for presurgical assessment. TEE provides superior imaging quality, but its incremental value is notable

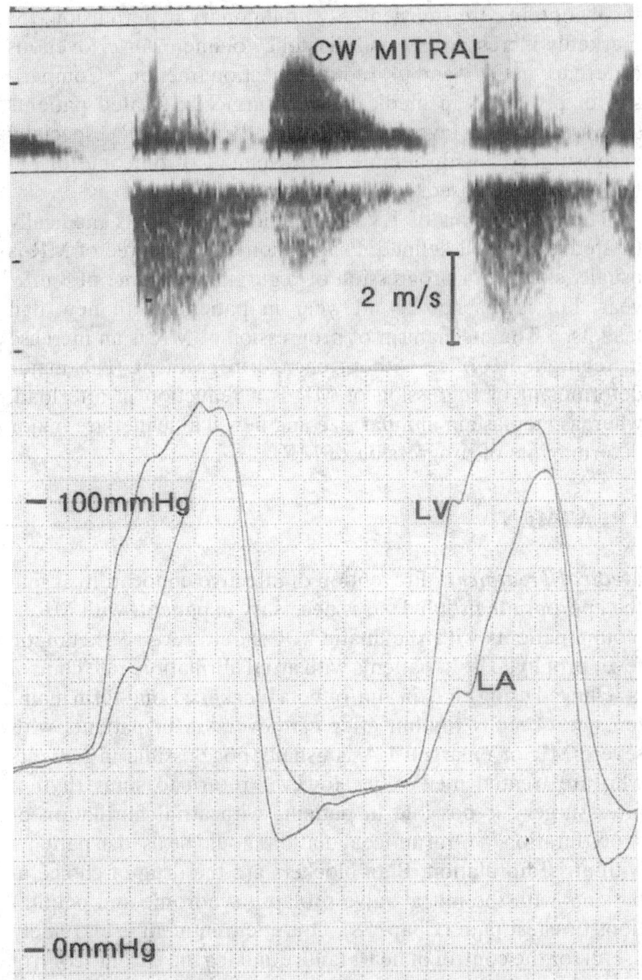

FIGURE 57-20 Simultaneous recording of LV and LA pressures and continuous-wave Doppler (CW) in a patient with severe MR. Note the large V wave on the left atrial pressure recording, with a triangular shape of the mitral regurgitant jet obtained by CW. (Courtesy of Dr. Rick Nishimura, Mayo Clinic.)

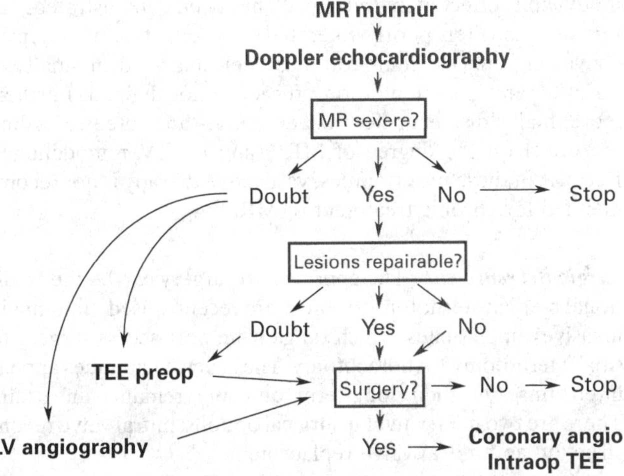

FIGURE 57-21 Strategy of utilization of tests in patients with mitral regurgitation.

only when the transthoracic information is incomplete.[92] In our practice it is reserved preoperatively to the patients in whom a doubt persists regarding the lesions (especially if endocarditis is suspected) or regarding the severity of regurgitation, but it is utilized on a large scale intraoperatively to monitor the results of valve repair.[113]

Coronary angiography is indicated as a presurgical procedure depending on age. LV angiography is not required unless there is concern regarding validity of echocardiographic studies.[114] Although color-flow Doppler showed a significant number of discrepancies as compared to angiography,[115] the understanding of its pitfalls[76] and more recently introduced quantitative methods have reduced the need for redundant tests. Also, the analysis of LV function provided by routine LV angiography does not appear to add significant information to the noninvasive data.[90] However, the utilization of tests should be individualized based on the patient's characteristics and the results of noninvasive studies.

Management

PRINCIPLES

Surgical treatment is reserved for patients with severe MR. Criteria most often used for severe MR are angiographic 4+ grade or color flow jet ≥8 cm^2,[96] with the intrinsic limitations of these definitions. Using quantitative techniques, thresholds for severe MR are 60 mL per beat for regurgitant volume, 50 percent for regurgitant fraction, and 40 mm^2 for effective regurgitant orifice.[116] Patients with severe MR will require surgery at some point during their follow-up. In these patients, the most relevant question is the timing of the surgical indication, which is influenced by the natural history of MR and by the outcome after surgical correction of MR. The determinants of outcome are listed in Table 57-14.

NATURAL HISTORY

Because of the qualitative and imprecise assessment of the degree of MR, the natural history of MR is ill defined. Patients with mild rheumatic MR appear to have a good prognosis,[117] whereas in those with more severe MR a higher mortality has been noted.[84,118] In patients with unoperated clinically significant MR, the late survival has been found as high 60 percent at 10 years[119] or as low as 46 percent[120] or even 27 percent[121] at 5 years. In our experience with flail mitral leaflets, at 10 years, survival was 57 percent, which represents an excess mortality as compared to the expected survival.[84]

The probability of sudden death is important to consider

TABLE 57-14 Determinants of Outcome

Unoperated Patients	Operated Patients
Symptoms	Age
Pulmonary hypertension	Preoperative symptoms
LV end-diastolic volume	Coronary disease
AV-O_2 difference	End-systolic dimensions
Ejection fraction	Ejection fraction
	LA size?
	Valve repair

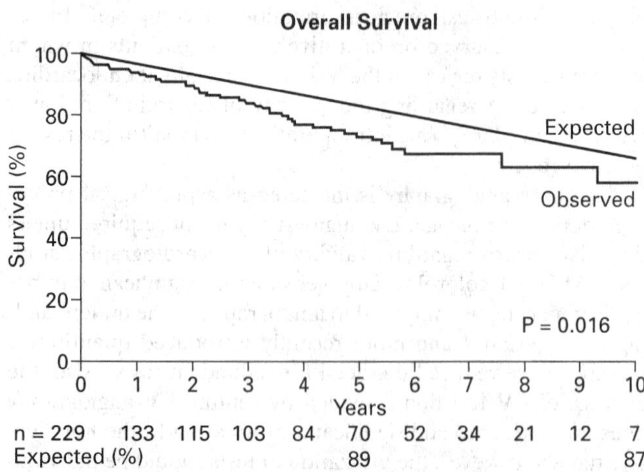

FIGURE 57-22 Survival with medical treatment of patients diagnosed with MR due to flail leaflets. Note the excess mortality in comparison to the expected survival. (Reprinted by permission of the *New England Journal of Medicine* from Ling LH, et al. 1996; 335:1417–1423. Copyright 1996, Massachusetts Medical Society.)

before delaying surgery. Such a devastating complication occurs more often if the ventricular function is decreased[84] but may also occur in patients with normal EF who are asymptomatic.[118] In our experience, sudden death in patients with MR due to flail leaflets occurs at a rate of 1.8 percent per year.[122] The rates are higher in patients with symptoms or reduced ejection fraction, but even in the absence of these risk factors the rate is 0.8 percent per year.[122]

Morbidity in patients with severe MR is also high. Of patients who are initially asymptomatic, approximately 10 percent per year develop symptoms,[123] which may be hastened by atrial fibrillation. In patients with flail leaflets 10 years after diagnosis, heart failure occurred in 63 percent, and permanent atrial fibrillation in 30 percent of those initially in sinus rhythm[84] (Fig. 57-22). Also at 10 years, 90 percent of the patients had either died or undergone surgery,[84] confirming that in these patients surgery is almost unavoidable (Fig. 57-23).

The predictors of poor outcome in patients medically treated are (1) severe symptoms (NYHA classes III to IV),[120] even if

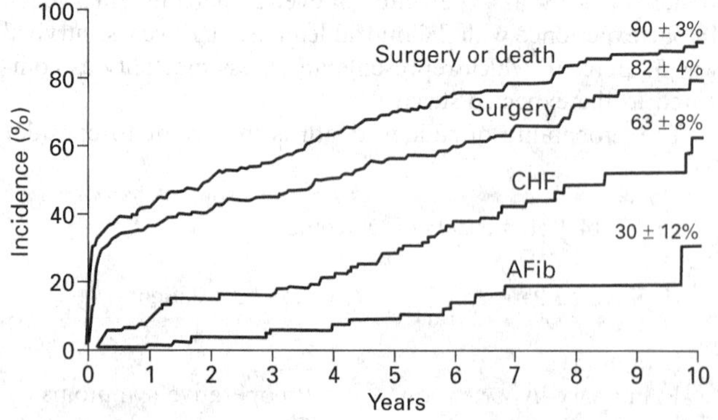

FIGURE 57-23 Cardiac morbidity with medical treatment in patients diagnosed with MR due to flail leaflets. CHF, congestive heart failure, Afib, atrial fibrillation. (Reprinted by permission of the *New England Journal of Medicine* from Ling LH, et al. 1996; 335:1417–1423. Copyright 1996, Massachusetts Medical Society.)

the symptoms are transient,[84] (2) pulmonary hypertension, (3) markedly increased LV end-diastolic volume or arteriovenous difference in O_2,[124] and (4) reduced ejection fraction.[84] Comparison of prognosis in medically and surgically treated patients shows a trend in favor of the surgical treatment,[118] especially early surgery,[84] with definite improvement of outcome of patients with decreased systolic LV function.[124]

The progression of LV dysfunction in patients medically treated is not well defined. Progression of the degree of MR is usually slow, with progression of regurgitant volume of 8 mL/year, but it reaches 20 mL/year in patients with new flail leaflets.[125] The mechanism of progression of MR is an increase in regurgitant orifice without change in gradient. The major determinant of regression of MR is a reduction in afterload, whereas increase in annular size and new flail leaflet are major determinants of progression of MR.[125]

TREATMENT

Medical Treatment Prevention of infective endocarditis using the appropriate prophylaxis is necessary in patients with MR.[126] Young patients with rheumatic MR should receive rheumatic fever prophylaxis. In patients with atrial fibrillation, rate control is achieved using digoxin and/or beta blockers. Long-term maintenance of sinus rhythm after cardioversion in patients with severe MR or enlarged LA is usually not possible in patients who are treated medically. However return to sinus rhythm after surgery is possible in patients with atrial fibrillation of short duration.[127] Oral anticoagulation should be used in patients with atrial fibrillation. Beta blockers are the drug of choice in patients with the mitral valve prolapse syndrome and palpitations or chest pain (Chap. 58). Diuretic treatment is extremely useful for the control of heart failure and for the chronic control of symptoms, especially dyspnea.

Acute afterload reduction may decrease the degree of MR.[59] This effect is achieved by reducing the LV systolic pressure but also by decreasing the effective regurgitant orifice area.[60] Acute utilization of sodium nitroprusside in unstable patients with severe MR, especially in the context of myocardial infarction, may be lifesaving in preparation for surgery.[60]

Chronic afterload reduction is more controversial. The hemodynamic effect of hydralazine,[128] has been demonstrated, but this drug is often poorly tolerated. The effect of angiotensin converting enzyme inhibitors has been analyzed in small series,[129–131] and their long-term efficacy is not defined. Furthermore, major discrepancies between series are noted regarding the effect on the degree of MR[132] and on LV remodeling.[133] Because of these uncertainties, vasoactive therapy is not recommended for chronic treatment of MR.[112]

Surgical Treatment The approach to surgery can be the traditional median sternotomy or the more recently used "minimally invasive" approaches, which range from port-access surgery to small sternotomy to thoracotomy. These new techniques appear interesting but their long-term outcome remains uncertain. There are two main valvular surgical options: mitral valve reconstruction and mitral valve replacement.

MITRAL VALVE RECONSTRUCTION Reconstruction of the incompetent mitral valve is almost always possible (approximately

90 percent of patients referred for primary correction of acquired MR at the Mayo Clinic). The frequency with which valve repair can be used varies with experience of the operating team and the spectrum of underlying valve disease; repair is more often feasible with degenerative valve disease than with rheumatic valvulitis or endocarditis.

The *valvular procedure* is as follows. With leaflet prolapse immobilization of this prolapsing section can be obtained by plicating or by excising it and then repairing the leaflet. This will overcome the problem of localized prolapse. However, the resulting reduction in area of the leaflet could reduce coaptation and induce residual MR; therefore, annuloplasty is a routine part of the repair. Resection or plication of prolapsing sections is most successful with posterior leaflet prolapse. With anterior leaflet prolapse the risk of residual MR is higher if the plication or resection is not combined with subvalvular procedures.[113] Other repairable leaflet abnormalities include congenital clefts and acquired perforation, which may be closed by using a patch of pericardium or synthetic material.

In the *subvalvular procedure,* chordal shortening may be necessary in patients with elongated chordae to ensure the appropriate coaptation of the leaflets, but the durability of this procedure has been criticized.[134] A major recent progress has been the introduction of transposition of chordae and of artificial chordae which have made the anterior leaflet prolapse as repairable as the posterior leaflet prolapse.[135,136]

Annular dilatation, almost constantly associated with MR, is treated by reduction of mitral circumference, i.e., *annuloplasty*. The annuloplasty should be placed in the region supporting the posterior leaflet to preserve the area of anterior leaflet. A cloth-covered rigid ring was originally developed by Carpentier. Recently, flexible annuloplasty rings have been developed to preserve the normal systolic contraction of the mitral annulus.[137] In general, results with the Carpentier ring annuloplasty have been favorable, but LV outflow obstruction associated with abnormal systolic anterior motion of the anterior mitral leaflet has been reported in 6 to 10 percent of patients.[138] This complication is mainly due to hypovolemia and excessive use of inotropes[113] but may be lower with flexible rings.[139]

It is important to assess the adequacy of mitral valve reconstruction before completion of the operation. When satisfactory repair cannot be achieved, it is preferable to replace the valve immediately. To assess adequacy of mitral repair (residual stenosis, regurgitation, or systolic anterior motion), TEE, which does not interfere with the surgical procedure, is performed routinely.[113]

Valve Replacement When mitral reconstruction is considered impossible or is unsuccessful, replacement must be performed. The dilemma is the choice between a mechanical valve of excellent durability but with the hazard of thromboembolism and a biological valve with undefined long-term durability[140] but less tendency to cause thromboembolism. With atrial fibrillation, chronic anticoagulant therapy is necessary even with a bioprosthesis, so that avoiding anticoagulation is not relevant in choosing a prosthesis.

Postoperative Outcome Valve repair, by preserving the normal valvular tissue, is preferable to valve replacement. Compared to prosthetic replacement, mitral valve reconstruction has a lower operative mortality.[141,142] Direct comparison of the results of valve repair and replacement is difficult[142] because the patients undergoing a valve repair are usually at a less advanced stage of the disease than patients undergoing valve replacement.[141] However, survival and LV function after valve repair are better than after insertion of a prosthetic valve.[141] Better ventricular function with valvuloplasty may be due to preservation of chordae and papillary muscles.[143] Durability of valve repair for degenerative disease is excellent if no more than mild residual MR is accepted.[134] Valve repair has the same low rate of reoperation than valve replacement.[141] MR postrepair is due in two-thirds of the cases to new lesions and in one-third to an inadequate primary correction.[144] *Therefore valve repair should be the preferred procedure for surgical correction of MR* (Fig. 57-24).

Operative mortality has been reported between 5 and 12 percent[140] in earlier series, but most patients had prosthetic valve replacement rather than reconstruction. The operative risk is lower in the current era, around 1 to 2 percent in patients younger than 75 years with organic MR operated on at the Mayo Clinic whether they had valve repair or replacement.[90] LV function is not a predictor of operative mortality and patients with organtic MR even with markedly depressed function have a reasonable chance of surviving surgery.[90] Age symptoms and coronary disease are the most important predictors of operative mortality.[90] Some important points should be noted: First,

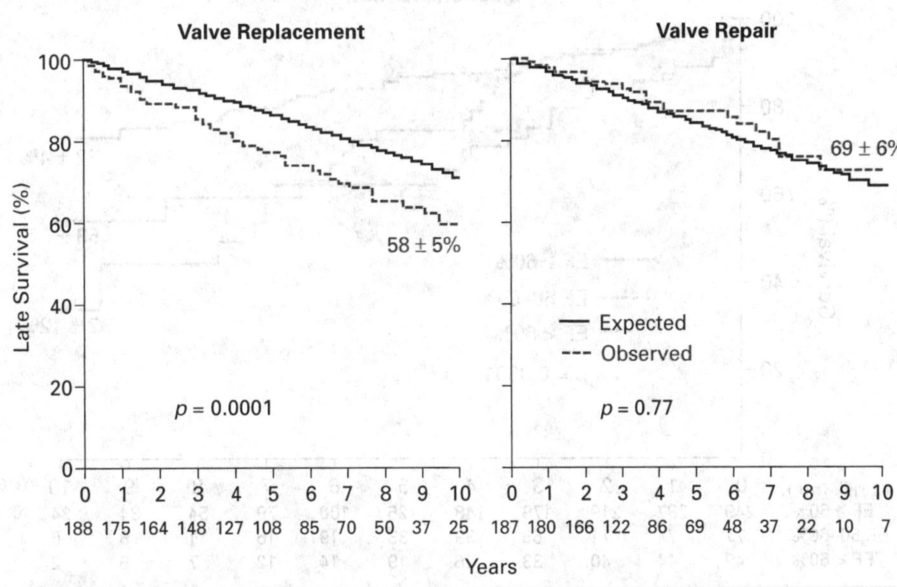

FIGURE 57-24 Late survival after surgical correction of organic MR. Note the excess mortality in comparison to the expected survival after valve replacement (*left*) in contrast to the survival identical to expected after valve repair (*right*). (From Enriquez-Sarano M, Schaff H, Orszulak T, et al. Valve repair improves the outcome of surgery for mitral regurgitation. *Circulation* 1995; 91:1264–1265, with the authorization of the American Heart Association.)

the risk of surgery has become progressively similar in patients 65 to 75 years old as compared to younger patients. Second, operative mortality has decreased recently in patients 75 and older but remains relatively high, around 5 percent. Third, in ischemic MR the operative mortality remains high, around 10 percent.

Postoperative survival has considerably improved and in our recent experience, with a population of mean age 62, the 5- and 10-year survivals were 83 and 68 percent after valve repair and 69 and 52 percent after valve replacement. Remarkably, the survival after valve repair is not different from the expected survival, whereas it represents 77 percent of the expected survival after valve replacement.[141]

A large majority of long-term survivors after mitral valve replacement for MR show a symptomatic improvement by at least one functional class and some become asymptomatic. However, with time postoperative heart failure and symptomatic deterioration tend to occur at a progressively increasing rate (38 percent at 10 years in operative survivors) and is most often (in two thirds of the cases) due to residual LV dysfunction.[145] Valvular or prosthetic dysfunction explain the heart failure in approximately one-third of the cases.[145] Postoperative congestive heart failure has a dismal prognosis and should be prevented as much as possible[145] by early correction of the MR.

The most frequent cause of mortality after surgical correction of MR is LV dysfunction[90] due to chronic irreversible myocardial damage.[66,69,70] LV dysfunction occurs, in our experience in 40 percent of patients overall and 32 percent of those with organic MR.[69] The majority of patients demonstrate a decrease in EF after successful valve replacement.[66,69] This decline may be the result of several factors: cumulative permanent myocardial damage, occasional myocardial insult sustained at the time of operation, diminished preload, and probably increase in impedance to ejection after elimination of the MR. However, the relationships between pre- and postoperative LV function[65,66,69,70,110] and between preoperative LV function and postoperative survival[68,90,105] underline the fact that LV dysfunction is most often already present preoperatively. Because of the modified loading conditions, multiple and complex indices of LV function have been proposed.[65,67,68] Despite these altered loading conditions preoperative EF is an acceptable independent predictor of postoperative EF[66,69,70] and survival.[90] In general, one can estimate that the postoperative EF likely will decrease by approximately 10 percent early after valve replacement.[66,69,70] However, there is a significant individual variation and more decline is observed with markedly increased end-systolic diameter,[69,105] volume,[70,110] or wall stress[69] or in patients with severe symptoms, prolonged duration of MR or coronary disease.[69] A markedly reduced preoperative EF (<50 percent) is associated with a high late mortality,[90] but nevertheless surgery provides a better outcome than medical treatment.[124] Even a "borderline" EF (50 to 60 percent) is associated with an excess late mortality.[90] Therefore, *currently the widely accepted signs of overt LV dysfunction in MR are LV diameter ≥45 mm or ejection fraction <60 percent.*[112] Nevertheless, the end-systolic diameter rarely and belatedly reaches 45 mm and the best outcome of surgery is obtained in patients with both end-systolic diameter <45 mm and ejection fraction ≥60 percent[69,90] (Fig. 57-25).

Another issue, which has been controversial, has been the impact on postoperative outcome of preoperative symptoms. Patients with severe preoperative symptoms, NYHA class III or IV, incur an excess postoperative mortality independently of all baseline characteristics, in particular age, EF, and the type of surgery performed.[146] Importantly, patients preoperatively in class I or II incur a very low operative risk,[146,147] and an excellent long term survival, identical to the expected survival.[146] These data suggest that *in centers and patients at low operative risk, timing of surgery when there are no or minimal symptoms offers distinctive advantages.*

Atrial fibrillation when present preoperatively usually persists postoperatively, unless of brief duration[127] but the excess risk due this arrhythmia appears modest,[90,127] although it requires anticoagulation. Conversely, the association of a Maze procedure to mitral valve repair can be accomplished with minimal risk.[148]

Late risk of thromboembolism after mitral replacement for MR is not different from it as in other mitral valve diseases. Differences in thromboembolic risk after valve repair and valve replacement have been variably estimated[141,142] but appear to favor valve repair. In addition, because following valve repair, anticoagulation is recommended permanently only if atrial

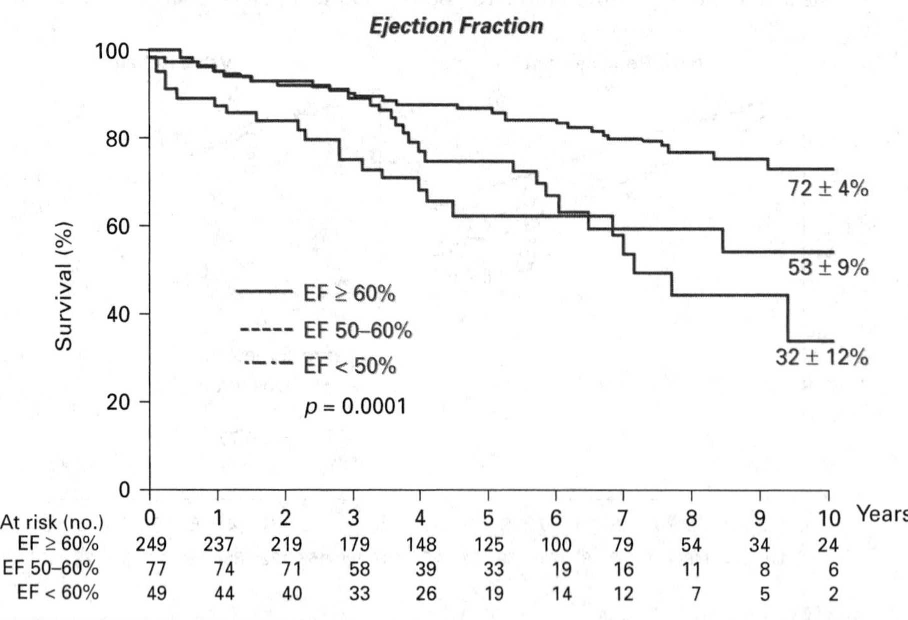

FIGURE 57-25 Survival after surgical correction of organic mitral regurgitation. Note the excess mortality in patients with preoperative ejection fraction above 50 percent but also in patients with preoperative ejection fractions of 50 to 60 percent. (From Enriquez-Sarano M, Tajik A, Schaff H, et al. Echocardiographic prediction of survival after surgical correction of organic mitral regurgitation. *Circulation* 1994; 90:830–837, with the authorization of the American Heart Association.)

fibrillation persists, the occurrence of bleeding is less common than following prosthetic replacement.[141]

Indications for Surgery Based on the most recent data regarding the natural history of MR treated with and without surgery, the indications for surgery have evolved[112] and can be outlined as follows:

TRADITIONAL INDICATIONS Patients with severe symptoms (functional NYHA class III or IV). Patients with transient severe symptoms even if they markedly improve with medical treatment should be considered at high risk and offered surgery within that category.

ADVANCED INDICATIONS These apply to patients with NYHA class II symptoms and to patients with no symptoms (class NYHA I) but with either signs of overt LV dysfunction (LV ejection fraction <60 percent, end-systolic diameter ≥45 mm) or with pulmonary hypertension or with atrial fibrillation.

EARLY INDICATIONS Patients with no symptoms (NYHA class I) and no sign of LV dysfunction (ejection fraction ≥60 percent). These patients can expect the best results of surgery and in particular, after the immediate postoperative phase, a survival identical to the expected survival.[90,146] Therefore, the authors consider surgery to be a reasonable option in this subgroup. However because surgery in these patients is justified neither by symptoms nor by LV dysfunction certain conditions should be fulfilled:

- *Low operative risk:* Both the operative mortality in the institution where such an indication is contemplated and the operative risk for the individual patient involved should be minimal (1 to 2 percent).
- *Reparability:* The valvular lesions as determined by echocardiography should be in all probability repairable and the surgeon performing the intervention should have a high degree of experience with all forms of valve repair.
- *Intraoperative TEE should be performed* by experienced physicians to monitor the repair procedure and help with decisions warranted by an imperfect result.
- *Quantitation of MR should be performed* systematically in these patients preoperatively using multiple noninvasive techniques to determine objectively the degree of MR and affirm that surgery is warranted.

Therefore, despite the considerable progress recently accomplished, currently *not all patients and not all institutions* are candidates for these early indications of surgical correction of MR, but surgery should be considered early in the course of MR when severe MR has been thoroughly documented.

References

1. Waller BE. Rheumatic and nonrheumatic conditions producing valvular heart disease. *Cardiovasc Clin* 1986; 16:3–104.
2. Rahimtoola SH. Valvular heart disease. In: Stein J, ed. *Internal Medicine*, 4th ed. St. Louis: Mosby-Year Book; 1994:202–234.
3. Braunwald E. Valvular heart disease. In: Braunwald E, ed. *Heart Disease*, 4th ed. Philadelphia: Saunders; 1992:1007–1018.
4. Davies JJ. *Pathology of Cardiac Valves*. London: Butterworth; 1980.
5. Fowler NO. Mitral stenosis and left atrial myxoma. In: *Diagnosis of Heart Disease*. New York: Springer-Verlag; 1991:146–159.
6. Osterberger LE, Goldstein S, Khaja F, Lakier JB. Functional mitral stenosis in patients with massive mitral annular calcification. *Circulation* 1981; 64:472–476.
7. Libman E, Sacks B. A hitherto undescribed form of valvular and mitral endocarditis. *Arch Intern Med* 1924; 33:701–737.
8. Galve E, Candell-Riera J, Pigrau C, et al. Prevalence, morphologic types, and evolution of cardiac valvular disease in systemic lupus erythematosus. *N Engl J Med* 1988; 319:817–823.
9. Schoen FJ, St. John Sutton M. Contemporary pathologic considerations in valvular disease. In: Virmani B, Atkinson JB, Feuoglio JJ, eds. *Cardiovascular Pathology*. Philadelphia: Saunders; 1991: 334–353.
10. Kawanishi DT, Rahimtoola SH. Mitral stenosis. In: Rahimtoola SH, ed. *Valvular Heart Disease II*. St. Louis: Mosby; 1996:8.1–8.24.
11. Leavitt JL, Coats MH, Falk RH. Effects of exercise on transmitral gradient and pulmonary artery pressure in patients with mitral stenosis or a prosthetic mitral valve: A Doppler echocardiographic study. *J Am Coll Cardiol* 1991; 17:1520–1526.
12. Selzer A. Effects of atrial fibrillation upon the circulation in patients with mitral stenosis. *Am Heart J* 1960; 59:518–526.
13. Wood P. An appreciation of mitral stenosis: Part 1. Clinical features. *BMJ* 1954; 1:1051–1063. An appreciation of mitral stenosis: Part 2. Investigations and results. *BMJ* 1954; 1:1113–1124.
14. Gash AK, Carabello BA, Cepin D, Spann JE. Left ventricular ejection performance and systolic muscle function in patients with mitral stenosis. *Circulation* 1983; 67:148–154.
15. Colle JP, Rahal S, Ohayon J, et al. Global left ventricular function and regional wall motion in pure mitral stenosis. *Clin Cardiol* 1984; 7:573–580.
16. Gaasch WH, Folland ED. Left ventricular function in rheumatic mitral stenosis. *Eur Heart J* 1991; 12(suppl B):66–69.
17. Harvey RM, Ferrer MI, Samet P, et al. Mechanical and myocardial factors in rheumatic heart disease in mitral stenosis. *Circulation* 1955; 11:531–551.
18. Mohan JC, Khalilullah M, Arora R. Left ventricular intrinsic contractility in pure rheumatic mitral stenosis. *Am J Cardiol* 1989; 64:240–242.
19. Bowe JC, Bland EF, Sprague HB, White PD. The course of mitral stenosis without surgery: 10 and 20 year perspective. *Ann Intern Med* 1960; 52:741–749.
20. Barrington WW, Bashore T, Wooley CE. Mitral stenosis: Mitral dome excursion at M_1 and the mitral opening snap—the concept of reciprocal heart sounds. *Am Heart J* 1988; 115:1280–1290.
21. Melhem RE, Dunbar JD, Booth RW. The "B" lines of Kerley and left atrial size in mitral valve disease: Their correlation with mean atrial pressure as measured by left atrial puncture. *Radiology* 1991; 76:65–69.
22. Reid CL, Chandraratna PAN, Kawanishi DT, et al. Influence of mitral valve morphology on double-balloon catheter balloon valvuloplasty in patients with mitral stenosis: An analysis of factors predicting immediate and 3-month results. *Circulation* 1989; 80:515–524.
23. Gordon PF, Douglas PS, Come PC, Manning WJ. Two-dimensional and Doppler echocardiographic determinants of the natural history of mitral valve narrowing in patients with rheumatic mitral stenosis: Implications for follow-up. *J Am Coll Cardiol* 1992; 19:968–973.
24. Shapiro ML. Echocardiography of the mitral valve. In: Wells PC, Shapiro LN, eds. *Mitral Valve Disease*, 2nd ed. London: Butterworth; 1996:47–50.
25. Khandheria BK, Tajik AJ, Reeder GS, et al. Doppler color flow imaging: A new technique for visualization and characterization of the blood flow jet in mitral stenosis. *Mayo Clin Proc* 1986; 61:623–630.

26. Rahimtoola SH. Perspective on valvular heart disease: An update. *J Am Coll Cardiol* 1989; 14:1–23.
27. Kawanishi DT, Kotlewski A, McKay CR, et al. The relative value of clinical examination, echocardiography with Doppler and cardiac catheterization with angiography in the evaluation of mitral valve disease. In: Bodnar E, ed. *Surgery for Heart Valve Disease.* London: ICR Publishers; 1990:73–78.
28. Olesen KH. The natural history of 271 patients with mitral stenosis under medical treatment. *Br Heart J* 1962; 24:349–357.
29. Roy SB, Gopinath N. Mitral stenosis. *Circulation* 1968; 38(suppl V):68–76.
30. Rowe JC, Bland EF, Sprague HB, White P. The course of mitral stenosis without surgery: Ten- and twenty-year perspectives. *Ann Intern Med* 1960; 52:741–749.
31. Prystowsky EN, Benson W Jr, Fuster V, et al. Management of patients with atrial fibrillation: A statement for healthcare professionals from the Subcommittee on Electrocardiography and Electrophysiology, American Heart Association. *Circulation* 1996; 93:1262–1277.
32. Kulick DL, Reid CL, Kawanishi DT, Rahimtoola SH. Catheter balloon commissurotomy in adults: Part II. Mitral and other stenoses. *Curr Probl Cardiol* 1990; 15:403–470.
33. Hickey MSJ, Blackstone EH, Kirklin JW, Dean LW. Outcome probabilities and life history after surgical mitral commissurotomy: Implications for balloon commissurotomy. *J Am Coll Cardiol* 1991; 17:29–42.
34. Scalia D, Rizzoli G, Campanile F, et al. Long-term results of mitral commissurotomy. *J Thorac Cardiovasc Surg* 1993; 105:633–642.
35. John S, Bashi VV, Jairaj PS, et al. Closed mitral valvotomy: Early results and long-term follow-up of 3724 consecutive patients. *Circulation* 1983; 68:891–896.
36. Crawford MH, Souchek J, Oprian CA, et al. Determinants of survival and left ventricular performance after mitral valve replacement. *Circulation* 1990; 81:1173–1181.
37. Rahimtoola SH. The problem of valve prosthesis—Patient mismatch. *Circulation* 1978; 58:20–24.
38. Turi ZG, Reyes VP, Raju S, et al. Percutaneous balloon versus surgical closed commissurotomy for mitral stenosis: A prospective, randomized trial. *Circulation* 1991; 83:1179–1185.
39. Patel JJ, Shama D, Mitha AS, et al. Balloon valvuloplasty versus closed commissurotomy for pliable mitral stenosis: A prospective hemodynamic study. *J Am Coll Cardiol* 1991; 18:1318–1322.
40. Arora R, Nair M, Kalra GS, et al. Immediate and long-term results of balloon and surgical closed mitral valvotomy: A randomized comparative study. *Am Heart J* 1993; 125:1091–1094.
41. Reyes VP, Raju BS, Wynne J, et al. Percutaneous balloon valvuloplasty compared with open surgical commissurotomy for mitral stenosis. *N Engl J Med* 1994; 331:961–967.
42. NHLBI Valvuloplasty Participants. Multicenter experience with balloon mitral commissurotomy—NHLBI Balloon Valvuloplasty Registry report on immediate and 30-day follow-up results. *Circulation* 1992; 85:448–461.
43. McKay CR, Kawanishi DT, Kotlewski A, et al. Improvement in exercise capacity and exercise hemodynamics 3 months after double-balloon catheter balloon valvuloplasty in the treatment of patients with symptomatic mitral stenosis. *Circulation* 1988; 77:1013–1021.
44. Cohen DJ, Kuntz RE, Gordon SPF, et al. Predictors of long-term outcome after percutaneous balloon mitral valvuloplasty. *N Engl J Med* 1992; 327:1329–1335.
45. Palacios I, Tuzcu ME, Weyman AE, et al. Clinical follow-up of patients undergoing percutaneous mitral balloon valvotomy. *Circulation* 1995; 91:671–676.
46. Dean LS, Mickel M, Bonan R, et al. Four year follow-up of patients undergoing percutaneous balloon mitral commissurotomy: A report from the National Heart, Lung and Blood Institute Balloon Valvuloplasty Registry. *J Am Coll Cardiol* 1996; 28:1452–1457.
47. Orrange SE, Kawanishi DT, Lopez BM, et al. Actuarial outcome after catheter balloon commissurotomy in patients with mitral stenosis. *Circulation* 1997; 95:382–389.
48. Bonow RO, Carabello B, de Leon AC Jr, et al. ACC/AHA Guidelines for the management of patients with valvular heart disease: A report of the American College of Cardiology/American Heart Association Task Force on Practice Guidelines (Committee on Management of Patients With Valvular Heart Disease). *J Am Coll Cardiol* 1998; 32:1486–1588.
49. Lam J, Ranganathan N, Wigle E, Silver M. Morphology of the human mitral valve: I. Chordae tendineae: A new classification. *Circulation* 1970; 41:449–458.
50. Ranganathan N, Lam J, Wigle E, Silver M. Morphology of the human mitral valve: II. The valve leaflets. *Circulation* 1970; 41:459–467.
51. Olson L, Subramanian R, Ackermann D, Orszulak T, Edwards W. Surgical pathology of the mitral valve: A study of 712 cases spanning 21 years. *Mayo Clin Proc* 1987; 62:22–34.
52. Hickey A, Wilcken D, Wright J, Warren B. Primary (spontaneous) chordal rupture: Relation to myxomatous valve disease and mitral valve prolapse. *J Am Coll Cardiol* 1985; 5:1341–1346.
53. Kishon Y, Oh J, Schaff H, Mullany C, Tajik A, Gersh B. Mitral valve operation in postinfarction rupture of a papillary muscle: Immediate results and long-term follow-up of 22 patients. *Mayo Clin Proc* 1992; 67:1023–1030.
54. Connolly H, Crary J, McGoon M, et al. Valvular heart disease associated with fenfluramine-phentermine. *N Engl J Med* 1997; 337:581–588.
55. Yellin E, Yoran C, Sonnenblick E, et al. Dynamic changes in the canine mitral regurgitant orifice area during ventricular ejection. *Circ Res* 1979; 45:677–683.
56. Schwammenthal E, Chen C, Benning F, et al. Dynamics of mitral regurgitant flow and orifice area. Physiologic application of the proximal flow convergence method: Clinical data and experimental testing. *Circulation* 1994; 90:307–322.
57. Enriquez-Sarano M, Sinak L, Tajik A, et al. Changes in effective regurgitant orifice throughout systole in patients with mitral valve prolapse: A clinical study using the proximal isovelocity surface area method. *Circulation* 1995; 92:2951–2958.
58. Enriquez-Sarano M, Seward J, Bailey K, Tajik A. Effective regurgitant orifice area: A noninvasive doppler development of an old hemodynamic concept. *J Am Coll Cardiol* 1994; 23:443–451.
59. Chatterjee K, Parmley W, Swan H, et al. Beneficial effects of vasodilator agents in severe mitral regurgitation due to dysfunction of subvalvular apparatus. *Circulation* 1973; 48:684–690.
60. Keren G, Bier A, Strom J, et al. Dynamics of mitral regurgitation during nitroglycerin therapy: A Doppler echocardiographic study. *Am Heart J* 1986; 112:517–525.
61. Yoran C, Yellin E, Becker R, et al. Dynamic aspects of acute mitral regurgitation: Effects of ventricular volume, pressure and contractility on the effective regurgitant orifice area. *Circulation* 1979; 60:170–176.
62. Grose R, Strain J, Cohen M. Pulmonary arterial V waves in mitral regurgitation: Clinical and experimental observations. *Circulation* 1984; 69:214–222.
63. Braunwald E, Awe W. The syndrome of severe mitral regurgitation with normal left atrial pressure. *Circulation* 1963; 27:29–35.
64. Wisenbaugh T, Spann J, Carabello B. Differences in myocardial performance and load between patients with similar amounts of chronic aortic versus chronic mitral regurgitation. *J Am Coll Cardiol* 1984; 3:916–923.
65. Starling M, Kirsch M, Montgomery D, Gross M. Impaired left ventricular contractile function in patients with long-term mitral regurgitation and normal ejection fraction. *J Am Coll Cardiol* 1993; 22:239–250.

66. Enriquez-Sarano M, Hannachi M, Jais J, Acar J. Résultats hémodynamiques et angiographiques après correction chirurgicale de l'insuffisance mitrale: A propos de 51 cathétérismes itératifs. *Arch Mal Coeur* 1983; 76:1194–1203.
67. Corin W, Monrad E, Murakami T, et al. The relationship of afterload to ejection performance in chronic mitral regurgitation. *Circulation* 1987; 76:59–67.
68. Carabello B, Nolan S, McGuire L. Assessment of preoperative left ventricular function in patients with mitral regurgitation: Value of the end-systolic wall stress-end-systolic volume ratio. *Circulation* 1981; 64:1212–1217.
69. Enriquez-Sarano M, Tajik A, Schaff H, et al. Echocardiographic prediction of left ventricular function after correction of mitral regurgitation: Results and clinical implications. *J Am Coll Cardiol* 1994; 24:1536–1543.
70. Crawford M, Souchek J, Oprian C, et al. Determinants of survival and left ventricular performance after mitral valve replacement. *Circulation* 1990; 81:1173–1181.
71. Urabe Y, Mann D, Kent R, et al. Cellular and ventricular contractile dysfunction in experimental canine mitral regurgitation. *Circ Res* 1992; 70:131–147.
72. Spinale F, Ishihra K, Zile M, et al. Structural basis for changes in left ventricular function and geometry because of chronic mitral regurgitation and after correction of volume overload. *J Thorac Cardiovasc Surg* 1993; 106:1147–1157.
73. Corin W, Murakami T, Monrad E, et al. Left ventricular passive diastolic properties in chronic mitral regurgitation. *Circulation* 1991; 83:797–807.
74. He S, Fontaine A, Schwammenthal E, et al. Integrated mechanism for functional mitral regurgitation. *Circulation* 1997; 96:1826–1834.
75. Otsuji Y, Handschumacher M, Schwammenthal E, et al. Insights from three dimensional echocardiography into the mechanism of functional mitral regurgitation. *Circulation* 1997; 96:1999–2008.
76. Enriquez-Sarano M, Tajik A, Bailey K, Seward J. Color flow imaging compared with quantitative doppler assessment of severity of mitral regurgitation: Influence of eccentricity of jet and mechanism of regurgitation. *J Am Coll Cardiol* 1993; 21:1211–1219.
77. Lamas G, Mitchell G, Flaker G, et al. Clinical significance of mitral regurgitation after acute myocardial infarction. *Circulation* 1997; 96:827–833.
78. Haggstrom J, Hansson K, Karlberg B, et al. Plasma concentration of atrial natriuretic peptide in relation to severity of mitral regurgitation in Cavalier King Charles spaniels. *Am J Vet Res* 1994; 55:698–703.
79. Brookes CI, Kemp MW, Hooper J, et al. Plasma brain natriuretic peptide concentrations in patients with chronic mitral regurgitation. *J Heart Valve Dis* 1997; 6:608–612.
80. Pedersen H, Koch J, Poulsen K. Activation of the renin-angiotensin system in dogs with asymptomatic and mildly symptomatic mitral valvular insufficiency. *J Vet Int Med* 1995; 9:328–331.
81. Dell'Italia L, Meng Q, Balcells E, et al. Increased ACE and chymase-like activity in cardiac tissue of dogs with chronic mitral regurgitation. *Am J Physiol* 1995; 269:H2065–H2073.
82. Dell'Italia L, Meng Q, Balcells E, et al. Compartmentalization of angiotensin II generation in the dog heart: Evidence for independent mechanisms in intravascular and interstitial spaces. *J Clin Invest* 1997; 100:253–258.
83. Singh J, Evans J, Levy D, et al. Prevalence and clinical determinants of mitral, tricuspid and aortic regurgitation *Am J Cardiol* 1999; 83:897–902.
84. Ling H, Enriquez-Sarano M, Seward J, et al. Clinical outcome of mitral regurgitation due to flail leaflets. *N Engl J Med* 1996; 335:1417–1423.
85. Kligfield P, Hochreiter C, Niles N, et al. Relation of sudden death in pure mitral regurgitation, with and without mitral valve prolapse, to repetitive ventricular arrythmias and right and left ventricular ejection fractions. *Am J Cardiol* 1987; 60:397–399.
86. Folland E, Kriegel B, Henderson W, et al. Implications of third heart sounds in patients with valvular heart disease: The Veterans Affairs Cooperative Study on Valvular Heart Disease. *N Engl J Med* 1992; 327:458–462.
87. Antman E, Angoff G, Sloss L. Demonstration of the mechanism by which mitral regurgitation mimics aortic stenosis. *Am J Cardiol* 1978; 42:1044–1048.
88. Desjardins V, Enriquez-Sarano M, Tajik A, et al. Intensity of murmurs correlates with severity of valvular regurgitation. *Am J Med* 1996; 100:149–156.
89. Forrester J, Diamond G, Freedman S, et al. Silent mitral insufficiency in acute myocardial infarction. *Circulation* 1971; 44: 877–883.
90. Enriquez-Sarano M, Tajik A, Schaff H, et al. Echocardiographic prediction of survival after surgical correction of organic mitral regurgitation. *Circulation* 1994; 90:830–837.
91. Glick B, Roberts W. Usefulness of total 12-lead QRS voltage in diagnosing left ventricular hypertrophy in clinically isolated, pure, chronic, severe mitral regurgitation. *Am J Cardiol* 1992; 70:1088–1092.
92. Enriquez-Sarano M, Freeman W, Tribouilloy C, et al. Functional anatomy of mitral regurgitation: Echocardiographic assessment and implications on outcome. *J Am Coll Cardiol* 1999; 34:1129–1136.
93. Shively B, Gurule F, Roldan C, et al. Diagnostic value of transesophageal compared with transthoracic endocardiography in infective endocarditis. *J Am Coll Cardiol* 1991; 18:391–397.
94. Izumi S, Miyatake K, Beppu S, et al. Mechanism of mitral regurgitation in patients with myocardial infarction: A study using realtime two-dimensional Doppler flow imaging and echocardiography. *Circulation* 1987; 76:777–785.
95. Boltwood C, Tei C, Wong M, Shah P. Quantitative echocardiography of the mitral complex in dilated cardiomyopathy: The mechanism of functional mitral regurgitation. *Circulation* 1983; 68: 498–508.
96. Spain M, Smith M, Grayburn P, et al. Quantitative assessment of mitral regurgitation by Doppler color flow imaging: Angiographic and hemodynamic correlations. *J Am Coll Cardiol* 1989; 13:585–590.
97. Pearson A, St. Vrain J, Mrosek D, Labovitz A. Color Doppler echocardiographic evaluation of patients with a flail mitral leaflet. *J Am Coll Cardiol* 1990; 16:232–239.
98. Tribouilloy C, Shen W, Quere J, et al. Assessment of severity of mitral regurgitation by measuring regurgitant jet width at its origin with transesophageal Doppler color flow imaging. *Circulation* 1992; 85:1248–1253.
99. Mele D, Vandervoort P, Palacios I, et al. Proximal jet size by Doppler color flow mapping predicts severity of mitral regurgitation. *Circulation* 1995; 91:746–754.
100. Klein A, Obarski T, Stewart W, et al. Transesophageal Doppler echocardiography of pulmonary venous flow: A new marker of mitral regurgitation severity. *J Am Coll Cardiol* 1991; 18:518–526.
101. Enriquez-Sarano M, Dujardin K, Tribouilloy C, et al. Determinants of pulmonary venous flow reversal in mitral regurgitation and its usefulness in determining the severity of the mitral regurgitation. *Am J Cardiol* 1999; 83:535–541.
102. Vandervoort P, Rivera J, Mele D, et al. Application of color Doppler flow mapping to calculate effective regurgitant orifice area. An in vitro study and initial clinical observations. *Circulation* 1993; 88:1150–1156.
103. Enriquez-Sarano M, Bailey K, Seward J, et al. Quantitative Doppler assessment of valvular regurgitation. *Circulation* 1993; 87:841–848.

104. Blumlein S, Bouchard A, Schiller N, et al. Quantitation of mitral regurgitation by Doppler echocardiography. *Circulation* 1986; 74:306–314.
105. Wisenbaugh T, Skudicky D, Sareli P. Prediction of outcome after valve replacement for rheumatic mitral regurgitation in the era of chordal preservation. *Circulation* 1994; 89:191–197.
106. Zile M, Gaasch W, Carroll J, Levine J. Chronic mitral regurgitation: Predictive value of preoperative echocardiographic indexes of left ventricular function and wall stress. *J Am Coll Cardiol* 1984; 3:235–242.
107. Sellers R. Left retrograde cardioangiography in acquired heart disease: Technic, indications and interpretations in 700 cases. *Am J Cardiol* 1964; 14:437–447.
108. Croft C, Lipscomb K, Mathis K, et al. Limitations of qualitative angiographic grading in aortic or mitral regurgitation. *Am J Cardiol* 1984; 53:1593–1598.
109. Sandler H, Dodge H, Hay R, Rackley C. Quantitation of valvular insufficiency in man by angiocardiography. *Am Heart J* 1963; 65:501–513.
110. Borow K, Green L, Mann T, et al. End systolic volume as a predictor of postoperative left ventricular performance in volume overload from valvular regurgitation. *Am J Med* 1980; 68:655–663.
111. Enriquez-Sarano M, Klodas E, Garratt KN, et al. Secular trends in coronary atherosclerosis—analysis in patients with valvular regurgitation. *N Engl J Med* 1996; 335:316–322.
112. Bonow R, Carabello B, DeLeon A, et al. ACC/AHA guidelines for the management of patients with valvular heart disease. *Circulation* 1998; 98:1949–1984.
113. Freeman W, Schaff H, Khanderia B, et al. Intraoperative evaluation of mitral valve regurgitation and repair by tranesophageal echocardiography: Incidence and significance of systolic anterior motion. *J Am Coll Cardiol* 1992; 20:599–609.
114. Leitch J, Mitchell A, Harris P, et al. The effect of cardiac catheterization upon management of advanced aortic and mitral regurgitation. *Eur Heart J* 1991; 12:602–607.
115. Slater J, Gindea A, Freedberg R, et al. Comparison of cardiac catheterization and Doppler echocardiography in the decision to operate in aortic and mitral valve disease. *J Am Coll Cardiol* 1991; 17:1026–1036.
116. Dujardin K, Enriquez-Sarano M, Bailey K, et al. Grading of mitral regurgitation by quantitative Doppler echocardiography—Calibration by left ventricular angiography in routine clinical practice. *Circulation* 1997; 96:3409–3415.
117. Wilson M, Lim W. The natural history of rheumatic heart disease in the third, fourth, and fifth decades of life. I. Prognosis with special reference to survivorship. *Circulation* 1957; 16:700–712.
118. Delahaye J, Gare J, Viguier E, et al. Natural history of severe mitral regurgitation. *Eur Heart J* 1991; 12(suppl B):5–9.
119. Rappaport E. Natural history of aortic and mitral valve disease. *Am J Cardiol* 1975; 35:221–227.
120. Munoz S, Gallardo J, Diaz-Gorrin J, Medina O. Influence of surgery on the natural history of rheumatic mitral and aortic valve disease. *Am J Cardiol* 1975; 35:234–242.
121. Horstkotte D, Loogen F, Kleikamp G, et al. Effect of prosthetic heart valve replacement on the natural course of isolated mitral and aortic as well as multivalvular diseases: Clinical results in 783 patients up to 8 years following implantation of the Björk-Shiley tilting disc prosthesis. *Z Kardiol* 1983; 72:494–503.
122. Grigioni F, Enriquez-Sarano M, Ling L, et al. Sudden death in mitral regurgitation due to flail leaflet. *J Am Coll Cardiol* 1999; 34:2078–2085.
123. Rosen S, Borer J, Hochreiter C, et al. Natural History of the asymptomatic/minimally symptomatic patient with severe mitral regurgitation secondary to mitral valve prolapse and normal right and left ventricular performance. *Am J Cardiol* 1994; 74:374–380.
124. Hammermeister K, Fisher L, Kennedy W, et al. Prediction of late survival in patients with mitral valve disease from clinical, hemodynamic, and quantitative angiographic variables. *Circulation* 1978; 57:341–349.
125. Enriquez-Sarano M, Basmadjian A, Rossi A, et al. Progression of mitral regurgitation: A prospective Doppler echocardiographic study. *J Am Coll Cardiol* 1999; 34:1137–1144.
126. Shulman S, Amren D, Bisno A, et al. Prevention of bacterial endocarditis: A statement for health professionals by the Committee on Rheumatic Fever and Bacterial Endocarditis of the Council on Cardiovascular Diseases in the Young of the American Heart Association. *Am J Dis Child* 1985; 139:232–235.
127. Chua Y, Schaff H, Orszulak T, Morriss J. Outcome of mitral valve repair in patients with preoperative atrial fibrillation: Should the maze procedure be combined with mitral valvuloplasty? *J Thorac Cardiovasc Surg* 1994; 107:408–415.
128. Greenberg B, Massie B, Brundage B, et al. Beneficial effects of hydralazine in severe mitral regurgitation. *Circulation* 1978; 58:273–279.
129. Tishler M, Rowan M, LeWinter M. Effect of Enalapril on left ventricular mass and volumes in asymptomatic chronic, severe mitral regurgitation secondary to mitral valve prolapse. *Am J Cardiol* 1998; 82:242–245.
130. Marcotte F, Honos G, Walling A, et al. Effect of angiotensin converting enzyme inhibitor therapy in mitral regurgitation with normal left ventricular function. *Can J Cardiol* 1997; 13:479–485.
131. Host U, Kelbaek H, Hildebrandt P, et al. Effect of Ramilpril on mitral regurgitation secondary to mitral valve prolapse. *Am J Cardiol* 1997; 80:655–658.
132. Rothlisberger C, Sareli P, Wisenbaugh T. Comparison of single dose nifedipine and captopril for chronic severe mitral regurgitation. *Am J Cardiol* 1994; 73:978–981.
133. Wisenbaugh T, Sinovich V, Dullbh A, Sareli P. Six month pilot study of captopril for mildly symptomatic, severe isolated mitral and isolated aortic regurgitation. *J Heart Valve Dis* 1994; 3:197–204.
134. Gillinov A, Cosgrove D, Blackstone E, et al. Durability of mitral valve repair for degenerative disease. *J Thorac Cardiovasc Surg* 1998; 116:734–743.
135. Frater R, Gabbay S, Shore D, et al. Reproducible replacement of elongated or ruptured mitral valve chordae. *Ann Thorac Surg* 1983; 35:14–28.
136. Lessana A, Escorsin M, Romano M, et al. Transposition of posterior leaflet for treatment of ruptured main chordae of the anterior mitral leaflet. *J Thorac Cardiovasc Surg* 1985; 89:804–806.
137. Duran C, Revuelta J, Gaite L, et al. Stability of mitral reconstructive surgery at 10–12 years for predominantly rheumatic valvular disease. *Circulation* 1988; 78:I91–I96.
138. Mihaileanu S, Marino J, Chauvaud S, et al. Left ventricular outflow obstruction after mitral valve repair (Carpentier's technique). Proposed mechanisms of disease. *Circulation* 1988; 78:I78–I84.
139. David T, Komeda M, Pollick C, Burns R. Mitral valve annuloplasty: The effects of the type on left ventricular function. *Ann Thorac Surg* 1989; 47:524–528.
140. Cohn IH, Allred E, Cohn IA, et al. Early and late risk of mitral valve replacement: A 12-year concomitant comparison of the porcine bioprosthetic and prosthetic disc mitral valves. *J Thorac Cardiovasc Surg* 1985; 90:872–880.
141. Enriquez-Sarano M, Schaff H, Orszulak T, et al. Valve repair improves the outcome of surgery for mitral regurgitation. *Circulation* 1995; 91:1264–1265.
142. Perier P, Deloche A, Chauvaud S, et al. Comparative evaluation of mitral valve repair and replacement with Starr, Bjork, and porcine valve prostheses. *Circulation* 1984; 70:I187–I192.

143. David T, Burns R, Bacchus C, Druck M. Mitral regurgitation with and without preservation of chordae tendinae. *J Thorac Cardiovasc Surg* 1984; 88:718–725.
144. Cerfolio R, Orszulak T, Pluth J, et al. Reoperation after valve repair for mitral regurgitation: Early and intermediate results. *J Thorac Cardiovasc Surg* 1996; 111:1177–1183.
145. Enriquez-Sarano M, Schaff H, Orszulak T, et al. Congestive heart failure after surgical correction of mitral regurgitation. A long-term study. *Circulation* 1995; 92:2496–2503.
146. Tribouilloy C, Enriquez-Sarano M, Schaff H, et al. Impact of preoperative symptoms on survival after surgical correction of organic mitral regurgitation: Rationale for optimizing surgical indications. *Circulation* 1999; 99:400–500.
147. Sousa Uva M, Dreyfus G, Rescigno G, et al. Surgical treatment of asymptomatic and mildly symptomatic mitral regurgitation. *J Thorac Cardiovasc Surg* 1996; 112:1240–1249.
148. Handa N, Schaff HV, Morris JJ, et al. Outcome of valve repair and the cox maze procedure for mitral regurgitation and associated atrial fibrillation. *J Thorac Cardiovasc Surg* 1999; 118:628–635.

CHAPTER 58

MITRAL VALVE PROLAPSE SYNDROME

Robert A. O'Rourke

The syndrome of mitral valve prolapse (MVP) is the most common form of valvular heart disease, occurring in 2 to 6 percent of the population, thus being more common than a bicuspid aortic valve. The incidence varies depending on the criteria used for its diagnosis.[1,2] MVP is commonly detected by cardiac auscultation, with one or more systolic clicks and/or a mid- to late-systolic murmur detected on a careful physical examination. Often the auscultatory complex is the only clinical manifestation of cardiac disease, and many patients are asymptomatic.

Midsystolic clicks were first described in the late nineteenth century and originally were attributed to a pericardial or extracardiac etiology. Subsequently, late-systolic murmurs were recognized to be present in apparently healthy people and were associated with a benign natural history. Thus the murmur also was considered to be extracardiac in origin.

In 1961, Reid[3] suggested that the midsystolic click and the late-systolic murmur were due to mitral regurgitation. In 1963, Barlow et al.[4] confirmed this hypothesis by left ventricular (LV) cineangiography. Subsequently, intracardiac phonocardiogram studies documented the mitral valve origin of a systolic click and late-systolic murmur.

During the past four decades, considerable new data obtained from pathologic studies, echocardiography, and cineventriculography have demonstrated that this common syndrome is associated with prolapse of one or both mitral valve leaflets into the atrium during LV systole.

Recognition of MVP (also known as the *systolic click–late systolic murmur syndrome*) is often difficult because of the extreme variability of its clinical manifestations. It is, however, an important cause of incapacitating chest pain and refractory arrhythmias in certain patients. The abnormal components of the mitral valve apparatus are a potential site for endocarditis, and some patients, particularly males in their sixties and seventies, can develop severe mitral regurgitation (MR) due to ruptured chordae tendineae.

DEFINITION, ETIOLOGY, AND TIMING

MVP refers to the systolic billowing of one or both mitral leaflets into the left atrium, with or without MR. MVP often occurs as a clinical entity with no or only mild MR, and it is frequently associated with unique clinical characteristics when compared with the other causes of MR.[5-9] Nevertheless, MVP is the most common cause of significant MR and the most frequent substrate for mitral valve endocarditis in the United States. The mitral valve apparatus is a complex structure composed of the mitral annulus, valve leaflets, chordae tendineae, papillary muscles, and the supporting left ventricle, left atrium, and aortic walls[10] (Fig. 58-1). Disease processes involving any one or more of these components may result in dysfunction of the valvular apparatus and prolapse of the mitral leaflets toward the left atrium during systole when LV pressure exceeds left atrial (LA) pressure.

The complexity of the mitral valve apparatus provides an explanation for the presence of secondary prolapse in many conditions that affect one or more of the components of the apparatus (e.g., ruptured mitral chordae). There is, however, considerable evidence that a disorder of the mitral valve leaflets exists in which there are specific pathologic changes causing redundancy of the mitral leaflets and their prolapse into the left atrium during systole. This is the primary form of MVP (Table 58-1).

In *primary* MVP, there is interchordal hooding due to leaflet redundancy that involves both the rough and clear zones of the involved leaflets[6] (Fig. 58-2). The height of the interchordal hooding usually exceeds 4 mm and involves at least one-half of the anterior leaflet or at least two-thirds of the posterior leaflet. The basic microscopic feature of primary MVP is marked proliferation of the *spongiosa,* the delicate myxomatous connective tissue between the *atrialis* (a thick layer of collagen and elastic tissue forming the atrial aspect of the leaflet) and the *fibrosa,* or *ventricularis,* which is composed of dense layers of

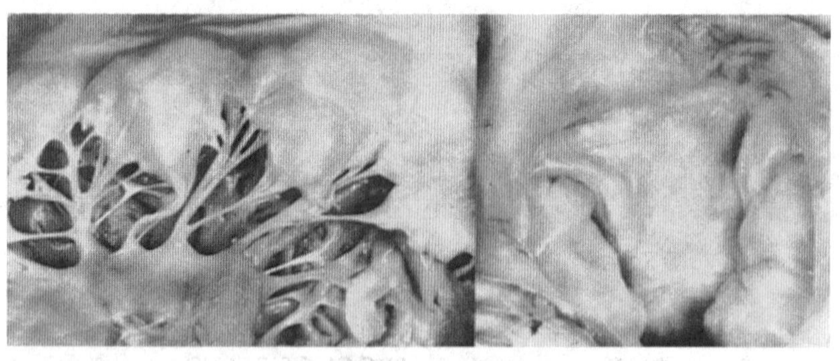

FIGURE 58-1 Myxomatous mitral valve. *A*. The opened mitral valve shows characteristic interchordal hooding and redundancy of the leaflets. *B*. The unopened mitral valve viewed from the left atrial side shows extensive scalloping that is characteristic of a myxomatous mitral valve. (From Guthrie and Edwards.[14] Reproduced with permission from the publisher and authors.)

TABLE 58-1 Classification of Mitral Valve Prolapse

Primary mitral valve prolapse
Familial
Nonfamilial
Marfan syndrome
Other connective tissue diseases
Secondary mitral valve prolapse
Coronary artery disease
Rheumatic heart disease
Cardiomyopathies
"Flail" mitral valve leaflet(s)
Normal variant
Inaccurate auscultation
"Echocardiographic heart disease"

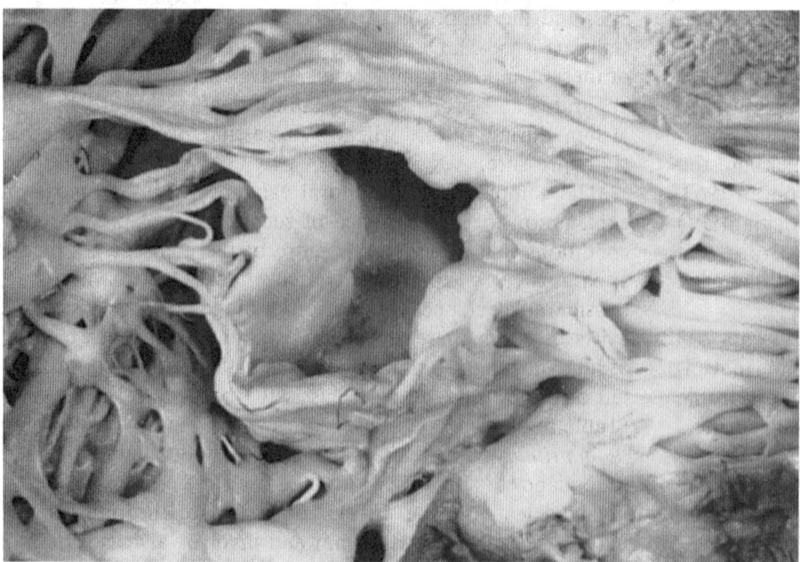

FIGURE 58-2 Myxomatous mitral valve with ruptured posterior leaflet chordae. The central part of the posterior leaflet (*lower center*) shows fragments of ruptured chordae. The intact chordae are elongated, and the leaflets show redundancy and fibrous thickening. (From Edwards F. Pathology of mitral incompetence. In: Silver MD, ed. *Cardiovascular Pathology*. New York: Churchill Livingstone; 1983. Reproduced with permission from the publisher and authors.)

collagen and forms the basic support of the leaflet.[6] In primary MVP, myxomatous proliferation of the acid mucopolysaccharide-containing spongiosa tissue causes focal interruption of the fibrosa. Secondary effects of the primary MVP syndrome include fibrosis of the surfaces of the mitral valve leaflets, thinning and/or elongation of chordae tendineae, and ventricular friction lesions. Fibrin deposits often form at the mitral valve–left atrial angle.

The primary form of MVP may occur in families, where it appears to be inherited as an autosomal dominant trait with varying penetrance.[11,12] No consistent chromosomal abnormalities have yet been identified in patients with MVP, which also often occurs in isolated cases.[13,14] Primary MVP has been found with increasing frequency in patients with Marfan syndrome, where it is almost always present, and in other heritable connective tissue diseases such as Ehlers-Danlos syndrome,[15] pseudoxanthoma elasticum,[16] and osteogenesis imperfecta.[17] Marfan syndrome also has an autosomal dominant mode of inheritance. It is possible that some genetic studies of MVP may have been tracking a more general connective tissue disorder such as Marfan syndrome (see also Chap. 76).

Many observers have speculated that primary MVP syndrome represents a generalized disorder of connective tissue. Thoracic skeletal abnormalities such as straight thoracic spine and pectus excavatum are commonly associated with this syndrome.[18] The mitral valve undergoes differentiation between the thirty-fifth and forty-second days of fetal life, when the vertebrae and thoracic cage are beginning chondrification and ossification.[19] Any adverse factors in this period may affect both the mitral valve and the bones of the thoracic cage. Of possible relevance, rats fed a diet containing large amounts of peas of the genus *Lathyrus* develop both bony abnormalities and myxomatous changes in their valve leaflets. Therefore, it has been postulated that the MVP syndrome is a connective tissue disorder resulting from fetal exposure to toxic substances during the early part of pregnancy.[20,21]

Others have suggested that MVP is a result of defective embryogenesis of cell lines of mesenchymal origin. The increased prevalence of primary MVP in patients with von Willebrand disease and other coagulopathies, primary hypomastia, and various connective tissue diseases has been used to support this concept.[21]

In *secondary* forms of MVP (see Table 58-1), myxomatous proliferation of the spongiosa portion of the mitral valve leaflet is absent. Tei et al.[22] were able to produce de novo echocardiographic evidence of MVP, often with MR, in closed-chest dogs undergoing transient coronary artery occlusion; MVP was attributed to relative displacement of ischemic papillary muscles. Also, serial studies in patients with known ischemic heart disease occasionally have documented unequivocal MVP following an acute coronary syndrome that was previously absent.[23] In most patients with coronary artery disease (CAD) and MVP, however, the two entities are coincident but unrelated.

More recent studies[24–26] indicate that MR caused by MVP may result from postinflammatory changes, including those following rheumatic fever. In histologic studies of surgically excised valves, fibrosis with vascularization and scattered infiltration of round cells, including lymphocytes and plasmacytes, was found *without myxomatous proliferation* of the spongiosa.[24] With rheumatic carditis, the anterior mitral leaflet is more likely to prolapse.[26]

MVP has been observed in patients with hypertrophic cardiomyopathy, in whom posterior MVP may result from a disproportionately small LV cavity, altered papillary muscle alignment, or a combination of factors.[21] The mitral valve leaflet is usually normal, but occasionally, the changes of primary MVP are present. Since LV segmental wall motion abnormalities and sometimes depressed global LV function occur in certain patients with echocardiographic and auscultatory evidence of MVP and MR, nonhypertrophic cardiomyopathy has been listed as a cause of mitral prolapse.[27] This is probably not the case; the ventricular wall motion abnormalities usually disappear when the mitral valve is repaired or replaced. In MVP patients, atrial septal defects, pulmonary hypertension, anorexia nervosa, dehydration, or straight-back syndrome may be secondary to the relatively small size of the left ventricle in this disorder, resulting in a mitral apparatus that is relatively large and redundant.[21,28] However, atrial septal defect may be associated with primary MVP.[16] Patients with primary and secondary MVP must be distinguished from those with normal variations on cardiac auscultation or echocardiography; these variations can result in an incorrect diagnosis of MVP, particularly in patients who are hyperkinetic or dehydrated during the physical examination or two-dimensional (2-D) echocardiography. Other auscultatory findings may be misinterpreted as midsystolic clicks or late-systolic murmurs.[8,21] Patients with mild to moderate billowing of one or more nonthickened leaflets toward the left atrium with the leaflet coaptation point on the ventricular side of the mitral annulus and no or minimal MR by Doppler echocardiography are probably normal. Unfortunately, many such patients with neither a nonejection click nor murmur of MR are frequently overdiagnosed as having the MVP syndrome.[1,2,29]

PATHOPHYSIOLOGY

In patients with MVP, there is frequently LA enlargement and LV enlargement, depending on the presence and severity of MR.[30] The supporting apparatus is often involved, and in patients with connective tissue syndromes such as Marfan syndrome, the mitral annulus is usually dilated, sometimes calcified, and does not decrease its circumference by the usual 30 percent during LV systole. The hemodynamic effects of mild to moderate MR are similar to those from other causes of MR.

Many studies suggest an increased prevalence of autonomic nervous system dysfunction in patients with primary MVP. In 1979, Gaffney et al.[31] reported a reduced heart rate slowing with intravenous phenylephrine and an abnormal diving reflex heart rate response in patients with MVP as compared with age-matched controls. Patients with MVP had a lesser lower extremity pooling of blood in response to lower body negative pressure. Increased vagal tone and prolonged QT intervals on the electrocardiogram (ECG) are more common in patients with MVP. Measurements of serum and 24-h urine epinephrine and norepinephrine levels are often increased in patients with symptomatic MVP as compared with controls.[32] Patients with MVP often have an increased heart rate and contractility response to intravenous isoproterenol.[33] An increased incidence of high-affinity beta receptors in the lymphocytes of patients with MVP has been reported, as well as greater than usual increases in cyclic adenosine monophosphate with isoproterenol stimulation as compared with normal individuals.[33] Patients with MVP often have postural phenomena such as orthostatic tachycardia and hypotension. Low intravascular volume and/or an abnormality in the renin-aldosterone axis may contribute to the orthostatic changes.[7,34]

ASSOCIATED CONDITIONS

Tricuspid valve prolapse, with similar interchordal hooding and histologic evidence of mucopolysaccharide proliferation and collagen dissolution, occurs in about 40 percent of patients with MVP.[6] Pulmonic valve prolapse and aortic valve prolapse occur in approximately 10 and 2 percent of patients with MVP, respectively.[6] The frequent findings of thoracic skeletal abnormalities in patients with MVP were noted earlier. There is an increased incidence of secundum atrial septal defect in patients with MVP and an increased incidence of MVP in patients with atrial septal defects that cannot be explained by a chance occurrence and does not represent only stretching of a patent fossa ovalis (see also Chaps. 63 and 64). An increased incidence of left-sided atrioventricular bypass tracts and supraventricular tachycardias also occurs in patients with MVP.[6,35]

CLINICAL MANIFESTATIONS

Symptoms

The diagnosis of MVP is most commonly made by cardiac auscultation in asymptomatic patients or by echocardiography being performed for some other purpose. The patient may be evaluated because of a family history of cardiac disease or occasionally may be referred because of an abnormal resting ECG. Some patients consult their physicians because of one or more of the common symptoms that occur in patients with this syndrome. The most common presenting complaint is *palpitation*. The source of palpitation is usually ventricular premature beats, but various supraventricular arrhythmias are also frequent, and the most common sustained tachycardia is paroxysmal reentry supraventricular tachycardia (see Chap. 24). Ventricular tachycardia occurs in some patients, and others have had symptomatic bradyarrhythmias. Palpitation is often reported by patients at a time when continuous ambulatory ECG recordings show no arrhythmias.

Chest pain is a frequent complaint in patients with MVP. It is atypical in most patients without coexisting ischemic heart disease and rarely resembles classic angina pectoris. Occasionally, it is recurrent and can be incapacitating. The etiology of the chest pain is unknown; sometimes it may represent true myocardial ischemia produced by abnormal tension on the papillary muscles and supporting ventricular wall by the prolapsing mitral leaflets.[36] Coronary artery spasm has been reported in patients with MVP, but it is unlikely to be the cause of most episodes of atypical chest pain.[37]

Dyspnea and *fatigue* are frequent symptoms in patients with MVP, including many without severe MR. Objective exercise testing often fails to show impaired exercise tolerance, and some patients exhibit distinct episodes of hyperventilation. Neuropsychiatric complaints occur in certain patients with MVP. Some have panic attacks (see Chap. 80), and others have frank manic-depressive syndromes. Transient cerebral ischemic episodes occur with increased incidence in patients with MVP, and some develop stroke syndromes.[38–42] One recent study showed no association between MVP and stroke.[43] Reports of amaurosis fugax, homonymous field loss, and retinal artery occlusion have been made; occasionally, the visual loss persists.[44] These signs likely are due to embolization of platelets and fibrin deposits that occur on the atrial side of the mitral valve leaflets.[45] *It is important to note that both MVP and panic attacks occur relatively frequently. Accordingly, the occurrence of the two syndromes in the same individual would be expected to occur frequently by chance, rather than panic attacks necessarily being part of the primary MVP syndrome.*

Physical Examination

The presence of thoracic skeletal abnormalities may suggest the diagnosis of MVP, the most common being scoliosis, pectus excavatum, straightened thoracic spine, and narrowed anteroposterior diameter of the chest.[16] Some patients with MVP may show signs, such as arachnodactyly, more typical of Marfan syndrome.

The principal cardiac auscultatory feature of this syndrome is the midsystolic click, a high-pitched sound of short duration (see Chap. 10). The click may vary considerably in intensity and location in systole according to LV loading conditions and contractility. It results from the sudden tensing of the mitral valve apparatus as the leaflets prolapse into the left atrium during systole. Multiple systolic clicks may be generated by different portions of the mitral leaflets prolapsing at varying times during systole.[46] The major differentiating feature of the midsystolic click of MVP from that due to other causes (e.g., aneurysm of the ventricular septum, atrial myxomas, or pericarditis) is that its timing during systole may be altered by maneuvers that change hemodynamic conditions (Table 58-2).

The midsystolic click is frequently followed by a late-systolic murmur, usually medium- to high-pitched and most audible at the apex. Occasionally, the murmur has a musical or honking quality. The character and intensity of the murmur also vary under certain conditions, from brief and almost inaudible to holosystolic and loud (Fig. 58-3).

Dynamic auscultation is often useful for establishing the clinical diagnosis of the MVP syndrome.[21] Changes in the LV end-diastolic volume lead to changes in the timing of the midsystolic click and murmur. When end-diastolic volume is decreased, the critical volume is achieved earlier in systole, and the click-murmur complex occurs shortly after the first heart sound (Fig. 58-4). In general, any maneuver that decreases the end-diastolic LV volume, increases the rate of ventricular contraction, or decreases the resistance to LV ejection of blood causes the MVP to occur early in systole, and the systolic click and murmur to move toward the first heart sound (see Table 58-2). By contrast, any maneuver that augments the volume of blood in the ventricle, reduces myocardial contractility, or increases LV afterload lengthens the time from the onset of systole to the initiation of MVP, and the systolic click and/or murmur move toward S_2. Maneuvers causing the click and/or murmur to occur earlier in systole include standing from the supine position, submaximal isometric handgrip exercise, the Valsalva maneuver, and amyl nitrite inhalation. Those which cause the click and murmur to move toward S_2 include squatting from the upright position and maneuvers that slow the heart rate.

TABLE 58-2 Response of the Murmur of Mitral Valve Prolapse to Interventions

Intervention	Timing	Intensity
Standing upright	←	↑
Recumbent	→	↓ or 0
Squatting	→	↓ or 0
Hand-grip	←	±
Valsalva	←	±
Amyl nitrite	±	↑

NOTE: ↑ = increase; ↓ = decrease; 0 = no change; ± = variable; ← = earlier; → = later.

Electrocardiogram

The ECG is usually normal in patients with MVP. The most common abnormality noted is the presence of ST-T-wave depression or T-wave inversion in the inferior leads (III, aV_F)[47] (Fig. 58-5). These changes may reflect ischemia of the inferior wall due to traction on the posteromedial papillary muscle by the prolapsing mitral leaflets. Sometimes ST-T-wave changes are present only during interventions that induce prolapse earlier in systole, as discussed earlier. More unusual electrocardiographic changes include prominent U waves, peaked T waves in the midprecordial leads, and prolongation of the QT interval.

MVP is associated with an increased incidence of false-positive exercise electrocardiographic results in patients with normal coronary arteries, especially females. Myocardial perfusion imaging with thallium or technetium sestamibi has been useful for differentiating false from true abnormal exercise electrocardiographic findings in patients with MVP (see Chap. 16).

Although arrhythmias may be observed on the resting ECG or during treadmill or bicycle exercise, they are detected more reliably by continuous ambulatory electrocardiographic recordings (see Chap. 13). The reported incidence of documented arrhythmias is higher in patients with MVP, ranging from 40 to 75 percent.[48] Most of the arrhythmias detected, however, are not life-threatening. Patients with ST-T-wave changes in the inferior electrocardiographic leads appear to have a higher incidence of serious ventricular arrhythmias on ambulatory recordings.[20]

Echocardiography

Echocardiography (see Chap. 13) is the most useful noninvasive test for defining MVP. The M-mode echocardiographic definition of MVP includes 2 mm or more of posterior displacement of one or both leaflets or holosystolic posterior "hammocking"

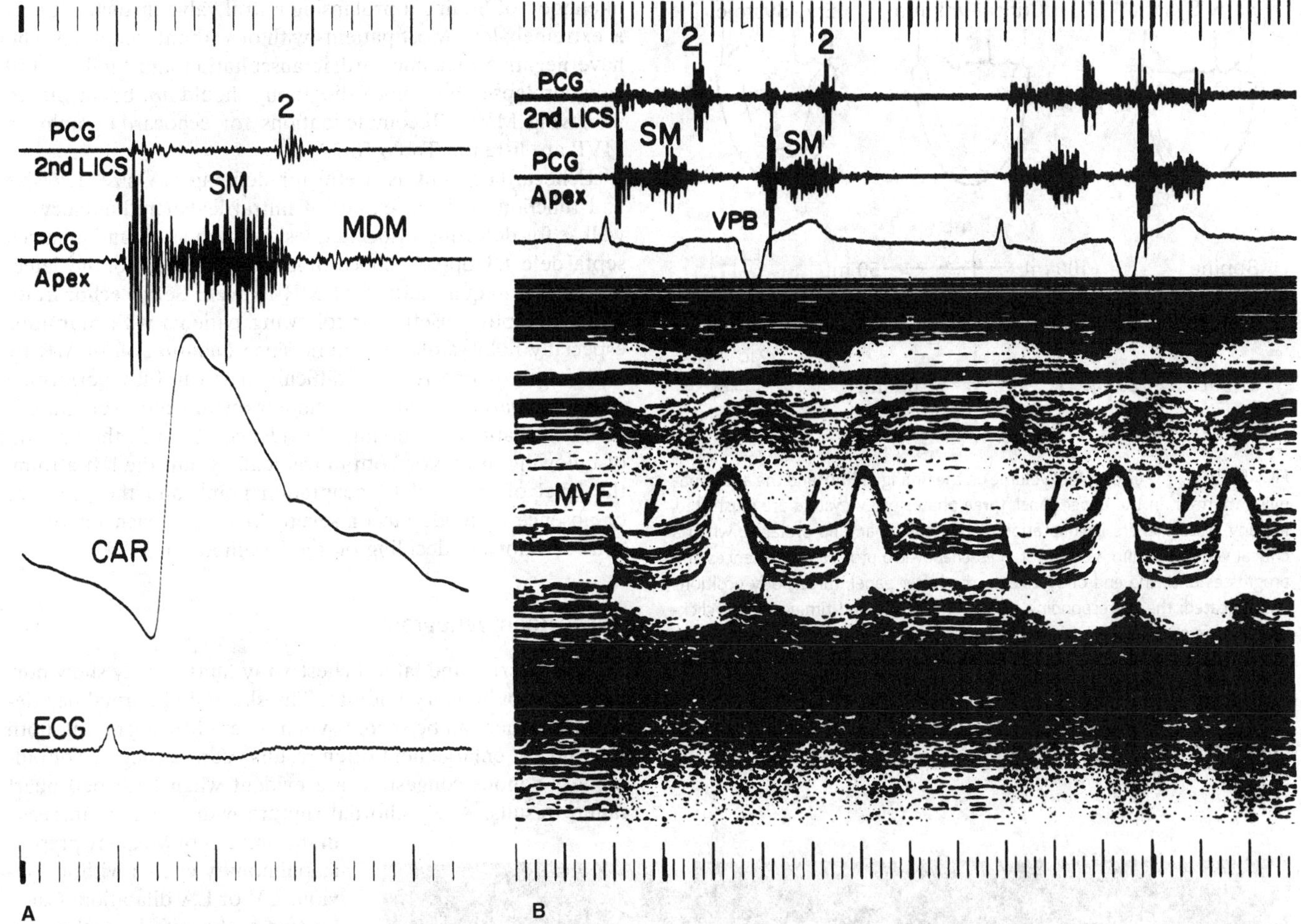

FIGURE 58-3 Phonocardiogram and echocardiogram in mitral valve prolapse. *A*. The phonocardiogram shows a high-frequency holosystolic murmur (HSM) with late-systolic accentuation. A low-frequency middiastolic murmur (MDM) is present at the apex. *B*. The echocardiogram demonstrates a hammock-shaped systolic motion of the valve leaflets. The rhythm is atrial fibrillation with bigeminy. 1, first heart sound; 2, second heart sound; MVE, mitral valve echogram. (Courtesy of Dr. Ernest Craige.)

of more than 3 mm (see Fig. 58-3). On 2-D echocardiography, systolic displacement of one or both mitral leaflets, particularly when they coapt on the LA side of the annular plane, in the parasternal long-axis view indicates a high likelihood of MVP[49] (see Fig. 58-5). There is disagreement concerning the reliability of an echocardiographic diagnosis of MVP when observed only in the apical four-chamber view. The diagnosis of MVP is even more certain when the leaflet thickness is greater than 5 mm during ventricular diastole. Leaflet redundancy is often associated with an elongated mitral annulus and elongated chordae tendineae. On Doppler velocity recordings, the presence or absence of MR is an important consideration, and MVP is more likely when the MR is detected as a high-velocity jet midway or more posterior in the left atrium.[29]

At present, there is no consensus on the 2-D echocardiographic criteria for MVP. Since echocardiography is a tomographic cross-sectional technique, no single view should be considered diagnostic. The parasternal long-axis view permits visualization of the medial aspect of the anterior mitral leaflet and middle scallop of the posterior leaflet. If the findings of prolapse are localized to the lateral scallop in the posterior leaflet, they would be best visualized by the apical four-chamber view.[49,50] All available echocardiographic views should be used, with the provision that anterior leaflet billowing alone in the four-chamber apical view is not evidence of prolapse; however, a displacement of the posterior leaflet or the coaptation point in any view including the apical views suggests the diagnosis of prolapse. The echocardiographic criteria for MVP should include structural changes such as leaflet thickening, redundancy, annular dilatation, and chordal elongation.

Patients with echocardiographic criteria for MVP but without evidence of thickened/redundant leaflets or definite MR are more difficult to classify. If such patients have auscultatory findings typical of MVP, the echocardiogram confirms the diagnosis. On the other hand, a patient with typical auscultatory findings but a negative echocardiogram likely also has MVP; in the past, as many as 10 percent of patients with MVP have had a nondiagnostic echocardiographic study. Currently, this percentage is lower because of more careful and complete echocardiographic studies. In clinical practice, a false diagnosis of MVP occurs too frequently. The use of echocardiography as a screening test for MVP in patients with and without symptoms who have no systolic click or murmur on serial, carefully performed auscultatory examinations *is not recommended*. The

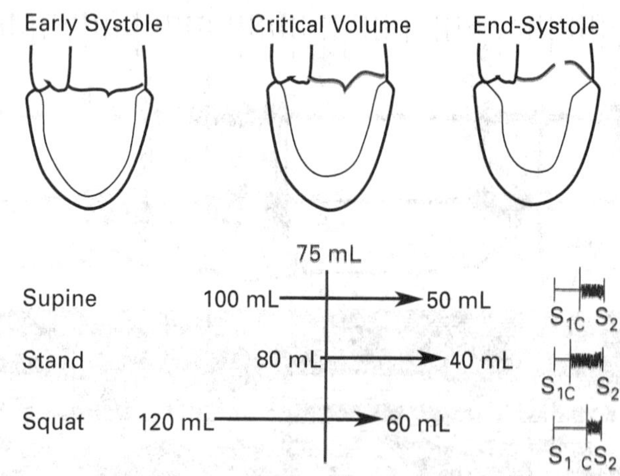

FIGURE 58-4 The effect of LV volume on the timing of MVP and the accompanying murmur. In the upper panel, three phases of LV systole are illustrated. In early systole, there is coaptation of the leaflets and no prolapse; when a critical ventricle volume of 75 mL is reached, valve prolapse commences and progresses until the end of systole. In the lower panel, three body positions are indicated; the corresponding change in volume and timing of the click-murmur are shown. The critical volume for prolapse remains constant. When the critical volume occurs earlier, the onset of the click-murmur is earlier. When the critical volume occurs later, the onset of the click-murmur is later. (From Crawford MH, O'Rourke RA. In: Isselbacher KJ et al., eds. *Harrison's Principles of Internal Medicine*, 9th ed. New York: McGraw-Hill; 1980:91–105. Reproduced with permission from the publisher, editors, and authors.)

likelihood of finding a prolapsing mitral valve in such patients is extremely low. Most patients with or without symptoms who have negative dynamic cardiac auscultation and "mild mitral valve prolapse" by echocardiography should not be diagnosed as having MVP. Recommendations for echocardiography in MVP are listed in Table 58-3.[51]

Echocardiography is useful for defining LA size, LV size and function, and the extent of mitral leaflet redundancy, as well as for detecting associated lesions such as secundum atrial septal defect. Doppler echocardiography is helpful for the detection and semiquantitation of MR as well. Serial echocardiograms are often useful for following patients with murmurs, especially holosystolic murmurs, since quantitation of MR by examination alone is more difficult. In a carefully performed study comparing auscultatory findings with echocardiographic results in patients with clinical evidence of MVP, the amount of billowing of one or both mitral leaflets into the left atrium, the level of the leaflets' coaptation point, and the presence or absence of moderate or severe MR were each important considerations in deciding on the likelihood of MVP.[29]

Chest Roentgenogram

Posteroanterior and lateral chest x-ray films usually show normal cardiopulmonary findings. The skeletal abnormalities described earlier can be seen.[19] When severe MR is present, both LA and LV enlargement often results. Various degrees of pulmonary venous congestion are evident when left-sided heart failure results. Acute chordal rupture with a sudden increase in the amount of MR may present as pulmonary edema without obvious LV or LA dilatation. Calcification of the mitral annulus may be seen, particularly in adults with Marfan syndrome (see Chap. 12).

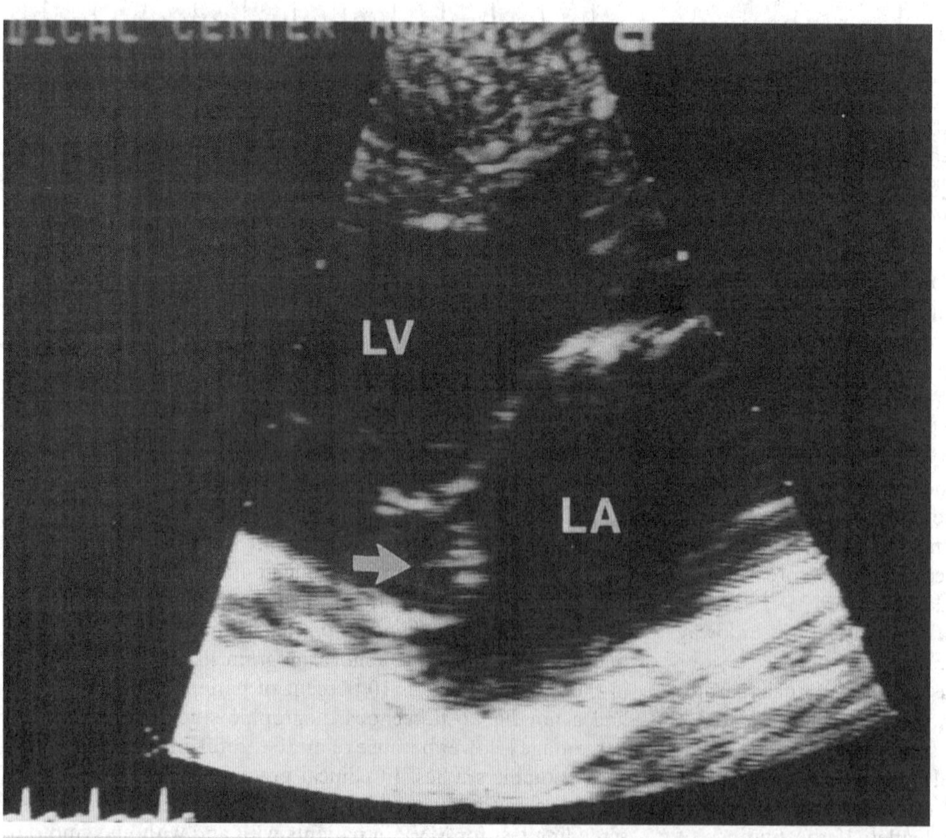

FIGURE 58-5 A parasternal 2-D echocardiographic view showing prolapse of a redundant posterior mitral leaflet toward the left atrium during systole. LV, left ventricle; LA, left atrium.

Myocardial Perfusion Scintigraphy

Exercise myocardial perfusion imaging with thallium or technetium sestamibi has been recommended as an adjunct to exercise ECG for determining the presence or absence of coexistent myocardial ischemia in patients with MVP.[52] Most MVP patients *with clinical evidence of CAD* have an abnormal exercise scintigram. On the other hand, a negative scintigram in these patients does not exclude ischemia as the basis for the chest pain, nor does it completely exclude CAD as the etiology (see Chap. 16).

Cardiac Catheterization

Cardiac catheterization is rarely used as a diagnostic technique for

MVP. Also, contrast ventriculography is unnecessary for determining LV function because it usually can be quantitated by 2-D echocardiography or radionuclide ventriculography. While contrast cineventriculography is often useful for assessing the severity of MR, cardiac catheterization and angiography are used most commonly in patients with MVP to exclude the possibility of CAD.

Intracardiac pressures and cardiac output are usually normal in uncomplicated MVP; however, these measurements become progressively more abnormal as MR becomes more severe.

LV cineangiography usually confirms the presence of prolapse of the mitral valve.[5,8] The right anterior oblique projection is best for observing prolapse of the three scallops of the posterior leaflet. The left anterior oblique view is necessary for the adequate evaluation of prolapse of the anterior leaflet.

LV wall motion is usually normal in patients with primary MVP, but some patients show abnormal contraction patterns in the absence of CAD.[5,27] These contraction abnormalities usually represent indentation of the left ventricle at the point of attachment of the papillary muscles; it is thought to be due to abnormal traction on the papillary muscles and buckling of the ventricular wall. Patients with the most severe prolapse more commonly exhibit misshapen ventricular cavities during systole, and wall motion abnormalities frequently disappear after successful mitral valve replacement or repair.[27]

Coronary arteriography is usually normal in patients with primary MVP, and no congenital anomalies of the coronary vessels have been associated with this syndrome.

TABLE 58-3 Recommendations for Echocardiography in Mitral Valve Prolapse

Indication	Class
1. Diagnosis, assessment of hemodynamic severity of MR, leaflet morphology, ventricular compensation in patients with physical signs of MVP.	I
2. To exclude MVP in patients who have been given the diagnosis where there is no clinical evidence to support the diagnosis.	I
3. To exclude MVP in patients with first-degree relatives with known myxomatous valve disease.	IIa
4. Risk stratification in patients with physical signs of MVP with no or mild regurgitation.	IIa
5. To exclude MVP in patients in the absence of physical findings suggestive of MVP a positive family history.	III
6. Routine repetition of echocardiography in patients with MVP with no MR and no changes in clinical signs or symptoms.	III

Class I: Conditions for which there is evidence and/or general agreement that a given procedure or treatment is useful and effective.

Class II: Conditions for which there is conflicting evidence and/or a divergence of opinion about the usefulness/efficacy of a procedure or treatment.

Class IIa: Weight of evidence/opinion is in favor of usefulness/efficacy.

Class IIb: Usefulness efficacy is less well established by evidence/opinion.

Class III: Conditions for which there is evidence and/or general agreement that the procedure/treatment is not useful/effective and in some cases may be harmful.

SOURCE: From ACC/AHA clinical practice guidelines for valvular heart disease. *J Am Coll Cardiol* 1998; 32:1486–1588.

Electrophysiologic Testing

The indications for electrophysiologic testing in a patient with MVP are similar to those in other patients (i.e., recurrent unexplained syncope, sudden death survivors, symptomatic complex ventricular ectopy, and the presence of the preexcitation syndromes) (see Chap. 26). Upright tilt studies with monitoring of blood pressure and rhythm may be valuable in patients with light-headedness or syncope and in diagnosing autonomic dysfunction (see Chap. 32).

NATURAL HISTORY, PROGNOSIS, AND COMPLICATIONS

In most patient studies, the MVP syndrome is associated with a benign prognosis[6,53–60] (Fig. 58-6). The age-adjusted survival rate for both males and females with MVP is similar to that

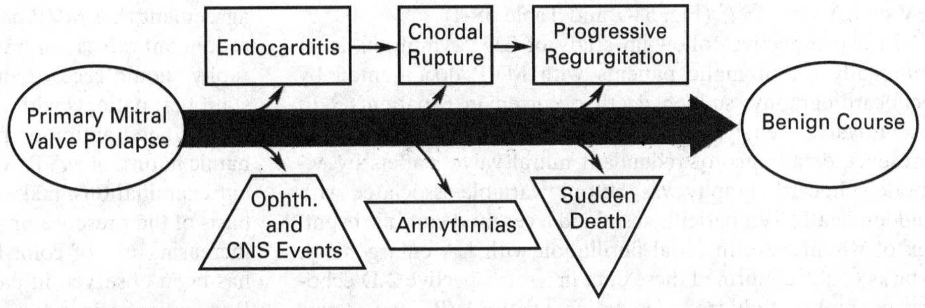

FIGURE 58-6 The course and possible complications of MVP. In most patients, the MVP syndrome is associated with a benign prognosis. CNS, central nervous system; Ophth, ophthalmologic. (From Crawford MH, O'Rourke RA. In: Isselbacher KJ et al., eds. *Harrison's Principles of Internal Medicine*, 9th ed. New York: McGraw-Hill; 1980:91–105. Reproduced with permission from the publisher, editors, and authors.)

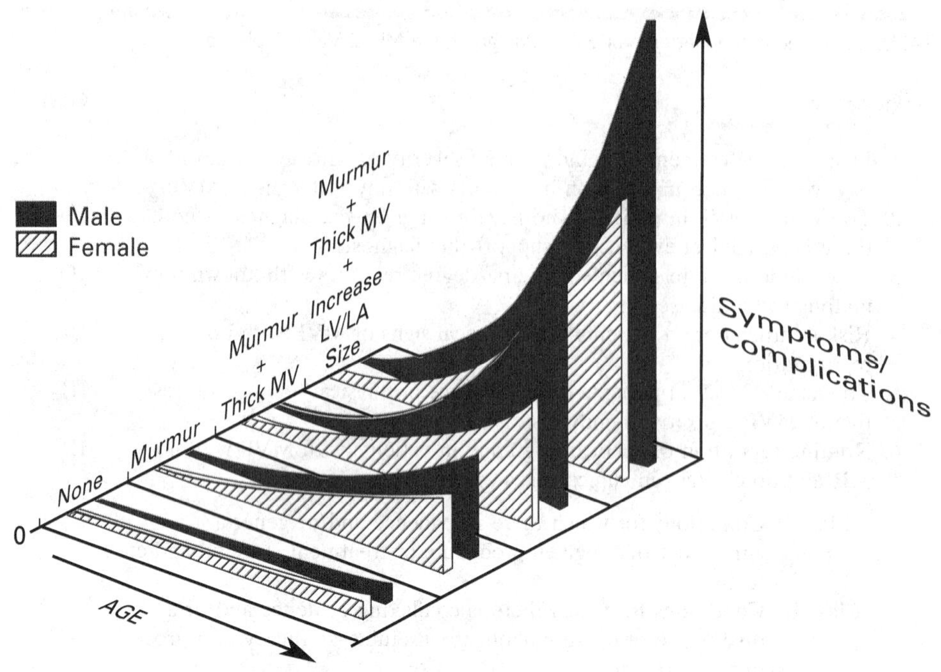

FIGURE 58-7 The relations between cardiac structure, age, and complications in the MVP syndrome. Patients with MVP, typical auscultatory findings, thickening of the valve leaflets, and LV or LA enlargement are at risk of developing complications. When two or more of these findings are present, the likelihood of complications is highest. By contrast, the absence of these features can be used to identify patients with MVP who have an exceedingly low risk. In general, complications increase with age and are more common in males than in females. (From Boudoulas et al.[57] Reproduced with permission from the publisher and authors.)

in patients without this common clinical entity. The gradual progression of MR in patients with mitral prolapse, however, may result in progressive dilatation of the left atrium and ventricle. LA dilatation often results in atrial fibrillation, and moderate to severe MR eventually results in LV dysfunction and the development of congestive heart failure. Pulmonary hypertension may occur with associated right ventricular dysfunction. In some patients with an initially prolonged asymptomatic interval, the entire process may enter an accelerated phase as a result of LA and LV dysfunction, atrial fibrillation, and in certain instances, ruptured mitral valve chordae. The latter occurs more commonly in males and with increasing age.[6,7]

Several long-term prognostic studies suggest that complications occur most commonly in patients with a mitral systolic murmur, thickened redundant mitral valve leaflets, or increased LV or LA size[30,57,58,62] (Fig. 58-7 and Table 58-4).

In a prospective follow-up study of 237 asymptomatic or minimally symptomatic patients with MVP documented by echocardiography, sudden death occurred in 6 patients.[55] In a multivariant analysis of the echocardiographic findings, the presence or absence of redundant mitral valve leaflets by M-mode echocardiography was the only variable associated with sudden death. Ten patients sustained a cerebral embolic event, six of whom were in atrial fibrillation with LA enlargement. Marks et al.[49] confirmed these data in a retrospective 2-D echocardiographic study from 456 patients with MVP. Two groups of patients were compared; those with thickening and redundancy of the mitral valve leaflet and those without leaflet thickening. Complications or a history of complications was more prevalent in those with leaflet thickening and redundancy compared with those without leaflet thickening. The incidence of stroke, however, was similar in the two groups. Long-term follow-up studies in patients with MVP associated with a floppy, myxomatous mitral valve permit several conclusions.[7] Serious complications occur in some patients with MVP, predominantly in those with diagnostic auscultatory findings. Also, redundant mitral valve leaflets and increased LV size are associated with a frequency of serious complications. Finally, men and those over 50 years of age are at increased risk of complications, including severe MR requiring surgery.

Sudden death is the least common but obviously the most severe complication of MVP (Table 58-5). While infrequent, the highest incidence of sudden death has been reported in the familial form of MVP. Some of these patients have been noted to have QT-interval prolongation. Also, patients with MVP with severe autonomic dysfunction and excessive vagotonia resulting in bradyarrhythmias and asystole have been reported.[63,64] Therefore, arrhythmias are likely to be the usual cause of sudden death in patients with MVP, so it seems prudent to limit ambulatory electrocardiographic recordings to those patients at highest risk. Many believe that patients with electrocardiographic ST-T-wave changes are more likely to have complex ventricular arrhythmias.[6,7] Certainly, any patients with symptoms suggestive of arrhythmia or who have arrhythmias noted during physical examination or on the resting ECG should be evaluated further (see Chap. 24).

Infective endocarditis is a serious complication of MVP, and MVP is the leading predisposing cardiovascular diagnosis in most series of patients reported with endocarditis.[6,7,65] Since the absolute incidence of endocarditis is extremely low for the entire MVP population, there has been much discussion concerning the risk of endocarditis in MVP.[66] While there is general agreement that MVP patients with murmurs and/or thickened redundant valves confirmed by echocardiography or cineangiography should receive antibiotic prophylaxis, some authorities state that patients with isolated systolic clicks and no murmurs do not need antibiotic prophylaxis for endocarditis.[67] The dynamic nature of MVP, with variable physical findings on different examinations, makes it difficult to make judgments on the basis of the presence or absence of a systolic murmur. With the increasing use of color-flow echo-Doppler studies, MR often has been observed in patients in whom no murmur is heard.[68] Recommendations for antibiotic endocarditis prophylaxis for patients with MVP undergoing procedures associated with bacteremia are listed in Table 58-6.

As indicated earlier, progressive MR occurs frequently in patients with long-standing MVP. Fibrin emboli are responsible

TABLE 58-4 Use of Echocardiography for Risk Stratification in Mitral Valve Prolapse

Study	No. of Patients	Features Examined	Outcome	p
Nishimura et al., 1985[55]	237	MV leaflet ≥5 mm	↑ sum of sudden death, endocarditis and cerebral embolus	P <0.02
		LVID ≥60 mm	↑ MVR (26 vs. 3.1%)	P <0.001
Zuppiroli et al., 1994[58]	119	MV leaflet >5 mm	↑ complex ventricular arrhythmia	P <0.001
Babuty et al., 1994[61]	58	Undefined MV thickening	No relation to complex ventricular arrhythmias	NS
Takamoto et al., 1991[59]	142	MV leaflet ≥3 mm redundant, low echo density	↑ ruptured chordae (48 vs. 5%)	NS
Marks et al., 1989[49]	456	MV leaflet ≥5 mm	↑ endocarditis (3.5 vs. 0%)	P <0.02
			↑ moderate-severe MR (11.9 vs. 0%)	P <0.001
			↑ MVR (6.6 vs. 0.7%)	P <0.02
			↑ stroke (7.5 vs. 5.8)	NS
Chandraratna et al., 1984[60]	86	MV leaflets >5.1 mm	↑ cardiovascular abnormalities (60 vs. 6%) (Marfan's syndrome, TVP, MR, dilated descending aorta)	P <0.001

NOTE: MV, mitral valve; LVID, left ventricular internal diameter; MVR, mitral valve replacement; MR, mitral regurgitation; TVP, tricuspid valve prolapse.
SOURCE: From ACC/AHA guidelines for the clinical application of echocardiography. *Circulation* 1997; 95:1686–1744.

in some patients for visual problems consistent with involvement of the ophthalmic or posterior cerebral circulation. Several studies have indicated an increased likelihood of cerebral vascular accidents of various types in patients under age 45 who have MVP than would have been expected in a similar population without MVP. Therefore, it has been recommended that antiplatelet drugs such as aspirin be administered to patients who have MVP and suspected cerebral nervous system emboli; however, neither antiplatelet drugs nor anticoagulants should be prescribed routinely for patients with MVP because the incidence of embolic phenomena is very low. Recommendations for aspirin and oral anticoagulants in MVP are listed in Table 58-7. *It is important to avoid the incorrect diagnosis of MVP syndrome. This mistake is especially likely to occur in patients with neuropsychiatric symptoms, in whom an incorrect diagnosis of MVP is made from the ECG. Such an improper diagnosis can form the foundation of a chronic, often disabling cardiac neurosis. Even if the diagnosis of MVP is properly made, it is not necessarily correct to attribute neuropsychiatric symptoms to the MVP* (see also Chap. 80).

TREATMENT

The majority of patients with MVP are asymptomatic and lack the high-risk profile described earlier. These patients with mild or no symptoms and findings of milder forms of prolapse should be assured of a benign prognosis. A normal lifestyle and regular exercise are encouraged.[5,7] For most patients in whom the *diag-*

TABLE 58-5 Mitral Valve Complications in 102 Hearts with Mitral Valve Prolapse

	No.	Percent
Sudden death	0	0
Primary rupture of chordae	7	7
Bacterial endocarditis	7	7
Mitral valve regurgitation	18	18
Primary rupture of chordae	(7)	—
Bacterial endocarditis	(4)	—
Severe prolapse	(4)	—
Entrapped chordae	(3)	—
Fibrin deposits	4	4

SOURCE; Modified from Lucas RV Jr, Edwards JE. The floppy mitral valve. *Curr Probl Cardiol* 1982; 7:1–48.

TABLE 58-6 Recommendations for Antibiotic Endocarditis Prophylaxis for Patients with Mitral Valve Prolapse Undergoing Procedures Associated with Bacteremia

Indication	Class
1. Patients with characteristic systolic click-murmur complex.	I
2. Patients with isolated systolic click and echo evidence of MVP and MR.	I
3. Patients with isolated systolic click, echo evidence of high-risk MVP.	IIa
4. Patients with isolated systolic click and no or equivocal evidence of MVP.	III

SOURCE: From ACC/AHA guidelines for the clinical application of echocardiography. *Circulation* 1997; 95:1686–1744.

TABLE 58-7 Recommendations for Aspirin and Oral Anticoagulants in Mitral Valve Prolapse

Indication	Class
1. Aspirin therapy for cerebral transient ischemic attacks (TIAs).	I
2. Warfarin therapy for patients in atrial fibrillation with age ≥65 yr, hypertension, MR murmur, or history of heart failure.	I
3. Aspirin therapy for patients in atrial fibrillation <65 years old with no history of MR, hypertension, or heart failure.	I
4. Warfarin therapy for poststroke patients.	I
5. Warfarin therapy patients for TIAs despite aspirin therapy.	IIa
6. Aspirin therapy in poststroke patients with contraindications to anticoagulants.	IIa
7. Aspirin therapy for patients in sinus rhythm with echocardiographic evidence of high-risk MVP	IIb

SOURCE: From ACC/AHA guidelines for the clinical application of echocardiography. *Circulation* 1997; 95:1686–1744.

nosis of MVP is definite, we recommend antibiotic prophylaxis for the prevention of infective endocarditis while undergoing procedures associated with bacteremia. Patients with MVP and palpitation associated with sinus tachycardia or mild tachyarrhythmias and those with chest pain, anxiety, or fatigue often respond to therapy with beta blockers.[5,7,69] In many cases, however, the cessation of catecholamine stimulants such as caffeine, alcohol, cigarettes, and certain drugs may be sufficient to control symptoms.

Orthostatic symptoms are best treated with volume expansion, preferably by liberalizing fluid and salt intake. Mineralocorticoid therapy may be needed in severe cases, and wearing support stockings may be beneficial.[7] In sudden death survivors and those patients with symptomatic complex arrhythmias, specific antiarrhythmic therapy should be guided by monitoring techniques, including electrophysiologic testing when indicated[7] (see Chap. 26).

Daily aspirin therapy (80–325 mg/day; see Table 58-7) is recommended for MVP patients with documented focal neurologic events. Such patients also should avoid cigarettes and oral contraceptives. Some clinicians use long-term anticoagulant therapy with warfarin in poststroke patients with prolapse, particularly when symptoms occur on aspirin therapy (see also Chap. 89).

Restriction from competitive sports is recommended when moderate LV enlargement, LV dysfunction, uncontrolled tachyarrhythmias, long QT interval, unexplained syncope, prior sudden death survival, or aortic root enlargement is present, individually or in combination.[7]

The familial occurrence of MVP should be explained to the patient and is particularly important in those with associated disease, who are at greater risk for complications. Screening relatives can uncover high-risk individuals and potentially prevent some complications. There is no contraindication to pregnancy based on the diagnosis of MVP alone.

Patients with severe MR with symptoms and/or impaired LV systolic function require cardiac catheterization studies and evaluation for mitral valve surgery.[70] The thickened, redundant mitral valve often can be repaired rather than replaced, with a low operative mortality and excellent long-term results.[71–79] Follow-up studies also suggest lower thromboembolic and endocarditis risk than with prosthetic valves.

Asymptomatic patients with MVP and no significant MR can be evaluated clinically every 2 to 3 years. Echocardiography has been suggested every 5 years in such patients to help determine the natural history and the likelihood of complications. Patients with MVP who have high-risk characteristics, including those with moderate to severe MR, should be followed more frequently, even if no symptoms are present.

Surgical Considerations

Management of the patient with MVP may require valve surgery, particularly in those patients who develop a flail mitral leaflet due to rupture of chordae tendineae or their marked elongation.[79] Most such valves can be repaired successfully by surgeons experienced with mitral valve repair, especially when the posterior leaflet valve is predominantly affected. Symptoms of heart failure, the severity of MR, the presence or absence of atrial fibrillation, LV systolic function, LV end-diastolic and end-systolic volumes, and pulmonary artery pressure (rest and exercise) all influence the decision to recommend mitral valve surgery. Recommendations for surgery in patients with MVP and MR are the same as for those with other forms of nonischemic severe MR and include class III–IV symptoms, LV ejection fraction less than 60 percent, and/or marked increases in LV end-diastolic and end-systolic volumes. If mitral repair is likely to be successful, severe MR with class II symptoms or atrial fibrillation may be an appropriate reason for surgical referral.[51]

References

1. Freed LA, Levy D, Levine RA, et al. Prevalence and clinical outcomes of mitral valve prolapse. *N Engl J Med* 1999; 341:1–7.
2. Nishimura R, McGoon MD. Perspectives on mitral-valve prolapse. *N Eng J Med* 1999; 341:48–58.
3. Reid JV. Mid-systolic clicks. *S Afr Med J* 1961; 35:353–357.
4. Barlow JB, Pocok WA, Marchand P, Denny M. The significance of late systolic murmurs. *Am Heart J* 1963; 66:443–452.
5. O'Rourke RA, Crawford MH. The systolic click-murmur syndrome: Clinical recognition and management. *Curr Probl Cardiol* 1976; 1(1):1.
6. Lucas RV Jr, Edwards JE. The floppy mitral valve. *Curr Probl Cardiol* 1982; 7:1–48.
7. Fontana ME, Sparks EA, Boudoulas H, Wooley CF. Mitral valve prolapse in the mitral valve prolapse syndrome. *Curr Probl Cardiol* 1991; 16:315–375.
8. O'Rourke RA. The mitral valve prolapse syndrome. In: Chizner MA, ed. *Classic Teachings in Clinical Cardiology*. Cedar Grove, NJ: Laennec; 1996:1049–1070.
9. Devereux RB. Recent developments in the diagnosis and management of mitral valve prolapse. *Curr Opin Cardiol* 1995; 10:107–116.
10. Perloff JK, Roberts WC. The mitral apparatus: Functional anatomy of mitral regurgitation. *Circulation* 1972; 46:227–239.
11. Devereux RB, Brown WT, Kramer-Fox R, Sachs I. Inheritance of mitral valve prolapse: Effect of age and sex on gene expression. *Ann Intern Med* 1982; 97:826–832.
12. Shell WE, Walton JA, Clifford ME, Willis PW III. The familial

occurrence of the syndrome of mid-late systolic click and late systolic murmur. *Circulation* 1969; 39:327–338.
13. Savage DD, Garrison RJ, Devereux RB, et al. Mitral valve prolapse in the general population: I. Epidemiologic features: The Framingham Study. *Am Heart J* 1983; 106:571–576.
14. Procacci PM, Savran SV, Schrieter SL, Bryson AL. Prevalence of clinical mitral valve prolapse in 1169 young women. *N Engl J Med* 1976; 294:1086–1088.
15. Leier CV, Call TD, Fulkerson PK, Wooley CF. The spectrum of cardiac defects in the Ehlers-Danlos syndrome, types I & III. *Ann Intern Med* 1980; 92:171–178.
16. Lebwohl MG, Distefano D, Prioleau PG, et al. Pseudoxanthoma elasticum and mitral valve prolapse. *N Engl J Med* 1982; 307:228–231.
17. Schwartz T, Gotsman MS. Mitral valve prolapse in osteogenesis imperfecta. *Isr J Med Sci* 1981; 17:1087–1088.
18. Udoshi MB, Shah A, Fisher VJ, Dolgin M. Incidence of mitral valve prolapse in subjects with thoracic skeletal abnormalities: A prospective study. *Am Heart J* 1979; 97:303–311.
19. Bon Tempo CP, Ronan JA Jr. Radiographic appearance of the thorax in systolic click: Late systolic murmur syndrome. *Am J Cardiol* 1975; 36:27–31.
20. Crawford MH, O'Rourke RA. Mitral valve prolapse syndrome. In: Isselbacher KJ, Adams RD, Braunwald E, et al, eds. *Update I: Harrison's Principles of Internal Medicine*. New York: McGraw-Hill; 1981:91–152.
21. O'Rourke RA. The syndrome of mitral valve prolapse. In: Albert JA, ed. *Valvular Heart Disease*. New York: Lippincott-Raven; 1999:157–182.
22. Tei C, Sakamaki T, Shah PM, et al. Mitral valve prolapse in short-term experimental coronary occlusion: A possible mechanism of ischemic mitral regurgitation. *Circulation* 1983; 68:183–189.
23. Crawford MH. Mitral valve prolapse due to coronary artery disease. *Am J Med* 1977; 62:447–451.
24. Tomaru T, Uchida Y, Mohri N. Post-inflammatory mitral and aortic valve prolapse: A clinical and pathological study. *Circulation* 1987; 76:68–76.
25. Lembo NJ, Dell'Italia LJ, Crawford MH, et al. Mitral valve prolapse in patients with prior rheumatic fever. *Circulation* 1988; 77:830–836.
26. Marcus RH, Sareli P, Pocock WA, et al. Functional anatomy of severe mitral regurgitation in active rheumatic carditis. *Am J Cardiol* 1986; 63:577–584.
27. Crawford MH, O'Rourke RA. Mitral valve prolapse: A cardiomyopathic state? *Prog Cardiovasc Dis* 1984; 27:133–139.
28. Lax D, Eicher M, Goldberg SJ. Mild dehydration induces echocardiographic signs of mitral valve prolapse in healthy females with prior normal cardiac findings. *Am Heart J* 1992; 124:1533–1540.
29. Krivokapich J, Child JS, Dadourian BJ, Perloff JK. Reassessment of echocardiographic criteria for the diagnosis of mitral valve prolapse. *Am J Cardiol* 1988; 61:131–135.
30. Fukuda N, Oki T, Iuchi A, et al. Predisposing factors for severe mitral regurgitation in idiopathic mitral valve prolapse. *Am J Cardiol* 1995; 76(7):503–507.
31. Gaffney FA, Karlsson ES, Campbell W, et al. Autonomic dysfunction in women with mitral valve prolapse. *Circulation* 1979; 59:894–899.
32. Boudoulas H, Reynolds JC, Mazzaferri E, Wooley CF. Metabolic studies in mitral valve prolapse syndrome. *Circulation* 1980; 61:1200–1205.
33. Anwar A, Kohn SR, Dunn JF, et al. Altered beta-adrenergic receptor function in subjects with symptomatic mitral valve prolapse. *Am J Med Sci* 1991; 302:89–97.
34. Santos AD, Puthenpurakal MK, Ahmad H, et al. Orthostatic hypotension: A commonly unrecognized cause of symptoms in mitral valve prolapse. *Am J Med* 1981; 71:746–750.
35. Betriu A, Wigle ED, Felderhof CH, McLoughlin MJ. Prolapse of the posterior leaflet of the mitral valve associated with secundum atrial septal defect. *Am J Cardiol* 1975; 35:363–369.
36. LeWinter MM, Hoffman JR, Shell WE, et al. Phuenylephrine-induced atypical chest pain in patients with prolapsing mitral valve leaflets. *Am J Cardiol* 1974; 34:12–18.
37. Sabom MB, Curry RC Jr, Pepine CJ, et al. Ergonovine testing for coronary artery spasm in patients with angiographic mitral valve prolapse. *Cathet Cardiovasc Diagn* 1978; 4:265–274.
38. Barnett HJM, Jones MW, Boughner DR, Kostuck WJ. Cerebral ischemic events associated with prolapsing mitral valve. *Arch Neurol* 1976; 33:777–782.
39. Barletta GA, Gagliardi R, Benvenuti L, Fantini F. Cerebral ischemic attacks as a complication of aortic and mitral valve prolapse. *Stroke* 1985; 16:219–223.
40. Barnett HJM, Boughner DR, Taylor DW, et al. Further evidence relating mitral valve prolapse to cerebral ischemic event. *N Engl J Med* 1980; 302:139–144.
41. Petty GW, Orencia AJ, Khandheria BK, Whisnant JP. A population-based study of stroke in the setting of mitral valve prolapse: Risk factors and infarct subtype classification. *Mayo Clin Proc* 1994; 69:632–634.
42. Orencia AJ, Petty GW, Khandheria BK, et al. Mitral valve prolapse and the risk of stroke after initial cerebral ischemia. *Neurology* 1995; 45:1083–1086.
43. Gilon D, Buonanno FS, Jaffee MM, et al. Lack of evidence of an association between mitral valve prolapse and stroke in young patients. *N Engl J Med* 1999; 341:8–13.
44. Wilson LA, Keeling PW, Malcolm AD, et al. Visual complications of mitral leaflet prolapse. *Br Med J* 1977; 2:86–88.
45. Chesler E, King RA, Edwards JE. The myxomatous mitral valve and sudden death. *Circulation* 1983; 67:632–639.
46. Weis AJ, Salcedo EE, Stewart WJ, et al. Anatomic explanation of mobile systolic clicks: Implications for the clinical and echocardiographic diagnosis of mitral valve prolapse. *Am Heart J* 1995; 129:314–320.
47. Bhutto ZR, Barron JT, Liebson PR, et al. Electrocardiographic abnormalities in mitral valve prolapse. *Am J Cardiol* 1992; 70:265–266.
48. Schaal SF. Ventricular arrhythmias in patients with mitral valve prolapse. *Cardiovasc Clin* 1992; 22(1):307–316.
49. Marks AR, Choong CY, Sanfilippo AJ, et al. Identification of high-risk and low-risk subgroups of patients with mitral valve prolapse. *N Engl J Med* 1989; 320:1031–1036.
50. Shah PM. Echocardiographic diagnosis of mitral valve prolapse. *J Am Soc Echocardiogr* 1994; 7(3 pt 1):286–293.
51. Bonow RO, Carabello B, De Leon AC Jr, et al. ACC/AHA guidelines for the management of patients with valvular heart disease. *J Am Coll Cardiol* 1998; 32:1486–1588.
52. Klein GJ, Kostuck WJ, Bougher DR, Chamberlain MJ. Stress myocardial imaging in mitral leaflet prolapse syndrome. *Am J Cardiol* 1978; 42:746–750.
53. Allen H, Harris A, Leatham A. Significance and prognosis of an isolated late systolic murmur: A 9- to 22-year follow-up. *Br Heart J* 1974; 36:525–532.
54. Mills P, Rose J, Hollingsworth J, et al. Long-term prognosis of mitral valve prolapse. *N Engl J Med* 1977; 297:13–18.
55. Nishimura RA, McGood MD, Shub C, et al. Echocardiographically documented mitral-valve prolapse: Long-term follow-up of 237 patients. *N Engl J Med* 1985; 313:1305–1309.
56. Düren DR, Becker AE, Dunning AJ. Long-term follow-up of idiopathic mitral valve prolapse in 300 patients: A prospective study. *J Am Coll Cardiol* 1988; 11:42–47.
57. Boudoulas H, Kolibash BH, Wooley CF. Mitral valve prolapse: A heterogenous disorder. *Prim Cardiol* 1991; 17:29–43.
58. Zuppiroli A, Rinaldi M, Kramer-Fox R, et al. Natural history of mitral valve prolapse. *Am J Cardiol* 1995; 75:1028–1032.
59. Takamoto T, Nitta M, Tsujibayashi T, et al. The prevalence and

clinical features of pathologically abnormal mitral valve leaflets (myxomatous mitral valve) in the mitral valve prolapse syndrome: An echocardiographic and pathologic comparative study. *J Cardiol Suppl* 1991; 25:75–86.
60. Chandraratna PAN, Nimalasuriya A, Kawanishi D, et al. Identification of the increased frequency of cardiovascular abnormalities associated with mitral valve prolapse by two-dimensional echocardiography. *Am J Cardiol* 1984; 54:1283–1285.
61. Babuty D, Cosnay P, Breuillac JC, et al. Ventricular arrhythmia factors in mitral valve prolapse. *PACE* 1994; 17:1090–1099.
62. Cheitlin MD, Alpert JS, Armstrong WF, et al. ACC/AHA guidelines for the clinical application of echocardiography. *Circulation* 1997; 95:1686–1744.
63. Cosgrove DM, Stewart WJ. Mitral valvuloplasty. *Curr Probl Cardiol* 1989; 14:359–415.
64. Kirklin JW. Mitral valve repair for mitral incompetence. *Mod Concepts Cardiovasc Dis* 1987; 56:7–11.
65. Marshall CE, Shappel SD. Sudden death and the ballooning posterior leaflet syndrome: Detailed anatomic and histochemical investigation. *Arch Pathol* 1974; 98:134–138.
66. Clemens JD, Horwitz RI, Jaffe CC, et al. A controlled evaluation of the risk of bacterial endocarditis in persons with mitral valve prolapse. *N Engl J Med* 1982; 307:776–781.
67. Devereux RB, Frary CJ, Kramer-Fox R, et al. Cost-effectiveness of infective endocarditis prophylaxis for mitral valve prolapse with or without a mitral regurgitant murmur. *Am J Cardiol* 1994; 74:1024–1029.
68. Dajani AS, Bisno AL, Chung KJ, et al. Prevention of bacterial endocarditis: Recommendations by the American Heart Association. *JAMA* 1990; 264:2919–2922.
69. Winkle RA, Lopes MG, Goodman DJ, et al. Propranolol for patients with mitral valve prolapse. *Am Heart J* 1977; 93:422–427.
70. Galloway AC, Colvin SB, Baumann FG, et al. Current concepts of mitral valve reconstruction for mitral insufficiency. *Circulation* 1988; 78:1087–1098.
71. Cheitlin MD. The timing of surgery in mitral and aortic valve disease. *Curr Probl Cardiol* 1987; 12:75–149.
72. Cosgrove DM, Stewart WJ. Mitral valvuloplasty. *Curr Probl Cardiol* 1989; 14:359–415.
73. Kirklin JW. Mitral valve repair for mitral incompetence. *Mod Concepts Cardiovasc Dis* 1987; 56:7–11.
74. Cohn LH, Couper GS, Aranki SF, et al. Long-term results of mitral valve reconstruction for regurgitation of the myxomatous mitral valve. *J Thorac Cardiovasc Surg* 1994; 107:143–150.
75. Eishi K, Kawazoe K, Sasako Y, et al. Comparison of repair techniques for mitral valve prolapse. *J Heart Valve Dis* 1994; 3:432–438.
76. Perier P, Clausnizer B, Mistarz K. Carpentier "sliding leaflet" technique for repair of the mitral valve: Early results. *Ann Thorac Surg* 1994; 57:383–386.
77. Eishi K, Kawazoe K, Sasako Y, et al. Comparison of repair techniques for mitral valve prolapse. *J Heart Valve Dis* 1994; 3:432–438.
78. Perier P, Clausnizer B, Mistarz K. Carpentier sliding leaflet technique for repair of the mitral valve: Early results. *Ann Thorac Surg* 1994; 57:383–386.
79. Ling LH, Enriquez-Sarano M, Seward JB, et al. Clinical outcome of mitral regurgitation due to flail leaflet. *N Engl J Med* 1996; 335;1417–1423.

C H A P T E R 59

TRICUSPID VALVE, PULMONIC VALVE, AND MULTIVALVULAR DISEASE

Robert A. O'Rourke

DEFINITION, ETIOLOGY, AND PATHOLOGY

Tricuspid Valve Disease

Tricuspid valve dysfunction can occur with normal or abnormal valves.[1] When normal tricuspid values develop dysfunction, the resulting hemodynamic abnormality is almost always pure regurgitation. Tricuspid regurgitation (TR) occurs when the tricuspid valve allows blood to enter the right atrium (RA) during a right ventricular (RV) contraction. Tricuspid stenosis (TS) results from obstruction to diastolic flow across the valve during filling of the RV. A diagrammatic illustration of tricuspid valve disease and the prevalence of various pathologic etiologies are shown in Fig. 59-1*A* and *B*.

Diseases causing TR are more numerous than those causing TS. It is important to note that the normal tricuspid valve often does not completely coapt in systole, as is shown by the frequent occurrence of TR jets on Doppler ultrasound. Usually the volume of regurgitant blood is so small that the TR is silent; this finding occurs in 24 to 96 percent of normal individuals by Doppler ultrasound and thus must be considered a variant of normal.[2–4] Pathologic TR is most commonly due to diseases that cause RV dilatation and failure;[5] left ventricular (LV) failure and/or pulmonary hypertension can result in tricuspid regurgitation (Table 59-1). Primary diseases of the tricuspid valve apparatus, which includes the tricuspid annulus, the leaflets, the chordae, the papillary muscle, and the RV wall, also cause TR (Table 59-1).[6–8] The most common etiology of isolated TR is infective endocarditis in drug addicts[9] (see Chap. 73). Less common causes include myocardial infarction, trauma, carcinoid, leaflet prolapse, and such congenital abnormalities as atrial septal defect and Ebstein's anomaly[10–15] (see Chap. 63). TR also occurs in patients with rheumatoid arthritis, radiation therapy, and Marfan's syndrome.[6] Primary involvement of the tricuspid valve due to rheumatic fever results in TS, usually in association with TR (Fig. 59-2).

The most common cause of TS is rheumatic fever. This is usually associated with concomitant mitral stenosis (MS). Isolated TS can be seen with the carcinoid syndrome, infective endocarditis, endocardial fibroelastosis, endomyocardial fibrosis, and systemic lupus erythematosus, among other conditions[6–8] (Table 59-2). It has also been reported to occur in patients with Fabry's disease, or Whipple's disease and in patients receiving methysergide therapy.[6] Mechanical obstruction of the valve can be due to a RA myxoma, tumor metastases, and thrombi in the RA, each resulting in the hemodynamic abnormalities of TS.[16,17] In addition, RV inflow tract obstruction can result from thrombosis endocarditis, degeneration, or calcification affecting a prosthetic tricuspid valve.

In rheumatic tricuspid valve disease, alterations in the valve are characterized by fibrosis, with contracture of the leaflets and commissural fusion. The former leads to TR and the latter to TS.[18] The stenotic component of rheumatic tricuspid valve disease is often minor and would go unrecognized clinically if it were not for the high flow across the valve caused by the coexistent regurgitation. Whenever the tricuspid valve is affected by rheumatic disease, there is also involvement of left-sided valves.[19] Flammang and associates observed that 9.5 per-

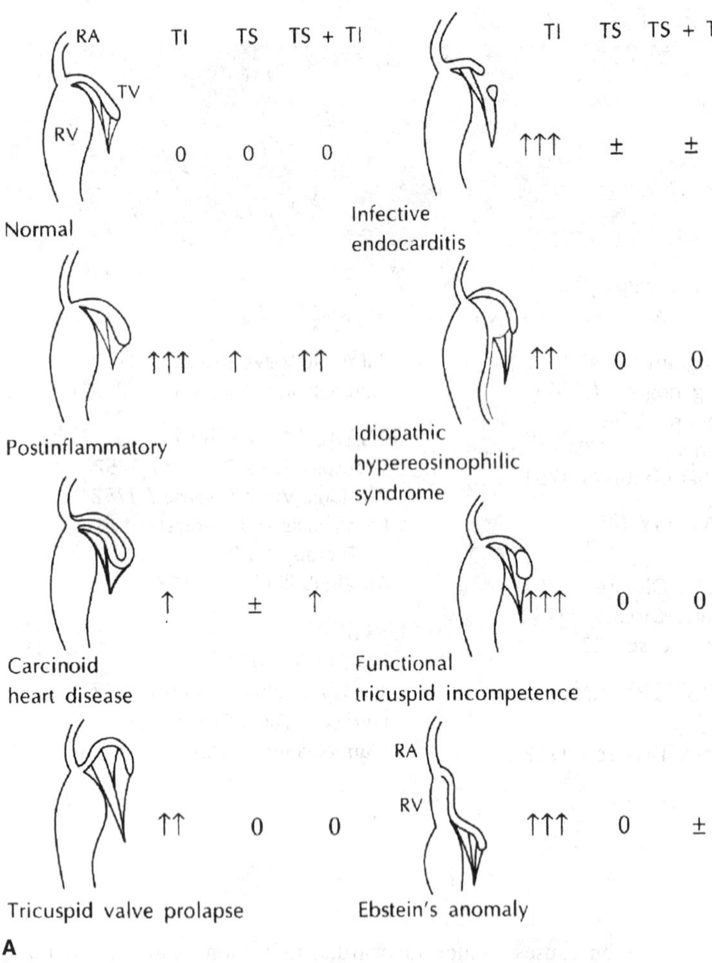

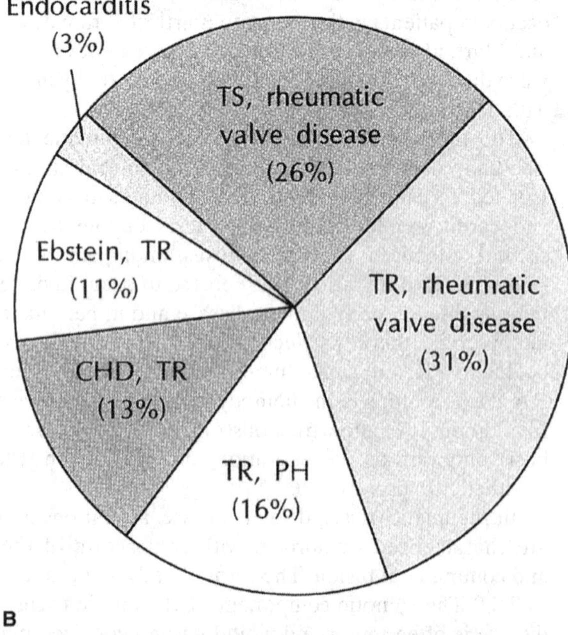

FIGURE 59-1 *A.* Tricuspid valve (TV) disease. Diagrammatic illustration of TV; TI, tricuspid insufficiency; TS, tricuspid stenosis; RA, right atrium; RV, right ventricle. *B.* Pathologic findings in TV. TR, tricuspid regurgitation; TS, tricuspid stenosis. [From Virmani R et al. Pathology of valvular heart diseases. In: Rahimtoola SH, ed. Philadelphia: Mosby (Current Medicine, Inc.), 1997:116, with permission.]

cent of cases requiring surgical replacement of *both* the mitral and aortic valves also had rheumatic involvement of the tricuspid valve.[20]

Carcinoid heart disease is present in up to 53 percent of patients with malignant carcinoid tumor (usually originating in the ileum) with extensive metastases[15] (see Chap. 77). Carcinoid usually causes TR and TS and, less often, pulmonic stenosis (PS) and pulmonic regurgitation (PR).[21,22] Changes include deposits of fibrous tissue on the surfaces of these valves. Fibrous plaques can also develop on the endocardial surfaces of the RA and RV as well as on the intima of the coronary sinus and the pulmonary artery.[23] The hemodynamic effects result from the rigidity and contracture of the fibrous tissues deposited on the valves. Although TS may result, the major functional abnormality is usually TR.

The most common type of TR is the secondary type that results from the enlargement of the orifice and annulus secondary to congestive heart failure with RV dilation due to LV disease (Table 59-1). TR may diminish when the heart failure is treated successfully but can be permanent with long-standing dilatation of the RV.[24–26] In infective endocarditis, the TR results from improper coaptation of the leaflets because of interposed vegetations (Table 59-1). Major degrees of regurgitation may be due to rupture of chordae tendineae of the RV or perforation of the valve leaflets.

Until recently, myocardial infarction was not considered a common cause of TR except when secondary to chronic congestive heart failure.[27] Rare cases have been described from rupture of an RV papillary muscle.[28,29] Currently, RV infarction is being recognized more often and is frequently associated with TR, as documented by echocardiography (see Chap. 42).

Various degrees of tricuspid valve prolapse are commonly present in the general population and may occur in 3 to 54 percent in patients with mitral valve prolapse[22] (see Chap. 58). The reported incidence of *severe* TR from prolapse is low.[30]

External blunt trauma, most often in motor vehicle accidents, is a classic cause of TR. Isolated instances of rupture of a tricuspid papillary muscle have been described from external cardiopulmonary resuscitation.[31] Traumatic TR usually results from rupture of one or more of the components of the tensor apparatus, with disruption of the papillary muscle occurring more often than rupture of the chordae.[13] Less frequently, there is a laceration of leaflet tissue.[32,33] Occasionally, traumatic TR and ruptured ventricular septum coexist[34] (Chap. 79). TR can also occur from iatrogenic trauma produced during an endomyocardial biopsy.[35,36] Mild TR often results when a pacemaker is placed across a normally functioning tricuspid valve or after extraction of permanent pacemaker leads.[37]

Tolerance to traumatic TR varies, with up to 39 years of survival reported.[38–40] Patients with rupture of a papillary muscle tend to tolerate the TR less well than do those in whom the trauma resulted in rupture of chordae.[39] Among reported cases of TR

TABLE 59-1 Diseases Causing Acquired Tricuspid Valve Regurgitation

Disease Causing Pulmonary Hypertension
All LV diseases with LV failure
Mitral stenosis or mitral regurgitation
Pulmonary venous obstruction
Diseases causing an increase in pulmonary vascular resistance
Primary pulmonary hypertension
Acquired pulmonary vascular disease (atrial septal defects), ventricular septal defects, and patent ductus arteriosus
Intrinsic pulmonary disease (chronic obstructive pulmonary disease, pulmonary fibrosis, and pulmonary resection)
Collagen vascular diseases
Pulmonary emboli, acute and chronic
Primary Diseases of the Tricuspid Valve
Rheumatic heart disease
Rheumatoid arthritis
Trauma, penetrating and nonpenetrating
Radiation therapy
Carcinoid heart disease
RA myxoma
Infective endocarditis
Eosinophilic myocarditis
Prosthetic and bioprosthetic valve malfunction, including thrombosis and calcification
RV myocardial infarction
Myxomatous tricuspid valve (tricuspid valve prolapse)

Source: Modified from Cheitlin and MacGregor,[22] with permission.

resulting from the rupture of the chordae, a traumatic etiology is more common than is infective endocarditis.[41] Primary congenital lesions of the tricuspid valve that cause regurgitation are Ebstein's malformation and valvular dysplasia, as discussed in Chap. 64.

Pulmonic Valve Disease

Acquired lesions of the pulmonic valve generally cause PR (Table 59-3). On rare occasions, an inflammatory process can create stenosis and regurgitation of the valve. Pulmonary hypertension from any cause, such as MS, chronic lung disease, or pulmonary emboli, can produce PR. Inflammatory diseases, such as endocarditis, rheumatic fever, and, rarely, tuberculosis, can result in PR.[42–45]

PS is created by obstruction of systolic flow across the valve and is most commonly congenital (Fig. 59-3; see Chaps. 63 and 64). Sarcomas and myxomas can sometimes extend to the pulmonic valve, causing PS.[46] Previous cardiac surgery on a congenital pulmonic valve lesion can result in PR. The carcinoid syndrome with cardiac involvement can create mild PS and associated PR[44] (Fig. 59-4). Compression of the pulmonary artery can stimulate valvular stenosis and is rarely produced by tumor, aneurysm, or even constrictive pericarditis.

Multivalvular Disease

Multivalvular disease includes mixed single valve disease [e.g., aortic stenosis (AS) plus aortic regurgitation (AR)] or combined disease affecting two or more values (e.g., MS plus TR). Rheumatic fever remains an important cause of combined disease of the mitral and aortic valves. Primary involvement of the tricuspid valve in the rheumatic process is unusual, and more commonly TR results from RV failure secondary to LV decompensation in valvular heart disease. A high prevalence of anatomic lesions involving two or more valves is present when the characteristic Aschoff body is observed at necropsy.[47] Connective tissue diseases (see Chap. 76) can affect both the aortic and the mitral valves. For example, in Marfan's syndrome mitral valve prolapse, resulting in MR, often occurs together with the frequently observed changes in the aortic valve and ascending aorta. In the aging patient, calcification can develop in the aortic valve and the mitral valve apparatus as well as in the mitral annulus. Finally, infective endocarditis of the aortic or mitral valve can extend to the adjacent valve apparatus. In an autopsy series, combined aortic and mitral valve disease was observed in 33 percent of 996 patients with rheumatic fever.[48] In a 30-year follow-up of 1042 children with a history of rheumatic fever, multiple-valve involvement became apparent in 50 percent of

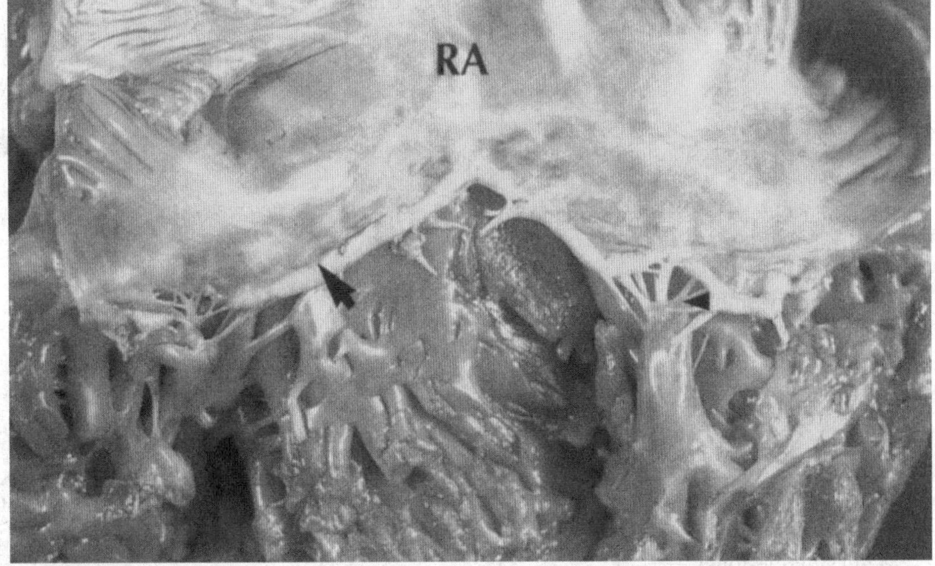

FIGURE 59-2 Heart displaying a tricuspid valve with fused, shortened chordae and rolled, thickened, fibrotic edge, consistent with chronic rheumatic heart disease. Isolated rheumatic TR or TS is very rare; it occurs almost always in the presence of concomitant MS. RA, right atrium. [From Farb A et al. Anatomy and pathology of the right ventricle (including acquired tricuspid and pulmonic valve disease). *Card Clin North Am* 1993; 10:1–2, with permission.]

TABLE 59-2 Diseases Causing Acquired Tricuspid Valve Stenosis

Rheumatic heart disease (usually with mitral stenosis)
Carcinoid heart disease
Fabry's disease
Whipple's disease
Endocardial fibroelastosis
Endomyocardial fibrosis
Methysergide therapy
Systemic lupus endocarditis
RA myxoma or thrombus
Prosthetic valve thrombosis
Prosthetic valve infective endocarditis
Paraprosthetic valve degeneration and calcification

SOURCE: Modified from Cheitlin and MacGregor,[22] with permission.

the individuals.[49] Bland and Jones followed 699 patients with cardiac involvement due to rheumatic fever for 20 years; 99 percent eventually exhibited aortic and mitral valve abnormalities.[50]

Rheumatic fever, myxomatous proliferation and prolapse, calcification in the aged, and infective endocarditis can impair both the aortic and mitral valves. The inflammatory process of rheumatic fever thickens and scars valve leaflets, which leads to fusion, fibrosis, and calcification (Fig. 59-5).

Myxomatous proliferation and valvular prolapse occur in the aortic, tricuspid, and pulmonic valves as well as in the mitral valve (Fig. 59-6). Fusiform aneurysms of the aortic sinus and ascending aorta can develop in Marfan's syndrome; a dilated annulus, prolapse, ruptured chordae, and annular calcification can affect the mitral valve (Fig. 59-7). Annular dilatation, with or without prolapse, is a major cause of mitral regurgitation (MR) in Marfan's syndrome,[51] and most of the patients with Marfan's syndrome have mitral valve prolapse (see Chaps. 60 and 76).

TABLE 59-3 Acquired Lesions of the Pulmonic Valve

Pulmonary hypertension with pulmonic regurgitation
Mitral stenosis
Chronic lung disease
Pulmonary emboli
Inflammatory lesions
Endocarditis
Rheumatic fever
Tuberculosis
Tumors
Sarcoma
Myxoma
Previous surgery or angioplasty for congenital lesions
Mediastinal lesions
Tumor
Aneurysm
Constrictive pericarditis
Miscellaneous
Carcinoid syndrome

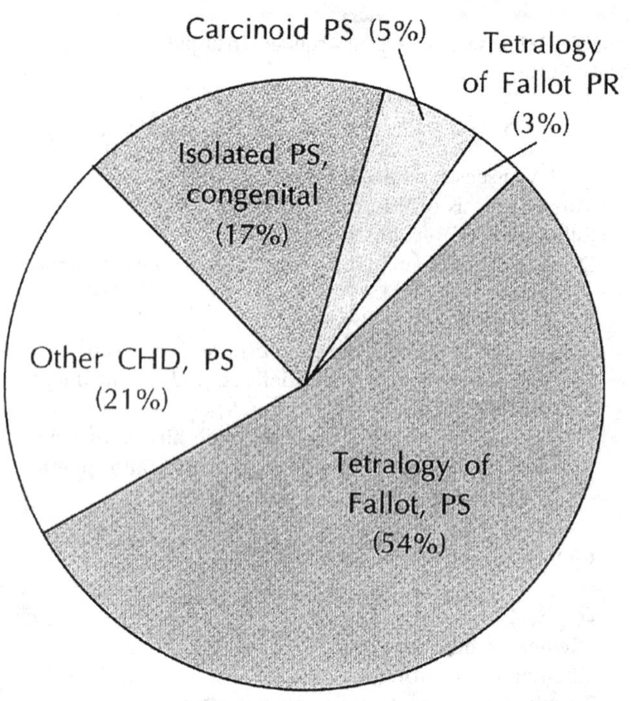

FIGURE 59-3 Pathologic findings in pulmonary valve (PV) replacement. CHD, congenital heart disease; PH, pulmonary hypertension; PR, pulmonary regurgitation; PS, pulmonary stenosis; TR, tricuspid regurgitation; TS, tricuspid stenosis. (Adapted from Altricher PM et al. Surgical pathology of the pulmonary valve; a study of 116 cases spanning 15 years. *Mayo Clin Proc* 1989; 64:1352–1360, with permission.)

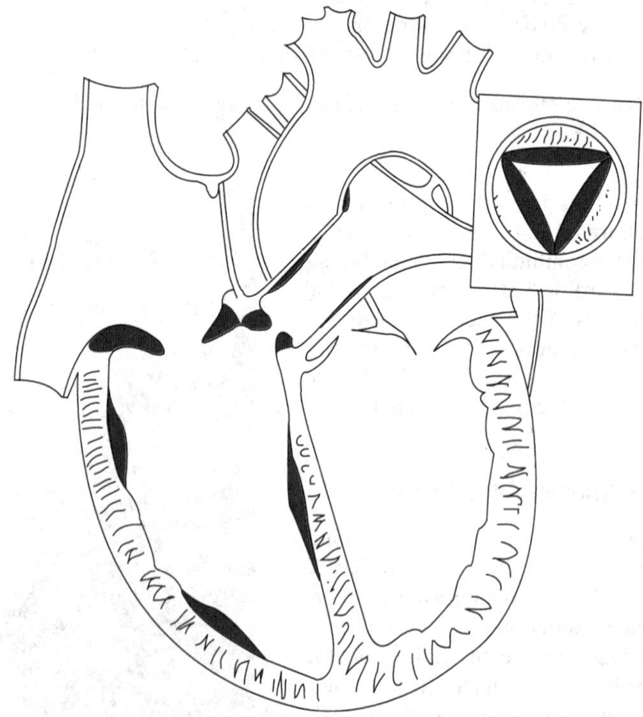

FIGURE 59-4 Carcinoid heart disease. The insert shows PS. The leaflets of the tricuspid valve are thickened. The valve is predominantly incompetent and causes PR. Fibrous plaques are deposited on the lining of the right ventricle and pulmonary trunk. (From Edwards JE. Effects of malignant noncardiac tumors upon the cardiovascular system. *Cardiovasc Clin* 1971; 4:282. Reproduced with permission from the publisher and author.)

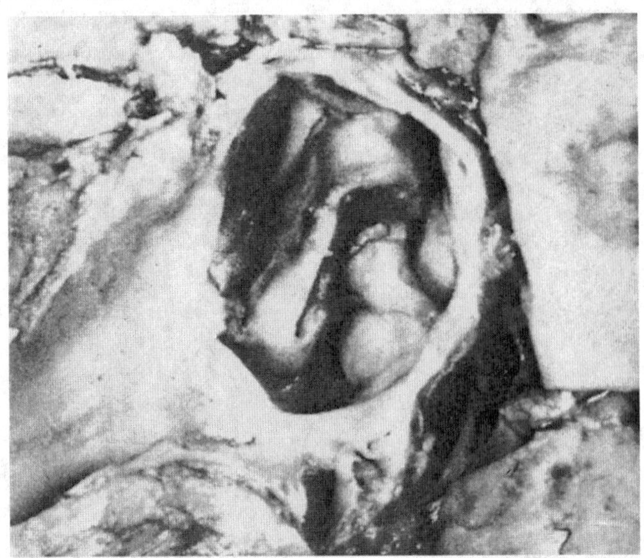

A

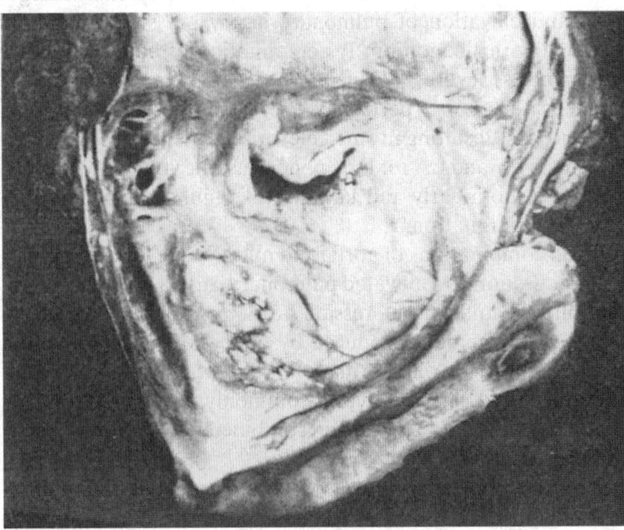

B

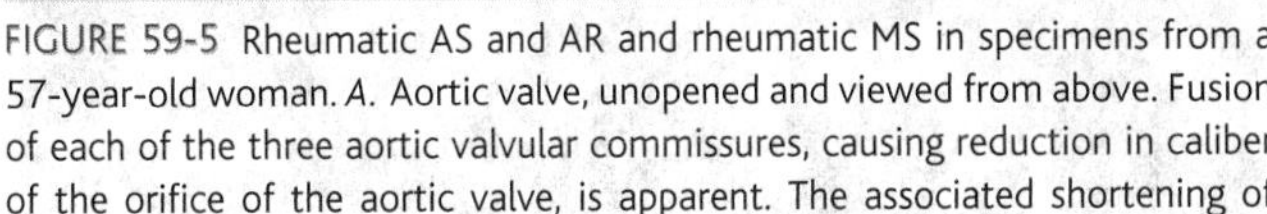

FIGURE 59-5 Rheumatic AS and AR and rheumatic MS in specimens from a 57-year-old woman. *A*. Aortic valve, unopened and viewed from above. Fusion of each of the three aortic valvular commissures, causing reduction in caliber of the orifice of the aortic valve, is apparent. The associated shortening of the cusps results in aortic regurgitation. *B*. Mitral valve, unopened and viewed from above, and opened LA. The mitral valve shows fusion at each of the commissures. The orifice is reduced in caliber. The LA is large, and calcification of the posterior part of the LA wall is present (lower part of figure).

In aging patients, calcification can involve the aortic and mitral valves. Aortic stenosis is common, whereas mitral annular calcification usually creates regurgitation (Fig. 59-8). Infective endocarditis can extend from either the aortic or the mitral valve to the adjacent valve through the inflammatory process (Fig. 59-9).

PATHOPHYSIOLOGY

Tricuspid Valve Disease

In TR, the systolic blood flow into the RA elevates the mean RA pressure.[52] Regurgitant flow produces a prominent *cv* wave reflected through the venous system. Diastolic volume overload of the RV causes further dilatation of the RV and movement of the intraventricular septum toward the LV during diastole. RV failure further raises the mean RA and vena caval pressures and results in systemic venous congestion and signs of RV failure.[22]

TR decreases diastolic flow across the valve, elevates the RA pressure, and reduces the cardiac output.[1,53,54] With TS, there is stiffening of the valve by fibrosis and commissural fusion, both of which narrow the effective valvular orifice.[1,22] Flow from systemic veins or RA into the RV is obstructed, and a pressure gradient develops in diastole between the RA and RV. The normal area of the tricuspid valve is 7 cm^2, and impairment of RV filling occurs when the valve area is reduced to less than 1.5 cm^2. Elevation of the mean RA pressure above 10 mmHg usually results in peripheral edema. Development of atrial fibrillation produces a higher RA pressure in TS than when sinus rhythm and normal RA contraction are present. The hemodynamic abnormalities in TS can be further influenced by coexisting MS. Reduced RV flow in tricuspid valve obstruction has been proposed as a mechanism for protection against severe pulmonary hypertension.

Pulmonic Valve Disease

Pulmonic regurgitation is the most frequently acquired lesion of the pulmonic valve (Table 59-3). Regurgitation may be secondary to pulmonary hypertension or may be caused by primary abnormalities in the leaflets. PR imposes a volume overload on the RV, and if pulmonic hypertension preexists, the overload is superimposed on hypertrophied myocardium. Volume overload of the RV may cause an increase in diastolic volume of the chamber, an increase in RV stroke volume, and subsequent RV failure, resulting in TR.[1,22] Fortunately, isolated PR can usually be tolerated for a long time without cardiac decompensation.[55]

Multivalvular Disease

Multiple valve diseases affecting the mitral and aortic valves can produce a pressure overload, volume overload, or combinations of the two.[1,22] In the presence of combined valvular lesions, the pressure overload will cause concentric LV hypertrophy, even if myocardial failure develops.[1,23] An LV volume overload will result from AR and MR, and further dilatation will follow, with development of heart failure.[1,22] The combination of MS and AR usually results in a volume overload on the LV associated with LV pressure-volume work and myocardial oxygen consumption.[56,57]

Important physiologic considerations in combined valvular disease are the predominance of a single valvular lesion in altering hemodynamics and the potential failure to identify the presence of a second abnormal valve. MS produces left atrial (LA) and pulmonary venous hypertension, with eventual pulmonary hypertension and RV failure, even though aortic stenosis may also be present. Despite the presence of MS, concomitant AS can create pressure overload and hypertrophy of the LV. When MR accompanies AS, the pressure and volume overloads create both LV dilatation and hypertrophy. LA enlargement and elevation of pulmonary artery pressure eventually accompany this condition. In regurgitation of both mitral and aortic valves, severe LV dilatation develops, accompanied by compensatory LV hypertrophy.[58] LV compliance increases in MR and AR, resulting in small elevations of end-diastolic pressure in the LV and LA for larger end-diastolic volumes.[59] Abnormalities in both early and late diastolic filling can accompany valvular regurgitation.[60]

In all combinations of aortic and mitral valve lesions, pulmonary congestion and elevated pulmonary capillary pressure usually follow significant depression of the contractile state of the LV. LA enlargement produced by either MS or MR is often associated with atrial fibrillation. Alterations in pulmonary blood flow and cardiac rhythm commonly accompany the LV pressure-volume overload in combined mitral and aortic valve disease.

TR usually accompanies RV dilatation secondary to pulmonary hypertension from any combination of mitral or aortic valve diseases. TS almost invariably is accompanied by disease of the mitral valve and can create significant elevations of the RA and central venous pressures.

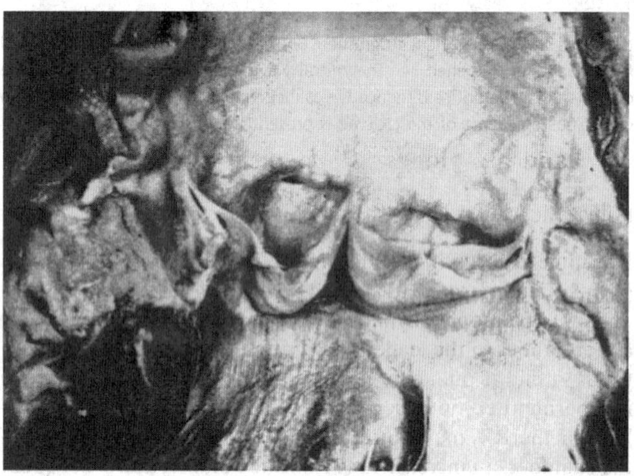

A

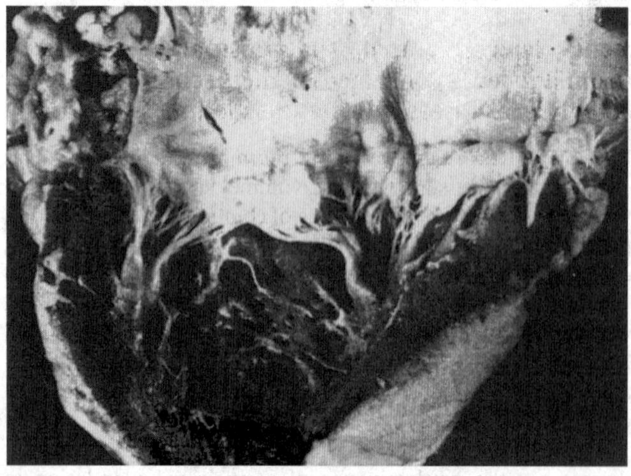

B

FIGURE 59-6 Prolapsed mitral valve and prolapsed aortic valve. *A*. Specimen of aortic valve from a 61-year-old man. The aortic valve shows redundance or prolapse of its right cusp. *B*. Specimen of mitral valve from a 73-year-old woman. The mitral valve shows prominent evidence of prolapse involving the posterior leaflet (right) and the posterior half of the anterior leaflet.

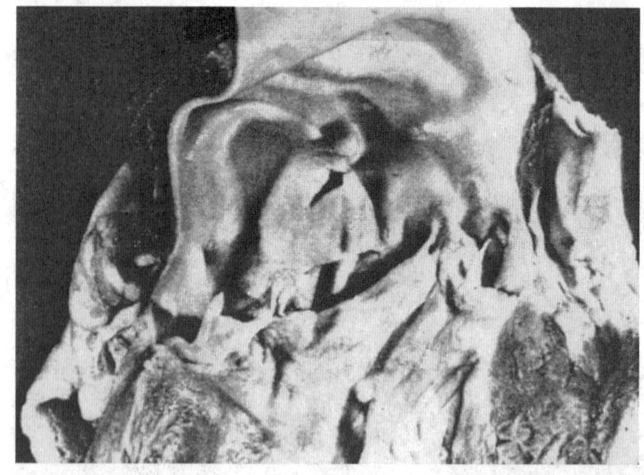

A

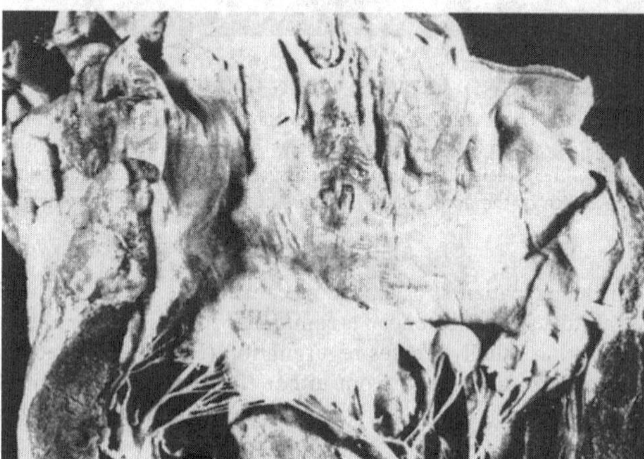

B

FIGURE 59-7 Floppy mitral valve and limited dissecting aneurysm of the ascending aorta, leading to aortic regurgitation, in a specimen from a 60-year-old man. *A*. Ascending aorta and aortic valve. The ascending aorta exhibits a laceration leading to a false channel within the aortic wall in which a hematoma is present (seen on each side of the opened aorta). Secondary distortion of the aortic valvular mechanism caused aortic regurgitation. *B*. Mitral valve, LA, and a portion of the LV. The posterior leaflet of the mitral valve (right) shows several areas of prolapse.

CLINICAL MANIFESTATIONS

Symptoms

TRICUSPID VALVE DISEASE

Since TR generally accompanies LV failure or MS, presenting symptoms include dyspnea, orthopnea, and peripheral edema.[61] Even though LV failure is usually present, paroxysmal nocturnal

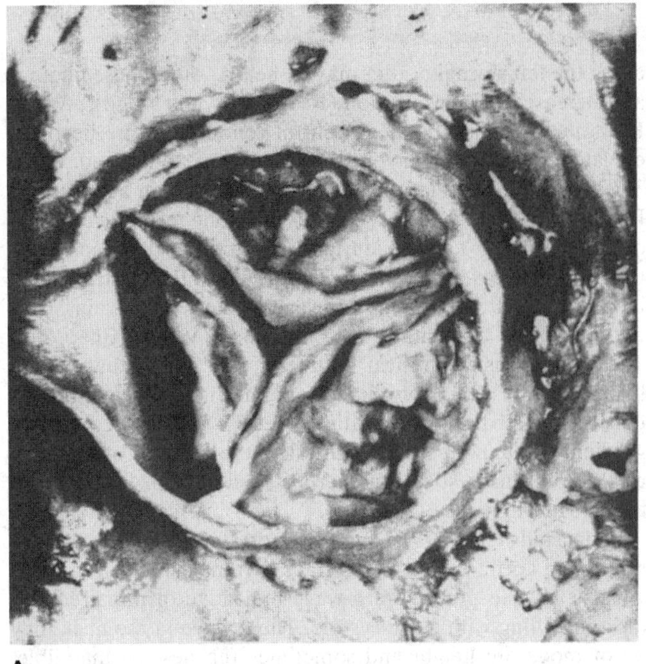

A

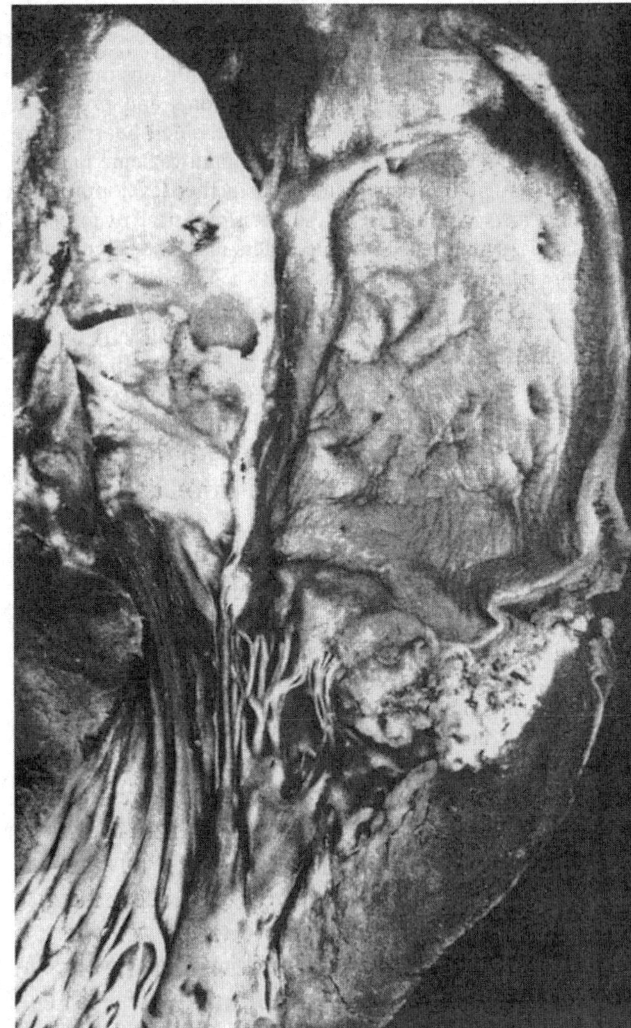

B

FIGURE 59-8 Senile calcific AS and calcification of the mitral ring in specimens from two individuals. *A.* Aortic valve. Classic example of senile calcific aortic stenosis in the unopened aortic valve viewed from above. *B.* LA, mitral valve, and lateral wall of LV. Sagittal section through LA and LV walls reveals a calcified mass at the junction of the LA, the LV, and the posterior mitral leaflet.

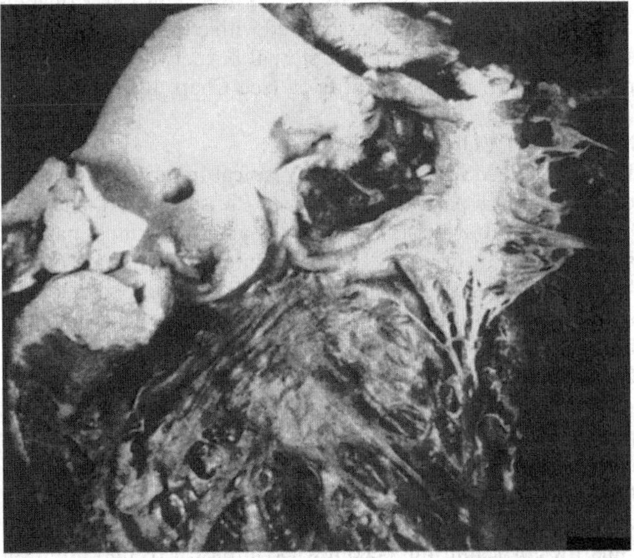

A

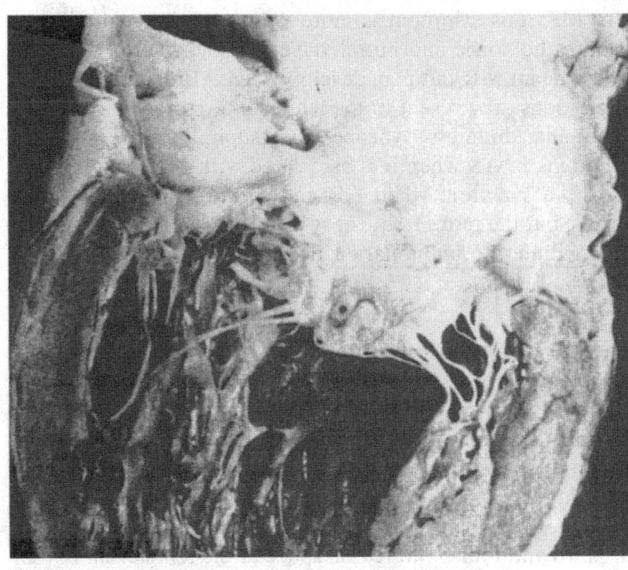

B

FIGURE 59-9 Bacterial endocarditis in specimens from a 36-year-old man. *A.* Aortic valve. The base of the aortic valve shows major destruction of a cusp with extension of inflammation onto the subjacent mitral valve. Near the free edge of the mitral valve, its ventricular aspect shows an ostium of a nonruptured mycotic aneurysm. *B.* Mitral valve, LA, and LV. The lobulated mycotic aneurysm of the mitral valve lies near its free edge.

dyspnea is often absent. TR under these conditions may occasionally ameliorate the pulmonary symptoms and provide a physiologic basis for the alleviation of left-sided heart failure by the development of right-sided heart failure. Some patients also have less pulmonary edema due to the development of pulmonary arteriolar disease. If the TR is produced by infective endocarditis, symptoms of febrile illness may be accompanied by fatigue and peripheral edema.

The most frequent symptoms in TS are dyspnea and fatigue. When MS coexists, the development of significant TS can diminish the paroxysmal symptoms of dyspnea, pulmonary congestion, and pulmonary hypertension.[16,17] Occasionally, patients with TS complain of prominent pulsations in the neck veins, which may precede the development of peripheral edema.

PULMONIC VALVE DISEASE

Clinical manifestations of acquired pulmonic valvular lesions depend on the severity of the hemodynamic impairment as well as on the extent of the underlying disease. Isolated PR can be tolerated without symptoms. Severe pulmonary hypertension may cause syncope in addition to shortness of breath and fatigue. With inflammatory lesions of the pulmonic valve, febrile manifestations and pulmonary infection may be present. The carcinoid syndrome is characterized by episodes of facial flushing, increased intestinal activity, diarrhea, and bronchospasm (see Chap. 77). Tumors involving the pulmonic valve may exert pressure from expansion and metastases that affect the heart and lungs.

MULTIVALVULAR DISEASE

Dyspnea is the most frequent complaint of patients with combined mitral and aortic valve disease.[1,22,62] With combined MS and AS, chest discomfort, palpitations, and syncope are frequent clinical manifestations. Symptoms of heart failure result from pulmonary congestion and usually include fluid retention. Although angina pectoris is uncommon in patients with predominant MR, this symptom is more frequent with regurgitation of both the aortic and mitral valves. Also, syncope is rare in predominant MR but may develop when AR and MR coexist; palpitations are present in the majority of patients.

Angina, dizziness, syncope, and palpitations are common symptoms in AS when it is associated with MR. Angina may also be a symptom when AR and MS are the predominant lesions; but the more frequent symptoms, dyspnea and fatigue, are attributed to pulmonary congestion and heart failure (see Chaps. 56 to 58).

Physical Examination

TRICUSPID VALVE DISEASE

In patients with primary TR not due to pulmonary hypertension, there are large *v* waves in the jugular venous pulse (JVP). There is a dilated RV with a precordial lift and right-sided third or fourth heart sounds. There is usually a long systolic murmur in the third and fourth intercostal space at the left sternal border that increases with inspiration. The murmur is often confined to early and mid-systole or may not be heard at all when there is small gradient between the RV and RA during systole and a large regurgitant orifice (see Chap. 10). When a large amount of blood returns to the RV in diastole, a short diastolic rumble along the left sternal border may be heard. All of these findings are increased with inspiration (Rivero Carvallo's sign).[63] When RV failure occurs, the mean central venous pressure becomes elevated, and the jugular veins are pulsatile and engorged. When TR is due to pulmonary hypertension, there is an accentuated P_2, and a high-pitched decrescendo diastolic murmur of PR is often heard that is louder during inspiration in the second and third left intercostal spaces. In patients with TR and atrial fibrillation, there is a prominent *cv* wave in the jugular veins, produced by the regurgitant flow into the RV (see Chap. 10). The characteristic physical finding of TR due to pulmonary hypertension is a holosystolic murmur at the left sternal border that increases during inspiration; there is a RV-RA pressure gradient throughout systole. Although the murmur of MR may also be present, respiration exerts a predominant influence on the TR murmur (see Chap. 10).

Tricuspid stenosis is frequently associated with lesions of the mitral and aortic valves. When sinus rhythm is present, the JVP will display the prominent *a* wave indicative of impaired RV diastolic filling with atrial systole. The *a* wave in the neck may be of moderate height and sometimes reaches the mandible. Auscultation of the heart is required to confirm that the rise of the venous *a* wave is simultaneous with the first heart sound. The *cv* wave is small, and the *y* descent is slow and insignificant (see Chap. 10).

PULMONIC VALVE DISEASE

If RV failure and TR have developed as a result of PR, a prominent *cv* wave will be present in the JVP. Increased RV activity may be visible and palpable along the left sternal border. If pulmonic hypertension is present, the pulmonic second sound will be accentuated over the left upper sternal border. The murmur of acquired PR is a high-pitched diastolic blow along the left sternal border. Thus, the murmur may be difficult to differentiate from the murmur of AR, but the absence of peripheral findings of AR is useful in identifying regurgitation of the pulmonic valve as the source of the diastolic murmur. Congenital PR characteristically is associated with a low-pitched, decrescendo murmur along the left sternal border, the peak of the murmur occurring shortly after P_2 (see Chap. 10).

MULTIVALVULAR DISEASE

In combined MS and AS, the LV apical impulse may not be displaced, but a palpable parasternal RV systolic lift is usually present. A mitral diastolic rumble is audible in most patients and can vary from grade I to III in intensity (on scale of I to VI). The aortic systolic murmur is usually loud, but occasionally may be faint with severe MS. A mitral opening snap may not be audible, and in some patients the diastolic rumble of MS cannot be heard.

When both AR and MR exist, the diastolic arterial blood pressure is usually less than 70 mmHg. In those with a diastolic blood pressure above 70 mmHg, there is usually a loud holosystolic mitral murmur. If AR is the dominant lesion, the early diastolic murmur is usually prominent, whereas when MR prevails, the aortic murmur becomes less intense. MR may diminish the AR due to the increased LV diastolic filling from the enlarged LA. Depending on the contractile state of the myocardium, loud regurgitant murmurs may be associated with mild regurgitation, whereas faint murmurs may accompany severe valvular regurgitation if myocardial failure has developed. A diastolic "flow murmur" across the mitral valve is heard in the majority of patients with combined MR and AR. If AR is important, a systolic murmur produced by the large forward flow across the aortic valve often is present (see Chap. 10).

When AR and MS are both present, the LV impulse is also displaced, sustained, and forceful. The early diastolic murmur at the apex may be prominent and may be accentuated by the AR flow striking the anterior leaflet of the stenotic mitral valve. Although the low-pitched diastolic murmur of MS and the diastolic flow murmur with AR are usually reliable diagnostic parameters, neither murmur correlates with the hemodynamic measurements when the two lesions coexist.

When AR is combined with MS, the systemic pulse pressure does not necessarily reflect the severity of AR. A prominent apical impulse in apparently pure MS indicates the likelihood of associated AR but may not indicate its severity. Finally, the intensity of the aortic diastolic murmur is of little value in predicting the severity of AR in the presence of MS (Chap. 10).

In the presence of AS and possible MR, an apical holosystolic murmur is reasonable evidence for associated MR, but the intensity of the murmur is not a reliable indicator in estimating severity.

While the murmur of TR often increases with inspiration, distinction from a concomitant MR murmur may be difficult. Identification of the rumble of TS requires careful auscultation during inspiration at the left lower sternal border. Detection by auscultation is more difficult because of the frequent association of MS and TS.

Electrocardiogram

TRICUSPID VALVE DISEASE

Atrial fibrillation is frequent in patients with TR. When TR results from myocardial infarction, acute or chronic electrocardiographic (ECG) changes will be seen in the inferior leads, and ST-segment elevation indicating RV infarction may be present in the right-sided precordial leads. The characteristic ECG finding in TS is a large P wave of RA enlargement in the absence of RV hypertrophy[1,22,64] (see Chap. 11).

PULMONIC VALVE DISEASE

Although there are no characteristic changes with pulmonic valvular lesions, preexisting pulmonary hypertension will produce RV hypertrophy, right-axis deviation, and changes in the *p* wave, suggesting RA enlargement. If pulmonary hypertension is secondary to mitral stenosis, P mitrale, with characteristic notches, will be present in lead II (see Chap. 11).

MULTIVALVULAR DISEASE

In combined MS and AS, ECG evidence of LV hypertrophy, LA enlargement, and atrial fibrillation is often present. Similar findings are observed in MR and AR, with a high likelihood of LA and LV enlargement along with atrial fibrillation. With AS and MR, LV hypertrophy is accompanied by a moderate incidence of atrial fibrillation. MS with severe AR also produces LV hypertrophy.

Chest Roentgenogram

TRICUSPID VALVE DISEASE

TR may produce some degree of RA enlargement, but there will usually be accompanying RV enlargement.[61] In TS, the most characteristic radiographic finding is prominence of the RA without significant pulmonary arterial enlargement or changes due to pulmonary hypertension[1,22] (see Chap. 12).

PULMONIC VALVE DISEASE

Patients with PR have pulmonary artery prominence along with an increase in RV dimensions. If PS is acquired, there may be poststenotic dilatation or prominence of the main pulmonary artery.

MULTIVALVULAR DISEASE

With combined MS and AS, the LA is always enlarged. LV chamber size may be significantly enlarged; however, prominent RV dimensions are usually present. Valvular calcification at either site is relatively uncommon. In AS accompanied by MR, heart size is increased, with both LV and LA enlargement. In MS with AR, marked LV enlargement is often present.

Echocardiogram

TRICUSPID VALVE DISEASE

With TR, there may be echocardiographic evidence of systolic prolapse, rupture of the chordae or papillary muscle, or vegetative lesions on the valve.[65] Increased RV dimensions indicate impaired RV function and the likelihood of secondary TR (see Chap. 13). Contrast echocardiography with peripheral venous injection can identify the back-and-forth flow across the valve.[66] The echo-Doppler technique can estimate the severity of the regurgitation and the systolic pressure in the RV[67] (Fig. 59-10). Color-flow Doppler imaging can delineate the patterns and sites of regurgitation across the valve apparatus[71] (see Chap. 13).

A characteristic pattern of TS can often be recorded with the echocardiogram. Fibrosis and calcification of the valve can be identified. Obstructive lesions, such as myxoma, thrombus, or other tumors, can be recognized echocardiographically. The two-dimensional echocardiogram of a patient with carcinoid syndrome with both TR and TS is shown in Fig. 59-11*A* and *B*. The echo-Doppler technique can be used to estimate the diastolic gradient across the valve with generally good accuracy (see Chap. 13).

PULMONIC VALVE DISEASE

Echocardiography can delineate the anatomy of the pulmonic valve as well as intrinsic or extrinsic lesions impinging on the valve apparatus. Sometimes a vegetative lesion or tumor can be detected in the pulmonic valve area. The echo-Doppler technique can estimate both the severity of both the regurgitation and the stenosis of the valve,[68] and analysis of echo-Doppler recordings can provide estimates of pulmonary artery pressure[69–71] (Fig. 59-12). Color-flow imaging can further confirm the patterns of regurgitation in the RV outflow tract (see Chap. 13).

MULTIVALVULAR DISEASE

Echocardiography provides information on valve anatomy, chamber dimensions, pressure gradients, valve size, patterns of regurgitation, and estimates of ventricular function. MS and AS produce characteristic echoes (see Chap. 13). Prolapse of mitral, aortic, and tricuspid valves can be characteristically recognized with echocardiography.[72] The number of aortic cusps can be identified, as can the presence of calcium in the aortic or mitral

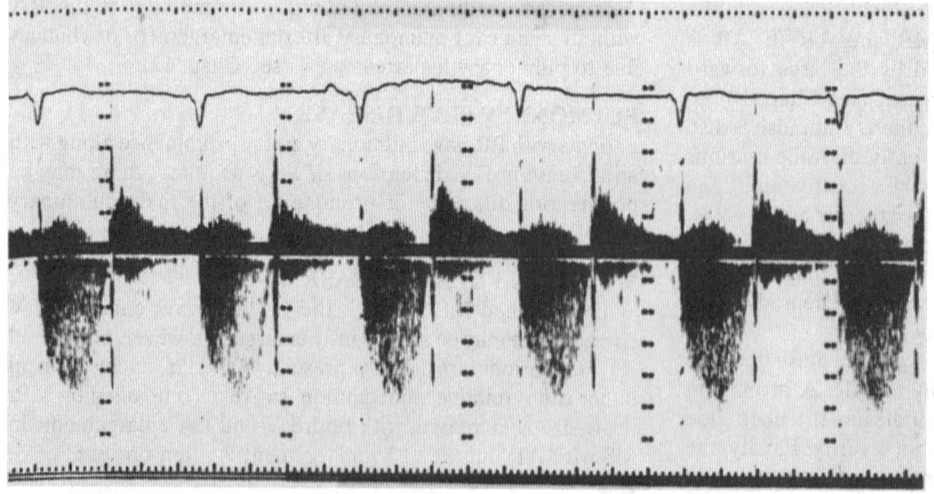

FIGURE 59-10 A continuous echo-Doppler recording in a patient with tricuspid valve disease illustrates TR in the lower portion and TS in the upper portion of the tracing. (Reproduced with permission from and courtesy of Dr. Pamela Sears-Rogan.)

valve apparatus. Dimensions of the LA, LV, and RV, together with LV wall thickness measurements and determinations of mass, are useful in estimating the extent of volume and pressure overload. Two-dimensional and Doppler echocardiographic techniques can assess the orifice size of the aortic and mitral valves and estimate the valve gradients accurately.[73,74] Even in the presence of AR, appropriate modifications in the mathematical analysis of the pressure gradient can yield reasonably accurate estimates of the aortic valve gradients (see Chap. 13). Color-flow Doppler readings can identify patterns and sites of valvular-regurgitation across the aortic and mitral valves.[75,76] Also, thrombus formation in the LA and LV can be detected with various echocardiographic methods. Transesophageal echocardiography can accurately assess prosthetic valve function and valvular repair during the operative procedures.

Nuclear Techniques

A radionuclide ventriculogram (RNV) can delineate dimensions of the RA and RV, which may help differentiate between TS and TR (see Chap. 16). RV size and function can be evaluated in stenotic and regurgitant lesions of the pulmonic valve. Myocardial perfusion imaging techniques are useful in detecting RV infarction as a cause of TR as well as in providing estimates of RV function. RV size and function can be evaluated in stenotic and regurgitant lesions of the pulmonic valve.

Quantitative information on LV function at rest and during exercise can be provided by RNV (see Chap. 16). Segmental wall motion can be assessed at rest and during exercise and

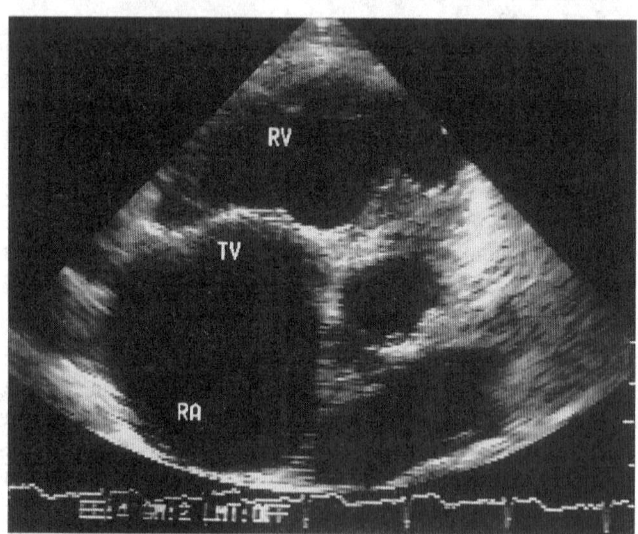

A

B

FIGURE 59-11 *A*. Two-dimensional echocardiogram of a 40-year-old patient, with carcinoid tumor of the testes without metastases. He presented with a testicular mass and was found to have a grade III/VI pansystolic murmur and grade III/VI diastolic murmur; both increased with inspiration. This four-chamber view shows a thickened stenotic tricuspid valve (TV) in diastole. The RA is enlarged, and the atrial septum bulges to the left, indicating a higher RA than LA pressure, which is consistent with tricuspid stenosis. The liver was normal because the humoral products of the carcinoid tumor bypassed the liver by the testicular venous drainage flowing directly to the inferior vena cava and renal veins. Carcinoid tumors arise from neuroendocrine cells known as enterochromaffin cells, which are found in organs derived from the embryonic gut. Because the liver detoxifies the humoral products of the carcinoid tumor, which most often arises in the ileum, it is extremely rare to see carcinoid heart disease in the absence of liver metastases, making this case extremely unusual.[4,5] Only about 20% of patients with carcinoid tumors develop cardiovascular symptoms. RV, right ventricle; SL, septal leaflet. *B*. Two-dimensional echocardiogram in diastole. This is from the same patient as in (*A*). Note the thickened tricuspid valve (TV) and the lack of excursion of the TV from diastole to systole. This washer-like, thickened TV is characteristic of carcinoid heart disease. It is common for a carcinoid TV to be both stenotic and insufficient. With carcinoid TV disease the valve becomes thickened, and its mobility and flexibility are reduced. RA, right atrium; RV, right ventricle. (From Cheitlin and MacGregor,[22] with permission.)

may assist in the recognition of underlying coronary artery disease. Since combined lesions of the aortic and mitral valves often create pulmonary hypertension and RV dysfunction, RNV is useful in estimating the RV ejection fraction[77] (see Chap. 16).

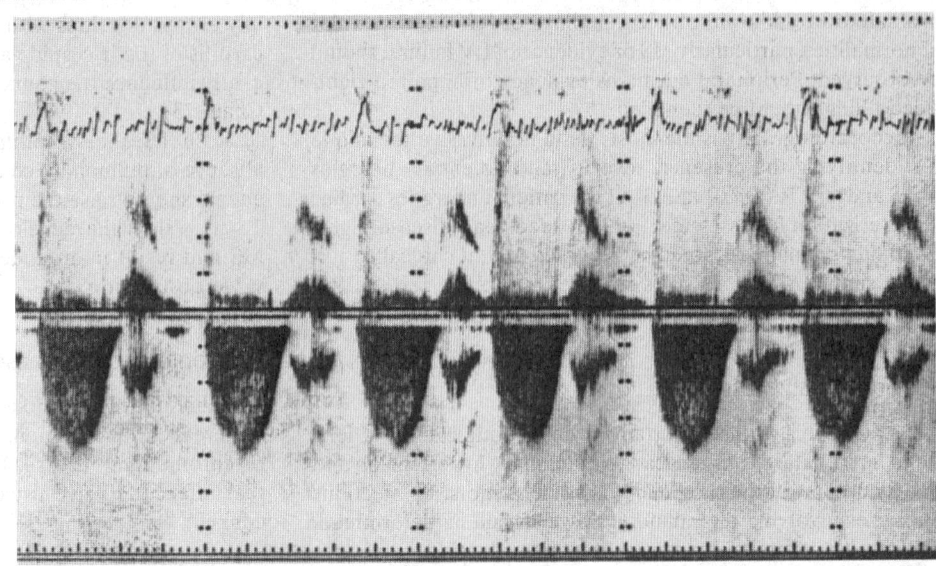

FIGURE 59-12 An echo-Doppler continuous tracing in a patient with TR. By employing the equation, the systolic gradient across the tricuspid valve can be calculated, and the addition of 10 mmHg yields an estimate of the pulmonary systolic pressure. Thus, in this patient, the level of pulmonary hypertension could be estimated from the echo-Doppler tracing of the TR. (Reproduced with permission from and courtesy of Dr. Pamela Sears-Rogan.)

Cardiac Catheterization

TRICUSPID VALVE DISEASE

Accurate angiographic documentation of TR is difficult to obtain because the catheter overrides the tricuspid valve, and ventricular irritability with an RV injection can induce TR. A prominent *cv* wave in the RA suggests TR, and an intracardiac phonocardiogram may record a regurgitation murmur in the absence of Rivero Carvallo's sign.[78]

If TS is clinically suspected, simultaneous pressures should be recorded in the RA and in the RV in order to measure the gradient across the valve accurately.[59] Since the normal gradient across the tricuspid valve is less than 1 mmHg, small gradients may not be detected if pullback pressure is recorded from the RV to the RA. The area of the tricuspid valve in TS is usually less than 1.5 cm^2; in severe TS, it is less than 1 cm^2.

PULMONIC VALVE DISEASE

PR is not readily demonstrated angiographically, but a right-sided injection can outline the pulmonary valve as well as show poststenotic dilatation. An aortic root injection can be helpful in the elimination of AR as the etiology of a diastolic murmur along the left sternal border. Nevertheless, this distinction is usually best made by echo-Doppler studies.

MULTIVALVULAR DISEASE

Cardiac catheterization is appropriate for most patients with combined valvular heart disease in order to calculate the stenotic and regurgitant status of each valve as well as to identify the predominant valvular lesion. Gradients across the valve can be measured with precision and the valve area calculated. Pulmonary hypertension is commonly present in these patients, and LV end-diastolic pressure is often elevated despite the presence of MS (see Chap. 15).

In MR plus AR, the LV end-diastolic pressure is elevated in most patients, and the central aortic pressure is generally greater than 40 mmHg. As noted, however, in approximately one-third of the patients the central aortic diastolic pressure may be above 70 mmHg. The *v* wave of MR can be recorded in the wedge position, and capillary and pulmonary arterial pressures are abnormally elevated in most of these patients.

In AS with MR, LV end-diastolic and pulmonary artery pressures are elevated; however, the extent of pressure elevation does not necessarily reflect the severity of the MR. When it is severe, forward cardiac output may be reduced; thus, a spuriously small pressure gradient may be recorded across a significantly stenotic aortic valve. In MS with AR, the LV end-diastolic pressure is abnormal and the central aortic diastolic pressure is usually less than 70 mmHg.

In combined valvular lesions, the measurement of total angiographic LV stroke volume is useful in calculating the regurgitant volume across each valve.[1,22] When both valves are regurgitant, it is more difficult to calculate the regurgitant volume across each valve.

Assessment of ventricular function is important in patients with combined valvular lesions; yet the ejection fraction may be spuriously normal or elevated in MR and, to a lesser extent, in AR. Measurements of LV end-systolic pressure, volume, and wall thickness permit calculation of end-systolic wall stress.[79] This parameter has been particularly helpful in pressure and volume overload conditions, since the end-systolic pressure-volume wall stress calculation is relatively independent of loading conditions.

Finally, coronary arteriography should be performed at the time of cardiac catheterization in patients above the age of 35, since coronary artery disease may be present without symptoms and may contribute to LV dysfunction. Coronary artery bypass grafting at the time of valve surgery is an important consideration.

USUAL STRATEGY OF WORKUP

Tricuspid Valve Disease

The history should identify underlying conditions, such as rheumatic fever, systemic disorders, and left-sided heart failure, as etiologies for tricuspid valve disease. The physical examination should carefully define the waveforms in the JVP. The auscultatory changes of systolic and diastolic murmurs at the left lower sternal border during the respiratory cycle should be carefully evaluated. In addition, physical findings of left-sided valvular abnormalities, particularly MS or evidence of LV failure, should be observed. Peripheral edema as evidence of impaired right-sided filling should be identified.

Echocardiography is the most useful noninvasive technique for identifying the presence, severity, and potential etiologies of TS and/or TR (see Chap. 13). If the patient undergoes cardiac catheterization for assessment of left-sided heart disease, right-sided hemodynamics should be recorded and, if clinically indicated, simultaneous pressures recorded in the RA and the RV (see Chap. 15).

Pulmonic Valve Disease

The clinical history is important in delineating causes of left-sided heart failure that can lead to pulmonary hypertension and PR. Symptoms of the carcinoid syndrome, tumors, or infectious etiologies involving the pulmonic valve should be determined. The physical examination is important in evaluating the venous pulsations in the neck veins as well as the pulmonic murmurs. RV prominence should be carefully evaluated, as should concomitant left-sided valve lesions and evidence of heart failure. Although an ECG and chest x-ray should be obtained to assess the pulmonic artery, RV outflow tract, and body of the RV, the most useful noninvasive technique is echocardiography. The anatomy, competence of the valve, extent of the regurgitation, and stenosis can be recognized and assessed by an echo-Doppler sudy. In addition, other valve lesions affecting the left side of the heart can be documented. Since PR can be relatively well tolerated, this specific lesion does not require such frequent follow-up, but underlying mechanisms for pulmonary hypertension or left-sided heart failure should be monitored closely.

Multivalvular Disease

Symptoms of dyspnea, exercise intolerance, chest discomfort, or syncope should be elicited during a carefully taken clinical history. On physical examination, special attention should be directed to the peripheral and central arterial pulses and the JVP. Heart size, precordial movement, and auscultatory findings should be carefully noted. A 12-lead ECG and posterior-anterior and lateral chest films should be obtained. Echocardiography is indicated to delineate valve anatomy, measure valve gradients, recognize regurgitant patterns, calculate orifice size, and estimate ventricular function and wall motion (see Chap. 13). A limited exercise test with or without radionuclide studies may help determine the exercise capacity as well as detect functional deterioration, chest pain, arrhythmias, deterioration of ventricular ejection fraction, or segmental wall motion abnormalities. If symptoms are atypical and the extent of valvular or LV function cannot be satisfactorily evaluated by noninvasive techniques, cardiac catheterization is indicated.

NATURAL HISTORY AND PROGNOSIS

Tricuspid Valve Disease

With TR due to RV hypertension, the symptoms and clinical course are primarily related to the left-sided heart conditions that produce a pressure-volume overload on the RV. TR virtually always develops with severe RV failure. In infective endocarditis of the tricuspid valve, the type of organism may significantly influence the course and the response to antibiotics (see Chap. 73).

With TS, the symptoms are usually those of MS, and the absence of pulmonary congestion in the presence of peripheral edema should raise the possibility of underlying TS. Significant TS may slow the development of characteristic symptoms of MS and result in an underestimation of the severity of mitral valve obstruction.

Pulmonic Valve Disease

In pulmonic valve lesions, the course will be more prolonged if there is chronic pulmonary hypertension due to mitral stenosis or chronic lung disease. Inflammatory conditions and tumors that affect the valve usually result in a much shorter clinical course.

Multivalvular Disease

When combined aortic and mitral valve disease are due to rheumatic fever, 10 years or more may elapse before the development of significant murmurs, and an additional decade (or more) may elapse before symptoms become manifest. If lesions of the aortic and mitral valves are due to degenerative collagen changes, symptoms may develop later in life. When combined lesions are due to calcific changes in the aortic valve and annulus as well as the mitral valve annulus, symptoms develop much later in life. There may, however, be rapid progression of degenerative aortic calcific stenosis over a 2- to 3-year period (see Chap. 56).

MEDICAL MANAGEMENT

Tricuspid Valve Disease

With TR, treatment of RV failure requires digitalis and diuretics, and vasodilating agents are also required for the management of LV failure (see Chap. 21). If failure of the right side of the heart is caused by MS, early intervention to enlarge or replace the mitral valve is appropriate (see Chap. 57).

In TS, the usual precautionary measures of antibiotic coverage and prevention of endocarditis apply. Peripheral edema may not respond well to administration of digitalis, diuretics, and vasodilator therapy, thus emphasizing the clinical importance of detecting underlying TS. Tricuspid balloon valvuloplasty has been used successfully in patients with predominant TS.[80]

Pulmonic Valve Disease

Patients with congenital pulmonic valve stenosis are usually best treated by catheter balloon valvotomy (see Chaps. 63 and 64).

Prophylaxis and Medical Therapy

Antibiotic prophylaxis against endocarditis (see Chap. 73) is appropriate for patients with either tricuspid or pulmonic valve lesions. If pulmonary emboli contribute to the pulmonary hypertension, anticoagulation is indicated (see Chap. 53). Further treatment of pulmonary hypertension may require managementof left heart failure, correction of MS, or the use of vasodilating agents that can lower pulmonary artery pressure. Vasodilating agents are often ineffective in treating primary pulmonary hypertension (see Chap. 52).

If rheumatic fever is the likely etiology of combined aortic and mitral valve disease, prophylactic penicillin should usually be continued until age 35 years (see Chap. 55). Dental prophylaxis with antibiotic coverage, using either amoxicillin or erythromycin, should be provided in all patient groups prior to dental procedures. For genitourinary or other abdominal procedures, gram-negative antibiotic coverage should be provided (see Chap. 82).

Atrial Fibrillation

If atrial fibrillation develops, chronic anticoagulation with low-dose warfarin [International Normalized Ratio (INR) 2.0 to 3.0] is warranted, since the accompanying incidence of systemic and cerebral emboli is estimated at 10 to 20 percent (see Chap. 61).

The early development of atrial fibrillation associated with hemodynamic deterioration warrants an initial attempt at electrical cardioversion. If this is successful, digitalis as well as antiarrhythmic preparations should be administered thereafter for prophylaxis against recurrence (see Chap. 24). Chronic atrial fibrillation should be controlled with digitalis, beta blockers, and calcium blockers as indicated. The development of symptoms, particularly dyspnea, limited exercise activity, chest pain, and syncope, warrants consideration for surgery. It is usually recommended for New York Heart Association (NYHA) class III symptoms despite adequate medical therapy.

SURGICAL MANAGEMENT

Tricuspid Valve Disease

The decision to proceed with valvular heart surgery is usually based on the severity of the aortic and mitral valve disease, rather than on the severity of the disease of the tricuspid valve. The usual decisions to be made regarding the tricuspid valve are (1) whether a procedure should be added to the mitral and/or aortic valve procedures and, (2) if so, which procedure—annuloplasty or valve replacement—should be performed. Patients may present with mild mitral valve disease but severe tricuspid valve dysfunction. Such patients may require an operation on the tricuspid valve only.

The severity of the symptoms and clinical signs of tricuspid valve disease are used to determine the indications for tricuspid valve surgery. If there are signs of TS and, particularly, if stenosis is demonstrated by cardiac catheterization and two-dimensional echocardiography, the tricuspid valve is directly visualized at operation with the anticipation of performing commissurotomy or valve replacement. Tricuspid valve balloon valvulotomy has been advocated for[80–84] TS of various etiologies.[82] However, severe TR is a common consequence of this procedure, and results are poor when severe TR develops.

When there are signs of severe TR secondary to MS, it is important to document the duration of the regurgitation and the severity and duration of pulmonary artery hypertension. If the TR is severe and long-standing and if there is chronic pulmonary artery hypertension, it is unlikely to resolve in the early postoperative period after mitral valve surgery alone. In this circumstance, tricuspid valve surgery is usually indicated. In contrast, if TR and pulmonary artery hypertension are of short duration, mitral valve replacement will usually reduce pulmonary artery pressure in the early postoperative period, and this will result in a decrease in the TR. Occasionally, severe TR will be present with only modest elevation of pulmonary artery pressure. In this circumstance, the tricuspid valve leaflets are usually deformed and valve replacement is necessary.[83]

The appearance of the heart at the time of surgery is helpful in assessing the severity of tricuspid valve disease. A thinned-out RA wall together with moderate to marked enlargement of the RA and venae cavae are indications of significant disease. The degree of stenosis and regurgitation can be estimated by palpation through the RA appendage. Intraoperative transesophageal echocardiography (see Chap. 13) provides more precise information as to the degree of residual valvular regurgitation after repair. The ACC/AHA guidelines recommendations for surgery for TR are listed in Table 59-4.

TS may be treated successfully by commissurotomy, which is usually performed under direct vision. The procedure may be combined with annuloplasty to correct valve regurgitation. Valve replacement is occasionally necessary if the changes in the leaflets and subvalvular structures are advanced or if severe TR cannot be relieved by annuloplasty. For TR, three basic reconstructive techniques have been described. The first procedure is used widely and consists of plication of the posterior leaflet,[84,85] thus converting the tricuspid valve into a functionally bicuspid valve.[84,85] De Vega described a second type of annuloplasty that narrows the annulus along the anterior and posterior leaflets with a pursestring suture.[86,87] The third major technique, described by Carpentier et al., consists of placing a carefully sized semiflexible ring along the anterior and posterior

TABLE 59-4 Recommendations for Surgery for Tricuspid Regurgitation

Indication	Class
Annuloplasty for severe TR and pulmonary hypertension in patients with mitral valve disease requiring mitral valve surgery	I
Valve replacement for severe TR secondary to diseased or abnormal tricuspid valve leaflets not amenable to annuloplasty or repair	IIa
Valve replacement of annuloplasty for severe TR with mean pulmonary artery pressure <60 mmHg when symptomatic	IIa
Annuloplasty for mild TR in patients with pulmonary hypertension secondary to mitral valve disease requiring mitral valve surgery	IIb
Valve replacement or annuloplasty for TR with pulmonary artery systolic pressure <60 mmHg in presence of a normal mitral valve in asymptomatic patients or in symptomatic patients who have not received a trial of diuretic therapy	III

aspects of the annulus.[88] It draws in and supports the tissue evenly. Follow-up studies have shown that annular dilatation occurs in these areas rather than along the leaflets.[89]

When the leaflets and subvalvular apparatus are severely deformed as a result of rheumatic fever, reconstruction may not be feasible. In such cases, replacement is performed with either a mechanical or tissue valve. Anticoagulation with warfarin (see Chap. 52) is generally advisable in patients with tricuspid valve replacement, and therefore the major advantage of a bioprosthetic valve is negated. If a mechanical valve is preferred and the cavity of the RV is not capacious, a low-profile, tilting disk-type prosthesis seems appropriate. Usually, however, if TR is severe, a ball-cage prosthesis functions better.

Mild TR does not seem to increase the risk of surgery involving the mitral valve or both aortic and mitral valves. When the TR is moderate to severe, however, the risk of operation is significantly increased. Although long-term improvement in TR after mitral valve replacement alone has been documented, a tricuspid procedure is generally employed in the setting of moderate to severe TR to enhance cardiac function in the critical early days after operation.[90] Mitral valve replacement alone does not invariably decrease TR, even several months after operation.[91]

In general, the early and late results of tricuspid annuloplasty have been superior to those of valve replacement, and valve replacement should be avoided when possible. There is a significant incidence of thrombosis with tricuspid prostheses, and the long-term functional results have been less favorable than those of aortic and mitral valve replacements.[92] Good early results have been obtained with all three methods of annuloplasty.[93–97] When tricuspid valve replacement is necessary, the 30-day perioperative mortality increases to 15 to 20 percent. Two preoperative factors—severity of edema and mean pulmonary artery pressure—as important predictors of long-term survival.[98] A variety of prostheses have been used for tricuspid valve replacement with variable results.[98–103]

Infective endocarditis of the tricuspid valve is relatively common because of the increased incidence of drug abuse. In general, the treatment of tricuspid valve endocarditis is medical. When septic pulmonary embolization occurs despite intensive antibiotic treatment, tricuspid valve surgery is indicated. Excision of the valve without replacement has been recommended, and reinfection of the new valve in intravenous drug users is an important risk.[104] Nevertheless, since valvulectomy alone carries an important risk of heart failure, tricuspid valve replacement has been recommended by others.[105]

The cardiac output is often marginal after tricuspid valve surgery, a reflection of persistent pulmonary arterial hypertension and long-standing RV dysfunction. Measurements of cardiac output and pulmonary artery pressure are used to guide postoperative care. If annuloplasty is performed, a pulmonary artery catheter can be used for such measurements (see Chap. 15). Nitroglycerin infused through a central venous catheter is a valuable adjunct in reducing pulmonary artery pressure. Prostaglandin E_1, in combination with pressor agents, may also be employed to treat severe postoperative pulmonary hypertension.[106] Intravenous dopamine and dobutamine may be used to enhance myocardial contractility. If cardiac output remains marginal, an intraaortic balloon pump may be used to reduce left-sided pressures. Pulmonary artery balloon counterpulsation has been employed for acute RV failure.[107] The use of a temporary circulatory assist device, such as a centrifugal pump, to bypass the RV may sustain adequate circulation when RV failure is unresponsive to other measures.

Digitalis and diuretics are usually employed for several months after tricuspid valve surgery. For patients with tricuspid valve replacement, warfarin and dipyridamole are used as anticoagulants.[108] The additional use of antiplatelet agents in this setting may improve the long-term results.[109] A serious late complication of tilting disk valves in the tricuspid position is thrombosis. Thrombolytic therapy with streptokinase has been used successfully to restore valve function.[110] Prophylaxis against infective endocarditis is also required (see Chap. 73).

Pulmonic Valve Disease

Pulmonic valve surgery for acquired disease is performed infrequently. PS on an acquired basis is rare. Although there are a variety of causes of PR, this hemodynamic condition is relatively well tolerated if pulmonary vascular resistance is normal. Pulmonic valve replacement may be performed for acquired conditions, such as carcinoid heart disease and infective endocarditis, but it usually is limited to cases where RV dysfunction has become severe after congenital heart disease surgery[111,112] (see Chaps. 63 and 64). In general, bioprosthetic valves have been preferred because of the tendency for mechanical valve thrombosis in this position. Pulmonic valve surgery is currently being performed earlier and more commonly, since studies indicate that RV dysfunction may be present in asymptomatic postoperative patients with PR.[113]

Infective endocarditis involves the pulmonic valve in about 1 percent of cases seen at autopsy. Isolated pulmonic valve infective endocarditis is even more uncommon but may be the cause of metastatic pulmonary infections. In a review of 28 cases of this entity, the overall mortality rate was 24 percent, with all those treated by operation surviving.[114] Valvulectomy in combination with antibiotic therapy is sometimes the most effective treatment (see Chap. 77).

Multivalvular Disease

Many patients with clinical evidence of combined disease of the mitral and aortic valves have severe and progressive symptoms. Experience indicates that both valves can be replaced, with a hospital mortality rate that is now between 5 and 10 percent.

Commonly, in the presence of aortic and mitral valve disease, repair, rather than replacement, of the stenotic or regurgitant mitral valve can be accomplished (see Chap. 57). Disease of the aortic valve in adults usually requires valve replacement. The combination of aortic valve replacement with mitral valve repair probably decreases early mortality rates and improves long-term survival. There have been marked subjective and objective improvements in surviving patients. When tricuspid valve replacement is added, the risk of the operation is higher (up to 20 percent), but even then the long-term results are considerably better than the life history of surgically untreated patients with triple-valve disease. The use, when possible, of tricuspid annuloplasty rather than replacement has greatly improved the early results of operation in this group of patients.

When hemodynamic derangement is significant at both mitral and aortic valves, the decision to repair or replace both is easily made, and the principles of surgical treatment are the same as when one valve alone requires operation.[115,116]

MULTIVALVULAR SURGERY

Combined MS and AR When mechanical correction is anticipated in predominant MS, balloon mitral valvotomy followed by aortic valve replacement (AVR) obviates the need for double-valve replacement, which has a higher risk of complications than does single-valve replacement.[117] In most cases, it is advisable to perform mitral valvotomy first and then follow the patient for symptomatic improvement. If symptoms disappear, correction of AR can be delayed.

Combined MS and TR If the mitral valve anatomy is favorable for percutaneous balloon valvotomy and there is concomitant pulmonary hypertension, valvotomy should be performed regardless of symptom status. After successful mitral valvotomy, pulmonary hypertension and TR almost always diminish.[118]

If mitral valve surgery is performed, concomitant tricuspid annuloplasty should be considered, especially if there are preoperative signs or symptoms of right-heart failure, rather than risking severe, persistent TR, which may necessitate a second operation. However, TR that seems severe on echocardiography but does not cause elevation of RA or RV diastolic pressure will generally improve greatly after mitral valve replacement (MVR). If intraoperative assessment suggests that TR is functional without significant dilatation of the tricuspid annulus, it may not be necessary to perform an annuloplasty.

Combined MS and AS If the degree of AS appears to be mild and the mitral valve is acceptable for balloon valvotomy, this should be attempted first. If mitral balloon valvotomy is successful, the aortic valve should then be reevaluated.

Combined AS and MR Noninvasive evaluation should be performed with two-dimensional and Doppler echocardiography to evaluate the severity of both AS and MR. Attention should be paid to LV size, wall thickness and function, LA size, right-heart function, and pulmonary artery pressure. Patients with severe AS and severe MR (with abnormal mitral valve morphology) with symptoms, LV dysfunction, or pulmonary hypertension should undergo combined AVR and MVR or mitral valve repair. However, in patients with severe AS and lesser degrees of MR, the severity of MR may improve greatly after isolated AVR, particularly when there is normal mitral valve morphology. Intraoperative transesophageal echocardiography and, if necessary, visual inspection of the mitral valve should be performed at the time of AVR to determine whether additional mitral valve surgery is warranted in such patients.

In patients with mild to moderate AS and severe MR in whom surgery on the mitral valve is indicated because of symptoms, LV dysfunction, or pulmonary hypertension, preoperative assessment of the severity of AS may be difficult because of reduced forward stroke volume. If the mean aortic valve gradient is greater than 30 mmHg, AVR should be performed. In patients with less severe aortic valve gradients, inspection of the aortic valve and its degree of opening on two-dimensional or transesophageal echocardiography as well as visual inspection by the surgeon may be important in determining the need for concomitant AVR.

References

1. Bonow RO, Carabello B, de Leon AC Jr, et al. ACC/AHA guidelines for the management of patients with valvular heart disease: A report of the American College of Cardiology/American Heart Association Task Force on Practice Guidelines (Committee on Management of Patients with Valvular Heart Disease). *J Am Coll Cardiol* 1998; 32:1486–1588.
2. Kostucki W, Vandenbossche JL, Friart A, Engbert H. Pulsed Doppler regurgitant flow patterns of normal valves. *Am J Cardiol* 1986; 58:309–313.
3. Sahn DJ, Maciel BC. Physiological valvular regurgitation: Doppler echocardiography and the potential for iatrogenic heart disease. *Circulation* 1988; 78:1075–1077.
4. Yoshida K, Yoshikawa J, Shakudo M. Color Doppler evaluation of valvular regurgitation in normals. *Circulation* 1988; 78: 840–847.
5. McMichael J, Shillingford JP. The role of valvular incompetence in heart failure. *Br Med J* 1957; 1:537–542.
6. Waller BF, Howard J, Fess S. Pathology of tricuspid valve stenosis and pure tricuspid regurgitation: III. *Clin Cardiol* 1995; 18: 225–230.
7. Waller BF, Howard J, Fess S. Pathology of tricuspid valve stenosis and pure tricuspid regurgitation: I. *Clin Cardiol* 1995; 18: 97–102.
8. Waller BF, Howard J, Fess S. Pathology of tricuspid valve stenosis and pure tricuspid regurgitation: II. *Clin Cardiol* 1995; 18: 167–174.
9. Glancy DL, Marcus FI, Cuadra M, et al. Isolated organic tricuspid valvular regurgitation. *Am J Med* 1969; 46:989–996.
10. Nishimura RA, Smith HC, Gersh BJ. Tricuspid regurgitation after myocardial infarction. *Am J Cardiol* 1994; 74:308.
11. Szyniszewski AM, Carson PE, Sakwa M, et al. Valve replacement for tricuspid regurgitation appearing late after healing of left ventricular posterior wall and right ventricular acute myocardial infarction. *Am J Cardiol* 1994; 73:616-617.
12. Chiu WC, Shindler DM, Scholz PM, Boyarsky AH. Traumatic tricuspid regurgitation with cyanosis: Diagnosis by transesophageal echocardiography. *Ann Thorac Surg* 1996; 63:992–993.
13. Chataline A, Agnew TM, Graham KJ, et al. Blunt chest trauma of the heart. *NZ Med J* 1999; 112:334–336.
14. Aziz TM, Burgess MI, Rahman AN, et al. Risk factors for tricuspid valve after orthotopic heart transplantation. *Ann Thorac Surg* 1999; 68:1247–1251.
15. Soga J, Yakyura Y, Osaka M. Carcinoid syndrome: A statistical evaluation of 748 reported cases. *J Exp Clin Cancer Res* 1999; 18:133–141.
16. Perloff JK, Harvey WP. Clinical recognition of tricuspid stenosis. *Circulation* 1960; 22:346–364.
17. Kitchin A, Turner R. Diagnosis and treatment of tricuspid stenosis. *Br Heart J* 1964; 26:354–379.
18. Edwards JE. The spectrum and clinical significance of tricuspid regurgitation. *Pract Cardiol* 1980; 6:86–90.
19. Roguin A, Reinkerich D, Milo S, et al. Long-term follow-up of patients with severe rheumatic tricuspid stenosis. *Am Heart J* 1998; 136:103–108.
20. Flammang D, Jaumin P, Kremer R. Organic tricuspid pathology in rheumatic valvulopathies. *Acta Cardiol* 1975; 30:155–170.
21. Pellikka PA, Tajik AJ, Khandheria BK, et al. Carcinoid heart disease: Clinical and echocardiographic spectrum in 74 patients. *Circulation* 1993; 87:1188–1196.
22. Cheitlin MD, MacGregor J. Acquired tricuspid and pulmonic

valve disease. In: Rahimtoola SH, ed. *Atlas of Heart Diseases: Valvular Heart Disease.* St. Louis: Mosby; 1997: 11.2–1.

23. Ludwig J. Cardiac vein involvement in carcinoid syndrome: Possible evidence of retrograde blood flow in cardiac veins in tricuspid insufficiency. *Am J Clin Pathol* 1971; 55:617–623.
24. McMichael J, Shillingford JP. The role of valvular incompetence in heart failure. *Br Med J* 1957; 1:537–541.
25. Boucek RJ Jr, Graham TP, Morgan JP, et al. Spontaneous resolution of massive congenital tricuspid insufficiency. *Circulation* 1976; 54:795–800.
26. Ajayi AA, Adigun AQ, Ojofeitim EO, et al. Arthrometric evaluation of cachexia in chronic congestive heart failure: The role of tricuspid regurgitation. *Int J Cardiol* 1999; 71:79–84.
27. Collins R, Daly JJ. Tricuspid incompetence complicating acute myocardial infarction. *Postgrad Med J* 1977; 53:51–52.
28. Zone DD, Botti RE. Right ventricular infarction with tricuspid insufficiency and chronic right heart failure. *Am J Cardiol* 1976; 37:445–448.
29. McAllister RG Jr, Friesinger GC, Sinclair-Smith BC. Tricuspid regurgitation following inferior myocardial infarction. *Arch Intern Med* 1976; 95:95–99.
30. Maranhao V, Gooch AS, Yang SS, et al. Prolapse of the tricuspid leaflets in the systolic murmur-click syndrome. *Cath Cardiovasc Diagn* 1975; 1:81–90.
31. Gerry JL Jr, Bulkley BH, Hutchins GM. Rupture of the papillary muscle of the tricuspid valve: A complication of cardiopulmonary resuscitation and a rare cause of tricuspid insufficiency. *Am J Cardiol* 1977; 40:825–828.
32. Jahnke EJ Jr, Nelson WP, Aaby GV, FitzGibbon GM. Tricuspid insufficiency: The result of nonpenetrating cardiac trauma. *Arch Surg* 1967; 95:880–886.
33. VanGilder JE, Jain AC, Weiss RB, et al. Traumatic right ventricular aneurysm presenting as tricuspid regurgitation. *WV Med J* 1979; 75:93–98.
34. Stephenson LW, MacVaugh H III, Kastor JA. Tricuspid valvular incompetence and rupture of the ventricular septum caused by nonpenetrating trauma. *J Thorac Cardiovasc Surg* 1979; 77: 768–772.
35. Williams MJ, Lee MY, DiSalvo TG, et al. Biopsy-induced flail tricuspid leaflet and tricuspid regurgitation following orthotopic cardiac transplantation. *Am J Cardiol* 1996; 77:1339–1344.
36. Hausen B, Albes JM, Rohde R, et al. Tricuspid valve regurgitation attributable to endomyocardial biopsies and rejection in heart transplantation. *Ann Thorac Surg* 1995; 59:1134–1140.
37. Marvin RF, Schrank JP, Nolan SP. Traumatic tricuspid insufficiency. *Am J Cardiol* 1973; 32:723–727.
38. Brandenburg RO, McGoon DC, Campeau L, Giuliani ER. Traumatic rupture of the chordae tendineae of the tricuspid valve: Successful repair twenty-four years later. *Am J Cardiol* 1966; 18:911–915.
39. Morgan JR, Forker AD. Isolated tricuspid insufficiency. *Circulation* 1971; 43:559–564.
40. Croxson MS, O'Brien KP, Lowe JB. Traumatic tricuspid regurgitation: Long-term survival. *Br Heart J* 1971; 33:750–755.
41. Grubier M, Denis B, Martin-Noel O. Les ruptures de cordages tricuspidiens. *Coeur Med Int* 1976; 15:215–222.
42. Espino Vela J, Contreras R, Rustrian Rosa F. Rheumatic pulmonary valve disease. *Am J Cardiol* 1969; 23:12–18.
43. Roberts WC, Buchbinder NA. Right-sided valvular infective endocarditis. *Am J Med* 1972; 53:7–19.
44. Levitt MA, Snoey ER, Tamkin GW, Gee G. Prevalence of cardiac value anomalies in afebril injection drug users. *Acad Emerg Med* 1999; 9:911–915.
45. Seymour J, Emanuel R, Patterson N. Acquired pulmonary stenosis. *Br Heart J* 1968; 30:776–785.
46. Rossignol B, Machecourt J, Denis B, et al. Cardiopathie carcinoide secondaire a une tumeur du grêle: A propos d'un cas associat insuffisance tricuspidienne et insuffisance pulmonaire. *Arch Mal Coeur Vaiss* 1977; 70:1221–1226.
47. Roberts WC, Virmani R. Aschoff bodies at necroposy in valvular heart disease. *Circulation* 1978; 57:803–815.
48. Clausen BJ. Rheumatic heart disease: An analysis of 796 cases. *Am Heart J* 1940; 20:454–474.
49. Wilson MG, Lubschez R. Longevity in rheumatic fever. *JAMA* 1948; 138:794–798.
50. Bland EF, Jones TD. Rheumatic fever and rheumatic heart disease: A twenty-year report on 1000 patients followed since childhood. *Circulation* 1951; 4:836–843.
51. Roberts WC, Honig HS. The spectrum of cardiovascular disease in the Marfan's syndrome: A clinico-pathologic study of 18 necropsy patients and comparison to 151 previously reported patients. *Am Heart J* 1982; 104:115–135.
52. Hansing CE, Rowe GG. Tricuspid insufficiency: A study of hemodynamics and pathogenesis. *Circulation* 1972; 45:793–799.
53. Killip T, Lukas DS. Tricuspid stenosis: Physiologic criteria for diagnosis and hemodynamic abnormalities. *Circulation* 1957; 16:3–13.
54. El-Sherif N. Rheumatic tricuspid stenosis: A hemodynamic correlation. *Br Heart J* 1971; 33:16–31.
55. Holmes JC, Flowler NO, Kaplan S. Pulmonary valvular insufficiency. *Am J Med* 1968; 44:851–862.
56. Rackley CE, Bechar VS, Whalen RE, McIntosh HD. Biplane cineangiographic determinations of left ventricular function: Pressure-volume relationships. *Am Heart J* 1967; 74: 766–779.
57. Baxley WA, Dodge HT, Rackley CE, et al. Left ventricular mechanical efficiency in man with heart disease. *Circulation* 1977; 55:564–568.
58. Jones JW, Rackley CE, Bruce RA, et al. Left ventricular volumes in valvular heart disease. *Circulation* 1964; 29:887–891.
59. Kern MJ, Aguirre F, Donohue T, Bach R. Interpretation of cardiac pathophysiology from pressure waveform analysis: Multivalvular regurgitant lesions. *Cath Cardiovasc Diagn* 1993; 28: 167–172.
60. Rousseau MF, Pouleur H, Charlier AA, Bruseur LA. Assessment of left ventricular relaxation in patients with valvular regurgitation. *Am J Cardiol* 1982; 50:1028–1036.
61. Salazar E, Levine HD. Rheumatic tricuspid regurgitation: The clinical spectrum. *Am J Med* 1962; 33:111–129.
62. Terzaki AK, Cokkinos DV, Leachman RD, et al. Combined mitral and aortic valve disease. *Am J Cardiol* 1970; 25: 588–601.
63. Rivero Carvallo JM. El diagnostica de la estenosis tricuspides. *Arch Inst Cardiol Mex* 1950; 20:1–11.
64. Killip T, Lukas DS. Tricuspid stenosis: Clinical features in twelve cases. *Am J Med* 1958; 24:836–852.
65. DePace NL, Ross J, Ashandrian AS, et al. Tricuspid regurgitation: Noninvasive techniques for determining causes and severity. *J Am Coll Cardiol* 1984; 3:1540–1550.
66. Meltzer RS, van Hoogenhuyze D, Serruys PW, et al. Diagnosis of tricuspid regurgitation by contrast echocardiography. *Circulation* 1981; 63:1093–1099.
67. Yock PG, Popp RL. Noninvasive estimation of right ventricular systolic pressure by Doppler ultrasound in patients with tricuspid regurgitation. *Circulation* 1984; 70:657–662.
68. Waggoner AD, Quinones MA, Young JB, et al. Pulsed Doppler echocardiographic detection of right-sided valve regurgitation: Experimental results and clinical significance. *Am J Cardiol* 1981; 47:279–286.
69. Masuyama T, Kodama K, Kitabatake A, et al. Continuous-wave Doppler echocardiographic detection of pulmonary regurgitation and its application to noninvasive estimation of pulmonary artery pressure. *Circulation* 1986;74:484–492.
70. Isobe M, Yazaki Y, Takaku F, et al. Prediction of pulmonary

arterial pressure in adults by pulsed Doppler echocardiography. *Am J Cardiol* 1986; 57:316–321.
71. Chan KL, Currie PJ, Seward JB, et al. Comparison of three Doppler ultrasound methods in the prediction of pulmonary artery pressure. *J Am Coll Cardiol* 1987; 9:549–554.
72. Ogawa S, Hayashi J, Sasaki H, et al. Evaluation of combined valvular prolapse syndrome by two-dimensional echocardiography. *Circulation* 1982; 65:174–180.
73. Otto CM, Pearlman AS, Comens KA, et al. Determination of the stenotic aortic valve area in adults using Doppler echocardiography. *J Am Coll Cardiol* 1986; 7:509–517.
74. Smith MD, Handshoe R, Handshoe S, et al. Comparative accuracy of two-dimensional echocardiography and Doppler pressure half-time methods in assessing severity of mitral stenosis in patients with and without prior commissurotomy. *Circulation* 1986; 78:100–107.
75. Perry GJ, Helmcke F, Nanda NC, et al. Evaluation of aortic insufficiency by Doppler color flow mapping. *J Am Coll Cardiol* 1987; 9:952–959.
76. Enriquez-Serano M, Bailey KP, Seward JB, et al. Quantitative Doppler assessment of valvular regurgitation. *Circulation* 1993; 87:841–848.
77. Winzelberg GG, Boucher CA, Pohost GM, et al. Right ventricular function in aortic and mitral valve disease: Relation of gated first-pass radionuclide angiography to clinical and hemodynamic findings. *Chest* 1981; 79:520–528.
78. Cha SD, Gooch AS, Maranhao V. Intracardiac phonocardiography in tricuspid regurgitation: Relation to clinical and angiographic findings. *Am J Cardiol* 1981; 48:573–583.
79. Rackley CE. Quantitative evaluation of left ventricular function by radiographic techniques. *Circulation* 1976; 54:862–879.
80. Patel TM, Sani SI, Shah SC, Patel TK. Tricuspid balloon valvuloplasty: A more simplified approach using Inoue balloon. *Cath Cardiovasc Diagn* 1996; 37:86–88.
81. Kratz J. Evaluation and management of tricuspid valve disease. *Cardiol Clin* 1991; 9:397–407.
82. Orbe LC, Sobrino N, Arcas R, et al. Initial outcome of percutaneous balloon valvuloplasty in rheumatic tricuspid valve stenosis. *Am J Cardiol* 1993; 71:353–354.
83. Onate A, Alcibar J, Inguanzo R, et al. Balloon dilatation of tricuspid and pulmonary valves in carcinoid heart disease. *Tex Heart Inst J* 1993; 20:115–119.
84. Kay JH, Maselli-Campagna G, Tsuji HK. Surgical treatment of tricuspid insufficiency. *Ann Surg* 1965; 162:53–58.
85. Boyd AD, Engelman RM, Isom OW, et al. Tricuspid annuloplasty: Five and one-half years' experience with 78 patients. *J Thorac Cardiovasc Surg* 1974; 68:344–351.
86. DeVega NF. La annulplastia selectiva: Reguable y permanente. *Rev Esp Cardiol* 1972; 25:55–60.
87. Abe T, Tsukamoto M, Morishita K, et al. 1989: De Vega's annuloplasty for acquired tricuspid disease: Early and late results in 110 patients, updated in 1996. *Ann Thorac Surg* 1996; 62:1876–1877.
88. Carpentier A, Deloche A, Hanania G, et al. Surgical management of acquired tricuspid valve disease. *J Thorac Cardiovasc Surg* 1974; 67:53–65.
89. Deloche A, Guerino J, Fabiani JN, et al. Étude anatomique des valvulopatheis rheumatismales tricuspidiennes. *Ann Chir Thorac Cardiovasc* 1973; 44:343–349.
90. Braunwald NS, Ross J, Morrow AG. Conservative management of tricuspid regurgitation in patients undergoing mitral valve replacement. *Circulation* 1967; 35(suppl 1):163–169.
91. Simon R, Oelert H, Borst HG, Lichtelen PR. Influence of mitral valve surgery on tricuspid incompetence concomitant with mitral valve disease. *Circulation* 1980; 62:1152–1157.
92. Thorburn CW, Morgan JJ, Shanahan MX, Chang VP. Long-term results of tricuspid valve replacement and the problem of prosthetic valve thrombosis. *Am J Cardiol* 1983; 51:1128–1132.
93. Grondin P, Meere C, Limet R, et al. Carpentier's annulus and De Vega's annuloplasty: The end of the tricuspid challenge. *J Thorac Cardiovasc Surg* 1975; 70:852–861.
94. Kay JH, Mendez AM, Zubiate P. A further look at tricuspid annuloplasty. *Ann Thorac Surg* 1976; 22:498–500.
95. Peterffy A, Jonasson R, Szamosi A, Henze A. Comparison of Kay's and De Vega's annuloplasty in surgical treatment of tricuspid incompetence. *Scand J Thorac Cardiovasc Surg* 1980; 14:249–255.
96. Rabago G, De Vega NG, Castillon L, et al. The new De Vega technique in tricuspid annuloplasty: Results in 150 patients. *J Cardiovasc Surg* 1980; 21:231–238.
97. Reed GE, Boyd AD, et al. Operative management of tricuspid regurgitation. *Circulation* 1976; 54(suppl 3):III96–III98.
98. Baughman K, Kallman C, Yurchak P, et al. Predictors of survival after tricuspid surgery. *Am J Cardiol* 1984; 54:137–141.
99. Breye RH, McClenathan JH, Michaelis LL, et al. Tricuspid regurgitation: A comparison of nonoperative management, tricuspid annuloplasty, and tricuspid valve replacement. *J Thorac Cardiovasc Surg* 1976; 72:867–874.
100. Jugdutt BI, Fraser RS, Lee SJK, et al. Long-term survival after tricuspid valve replacement: Results with seven different prostheses. *J Thorac Cardiovasc Surg* 1977; 74:20–27.
101. Kouchoukos NT, Stephenson LW. Indications for and results of tricuspid valve replacement. *Adv Cardiol* 1976; 17:199–206.
102. Sanfelippo PM, Giuliani ER, Danielson GK, et al. Tricuspid valve prosthetic replacement: Early and late results with the Starr-Edwards prosthesis. *J Thorac Cardiovasc Surg* 1976; 71: 441–445.
103. Singh AK, Christian FD, Williams DO, et al. Follow-up assessment of St. Jude medical prosthetic valve in the tricuspid position: Clinical and hemodynamic results. *Ann Thorac Surg* 1984; 37:324–327.
104. Arbulu A, Asfaw I. Tricuspid valvulectomy without prosthetic replacement: Ten years of clinical experience. *J Thorac Cardiovasc Surg* 1981; 82:684–691.
105. Stern H, Sisto D, Strom J, et al. Immediate tricuspid valve replacement for endocarditis. *J Thorac Cardiovasc Surg* 1986; 91: 163–167.
106. D'Ambra M, LaRaia P, Philbin D, et al. Prostaglandin E1: A new therapy for refractory right heart failure and pulmonary hypertension after mitral valve replacement. *J Thorac Cardiovasc Surg* 1985; 89:567–572.
107. Miller DD, Moreno-Cabral RJ, Stinson EB, et al. Pulmonary artery balloon counterpulsation for acute right ventricular failure. *J Thorac Cardiovasc Surg* 1980; 80:760–763.
108. Cannegieter SC, Rosendaal FR, Wintzen AR, et al. Optimal oral anticoagulant therapy in patients with mechanical heart valves. *N Engl J Med* 1995; 333:11–17.
109. Chesebro JH, Fuster V, Elveback LR, et al. Trial of combined warfarin plus dipyridamole of aspirin therapy in prosthetic heart valve replacement: Danger of aspirin compared with dipyridamole. *Am J Cardiol* 1983; 51:1537–1541.
110. Boskovic D, Elezovic I, Boskovic D, et al. Late thrombosis of the Björk-Shiley tilting disc valve in the tricuspid position. *J Thorac Cardiovasc Surg* 1986; 91:1–8.
111. DePace NL, Iskandrian AS, Morganroth J, et al. Infective endocarditis involving a presumably normal pulmonic valve. *Am J Cardiol* 1984; 53:385–387.
112. Misbach GA, Turley K, Ebert PA. Pulmonary valve replacement for regurgitation after repair of tetralogy of Fallot. *Ann Thorac Surg* 1983; 36:684–691.
113. Wessel HU, Cunningham WJ, Paul MH, et al. Exercise performance in tetralogy of Fallot after intracardiac repair. *J Thorac Cardiovasc Surg* 1980; 80:582–593.

114. Cassling R, Rogler W, McManus B. Isolated pulmonic valve infective endocarditis: A diagnostically elusive study. *Am Heart J* 1985; 109:558–567.
115. Stephenson LW, Edic RN, Harken AH, Edmunds H Jr. Combined aortic and mitral valve replacement: Changes in practice and prognosis. *Circulation* 1984; 69:640–644.
116. Kumar AS, Chander H, Trehan H. Surgical technique of multiple valve replacement with biological valves. *J Heart Valve Dis* 1995; 4:45–46.
117. Blackstone EH, Kirklin JW. Death and other time-related events after valve replacement. *Circulation* 1985; 72:753–767.
118. Skudicky D, Essop MR, Sareli P. Efficacy of mitral balloon valvotomy in reducing the severity of associate tricuspid valve regurgitation. *Am J Cardiol* 1994; 73:209–211.

CHAPTER 60

CLINICAL PERFORMANCE OF PROSTHETIC HEART VALVES

Gary L. Grunkemeier / Albert Starr / Shahbudin H. Rahimtoola

A heart valve functions as a check valve: opening to permit forward blood flow and closing to prevent retrograde flow, about 40 million times per year. Heart valve prostheses consist of an orifice, through which blood flows, and an occluding mechanism that closes and opens the orifice. There are two classes of heart valves: *mechanical prostheses,* with rigid, manufactured occluders, and *biological* or *tissue valves,* with flexible leaflet occluders of animal or human origin. Among the mechanical valves there are three basic types, depending on whether the occluding mechanism is (1) a reciprocating ball, (2) a tilting disk, or (3) two semicircular hinged leaflets. The biological valves include those whose origin is from (1) the patient, (2) another human, or (3) another species. For each type there are several models available from different manufacturers. Selected frequently used valves are described.

PROSTHETIC HEART VALVES

Mechanical Valves

Ball valves appeared in the early 1960s, disk valves in the early 1970s, and bileaflet valves predominantly during the 1980s.

BALL VALVES

The first successful valve replacement devices, which led to long-term survivors and a design that has endured until today, used a ball-in-cage design.[1,2] Several modifications of this design have been used, but only the *Starr-Edwards* valve (Fig. 60-1, Plate 94) has endured; it has been used about 200,000 times.

DISK VALVES

Improvement on the clinical success of the ball valves was sought by developing designs with reduced height. The first successful low-profile design was the *Björk-Shiley* tilting-disk valve, introduced in 1969.[3] It evolved through several design refinements,[4] and about 360,000 valves were implanted. These refinements also introduced a structural failure mode caused by strut fracture in the Convexo-Concave model. Some results with the discontinued Björk-Shiley models are included because many patients are still alive with these valves. Tilting-disk valves employ a circular disk as an occluder. It is retained by wirelike arms or closed loops that project into the orifice. The disks are graphite with a coating of pyrolytic carbon, and the housings are stainless steel or titanium. With the disk open, the primary orifice is separated into two unequal (major and minor) orifices. The *Medtronic Hall* valve has been used clinically since 1977.

BILEAFLET VALVES

Current development in mechanical valves is based on the bileaflet design, introduced by St. Jude Medical in 1977. Unlike the free-floating occluders in ball and disk valves, the two semicircular leaflets of a bileaflet valve are connected to the orifice housing by a hinge mechanism. The leaflets swing apart during opening, creating three flow areas: one central and two peripheral. The *St. Jude* bileaflet valve (Fig. 60-2, Plate 95) has been used over 900,000 times and the *Carbomedics* valve has been used about 300,000 times since its clinical introduction in 1986.

Biological Valves

Biological valves include as wide a variety of models, as do mechanical valves:

1. An *autograft* valve is one that is translocated within the same individual—e.g., the pulmonary valve in the aortic valve position.
2. A *homograft* (or allograft) valve is one that has been transplanted from a donor of the same species—when, for example, a donor's aortic or pulmonary valve has been placed in a recipient's aortic or pulmonary position.

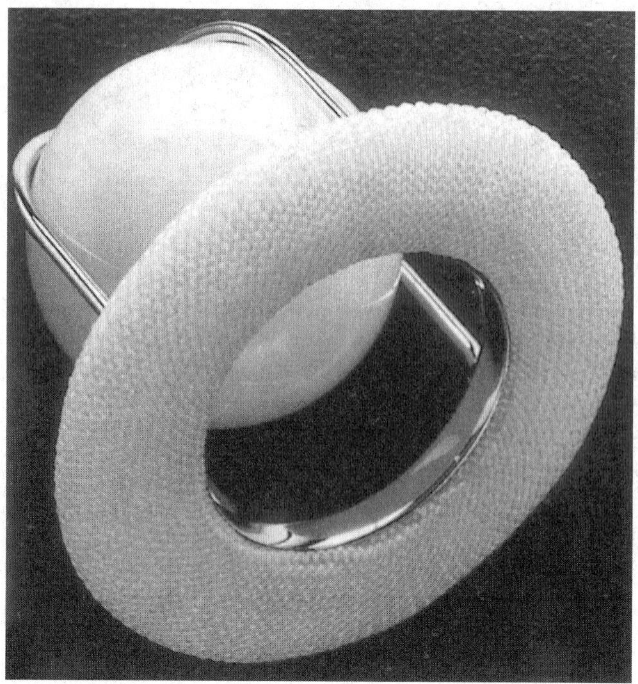

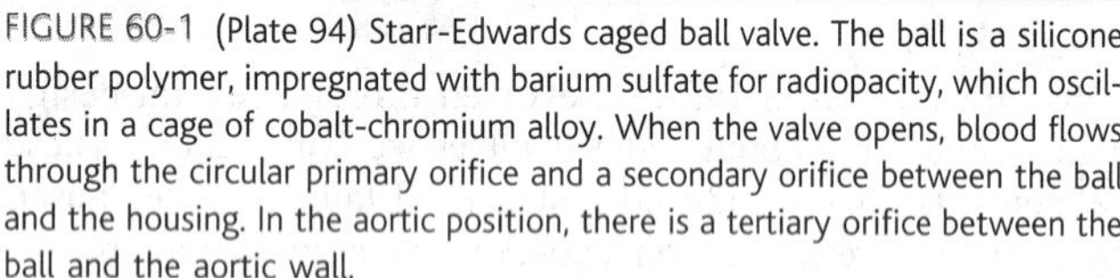

FIGURE 60-1 (Plate 94) Starr-Edwards caged ball valve. The ball is a silicone rubber polymer, impregnated with barium sulfate for radiopacity, which oscillates in a cage of cobalt-chromium alloy. When the valve opens, blood flows through the circular primary orifice and a secondary orifice between the ball and the housing. In the aortic position, there is a tertiary orifice between the ball and the aortic wall.

3. *Heterograft* (or xenograft) valve is a transplant from another species, either an intact valve (e.g., a porcine aortic valve) or a valve fashioned from heterologous tissue (e.g., bovine pericardium).

The point of using biological valves is to reduce the complications associated with thromboembolism and the need for anticoagulation. The first successful biological valves were homografts, pioneered by Ross[5] and Barratt-Boyes[6] in 1962.

AUTOGRAFT

The pulmonary autograft procedure consists of an autotransplant of the pulmonary valve to the aortic position; the pulmonary valve is then replaced by an aortic or pulmonary homograft. This operation was first described in 1967[7] and is called the Ross procedure; it is currently undergoing increased popularity,[8–12] but this operation involves a double valve replacement, with the attendant early and late risks. This procedure uses double valve replacement to solve a single valve problem; however, subsequent problems with pulmonary valve replacement may be easier to remedy and those related to autograft will be similar to those of aortic valve re-replacement.

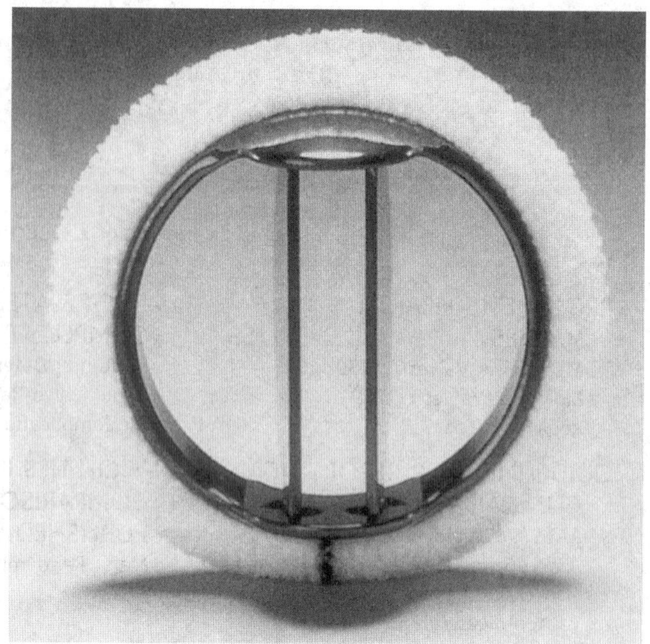

A

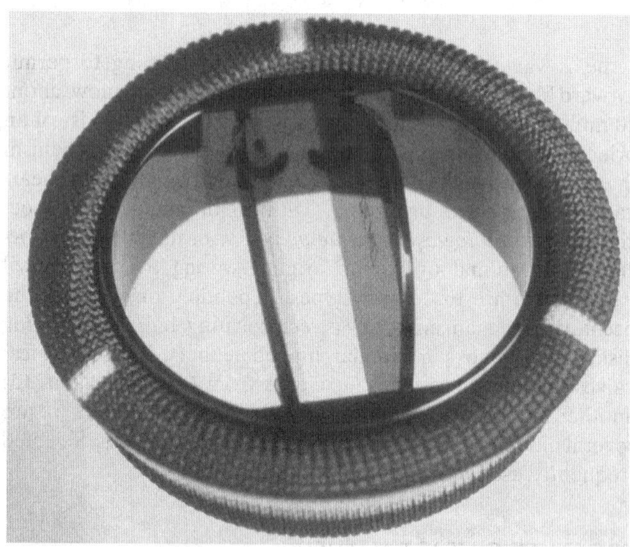

B

FIGURE 60-2 (Plate 95) Bileaflet valves. The St. Jude Medical valve (*A*) has leaflets that open to an angle of 85 degrees from the plane of the orifice and travel from 55 to 60 degrees to the fully closed position, depending on valve size. The original version, whose housing did not rotate within the sewing ring, has been supplemented by a model that does rotate for intraoperative adjustment. The Carbomedics valve (*B*) has flat leaflets that open to 78 to 80 degrees and close at an angle of 25 degrees with the horizontal and has a carbon-coated surface on the sewing ring to inhibit thrombus formation.

HOMOGRAFT

The homograft valve is considered to be a preferred substitute for aortic valve replacement, especially in younger patients. It achieves excellent hemodynamics; there is no need for anticoagulation and it has low thrombogenicity. The drawbacks are a more technically demanding operation and a low availability; however, the latter drawback has been alleviated by its commercial availability from cryopreservation services. Several methods of procurement, sterilization, and preservation have been used.[13] Three surgical techniques are used for aortic valve replacement: (1) replacement of the valve only into the subcoronary position, (2) complete aortic root replacement with reimplantation of

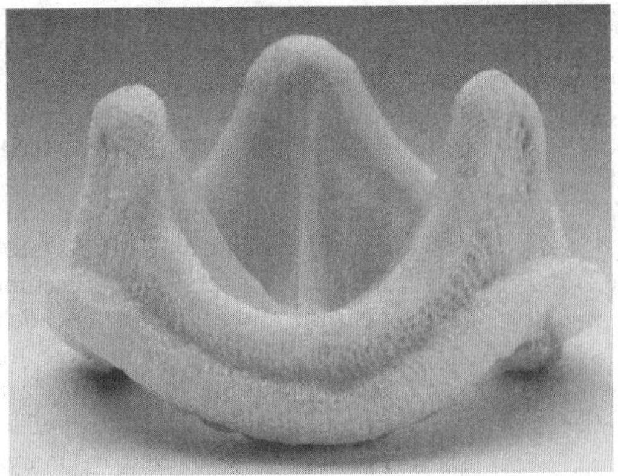

FIGURE 60-3 (Plate 96) Stented porcine valves. The Carpentier-Edwards SupraAnnular Valve is designed to be implanted above rather than within the aortic annulus. It has low-pressure fixation and a cone-shaped stent which flares out at the top to improve leaflet durability.

the coronary arteries, and (3) miniroot replacement with part of the donor aortic wall inserted within the host aorta.

PORCINE HETEROGRAFT

Glutaraldehyde sterilizes valve tissue, renders it bioacceptable by destroying antigenicity, and stabilizes the collagen cross-links for durability. The use of glutaraldehyde for tissue preservation was pioneered by Carpentier,[14] who introduced the term *bioprosthesis*[15] for nonviable valves of biological origin, such as the *Hancock II* and *Carpentier-Edwards SupraAnnular* (SAV) porcine valves (Fig. 60-3, Plate 96).

Most porcine valves are mounted on rigid or flexible stents, to which the leaflets and the sewing ring are attached. Unstented versions have also been devised by several manufacturers.[16–20] Their goal is to achieve some of the potential benefit of a homograft valve, especially hemodynamics and perhaps durability, with an easily available commercial product. The valve, however, is porcine and can be expected to have the same problems of primary valve failure as the stented porcine valve. As with homografts, there are potentially three ways of implanting a stentless porcine valve (valve only, aortic root replacement, and cylinder inclusion). The St. Jude Medical Toronto SPV (Fig. 60-4, Plate 97) and the Medtronic Freestyle (Fig. 60-5, Plate 98) stentless porcine valves were approved for marketing by the FDA in 1997.

BOVINE PERICARDIAL VALVE

Pericardial valves that are tailored and sewn into a valvular configuration using bovine pericardium as a fabric result in a valve that opens more completely than a porcine valve, providing better hemodynamics. They might also be expected to have better durability, because there is extra tissue to allow for shrinkage and a higher percentage of collagen to be cross-linked during fixation. Unfortunately, the Ionescu-Shiley, the first commercially available pericardial valve, did not bear out this promise and was taken off the market, as was the Hancock pericardial valve. These failures were due to aspects of the design, however, rather than to an intrinsic problem with pericardial tissue. The Carpentier-Edwards Perimount pericardial bioprosthesis (Fig. 60-6) has a method of construction that overcomes these design issues. It has been used clinically since 1982 and received FDA approval, for the aortic position only, in 1991.

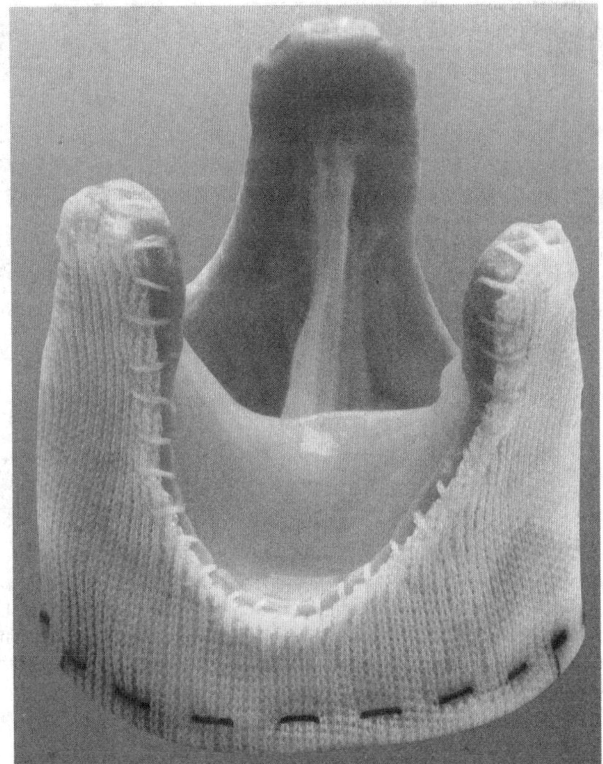

A

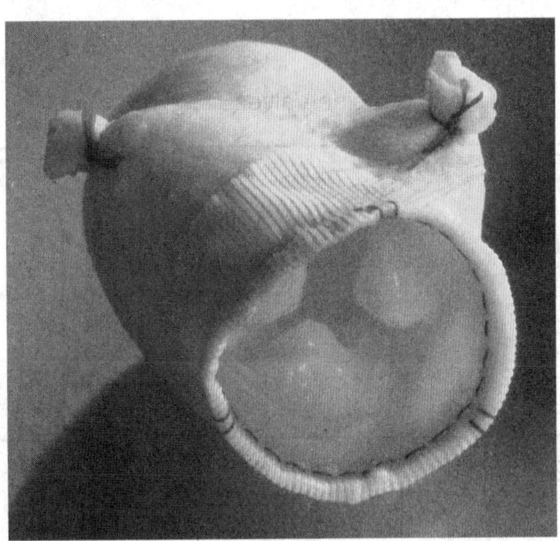

B

FIGURE 60-4 (Plate 97) St. Jude Toronto SPV (*A*) and Medtronic Freestyle (*B*) stentless porcine valves. The Toronto SPV is designed to be used as a subcoronary valve replacement. The Freestyle can be implanted using any of the methods of implantation used for homografts: subcoronary implantation of the valve alone, aortic root replacement, or cylinder (root) inclusion.

Repair

When possible, valve repair[21–23] is generally preferable to replacement (see discussion below).

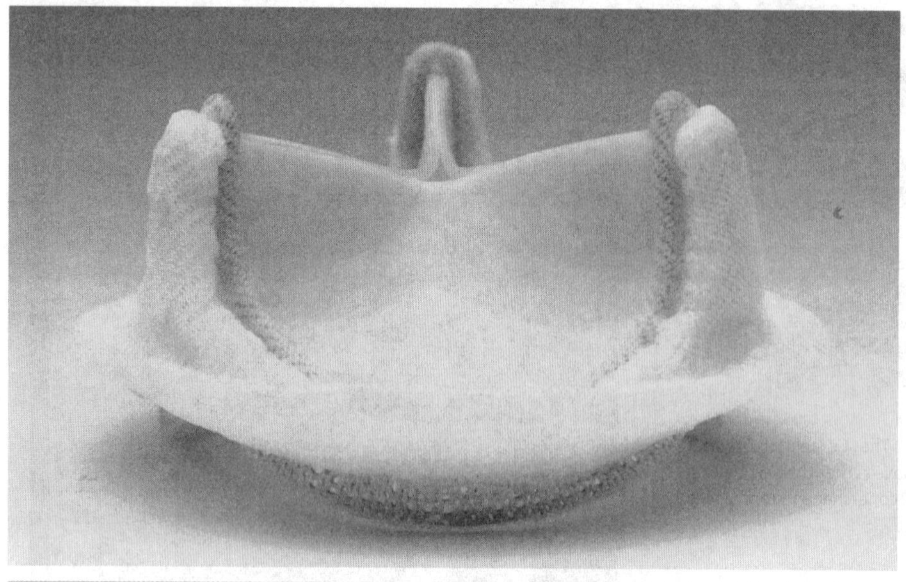

FIGURE 60-5 (Plate 98) The Carpentier-Edwards Perimount pericardial bioprosthesis uses a method of mounting the leaflets to the stent, which does not depend on retaining stitches passed through the pericardium—a design weakness of previous pericardial valves. Instead, the leaflets are anchored behind the stent pillars.

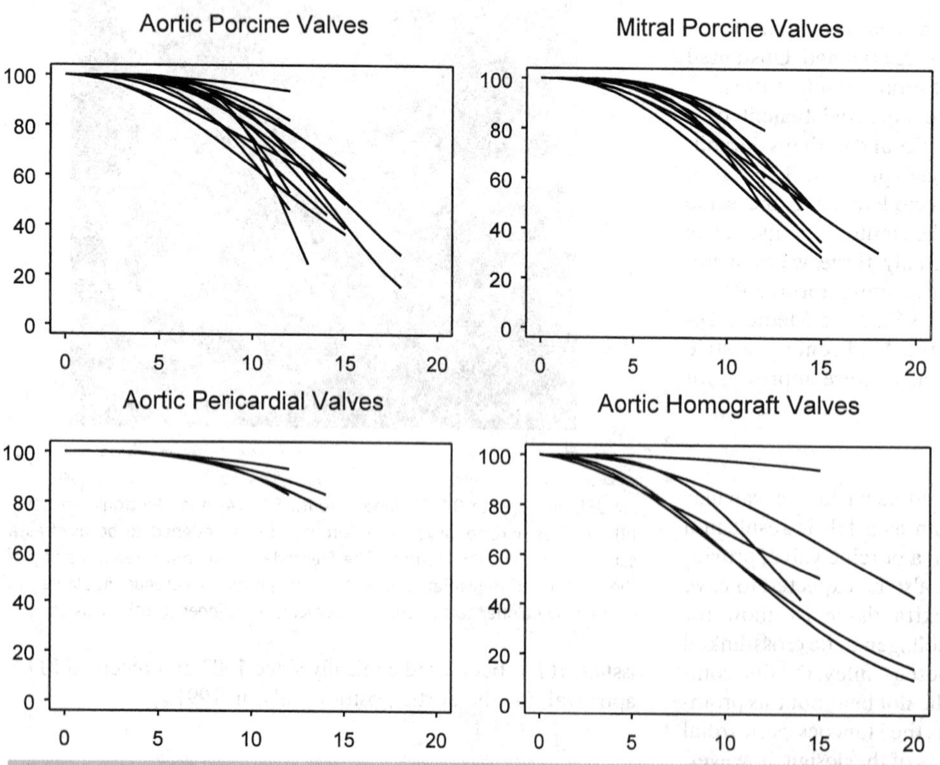

FIGURE 60-6 Structural valve deterioration with four types of biological valves. The vertical axes represent percent freedom from SVD; horizontal axes represent years after implant. These follow-up data relates to studies with minimum follow-up to 400 valve-years and conform to the FDA requirements for each location of valve. (From Grunkemeier et al.[61] Reproduced by permission of the publisher and authors.)

GUIDELINES FOR REPORTING CLINICAL RESULTS

The analytic aspects of the reporting of clinical results of heart valves have evolved consistently since the first successful implants in 1960. As late (posthospital) experience accumulated near the end of the first decade of implants, the need to analyze time-related events resulted in the introduction of actuarial analysis,[24] which had previously been used to analyze the results of cancer therapy.[25] Later, the use of linearized (constant hazard) rates,[26,27] Cox regression,[28] and multivariable parametric models[29] was advocated. The effectiveness of these refined statistical methods in comparing results from different series, however, was limited by the lack of standardization in definitions and follow-up methods.

AATS/STS Guidelines for Clinical Reporting

In 1988, standards that specified which complications should be collected and how they should be defined were proposed by the Ad Hoc Liaison Committee for Standardizing Definitions of Prosthetic Heart Valve Morbidity, a joint committee of the American Association for Thoracic Surgery (AATS) and the Society of Thoracic Surgeons (STS).[30] These guidelines were revised in 1996.[31,32] The complications that were determined to be of critical importance by these guidelines are as follows:

1. *Structural valvular deterioration,* or any change in function of an operated valve resulting from an intrinsic abnormality that causes stenosis or regurgitation.
2. *Nonstructural dysfunction,* a composite category that includes any abnormality that results in stenosis or regurgitation of the operated valve that is not intrinsic to the valve itself, exclusive of thrombosis and infection. This includes inappropriate sizing, also called *prosthesis-patient mismatch.*[33]

3. *Valve thrombosis* is any thrombus, in the absence of infection, attached to or near an operated valve that occludes part of the blood flow path or that interferes with the function of the valve.
4. *Embolism* is any embolic event that occurs in the absence of infection after the immediate perioperative period (when anesthesia-induced unconsciousness is completely reversed). These include any new, temporary or permanent, focal or global neurologic deficits and peripheral embolic events; emboli proven to consist of nonthrombotic material are excluded.
5. *Bleeding event (formerly anticoagulant hemorrhage)* is any episode of major internal or external bleeding that causes death, hospitalization, or permanent injury (e.g., vision loss) or requires transfusion. The complication "bleeding event" applies to all patients, whether or not they are taking anticoagulants or antiplatelet drugs.
6. *Operated valvular endocarditis* is any infection involving an operated valve. Morbidity associated with active infection—such as valve thrombosis, thrombotic embolus, bleeding event, or paravalvular leak—is included under this category but is not included in other categories of morbidity.

TABLE 60-1 Complications for Evaluating Clinical Performance of Replacement Heart Valves and Objective Performance Criteria (OPC)[a] Values for Complication Rates (Percent/Year)

Definitions of Morbidity	OPC, %/YEAR Mechanical	Biological
1. *Structural deterioration:* Valve deterioration, wear, stress fracture, poppet escape, clacification, leaflet tear, stent creep; *excludes* infected or thrombosed valves		
2. *Nonstructural dysfunction:* Entrapment by pannus or suture, leak, inappropriate sizing, hemolytic anemia; excludes thromboembolism and infection	(leak) 1.2 (major 0.6)	(leak) 1.2 (major 0.6)
3A. *Valve thrombosis:* Thrombosis proved by operation, autopsy, or clinical investigation; *excludes* infection	0.8	0.2
3B. *Thromboembolism:* Neurologic deficit, peripheral arterial emboli, acute myocardial infarction *after* operation in patients with known normal coronary arteries or those <40 years of age; *excludes* septic emboli, hemorrhage, immediate surgical events	3.0	2.5
4. *Anticoagulant-related hemorrhage:* Bleeding that causes death, stroke, operation, hospitalization, or transfusion in patients receiving anticoagulants and/or antiplatelet drugs	3.5 (major 1.5)	1.4 (major 0.9)
5. *Prosthetic valve endocarditis:* Based on blood cultures, clinical signs, and/or histologic evidence at reoperation or autopsy; *includes* valve thrombosis, embolus, or paravalvular leak associated with active infection	1.2	1.2

[a]Please see text for definition of OPC.
SOURCE: The complications and their definitions are adapted from Ref. 30, the OPC values are taken from Appendix K of Ref. 35.

The *consequences* of the above morbid events include reoperation, valve-related mortality, sudden unexpected unexplained death, cardiac death, total deaths, and permanent valve-related impairment.[31,32]

FDA Guidelines for New Valve Approvals

In 1976, medical devices including prosthetic heart valves came under the jurisdiction of the FDA,[34] which subsequently issued various guidelines for submission of premarket approval (PMA) applications for heart valves. The FDA issued a guidance document in December 1993[35] that used the analytical approach to clinical studies adapted from the work of Gersh et al.[36] These authors proposed a method for premarket clinical testing of heart valves that emphasizes confidence interval estimation and comparisons to objective performance criteria (OPC). *OPC are linearized rates for critical complications, representing averages achieved by the best currently used valves.* A *linearized rate* is calculated as the number of events divided by total patient-years and multiplied by 100 to convert it to units of "events per 100 years" or "percent per year."[27]

To determine OPC for contemporary use, the FDA screened the literature plus data submitted by clinical investigators of approved devices and identified OPC for the major morbidity categories.[35] They determined that these rates were similar for aortic and mitral positions but varied for some complications between mechanical and biological valves. The OPC for complications are given in Table 60-1 for mechanical and biological replacement heart valves. Several observations on these data are significant.

The category *Structural deterioration* was not included in the list of OPC because the clinical PMA investigation is not designed to detect intrinsic valve failure. Structural durability should be evaluated by in vitro testing, and the clinical realization of structural failure should be so small (mechanical valves) that the clinical study is of insufficient size or so long-term (tissue valves) that the clinical study is of insufficient duration to assess it adequately.

From the *Nonstructural dysfunction* category, the FDA included only leak, the most common and the most frequently reported subcategory, and derived OPC for major leaks ("as defined by AATS/STS, 1988")[30] and for all leaks.

The FDA separated *Thromboembolism* into the separate categories of valve thrombosis and thromboembolism, as had been strongly advocated,[37,38] and the FDA derived OPC both for major *Anticoagulant-related hemorrhage* events ("as defined by AATS/STS, 1988")[30] and for all bleeding events.

Based on the OPC values given in Table 60-1, the FDA has set the minimum amount of follow-up required for a PMA study at 800 valve-years.[39] The assumption of constant risk for heart valve complications, as embodied by the OPC formulation, is only an approximation; but if operative events are excluded (the intent of the FDA guidelines) and maximum follow-up is in the 2- to 3-year range, this assumption may be acceptable, at least for the purpose of sample size estimation.

VALVE-RELATED COMPLICATIONS

Actuarial valve failure–free curves[25] are used to describe tissue valve durability, and linearized rates[27] are used for all other complications.

Structural Deterioration

This category, the first one considered in the guidelines for reporting, virtually always results in death or valve explant. There is a dual standard with regard to this complication: for biological valves, structural deterioration is probably inevitable if the patient lives long enough; whereas for mechanical valves, the only acceptable rate is a very low one (near zero).

MECHANICAL VALVES

The durability of currently used mechanical valves is remarkable, given the harsh biological environment in which the valve must perform. For example, the current Starr-Edwards ball valve, now in use for 35 years and in over 200,000 patients, has had fewer than a dozen structural problems reported to the manufacturer, most of which did not cause clinical problems. Even the discontinued Björk-Shiley Convexo-Concave valve, whose strut fracture failures have been highly publicized, had fewer than 1 percent failures reported after 15 years of experience.[40] The Medtronic Hall valve had three leaflet fractures in a version that is not used in the United States. The problem was determined to be related to unequal coatings of pyrolytic carbon on the two faces of the leaflet and to be limited to a very small subset of valves. Since the manufacturing specifications were changed to ensure more equal coatings, the problem has not recurred. The St. Jude valve has had only 12 reported postoperative fractures of the disk or housing, which resulted in leaflet escape reported to the FDA—an excellent record considering that over 900,000 valves have been implanted.

BIOLOGICAL VALVES

Data on freedom from structural deterioration for several series of aortic porcine and pericardial bioprostheses and homografts are shown in Fig. 60-6. The mean age of patients in these older series is around 50 years. The current series of porcine valves, together with the tendency to select older patients,[41–44] should have improved durability. Design changes in some porcine valves,[45,46] such as stentless configurations,[16–20] may possibly improve durability.

Although the Carpentier-Edwards pericardial valve has been available for over 15 years, relatively few long-term results on the valve are available. Those that have been reported, however, show improved durability in the aortic position, as compared with the previously discontinued Ionescu-Shiley pericardial valve. The durability of the Carpentier-Edwards pericardial valve also compares favorably with that of porcine valves (Fig. 60-6; Table 60-2). The patients in the Carpentier-Edwards pericardial valve series were older than patients in previous series of pericardial and porcine valves, however, and it is unknown to what extent this has resulted in apparent improvement in the durability of the Carpentier-Edwards pericardial valve.

Structural durability is considered to be better with *homografts* than with other bioprostheses. From various published reports[13] for homografts used primarily in the aortic position, it is apparent that the variation among series is wide, the current methods of sterilization/preservation provide better results than those which have been discontinued, and the results do not appear better than those for porcine bioprostheses (Fig. 60-6).

The pulmonary autograft is considered an excellent aortic valve substitute, especially for young patients[10] and in the treatment of patients with endocarditis.[47] Freedom from reoperation has been reported as 100 percent in 33 patients from 8 to 47 years old followed to a maximum of 48 months[11] and 93 percent at 5.5 years in 51 patients from 2 to 21 years old.[10] Data from one center showed 48.5 percent freedom from reoperation at 19 years[47] and, after excluding patients from three hospitals, 85 percent freedom from reoperation at 20 years.[48] To evaluate complications of this procedure fully, problems with the valve used to replace the pulmonary valve must be combined with complications of the pulmonary autograft itself.

TABLE 60-2 14-Year Results with Carpentier-Edwards Pericardial Valve

		FDA-Mandated Patients[a] (n = 267) Actuarial (%)
Thromboembolism/thrombosis		19 ± 4
Anticoagulant-related bleeding		6 ± 2
Endocarditis/sepsis		7 ± 2
Valve dysfunction		70 ± 4
Explant due to structural valve deterioration:	Total	15 ± 3
	≤65 years of age	24 ± 5
	>65 years of age	4 ± 2
Mortality:	Total	60 ± 3.1
	Valve-related	21 ± 3.2

[a]FDA approval was based on 719 patients at 7 years. Data from FDA-mandated longer follow-up of selected patients are from Frater et al.[85]

VALVE REPAIR

Mitral valve repair is considered preferable to replacement, when practicable. It has been shown to improve ejection fraction[49] and to provide good results for treating bacterial endocarditis[50] and valve problems in elderly patients.[51,52] It has been strongly suggested that it improves survival; however, there are problems associated with the comparisons.[53]

The weakness of valve repair is durability. The 10-year actuarial reoperation rate has been reported to be 15 percent in nonrheumatic mitral disease.[54] The reoperation rate for patients with rheumatic mitral disease varies from 25 percent reoperation at 5 years[55] to 17 percent at 10 years in a large series in which calcium debridement[56] and anterior leaflet procedures were performed.[57] The reoperation rate at 10 years was 24 percent for patients less than 20 years of age and 9 percent at 10 years for patients over 20 years of age.[58]

Early results of aortic valve repair have been published,[23,59,60] but further follow-up is needed to assess the long-term results.

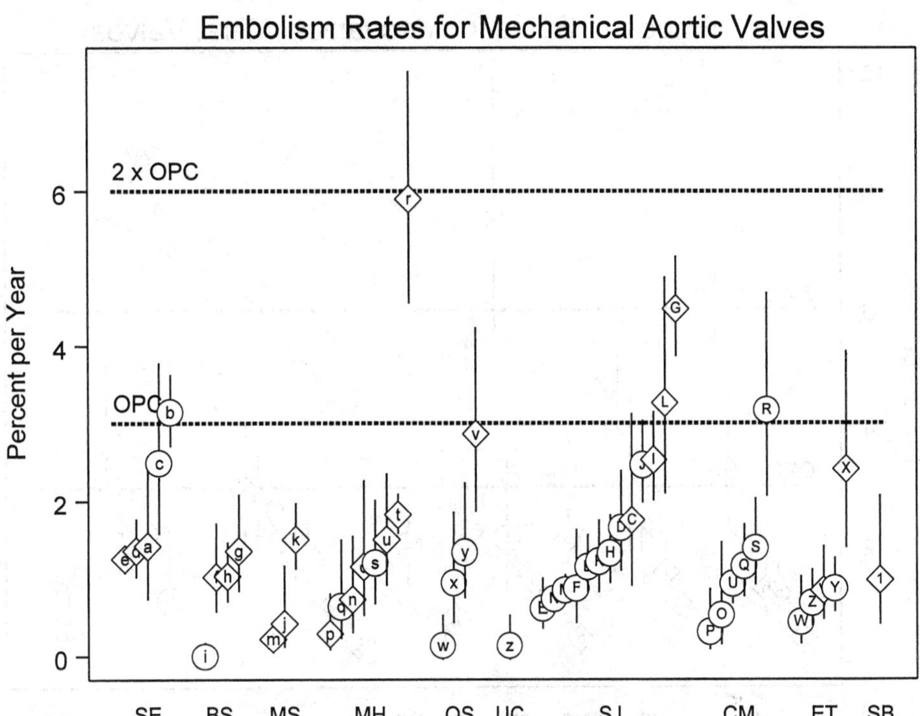

FIGURE 60-7 Embolism rates for mechanical aortic valves. Each open symbol represents a different series, and the height of the symbol is the linearized rate for the series. The vertical bar indicates the 95 percent confidence interval. There is a dashed line at the height of the FDA objective performance criteria (OPC); for approval of a new valve, the upper confidence limit should be less than twice the OPC (*upper dashed line*). Diamonds indicate that both early and late events were used to calculate the rates, circles indicate that only late events were used. Letters inside the symbols correspond to the cited references for the series in the original publication. The series are grouped by valve model, shown below the horizontal axis by two-letter abbreviations: SE = Star-Edwards caged-ball; BS = Björk-Shiley tilting disk; MS = Monostrut tilting disk; MH = Medtronic Hall tilting disk; OS = Omniscience and Omnicarbon tilting disk; UC = Ultracor tilting disk; SJ = St. Jude bileaflet; CM = Carbomedics bileaflet; ET = Edwards Tekna and Duromedics bileaflet; SB = Sorin Bicarbon bileaflet. (From Grunkemeier et al.[61] Reproduced by permission of the publisher and authors.)

Other Valve-Related Complications

Linearized rates are often used to describe the complications required by the AATS/STS guidelines for reporting.[30–32] The use of such rates assumes that the risks are constant, which is usually only approximately true. A review of a large number of published reports of the performance of prosthetic heart valves reveals a wide spread of results for every complication for every valve. In 172 series of heart valves covering 335,485 valve-years accumulated by 63,531 valves of 20 different models implanted in two positions (aortic, mitral), the linearized event rates ranged from 0 to 7.5 percent per year for thromboembolism, 0 to 0.6 percent per year for thrombosis, 0 to 9.3 percent per year for bleeding, 0 to 1.7 percent per year for infection, and 0 to 2.8 percent per year for paravalvular leak.[61] Caution must be exercised in directly comparing event rates among valves for many reasons, including the simplifications involved in the use of linearized rates, varying definitions of complications (many of these reports predate the standardized definitions), and differences in patient characteristics between series.[53,62]

DIFFICULTIES IN MAKING COMPARISONS BETWEEN PUBLISHED SERIES

As noted above, there is wide variation in the reported complication rates of series using the same valves. Figures 60-7 to 60-10 illustrate the wide range of embolism with use of the same heart valve in different series. This variation must be due to variations between series other than the *valve model.* These include factors associated with the following:

1. *Patients*—age, ventricular function, comorbidities, etc.
2. *Reporting center*—surgical variables, postoperative medical management, method, frequency and thoroughness of follow-up, definitions of complications, etc.
3. Problems with *data analysis*[63,64]—many patient-related factors are known to influence thromboembolism,[53,65] stroke rates in patients with atrial fibrillation and in the elderly are equal to those observed in prosthetic valve series,[66] and standardized definitions[30–32] were not in effect or were not employed when many of the available series were reported, etc.
4. *Published data*—these reports describe only a small fraction of the valves implanted and are probably not a representative subset.

Several types of bias can affect reported results. As examples, selection bias occurs in the collection and analysis of data and the decision to report them;[63] publication bias describes the fact that published series tend to be those with the best (or worst, but

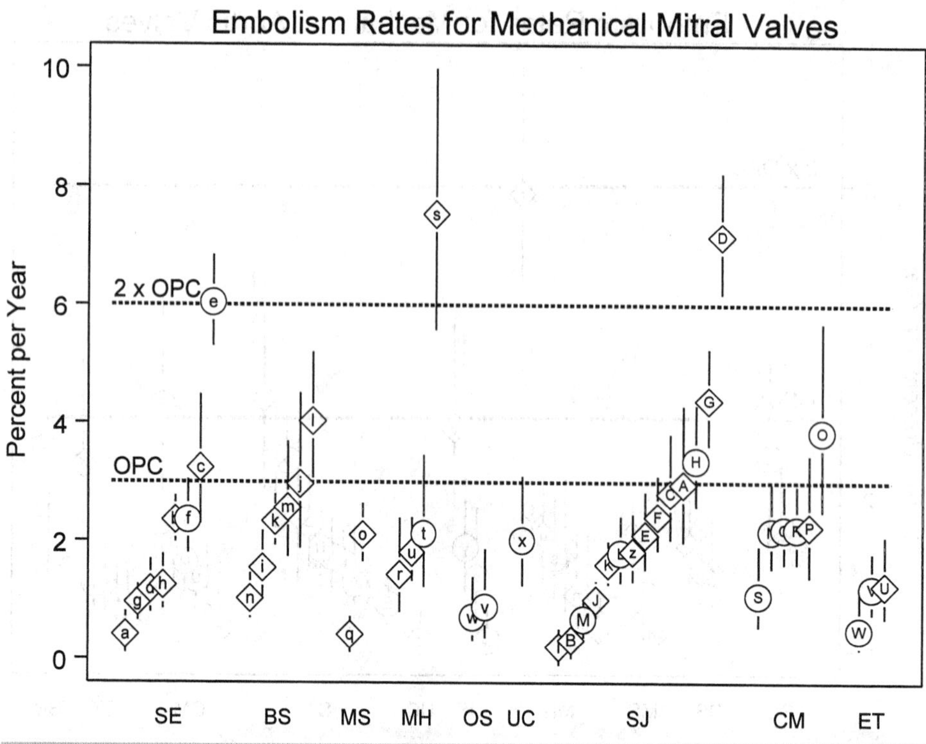

FIGURE 60-8 Embolism rates for mechanical mitral valves. For explanation of symbols and valve model abbreviations, see Fig. 60-7. (From Grunkemeier et al.[61] Reproduced by permission of the publisher and authors.)

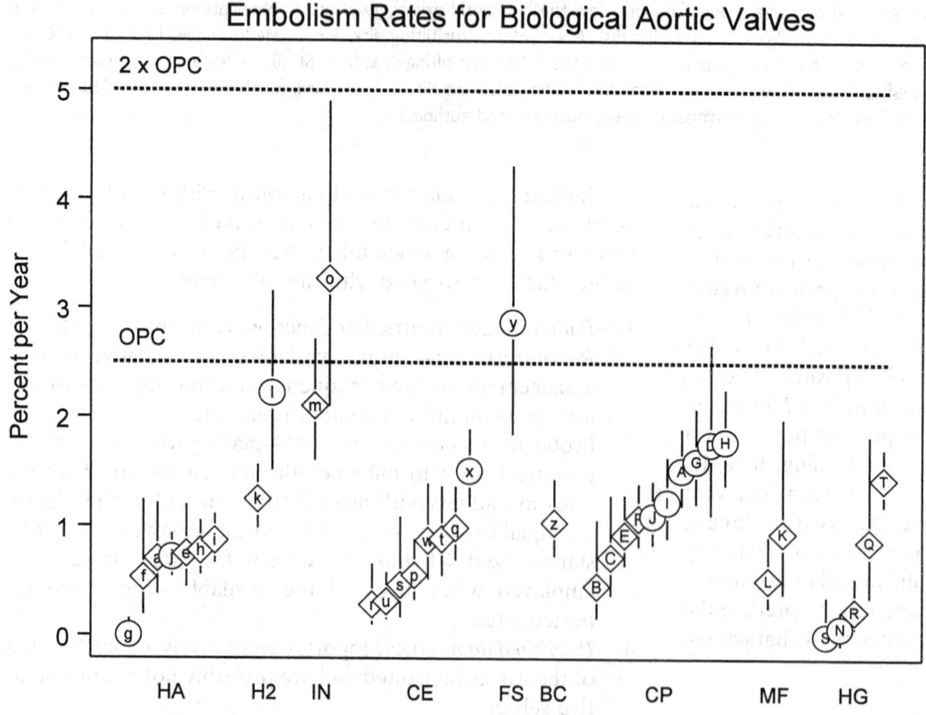

FIGURE 60-9 Embolism rates for biological aortic valves. For explanation of symbols, see Fig. 60-7. Valve model abbreviations: HA = Hancock I and Modified Orifice porcine; H2 = Hancock II porcine; IN = Intact porcine; CE = Carpentier-Edwards porcine; FS = Freestyle stentless porcine; BC = Biocor stentless porcine; CP = Carpentier-Edwards Perimount pericardial; MF = Mitroflow pericardial; HG = homograft. (From Grunkemeier et al.[61] Reproduced by permission of the publisher and authors.)

not typical) results.[67] If a random allocation of valves had been made among patients within a center, statistical methods could theoretically assess the effect on complication rates due to valve model. For logistic, financial, and ethical reasons, however, the number of randomized studies of valves is small, and the available studies are usually of insufficient size to show differences among valves. Although randomized studies provide the best internal validity or valve-specific comparison within centers, they may lack external validity or generalizability to patients outside of the study.[68]

A theoretically preferable way to answer this bias is to allocate patients randomly to different treatments (valves). Randomized trials, however, also have difficulties,[69] and as noted, there are logistic, financial, and ethical arguments against randomization of patients to different heart valves.[70] Consequently, the number of randomized studies of valves is small, and those that exist are usually of insufficient size to add to the knowledge already obtained from careful observational studies except for comparison of survival data with use of different types of prosthesis.

Major Randomized Trials

The two major randomized clinical trials that have been reported are the Edinburgh Heart Valve Trial[71] and the Veterans Administration (VA) Cooperative Study on Valvular Heart Disease.[72] Both studies compared mechanical valves to porcine bioprostheses.

The Edinburgh trial compared the Björk-Shiley Standard valve to porcine valves—initially the Hancock and later the Carpentier-Edwards.[71] It contains actuarial comparisons at 5 and 12 years for the 211 aortic and 261 mitral valve patients. The authors concluded that survival with a mechanical valve was better than with the bioprosthetic valve, but that this was somewhat offset by the increased risk of bleeding.

The VA trial compared the

standard Björk-Shiley valve to the Hancock Modified Orifice (size 21 to 23 mm aortic) or Hancock Standard (other sizes) porcine valves.[72] Table 60-3 contains actuarial comparisons of the endpoint variables at 15 years. The principal long-term findings of this randomized trial[73] are: (1) Use of a mechanical valve resulted in a lower mortality and a lower reoperation rate after aortic valve replacement (AVR); (2) The mortality after mitral valve replacement (MVR) was similar with use of the two prosthetic valve types; (3) There were virtually no primary valve failures with use of a mechanical valve; (4) Primary valve failure after AVR and MVR occurred more frequently in patients with a bioprosthetic valve especially in patients aged <65 years; (5) The primary valve failure rate between bioprosthesis and mechanical valve was not significantly different in those aged ≥65 years; (6) Use of a bioprosthetic valve resulted in a lower bleeding rate; and (7) There were no significant differences between the two valve types with regard to other valve related complications including thromboembolism, and all complications.

Comparison of the 12-year actuarial event rates between these two trials[72] showed that the bleeding and thromboembolism rates were higher in the VA study but that reoperation rates were higher in the Edinburgh study. These differences could be partially accounted for by the composition of the two patient populations: The Edinburgh patients (1) were younger and less heavily anticoagulated, (2) included women and those with double valve replacements, and (3) had a higher percentage of porcine valves in the mitral position. Late results show a better survival with mechanical valves than with bioprostheses in the mitral position with the original valve in the Edinburgh trial (42 versus 24 percent, $p < .05$), probably because of the high rate of bioprosthetic degeneration, and in the aortic position in the VA trial (23 versus 0 percent; $p = 0.0001$).

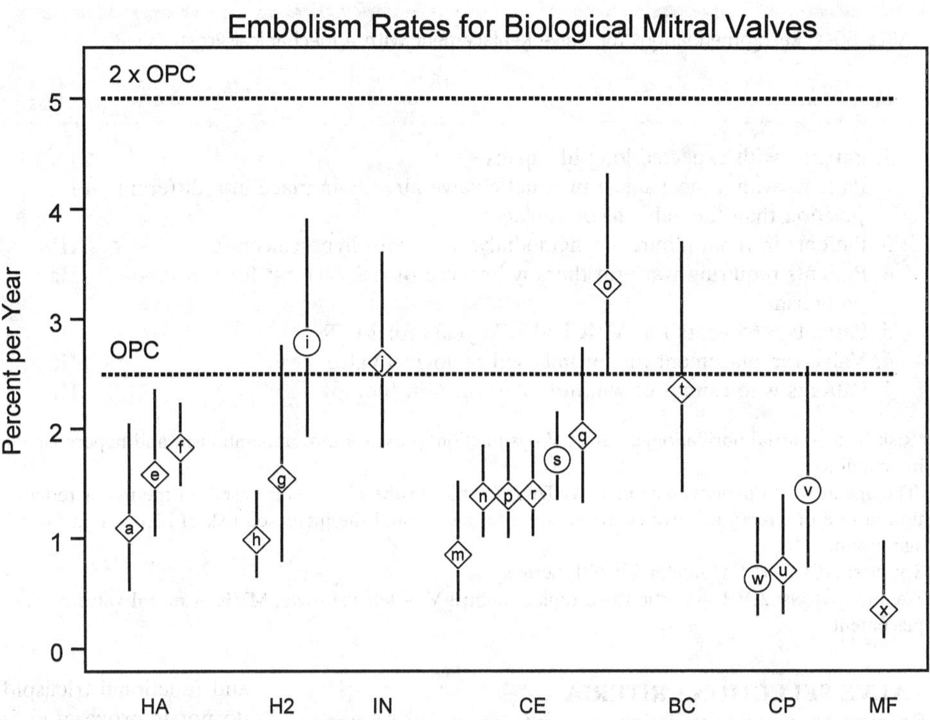

FIGURE 60-10 Embolism rates for biological mitral valves. For explanation of symbols, see Fig. 60-7. Valve model abbreviations: see Fig. 60-9. (From Grunkemeier et al.[61] Reproduced by permission of the publisher and authors.)

TABLE 60-3 Probability of Death due to Any Cause, Any Valve-Related Complication and Individual Valve-Related Complications 15 Years after Randomization[a]

	Aortic Valve Replacement			Mitral Valve Replacement		
Outcome Event	Mechanical $n = 198$	Bioprosthetic $n = 196$	p	Mechanical $n = 88$	Bioprosthesis $n = 93$	p
Death from any cause	66 ± 3%	79 ± 3%	0.02	81 ± 4%	79 ± 4%	0.30
Any valve-related complication	65 ± 4%	66 ± 5%	0.26	73 ± 6%	81 ± 5%	0.56
Systemic embolism	18 ± 4%	18 ± 4%	0.66	18 ± 5%	22 ± 5%	0.96
Bleeding	51 ± 4%	30 ± 4%	0.0001	53 ± 7%	31 ± 6%	0.01
Endocarditis	7 ± 2%	15 ± 5%	0.45	11 ± 4%	17 ± 5%	0.37
Valve thrombosis	2 ± 1%	1 ± 1%	0.33	1 ± 1%	1 ± 1%	0.95
Perivalvular regurgitation	8 ± 2%	2 ± 1%	0.09	17 ± 5%	7 ± 4%	0.05
Reoperation	10 ± 3%	29 ± 5%	0.0004	25 ± 6%	50 ± 8%	0.15
Primary valve failure	0 ± 0%	23 ± 5%	0.0001	5 ± 4%	44 ± 8%	0.0002

n = number of patients randomized.
*Values given are actuarial percentages ± standard error.
NOTE: p values are for differences between mechanical and porcine valves.
SOURCE: From Hammermeister et al.[73]

TABLE 60-4 Recommendations for Valve Replacement with a Mechanical Prosthesis

Indication	Class
1. Patients with expected long life spans	I
2. Patients with a mechanical prosthetic valve already in place in a different position than the valve to be replaced	I
3. Patients in renal failure, on hemodialysis, or with hypercalcemia	II
4. Patients requiring warfarin therapy because of risk factors[a] for thromboembolism	IIa
5. Patients ≤65 years for AVR and ≤70 years for MVR[b]	IIa
6. Valve rereplacement for thrombosed biological valve	IIb
7. Patients who cannot or will not take warfarin therapy	III

[a]Risk factors: atrial fibrillation, severe LV dysfunction, previous thromboembolism and hypercoagulable condition.
[b]The age at which patients may be considered for bioprosthetic valves is based on the major reduction in rate of structural valve deterioration after age 65 and the increased risk of bleeding in this age group.
SOURCE: ACC/AHA Guidelines,[74] with permission.
ABBREVIATIONS: AVR = aortic valve replacement; LV = left ventricle; MVR = mitral valve replacement.

VALVE SELECTION CRITERIA

Because of the wide variation in results among and between various valve models, it is impossible to rank valves within valve types on the basis of complication rates. Some general recommendations, however, can be made with regard to valve selection (Table 60-4).[74]

A biological valve should be used when the patient cannot or will not take anticoagulants or has a short life expectancy. Its use in relation to subsequent pregnancy is controversial (see Chap. 61). A mechanical valve should be used if the patient needs anticoagulant therapy (e.g., because of atrial fibrillation), has a mechanical valve in another position, previously had a stroke, requires double valve replacement, or has a long life expectancy. Mechanical valves should be considered for double valve replacement because the risk of structural deterioration for two porcine valves is additive,[75] whereas the thromboembolic risk of two mechanical valves is not additive.[76]

MANAGEMENT OF PATIENTS WITH PROSTHETIC HEART VALVES

Patients who have undergone valve replacement are *not* cured but still have serious heart disease. They have exchanged native valvular disease for prosthetic valvular disease and must be followed with the same care as patients with native valvular disease.[77] The clinical course of patients with prosthetic heart valves is influenced by several factors.[78]

Ventricular Dysfunction

Despite relief of valvular obstruction or regurgitation, some patients fail to improve after valve replacement or even deteriorate because of ventricular dysfunction. The cause of dysfunction may be carditis associated with rheumatic disease, myocardial degeneration and fibrosis from long-standing pressure or volume overload, ischemic damage at the time of valve replacement, coronary artery disease, or other associated diseases such as systemic hypertension or idiopathic dilated cardiomyopathy. Perioperative myocardial damage is an important cause of postoperative ventricular dysfunction. The importance of myocardial protection at the time of valve surgery is now recognized, and current operative techniques reduce myocardial oxygen consumption by hypothermic cardioplegia and use a variety of means for maintaining adequate myocardial perfusion and protection.

Other Cardiac Lesions

Cardiac diseases affecting primarily one valve often affect other valves, the conduction system, the coronary arteries, and the pulmonary vasculature. With the exception of pulmonary hypertension and functional tricuspid regurgitation, these disorders usually do not improve after isolated valve replacement. Rheumatic disease typically affects both mitral and aortic valves but not necessarily with the same severity at the same time. Therefore, patients who have mitral valve replacement may subsequently, years later, require aortic valve replacement, or vice versa. Calcification of the aortic and mitral valve annuli may extend to the conduction system. High-degree or complete atrioventricular block may occur at the time of surgery or during the late postoperative period, requiring pacemaker implantation. Coronary artery disease is very common in the age range of patients requiring valve replacement. Preoperative coronary arteriography should be performed in all patients with myocardial ischemic pain, in those with left ventricular dysfunction, in those with risk factors for coronary artery disease, and in those about 35 years of age or older.[78,79] Coronary bypass surgery of technically suitable vessels should be performed at the time of valve surgery if the patients have associated significant coronary artery disease.

Prosthesis-Related Problems

The incidence of problems with each prosthesis (see Tables 60-5 and 60-6) was discussed earlier. *Operative mortality* is related to older age of patient, New York Heart Association functional class III or IV, increased left ventricular size, left ventricular dysfunction, heart failure, pulmonary hypertension, low cardiac output, and presence of associated diseases such as systemic arterial hypertension, diabetes mellitus, peripheral and cerebral vascular disease, prior heart surgery, prior myocardial infarction, chronic obstructive pulmonary disease, and renal and hepatic failure. Coronary bypass surgery performed at the same time as valve replacement increases the operative mortality modestly (from 1.4 to 4.0 percent), but associated coronary artery disease, if not bypassed, significantly increases the operative mortality to 9.4 percent and the 10-year mortality to 64 percent.[80] Other very important factors include the occurrence of perioperative myocardial infarction, the duration of the operation, aortic cross-clamp time, and whether or not the patient needed reoperation within 1 to 2 weeks after the initial operation, and on an elective or emergency basis.

The risk of *prosthetic endocarditis* is about 3 percent in the first year and 0.5 percent in subsequent years. Infections in the early postoperative period (up to 2 to 12 months) are due to hospital-based organisms. Despite therapy, the infections are difficult to cure and have a high mortality (about 80 percent);[81,82] early reoperation is usually recommended. The mortality rate from late (2 to 12 months or later) postoperative infection is approximately 40 percent;[81,82] about half the patients can be treated successfully with medication alone. The infected valve should be replaced in patients who do not respond to medical treatment or who have evidence of heart failure, annular invasion, embolism, prosthetic dysfunction, unstable prosthesis, or gram-negative, staphylococcal, or fungal infection.[64] The importance of adequate antibiotic prophylaxis for the prevention of endocarditis cannot be overemphasized; the prevention and treatment of prosthetic valve endocarditis are discussed in Chap. 82.

Long-term anticoagulant therapy is associated with *bleeding* episodes. The incidence of minor bleeding is about 2 to 4 percent per year or less. The incidence of major bleeding is about 1 to 2 percent per year or less, with a mortality rate of about 0.5 percent per year or less. The incidence of these complications is lower in patients who take their medications reliably, in those in whom smooth long-term anticoagulation can be achieved, and in those who receive low-dose warfarin therapy (INR 2 to 3 versus >3). With oral anticoagulants, low- or mid-dose warfarin therapy is combined with low-dose aspirin. Higher degrees of anticoagulation increase the incidence of bleeding without reducing the incidence of thromboembolism. The management of antithrombotic therapy is discussed in Chap. 68.

Prosthetic dehiscence is the result of sutures pulling out of the cardiac tissues. It may result from infection, inadequate surgical technique, or diseased cardiac tissue (e.g., edema, necrosis, calcification).

Because of the continued proliferation of new types and models of prostheses and their relatively brief history of clinical use, the natural history of *structured valve deterioration* is incompletely determined. Although some mechanical prostheses had initial problems with component failure, the most common cause for dysfunction of mechanical prosthetic valves is thrombotic obstruction. The incidence of thrombotic obstruction with the Björk-Shiley spherical occluder valve is higher than that seen with the Starr-Edwards or St. Jude valves, particularly in the mitral position. Failure of biological valves is more common than failure of mechanical prostheses because of leaflet deterioration or calcification; progressive prosthetic regurgitation and/or stenosis is the rule. Bioprosthesis failure is greater in younger patients, in older patients with chronic renal insufficiency, and in the mitral position. In younger patients (average age <60 years), failure of mitral prostheses usually starts at 5 to 8 years and of aortic prostheses at 8 to 10 years. It is unlikely that the tissue valves currently in use will be able to provide the long-term performance demonstrated by the ball-valve mechanical prosthesis.

Red cells are fractured by turbulence and contact with foreign surfaces. Some degree of *hemolysis* is present with all mechanical prostheses but not with bioprostheses. Important hemolysis, however, may occur with a perivalvular leak or severe prosthetic obstruction regardless of prosthesis type. Serum

TABLE 60-5 Recommendations for Valve Replacement with a Bioprosthesis

Indication	Class
1. Patients who cannot or will not take warfarin therapy	I
2. Patients ≥65 years[a] needing AVR who do not have risk factors for thromboembolism[b]	I
3. Patients considered to have possible compliance problems with warfarin therapy	IIa
4. Patients >70 years[a] needing MVR who do not have risk factors for thromboembolism[b]	IIa
5. Valve rereplacement for thrombosed mechanical valve	IIb
6. Patients <65 years[a]	IIb
7. Patients in renal failure, on hemodialysis, or with hypercalcemia	III
8. Adolescent patients who are still growing	III

[a]The age at which patients should be considered for bioprosthetic valves is based on the major reduction in rate of structural valve deterioration after age 65 and increased risk of bleeding in this age group.

[b]Risk factors: atrial fibrillation, severe LV dysfunction, previous thromboembolism, and hypercoagulable condition.

SOURCE: ACC/AHA Guidelines,[74] with permission.

ABBREVIATION: AVR = aortic valve replacement; LV = left ventricle; MVR = mitral valve replacement.

TABLE 60-6 Major Complications of Valve Replacement

1. Operative mortality
2. Perioperative myocardial infarction
3. Prosthetic endocarditis
4. Prosthetic dehiscence
5. Prosthetic dysfunction
   a. Obstruction: Usually thrombotic, occasionally due to item 3, 4, or 8
   b. Regurgitation
   c. Hemolysis
   d. Structural failure
6. Thromboemboli
7. Hemorrhage with anticoagulant therapy
8. Valve prosthesis-patient mismatch
9. Prosthetic replacement often caused by item 3, 4, or 5, occasionally caused by item 6, 7, or 8
10. Late mortality, including sudden, unexplained death

SOURCE: Rahimtoola.[64] Reproduced with permission of the publisher and author.

lactic dehydrogenase (LDH) is usually the simplest and most reliable index of hemolysis to follow in patients with prosthetic valves. A sudden increase in LDH may indicate prosthesis dysfunction, perivalvular leak, or cloth tear. Iron and folate therapy usually correct the anemia. Valve rereplacement may be required for severe, refractory hemolytic anemia.

Important *systemic embolization* is an unfortunate complication of prosthetic valve replacement. Anticoagulation is recommended for all patients with mechanical prostheses. *Despite long-term anticoagulation, patients with prosthetic valves face an embolic rate from aortic prostheses of 1 to 2 percent or less per year and from mitral prostheses of 3 to 4 percent or less per year.*

No prosthesis currently employed has an effective orifice as large as that of the native valve, and valve prosthesis-patient mismatch[33] may occur. *All patients with prosthetic heart valves have mild to moderate stenosis.* Patients with aortic valve prostheses have obstruction to left ventricular outflow (aortic stenosis), and patients with mitral valve prostheses have obstruction to left atrial emptying (mitral stenosis). This is most important in a large patient in whom a prosthesis that is considered "small" in relation to body size must be placed for technical reasons. The resulting patient-prosthesis mismatch[33] contributes to incomplete relief of symptoms. The long-term effect of intrinsic prosthetic stenosis on survival and ventricular dysfunction is unknown but may lead to long-term effects similar to those of aortic or mitral stenosis.[83] The presence of intrinsic prosthetic stenosis must be considered when patients with prosthetic heart valves are being advised concerning activity.

Reoperation to replace a prosthetic heart valve is a serious complication. It is usually required for moderate to severe prosthetic dysfunction and dehiscence, prosthetic valve endocarditis, and occasionally recurrent thromboembolism, severe recurrent bleeding from anticoagulant therapy, or valve prosthesis–patient mismatch.

Late cardiac death may result from ventricular dysfunction, other cardiac lesions, or prosthesis-related causes. Late, sudden death is not uncommon. It may result from a bradyarrhythmia; a tachyarrhythmia that is often associated with ventricular dysfunction, prosthetic dysfunction, or mismatch; coronary artery disease; or a combination of these.

Management[78]

All patients with prosthetic valves need appropriate antibiotics for prophylaxis against infective endocarditis (Chap. 82). Patients with rheumatic heart disease continue to need antibiotics as prophylaxis against the recurrence of rheumatic carditis (Chap. 62). Adequate antithrombotic therapy is needed for appropriate patients (Chap. 68).

During the first 4 to 6 weeks after surgery, the physician and surgeon jointly manage the patient, directing their attention toward relieving postoperative discomfort, readjusting cardiac medications, and instituting anticoagulation if not contraindicated. A graduated plan of activity is started that, in most cases, enables the patient to return to full activity in 4 to 6 weeks.

Several syndromes are peculiar to the postoperative period. The *postperfusion syndrome* usually appears in the third or fourth postoperative week. It is characterized by fever, splenomegaly, and atypical lymphocytes; it is benign and self-limited. The *postpericardiotomy syndrome* is characterized by fever and pleuropericarditis. It usually develops in the second or third postoperative week but can appear as late as 1 year after surgery and sometimes recurs. Although this syndrome is usually self-limited, most patients benefit from taking anti-inflammatory drugs, such as aspirin or indomethacin; a short course of glucocorticoids is also occasionally required.

Even though the pericardium is left open at the end of surgery, *cardiac tamponade* has been known to occur during the first 6 weeks. The fact that a critically ill patient may improve promptly with pericardial drainage underscores the need to consider this uncommon postoperative complication. Usually, anticoagulants have been given and the fluid is hemorrhagic.

The *4- to 6-week postoperative visit* is critical, because by this time the patient's physical capabilities and expected improvement in functional capacity can usually be assessed. At this time, the physician should assemble essential records and data for the subsequent office follow-up, including the preoperative history, physical examination, chest roentgenogram, electrocardiogram (ECG) and indication for surgery, preoperative echocardiographic/Doppler ultrasound and cardiac catheterization/angiographic reports, surgeon's operative report, postoperative complications, and hospital discharge summary. The prosthesis model, serial number, and size should be recorded.

The workup on this visit should include an interval or complete initial history and physical examination, ECG, chest x-ray, echocardiography/Doppler ultrasound, complete blood count, and measurement of electrolytes, LDH, and international normalized ratio (INR) if indicated (Table 60-7). The examination's main focus is on physical signs that relate to functioning of the prosthesis or suggest the presence of a myocardial, conduction, or valvular disorder. The auscultatory findings to expect with some normally functioning prostheses have been described.[84]

TABLE 60-7 Recommendations for Follow-up Strategy of Patient with Prosthetic Heart Valves

Indication	Class
1. History, physical exam, ECG, chest x-ray, echocardiogram, complete blood count, serum chemistries, and INR (if indicated) at first postoperative outpatient evaluation[a]	I
2. Radionuclide angiography or magnetic resonance imaging to assess LV function if result of echocardiography is unsatisfactory	I
3. Routine follow-up visits at yearly intervals with earlier reevaluations for change in clinical status	I
4. Routine serial echocardiograms at time of annual follow-up visit in absence of change in clinical status	IIb
5. Routine serial fluoroscopy	III

[a]This evaluation should be performed 3 to 4 weeks after hospital discharge. In some settings, the outpatient echocardiogram may be difficult to obtain: if so, an inpatient echocardiogram may be obtained before hospital discharge.

SOURCE: ACC/AHA Guidelines,[73] with permission.

ABBREVIATIONS: INR = international normalized ratio; LV = left ventricle.

Severe perivalvular mitral regurgitation can be inaudible on physical examination, a fact to remember when considering possible causes of functional deterioration in a patient.

The interval between routine follow-up visits depends on the patient's needs. Anticoagulant regulation usually does not require office visits.

Multiple noninvasive tests have emerged for assessing valvular and ventricular function. Fluoroscopy can reveal abnormal rocking of a dehiscing prosthesis or limitation of the occluder if the latter is opaque as well as strut fracture of a Björk-Shiley valve. Radionuclide angiography, which is useful for determining whether or not functional deterioration is the result of reduced ventricular function, is performed if the same data cannot be obtained by echocardiography.

Echocardiography/Doppler ultrasound is the most useful noninvasive test. It provides information about prosthesis stenosis/regurgitation, valve area, assessment of other valve disease(s), pulmonary hypertension, atrial size, left ventricular hypertrophy, left ventricular size and function, and pericardial effusion/thickening. It is essential at the first postoperative visit because it allows an assessment of the effects and results of surgery and serves as a baseline for comparison should complications and/or deterioration occur later. Subsequently, it is performed as is needed in both symptomatic and asymptomatic patients at 1- to 2-year intervals. We recommend that in patients with a bioprosthesis in the mitral position, echocardiography/Doppler ultrasound should be performed annually after 5 years and in the aortic position annually after 8 years because of the increasing incidence of bioprosthetic structural valve deterioration.

"Heart failure" after valve replacement may be the result of (1) preoperative left ventricular dysfunction that improved partially or not at all, (2) perioperative myocardial damage, (3) progression of other valve disease, (4) complications of prosthetic heart valves, and (5) associated heart disease such as coronary artery disease and systemic arterial hypertension.

Any patient with a prosthetic heart valve who does not improve after the surgery or who later shows deterioration of functional capacity should undergo appropriate testing to determine the cause. Such studies are also usually necessary for patients who require reoperation for endocarditis or repeated embolism to determine the hemodynamics and anatomy.

The indications for reoperating on a patient with prosthetic valve endocarditis have already been discussed. A patient in stable condition, without prosthetic valve endocarditis, can usually undergo reoperation with only slightly greater risk than that of the initial surgery. For the patient with catastrophic dysfunction, surgery is clearly indicated and urgent. The patient without endocarditis or severe dysfunction requires careful hemodynamic evaluation; the decision about reoperation should then be based on the hemodynamic abnormalities, the symptoms, ventricular function, and current knowledge of the natural history of the particular prosthesis.

ACKNOWLEDGMENT

The authors wish to thank Hui-Hua Li, MD, and K. Jeanne Zerr, RN, MBA, for valuable assistance in the preparation of this chapter. We are also grateful to the heart valve manufacturers for supplying information about their products.

References

1. Harken D, Soroff HS, Taylor WJ. Partial and complete prosthesis in aortic insufficiency. *J Thorac Cardiovasc Surg* 1960; 40:744–762.
2. Starr A, Edwards M. Mitral replacement: Clinical experience with a ball valve prosthesis. *Ann Surg* 1961; 154:726–740.
3. Björk VO. A new tilting disc valve prosthesis. *Scand J Thorac Cardiovasc Surg* 1969; 3:1–10.
4. Björk VO. The improved Björk-Shiley tilting disc valve prosthesis. *Scand J Thorac Cardiovasc Surg* 1978; 12:81–84.
5. Ross DN. Homograft replacement of the aortic valve. *Lancet* 1962; 2:487.
6. Barratt-Boyes BG. Homograft aortic valve replacement in aortic incompetence and stenosis. *Thorax* 1964; 19:131–135.
7. Ross DN. Replacement of aortic and mitral valves with a pulmonary autograft. *Lancet* 1967; 2:956–958.
8. Elkins RC. Pulmonary autograft—The optimal substitute for the aortic valve? *N Engl J Med* 1994; 330:59–60.
9. Oury JH, Eddy AC, Cleveland JC. The Ross procedure: A progress report. *J Heart Valve Dis* 1994; 3:361–364.
10. Elkins RC, Santangelo K, Randolph JD, et al. Pulmonary autograft replacement in children. The ideal solution? *Ann Surg* 1992; 216:363–370; discussion, 370–371.
11. Kouchoukos NT, Davila-Román VG, Spray TL, et al. Replacement of the aortic root with a pulmonary autograft in children and young adults with aortic-valve disease. *N Engl J Med* 1994; 330:1–6.
12. Chambers JC, Somerville J, Stone S, Ross DN. Pulmonary autograft procedure for aortic valve disease: Long-term results of the pioneer series. *Circulation.* 1997; 96:2206–2214.
13. Grunkemeier GL, Bodnar E. Comparison of structural valve failure among different "models" of homograft valves. *J Heart Valve Dis* 1994; 3:556–560.
14. Carpentier A, Lemaigre G, Robert L. Biological factors affecting long-term results of valvular homografts. *J Thorac Cardiovasc Surg* 1969; 58:467–483.
15. Carpentier A, Dubost C. From xenograft to bioprosthesis. In: Ionescu MI, Ross DN, Wooler GH, eds. *Biological Tissue in Heart Valve Replacement.* London: Butterworth; 1971:515–541.
16. Hazekamp MG, Goffin YA, Huysmans HA. The value of the stentless biovalve prosthesis: An experimental study. *Eur J Thorac Cardiovasc Surg* 1993; 7:514–519.
17. Konertz W, Hamann P, Schwammenthal E, et al. Aortic valve replacement with stentless xenografts. *J Heart Valve Dis* 1992; 1:249–252.
18. David TE, Bos J, Rakowski H. Aortic valve replacement with the Toronto SPV bioprosthesis. *J Heart Valve Dis* 1992; 1:244–248.
19. Vrandecic MP, Gontijo BF, Fantini FA, et al. The new stentless aortic valve: Clinical results of the first 100 patients. *Cardiovasc Surg* 1994; 2:407–414.
20. Hvass U, Chatel D, Ouroudji M, et al. The O'Brien-Angell stentless valve: Early results of 100 implants. *Eur J Cardiothorac Surg* 1994; 8:384–387.
21. Carpentier A. Mitral reconstruction in predominant mitral incompetence. In: Duran C, Angell WW, Johnson AD, Oury JH, eds. *Recent Progress in Mitral Valve Disease.* London: Butterworth; 1984:265–276.
22. Duran C. Mitral reconstruction in predominant mitral stenosis. In: Duran C, Angell WW, Johnson AD, Oury JH, eds. *Recent Progress in Mitral Valve Disease.* London: Butterworth; 1984: 255–264.
23. Cosgrove DM, Rosenkranz ER, Hendren WG, et al. Valvuloplasty for aortic insufficiency. *J Thorac Cardiovasc Surg* 1991; 102:571–576; discussion, 576–577.
24. Duvoisin GE, Brandenburg RO, McGoon DC. Factors affecting

thromboembolism associated with prosthetic heart valves. *Circulation* 1967; 35,36(suppl I):70–76.

25. Kaplan EL, Meier P. Nonparametric estimation from incomplete observations. *J Am Stat Assn* 1958; 53:457–481.
26. Stinson EB, Griepp RB, Oyer PE, Shumway NE. Long-term experience with porcine xenografts. *J Thorac Cardiovasc Surg* 1977; 73:54–63.
27. Grunkemeier GL, Thomas DR, Starr A. Statistical considerations in the analysis and reporting of time-related events: Application to analysis of prosthetic valve-related thromboembolism and pacemaker failure. *Am J Cardiol* 1977; 39:257–258.
28. Grunkemeier GL, Macmanus Q, Thomas DR, Starr A. Regression analysis of late survival following mitral valve replacement. *J Thorac Cardiovasc Surg* 1978; 75:131–138.
29. Blackstone EH, Naftel DC, Turner ME Jr. The decomposition of time-varying hazard into separate phases, each incorporating a separate stream of concomitant information. *J Am Stat Assoc* 1986; 81:615–624.
30. Edmunds LH Jr, Clark RE, Cohn LH, et al. Guidelines for reporting morbidity and mortality after cardiac valvular operations. *Ann Thorac Surg* 1988; 46:257–259.
31. Edmunds LH Jr, Clark RE, Cohn LH, et al. Guidelines for reporting morbidity and mortality after cardiac valvular operations. *Ann Thorac Surg* 1996; 62:932–935.
32. Edmunds LH Jr, Clark RE, Cohn LH, et al. Guidelines for reporting morbidity and mortality after cardiac valvular operations. *J Thorac Cardiovasc Surg* 1996; 112:708–711.
33. Rahimtoola SH. The problem of prosthesis-patient mismatch. *Circulation* 1978; 58:20–24.
34. Rahimtoola SH, Rahmoeller GA. The law on cardiovascular devices: The role of the Food and Drug Administration and of physicians in its implementation. *Circulation* 1980; 62:919–924.
35. *Draft Replacement Heart Valve Guidance.* Rockville, MD: Prosthetic Devices Branch, Division of Cardiovascular, Respiratory and Neurological Devices, Office of Device Evaluation, Center of Devices and Radiological Health, Food and Drug Administration. December 7, 1993.
36. Gersh BJ, Fisher LD, Schaff HV, et al. Issues concerning the clinical evaluation of new prosthetic valves. *J Thorac Cardiovasc Surg* 1986; 91:460–466.
37. Nashef SAM. Reporting the results of heart valve operations (letter). *Ann Thorac Surg* 1989; 47:949–950.
38. Bodnar E, Butchart EG, Bamford J, et al. Proposal for reporting thrombosis, embolism and bleeding after heart valve replacement. *J Heart Valve Dis* 1994; 3:120–123.
39. Grunkemeier GL, Johnson D, Naftel DC. Sample size requirements for studying heart valves with constant risk events. *J Heart Valve Dis* 1994; 3:53–58.
40. Grunkemeier GL, Anderson WN. Passive surveillance of heart valve devices: Björk-Shiley outlet strut fracture rates. *J Long-Term Effects Med Implants* 1995; 5:155–168.
41. Jones LE, Weintraub WS, Craver JM, et al. Ten-year experience with the porcine bioprosthetic valve: Interrelationship of valve survival and patient survival in 1,050 valve replacements. *Ann Thorac Surg* 1990; 49:370–383; discussion, 383–384.
42. Jamieson WR, Tyers GF, Janusz MT, et al. Age as a determinant for selection of porcine bioprostheses for cardiac valve replacement: Experience with Carpentier-Edwards standard bioprosthesis. *Can J Cardiol* 1991; 7:181–188.
43. al-Khaja N, Belboul A, Rashid M, et al. The influence of age on the durability of Carpentier-Edwards biological valves: Thirteen years' follow-up. *Eur J Cardiothorac Surg* 1991; 5:635–640.
44. Pelletier LC, Carrier M, Leclerc Y, et al. Influence of age on late results of valve replacement with porcine bioprostheses. *J Cardiovasc Surg* 1992; 33:526–533.
45. Barratt-Boyes BG, Jaffe WM, Ko PH, Whitlock RM. The zero pressure, fixed Medtronic Intact porcine valve: An 8.5 year review. *J Heart Valve Dis* 1993; 2:604–611.
46. Munro AI, Jamieson WR, Tyers GF, Burr LH. The Medtronic Intact porcine bioprosthesis: Clinical performance to eight years. *J Heart Valve Dis* 1994; 3:634–640.
47. Matsuki O, Okita Y, Almeida RS, et al. Two decades' experience with aortic valve replacement with pulmonary autograft. *J Thorac Cardiovasc Surg* 1988; 95:705–711.
48. Ross D, Jackson M, Davies J. Pulmonary autograft aortic valve replacement: Long-term results. *J Cardiac Surg* 1991; 6(suppl 4):529–533.
49. Enriquez-Sarano M, Schaff HV, Orszulak TA, et al. Valve repair improves the outcome of surgery for mitral regurgitation: A multivariate analysis. *Circulation* 1995; 91:1022–1028; comments, 1264–1265.
50. Hendren WG, Morris AS, Rosenkranz ER, et al. Mitral valve repair for bacterial endocarditis. *J Thorac Cardiovasc Surg* 1992; 103:124–128; discussion, 128–129.
51. Azar H, Szentpetery S. Mitral valve repair in patients over the age of 70 years. *Eur J Cardiothorac Surg* 1994; 8:298–300.
52. Jebara VA, Dervanian P, Acar C, et al. Mitral valve repair using Carpentier techniques in patients more than 70 years old: Early and late results. *Circulation* 1992; 86(suppl II):53–59.
53. Rahimtoola SH. Lessons learned about the determinants of the results of valve surgery. *Circulation* 1988; 78:1503–1507.
54. Aoyagi S, Tanaka K, Kawara T, et al. Long-term results of mitral valve repair for non-rheumatic mitral regurgitation. *Cardiovasc Surg* 1995; 3:387–392.
55. Skoularigis J, Sinovich V, Joubert G, Sareli P. Evaluation of the long-term results of mitral valve repair in 254 young patients with rheumatic mitral regurgitation. *Circulation* 1994; 90(suppl II):167–174.
56. Grossi EA, Galloway AC, Steinberg BM, et al. Severe calcification does not affect long-term outcome of mitral valve repair. *Ann Thorac Surg* 1994; 58:685–687.
57. Grossi EA, Galloway AC, LeBoutillier M III, et al. Anterior leaflet procedures during mitral valve repair do not adversely influence long-term outcome. *J Am Coll Cardiol* 1995; 25:134–136.
58. Duran CM, Gometza B, Saad E. Valve repair in rheumatic mitral disease: An unsolved problem. *J Cardiac Surg* 1994; 9(suppl 2):282–285.
59. Cosgrove DM, Lytle BW, Taylor PC, et al. The Carpentier-Edwards pericardial aortic valve: Ten year results. *J Thorac Cardiovasc Surg* 1995; 110:651–662.
60. Waller DA, Essop AR, Scott PJ, Nair RU. Repair of asymptomatic aortic valve disease during other cardiac surgery. *Int J Cardiol* 1992; 36:309–314.
61. Grunkemeier GL, Li H-H, Starr A, Rahimtoola SH. Long-term performance of heart valve prostheses. *Curr Probl Cardiol* 2000; 25:75–154.
62. Grunkemeier GL, London MR. Reliability of comparative data from different sources. In: Butchart E, Bodnar E, eds. *Current Issues in Heart Valve Disease: Thrombosis, Embolism and Bleeding.* London: ICR; 1992:464–475.
63. Sackett DL. Bias in analytic research. *J Chronic Dis* 1979; 32:51–63.
64. Rahimtoola SH. Valvular heart disease: A perspective. *J Am Coll Cardiol* 1983; 3:199–215.
65. Edmunds LH Jr. Thrombotic and bleeding complications of prosthetic heart valves. *Ann Thorac Surg* 1987; 44:430–445.
66. Bamford J, Warlow C. Stroke and TIA in the general population. In: Butchart EG, Bodnar E, eds. *Thrombosis, Embolism and Bleeding.* London: ICR; 1992:3–15.
67. Berlin JA, Begg CB, Louis TA. An assessment of publication bias using a sample of published clinical trials. *J Am Stat Assoc* 1989; 84:381–392.

68. Kramer MS, Shapiro SH. Scientific challenges in the application of randomized trials. *JAMA* 1984; 252:2739–2745.
69. Rahimtoola SH. Some unexpected lessons from large multicenter randomized clinical trials. *Circulation* 1985; 72:449–455.
70. Grunkemeier GL, Starr A. Alternatives to randomization in surgical studies. *J Heart Valve Dis* 1992; 1:142–151.
71. Bloomfield P, Wheatley DJ, Prescott RJ, Miller HC. Twelve-year comparison of a Björk-Shiley mechanical heart valve with porcine bioprostheses. *N Engl J Med* 1991; 324:573–579.
72. Hammermeister KE, Sethi GK, Henderson WG, et al. A comparison of outcomes in men 11 years after heart-valve replacement with a mechanical valve or bioprosthesis. Veterans Affairs Cooperative Study on Valvular Heart Disease. *N Engl J Med* 1993; 328:1289–1296.
73. Hammermeister K, Sethi GK, Henderson WG, Grover FL, et al. Outcomes 15 years after valve replacement with a mechanical vs bioprosthetic valve: Final report of the VA randomized trial. *J Am Coll Cardiol.* In press, October 2000.
74. Bonow RO, Carabello B, de Leon AC Jr, et al. ACC/AHA guidelines for the management of patients with valvular heart disease: A report of the American College of Cardiology/American Heart Association Task Force on Practical Guidelines (Committee on Management of Patients with Valvular Heart Disease). *J Am Coll Cardiol* 1998; 32:1486–1588.
75. Grunkemeier GL, Jamieson WR, Miller DC, Starr A. Actuarial versus actual risk of porcine structural valve deterioration. *J Thorac Cardiovasc Surg* 1994; 108:709–718.
76. Starr A, Grunkemeier GL. Recurrent thromboembolism: Significance and management. In: Butchart EG, Bodnar E, eds. *Current Issues in Heart Valve Disease: Thrombosis, Thromboembolism and Bleeding*. London: ICR; 1992:402–415.
77. Rahimtoola SH. Valvular heart disease. In: Stein J, ed. *Internal Medicine*, 4th ed. *Cardiology*, O'Rourke RA, section ed. St. Louis: Mosby-Year Book; 1994:202–234.
78. Grunkemeier GL, Rahimtoola SH, Starr A. Prosthetic heart valves. In: Rahimtoola SH, ed. *Atlas of Heart Diseases, 11*. Philadelphia: Current Medicine; 1997:13.1–13.27.
79. Rahimtoola SH. Aortic valve stenosis. In: Rahimtoola SH, ed. *Valvular Heart Disease, II.* St. Louis: Mosby; 1997:7.02–7.26.
80. Mullany CJ, Elveback LR, Frye RL, et al. Coronary artery disease and its management: Influence on survival in patients undergoing aortic valve replacement. *J Am Coll Cardiol* 1987; 10:66–72.
81. Kloster FE. Infective prosthetic valve endocarditis. In: Rahimtoola SH, ed. *Infective Endocarditis*. New York: Grune & Stratton; 1978:291–305.
82. Douglas JL, Cobbs CG. Prosthetic valve endocarditis. In: Kaye D, ed. *Infective Endocarditis*, 2d ed. New York: Raven Press; 1992:375–396.
83. Rahimtoola SH, Murphy E. Valve prosthesis-patient mismatch: A long-term sequela. *Br Heart J* 1981; 45:331–335.
84. Vongpatawasin W, Hillis LD, Lange RA. Prosthetic heart valves. *N Engl J Med* 1996; 335:407–416.
85. Frater RWM, Furlong P, Cosgrove DM, et al. Long-term durability and patient functional status of the Carpentier-Edwards Perimount pericardial bioprosthesis in the aortic position. *J Heart Valve Dis* 1998; 7:48–53.

CHAPTER 61

ANTITHROMBOTIC THERAPY FOR VALVULAR HEART DISEASE

John H. McAnulty / Shahbudin H. Rahimtoola

INTRODUCTION

The most important reason to address the issue of protection against thromboemboli in every patient with valve disease is the risk of a stroke. In addition, the consequences of valve thrombosis and of emboli to other organs make the risk of antithrombotic therapy reasonable to assume in many patients with valve disease. Treatment has to be individualized, but some issues and principles are widely applicable (Table 61-1).[1,2] Although some recommendations are appropriate for affluent American communities, the risk, benefit, and cost ratio may not be applicable in poorer areas, where the resources are simply not available. Thromboemboli are not ignored, but alternative therapy—for example, a greater use of antiplatelet agents, in particular aspirin—may, on balance, be more appropriate.

Intracardiac thrombosis most often presents as an embolic cerebrovascular event in over 80 percent of cases. Rarely, thrombosis becomes manifest by causing valve dysfunction. The physical examination should include careful attention to the peripheral pulses and to the skin, fundi, and soft tissues (mouth, conjunctiva), looking for clues of an embolus. A detailed neurologic assessment for focal deficits is essential. Although thrombosis most often occurs without any change in the cardiac examination, auscultation to assess for a change in a murmur or in the quality of heart sounds is important. Intracardiac thrombosis often is first diagnosed when cardiac catheterization or echocardiography is performed for other reasons.

Thrombus is the most common but not the exclusive cause of an embolus. Infective endocarditis must be considered and excluded as a cause, particularly in individuals with valve disease. Disruption of a vascular plaque in the ascending aorta, arch, or descending aorta and in the cerebral vessels may be a common cause of peripheral and cerebral emboli in patients with atherosclerotic disease. Intracardiac tumors or calcified emboli from the heart or aorta are other rare causes.

NATIVE VALVE DISEASE

The risk of thromboembolism in patients with native valve disease is most directly related to certain risk factors, including atrial fibrillation, a history of thromboembolism, left ventricular (LV) dysfunction, and known hypercoagulability. The risk is increased by the presence of certain types of native valve disease (e.g., mitral stenosis) and with prosthetic heart valves, particularly mechanical prostheses, which put a patient at risk even without other associated risk factors (Fig. 61-1).

Risk Factors for Thromboemboli with Native Valve Disease

ATRIAL FIBRILLATION

Most is known about the stroke risk with atrial fibrillation, which is common even without valve disease. Six recent large prospective randomized trials have assessed the value of antithrombotic therapy for primary prevention in patients with nonvalvular atrial fibrillation.[3-8] The term *nonvalvular* is not completely accurate, as at least some patients with aortic valve disease and with mitral regurgitation were included in the studies if the valve lesions were considered hemodynamically "insignificant."

In these trials, the embolic rate (essentially the rate of a stroke in untreated patients with nonvalvular atrial fibrillation) ranged from 3 to 8 percent per year. This was true whether the atrial fibrillation was constant or paroxysmal. Importantly, these trials indicated that warfarin therapy reduced the stroke rate to approximately 0.5 to 2 percent per year. One study, SPAF II,[7] demonstrated equal protection against an adverse neurologic event when aspirin (325 mg daily) was compared to warfarin. In SPAF III,[8] the aspirin was less protective if atrial fibrillation occurred in association with LV dysfunction or uncontrolled

TABLE 61-1 Valve Disease and Antithrombotic Therapy[a,b]

1. Prevention of thromboemboli should be addressed each time a patient with valve disease is seen.
2. Lifelong antithrombotic therapy is required in patients with atrial fibrillation (paroxysmal or persistent) (Table 61-2).
3. Warfarin therapy is required in all patients with a mechanical prothesis (Table 61-3).
4. Antithrombotic therapy should be started early after valve surgery.
5. Warfarin should be avoided in the first trimester of pregnancy.
6. Antithrombotic therapy should be individualized during noncardiac surgery and cardiovascular procedures (Table 61-5).

[a]See text for discussion.
[b]In general, whenever warfarin/aspirin therapy is recommended it is assumed that there is no specific contraindication to its use.

hypertension, if the patient was a woman over age 75, and most importantly, if the patient had had a previous thromboembolic event. Warfarin is indicated in these patients if they are reasonable candidates for the drug, with particular emphasis on its role in those who have had a previous embolic event, as secondary prevention;[6,8] the International Normalized Ratio (INR) should be in the 2.0 to 3.0 range (see also Chap. 44).

The exclusion of mitral stenosis in these prospective trials implies that the risks of emboli and the benefits of warfarin in these patients with associated atrial fibrillation are well understood; however, these are not thoroughly documented or proven. Retrospective assessment, however, suggests that such patients may have an embolic rate >5 percent per year. Until the role of warfarin is better defined, the authors recommend its use in patients with mitral stenosis and one or more risk factors.

LEFT VENTRICULAR DYSFUNCTION

Systemic or pulmonary thromboemboli occur at a rate of over 5 percent per year in patients with LV dysfunction. The type and degree of dysfunction indicating risk are not well defined, but LV systolic abnormalities have been related to emboli most often. However, antithrombotic therapy is of unproven value in preventing or reducing the embolic rate.[9,10] Still, the risk is sufficient that, with or without valve disease, consideration should be given to treatment. One approach (including the authors') is to use warfarin if the LV ejection fraction (EF) ≤0.30 and the patient is a reasonable candidate for this treatment.

PREVIOUS THROMBOEMBOLI

In other clinical situations (e.g., in patients with atrial fibrillation[6,8] or with a prosthetic valve[11–13]), a thromboembolic event defines patients at high risk for having an embolic event—i.e., a recurrent event. It is unclear whether this is true in patients with native valve disease, but we recommend lifelong warfarin therapy.

HYPERCOAGULABLE CONDITIONS

Reasons to consider anticoagulant therapy are the presence of protein C, protein S, or antithrombin III deficiencies; the anticardiolipin antibody syndrome; resistance to activated protein C; or an associated malignancy. This is also true in patients with native valve disease (see also Chap. 44).

Screening for Patients at High Risk for Thromboemboli

The risk factors described above define patients requiring antithrombotic therapy. Transthoracic (TTE) and transesophageal echocardiography (TEE) are often performed in patients with valvular heart disease and in those who have had a systemic embolic episode. The use of these procedures in determining which patients are at risk of thromboemboli is not yet well defined; left atrial (LA) thrombi, a patent foramen ovale, an atrial septal aneurysm, or spontaneous echo contrast are occasional findings of concern, but the value of treatment is unproven. Until more is known, it may not be appropriate to screen patients with native valve disease who do not have one of the obvious clinical risk factors listed above.

Risk of Thromboembolism

High (>2% per year)	Atrial fibrillation LV dysfunction Previous thromboembolism Hypercoagulable condition Mechanical prosthesis	i.e., **"risk factors"** for thromboemboli
↓		
Low (<1% per year)	Normal sinus rhythm Normal LV function No previous thromboembolism Tissue prosthesis	

FIGURE 61-1 Risk of thromboembolism. Clinical variables define valve disease patients as being at high or low risk of thromboembolic events.

Antithrombotic Treatment for Native Valve Disease

Antithrombotic therapy is not required in patients with native valve disease (Table 61-2) unless there is an associated risk factor.[2,14] Theoretically, the risk of thrombosis is greater with mitral valve disease as compared to aortic valve disease: there is more blood stasis, the LA may be larger, and the frequency of atrial fibrillation is greater. Still, the presence of mitral valve stenosis or regurgitation by itself is not a reason to initiate antithrombotic therapy. If there is a risk factor, antithrombotic therapy should be considered as defined in Table 61-2. If the patient is a reasonable candidate for war-

TABLE 61-2 Antithrombotic Therapy—Native Valve Disease

I. *No therapy* if no thrombosis risk factor
II. *Therapy* if thrombosis risk factor present
   A. *Atrial fibrillation*
      1. Warfarin (INR 2–3) if congestive heart failure, hypertension, or previous thromboembolism
      2. Warfarin (INR 2–3) if valve lesion is mitral stenosis
      3. Aspirin (325 mg/day) or warfarin (INR 2–3) if valve lesion other than mitral stenosis
   B. *Previous thromboembolism*—warfarin (INR 2–3)
   C. *LV dysfunction* (ejection fraction ≤0.30—warfarin (INR 2–3)
   D. *Hypercoagulable state*—warfarin (INR 2–3)

Abbreviation: INR = International Normalized Ratio.

farin therapy, the use of warfarin (maintaining an INR of 2 to 3) is appropriate if a patient with valve disease has atrial fibrillation (constant or paroxysmal) in combination with reduced LV function (heart failure or LV EF ≤0.30) or with associated severe hypertension or if there is a history of thromboemboli. There is a suggestion that women over the age of 75 with atrial fibrillation might be better protected by warfarin than aspirin,[8] but the bleeding rate on warfarin is significant in this patient population; treatment should be individualized and the INR more closely monitored. If a patient with atrial fibrillation has reasonable LV function, has not had a previous thromboembolism, and does not have other risk factors, aspirin (325 mg/day) is just as likely as warfarin to be protective against thromboemboli, without the associated expense and risk of warfarin therapy.[7,15] Unrelated to atrial fibrillation, warfarin therapy is recommended if a patient has had a previous thromboembolism or has LV dysfunction (heart failure and an ejection fraction ≤0.30).

PROSTHETIC HEART VALVES

All patients with mechanical valves require warfarin therapy. Even with the use of warfarin, the risk of thromboemboli in these patients is 1 to 2 percent per year;[16–19] the risk is *considerably higher* without treatment with warfarin.[11] The risk of an embolus in patients with biological valves in sinus rhythm has been approximately 0.6 to 0.7 percent per year, and most of those patients were not on warfarin therapy.[16,17,19–21] Almost all studies have shown that the risk of embolism is greater with a valve in the mitral position (mechanical or biological) as compared to a valve in the aortic position;[11,16] however, this was not found in one study.[17] With either type of prosthesis or valve location, the risk of emboli is probably higher in the first few days and months after valve insertion,[20] before the valve is fully endothelialized.

Antithrombotic Treatment for Prosthetic Valves (Table 61-3)

MECHANICAL VALVES

All patients with mechanical valves require warfarin, and the INR should be maintained between 2.0 and 3.5.[16,17,22–24] In patients with an aortic prosthesis without risk factors for emboli the INR should be between 2.0 and 3.0; in those with risk factors and in those with a mitral prosthesis the INR should be between 2.5 and 3.5.[2] Some valves are thought to be more thrombogenic than others (particularly the tilting-disk valves), and a case could be made for increasing the INR to between 3 and 4.5, but this would be associated with an increased risk of bleeding.[22,25,26] The addition of low-dose aspirin (50 to 100 mg/day) to warfarin therapy may further decrease the risk of thromboembolism.[27,28] The authors recommend the addition of aspirin (50 to 100 mg/

TABLE 61-3 Antithrombotic Therapy[a]—Prosthetic Heart Valves

	Mechanical Prosthetic Valves			Biological Prosthetic Valves		
	Warfarin, INR 2–3	Warfarin, INR 2.5–3.5	Aspirin, 50–100 mg	Warfarin, INR 2–3	Warfarin, INR 2.5–3.5	Aspirin, 50-100 mg
First 3 months after valve replacement		+	+		+	+
After first 3 months						
Aortic valve	+		+			+
Aortic valve + risk factor[b]		+	+	+		
Mitral valve		+	+			+
Mitral valve + risk factor		+	+		+	+

[a]Depending on the clinical status of patient, antithrombotic therapy must be individualized (see special situations in text).
[b]Risk factors (see Fig. 61-1): atrial fibrillation, previous thromboembolus, LV dysfunction, hypercoagulable state.

day) to warfarin unless there is a contraindication to the use of aspirin (i.e., bleeding or aspirin intolerance). This combination is particularly appropriate in patients who have had an embolus while on warfarin therapy and/or who are known to be particularly hypercoagulable; for example, it is recommended by a committee addressing antithrombotic therapy in women during pregnancy.[29] It is important to note that the thromboembolic risk increases early after the insertion of the prosthetic valve; this is a reason to initiate heparin therapy within the first 24 to 48 h of surgery, with maintenance of the *activated partial thromboplastin time* (aPTT) at a "therapeutic effect" level (Table 61-4) until warfarin therapy has achieved the recommended INR level.

BIOLOGICAL (TISSUE) VALVES

Because of an increased risk of thromboemboli during the first 3 months after implantation of a biological prosthetic valve, anticoagulation with warfarin is indicated.[20] The risk is particularly high in the first few days after surgery, and heparin therapy should be started within 24 to 48 h, with maintenance of the aPTT at a "therapeutic effect" level (Table 61-4) until an INR of 2.0 to 3.0 is achieved with warfarin. After 3 months, the tissue valve can be treated like native valve disease (see Table 61-2), and warfarin can be discontinued in approximately two-thirds of patients with biological valves.[16,17,20,30] Associated atrial fibrillation or an LV EF ≤0.30 are reasons for lifelong warfarin therapy.

TABLE 61-4 "Therapeutic Effect" of Heparin

Unfractionated heparin	An aPTT at 8 h after a dose that has been calibrated[a] to reflect a heparin level of 0.35 to 0.70 anti-Xa units
Low-molecular-weight heparin	An aPTT at 8 h after a dose that has been calibrated[a] reflect a heparin level of 0.7 to 1.1 anti-Xa units
During pregnancy	A heparin level of 0.6 to 0.7 anti-Xa units with unfractionated heparin or 0.10 to 0.11 anti-Xa units with low-molecular-weight heparin[b] (aPTT measurements do not accurately reflect heparin levels during pregnancy)

[a]Calibration of aPTT to heparin levels is performed in each clinical laboratory; thus the time (number of seconds) of the aPTT reflecting the "therapeutic effect" levels will vary.

[b]*Important Note:* Although low-molecular-weight heparin is increasingly being utilized in many disorders, it is reemphasized here (see text) that its value in protecting against thromboemboli in patients with valve disease has *not* been proven. Therefore its use in patients with valve disease *cannot* be recommended at the present time.

SPECIAL CLINICAL SITUATIONS

Altered Native Valves

Valve disease is increasingly being treated by interventional catheter techniques or surgical valve repair. It is difficult to give firm recommendations about antithrombotic therapy in these patients, but the recommendations given for treatment of native valve disease would seem most applicable in patients who have had surgical valve repair or catheter valve procedures (see Table 61-2).

Pregnancy

Pregnancy makes decisions regarding antithrombotic therapy for valve disease more difficult. Warfarin should be avoided in the first trimester of pregnancy, particularly in weeks 6 through 12.[29,31,32] It crosses the placental barrier and is associated with, and is the clear cause of, an embryopathy manifest in the live born as mental impairment, ocular atrophy, and facial and digital abnormalities. Therefore, warfarin should be discontinued immediately when pregnancy is recognized and heparin therapy should be initiated. The value of switching from warfarin to heparin *before* conception is uncertain. We suggest this when pregnancies are planned, since little is known about the consequences of warfarin taken in the first 6 weeks of pregnancy; however, this is often not clinically practical or feasible. Currently, the estimated risk of an embryopathy in well-managed warfarin therapy is ≤5 percent. While a return to warfarin during the second and third trimesters is recommended, there is concern that this drug may continue to endanger the fetus.

Heparin does not cross the placenta. While not devoid of problems (maternal bleeding, heparin-initiated thrombocytopenia, an increased risk of osteoporosis when used for longer than 1 month), successful pregnancies have occurred when adequate doses of the drug are administered subcutaneously at home throughout gestation.[33] Thromboembolic complications have occurred with heparin use during pregnancy in women with a mechanical prosthesis.[34,35] To minimize this, it is important to give a dose that will result in high "therapeutic effect" heparin levels (Table 61-4) prior to the next dose (this usually requires 15,000 to 30,000 units every 12 h).[29,36] Activated PTT measurements do not accurately reflect heparin levels during pregnancy.

Low-molecular-weight heparin (LMWH) is currently approved *only* for treatment of venous thrombosis. Still, there is no reason to suspect that it will not result in effective anticoagulation in patients with valve disease. It has been used safely in pregnancy,[37,38] does not cross the placenta, can be given once or twice daily, does not require regular blood test monitoring, and is associated with less thrombocytopenia and osteoporosis. More studies are needed.[39] Since there are *no* data about use of LMWH in patients with native valve disease or with prosthetic heart valves, LMWH cannot be recommended in such patients at this time.

Aspirin crosses the placenta and has been implicated as a cause of abortion and fetal growth retardation,[40] but it has been used so frequently without problems and has even been considered for use in all pregnant women as prophylaxis against preclampsia[41] that, when required for valve disease (see Table 61-2), it should be continued.

The concern about the use of antithrombotic therapy during pregnancy makes the decision about management of valve disease more difficult in women of childbearing age. If valve surgery is required, commissurotomy or valve repair is preferable because subsequent antithrombotic therapy is not required unless the woman has one of the risk factors for thrombosis (see Fig. 61-1). If a prosthetic valve is required in a woman of childbearing age, the advantage of a mechanical prosthesis is its durability. On the other hand, it obligates the woman of childbearing age to anticoagulation with warfarin because aspirin therapy itself does not offer adequate protection against thromboembolism. The theoretical advantage of a biological prosthesis is that, except for the first 3 months after valve replacement, warfarin therapy is not required. However, as many as one-third of patients with biological valves have associated atrial fibrillation and require warfarin antithrombotic therapy. In addition, the rate of degeneration of biological valves accelerates dramatically in young patients and thus also in women of childbearing age.[42] Furthermore, some data suggest that the rate of structural valve degeneration is increased in pregnant women. The choice of a prosthesis should be individualized. A young woman capable of safely using warfarin when not pregnant and warfarin/heparin during pregnancy is best treated with a mechanical valve. If a woman's social situation or attention to her health is questionable in regard to the safe use of anticoagulation therapy, a biological valve may be considered. In young women needing aortic valve replacement, the Ross procedure should be considered (see also Chap. 60).

Surgery and Dental Care (Table 61-5)

The risk of increased bleeding during a procedure performed with a patient on antithrombotic therapy has to be weighed against the increased risk of a thromboembolism caused by stopping the therapy.

The risk of stopping warfarin can be estimated and is relatively low if the drug is withheld for only a few days. As an example, and using a *worst case* scenario (e.g., a patient with a mechanical prosthesis with previous thromboemboli), the risk of a thromboembolus off warfarin could be as high as 10 to 20 percent per year. Thus, if the therapy were stopped for 3 days, the risk of an embolus would be 3/365 times 0.10 to 0.20, which equals 0.08 to 0.16 percent. There are theoretical concerns that stopping the drug and then reinstituting it might result in hypercoagulability—with a thrombotic "rebound." An increase in markers for activation of thrombosis with abrupt discontinuation of warfarin therapy has been observed,[43] but it is not clear that these increase the clinical risk of thromboembolism.[44] In addition, when reinstituting warfarin therapy, there are theoretical concerns of a hypercoagulable state caused by suppression of proteins C and S before the drug affects the thrombotic factors. Although the risks are only hypothetical, this is a reason to treat individuals at very high risk with heparin therapy until the INR returns to the desired range.

Although antithrombotic therapy must be individualized, some generalizations apply (see Table 61-6). For procedures where bleeding is unlikely or would be inconsequential if it occurred, antithrombotic therapy should not be stopped. This can apply to surgery on the skin, dental prophylaxis, or simple treatment for dental caries. Eye surgery, in particular surgery for cataracts or glaucoma, is usually associated with very little bleeding; when bleeding is likely or its potential consequences are severe, antithrombotic treatment should be altered. If a patient is on aspirin, it should be discontinued 1 week before the procedure and restarted as soon as it is considered safe by the surgeon or dentist.

For most patients on warfarin, the drug should be stopped 48 to 72 h before the procedure to ensure the INR is ≤1.5 and restarted within 24 h after a procedure; admission to the hospital or a delay in discharge to give heparin is usually unnecessary.[2,27,44–47] Deciding who is at very high risk of thrombosis and thus should require heparin until warfarin can be reinstated may be difficult; clinical judgment is required. Heparin can usually be reserved for those who have had a recent thrombosis or embolus (arbitrarily within 1 year), those with demonstrated thrombotic problems when previously off therapy, and those with three or more risk factors. When used, unfractionated heparin should be started 24 h after warfarin is stopped (i.e., 48 h before surgery) and stopped 4 to 6 h before the procedure. The heparin should be restarted as early after surgery as bleeding stability allows and the aPPT maintained at a "therapeutic level" (Table 61-4) until warfarin is restarted and the desired INR can be achieved. Home administration and management of heparin (and warfarin) can be arranged to minimize time in the hospital. LMWH is even more easily utilized outside of the hospital (see also Chap. 48); however, there are no data with its use in patients with valve disease.

TABLE 61-5 Antithrombotic Therapy at the Time of Surgery

I. Usual approach
- A. If patient on warfarin
  - Stop 72 h before procedure
  - Restart on day of procedure or after control of active bleeding
- B. If patient on aspirin
  - Stop 1 week before procedure
  - Restart the day after procedure or after control of active bleeding

II. Unusual circumstances
- A. Very high risk of thrombosis if off warfarin[a]
  - Stop warfarin 72 h before procedure
  - Start heparin 48 h before procedure[b]
  - Stop heparin 6 h before procedure
  - Restart heparin within 24 h of procedure and continue until warfarin can be restarted and the INR is 2–3
- B. Surgery complicated by postoperative bleeding
  - Start heparin as soon after surgery as deemed safe and maintain aPTT of 60–80 s until warfarin restarted and the INR is 2–3
- C. Very low risk from bleeding[c]
  - Continue antithrombotic therapy

[a]Clinical judgment: consider this approach if recent thromboembolus or if three risk factors are present.
[b]Heparin can be given in outpatient setting before and after surgery.
[c]For example, local skin surgery, dental prophylaxis, and treatment for caries.
Abbreviation: aPTT = activated partial thromboplastin time.

TABLE 61-6 Antithrombotic Therapy at the Time of a Thromboembolic Event

I. Acute management
  A. *No* antithrombotic treatment for 72 h
  B. CT scan at 72 h
    1. *No (or little) hemorrhage* on CT:
      a. Heparin: aPTT in low "therapeutic effect" (Table 61-4)
      b. Warfarin: continue heparin until INR in desired range[a]
    2. *Hemorrhage* on CT:
      a. No treatment until bleed stabilized or treated (7–14 days), then heparin and warfarin as above
II. Chronic management
  A. If embolus occurred *off* antithrombotic therapy:
    1. Treat with warfarin[a]
  B. If embolus occurred *on* antithrombotic therapy:
    1. If patient was on aspirin, switch to warfarin[a]
    2. If patient was on warfarin but INR was low, increase dose until INR in high desired range[a]
    3. If patient was on warfarin and INR was in desired range, add aspirin 80–325 mg/day
    4. If recurrent embolus or bleed on warfarin plus aspirin, assess valve for possible surgery

[a]See Tables 61-2 and 61-3.
Abbreviation: CT = computed tomography.

Cardiac Catheterization and Angiography

Antiplatelet therapy or heparin need not be stopped for these procedures. Protamine can be given to the patient on heparin if bleeding occurs. In an emergent or semiemergent situation, cardiac catheterization can be performed with a patient on warfarin, but, preferably, the drug should be stopped 72 h before the procedure and restarted the day of the procedure. This is also true for most patients with prosthetic heart valves (mechanical as well as biological). If a patient is at very high risk of thromboembolism, heparin should be started 48 h before the procedure and continued until warfarin is restarted and the desired INR is achieved. If the catheterization procedure is to include a transseptal puncture (especially in a patient who has not had previous opening of the pericardium), patients should be off all antithrombotic therapy and the INR should be <1.2—the same is also true if an LV puncture is to be performed.[48]

Therapy at the Time of an Active Thromboembolic Event

VALVE THROMBOSIS

Thrombosis of a valve, usually a prosthetic valve, can result in severe hemodynamic compromise. If recognized (TEE can be diagnostic[49]), this complication may be treated with thrombolytic therapy, although the risk of bleeding and of emboli at the time of treatment is high.[50,51] Thrombolytic therapy is most effective for a "young thrombus." Many valves, however, have pannus formation and tissue ingrowth on the valve, which is not amenable to thrombolytic therapy. Therefore, we recommend emergency surgery rather than thrombolytic therapy in the patient with severe hemodynamic compromise. If a patient is not a surgical candidate, thrombolysis should be attempted.[2,52] Streptokinase or urokinase should be initiated but stopped at 24 h if there is no improvement by Doppler echocardiography and at 72 h even if hemodynamic recovery is incomplete.[2] This should be followed by heparin until high INR levels are achieved with concomitant warfarin therapy (INR 3 to 4 for aortic prostheses or 3.5 to 4.5 with mitral prostheses).

THROMBOEMBOLIC EVENT

An embolic event often indicates inadequate therapy for that patient's circumstances. Data and opinions about optimal timing for initiating or continuing anticoagulants in patients in whom an embolus is the presumed cause of a stroke are conflicting.[2,53–55] Ideally, treatment would be started early to prevent recurrent emboli, but the early use of heparin (within 72 h) is associated with a 15 to 25 percent chance of converting a nonhemorrhagic into a hemorrhagic stroke.[54] While a case can still be made for immediate use of heparin,[53,54] the early recurrence of an embolus in patients with valve disease while off anticoagulants has not been clearly documented. Data are insufficient to provide definitive treatment outlines, but the authors' practice is listed in Table 61-6.

ACUTE MANAGEMENT OF AN EMBOLIC EVENT

Antithrombotic therapy should be withheld or stopped for 72 h. If a computed tomography (CT) scan at that time reveals little or no hemorrhage, heparin should be administered to maintain an aPPT at the lower end of the therapeutic level (Table 61-4) until warfarin, started at the same time, results in the desired INR (see Tables 61-2 and 61-3). If the CT scan demonstrates significant hemorrhage, antithrombotic therapy should be withheld until the bleed is treated or has stabilized (7 to 14 days). Anticoagulation can then be started as just described.

LONG-TERM MANAGEMENT

If the embolic event occurs when a patient is *off* antithrombotic therapy, long-term warfarin therapy is required (see Tables 61-2 and 61-3). An exception may be those with mitral valve prolapse; aspirin (325 mg/day) is recommended for those who are judged to have had a minor event. If the embolic event occurs while the patient is *on* antithrombotic treatment, therapy should be individualized. Those who are on warfarin but in whom the INR was low at the time of the embolus should have the dose increased into the high end of the desired range (see Tables 61-2 and 61-3). If the embolus occurs in a patient despite an INR in the desirable range, aspirin (50 to 100 mg/day) should be added to the warfarin. Embolism recurring with this combination should lead to consideration of possible valve surgery if the valve is the likely source of the thrombus.

Therapy at the Time of a Bleed

With significant bleeding, antithrombotic therapy should be stopped and, if the patient is at risk, drug effects should be reversed. If possible, the site of bleeding should be corrected and antithrombotic therapy restarted as soon as possible. If this is not possible, treatment decisions are difficult. In patients with a mechanical prosthesis or multiple risk factors for thromboemboli, acceptance of intermittent bleeding with acute management for the bleeds may be necessary. In valve patients who are at lower risk of emboli or in whom the role of antithrombotic treatment is less clear (e.g., LV dysfunction), it may be optimal to withhold chronic therapy or, if a patient is on warfarin, to switch to aspirin. In some patients with mechanical valves, consideration should be given to replacing the mechanical valve with a biological valve, for example, in those who have had multiple, large life- or organ-threatening bleeds.

Antithrombotic Therapy in the Patient with Endocarditis

If a patient with valve disease develops endocarditis, antithrombotic therapy should be continued.[2,56] If the patient presents with or develops an embolic event involving the central nervous system, therapy should be as described above for acute embolic events. Additionally, the issue of whether or not the embolus is due to thrombus or infected vegetation should be addressed. If thrombus is likely, the chronic anticoagulation program will also require alteration.

References

1. Rahimtoola S. Lessons learned about the determinants of the results of valve surgery. *Circulation* 1988; 78:1503–1506.
2. Bonow RO, Carabello B, deLeon AC Jr, et al. ACCAHA guidelines for the management of patients with valvular heart disease: A report of the American College of Cardiology American Heart Association Task Force on Practice Guidelines (Committee on Management of Patients with Valvular Heart Disease). *J Am Coll Cardiol* 1998; 32:1486–1588.
3. Petersen P, Boysen G, Godtfredsen J, et al. Placebo controlled, randomized trial of warfarin and aspirin for prevention of thromboembolic complications in chronic atrial fibrillation. *Lancet* 1989; 1:175–179.
4. The Boston Area Anticoagulation Trial for Atrial Fibrillation Investigators. The effect of low-dose warfarin on the risk of stroke in patients with nonrheumatic atrial fibrillation. *N Engl J Med* 1990; 323:1505–1511.
5. Ezekowitz MD, Bridgers SL, James KE, et al. Warfarin in the prevention of stroke associated with nonrheumatic atrial fibrillation. *N Engl J Med* 1992; 327:1406–1412.
6. EAFT (European Atrial Fibrillation Trial) Study Group. Secondary prevention in nonrheumatic atrial fibrillation after transient ischemic attack or minor stroke. *Lancet* 1993; 342:1255–1262.
7. Stroke Prevention in Atrial Fibrillation Investigators. Warfarin versus aspirin for prevention of thromboembolism in atrial fibrillation: Stroke Prevention in Atrial Fibrillation II Study. *Lancet* 1994; 343:687–691.
8. Stroke Prevention in Atrial Fibrillation Investigators. Adjusted-dose warfarin versus low-intensity, fixed dose warfarin plus aspirin for high-risk patients with atrial fibrillation: Stroke Prevention in Atrial Fibrillation III randomized clinical trial. *Lancet* 1996; 348:633–638.
9. ACCAHA Task Force. Guidelines for the evaluation and management of heart failure. *Circulation* 1999; 92:2764–2784.
10. Al-Khadra AS, Salem DN, Rand WM, et al. Warfarin anticoagulation and survival: A cohort analysis from the Studies of Left Ventricular Dysfunction. *J Am Coll Cardiol* 1998; 31:749–753.
11. Cannegieter SC, Rosendaal FR, Briet E. Thromboembolic and bleeding complications in patients with mechanical heart valve prostheses. *Circulation* 1994; 89:635–641.
12. Starr A, Grunkemeier GL. Recurrent thromboembolism: Significance and management. In: Butchart EG, Bodnar E, eds. *Thrombosis, Embolism and Bleeding.* London: ICR; 1992: 402–415.
13. Blackstone EH. Analyses of thrombosis, embolism and bleeding as time-related outcome events. In: Butchart EG, Bodnar E, eds. *Thrombosis, Embolism and Bleeding.* London: ICR; 1992: 445–463.
14. Levin HJ, Pauler SG, Eckman MH. Antithrombotic therapy in valve disease: Fourth ACCP conference on antithrombolic therapy. *Chest* 1995; 108(suppl):360S–370S.
15. The SPAF III Writing Committee for the Stroke Prevention in Atrial Fibrillation Investigators. Patients with nonvalvular atrial fibrillation at low risk of stroke during treatment with aspirin: Stroke Prevention in Atrial Fibrillation III Study. *JAMA* 1998; 279:1273–1277.
16. Bloomfield P, Wheatley DJ, Prescott RJ, Miller HC. Twelve-year comparison of a Bjork-Shiley mechanical heart valve with porcine bioprostheses. *N Engl J Med* 1991; 324:573–579.
17. Hammermeister KE, Sethi GK, Henderson WG, et al. A comparison of outcomes in men 11 years after heart-valve replacement with a mechanical valve or bioprosthesis. *N Engl J Med* 1993; 328:1289–1296.
18. Cobanoglu A, Fessler CL, Guvendik L, et al. Aortic valve replacement with the Starr-Edwards prosthesis: A comparison of the first and second decades of follow-up. *Ann Thorac Surg* 1988; 45:248–252.
19. Vongpatanasin W, Hillis D, Lange RA. Prosthetic heart valves. *N Engl J Med* 1996; 335:407–416.
20. Geras M, Chesebro JH, Fuster V, et al. High risk of thromboemboli early after bioprosthetic cardiac valve replacement. *J Am Coll Cardiol* 1995; 25:1111–1119.
21. North RA, Sadler L, Stewart AW, et al. Long-term survival and valve-related complications in young women with cardiac valve replacements. *Circulation* 1999; 99:2669–2676.
22. Cannegieter SC, Rosendaal FR, Wintzen AR, et al. Optimal oral anticoagulant therapy in patients with mechanical heart valves. *N Engl J Med* 1995; 333:11–17.
23. Jegaden O, Eker A, Delahaye F, et al. Thromboembolic risk and late survival after mitral valve replacement with the St. Jude medical valve. *Ann Thorac Surg* 1994; 58:1721–1728.
24. Saour JN, Sieck JO, Mamo LAR, Gallus AS. Trial of different intensities of anticoagulation in patients with prosthetic heart valves. *N Engl J Med* 1990; 322:428–432.
25. Hylek EM, Skates SJ, Sheehan MA, Singer DE. An analysis of the lowest effective intensity of prophylactic anticoagulation for patients with nonrheumatic atrial fibrillation. *N Engl J Med* 1996; 335:540–546.
26. Acar J, Iung B, Boissel JP, et al. AREVA: Multicenter randomized comparison of low-dose versus standard-dose anticoagulation in patients with mechanical prosthetic heart valves. *Circulation* 1996; 94:2107–2112.
27. Hyashi J, Nakazawa S, Oguma F, et al. Combined warfarin and antiplatelet therapy after St. Jude medical valve replacement for mitral valve disease. *J Am Coll Cardiol* 1994; 23:672–677.
28. Turpie AG, Gent M, Laupacis A, et al. A comparison of aspirin with placebo in patients treated with warfarin after heart-valve replacement. *N Engl J Med* 1993; 329:524–529.
29. Ginsberg JS, Hirsh J. Use of antithrombotic agents during pregnancy. Fourth ACCP conference on antithrombolic therapy. *Chest* 1995; 108 (suppl):305S–311S.
30. Turpie AGG, Gunstensen J, Hirsh J, et al. Randomized comparison of two intensities of oral anticoagulant therapy after tissue heart valve replacement. *Lancet* 1988; 1:1242–1245.
31. Hall JR, Pauli RM, Wilson KM. Maternal and fetal sequelae of anticoagulation during pregnancy. *Am J Med* 1980; 68:122.
32. Iturbe-Alessio I, del Carmen Fonseca M, Mutchinick O, et al.

Risks of anticoagulant therapy in pregnant women with artificial heart valves. *N Engl J Med* 1986; 315:1390–1393.
33. Ginsberg JS, Kowalchuk G, Hirsh J, et al. Heparin therapy during pregnancy. *Arch Intern Med* 1989; 149:2233–2236.
34. Hanania G, Thomas D, Michel PL, et al. Pregnancy and prosthetic heart valves: A French cooperative retrospective study of 155 cases. *Eur Heart J* 1994; 15:1651–1658.
35. Salazar E, Iazguirre R, Verdejo J, Mutchinick O. Failure of adjusted doses of subcutaneous heparin to prevent thromboembolic phenomena in pregnant patients with mechanical cardiac valve prostheses. *J Am Coll Cardiol* 1996; 27:1698–1703.
36. Elkayam U. Anticoagulation in pregnant women with prosthetic heart valves: A double jeopardy (editorial). *J Am Coll Cardiol* 1996; 27:1704–1706.
37. Sturridge F, DeSwiet M, Letsky E. The use of low molecular weight heparin for thromboprophylaxis in pregnancy. *Br J Obstet Gynaecol* 1994; 101:69–71.
38. Nelson-Piercy C, Letsky EA, DeSweit M. Low-molecular weight heparin for obstetric thromboprophylaxis: Experience of sixty-nine pregnancies in sixty-one women at high risk. *Am J Obstet Gynecol* 1997; 176:1062–1068.
39. Sanson BJ, Lensing AW, Prins MH, et al. Safety of low-molecular-weight heparin in pregnancy: A systematic review. *Thromb Haemost* 1999; 81:668–672.
40. Corby DG. Aspirin in pregnancy and fetal effects. *Pediatrics* 1978; 62:930–937.
41. DuBard MB, Cutter GR. Low-dose aspirin therapy to prevent preeclampsia. *Am J Obstet Gynecol* 1993; 168:1083–1091.
42. Jamieson WR, Miller DC, Akins CW, et al. Pregnancy and bioprostheses: Influence on structural valve deterioration. *Ann Thorac Surg* 1995; 60:S282–S286.
43. Genewein U, Hasberli A, Werner S, Beer J. Rebound after cessation of oral anticoagulant therapy: The biochemical evidence. *Br J Haematol* 1996; 92:479–485.
44. Eckman MH, Beshansky JR, Durand-Zaleski I, et al. Anticoagulation for noncardiac procedures in patients with prosthetic heart valves: Does low risk mean high cost? *JAMA* 1990; 263:1513–1521.
45. Bryan AJ, Butchart EG. Prosthetic heart valves and anticoagulant management during non-cardiac surgery. *Br J Surg* 1995; 82: 577–578.
46. Busuttil WJ, Fabr BMI. The management of anticoagulation in patients with prosthetic heart valves undergoing non-cardiac operations. *Postgrad Med J* 1995; 71:390–392.
47. Tinker JH, Tarhan S. Discontinuing anticoagulant therapy in surgical patients with cardiac valve prostheses: Observations in 180 operations. *JAMA* 1978; 239:738–739.
48. Morton MJ, McAnulty JH, Rahimtoola SH, Ahuja N. Risks and benefits of postoperative cardiac catheterization in patients with ball-valve prostheses. *Am J Cardiol* 1977; 40:870–875.
49. Gueret P, Vignon P, Fournier P, et al. Transesophageal echocardiography for the diagnosis and management of nonobstructive thrombosis of mechanical mitral valve prosthesis. *Circulation* 1995; 91:103–110.
50. Silber H, Khan SS, Matloff JM, et al. The St. Jude valve: Thrombolysis as the first line of therapy of cardiac valve thrombosis. *Circulation* 1993; 887:30–37.
51. Reddy NK, Padmanabhan TNC, Singh S, et al. Thrombolysis in left-sided prosthetic valve occlusion: Immediate and follow-up results. *Ann Thorac Surg* 1994; 58:462–471.
52. Lengyel M, Fuster V, Keltai M, et al. Guidelines for management of lift-sided prosthetic valve thrombosis: A role for thrombolytic therapy: Consensus Conference on Prosthetic Valve Thrombosis. *J Am Coll Cardiol* 1997; 30:1521–1526.
53. Pessin MS, Estol CJ, Lafranchise F, Chaplan LR. Safety of anticoagulation after hemorrhagic infarction. *Neurology* 1994; 43:1289–1303.
54. Chamorro A, Vila N, Saiz A, et al. Early anticoagulation after large cerebral embolic infarction: A safety study. *Neurology* 1995; 45:861–865.
55. Sherman DJ, Dyken ML, Gent M, et al. Antithrombotic therapy for cerebrovascular disorders: Fourth ACCP consensus conference on antithrombolic therapy. *Chest* 1995; 108(suppl):444s–456s.
56. Wilson WR, Geraci JE, Danielson GK, et al. Anticoagulant therapy and central nervous system complication in patients with prosthetic valve endocarditis. *Circulation* 1978; 57:1004–1007.

PART TEN

CONGENITAL HEART DISEASE

C H A P T E R 62

CARDIOVASCULAR DISEASES DUE TO GENETIC ABNORMALITIES

Jeffrey A. Towbin / Robert Roberts

Genetic factors play a significant role in the pathogenesis of many if not all cardiovascular disorders. Malformations of the heart and blood vessels account for the largest number of human birth defects, occurring in about 1 percent of all live births; among stillbirths, the prevalence is estimated to be tenfold higher.[1,2] In conjunction with cytogenetics (the study of chromosomes and their abnormalities), molecular genetics provides an opportunity to decipher the genetic basis of cardiovascular diseases. Genetic diagnosis and screening for genetic disorders will soon be incorporated into standard practice.[3] The goal of the Human Genome Project[4] is to identify all of the genes by the year 2001 (see Chap. 7).[5] The challenge for the clinical and investigative cardiologist is to link these genes to their specific physiologic or pathologic function.[6] It is thus imperative that the cardiologist understand the basis for genetic disorders so as to have a better appreciation of the medical, ethical, and moral implications.[7]

BASIS FOR GENETIC TRANSMISSION

All hereditary information is transmitted through DNA, a linear polymer composed of purine (adenine, guanine) and pyrimidine (cytosine, thymine) bases (see Chap. 4). The basic hereditary unit is the gene, which consists of a distinct fragment of DNA that encodes for a specific polypeptide (protein). It is estimated there are only about 100,000 genes, although there is enough DNA to code for several hundred thousand genes. However, less than 5 percent of the DNA is used to code for genes. Each individual has two copies of each gene—called alleles. The genes are localized in linear sequence along 23 pairs of chromosomes, the rod-shaped bodies derived from the parents of each individual. Each parent contributes one member of each chromosome pair (the pair is referred to as *homologous chromosomes*) and thus one copy of each gene. The site at which a gene is located on a particular chromosome is called the *genetic locus*. A given gene always resides at the same specific locus on a particular chromosome, so the loci on homologous chromosomes are identical but the alleles residing at these loci may be the same or different. When the same loci on two homologous chromosomes have identical alleles, the individual is homozygous. When the two genes differ (i.e., two different alleles present at the locus), the individual is heterozygous at that locus. Each individual is homozygous at some loci and heterozygous at others, and, based on present knowledge, at least one-third of human genes have polymorphic forms. The gene, transmitted to each offspring during the union of sperm and ova, passes on the genetic information to the offspring (genotype), which, through the synthesis of their corresponding proteins, determines the observable characteristics of an individual (phenotype). The genetic information carried in the gene's DNA is coded by the sequence of the four bases. Translation of this information into protein is through a translational code passed on through messenger ribonucleic acid (mRNA), whereby each specific amino acid is encoded by three bases referred to as a *codon* (Chap. 4). The mRNA transcribed from the gene serves as the template that determines which amino acids are included and their sequence in the resulting polypeptide. Although it is true each gene encodes for a unique protein, it is preferable to use polypeptide, since many proteins are single polypeptides and other proteins consist of several polypeptides which may be from a single gene or multiple genes. The 23 pairs of chromosomes include 22 pairs of autosomes (chromosomes 1 to 22) and one pair of sex chromosomes, X and Y. Females have two X chromosomes, while males carry one X and one Y chromosome. Both autosomal alleles are potentially active in specifying RNA copies of their DNA sequences, but the expression of each gene depends on the cell type, developmental stage, and regulatory molecules that interact with promoter sequences, and enhancer sequences that control gene transcription. In cells that carry two X chromosomes, whether these are derived from normal females or XXY individuals with Klinefelter syndrome, only one X is active after early embryogenesis.

ORIGIN OF GENETIC DISEASE

The three broad categories of inherited diseases are chromosomal abnormalities, single gene disorders, and polygene disorders (Table 62-1). Thus, hereditary and congenital diseases may be due to chromosomal abnormalities or mutations within a single gene or multiple genes. A mutation is a stable, heritable alteration in DNA caused by a number of factors, including environmental agents such as radiation, chemicals, and viruses as well as baseline changes in the fidelity of transfer of sequences. Since offspring typically resemble their parents, it is assumed that the DNA nucleotide sequences remain stable. Base sequence changes do occur, however, albeit at a slow rate compared to the overall life span of humans, and these changes occur by a number of different mechanisms. Mutations can involve a visible alteration at the level of the chromosome, such as deletion or translocation of a portion of the chromosome, whereby often several genes are eliminated or altered. Chromosome alterations (discussed later), especially those involving too many or too few chromosomes (called an euploidy), are quite common in human development. The sequence of each codon determines the amino acid, and the linear sequence of the codons in the mRNA is collinear with the linear sequence of the amino acids in the protein. A change in even one amino acid, if critical to the function of the protein, will result in altered function or lack of function, with a concomitant change in the phenotype. Since proteins are the working molecules derived from genes, mutations in genes exert their deleterious effects via structural alteration of the proteins, whether they be enzymes, regulatory proteins, or structural proteins. On the average, a mutation occurs every 106 cell divisions, and, obviously, only mutations occurring in the gametes are transmitted. On the average, a gene undergoes one mutation per 200,000 years.

TABLE 62-1 Inherited Disorders

Chromosomal abnormalities	Polygene disorders
Single-gene disorders	

GENETICS OF SINGLE-GENE DISORDERS

Inherited disorders due to a single abnormal gene are transmitted to offspring in a predictable fashion termed *mendelian transmission*. These inheritance patterns produce phenotypes that are inherited according to Mendel's laws of inheritance. As previously noted, in each individual there exists two copies of each gene, referred to as alleles, one obtained from the mother and one from the father. Mendel's first law states that each of the two alleles located on separate chromosomes segregates independently and is passed unchanged into different gametes at the formation of the next generation. Thus, the odds of getting the mother's allele versus the father's are by chance alone, namely, 50 percent. Mendel's second law states that genes on the same chromosome also assert themselves independently through the process of crossover between chromosomes (discussed below). The greater the distance between two loci, the more likely they are to be separated during genetic transmission. As a result of gene mutations, abnormal genes located on any of the 22 autosomal pairs or the two sex chromosomes may produce phenotypes inherited by simple patterns classified as autosomal (dominant or recessive) or X-linked, respectively. When different genes induce the same phenotype, it is referred to as *genetic heterogeneity*, and most diseases in humans exhibit genetic heterogeneity. The same disease may be due to multiple mutations in the same gene (*allele heterogeneity*) or it may be due to a single or multiple mutations in two or more genes (*locus heterogeneity*). Within any one family, however, the gene and the mutation responsible for the disease are the same and only rarely would two genes be transmitted for the same disease. A good example is familial hypertrophic cardiac myopathy (HCM), in which eight different genes have been recognized with multiple mutations in each. Genetic heterogeneity is to be distinguished from polygenic disorders, such as atherosclerosis, which are due to the interaction of several genes. As noted above, mutations can involve a microscopically visible alter-

TABLE 62-2 Single-Gene Disorders

Alteration of a single nucleotide (point mutation)
Missense
Truncated
Elongated
Nonsense
Synonomous
Deletion of several nucleotides
Addition of several nucleotides

ation, such as deletion or translocation of a portion of the chromosome, or they can involve a minute change in one purine or pyrimidine base in the DNA sequence of a single codon. Mutations involving only a single nucleotide are known as point mutations and are responsible for 70 percent or more of all adult single gene disorders (Table 62-2). A point mutation may be a substitution of one nucleotide for another, resulting in a different amino acid being encoded (missense mutation); or it may change the codon from encoding for an amino acid to that of a stop codon, which will truncate the protein (truncated mutant); or it may eliminate a stop codon so the protein is elongated (elongated mutant). Finally, a nucleotide may be deleted or added, which results in a frame shift, and the gene is read entirely differently (nonsense mutation), resulting in a nonfunctioning protein. If a purine nucleotide is substituted for a pyrimidine, the mutation is referred to as a *transversion,* while if purine or pyrimidine substitutes for another purine or pyrimidine, respectively, it is called a *transition*. Other mutations may result from deletion or addition of several nucleotides. An example of the latter is the defect responsible for myotonic dystrophy, where a triplet repeat of several thousand nucleotides in length is inserted into the 3′ end of the gene. Another type of mutation is known as *gene conversion,* where two genes interact and part of the nucleotide sequence of one gene becomes incorporated into the other. Mutations in genes exert their deleterious effects via structural alteration of enzymes, regulatory proteins, or structural proteins. The terms *dominant inheritance* and *recessive inheritance* refer to characteristics of the phenotype and are not characteristics of the gene per se. Dominant inheritance implies that a person with one copy of a mutant allele and one copy of the normal allele develops a phenotype of the mutant allele. Recessive traits, on the other hand, require both alleles to be mutant to develop a phenotype. This situation usually occurs when the patients are consanguineous, with each carrying mutant alleles, or when the mutant allele is common in the population, as is seen in sickle cell anemia.

Genetic Penetrance and Expressivity

The percentage of individuals with a disease-related gene who have one or more features of the disease is referred to as *penetrance*. Penetrance is an all-or-none phenomenon, and any manifestation, however minute, indicates that the gene has full penetrance in that individual. Nonpenetrance refers to lack of any observable phenotype. This feature is to be distinguished from *expressivity,* which refers to the variable nature of the clinical features. Thus, by definition, to have expressivity, the trait must be penetrant. Numerous genetic and environmental factors can affect expression of a gene, making it nearly impossible to determine which factor is most important in a specific individual or specific disease. These factors include (1) genetic background, (2) age-dependency, (3) sex influence and sex limitation, (4) exogenous factors, (5) maternal factors, (6) modifying loci, and (7) gene alterations.

Patterns of Inheritance

AUTOSOMAL DOMINANT INHERITANCE

Dominant disorders are those that have phenotypic manifestations (disease) in heterozygous individuals—persons carrying only one abnormal allele, with the other allele on the homologous chromosome being normal. In autosomal dominant disorders, both males and females can be affected, and since alleles segregate independently at meiosis, there is a 50-50 chance that the offspring of an affected heterozygote will inherit the mutant allele. Not all affected individuals, however, must have an affected parent because, in all autosomal dominant diseases, a certain proportion of cases occur due to a new mutation (i.e., they are sporadic). The parent whose germ cells contain the new mutation will be clinically normal, since the mutation affects only a single germ cell, but will transmit the disease-causing allele to half of his or her offspring. Autosomal dominant inheritance can be misdiagnosed as sporadic if there is low expressivity in the phenotypically normal parent carrying the mutant allele or if extramarital paternity has occurred. The following features are characteristic of autosomal dominant inheritance (Fig. 62-1): (1) each affected individual has an affected parent unless the disease occurred due to a new mutation or the heterozygous parent has low expressivity; (2) equal proportions (i.e., 50-50) of normal and affected offspring are likely statistically to be born to an affected individual; (3) normal children of an affected individual bear only normal offspring; (4) equal proportions of males and females are affected; (5) both sexes are equally likely to transmit the abnormal allele to male and female offspring, and male-to-male transmission occurs; and (6) vertical transmission through successive generations occurs. Two other features are characteristically seen in autosomal dominant diseases that help to differentiate this type of inheritance from autosomal recessive disorders: delayed age of onset and variable clinical expression. The former is commonly seen in such disorders as familial HCM, while the latter may occur in Holt-Oram syndrome, in which the patient may present with an atrial septal defect (ASD) and skeletal abnormality of the upper extremity in combination or with either of these abnormalities individually. Examples of autosomal dominant primary heart disease include HCM and Romano-Ward long-QT syndrome.

AUTOSOMAL RECESSIVE INHERITANCE

Autosomal recessive phenotypes are clinically apparent when the patient carries two mutant alleles (i.e., is homozygous) at the locus responsible for the disease state. The disease-causing gene is found on one of the 22 autosomes, and thus both males and females will be equally affected. Clinical uniformity is typical, and disease onset generally occurs early in life. Recessive disorders are more commonly diagnosed in childhood than are dominant diseases. Only one in four children (25 percent) on average, will be affected. The following are characteristics of

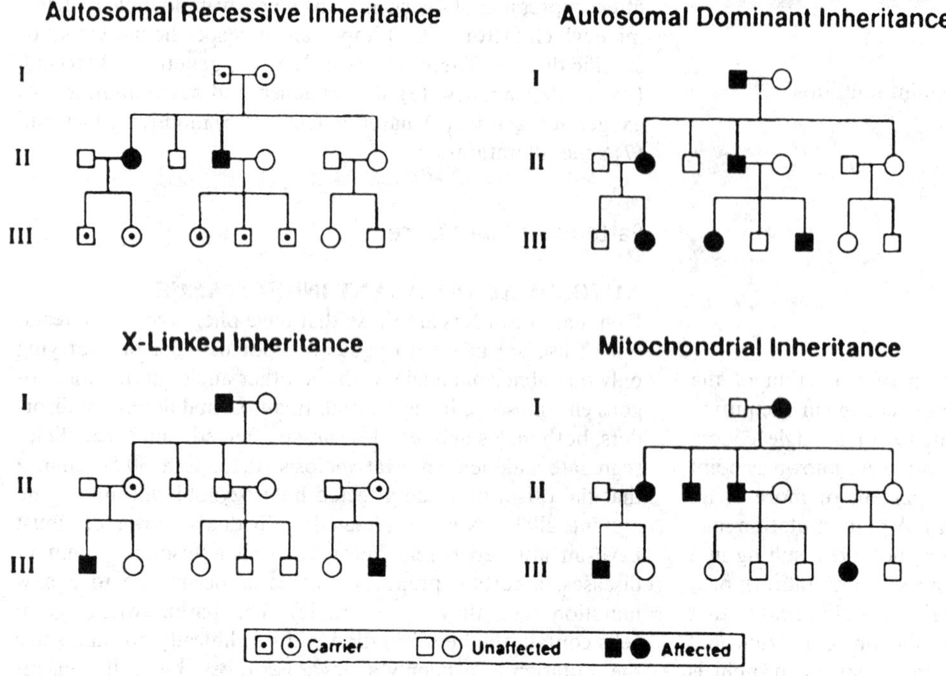

FIGURE 62-1 This typical set of pedigrees outlines the usual inheritance patterns for autosomal dominant and recessive traits, X-linked inheritance, and mitochondrial inheritance. Squares signify males and circles, females. Filled-in circles and squares are affected females and males, respectively. A slash line through a circle or square designates a deceased individual.

autosomal recessive disorders (Fig. 62-1): (1) parents are clinically normal heterozygotes; (2) alternate generations are affected, with no vertical transmission; (3) both sexes are affected with equal frequency; and (4) each offspring of heterozygous carriers has a 25 percent chance of being affected, a 50 percent chance of being an unaffected carrier, and a 25 percent chance of inheriting only normal alleles. Examples of autosomal recessive disorders affecting the heart include Jervell and Lange-Nielsen long-QT/deafness syndrome and Pompe's (type II glycogen storage) disease.

X-LINKED INHERITANCE

X-linked inherited disorders are caused by genes located on the X chromosome; therefore the clinical risk and severity of disease differ between the sexes. Since a female has two X chromosomes, she may carry either one mutant allele (heterozygote) or two mutant alleles (homozygote); the trait may therefore display dominant or recessive expression. Males have a single X chromosome (and one Y chromosome); therefore they are expected to display the full syndrome whenever they inherit the abnormal gene from their mother. This development of the trait occurs regardless of whether the mother carrying the mutant allele exhibits a recessive (i.e., clinically silent) or dominant (i.e., clinically apparent) trait. Hence, the terms *X-linked dominant* and *X-linked recessive* apply only to the expression of the gene in females. Since males must pass on their Y chromosome to all male offspring, they cannot pass on mutant X alleles to their sons; therefore no male-to-male transmission of X-linked disorders can occur. On the other hand, males must contribute their one X chromosome to all daughters. All females receiving a mutant X chromosome are known as *carriers,* and those who become affected clinically with the disease are known as *manifesting female carriers*. The characteristic features of X-linked inheritance (Fig. 62-1) include (1) no male-to-male transmission; (2) all daughters of affected males are carriers; (3) sons of carrier females have a 50 percent risk of being affected, and daughters have a 50 percent chance of being carriers; (4) affected homozygous females occur only when an affected male and carrier female have children; and (5) the pedigree pattern in X-linked recessive traits tends to be oblique because of the occurrence of the trait in the sons of normal carriers sisters of affected males (i.e., uncles and nephews affected). Examples of X-linked disorders of the heart include X-linked cardiomyopathy, X-linked cardioskeletal myopathy (Barth's syndrome) and those X-linked diseases in which the heart is affected, such as muscular dystrophy (MD) (e.g., Duchenne/Becker and Emery-Dreifuss MD).

MITOCHONDRIAL INHERITANCE

Another inheritance pattern described in patients with cardiovascular anomalies occurs because of abnormalities of the mitochondrial genome. Generation of energy is dependent on the oxidative phosphorylation process within the mitochondria. Within many mitochondria is a single chromosome that encodes for a number of the enzymes of oxidative phosphorylation (i.e., encodes for 13 of the 69 proteins required for oxidative metabolism) and the transfer RNAs (tRNAs) and ribosomal RNAs (rRNAs) required for their translation. The remaining enzymes of the oxidative-phosphorylation pathway are encoded by genes on the nuclear chromosomes, and the resultant proteins are transported into the mitochondrion. Genetic defects of oxidative phosphorylation, therefore, can be due either to gene mutations within the X chromosome or autosomes (i.e., nuclear chromosomes), resulting in diseases that behave as Mendelian recessive traits, or to mitochondrial genome defects that cause diseases with nonmendelian traits. These differences may be explained by events of conception, since the spermatocyte contributes few or no mitochondria to the zygote (Fig. 62-2). The entire mitochondrial complement present in a fetus must therefore be derived from the mitochondria already present in the cytoplasm of the oocyte. Thus, phenotypes due to mitochondrial DNA mutations demonstrate maternal inheritance only. The characteristic features of mitochondrial inheritance of disease (Fig. 62-1) include (1) equal frequency and severity of disease for each sex; (2) transmission through females only, with offspring of affected males being unaffected; (3) all offspring of affected females may be affected; (4) extreme variability of expression of disease within a family (may include apparent nonpenetrance); (5) phenotypes may be age-dependent; (6) or-

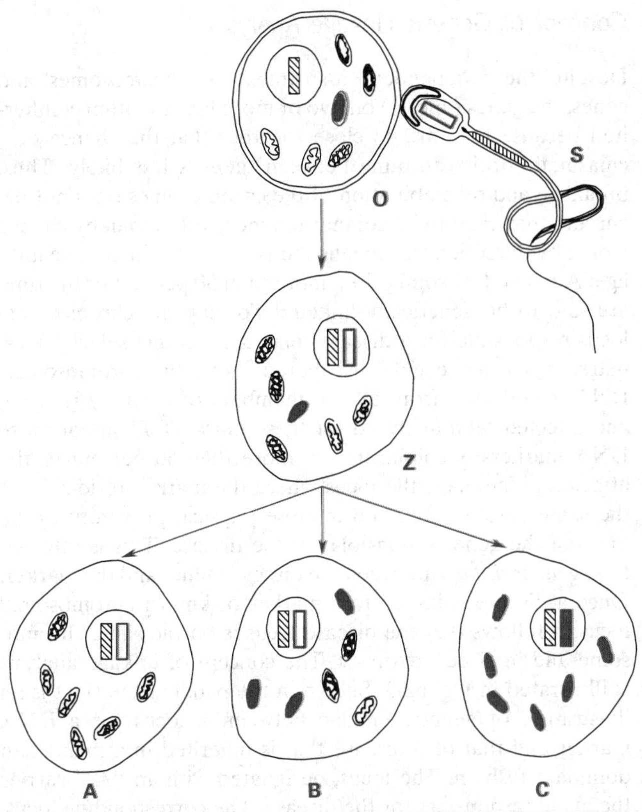

FIGURE 62-2 Cartoon (not to scale) illustrating maternal inheritance of mtDNA, compared with biparental inheritance of nuclear genes, and the random distribution of normal and mutant mitochondrial genomes in daughter cells of the zygote. It is assumed for simplicity that individual mitochondria contain either normal (open mitochondria) or mutant (filled mitochondria) mtDNA, not both. O = oocyte; S = sperm; Z = zygote; A, B, C = daughter cells of zygote, representing stem cells of different tissues. (Reprinted with permission from DiMauro S et al. Mitochondrial encephalomyopathies. *Neurol Clin* 1990; 8:494.)

gan mosaicism is common. An example of mitochondrial inherited cardiac disease is the cardiomyopathy of Kearns-Sayre syndrome.

POLYGENIC INHERITANCE OF CARDIAC DISEASE

Disorders such as hypertension or ischemic heart disease are believed to require concomitant mutations in several genes—i.e., they are polygenic hereditary disorders (discussed in Chap. 7). The genes responsible for polygenic hereditary disorders are difficult to map, since computational methods to describe their mode of inheritance are only now being explored.[8] Over the past two decades, this type of inheritance has been invoked for a large number of disorders, including coronary artery disease and congenital heart disease. In multifactorial, or polygenic, genetic diseases, multiple genes interact in a cumulative fashion to induce the disease or provide an increased risk of developing the disease. This multifaceted process is illustrated by coronary artery disease, in which one common phenotype is myocardial infarction due to thrombosis superimposed on atherosclerosis. There are many single-gene disorders that alter plasma lipoproteins and contribute to atherosclerosis (see Chaps. 7, 35, and 38). Several other genetic risk factors have been identified that predispose to atherosclerosis, such as the paraoxonase gene or homocysteine gene.[9] The phenotype of acute myocardial infarction is more likely if the individual, in addition to atherosclerosis, has a mutant form of fibrinogen[10] or mutant forms of other clotting factors, discussed in detail in Chap. 7.

OVERVIEW OF CHROMOSOMAL MAPPING AND IDENTIFICATION OF A DISEASE-RELATED GENE

Identification of a disease-causing gene, in the setting where the protein is unknown, was until the 1980s nearly impossible. Familial hypercholesterolemia and some of the thalassemias are disorders in which genes were isolated and cloned, knowing the protein. For the majority of diseases, however, neither the defect nor the protein is known. Technical advances[11] aiding chromosomal mapping include (1) computerized linkage analysis, (2) development of highly informative DNA markers, and (3) detection of markers by polymerase chain reaction (PCR).[11] The 46 chromosomes of the human genome contain 3 billion base pairs (bp). To locate a particular gene, one must first map the chromosomal location and its relative position. This process requires certain chromosomal landmarks. Identification of a particular locus is made possible by showing that the disease-related gene of interest is on the same chromosome and in close proximity to one of these landmarks, a method referred to as *genetic linkage analysis*. This technique requires a family with a disease that is transmitted over at least two generations (and preferably three) with at least 10 affected individuals, although even 6 or 7 affected individuals may be adequate, depending on the structure of the family. A landmark, referred to as a DNA or chromosomal *marker*, is a polymorphic sequence of DNA, the chromosomal position of which is known and can be detected by analyzing an individual's DNA (discussed in detail below). A major limitation until recently was the lack of markers evenly distributed across each of the chromosomes. Today there is a marker available at least every 1 million base pairs on all chromosomes.[12,13] Genetic distance is measured in terms of centimorgans (cM), named after the geneticist T. H. Morgan, and 1 cM approximates 1 million bp. Markers, like genes, have two alleles and are transmitted to offspring according to Mendel's law, with the individual being heterozygous or homozygous for that marker. If a marker is homozygous, it is not informative for genetic linkage. Hence, several markers in the same region may have to be analyzed to find one that is heterozygous in that individual. When all of the markers are placed together on each chromosome and the genetic distance between them is estimated, a *genetic map* is produced. A map of over 5000 highly informative markers has been developed, which has significantly accelerated the mapping of disease-related genes—an achievement that provides the foundation for genetic linkage analysis.[13] Each gene, allele, or marker is transmitted independently; thus, the odds of any two genes (or a marker and a gene) being coinherited are by chance alone (50 percent), even though they are on the same chromosome. The homologous pairs of chromosomes are assorted, and one from each parent is transmitted to the offspring by chance. Genetic diversity from homologous chromosomes segregating independently would produce 223 types of gametes; in other words, the probability of an offspring inheriting a set of chromosomes identical to those of a parent is one in 8,388,608.[14] If this were the only mechanism for diversity, all of the genes on a particular chromosome would be coinherited in the next progeny. This does not happen. Genes on the same chromosome are transmitted independently unless they are in close physical proximity to each other. Genes on the same chromosome are transmitted independently by the mechanism of crossover between homologous chromosomes (Fig. 62-3), which provides continual mixing of the genes during every meiosis and is the predominant reason why no two individuals have the same genotype unless they are identical twins. Prior to meiosis, the two homologous chromosomes come together and form bridges (*chiasmata*) such that segments of equal proportion are exchanged between them, giving rise to crossover of various genes. There is no net loss of chromosomal material or genes, but crossover leads to a constant intermixing of the chromosomes such that no two offspring will ever be identical. Crossovers occur only between homologous chromosomes. The loci occupy the same chromosomal position on the homologous chromosome on which they are combined as they had on their original homologous chromosome. On average there are 33 crossovers between homologous chromosome pairs per meiosis.[14] In genetic parlance, crossing over is referred to as recombination.

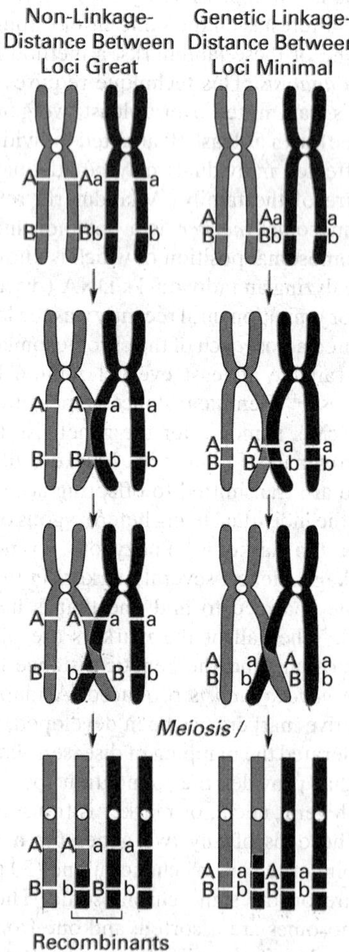

FIGURE 62-3 Comparison of nonlinked genes (*left*) and linked genes (*right*). In nonlinkage, the distance between loci is large, allowing crossing over to occur and resulting in recombinants after meiosis. The distance between linked genes is comparatively small, thereby minimizing the chance for recombinants.

Concept of Genetic Linkage Analysis

Despite the independent assortment of chromosomes and genes, the genes (alleles) on two or more loci are often coinherited because they are so close together that the chance of a chiasmatic bridge forming between them is less likely. Thus, breakage and recombination of the chromosomes does not occur and they tend to be coinherited more often than by chance alone; by definition this means the two loci are in genetic linkage. Any two loci coinherited more than 50 percent of the time are said to be genetically linked.[15] To map the chromosomal locus responsible for a disease-related gene, one selects DNA markers that are evenly distributed across the chromosomes. DNA is collected from all the members of a family (normal and affected) and analyzed for these markers. If one or more DNA markers is coinherited in more than 50 percent of the affected individuals, the locus where the marker resides is on the same chromosome and in close physical proximity to the locus of the gene responsible for the disease. This is referred to as *genetic linkage* between the disease (gene) and the marker. Once a disease is linked to a marker of known chromosomal locus, it follows that the disease locus is on the same chromosome and in close proximity. The concept of linkage analysis is illustrated in Fig. 62-3. Shown in the panel at the right is an illustration of genetic linkage between a locus for a DNA marker and that of a disease that is inherited in a mendelian dominant fashion. The locus, designated with an "A," carries the allele responsible for the disease. The corresponding locus, "a," on the homologous chromosome has the allele that codes for the same protein but has not undergone a mutation and is thus the normal allele. The loci designated "B" and "b" represent alleles of a DNA marker of known location that has nothing to do with the disease. In the panel on the right, the disease and the marker loci are so close that they tend to be coinherited within the family, whereas in the panel on the left, the DNA marker of known location is so far from the locus carrying the disease allele it is not coinherited but separate by chance. The calculation necessary to prove definitively that genetic linkage exists between a marker and a disease-related locus is sophisticated and requires advanced computer programs. The odds for and against linkage are calculated, and linkage exists if the odds in favor of linkage are at least 1000:1. To avoid the cumbersome ratio (1000:1), the logarithm to base 10 is derived, which is 3 (i.e., 10^3), and is referred to as the LOD score (log of the odds). If the LOD score is -2 (i.e., 10^{-2} or 100:1 odds against linkage), it excludes linkage. The likelihood of two genes being separated by recombination increases in proportion to the distance between them. The distance between a marker and a disease-causing gene when genetically linked is quite variable and may be anywhere from 1000 kilobase pairs (kbp) to 50,000 kbp but is usually within 1000 to 10,000 kbp.[16] The inherent resolution of genetic linkage analysis is never better than 1000 kbp. It is possible on the basis of linkage analysis alone to construct a chromosomal map of all the markers, with the distance between the various markers estimated in centimorgans. This is a complex calculation derived from the number of recombinations between the markers during meioses. The recombination frequency between two markers, two genes, or a gene and a marker is the ratio of the number of crossover events to the total number of meioses. The lower the recombination frequency between the locus of a marker and that of a disease-related gene, the closer those two must be in physical distance on the chromosome. Even though the locus of the marker and that of the disease-related gene are in close enough proximity to be genetically linked, recombination may occur, and the extent to which recombination does occur reflects roughly the physical distance between the two loci. The recombination fraction (or *theta*) is used to develop a means of estimating the genetic distance (in centimorgans) between genetically linked loci. A recombination frequency or crossover of 1 percent between two loci, whether occupied by two genes or one gene and a marker, reflects a physical distance between them of approximately 1 million bp (1 cM).[16] For a marker and a gene separated by 1 cM, this means the chance of a crossover between them during meiosis is only 1 percent; thus, the chance of being coinherited is 99 percent. This is a statistically derived genetic map, however, and the distances are only approximate. The correlation between the percent crossover and the physical distance in base pairs varies somewhat from chromosome to chromosome and from region to region even on the same chromosome. For example, recombination is more frequent in the telomeric than in the centromeric portion of the chromosome and is also more frequent in females. If the marker locus and the disease-related locus are close, such as 5 to 10 cM, then a single crossover may be uncommon and a double crossover rare. Two loci may be 20 to 40 cM apart, however, and a double crossover occurs, which recombines the locus with the original chromosome and leads to coinheritance of the two (linkage of the two loci). When this occurs, the genetic distance is misleading and represents a gross underestimation of the true physical distance between the two loci.

Chromosomal Markers and Their Identification

A chromosomal marker (as defined above) is any DNA sequence of known chromosomal location that is polymorphic for the population (two or more alleles). The greater the number of alleles, the more informative the marker. When compared between individuals in the population, the DNA of the human genome shows a difference in the nucleotide sequence (polymorphism) every 300 to 500 bp. Polymorphisms occur more frequently in the sequence of the unexpressed DNA (intron) than in DNA coding for proteins (exon). Until recently, the most common chromosomal marker was that of restriction fragment length polymorphism (RFLP)[17] identified by Southern blotting. These markers have been replaced by what are referred to as short tandem repeat polymorphisms (STRP),[18] which occur more frequently, are more informative, and are more conveniently and rapidly detected than are RFLPs[19] (Fig. 62-4). Distributed throughout the human genome are repeats of dinucleotides, trinucleotides, or tetranucleotides that are repeated in tandem (microsatellites) and may vary anywhere from 60 to 300 repeats. The number of tandem repeats of STRPs, which provide for marked polymorphism, occur about every 500 bp throughout the human genome. The dinucleotide repeats of cytosine-adenosine are more common than trinucleotide or tetranucleotide repeats. A major advantage of STRPs is rapid and convenient detection by PCR rather than requiring Southern blotting, as is necessary for RFLPs. PCR requires only a nanogram of DNA as opposed to a milligram for RFLPs, and results are available in only 1 to 24 h as opposed to 9 to 10 days for Southern blotting. The resolution of STRPs detected by PCR is much better than by Southern blotting and, since STRPs have multiple alleles (as opposed to RFLPs, which have only two alleles), they are much more informative for genetic linkage. A more recent marker is that of single nucleotide polymorphism, which may represent the markers of the future.[17–19]

Identification of the Gene

Once the chromosomal location of a gene has been mapped, the first technique in attempting to identify the gene is referred to as the *candidate gene approach.* Over 5000 loci have now been mapped for human genes and over 1000 genes recorded in a gene bank. In addition, there are over 50,000 expressed sequenced tags (ESTs) mapped. The ESTs are unique DNA sequences of 100 to 200 bp, each of which is believed to represent a unique gene.[20] These genes and ESTs are entered through a worldwide network of databases[21] in the United States, Europe, and Japan that is updated on a daily basis. Once a locus is identified on a chromosome, genes previously known to be localized to that region become candidate genes for the newly mapped locus. These genes are amplified, usually by PCR, to determine if there is a mutation that segregates with the disease. If none of the candidate genes in the region is shown to have a mutation that cosegregates with the disease, it may be necessary to clone the region. This approach is referred to as *posi-*

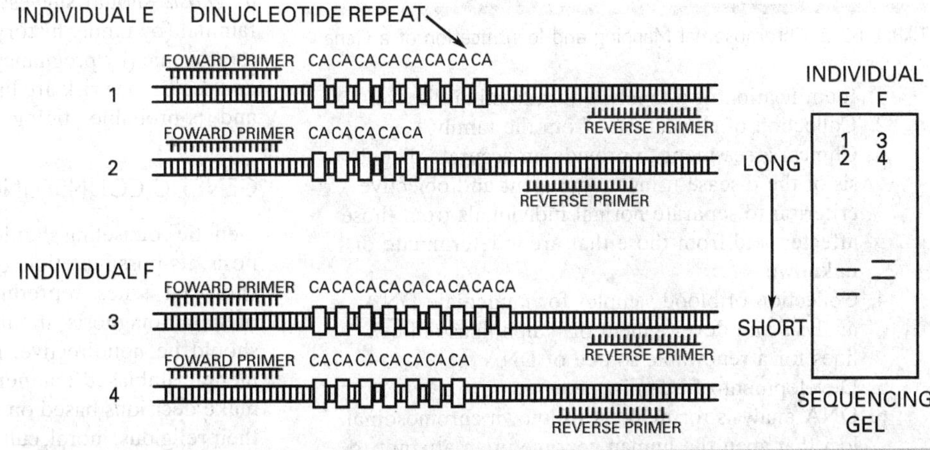

FIGURE 62-4 Sequence-based polymorphisms. This type of polymorphism is based on sequence variations caused by variable numbers of repeat sequence within a population. In this case, variable numbers of CA dinucleotide repeats are shown at one locus. These polymorphisms can be detected by use of specific oligonucleotide primers and the polymerase chain reaction (PCR). The resultant PCR products will vary in size and can be detected by polyacrylamide gel electrophoresis. These sequence-based PCR polymorphisms may be highly polymorphic, thus providing increased statistical strength to linkage analysis over two-allele polymorphisms seen in Southern blot restriction fragment length polymorphisms (RFLPs). (Reprinted with permission from Keating M. Linkage analysis and long QT syndrome. Using genetics to study cardiovascular disease. *Circulation* 1992; 85:1973–1986.)

tional cloning, so named because a region is cloned knowing only its position relative to the genetically linked marker. Positional cloning is usually not attempted unless the region (containing the gene) between the flanking markers is 1 cM or less. To reduce the region for cloning, it is necessary to expand the family with the hope of finding crossovers such that markers common to all affected would span only a short distance (<1 cM). This collection of markers in a region would represent the haplotype being inherited by the affected individual and contains the responsible gene. To prove that the gene causes the disease, the mutation must be identified and shown to co-segregate with the disease and not with the unaffected members in the family. The remaining task would be to determine the gene product (protein) and the pathophysiology of how the mutation induces the disease. In attempting to decipher the pathophysiology, one may transfect cells in culture with normal and mutant forms of the gene and compare the resulting phenotype. The other definitive approaches for determining causality are to overexpress the gene as a transgene in animals such as mice or to do homologous knockout, replacing the normal with the mutant gene to determine whether the disease phenotype is induced as have been done for familial hypertrophic cardiomyopathy (FHCM).[22–24] Chromosomal mapping of hereditary diseases by linkage analysis and subsequent isolation of the gene[25] are summarized in Table 62-3.

Family History and Evaluation

The most important part of an evaluation for genetic disease is the family history. First, the family history may give clues to the diagnosis of a particular disorder, information about possible inheritance patterns within an individual family, and information about conditions for which family members may be at an increased risk. An individual's ethnic background may, for instance, suggest the need for specific types of genetic screening such as for hemoglobinopathies in individuals of African or Mediterranean ancestry or for Tay-Sachs disease in individuals of eastern European (Ashkenazi) Jewish ancestry. The individual with the medical problem who brought the family to the attention of the physician is referred to as the *proband,* or *propositus* (proposita for females). Information generally should be collected on all individuals who are first-, second-, or third-degree relatives of the proband. First-degree relatives of the proband are the parents and children. Second-degree relatives are aunts and uncles, grandparents, and grandchildren of the proband. Third-degree relatives are first cousins, great aunts and uncles, great-grandparents, and great-grandchildren. A pedigree chart (as shown in Fig. 62-1) is useful in this task. This information should include medical problems and pregnancies. If relatives are deceased, the age at death and the cause of death should be recorded. With a pedigree chart and specific family information, more general questions are asked, including whether other family members have the same or similar problems. Information about various types of birth defects, mental retardation, early infant deaths, miscarriages, stillbirths, or other diseases or handicaps in the family is sought. With some disorders, there may be a variability of a particular condition (i.e., clinical heterogeneity), even within a family. For example, with a possible diagnosis of FHCM, one should ask about premature death or syncope. A pregnancy history may provide information to support a possible teratogenic exposure. The date of the last menstrual period, whether the pregnancy was planned, whether contraception was used immediately prior to pregnancy, the time when the pregnancy was recognized, and when the mother sought prenatal care should be noted. Problems during the pregnancy, such as bleeding, spotting, cramping, fevers, rashes, or illnesses; drug exposures (both prescribed and nonprescribed), alcohol intake, or "recreational" drug use; and exposures to potent chemicals in the workplace or while involved in various hobbies should be explored. Pregnancy and family histories can then be used in conjunction with the findings on physical examination to derive a potential etiologic diagnosis and to plan for further diagnostic studies. The term *etiologic diagnosis* should suggest whether a specific cardiac defect is familial (by family history), genetic but not familial (sporadic), teratogenic (by pregnancy history), or multifactorial. Prognosis and recurrence risk are linked strongly to an accurate diagnosis and its probable etiology.

TABLE 62-3 Chromosomal Mapping and Identification of a Gene

1. Identification of a family with a familial disease
2. Collection of clinical data from the family
3. Clinical assessment to provide an accurate diagnosis of the disease using a consistent and objective criterion to separate normal individuals from those affected and from those that are indeterminate or unknown
4. Collection of blood samples for immediate DNA analysis and development of lymphoblastoid cell lines for a renewable source of DNA
5. Development of a family pedigree
6. DNA analysis for markers of known chromosomal loci that span the human genome in an attempt to find a marker locus linked to the disease
7. Identification of the gene
8. Identification of mutation(s) causing the disease
9. Demonstration of a causal relationship between the mutant gene and the disease
10. Development of a convenient test to screen for the mutations

GENETIC COUNSELING PRINCIPLES

Genetic counseling should provide information about the diagnosis, its possible etiology, and its prognosis. In addition, psychosocial issues, reproductive options, and the availability of prenatal diagnosis should be discussed. Genetic counseling should be nondirective, providing information in a nonjudgmental, unbiased manner. The family should then be able to make decisions based on medical information in the context of their religious, moral, cultural, and social backgrounds and their financial situation. Although a genetic counselor may occasionally feel frustrated with a specific couple's decision, an effective counselor does not let personal biases interfere with the counseling role. Conflicts leading to major ethical issues and disputes may arise, however, and may be particularly apparent regarding issues of nonpaternity, sex selection, pregnancy termination, and selective nontreatment of malformed infants. Couples have many reproductive options, but not all may be acceptable religiously or culturally. Nevertheless, potential options should be mentioned in a sensitive manner. A common misunderstanding among families in genetic counseling is the issue of prenatal diagnosis and its relationship to abortion. Prenatal diagnosis does not imply that a parent should or would terminate the pregnancy. In many circumstances, the information from prenatal diagnosis may help to reassure a couple that their risk of having another handicapped child is in fact much lower than expected. Conversely, if defects are found, the subspecialist may use more diagnostic approaches to make rational decisions about medical management of the infant prior to or immediately after delivery.

Genetic Diagnosis and Health Insurance

The accelerated pace of gene discovery, molecular medicine, and molecular diagnostics has begun to allow for improved genetic counseling and portends the possibility of future genetic therapy. As knowledge about the genetic basis of disease grows, however, so does the potential for health insurance coverage discrimination to be used to exclude individuals at risk or to change prohibitively high rates on the basis of predetermined illness. For this reason, planners of the Human Genome Project recognized the need to protect individuals who volunteered for genetic study as well as those diagnosed by molecular methods in the future. Also for this reason, the National Institutes of Health–Department of Energy (NIH-DOE) Working Group on Ethical, Legal, and Social Implications (ELSI) of the Human Genome Project was developed. The Congress has passed a bill prohibiting companies from using DNA analysis to assess genetic risk as a basis for hiring. Only 11 states, however, prohibit the use of DNA analysis to determine who should get medical insurance or whether they qualify for high- or low-risk premiums.[7]

CARDIOVASCULAR DISEASE DUE TO SINGLE-GENE MUTATIONS

Compensatory Response of the Heart Is Limited to Hypertrophy, Dilatation, or a Combination

The heart responds to stimuli, physiologic or pathologic, which may be inherited or acquired, with hypertrophy, dilation, or a combination of the two.[26] The same mechanisms mediate the growth response to pressure overload, volume overload, or loss of contractile mass (myocardial infarction). In FHCM, hypertrophy occurs without altered workload. In familial dilated cardiomyopathy (DCM), the heart responds predominantly by dilatation, generally in association with diffuse loss of myocytes and fibrosis. Most inherited defects are associated with hypertrophy. Several mutations in the mitochondrial genome have been associated with cardiac hypertrophy or dilatation.[27,28] In mitochondrial DNA mutations, HCM or DCM is usually part of a general phenotypic expression of a systemic disease that is characterized by metabolic disorders and involving the central nervous and the skeletal muscle systems. Three clinical categories of primary cardiomyopathies exist: (1) hypertrophic, (2) dilated, and (3) restrictive forms. Most of the cardiomyopathies other than those caused by infection have a genetic basis, although many of the mutations may occur de novo and are not necessarily familial. Only when a genetic defect is present in the germline and transmitted to one or more generations is it familial. For a detailed discussion of the clinical features, diagnosis, and treatment of the cardiomyopathies refer to Chaps. 64 to 69.

Familial Hypertrophic Cardiomyopathy (FHCM)

GENETIC BASIS

Familial HCM is an autosomal dominant disorder characterized by myocardial hypertrophy with a wide spectrum of symptoms, including dyspnea, chest pain, and syncope. The annual mortality rate of 2 to 4 percent is primarily due to sudden death, which often occurs in asymptomatic individuals (see Chap. 67). This disorder is the leading cause of sudden death in the young and in athletes. The annual incidence of sudden death is higher in younger patients with FHCM (about 6 percent) than in the elderly (1 percent). The diagnosis is based on typical clinical features and the demonstration of unexplained left ventricular, right ventricular, or biventricular hypertrophy on two-dimensional echocardiography. The left ventricular hypertrophy is commonly asymmetrical, localized to the septum, but it may involve the entire ventricle in a concentric pattern. Isolated right ventricular hypertrophy occurs in fewer than 5 percent. Isolated apical hypertrophy is rare except in Japan, where it is claimed to account for 20 to 30 percent of the cases. Dynamic outflow tract obstruction occurs in about 30 percent.[29,30] Histologically, the myocardial hypertrophy consists of myocyte hypertrophy, cellular and myofibrillar disarray, and myocardial fibrosis. The literature suggests that the hallmark of FHCM is myocyte and myofibrillar disarray (see Chap. 66). The disorder exhibits marked variability of expressivity, even in the same family. FHCM was the first primary cardiomyopathy to yield to molecular genetics. Jarcho et al. in 1989 showed genetic linkage of the disease to the chromosomal locus of 14q1 in a large French/Canadian family.[31] The 14q1 locus subsequently was shown to be involved in FHCM in several families throughout North America.[32] The β-myosin heavy chain (βMHC) gene was identified as the responsible gene (Fig. 62-5), and over 50 mutations have been detected.[11,33,34] A total of eight genes have now been identified responsible for FHCM and a brief description of the loci and the proteins they encode, together with their function, is summarized in Table 62-4. Mutations in the βMHC gene may account for 30 to 50 percent of the families with FHCM.[33] While it remains to be determined for certain, these eight genes probably account for 80 to 90 percent of the disease of FHCM. Two other loci have been identified, one in a family with HCM and Wolff-Parkinson-White (WPW) syndrome mapped to 7q3[35] and the other to chromosome 11q in a Japanese family.[36] Since all of the genes identified to date involve the sarcomere, it has been proposed that FHCM is a disease of the sarcomere and perhaps should be referred to as *sarcomeropathy*.[34]

The βMHC is the most common gene for FHCM and over 50 mutations have been described. Almost all of the mutations are point mutations (a single base nucleotide) that result in substitution of one amino acid for another and are located in the globular head of the myosin molecule. These mutations appear to arise independently.[37] The frequency of each particular mutation is low. Two hot spots, codons 403 and 719, have been identified for mutations in the βMHC in patients with

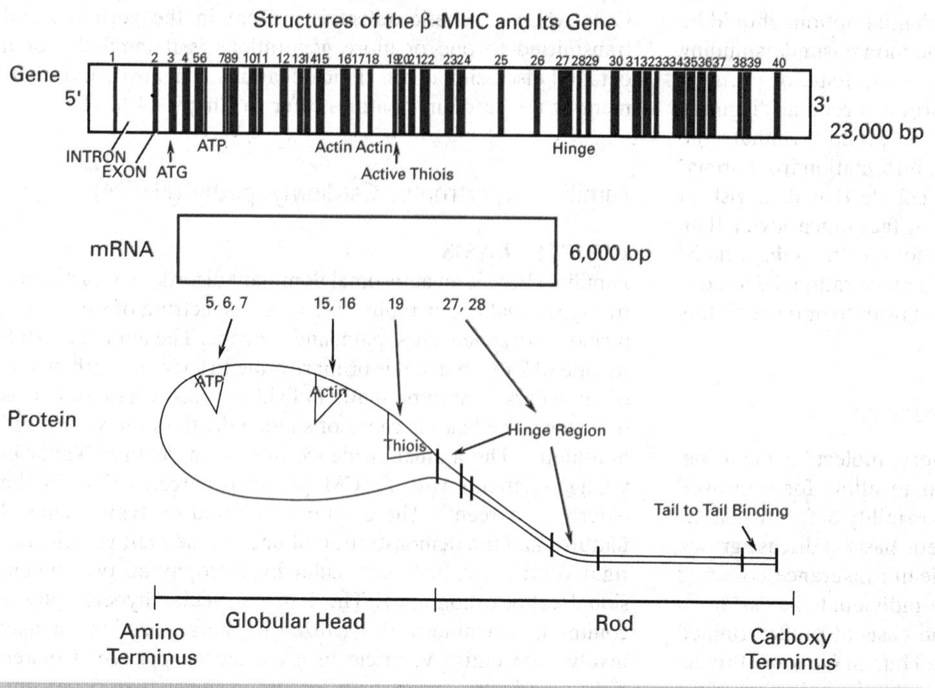

FIGURE 62-5 Structure of β-myosin heavy chain (β-MHC) and its gene.

with a high incidence of sudden death, yet there is often minimal hypertrophy.[44] The occurrence of palpitations, arrhythmias, or syncope are poor predictors of sudden death. A family history of sudden death usually indicates that the affected individuals in the family are at risk for sudden death. Several studies have now been performed correlating the genotype to the phenotype and several interesting observations have evolved pertinent to the diagnosis and treatment and future genetic screening. Results of these studies[45] have shown that the majority of families with the βMHC mutations Arg^{403}Gln, Arg^{453}Cys, and Arg^{719}Trp are associated with a poor prognosis and a high incidence of sudden cardiac death[34,42,43,46] (Fig. 62-6). In contrast, the βMHC mutations Leu^{908}-Val, Gly^{256}Glu, and Val^{606}Met are associated with near-normal life

HCM.[38,39] Mutations in the rod region of the βMHC molecule have also been described but are uncommon and appear to induce a mild phenotype.[40]

PROGNOSIS FROM GENOTYPE-PHENOTYPE CORRELATIONS

The hypertrophy of FHCM is markedly variable in its degree, distribution, and age at onset as well as in the type and severity of its associated clinical manifestations.[41–43] The natural course of FHCM in certain families is riddled with sudden cardiac death, whereas in others, sudden cardiac death is almost absent and the life span is essentially normal.[34] None of the clinical features are reliable predictors of sudden death. Hypertrophy, while present in all individuals, since it is required for the clinical diagnosis, does not correlate with the incidence of sudden death. FHCM due to mutations in the troponin T gene is associated

expectancy, and mutations Glu^{930}Lys and Arg^{249}Gln are associated with an intermediate risk of sudden cardiac death.[47] The incidence of premature death in affected individuals with Arg^{403}Gln is approximately 50 percent,[34] and the mean age of sudden cardiac death is 33 years. The life expectancy of affected individuals with the βMHC mutation Arg^{719}Gln appears to be about 38 years and in those with Arg^{453}Cys about 30 years. In contrast, the mutation Leu^{908}Val is associated with low penetrance, a benign course, and a low incidence of sudden cardiac death.[46] The cumulative survival rate at 60 years of age was 92 percent with this mutation. Similarly, the Gly^{256}Glu and Val^{606}-Met mutations are associated with a relatively benign course, with most individuals having a near-normal life span. In contrast, the two mutations Glu^{930}Lys and Arg^{249}Gln[46,47] show an intermediary prognosis, with an average age of onset of cardiac failure and severe symptoms around 49 years. These correla-

TABLE 62-4 Hypertrophic Cardiomyopathy (HCM) Genes, mRNA, and Proteins

Gene	Chromosomal Locus	Frequency	Number of Mutations	Function and Location
β-MyHC	14q1	35–50%	>50	Contractile molecule that forms a thick filament of the sarcomere
MyBP-C	11q11	15–20%	>15	Binds to myosin and titin
Cardiac troponin T (cTnT)	1q3	15–20%	>20	Regulation of contraction via calcium binding
α-Tropomyosin	15q2	<5%	3	Binds the troponin complex to actin
Cardiac troponin 1	19q13	<1%	3	Inhibits contractility
MLC-1	3p	<1%	2	Unknown
MLC-2	12q	<1%	2	Unknown
α-Cardiac actin	15q11	?	2	Forms the actin thin filament of the sarcomere
Unknown	7q3	?	?	Unknown
Unknown	11q	?	?	Unknown

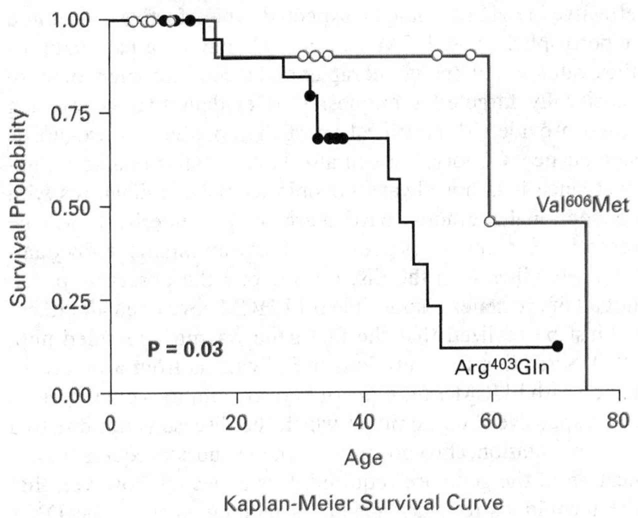

FIGURE 62-6 Kaplan-Meier survival curve in patients with hypertrophic cardiomyopathy depending on myosin heavy chain mutation.

tions must be interpreted with caution, however, as the number of families studied remains too small for definitive generalizations to be made. Although most individuals affected with FHCM due to the βMHC mutation manifest the disease in the second or third decade of life, those with FHCM due to myosin-binding protein C mutations frequently do not develop any evidence of the disease until the fourth or fifth decade.[48] This is a striking example of age-dependent penetrance based on 16 families involving over 500 individuals. However, once the disease develops, the particular mutation is highly predictive of risk for sudden death. Mutations in the essential light chain (3p) and the regulatory light chain of myosin (12q23-q24.3) of patients is associated with a peculiar form of HCM in which mid–left ventricular chamber thickening occurs due to massive hypertrophy of the papillary muscles and adjacent ventricular tissue, resulting in mid-cavitary obstruction.[49] In addition to the cardiac abnormalities described, the skeletal muscles of these patients were histologically abnormal and appeared as ragged-red fibers.

INFLUENCE OF OTHER GENES AND THE ENVIRONMENT

While a single-gene mutation appears to be the primary cause of the disease, there remain significant environmental and other genetic influences that determine whether or not the phenotype develops (penetrance) and its expressivity. A striking example of the influence of environment on FHCM is the observation that hypertrophy seldom develops in the right ventricle, yet the defective genes and their mutations are present to the same extent in the right as in the left ventricles.[34] Presumably, the increased workload and pressure in the left ventricle stimulate the development of the hypertrophy and phenotypic expression. There also appears to be more hypertrophy in males than females who have FHCM. βMHC is the major myosin and contractile unit of many skeletal muscles, yet the latter do not appear to be affected by this disease, again emphasizing the influence of either the environment or other genes.[50] Another example of presumably environmental or other genetic influences is the marked variability of the extent and degree of left ventricular hypertrophy that occurs even within the same family with the same mutation. In addition, there is a significant effect from other genes that predispose to features such as hypertrophy. An example of the influence of another gene on FHCM is afforded by the angiotensin converting enzyme (ACE) DD genotype. Patients with FHCM who also have the ACE DD genotype have a much higher incidence of sudden death[51] and more extensive hypertrophy,[52] which may be mediated through the mitogenic effect of angiotensin II. Individuals with FHCM who participate in combative reports seem to be more prone to develop hypertrophy and sudden death.[53] A similar effect is observed if they have a variance of the endothelin I gene.[54] It is not surprising that the phenotype of cardiac hypertrophy requires the coordination of probably hundreds of genes, and thus it is highly likely that other genes in addition to ACE will exert a minimal, yet significant influence on either the penetrance or expressivity of the primary genetic defect.

ELUCIDATION OF THE PATHOGENESIS FROM GENETIC MODELS

Based on in vitro and in vivo studies in genetic animal models of HCM, it now appears that the primary defect is impaired contractility. Analysis of a human heart from a patient with the Arg^{403}Gln mutation showed the ratio of myosin to actin was normal,[55] indicating there is no deficiency of the βMHC protein. All of the responsible mutant genes encode for a sarcomeric protein and appear in some way to impair systolic contraction or diastolic relaxation. In feline adult cardiac myocytes, in which βMHC is the predominant myosin form, expression of human mutant βMHC gene, Arg^{403}Gln, was associated with sarcomere disassembly.[56] Expression of the human mutant troponin T in this model also induced sarcomere disassembly and was associated with impaired rate of cell shortening as detected by laser.[24] Furthermore, it was shown the expressed mutant protein was incorporated into the sarcomere. In a transgenic mouse, expression of troponin T gene (cTnT-Gln^{92})[57] exhibited sarcomere disarray, increased fibrous tissue, and sudden death, but only minimal hypertrophy. In this model it was also shown that increased expression of the mutant protein was associated with a more severe phenotype, confirming the mutant protein has a dominant-negative effect as expected. These results have been confirmed by several investigators.[56,58-60] Expression of the mutant myosin heavy chain gene or the troponin gene in the mouse has, in general, been associated with less hypertrophy than expected.[57] Recently, a transgenic rabbit model (rabbit has βMHC as its cardiac myosin) has been developed expressing the βMHC (Arg^{403}Gln) mutation, which exhibits sarcomere disarray, hypertrophy, and increased fibrous tissue virtually identical to that observed in humans.[61] Thus, the overall postulated pathogenesis of FHCM may be summarized briefly as follows: The mutant protein is incorporated into the sarcomere and acts as a poison peptide which impairs contractility of that particular cell which, in turn, provides the stimulus for the mitogenic response (probably several growth factors) of compensatory hypertrophy. The growth stimulus, as in acquired disorders, appears highly localized and mediated by autocrine or intracrine factors, given that the hypertrophy is localized in many patients, primarily to the interventricular septum. The growth factors also stimulate fibroblast proliferation and increased matrix formation. The relationship between the hypertrophy and increased fibrous tissue response to sudden death and arrhythmias remains to be determined. It is postulated that the fibrous tissue leads to delayed electrical conduction and predisposes to arrhythmias and sudden death.[62,63] The future elucidation of the molecular basis for the pathogenesis of this disease, however, must provide a rationale for three puzzling, consistent features of the pathology of FHCM: (1) predominance of hypertrophy in the septum, (2) sarcomere and myocyte disarray, and (3) the supernormal systolic function. The diastolic stiffness or decreased compliance is expected with hypertrophy, whether it is primary or compensatory, but these other features are not seen in compensatory hypertrophy associated with myocardial infarction or pressure overload.

IMPLICATIONS FOR FUTURE THERAPIES

Based on clinical studies and experimental genetic models, certain important observations have evolved. FHCM is seldom manifested before puberty and when due to certain genes may not be manifested until the fourth or fifth decade. This provides a window for future therapeutic intervention as therapies become available. The observation that the DD genotype increases the extent of hypertrophy and the risk for sudden death in individuals with FHCM is of considerable therapeutic interest.[51] ACE inhibitors have been shown to either induce regression or prevent progression of hypertrophy due to pressure overload, in part due to a direct effect on the growth response. Therefore, it would be intriguing to know whether or not ACE inhibitors induce regression of hypertrophy in patients with FHCM and, perhaps more importantly, prevent hypertrophy in children genetically affected who are identified by genetic testing prior to the development of hypertrophy. There is no evidence to recommend such therapy for FHCM at this time. Elucidation that the hypertrophy is secondary and similar to the hypertrophy developed in response to pressure overload also has important implications; hence, therapies shown to be effective in FHCM would be expected to be effective in acquired hypertrophy. Thus, HCM, as a model, may be a paradigm for the evaluation of known therapies and the development of more specifically targeted therapies. It is evident that genotyping could provide risk stratification of therapeutic and prognostic significance. Genotyping will also have a major diagnostic impact since it is not always possible to make a diagnosis with conventional methods, particularly in the elderly. It will be essential for genetic screening of asymptomatic individuals within families with the disease. Despite the observation that not all of the genes responsible for FHCM have been identified, it must be realized that the first gene was not identified until 1990. Screening for mutations in individuals from a family affected with FHCM is feasible for known mutations but is tedious and expensive. In a family in which the disease is not due to a known mutation, chromosomal mapping and subsequent identification of the gene are required. It is expected, however, that the techniques for mass genetic screening, such as the DNA chip array, will make it possible to do routine genetic screening.[64] Ultimately, if gene therapy becomes available, genotyping will, of course, be essential. It is conceivable that regression of cardiac hypertrophy can be induced by inhibiting transcription of the mutant allele or translation of the mutant mRNA, thus abolishing synthesis of the mutant peptide. Thus, not only genetic diagnosis but also curative therapy may be possible. Since the heart, even in an adult, is renewed every 2 to 3 weeks, there is a tremendous potential for a cure with subsequent remodeling to normal.

Pompe's Disease (Type II Glycogen Storage Disease)

Genetic deficiency of acid α-1,4-glucosidase production results in a wide clinical spectrum ranging from the rapidly fatal infantile-onset of type II glycogen storage disease (GSD) to a slowly progressive adult-onset myopathy. The infantile-onset form (Pompe disease) typically manifests during the first months of life and patients usually die before their second year.[65] This rare inborn error of glycogen metabolism occurs in less than 1 per 100,000 persons. Massive glycogen accumulation occurs, leading to the clinical findings of enlarged tongue, striking hepatomegaly, hypotonia with decreased deep tendon reflexes, and hypertrophic cardiomyopathy[65] with cardiac failure (Table 62-5). The diagnosis may be predicted from the electrocardiogram (ECG), which demonstrates striking QRS complex voltage.[65] The diagnosis can also be made by analysis of α-glucosidase in blood lymphocytes or skin fibroblasts. Recently, urinary oligosaccharide identification using matrix-assisted laser desorption ionization time-of-flight mass spectrometry

TABLE 62-5 Cardiovascular Anomalies Associated with Selected Autosomal Recessive Syndromes

Syndrome	Cardiovascular Anomaly
Carpenter's syndrome	Patent ductus arteriosus
Cockayne's syndrome	Atherosclerosis
Cutis laxa	Pulmonary hypertension
Cystic fibrosis	Cor pulmonale
Ellis–van Creveld syndrome	Atrial septal defect
Friedreich's ataxia	Hypertrophic cardiomyopathy
Homocystinuria	Thromboses
MPS IH (Hurler's syndrome)	Coronary artery disease, aortic and mitral insufficiency, hypertrophic cardiomyopathy
MPS IS (Scheie's syndrome)	Aortic valve disease
MPS IV (Morquio's syndrome)	Aortic valve disease
MPS VI (Maroteaux-Lamy syndrome)	Aortic valve disease
Pompe's disease (GSD II)	Hypertrophic cardiomyopathy
Pseudoxanthoma elasticum	Coronary artery disease, mitral insufficiency
Refsum disease	Arrhythmias
Smith-Lemli-Opitz syndrome	Ventricular septal defect, patent ductus arteriosus
Thrombocytopenia–absent radii (TAR) syndrome	Atrial septal defect, tetralogy of Fallot

has been shown to allow facile and sensitive identification of the pathognomonic oligosacchariduria of this disorder.[66] The disease has autosomal recessive inheritance and is caused by mutations in this lysosomal gene found on chromosome 17q23-q25. Recently, the lysosomal-associated membrane protein (LAMP-1) was shown to be elevated in Pompe disease, which occurs due to altered trafficking and turnover of LAMP-1.[67]

In an attempt to better understand this metabolic disorder, animal models have been developed using targeted disruption of the murine acid α-glucosidase gene.[68,69] This model closely mimics the human disorder, particularly the cardiac phenotype. Also, using animal models such as quail and rat, gene therapy using recombinant α-glucosidase has been shown to correct the enzyme levels and clinical phenotype, suggesting that enzyme replacement by this method is promising therapy in humans.[70–72]

Beckwith-Wiedemann Syndrome (BWS)

The combination of macroglossia, exophthalmos, and visceromegaly has been designated the BWS.[73,74] Multiple other abnormalities have also been described, including fetal adrenocortical cytomegaly, hypoglycemia due to pancreatic islet hyperplasia, transverse linear creases of the ear lobules, hemihypertrophy, and accelerated osseous maturation. Infants with this syndrome are at particularly high risk, cumulatively estimated at between 5 and 20 percent, for development of Wilms' tumor, adrenocortical carcinomas, hepatoblastomas, and rhabdomyosarcomas.[75] The cardiovascular system is also commonly affected with the development of HCM. The BWS occurs with an incidence of 1 in 13,700 live births. Cases (about 85 percent) are generally sporadic, but familial disease (15 percent) has been described. Most of these familial cases have apparent autosomal dominant inheritance,[76] albeit with reduced, sex-dependent penetrance and variable expressivity. A variety of structural abnormalities of chromosome 11 have been shown, including partial duplication of 11p13, duplication of 11p15 only, deletion of 11p11-13, or deletion of 11p11. The extra chromosomal material is usually of paternal origin. The breakpoints found in BWS patients with balanced chromosomal translocation or inversion involving chromosome 11 lie in two regions: (1) close to the insulin/insulin-like growth factor II (INS/IGF2) genes in 11p15.5 or (2) proximal to β-hemoglobin (HBB). The recombinant chromosome was shown to be of maternal origin. Family studies showed that the gene responsible for familial BWS mapped to 11p15.5. For sporadic BWS, uniparental paternal disomy for 11p15.5 markers was found in approximately 20 percent of cases analyzed. Mutations in p57KIP2, a potent tight-binding of several G1 cyclin/cyclin-dependent kinase complexes, have been identified in cases of BWS,[77–80] and mice lacking this gene have been shown to have a phenotype similar to that seen in humans.[81] Clinical heterogeneity exists, however; potential mechanisms include a possible role for genomic imprinting (i.e., an epigenetic chromosomal modification in the gamete or zygote causing preferential expression of a specific parental allele in the somatic cells of the offspring) in 11p15, and this was later shown to occur with KVLQT1, a cardiac potassium channel gene known to cause long-QT syndrome when mutated.[82,83] This region of 11p15.5 has a cluster of imprinted genes, in fact, such as insulin-like growth factor II (IGF2),[84] HI9,[85] LIT1,[86] and p57KIP2.[77–80] Animal models have been created using these as transgenes.[84]

Leopard Syndrome

This rare autosomal dominant disorder is characterized by the cardinal features leading to the pneumonic L (lentigenes), E (ECG conduction defects), O (ocular hypertelorism), P (pulmonic valve stenosis), A (abnormalities of genitals), R (retardation of growth), and D (deafness, sensorineural). Cardiac abnormalities are common and include both anatomic as well as conduction defects. Anatomically, PS is the most frequent, followed by HCM and endocardial fibroelastosis (Table 62-6). The most common ECG defects include first-degree AV block, left anterior hemiblock, and complete heart block. No cytogenetic or molecular genetic abnormalities have been identified.

Friedreich's Ataxia (FA)

FA is the most common of the hereditary spinal cerebellar degenerations, with an incidence of 1 in 50,000 and carrier frequency of 1 in 110.[87] This autosomal recessive form of spinocerebellar degeneration is characterized by progressive limb ataxia, loss of deep tendon reflexes, sensory abnormalities, and musculoskeletal deformities. The symptoms of FA usually appear insidiously during childhood or early adolescence. Progres-

TABLE 62-6 Cardiovascular Anomalies Associated with Selected Autosomal Dominant Syndromes

Syndrome	Cardiovascular Anomaly
Albright's hereditary osteodystrophy	Cardiomyopathy
Ehlers-Danlos syndrome	Rupture of large vessels
Holt-Oram syndrome	Atrial and ventricular septal defects
Leopard syndrome	Pulmonic stenosis, hypertrophic cardiomyopathy, prolonged PR interval
Marfan syndrome	Aortic aneurysm, aortic insufficiency, mitral valve prolapse
Myotonic dystrophy	Dilated cardiomyopathy, conduction abnormalities
Neurofibromatosis	Coarctation of the aorta, renal artery Stenosis
Treacher Collins syndrome	Atrial and ventricular septal defects, patent ductus arteriosus
Tuberous sclerosis	Myocardial rhabdomyoma, Wolff-Parkinson-White syndrome
Noonan's syndrome	Pulmonic stenosis, hypertrophic cardiomyopathy, atrial septal defect, aortic stenosis

sive weakness of the upper and lower extremities gradually becomes obvious. Gait difficulties are often the first symptom; they progress slowly, followed by unsteadiness in the arms and hands. Difficulty in writing and handling eating utensils subsequently becomes apparent.

Cardiac involvement[87] occurs in 50 to 90 percent of patients. The most common abnormality is hypertrophic cardiomyopathy (Table 62-5); dilated cardiomyopathy occurs rarely. Thus, the most common cardiac symptoms relate to cardiac failure and arrhythmias. Left ventricular outflow tract obstruction due to asymmetrical septal hypertrophy may be evident, and approximately 50 percent of patients die of cardiac disease. Patients are followed for development of arrhythmias and the signs and symptoms of cardiac failure. Treatment consists primarily of conventional drugs to relieve the symptoms and signs of heart failure.

Involvement of the heart is readily detected by electrocardiography and echocardiography. The electrocardiographic abnormalities are found in 90 percent of patients and include repolarization abnormalities manifesting as inverted or biphasic T waves in the inferior limb leads and left precordial leads, a short PR interval, left and right ventricular hypertrophy, as well as left and right axis deviation. Premature atrial contractions, atrial flutter/fibrillation, and premature ventricular contractions are common. Echocardiography detects cardiac involvement in 60 to 100 percent of patients with the most common finding of concentric hypertrophy, but asymmetrical septal hypertrophy accompanied by systolic anterior motion (SAM) of the mitral valve is also common. Left ventricular chamber diameter may be normal or decreased and fractional shortening or ejection fraction is usually normal, although dilated cardiomyopathy (left ventricular dilation and reduced contractility) is seen occasionally (see Chap. 10). There is no specific treatment for the cardiac manifestations except symptomatic treatment if cardiac failure ensues (see Chap. 23).

Friedreich's ataxia is inherited as an autosomal recessive disorder, and parental consanguinity has been noted in some cases. The gene was initially mapped to chromosome 9q13-31.1,[88] and in 1996 the gene was identified.[89] This gene is 40 kb, contains five exons, has a 1.3-kb transcript, and encodes a 210–amino acid protein called frataxin. The highest level of expression is within the heart, while intermediate levels are seen in liver, skeletal muscle, and pancreas; minimal levels are identified in other tissues, including the brain. Although a few affected patients were found to have a point mutation of frataxin, the majority (about 95 percent) are homozygous for an unstable GAA trinucleotide expansion in the first intron.[89] The remainder of patients are compound heterozygotes for the expansion. In patients homozygous for the expansion, there is a correlation between the number of GAA repeats on the smaller allele, age of onset, disease progression, and cardiomyopathy,[87,90–93] confirming that the expansion is the primary cause of disease. The expansion results in severely reduced levels of mature frataxin mRNA.[89]

Campuzano et al.[94] demonstrated that frataxin is localized to the mitochondria associated with the mitochondrial membranes and crests using immunocytofluorescence and immunocytoelectron microscopic evaluation. They suggested that reduction in frataxin results in oxidative damage. Subsequently, Rotig and colleagues[95] suggested that frataxin regulates mitochondrial iron transport and that deficiency of iron-sulfur cluster-containing subunits of mitochondrial respiratory complexes I and II and the iron-sulfur protein aconitase occurs. Hence, it appears that Friedreich's ataxia is a mitochondrial disorder.[96,97] As these patients have HCM, diabetes, ataxia, and apparent free radical toxicity, the mitochondrial basis of this disorder clarifies the clinical features.

Dilated Cardiomyopathy

IDIOPATHIC DILATED CARDIOMYOPATHY

Idiopathic DCM (DCM) is a disease of unknown etiology characterized by increased ventricular chamber size, decreased wall thickness, and impaired systolic ventricular function. The prevalence of idiopathic DCM has been estimated to be approximately 40 cases per 100,000.[98] The diagnosis of DCM is typically made by echocardiography (see Chap. 65), and symptoms usually are those of sudden death and heart failure. Familial DCM (FDCM) is estimated to account for 30 percent of patients with idiopathic DCM. In a large family with idiopathic DCM, an autosomal dominant pattern was determined and the disease was linked to chromosome 1q32.[99] Three other chromosomal loci have been identified: 9q13,[100] 2q31,[101] and 10q21-23.[102] Three additional chromosomal loci have been mapped—to 1p1-1q1,[103] 3p22-25,[104] and 6q23[105]—in families having DCM in association with conduction defects and 6q23 also has limb girdle dystrophy. In the family mapped to 1p1-1q1, transient arrhythmias, which presented in the second or third decade, become sustained and commonplace by the third or fourth decade. The abnormal rhythms included second- or third-degree AV block, atrial fibrillation, or marked bradycardia, commonly requiring a pacemaker. DCM usually developed in the fourth or fifth decade, generally out of proportion to the severity of the rhythm disturbance. Sudden death commonly occurred in the late stages of the disease. On autopsy, marked right and left ventricular dilatation, interstitial fibrosis, myocyte degeneration characterized by cytoplasmic vacuolization, and AV nodal cell replacement by fibrous tissue were noted. The gene and its characteristics have recently been described as lamin A/C, the same gene identified for autosomal dominant Emery-Dreifuss muscular dystrophy. None of the other genes residing at these loci responsible for FDCM have yet been identified. However, two genes have now been identified responsible for FDCM—actin[106] and desmin.[107] Three missense mutations have been identified in actin. Actin, in addition to forming the thin filaments of the sarcomere, essential to the generation of force, is also an important cytoskeletal protein involved in structural integrity and the transmission of force. Mutations in actin responsible for FDCM are located in the domain which is immobilized and attached to the Z-band or intercalated disk and involved with transmitting force. In contrast, it was recently shown that mutations in the actin domain affecting the myosin cross bridges and the generation of force (sarcomere) give rise to FHCM.[108] Desmin is the specific intermediate filament for muscle and an essential cytoskeletal protein for maintaining cardiac structure and for the transmission of force and other signals to the cytoplasm and the nucleus of the cell. Desmin stretches from its attachment to the sarcomere Z-band to the nuclear membrane and other organelles.[109] Mutations in desmin have been shown to be associated with cardiac and skeletal abnormalities.[110] A missense mutation ($Ile^{451}Met$) was recently found to be responsible for DCM in a family without any skeletal or smooth muscle abnormalities. Mutations leading to combined skeletal and cardiac abnormalities have all been in the rod region of desmin. In contrast, the Ile[451]Met mutation responsible for the restricted cardiac phenotype of DCM encodes for the tail domain of human desmin, located in codon 451 with cytosine substituting for guanine. This would suggest a possible unique cardiac function for the domain in this region. Elimination of the desmin gene in a knockout mouse was associated with a phenotype of DCM exhibiting impaired cardiac function and myocyte necrosis.[110] It is of note that DCM associated with musculoskeletal disorders such as Duchenne muscular dystrophy are due to dystrophin, α-dystroglycan, and α-sarcoglycan, all of which are cytoskeletal proteins[111] (Fig. 62-7). There is thus the strong suggestion that familial DCM may be a disease of the cytoskeletal proteins[107,112–114] analogous to HCM being a disease of the sarcomere. This has been termed by Towbin as the "final common pathway hypothesis"[113,114] (Fig. 62-8).

X-LINKED DILATED CARDIOMYOPATHY (XLCM)

Berko and Swift[2] reported a five-generation kindred with DCM and no clinical evidence of skeletal myopathy. Males presented in their teens or early twenties with clinical evidence of mitral regurgitation and an echocardiographic diagnosis of DCM. Episodes of ventricular tachycardia were noted in several patients. The males progressed rapidly (within 1 or 2 years) to death or cardiac transplantation. Manifesting female carriers developed mild cardiomyopathy in the fourth or fifth decade and progressed slowly. Right ventricular endomyocardial biopsy revealed minimal interstitial fibrosis, while postmortem evaluation showed marked dilatation, widespread patchy fibrosis (worst in the posterior wall), and normal mitochondria on electron microscopy. There were no pathognomonic findings differentiating this cardiomyopathy from other dilated forms except for the apparent X-linked inheritance and elevation of the muscle isoform of creatine kinase (CK-MM) in the serum of affected males and female carriers.

Towbin and colleagues[115] demonstrated linkage of XLCM to the dystrophin locus at Xp21 (i.e., the gene responsible for Duchenne and Becker muscular dystrophy) in the family described above as well as in a second family. Evaluation of the protein defect in XLCM showed absence (or low abundance) of the *N*-terminal and rod portion of the dystrophin protein, while skeletal muscle total protein was normal.[115] The 156-kDa dystrophin-associated glycoprotein (known as α-dystroglycan),[116,117] a membrane-bound constituent of the dystrophin-associated glycoprotein complex, was decreased in cardiac tissue as well.[116] This was later confirmed.[118] Diverse mutations leading to XLCM have been shown by Towbin and Ortiz-Lopez,[119,120] Yoshida et al.,[121] Muntoni et al.,[122] and Milasin et al.,[123] with most mutations residing in the 5′ portion of the gene. It appears that the DCM occurs due to mechanical destablization of the muscle membrane. Recently, novel mutations in the 5′ end of dystrophin, including a transposon[124] insertion and an *Alu*-rearrangement[125] were found to result in XLCM. Treatment of congestive heart failure and ventricular arrhythmias is necessary and transplantation is common (see Chap. 23).

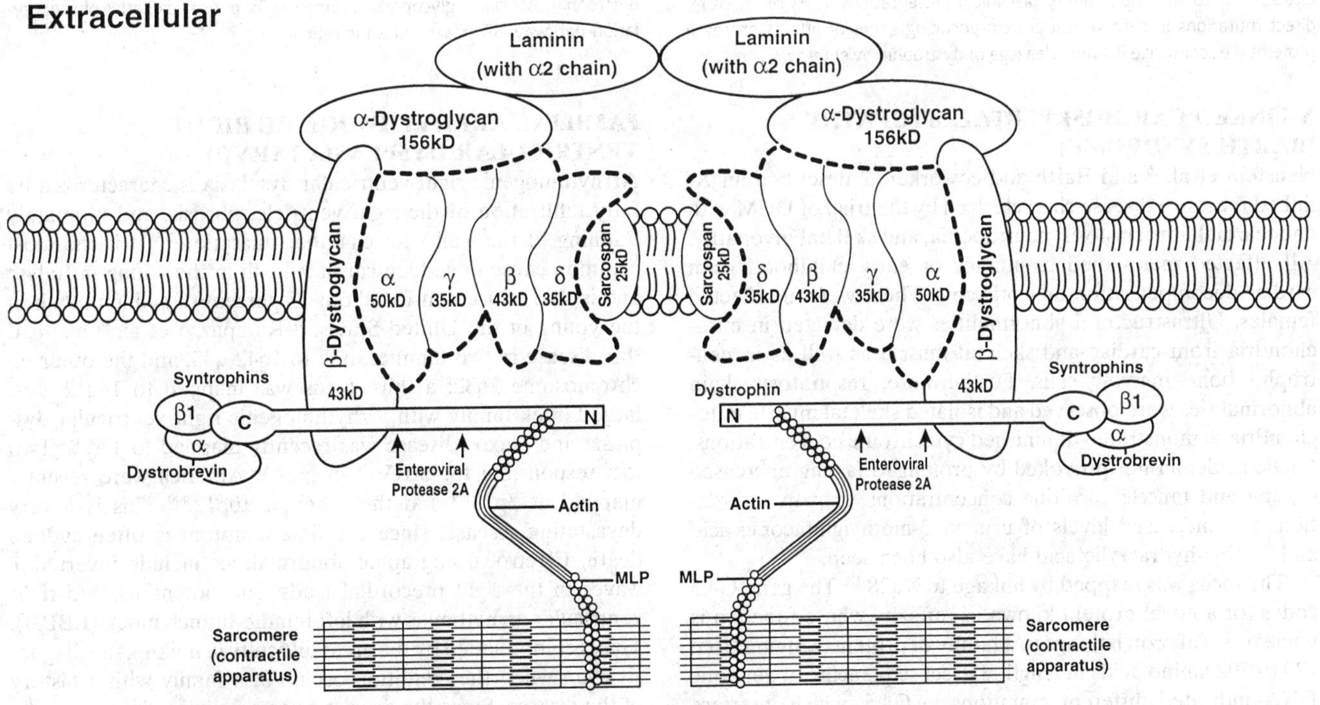

FIGURE 62-7 Schematic representation of the proteins of the cytoskeleton involved in development of dilated cardiomyopathy with or without skeletal myopathy and/or conduction defect. Note that dystrophin links the sarcomere to the sarcolemma and extracellular matrix. Mutations in dystrophin, actin, MLP, and the dystroglycan and sarcoglycan complexes have resulted in dilated cardiomyopathy in patients and animal models.

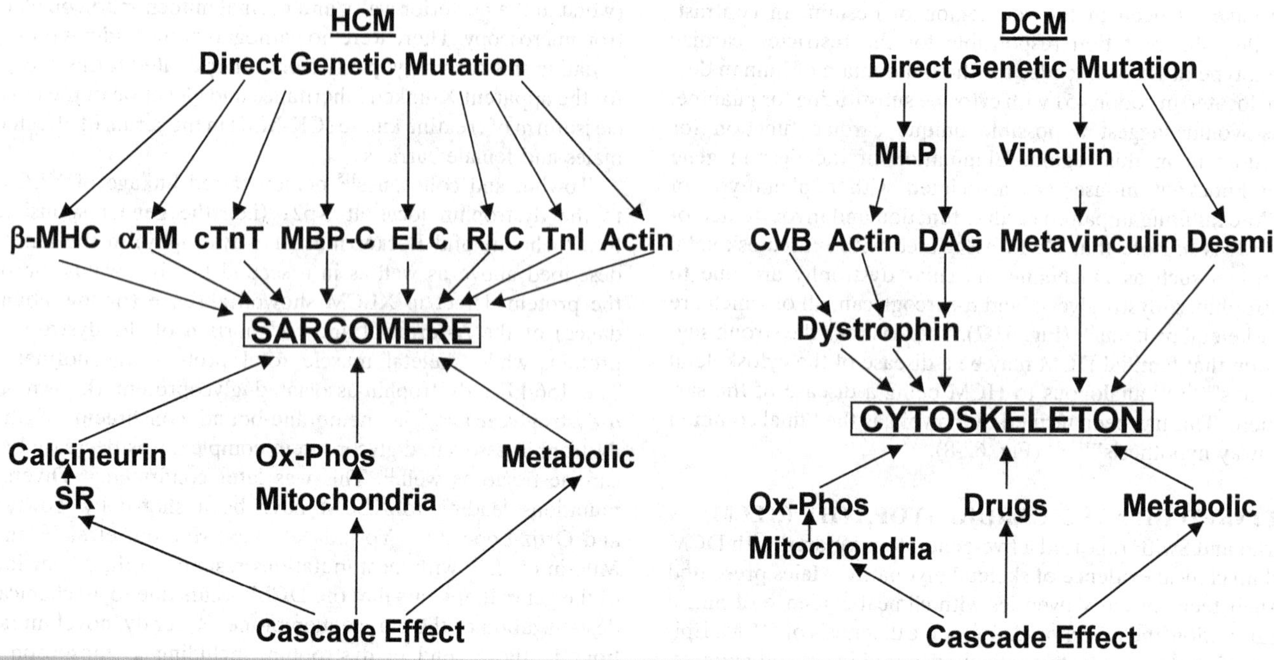

FIGURE 62-8 The "final common pathway hypothesis" described by Towbin, showing the pathways involved in development of hypertrophic (HCM) and dilated cardiomyopathy (DCM). In HCM, mutations in the sarcomeric protein-encoding genes result in the phenotype. In addition, the phenotype may be altered or modified by metabolic or mitochondrial derangements as well as by activation of a molecular pathway such as calcineurin. These cascade effects lead to the wide variety of clinical presentations in HCM. In DCM, direct mutations in cytoskeletal protein-encoding genes or effects on these proteins (i.e., coxsackie B3 virus cleavage of dystrophin by enteroviral protease 2A) also modify the clinical phenotype. Cascade effects via metabolism, mitochondrial abnormalities, or drug interactions are also influential in the severity of disease. HCM/DCM abbreviations: β-MHC = β-myosin heavy chain; αTM = α tropomyosin; cTnT = cardiac troponin T; MBP-c = myosin binding protein C; ELC = essential light chain; RLC = regulatory light chain; TNI = troponin I; CVB = coxsackie virus B; MLP = muscle LIM protein; DAG = dystrophin-associated glycoprotein complex; Ox-phos = oxidative phosphorylation pathway; SR = sarcoplasmic reticulum.

X-LINKED CARDIOSKELETAL MYOPATHY (BARTH SYNDROME)

Neustein et al.[126] and Barth and coworkers[127] described an X-linked recessive disease characterized by the triad of DCM with endocardial fibroelastosis, neutropenia, and skeletal myopathy. All affected males died in infancy or early childhood from cardiac decompensation or septicemia. There were no affected females. Ultrastructural abnormalities were detected in mitochondria from cardiac and skeletal muscle as well as in neutrophil bone marrow cells. Furthermore, respiratory chain abnormalities were observed and isolated skeletal muscle mitochondria demonstrated diminished cytochrome concentrations. Lactic acidemia not provoked by prolonged fasting, increased plasma and muscle carnitine concentrations, growth retardation, and increased levels of urinary 3-methylglutaconic acid and 2-ethyl-hydracrylic acid have also been seen.

The locus was mapped by linkage to Xq28.[128] The gene G4.5 codes for a novel protein known as taffazin, whose function is unclear.[129] Tafazzin belongs to a family of proteins ranging from 129 to 292 amino acids in length. Direct sequencing of genomic DNA indicated different mutations in G4.5, which interfere with translation of the putative protein. Mutations in G4.5 have also been shown to cause other infantile cardiomyopathies, including isolated left ventricular noncompaction[130–132] and dilated hypertrophic cardiomyopathy. Treatment is that for cardiac failure (see Chap. 23).

FAMILIAL ARRHYTHMOGENIC RIGHT VENTRICULAR DYSPLASIA (ARVD)

Arrhythmogenic right ventricular dysplasia is characterized by fatty infiltration of the right ventricle, fibrosis, and ultimately thinning of the wall with chamber dilatation.[133] It is the most common cause of sudden cardiac death in the young in Italy[134] and is said to account for about 17 percent of sudden death in the young in the United States.[135] Rampazzo et al.[136] mapped this disease in two families, one to 1q42-q43, and the other on chromosome 2q32; a third locus was mapped to 14q12.[137] A large Greek family with arrhythmogenic right ventricular dysplasia and Naxos disease was recently mapped to 17q.[138] Two loci responsible for ARVD in North America were recently mapped at 3p23[139] and the other at 10p12.[140] This is a very devastating disease, since the first symptom is often sudden death. Electrocardiographic abnormalities include inverted T waves in the right precordial leads, late potentials, and right ventricular arrhythmias with left bundle-branch block (LBBB). This is compounded by the great difficulty in making the diagnosis even when the condition occurs in a family with a history of the disease. Since the disease affects only the right ventricle, it is difficult to detect.[106] There is no definitive diagnostic standard. The right ventricular biopsy is definitive when positive but often produces a false-negative result, since the disease initiates in the epicardium and spreads to the endocardium of the right ventricular free wall, making it inaccessible to biopsy.

Consensus diagnostic criteria was developed that include right ventricular biopsy, magnetic resonance imaging (MRI), echocardiography, and electrocardiography.[141] Identification of the gene will have tremendous diagnostic impact and hopefully will provide an explanation as to why ARVD is restricted to the right ventricle. Is it a specific right ventricular chamber gene? Is there a stimulus that is unique or predominates in the right ventricle that precipitates the phenotype? What is the stimulus? There are data suggesting that apoptosis is the process leading to the development of fat and fibrosis in ARVD. Discovery of a gene should shed light on the apoptosis pathway.

RESTRICTIVE CARDIOMYOPATHY

In the western countries, restrictive cardiomyopathy (RCM) is the least common of the three major categories of cardiomyopathy (see Chap. 75). The most common cause of secondary restrictive cardiomyopathy in adults is myocardial amyloid. Patients manifest exercise intolerance due to their inability to increase cardiac output by tachycardia without further compromising ventricular filling. Weakness and dyspnea are often prominent, and chest pain may also occur. At end stage, the findings are those of cardiac failure with anasarca. Mutations in the transthyretin (TTR) gene[142,143] which codes for the TTR serum protein, has been found associated with RCM. This protein contains four subunits, each with 127 amino acids, encoded by four exons within a 7-kb gene. Many TTR point mutations cause TTR to form amyloid, which occurs primarily in the heart, leading to heart failure. The diagnosis is suspected by echo and confirmed by genetic analysis. Treatment is that of cardiac failure.

Familial forms of restrictive cardiomyopathy have also been seen. One such family was found to have mutations in the desmin gene[144] and mice have been created with desmin mutations that have a similar phenotype as the clinical condition.[110]

Mucopolysaccharidoses

The mucopolysaccharidoses (MPS) are a group of diseases caused by deficiency of lysosomal enzymes involved in the degradation of glycosaminoglycans.[145] Undegraded glycosaminoglycans accumulate in lysosomes and affect tissue function. MPS have been divided into seven major types. The classification (types I to VII) is based on the deficient enzyme responsible for the disorder. These disorders carry such eponyms as *Hurler, Scheie, Hurler-Scheie, Hunter, Sanfilippo, Morquio, Maroteaux-Lamy,* and *Sly*. They share many clinical features, including multiple system involvement, organomegaly, dysostosis multiplex, facial abnormalities, loss of hearing and vision, joint involvement, cardiac involvement, and central nervous system (CNS) involvement. Cardiac disease includes myocardial hypertrophy, pulmonary and systemic hypertension, valvular disease, coronary occlusion, and myocardial infarction. Congestive heart failure and sudden death are relatively frequent. The most common mucopolysaccharidosis with cardiac involvement is MPS I (Hurler syndrome). Valvular disease is prominent in the Scheie's syndrome (late-onset form). Less commonly, heart disease has been noted in Sanfilippo A syndrome with aortic regurgitation, as well as in severe Maroteaux-Lamy syndrome with valvular heart disease (Table 62-5). The diagnosis for either of these disorders is made by assaying the enzyme activity in cultured skin fibroblasts or leukocytes.

Hurler's Syndrome

Hurler's syndrome (MPS-I) is an autosomal recessive trait found on chromosome 22 (22q11), which occurs in approximately 1 of 40,000 people. It is caused by a deficiency of α-iduronidase (IDUA), which is required for the degradation of both heparan sulfate and dermatan sulfate.[146] The result is similar to that of Hunter's syndrome, with both dermatan and heparan sulfate in high concentrations in the urine. Myocardial infarction occurs in childhood (Table 62-5). *Severe* (Hurler, MPS-IH), *intermediate* (Hurler/Scleie, MPS-IH/S), and *mild* (Scheie) clinical subtypes of MPS-I occur.[145] MPS-IH patients usually present within the first year of life and progress with a combination of hepatosplenomegaly, skeletal deformities, corneal clouding, and severe mental retardation. Obstructive airway disease, respiratory infection, and cardiac complications usually result in death before age 10 years. Dangel[147] reported on 64 children with mucopolysaccharidoses, noting 72 percent with cardiac disease (valvular lesions, cardiomyopathy). Mitral valve thickening with regurgitation or stenosis, hypertrophic cardiomyopathy, aortic stenosis, and EFE were most common. MPS-IH/S is characterized by little neurologic involvement but most of the somatic involvement described for MPS-IH develops early in the teenage years, causing considerable loss of mobility. MPS-IS patients, those with the mildest symptoms, have little or no neurologic involvement, normal stature, and normal life span but do develop stiff joints, mild hepatosplenomegaly, aortic valve disease, and corneal clouding.[145] Diagnosis is confirmed in MPS-I by demonstration of mucopolysacchariduria and absence of IDUA activity in leukocytes and fibroblasts. Biochemical differentiation between subtypes is difficult. Gene identification[148] has allowed for mutation analysis; the broad range of clinical phenotypes is related to the types of mutations in the IDUA gene.[149] Allogenic bone marrow transplantation is the most effective treatment for Hurler's syndrome[150] and gene transfer is being evaluated.[151] Animal models are now available[152–154] for study.

Hunter's Syndrome

Hunter's syndrome, an X-linked disorder mapped to the Xq26-Xq28 region, is found in approximately 1 of 30,000 people.[145] It is caused by a deficiency of the enzyme iduronate sulfatase and results in excessive urinary excretion of dermatan and heparan sulfate and accumulation of mucopolysaccharides, which can result in coronary obstruction and subsequent myocardial infarction in childhood. Most patients die before the third decade. Mutations in this gene are heterogeneous, ranging from small microlesions to gross deletions and inversions[155–157] and, in some cases, involves neighboring genes. Therefore, wide clinical variation is common. Gene therapy has been reported.[158–160]

Morquio's Disease

Morquio's disease (MPS-IVA), an autosomal recessive disorder caused by a genetic deficiency in *N*-acetyl-galactosamine-6-sulfatase, is a prototypical chondroosteodystrophy.[145] The disorder is characterized by specific spondyloepiphyseal dysplasia, short-trunk dwarfism, coxa valga, odontoid hypoplasia, corneal opacities, normal intelligence, and excessive urinary excretion of keratan sulfate and chondroitin 6-sulfate. The deficient *N*-acetyl-galactosamine-6-sulfatase results in progressive accumulation of mucopolysaccharides in lysosomes of various tissues, leading to vertebral involvement and cardiac disease (Table 62-5) in the second decade of life. Tomatsu et al.[161] isolated and characterized the full-length cDNA of the gene and it was localized to chromosome 16q24.[162] This gene is approximately 50 kb in size and has 14 exons; mutations have been described.[163,164]

Maroteaux-Lamy Disease

The Maroteaux-Lamy syndrome is caused by the deficiency of the enzyme arylsulfatase B, which is required for degradation of the glycosaminoglycans, dermatan sulfate, and chondroitin 4-sulfate.[165] It is associated with aortic valve disease. This gene, located on 5q13-q14,[165] has been isolated and characterized.[166] Mutations have been identified, and different mutations cause different clinical phenotypes.[167] The clinical features are quite variable, occurring in infancy and consist of growth retardation, coarse facies, corneal clouding, and multiple skeletal changes, together with dilated cardiomyopathy and aortic or mitral value stenosis or insufficiency. Cardiac manifestations usually appear after the neurologic features but are usually present by adolescence. Molecular diagnosis is currently available. Bone marrow transplants are currently the treatment of choice.[150] All of these disorders can be diagnosed prenatally by enzyme assay in at-risk pregnancies.

MUSCULAR DYSTROPHIES WITH CARDIAC INVOLVEMENT

The muscular dystrophies are a heterogeneous group of diseases, the primary manifestations of which include progressive muscle wasting secondary to intrinsic defects of the muscle fiber. These defects have a wide spectrum of clinical expression and include Duchenne's muscular dystrophy, Becker's muscular dystrophy, Emery-Dreifuss muscular dystrophy, the limb-girdle muscular dystrophies, and myotonic dystrophy. Cardiac disease, especially DCM, is central to the morbidity and mortality associated with these disorders (Table 62-7).

Duchenne Muscular Dystrophy (DMD)

DMD is an X-linked disorder characterized by the early onset of progressive, generalized muscle weakness and "pseudohypertrophy" of certain muscle groups.[168] The incidence of DMD is estimated to be 1 in 3300 live male births with little ethnic variation, and the calculated mutation rate of 10^4 is an order of magnitude higher than for most other genetic diseases. About one-third of cases arise by spontaneous mutation, with the remaining two-thirds occurring by inheritance of the disease-causing gene from the carrier mother. Female carriers of DMD are usually asymptomatic but occasionally have a slowly progressive myopathy of moderate severity. This "manifesting female carrier" state occurs in approximately 8 percent of carriers and is thought to occur due to random X-inactivation. The disease may also be expressed in females with Turner syndrome having a single X chromosome and in females with X-autosome translocations that disrupt the DMD gene. In the latter case, the translocation not only disrupts the DMD gene but also causes the nonrandom inactivation of the normal allele on the other X chromosome, resulting in the expression of the disease phenotype.

Although evidence of skeletal muscle disease in boys with DMD is evident in the neonatal period, as seen by high serum muscle enzymes (particularly CK-MM), clinical disease is not. There may be mild developmental delay, walking later than expected, but weakness is usually not appreciated until at least 2 or 3 years of age. Early symptoms reported by parents include difficulty in running or climbing stairs, frequent falling, and enlargement of calf muscles. Pelvic-girdle weakness is more obvious than shoulder-girdle weakness in the early stages. The gait becomes lordotic and waddling, and the child usually walks with the heels raised slightly off the ground (i.e., toe walking). As pelvic girdle weakness increases, the child has increasing difficulty rising from a seated position. In order to rise from the floor to a standing position, the child must brace the arms against the front of the thigh and climb up the legs, the so-called Gowers sign. Muscle pseudohypertrophy usually appears by 5 to 6 years of age, with muscle enlargement most commonly occurring in the calf muscles; the quadriceps, infraspinatus, deltoid, and gluteal muscles may also be involved, however. The upper and lower extremities become progressively weaker with age, and joint contractures may appear due to uneven weakness of agonist and antagonist muscles. Contractures of the hip flexors, iliotibial bands, and heel cords develop in 70 percent of patients between 6 and 10 years of age. Most patients are wheelchair-bound by the end of the first decade of life. After ambulation is lost, fixed contractures occur and paraspinal muscle weakness leads to progressive kyphoscoliosis. Significant weakness of the respiratory muscles occurs early in the second decade and is a common cause of demise.

Although most cases of DMD can be recognized on the basis of the patient's history and clinical signs alone, laboratory evaluation is important to confirm the diagnosis.[168] As previously noted, extremely high levels of CK-MM are found in the early stages of disease, as early as birth, and precede evidence of clinical involvement. Other muscle enzymes—including aldolase, SGOT, lactic dehydrogenase (LDH), and pyruvate kinase—are also grossly elevated. In the end stages of the disease, enzyme levels fall but do not reach normal values. Electromyographic examination may also be useful, demonstrating the characteristic features of a myopathy. Insertional activity is normal or increased initially but decreases in the advanced stages of the disease, when fibrosis replaces muscle fibers. Fibrillation potentials and positive sharp waves occur in the early stages of the disease due to the splitting of muscle fibers. The motor unit potentials are small and polyphasic, and an early recruitment pattern with minimal effort is present. Mild intellectual impairment is common in patients with DMD. The retardation is present at an early age, is nonprogressive, and does not correlate well with the stage of the disease. Approximately one-third of patients have IQs below 75, characterized primarily by impaired verbal ability.

The heart is commonly involved in DMD, with electrocardiographic abnormalities and dilated cardiomyopathy being most typical.[168] Cardiac symptoms, however, are unusual before the terminal stages of the disease. Congestive heart failure tends to occur. A midsystolic click and late systolic murmur associated with mitral valve prolapse are also common. In addition, an S3 or S4 gallop, sinus tachycardia, and a mitral regurgitation murmur are usually heard; cardiomegaly and increased pulmonary vascular markings appear at this stage, and bilateral diaphragmatic elevations may be seen owing to diaphragmatic dystrophy. Unlike the late-onset findings of dilated cardiomyopathy, the electrocardiogram is abnormal early in the course of DMD, with a tall R-wave and an abnormally increased R/S ratio in the right precordial chest leads and a deep, narrow Q-wave in leads I, aV_L, V_5, and V_6. These abnormalities progress over time and are attributed to the finding of that the greatest dystrophic myocardial changes in the posterobasal and contiguous lateral left ventricular myocardium. In addition, P waves with negative terminal deflections in V_1 exceeding 20 ms and 0.1 mV appear in 20 to 45 percent of patients and, in the absence of left atrial enlargement on echocardiogram, are attributed to an intrinsic disorder of left atrial or intraatrial conduction. A short PR interval may be seen in up to 50 percent of patients but is not thought to be due to a bypass tract, as seen in Wolff-Parkinson-White syndrome. Infranodal conduction abnormalities, however, may be seen in patients with DMD, and these include complete or incomplete bundle-branch block, and left anterior or posterior fascicular block. Atrial and ventricular premature beats and atrial flutter are seen in some patients.

Echocardiography reveals left ventricular dilatation and dysfunction, with significantly reduced ejection fraction, and LV hypokinesis of the posterobasal ventricular wall is identified. Doppler and color Doppler commonly demonstrate mitral regurgitation, either secondary to the dilated cardiomyopathy or to the associated mitral valve prolapse, which occurs secondary to papillary muscle dysfunction. In some patients systolic function appears normal but diastolic dysfunction is present.

Histopathologic abnormalities of the heart and skeletal muscle are universal in patients with DMD, and those of skeletal muscle are widespread even in the early stages of disease.[168] Typical findings are rounding of the muscle fibers, increased variability in fiber size, increased central nucleation, and fiber splitting. Necrotic and regenerating fibers are present along with large, round hyaline fibers. In the late stages, muscle may be virtually replaced by fat and fibrous tissue. In the heart, degenerative changes in muscle fibers and areas of fibrosis in the ventricles, atria, and conduction system occur, with most pronounced changes in the posterobasal region and adjacent lateral wall of the left ventricle. The underlying cause of cardiac disease is not currently known, but it is speculated that the gene defect in DMD leads to instability of the translated cytoskeletal protein, leading to weakening of the myocyte membrane and subsequent myocyte death due to mechanical stress.

The dystrophin gene, on the short arm of the X chromosome,[168,169] is responsible for these disorders and when dystrophin abnormalities occur due to mutations, may cause either low level production of a nonfunctional protein or complete absence of dystrophin in the heart and skeletal muscle of affected patients. It is among the largest genes discovered thus far, comprising approximately 2.5 Mbp and transcribing a 14-kb mRNA molecule. This cytoskeletal protein-encoding gene is normally expressed in striated and smooth muscle as well as in brain. In muscle tissue, the dystrophin protein has been localized to the cytoplasmic surface of the sarcolemma and is associated with several integral membrane glycoproteins.[170] This glycoprotein/dystrophin complex—which involves the sarcoglycans, dystroglycans, syntrophins, and dystrobrevins—connects dystrophin to the sarcolemma and links to the extracellular matrix; it may be involved in the regulation of intracellular calcium, which is increased in dystrophin-deficient muscle, along with increased calcium channel transport.

The diagnostic approaches to DMD have changed dramatically over the past decade. Previously, serum CK-MM level and muscle biopsy were the standard approaches. Today DMD is diagnosed primarily by molecular analysis, which is rapid and accurate and may predict clinical course. Most commonly, dystrophin mutations that cause a frameshift[171] of the nucleotide sequence result in the severe form of muscular dystrophy, DMD.

Management of the congestive heart failure associated with the DCM seen in DMD is identical to that used for patients with other causes of heart failure and arrhythmias. Pacing is not usually necessary.

Becker's Muscular Dystrophy (BMD)

BMD is an X-linked disorder that differs in both severity and time of onset from DMD,[168] despite being due to allelic mutations in dystrophin, the gene responsible for DMD. BMD appears later and progresses more slowly than DMD, so that survival to middle age is seen. The pattern of muscle weakness, however, is identical to that in DMD, with early involvement of the pelvic girdle and proximal lower extremities.[168] The initial signs of weakness usually appear during the second decade but may be seen as late as the third decade. The weakness gradually progresses, with the upper extremities becoming involved after 5 to 10 years. Patients generally remain ambulatory until their mid-thirties. As in DMD, muscle hypertrophy is common; intellectual impairment, however, is less common and less severe. As in DMD, life expectancy is also reduced in BMD, with only 50 percent of patients surviving to 40 years of age.

Cardiac involvement may be seen in adolescence and ultimately affects 80 percent of patients.[172] As in DMD, dilated cardiomyopathy and cardiac failure are the usual abnormalities encountered (Table 62-7) and are often the ultimate cause of death. Conduction abnormalities manifesting as fascicular block or complete heart block are also seen. As in DMD, muscle enzyme activity is markedly elevated in BMD, and preclinical cases may be detected by elevated CK-MM. Electromyographic examination shows a "myopathic" pattern with small, polyphasic motor units and early recruitment of motor units. The histology of BMD is similar to that of other forms of muscular dystrophy. In contrast to DMD, hyaline fibers are rarely seen. Electrocardiographic changes are similar to those seen in DMD. Other electrocardiographic abnormalities encountered include left axis deviation, right bundle-branch block, left bundle-branch block, and complete heart block. The echocardiogram may demonstrate the features of dilated cardiomyopathy.

BMD is also due to mutations within the dystrophin gene; i.e., it is allelic with DMD. As is the case with DMD, more than 30 percent of patients with BMD have no family history of the disease, an indication that they represent spontaneous mutations. The phenotypic difference between DMD and BMD patients has been speculated to be due to frameshift mutations leading to more severe disease (DMD) while out-of-frame mutations cause less severe (BMD) disease.[171] The frameshift hypothesis explains more than 90 percent of the cases of DMD versus BMD. The cardiac abnormalities in BMD, like those

TABLE 62-7 Manifestations of Neurologic Cardiac Disorders

Neuromuscular Disorder	Mode of Inheritance	Incidence per 100,000	Age of Onset	Pathology		Clinical	
				Cardiac	Musculoskeletal	Cardiac	Musculoskeletal
Myotonic dystrophy	Autosomal dominant	10	Third to fourth decade	Atrophy, interstitial fibrosis and fatty infiltration of the conduction system	Atrophy, interstitial fibrosis and fatty infiltration	AV block, atrial arrhythmias, CHF (rare)	Myotonia, atrophy of strap muscles
Friedreich's ataxia	Autosomal recessive	2.0	Child/adolescent	Interstitial fibrosis, myocyte hypertrophy	Normal	Abnormal ECG axis and Q waves, atrial arrhythmias, hypertrophic cardiomyopathy (concentric, asymmetrical), dilated cardiomyopathy	Ataxia, kyphoscoliosis
Duchenne's muscular dystrophy	X-linked recessive	2.0	2–5 years	Myocardial fibrosis in posterobasal LV free wall, degeneration of conducting fibers, noninflammatory arteriopathy	Myofibril necrosis, interstitial accumulation of fat and fibrous tissue	Dysrhythmias, ECG abnormalities, dilated cardiomyopathy	Pseudohypertrophy, proximal limb and neck weakness, contractures, scoliosis and chest cage deformities
Becker's muscular dystrophy	X-linked recessive	0.4	Second to third decade	Focal areas of fatty infiltration and proliferating connective tissue	Same as Duchenne's	Dilated cardiomyopathy	Pseudohypertrophy, proximal limb-girdle weakness and atrophy

Kearns-Sayre syndrome	Maternal, nonmedelian (i.e., mitochondrial)	Rare	Childhood/adolescence	Ragged-red fibers	Ragged-red fibers, glycogen accumulation, proliferation of abnormal mitochondria	Progressive AV block, dilated cardiomyopathy, hypertrophic cardiomyopathy	Ptosis, ataxia
Emery-Dreifuss syndrome	X-linked recessive (? autosomal dominant)	Rare	Second to third decade	Focal myocardial fibrosis	Same as Duchenne's	Atrial standstill, progressive conduction block, malignant ventricular arrhythmias, dilated cardiomyopathy	Contractures of elbows, pericervical muscles, and Achilles tendon; humeroperoneal muscle weakness and atrophy
Fascioscapulohumeral muscular dystrophy	Autosomal dominant	0.6	Second to third decade	Unknown	Same as Duchenne's	Atrial abnormalities, conduction delays, atrial fibrillation/flutter	Proximal shoulder and facial weakness and atrophy; lower extremity weakness
Myotubular (centronuclear) myopathy	X-linked recessive	Rare	Variable	Myocardial fibrosis	Hypertrophic fibers with central nuclei	Dilated cardiomyopathy	Respiratory difficulty and hypotonia
Nemaline myopathy	Autosomal dominant with reduced penetrance	Rare	Birth/infancy	Nemaline bodies	Nemaline bodies	Dilated cardiomyopathy	Diffuse muscle weakness and hypotonia

SOURCE: From Berko and Swift,[2] Collins et al.,[3] and Brower,[4] with permission.

described for DMD, require further study.[173] The treatment of CHF and arrhythmias is similar to that of other patients with these signs and symptoms.

Animal models have been created during the past several years that help to characterize the roles of dystrophin and the associated complexes.[174–180] Loss-of-function mutations of dystrophin lead to a DMD or BMD phenotype, while utrophin-deficient mice have defects in the postsynaptic membrane folds at the neuromuscular junction. Mice lacking both dystrophin and utrophin display a severe muscular dystrophy with premature death.[177–180] Sarcoglycan-deficient mice also demonstrate severe muscular dystrophy but, in addition, severe hypertrophic and/or dilated cardiomyopathy has been seen.[174,175]

Various methods evaluating the possibility of gene therapy for dystrophinopathies have been reported over the past several years in mice, with varying degrees of success. Minigene and stem-cell transplantation have both been considered promising using dystrophin and utrophin.[181,182]

Emery-Dreifuss Muscular Dystrophy (EDMD)

EDMD is a relatively rare disorder[168] characterized by weakness in the humeroperoneal distribution, early joint contractures, and dilated cardiomyopathy, with X-linked (occasionally, autosomal dominant) inheritance. The onset of disease in these patients occurs between 2 and 10 years of age, with weakness initially noted in the shoulder girdles and upper extremities. Contractures of the elbows and posterior cervical muscles appear early. The disease is slowly progressive, with involvement of the distal leg musculature following that of the upper extremities; contractures of the knees and ankles follow contractures of the elbows. Unlike the case in DMD and BMD, muscle pseudohypertrophy does not occur. The disease evolves slowly and usually stabilizes in the third decade, with most patients remaining ambulatory. Dilated cardiomyopathy is a common occurrence, but the severity of disease varies from family to family. Varying degrees of atrioventricular block are common (Table 62-7) and atrial standstill may occur. These electrical abnormalities may lead to episodes of syncope, transient ischemic attacks, stroke, and sudden death. A pacemaker is commonly required. Atrial fibrillation has also been observed. As in DMD and BMD, muscle enzyme activity is elevated, albeit to a lesser extent. Skeletal muscle biopsy histopathologic findings are similar to those associated with other forms of muscular dystrophy. Type I fiber atrophy has been described in some cases (Fig. 62-9). The gene responsible for X-linked EDMD was localized to Xq28[184] before being cloned. The gene called emerin (or STA) was shown to have an open reading frame of 762 nucleotides that encodes a serine-rich 254–amino acid protein with probable mechanical/structural function.[185] Emerin mRNA shows ubiquitous tissue distribution, with the highest expression in skeletal and cardiac muscles. The cDNA sequence of emerin predicts a tail-anchor membrane protein with an amino acid sequence similar to that of the thymopoietins, a group of nuclear lamina-associated proteins.[186] Nagano et al.[187] and Manilal et al.[188] both showed that emerin is a 34-kDa nuclear membrane protein in skeletal and cardiac muscle, which is absent in EDMD.

The autosomal dominant form of EDMD was initially mapped to chromosome 1, and recently the gene was identified as lamin A/C.[189] The encoded protein is also thought to be a nuclear lamina-associated protein. The phenotypic spectrum of this gene appears to be broad when mutated. In some cases, only a DCM phenotype with conduction disease occurs in the absence of skeletal muscle disease clinically, similar to what is seen with dystrophin.

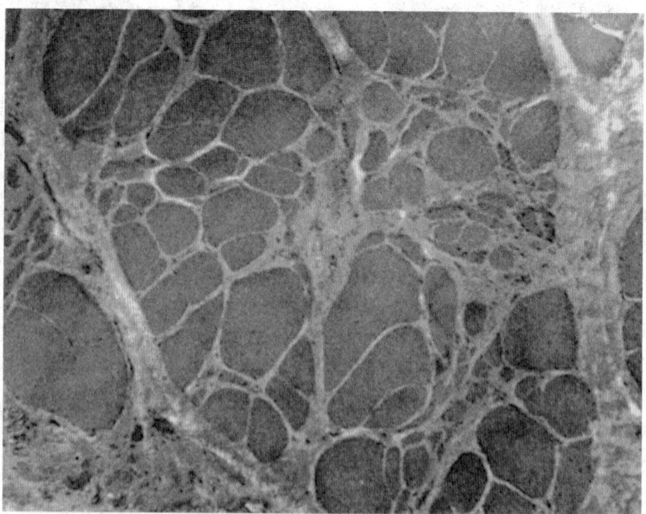

FIGURE 62-9 Skeletal muscle biopsy in Emery-Dreifuss muscular dystrophy. Increased endomysial and perimysial connective tissue, with marked variation in myofiber size, internal nuclei, and myofibers splitting (×153). (Reprinted with permission from Specht LA, McKee AC. MGH Case Records (case 34-1992): A 19-year-old man with progressive proximal muscle weakness, contractures, and cardiac abnormalities. *N Engl J Med* 1992; 327:558.)

Myotonic Dystrophy (Steinert's Disease)

Myotonic dystrophy (DM) is the most common form of inherited muscular dystrophy in adults, with an incidence of 1 in 8000 to 10,000 persons.[168] This autosomal dominant disorder affects multiple organ systems and its name is derived from the combined myopathy, dystrophy, and myotonia of skeletal muscle. Myotonia, an abnormality in relaxation after muscle contraction, is the primary feature of this disease. DM is variably expressed, and individuals may present with signs and symptoms involving many different organ systems. Penetrance varies with age and the disease may affect different tissues at different periods of life; a severe form of DM exists with symptoms at birth.

Classically, DM presents in a young adult with new-onset weakness of the hands or mild foot drop. Asymptomatic myotonia—namely, sustained contraction and depolarization of skeletal muscle in response to a percussive or electrical impulse—may be elicited. Myotonia is usually in the hands and tongue, while weakness involves the distal extremities predominantly. A typical facies usually accompanies these findings, including loss of temporal muscle and slight weakness of the lips and mouth with a "hatchet-like" shape, frontal balding, and ptosis (Fig. 62-10). Other systems including heart, eyes, CNS, endocrine system, gastrointestinal system and respiratory system may be involved (Table 62-5). Electromyographic abnormalities are frequent and subcapsular; punctuate iridescent cataracts are common in middle-aged patients.

Myotonia is best seen in the small muscles of the hand and in the tongue. There are repetitive discharges with gradual and

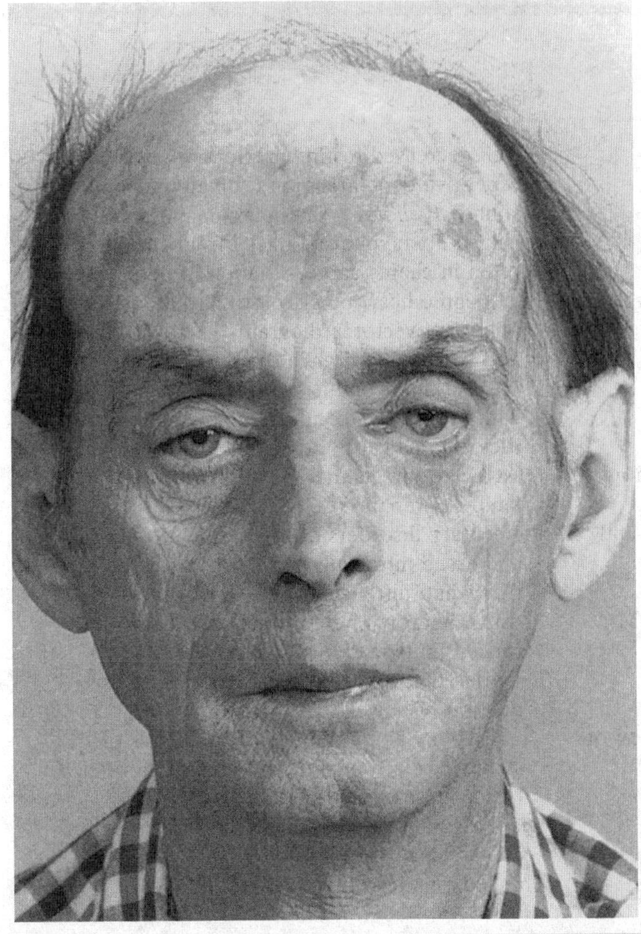

FIGURE 62-10 A 41-year-old man with myotonic dystrophy (DM). Muscle wasting of temporalis muscles with narrow small chin produces a "hatchet-like" facies. Baldness and ptosis (note droopy eyelids with pupils partially covered and sclerae visible) contribute to characteristic appearance. (Reprinted with permission from Roses AD, Pericak-Vance MA. In: *Molecular Basis of Neurology*. Cambridge, MA: Blackwell; 1993:147–159.)

uneven decay of amplitude on electromyography. Myotonic muscles undergo dystrophic changes, which may take years to several decades. In general, the younger the presentation, the more rapid the progression. Only a small percentage of affected individuals, probably less than 10 percent, progress to requiring a wheelchair for ambulation; many require a brace worn in the shoes to control foot drop.

Serious complications of DM involve the heart.[189] Cardiac conduction abnormalities are common (Tables 62-7 and 62-8) and may be progressive, particularly in younger patients. These are identified by periodic ECG monitoring and usually occur without obvious cardiac complaints. Sudden cardiac death in athletically inclined adolescents is relatively frequent. In studies of families with DM, cardiac findings may be the initial clinical manifestation of the disease, with bradycardia and first-degree heart block being common. Progression to complete heart block may occur over time and is not well tolerated, potentially ending in death and frequently requiring pacing. In some cases, ventricular tachycardia or dilated cardiomyopathy may also occur (Table 62-8). Typically, however, systolic function is preserved but diastolic dysfunction occurs.

DM patients may have a particular psychological profile that includes indifference, reticence, and hostility. Mild mental retardation may be seen, particularly in patients with congenital DM. Young and middle-aged patients may be hypersomnolent and indolent, sometimes sleeping up to 20 h daily. Testicular atrophy is common in males and amenorrhea and ovarian cysts may occur in females (Table 62-8). Increasing debilitation, handicap, and disability may occur in subsequent generations of a family; this increasing disease severity is known as *anticipation*.

The gene for myotonic dystrophy was localized to 19q13.3[190] and encodes for myotonin protein kinase (DMPK), a serine-threonine protein kinase.[191] The genetic basis for myotonic dystrophy consists of long stretches of three bases repeated in tandem. The triplet repeat present in the DMPK gene is CTG, which in the mRNA is CUG and is located in the 3′ end of the gene beyond the protein coding region. The severity of disease (neuromuscular, cardiac, and CNS) relates to the length of the repeats. Less than 50 triplet repeats is usually associated with no disease. Usually 100 to 250 repeats are required to cause disease and, if more than 250 repeats are present, the disease is usually seen at birth and reflects genetic anticipation (increasingly severe expression and earlier onset of disease through generations as a result of the increase in the number of CTG repeats with subsequent generations). Clinical cardiac symptoms (i.e., syncope) and ECG abnormalities (i.e., left bundle-branch block) correlate directly with CTG expansion size.[189] In addition, the incidence of malignant ventricular arrhythmias also correlate directly with the size of CTG expansion.

Myotonic dystrophy is one of the many familial neuromuscular diseases due to the genetic defect of multiple triplet repeats.[189] However, the mechanisms whereby the triplet repeats induce the disease remains an enigma. Myotonic dystrophy is somewhat unique since the triplet repeats are in the 3′ end of the gene beyond the protein coding region. DMPK levels are reduced in patients with myotonic dystrophy; when the gene for DMPK is eliminated in knockout mice, muscle weakness results, but none of the other organs are involved, such as the eyes or testes, as observed in myotonic dystrophy. This has led to an extensive search for other explanations, including adjacent genes. One by-product of this research was identification of a novel group of proteins that bind specifically to triplet repeats in DNA and RNA[192]; binding is determined by the sequence of the triplet repeat. A specific protein was identified that binds only to the CUG sequence in the mRNA of DMPK. The CUG-BP protein has a molecular weight of 52 kDa and three binding sites for CUG repeats.[192] The protein has several serine and threonine phosphorylation sites, which appear to be regulated by DMPK. Further studies indicated that this protein is identical to another protein (NB50) that is known to be responsible for mRNA transport from the nucleus to the cytoplasm.[193] This has given rise to the hypothesis that the CUG-BP is sequestered by the multiple CUG repeats and not available to other mRNAs for processing or transport from the nucleus. The involvement of several mRNAs would explain the multiple organs involved. This would also explain why, in the mouse with the DMPK gene knocked out, one observes only muscle weakness because in the absence of the multiple triplet repeats, the other mRNAs are properly transported by the CUG-BP protein and function

TABLE 62-8 Systemic Involvement in Myotonic Dystrophy

Organ or System	Clinical	Diagnostic Signs
Muscle	Myotonia, weakness, dystrophy	*EMG:* decreased resting membrane potential, repetitive depolarization ("dive bomber" sound) *Pathology:* sarcoplasmic masses, ringed fibers, internal nuclei frequent; nuclei often in chains; large variation in fiber size
Cardiac	Bradycardia common, complete heart block frequent, prolonged PR interval, dilated cardiomyopathy	First-degree heart block, bradycardia on ECG; abnormal vectorcardiogram; SA node, right and left bundle branch dysfunction; increased His-Purkinje conduction (His bundle studies) with progressive conduction system abnormalities; dilated cardiomyopathy
Lens	Posterior subcapsular, iridescent, or scintillating cataracts	Dust-like cataracts may be visible only on slit lamp examination
Eye	Decreased vision (independent of cataracts and diabetic retinopathy); diplopia	Pigmentary disorders of macula keratosis sicca; decreased intraocular pressure; frequent ptosis and ultraocular muscle weakness
CNS	Mental retardation (especially congenital DM); hypersomnia	Possible neuronal heterotopias; suspicious, reticent personality characteristics
Gastrointestinal	Dysphagia, abdominal pain	Disordered esophageal and gastric peristalsis; dilation of bowel
Skeletal	Cranial and facial abnormalities, malocclusion of dentition	Cranial bony abnormalities, hyperostosis of skull (localized or diffuse), small sella turcica, large sinuses, micrognathia
Respiratory	Hypoventilation, postanesthesia respiratory failure	Diaphragmatic and intercostal muscle weakness
Smooth muscle	Dilation of hollow-viscus organs and ureters, abnormal bowel motility	Thinned or interrupted smooth muscle

normally.[194,195] This hypothesis is now actively pursued by many investigators. Preliminary findings show an accumulation of the CUG-BP in the nuclei of cells from DM.[196,197] Another possible mechanism is variations in gene levels in the immediate vicinity, such as the homeobox gene DMPHP.

Relative to therapy, conduction disturbances typically require permanent pacemaker implantation and dilated cardiomyopathy requires treatment for heart failure.

Fascioscapulohumeral Dystrophy

Fascioscapulohumeral,[198] or Landouzy-Dejerine, muscular dystrophy exists as two clinical types. One type has autosomal dominant inheritance with onset at the end of the first or the beginning of the second decade. The weakness of the facial, shoulder, and upper arm muscles is slowly progressive, but wide variability is seen. The second clinical type of fascioscapulohumeral dystrophy is the infantile form. Onset is within the first 2 years of life, and many patients are wheelchair-bound by 1 year of age. Clinical manifestations of muscular dystrophy generally are absent in the parents.

The cardiac involvement involves progressive atrial dysfunction resulting in permanent paralysis of the atria, beginning with sinus bradycardia, junctional escape rhythm, and AV block (Table 62-7). Criteria for diagnosis of permanent paralysis of the atria include absence of P waves on surface ECG, esophageal electrogram, and intracardiac electrocardiogram, unresponsiveness of the atrium to electrical stimulation, and immobility of the atria on fluoroscopy and echocardiography. Focal abnormalities of the atria precede these events. Nonparalytic regions of the atrium may demonstrate enhanced activity, apparent clinically as atrial tachycardia or flutter. Therapy depends on the clinical features. The chromosomal locus has been identified on chromosome 4q35,[199] but the responsible gene(s) are unknown.

Nemaline Myopathy

Nemaline myopathy is named for the small rod-like particles found in striated muscle. Inheritance is probably autosomal dominant, although autosomal recessive inheritance may occur.[200] Clinical features include hypotonia with truncal and extremity weakness from an early age and a narrow arched palate. Conduction abnormalities and cardiac dilatation have been described[200,201] but are unusual (Table 62-7). Nemaline rods are demonstrable in the myocardium and conduction tissues. The genetic cause of this disease was recently discovered by Nowak et al.,[202] who identified mutations in the human skeletal muscle α-actin gene (ACTA1), all missense mutations. Interestingly, the clinical phenotype varied significantly, from mild disease to severe, infantile-onset disease. In addition, a different clinical disorder, actin myopathy (i.e., congenital myopathy with excessive thin filaments), was also found to carry mutations in ACTA1.[202,203]

Two other forms of nemaline myopathy have also been identified. Mutations in TPM3, encoding α-tropomyosin slow, has been found mutated in both dominant and recessive nemaline myopathy.[204] In addition, mutations in NEB, encoding nebulin, has been seen in slowly progressive congenital nemaline myopathy.[205] Therefore, the underlying cause for this phenotype are mutations in skeletal muscle sarcomeric genes, similar to that seen in HCM and cardiac sarcomeric genes. Therapy is required when the conduction abnormalities or cardiac dilatation causes clinical symptoms.

Endocardial Fibroelastosis (EFE)

This disorder is characterized by endocardial thickening, which leads to decreased compliance and impaired diastolic function. Primary forms are typically unassociated with other cardiac anomalies. Most commonly, this disease presents in infancy and early childhood with signs and symptoms of congestive heart failure.[206] The diagnosis is usually made by biopsy. The incidence of primary EFE in the United States in the past was relatively high—approximately one case in 5000 live births.[207] During the past decade, however, this incidence has decreased markedly, for unknown reasons. Treatment of children with primary EFE with anticongestive and inotropic measures has been ineffective, and the clinical course usually results in either death or transplantation. Postmortem examination typically demonstrates enlargement of the left ventricle. Histopathology commonly reveals extensive deposition of extracellular matrix, primarily collagen and elastic fibers, in the endocardium. Three inherited forms of EFE have been described: autosomal recessive, autosomal dominant, and an X-linked recessive disorder. The majority of cases, however, occur sporadically. The X-linked form shows mitochondrial abnormalities similar to Barth syndrome[127,128] with the exception that EFE patients have endocardial scarring. It is likely, however, that this form is caused by mutations in the G4.5 gene found in Barth syndrome and LV noncompaction.[129] It was hypothesized in the 1950s and 1960s that EFE is secondary to intrauterine myocarditis in sporadic cases, particularly as a result of mumps or Coxsackievirus. Ni et al.[208] recently identified mumps viral genome in the majority of autopsy specimens retrieved from infants dying between the 1950s and 1980s. This disease essentially disappeared after the program of vaccination (mumps-measles-rubella or MMR) began in the United States.

DEFECTS OF METABOLISM CAUSING CARDIOMYOPATHY

Carnitine Deficiency

L-Carnitine is a small, water-soluble molecule containing seven carbon atoms and is important in the shuttling of long-chain fatty acids and activated acetate across the inner mitochondrial membrane. A specific translocase facilitates the exchange of long-chain acylcarnitine and acetylcarnitine. Carnitine also serves as the shuttle for the end products of peroxisomal fatty acid oxidation and for α-ketoacids derived from branched chain amino acids. These metabolites are transferred into the mitochondrial matrix for terminal oxidation.

Primary carnitine deficiency syndrome is characterized by a profound decrease in carnitine in affected tissues. The mechanism underlying the primary disorder is defective transport of carnitine from the serum into the affected cells.[209] End-stage disease of many different organs, including the heart, may induce depletion of carnitine stores and must be differentiated from the chronic inherited type. Based on carnitine levels, carnitine defiency is usually divided into two forms: a myopathic form and a systemic form. In the myopathic form, carnitine levels are decreased only in muscle tissue; in the systemic form, multiple tissues are affected, including muscle, liver, and plasma.[209] The systemic form presents in infancy or early childhood with episodes of hypoglycemia, ammonemia, acidemia, hepatomegaly, and EFE. A gene for primary systemic "carnitine" deficiency was recently mapped to chromosome 5q31.1-5q32,[210] the SCD locus. A murine model with juvenile visceral steatosis (*jvs*) has been identified[211] in which homozygotes have low serum total and free carnitine levels but no reduction in urinary excretion of carnitines.[212] This gene was mapped to the *jvs* locus on chromosome 11 of the mouse, which is syntenic to human 5q.[213] The human gene was recently found to be a novel sodium ion-dependent carnitine transporter, OCTN2.[214]

Therapy includes oral carnitine, occasionally reversing the cardiomyopathy. Additional therapy includes bicarbonate to reverse the acidemia, intravenous glucose, and anticongestive measures. Intercurrent illness commonly causes acute decompensation and death.

Medium Chain Acyl-CoA Dehydrogenase (MCAD) Deficiency

This disorder appears to be the most common inborn error of fatty acid oxidation, estimated to occur in one per 6000 to 10,000 live Caucasian births. It is characterized by recurrent episodes of illness, provoked by fasting more than 12 h, with the first episode generally occurring between 6 and 24 months of life. The most common symptoms include vomiting and severe lethargy that can progress to coma, as well as the less striking symptoms of muscle weakness and exercise intolerance. Hypoglycemia is often present between episodes, when patients appear normal. Hepatomegaly and DCM (rarely) are also seen. Liver biopsy can show marked fatty infiltrate ranging from predominantly microvesicular to a macrovesicular pattern. This autosomal recessive disorder was localized to chromosome 1p31 and human and rat MCAD cDNAs were cloned and sequenced.[215] The coding region is 1263 bp and encodes a precursor protein containing 421 amino acids. A variety of mutations have been reported. An A-to-G nucleotide replacement at position 985 of MCAD cDNA appears to be the most prevalent mutation responsible for MCAD deficiency (greater than 90 percent).[216] This deletion is predicted to result in a truncated protein of 385 amino acids instead of the normal 421–amino acid product. The common A-to-G 985 mutation appears to be due to a founder effect. Poor genotype-phenotype correlation exists.[217]

The therapy for these patients includes treatment of the acidosis and, when present, treatment of heart failure. Glucose therapy is indicated for hypoglycemia while intravenous fluids are needed during episodes of vomiting.

Long-Chain Acyl-CoA Dehydrogenase (LCAD) Deficiency/Very Long Chain Acyl-CoA Dehydrogenase (VLCAD) Deficiency

First described in 1985, LCAD manifests itself as recurrent episodes of coma, vomiting, and hypoglycemia triggered by fasting. Some patients have much more severe illness with notable involvement of cardiac and skeletal muscle.[28] Both DCM and HCM have been seen. Like MCAD, LCAD patients have secondary carnitine deficiency, and their fasting urine organic acid profile is abnormal, with low ketones and increased levels of dicarboxylic acids. The LCAD gene was identified[218] in 1991. In addition to the well-known β-oxidation enzymes in the mitochondrial matrix, there are two additional membrane-bound enzymes of β-oxidation.[219,220] One of these has been called "very long chain acyl-CoA dehydrogenase" (VLCAD), while the other is known as the "trifunctional protein." VLCAD is a membrane-bound homodimer with monomers of larger size than the other enzymes of the complex. It catalyzes the initial rate limiting step in mitochondrial fatty acid β-oxidation. The human VLCAD cDNA[221,222] and genomic sequence[210] were identified over the past several years, with multiple mutations subsequently identified.[224] Andresen et al.[225] recently showed that clear correlation of genotype with disease phenotype exists. Patients with severe childhood phenotype, which has a high incidence of cardiomyopathy and mortality, have mutations that result in no residual enzyme activity. Those with milder childhood and adult phenotypes have mutations that may result in residual enzyme activity. This clear genotype-phenotype correlation sharply contrasts that seen in MCAD deficiency, in which no correlation has been established. This new understanding of the mitochondrial β-oxidation pathway has led to new insights of the disorder once thought to be due to LCAD deficiency but now thought to be VLCAD deficiency.

Therapy for these patients includes aggressive treatment with glucose and hemodynamic support. When cardiac disease persists, chronic therapy for the dilated or hypertrophic heart disease should be instituted.

Fabry's Disease

An X-linked recessive disorder with complete penetrance and variable clinical expressivity, this entity is due to a deficiency of the enzyme α-galactosidase A, a lysosomal enzyme that participates in the catabolism of neutral glycosphingolipids, and is found in one in 40,000 live births. The disease frequently has its onset in adolescence and typically manifests with sensations of burning pain in the hands and feet. These sensations tend to be associated with fever, heat, cold, and exercise. Multiple angiokeratomas are noticeable with increasing age, with the umbilical area and genitalia the sites most commonly affected. Progressive renal failure develops with age, and CNS manifestations commonly include seizures, headaches, hemiplegia, and stroke. Corneal opacities are also frequently seen.

The cardiac manifestations of Fabry's disease generally appear in young adulthood. Aortic root dilation, dilated or hypertrophic cardiomyopathy,[226] valve dysfunction (especially mitral valve),[227] and myocardial infarction occur in these patients. Recently, association with tetralogy of Fallot was reported,[228] as was restrictive cardiomyopathy.[229] Electrocardiographic abnormalities commonly include atrial fibrillation, intraventricular conduction delay, right bundle-branch block, ST-T wave changes, short PR interval, and left ventricular hypertrophy. The short PR interval can progressively shorten over time probably secondary to lipid deposition in the atrioventricular node. Chamber thickness and mitral valve prolapse are evident on echocardiographic examination. Light microscopy shows lipid accumulation in nearly all cardiac tissue. Concentric lamellae are seen within cells and contain the neutral glycophospholipid. Therapy for these cardiac abnormalities does not differ from that typically used for HCM, myocardial ischemia or infarction, or mitral insufficiency found in patients without Fabry's disease. Recently, cardiac transplantation has been reported.[230]

The disease-causing gene, lysosomal-galactosidase A (GLA), is localized to Xq12.1-Xq12.2. The full-length cDNA has 1393 bp with a 60-nucleotide 5′ untranslated region, encoding for a precursor peptide of 429 amino acids.[231] The gene was found to contain seven exons. Mutations have been described[232,233] and genotype-phenotypic correlation performed. Mouse models have been developed which closely mimic the human disorder.[234] Antenatal and postnatal diagnosis is available. Therapy is symptomatic at present, but enzyme replacement therapy is likely in the future. Recently, gene transfer studies have been reported that correct the enzymatic and lysosomal storage defects in Fabry-like mice.[235]

Homocystinuria

Homocystinuria, inherited as an autosomal recessive defect, occurs with a frequency of 1 in 75,000. There is a deficiency of cystathionine β-synthase (CBS), which leads to elevated methionine in the blood and homocystine and methionine in the urine[236] (see Chaps. 39 and 41). In the homozygous individuals, major clinical features include a marfanoid habitus with a thin, tall body build and arachnodactyly, pectus excavatum, kyphoscoliosis, and osteoporosis. Subluxation of the lens, usually in a downward position, is frequently seen by 10 years of age, and myopia is common. Approximately 60 percent of affected individuals are mentally retarded to some degree. Schizophrenic behavior has also been noted in some patients. Cardiovascular abnormalities consist primarily of arterial and venous thrombosis (Table 62-5), with medial degeneration of the aorta and large arteries and intimal hyperplasia and fibrosis. It is estimated that about one-third of patients with familial homocystinuria will experience arterial or venous thrombosis. It is interesting that even within the same family with the same mutation there is marked variability among affected siblings.[237] The thrombotic episodes usually occur before the age of 30 years and include deep vein thrombosis, pulmonary embolism, and arterial thrombosis in the cerebral, peripheral, and coronary arteries.[237] However, when this disease occurs in individuals with other thrombogenic risk factors such as factor V Leiden,[238] the incidence of thrombosis, both arterial and venous, is significantly increased. An increased risk of cardiovascular disease has also been observed in carriers of the gene for homocystinuria. The gene was initially assigned to the subtelomeric region of band 21q22.3 by in situ hybridization studies.[239] Three types of cDNAs differing in both their translated and untranslated regions were isolated, with the resultant differences due to alternative splicing. The human gene was cloned and complete-sequence, alternatively spliced forms, and mutations described.[240] Numerous mutations have now been identified and correlated with the phenotype. The gene is 28 kb in size, contains 23 exons, and contains many *alu* repeat sequences which predisposes the gene to rearrangements.[241] The defect can be treated in some cases by pyridoxine supplementation. The percentage of pyridoxine responders ranges between 13 and 47 percent. Betaine, low-methionine diet, and aspirin treatments have also been tried with varying success. Prenatal diagnosis is available by an enzyme assay and gene analysis. Recently, tandem spectrometry has been used in the diagnosis.[241]

Homocystinuria, while a rare disease, has received increased attention recently because of several studies indicating that homocysteine is an important and independent risk factor for atherosclerosis and thrombosis.[242,243] In one such study performed recently, of 269 patients with the first episode of deep vein thrombosis, 10 percent had elevated plasma homocysteine levels, compared with 4 percent in 269 matched controls.[243] Homocystinuria results from impaired enzyme activity in the metabolism of cobalamin, but may also occur from a deficiency of vitamin B_6, folate, or vitamin B_{12}. The mechanism whereby homocysteine induces atherosclerosis is postulated to be through induction of the cyclin A gene which induces vascular smooth muscle proliferation, a major component of atherosclerosis.[244] The mechanism whereby homocysteine induces thrombosis is probably through its known effect on activation of factor V in endothelial cells, inhibition of protein C, and decreased antithrombin III activity. It remains somewhat controversial as to how common hyperhomocysteinemia is as a risk factor for atherosclerosis and/or thrombosis. It is, however, very important to exclude hyperhomocysteinemia in patients with vascular disease such as myocardial infarction, strokes, or systemic thrombosis, particularly if these are occurring prematurely or there are no other risk factors, since, in the acquired form, the condition is relatively easy to treat by the administration of vitamins.

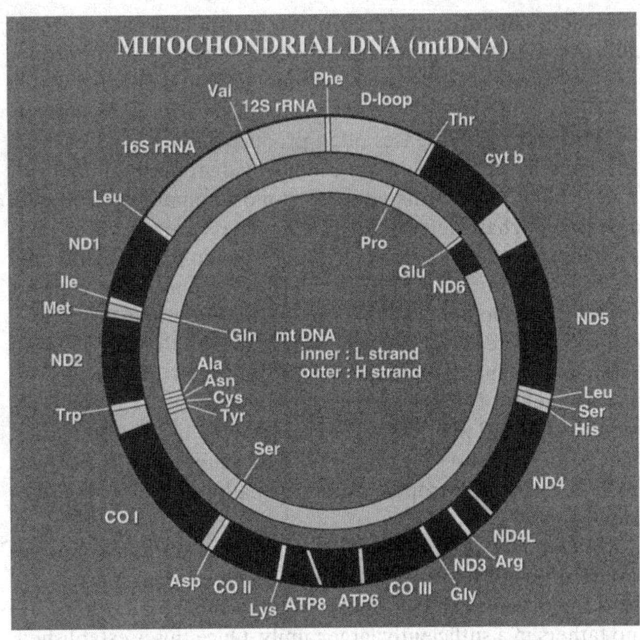

FIGURE 62-11 Mitochondrial genome. This small, circular DNA molecule encodes 13 enzymes of the respiratory chain, 22 tRNAs, and 2 rRNAs. When it is mutated, cardiac, neurologic, and myopathic disorders develop.

Mitochondrial Cardiomyopathies

The human mitochondrial genome[245] is a small, circular DNA molecule (Fig. 62-11) that is maternally inherited. Mitochondrial DNA (mtDNA) encodes 13 of the 69 proteins required for oxidative metabolism, 22 transfer RNAs (tRNAs), and 2 ribosomal RNAs (rRNAs) required for their translation. Since mtDNA has much less redundancy than the nuclear genome (in which essentially identical information is received from both parents), and tRNAs and rRNAs are present in multiple copies, the mitochondrial genome is an excellent target for mutations giving rise to human disease.[246,247] Mitochondria are dependent on nucleocytoplasmic mechanisms for most structural components, but do contribute vital peptides that are central to cellular respiration. The electron transport chain, which generates cellular ATP, is organized into complexes I to IV and the ATP synthase (complex V) (Fig. 62-12). The 13 mtDNA genes that encode enzymes in the respiratory chain include 7 complex I[246,248] subunits (ND1, 2, 3, 4L, 4, 5, and 6); 1 complex III subunit (cytochrome b); 3 complex IV subunits (COI, II, III); and 2 complex V subunits (ATPase 6 and 8). Each cell contains numerous mitochondria and each mitochondrion contains multiple copies of mtDNA. In most mitochondrial

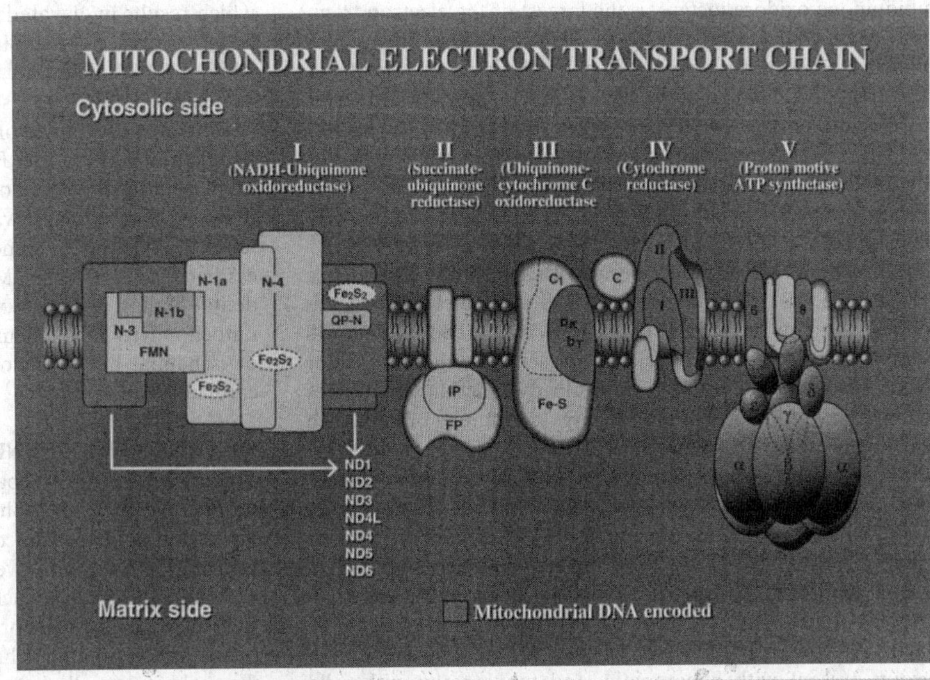

FIGURE 62-12 The electron transport chain enzyme complex (complexes I to V).

disorders, patients carry a mix of mutant and normal mitochondria—a condition known as *heteroplasmy,* with the proportions varying from tissue to tissue and individual to individual within a pedigree, in a manner correlating with severity of phenotype.

Mitochondrial diseases often produce disturbances of brain and muscle function and are usually evident during infancy or early childhood. Cardiac disease is most commonly seen with respiratory chain defects. Ragged-red fibers are present in muscle biopsy specimens almost invariably when the molecular defect involves mtDNA.[249] These defects represent the genetics of ATP production. The diverse clinical syndromes associated with various respiratory chain complexes are thought to result from involvement of tissue-specific isoforms in some cases, involvement of tissue-nonspecific (generalized) subunits in other cases, and the residual enzyme activity in affected tissues. The cardiac diseases seen associated with mitochondrial defects include both hypertrophic cardiomyopathy and dilated cardiomyopathy.[246]

Mitochondrial gene mapping, in contrast to the nuclear genome, does not require genetic linkage. One simply has to show that the disease exhibits transmission through all mothers and no fathers in a sufficiently large family. Once this is established, the mitochondrial genome can be sequenced to identify the mutation, which must be shown to segregate with the disease since there are many harmless polymorphisms.

Therapy for these disorders is generally symptom-based. Conduction disturbance generally requires placement of a permanent pacemaker, and heart failure is treated with the usual therapy. In some patients, beta-blockers may be useful. Hypertrophic heart disease is usually treated in a fashion similar to that of other forms of HCM. Mitochondrial-based therapy may include coenzyme Q10, carnitine, or vitamins, but these therapeutic approaches typically do not alter the clinical course.

COMPLEX I DEFICIENCY

Complex I, or nicotinamide adenine dinucleotide (NADH): ubiquinone oxidoreductase, is the largest of the electron transport chain complexes[250,251] (Fig. 62-12) with at least 35 complex I nuclear gene products and 7 mitochondrially encoded proteins. It is embedded in the inner mitochondrial membrane and serves to dehydrogenate NADH and shuttle electrons to coenzyme Q. This electron transport generates a protein gradient across the inner mitochondrial membrane, helping to synthesize ATP. When complex I abnormalities occur, significant health problems arise.

Mitochondriocytopathies occur with an estimated incidence of 1 per 10,000 live births, and isolated complex I deficiency is one of those most frequently encountered.[248] The first clinical symptoms of complex I deficiency, presenting either at birth or in early childhood, result from brain dysfunction, sometimes combined with defects in other energy-consuming organs, such as skeletal muscle and the heart. For this reason, complex I deficiencies are grouped among the mitochondrial encephalomyopathies.

Robinson[248] categorized complex I–deficient patients into three major clinical groups. The most common presentation is Leigh syndrome, with cardiomyopathy occuring in about 40 percent of cases.[252] A second category often seen is fatal neonatal lactic acidosis (MELAS—see below). A third but uncommon group present with hepatopathy and tubulopathy with mild symptoms, such as exercise intolerance, or with cataracts and cardiomyopathy. The most frequently observed pathologic mtDNA mutations are found in genes for mitochondrial tRNAs for leucine (T3271C, A3243G) and lysine (A8344G, T8356C) and in the protein-encoding subunits ND1 (T4160A, G3460A), ND4 (G11778A), and ND6 (T14484C, G14459A).

Treatment of these disorders is limited. Riboflavin, succinate supplements (since the metabolite enters the respiratory chain at complex II), ubiquonone, and idebanone have been recommended for therapy in patients with MELAS. Carnitine and coenzyme Q10 have also been used.

COMPLEX III DEFECTS

This results in a myopathic or multisystem disorder. Cardiomyopathy has been found both alone or in conjunction with skeletal myopathy. Encephalomyopathy also presents with retinopathy, ataxia, spasticity, dementia, weakness, sensorineural hearing loss, and exercise intolerance.

COMPLEX IV DEFECTS

This abnormality is similar clinically to complex I defects. The mitochondrial genome encodes for three subunits of cytochrome C oxidase, which represents the terminal portion of the respiratory chain (Fig. 62-12) and catalyzes conversion of molecular oxygen to water. A benign reversible infantile myopathy which normalizes by early childhood may occur, as may a fatal infantile myopathy manifested by profound weakness, hypotonia, respiratory insufficiency, and death. This myopathy may occur alone, or in association with severe renal tubular dysfunction or cardiomyopathy with red ragged fibers.

HYPOXEMIA, mtDNA DAMAGE, AND CARDIAC DISEASE

Since cardiac tissue relies on mitochondrial oxidative phosphorylation (ox-phos) for energy production, deficiency of portions of this system or its end-product may cause cardiac abnormalities.[248] Hypoxemia can increase oxygen radical production, which results in elevated mtDNA damage and altered ox-phos gene expression. In addition, these enzymes decline with age while mtDNA deletions increase with age, especially deletion at nucleotide 4977 bp. Ischemic hearts may be more likely to have increased chances of mtDNA deletion due to the effect of hypoxemia[253] and, using PCR amplification across the deletion breakpoint of the common mtDNA4977 deletion, it was found that mtDNA damage was increased in chronically ischemic hearts, as well as in some hearts with other forms of chronic cardiac disease (i.e., DCM, HCM), but this is probably an incidental finding and has no effect on cardiac function. Similarly, mitochondrial DNA damage increases with age independent of ischemia, but it is doubtful whether it in any way alters cardiac function.

KEARNS-SAYRE SYNDROME (KSS)

This mitochondrial myopathy is characterized by ptosis, chronic progressive external ophthalmoplegia, abnormal retinal pigmentation, and cardiac conduction defects as well as DCM.[255] Hearing loss and limb weakness are frequently associated, as are endocrinopathies such as diabetes mellitus, hypoparathyroidism, and growth hormone deficiency. Approximately 20 percent of KSS patients have cardiac involvement and of these, the majority usually have conduction defects causing progressive heart block (Table 62-7). These patients generally have large heterogeneous deletions in the mitochondrial genome, of which tRNA$^{leu(UUR)}$-3243 is most common.

Clinically, conduction abnormalities, bifascicular block, or progressive high-grade block may define the requirement for permanent pacemaker implantation. Symptomatic improvement using mitochondrial therapies may occasionally be seen with coenzyme Q10 therapy. The major function of coenzyme Q10 in mitochondria is to shuttle electrons from complexes I and II to complex III, while stabilizing the respiratory chain complexes. Vitamins such as phylloquinone (vitamin K_1), menadione (vitamin K_3), and ascorbic acid (vitamin C) have been used to donate electrons directly to cytochrome *c*. In addition, the endocrine abnormalities and heart failure should be treated in the usual way.

MERRF SYNDROME

This syndrome is characterized by *m*yoclonic *e*pilepsy with *r*agged-*r*ed muscle *f*ibers (MERRF) and is caused by a single nucleotide substitution in tRNA^{Lys}, which apparently interferes with mitochondrial translation.[256] The defining clinical features are myoclonus, generalized seizures, ataxia, and hypertrophic cardiomyopathy. Skeletal muscle biopsy demonstrates ragged-red fibers on microscopy. Symptoms usually begin in childhood, but adult onset has been described. Other common manifestations include impaired hearing, demential neuropathy, short stature, optic atrophy, lactic acidosis, and lipomas.

Shoffner et al.[256] showed an A-to-G transition mutation (position 8344) as the cause of the disease and associated with defects in complexes I and IV. This abnormality causes decline in ATP-generating capacity, with a resultant cardiomyopathy. Other reports have outlined various disease-causing mutations. Therapy is similar to other mitochondrial myopathies; anticonvulsant medications may also be indicated.

MELAS SYNDROME

*M*itochondrial *e*ncephalomypathy and *l*actic *a*cidosis with *s*troke-like episodes (MELAS) is clinically characterized by stroke before age 40 years; encephalopathy with seizures, dementia, or both; and lactic acidosis, ragged-red fibers, or both.[257] Recurrent headaches and recurrent vomiting are common. Other frequent manifestations include exercise intolerance, limb weakness, short stature, and elevated CSF protein. Hypertrophic cardiomyopathy or dilated cardiomyopathy may occur.

Variable respiratory chain defects have been described, but complex I abnormalities are most common. Between 80 and 90 percent of patients have an adenine-to-guanine point mutation in tRNA$^{Leu(UUR)}$ at position 3243. Therapy is similar to that described for MERRF.

THERAPY

Medical therapy for mitochondrial disorders has been disappointing and for that reason newer approaches have been sought. As most pathologic mtDNA mutations are heteroplasmic and there is a threshold whereby a certain level of mutated mtDNA is necessary before a disease becomes biochemically or clinically apparent, any approach that increases the proportion of wild-type to mutated mtDNA will reverse the phenotype and thus be a potentially useful treatment. When there is an extremely high level of the pathogenetic mutation in cells, as occurs with muscle necrosis, these necrotic cells form regenerated muscle. Clark et al.[258] took advantage of this phenomenon by inducing necrosis and regeneration in muscle by performing a muscle biopsy, which resulted in the absence of mutated mtDNA in the biopsied muscle. Due to the invasiveness of this approach, reduced utility of the therapy is anticipated unless other methods of inducing necrosis can be developed.

More recently, Taivassalo et al.[259] developed a novel therapy that they called *gene shifting,* which is similar to that described by Clark et al.[258] These authors enhanced the incorporation of new (satellite) cells through regeneration following injury or muscle hypertrophy induced by eccentric or concentric resistance exercise training. They were able to show a remarkable increase in the ratio of wild-type to mutant mtDNAs, and in the proportion of muscle fibers with normal respiratory chain activity. This work suggests that it might be possible to reverse the molecular events that led to the expression of metabolic myopathy and demonstrates that this form of "gene shifting" therapy could be effective.

Connective Tissue Disorders

The composition, structure, and function of normal and abnormal connective tissues are gradually being elucidated[260,261] (see Chap. 85). The annuli fibrosis that separate the atria and ventricles and support the two atrioventricular valves are largely type I collagen fiber bundles, while the blood vessel walls are elastin and collagen types I and III (50 percent), with lesser contributions from types IV, V, and VI collagen. Elastin in located at 7q11; collagen 1A1, at 17q21.13-17q22.05; collagen 1A2, at 7q21.3-7q22.1; collagen 2A1, at 12q13.1-12q13.3; collagen 3A1, at 2q31; and collagen 5A2, at 2q31.

MARFAN SYNDROME

Marfan syndrome is a heritable disorder of connective tissue caused by a defect in fibrillin protein encoded by the fibrillin-1 gene on chromosome 15 at 15q15-q20 (see Chap. 98). The Marfan syndrome occurs in approximately 1 in 10,000 individuals and is equally common in males and females. There is marked variation in clinical expression, and the diagnosis can be made at any age from the newborn period through adulthood.[263] Because of the variability in expression, overlap with nonpathologic features (such as tall stature) can be observed in the general population. Since fibrillin[264] is diffuse, Marfan syndrome affects skeletal, ocular, cardiovascular, skin, pulmonary, and central nervous system.[260,261] The skeletal manifestations of Marfan syndrome include tall stature, thin body build, long arms and legs (dolichostenomelia), long fingers and toes (arachnodactyly), hyperextensibility, pectus deformity, scoliosis, joint contractures, and narrow, high-arched palate. Cardiovascular abnormalities, particularly affecting the mitral apparatus and aorta, are also common. There may also be overlap with other disorders that share some of the same phenotypic features, such as the condition termed *congenital contractual arachnodactyly* (CCA).[265] Clinical manifestations of CCA include dolichostenomelia and arachnodactyly, contractures of large joints, and abnormal pinnae formation. In 1990, Marfan syndrome was mapped to the long arm of chromosome 15(15q15q-q20).[266] Subsequently, a defect in the gene for fibrillin-1 (FBN1)[267] was found to be the cause of Marfan syndrome. This large glycoprotein has a molecular weight of 350 kDa[264] and is a component of microfibrils that are ubiquitous in the connective frequently occurs or increases during adolescence. The mRNA transcript of this gene is approximately 10 kb. Not only do defects in this gene cause Marfan syndrome, but Milewicz and Duvic[268] also showed that severe neonatal Marfan syndrome is due to a specific 3-bp insertion in the fibrillin-1 cDNA. Furthermore, fibrillin defects have been found in patients with atypical phenotypes including autosomal dominant ectopia lentis with skeletal features[269] and milder forms such as the MASS phenotype (mitral valve, aorta, skeleton, and skin)[269] or isolated ascending aortic aneurysm with dissection.[270,271] Unfortunately, each family appears to have an individual mutation in the gene, making screening difficult and requiring that each new mutation case be studied individually.[272] This high impact disorder is estimated to be responsible for 1 to 2 percent of the deaths in industrialized societies, with death usually caused by rupture of an asymptomatic, undiagnosed aneurysm. Mutations in FBN1 also have been associated with the marfanoid craniosynostosis (Shprintzen-Goldberg) syndrome.[273] Recent data suggest that CCA is a separate disorder due to a fibrillin-2 gene (FBN2) defect on chromosome 5 (5q23-q31).[274]

Another locus for Marfan syndrome has also been mapped to 3p24.2-p25.[275] Marfan syndrome has been observed in all racial and ethnic groups, and approximately 55 percent are sporadic cases with no family history. There appears to be an increased effect of paternal age, with the mean age of fathers of sporadic cases being increased.

Some of the skeletal features can be analyzed anthropometrically. For example, the increased limb length can be measured by the length of the upper and lower segments and by the upper-lower segment ratio (US/UL). The lower segment is measured from the top of the pubic ramus to the floor, and the upper segment is measured from the pubic ramus to the top of the head. US/UL is reduced for classic Marfan syndrome at all ages. The ratio of arm span to height is usually increased in Marfan syndrome, although scoliosis may complicate the calculation of both ratios. Arachnodactyly can be assessed by the ratio of the middle finger length to total hand length or by analysis of the metacarpal index on hand radiographs.

Hyperextensibility can be assessed by several simple maneuvers. The Steinberg (thumb) sign is positive when the thumb projects through the clenched hand on the ulnar side. The Walker-Murdock (wrist) sign is positive when the first and fifth digit of one hand wrap completely around the wrist of the other hand. Pectus excavatum of variable severity is fairly common. Scoliosis can occur at any age. The ocular findings of Marfan syndrome classically include subluxation of the lenses (ectopia lentis), usually but not always in an upward direction. This occurs in 50 to 60 percent of patients. Myopia is very common, and retinal detachments have also occurred, especially after surgical removal of the lenses. Corneal flattening is also described. Loss of vision occurs in a significant number of patients. Other manifestations include an increase in the occurrence of inguinal hernias, which may recur, and the development of spontaneous pneumothorax and lung abnormalities in some patients. Sacral meningoceles and dilated cisterna magna have also been reported. A severe neonatal form of the Marfan syndrome has cardiovascular, skeletal, and ocular complications present at birth,[261] and patients typically succumb within the first year of life, often from congestive heart failure.

The majority of cardiac abnormalities associated with Marfan syndrome affect the ascending aorta, the aortic valve, and the mitral valve (Table 62-6). Physical examination alone is insufficient to detect subtle changes in the heart and in the aorta. The dilation of the ascending aorta may occur gradually before physical findings occur. Echocardiograms are recommended annually and beta-blocker therapy should be considered.[276] If the diameter of the aorta corrected for body surface area exceeds the upper limits of normal by 50 percent, the frequency of evaluations should be increased to at least every 6 months. Prophylactic repair with composite graft including aortic valve should be performed when ascending aortic dilation reaches a diameter of 6 cm[277] (see Chap. 98). Repair of a severe pectus excavatum may be indicated at an earlier stage, not only for cosmetic reasons, but to allow easier and safer aortic surgery, should it be indicated. After surgery, the use of beta blockers and anticoagulants should be maintained, and individuals should avoid contact sports and marked physical exertion. Surveillance of the aorta should continue after surgery. Some evidence suggests that beta blockers may reduce the rate of aortic dilation and the risk of serious complications.[276] Prophylactic antibiotics should be used on all patients to decrease the risk of bacterial endocarditis. In general, contact sports (e.g., football, basketball) should be avoided—along with isometric exercises, weight lifting, and extreme physical activity—and replaced with noncompetitive sports such as swimming and bicycling. Other abnormalities include mitral valve prolapse, mitral regurgitation, and aortic regurgitation. The cardiovascular abnormalities in neonatal Marfan syndrome differs somewhat from that seen in older patients, demonstrating significant mitral regurgitation as well as tricuspid and pulmonary valve regurgitation. In addition, these children have significant heart failure, as previously noted.

A special issue involves Marfan syndrome and pregnancy (see Chap. 92). In addition to the 50 percent recurrence risk in offspring, there is also a concern about the stress that pregnancy will put on the aorta. There are at least two dozen case reports of aortic dissection during pregnancy or shortly after delivery,[278] generally occurring with aortic regurgitation or other evidence of aortic dilatation. Pregnant women with Marfan syndrome should have echocardiograms every 6 to 8 weeks during pregnancy and should be followed as high-risk obstetrical patients.

The diagnosis of Marfan syndrome is currently made primarily on clinical grounds although molecular diagnosis is now feasible (although not useful).[279] Suspected patients with a positive family history should have positive clinical features in at least two organ systems. If the family history is negative for Marfan syndrome, positive findings should be present in the skeletal system and in at least two other organ systems. Suspected patients should also have a negative urine nitroprusside test to rule out homocystinuria, one of the disorders in the differential diagnosis. Management of patients with a negative family history and only suggestive skeletal features is unclear. In view of its implications, it may be unwise to inform such patients with minimal features that they have Marfan syndrome. Nonetheless, they should be followed clinically with perhaps periodic echocardiograms and ophthalmologic exams. In these individuals, strong consideration for molecular genetic evaluation is wise.

In terms of genetic counseling, families should be informed of the autosomal dominant inheritance pattern, with 50 percent recurrence in offspring. The rationale for patient follow-up and management should also be explained, along with psychosocial support and medical follow-up. Prenatal diagnosis may be possible.[263,268]

EHLERS-DANLOS SYNDROMES

There are at least 11 different forms of Ehlers-Danlos syndrome (EDS), which are generally given numerical designations.[279] The most common forms are types I through IV, as discussed here. Types II and III overlap with the features of type I, but both are progressively less severe; type III is sometimes known as *benign hypermobility syndrome*. The features of Ehlers-Danlos type I include hyperextensible and fragile skin with poor wound healing and "cigarette paper" scarring. Hyperextensibility of the joints increases susceptibility to dislocation of the hips, shoulders, elbows, knees, and clavicles. The ears tend to be hypermobile and are sometimes described as "lop ears." Scoliosis is a relatively common finding, as are clubfeet in infancy. There is an increased risk of premature birth resulting from premature rupture of membranes. Umbilical and diaphragmatic hemias tend to be relatively common.

The most common cardiac features include mitral valve prolapse, tricuspid valve prolapse, and dilation of the aortic root and/or sinus of Valsalva.[279] Atrial septal defects and other abnormalities of the aortic arch and mitral valve have also been seen. Probably the most significant cardiovascular defect is the increased susceptibility to dissecting aortic aneurysm (Table 62-6), which can lead to death. Poor wound healing and decreased vascular integrity have been noted. Surgical procedures are freqeuntly not tolerated well, and patients should probably avoid unnecessary surgery. In addition, patients should be cautioned to avoid tauma as much as possible. Type I Ehlers-Danlos is inherited as an autosomal dominant disorder with variability in expression. The presumed defect in this disorder involves synthesis of normal collagen with mutations identified in the $\alpha 2$ (V) chain of type V collagen.[279,280]

Ehlers-Danlos type IV is sometimes referred to as the "malignant" form of Ehlers-Danlos syndrome,[281] since there is marked susceptibility to spontaneous rupture of large blood vessels or bowel. The hyperelasticity and hyperextensibility tend to be less obvious than in type I. Easy bruisability and susceptibility to bleeding, however, are very prominent. Spontaneous rupture of any of the major vessels has been reported. Pregnancy-related complications are particularly striking, the overall risk of death with pregnancy being 25 percent. The basic defect in this autosomal dominant disorder is in the type III collagen gene located on chromosome 2 (2q31),[282] and defects have been reported.[283] Other Ehlers-Danlos genes thus far identified include types VI (1p36.3-1p36.2; lysyl hydroxylase),[284,285] VII A1 (17q21.31-q22), and VII A2 (7q22.1),[286] with mutations of the COLIA2 gene,[281] and the progeroid variant,[287] which is caused by galactosyl-transferase mutations.

Patients with types I and IV EDS require yearly cardiac examinations. Initial evaluation with chest radiography and echocardiography will enable the cardiologist to decide the frequency of follow-up and repeat echocardiograms depending on the level of aortic dilatation and mitral valve prolapse (MVP). Annual chest x-rays are cost-effective as a minimal approach, with echocardiograms necessary every 1 to 2 years. Antibiotic prophylaxis for subacute bacterial endocarditis (SBE) is also needed in patients with MVP or aortic abnormalities.

FAMILIAL ANEURYSMS

It has been recognized for some time that certain aneurysms in peripheral and central arteries (see Marfan's syndrome above) have a familial tendency.[288] As data accumulates on genetic defects in fibrillin[261,279] (Marfan's syndrome) and in the collagen disorders,[289,290] there appears to be overlap in the genetic defects of fibrilin and procollagen, particularly type III, as causes for aneurysms. Some have a defect in type II procollagen (COL3A1) similar to defects that have been reported in Ehlers-Danlos syndrome (EDS) type IV.[283] Familial incidence of aneurysms is said to account for 7 percent of aneurysms.[291] Since EDS is relatively rare, many of the more common familial procollagen abnormalities may represent phenotypic overlap. These findings have resulted in a reassessment of the traditional teaching that most aortic aneurysms result from atherosclerosis. Family history should be carefully assessed in all patients with aortic or cerebral aneurysms, and, if it is positive, other family members should be assessed. Many should be followed with noninvasive evaluation in a fashion similar to that described for Marfan's syndrome.

PSEUDOXANTHOMA ELASTICUM (PXE)

This is a genetic disease of the elastic tissue which involves the skin, eyes, and cardiovascular system.[292] The characteristic lesion is that of the skin consisting of a highly raised, yellowish papule known as a *pseudoxanthoma,* overlying areas of flexural stress such as the neck, cubital and popliteal fossae, and groin. The eye changes are slate-gray linear bands representing tears in Bruch's membrane and subsequent fibrosis leading to loss of central vision in 70 to 80 percent of cases. Calcification of peripheral arteries occurs frequently, most commonly in the femoral artery, but also in the coronary arteries. The heart is affected by myocardial ischemia and infarction, secondary to the coronary disease, which is the major cause of morbidity and mortality (Table 62-5). A restrictive cardiomyopathy is common due to endocardial fibrosis with mitral valve prolapse (MVP).[293,294] Two genetic variants having autosomal dominant inheritance and two others with autosomal recessive inheritance occur. The only difference between the recessive and dominant forms is the presence of affected parents and offspring. Bale recently mapped a gene to 16p13.1, but the gene remains unknown.[281] Because the basic defect is unknown, no specific treatment is available.

The cardiac features should be followed closely once abnormalities are noted. In stable patients, yearly examinations are required at a minimum. Myocardial dysfunction with or without heart failure requires anticongestive and inotropic support, while SBE prophylaxis is needed for those patients with MVP. Symptoms should be used to direct therapy.

CUTIS LAXA

This designation refers not only to a specific dermatologic sign but also to a variety of mendelian and nonmendelian congenital and acquired syndromes sharing the characteristic feature of lax, nonresilient skin. Two varieties of autosomal recessive cutis laxa exist. Death from pulmonary complications may occur in the first months of life and most patients die by the third year. Signs of right-sided heart failure are often seen in infancy and are generally due to pulmonary disease, although pulmonary artery stenosis also occurs[295] (Table 62-5). Histopathologically, the pulmonary artery lesions are due to medioelastic fiber paucity. MVP has also been notable. A gene that causes this spectrum of disease has been identified as elastin (ELN), the same gene previously shown to cause supravalvular aortic stenosis (SVAS).[296–298] As increased fibroblast activity in acquired cutis laxa has also been noted,[299] there is molecular and biochemical correlation. In addition, ultrastructural alterations of skin elastic fibers has been reported.[300]

Primary Disorders of Rhythm and Conduction

Virtually all rhythm and conduction abnormalities have been reported to be familial. However, many families have been small so that the mode of inheritance (or even whether the inheritance is mendelian) is uncertain. In many cases, these conduction defects have been associated with other cardiac and systemic disorders. For a detailed clinical discussion of arrhythmia and conduction disorders, see Chap. 27.

ROMANO-WARD LONG-QT SYNDROME (LQTS)

The association of stress-induced syncope, sudden death, and ventricular arrhythmias in families has long been noted, including a distinct syndrome[301] having prolongation of the QT interval and abnormal T waves on ECG. Multiple families with this syndrome have demonstrated autosomal dominant inheritance, with torsade de pointes polymorphic ventricular tachycardia, bradycardia and T-wave alternans (see Chap. 36). The diagnosis is made when the QT interval corrected for heart rate (QTc) is greater than 480 ms using Bazzett's formula; T-wave abnormalities are usually seen. In symptomatic patients (i.e., patients with syncope or "seizures"), the diagnosis may be made with shorter QTc (i.e., 470 ms). A diagnostic algorithm has been useful.[302] Two likely hypothetical pathogenetic mechanisms for Romano-Ward LQTS was proposed by Schwartz.[303] They include (1) sympathetic nervous system abnormalities and (2) potassium channel (or other ion channel) abnormalities.

In 1991, Keating and coworkers[304] provided evidence for tight molecular genetic linkage to chromosome 11p (11p15.5). Shortly thereafter, Towbin and colleagues demonstrated genetic heterogeneity in families with Romano-Ward LQTS.[305] Linkage evidence was found for loci on chromosome 7 (LQT2)[301] and chromosome 3 (LQT3) and another gene was linked to chromosome 4 (LQT4).[301] More recently, two other genes have been mapped for LQT5 and LQT6, both found on chromosome 21q22.[306]

The chromosome 11–linked (LQT1) gene was discovered to be KCNQ1, which encodes a potassium channel known as KVLQT1,[301] the slowly activated, delayed rectifier potassium channel I_{Ks}. Multiple mutations in KVLQT1 have been identified and this gene appears to be the most commonly mutated gene in LQTS. KVLQT1 was later shown to require a β-subunit to function normally. This β-subunit gene, KCNE1, encodes minK, which regulates the function of these combined channels, resulting in normal function of this slowly activated delayed rectifier potassium (I_{Ks}) channel. This gene, now also called LQT5, maps to chromosome 21q22. Mutations in either KVLQT1 or minK result in LQTS. The HERG gene, an I_{Kr} potassium channel, has been mapped to chromosome 7q35-q36 and mutations in a variety of domains of this channel were shown to be responsible for the disease in LQT2 families.[301] Another channel gene, the cardiac sodium channel called SCN5A, mapped to 3p21, was shown to be responsible for LQT3. Recently, LQT6 was discovered by Abbott and coworkers[306] to be the β-subunit, MiRP1 or KCNE2. This small channel protein regulates I_{Kr}, the rapidly activated delayed rectifier potassium channel, by interacting with HERG. Mutations in either MiRP1 or HERG result in the LQTS phenotype although the mutations in MiRP1 have been shown to also cause drug-induced (i.e., clarithromycin) VT or VF. The chromosome 4-linked (LQT4) gene remains undiscovered presently. The long-QT syndrome, therefore, appears to be an ion channelopathy, and multiple different ion-channel mutations could result in the long-QT syndrome (Fig. 62-13).

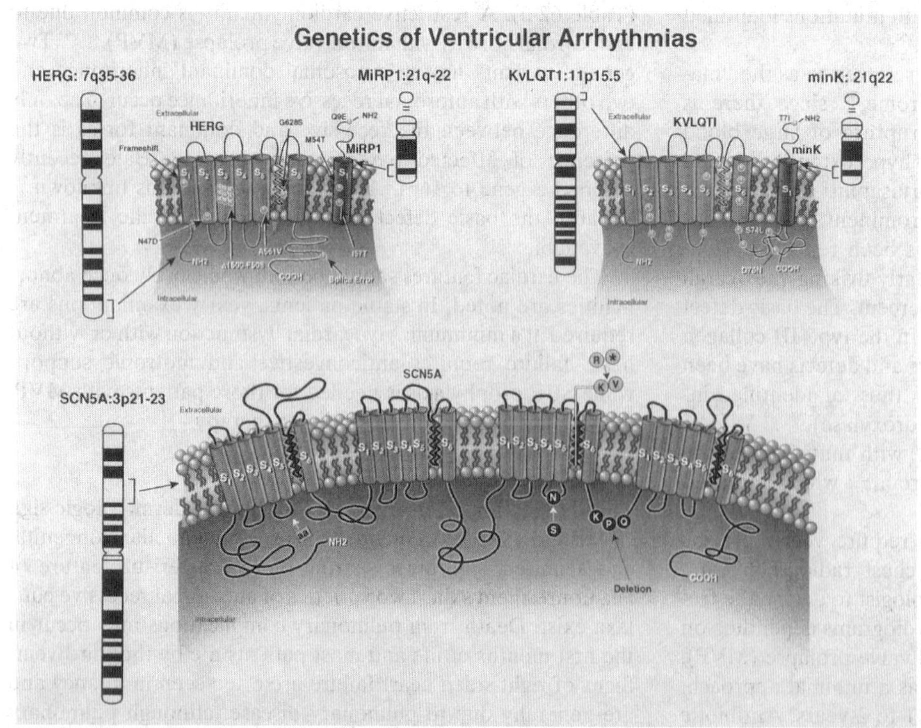

FIGURE 62-13 Genetic loci and ion channels encoded by the genes responsible for long-QT syndrome.

Phenotype-genotype studies have been reported in LQTS. Distinct ECG differences between patients have been demonstrated with mutations of different genes (LQT1-LQT3).[307] Important prognostic differences appear to occur with various mutations of the different genes.[301,308] Zareba et al.[308] recently provided genotype-phenotype correlation of mutations in LQT1, LQT2, and LQT3. In this study, mutations in LQT1 and LQT2 resulted in earlier onset of syncope than LQT3 (usually by age 15 years) and more frequent episodes of syncope. However,

LQT3 patients appeared to be at higher risk of death than either LQT1 or LQT2. The mode of symptoms and death also appears to be gene-specific to some extent. LQT1 mutations have been associated with episodes of syncope, seizures, or sudden death during diving/swimming or emotional upset. LQT2 also appears to be triggered by emotions but auditory triggers (i.e., phone or alarm clock ringing) are also important. LQT3, on the other hand, has a high incidence of events during sleep. LQT3 patients appear to shorten their QT intervals with exercise, while exercise seems to trigger events in LQT1 and LQT2 patients.

Recently, Schwartz et al.[309] have provided evidence that sudden infant death syndrome (SIDS) could be due to QT prolongation. Using ECGs on the third or fourth day of life in over 34,000 infants over a >20 year period, they found 34 infants died prior to their first birthday. In 24 of these cases, SIDS was diagnosed. Retrospective ECG analysis demonstrated that one-half of these infants had QTc prolongation on the initial screening ECG. Although no molecular analysis exists, it is speculated that ion channel mutations could be at play for a group of children with SIDS.[309,310]

Gene based therapy has been reported to improve the ECG features of LQTS, including QTc shortening and T-wave normalization. Schwartz et al.[311] treated patients with LQT2 and LQT3 with the sodium channel blocker mexiletine and showed significant QTc shortenting. Compton et al.[312] used exogenous potassium to increase the serum potassium in LQT2 patients with QTc shortening noted, while Shimizu et al.[313] used potassium channel openers to achieve similar results. However, no long-term results or outcomes have been reported with any of these therapies.

JERVELL AND LANGE-NIELSEN LONG-QT SYNDROME

This syndrome, described in 1957, is characterized by congenital deafness, syncope, prolonged QT interval, sudden death, and autosomal recessive inheritance[301] (see Chap. 36). Affected individuals are usually diagnosed in childhood with congenital, severe high-tone perceptive bilateral deafness; fainting spells precipitated by exertion, rage or fright; and ECG evidence of QT interval prolongation and T-wave abnormalities. As would be expected for rare autosomal recessive traits, the parents of affected individuals are more likely than usual to be consanguineous. Homozygous mutations or compound heterozygous mutations in either KVLQT1 or *minK* (i.e., I_{Ks}) have been shown to result in Jervell and Lange-Nielsen syndrome.[314–317] In this circumstance, the deafness requires a homozygous mutation, which results in abnormal production of endolymph, a potassium-rich fluid, in the inner ear. Thus, deafness is autosomal recessive while LQTS is autosomal dominant (i.e., heterozygous mutation results in LQTS; homozygous mutation results in longer QTc and worse outcome).

BRUGADA SYNDROME (IDIOPATHIC VENTRICULAR FIBRILLATION)

First described in detail in 1992, the Brugada syndrome is characterized by ST-segment elevation in leads V_1–V_3, with or without right bundle-branch block[318,319] (Fig. 62-14). Clinical symptoms occur due to ventricular fibrillation. In many patients, spontaneous resuscitation occurs. In others, sudden death occurs, particularly during sleep. This disorder appears to be relatively common in Europe and Southeast Asia and commonly is

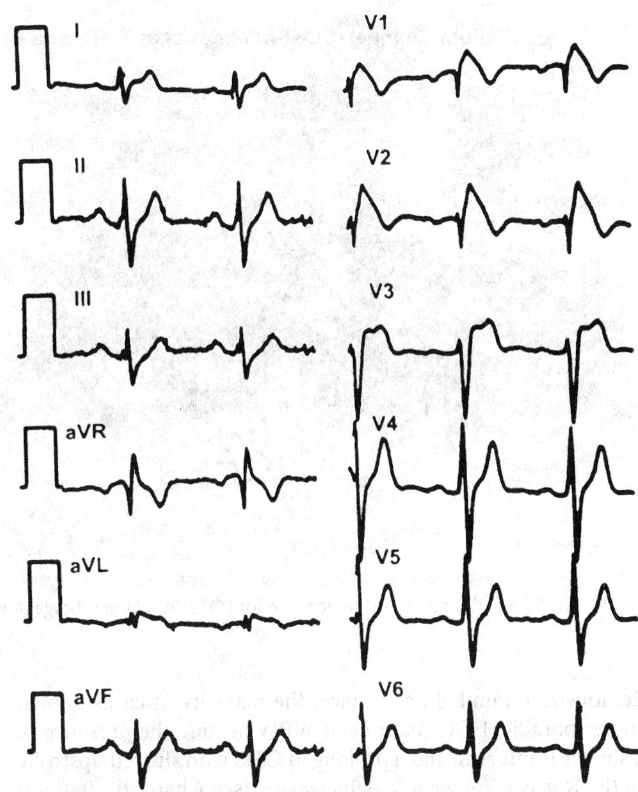

FIGURE 62-14 Electrocardiographic characteristics of Brugada syndrome. Note the ST-segment elevation in V_1 to V_3.

familial, usually with autosomal dominant inheritance.[320] Some patients do not have overt ECG manifestations and provocation studies in the catheterization laboratory using procainamide, flecainide, or ajmaline may be necessary for diagnosis.

The genetics of Brugada syndrome appear to involve mutations in ion channels as well. Mutations in SCN5A, the cardiac sodium channel gene previously shown to cause LQT3, have been identified[320,321] (Fig. 62-15). Although the surface ECG and biophysical characteristics of these patients differ from LQT3, it is interesting that symptoms occur during sleep in both disorders. There also appears to be a temperature-dependent effect on the electrophysiologic properties of some of these mutations.[322] Genetic heterogeneity appears to occur, but no other genes have been reported to date.

FAMILIAL ATRIAL FIBRILLATION

Familial atrial fibrillation appears to be rare, but a moderately sized family was identified and the gene responsible for the disease mapped to 10q22.[323] This family inherited the disease as an autosomal dominant trait, with the average age of onset of atrial fibrillation being 17 years. This family has a highly penetrant form of the disease, with most affected developing atrial fibrillation very early in childhood. The signs and symptoms are those related to atrial fibrillation which include palpitations, syncope, and dyspnea. Several other families with familial atrial fibrillation have since been identified due to the same locus.

WOLFF-PARKINSON-WHITE SYNDROME (WPW)

The preexcitation syndromes, including WPW, have been considered to be congenital, but only a small number of patients

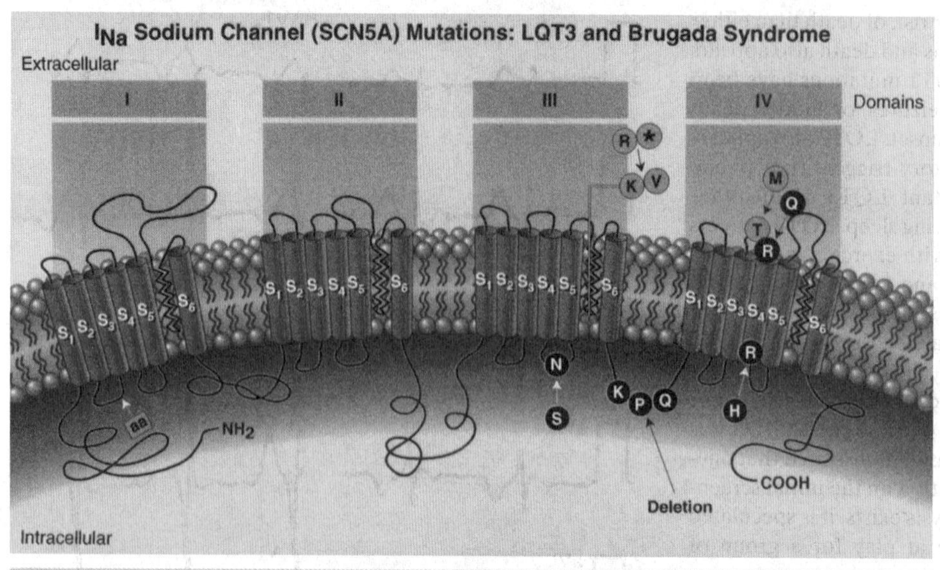

FIGURE 62-15 SCN5A mutations responsible for LQT3 (*black*) and Brugada syndrome (*gray*).

genetically heterogeneous and search for other disease-causing genes is being pursued. The more common form of familial secundum ASD is associated with atrioventricular conduction delay, which rarely progresses to heart block. In these patients, attention should be directed to the upper limbs, particularly the thumbs, to rule out the Holt-Oram syndrome, which will be described below. Another form of familial ASD has also been described which is thought to be mitochondrially inherited.

demonstrate familial occurrence; the majority of cases appear to be sporadic. ECG features of WPW include the presence of a short PR interval, and a prolonged QRS with slurred upstroke of the R wave, known as a delta wave[324] (see Chap. 26). Patients with WPW are prone to episodes of paroxysmal supraventricular tachycardia (see Chap. 27). An autosomal dominant pattern of inheritance of accessory pathways has been reported.[35] In a family with FHCM and WPW the locus was mapped to chromosome 7 (7q3) has been shown in patients with both FHCM and WPW.[35]

Autosomal Dominant Atrioventricular Block This disorder, when familial, presents with adult onset (age 20 to 50 years) and has an autosomal dominant inheritance pattern.[301,325] Approximately 50 families have been identified with this disorder which, in each transmission, is consistent with autosomal dominant inheritance with full penetrance and variable expression. Whether all of these conditions represent a single disorder is not known. The common presentation of this disease includes one of the following: (1) right bundle-branch block (RBBB) alone; (2) left axis deviation (LAD) alone; (3) RBBB plus LAD; or (4) complete heart block. In addition, atrioventricular block has been associated with DCM and skeletal myopathy, and several genetic loci have been identified.[105,326,327] Another gene has been mapped to chromosome 19q13 in a family with AV block but without DCM.[326]

Congenital Heart Disease with or without Genetic Syndromes

FAMILIAL ATRIAL SEPTAL DEFECT (ASD)

Two mendelian forms of ASD exist as autosomal dominant traits. One form has no other associated abnormalities and was initially speculated to be on chromosome 6p, linked to the HLA complex, as yet unconfirmed by genetic linkage analysis. Further analysis identified mutations in the transcription factor Nkx2.5 in families and sporadic cases of ASD.[327] This is likely to be genetically heterogeneous and search for other disease-causing genes is being pursued.

HOLT-ORAM SYNDROME (HOS)

The cardinal manifestations of this autosomal dominant condition include upper limb dysplasia, ASD, and marked variability within families. The abnormalities of the arm demonstrate a wide spectrum in heterozygous individuals, ranging from undetectable, to distally placed thumbs and hypoplastic thenar eminences, triphylangeal thumbs, anomalies of the carpus, and radial aplasia, to phocomelia and hypoplasia of the clavicles and shoulders. The upper extremity deformity is typically bilateral, but the left side commonly is more severe than the right. In addition to the ASD, other cardiac malformations are occasionally found, the most frequent of which is a ventricular septal defect (VSD). Cardiac conduction disturbances, usually involving the AV node in patients with septal defects and hypoplastic peripheral arteries, are also found (Table 62-6). Other noncardiac manifestations include dermatoglyphic abnormalities and pectus excavatum. Since the noncardiac abnormalities have a very wide spectrum, all patients with ASD should be evaluated closely for upper limb deformities.

A male with features consistent with Holt-Oram syndrome in addition to mental retardation and other anomalies was found to have a deletion of chromosome 14 in the q23-q24.2 region. Linkage to chromosome 12 (12q213-q22) was later demonstrated in one family with Holt-Oram syndrome, while other families did not link to this region, indicative of heterogeneity.[328,329] The responsible gene for 12q21.3 was subsequently identified.[330,331] The chromosome 12–linked HOS was concomitantly reported by Basson et al.[330] and Li et al.[331] as TBX5, a member of the Brachyury (T) gene family, located at 12q24.1. This gene is a member of the T-box transcription factor family,[332,333] a group of genes that share a common DNA-binding motif (T box). Basson et al.[330] identified mutations in two families (nonsense, missense mutations) and suggested that haplo-insufficiency was the mechanism at play. Li et al.[331] identified mutations in three families and three sporadic cases, four of which encoded premature stop codons and two reading frame shift mutations. The authors pointed out that no obvious phenotype-genotype correlations existed. In fact, individuals with identical mutations had widely different skeletal and cardiac features. They also suggested that haplo-insufficiency was at play and occurred between days 26 and 52 of gestation.

SUPRAVALVULAR AORTIC STENOSIS (SVAS) AND WILLIAMS SYNDROME

SVAS occurs in three different situations, occurring with an estimated incidence of 1 in 20,000 births. The most common is associated with the Williams syndrome which is usually sporadic but may be a highly variable autosomal dominant condition. The full spectrum of Williams syndrome[334,335] includes dysmorphic facies, often called "elfin" facies, infantile hypercalcemia, mental retardation, short stature, SVAS, and multiple peripheral pulmonic stenoses.[279,334] Many of these individuals have robust (so-called cocktail party) personalities. Late-onset problems may include progressive joint contractures, gastrointestinal dysfunction, and genitourinary dysfunction.

Cardiovascular features of Williams syndrome are present in about 75 percent of patients,[279,335] the most characteristic of which is supravalvular aortic stenosis. Other findings include peripheral pulmonic arterial stenosis and pulmonic valvular stenosis. Occasionally, VSD or ASD may be present. Peripheral vascular anomalies, including renal arterial stenosis, diffuse narrowing of the aorta, and coarctation of the aorta, may be present and may be associated with systemic hypertension. Sudden death has occurred in children with Williams syndrome, especially after cardiac catheterization. Coronary arterial stenosis may occur and lead to myocardial infarction. Histopathology in these patients suggests the possibility of abnormal elastic fibers.[336]

A second setting for SVAS is the autosomal dominant entity which is distinct from that of Williams syndrome (WS). Mental retardation and abnormal facies are not found and these individuals present with SVAS and/or peripheral pulmonary artery stenoses.[279,334] In some cases, family members present with moderate pulmonic valve and branch pulmonary artery stenoses but without SVAS. Later, the valvular and branch pulmonary stenoses may disappear while SVAS becomes evident. The stenotic aortic lesion requires surgery in less than one-half of these patients. The diagnosis relies on echocardiography, but cardiac catheterization is sometimes required. Finally, SVAS may present as sporadic cases. Many investigators have long believed that the sporadic SVAS, WS, and autosomal dominant SVAS are all interrelated.

In 1993, WS was shown to result from a submicroscopic deletion involving chromosome 7q11.23 in the region of the elastin gene,[337] and subsequently confirmed.[338] Inherited or de novo deletion of one elastin allele was identified in each of the patients studied and suggested that hemizygosity at the elastin locus is responsible for the vascular pathology in WS. Concordance in monozygotic twins and occurrence in second cousins has been described and anecdotal reports of parent and child with WS have been reported. In addition, familial supravalvular aortic stenosis (SVAS) without WS, which appears to be inherited as an autosomal dominant trait, is well known. This autosomal dominant form of SVAS was found to be linked to the elastin gene at 7q11.23[334] as well, and deletions were identified. Baumer et al.[339] suggested that WS results from this deletion at 7q11.23 that arises from recombination between misaligned repeat sequences flanking the WS region. It is currently believed that this syndrome is a contiguous gene syndrome. The first deleted gene identified in the critical region, elastin (ELN), has been shown to cause the SVAS phenotype but not any of the other features of Williams syndrome (Fig. 62-16, Plate 99). Elastin gene (ELN) deletion is seen in 90 to 95 percent of WS patients and translocations also occur. ELN rearrangements, point mutations, splice mutations, and nonsense mutations have been found in families and sporadic cases of SVAS or Williams syndrome. However, a few patients with classic features of WS, usually without cardiac defects, do not have a deletion involving elastin. This fact suggests that, while deletion of elastin is necessary for the SVAS phenotype, it may not be necessary for Williams syndrome. Elastin is an extracellular matrix protein that comprises 90 percent of the elastic matrix that restores a vessel's shape after it has been stretched. Intense efforts to identify other deleted genes that contribute to the phenotype subsequently identified deletions of LIMK1 (a protein tyrosine kinase expressed in developing brain), syntaxin IA (a component of the synaptic apparatus), WBSCR1 (containing an RNA-binding motif), RFC2 (a subunit of the replication factor C complex involved in DNA replication), FKBP6 (a FK506-binding protein immunophilin which is thought to play a role in the calcium metabolism abnormalities and growth delay in these patients), WSTF (a putative transcription factor), WS-TRP (considered as playing a role in signal transduction), FZD3 (a gene homologous to *Drosophila* tissue polarity gene *frizzled*), and GTF21 (a multifunctional member of a widely expressed transcription factor complex that is phosphorylated by Bruton tyrosine kinase).[340–348] The roles of these genes in the Williams syndrome phenotype, however, is not known. In order to localize, isolate, and characterize the genes that contribute to the Williams syndrome phenotype, Hockenhull et al.[349] constructed a high-resolution integrated map of the critical region, established a panel of somatic cell hybrids from patients with classic clinical features, and defined deletion breakpoints and estimated the size of the deletions with classical Williams syndrome. They also identified two new genes, CPETR1 and CPETR2, which are deleted in these patients. A mouse knockout model has been created and is being studied.

NOONAN SYNDROME

In 1963, nine patients with valvular pulmonic stenosis, short stature, mild mental retardation, hypertelorism, and unusual facial features were described.[350] This disorder, sometimes confused with Turner syndrome, is distinct and females and males are equally affected. Noonan syndrome is relatively common, with an incidence of 1 in 1000 to 2500 live births. The diagnosis can sometimes be made prenatally. Postnatal growth, however, is generally delayed and tends to parallel the third percentile with normal growth velocity, although the adolescent growth spurt is usually blunted or absent. Facial features appear to change with age. The main features of the newborn period are hypertelorism with down-slanted palpebral fissures; low-set, posteriorly rotated ears with thickened helices; deeply grooved philtrum; micrognathia; and excess neck skin with low posterior hairline. As the infant ages, the head appears larger, with prominent eyes and thinning of the palpebral fissures and depression of the nasal root. The face appears more myopathic and becomes more triangular in shape. In some young adults, the eyes become less prominent. The neck length is relatively short, which exaggerates the webbing. Individuals tend to have prominent nasolabial folds, a high anterior hairline, and transparent, wrinkled skin. The hair is generally described as being curly

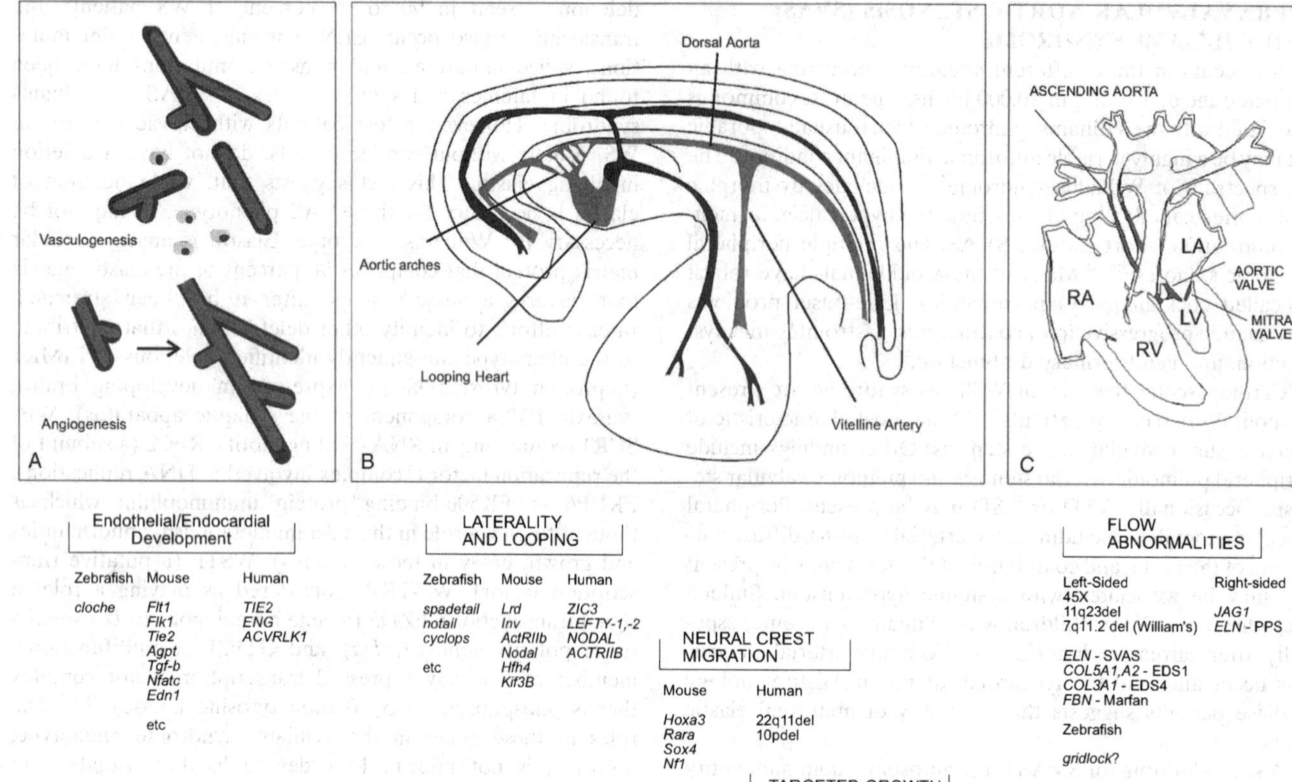

FIGURE 62-16 (Plate 99) Genetic defects causing congenital heart disease with or without genetic syndromes. Mutants from zebrafish, mouse, and human relating to primary developmental processes or maintenance of the vascular system are illustrated, including those of vasculogenesis and angiogenesis (*A*), embryonic development of the vascular system (*B*), and LV outflow tract obstruction (*C*).

or woolly in older children and adolescents. Approximately 60 percent of males have cryptorchidism. Sexual development is variable and may be delayed. Most females appear to be fertile. Pectus carinatum superiorly and pectus excavatum inferiorly appears to be present in about 70 percent of individuals. The chest appears to lengthen with age, giving the appearance of relatively low-set nipples. Other features include cubitus valgus, clinodactyly, vertebral anomalies, dental malocclusion, café-au-lait spots, pigmented nevi, bleeding disorders, lymphatic dysplasia, and pulmonary and intestinal lymphangiectasia. Mental retardation is present in 35 percent of cases.[351]

It appears that about two-thirds of patients with Noonan syndrome have some type of cardiac defect. Approximately half of these patients have valvular pulmonic stenosis. Other relatively common cardiac anomalies include hypertrophic cardiomyopathy, ASDs, VSDs, and persistent patent ductus arteriosus. Pulmonic arterial branch stenosis, mitral valve prolapse, Ebstein's anomaly, and single ventricle have also been reported (Table 62-6).

The clinical features of Noonan syndrome can overlap with a number of other conditions. Chromosome studies should be done in females to rule out Turner syndrome. Phenotypic overlap with WS, primidone teratogenicity syndrome, fetal alcohol syndrome, Aarskog syndrome, Leopard syndrome, neurofibromatosis, and malignant hyperthermia (King syndrome) have been reported.

Most cases of Noonan syndrome appear to be sporadic. Thus, the percentage of inherited cases may actually be much higher than the 30 percent previously reported. The majority of inherited cases are apparently inherited from the mother, thought to be the result of decreased fertility in males. Therefore, although the recurrence risk for offspring is expected to be 50 percent, it might actually be somewhat lower. A gene causing Noonan syndrome has been mapped to chromosome 12(12q22-qter),[352] but the gene has remained elusive. Genetic heterogeneity has also been demonstrated.

TUBEROUS SCLEROSIS (TS)

Classically, tuberous sclerosis consists of the triad of mental retardation, seizures, and adenoma sebaceum. These features, however, may not be present in all patients. The term *tuberous sclerosis* primarily refers to hamartomatous lesions in the brain as well as intracranial calcifications primarily in the area of the basal ganglia. These lesions appear to be present in about 90 percent of patients. Seizures are a frequent finding, being seen in about 90 percent, and have some correlation with mental retardation. About 60 percent of tuberous sclerosis patients are mentally retarded, close to 100 percent of whom have seizures; of those without mental retardation, only 75 percent have seizures. Seizures tend to occur earlier in patients with mental retardation than those without mental retardation. Ocular lesions, particularly benign astrocytoma, occur in about 50 percent of patients. Cutaneous lesions are common; 80 percent of patients develop angiofibromas of the face, usually referred to by the misnomer adenoma sebaceum. Depigmented skin patches that are especially apparent by Wood's light examination are seen in about 80 percent of patients, frequently from birth. Pulmonary disease may occur primarily in adult females and is likely to be severe and life-threatening. The primary cardiac finding is the presence of rhabdomyomata.[353,354] Wolff-Parkinson-White (WPW) syndrome and supraventricular tachycardia have also been reported.[354,355]

Tuberous sclerosis is an autosomal dominant condition in which about 80 percent of cases are suspected as resulting from new mutations with unaffected parents. A child diagnosed with tuberous sclerosis should be evaluated by computed tomography (CT) of the brain and electroencephalography for the presence of CNS lesions and also have renal ultrasound. Parents should be examined for the presence of depigmented patches (by Wood's light), dental abnormalities, retinal findings, and abdominal ultrasound for renal cysts. It is now apparent that there are at least two genes causing tuberous sclerosis: TSC1 on chromosome 9 at 9q34 (hamartin)[356] and TSC2 (tuberin) on chromosome 16 at 16p13. These two protein products co-localize to cytoplasmic vesicles[357] and interact with each other. TSC2 spans 43 kb of genomic DNA and encodes a number of alternatively spliced transcripts of 16 kb. Constitutional inactivating mutations of the TSC2 gene, including complete deletion, have been detected in patients with TS and the associated hamartomas show loss of heterozygosity for markers in the TSC2 region, indicating that TSC2 functions as a tumor suppressor gene and that loss of function of both alleles is normally required before cellular growth becomes dysregulated. Various cancers[358] have been found to occur due to mutations in the TS complex. In addition, large deletions in TSC2 and its neighboring gene PKD1 have been seen in children with polycystic kidney disease.[359] Genotype-phenotype correlations are not helpful.[360,361] Animal models have been developed with resultant tumors noted.[362–365]

FAMILIAL COARCTATION OF THE AORTA

Familial coarctation of the aorta (usually with autosomal dominant transmission) has been described but no locus or gene has been identified. This congenital lesion is the most common congenital anomaly of the aortic arch in humans, occurring in 5 to 8 percent of children with congenital heart defects. A recessive mutation, *gridlock,* in the zebrafish (*Danio rerio*) has been identified in which blood flow to the tail is impeded by a localized vascular defect.[366] There is some question as to whether this mutation is a model for human aortic coarctation,[367] but it may aid in learning about vascular obstruction. As coarctation of the aorta occurs in association with other left heart obstructive lesions in an individual or in members of a family with other left heart obstructive lesions, it is likely that the mechanism causing disease is complex. Other mutations, such as those of endothelin1, endothelin A receptor, Hand2, MFH-1, and retinoid receptor genes have been shown to lead to aortic arch malformations in mice (Fig. 62-16).

IVEMARK SYNDROME (ASPLENIA/POLYSPLENIA) OR HETEROTAXY SYNDROMES

Ivemark syndrome represents a group of defects that interferes with the normal establishment of laterality.[279,368] The more severe asplenia and polysplenia syndromes have an estimated incidence of 1 in 10,000 to 20,000 live births. The occurrence is usually sporadic, but familial cases have been described with autosomal recessive and X-linked transmission; chromosomal translocations (i.e., between chromosomes 12 and 13) and deletions (involving chromosomes 10 and 13) have been described, as has monozygotic twinning. Both forms tend to have similar cardiac defects, including ASDs, VSDs, endocardial cushion defects, and pulmonic stenosis as well as other defects.[369,370] Asplenia, however, tends to be more commonly associated with severe defects of the atrioventricular canal and VSDs, while polysplenia tends to be more associated with ASDs. In many cases, complex cardiac malformations occur, including single ventricle physiology. A total of 32 cases of asplenia were identified in 4059 autopsies, and all cases were sporadic with a male excess.

Rightward looping of the midline heart tube is the first overt manifestation of anatomic left-right differences, which eventually come to include the asymmetry of the lungs and most malformations associated with abnormal looping; therefore, they usually occur as one manifestation of a more global abnormality of left-right heart anomalies, abnormalities of spleen position and/or number, and some degree of malrotation of the gut. The overall left-right axis of the individual may be situs ambiguus (i.e., indeterminate sidedness) or situs inversus (complete left-right reversal), compared to normal sidedness (situs solitus).

Cardiac malformations attributable to abnormal laterality represent 3.4 percent of all heart defects.[371] Since there is familial clustering of situs, it appears that genetics contributes significantly to these abnormalities. This is supported by mutant mouse models with similar defects,[371] as well as gene defects in some humans.

The first gene locus for human situs defects was mapped to Xq26.2 in families with X-linked disease.[372] This gene was later shown to be a zinc-finger transcription factor Z1C3, and mutations were found in sporadic and familial cases.[371,372] Studies in other vertebrates yielded additional candidate genes as well. Several genes were found to be asymmetrically expressed along the left-right axis in chick prior to development of anatomic left-right asymmetry[274,368] and some of these same genes were also found to be asymmetrically expressed in the mouse (Fig. 62-16). These genes included nodal, pitx2, lefty-1 and lefty-2. Genetic studies in mice also implicated several additional genes that did not have asymmetric expression, such as HNF3, Actrllb, and Smad.[373–375] Mutation analysis in patients have identified a small number of mutations in all of these genes.[376,377]

Other Genetic Syndromes

A variety of other genetic syndromes with associated cardiovascular disease occur primarily in childhood. These include Ellis-Van Crevald syndrome, Treacher Collins syndrome, Alagille syndrome, Smith-Lemli-Opitz syndrome, thrombocytopenia-absent radii (TAR) syndrome, Goldenhar syndrome, Cornelia de Lange syndrome, Rubinstein-Taybi syndrome, VACTERL association, and CHARGE association. Since these are primarily pediatric diseases, they are not included in this discussion. For detailed descriptions of these and other pediatric genetic syndromes with cardiovascular abnormalities, see current reviews of this topic.[378]

CARDIOVASCULAR DISORDERS ASSOCIATED WITH CHROMOSOME ABNORMALITIES

Chromosomal Nomenclature

Cytogenetics is the study of chromosomes and chromosomal abnormalities. Chromosomes are classified according to their size and shape. Chromosomes have two arms, one long and one short. The short arm is usually referred to as the "p" arm, and the long arm is usually referred to as the "q" arm. For instance, the long arm of chromosome 22 is designated 22q and the short arm 22p. The arms of the chromosomes meet at the centromere or primary constriction, which is responsible for division of chromosome pairs during meiosis and mitosis. There are three shapes of human chromosomes based on the position of the centromere. Metacentric chromosomes have the centromere in a central position and the long and short arms are approximately equal. Submetacentric chromosomes have an eccentric centromere, producing arms of unequal lengths. Acrocentric chromosomes have a centromere close to one end of the chromosome. Acrocentric chromosomes have small pieces of chromatin known as satellites attached to their short arms.

Since 1971, banding of chromosomes has become routine and the banding patterns of each chromosome can be distinguished separately. For this reason, chromosome abnormalities are designated by the actual chromosome number rather than the chromosome group (e.g., trisomy 18 rather than trisomy E).

Classification of Chromosomal Alterations

Chromosome alterations, especially those involving too many or too few chromosomes (called aneuploidy), are quite common in human development. Chromosome aberrations most commonly cause structural defects of the cardiovascular system, and typically these are evident at birth. Approximately 50 percent of all fetuses conceived are spontaneously aborted (usually in the first trimester), with one-half of these being aneuploid. Among live-born infants, about 1 in 200 (0.5 percent) have a chromosome abnormality. The frequency of chromosome abnormalities among live-born children with congenital heart defects is in the range of 5 to 13 percent.[378] Hence, the vast majority of chromosomal aberrations are lost in early fetal life and, in most instances, occur as new mutations. For this reason, with both parents being normal, the risk of recurrence to relatives is usually low.

1. Aneuploidy, defined as the gain or loss of chromosomes resulting in too many or too few chromosomes, occurs most commonly by nondysjunction (failure of a homologous pair of chromosomes to separate). Nondisjunction occurs during meiosis in one parent (i.e., in spermatogenesis or oogenesis) or in the first mitotic cleavage of the zygote. In meiotic nondysjunction, when a pair of chromosomes does not normally separate, both members of the pair (or neither member of the pair) pass into one gamete. When an additional copy of the chromosome is added during fertilization, three copies of the same chromosome (or only one copy) are found in the new zygote instead of the chromosome pair. Two of the most common chromosomal disorders causing heart disease, Down syndrome (trisomy 21) and Turner syndrome (XO), are due to nondisjunction. Absence of one chromosome is called *monosomy;* all autosomal monosomies, as well as those containing only a Y sex chromosome, are lethal for the embryo. The presence of three chromosomes is called *trisomy,* as seen in Down syndrome, while the presence of an entire extra set of chromosomes is known as *triploidy.*

2. Chromosomal rearrangements occur when a chromosome breaks and rejoins within itself differently than normally occurs. This can potentially result in an inversion of genetic material. Typically there is no apparent phenotypic effect in persons carrying an inversion but their offspring may have severe abnormalities due to the disruption in chromosome pairing during meiosis that can take place.

3. Chromosome deletions, or loss of chromosomal material, may be seen by light microscopy and consists of deletion of 10^6 bp or greater. If there is a large amount of DNA lost, more than one gene may be affected (disrupted or lost), a series of abnormalities in a single individual may result due to interruptions in a series of genes within the loci of a single chromosome. These contiguous gene deletion syndromes[379] may be heritable and the occurrence of the disorder in a family behaves as a dominant disorder (X-linked or autosomal dominant). Most deletions occur de novo. Two breaks in the same chromosome that reunite with the intermediate segment being inverted is referred to as an inversion. Isochromes are formed when two short or long arms join with loss of the other arm. Chromosomal translations occur when breaks occur in two chromosomes and reunite after exchange of segments. These deletions are best appreciated at the DNA level by Southern analysis or polymerase chain reaction (PCR) analysis.

4. Chromosome duplications or gains of chromosomal material may also be associated with phenotypic abnormality but most commonly cause no obvious aberration.

Cytogenetics and Techniques

High-resolution cytogenetic techniques allow unambiguous identification of each human chromosome and detection of most structural abnormalities of the chromosomes. These structural abnormalities include translocations, deletions, and duplications. High-resolution chromosome analysis involves synchronization of lymphocyte cultures in order to accumulate all cells at one point in the cell cycle. Other cells that may be used include skin, fibroblasts, and amniotic cells. Enrichment of this cell population in prophase and prometaphase rather than the middle to late stages of metaphase, which is characteristic of conventional harvesting techniques, allows improved visualization of the subbanding patterns of chromosomes. Each band seen at metaphase actually represents multiple subbands in earlier stages that have fused together as the chromosome contracts. Whereas a typical metaphase cell contains 300 to 400 bands per haploid genome, synchronized chromosome preparations make it possible to visualize 500 to 1000 bands per haploid set. With the development of banding methods, the human karyotype could be divided into 300 to 400 descrete bands or approximately 7 to 10 $\times$ 10^6 bp per band, and a much greater number of deletions, duplications, and translocations could be detected. High-resolution techniques allow visualization of from 500 to 2000 bands per haploid genome, and have enabled the delineation of a number of microdeletion or microduplication syndromes (also known as contiguous gene syndromes), including the DiGeorge syndrome and Beckwith-Wiedemann syndrome.

FLUORESCENCE IN SITU HYBRIDIZATION (FISH)

Fluorescence in situ hybridization or FISH provides for the detection of submicroscopic chromosomal deletions or duplications. This technique uses DNA probes conjugated with a fluorescent dye visible under a fluorescence microscope derived from chromosomal regions that hybridize to the specific chromosomes. This method makes possible direct visualization of single sequences not only on chromosomes but also within decondensed interphase nuclei, providing a high-resolution (<1 mb) approach to gene mapping and analysis of nuclear organization.

INDICATIONS FOR CHROMOSOMAL ANALYSIS

Chromosomal studies can provide valuable information to the family and the physician and should be considered in any child who has a heart defect with (1) minor dysmorphic features, (2) growth retardation that cannot be explained by the heart defect, or (3) developmental delay. In addition, the practitioner might more strongly consider chromosome studies if there is a family history of multiple miscarriages or other infants with birth defects or mental retardation. A genetic consultant can help determine whether or not chromosome studies should be performed, and they can help to integrate the findings of the chromosome analysis with the clinical picture. The major disadvantage of doing chromosomal studies is the cost (generally between $300 to $500).

Chromosomal Disorders

Many chromosomal disorders have associated cardiovascular disease. The most common of these include Down's syndrome (trisomy 21), Patau syndrome (trisomy 13), Edwards syndrome (trisomy 18), and Turner syndrome. Since trisomy 13 and 18 usually result in death during infancy, these are not described. A significant number of other chromosomal abnormalities are also associated with cardiovascular disease and are seen primarily as pediatric disorders. These abnormalities include triploidy, aneuploidy (other than trisomy 21, trisomy 18, trisomy 13, and Turner syndrome), deletions, and duplications. The triploidy syndromes—which include 69,XXX, 69,XXY, or 69,XYY—have a greater than 50 percent incidence of congenital heart disease, the vast majority of which are atrial and ventricular septal defects (ASD, VSD). The aneuploidy syndromes, not discussed thus far, are varied and uncommon. These include mosaicism of chromosome 8 and chromosome 9, which clinically present with VSDs with or without other associated complex defects. Aortic root dilatation and MVP occur with partial monosomy of chromosome 22. Other cardiovascular abnormalities associated with partial trisomy of chromosome 7q includes VSD, pulmonic stenosis (PS), patent ductus arteriosus (PDA), coarctation of the aorta (CoA), and L-transposition of the great vessels. Partial trisomy of chromosome 7p also occurs and most commonly is associated with VSD, PS, or AV canal.

DOWN'S SYNDROME (TRISOMY 21)

Chromosome 21 is the smallest of all human chromosomes, containing less than 2 percent of the genomic DNA. Down's syndrome, however, is the most common phenotype caused by a human chromosome abnormality, occurring approximately once in every 500 to 600 births. This disorder is usually due to the presence of an extra chromosome 21 (i.e., trisomy 21), but in some cases it is caused by the presence of only the distal half of chromosome 21, band q22 (i.e., 21q22)—the "Down's syndrome critical region"—so-called due to the presence of a subset of major phenotypic features of Down's syndrome including mental retardation, congenital heart disease, characteristic facial appearance, hand and dermatoglyphic changes.[380–382] In order to produce this syndrome, the region of 21q22 must be triplicated. The gene or genes responsible for manifesting Down's syndrome are unknown, but the severity of the disease is believed to depend on the extent of the region q22 and beyond that is triplicated. Creation of a linkage map of chromosome 21 has allowed for consideration of potential candidate genes. Recently, several genes have been implicated in some of the phenotypic features, but the cardiac features currently have no known cause.

The typical trisomy 21 occurs in 95 percent of cases of Down's syndrome and results from chromosomal nondisjunction. Some 2 to 3 percent of Down's syndrome cases are mosaics, having one trisomy cell line and one normal cell line, and the remainder (1 to 4 percent) are due to an extra copy of all or part of the long arm of chromosome 21 being translocated to another chromosome. The risk of trisomy 21 is exponentially related to maternal age, with the lowest risk for young women, rising steeply after age 35 years, and reaching 4 percent for women older than 45 years.

The recurrence risk is generally quoted at 1 to 2 percent. When a child with a translocation type of Down's syndrome is discovered, parental chromosomal analysis should always be performed to determine whether the translocation was inherited. If the translocation was not inherited and both parents have normal chromosomes, the recurrence risk is probably low, although prenatal chromosome diagnosis may be considered for future pregnancies. If the mother carries translocation of chromosome 21, the recurrence risk is approximately 10 percent. If the father is determined to be the carrier of a D;21 translocation, the recurrence risk is about 2 percent.[378] If one of the parents is determined to specifically be a 21;21 translocation carrier, the parents have a 100 percent chance of recurrence of Down's syndrome and no possibility of having normal offspring.[378] Luckily, the latter occurs in only about 1 in every 2000 cases of Down's syndrome but clearly has a significant impact on family planning.

Some 40 to 50 percent of patients with Down's syndrome have congenital heart disease (40 to 60 percent of these are atrioventricular septal defects, AVSDs) and this, along with hematologic malignant disease and duodenal atresia, are among the most common causes of morbidity and mortality.[378] Patients who escape these problems generally survive into the fifth decade and beyond. The most characteristic cardiac defect in

TABLE 62-9 Chromosomal Abnormalities Associated with Specific Types of Congenital Heart Defects

Endocardial cushion defect	Trisomy 21
Coarctation of the aorta	Turner syndrome
Total anomalous pulmonary venous return	Partial trisomy 22q 49,XXXXX; 49,XXXXX
Patent ductus arteriosus	Partial trisomy 8q
Tetralogy of Fallot	Monosomy 22q11
Conotruncal abnormalities	Partial trisomy 5q
Conduction defect	Turner syndrome
Hypoplastic left heart	

Down's syndrome is the AVSD (also called *endocardial cushion defect* or *atrioventricular canal defect*) (Table 62-9).[378] In addition to problems of volume overload secondary to left-to-right shunting, these patients are predisposed to early pulmonary hypertension. Elevated pulmonary vascular resistance becomes a significant risk beyond 1 year of age. Once this occurs, these patients become unsuitable for surgical repair. Approximately one-third of patients with Down's syndrome and congenital heart defects have complex heart disease, increasing the morbidity and mortality further. Other clinical features of Down's syndrome include hypotonia and decreased Moro reflex with joint hyperextensibility in the newborn period, a flat facial profile with excessive, redundant skin in the posterior neck, antimongoloid slant (upward) of palpebral fissures, and small white Brushfield spots around the circumference of the irides in children with blue irides. The hands and feet may reveal a simian crease (50 percent), clinodyactyly, or incurving of the fifth finger, brachydactyly with short metacarpals and phalanges, and a wide gap between the first two toes. Individuals are mentally retarded to varying degrees, with IQs ranging from 25 to 70. Generally, males are infertile.

TURNER SYNDROME

This disorder, which is due to a single X chromosome in females (i.e., XO genotype), occurs in approximately 1 female in 2500.[378] The frequency of nonmosaic XO karotypes is significantly higher in spontaneous abortuses than in liveborns, with less than 2 percent of such conceptuses reaching term. Clinically, there is a variable and often mild phenotype, and the diagnosis may go unsuspected until a child's short stature is evaluated or a women complains of amenorrhea. The clinical findings[378] of patients with Turner syndrome includes lymphedema of hands and feet, inguinal hernias, short stature, primary amenorrhea, facial features including a slightly traingular face with downslated palpebral fissures, epicanthal folds, and ptosis. Ears are frequently low-set and posteriorly rotated, and the mandible is commonly micrognathic. The neck is typically short with marked webbing and the posterior hairline may be low, extending to the upper shoulders. A broad thorax with widely spaced nipples is common, as is cubitus valgus and shortening of fourth and fifth metacarpals. Abnormalities of sexual development are usually associated, including hypogonadotropic hypogonadism with ovarian dysgenesis. Intelligence is normal. Many cases are mosaic for cell lines with the normal 46XX or 46XY makeup. The frequency of congenital cardiac disease varies from 20 to 50 percent, with at least one-half of these having CoA. A variety of other cardiac defects may also occur either singly or in combination with CoA. The majority of these include other left heart abnormalities including bicuspid aortic valve, aortic stenosis, dilated ascending aorta,[378] and hypoplastic left heart syndrome (HLHS). ASD and VSD as well as partial anomalous pulmonary venous return have also been reported (Table 62-9).

Coarctation of the aorta can usually be diagnosed clinically due to poor femoral pulses and differential blood pressure, with the arm blood pressure being consistently hypertensive, while the leg pressures are typically very low. Echocardiography or magnetic resonance imaging will confirm the diagnosis. Therapy may include surgical repair or, in some cases, balloon angioplasty. Infants may require prostaglandin E therapy to keep the ductus arteriosis patent; these young patients may present in heart failure or cardiac collapse if duct-dependent. Those patients with HLHS are duct-dependent and will die unless a Norwood operation or cardiac transplant is performed. Bicuspid aortic valves do not usually require therapy unless stenosis occurs. All cardiac defects require prophylaxis for subacute bacterial endocarditis (SBE). Chromosomal studies are recommended in all cases of Turner syndrome, since only about 60 percent of cases will have monosomy X. The remaining cases have mosaicism or various abnormalities of the X chromosome. Most cases of Turner syndrome are sporadic and the recurrence risk appears to be relatively low. However, parents may choose to have prenatal chromosomal diagnosis in subsequent pregnancies.

CATCH-22 Syndromes

DIGEORGE ANOMALY

First described in 1965,[383] the combination of thymic hypoplasia, parathyroid hypoplasia, and cardiac defects has been termed DiGeorge syndrome or DiGeorge anomaly. Because the disorder is of heterogeneous etiology, the term *DiGeorge anomaly* is currently preferred to *DiGeorge syndrome*. These thymic, parathyroid, and cardiac defects all result from developmental abnormalities of the third and fourth branchial arches.

Eighty percent of affected infants present with congenital heart defects within the first 48 h of life. According to the classification system of Clark,[384] the two types of defects associated with DiGeorge anomaly are conotruncal defects and branchial arch mesenchymal tissue defects. Among conotruncal defects, truncus arteriosus is the most common type. Among the branchial arch mesenchymal tissue defects, interrupted aortic arch type b and right aortic arch are the most common.[378]

The second key feature is persistent hypocalcemia, occurring either as the initial presenting feature or in combination with the cardiac defect. Parathyroid glands may be absent or reduced in size and number, and serum parathyroid hormone levels are decreased. Hypocalcemia may require continuous calcium infusions and/or frequent calcium supplementation. In cases of partial defect, the hypocalcemia may improve over time.

There are multiple etiologies for DiGeorge which include chromosome abnormalities, single-gene defects, teratogenic exposures, and association with other defects.[384] Approximately 5 to 10 percent of infants with features of DiGeorge anomaly will have an obvious abnormality of chromosome 22 with monosomy of the proximal portion of the long arm. However, approximately 70 percent of patients will have submicroscopic deletions of 22q11 detectable only by FISH.[384,385] In addition, many of these patients have features of the Sprintzen velocardiofacial (VCF) syndrome and the Takao conotruncal face syndrome.[386,387] These syndromes are currently referred to as a group by the mnemonic of CATCH-22 syndrome for the associated defects: *c*ardiac, *a*bnormal facies, *t*hymic hypoplasia, *c*left platate, *h*ypocalcemia, *22*q11 deletions). Approximately 15 percent of infants with DiGeorge anomaly can be found to have obvious chromosome abnormalities of which about two-thirds involve a monosomy 22q11.[388] This usually results from an unbalanced translocation involving chromosome 22 and another chromosome. More recent studies using fluorescence in situ hybridization (FISH) with probes from the critical region have shown that a total of about 85 percent of DiGeorge anomaly patients are deleted, with about 70 percent of patients having submicroscopic, molecular deletions, del22 (q11.21 q11.23). Although patients have different deletion endpoints, a 1.5-Mb region is deleted in most. Rarely, a syndrome of "partial" DiGeorge syndrome due to balanced translocation has been described. This translocation was cloned and a disrupted gene DNA-binding protein.[389] More recently, a variety of candidate genes have been identified, including the human homolog of the *Drosophila disheveled* segment-polarity gene,[390] the *clathrin heavy chain-like* gene (CLTCL),[391] *UFD1L* (a developmentally expressed ubiquitination gene),[392] *HIRA*,[393] *DGSI*,[394] and the *goosecoid-like* (GSCL) homeobox gene[395] (Fig. 62-16). The best of these candidate genes, fulfilling most of the criteria necessary to cause this complex, are *HIRA* and *UFD1L*. *HIRA* is a mammalian homolog of yeast proteins, which are corepressors of cell cycle–dependent histone gene transcription, expressed in neural crest and neural crest–derived tissues.[396] This gene has been shown to be required for outflow tract septation. However, mice with haploinsufficiency are normal. *UFD1L*, the homolog of a highly conserved yeast gene involved in degradation of ubiquinated proteins, results in the same craniofacial and cardiac defects seen in CATCH-22 when mutated.[397] Recently, Lindsay et al.[398] engineered a chromosomal deletion (Dfl) in mice that spanned the critical region. The heterozygous deleted animals developed heart disease identical to that seen in humans. They suggested that the cardiovascular lesions occurred due to inadequate formation, early regression, or growth failure of the fourth aortic arch arteries. It should be noted that Yamagishi et al.[397] reported a DGS and/or VCFS patient who is heterozygous for a de novo deletion spanning 20 kb of DNA, disrupting *CDC45L* and *UFD2L*, both candidate genes. The authors suggested these genes to be involved in the development of these syndromes and argued that these genes were regulated by dHAND, a basic helix-loop-helix transcription factor. They proposed a model whereby downregulation of UFD1L activity results in accumulation of certain proteins and excessive apoptosis or maldevelopment of neural crest cells. Based on their view, they suggested disruption of UFD1L function alone, or in combination with CDC45L and/or HIRA is the most likely etiology for most defects seen in DGS. This is currently being carefully studied.

Several therapies have been used to treat the profound T-cell immunodeficiency associated with the DiGeorge syndrome. These therapies have included bone-marrow transplantation. Recently, Market et al.[399] described use of cultured postnatal thymus tissue transplantation in five infants, with good results.

SHPRINTZEN VELOCARDIOFACIAL (VCF) SYNDROME

This condition was first recognized in 1978 with ascertainment primarily in children with palatal defects[386]; this is the most common syndrome associated with cleft palate and appears to be the same disorder as the Takao conotruncal anomaly face syndrome.[387] The clinical features include mild short stature, cleft palate especially of the secondary palate with submucous clefts, pharyngeal incompetence leading to speech disorders, and speech delay. Most cases are sporadic but some autosomal cases have been reported.

Cardiac defects are prominent in this disorder, the majority being conotruncal-type defects.[400–403] Ventricular septal defect occurs in 70 to 75 percent, while right-sided aortic arch occurs in about 50 percent and tetralogy of Fallot is found in 15 to 20 percent of children. Partial DiGeorge anomaly seems to be present in some cases. About 85 percent of VCF syndrome patients have deletions of chromosome 22q11, usually submicroscopic and visible only by FISH techniques.

Takao syndrome (conotruncal face anomaly syndrome) first described in 1976, has similarities to both DiGeorge and Shprintzen syndromes clinically,[387,402] hence its incorporation in the CATCH-22 association. These Japanese children were noted to have a specific dysmorphic facial appearance in association with conotruncal malformations. Deletions within the 22q11 region in these patients have been found,[402] confirming its similarity to the DiGeorge syndrome and VCF syndrome.

References

1. Hoffman JIE. Incidence of congenital heart disease: II. Prenatal incidence. *Pediatr Cardiol* 1995; 16:155–165.
2. Berko BA, Swift M. X-linked dilated cardiomyopathy. *N Engl J Med* 1987; 316:1186–1190.
3. Collins FS, Patrinos A, Jordan E, et al. New goals for the U.S. Human Genome Project: 1998–2003. *Science* 1998; 282:682–689.
4. Brower V. News in science. *Nature Biotech* 1998; 16:895.
5. Brower V. Genome II: The next frontier. *Nature Biotech* 1998; 16:104.
6. Roberts R. A glimpse of the future from present day molecular genetics. In Opie LH, Yellon DM, eds. *Cardiology at the Limits III*. Cape Town: Stanford Writers; 1999:105–120.
7. Roberts R, Ryan TJ. 29th Bethesda Conference-Task Force 3: Clinical research in a molecular era and the need to expand its ethical imperatives. *J Am Coll Cardiol* 1998; 31:917–949.
8. Haines JL, Perricak-Vance MA. Sibpair analysis. In Haines JL, Perricak-Vance MA, eds. *Approaches to Gene Mapping in Complex Human Diseases*. New York: Wiley-Liss; 1998:273–303.
9. Serrato M, Marian AJ. A variant of human paraoxonase/arylesterase (HUMPONA) gene is a risk factor for coronary artery disease. *J Clin Invest* 1995; 96:3005–3008.
10. Yu QT, Safavi F, Roberts R, et al. A variant of β-fibrinogen is a genetic risk factor for coronary artery disease and myocardial infarction. *J Invest Med* 1996; 44:154–159.
11. Roberts R, Marian AJ, Bachinski LL. Overview: Application of molecular biology to medical genetics. In Markwald RR, Clark EB, Takao A, eds. *Inborn Heart Disease—Developmental Mechanisms*. Mount Kisco, NY: Futura Press; 1994:87–111.
12. Weissenbach J. A second generation linkage map of the human genome based on highly informative microsatellite loci. *Gene* 1994; 135:275–278.
13. Cooperative Human Linkage Center (CHLC). A comprehensive human linkage map with centimorgan density. *Science* 1994; 265:2049–2054.

14. Cooper NG, ed. *The Human Genome Project: Deciphering the Blueprint of Heredity*. Mill Valley, CA: University Science Books; 1994.
15. Haines JL, Perricak-Vance MA. Lod score analysis. In: Haines JL, Perricak-Vance MA, eds. *Approaches to Gene Mapping in Complex Human Diseases*. New York: Wiley-Liss; 1998:253–272.
16. Roberts R, Towbin J. Principles and techniques of molecular biology. In: Roberts R, ed. *Molecular Basis of Cardiology*. Cambridge, MA: Blackwell; 1993:15–112.
17. Hagmann M. A good SNP may be hard to find. *Science* 1999; 285:21–22.
18. Halushka MK, Fan J-B, Bentley K, et al. Patterns of single-nucleotide polymorphisms in candidate genes for blood-pressure homeostasis. *Nature Genet* 1999; 22:239–247.
19. Cargill M, Altshuler D, Ireland J, et al. Characterization of single-nucleotide polymorphisms in coding regions of human genes. *Nature Genet* 1999; 22:231–238.
20. Adams MD, Kelley JM, Gocayne JD, et al. Complementary DNA sequencing: Expressed sequence tags and Human Genome Project. *Science* 1991; 252:1651–1656.
21. Collins FS. Shattuck lecture: Medical and societal consequences of the Human Genome Project. *N Engl J Med* 1999; 341:28–37.
22. Oberst L, Zhao G, Park JT, et al. Dominant-negative effect of a mutant cardiac troponin T on cardiac structure and function in transgenic mice. *J Clin Invest* 1998; 102:1498–1505.
23. Blanchard EM, Lizuka K, Christe M, et al. Targeted ablation of the murine α-tropomyosin gene. *Circ Res* 1997; 81:1005–1011.
24. Marian AJ, Zhao G, Seta Y, et al. Expression of a mutant (Arg92Gln) human cardiac troponin T, known to cause hypertrophic cardiomyopathy, impairs adult cardiac myocytes contractility. *Circ Res* 1997; 81:76–85.
25. Hejtmancik JF, Roberts R. Molecular genetics and the application of linkage analysis. In: Roberts R, ed. *Molecular Basis of Cardiology*. Cambridge, MA: Blackwell; 1993:355–381.
26. Roberts R, Bachinski LL, Yu QT, et al. Molecular analysis of genotype/phenotype correlations of hypertrophic cardiomyopathy. In: Dhalla NS, Singal PK, Beamish RE, eds. *Heart Hypertrophy and Failure*. Boston: Kluwer; 1995:3–19.
27. Ozawa T, Tanaka M, Sugiyama S, et al. Multiple mitochondrial DNA deletions exist in cardiomyocytes of patients with hypertrophic or dilated cardiomyopathy. *Biochem Biophys Res Comm* 1990; 170:830–836.
28. Kelly DP, Strauss AW. Inherited cardiomyopathies. *N Engl J Med* 1994; 330:913–919.
29. Lakkis NM, Nagueh SF, Kleiman NS, et al. Echocardiography guided ethanol septal reduction for hypertrophic obstructive cardiomyopathy. *Circulation* 1998; 98:1750–1755.
30. Nagueh SF, Lakkis NM, He Z-X, et al. Role of myocardial contrast echocardiography during nonsurgical septal reduction therapy for hypertrophic obstructive cardiomyopathy. *J Am Coll Cardiol* 1998; 32:225–229.
31. Jarcho JA, McKenna W, Pare JAP, et al. Mapping a gene for familial hypertrophic cardiomyopathy to chromosome 14q1. *N Engl J Med* 1989; 321:1372–1378.
32. Hejtmancik JF, Brink PA, Towbin J, et al. Localization of the gene for familial hypertrophic cardiomyopathy to chromosome 14q1 in a diverse U.S. population. *Circulation* 1991; 83:1592–1597.
33. Marian AJ, Roberts R. Familial hypertrophic cardiomyopathy: A paradigm of the cardiac response to injury. *Ann Med* 1998; 30:24–32.
34. Marian AJ, Roberts R. Recent advances in the molecular genetics of hypertrophic cardiomyopathy. *Circulation* 1995; 92:1336–1347.
35. MacRae C, Ghasia N, Kass S, et al. Familial hypertrophic cardiomyopathy with Wolfe-Parkinson-White syndrome maps to a locus on chromosome 7q3. *J Clin Invest* 1995; 96:1216–1220.
36. Ko Y-L, Chen J-J, Tang T-K, et al. Mapping the locus for familial hypertrophic cardiomyopathy to chromosome 11 in a family with a case of apical hypertrophic cardiomyopathy of the Japanese type. *Hum Genet* 1996; 97:457–461.
37. Watkins H, Thierfelder L, Anan R, et al. Independent origin of identical β-cardiac myosin heavy-chain mutations in hypertrophic cardiomyopathy. *Am J Hum Genet* 1993; 53:1180–1185.
38. Dausse E, Komajda M, Fetler L, et al. Familial hypertrophic cardiomyopathy: Microsatellite haplotyping and identification of a hot spot for mutations in the β-myosin heavy chain gene. *J Clin Invest* 1993; 92:2807–2813.
39. Consevage MW, Salada GC, Baylen BG, et al. A new missense mutation, Arg^{719}Gln, in the β-cardiac heavy chain myosin gene of patients with familial hypertrophic cardiomyopathy. *Hum Mol Genet* 1994; 3:1025–1026.
40. Marian AJ, Yu QT, Mares A Jr, et al. Detection of a new mutation in the β-myosin heavy chain gene in an individual with hypertrophic cardiomyopathy. *J Clin Invest* 1992; 90:2156–2165.
41. Abchee AB, Lechin M, Quinones MA, et al. The severity of left ventricular hypertrophy is greater in patients with hypertrophic cardiomyopathy due to malignant mutations (abstr). *J Am Coll Cardiol* 1995; 25:415A.
42. Marian AJ. Sudden cardiac death in patients with hypertrophic cardiomyopathy: From bench to bedside with an emphasis on genetic markers. *Clin Cardiol* 1995; 18:189–198.
43. Anan R, Greve G, Thierfelder L, et al. Prognostic implications of novel β-cardiac myosin heavy chain gene mutations that cause familial hypertrophic cardiomyopathy. *J Clin Invest* 1994; 93: 280–285.
44. Moolman J, Corfield VA, Rosen B, et al. Sudden death due to troponin T mutations. *J Am Coll Cardiol* 1997; 29:549–555.
45. Roberts R. Molecular genetics: Therapy or terror? *Circulation* 1994; 89:499–502.
46. Epstein ND, Cohn GM, Cyran F, et al. Differences in clinical expression of hypertrophic cardiomyopathy associated with two distinct mutations in the β-myosin heavy chain gene: A 908 Leu-Val mutation and a 403 Arg-Gln mutation. *Circulation* 1992; 86:345–352.
47. Watkins H, Rosenzweig A, Hwang D, et al. Characteristics and prognostic implications of myosin missense mutations in familial hypertrophic cardiomyopathy. *N Engl J Med* 1992; 326:1108–1114.
48. Watkins H, McKenna W, Thierfelder L, et al. Mutations in the genes for cardiac troponin T and α-tropomyosin in hypertrophic cardiomyopathy. *N Engl J Med* 1995; 332:1058–1064.
49. Poetter K, Jiang H, Hassenzadeh S, et al. Mutations in either the essential or regulatory light chains of myosin are associated with a rare myopathy in human heart and skeletal muscle. *Nature Genet* 1996; 13:63–69.
50. Perryman MB, Yu QT, Marian AJ, et al. Expression of a missense mutation in the mRNA for β-myosin heavy chain in myocardial tissue in hypertrophic cardiomyopathy. *J Clin Invest* 1992; 90:271–277.
51. Marian AJ, Yu QT, Workman R, et al. Angiotensin converting enzyme polymorphism in hypertrophic cardiomyopathy and sudden cardiac death. *Lancet* 1993; 342:1085–1086.
52. Lechin M, Yu QT, Roberts R, et al. Angiotensin I converting enzyme geneotypes and left ventricular hypertrophy in patients with hypertrophic cardiomyopathy. *Circulation* 1995; 92:1808–1812.
53. Maron BJ. Cardiovascular preparticipation screening of competitive athletes. In: Williams RA, ed. *The Athlete and Heart Disease: Diagnosis, Evaluation & Management*. Philadelphia: Lippincott Williams & Wilkins; 1999:273–285.
54. Beohar N, Damaraju S, Prather A. Angiotensin-I converting enzyme genotype DD is a risk factor for coronary artery disease. *J Invest Med* 1995; 43:275–280.
55. Vybiral T, Roberts R, Deitiker PR, et al. Accumulation and

assembly of myosin in the Arg-Gln β-MHC hypertrophic cardiomyopathy mutant. *Circ Res* 1992; 71:1404–1409.
56. Marian AJ, Yu QT, Mann DL, et al. Expression of a mutation causing hypertrophic cardiomyopathy in adult feline cardiocytes disrupts sarcomere assembly in adult feline cardiac myocytes. *Circ Res* 1995; 77:98–106.
57. Oberst L, Zhao G, Park JT, et al. Dominant-negative effect of a mutant cardiac troponin T on cardiac structure and function in transgenic mice. *J Clin Invest* 1998; 102:1498–1505.
58. Vikstrom KL, Factor SM, Leinwand LA. Mice expressing mutant myosin heavy chains are a model for familial hypertrophic cardiomyopathy. *Mol Med Today* 1996; 2:556–567.
59. Geisterfer-Lowrance AA, Christe M, Conner DA, et al. A mouse model of familial hypertrophic cardiomyopathy. *Science* 1996; 272:731–734.
60. Becker KD, Gottshall KR, Hickey R, et al. Point mutations in human cardiac myosin heavy chain have differential effects on sarcomeric structure and assembly: An ATP binding site change disrupts both thick and think filaments, whereas hypertrophic cardiomyopathy mutations display normal assembly. *J Cell Biol* 1997; 137:137–140.
61. Marian J, Wu Y, McCluggage M. A transgenic rabbit model for human hypertrophic cardiomyopathy. *J Clin Invest* 1999; 104:1683–1692.
62. Berenfeld O, Jalife J. Purkinje-muscle reentry as a mechanism of polymorphic ventricular arrhythmias in a 3-dimensional model of the ventricles. *Circ Res* 1998; 82:1063–1077.
63. Pogwizd SM, McKenzie JP, Cain ME. Mechanisms underlying spontaneous and induced ventricular arrhythmias in patients with idiopathic dilated cardiomyopathy. *Circulation* 1998; 98:2404–2414.
64. Service R. DNA chips survey an entire genome. *Science* 1998; 281:1122.
65. Towbin JA. Molecular genetic aspects of cardiomyopathy. *Biochem Med Metab Biol* 1993; 49:285–320.
66. Klein A, Lebreton A, Lemoine J. Identification of urinary ligosaccharides by matrix-assisted laser desorption ionization time-of-flight mass spectrometry. *Clin Chem* 1998; 44:2422–2428.
67. Meikle PJ, Yan M, Ravenscroft EM, et al. Altered trafficking and turnover of LAMP-1 in Pompe disease-affected cells. *Mol Genet Metab* 1999; 66:179–188.
68. Bijvoet AJ, van de Kamp EH, Kroos MA, et al. Generalized glycogen storage and cardiomegaly in a knockout mouse model of Pompe disease. *Hum Mol Genet* 1998; 7:53–62.
69. Raben N, Nagaraju K, Lee E, et al. Targeted disruption of the acid α-glucosidase gene in mice causes an illness with critical features of both infantile and adult human glycogen storage disease type II. *J Biol Chem* 1998; 273:19086–19092.
70. Yang HW, Kikuchi T, Hagiwara Y, et al. Recombinant human acid α-glucosidase-deficient human fibroblasts, quail fibroblasts, and quail myoblasts. *Pediatr Res* 1998; 43:374–380.
71. Kikuchi T, Yang HW, Pennybacker M, et al. Clinical and metabolic correction of Pompe disease by enzyme therapy in acid maltase-deficient quail. *J Clin Invest* 1998; 101:827–833.
72. Pauly DF, Johns DC, Matelis LA, et al. Complete correction of acid α-glucosidase deficiency in Pompe disease fibroblats in vitro, and lysosomally targeted expression in neonatal rat cardiac and skeletal muscle. *Gene Ther* 1998; 5:473–480.
73. Wiedemann HR. Complexo malformatif familial avec hernie unbilicate et macroglossie: Un "syndrome nouveau"? *J Genet Hum* 1964; 13:223–232.
74. Beckwith JB. Macroglossia, omphalocele, adrenal cytomegaly, gigantism and hyperplastic visceromegaly. *Birth Defects* 1969; 2:188–196.
75. Sotelo-Avila C, Gonzalez-Crussi F, Fowler JW. Complete and incomplete forms of Beckwith-Wiedemann syndrome: Their oncogenic potential. *J Pediatr* 1980; 96:47–50.
76. Best LG, Hoekstra RE. Wiedemann-Beckwith syndrome: Autosomal dominant inheritance in a family. *Am J Med Genet* 1981; 9:291–299.
77. Bhuiyan ZA, Yatsuki H, Sasaguri T, et al. Functional analysis of the p57KIP2 gene mutation in Beckwith-Wiedemann syndrome. *Hum Genet* 1999; 104:205–210.
78. Hatada I, Nabetani A, Morisaki H, et al. New p57KIP2 mutations in Beckwith-Wiedemann syndrome. *Hum Genet* 1997; 100: 681–683.
79. Lam WW, Hatada I, Ohishi S, et al. Analysis of germlinie CDKNIC (p57KIP2) mutations in familial and sporadic Beckwith-Wiedemann syndrome (BWS) provides a novel genotype-phenotype correlation. *J Med Genet* 1999; 36:518–523.
80. Lee MP, De Baun M, Randhawa G, et al. Low frequency of p57KIP2 mutation in Beckwith-Wiedemann syndrome. *Am J Hum Genet* 1997; 61:304–309.
81. Zhang P, Liegeois NJ, Wong C, et al. Altered cell differentiation and proliferation in mice lacking p57KIP2 indicates a role in Beckwith-Wiedemann syndrome. *Nature* 1997; 387:151–158.
82. Lee MP, Hu RJ, Johnson LA, Feinberg AP. Human KVLQT1 gene shows tissue-specific imprinting and encompasses Beckwith-Wiedemann syndrome chromosomal rearrangements. *Nature Genet* 1997; 15:181–185.
83. Smilinich NJ, Day CD, Fitzpatrick GV, et al. A maternally methylated CpG island in KVLQT1 is associated with an antisense paternal transcript and loss of imprinting in Beckwith-Wiedemann syndrome. *Proc Natl Acad Sci USA* 1999; 96:8064–8069.
84. Sun FL, Dean WL, Kelsey G, et al. Transactivation of lgf2 in a mouse model of Beckwith-Wiedemann syndrome. *Nature* 1997; 389:809–815.
85. Catchpoole D, Lam WW, Valler D, et al. Epigenetic modification and uniparental inheritance of H19 in Beckwith-Wiedemann syndrome. *J Med Genet* 1997; 34:353–359.
86. Mitsuya K, Megura M, Lee MP, et al. LIT1, an imprinted antisense RNA in the human KVLQT1 locus identified by screening for differentially expressed transcripts using monochromosomal hybrids. *Human Mol Genet* 1999; 8:1209–1217.
87. Durr A, Cossee M, Agid Y, et al. Clinical and genetic abnormalities in patients with Friedreich's ataxia. *N Engl J Med* 1996; 335:1169–1175.
88. Chamberlain S, Shaw J, Rowland A, et al. Mapping of mutation causing Friedreich's ataxia to human chromosome 9. *Nature* 1988; 334:248–250.
89. Campuzano V, Montermini L, Mooto MD, et al. Friedreich's ataxia: 81. Autosomal recessive disease caused by an intronic GAA triplet repeat expansion. *Science* 1996; 271:1423–1427.
90. Filla A, De Michele G, Cavalcanti F, et al. The relationship between trinucleotide (GAA) repeat length and classical features in Friedreich ataxia. *Am J Hum Genet* 1996; 59:554–560.
91. Montermini L, Richter A, Morgan K, et al. Phenotypic variability in Friedreich ataxia: Role of the associated GAA triplet repeat expansion. *Ann Neurol* 1997; 41:675–682.
92. Lamont PJ, Davis MB, Wood NW. Identification and sizing of the GAA triplet repeat expansion of Friedreich ataxia in 56 patients: Clinical and genetic correlates. *Brain* 1997; 120:672–680.
93. Monros E, Molto MD, Martinez F, et al. Phenotype correlation and intergenerational dynamics of the Friedreich ataxia GAA trinucleotide repeat. *Am J Hum Genet* 1997; 61:101–110.
94. Campuzano V, Montermini L, Lutz Y, et al. Frataxin is reduced in Friedreich ataxia patients and is associated with mitochondrial membranes. *Hum Mol Genet* 1997; 11:1771–1780.
95. Rotig A, de Lonlay P, Chretien D, et al. Aconitase and mitochondrial iron-sulphur protein deficiency in Friedreich ataxia. *Nature Genet* 1997; 17:215–217.
96. Knight SAB, Kim R, Pain D, Dancis A. the yeast connection to Friedreich ataxia. *Am J Hum Genet* 1999; 64:365–371.
97. Koutnikova H, Campuzano V, Foury F, et al. Studies of human,

mouse and yeast homologues indicate a mitochondrial function for frataxin. *Nature Genet* 1997; 16:345–351.
98. Codd MB, Sugrue DD, Gersh BJ, et al. Epidemiology of idiopathic dilated and hypertrophic cardiomyopathy: A population-based study in Olmsted County, Minnesota, 1975–1984. *Circulation* 1989; 80:564–572.
99. Durand JB, Bachinski LL, Beiling L, et al. Localization of a gene responsible for familial idiopathic dilated cardiomyopathy to chromosome 1q32. *Circulation* 1995; 92:3387–3389.
100. Krajinovic M, Pinamonti B, Sinagra G, et al. Linkage of familial dilated cardiomyopathy to chromosome 9. *Am J Hum Genet* 1995; 57:846–852.
101. Siu BL, Nimura H, Osborne JA, et al. Familial dilated cardiiomyopathy locus maps to chromosome 2q31. *Circulation* 1999; 99:1022–1026.
102. Bowles KR, Gajarski R, Porter P, et al. Gene mapping of familial autosomal dominant dilated cardiomyopathy to chromosome 10q21-23. *J Clin Invest* 1996; 98:1355–1360.
103. Kass S, MacRae C, Graber HL, et al. A gene defect that causes conduction system disease and dilated cardiomyopathy maps to chromosome 1p1-1q1. *Nature Genet* 1994; 7:546–551.
104. Olson TM, Keating MT. Mapping a cardiomyopathy locus to chromosome 3p22-25. *J Clin Invest* 1996; 97:528–532.
105. Messina DN, Speer MC, Pericak-Vance MA, et al. Linkage of familial dilated cardiomyopathy with conduction defect and muscular dystrophy to chromosome 6q23. *Am J Hum Genet* 1997; 61:909–917.
106. Olson T, Michels VV, Thibodeau, SN, et al. Actin mutations in dilated cardiomypathy, a heritable form of heart failure. *Science* 1998; 280:750–752.
107. Li D, Tapscott T, Gonzalez O, et al. Desmin mutation responsible for idiopathic dilated cardiomyopathy. *Circulation* 1999; 100:461–464.
108. Morgensen J, Klausen C, Pedersen AK, et al. α-Cardiac actin is a novel disease gene in familial hypertrophic cardiomyopathy. *J Clin Invest* 1999; 103:R39–R43.
109. Fuchs E. Intermediate filaments and disease: Mutations that cripple cell strength. *J Cell Biol* 1994; 125:511–516.
110. Milner DJ, Weitzner G, Tran D, et al. Disruption of muscle architecture and myocardial degeneration in mice lacking desmin. *J Cell Biol* 1996; 1343:1255–1270.
111. Maeda M, Holder E, Lowes B, et al. Dilated cardiomyoapthy associated with deficiency of the cytoskeletal protein metavinculin. *Circulation* 1997; 95:17–20.
112. Marian AJ, Roberts R. Molecular pathophysiology of cardiomyopathies. In: Sperelakis N, ed. *Cardiac Physiology*. San Diego, CA: Academic Press; 1999.
113. Towbin JA. The role of cytoskeletal proteins in cardiomyopathies. *Curr Opin Cell Biol* 1998; 10:131–139.
114. Towbin JA, Bowles KR, Bowles NE. Etiologies of cardiomyopathy and heart failure: Evidence for a final common pathway for disorders of the myocardium. *Nature Med* 1999; 5:266–267.
115. Towbin JA, Hejtmancik JF, Brink P, et al. X-linked dilated cardiomyopathy (XLCM): Molecular genetic evidence of linkage to the Duchenne muscular dystrophy gene at the Xp21 locus. *Circulation* 1993; 87:1854–1865.
116. Towbin JA. Biochemical and molecular characterization of X-linked dilated cardiomyopathy. In: Clark EB, Markwald RR, Takao A, eds. *Developmental Mechanisms of Heart Disease*. New York: Futura; 1995:121–132.
117. Ohlendieck K, Matsumura K, lonasescu W, et al. Duchenne muscular dystrophy: Deficiency of dystrophin-associated proteins in the sarcolemma. *Neurology* 1993; 43:795–800.
118. Bies RD, Maeda M, Roberds SL, et al. A 5′ dystrophin duplication mutation causes membrane deficiency of alpha-dystroglycan in a family with X-linked cardiomyopathy. *J Mol Cell Cardiol* 1997; 29:3175–3188.
119. Towbin JA, Ortiz-Lopez R. X-linked dilated cardiomyopathy is not due to a muscle promoter deletion in dystrophin in 3 families. *N Engl J Med* 1994; 330:369–370.
120. Ortiz-Lopez R, Li H, Su J, et al. Evidence for a dystrophin missense mutation as a cause of X-linked dilated cardiomyopathy (XLCM). *Circulation* 1997; 95:2434–2440.
121. Yoshida K, Ikeda S, Nakamura A, et al. Molecular analysis of the Duchenne muscular dystrophy gene in patients with Becker muscular dystrophy presenting with dilated cardiomyopathy. *Muscle Nerve* 1993; 16:1161–1166.
122. Muntoni F, Cau M, Ganau A, Congi R, et al. Brief report: Deletion of the dystrophin muscle-promoter region associated with X-linked dilated cardiomyopathy. *N Engl J Med* 1993; 329:921–925.
123. Milasin J, Muntoni F, Severini GM, et al. A point mutation in the 5′ splice site of the dystrophin gene first intron responsible for X-linked dilated cardiomyopathy. *Hum Mol Genet* 1996; 5:73–79.
124. Yoshida K, Nakamura A, Yazaki M, et al. Insertional mutation by transposable element L1, in the DMD gene results in X-linked dilated cardiomyopathy. *Hum Mol Genet* 1998; 7:1120–1132.
125. Ferlini A, Galie N, Merlini L, et al. A novel Alu-like element rearranged in the dystrophin gene causes a splicing mutation in a family with X-linked dilated cardiomyopathy. *Am J Hum Genet* 1998; 63:436–446.
126. Neustein HB, Lurie PR, Dahms B, et al. An X-linked recessive cardiomyopathy with abnormal mitochondria. *Pediatrics* 1998; 64:24–29.
127. Barth PG, Schotte HR, Berden JA, et al. An X-linked mitochondrial disease affecting cardiac muscle skeletal muscle and neutrophil leukocytes. *J Neurol Sci* 1983; 62:327–355.
128. Bolhuis PA, Hensels GW, Hulsebos TJM, et al. Mapping of the locus for X-linked cardioskeletal myopathy with neutropenia and abnormal mitochondria (Barth syndrome) to Xq28. *Am J Hum Genet* 1991; 48:481–485.
129. Bione S, D'Adamo P, Maestrini E, et al. A novel X-linked gene, G4.5, is responsible for Barth syndrome. *Nature Genet* 1996; 12:385–389.
130. Bleyl SB, Mumford Thompson V, et al. Neonatal lethal noncompaction of the left ventricular myocardium is allelic with Barth syndrome. *Am J Hum Genet* 1997; 61:868–872.
131. Johnston J, Kelley, RI, Feigenbaum A, et al. Mutation characterization and genotype-phenotype correlation in Barth syndrome. *Am J Med Genet* 1997; 61:1053–1058.
132. D'Adamo P, Fassone L, Patton MA, et al. The X-linked gene G4.5 is responsible for different infantile dilated cardiomyopathies. *Am J Hum Genet* 1997; 61:862–867.
133. Thiene G, Basso C, Danieli G, et al. Arrhythmogenic right ventricular cardiomyopathy. *Trends Cardiovasc Med* 1997; 7:84–90.
134. Thiene G, Nava A, Corrado D, et al. Right ventricular cardiomyopathy and sudden death in young people. *N Engl J Med* 1988; 318:129–133.
135. Shen WK, Edwards WD, Hammill SC, et al. Right ventricular dysplasia: A need for precise pathological definition for interpretation of sudden death. *J Am Coll Cardiol* 1994; 23:34.
136. Rampazzo A, Nava A, Erne P, et al. A new locus for arrhythmogenic right ventricular cardiomyopathy (ARVD2) maps to chromosome 1q42-q43. *Hum Mol Genet* 1995; 4:2151–2154.
137. Severini GM, Krajinovic M, Pinamonti B, et al. A new locus for arrhythmogenic right ventricular dysplasia on the long arm of chromosome 14. *Genomics* 1996; 31:193–200.
138. Coonar AS, Protonotarios N, Tsatsopoulou A, et al. Gene for arrhythmogenic right ventricular cardiomyopathy with diffuse nonepidermolytic palmoplantar keratoderma and woolly hair wooly hair (Naxos disease) maps to 17q21. *Circulation* 1998; 97:2049–2058.
139. Ahmad F, Li D, Karibe A, et al. Localization of a gene responsible for arrhythmogenic right ventricular dysplasia to chromosome 3p23. *Circulation* 1998; 98:2791–2795.

140. Li D, Ahmad F, Gardner MJ, Weilbaecher D, et al. The locus of a novel gene responsible for arrhythmogenic right ventricular dysplasia characterized by early onset and high penetrance maps to chromosome 10p12-p14. *Am J Hum Genet* 2000; 66:148–156.
141. McKenna WJ, Thiere G, Nava AA, et al. Diagnosis of arrhythmogenic right ventricular dysplasis/cardiomyopathy. *Br Heart J* 1994; 71:215–218.
142. Jacobson DR, Pastore R, Yaghoubian R, et al. Variant-sequence transthyretin (isoleucine 122) in late-onset cardiac amyloidosis in black Americans. *N Engl J Med* 1997; 336:466–473.
143. Jacobson DR, Ittmann M, Buxbaum JN, et al. Transthyretin Ile 122 and cardiac arryloidosis in African-Americans; 2 case reports. *Tex Heart Inst J* 1997; 24:45–52.
144. Goldfarb LG, Park K-Y, Cervenakova L, et al. Missense mutations in desmin associated with familial cardiac and skeletal myopathy. *Nature Genet* 1998; 19:402–403.
145. Neufeld EF, Muenzer J. The mucopolysaccharidoses. In: Scriver CR, Beaudet AL, Sly NS, Valle D, ed. *The Metabolic and Molecular Basis of Inherited Disease*. New York: McGraw-Hill; 1995: 2465–2494.
146. Bach G, Freidman R, Weissmann B, et al. The defect in Hurler and Scheie syndromes: Deficiency of α-L-iduronidase. *Proc Natl Acad Sci USA* 1972; 69:2049–2051.
147. Dangel JH. Cardiovascular changes in children with mucopolysaccharide storage diseases and related disorders—Clinical and echocardiographic findings in 64 patients. *Eur J Pediatr* 1998; 157:534–538.
148. Scott HS, Guo X, Hopwood JJ, et al. Structural and sequence of the human α-L-iduronidase gene. *Genomics* 1992; 13:1311–1313.
149. Scott HS, Litjens T, Nelson PV, et al. Identification of mutations in the α-L-iduronidase gene (IDUA) that cause Hurler and Scheie syndromes. *Am J Hum Genet* 1993; 53:973–986.
150. Krivit W, Peters C, Shapiro EG. Bone marrow transplantation as effective treatment of central nervous system disease in globoid cell leukodystrophy, metachromatic leukodystrophy, adenoleukodystrophy, mannosidosis, fucosidosis, aspartylglucosaminuria, Hurler, Maroteaux-Lamy, and Sly syndromes, and Gaucher disease type III. *Curr Opin Neurol* 1999; 12:167–176.
151. Huang MM, Wong A, Yu X, et al. Retrovirus-mediated transfer of the human α-L-iduronidase cDNA into human hematopoietic progenitor cells leads to correction in trans of Hurler fibroblasts. *Gene Ther* 1997; 4:1150–1159.
152. Russell C, Hendson G, Jevon G, et al. Murine MPS1: Insights into the pathogenesis of Hurler syndrome. *Clin Genet* 1998; 53:349–361.
153. Clarke LA, Russell CS, Pownall S, et al. Murine mucopolysaccharidoses type I: Targeted disruption of the murne α-L-iduronidase gene. *Hum Mol Genet* 1997; 6:503–511.
154. He X, Li CM, Simonaro CM, et al. Identification and characterization of the molecular lesion causing mucopolysaccharidoses type I in cats. *Mol Genet Metab* 1999; 67:106–112.
155. Hartog C, Fryer A, Upadhyaya M. Mutation analysis of iduronate-2-sulphatase gene in 24 patients with Hunter syndrome: characterization of 6 novel mutations. *Hum Mutat* 1999; 14:87.
156. Timms KM, Bondeson ML, Ansari-Lari MA, et al. Molecular and phenotypic variation in patients with severe Hunter syndrome. *Hum Mol Genet* 1997; 6:479–486.
157. Li P, Bellows AB, Thompson JN. Molecular basis of iduronate-2-sulphatase gene mutations in patients with mucopolysaccharidosis type II (Hunter syndrome). *J Med Genet* 1999; 36:21–27.
158. DiFrancesco C, Cracco C, Tomanin R, et al. In vitro correction of iduronate-2-sulphatase deficiency by adenovirus gene transfer. *Gene Ther* 1997; 4:442–448.
159. Marra BL, Medina CD, Hoang GKB, et al. Gene therapy for neurologic disease: Benchtop discoveries to bedside applications. 2. The bedside. *J Child Neurol* 1997; 12:77–84.
160. Stroncek DF, Hubel A, Shankar RA, et al. Retroviral transduction and expansion of peripheral blood lymphocytes for the treatment of mucopolysaccharidosis type II, Hunter's syndrome. *Transfusion* 1999; 39:343–350.
161. Tomatsu S, Fukuda S, Masue M, et al. Morquio disease: Isolation, characterization and expression of full-length cDNA for human N-acetyl-galactosamine-6-sulfate sulfatase. *Biochem Biophys Res Comm* 1991; 1871:677–683.
162. Masuno M, Tomatsu S, Nakashima Y, et al. Mucopolysaccharidosis IVA: Assignment of the human N-acetylgalactosamine-6-sulfatase (GALNS) gene to chromosome 16q24. *Genomics* 1993; 16:777–778.
163. Fukuda S, Tomatsu S, Masue M, et al. Mucopolysaccharidosis type IVA N-acetyl galactosamine-6-sulfate sulfatase exonic point mutations in classical Morquio and mild cases. *J Clin Invest* 1992; 90:1049–1053.
164. Yamada N, Fukuda S, Tomatsu S, et al. Molecular heterogeneity in mucopolysaccharidosis IVA in Australia and Northern Ireland: Nine novel mutations including T312S, a common allele that confers a mild phenotype. *Hum Mutat* 1998; 11:202–208.
165. Jackson CE, Yuhki N, Desnick RJ, et al. Feline arylsulfatase B (ARSB): Isolation and expression of the cDNA, comparison with human ARSB, and gene localization to feline chromosome A1. *Genomics* 1992; 14:403–411.
166. Mondaressi S, Rupp K, Von Figura K, et al. Structure of the human arylsulfatase B gene. *Biol Chem Hoppe Seyler* 1993; 374:327–335.
167. Voskoboeva E, Isbrandt D, Von Figura K, et al. Four novel mutant alleles of the arylsulfatase B gene in two patients with intermediate form of mucopolysaccharidosis VI (Maroteaux-Lamy syndrome). *Hum Genet* 1994; 93:259–264.
168. Cox GF, Kunkel LM. Dystrophies and heart disease. *Curr Opin Cardiol* 1997; 12:329–343.
169. Sadoulet-Puccio HM, Kunkel LM. Dystrophin and its isoforms. *Brain Pathol* 1996; 6:25–35.
170. Bonnemann CG, McNally EM, Kunkel LM. Beyond dystrophin: Current progress in the muscular dystrophies. *Curr Opin Pediatr* 1997; 8:569–582.
171. Malhotra SB, Hart KA, Klamut HJ, et al. Frame-shift deletions in patients with Duchenne and Becker muscular dystrophy. *Science* 1988; 242:755–759.
172. Melacini P, Fanin M, Danieli GA, et al. Myocardial involvement is very frequent among patients affected with subclinical Becker muscular dystrophy. *Circulation* 1996; 94:3168–3175.
173. Yoshida K, Ikeda S, Nakamura A, et al. Molecular analysis of the Duchenne muscular dystrophy gene in patients with Becker muscular dystrophy presenting with dilated cardiomyopathy. *Muscle Nerve* 1993; 16:1161–1166.
174. Nigro V, Okazaki Y, Belsito A, et al. Identification of the Syrian hamster cardiomyopathy gene. *Hum Mol Genet* 1997; 6:601–607.
175. Sakamoto A, Ono K, Abe M, et al. Both hypertrophic and dilated cardiomyopathies are caused by mutation of the same gene, α-sarcoglycan in hamsters: An animal model of disrupted dystrophin-associated glycoprotein complex. *Proc Natl Acad Sci USA* 1997; 94:13873–13878.
176. Deconinck KAE, Potter AC, Tinsley JM, et al. Postsynaptic abnormalities in the neuromuscular junctions of utrophin-deficient mice. *J Cell Biol* 1997; 136:883–894.
177. Grady RM, Merlie JP, Sanes SR. Subtle neuromuscular defects in utrophin-deficient mice. *J Cell Biol* 1997; 136:871–882.
178. Deconinck AE, Rafael JA, Skinner JA, et al. Utrophin-dystrophin-deficient mice as a model for Duchenne muscular dystrophy. *Cell* 1997; 90:717–727.
179. Grady RM, Teng HB, Nichol MC, et al. Skeletal and cardiac myopathies in mice lacking utrophin and dystrophin: A model for Duchenne muscular dystrophy. *Cell* 1997; 90:729–738.
180. Lumeng CN, Phelps SF, Rafael JA, et al. Characterization of

dystrophin and utrophin diversity in the mouse. *Hum Mol Genet* 1999; 8:593–599.

181. Tinsley JM, Potter AC, Phelps SR, et al. Amelioration of the dystrophic phenotype of *mdx* mice using a truncated utrophin transgene. *Nature* 1996; 384:349–353.
182. Rafael JA, Sunada Y, Cole NM, et al. Prevention of dystrophic pathology in *mdx* mice by a truncated dystrophin isoform. *Hum Mol Genet* 1994; 3:1725–1733.
183. Gussoni E, Soneoka Y, Strickland CD, et al. Dystrophin expression in the *mdx* mouse restored by stem cell transplantation. *Nature* 1999; 401:390–394.
184. Consalez GG, Thomas NST, Stayton CL, et al. Assignment of Emery-Dreifuss muscular dystrophy to the distal region of Xq28: The results of a collaborative study. *Am J Hum Genet* 1991; 48:468–480.
185. Bione S, Maestrini E, Rivella S, et al. Identification of a novel X-linked gene responsible for Emery-Dreifuss muscular dystrophy. *Nature Genet* 1994; 8:323–327.
186. Harris CA, Andryuk PJ, Cline SW, et al. Structure and mapping of the human thymopletin (TMPO) gene and relationship of the human TMPO-b to rat lamin-associated polypeptide-2. *Genomics* 1995; 28:198–205.
187. Nagano A, Koga R, Ogawa M, et al. Emerin deficiency at the nuclear membrane in patients with Emery-Dreifuss muscular dystrophy. *Nature Genet* 1996; 12:254–259.
188. Manilal S, thi Man N, Sewry CA, et al. The Emery-Dreifuss muscular dystrophy protein, emerin, is a nuclear membrane protein. *Hum Mol Genet* 1996; 5:801–808.
189. Bonne G, DiBarletta MR, Varnous S, et al. Mutations in the gene encoding lamin A/C cause autosomal dominant Emery-Dreifuss muscular dystrophy. *Nature Genet* 1999; 21:285–289.
190. Brunner H, Korneluk R, Coerwinkel-Driessen M, et al. Myotonic dystrophy is closely linked to the gene for muscle-type creatine kinase (CKMM). *Hum Genet* 1989; 81:308–310.
191. Timchenko LT. Myotonic dystrophy: The role of RNA CUG triplet repeats. *Am J Hum Genet* 1999; 64:360–364.
192. Timchenko LT, Timchenko NA, Caskey CT, et al. Novel proteins with binding specificity for DNA CTG repeats and RNA CUG repeats: Implications for myotonic dystrophy. *Hum Mol Genet* 1996; 5:115–121.
193. Timchenko LT, Miller JW, Timchenko NA, et al. Identification of a (CUG)n triplet repeat RNA-binding protein and its expression in myotonic dystrophy. *Nucleic Acids Res* 1996; 24:4407–4414.
194. Roberts R, Timchenko NA, Miller JW, et al. Altered phosphorylation and intracellular distribution of a (CUG) triplet repeat RNA-binding protein in patients with myotonic dystrophy and in myotonic protein kinase knock out mice. *Proc Natl Acad Sci USA* 1997; 94:13221–13226.
195. Jansen G, Groenen PJ, Bachner D, et al. Abnormal myotonic dystrophy protein kinase levels produce only mild myopathy in mice. *Nature Genet* 1996; 13:316–324.
196. Philips AV, Timchenko LT, Cooper T. Disruption of splicing regulated by a CUG-binding protein in myotonic dystrophy. *Science* 1998; 280:737–740.
197. Lu X, Timchenko NA, Timchenko LT. Cardiac elav-type RNA-binding protein (ETR-3) binds to RNA CUG repeats expanded in myotonic dystrophy. *Hum Mol Genet* 1999; 8:53–60.
198. Hanson PA, Rowland LP. Mobius syndrome and facioscapulohumeral muscular dystrophy. *Arch Neurol* 1971; 24:31–39.
199. Galluzzi G, Deidda G, Cacurri S, et al. Molecular analysis of 4q35 rearrangements in fascioscapulohumeral muscular dystrophy (FSHD): application to family studies for a correct genetic advice and a reliable prenatal diagnosis of the disease. *Neuromusc Disord* 1999; 9(3):190–198.
200. North KN, Laing NG, Wallgren-Pettersson C, et al. Nemaline myopathy: Current concepts. *J Med Genet* 1997; 34:705–713.
201. Wallgren-Patterson C. Congenital nemaline myopathy: A clinical follow-up study of twelve patients. *J Neurol Sci* 1989; 89:1–14.
202. Nowak KH, Wattansirichaigoon D, Goebel HH, et al. Mutations in the skeletal muscle α-actin gene in patients with actin myopathy and nemaline myopathy. *Nature Genet* 1999; 23:208–212.
203. Goebel HH, Anderson JR, Hubner C, et al. Congenital myopathy with excess of thin filaments. *Neuromusc Disord* 1997; 7:160–168.
204. Laing NG, Wilton SD, Akkari PA, et al. A mutation in the α-tropomyosin gene TPM3 associated with autosomal dominant nemaline myopathy. *Nature Genet* 1995; 9:75–79.
205. Pelin K, Hilpelä P, Donner K, et al. Mutations in the nebulin gene associated with autosomal recessive nemaline myopathy. *Proc Natl Acad Sci USA* 1999; 96:2305–2310.
206. Sellers FJ, Keith JD, Manning JA. The diagnosis of primary endocardial fibroelastosis. *Circulation* 1994; 29:49–59.
207. Opitiz JM. Genetic aspects of endocardial fibroelastosis. *Am J Med Genet* 1982; 11:92–96.
208. Ni J, Bowles NE, Kim Y, et al. Viral infection of the myocardium in endocardial fibroelastosis: Molecular evidence for the role of mumps virus as an etiological agent. *Circulation* 1997; 95:133–139.
209. Waber LJ, Valle D, Neill C, et al. Carnintine deficiency presenting as familial cardiomyopathy: A treatable defect in carnitine transport. *J Pediatr* 1982; 101:700–705.
210. Shoji Y, Koizumi A, Kayo T, et al. Evidence for linkage of human primary systemic carnitine deficiency with D5S436: A novel gene locus on chromosome 5q. *Am J Hum Genet* 1998; 63:101–108.
211. Koizumi T, Nikaido H, Hayakawa J, et al. Infantile disease with microvascular fatty infiltration of viscera spontaneously occuring in C3H-H2-2 strain of mouse with similarities to Reye's syndrome. *Lab Anim* 1988; 22:83–87.
212. Kuwajima M, Kono N, Horiuchi M, et al. Animal model of systemic carnitine deficiency: Analysis in C3H-H-2° strain of mouse associated with juvenile visceral steatosis. *Biochem Biophys Res Commun* 1991; 174:1090–1094.
213. Nikaido H, Horiuchi M, Hashimoto N, et al. Mapping the *jvs* (juvenlie steatosis) gene, which causes systemic carnitine deficiency in mice of chromosome 11. *Mamm Genome* 1995; 6:369–370.
214. Nezu J-i, Tamai I, Oku A, et al. Primary systemic carnitine deficiency is caused by mutations in a gene encoding sodium ion-dependent carnitine transporter. *Naure Genet* 1999; 21:91–94.
215. Kelly JP, Kim J, Billadello JJ, et al. Nucleotide sequence of medium-chain acyl-CoA dehydrogenase mRNA and its expression in enzyme-deficient human tissue. *Proc Natl Acad Sci USA* 1987; 84:4068–4072.
216. Romppanen EL, Mononen T, Monenen I. Molecular diagnosis of medium-chain acyl-CoA dehydrogenase deficiency by oligonucleotide ligation assay. *Clin Chem* 1998; 44:68–71.
217. Andresen BS, Bross P, Udvari S, et al. The molecular basis of medium-chain acyl-CoA dehydrogenase (MCAD) deficiency in compound heterozygous patients: Is there correlation between genotype and phenotype? *Hum Mol Genet* 1997; 6:695–707.
218. Indo Y, Yang-Feng T, Glassberg R, et al. Molecular cloning and nucleotide sequence of cDNAs encoding human long-chain acyl-CoA dehydrogenase and assignment of the location of its gene (ACADL) to chromosome 2. *Genomics* 1991; 11:609–620.
219. Izai K, Uchida Y, Orii T, et al. Novel fatty acid β-oxidation enzymes in rat liver mitochondria: I. Purification and properties of very long-chain acyl-coenzyme A dehydrogenase. *J Biol Chem* 1992; 267:1027–1033.
220. Uchida Y, Izai K, Orii T, et al. Novel fatty acid β-oxidation enzymes in rat liver mitochondria. II. Purification and properties of enoyl-coenzyme A (CoA) hydratase/3-hydroxyacyl-CoA dehydrogenase 3-ketoacyl-CoA thiolase trifunctional protein. *J Biol Chem* 1992; 267:1034–1041.
221. Andresen BS, Bross P, Vianey-Saban C, et al. Cloning and characterization of human very-long-chain acyl-CoA dehydrogenase

cDNA, chromosomal assignment of the gene and identification in four patients of nine different mutations within the VLCAD gene. *Hum Mol Genet* 1996; 5:461–472.
222. Aoyama T, Souri M, Ueno I, et al. Cloning of human very-long-chain acyl-coenzyme A dehydrogenase and molecular characterization of its deficiency in two patients. *Am J Hum Genet* 1995; 57:273–283.
223. Strauss AS, Powell CK, Hale DE, et al. Molecular basis of human mitochondrial very-long-chain acyl-CoA dehydrogenase deficiency causing cardiomyopathy and sudden death in childhood. *Proc Natl Acad Sci USA* 1995; 92:10196–10500.
224. Andresen BS, Vianey-Saban C, Bross P, et al. The mutational spectrum in very-long-chain acyl-CoA dehydrogenase (VLCAD) deficiency. *J Inherit Metab* 1996; 19:169–172.
225. Andresen BA, Olpin S, Poorthuis BJHM, et al. Clear correlation of genotype with disease phenotype in very-long chain acyl-CoA dehydrogenase deficiency. *Am J Hum Genet* 1999; 64:479–494.
226. Colucci WS, Lorell BH, Schoen FJ, et al. Hypertrophic obstructive cardiomyopathy due to Fabry's disease. *N Engl J Med* 1982; 307:926–928.
227. Becker AE, Schoorl R, Balk AG, van der Heide RM. Cardiac manifestations of Fabry's disease: Report of a case with mitral insufficiency and electrocardiographic evidence of myocardial infarction. *Am J Cardiol* 1975; 36:829–835.
228. Lewin MB, Belmont J, McNamara DG, et al. Further associations of congenital heart disease and genetic syndromes: Report of a case of tetralogy of Fallot and Fabry's disease. *Pediatr Cardiol* 1999; 20:236–237.
229. Cantor WJ, Butany J, Iwanochko M, et al. Restrictive cardiomyopathy secondary to Fabry's disease. *Circulation* 1998; 98:1457–1459.
230. Cantor WJ, Daly P, Iwanochko M, et al. Cardiac transplantation for Fabry's disease. *Can J Cardiol* 1998; 14:81–84.
231. Bishop DF, Calhoun DH, Bernstein HS, et al. Human alpha-galactosidase A: Nucleotide sequence of a cDNA clone encoding the mature enzyme. *Proc Natl Acad Sci USA* 1986; 83:4859–4863.
232. Eng CM, Desnick RJ. Molecular basis of Fabry disease: Mutations and polymorphisms in the human alpha-glactosidase A gene. *Proc Natl Acad Sci USA* 1994; 3:103–111.
233. Germain DP, Poenaru L. Fabry disease: Identification of novel α-galactosidase A mutations and molecular carrier detection by use of fluorescent chemical cleavage mismatches. *Biochem Biophys Res Commun* 1999; 257:708–713.
234. Suzuki K, Proia RL, Suzuki K. Mouse models of human lysosomal diseases. *Brain Pathol* 1998; 8:195–215.
235. Ziegler RJ, Yew NS, Li C, et al. Correction of enzymatic and lysosomal storage defects in Fabry mice by adenovirus-mediated gene transfer. *Hum Gene Ther* 1999; 10:1667–1682.
236. Skovby P. Homocystinuria: Clinical, biochemical and enetic aspects of cystathionine beta-synthase and its deficiency in man. *Acta Paediatr Scand* 1985; 321:14–21.
237. Mudd SH, Skovby F, Levy HL, et al. The natural history of homocystinuria due to cystathionine β-synthase deficiency. *Am J Hum Genet* 1985; 37:1–31.
238. Mandel H, Brenner B, Berant M, et al. Coexistence of hereditary homocystinuria and factor V Leiden: Effect on thrombosis. *N Engl J Med* 1996; 334:763–768.
239. Munke M, Kraus JP, Ohura T, Francke U. The gene for cystathionine beta-synthase (CBS) maps to the subtelomeric region on human chromosome 21q and to proximal mouse chromosome 17. *Am J Hum Genet* 1988; 42:550–559.
240. Kraus JP, Oliverusova J, Sokolova J, et al. The human cystathionine β-synthase (CBS) gene: Complete sequence, alternative splicing, and polymorphisms. *Genomics* 1998; 52:312–324.
241. Seashore MR. Tandem spectrometry in newborn screening. *Curr Opin Pediatr* 1998; 10:609–614.
242. Mayer EL, Jacobsen DW, Robinson K. Homocysteine and coronary atherosclerosis. *J Am Coll Cardiol* 1996; 27:517–527.
243. den Heijer M, Koster T, Blom HJ, et al. Hyperhomocysteinemia as a risk factor for deep-vein thrombosis. *N Engl J Med* 1996; 334:759–762.
244. Tsai J, Wang H, Perrella MA, et al. Induction of cyclin a gene expression by homocysteine in vascular smooth muscle cells. *J Clin Invest* 1996; 97:146–153.
245. Attardi G. The elucidation of human mitochondrial genome: A historical perspective. *Bioessays* 1994; 5:34–39.
246. Smeitink J, van den Heuvel L. Human mitochondrial complex I in health and disease. *Am J Hum Genet* 1999; 64:1505–1510.
247. Liang MH, Wong L. Yield on mtDNA mutation analysis in 2000 patients. *Am J Med Genet* 1998; 77:395–400.
248. Robinson BH. Human complex I deficiency: Clinical spectrum and involvement of oxygen free radicals in the pathogenicity of the defect. *Biochem Biophys Acta* 1998; 1364:271–286.
249. Chomyn A. The myoclonic epilepsy and ragged-red fiber mutation provides new insights into human mitochondria function and genetics. *Am J Hum Genet* 1998; 62:745–751.
250. Smeitink JAM, Loeffer JLCM, Triepels RH, et al. Nuclear genes of human complex I of the mitochondrial electron transport chain: State of the art. *Hum Mol Genet* 1998; 7:1573–1579.
251. Loeffen JL, Triepels RH, van den Heuvel LP, et al. cDNA of eight nuclear encoded subunits of NADH: Ubiquinone oxidoreductase: Human complex I cDNA characterization completed. *Biochem Biophys Res Commun* 1998; 253:415–422.
252. Morris AA, Leonard JV, Brown GK, et al. Deficiency of respiratory chain complex I is a common cause of Leigh disease. *Ann Neurol* 1996; 40:25–30.
253. Carral-Debrinski M, Stepien G. Shoffner JM, et al. Hypoxemia is associated with mitochondrial DNA damage and gene induction: Implications for cardiac disease. *JAMA* 1991; 266:1812–1816.
254. Rowland LP, Blake D, Kirano M, et al. Clinical syndromes associated with ragged-red fibers. *Rev Neurol* 1991; 147:467–473.
255. Tveskov C, Angelo-Nielsen K. Kearns-Sayre syndrome and dilated cardiomyopathy. *Neurology* 1990; 40:553–554.
256. Shoffner JM, Lott MI, Lezza AMS, et al. Myotonic epilepsy and ragged-red fiber disease (MERRF) is associated with a mitochondrial DNA tRNA^{LYS} mutation. *Cell* 1990; 61:931–937.
257. Pavalakis SG, Phillips PC, DiMauro S, et al. Mitochondrial myopathy, encephalopathy, lactic acidosis, and strokelike episodes: A distinctive clinical syndrome. *Ann Neurol* 1984; 16:481–487.
258. Clark KM, Bindoff LA, Lightowlers RN, et al. Reversal of a mitochondrial DNA defect in human skeletal muscle. *Nature Genet* 1997; 16:222–224.
259. Taivassalu T, Fu K, Johns T, Arnold D, et al. Gene shifting: a novel therapy for mitochondrial myopathy. *Hum Mol Genet* 1999; 8:1047–1052.
260. Byers PH. Disorders of collagen biosynthesis and structure. In: Scriver CR, Beaudett AL, Sly NS, Valle D, eds. *The Metabolic and Molecular Basis of Inherited Disease*. New York: McGraw-Hill; 1995:4029–4077.
261. Milewicz DM, Molecular genetics of Marfan syndrome and Ehlers-Danlos type IV. *Curr Opin Cardiol* 1998; 13:198–204.
262. Tsipouras P, del Mastro R, Sarfarazi M, et al. Genetic linkage of the Marfan syndrome, ectopia lentis, and congential contractural arachnodatyly to the fabrillin genes on chromosomes 15 and 5. *N Engl J Med* 1992; 326:905–909.
263. Geva T, Sanders SP, Diogenes MS, et al. Two-dimensional and Doppler echocardiographic and pathologic characteristics of the infantile Marfan syndrome. *Am J Cardiol* 1990; 65:1230–1237.
264. Sakai LY, Keene DR, Engvall E. Fibrillin. a new 250-kD glycoprotein, is a component of extracellular microfibrils. *J Cell Biol* 1986; 103:2499–2509.
265. Huggon IC, Burke JP, Talbot JF. Contractural arachnodactyly

with mitral regurgitation and iridodonesis. *Arch Dis Child* 1990; 65:317–319.
266. Kainulainen K, Pulkkinen L, Savolainen A, et al. Location on chromosome 15 of the gene defect causing Marfan's syndrome. *N Engl J Med* 1990; 323:935–939.
267. Dietz HC, Cutting GR, Pyeritz RE, et al. Marfan syndrome caused by a recurrent de novo missense mutation in the fibrillin gene. *Nature* 1991; 352:337–339.
268. Milewicz DM, Duvic M. Severe neonatal Marfan syndrome resulting from a de novo three base pair insertion into the fibrillin gene on chromosome 15. *Am J Hum Genet* 1994; 54:447–453.
269. Lonnqvist L, Child A, Kainulainen K, et al. A novel mutation of the fibrillin gene causing ectopia lentis. *Genomics* 1994; 19:573–576.
270. Boileau C, Jondeau G, Babron M, et al. Autosomal dominant Marfan-like connective tissue disorder with aortic dilation and skeletal anomalies not linked to the fibrillin genes. *Am J Hum Genet* 1993; 53:46–54.
271. Francke U, Berg MA, Tynan K, et al. A Gly1127Ser mutation in an EGF-like domain of the fibrillin-1 gene is a risk factor for ascending aortic aneurysm and dissection. *Am J Hum Genet* 1994; 45:1287–1296.
272. Milewicz DM, Michael K, Fisher N, et al. Fibrillin-1 (FNB1) mutations in patients with thoracic aortic aneurysms. *Circulation* 1996; 94:2708–2711.
273. Sood SR, Eldadah ZA, Krause WL, et al. Mutation in fibrillin-1 and the marfanoid-craniosynostosis (Sprintzen-Goldberg) syndrome. *Nature Genet* 1996; 12:209–211.
274. Putnam EA, Zhang H, Ramirez F, Milewicz DM. Fibrillin-2 (RBN2) mutations result in the Marfan-like disorder, congenital contractural arachnodactyly. *Nature Genet* 1995; 11:456–458.
275. Collod G, Babron M, Jondeau G, et al. A second locus for Marfan syndrome maps to chromosome 3p24.2-p25. *Nature Genet* 1994; 8:264–268.
276. Shores J, Berger KR, Murphy EA, Pyeritz RE. Progression of aortic dilatation and the benefit of long-term beta-adrenergic blockade in Marfan's syndrome. *N Engl J Med* 1994; 330:1335–1341.
277. Gott VL, Gillinov AM, Pyeritz RE, et al. Aortic root replacement. Risk factor analysis of a seventeen-year experience with 270 patients. *J Thorac Cardiovasc Surg* 1995; 109:536–544.
278. Pyeritz RE. Maternal and fetal complications in pregnancy in the Marfan syndrome. *Am J Med* 1981; 71:784–790.
279. Towbin JA, Casey B, Belmont J. The molecular basis of vascular disorders. *Am J Hum Genet* 1999; 64:678–684.
280. Michalickova K, Susic M, Willing MC, et al. Mutations of the α-2(v) chain of type V collagen impair matrix assembly and produce Ehlers-Danlos syndrome type I. *Hum Mol Genet* 1998; 78: 249–255.
281. Giunta C, Superti Furga A, Spranger S, et al. Ehlers-Danlos type VII: clinical features and molecular defects. *J Bone Joint Surg Ann* 1999; 81:225–238.
282. Emanuel BS, Cannizzaro LA, Seyer JM, et al. Human A1 (III) and A2 (V) procollagen genes are located on the long arm of chromosome 2. *Proc Natl Acad Sci USA* 1985; 82:3385–3389.
283. Burrows NP. The molecular genetics of the Ehlers-Danlos syndrome. *Clin Exp Dermatol* 1999; 24:99–106.
284. Walker LC, Marini JC, Grange DK, et al. A patient with Ehlers-Danlos syndrome type VI is homozygous for a premature termination codon in exon 14 of the lysyl hydroxylase I gene. *Mol Genet Metab* 1999; 67:74–82.
285. Passoja K, Rautavuoma K, Ala-Kokko L, et al. Cloning and characterization of a third human lysyl hydroxylase isoform. *Proc Natl Acad Sci USA* 1998; 95:10482–10486.
286. Prockop DJ. Mutations in collagen genes as a cause of connective-tissue diseases. *N Engl J Med* 1992; 326:540–546.
287. Okajima T, Fukumoto S, Furukawa K, et al. Molecular basis for the progeroid variant of Ehlers-Danlos syndrome: Identification and characterization of two mutations in galactosyl transferase I gene. *J Biol Chem* 1999; 274:28841–28844.
288. Kontusaari S, Tromp G, Kuivaniemi H, et al. A mutation in the gene for type II procollagen (COL3AI) in a family with aortic aneurysms. *J Clin Invest* 1990; 86:1465–1473.
289. MacSweeney ST, Skidmore C, Turner RJ, et al. Unravelling the familial tendency to aneurysmal disease: Popliteal aneurysm, hypertension and fibrillin genotype. *Eur J Vasc Endosc Surg* 1996; 12:162–166.
290. McMillan WD, Patterson BK, Keen RR, et al. In situ localization and quantification of mRNA for 92-kD bype IV collagenase and its inhibitor in aneurysmal, occlusive, and normal aorta. *Athers Thromb Vasc Biol* 1995; 15:1139–1144.
291. Kuivaniemi H, Tromp G, Prockop DJ. Genetic causes of aortic aneurysms: Unlearning at least part of what the textbooks say. *J Clin Invest* 1991; 88:1441–1444.
292. Sherer DW, Sapadin AN, Lebwohl MG. Pseudoxanthoma elasticum: An update. *Dermatology* 1999; 199:3–7.
293. Challenor VF, Conway N, Munro JL. The surgical treatment of restrictive cardiomyopathy in pseudoxanthoma elasticum. *Br Heart J* 1988; 59:266–269.
294. Pyeritz RE, Weiss JL, Renie WE, et al. Pseudoxanthoma elasticum and mitral-valve prolapse. *N Engl J Med* 1982; 307:1451–1452.
295. Weir EK, Joffe HS, Blaufuss AH, Beighton P. Cardiovascular abnormalities in cutis laxa. *Eur J Cardiol* 1977; 5:255–261.
296. Bale SJ. Recent advances in gene mapping of skin diseases pseudoxanthorna elasticum: A satisfying sibling study. *J Cutan Med Surg* 1999; 3:154–156.
297. Zhang MC, He L, Giro M, et al. Cutis laxa arising from frameshift mutations in exon 30 of the elastin gene (ELN). *J Biol Chem* 1999; 274:981–986.
298. Tassabehji M, Metcalfe K, Hurst J, et al. An elastin gene mutation producing abnormal tropelastin and cutis laxa. *Hum Mol Genet* 1998; 7:1021–1028.
299. Bouloc A, Godeau G, Zeller J, et al. Increases fibroblast elastase activity in acquired cutis laxa. *Dermatology* 1999; 198:346–350.
300. Boente MC, Winik BC, Asial RA. Wrinkly skin syndrome: Ultrastructural alterations of the elastic fibers. *Pediatr Dermatol* 1999; 16:113–117.
301. Priori SG, Barhanin J, Hauer RNW, et al. Genetic and molecular basis of cardiac arrhythmias: Impact on clinical management (Parts I and II). *Circulation* 1999; 99:518–528.
302. Schwartz PJ, Moss AJ, Vincent GM, et al. Diagnostic criteria for the long QT syndrome: An update. *Circulation* 1993; 88:782–784.
303. Schwartz PJ, Locati EH, Napolitano C, et al. The long QT syndrome. In: Zipes DP, Halife J, eds. *Cardiac Electrophysiology: From Cell to Bedside.* Philadelphia: Saunders; 1996:788–811.
304. Keating M, Dunn C, Atkinson D, et al. Linkage of a cardiac arrhythmia, the long QT syndrome, and the Harvey ras-1 gene. *Science* 1991; 252:704–706.
305. Towbin JA, Li H, Taggart RT, et al. Evidence of genetic heterogeneity in Romano-Ward long QT syndrome: Analysis of 23 families. *Circulation* 1994; 90:2635–2644.
306. Abbott GW, Sesti F, Splawski I, et al. MiRP1 forms I_{Kr} potassium channels with HERG and is associated with cardiac arrhythmia. *Cell* 1999; 97:175–187.
307. Moss AJ, Zareba W, Benhorin J, et al. Electrocardiographic T-wave patterns in genetically distinct forms of the hereditary long-QT syndrome. *Circulation* 1995; 92:2929–2934.
308. Zareba W, Moss AJ, Schwartz PJ, et al. ECG T-wave patterns in genetically distinct forms of the hereditary long QT syndrome. *Circulation* 1995; 92:2929–2934.
309. Schwartz PJ, Stramba-Badiale M, Segantini A, et al. Prolongation of the QT interval and the sudden infant death syndrome. *N Engl J Med* 1998; 338:1709–1714.

310. Towbin JA, Friedman RA. Prolongation of the long QT syndrome and sudden infant death syndrome. *N Engl J Med* 1998; 338:1760–1761.
311. Schwartz PJ, Priori SG, Locati EH. Long QT syndrome patients with mutations of the SCN54 and HERG genes have differential response to Na+ channel blockade and to increases in heart rate: Implications for gene-specific therapy. *Circulation* 1995; 92:3373–3375.
312. Compton SJ, Lux RL, Ramsey MR, et al. Genetically defined therapy of inherited long-QT syndrome: Correction of abnormal repolarization by potassium. *Circulation* 1996; 94:1018–1022.
313. Shimzu W, Kurita T, Matsuo K, et al. Improvement of repolarization abnormalities by a K+ channel opener in LQT1 form of congenital long-QT syndrome. *Circulation* 1998; 97:1581–1588.
314. Neyroud N, Tesson F, Denjoy I, et al. A novel mutation on the potassium channel gene *KVLQT1* causes the Jervell and Lange-Nielsen cardioauditory syndrome. *Nature Genet* 1997; 15: 186–189.
315. Splawski I, Timothy KW, Vincent GM, et al. Brief report: Molecular basis of the long-QT syndrome associated with deafness. *N Engl J Med* 1997; 336:1562–1567.
316. Chen Q, Zhang D, Gingell RL, et al. Homozygous deletion in KVLQT1 associated with Jervell and Lange-Nielsen syndrome. *Circulation* 1999; 99:1344–1347.
317. Tyson J, Tranebjaerg L, Bellman S, et al. IsK and *KVLQT1:* mutation in either of the two subunits of the slow component of the delayed rectifier potassium channel can cause Jervell and Lange-Nielsen syndrome. *Hum Mol Genet* 1997; 12:2179–2185.
318. Brugada P, Brugada J. Right bundle-branch block, persistent ST segment elevation and sudden cardiac death: A distant clinical and electrocardiographic syndrome—A multicenter report. *J Am Coll Cardiol* 1992; 20:1391–1396.
319. Gussak I, Antzelevitch C, Bjerregaard P, et al. The Brugada syndrome: Clinical, electrophysiological, and genetic considerations. *J Am Coll Cardiol* 1999; 33:5–15.
320. Nademanee K, Veerakul G, Nimmannit S, et al. Arrhythmogenic marker for the sudden unexplained death syndrome in Thai men. *Circulation* 1997; 96:2595–2600.
321. Chen Q, Kirsch GE, Zhang D, et al. Genetic basis and molecular mechanism for idiopathic ventricular fibrillation. *Nature* 1998; 392:293–296.
322. Dumaine R, Towbin JA, Brugada P, et al. Ionic mechanisms responsible for the electrocardiographic phenotype of the Brugada syndrome are temperature dependent. *Circ Res* 1999; 85:803–809.
323. Brugada R, Tapscott T, Czernuszewicz GZ, et al. Identification of a genetic locus for familial atrial fibrillation. *N Engl J Med* 1997; 336:905–911.
324. Wolff L, Parkinson J, White PD. Bundle branch block with short PR interval in healthy young people prone to paroxysmal tachycardia. *Am Heart J* 1930; 5:686–704.
325. Waxman MB, Catching JD, Felderhof CH, et al. Familial atrioventricular heart block: An autosomal dominant trait. *Circulation* 1975; 51:226–233.
326. Brink PA, Ferreira A, Moolman JC, et al. Gene for progressive familial heart block type I maps to chromosome 19q13. *Circulation* 1995; 91:1633–1640.
327. Schott J-J, Benson DW, Basson CT, et al. Congenital heart disease caused by mutations in the transcription factor NKX2-5. *Science* 1998; 281:108–111.
328. Bonnet D, Pelet A, Legeai-Mallet L, et al. A gene for Holt-Oram syndrome maps to the distal long arm of chromosome 12. *Nature Genet* 1994; 6:405–408.
329. Basson CT, Cowley GS, Solomon SD, et al. The clinical and genetic spectrum of the Holt-Oram syndrome (heart-hand syndrome). *N Engl J Med* 1994; 330:885–891.
330. Basson CT, Bachinski DR, Lin RC, et al. Mutations in human cause limb and cardiac malformation in Holt-Oram syndrome. *Nature Genet* 1997; 15:30–35.
331. Li QY, Newbury-Ecog RA, Terrett JA, et al. Holt-Oram syndrome is caused by mutations in TBX5, a member of the *Brachyury* (*T*) gene family. *Nature Genet* 1997; 15:21–29.
332. Manouvrier-Hanu S, Holder-Espinasse M, Lyonnet S. Genetics of limb anomalies in humans. *Trends Genet* 1999; 15:409–417.
333. Smith J. T-box genes: What they do and how they do it? *Trends Genet* 1999; 15:154–158.
334. Morris CA. Genetic aspects of supravalvular aortic stenosis. *Curr Opin Cardiol* 1998; 13:214–219.
335. Hallidie-Smith KA, Karas S. Cardiac anomalies in Williams-Beuren syndrome. *Arch Dis Child* 1988; 63:809–813.
336. O'Connor WN, Davis JB, Geissler R, et al. Supravalvular aortic stenosis: Clinical and pathological observations in six patients. *Arch Pathol Lab Med* 1985; 109:179–185.
337. Ewart AK, Morris CA, Atkinson D, et al. Hemizygosity at the elastin locus in developmental disorders, Williams syndrome. *Nature Genet* 1993; 5:11–16.
338. Nickerson E, Greenberg F, Keating MT, et al. Deletions of the elastin gene at 7q11.23 occur in about 90% of patients with Williams syndrome. *Am J Hum Genet* 1995; 56:1156–1161.
339. Baumer, A, Dutly F. Balmer D, et al. High level of unequal meiotic crossovers at the origin of 22q11.2 and 7q11.23 deletions. *Hum Mol Genet* 1998; 7:887–894.
340. Frangiskakis JM, Ewart AK, Morris CA, et al. LIM-kinase I hemizygosity implicated in impaired visuospatial constructive cognition. *Cell* 1996; 86:59–69.
341. Tassabehji M, Metcalfe K, Ferguson WD, et al. LIM-kinase deleted in Williams syndrome. *Nature Genet* 1996; 13:272–273.
342. Osborne LR, Soder S, Shi X-M, et al. Hemizygous deletion of the syntaxin IA gene in individuals with Williams syndrome. *Am J Hum Genet* 1997; 61:449–452.
343. Meng X, Lu X, Li Z, Green ED, et al. Complete physical map of the common deletion region in Williams syndrome and identification and characterization of three novel genes. *Hum Genet* 1998; 103:590–599.
344. Osborne LR, Martindale D, Sherer SW, et al. Identification of genes from a 500-kb region at 7q11.23 that is commonly deleted in Williams syndrome patients. *Genomics* 1996; 36:328–336.
345. Peoples R, Perez-Jurado L, Wang Y-K, et al. The gene of replication factor C subunit 2 (RFC-2) is within the 7q11.23 Williams syndrome deletion. *Am J Hum Genet* 1996; 58:1370–1373.
346. Perez-Jurado LA, Wang Y-K, Peoples R, et al. A duplicated gene in the breakpoint regions of the 7q11.23 Williams-Beuren syndrome encodes the initiator binding protein TFII-I and BAP-135, a phosphorylation target of BTK. *Hum Mol Genet* 1998; 7:325–334.
347. Wang Y-K, Samos CH, Peoples R, et al. A novel human homologue of the *Drosophila frizzled wnt* receptor gene binds wingless protein and is in the Williams syndrome deletion at 7111.23. *Hum Mol Genet* 1997; 6:465–574.
348. Lu X, Meng X, Morris CA, et al. A novel human gene, WSTF, is deleted in Williams syndrome. *Genomics* 1998; 54:241–249.
349. Hockenhull EL, Carett MJ, Metcalfe K, et al. A complete physical contig and partial transcript map of the Williams syndrome critical region. *Genomics* 1999; 58:138–145.
350. Noonan JA, Ehmke DA. Associated noncardiac malformations in children with congenital heart disease. *J Pediatr* 1963; 63:468–470.
351. Sharland M, Burch M, McKenna WM, et al. A clinical study of Noonan syndrome. *Arch Dis Child* 1992; 67:178–183.
352. Jamieson CR, van der Burgt I, Brady AF, et al. Mapping a gene for Noonan syndrome to the long arm of chromosome 12. *Nature Genet* 1994; 8:357–360.
353. Quek SC, Yip W, Quek ST, et al. Cardiac manifestations in tuberous sclerosis: A 10-year review. *J Pediatr Child Health* 1998; 34:283–287.

354. Smith M, Sperling D. Novel 23-base-pair duplication in TSC1 exon 15 in an infant presenting with cardiac rhabdomyomas. *Am J Med Genet* 1999; 84:346–349.
355. O'Callaghan FJ, Clarke AC, Jaffe H, et al. Tuberous sclerosis complex and Wolff-Parkinson-White syndrome. *Arch Dis Child* 1998; 78:159–162.
356. Povey S, Burley MW, Attwood J, et al. Two loci for tuberous sclerosis: one on 9q34 and one on 16q13. *Ann Hum Genet* 1994; 58:107–127.
357. Plank TL, Yeung RS, Henske EP. Hamartin, the product of the tuberous sclerosis 1 (TSC1) gene, interacts with tuberin and appears to be localized to cytoplasmic vesicles. *Cancer Res* 1998; 58:4766–4770.
358. Hornigold N, Devlin J, Davies AM, et al. Mutation of the 9q34 gene TSC1 in sporadic bladder cancer. *Oncogene* 1999; 18:2657–2661.
359. Longa L, Scolari F, Brusco A, et al. A large TSC2 and PKD1 gene deletion is associated with renal and extrarenal signs of autosomal dominant polycystic kidney disease. *Nephrol Dial Transplant* 1997; 12:1900–1907.
360. Van Slegtenhorst M, et al. Mutational spectrum of the TSC1 gene in a cohort of 225 tuberous sclerosis complex patients: No evidence for genotype-phenotype correlation. *J Med Genet* 1999; 36:285–289.
361. Jones AC, Shyamsunder MM, Thomas MW, et al. Comprehensive mutation analysis of TSC1 and TSC2 and phenotypic correlatives in 150 families with tuberous sclerosis. *Am J Hum Genet* 1999; 64:1305–1315.
362. Onda H, Lueck A, Marks PW, et al. Tsc 2(+/−) mice develop tumors in multiple sites that express gelsolin and are influenced by genetic background. *J Clin Invest* 1999; 104:687–695.
363. Hino O, Fukuda T, Satake N, et al. TSC2 gene mutant (Eker) rat model of a dominantly inherited cancer. *Prog Exp Tumor Res* 1999; 35:95–108.
364. Yeung RS, Katsetos CD, Klein-Szanto A, et al. Subependymal astrocytic hamertome, in the Eker rat model of tuberous sclerosis. *Am J Pathol* 1997; 151:1477–1486.
365. Satake N, Kobayashi T, Kobayashi E, et al. Isolation and characterization of a rat homologue of the human tuberous sclerosis 1 gene (TSC1) and analyses of its mutations in rat renal carcinomas. *Cancer Res* 1999; 59:849–855.
366. Weinstein BM, Stemple DL, Driever W, et al. Gridlock, a localized heritable vascular patterning defect in the zebrafish. *Nature Med* 1995; 1:1143–1147.
367. Towbin JA, McQuinn TC. Gridlock: A model for coarctation of the aorta? *Nature Med* 1995; 1:1141–1142.
368. Yost HJ. The genetics of midline and cardiac laterality defects. *Curr Opin Cardiol* 1998; 13:185–189.
369. Rose V, Izukawa T, Moes CA. Syndromes of asplenia and polysplenia: A review of cardiac and noncardiac malformations in 60 cases with special references to diagnosis and prognosis. *Br Heart J* 1987; 37:840–852.
370. Seo J, Brown NA, Ho SY, et al. Abnormal laterality and congenital cardiac anomalies: Relations of visceral and cardiac morphologies in the *iv/iv* mouse. *Circulation* 1992; 86:642–650.
371. Casey B. Two rights make a wrong: human left-right malformations. *Hum Mol Genet* 1998; 7:1565–1571.
372. Gebbia M, Ferrero GB, Pilia G, et al. X-linked situs abnormalities result from mutations in *ZIC3*. *Nature Genet* 1997; 17:305–308.
373. Meno C, Saijoh Y, Fujii H, et al. Left-right asymmetric expression of the TGF β-family member lefty in mouse embryos. *Nature* 1996; 381:151–155.
374. Meno C, Shimono A, Saijoh Y, et al. Lefty-1 is required for left-right determination as a regulator of lefty-2 and nodal. *Cell* 1998; 94:287–297.
375. Nomura M, Li E, Smadz role in mesoderm formation, left-right patterning, and cranofacial development. *Nature* 1998; 393:786–790.
376. Kosaki K, Bassi MT, Kosaki R, et al. Characterization and mutation analysis of human LEFTY A and LEFTY B, homologues of murine genes implicated in left-right axis development. *Am J Hum Genet* 1999; 64:712–721.
377. Kosaki R, Gebbia M, Kosaki K, et al. Left-right axis malformations associated with nucleotide substitutions in ACVR2B, the gene for human activin receptor type IIB. *Am J Med Genet* 1999; 82:70–76.
378. Towbin JA, Greenberg F. Genetic syndromes and clinical molecular genetics. In: Bricker JT, Garson A Jr, Fisher DJ, Neish SR, eds. *The Science and Practice of Pediatric Cardiology*. Baltimore: Williams & Wilkins; 1998:2627–2700.
379. Emanuel BS. Molecular cytogenetics: Toward dissection of the contiguous gene syndromes. *Am J Hum Genet* 1988; 43:575–578.
380. Korenberg JR, Kawashima H, Pulst S-M, et al. Molecular definition of a region of chromosome 21 that causes features of the Down syndrome phenotype. *Am J Hum Genet* 1990; 47:236–246.
381. Korenberg JR, Bradley C, Disteche CM. Down syndrome: Molecular mapping of the congenital heart disease and duodenal stenosis. *Am J Hum Genet* 1992; 50:294–302.
382. Hubert R, Mitchell S, Chen XN, et al. BAC and PAC contig covering 3.5 Mb of the Down syndrome congenital heart disease region between DZIS5S and MX1 on chromosome 21. *Genomics* 1997; 41:218–226.
383. DiGeorge AM. Discussions on a new concept of the cellular base of immunology. *J Pediatr* 1965; 67:907–908.
384. Clark EB. Mechanisms in the pathogenesis of congenital heart defects. In: Pierpont ME, Moller JM, eds. *The Genetics of Cardiovascular Disease*. Boston: Martinus Nijhoff; 1985:3–36.
385. Emanuel BS, Budarf ML, Scambler PJ. The genetic basis of conotruncal cardiac defects: The chromosome 22q11.2 deletion. In: Harvey RP, Rosenthal N, eds. *Heart Development.* San Diego, CA: Academic Press; 1999:463–478.
386. Shprintzen RJ, Goldberg RB, Young D, et al. The velo-cardio-facial syndrome: A clinical and genetic analysis. *Pediatrics* 1981; 67:167–172.
387. Burn JA, Takao A, Wilson D, et al. Conotruncal anomaly face syndrome is associated with a deletion within chromosome 22q11. *J Med Genet* 1993; 30:822–824.
388. Greenberg F, Elder FFB, Haffner P, et al. Cytogenetic findings in a prospective series of patients with DiGeorge anomaly. *Am J Hum Genet* 1988; 43:605–611.
389. Budarf ML, Collins J, Gong W, et al. Cloning a balanced translocation associated with DiGeorge syndrome and identification of a disrupted candidate gene. *Nature Genet* 1994; 10:269–278.
390. Pizzuti A, Novelli G, Mari A, et al. Human homologue sequences to the *Drosophila disheveled segment-polarity* gene are deleted in the DiGeorge syndrome. *Am J Hum Genet* 1996; 58:722–729, 1996.
391. Holmes SE, Riazi MA, Gong W, et al. Disruption of the clathrin heavy chain-like gene (*CLTCL*) associated with features of DGS/VCFS: A balanced (21;22)(p12;q11) translocation. *Hum Mol Genet* 1997; 6:357–367.
392. Puzzuti A, Novelli G, Ratti A, et al. UFD1L, a developmentally expressed ubiquitination gene, is deleted in CATCH 22 syndrome. *Hum Mol Genet* 1997; 6:259–265.
393. Wilming LG, Snoeren CAS, Van Rijswijk A, et al. The murine homologue of HIRA, a DiGeorge syndrome candidate gene, is expressed in embryonic structures affected in human CATCH 22 patients. *Hum Mol Genet* 1997; 6:247–258.
394. Gong W, Emanuel BS, Galili N, et al. Structural and mutational analyses of a conserved gene (*DGSI*) from the minimal DiGeorge syndrome critical region. *Hum Mol Genet* 1997; 6:267–276.
395. Wakamiya M, Lindsay EA, Rivera-Perez JA, et al. Functional

analysis of *Gscl* in the pathogenesis of the DiGeorge and velocardiofacial syndromes. *Hum Mol Genet* 1998; 7:1835–1840.

396. Farrell MJ, Stadt H, Wallis KT, et al. HIRA, a DiGeorge syndrome candidate gene, is required for cardiac outflow tract septation. *Circ Res* 1999; 84:127–135.

397. Yamagishi H, Garg V, Matsuko R, et al. A molecular pathway revealing a genetic basis for human cardiac and craniofacial defects. *Science* 1999; 283:1158–1161.

398. Lindsay EA, Botta A, Jurecic V, et al. Congenital heart disease in mice deficient for the DiGeorge syndrome region. *Nature* 1999; 401:379–383.

399. Markert ML, Boeck A, Hale LP, et al. Transplantation of thymus tissue in complete DiGeorge syndrome. *N Engl J Med* 1999; 341:1180–1189.

400. Recto MR, Parness IA, Gelb BD, et al. Clinical implications and possible association of malposition of the branch pulmonary arteries with DiGeorge syndrome and microdeletion of chromosomal region 22q11. *Am J Cardiol* 1997; 80:1624–1627.

401. Lu J-H, Chung M-Y, Hwang B, et al. Prevalence and parental origin in tetralogy of Fallot associated with chromosome 22q11 microdeletion. *Pediatrics* 1999; 104:87–90.

402. Wulfsberg EA, Leara-Cox J, Neri G. What's in a name? Chromosome 22q11 abnormalities and the DiGeorge, velocardiofacial, and conotruncal anomalies face syndromes. *Am J Med Genet* 1997; 65:317–319.

403. Goldmuntz E, Clark BJ, Mitchell LE, et al. Frequency of 22q11 deletions in patients with conotruncal defects. *J Am Coll Cardiol* 1998; 32:492–498.

CHAPTER 63

THE PATHOLOGY, PATHOPHYSIOLOGY, RECOGNITION, AND TREATMENT OF CONGENITAL HEART DISEASE

Michael D. Freed

INCIDENCE AND ETIOLOGY

The incidence of congenital heart disease in the United States is approximately 8 per 1000 live births.[1,2] Many infants who are born alive with cardiac defects have anomalies that do not represent a threat to life, at least during infancy. Almost one-third of those infants, or 2.6 per 1000 live births, however, have critical disease, which is defined as a malformation severe enough to result in cardiac catheterization, cardiac surgery, or death within the first year of life.[3] Today, with early detection and proper management, the majority of infants with critical disease can be expected to survive the first year of life.[3] Most who now survive infancy will join the increasingly large cohort of adults with congenital heart disease.

Estimates of the incidence of specific lesions vary, depending on whether the data are drawn from infants or older children and whether the diagnosis is based on clinical, echocardiographic, catheterization, surgical, or postmortem studies.[1-4] The incidence in other countries is remarkably similar to that reported for the United States.[5,6]

Despite these differences in case material, except for bicuspid aortic valve and mitral valve prolapse, it is apparent that ventricular septal defect (VSD) is the most common malformation, occurring in 28 percent of all patients with congenital heart disease (Table 63-1).

Among 2251 infants with critical congenital heart disease in the New England Regional Infant Cardiac Program,[3] 53.7 percent were male. Certain defects, however, are considerably more common in one sex than in the other. Aortic stenosis occurs more commonly in boys (4:1), and atrial septal defects occur more frequently in girls (2.5:1).

Although earlier theories concerning the etiology of congenital heart diseases suggested that most defects were multifactorial—that is, the malformations are caused by a combination of a hereditary predisposition (presumably caused by abnormalities in the genetic code) and an environmental trigger[7]—more recent advances in molecular biology suggest that a much higher percentage are caused by point mutations.[8]

Some abnormalities are caused by chromosomal aberrations (see Chap. 62). Trisomy 21 (Down's syndrome) is highly associated with complete atrioventricular (AV) canal, VSDs, and tetralogy of Fallot, and children with Turner's syndrome (XO) frequently have coarctation of the aorta. Other anomalies are caused by teratogens: VSD in fetal alcohol syndrome, Ebstein's anomaly in a fetus with prenatal exposure to lithium, and patent ductus arteriosus (PDA) in mothers who contracted rubella during the first trimester are examples.

Some syndromes are inherited as single-gene defects and have congenital heart disease as one of their manifestations. Holt-Oram syndrome, an association of radial limb abnormalities and atrial septal defects (ASDs), is caused by an abnormality of a T-box transcription factor Tbx5, and the cardio-velo-facial syndrome, associated with abnormalities of the conotruncus, resulting in a high proportion of infants born with truncus arteriosus or interrupted aortic arch, is a result of a deletion on chromosome 22 (22 q 11)[9] (see Chap. 62).

It is clear now that a higher proportion of congenital heart disease than previously thought is due to single-gene defects and that the same malformation may be caused by mutant genes at different loci.[8] With increasing knowledge of molecular mechanisms, it seems inevitable that the etiology and pathogenesis of congenital heart disease will be clarified increasingly in the years ahead.

TABLE 63-1 Incidence of Specific Congenital Heart Defects

Defect	Percentage of Cases[a] Averaged
Ventricular septal defect	28.3
Pulmonary stenosis	9.5
Patent ductus arteriosus	8.7
Ventricular septal defect with pulmonary stenosis[b]	6.8
Atrial septal defect, secundum	6.7
Aortic stenosis	4.4
Coarctation of aorta	4.2
Atrioventricular canal[c]	3.5
Transposition of great arteries	3.4
Aortic atresia	2.4
Truncus arteriosus	1.6
Tricuspid atresia	1.2
Total anomalous pulmonary venous connection	1.1
Double-outlet right ventricle	0.8
Pulmonary atresia without ventricular septal defect	0.3

[a]Total number of cases = 103,590.
[b]Includes tetralogy of Fallot.
[c]Includes partial and complete.
SOURCE: References 1–3, 5, 6.

FETAL CIRCULATION AND THE TRANSITION TO NEONATAL AND ADULT CIRCULATION

The fetus obtains all metabolic necessities, including oxygen, from the placenta. The fetal circulation is an adaptation to allow most of the right ventricular output to bypass the lungs and go instead to the placenta to pick up oxygen. Most of the understanding of this adaptation comes from more than 40 years of research,[10–18] primarily on fetal lambs. The fetal circulation is arranged in parallel rather than in series, with mixing at the atrial (foramen ovale) and great vessel (ductus arteriosus) level (Fig. 63-1). Normally, blood returning from the body goes into the right atrium via the superior vena cava or inferior vena cava. Inferior vena cava blood is diverted by the crista dividens so that approximately 27 percent of combined ventricular output passes through the foramen ovale into the left atrium, with the remainder passing through the tricuspid valve to the right ventricle. Left atrial return is mixed with blood returning from the lungs into the left ventricle and then to the ascending aorta, where it goes to the coronary arteries, head, and upper body vessels, with a small proportion going across the arch into the descending aorta. Right ventricular blood passes out of the pulmonary artery, where approximately 90 percent (59 percent of combined ventricular output) is diverted through the ductus arteriosus into the descending aorta by the elevated pulmonary vascular resistance. Thus, approximately two-thirds of the blood passes through the right side of the heart and one-third passes through the left side of the heart.

The oxygen saturation of fetal blood is considerably lower than that in a newborn or infant because of the lower efficiency of the placenta compared with the lungs for oxygen exchange (Fig. 63-2). The blood with the highest saturation (approximately 70 percent) is that returning from the placenta. Some of this higher-saturation blood is diverted across the foramen ovale so that saturation on the left side of the heart (65 percent) is somewhat higher than it is on the right side (55 percent). This allows diversion of the lowest-saturation blood (~55 percent) through the ductus arteriosus to the placenta, increasing the efficiency of oxygen pickup. An additional fetal adaptation to oxygen transport at low oxygen saturation is the presence of high levels of fetal hemoglobin with a higher affinity for oxygen than normal hemoglobin. This leftward shift of the oxygen dissociation curve facilitates oxygen uptake at the relatively low P_{O_2} of the placenta vasculature.

The wide communication at the atrial level (foramen ovale) allows for near equalization of atrial and ventricular end-diastolic pressures. The wide communication at the great vessel level (ductus arteriosus) allows equalization of systolic pressures in the aorta and the pulmonary artery and, in the absence of aortic or pulmonic stenosis, at the ventricular level (Fig. 63-3).

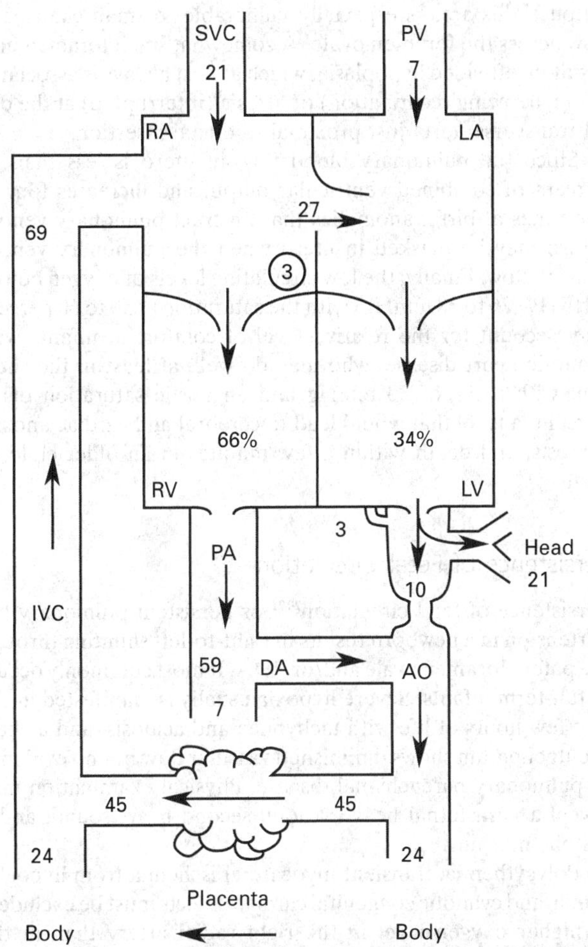

FIGURE 63-1 The course of the circulation in a late-gestation fetal lamb. *The numbers represent the percentage of combined ventricular output.* Some of the return from the inferior vena cava (IVC) is diverted by the crista dividens in the right atrium (RA) through the foramen ovale into the left atrium (LA), where it meets the pulmonary venous return (PV), passes into the left ventricle (LV), and is pumped into the ascending aorta. Most of the ascending aortic flow goes to the coronary, subclavian, and carotid arteries, with only 10 percent of combined ventricular output passing through the aortic arch (indicated by the narrowed point in the aorta) into the descending aorta (AO). The remainder of the inferior vena cava flow mixes with the return from the superior vena cava (SVC) and coronary veins, passes into the right atrium and right ventricle (RV), and is pumped into the pulmonary artery (PA). Because of the high pulmonary resistance, only 7 percent passes through the lungs (PV), with the rest going into the ductus arteriosus (DA) and then to the descending aorta (AO), the placenta, and the lower half of the body. (From Freed MD. Fetal and transitional circulation. In: Fyler DC, ed. *Nadas' Pediatric Cardiology*. Philadelphia: Hanley & Belfus; 1992. Reproduced with permission from the publisher and author.)

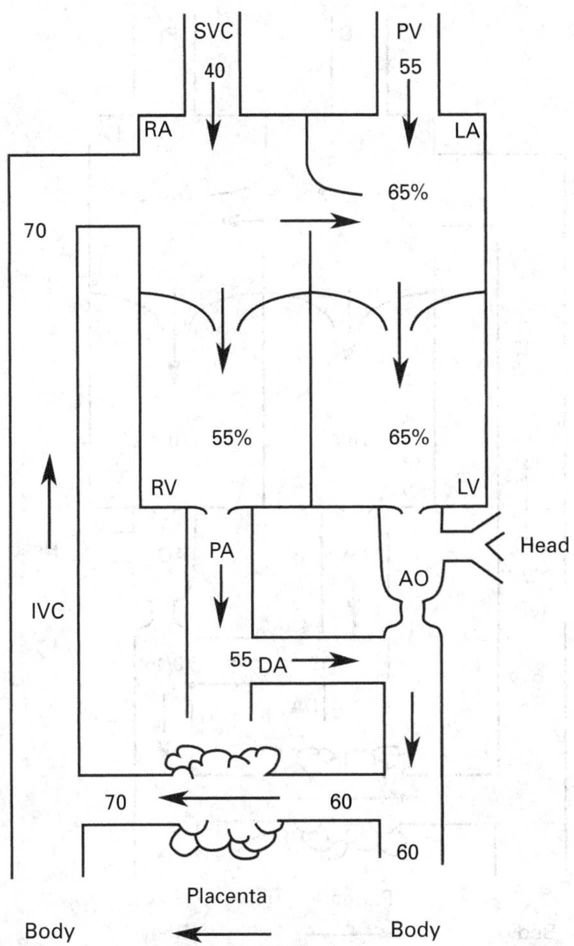

FIGURE 63-2 *The numbers indicate the percent of oxygen saturation in a late-gestation lamb.* The oxygen saturation is highest in the inferior vena cava, representing that primarily from the placenta. The saturation of blood in the heart is slightly higher on the left side than on the right side. The abbreviations in this diagram are the same as those in Fig. 63-1. (From Freed MD. Fetal and transitional circulation. In: Fyler DC, ed. *Nadas' Pediatric Cardiology*. Philadelphia: Hanley & Belfus; 1992. Reproduced with permission from the publisher and author.)

Within a few moments after birth, the circulatory physiology must switch rapidly from the placenta to the lung as the organ of oxygen exchange. Failure of any one of a number of a complex series of pulmonary and cardiac events may result in cerebral and then generalized hypoxemia, with lasting damage or death. With the onset of spontaneous respiration, the lungs are expanded and the pulmonary arterioles, which probably have been actively vasoconstricted, dilate. The reduction in pulmonary vascular resistance results from both simple physical expansion of the lung with the onset of respiration and the vasodilation of the pulmonary resistance vessels, probably partly as a result of the high level of oxygen in alveolar gas. Simultaneously, the placenta is removed from the circulation either by clamping the umbilical cord or by constriction of the umbilical arteries. This sudden increase in systemic vascular resistance and drop in pulmonary vascular resistance cause blood leaving the right ventricle to go out into the lung rather than through the ductus arteriosus. The sudden increase in left atrial return of blood now going through the lung increases left ventricular end-diastolic and left atrial pressure, shutting the flap valve of the foramen ovale against the edge of the cristae dividens, eliminating the atrial-level shunt.

With pulmonary vascular resistance lower than systemic vascular resistance, there may be some left-to-right (aorta to pulmonary artery) shunting through the ductus arteriosus. The mechanism for closure of the ductus arteriosus is not completely understood. The increased level of oxygen probably causes vasoconstriction of the ductus musculature, but there are strong

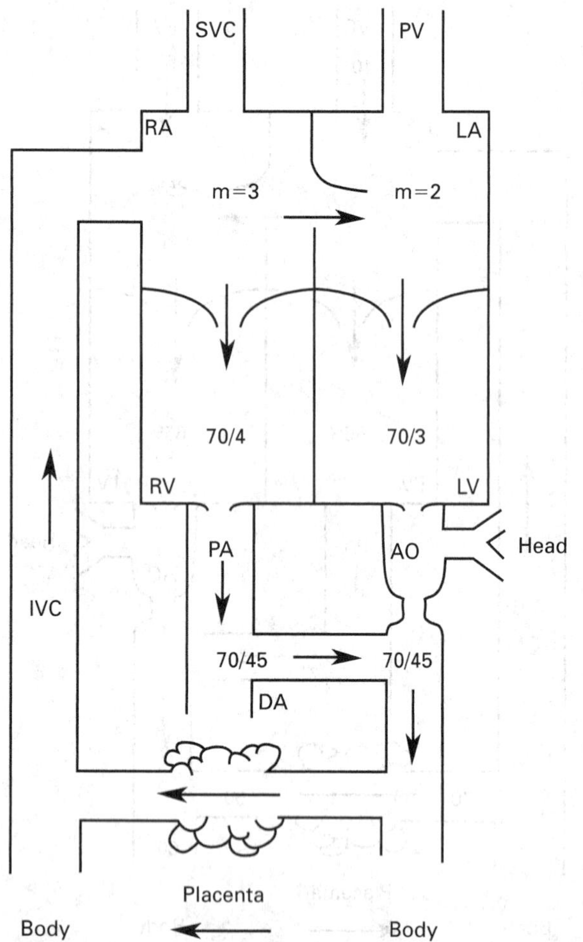

FIGURE 63-3 The numbers indicate the pressures observed in late-gestation lambs. Because large communications between the atrium and the great vessels are present, the pressures on both sides of the heart are virtually identical. The abbreviations are the same as those in Fig. 63-1. (From Freed MD. Fetal and transitional circulation. In: Fyler DC, ed. *Nadas' Pediatric Cardiology*. Philadelphia: Hanley & Belfus; 1992. Reproduced with permission from the publisher and author.)

suggestions that a reduction in circulating prostaglandins (PGs) of the E series plays a role. Within 3 or 4 days, the biochemical closure becomes irreversible when cellular necrosis of the endothelium leads to obliteration of the lumen. The pulmonary artery pressure drops to approximately half systemic levels within a day or so but takes another 2 to 6 weeks to drop down to adult levels.

The structure and hemodynamics of the field circulation have significant consequences in a neonate with congenital heart disease.[19] The parallel circulation with connections at the atrial and great vessel level allows a wide variety of congenital cardiac malformations to exist while still picking up oxygen at the placenta and delivering it to the tissues. For example, atresia of the tricuspid or mitral valve, while devastating after birth, does not have a significant effect in utero. Furthermore, since the right ventricle performs two-thirds of the cardiac work before birth, the left ventricle is underloaded; this may explain why congestive heart failure is seen not uncommonly with congenital defects. Because the normal flow across the aortic isthmus is relatively low (only about 10 percent of combined ventricular output), this area is especially vulnerable to small changes in flow across the foramen ovale. A somewhat small foramen may result in left-sided hypoplasia, which almost always is associated with narrowing (coarctation) or atresia (interrupted) at the distal transverse aorta just proximal to ductal insertion.

Since the pulmonary blood flow in utero is less than 10 percent of combined ventricular output and increases four to five times at birth, anomalies that obstruct pulmonary venous return may be masked in utero when the pulmonary venous return is low. Finally, the low circulating levels of oxygen before birth (P_{O_2} 26 to 38 mmHg) with the saturation at 50 to 60 percent may account for the relative level of comfort in infants with cyanotic heart disease, who may do well, at least in the short run, with a P_{O_2} of 30 mmHg and an aortic saturation of 50 percent, a level that would lead to cerebral and cardiac anoxia, acidosis, and death within a few minutes in an older child or adult.

Persistence of Fetal Circulation

Persistence of fetal circulation[20,21] or persistent pulmonary hypertension in a newborn results in right-to-left shunting through the patent foramen ovale and/or PDA. It most commonly occurs in full-term infants. Severe hypoxia usually is manifested in the first few hours of life with tachypnea and acidosis, and a chest roentgenogram shows diminished vascular flow but no evidence of pulmonary parenchymal disease. Physical examination may reveal a parasternal heave, a loud second heart sound, and a systolic murmur.

Polycythemia, transient myocardial ischemia from hypoglycemia, and cyanotic congenital cardiac defects must be excluded. A higher oxygen level in the right radial artery than in the umbilical artery confirms right-to-left shunting through the ductus arteriosus. Echocardiography and Doppler evaluation are of the utmost importance to rule out structural heart disease, especially total anomalous pulmonary venous connection.

The initial treatment[21] includes an increase in the inspired oxygen level and correction of acidosis with sodium bicarbonate. Frequently, artificial ventilation is required. Hyperventilation to diminish the partial pressure of carbon dioxide often is successful in lowering the pulmonary pressure and diminishing the right-to-left shunt. Recently, inhaled nitric oxide to reduce pulmonary vascular resistance has been found to be a useful adjunct to other therapies.[22] Treatment of severe disease with an extracorporeal membrane oxygenator is successful in a significant number of patients.[23] Similar hemodynamic alterations also may be seen in newborns with parenchymal lung disease.

COMPLICATIONS OF CONGENITAL HEART DISEASE

Complications associated with congenital heart disease are listed in Table 63-2.

TABLE 63-2 Complications of Congenital Heart Disease in Children

Congestive heart failure	Growth retardation
Hypoxemia	Pulmonary vascular disease

Congestive Heart Failure

Congestive heart failure is a potentially lethal complication of congenital heart disease and occurs in over 80 percent of infants who have malformations severe enough to require cardiac catheterization or surgery within the first year of life.[24] Its onset is usually a phenomenon of the first 6 months of life. Onset after 1 year of age is rare without a serious intercurrent problem such as infective endocarditis, pneumonia, or anemia.

Heart failure within the first 12 to 18 h of life usually is due to malformations that involve pressure or volume overload independent of pulmonary flow, as occurs with severe valvular regurgitation or a systemic arteriovenous fistula. Rarely, myocarditis may produce failure from the time of birth, as may congenital complete heart block or supraventricular tachycardia. Other causes in this age group include primary cardiomyopathy, severe polycythemia or anemia, and depressed myocardial contractility from neonatal asphyxia, hypocalcemia, hypoglycemia, or sepsis.

A majority of full-term infants presenting with severe heart failure during the remainder of the first week have critical obstruction to systemic arterial flow, which in virtually all cases has been unmasked by narrowing or closure of the ductus arteriosus. Examples are aortic atresia, coarctation of the aorta, interruption of the aortic arch, and critical aortic stenosis. *During the second week of life, aortic atresia and coarctation remain the most common causes of heart failure, but left ventricular volume overload from VSD, transposition of the great arteries with a VSD, and truncus arteriosus make their appearance.* These malformations present as the pulmonary vascular resistance falls, increasing the left-to-right shunt. *Statistically, VSD is the primary cause of congestive failure, followed by transposition, coarctation, complete AV canal, and PDA.*

The most common symptom of congestive heart failure is difficulty in breathing, with rapid, grunting, or gasping breathing or breathlessness with feeding. Observation of an undisturbed infant reveals dyspnea, the signs of which are nasal flaring and subcostal or intercostal retractions. A respiratory rate consistently above 60 is to be expected, and rates in the range of 90 to 100 are not uncommon. Poor weight gain is the rule. Cool moist skin, a subdued and rapid arterial pulse, and hepatic enlargement are common accompanying signs. A gallop rhythm, pulmonary rales, and expiratory wheezes may be present. It may be difficult to distinguish the pulmonary findings of heart failure from those of pneumonia or bronchiolitis; indeed, many infants develop heart failure during an intercurrent pulmonary infection. Edema, if present, usually is found in the periorbital area and on the dorsa of the feet and hands. Cardiac enlargement is confirmed by chest roentgenography. Infants with malformations such as coarctation of the aorta and total anomalous pulmonary venous connection, abnormalities that usually are not characterized by an impressive murmur, sometimes are referred only after weeks of tachypnea and failure to thrive, when a chest roentgenogram taken to explore the possibility of lung disease has revealed cardiac enlargement.

When a sizable systemic-to-pulmonary communication exists in a premature infant, usually as a result of a PDA, signs of heart failure usually are associated with signs of ventilatory failure.

Hospitalization is recommended for all infants with heart failure. Elevation of the head and chest to an angle of approximately 30° and administration of humidified oxygen by techniques that do not disturb the infant help relieve dyspnea and systemic arterial hypoxia as determined by pulse oximetry. Arterial oxygen saturation levels should be monitored in newborns, particularly the premature, to avoid the risk of retrolental fibroplasia. Rest, aided by sedation, is beneficial. With severe failure, oral feedings should be suspended temporarily to prevent aspiration and fluid intake should be restricted to 65 mL/kg per day intravenously for at least the first 24 h. Anemia, acidosis, hypoxia, hypercarbia, hypoglycemia, or hypocalcemia should be corrected; serum sodium, potassium, blood urea nitrogen, and creatinine concentrations should be monitored. A low threshold for the administration of antibiotics is appropriate.

Digoxin is recommended for the management of congestive failure in infants and children, especially those with decreased ventricular systolic function, because of its excellent absorption when given orally, rapid onset of action, relatively rapid excretion, and convenience of administration. The recommended oral maintenance doses of digoxin for the different age ranges of children, expressed in μg/kg per day, are as follows: for the premature, 5; for neonates, 10; for infants between 4 and 24 months of age, 15; for older children, 10; and for adolescents, 5. The daily maintenance dose usually is given in two divided doses approximately 12 h apart. The total digitalizing dose is three times the daily maintenance dose. Parenteral doses of digoxin are approximately 75 percent of oral doses for digitalization and maintenance. Half the digitalizing dose may be given initially, followed by the remaining two quarter doses at 4-, 8-, or 12-h intervals, depending on the desired speed of total digitalization. Maintenance therapy should be started 8 to 12 h after the last digitalizing dose. In a severely ill infant with decreased perfusion and unpredictable absorption, digitalization by the intravenous route is recommended. Impaired renal function leads to digoxin accumulation and toxicity, and so the initial and maintenance doses should be adjusted accordingly. Toxicity, if it is to occur, usually appears within the first week of therapy. If anorexia, nausea or vomiting, or electrocardiographic evidence of either atrial or ventricular ectopy or AV block appears, digoxin should be stopped and the serum digoxin level should be determined. Toxicity is probable if the level exceeds 3.0 ng/mL in an infant less than 6 months of age or 2.0 ng/mL in an older infant or child. If the need for digoxin continues, the dose is adjusted as the patient grows and gains weight.

The diuretic furosemide used intravenously in doses of 1.0 to 2.0 mg/kg or orally in doses of 1.5 to 2.0 mg/kg is very effective in the acute management of congestive heart failure. With severe failure, the dose may be increased by increments of 1.0 mg/kg intravenously if no urinary response has been achieved after 45 min. For long-term oral diuretic therapy, 1.5 to 2.0 mg/kg once daily or, if necessary, twice daily is recommended. Chlorothiazide, a slightly less potent diuretic but one with a longer duration of action, may be given orally in a dose of 20 to 50 mg/kg per day. Hypokalemia and hypochloremia can be induced with these potent diuretics, and a daily oral supplement of potassium chloride in the range of 1.0 to 1.5 meq/kg, with adjustment depending on the serum level, is recommended. Spironolactone, an aldosterone antagonist, has proved useful in supplementing the diuresis and preventing the hypokalemia induced by the diuretics described above. It may be given orally in a single daily dose of 2 to 3 mg/kg. A regimen of spironolactone 2 mg/kg given every day and furosemide

1 mg/kg is usually adequate for long-term diuretic therapy for mild to moderate heart failure and usually does not require potassium supplementation.

In emergency situations, it may be necessary to provide an immediate inotropic stimulus in the form of intravenous sympathomimetic amines administered by constant infusion pump. Isoproterenol in a dose of 0.1 μg/kg per minute exerts a powerful inotropic effect, but its usefulness may be limited by induced tachycardia and peripheral vasodilation, sometimes to the detriment of renal perfusion. Epinephrine in a dose of 0.1 to 1.0 μg/kg per minute or dobutamine or dopamine in a dose of 5 to 15 μg/kg per minute generally has been more helpful, with dopamine providing more adequate renal flow. The systemic arterial blood pressure, urinary output, and electrocardiogram (ECG) should be monitored continuously. Vasodilator therapy in the form of intravenous sodium nitroprusside may be of considerable help in patients with severe congestive failure that is not associated with large left-to-right shunts. The infusion rate at the start should be no higher than 0.5 μg/kg per minute, but it may be increased gradually to 4.0 μg/kg per minute to achieve the desired effect. Systemic arterial pressure should be monitored continuously to detect serious hypotension. The angiotensin-converting enzyme inhibitors captopril, enalapril, and lisinopril given orally have proved effective in selected patients: captopril starting at 0.1 to 0.4 mg/kg per dose in a neonate and 0.3 to 0.6 mg/kg per dose in an older child given one to four times per day, enalapril 0.16 to 0.25 mg/kg per day in two divided doses, or lisinopril 0.16 to 0.25 mg/kg per day in a single daily dose. Hypotension and/or hyperkalemia are the primary adverse effects of these agents.[25]

Infants with potentially exhausting respiratory effort or with hypoxia or hypercapnia secondary to pulmonary edema or respiratory failure benefit from endotracheal intubation and ventilation on a volume-controlled, positive-pressure respirator, usually with the addition of positive end-expiratory pressure. These measures may permit additional therapy, cardiac catheterization, and surgical intervention with a much greater margin of safety.

In newborns who have failure as a result of narrowing or closure of the ductus arteriosus in the presence of critical obstruction to flow from the left side of the heart, dramatic and lifesaving relief can be expected with reopening of the ductus by the infusion of PGE_1 at a dose of 0.1 μg/kg per minute.

Finally, infants or children in whom medical therapy is clearly inadequate or only temporarily successful may require prompt surgical intervention for control of heart failure. *As a rule, the earlier the onset of congestive failure, the more likely the need for surgery.*

Hypoxemia

The sequelae of hypoxemia are listed in Table 63-3. *Cyanosis,* a bluish tinge to the color of the skin caused by the presence of at least 3 to 5 g/dL of reduced hemoglobin, is frequently the initial sign of congenital heart disease in an infant. It also may be an early sign of pulmonary, central nervous system, or metabolic disease or methemoglobinemia. Nonsurgical palliation with PGE_1 and the rapid development of surgical techniques for infants make a prompt distinction between cardiac and noncardiac cyanosis, usually by echocardiography, extremely important.

TABLE 63-3 Sequelae of Hypoxemia

Cyanosis	Exercise intolerance
Clubbing	Hypoxic spells
Polycythemia	Brain abscess
Squatting	Cerebrovascular accidents

Hypoxia leading to cyanosis in congenital heart disease may be due to heart failure with pulmonary edema and pulmonary venous desaturation or to intracardiac right-to-left shunting. The hypoxia that is due either to heart failure or to lung disease with intrapulmonary shunting usually responds dramatically to oxygen administration, whereas hypoxia that is due to cyanotic defects does not. Since many infants are relatively anemic during the first few months of life (hemoglobin concentration, 10.4 to 12 g/dL), cyanosis may be subtle.

When cyanosis has been present in older children for several months, the distal tips of the fingers and toes become hyperemic. Eventually, the capillary end loop dilation causes *clubbing* of the fingers and toes with a loss of the normal angle of the base of the nail and fingers. Also, with long-standing hypoxemia, the hematocrit increases to maintain the oxygen-carrying capacity of the blood (*polycythemia*). The increased hemoglobin concentration at any given oxygen saturation will result in more reduced hemoglobin, exaggerating the cyanosis.

The central nervous system may be the target organ of cerebrovascular accidents or brain abcess. *Brain abcess* probably is due to bacteremia primarily with mouth organisms that cross from the venous system to the arterial system right-to-left from shunting. The incidence seems to be directly related to arterial saturation and occurs mostly in older children and adolescents.[26]

Cerebrovascular accidents are due directly to hypoxemia or indirectly in children who are polycythemic presumably secondary to sludging.[27] The former group usually consists of infants less than 2 years old who are anemic and thus may have markedly reduced oxygen levels. The latter group consists of children or young adults who are polycythemic and have sludging or in situ microthrombosis. Interestingly, iron deficiency leads to stiff red cells, and so sludging may occur with modest levels of polycythemia (hematocrit 55 to 60 percent) in the presence of iron deficiency. With hematocrits in the range of 65 percent or higher, increased viscocity may lead to a cerebrovascular accident. Maintaining a proper level of hemoglobin has a salutory effect on hemodynamics and oxygen delivery in the presence of significant hypoxemia.[28,29]

Other systems also may be affected by hypoxemia or polycythemia. In older adolescents, the increase in hemoglobin breakdown may result in hyperuricemia and can precipitate a secondary form of gout.[30]

Disturbances in hemostasis also occur with polycythemia. Coagulation factors are commonly abnormal in patients with hematocrits in excess of 60 percent.[31] Actual platelet counts may be normal but can be increased initially in some patients, with subsequent decreases related to persistent and worsening desaturation. There is evidence of shortened platelet survival time in patients with cyanotic heart disease.[32] Laboratory evaluation of coagulation status requires that correction be made for the diminished volume of plasma and for the volume of anticoagulant used in blood samples to avoid false results. Hematologic management of adults with cyanotic congenital heart disease requires special experience and knowledge.[33]

The major consequences of cyanosis can be avoided in many instances, although differences in intelligence have been demonstrated between cyanotic and acyanotic children.[34]

Retardation of Growth and Development

Children with severe cardiac malformations frequently exhibit retardation of growth and development, with height and weight near or below the third percentile or weight 20 percentile points below the mean percentile for height.[35]

Growth retardation is most severe among children with overt cyanosis and those with large left-to-right shunts that cause heart failure. Heart failure tends to cause a greater retardation of weight than of height. Skeletal retardation, reflected by bone age, usually occurs with height and weight retardation and, among children with cyanotic heart disease, correlates with the severity of hypoxemia.

Other factors contribute to growth retardation, including insufficient caloric intake, dyspnea, frequent infections, psychological disturbances, malabsorption, and hypermetabolism. Among infants with severe congenital heart disease recognized within the first year of life, there is a significantly increased incidence of subnormal birth weight, intrauterine growth retardation, and major extracardiac anomalies.[3] Finally, a relatively small number of children have associated syndromes known to be characterized by growth retardation, such as rubella and Noonan's, Turner's, and Down's syndromes.

Growth retardation related primarily to congenital heart disease usually responds to surgical correction or palliation, with an impressive acceleration of growth and a return to or toward normal.

Although cardiac surgery seldom is recommended on the basis of growth failure alone, decelerated growth should be recognized early and, until proved otherwise, considered an index of the severity of heart disease. In general, the more successful the surgery is, the less will be the retardation of growth and development, with its sequelae of physical, psychological, and intellectual problems.[36]

Pulmonary Arterial Hypertension and Pulmonary Vascular Obstructive Disease

Pulmonary arterial hypertension (PAH) and pulmonary vascular obstructive disease (PVOD) are serious complications of congenital heart disease. PAH usually results from direct transmission of systemic arterial pressure to the right ventricle or pulmonary arteries via a large communication. Less frequently, it is due to severe obstruction to blood flow through the left side of the heart at the pulmonary venous level or beyond. PVOD refers to a process involving structural and developmental changes in the smaller muscular arteries and arterioles of the lung that gradually diminishes and eventually destroys the ability of the pulmonary vascular bed to transport blood from the larger pulmonary arteries to the pulmonary veins without an abnormal elevation of proximal pulmonary arterial pressure.

Pulmonary resistance (R_p) may be as high as 8 to 10 Wood units immediately after birth but falls rapidly throughout the first week of life. Indexed Wood units, as a measure of resistance to flow across either the pulmonary or the systemic vascular bed, are obtained by dividing the mean pressure difference (in millimeters of mercury) across the pulmonary or systemic vascular beds by the blood flow index (expressed in liters per minute per square meter) across those respective beds. By 6 to 8 weeks, it usually has reached the normal adult level (1 to 3 Wood units). These changes are accompanied by a gradual dilatation of first the smaller and then the larger muscular pulmonary arteries and then, in the weeks and months that follow, a thinning of their muscular walls, the growth of existing arteries, and the development of new arteries and arterioles. The latter process contributes over 90 percent of the smaller or intraacinar pulmonary arterial vessels present in older children and adults.[37]

Increased pulmonary arterial pressure has an adverse effect on the normal maturation of the pulmonary vascular bed. Such pressure encourages a persistence of the thick muscular medial layer present in the smaller pulmonary arteries of term newborns, stimulates an extension of smooth muscle into smaller and more peripheral arteries than normal for age, and retards the growth of existing acinar arteries and the development of new ones.

In the presence of a large systemic-to-pulmonary communication, pulmonary arterial pressures remain at or near systemic levels, with the result that the diminution in pulmonary muscle mass and pulmonary resistance is less rapid and of a lesser magnitude than it is in a normal infant. Nevertheless, the diminution is usually sufficient to permit a large pulmonary blood flow and, as a result, congestive failure by the end of the first month. Exceptions are found among infants with a large systemic-to-pulmonary communication but with alveolar hypoxia, a stimulus for pulmonary vasoconstriction, in whom there is less than normal involution of the medial musculature and a diminution in pulmonary vascular resistance. Clinically, this is expressed by the lower incidence of congestive failure observed among infants with large VSDs born and living at high altitude and in some children with Down's syndrome and a large VSD or atrioventricular canal who may hypoventilate or have upper airway obstruction. Rarely, an infant will maintain a very high pulmonary vascular resistance in the face of an anatomically large systemic-to-pulmonary communication without evidence of significant hypoxemia or acidemia and remain free of the signs and symptoms of congestive failure. Conversely, in a premature infant in whom the medial muscle mass is less at birth than it is in a full-term infant, the fall in pulmonary vascular resistance is usually much more rapid than normal.

Chronic PAH, increased flow, or both produce a characteristic series of histologic changes in the smaller pulmonary arteries and arterioles originally described and graded by Heath and Edwards (grades I through VI below)[38] (Fig. 63-4, Plate 100) and, more recently, by Rabinovitch[37] (grades A through C below):

- Grade I—medial hypertrophy
- Grade II—concentric or eccentric cellular intimal proliferation
- Grade III—relatively acellular intimal fibrosis with occlusion of the smaller pulmonary arteries and arterioles
- Grade IV—progressive, generalized dilatation of the distal muscular arteries and the appearance of plexiform lesions, complex vascular structures composed of a network or plexus

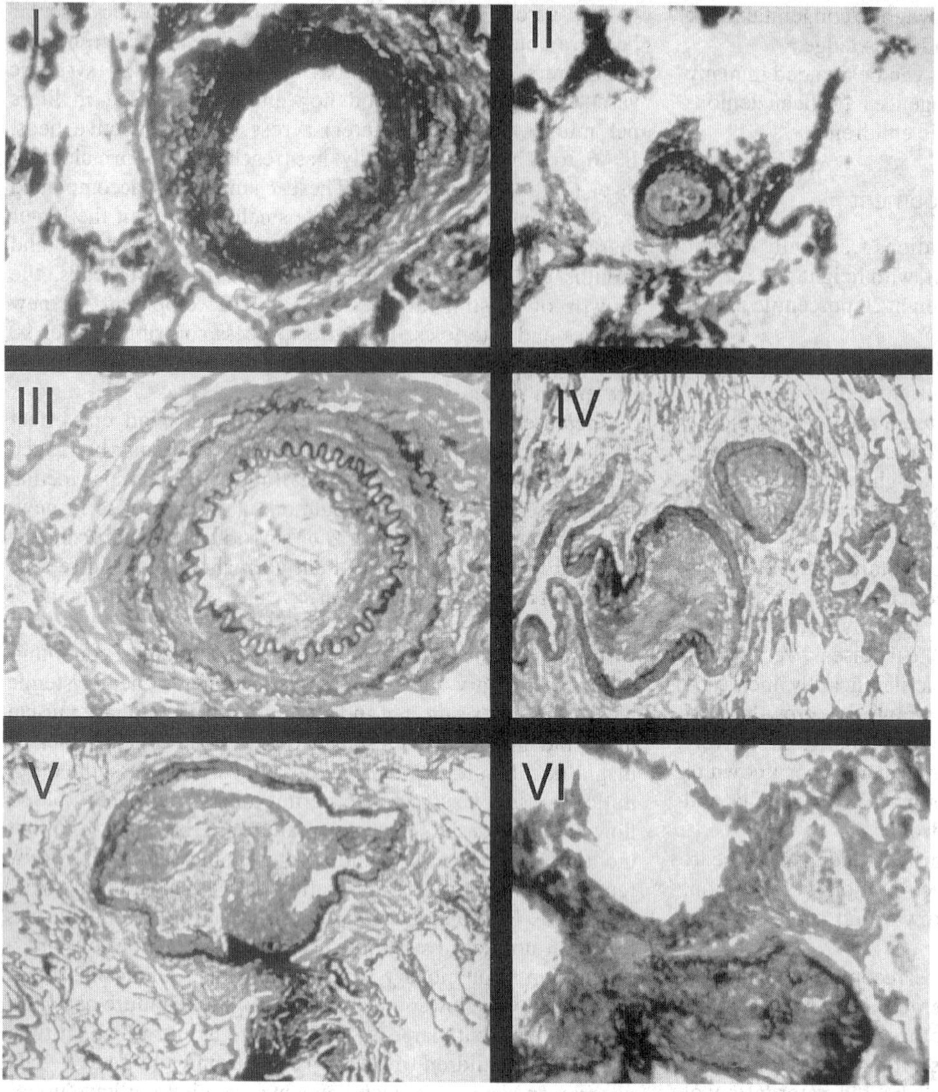

FIGURE 63-4 (Plate 100) Pulmonary vascular changes by the Heath and Edwards criteria (see text). Grades 1–6 are represented by panels I–VI, respectively.

of proliferating endothelial tissue, frequently accompanied by thrombus, within a dilated thin-walled sac

- Grade V—thinning and fibrosis of the media superimposed on the plexiform lesions
- Grade VI—necrotizing arteritis within the media
- Grade A—extension of muscle into normally nonmuscular peripheral arteries with or without a mild increase in medial wall thickness of normally muscular arteries (less than 1.5 times normal)
- Grade B—extension of muscle as described above with an even greater increase in medial wall thickness of normally muscular arteries (mild, 1.5–2 × normal; severe, >2 × normal)
- Grade C—changes seen in grade B (severe) but with a decreased arterial concentration relative to alveoli (mild, ≥1/2 normal; severe, <1/2 normal)

Grades A and B are partitions of Heath-Edwards grade I and may be seen with large left-to-right shunts with (B) or without increased pressure (A). Grade C criteria may be found with grades I and II, are invariable with grade III, and usually preclude a complete return to normal of pulmonary arterial pressures and resistance despite successful surgical correction of the systemic-to-pulmonary communication.

Estimation of pulmonary vascular resistance from data obtained at cardiac catheterization remains the most widely used means of assessing the state of the pulmonary vascular bed. Hypoxemia from oversedation, atelectasis, or pneumonitis at the time of study should be avoided scrupulously. If pulmonary vascular resistance is elevated, its responsiveness to vasodilation induced by the inhalation of 100% oxygen, the pulmonary arterial administration of prostacyclin, or the inhalation of nitric oxide should be tested.[39]

Values of $R_p \leq 3$ Wood units are considered normal. The status of the pulmonary vasculature also can be expressed as a ratio of pulmonary vascular resistance to systemic vascular resistance (R_p/R_s). *Pulmonary/systemic resistance ratios less than 0.2:1 are considered normal.*

As pulmonary vascular resistance increases, pulmonary blood flow generally decreases. Eventually, a point is reached where surgical closure of the defect will produce only a small diminution of blood flow, a proportionately small decrease in pulmonary arterial pressure, and no significant change in the factors contributing to the progression of vascular disease. At this point surgery usually is not recommended, since the benefits are minimal and closure of the defect may eliminate a useful "blow-off" for increasing resistance. *An R_p/R_s ratio of 0.7:1 or an R_p of 11 Wood units with a pulmonary/systemic blood flow ratio of 1.5:1 is the criterion generally used to define this situation.* Without surgery, these patients survive as examples of the Eisenmenger syndrome, in which $R_p \geq R_s$ and at least some right-to-left shunting occurs at rest or with exercise. Some of these patients can survive for several decades and lead productive lives, with relatively mild symptoms and few limitations.[40]

The decision regarding surgery for patients with less severe PVOD is a clinical one. The higher the calculated resistance is and the greater the structural changes in the pulmonary vasculature are, as judged by lung biopsy or quantitative pulmonary arterial wedge angiography, and the older the patient is with any given level of elevated resistance or grade of structural change, the less likely it is that the outcome will be satisfactory.[37]

The prevention of PVOD requires the identification of the patients at risk, i.e., all patients with a systemic-to-pulmonary communication and a pulmonary arterial systolic pressure higher than half the systemic arterial systolic pressure. Also included are all patients with transposition, regardless of pressure or flow, with the possible exception of those with severe pulmonary stenosis. Ideally, all patients at risk should undergo correction or pulmonary arterial banding unless there is proof that the pulmonary arterial systolic pressure has fallen to or is less than half the systemic systolic pressure before the end of the first year of life among those with normally related great arteries. Among patients with transposition with a large VSD or patent ductus arteriosis, action must be taken within the first 3 months of life.

Long-Term Problems with Surgically Corrected Defects

With the advances that have occurred in the surgical treatment of congenital heart defects, more of these patients are living to adulthood. This discussion of potential long-term problems is intended for those who follow these children after surgery and through adult life[41] (see Chap. 64).

There are residua, sequelae, and complications that result from most surgical procedures for congenital heart defects. A residual part of the original defect, such as mitral prolapse in repaired ASD, may purposefully not have been approached surgically. Some sequelae are unavoidable consequences of the surgery, such as pulmonary regurgitation after pulmonary valvotomy. There are also complications that occur as unexpected but related events after successful surgery, such as late complete heart block. When viewed with these possibilities in mind, only surgical correction of a PDA is likely to result in no long-term problems.

Most patients have residual murmurs after surgery for congenital heart defects. Determination of the origin of these murmurs and evaluation of the severity of the hemodynamic abnormalities they represent are important. Noninvasive diagnostic tools, especially Doppler and two-dimensional echocardiography, are often useful.

The risk of infective endocarditis to patients persists after surgery, with the exception of those who have undergone patent ductus ligation or division or repair of an ASD or VSD in whom there is no residual shunt. Patients in whom it has been necessary to place an artificial valve are at increased risk of endocarditis.[42,43]

There are specific problems related to some of the more common defects. For those with repaired ASDs, VSDs, and AV (canal) septal defects, a residual shunt may be present, but ordinarily it is small and not of hemodynamic significance. Those with repaired AV canal defects may have important AV valvular regurgitation. Repaired coarctation of the aorta can gradually become narrowed again, or patients may develop idiopathic hypertension. Surgery for valvular pulmonary stenosis usually results in mild residual stenosis and regurgitation, which are well tolerated and have little tendency to progress with time. The natural history of valvular aortic stenosis after surgery is not as benign.[44] Because significant regurgitation must be avoided, the initial results may not be as good in terms of the severity of residual stenosis. In addition, aortic stenosis tends to worsen with time; thus, proper follow-up is mandatory for these patients.

Few patients enter adulthood with the continued problem of cyanosis. Since those with residual defects amenable to surgical correction should have had surgery well before this time, only patients with complex and uncorrectable defects and those with pulmonary vascular disease should have problems of cyanosis during the adult years. Particularly important among these patients is management of any attendant psychosocial problems (employment, insurability,[45] and learning disabilities) and difficulties related to pregnancy.[46]

Those who have had surgery for cyanotic defects are more likely to have sequelae and complications. Some degree of exercise intolerance is not unusual in this group of patients, and exercise stress testing aids in their management.[47]

Dysrhythmias are particularly common among these patients. *In those who have had intraventricular repairs, most commonly for tetralogy of Fallot, late complete heart block and serious ventricular arrhythmias can occur and may result in sudden death.*[48] This risk appears to be highest in those who had transient complete heart block at the time of surgery and who develop right bundle branch block with left anterior hemiblock after surgery. Extensive interatrial surgical procedures for transposition of the great arteries also frequently lead to dysrhythmias, most commonly sick sinus syndrome with bradytachyarrhythmias and atrial flutter, with a high incidence of sudden death.[49] Ambulatory 24-h electrocardiographic monitoring (see Chap. 25) and stress testing (see Chap. 14) and intracardiac electrophysiologic studies are important in following patients who have had complex repairs. Atrial dilation after the Fontan operation has resulted in atrial flutter and/or fibrillation, which are frequently problematic therapeutically.[50]

Serious ventricular dysfunction[51] and venous obstructions also may occur, usually in those who had severe defects. Interatrial repairs for transposition of the great arteries leave the anatomic right ventricle to do the work of the systemic ventricle.[52] In addition, these repairs may lead to pulmonary and/or systemic venous obstruction. Atriopulmonary connections for the repair of tricuspid atresia and many types of univentricular hearts frequently leave an anatomically abnormal ventricle as the systemic ventricle. In this group of patients, the right atrium has become the "pulmonary ventricle," with an elevated right atrial pressure that may lead to problems of systemic venous hypertension such as protein-losing enteropathy.[53]

Finally, some children have had repairs in which synthetic prostheses were utilized. Artificial valves do not grow as the child does, and they must be much more durable in view of the child's life expectancy. There are also some surgical procedures that require the placement of conduits, with or without valves, that can degenerate and become obstructive with time. *Bioprosthetic valves undergo accelerated fibrosis and calcification in patients less than about 30 to 35 years of age.*

It should be kept in mind that in spite of these problems, the majority of patients who reach adulthood after surgical repair of congenital defects are relatively asymptomatic; they can and do lead productive lives.

INTRACARDIAC COMMUNICATIONS BETWEEN THE SYSTEMIC AND PULMONARY CIRCULATIONS, USUALLY WITHOUT CYANOSIS

Ventricular Septal Defect

PATHOLOGY AND INCIDENCE

A ventricular septal defect is the most common congenital cardiac anomaly (Table 63-4). It may be an isolated defect or part of a complex malformation. Approximately 80 percent of these defects are paramembranous but may extend into the inlet, trabecular, or outlet sections of the muscular septum. Less common are conal septal or subarterial doubly committed defects (5 to 7 percent), inlet defects lying beneath the septal leaflet of the tricuspid valve in the region of the atrioventricular canal (5 to 8 percent), and defects in the muscular septum that may be in the inlet, trabecular, or outlet area[54] (Fig. 63-5). Multiple muscular defects are not infrequently seen.

The incidence of VSDs is about 2 per 1000 live births, and its prevalence among school-age children has been estimated as 1 per 1000, constituting about one-quarter of the congenital cardiac malformations in combined series (Table 63-1). Males and females are affected equally.

VSDs may be isolated or associated with other congenital cardiac abnormalities. Malformations associated with VSD are, in order of decreasing frequency: (1) coarctation of the aorta, (2) additional shunts, most commonly ASD and PDA, (3) intracardiac obstructions such as subpulmonary or subaortic stenosis, mitral stenosis, and anomalous muscle bundle of the right ventricle, and (4) incompetent atrioventricular valves.

ABNORMAL PHYSIOLOGY

The consequences of a VSD depend on the size of the defect and the pulmonary vascular resistance. A small defect offers a large resistance to flow. There is no elevation of right ventricular or pulmonary arterial pressure, and the left-to-right shunt may be so small that it can be detected only by selective left ventricular angiography or two-dimensional imaging with Doppler color flow mapping. This type of defect imposes little physiologic burden on the heart, although there is always the danger of infective endocarditis.

A defect of moderate size still permits a difference between the right and left ventricular systolic pressures but may allow a large left-to-right shunt with resulting left atrial hypertension and dilatation and left ventricular volume overload. The development of pulmonary vascular disease among these patients is unusual but possible.

When the effective area of the defect is large, approximately equal to or greater than the aortic valve orifice, the defect offers

TABLE 63-4 Communications with Predominant Left-to-Right Shunting

Ventricular septal defect	Atrioventricular canal
Atrial septal defect	Patent ductus arteriosus
Partial anomalous pulmonary venous connection	Sinus of Valsalva fistula

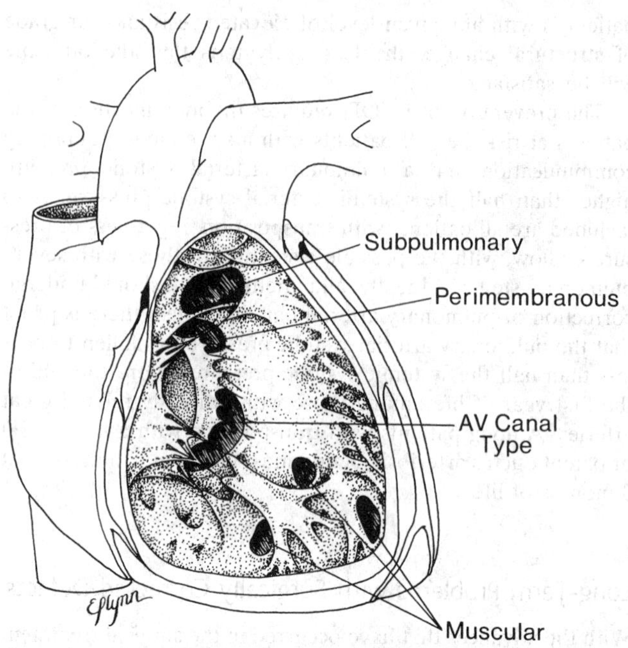

FIGURE 63-5 Different types of ventricular septal defects when viewed from the right ventricle. (From Fyler DC, ed. *Nadas' Pediatric Cardiology*. Philadelphia: Hanley & Belfus; 1992. Reproduced with permission from the publisher and author.)

virtually no resistance to flow and the systolic pressures in both ventricles, the aorta, and the pulmonary artery are essentially the same. The relative proportion of blood going to the two circulations is directly governed by the relative resistance of the two vascular beds.

At birth, pulmonary vascular resistance is high and there is little, if any, left-to-right shunt despite the presence of a large defect. This resistance to flow gradually falls over the first few weeks of life, permitting a progressively greater amount of blood to flow through the defect, through the lungs, and back to the left atrium and left ventricle. In most infants, the left ventricular volume overload eventually leads to left ventricular "failure" with elevated left ventricular end-diastolic and left atrial pressures and pulmonary congestion.

In term infants born at sea level with a large VSD, clinical deterioration may occur at any time from about 3 to 12 weeks after birth. In premature infants, in whom the less well developed pulmonary vascular hypertrophy regresses more rapidly, failure frequently is noted at 1 to 4 weeks.

History Infants or children with a small isolated defect are asymptomatic. The murmur of a small defect may be detected within the first 24 to 36 h of life, since the very restrictive opening permits the normal rapid fall in pulmonary arterial resistance and pressures. Infants with larger defects usually present between 3 and 12 weeks of age with congestive failure, frequently with associated lower respiratory tract infections. Parents describe tachypnea, grunting respirations, and fatigue, particularly with feedings. Weight gain is slow, and excessive sweating is common.

Physical Examination A child with a small defect is comfortable. With moderate holes, a systolic thrill at the lower left sternal border is common. If the defect is small, the pulmonary artery pressure is normal and so the second heart sound is not accentuated. The systolic murmur along the lower left sternal border is characteristically holosystolic but may be limited to early or midsystole. This latter feature suggests a defect in the muscular septum rather than the membranous septum.

Infants with large defects, large left-to-right shunt, and PAH tend to be restless, irritable, and underweight. Moderate respiratory distress may be present. Both the right and the left ventricular systolic impulses are impressively hyperdynamic to palpation. A thrill at the lower left sternal border is common. The second heart sound is narrowly split, with a loud, frequently palpable pulmonary component. Third heart sound gallops at the apex are common. Characteristically, the systolic murmur is holosystolic at the lower left sternal border and is accompanied by a middiastolic rumble of grade 2 to 3 intensity at the apex, with the latter indicating a pulmonary/systemic blood flow ratio (Q_p/Q_s) of 2:1 or greater. Hepatic enlargement can be identified below the right costal margin. Pulmonary rales may be seen with severe failure.

With the passage of time, one may observe signs of a diminishing left-to-right shunt with an improved rate of weight gain, less dyspnea, a diminution of the precordial hyperactivity, and disappearance of the apical diastolic flow rumble. This clinical improvement may be a result of the defect becoming smaller, the development of subvalvular pulmonary stenosis with little or no appreciable change in the size of the defect, or, most worrisome, the development of PVOD with continued severe PAH. With developing subpulmonary stenosis, the systolic murmur radiates more and more impressively to the upper left sternal border and the second heart sound becomes more widely split, with a progressive diminution in the intensity of the pulmonary component. Decreased flow resulting from pulmonary vascular disease is characterized by a gradual reduction in the intensity and duration of the systolic murmur, more narrow splitting of the second heart sound, and marked accentuation of the pulmonary component.

The clinical picture of advanced pulmonary vascular disease secondary to a congenital left-to-right shunt, or Eisenmenger's syndrome, is that of a relatively comfortable older child, adolescent, or young adult with mild cyanosis and clubbing in whom one finds a prominent a wave in the jugular venous pulse, a mild right ventricular lift, and a second heart sound that is narrowly split or virtually single with a very loud, usually palpable pulmonary component. An early pulmonary systolic ejection sound, reflecting dilatation of the main pulmonary artery, may be heard, and there may be no systolic murmur at all. In older adolescents and adults, an early diastolic murmur of pulmonary regurgitation or a holosystolic murmur of tricuspid regurgitation may appear.

Chest Roentgenogram In the presence of a small defect, the heart size and shape and the pulmonary blood flow are barely altered. With large defects, there is moderate to marked enlargement of the heart, with prominence of the main pulmonary arterial segment and impressive overcirculation in the peripheral lung fields. The left atrium is dilated unless an associated ASD is present, allowing decompression of the left atrium. With increasing pulmonary vascular disease, there is diminution in heart size toward normal while the central pulmonary arteries remain dilated. The peripheral pulmonary arterial markings become attenuated, and a "pruned" effect is produced in the outer third of the lung fields.

Electrocardiogram With a small defect, one can expect the normal progression of the mean QRS axis from right to left and the normal gradual diminution of the prominent right ventricular voltages characteristic of newborns. The left ventricular forces remain within normal limits or become slightly augmented as a reflection of the mild left ventricular volume overload. With large defects, the mean QRS axis tends to remain oriented to the right and there is little or no regression in right ventricular voltage. The left ventricular forces gradually increase, resulting in a pattern of biventricular hypertrophy within the first few weeks of life. Left atrial hypertrophy is usually present, and frequently right atrial hypertrophy as well. With the development of pulmonary vascular disease or significant pulmonary stenosis, the mean QRS axis tends to remain oriented to the right; there is no regression in right ventricular voltage, but the evidence of left ventricular and left atrial hypertrophy lessens or disappears.

Echocardiogram Two-dimensional imaging can distinguish an uncomplicated VSD from more complex malformations and is capable of imaging most defects directly when multiple transducer positions are used. The addition of pulsed-wave Doppler with color flow mapping permits the identification of small, multiple, muscular, and other less easily visualized defects. The position and size of the opening can be determined as well as its relationships to the aorta, pulmonary artery, and AV valves. Continuous-wave Doppler echocardiography can predict the systolic right ventricular pressure from the difference between the systolic pressure measured by a blood pressure cuff if there is no aortic stenosis and the Doppler gradient (Fig. 63-6). In the absence of associated pulmonic stenosis, the right ventricular

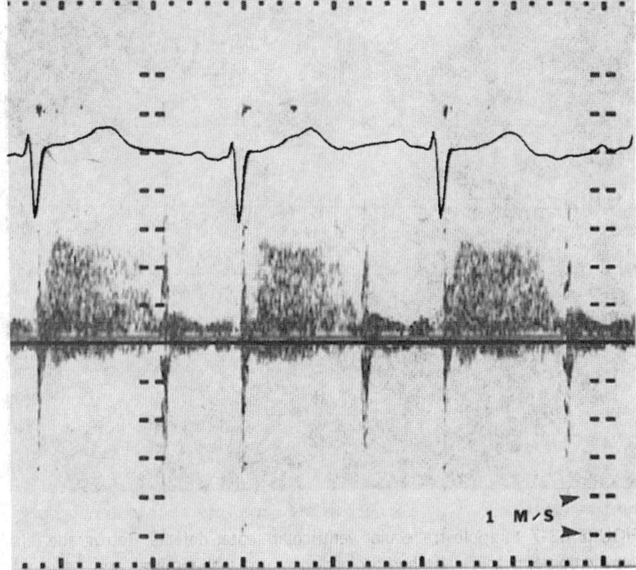

FIGURE 63-6 Continuous-wave Doppler with spectral display from the left lower sternal border of a child with a ventricular septal defect that demonstrates holosystolic turbulence with peak velocity = 2.8 m/s across the defect, compatible with an instantaneous systolic pressure difference of 31 mmHg between the right and left ventricles.

systolic pressure provides an estimate of the pulmonary artery pressure. An accurate approximation of right ventricular systolic pressure also can be made by estimating the right ventricular to right atrial systolic pressure gradient across the tricuspid valve if tricuspid regurgitation is present.

Cardiac Catheterization Cardiac catheterization is being done less commonly in VSDs not associated with other cardiac malformations. When it is performed, an increase in oxygen saturation at the right ventricular level reflects the left-to-right shunt via the VSD. With small defects, the right ventricular and pulmonary arterial systolic pressures are normal. With large defects, these pressures are at or near systemic levels, and the mean left atrial pressure may be elevated to the range of 10 to 15 mmHg.

Selective left ventricular angiography in the anteroposterior, lateral, and oblique views with craniocaudal angulation can be done to establish the spatial relations of the great arteries to each other and to the ventricles and also to determine the exact site, size, and number of septal defects (Fig. 63-7). Aortography is helpful in eliminating the possibility of an associated ductus arteriosus or unsuspected coarctation of the aorta if the arch cannot be well imaged by echocardiography.

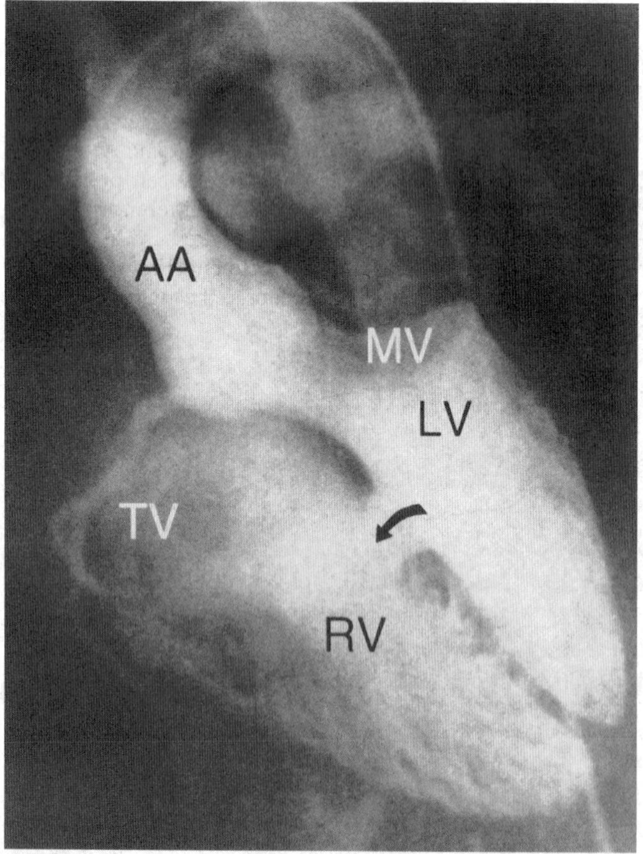

FIGURE 63-7 Multiple trabecular ventricular septal defects. Retrograde left ventriculogram, four-chamber projection, profiles the mitral and tricuspid valves and the midtrabecular VSD (*arrow*). Additional VSDs closer to the apex are more anterior in location and are not profiled in this projection. AA = ascending aorta; LV = left ventricle; MV = mitral valve; RV = right ventricle; TV = tricuspid valve. (From Lock JE, Keane JF, Perry SB. *Diagnostic and Interventional Catheterization in Congenital Heart Disease*, 2d. ed. Boston: Kluwer; 2000.)

NATURAL HISTORY AND PROGNOSIS

Fortunately, the majority of VSDs are small and do not present a serious clinical problem. Approximately 24 percent of these small defects close spontaneously by 18 months, 50 percent by 4 years, and 75 percent by 10 years.[55] A spontaneous closure rate approaching 45 percent within the first 12 to 14 months has been observed among infants with an uncomplicated paramembranous or muscular VSD in the neonatal period.[56] Even large defects tend to become smaller, but the likelihood of eventual spontaneous closure is much lower (probably in the range of 60 percent if judged large at 3 months of age and only 50 percent if it is still large at 6 months).[55]

Congestive failure is a threatening and almost inevitable complication of a large VSD. Almost 80 percent of infants with large defects require hospitalization by age 4 months.[3] The risk of death with congestive failure is in the range of 11 percent. Significant subvalvular pulmonary stenosis develops in approximately 3 percent of these individuals and may progress to the point of severe tetralogy of Fallot. PVOD is seldom severe and rarely is irreversible in the first 12 months of life, but thereafter it becomes progressively more common and less likely to regress. At risk of this complication are infants and children with a pulmonary systolic pressure in excess of 50 percent of the systemic arterial systolic pressure beyond the first year of life.[57] A very small number of infants with large VSDs maintain a high level of pulmonary vascular resistance throughout the first year of life and remain almost entirely free of symptoms and congestive heart failure. In these patients, irreversible pulmonary vascular disease may develop without the usual and expected clinical signs and symptoms described above.

A small number of children, 0.6 percent in a large group of carefully followed patients, will develop aortic regurgitation as a result of prolapse of the right, the posterior, or both aortic valve leaflets into the defect.[58] This complication is more prevalent among males, in a ratio of 2:1, and seems particularly likely to occur with defects of the subpulmonary type. Shunt size appears not to be related to the development of this complication. The characteristic aortic diastolic murmur may appear at any time between ages 6 months and 20 years. Regurgitation is usually progressive, sometimes rapidly so, and predisposes these individuals to infective endocarditis.

The risk of infective endocarditis in patients with an uncomplicated VSD that is managed medically lies somewhere between 4 and 10 percent for the first 30 years of life.[59] The development of aortic regurgitation more than doubles this risk. Attempts at surgical closure of the defect with or without aortic regurgitation reduce the risk to less than half that of unoperated patients.[60]

MEDICAL MANAGEMENT

The basis of the medical management of children with ventricular septal defects is an understanding that defects frequently get smaller and may close spontaneously. Approximately 70 percent of small ventricular septal defects probably close.[55] Even large muscular defects may get significantly smaller, and up to 25 percent of them will become hemodynamically insignificant if one can wait long enough. Nevertheless, significant complications can occur, and the decision whether to proceed with medical or surgical management must be reevaluated constantly.

For children with a large ventricular septal defect, the first decision point usually occurs before 8 to 12 weeks of age. Infants with large septal defects usually develop significant left-to-right shunts as the pulmonary resistance drops. Congestive heart failure ensues with tachypnea, tachycardia, and difficulty feeding. Digoxin and diuretics are occasionally useful, but if the left-to-right shunt is very large, feeding may be problematic. For children who cannot gain at least 15 g per day (30 g per day is normal) in whom no other cause is found for failure to thrive, surgical repair is indicated. Occasionally, in marginal cases, increasing the caloric density of the formula from 20 calories per ounce up to 30 to 32 calories per ounce may be useful. In children whom the increased work prevents from taking more than 10 to 12 ounces per day, however, caloric supplementation is unlikely to be sufficient and surgical repair is necessary.

The second decision point in children who do not fail to thrive occurs between 9 and 12 months of age. Children with unrestrictive or mildly restrictive ventricular septal defects have pulmonary artery hypertension that may lead to irreversible pulmonary vascular obstructive disease. If the pulmonary artery pressure is elevated at 9 to 12 months of age, surgery is indicated to prevent this serious life-shortening complication. In some children, the high-pitched nature of the murmur, the normal pulmonary component of the second heart sound, the absence of right ventricular hypertension on ECG, and the large intraventricular pressure gradient on echocardiography make the estimation of normal pulmonary artery pressure firm. Occasionally in children in whom the signs, symptoms, and laboratory findings are ambiguous or conflicting, cardiac catheterization may be necessary to assure that the pulmonary artery pressure is normal and that pulmonary vascular obstructive disease is not a risk.

The third decision point occurs somewhere in midchildhood (5 to 10 years of age). If the defect has not caused failure to thrive and is not associated with pulmonary hypertension, it still may be associated with a significant left-to-right shunt, causing a volume overload to the left ventricle. Eventually, congestive heart failure is possible, and some recommend surgical closure during childhood if there is a significant volume overload. There is no firm number that suggests a dangerous level of left ventricular volume overload. Some centers close the ventricular septal defect when the pulmonary-to-systemic flow ratio (measured by cardiac catheterization, radionuclide angiography, echocardiography or magnetic resonance imaging) is more than 2 to 1. Others use significant left atrial and left ventricular dilation by echo. A minority of centers do not recommend surgical closure as long as the pulmonary artery pressure is normal since there are few adults with a ventricular septal defect who develop problems with late congestive heart failure.

Unfortunately, not all patients with a large defect are encountered during the first or second year of life, when it is possible to prevent injury to the pulmonary vascular bed. If significant PAH is allowed to persist, one can expect progression to irreversible pulmonary obstructive disease. For this reason, *prompt surgical closure of defects is recommended in all individuals beyond the age of 2 years if the pulmonary arterial systolic pressure is greater than half the systemic arterial systolic pressure, the mean pulmonary pressure exceeds 25 mmHg, or the R_p/R_s ratio is higher than 0.3:1.* With severe pulmonary vascular disease, a point eventually is reached where the risk of death at operation or in the months or years immediately after the operation as a result of progressive vascular disease more than offsets the possible benefits from surgical closure. At present, surgery is recommended if the calculated R_p is less than 10 Wood units/m^2 or the R_p/R_s ratio is 0.7:1, provided that the Q_p/Q_s ratio is still 1.5:1. In adults, the upper limit of pulmonary vascular resistance for surgery is approximately 800 dynes, or 10 Wood units.

Patients in whom the defect is judged clinically to be small at 6 months of age may be reexamined at 1- or 2-year intervals to reassure the patient and family, reemphasize the importance of antibiotic protection against infective endocarditis, document further narrowing or closure of the defect, and (in a very small number of patients) detect the first signs of aortic valve prolapse.

In patients with Eisenmenger's complex,[40] stamina is limited by systemic arterial hypoxemia and, in some, right-sided heart failure. Complications to be anticipated include syncope, hemoptysis, brain abscess, hyperuricemia, and congestive failure. Pregnancy, with a maternal mortality of 30 to 60 percent, and oral contraceptives are contraindicated. Transient symptomatic relief from extreme polycythemia (usually >68 percent) may be achieved with careful erythropheresis. Travel to or living at high altitudes is poorly tolerated, and supplemental oxygen should be provided and used during air travel. The average age of death for individuals with Eisenmenger's complex is 33 years, with sudden death the mode of exit in the majority.

The risk of congenital heart disease for a subsequent sibling of a single affected child is on the order of 1 to 2 percent. The risk to a newborn who has one parent with VSD is approximately 3 percent.[61] Pregnancy in the presence of a small defect and normal pulmonary vascular resistance does not appear to carry an increased risk to the patient or infant, although precautions against infective endocarditis should be taken.

SURGICAL MANAGEMENT

Banding of the pulmonary artery to reduce pulmonary blood flow and pressures played an important role in the management of congestive heart failure and the prevention of PVOD before the era of predictably successful closure of VSDs in infants but now is used rarely. Complications of pulmonary arterial banding include deformity of the pulmonary arteries and/or pulmonary valve, progressive right ventricular hypertrophy with loss of ventricular compliance, and the development of subaortic left ventricular outflow tract obstruction.

VSDs are closed during a total cardiopulmonary bypass with cardioplegic arrest and moderate systemic hypothermia. Total circulatory arrest or minimal perfusion with profound hypothermia (18°C) is sometimes necessary in infants who weigh less than 5 kg.[62]

Paramembranous VSDs may be exposed through the right atrium and the tricuspid valve orifice. A transverse or longitudinal right ventriculotomy may be necessary for closure of high conal septal defects associated with aortic valve leaflet prolapse.

Care is required to prevent injury to the AV node near the ostium of the coronary sinus and to the bundle of His as it courses inferiorly, passing on the left side of the ventricular septum near the posterocaudal margin of the septal defect. Interoperative transesophageal echocardiography with Doppler color flow assessment can be used for the detection of significant residual or previously unsuspected problems that may be corrected in the operating room.

Results from primary surgical closure of VSDs are generally excellent, with surgical mortality less than 1 percent in centers with extensive experience, when surgery is performed during the early months of life before the evolution of PVOD. Operative risk should be even lower in older children if the pulmonary vascular resistance remains low. The pulmonary vascular bed responds favorably when the systemic-to-pulmonary shunt is eliminated before age 2 years. Normal life expectancy and functional capabilities should be anticipated postoperatively. Survival 25 years after the closure of a VSD is approximately 95 percent.[63] The mortality rate is unquestionably higher among patients who are operated on with $R_p > 7$ Wood units.

The surgical repair of a multiple muscular VSD has been problematic. The highly trabecular right ventricular septal surface can make the localization of all the defects difficult. Recently, techniques have become available to close these defects in the catheterization laboratory.[64] A device that can be anchored on the left ventricular and right ventricular septal surface was approved by the U.S. Food and Drug Administration in 1999 for this indication. Other devices are now in phase 2 testing.

Between February 1989 and July 1998, 148 transcatheter closures were preformed at Children's Hospital in Boston with no deaths or late morbidity resulting from catheter-related events. By echocardiography, 83 percent of the defects were closed or had trivial residual leaks.[64] The relative role of surgery versus interventional catheterization closure remains to be determined in this subset with multiple trabeculated septal defects.

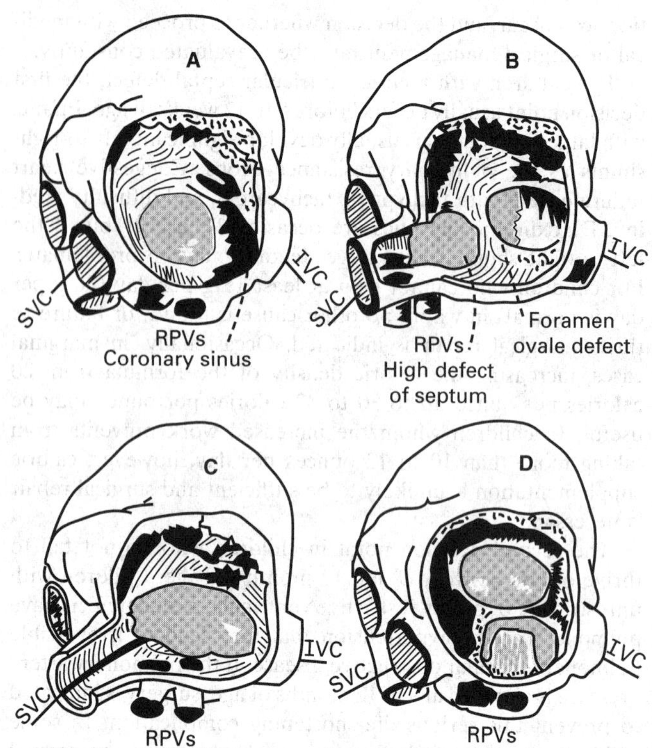

FIGURE 63-8 Types of interatrial communications. *A*. Large ostium secundum type of atrial septal defect. *B*. So-called sinus venosus type of defect—one high in the atrial septum associated with anomalous connection of the right superior pulmonary vein to the junctional area of the superior vena cava and right atrium. *C*. Very large ostium secundum type of atrial septal defect with absence of the posterior rim. *D*. Partial form of common atrioventricular canal with cleft mitral valve. SVC = superior vena cava; RPVs = right pulmonary veins; IVC = inferior vena cava. (From Lewis FJ et al.[65] Copyright 1957, American Medical Association. Reproduced with permission from the publisher and authors.)

Atrial Septal Defect

DEFINITION

An ASD is a through-and-through communication between the atria at the septal level. It is to be distinguished from a valvular-competent foramen ovale, which may persist into adulthood.

PATHOLOGY

ASDs are usually sufficiently large to allow free communication between the atria. They may be subdivided according to anatomic location[65] (Fig. 63-8).

ANATOMIC TYPES

Defect at the Fossa Ovalis (Ostium Secundum) This defect classically involves the region of the fossa ovalis and is the most common type (70 percent)[65,66] (Fig. 63-8*A* and *C*). Atrial septal tissue separates the inferior edge of the defect from the AV valves. Associated partial anomalous pulmonary venous connections are not uncommon, with one or more of the right pulmonary veins draining into the right atrium or one of its tributaries. Mitral valve prolapse is present in some cases.

Partial Atrioventricular Canal Defects Defects of the AV septum, which lies inferior to the fossa ovalis, constitute approximately 20 percent of ASDs and are part of a complex malformation known as *common atrioventricular canal defects*, which are considered below (Fig. 63-8*D*).

Sinus Venosus Defects These defects, accounting for approximately 6 percent of the total, appear to represent a biatrial connection of the superior vena cava (or, in rare instances, the inferior vena cava), which straddles the otherwise normal intact atrial septum. Also involved is an anomalous termination of one or more of the right-sided pulmonary veins either into the vena cava or into the right atrium near its junction with the vena cava (Fig. 63-8*B*).

Coronary Sinus Defects A coronary sinus defect is an uncommon type of ASD located in the position normally occupied by the ostium of the coronary sinus. This defect is part of a developmental complex consisting of the absence of the coronary sinus and entry of the left superior vena cava directly into the left atrium.

Conditions Common to All Anatomic Types The right atrial and ventricular chambers as well as the central pulmonary arteries become enlarged. When pulmonary hypertension intervenes, it usually does not do so before the third decade. The earliest lesion is cellular fibrous intimal thickening in the proximal segments of arterioles. The pulmonary arterial pressure then rises, followed by the development of medial hypertrophy of muscular arteries and the appearance of plexiform lesions. The right ventricular wall hypertrophies, and atherosclerosis may occur in the major pulmonary arteries. Saccular aneurysm and thrombosis with dissecting aneurysm or rupture may occur (see above, "Pulmonary Arterial Hypertension and Pulmonary Vascular Obstructive Disease"). In the final state, the pulmonary vascular bed may be difficult to distinguish from that in VSD with PVOD.

ABNORMAL PHYSIOLOGY

Usually there is no resistance to blood flow across the defect and no significant pressure difference between the two atria. A left-to-right shunt of blood occurs (Fig. 63-9) because (1) the right atrial system is more distensible than the left, (2) the tricuspid valve is normally more capacious than the mitral valve, and (3) the thinner-walled right ventricular chamber more readily accommodates a larger volume of blood at the same filling pressure than does the left ventricle. A large left-to-right shunt may be found in a neonate or young infant before the right ventricular compliance has had time to change appreciably from that of the left ventricle. Presumably, this occurs because a rapid fall in pulmonary vascular resistance encourages a larger right ventricular stroke volume, a smaller end-systolic volume, and hence an increased ability of the right ventricle to accept a larger volume of blood during the diastolic filling phase of the cardiac cycle.[67]

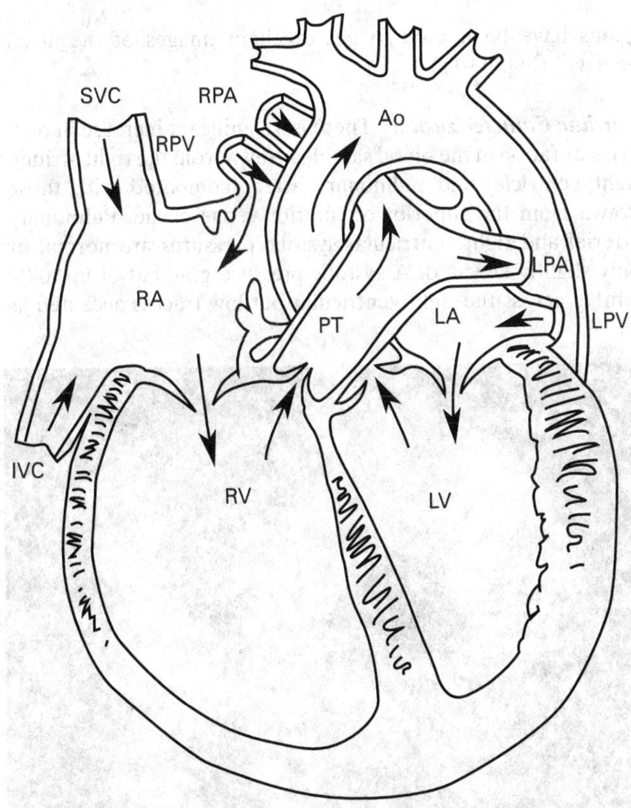

FIGURE 63-9 Atrial septal defect at fossa ovalis with left-to-right shunt. SVC = superior vena cava; IVC = inferior vena cava; RA = right atrium; RV = right ventricle; PT = main pulmonary arterial trunk; RPA = right pulmonary artery; LPA = left pulmonary artery; RPV = right pulmonary vein; LPV = left pulmonary vein; LA = left atrium; LV = left ventricle; AO = aorta. (From Edwards JE.[66] Reproduced with permission from the publisher and author.)

The pulmonary arterial system undergoes normal maturation after birth, with most patients tolerating the large volume load on the right ventricle and pulmonary circuit quite well for many years. With the development of pulmonary vascular disease and PAH, the left-to-right shunt decreases, largely because of the increased thickness and decreased compliance of the right ventricle. In some patients, this process continues until there is eventually shunt reversal, with arterial desaturation and cyanosis.

CLINICAL MANIFESTATIONS

ASD is found in approximately 6 percent of children who survive beyond the first year of life with congenital heart disease.[5] *If one excludes mitral valve prolapse and a congenitally bicuspid aortic valve, it is the most common form of congenital heart disease among adults.*

ASDs are more common among females, with a female/male ratio of approximately 2:1. The mode of transmission is best explained in most instances on a multifactorial basis, in which the risk would be approximately 2.5 percent for first-degree relatives of a single affected family member. However, examples of autosomal dominant transmission are recognized[68] either as an isolated entity associated with severe AV conduction disturbances or with upper extremity malformations as in the Holt-Oram syndrome. Examples of mendelian autosomal recessive transmission are found in the Ellis–van Creveld syndrome (see Chap. 62).

History The majority of these children are considered asymptomatic but probably most have some mild diminution of stamina, since it is not unusual for the patient or the parents to comment on the increased endurance that follows surgical correction. Symptoms of mild fatigue and dyspnea tend to be recognized in the late teens and early twenties, and at least three-quarters of these individuals will be definitely symptomatic as adults. Congestive heart failure is rare in childhood, but a few infants, perhaps 5 percent, have heart failure in the first year of life. Failure becomes more common again in the fourth and fifth decades, usually associated with the onset of arrhythmias.[69]

Physical Examination Many of these children have a slender habitus, but normal growth and development are the rule. Prominence of the left anterior chest is common, and a hyperdynamic right ventricular systolic lift usually can be felt. Looking at the jugular venous pulse demonstrates that the v wave is equal to the a wave instead of revealing the normal a wave predominance. The first heart sound may be slightly accentuated at the lower left sternal border. The two components of the second heart sound are characteristically widely split, with the interval of splitting fixed despite expiration or the Valsalva maneuver. The pulmonary component of the second heart sound may be accentuated even in the absence of PAH. With increasing pulmonary arterial pressure and resistance, the interval between the aortic and pulmonary components of the second heart sound narrows and the pulmonary component becomes louder, but the lack of respiratory influence on the interval between the two components persists. A midsystolic spindle-shaped murmur of grade 2 to 3 intensity at the left upper sternal border, reflecting increased right ventricular stroke volume and relative

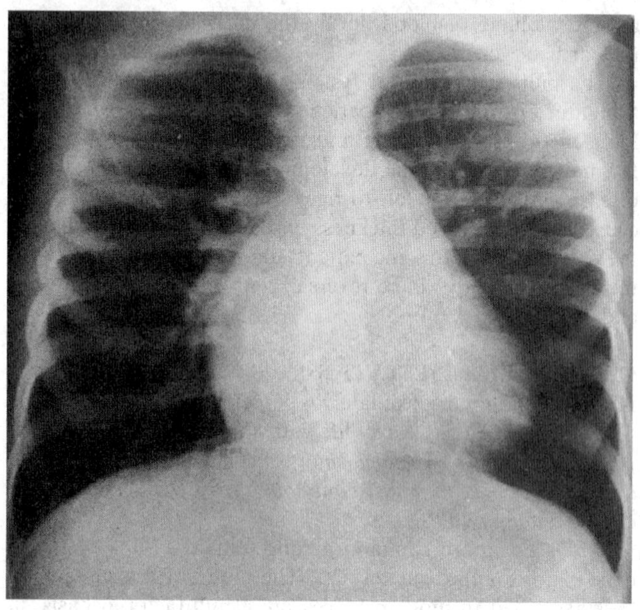

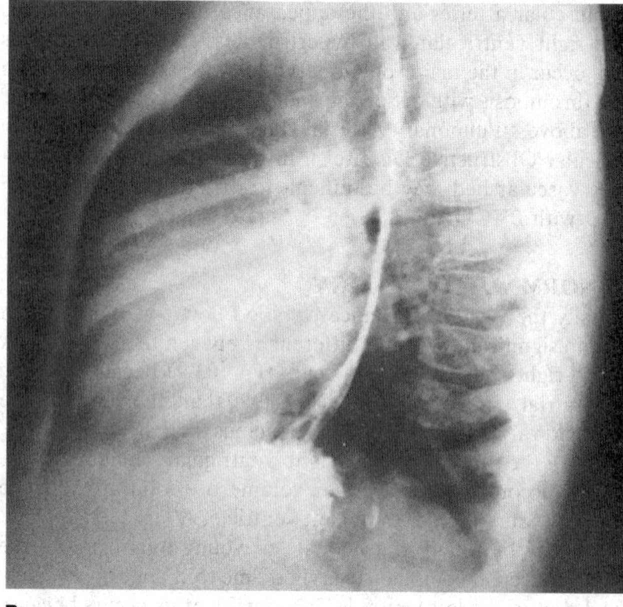

FIGURE 63-10 Chest roentgenogram of a 4-year-old child with a secundum atrial septal defect, a large left-to-right shunt, and normal pulmonary arterial pressures. *A*. Frontal. *B*. Lateral. Right ventricular enlargement (seen in the lateral view) accompanies prominence of the main pulmonary arterial segment and increased blood flow. No left atrial dilation is present.

pulmonary stenosis, is to be expected. A low- to medium-pitched early diastolic murmur over the lower left sternal border, denoting increased diastolic flow across the tricuspid valve, is present in most individuals with large shunts (see Chap. 10). Cyanosis and clubbing reflect right-to-left shunting. In this setting, the murmurs of tricuspid and pulmonary regurgitation are not uncommon.

Chest Roentgenogram Mild to moderate cardiac enlargement and prominence of the main and branch pulmonary arteries are characteristic. The absence of left atrial displacement of the barium-filled esophagus in the lateral view helps distinguish ASD from large left-to-right shunts at other levels (Fig. 63-10).

Electrocardiogram An rsR′ pattern over the right precordium indicating mild right ventricular conduction delay or mild right ventricular hypertrophy is characteristic in secundum-type ASD. The mean QRS axis in the frontal plane is 90° or greater in 60 percent of patients. Left-axis deviation is common in primum-type ASD. Abnormal leftward p axis is common in sinus venosus–type ASD. Serious arrhythmias are usually, though not invariably, limited to adults; atrial fibrillation and atrial flutter are the most common arrhythmias.

Echocardiogram M-mode studies reflect volume overload of the right side of the heart with increased right atrial and right ventricular dimensions and paradoxical ventricular septal motion. Two-dimensional and Doppler echocardiography with color flow mapping (see Chap. 13) permit identification and visualization of secundum, AV canal, and sinus venosus defects. Visualization of anomalous draining pulmonary veins is slightly more difficult. The transesophageal approach offers excellent images for those patients in whom the transthoracic approach is inadequate.[70] Recently three-dimensional (3-D) echocardiograms have been used to get excellent images of the atrial defects[71] (Fig. 63-11).

Cardiac Catheterization There is a significant increase in oxygen saturation in the blood samples drawn from the right atrium, right ventricle, and pulmonary artery compared with those drawn from the superior or inferior venae cavae. Pulmonary arterial and right ventricular systolic pressures are normal or only slightly elevated. A systolic pressure gradient of up to 20 mmHg across the right ventricular outflow tract is accepted as

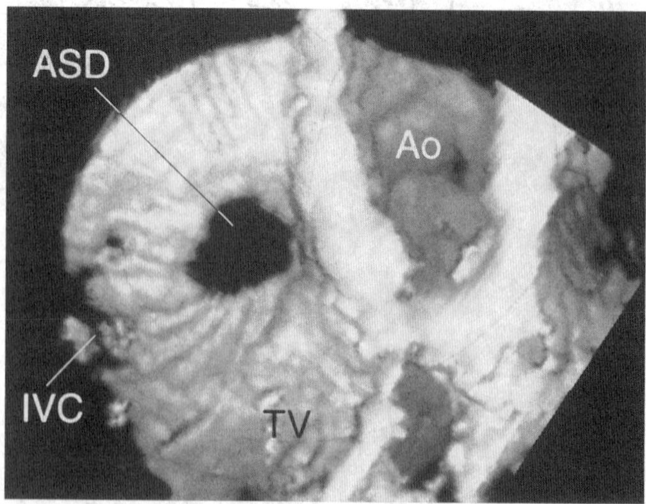

FIGURE 63-11 Three-dimensional echocardiogram of a secundum atrial septal defect (ASD). This is a right atrial en-face view that shows the size, shape, and position of the defect in relation to the right atrial septal surface. Ao = aortic valve; TV = tricuspid valve; IVC = inferior vena cava. Courtesy of Dr. Gerry Marx.

being secondary to flow rather than to organic obstruction. The right and left atrial mean and phasic pressures are virtually identical, with little, if any, elevation above normal (mean pressure gradient <3 mmHg) unless there are associated abnormalities.

NATURAL HISTORY AND PROGNOSIS

Defects of the secundum type usually go undetected in the first year or two of life because of the lack of symptoms and the unimpressive auscultatory findings. A soft systolic murmur is the usual reason for referral. Symptoms become more common in persons in their late teens and twenties, and by age 40 the majority of these individuals are symptomatic, some severely so.[72] Pulmonary vascular disease with serious pulmonary hypertension begins to make its appearance in the early twenties. *It affects approximately 15 percent of young adults, particularly women, and may be rapidly progressive, especially with pregnancy.* The incidence of atrial fibrillation or flutter also increases with each decade and is closely linked to the onset of congestive failure. Spontaneous closure of secundum defects is rare beyond the first 2 years of life.[69] Congestive heart failure is the most common cause of death among unoperated patients. Other causes of death include pulmonary embolism or thrombosis, paradoxical emboli, brain abscess, and infection.

MEDICAL MANAGEMENT

The few infants who present with symptoms of congestive failure are treated with digoxin and, if necessary, diuretics and are studied by cardiac catheterization. If the defect is uncomplicated and the symptoms persist despite a trial of therapy, surgical closure is advised without further delay. For asymptomatic infants and children, closure is recommended just before entry into school. Restrictions of activity or exercise are unnecessary. If the physical, laboratory, and echocardiographic findings are completely characteristic, preoperative catheterization is not necessary. Closure is recommended if the defect is large and if there is right ventricular volume overload on echocardiography. In those with pulmonary hypertension closure is recommended for patients with Q_p/Q_s ratios >1.5:1 by catheterization provided that the systemic arterial saturation is >92 percent and total $R_p < 15$ Wood units.[73] Closure would seem prudent before pregnancy or the use of contraceptives in view of the tendency to develop rapidly progressive PVOD in this setting. Transcatheter closure of centrally located secundum in selected older infants, children, and adults using a double-umbrella ("clamshell") or a buttoned device appears to be an acceptable alternative to surgical closure.[74–76] *Infective endocarditis is rare, and antibiotic coverage at times of possible bacteremia is recommended only if associated mitral valve disease is suspected.*

SURGICAL MANAGEMENT

Defects of the interatrial septum are exposed through the lateral wall of the right atrium.

Ostium secundum (fossa ovalis) defects frequently are closed by direct suturing; a very large defect or one with tenuous margins is closed with a patch, usually glutaraldehyde-treated autologous pericardium. Anomalous pulmonary veins are sought along the posterolateral aspect of the superior or inferior vena cava and from within the right atrium before closure of the defect. Sutures are placed with care along the posterior rim of the inferior vena caval orifice to prevent the creation of a tunnel from the inferior vena cava into the left atrium, which would cause postoperative hypoxemia.

High ASDs of the sinus venosus type, which often are associated with anomalous drainage of one or more right pulmonary veins into the superior vena cava, are corrected by means of the placement of a pericardial or tubular Dacron patch from above the abnormally draining vein or veins down to and around the ASD (Fig. 63-12). Pulmonary venous blood thus is diverted through the ASD into the left atrium. Pericardial gusset enlargement of the superior vena cava at the cavoatrial junction may be required. Anomalous right pulmonary veins draining to the right atrium are diverted into the left atrium by placement of a patch baffle well anterior and to the right of the pulmonary vein orifices. The risks of surgery are minimal (less than 0.5 percent), with virtually all these children home by the fourth postoperative day.

In adults, clinical benefit after closure of ASDs can be anticipated even in those with significant physiologic compromise,

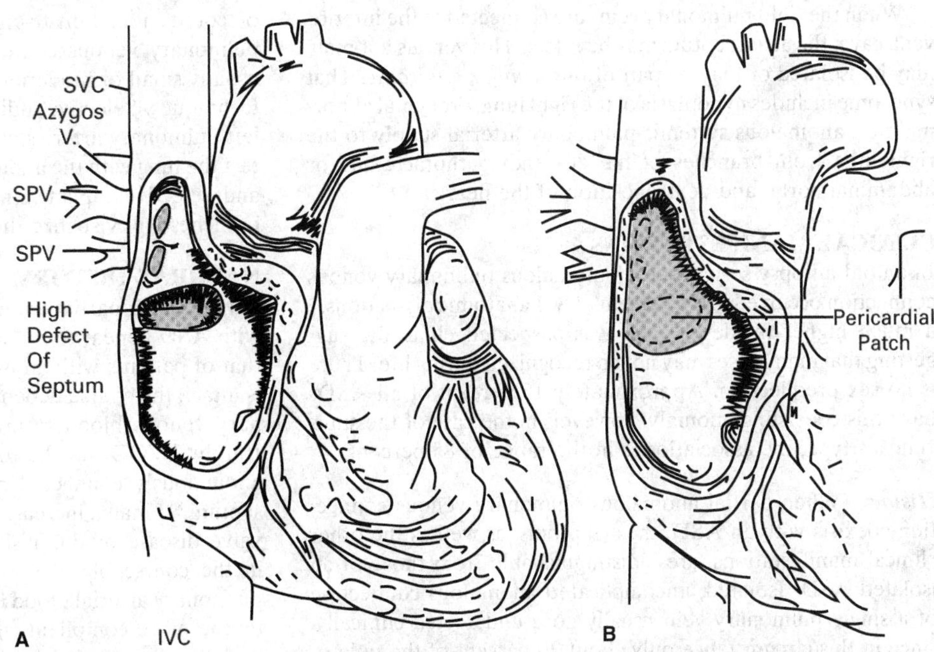

FIGURE 63-12 *A.* Sinus venosus type of atrial septal defect, with its constantly accompanying anomalous pulmonary venous connection of superior pulmonary vein (SPV) to superior vena cava (SVC). *B.* Repair is effected with a pericardial patch placed to divert pulmonary venous blood across the defect into the left atrium and to divert superior vena caval blood to the right atrium. (This illustration appeared originally in the first edition of *The Heart,* in 1966, and in all subsequent editions. It is reproduced here by courtesy of Dr. John W. Kirklin, Birmingham, Alabama.)

but mortality is higher than it is in the young and the magnitude of improvement is less certain. Nonetheless, surgical closure of ASDs is advised even when R_p approaches 15 Wood units because of the excessive morbidity and mortality associated with a persistent interatrial communication.[77] *Morbidity in adults and the low risk of surgical closure in young children mandate surgery in the preschool or preadolescent years.*

Although life-threatening complications after closure of ASDs in children are rare, transient postoperative atrial arrhythmias and postpericardiotomy syndrome with pericardial effusions occasionally are seen. The long-term prognosis for a normal life expectancy and functional capability is excellent for patients who have closure of an uncomplicated ASD during the first two decades of life.

Partial Anomalous Pulmonary Venous Connection

PATHOLOGY

In partial anomalous pulmonary venous connection, one or more, but not all, of the pulmonary veins enter the right atrium or its venous tributaries. The atrial septum may rarely be intact, but an ASD is usually present. There are many patterns of anomalous pulmonary venous connection, but the four most common, in order of decreasing frequency, are (1) pulmonary veins from the right upper and/or middle lobe to the superior vena cava, usually with a sinus venosus ASD, (2) all the right pulmonary veins to the right atrium, usually in the polysplenia syndrome, (3) all the right pulmonary veins to the inferior vena cava, entering this systemic vein just above or below the diaphragm, and (4) the left upper or both left pulmonary veins to an anomalous vertical vein draining to the left brachiocephalic vein.

When the right pulmonary veins are connected to the inferior vena cava, the atrial septum may be intact. This venous anomaly may be isolated or may be part of the *scimitar syndrome*. That syndrome includes hypoplasia of the right lung, bronchial abnormalities, anomalous systemic pulmonary arterial supply to the right lung from branches of the descending thoracic and/or abdominal aorta, and dextroposition of the heart.

CLINICAL MANIFESTATIONS

In an old autopsy series, partial anomalous pulmonary venous connection occurred in 0.6 percent of 801 anatomic dissections,[78] a much higher incidence than was suspected clinically, suggesting that many cases may not be recognized during life. There is no sex predilection. Approximately 15 percent of all ASDs have this coexisting anomaly; however, in the case of the sinus venosus type, the association is in the range of 85 percent.

History When partial anomalous pulmonary venous connection coexists with an ASD, the symptoms, as well as the other clinical manifestations, are indistinguishable from those of an isolated ASD. Isolated, uncomplicated anomalous connection of a single pulmonary vein usually goes undetected clinically, since in this circumstance only about 20 percent of the pulmonary venous flow returns to the right atrium or its tributaries. When the entire venous return from one lung or two pulmonary veins is connected anomalously, approximately 65 percent of the pulmonary venous flow returns to the right side of the heart and the symptoms are similar to those of an ASD with a comparable increase in pulmonary blood flow.

Physical Examination The findings are the same as those in patients with an ASD with the exception that *the two components of the second heart sound, though usually widely split, move normally with respiration if the atrial septum is intact.*

Chest Roentgenogram Right ventricular enlargement, pulmonary arterial dilatation, and increased pulmonary blood flow are characteristic when more than one pulmonary vein connects anomalously. With anomalous connection of the right pulmonary veins to the inferior vena cava, the pulmonary venous pattern may assume a crescent-shaped or scimitar curve in the right lower lung field along the right lower heart border (scimitar).

Electrocardiogram The ECG is normal (in the case of anomalous connection of a single pulmonary vein) or reflects volume overload of the right side of the heart, as was described above in "Atrial Septal Defect."

Echocardiogram If more than one pulmonary vein drains anomalously, the volume usually is sufficient to produce the characteristic pattern of right ventricular diastolic overload. Failure to visualize an atrial septal opening with two-dimensional imaging and color flow mapping from a subcostal coronal or high right-sided parasternal longitudinal view should arouse suspicion of an intact atrial septum. A variety of views supplemented by color flow mapping may be necessary to identify the anomalous connection.[79]

Cardiac Catheterization Anomalously connected pulmonary veins may be entered directly with the venous catheter. Selective biplane angiograms in these vessels will document their site of connection. Left-to-right shunting with partial anomalous pulmonary venous connection and an intact atrial septum is usually small or moderate and may go undetected by oximetry techniques. Selective indicator dilution curves in the right and left pulmonary arteries with systemic arterial sampling can detect the lung with the anomalous pulmonary venous connection, and selective biplane angiograms in the pulmonary arterial branches will visualize these connections.

NATURAL HISTORY AND PROGNOSIS

Patients with partial anomalous pulmonary venous connection with ASD appear to follow a course similar, if not identical, to that of patients with an isolated ASD. When the atrial septum is intact, the course depends primarily on the volume of pulmonary venous blood returning to the right side of the heart. Rarely, PVOD may be found even in the presence of a single anomalously connected pulmonary vein and an intact atrial septum.[80] Finally, increasing left atrial pressure caused by mitral valve disease or diminishing left ventricular compliance will, in the course of time, encourage a greater redistribution of pulmonary arterial blood flow to the portion of the lung drained by the more compliant right atrium. Thus, patients who were initially asymptomatic and had a very modest volume of anomalous pulmonary venous return in youth may become symptomatic and even develop congestive failure in adult life.

MEDICAL MANAGEMENT

Asymptomatic patients with small shunts require no treatment. Those with symptoms, larger pulmonary blood flows, congestive failure, or PAH require surgical correction. With an intact atrial septum, precise preoperative identification of the site of the anomalous venous connection is essential. Long-term follow-up in patients who have not had surgery is indicated to detect increasing flow or the appearance of PAH.

SURGICAL MANAGEMENT

Anomalous connection of a right pulmonary vein or veins to the superior vena cava usually is associated with a sinus venosus ASD (Fig. 63-12). (see "Atrial Septal Defect, Surgical Management," above.) Partial anomalous pulmonary veins draining to the superior vena cava, inferior vena cava, or right atrium are repaired by being diverted through the ASD into the left atrium, using an appropriately placed patch baffle. Isolated left-sided anomalous pulmonary veins draining to the left ascending vertical vein or the left superior vena cava are detached and anastomosed directly to the left atrial appendage. Long-term morbidity and mortality are minimal among patients with uncomplicated partial pulmonary venous connections, equivalent to those observed after closure of an ASD.

Common Atrioventricular Canal Defects

DEFINITION

Atrioventricular canal defects are characterized by an ASD in the lowermost part of the atrial septum (ostium primum), a cleft of the mitral valve (either alone or in combination with a cleft of the tricuspid valve), or deficiency of ventricular septal tissue or some combination. In the most severe form (complete AV canal defect), there is a large deficiency of the lower part of the atrial septum and the upper muscular portion of the ventricular septum and a common AV valve that straddles the ventricular septum. The condition appears to result from incomplete growth of the AV endocardial cushions and the AV septum.

PATHOLOGY

The ostium primum type of ASD is characterized by a crescent-shaped upper border and no septal tissue forming the lower border. The lower aspect of the defect is bounded by the atrial surfaces of the AV valves and, in the complete type (see below), in part by the upper edge of the ventricular septum. A small amount of septal tissue separates the defect from the posterior atrial wall.

ANATOMIC TYPES

Variations occur with respect to the nature of the AV valves. The terms *partial* and *complete* were first introduced to describe these types by Rogers and Edwards.[81]

Partial Type The ostium primum ASD is associated with a "cleft" in the anterior mitral leaflet or, probably more accurately, a septal commissure between the superior and inferior leaflets of the left AV valve (Figs. 63-8*D* and 63-13).[66] The tricuspid valve is not cleft or shows a minor central deficiency. The ventricular aspects of the anterior mitral valve elements are fused to the upper edge of the deficient ventricular septum, precluding an interventricular communication. If there is no atrial septal tissue or if the atrial septum is so rudimentary that it produces a common chamber involving both atria, the term *common atrium* or *single atrium* is applied.

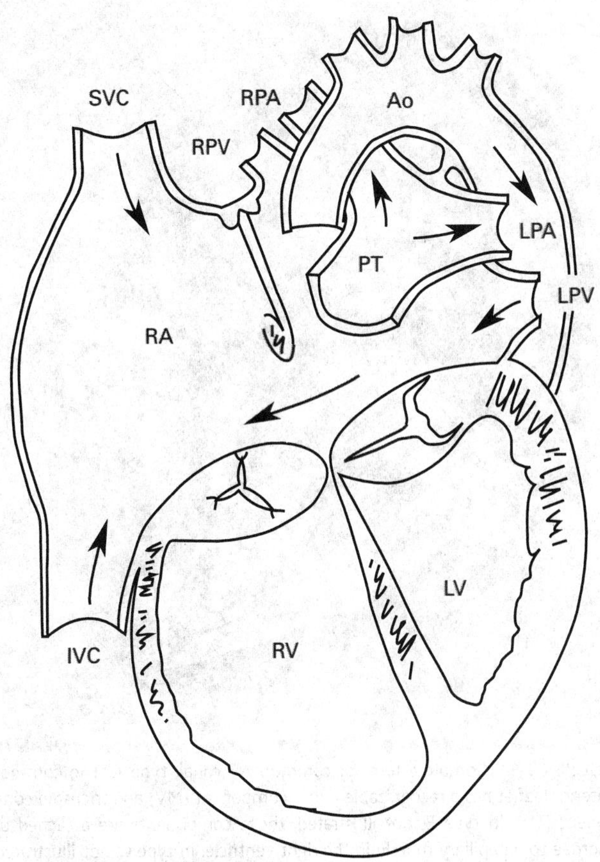

FIGURE 63-13 Common AV canal of the partial type. The mitral valve shows a cleft in its anterior leaflet, while the tricuspid valve is undisturbed. SVC = superior vena cava; IVC = inferior vena cava; RA = right pulmonary artery; LPA = left pulmonary artery; RPV = right pulmonary vein; LPV = left pulmonary vein; LV = left ventricle; Ao = aorta. (From Edwards JE.[66] Reproduced with permission from the publisher and author.)

Complete Type The complete type of common AV canal is characterized by failure of partitioning of the primitive canal into separate AV orifices. The orifice between the atria and the ventricles is guarded by a common valve, of which the anterior leaflet is derived from the ventral AV endocardial cushion and represents the anterior halves of the anterior mitral and septal tricuspid leaflets. The posterior leaflet is derived from the dorsal AV endocardial cushion and represents the posterior halves of the anterior mitral and septal tricuspid leaflets.

Usually, considerable space exists between the anterior and posterior leaflets above and the ventricular septum below; thus, in most cases of the complete type, there is free communication between the ventricles.

Rastelli and associates[82] subdivided the complete variety into three subgroups—types A, B, and C—on the basis of the structure of the common anterior leaflet and its chordal attachments to the ventricular septum and/or papillary muscles (Fig. 63-14). With regard to the posterior common leaflet, there is variation among the three types in regard to the presence or absence of subdivision and whether the posterior leaflet is attached to the ventricular septum by chordae or by an imperforate membrane.

Variations from the classic types of AV canal defects are recognized, the most common being the AV canal type of iso-

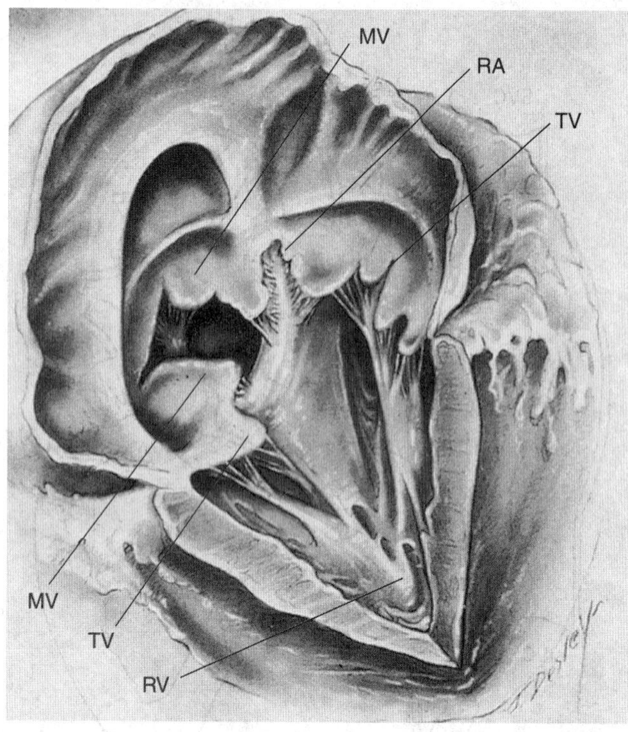

FIGURE 63-14 Complete form of common AV canal, type A. The common anterior leaflet has a recognizable mitral component (MV) and tricuspid component (TV). In type B, not illustrated, those components are attached by chordae to a papillary muscle in the right ventricle. In type C, not illustrated, the common anterior leaflet is a single unit without any attachment to the underlying ventricular septum. Type A is most amenable to repair. RV = right ventricle; RA = right atrium. (From Rastelli GC et al.[82] Reproduced with permission from the publisher and authors.)

lated VSD, isolated ostium primum ASD without malformed AV valves, and isolated cleft of the anterior mitral or septal tricuspid valve leaflets.

ASSOCIATED CONDITIONS

In the asplenia syndrome, the complete variety is almost universal; with polysplenia, it occurs in about one-quarter of cases.[83] An ASD of the secundum type is present in about half the cases. Double orifice of the mitral valve may be associated with the incomplete type, and tetralogy of Fallot may be associated with the complete type.

ABNORMAL PHYSIOLOGY

If the communication at the ventricular level is large, the right ventricular and pulmonary artery pressures will be elevated. These patients are similar to those with large VSDs. Patients with a communication at the atrial level usually have only normal or slightly elevated systolic pressures in the right side of the heart and a large pulmonary blood flow, as in the secundum type of ASD. Defects in the tricuspid valve, mitral valve, or both may result in severe regurgitation or direct shunting of blood from the left ventricle to the right atrium.

CLINICAL MANIFESTATIONS

Approximately 3 percent of infants and children with congenital heart disease have AV canal defects. The majority, some 60 to 70 percent, have the complete form. The female/male ratio is approximately 1.3:1. Well over half the patients with the complete form have associated Down's syndrome. Among children with Down's syndrome, 45 percent have some form of congenital heart disease. Malformations of the AV canal type, usually of the complete variety, account for approximately 50 percent of these abnormalities.[84]

History Only if the mitral valve is incompetent do the symptoms of patients with partial AV canal differ from those associated with a secundum type of ASD. The complete form of AV canal or the partial form connected with significant mitral regurgitation may be associated with poor weight gain, easy fatigue, dyspnea, repeated respiratory infections, and congestive heart failure. Patients with complete AV canal are almost invariably very sick.

Physical Examination The findings with a partial defect are those of an ASD. If the cleft anterior mitral leaflet is incompetent, the findings of mitral regurgitation also will be present.

The physical findings with the complete AV canal defect are those of a very large VSD, usually with full-blown congestive failure, but the second heart sound is split and fixed. The murmur of mitral regurgitation may not be heard or recognized as such.

Chest Roentgenogram Overall cardiac enlargement that is out of proportion to the degree of pulmonary plethora or a cardiac silhouette suggesting combined ventricular dilatation may serve to distinguish an uncomplicated secundum ASD from a primum defect with significant mitral regurgitation. Marked cardiac enlargement and severe pulmonary overcirculation are features of the complete AV canal defect.

Electrocardiogram One of the most helpful diagnostic features in distinguishing individuals with AV canal defects from those with isolated ASDs or VSDs is the characteristic superior orientation of the mean QRS axis in the frontal plane, with a right bundle branch delay in the precordial leads. Between 92 and 95 percent of both types of canal have a QRS axis lying between 0 and −150°. The patterns of atrial and ventricular hypertrophy reflect the underlying hemodynamic abnormalities.

Echocardiogram Two-dimensional echo is capable of visualizing the extent of septal defects and, with Doppler study and color flow mapping, left-to-right shunting at the atrial and/or ventricular level and associated mitral and/or tricuspid valvular regurgitation (Fig. 63-15). The anatomic features of the anterior AV leaflet and its connections may be visualized with sufficient clarity to permit subdivision of complete AV canal defects into types A, B, and C (Fig. 63-14). Straddling AV valves, a double-orifice mitral valve, single papillary muscles, and hypoplasia or outflow obstruction of the right or left ventricle also can be determined with this technique.[85]

Cardiac Catheterization Cardiac catheterization rarely is performed if the echocardiogram is characteristic and if the history, clinical examination, and echo suggest a large left-to-right shunt and low pulmonary resistance. When it is performed, a significant increase in oxygen saturation between the superior vena cava and the right atrium is present. A right ventricular or pulmonary arterial systolic pressure in excess of 60 percent of the systemic systolic pressure favors the presence of a complete canal. With a large communication between the two ventricles

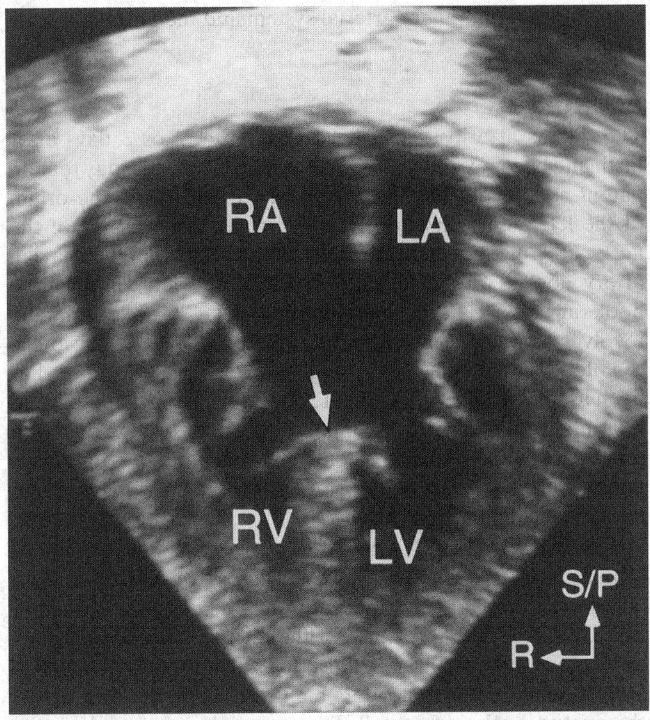

FIGURE 63-15 Apical four-chamber view of complete common AV canal. Note the large deficiency of both atrial and ventricular septa as well as apical displacement of the AV valves. The arrow points to the attachment of the inferior bridging leaflet to the ventricular septal crest. (From Levine J and Geva T.[85] Reproduced with permission.)

below the AV valves, the right ventricular, pulmonary arterial, and systemic arterial systolic pressures are virtually identical. Left ventricular angiography in the frontal view demonstrates the "gooseneck deformity" of the left ventricular outflow tract that is characteristic of AV canal malformations and allows a semiquantitative assessment of the degree of mitral regurgitation and shunting from the left ventricle to the right atrium. The left anterior oblique view with craniocaudal angulation is recommended for visualizing the interventricular defect and judging the extent of ventricular septal deficiency. Aortography is essential to eliminate the possibility of a PDA if the echocardiogram was not diagnostic.

NATURAL HISTORY AND PROGNOSIS

Partial defects without significant mitral regurgitation follow a course similar to that described for the secundum type of septal defects. An exception would be the greater likelihood of infective endocarditis because of the mitral valve deformity. Moderate or severe mitral regurgitation produces heart failure with resulting symptoms and growth retardation. Infants with a complete AV canal without protective pulmonary stenosis quickly develop and continue to have congestive failure until the course is altered by death, the development of PVOD, or surgical intervention.

MEDICAL MANAGEMENT

Children with an uncomplicated partial defect are managed in the same manner as children with an uncomplicated ASD. Those who are symptomatic should undergo early surgical closure of the primum ASD and, if possible, plication of the cleft in the septal commissure of the left AV ("mitral") valve. The few patients with significant residual mitral regurgitation after surgery are managed medically until mitral valve replacement is appropriate. Those without symptoms are repaired before they start school.

The approach to an infant with complete AV canal is the same as that for an infant with a large VSD but is tempered by the knowledge that spontaneous improvement is very unlikely except at the expense of the pulmonary vascular bed. Repair is recommended early if there is significant congestive heart failure or between 4 and 6 months of age if the pulmonary arterial systolic pressure is greater than half the systemic arterial systolic pressure. Elevation of pulmonary vascular resistance in the first year of life warrants surgical intervention without delay.

With regard to genetic counseling, the risk of a subsequent sibling having heart disease in the presence of a single affected family member is in the range of 2 percent; it is probably higher for the offspring of an affected parent, particularly if that parent is the mother.[86] Concordance for AV canal defects among affected siblings or offspring is much higher than it is with other forms of congenital heart disease and approaches 90 percent.

SURGICAL MANAGEMENT

The remarkable clinical improvement that follows anatomic repair of complete common AV septal defects in infancy encourages early correction within the first year of life. Banding of the pulmonary artery in a critically ill infant with a large interventricular defect was used in the past but has been replaced by a more reparative operation in most centers. The specifics of repair are dictated by anatomic detail: Individual variation is considerable (Fig. 63-16), but the creation of a competent, nonstenotic left-sided AV ("mitral") valve is essential for an acceptable early and long-term prognosis.

A patch usually is sutured to the right side of the ventricular septum to obliterate the interventricular communication. The anterior and posterior components of the common valve are divided, and the mitral valve is sutured to the patch at an appropriate level. The "cleft" between the left anterior and left posterior leaflets should be closed by suturing if approximation of these edges appears to increase competence without the creation of stenosis. Prosthetic valve implantation rarely is required during primary anatomic repair.[87] The right-sided AV ("tricuspid") apparatus, although less critical to survival, is repaired using the same principles. The interatrial communication usually is closed with a separate piece of pericardium to minimize hemolysis in the presence of residual mitral regurgitation.[87] Mitral valve competence is assessed by gentle distention of the left ventricle with cold saline.

A partial AV canal is repaired through a right atriotomy. The cleft may be closed with a few simple interrupted sutures to encourage inversion and coaptation of the leaflet margins. The ASD usually is closed with a pericardial patch.

Permanent complete heart block once contributed substantially to early mortality and morbidity but is now rare. Patients undergoing repair of a partial AV canal should be observed for the possible development of subaortic left ventricular outflow tract obstruction caused by redundant or residual endocardial cushion tissue.

In-hospital mortality after correction of a complete AV canal in infancy ranges from 3 to 10 percent;[88,89] the highest mortality is encountered during the first few months of life and in infants with severe AV valve regurgitation, elevated pulmonary vascular resistance, hypoplasia of the left or right ventricle, or other

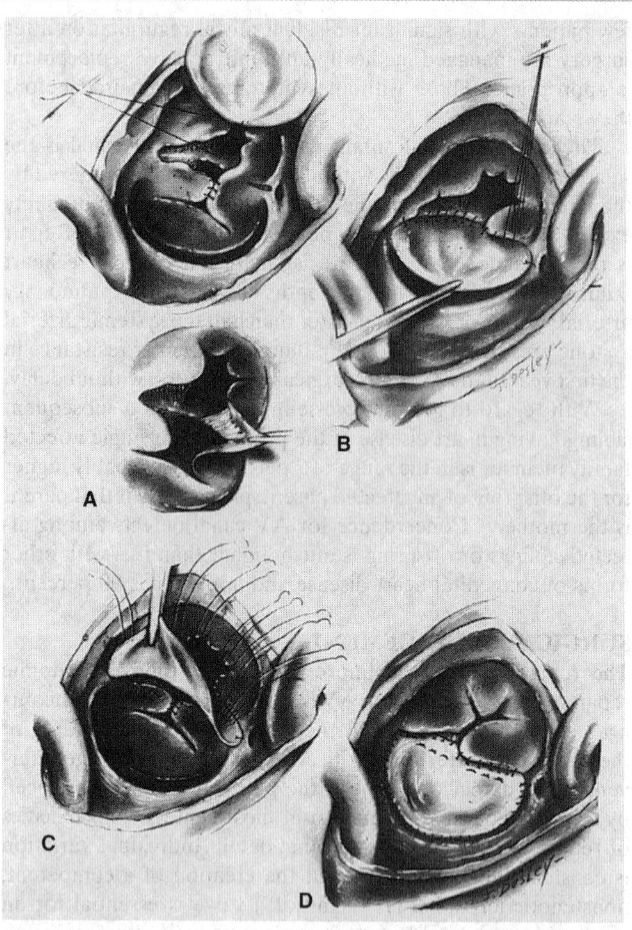

FIGURE 63-16 Steps in the repair of the complete form of common AV canal, type A. *A* and *B*. A pericardial patch is sutured to the ventricular septum. *C* and *D*. The anterior leaflet of the mitral valve is reconstructed and attached to the patch. A portion of the tricuspid leaflet is attached to the patch. (From Rastelli GC et al.[82] Reproduced with permission from the publisher and authors.)

cardiac malformations. At Children's Hospital in Boston, 191 children with a median age of 4.6 months were repaired between January 1990 and December 1998 with an operative mortality of 1.5 percent. Reoperation was necessary in 22 patients (11.7 percent), a mean of 20 months later: 18 for residual mitral regurgitation and 4 for left ventricular outflow tract obstruction.[90] Successful correction of a complete AV canal can be accomplished despite associated tetralogy of Fallot, double-outlet ventricle, and other complex anomalies.[87]

EXTRACARDIAC COMMUNICATIONS BETWEEN THE SYSTEMIC AND PULMONARY CIRCULATIONS, USUALLY WITHOUT CYANOSIS

Patent Ductus Arteriosus

DEFINITION

Patent ductus arteriosus, the most common type of extracardiac shunt, represents persistent patency of the vessel that normally connects the pulmonary arterial system and the aorta in a fetus (Fig. 63-17).

PATHOLOGY

The ductus arteriosus usually closes within 2 or 3 days after birth and becomes the *ligamentum arteriosum*, but it may remain patent as long as 8 weeks postnatally. It runs from the origin of the left pulmonary artery below to the lower aspect of the aortic arch just beyond the level of origin of the left subclavian artery above. The recurrent branch of the left vagus nerve hooks around its lateral and inferior aspects. Closure postnatally involves a complex interaction of increased oxygen tension in the blood and circulating prostaglandins. Exogenous PGE_1 has been used extensively to keep the ductus open postnatally,[91] and indomethacin, a prostaglandin inhibitor, can close the ductus in many premature infants in whom persistent patency is disadvantageous.[92]

ABNORMAL PHYSIOLOGY

Patients with PDA may be divided into groups according to whether the vascular resistance through the ductus is low, moderate, or high. The resistance of the ductus is related not only to its cross-sectional area but also to its length. In patients with a very small ductus that offers high resistance, the flow across the ductus is relatively small. The extra volume of work on the left ventricle is small, and the pulmonary pressure and resistance are not elevated. Patients with only moderate resistance in the

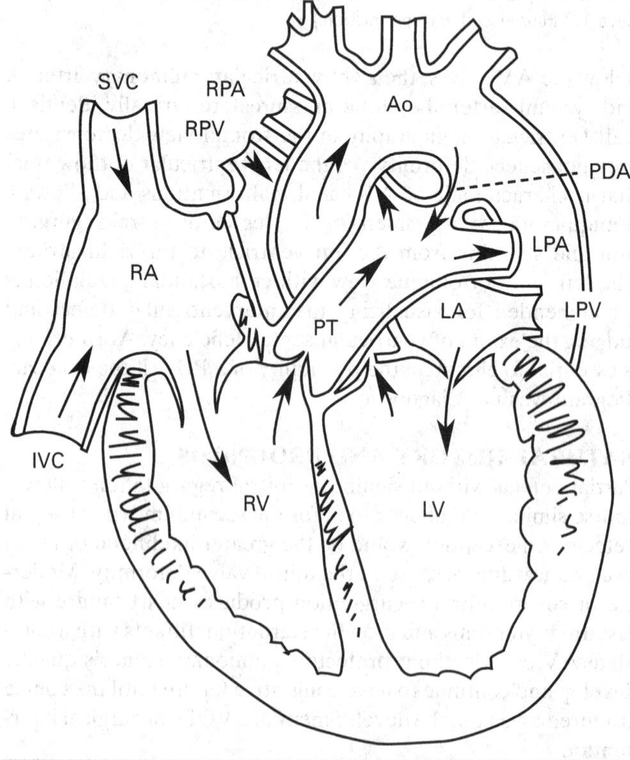

FIGURE 63-17 Patent ductus arteriosus (PDA). SVC = superior vena cava; IVC = inferior vena cava; RA = right atrium; RV = right ventricle; PT = main pulmonary arterial trunk; RPA = right pulmonary artery; LPA = left pulmonary artery; RPV = right pulmonary vein; LPV = left pulmonary vein; LA = left atrium; LV = left ventricle; Ao = aorta. (From Edwards JE.[66] Reproduced with permission from the publisher and author.)

ductus have some increase in pulmonary artery pressure, with a moderately greater volume of shunting across the ductus.

In patients with a large patent ductus, the aorta and pulmonary artery are essentially in free communication; the systolic pressure in the pulmonary artery is equal to that in the aorta. The volume load of blood recirculating through the lungs is on the left ventricle, with pulmonary congestion resulting from increased pulmonary flow and/or left ventricular failure. With time, the left ventricle compensates with dilation and hypertrophy to carry the volume load, and the pulmonary vasculature may respond to the high pressure (see the section on PAH, above). The right ventricle is burdened mainly by a pressure load.

If the pulmonary resistance equals or exceeds the resistance of the systemic circulation, there is shunting of unsaturated blood from the pulmonary artery to the aorta, resulting in hypoxemia, especially in the lower body and legs.

CLINICAL MANIFESTATIONS

History The history of the mother's pregnancy and of perinatal events may provide clues that are associated with a high incidence of PDA, such as exposure to rubella in the first trimester in a nonimmunized mother. PDA is also more common in premature infants, especially those with birth asphyxia or respiratory distress.[93]

Symptoms usually are restricted to patients with large shunts that produce heart failure or with other complicating problems, such as respiratory distress in a premature infant. The symptoms related to heart failure were discussed above. Heart failure is most likely to develop in the first few weeks or months of life. If it does not appear during infancy, it is unlikely to occur before the third decade. Growth may be affected in those with large shunts and failure. The clinical presentation in a premature infant is usually very different from that in a full-term infant, particularly in those with a birth weight under 1.5 kg, who are more likely to have moderate to severe respiratory distress. In these infants, the clinical features of respiratory distress often blend over the course of several days into those of heart failure. Increasing ventilatory or oxygen requirements with carbon dioxide retention or episodic apnea and bradycardia are often the first signs that a PDA may be complicating the picture.

Physical Examination In a full-term infant or child with PDA, there is frequently a systolic thrill over the pulmonary artery and in the suprasternal notch. The peripheral pulses are generally brisk and bounding, especially with the larger shunts secondary to runoff from the aorta to the pulmonary artery in diastole. A patient with elevated pulmonary vascular resistance and a right-to-left shunt will have "differential cyanosis," with cyanosis and clubbing of the toes but not the fingers, from shunting of hypoxemic blood from the pulmonary artery into the descending aorta. The apex impulse may be increased or displaced in those with large shunts. The right ventricular impulse is increased in a premature infant with respiratory distress and in infants and children with significant pulmonary hypertension. The typical murmur is a continuous, or "machinery," murmur that is best heard at the left upper sternal border and below the left clavicle. It is usually a rough murmur with eddy sounds, which are helpful in making the diagnosis, and it peaks at or near the second heart sound. In patients with at least a moderate shunt, there is a middiastolic rumble at the apex as a result of relative mitral stenosis from increased flow across the mitral valve. The second heart sound may be difficult to hear because of the continuous murmur, but it is usually normal. The pulmonary component is accentuated in those with pulmonary hypertension.

Chest Roentgenogram Findings on chest roentgenography also are dependent on the magnitude of the shunt. In patients with a small shunt, the chest roentgenogram is normal. With larger shunts, the left atrium and left ventricle are enlarged. Increases in pulmonary arterial flow on x-ray parallel the magnitude of the shunt. In the presence of heart failure, there are signs of pulmonary edema. In older patients who have developed Eisenmenger physiology, the only abnormality may be marked prominence of the central pulmonary arteries, with rapid tapering to the periphery of the lung fields.

Electrocardiogram With a small shunt, the ECG is normal. Left atrial hypertrophy is probably the most common abnormality found, but left ventricular hypertrophy of the volume overload type, with deep Q waves and increased R-wave voltage in the left precordial leads, is also common as the shunt size increases and left ventricular dilation occurs. Right ventricular hypertrophy is seen with pulmonary hypertension.

Echocardiogram There is left atrial enlargement, and the left ventricular end-diastolic dimension and mean velocity of circumferential fiber shortening are increased significantly. Small shunts can be detected with color Doppler imaging with a typical spectral flow pattern into the pulmonary artery, while a larger ductus can be visualized with two-dimensional echocardiography. Occasionally, a trivial amount of flow is seen through the ductus as an incidental finding in those with or without associated heart disease.

Cardiac Catheterization In those with typical, uncomplicated PDA, cardiac catheterization is not necessary. When catheterization is performed, the catheter usually passes preferentially from the left pulmonary artery into the descending aorta, except when the ductus is too small. The saturation is increased in the pulmonary artery compared with the right atrium and ventricle to a degree relative to the size of the shunt. The pulmonary arterial and right ventricular pressures are elevated in those with a large ductus. The pulmonary vascular resistance is elevated in older patients who have developed changes in the pulmonary vascular bed. These patients also have diminished saturation in the descending aorta once the pulmonary resistance reaches a level that will reverse the shunt. Aortography will opacify the ductus and pulmonary arteries.

NATURAL HISTORY AND PROGNOSIS

The complications related to PDA include infective endarteritis, heart failure, and pulmonary hypertension with vascular damage. Infection of the ductus is a risk regardless of its size. This risk increases with the length of survival. This can lead to the development of a mycotic aneurysm with the potential to compress the recurrent laryngeal nerve, embolize septic material to the lungs, or rupture. Calcification of the ductal wall is common in adults.

In patients with large shunts, heart failure can cause significant morbidity and mortality, particularly in a premature and young infant, and sudden death can occur. Progressive damage to the pulmonary vascular bed can occur in some, but it rarely occurs to an irreversible degree in the first year of life. Once irreversible damage occurs, premature death in late adolescence or early adulthood can be anticipated.

With improved technology, children without associated heart disease are noted to have a trivial amount of flow through a very small (<1 mm) patent ductus. Frequently, the shunt is too small to produce an audible murmur. The natural history of this echo-Doppler-discovered ductus arteriosus without clinical findings is unknown, but most think it is benign since cardiologists have not noted patients with endarteritis in a "silent" ductus.

MEDICAL MANAGEMENT

Interruption of flow through the PDA is the ultimate goal of management. For those in congestive heart failure, usually premature infants, medical management with digoxin and diuretics with fluid restriction may play a minor role, but the ultimate aim is closure to prevent heart failure and promote growth in infants and prevent infective endarteritis and pulmonary vascular disease in older children.

For premature infants, treatment with indomethacin is usually the first-line therapy.[94] Successful closure depends on both the dosage and the timing of treatment, although the major determinants seem to be gestational and postnatal age rather than the concentration of the drug. Because of ductal reopening, serial treatment regimens may be necessary, especially in those weighing less than 1000 g at birth. There is increasing evidence that the administration of "prophylactic" indomethacin in infants weighing less than 1000 g at birth may be associated with a higher closure rate and a better outcome.[92] Indomethacin therapy has been associated with an increased bleeding tendency resulting from platelet dysfunction, decreased urine output secondary to renal dysfunction, and necrotizing enterocolitis.[92] For the very premature with a PDA, however, a trial of indomethacin is preferable to the other options.

For premature infants who failed to close their PDA with a course of indomethacin or for term infants with a persistent PDA, closure has been recommended. If the PDA is large, there is usually a large left-to-right shunt with congestive heart failure. In these infants, the indication for closure is heart failure and usually failure to thrive. Even in the absence of these indications, when a large PDA is associated with PAH, closure is recommended to prevent PVOD. In children with a smaller PDA with an audible murmur but no evidence of significant hemodynamic embarrassment, closure usually is recommended because of the incidence of bacterial endarteritis, which over a lifetime is in the range of 30 percent. For children with a PDA without a heart murmur, which usually is discovered incidentally when an echocardiogram is performed for other reasons, the author does not currently recommend closure.

SURGICAL AND INTERVENTIONAL CATHETER CLOSURE

Surgery for a persistent PDA was first reported more than 60 years ago and is now done routinely in most centers. The safety and efficacy of this procedure even in very young children are well established, with risks that are very low (well under 1 percent), and success at interrupting flow is almost universal.

The PDA is exposed and mobilized through a small left thoracotomy in the fourth intercostal space.[95] Ductus obliteration is accomplished by division or ligation. A short, broad, or thin-walled ductus is divided between vascular clamps. The ends are closed with a continuous suture. A long, narrow, thick-walled ductus can be divided or ligated with two or three sutures spaced a few millimeters apart. The suture ligatures at each end are anchored superficially in the ductus wall to prevent migration and assure thrombosis and obliteration.

The fragile and thin-walled PDA of a premature infant is obliterated by gentle ligation with a thick suture to minimize disruption or, if small, by occlusion using metallic surgical clips. Extrapleural exposure is preferred by some surgeons. Ligation in the neonatal intensive care unit, avoiding transport to the operating room, is common. Transport from a remote intensive care unit to a cardiac surgical unit for ductus ligation on a "day-stay" basis is also efficacious.[96] Ductus obliteration offers clinical improvement in infants weighing as little as 500 g, with minimal operative risk, a reduced incidence of necrotizing enterocolitis, a reduced duration of intubation, and improvement in late survival.

Closure of a PDA in an adult requires particular caution; calcification and rigidity of the ductus wall complicate clamping. Placement of a Dacron patch over the aortic orifice of the ductus from within the aorta may be advisable.[97]

Recently, advances in less invasive surgery have been applied to the closure of a PDA using video-assisted thoracoscopic surgery. A miniaturized camera is inserted into the thorax, and through a separate tiny incision, a surgical stapler is inserted and a clip is placed across the PDA, interrupting flow. Among 230 patients, there was only 1 with minimal residual flow, 1 with persistent recurrent laryngeal nerve dysfunction, and no deaths, transfusions, or chylothoraces. The mean operating time was 20 min, and the hospital stay lasted only a couple of days.[98] At Children's Hospital in Boston, this procedure has been applied to premature infants as small as 575 g, with discharge from the hospital the day after the procedure in full-term infants and children.[99]

The PDA sometimes can be closed by interventional catheterization techniques. In 1971, Portsmann and Wierny introduced a rather complex methodology to plug a PDA by using a transarterial and transvenous approach employing very large catheters.[100] More recently, Rashkind and Cuaso introduced and others have since popularized the use of a double-umbrella device to plug a PDA,[101] but the large size of the delivery sheath of the Rashkind device makes it inapplicable to young and very small children. Gianturco coils—thin metallic wires glossed with Dacron that assume a coil configuration when released from a catheter—have become an attractive alternative (Fig. 63-18). They can be delivered through relatively small catheters and have been found to be quite effective, although their utility is limited in those <8 months of age with PDAs that are more than 3.5 or 4.0 mm at the narrowest point.[102] In the others using these coils, the results have been very promising, with a 90 percent success rate.

With several highly successful, low-risk, inexpensive, and minimally traumatic procedures available to close a persistent PDA in a neonate, child, adolescent, or adult without pulmonary vascular disease, local experience is likely to be the best guide to which option is preferable in an individual child.

Sinus of Valsalva Fistula

PATHOLOGY

Sinus of Valsalva fistula is uncommon; it also is referred to as *aortic sinus aneurysm* (see also Chap. 88). Because of an assumed intrinsic weakness at the union of the aorta with the heart, the aortic media may separate from the aortic annulus and retract upward. The structure that lies between becomes aneurysmal and may rupture to form a fistula. The usual sites of the defects are the posterior (noncoronary) sinus aneurysms that rupture through the atrial septal wall into the right atrium (Fig. 63-19*A*) and those of the right sinus that rupture into the right ventricular infundibulum (Fig. 63-19*B*).[103] The aneurysm is represented by a colored pouch with multiple perforations in the wall. The principal associated condition is a supracristal VSD in cases with aneurysms of the right sinus (about 50 percent).

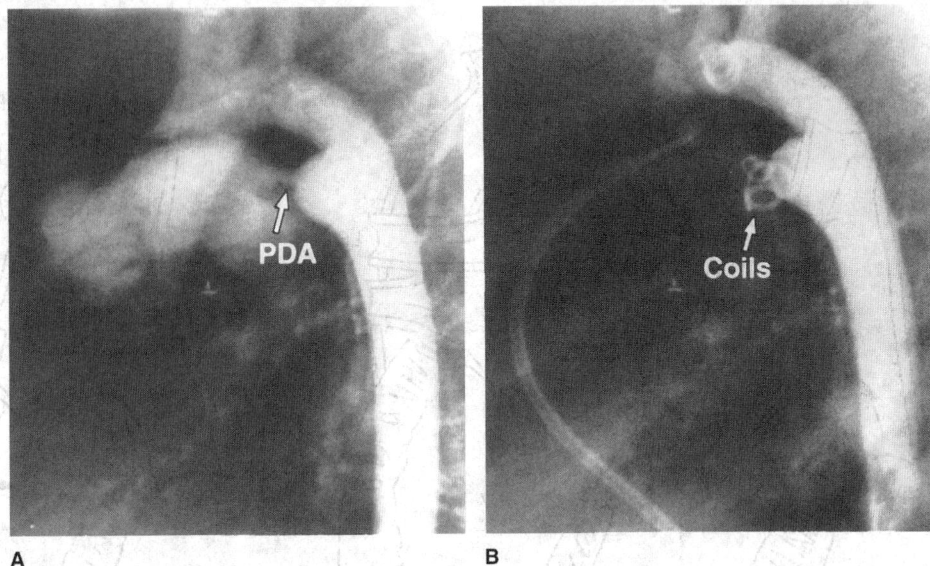

FIGURE 63-18 Lateral angiogram showing coil occlusion of a patent ductus arteriosus. *A*. Small PDA allows shunting from descending aorta to pulmonary artery. *B*. Shunting is eliminated by a coil placed in the ductus arteriosus. (Courtesy of John F. Keane, MD.)

CLINICAL MANIFESTATIONS

Sinus of Valsalva fistulas are most common in adults.[104] When the rupture is secondary to bacterial endocarditis, evidence of a preceding infection is found. If the rupture occurs slowly, a small fistulous tract into the right atrium or ventricle develops and presents recent-onset findings of a small left-to-right shunt. With sudden rupture, there is usually a tearing pain in the midchest associated with the dramatically rapid development of pulmonary congestion caused by the sudden onset of a large shunt. Characteristically, the murmur is loud and continuous but is heard lower on the chest than is the murmur of PDA. A to-and-fro murmur rather than a continuous one may be heard at times. The apex impulse is hyperdynamic, and the pulse pressure is widened. VSD may complicate the clinical picture. Cardiac catheterization will confirm the level of the shunt. A pressure difference across the right ventricular outflow tract may be present if the right sinus is involved. Aortography or Doppler echocardiography[105] will confirm the diagnosis.

NATURAL HISTORY AND PROGNOSIS

With slow rupture and a small shunt, the major risk is infective endocarditis or extension of the rupture with an increasing shunt. With a large shunt, the heart failure is usually rapidly progressive and may result in death very quickly. A few patients seem to stabilize in this situation.

MEDICAL MANAGEMENT

Appropriate cultures should be drawn and antibiotics should be begun if endocarditis is suspected. Treatment of heart failure should be instituted rapidly. *Because of the natural history, all patients should have this condition corrected surgically.*

SURGICAL MANAGEMENT

Aneurysms or fistulas from the noncoronary or right coronary sinuses are repaired through the aortic root while the patient is supported on total cardiopulmonary bypass with moderate hypothermia, using techniques similar to those employed for aortic valve replacement. The aortic valve leaflets, the margins of the aneurysm, and the coronary arterial orifices must be visualized precisely. Aneurysms of the noncoronary sinus can be repaired through the right atrium; those arising from the right coronary sinus are accessible through the right ventricle. In most cases, the orifice of the aneurysmal fistula is surgically obliterated, using a Dacron patch. In a recent series of 129 patients, reparative methods included plication (47 percent), patch repair (40 percent), and aortic root replacement (12 percent). Sixty percent of those patients needed aortic valve replacement at the same time.[104]

A conal, or supracristal (type I), VSD must be sought and closed through either the aortic valve or the right ventricular outflow tract when an aneurysm of the right coronary sinus extends into the right ventricle.

Surgical results are usually quite good. In the large series cited above, the operative survival was 96 percent with no late deaths in an average of 5.9 years of follow-up.[104]

VALVULAR AND VASCULAR MALFORMATIONS OF THE LEFT SIDE OF THE HEART WITH RIGHT-TO-LEFT, BIDIRECTIONAL, OR NO SHUNT

Coarctation of the Aorta

PATHOLOGY

Coarctation of the aorta is a discrete narrowing of the distal segment of the aortic arch. The characteristic lesion is a deformity of the media of the aorta that involves the anterior, supe-

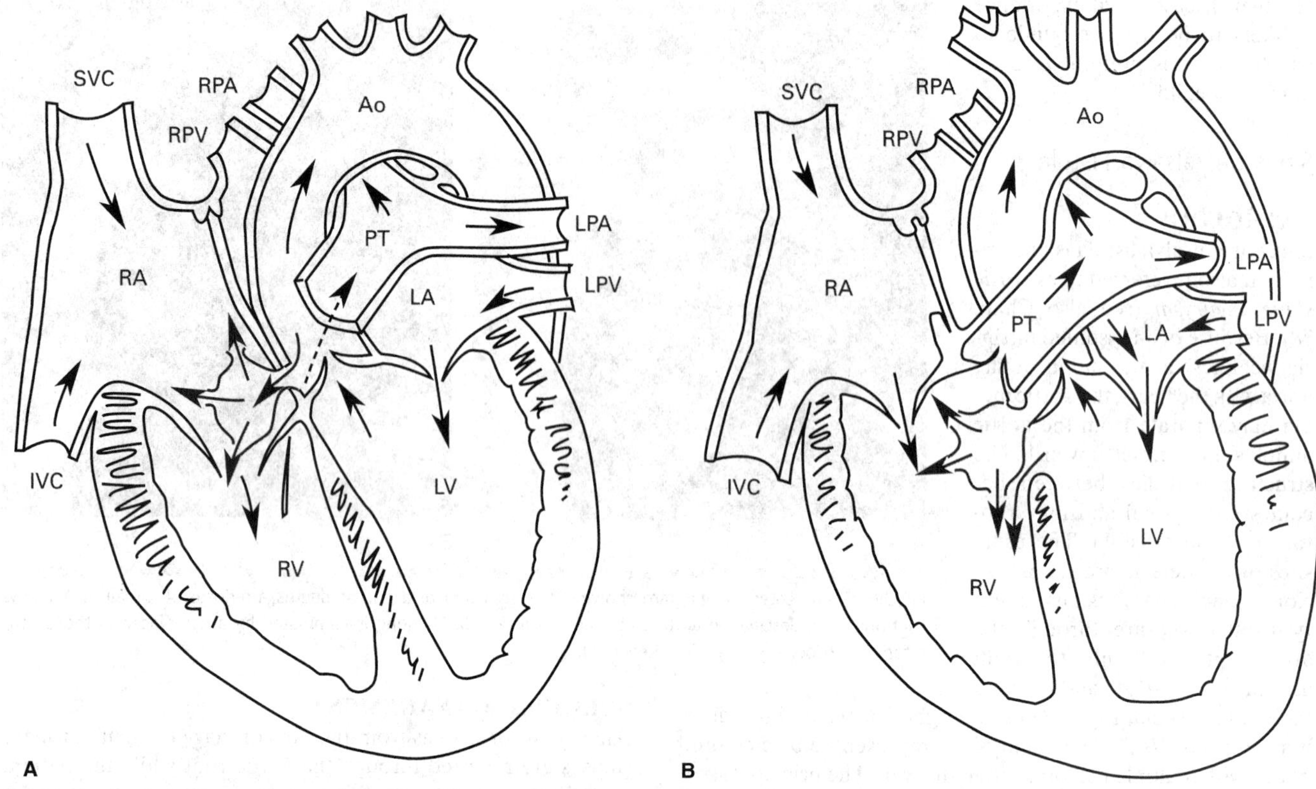

FIGURE 63-19 Sinus of Valsalva fistula. *A.* Aneurysm involves the posterior sinus and ruptures into the right atrium. *B.* Aneurysm involves the right aortic sinus and ruptures into the right ventricle. A ventricular septal defect is commonly associated, as illustrated. SVC = superior vena cava; IVC = inferior vena cava; RA = right atrium; RV = right ventricle; PT = main pulmonary arterial trunk; RPA = right pulmonary artery; LPA = left pulmonary artery; RPV = right pulmonary vein; LPV = left pulmonary vein; LA = left atrium; LV = left ventricle; Ao = aorta. (From Edwards JE.[66] Reproduced with permission from the publisher and author.)

rior, and posterior walls and is represented by a curtain-like infolding of the wall that causes the lumen to be narrowed and eccentric[106] (see Chap. 88).

In infants, the lesion lies either opposite the ductus or in a preductal location. In adolescents and adults, it is usually at the ligamentum arteriosum. An aberrant right subclavian artery may be associated. In rare cases, the narrowing lies proximal to the origin of the left common carotid artery or involves a segment of the abdominal aorta.

The principal cardiac abnormality is left ventricular hypertrophy. In some infants, left ventricular endocardial fibroelastosis may be associated. Tubular hypoplasia of the distal aortic arch and isthmus is very common, especially with associated cardiac abnormalities involving left heart obstruction.[107] The proximal aorta may show a moderate degree of cystic medial necrosis. Beyond the coarctation, the lining may show a localized jet lesion.

Prominent collaterals are characteristic in older infants, children, and adolescents. They may be divided into anterior and posterior systems, with the anterior system originating with the internal mammary arteries and making use of the epigastric arteries in the abdominal wall to supply the lower extremities. The posterior system involves parascapular arteries connected with the posterior intercostal arteries and carries blood to the distal aortic compartment principally for supply of the abdominal viscera. The anterior spinal artery, receiving branches from the proximal and distal compartments of the aorta, is also dilated and tortuous.

ASSOCIATED CONDITIONS

The most commonly associated defects are tubular hypoplasia of the aortic arch, PDA, VSD, and aortic stenosis (valvular and/or subvalvular). A bicuspid aortic valve is present in 46 percent of autopsy cases.[106]

ABNORMAL PHYSIOLOGY

In most instances, both the systolic and diastolic arterial pressures above the coarctation are elevated above normal levels. Below the coarctation, the systolic pressure is lower than that in the upper extremities, and the diastolic pressure is usually near or only slightly below the normal range. The mechanism of upper extremity hypertension appears to involve the increased resistance to aortic flow produced by the coarctation itself, the decreased capacity and distensibility of the vessels into which the left ventricle ejects, and humoral factors.[108]

CLINICAL MANIFESTATIONS

Coarctation of the aorta occurs in approximately 4 percent of all infants and children with congenital heart disease and is the predominant lesion in approximately 8 percent of infants presenting with critical heart disease in the first year of life. It ranks behind only VSD, dextrotransposition of the great arteries, and tetralogy of Fallot.[3] Among all individuals born with coarctation, approximately half present within the first month or two of life with heart failure. About 50 percent of infants so admitted have uncomplicated coarctation; the remaining half can be expected to have at least one complicating cardiac abnormality. VSD is the most common (64 percent), followed by left ventricular outflow tract obstruction (31 percent).[109] The timing of ductal tissue constriction in terms of both ductal closure and perhaps aortic constriction appears to play a decisive role in the onset or worsening of symptoms in most of these patients. The male/female ratio is approximately 3:1 for isolated coarctation but is only 1.1:1 for complicated coarctation. Approximately 45 percent of children with Turner's syndrome have coarctation.

History The clinical picture in a symptomatic infant is one of dyspnea, difficulty in feeding, and poor weight gain. Older children are for the most part asymptomatic, although a few complain of mild fatigue, dyspnea, or symptoms of claudication in the legs when running.

Physical Examination In a symptomatic infant, signs of congestive heart failure are characteristic. A gallop rhythm is common, and a murmur from associated defects or from the coarctation itself (posteriorly in the interscapular area) may be heard. Frequently, these murmurs are either inaudible or nondescript on admission and become characteristic only when congestive failure is brought under control. Prominent arterial pulsations may be visible in the suprasternal notch and carotid arteries, and the left ventricular impulse is forceful. An early systolic ejection click at the apex suggests the presence of a bicuspid aortic valve. The murmur from the coarctation is medium-pitched, systolic, and blowing in quality. It is best heard posteriorly in the interscapular area, usually with some degree of radiation to the left axilla, apex, and anterior precordium. Low-pitched, continuous murmurs of collateral circulation may be heard over the chest wall, particularly posteriorly, but seldom before adolescence. A short middiastolic rumble at the apex without clinical evidence of mitral disease is relatively common.

The characteristic systolic blood pressure difference between the upper and lower extremities may be difficult to appreciate or measure in infants with severe congestive failure or with a large VSD or PDA. With improved compensation, pulses in the upper extremities become readily palpable. The femoral pulses remain weak, delayed, or absent. In these very young infants, it is important that the pulses in both brachial and carotid arteries be assessed. Weak or absent pulses in all sites are more characteristic of critical aortic stenosis or aortic atresia.

In older children and adults, the radial arterial pulses typically are strong; those in the femoral arteries are diminished, delayed, or absent. A repeatedly measured systolic or mean pressure difference between the upper and lower extremities greater than 10 mmHg is diagnostic. The pulse pressure in the leg is reduced, and in some patients no pressure can be measured by auscultation or Doppler. Approximately one-third of older children have mild to severe hypertension, with severe hypertension defined as a systolic pressure above 150 mmHg, a diastolic pressure above 100 mmHg, or both. Some patients have only a mild pressure difference between the arms and the legs at rest but a much larger difference during treadmill exercise. A systolic pressure difference between the two arms suggests that the origin of one subclavian artery is at or below the obstruction, e.g., aberrent right subclavian from the descending aorta.

In light of the simplicity of measuring blood pressure in the upper and lower extremities of children and the importance of early detection, it is surprising and disappointing that approximately 95 percent of children and adolescents with coarctation are referred by pediatricians and other health care providers to a pediatric cardiologist for evaluation of a heart murmur and/or hypertension without this serious underlying malformation being recognized.[110]

Chest Roentgenogram For a symptomatic infant, the pattern is one of impressive cardiac enlargement and venous congestion. In an older and asymptomatic child, the heart size is generally at the upper limits of normal with a left ventricular prominence. A figure-three configuration of the left margin of the aorta at the level of the coarctation may be seen in overpenetrated films, with the upper curve formed by the slightly dilated aorta just above the coarctation, the central indentation by the coarctation itself, and the lower curve by the poststenotic dilatation below the coarctation. Notching of the inferior margin of the ribs by tortuous intercostal arteries acting as collaterals is seldom present before 7 or 8 years of age.

Electrocardiogram The ECG of a symptomatic infant reflects right or biventricular hypertrophy during the first 3 months of life. T-wave inversion in the left precordial leads is common. In older children, the ECG is usually normal or may indicate mild left ventricular and left atrial hypertrophy.

Echocardiogram Two-dimensional echocardiographic imaging of the aortic arch from the suprasternal notch permits visualization of the coarctation and detection of anatomic variations such as isthmic or transverse arch hypoplasia. The precordial and subxiphoid views are of great value in assessing the presence and severity of associated defects. Doppler flow studies are helpful for diagnostic confirmation. In infants with heart failure, left ventricular dilation and decreased contractility are common. The severity of the coarctation can be evaluated by Doppler gradients and the diminished pulsatile flow in the abdominal aorta.

Cardiac Catheterization Study of symptomatic infants characteristically reveals left atrial and left ventricular hypertension and a significant systolic pressure difference between the left ventricle and the femoral artery, particularly if the coarctation is isolated. In the presence of a large VSD and PDA, the left ventricular hypertension and the systolic pressure difference between the left ventricle and the femoral artery are less impressive and may not exist at all. Every attempt should be made to define the nature and severity of associated defects. Imaging is recommended in older children to demonstrate the exact site and length of the coarctation as well as to show unusual features of the collateral circulation that may be of importance to the surgeon. Magnetic resonance imaging is an excellent and in most instances preferable alternative to angiography today for demonstrating the site and length of the coarctation (Fig. 63-20).

NATURAL HISTORY AND PROGNOSIS

Approximately one-half of infants admitted with heart failure within the first weeks of life have coarctation without significant

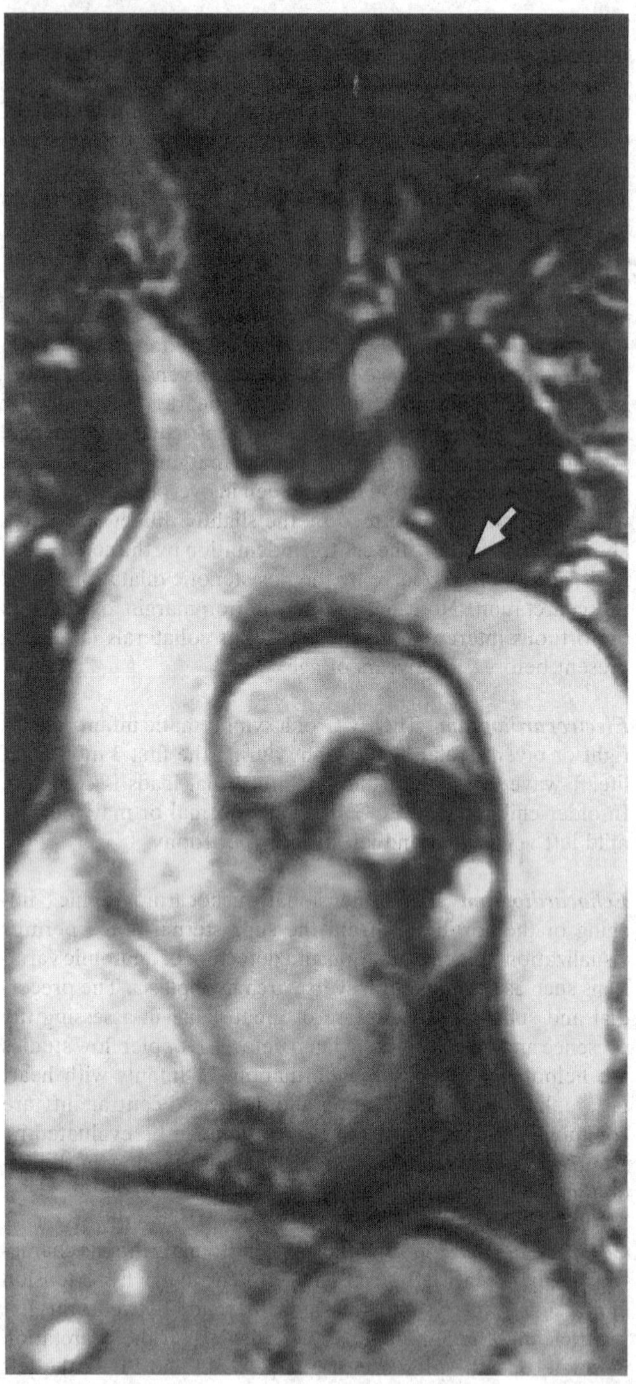

FIGURE 63-20 Selected frame from magnetic resonance angiogram in a child with discrete coarctation (*arrow*) distal to an enlarged left subclavian artery. (Courtesy of Andrew Powell, MD.)

associated defects.[109] The majority of these infants respond well to medical management and, if no repair is performed, reach a stage at 2 or 3 years of age where they are indistinguishable from asymptomatic children of the same age whose coarctation is first detected during a routine physical examination. Upper extremity hypertension usually increases during the first several months of life and then tends to diminish again as collateral circulation improves, while signs of failure diminish at the same time. For infants with severe failure and any serious associated defects, balloon dilation or surgery provides virtually the only chance of survival.

The consequences of persistent hypertension in an individual who has not undergone surgery appear in the second and third decades in the form of severe hypertension, aortic rupture, or intracranial hemorrhage from an aneurysm of the circle of Willis. Congestive heart failure that often is complicated by mitral or aortic valve disease, a dissecting aneurysm of the aorta, or atherosclerosis is seen in the fourth decade. The risk of endocarditis on the aortic or mitral valves or endarteritis at the site of coarctation appears to be spread relatively evenly over the years. The average age of death of patients who survive childhood with coarctation without surgery is 34 years.[111]

MEDICAL MANAGEMENT

Vigorous medical treatment is indicated for infants with severe heart failure. A newborn with severe failure may experience dramatic relief from the intravenous infusion of PGE_1 to reopen the closing ductus.[91] Prompt correction of the coarctation is recommended for all infants in whom there are one or more associated defects and for all infants with isolated coarctation unless the response to medical management has been dramatic and sustained.

The timing and type of correction of isolated discrete coarctation of the aorta remain a topic of some dispute. There is general agreement that all children with congestive heart failure should be repaired after a brief period of stabilization and treatment of the failure. Since heart failure usually is limited to infants in the first few months of life and since balloon dilation of native coarctation in children under 6 months of age has had an unacceptable restenosis rate of up to 75 percent,[112] virtually all physicians would consider surgical repair the favored approach. For infants and children without congestive heart failure, the timing has been somewhat more problematic. Historically, the preferred approach was waiting until age 1 to 4 to avoid the problem of recoarctation that was found occasionally among patients corrected before 1 year of age[113] and residual or recurrent hypertension among patients without demonstrable recurrent coarctation, renal disease, or significant aortic regurgitation, which appears to be related to the duration of hypertension before surgery. More recently, the ability to reduce the restenosis rate has led some centers to reduce the age of elective surgical repair of coarctation to 3 to 6 months. For those in whom balloon dilation is contemplated, waiting until age 1 to 4 still seems appropriate.

Although there is general agreement that symptomatic children under 6 months of age with coarctation ought to be repaired surgically and that the first approach to those who develop restenosis at virtually any age should be balloon dilation or stent placement, the proper therapy for the treatment of native coarctation in children older than 1 year of age remains somewhat controversial. For balloon dilation, immediate success (defined as an increase in the coarctation diameter with a residual gradient of less than 20 mmHg) occurs in 80 to 95 percent of patients who are dilated, with the gradient reduction averaging 75 percent. However, long-term gradient relief after angioplasty has been somewhat less than that with surgery. Restenosis rates in the intermediate term seem to be directly related to the age at dilation, with 85 percent of neonates, 35 percent of infants, and 10 percent of children over 2 years of age developing restenosis.[112] Repeat dilation is almost invariably successful, and many advocate this approach even if it requires two dilations rather than a one-step surgical approach. Occasionally in older children a stent can be placed if the balloon dilation fails to persistently increase the luminal diameter (Fig. 63-21). In selected older children and adults, this has been very successful, with an average reduction in the gradient from 25 to 5 mm in 32 patients at Children's Hospital in Boston.[114] Complications usually have been related to associated diseases, although aneurysms, usually small, at the site of dilation have been reported in about 5 percent of cases. Large catheters are necessary, and trauma to the femoral artery is not uncommon.

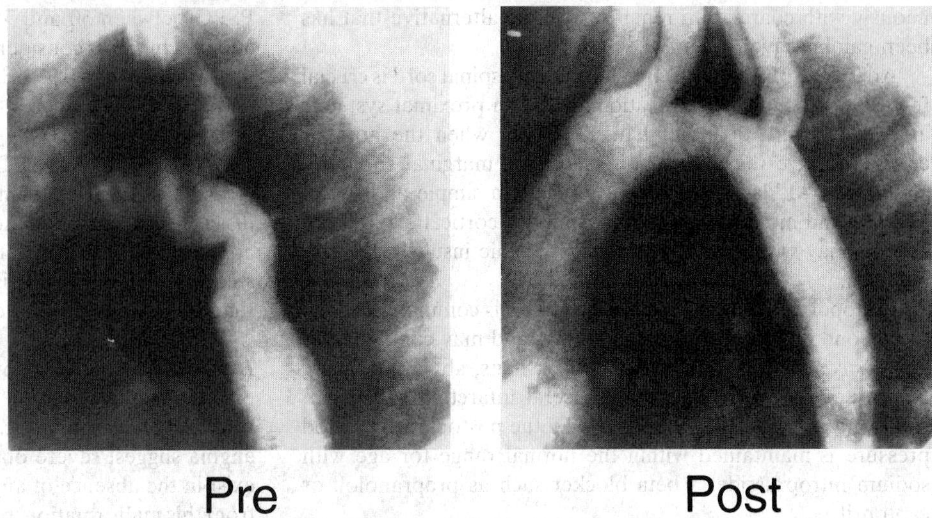

FIGURE 63-21 Repair of coarctation with a stent. *Left panel:* coarctation caused by kink with anterior indentation. *Right panel:* narrowing eliminated with stent. (Courtesy of Audrey Marshall, MD.)

Patients who have repaired coarctation need to be followed indefinitely. For those with significant recoarctation, expressed as a systolic pressure gradient between the upper and lower extremities of 20 mm or more at rest, balloon angioplasty and/or stent placement are recommended. Repeat surgery for recurrent coarctation is rarely necessary. Occasionally, patients are seen who have insignificant or small resting gradients but manifest abnormal upper extremity hypertension and significant gradients with exercise.[109] These patients probably should undergo balloon angioplasty and stent replacement with pharmacologic control of their hypertension if it is present at rest and beta blockade if the hypertension becomes significant with exercise.

SURGICAL MANAGEMENT

The coarctation is exposed and mobilized through a left posterolateral thoracotomy. It is usually possible to resect the narrow segment and restore continuity with a direct end-to-end anastomosis (Fig. 63-22). When the narrowed segment is longer, repair by subclavian flap aortoplasty or rarely a tubular vascular prosthesis to bridge the gap between the two ends of the aorta may be necessary. In adults with a relatively nonelastic or calcified aorta, a tubular vascular prosthesis can be used to bypass the unresected coarctation or the previous repair. Dacron patch repair of coarctation has an unacceptably high incidence of late aneurysm formation and is no longer advised.[115] Tension-free suture lines are essential. Postoperative bleeding, chylothorax, paraplegia, and injury to the phrenic and recurrent laryngeal nerves remain potential complications.[116]

If a significant VSD is also present, a pulmonary arterial band is placed at the time of coarctation repair during infancy. The VSD then may be repaired electively during the next several months, when the child's congestive heart failure is well controlled. Primary repair of the VSD shortly after or simulta-

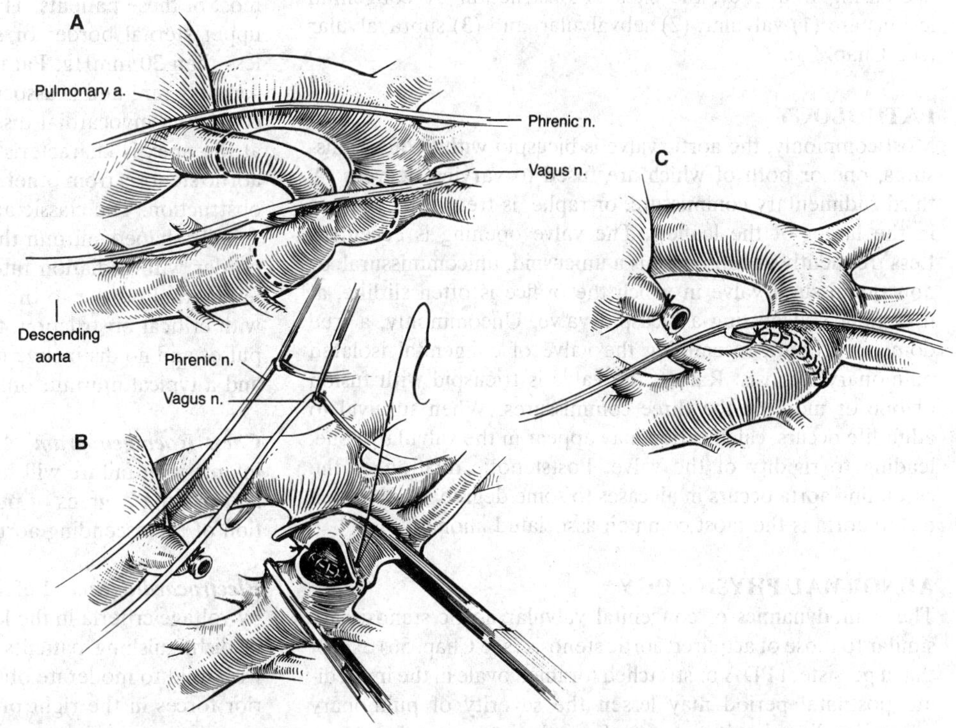

FIGURE 63-22 Repair of coarctation surgically. *A.* Discrete aortic coarctation in an infant with a small ductus arteriosus seen via left thoracotomy exposure. *B.* Repair technique using resection with end-to-end anastomosis. C. Complete repair. (From Castaneda AR, Jonas RA, Mayer JE Jr, Hanley FL. *Cardiac Surgery of the Neonate and Infant.* Philadelphia: Saunders; 1994: 333. Reproduced with permission from the publisher and author.)

neously with coarctation repair is a viable alternative that has been gaining favor recently.[117]

Adequacy of collateral circulation to the spinal cord is crucial for the safe repair of coarctation. A rise in proximal systemic arterial pressure of more than 20 mmHg when the aorta is clamped above the coarctation suggests a marginal collateral circulation. Mild systemic hypothermia is a simple and useful adjunct, and monitoring of somatosensory cortical evoked potentials may warn of an impending ischemic insult to the spinal cord.[118]

Postoperative paradoxical hypertension is common between the second and fifth postoperative days and may contribute to the *postcoarctation syndrome*, in which ileus, abdominal pain, mesenteric vasculitis, and even visceral infarction can occur. This syndrome rarely is encountered if the postoperative blood pressure is maintained within the normal range for age with sodium nitroprusside, a beta blocker such as propranolol, or captopril.

Operative mortality for infants with isolated coarctation is in the range of 0 to 3 percent [113,116,117] but is 10 percent or higher when other cardiovascular defects are present. Subsequent deaths are uncommon in surviving infants with isolated coarctation but are more likely in those with complicated associated defects.

Valvular Aortic Stenosis

DEFINITION

Aortic stenosis is defined as subtotal obstruction of varying severity in the channel of left ventricular outflow. In order of decreasing frequency, the sites of obstruction by congenital lesions are (1) valvular, (2) subvalvular, and (3) supravalvular (see Chap. 56).

PATHOLOGY

Most commonly, the aortic valve is bicuspid with two commissures, one or both of which are fused to varying degrees. A third rudimentary commissure, or raphe, is frequently present in the larger of the leaflets. The valve opening is eccentric. Less frequently encountered is a unicuspid, unicommissural, or noncommissural valve in which the orifice is often slitlike, at first glance suggesting a bicuspid valve. Uncommonly, a true dome is present, resembling the valve of congenital isolated pulmonary stenosis. Rarely, the valve is tricuspid with fusion of one or more of the three commissures. When survival to adult life occurs, calcification may appear in the valvular tissue, leading to rigidity of the valve. Poststenotic dilation of the ascending aorta occurs in all cases to some degree. Coarctation of the aorta is the most common associated anomaly.

ABNORMAL PHYSIOLOGY

The hemodynamics of congenital valvular aortic stenosis are similar to those of acquired aortic stenosis (see Chap. 56) except that a persistent PDA or stretched foramen ovale in the immediate postnatal period may lessen the severity of pulmonary edema by diverting blood away from the left ventricle.

Severity usually is judged by the peak systolic pressure gradient (PSPG) across the aortic valve, which is determined at cardiac catheterization, and the calculated aortic valve area. In the presence of a normal cardiac output, a PSPG $\geq$75 mmHg or an aortic valve area <0.5 cm^2/m^2 is considered severe, a PSPG between 50 and 75 mmHg or a valve area between 0.5 and 0.8 cm^2/m^2 is considered moderate, and a PSPG <50 mmHg or a valve area >0.9 cm^2/m^2 is considered mild (see Chaps. 15 and 56).

CLINICAL MANIFESTATIONS

About 7 percent of infants and children with congenital heart disease have aortic stenosis in one of its several forms, and approximately 80 percent of these patients have valvular aortic stenosis. Valvular stenosis is much more common among males than females, with a ratio of 4:1.

History The detection of a systolic murmur leads to the discovery of this malformation in most patients, the vast majority of whom are asymptomatic. Easy fatigue, dyspnea, syncope, and angina suggest severe obstruction, but severe obstruction may exist in the absence of any symptoms. Sudden death may occur from this malformation, but in most such cases death is preceded by either symptoms or ECG changes. Infants with critical stenosis from birth present with congestive failure within the first week or two of life and represent true emergencies. A similar small number of patients with less critical but still very severe obstruction are detected over the course of the next 4 to 6 months.

Physical Examination The arterial blood pressure and the quality of the peripheral arterial pulses of older infants and children are usually normal. A measured pulse pressure <20 mmHg suggests severe stenosis. The cardiac apex impulse may be forceful and sustained, and a systolic thrill along the right upper sternal border and over the carotid arteries is present in most of these patients. The absence of such a thrill at the right upper sternal border or suprasternal notch suggests a PSPG less than 30 mmHg. Paradoxical splitting of the second heart sound is rare and is associated with very severe obstruction or coexisting myocardial disease. An early systolic ejection click at the apex is characteristic and serves to distinguish valvular aortic stenosis from other forms of left ventricular outflow tract obstruction. The classic auscultatory finding is a harsh systolic spindle-shaped murmur that is loudest at the right upper sternal border with radiation into the carotid arteries and down the left sternal border to the apex (see Chap. 56). Among infants with critical obstruction, there may be no palpable peripheral pulses and no distinctive murmur, with a return of weak pulses and a typical murmur only after decongestive therapy.

Chest Roentgenogram The overall heart size is normal, but infants with failure will have generalized cardiac enlargement and varying degrees of pulmonary edema. Poststenotic dilatation of the ascending aorta is characteristic.

Electrocardiogram Left ventricular hypertrophy, as indicated by voltage criteria in the left precordial leads, is seldom helpful in distinguishing patients with severe obstruction from those with mild to moderate obstruction. However, diminished anterior forces in the right precordial leads and a deep $SV_1 \geq 30$ mm suggest severe stenosis, as does absence of the Q wave in V_6. Fifty percent of patients with severe obstruction have a flat, biphasic, or inverted T wave in V_6 (Fig. 63-23). Severe and even critical obstruction may be present with none of the ECG abnormalities mentioned above. Monitoring of the ST segment in leads V_5 through V_7 during cautious exercise testing appears to be a reliable method of detecting children in whom a significant PSPG (>50 mmHg) has developed and in whom that gradient may represent a threat of sudden death.[119] Symptomatic infants may show right, left, or biventricular hypertrophy, frequently with T-wave inversion over the left precordium.

Echocardiogram Continuous-wave Doppler echocardiography guided by two-dimensional echocardiographic imaging predicts very accurately the peak and mean instantaneous systolic pressure gradient across discrete forms of left ventricular outflow tract obstruction (see Chap. 13) (Fig. 63-24). Two-dimensional echocardiography can distinguish valvular from supravalvular or subvalvular obstruction and identify critically ill infants in whom the size of the left ventricle, mitral valve annulus, or aortic root is hypoplastic to a degree that would preclude survival.[120,121]

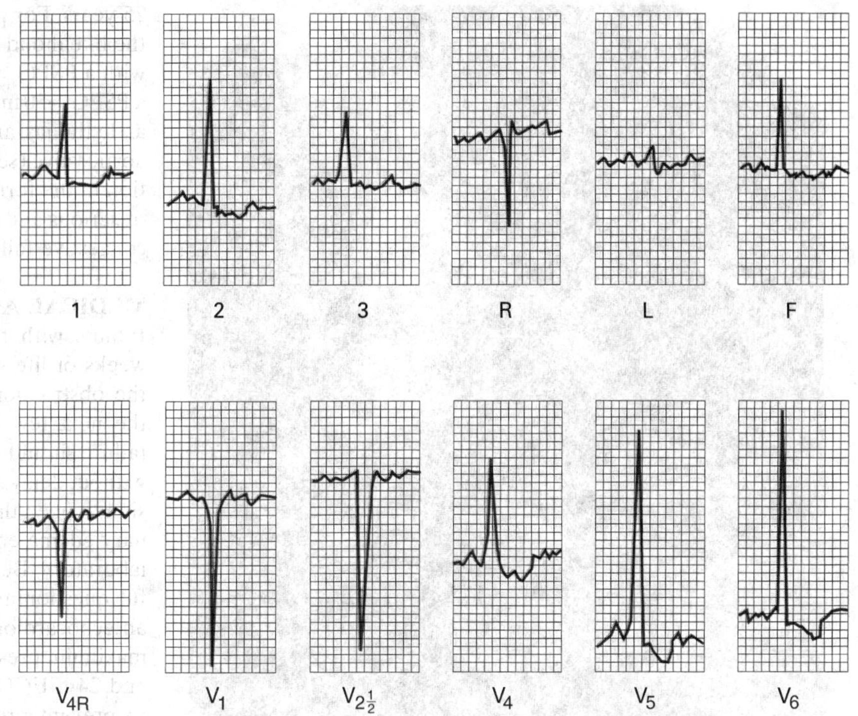

FIGURE 63-23 Electrocardiogram from an 8-year-old boy with valvular aortic stenosis and a 94-mmHg peak systolic pressure gradient. The small anterior QRS forces, abnormally large posterior forces, absent Q waves in leads V_5 and V_6, and abnormal T waves and ST segments reflect severe left ventricular systolic pressure overload with ischemia.

Cardiac Catheterization Infants symptomatic with severe aortic obstruction often have a left-to-right shunt through a stretched foramen ovale, PAH, and a right-to-left shunt through a PDA. A marked increase in left ventricular end-diastolic pressure is usually present. The PSPG between the left ventricle and the central aorta should be documented whenever possible. If left ventricular output is markedly diminished, this gradient may be relatively small even in the presence of severe obstruction. Left ventricular angiography will confirm the site of obstruction and outline the size of the left ventricular cavity (Fig. 63-25*A*).

In older infants and children, pressures on the right side of the heart are usually normal. Simultaneous recording of central aortic and left ventricular pressures or a pressure tracing upon catheter withdrawal from the left ventricle to the aorta, coupled with an accurate estimate of cardiac output, is necessary for reliable assessment of severity. Left ventricular angiography will document the site of obstruction. The aortic leaflets typically are thickened and domed, with a central or eccentric jet of contrast material entering the ascending aorta. Poststenotic dilatation is characteristic. Supravalvular aortography is recommended to assess the presence and severity of aortic regurgitation.

NATURAL HISTORY AND PROGNOSIS

About half the infants born with severe valvular aortic stenosis are symptomatic enough to require hospitalization within the first week of life. Not uncommonly, the murmur is mistaken for that of a VSD. Congestive heart failure beyond infancy and before adolescence usually is not seen without the presence of complicating factors. Symptomatic infants require prompt relief of obstruction by balloon or surgical valvotomy, but the mortality rate remains significant. Endocardial fibroelastosis, papillary muscle necrosis, associated intra- and extracardiac deformities, and a small left ventricular cavity contribute to this mortality rate. Survivors may have significant aortic regurgitation, but the majority can be managed medically until valve replacement is feasible.

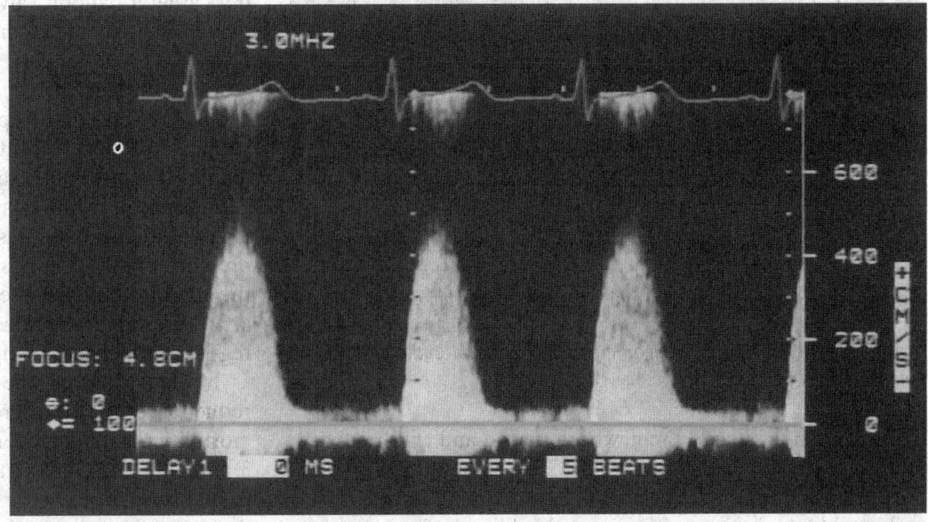

FIGURE 63-24 Doppler interrogation in the ascending aorta in a patient with valvar aortic stenosis. The peak velocity of 4.8 m/s correlates with a maximum instantaneous gradient of 92 mmHg across the aortic valve.

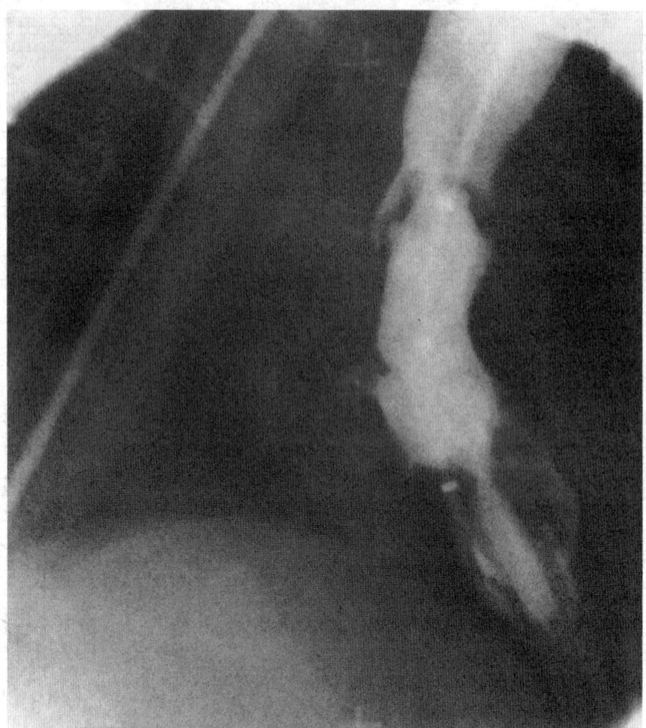

A

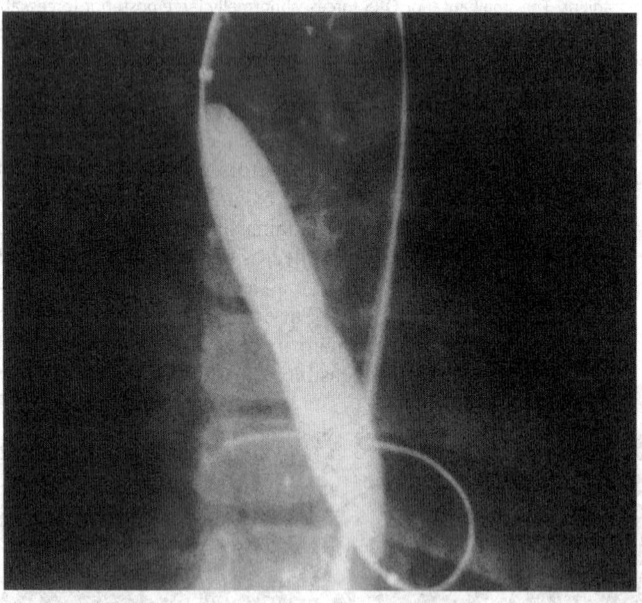

B

FIGURE 63-25 Balloon aortic valvuloplasty. *A.* Left ventricular angiogram showing a domed, thickened aortic valve with fusion of the right and left commissures. *B.* Balloon dilation using a retrograde technique. A waist is demonstrated in the midportion of the balloon before full inflation. (From Lock JE, Keane JF, Perry SB. *Diagnostic and Interventional Catheterization in Congenital Heart Disease.* Boston: Kluwer; 2000: 151.)

Most infants beyond the newborn period and children with mild aortic valvular stenosis (PSPG at catheterization <25 mmHg or a Doppler mean pressure gradient <25 mmHg) remain stable, with only a 21 percent likelihood of progression in severity and the need for intervention within the subsequent 25 years. For patients with a PSPG between 25 and 49 mmHg, the likelihood of significant progression rises to 41 percent, and with a PSPG >50 mmHg, it rises to 71 percent.[122] Patients with a PSPG >50 mmHg are judged to be at risk of serious ventricular arrhythmias and sudden death. Infective endocarditis on the aortic valve (see Chap. 73) poses an extremely serious complication in the form of systemic arterial emboli and the production of serious and sometimes catastrophic aortic regurgitation with congestive failure, shock, and death.[60]

MEDICAL AND SURGICAL MANAGEMENT

Infants with the characteristic murmur detected in the first weeks of life should be evaluated very carefully to be certain the obstruction is not severe and does not become severe in the next few weeks or months.[123] Those who develop heart failure should be operated on or undergo balloon valvuloplasty without delay. In a critically ill neonate, intravenous PGE_1 infusion to open the ductus may provide temporary relief of pulmonary edema en route to the operating room or catheterization laboratory. Beyond infancy, a plan of reexamination with careful questioning regarding symptoms and an ECG each year, an echocardiogram with Doppler assessment of the mean and maximum pressure gradient every year or two, exercise testing, and 24-h ECG monitoring about every 3 years should suffice to prevent progression from going unrecognized. Indications for cardiac catheterization for gradient assessment and possible balloon dilation include the appearance of symptoms or syncope, decreased anterior forces with an SV_1 ≥30 mm or flattening or inversion of the T wave in V_6 in the resting ECG, abnormal ST-T segments on exercise testing, or an estimated maximum instantaneous gradient of 65 mmHg or a mean pressure gradient >60 mmHg by echocardiographic Doppler techniques.

Transluminal catheter balloon valvuloplasty has become the acceptable alternative to surgery. In skilled hands, it can provide effective reduction of the transvalvular gradient while producing only a mild increment in aortic regurgitation in most instances.[124,125] Elective balloon dilation is recommended if the PSPG is >50 mmHg at catheterization and aortic regurgitation is mild or nonexistent. For a neonate with critical valvular obstruction, some centers continue to rely on surgical intervention, but catheter balloon valvuloplasty has become a very competitive alternative and in the author's institution is the procedure of choice for these very sick infants.

Balloon dilation has been performed since the mid-1980s, and long-term follow-up studies are not yet available. Early studies and more recent experience suggest that the balloon diameter should not exceed that of the valve ring, and most centers now use balloons that are 85 to 90 percent of the diameter of the aortic annulus. The balloon usually is inflated to a pressure of 4 to 6 atmospheres until the "waist" produced by the stenotic valve has been abolished (Fig. 63-25*B*). Transient arrythmias are seen occasionally, but other than creating aortic regurgitation, other complications are uncommon.

In older children, the results are usually quite good, with a reduction of the peak gradient of approximately 60 percent, a mortality rate under 2 percent, and a complication rate of about 3 percent.[124,125] In neonates, the results are more problematic, probably because of severity of disease, unstable conditions, and the size of the patient, with 12 percent early and late mortality in one series. In this center, reintervention (usually repeat balloon dilation) was necessary in 40 percent with a mean follow-up of 4.3 years.[126]

When surgical intervention is required for critical aortic stenosis during infancy, the heart is exposed through a median sternotomy and the aortic valve is visualized through the ascending aorta during a brief period of low-flow perfusion with mild hypothermia. Standard cardiopulmonary bypass, mild hypothermia, and cardioplegia are used in older children.[127] The surgeon must discriminate between true commissures and abnormal raphes because incision of the latter produces intolerable aortic valvular regurgitation. Relief of valvular stenosis is accomplished with a carefully placed incision in the middle of each fused but well-supported true commissure.

A conservative attitude is essential during operation for aortic stenosis in an infant or small child. Mild valvular regurgitation almost always occurs consequent to commissurotomy but is usually well tolerated. Moderate residual stenosis is preferred to intolerable aortic valvular regurgitation, especially in infants in whom valve implantation is technically difficult. If valve replacement is necessary in an infant or small child, use of the autograft pulmonary valve in the aortic position offers the attractive possibility of continuing growth of this neoaortic valve that may parallel that of the patient.[128]

The risk of operation is high in critically ill infants, in the range of 10 to 15 percent, particularly in those with a low ejection fraction, high left ventricular end-diastolic pressure, endocardial fibroelastosis, marked congestive failure, or features of left ventricular hypoplasia.[129] Morbidity after aortic valvotomy in an older child is rare, and the likelihood of relief of left ventricular outflow tract obstruction and survival is good. The Natural History Study of Congenital Heart Defects, reporting on 133 children undergoing aortic commissurotomy after age 2 years, found that only 27 percent required a second operation in the subsequent 20 years, with 78 percent of those operations consisting of valve replacement. Aortic regurgitation was the indication for operation in 14 percent of those with valve replacements.[122]

Relief of aortic valve obstruction, whether by balloon valvuloplasty or surgical valvotomy, is palliative rather than curative. Gradual restenosis is the rule, with almost one-third of infants who undergo valvotomy requiring a second operation, usually valve replacement, within the next two decades. Aortic regurgitation, a well-recognized complication of valvuloplasty, valvulotomy, and/or infective endocarditis, may require surgical intervention as well. Endocarditis is a serious and lifelong hazard, with an incidence among patients followed for 20 years of approximately 5 percent, a mortality rate of just over 25 percent, and a predilection for patients in the second, rather than first, decade of life and with PSPGs >50 mmHg.[60,122]

Secondary valvulotomy by balloon or surgery for recurrent or residual stenosis can be attempted, but calcification and restenosis eventually force aortic valve replacement in almost all those requiring surgery on the aortic valve in infancy or childhood. A small aortic annulus severely limits the relief of left ventricular hypertension unless one resorts to Konno's operation, in which the annulus is divided, the upper ventricular septum resected creating a VSD, patching the VSD with prosthetic material, and replacing the valve (a homograft or pulmonary autograft) into the enlarged annulus. The ascending aorta and anterior right ventricular wall are reconstructed using a prosthetic graft, and in the case of an autograft, the main pulmonary artery and pulmonary valve are replaced with a cryopreserved pulmonary homograft.[130]

Children with more than mild aortic stenosis are restricted from strenuous organized athletics, isometric exercises, and activities that require a good deal of stamina and produce shortness of breath.[131]

Supravalvular Aortic Stenosis

PATHOLOGY

The obstruction in the ascending aorta includes the following three types: (1) hourglass (discrete), (2) hypoplastic (diffuse), and (3) membranous. Associated obstructions in the pulmonary trunk, peripheral pulmonary arteries, and branches of the aortic arch are common.[132] Hypertrophy of the coronary arterial walls and premature coronary atherosclerosis have been described.[133]

CLINICAL MANIFESTATIONS

Supravalvular stenosis may be familial, associated with characteristic facies and mental retardation, sporadic, or (rarely) the result of congenital rubella. All forms may be and usually are associated with varying degrees of peripheral or branch pulmonary arterial stenosis. The familial form is transmitted as an autosomal dominant trait with variable expression (see Chap. 62). Mental retardation is not present, and there are no characteristic facial features.[134] Supravalvular aortic stenosis associated with mental retardation, frequently called *Williams' syndrome*, is associated with a high and prominent forehead, epicanthal folds, underdevelopment of the bridge of the nose and mandible, and a broad, overhanging upper lip. It is due to a deletion of the elastin gene on chromosome 7 and can now be identified by florescent in situ hybridization studies. It has been linked with idiopathic hypercalcemia of infancy, but in the majority of patients recognized beyond infancy, hypercalcemia is not present.[135]

The symptoms of supravalvular aortic stenosis are similar to those of subvalvular aortic stenosis (see below). Patients with the familial form usually have a distinctive family history but one that seldom emerges in its entirety on initial questioning. The physical findings are also similar to those of subvalvular aortic stenosis, although a systolic blood pressure difference may be recorded between the two arms on occasion, with the right arm pressure being greater than the left (Coanda effect).[136] Chest roentgenography and ECG are not distinctive unless associated pulmonary arterial stenosis leads to right ventricular hypertrophy. Echocardiography can identify the narrowed aortic lumen just above the aortic valve and provide an estimate of the severity of the obstruction by the Doppler-derived instantaneous pressure gradient.

At cardiac catheterization, a systolic pressure gradient can be demonstrated just above the aortic valve by careful pullback. Supravalvular aortography or left ventricular angiography will visualize the supravalvular narrowing (Fig. 63-26). Pressure recordings in the branch pulmonary arteries should be obtained, and pulmonary arterial angiography should be performed in the presence of any significant stenoses. Narrowing at the branch points of major arteries (coronary, carotid, mesenteric, renal, etc.) is seen occasionally.

NATURAL HISTORY AND PROGNOSIS

The sequence of progressive obstruction, the appearance of symptoms and ECG changes, and the possibility of sudden

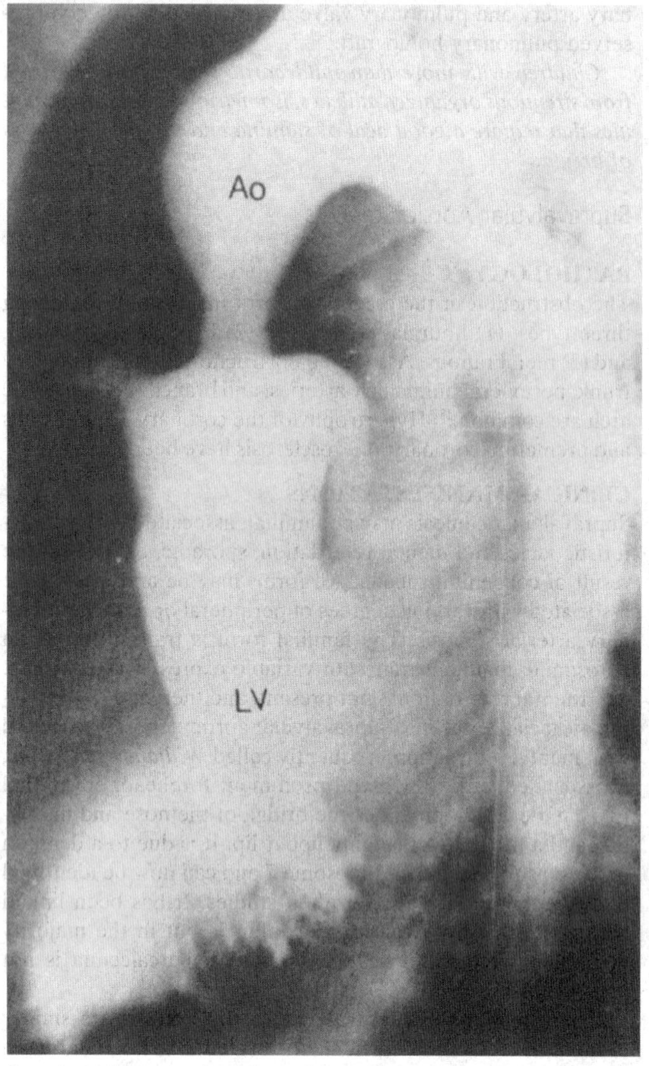

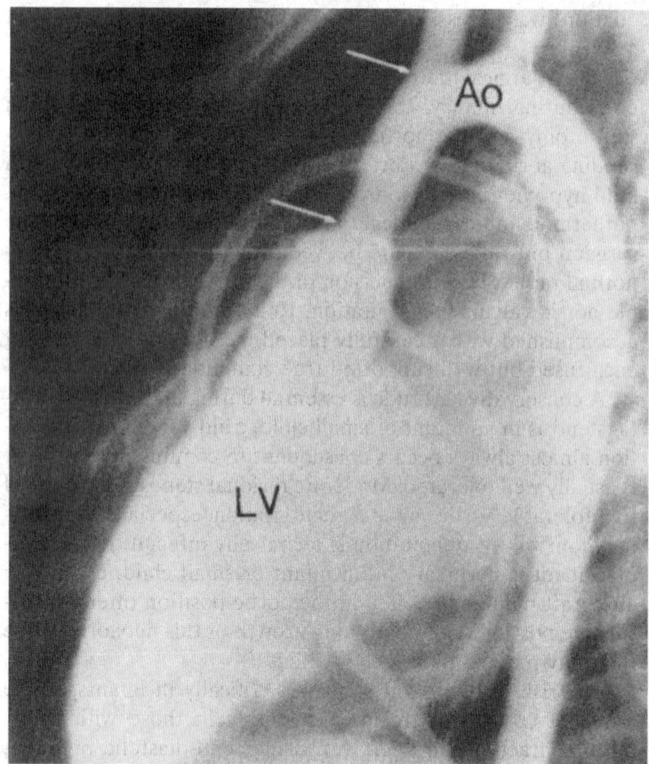

FIGURE 63-26 *A.* Supravalvar aortic stenosis, discrete type. The stenotic segment is located immediately above the aortic sinuses of Valsalva. The distal ascending aorta (Ao) is normal in size. LV = left ventricle. *B.* Supravalvar aortic stenosis, diffuse type. Narrowing in the ascending aorta begins above the aortic valve (*lower arrow*) and extends throughout the ascending aortic segment to the origin of the brachiocephalic vessels (*upper arrow*). In this patient, the aortic arch and descending aorta also appear hypoplastic. (Keane JF, Fellows KE, La Farge G, et al. The surgical management of discrete and diffuse supravalvar aortic stenosis. *Circulation* 1976; 54:112–117. Reproduced with permission of the author and publisher.)

death appear to apply for supravalvular aortic stenosis as well as for valvular aortic stenosis. Infective endocarditis represents a threat to these patients throughout life.

MANAGEMENT

The indications for cardiac catheterization and follow-up are the same as those with valvular aortic stenosis. Noninvasive imaging frequently suffices, but angiography may be necessary to evaluate the gradient and rule out arterial narrowing. Surgery usually is recommended if the gradient across the narrowing exceeds 40 mmHg.

Discrete supravalvular aortic stenosis is relieved by one or more incisions through the narrow segment of the ascending aorta, usually at the level of the sinotubular ridge at the top of the commissures. Incisions are extended well down into the aortic sinuses. Ridges of obstructing fibrous tissue are excised. The aorta is enlarged by the insertion of a gusset of prosthetic vascular graft material or pericardium to increase the circumference.[127] A favorable outcome can be anticipated postoperatively in most patients with supravalvular aortic stenosis if the arterial wall abnormality is localized.[137] Intimal obstruction of the coronary arterial ostia may require debridement, dilation, or even saphenous vein or internal mammary bypass grafting.

Diffuse tubular hypoplasia of the ascending aorta is a technically challenging problem that is associated with a higher mortality rate and usually poor postoperative hemodynamic results.

Subvalvular Aortic Stenosis

PATHOLOGY

Three classic varieties of subvalvular aortic stenosis involve the left ventricular outflow tract: the discrete, tunnel, and muscular types. The discrete type is characterized by a localized fibrous encirclement of the left ventricular outflow tract a short distance below the aortic valve (Fig. 63-27) or fibromuscular tissue that extends onto the mitral leaflet and also may attach to the aortic cusps. The tunnel type involves hypoplasia of the aortic annulus and a channel with a fibrous lining in the subjacent left ventricular outflow tract.[138,139] The muscular type also is known as *hypertrophic cardiomyopathy* (or idiopathic hypertrophic subaortic stenosis) and is discussed in Chap. 67.

More than half these patients have associated malformations, of which PDA, VSD, or coarctation are the most common.

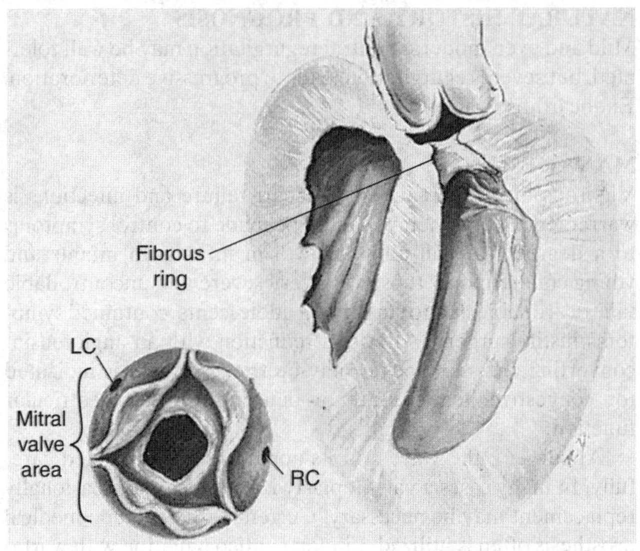

FIGURE 63-27 Localized subvalvular aortic stenosis. Obstruction is immediately upstream from the aortic valve. LC and RC = left and right coronary arteries. (From Kirklin JW and Ellis FH Jr.[144] Reproduced with permission from the publisher and authors.)

CLINICAL MANIFESTATIONS

Discrete stenosis is more common among males, with a male/female ratio of approximately 2.5:1. In the isolated forms, the majority of patients are referred because of the detection of a murmur that not uncommonly is mistaken initially for that of a VSD. The symptoms have the same implications as they do for valvular aortic stenosis.

The physical examination is similar to that of valvular aortic stenosis, with two exceptions: An early systolic ejection click is not heard, and an early diastolic murmur of aortic regurgitation is present in approximately one-half of these patients.

The roentgenographic features and ECG are also similar to those of valvular aortic stenosis except for the absence of poststenotic dilatation of the ascending aorta. Two-dimensional echocardiography permits excellent visualization of the anatomy of the obstruction. Estimation of the systolic pressure gradient can be obtained from Doppler echocardiographic studies.

When catheterization is performed, a careful pullback pressure tracing across the left ventricular outflow tract will document the severity of the gradient and establish the site of the obstruction. Left ventricular biplane angiography will outline the nature of the obstruction. Aortography is recommended to evaluate the degree of aortic regurgitation.

NATURAL HISTORY AND PROGNOSIS

Severe congestive failure in infancy is unusual and, if present, is almost invariably associated with complicating defects.[138] The obstruction is progressive in most instances, sometimes rapidly so. In one study, 75 percent of patients showed an increase of 25 mmHg or more in a 5-year period.[140] The cause of the progression is not known, but an intriguing theory suggests that distorted anatomy increases shear stress, leading to a stimulation of growth factors and cellular proliferation.[141] Associated aortic regurgitation also tends to be progressive and appears to result from damage from the jet of blood through the obstruction, with secondary thickening and deformity of the valve leaflets. The results of surgery depend on the extent of involvement of the left ventricular outflow tract, with the best results being obtained in patients with a thin, discrete subvalvular membrane. The least satisfactory results occur in patients with tunnel obstruction.

MANAGEMENT

Medical management is similar to that of patients with valvular aortic stenosis, but surgery for the discrete type usually is recommended for pressure gradients ≥30 mmHg because of the possibility of progression of obstruction, and the likelihood of progressive aortic valvular deformity and regurgitation.[142]

Continued follow-up for assessment of reobstruction and progression of aortic regurgitation and for reemphasis of the precautions against infective endocarditis is essential in all patients.[143]

Subvalvular fibromuscular (membranous) left ventricular outflow tract obstruction is exposed through the aortic root as was described for aortic valvular stenosis (Fig. 63-27). Small half-circle needles and sutures or hooks are placed into the abnormal fibromuscular tissue, pulling it into view for precise excision from the underlying ventricular septum and the anterior mitral valve leaflet. The area of the bundle of His, which usually is just beneath the anterior commissure between the right and noncoronary leaflets, is avoided. An additional septal myectomy or myotomy beneath and to the left of the commissure between the right and left leaflets may be required if secondary hypertrophy is significant. Immediate and early operative outcome is generally good, but *residual, recurrent, and progressive subaortic obstruction occurs in up to 25 percent of these patients, requiring long-term follow-up.*[144,145]

Diffuse tunnel obstruction in the left ventricular outflow tract poses a difficult technical problem that requires aortoseptoplasty, reconstruction of the left ventricular outflow (Konno's operation or a modification of it).[130,142]

Bicuspid Aortic Valve

PATHOLOGY

Classically, the two cusps are oriented anteriorly and posteriorly, with the anterior or conjoined cusp being the larger. A raphe, or ridge, is present along the aortic aspect of the larger cusp, running from the aortic wall to the free edge of the cusp. The most common associated condition of significance is coarctation of the aorta. The most common complication is calcification of the valve. *In about 85 percent of cases of calcific aortic stenosis in patients below age 70, the valve is congenitally bicuspid.* Aortic regurgitation from prolapse of the larger cusp is a less common complication and is usually not evident until adolescence or adult life.

CLINICAL MANIFESTATIONS

The incidence in the general population approaches 2 percent; therefore, it is the most common congenital abnormality of the heart or great vessels except possibly for mitral valve prolapse (see Chap. 58). Its importance lies in its frequent association with other forms of congenital heart disease: the predisposition of the valve to become stenotic as a result of fibrosis and deposition of calcium over the course of years, the tendency of the valve to become regurgitant, its association with aortic root dilatation and dissection,[146] and finally, the susceptibility of the valve to infective endocarditis. It is also common among patients with isolated or dominant aortic regurgitation, patients with infective endocarditis with or without a history of predisposing heart disease, and, probably most frequently, otherwise normal individuals who come to the physician's attention because of unrelated illnesses. Patients with uncomplicated bicuspid aortic valve are asymptomatic. The incidence among males is approximately 2.5 times that among females (see Chap. 56).

The characteristic feature is auscultatory and consists of an early systolic ejection click, which is best heard at the apex and does not vary with respiration. A soft, early, or midsystolic murmur is frequently present at the right upper sternal border. Less commonly, a soft murmur of aortic regurgitation may be heard. Two-dimensional echocardiography with adequate images can identify the bicuspid valve with a high degree of sensitivity and diagnostic accuracy.

NATURAL HISTORY AND PROGNOSIS

The majority of congenitally bicuspid aortic valves are nonobstructive at birth, but with the passage of time, a few of these valves become fibrotic, stiffer, and more obstructive and eventually become the site of calcium deposition, primarily among individuals between ages 15 and 65. Important calcium deposition is unusual before age 30, whereas grossly visible deposits of calcium are present in the valves of virtually all patients with severe stenosis beyond that age. A much smaller number of individuals born with a bicuspid aortic valve develop isolated aortic regurgitation. In approximately one-third, this is the result of fibrosis, prolapse, or retraction of one or both of the leaflets; in the remainder, regurgitation results from infective endocarditis on an apparently functionally normal bicuspid valve (see Chaps. 56 and 73).

Congenital Mitral Regurgitation

PATHOLOGY

Mitral regurgitation may be due to a primary valve abnormality or secondary to a more complex defect (see "Common Atrioventricular Canal Defects," above). There are a variety of rare primary malformations, including isolated cleft, fenestration, and double orifice. Mitral regurgitation also occurs frequently with conditions that cause left ventricular dilatation and failure.

CLINICAL MANIFESTATIONS

Poor growth, frequent respiratory infections, and failure occur with significant mitral regurgitation. The physical findings are generally similar to those with mitral regurgitation of other causes (see Chap. 10). There may be a prominent left precordial bulge if cardiomegaly has been present from infancy. The systolic murmur may radiate to the base of the heart. Left atrial and left ventricular enlargement correlate with the degree of volume overload. Echocardiography with Doppler color flow mapping will demonstrate these as well as left ventricular function and the severity of regurgitation. The specific defect may be outlined, such as an isolated cleft or a double-orifice valve. Findings at cardiac catheterization substantiate the hemodynamic alterations (see Chap. 15).

NATURAL HISTORY AND PROGNOSIS

Mild and even moderate mitral regurgitation may be well tolerated, but severe regurgitation leads to progressive deterioration. Endocarditis is a risk.

MANAGEMENT

Vigorous medical treatment of heart failure and infections is warranted. Every attempt should be made to control symptoms to a degree that will allow growth in infants. In infants and young children, only those with very severe and uncontrollable failure are subjected to surgery. In adolescents, continued symptoms justify surgery. Afterload reduction with an angiotensin-converting enzyme blocker may be tried. Surgery is indicated for congestive heart failure or deteriorating left ventricular function.

At surgery, the valve and its apparatus are inspected carefully. In many cases a valvuloplasty is possible, but occasionally replacement may be necessary. Currently, the St. Jude medical prosthesis often is utilized. Lifelong anticoagulation with warfarin (see Chap. 44) is required. With body growth, replacement with a larger prosthesis may be difficult, and no good annular enlarging operation exists.

VALVULAR AND VASCULAR MALFORMATIONS OF THE RIGHT SIDE OF THE HEART WITH RIGHT-TO-LEFT, BIDIRECTIONAL, OR NO SHUNT

Pulmonary Stenosis with Intact Ventricular Septum

PATHOLOGY

Valvular pulmonary stenosis with an intact ventricular septum usually is characterized by a dome-shaped stenosis of the pulmonary valve and less commonly by dysplasia of the valve. The valve may be unicuspid, bicuspid, or tricuspid. The annulus also may be narrow. The pulmonary trunk exhibits poststenotic dilatation. In adult patients, calcification of the valve may appear.

In pulmonary valvular dysplasia, the annulus of the valve may be abnormally narrow, but the most dramatic changes are related to the cusps, of which three are identifiable. The cusps are exceedingly thickened by mucoid and dense connective tissue.[147]

Concentric hypertrophy of the right ventricle is present, with its degree reflecting the degree of obstruction at the valve level. *The hypertrophy of the infundibular musculature may cause secondary infundibular stenosis.*

Less commonly, there may be isolated subvalvular pulmonary stenosis caused by infundibular narrowing or an anomalous muscle bundle across the middle of the right ventricle.[148] Both types may be associated with a VSD.

Isolated supravalvular pulmonary stenosis, or pulmonary arterial coarctations, also may occur. From angiographic studies, these are classified into four types: (1) *localized stenosis with poststenotic dilatation*, (2) *segmental stenosis*, (3) *diffuse hypoplasia*, and (4) *multiple peripheral stenoses*. The stenosis may be localized to any segment of the pulmonary arterial system. The process is unilateral in about one-third of cases and bilateral in two-thirds. Pulmonary arterial stenosis is commonly (about

75 percent), though not universally, associated with other cardiovascular abnormalities, such as tetralogy of Fallot. It also may be seen as a sequela of congenital rubella, Williams', Noonan's,[149] or Alagille's syndrome.

ABNORMAL PHYSIOLOGY

There is a pressure difference during systole between the main right ventricular cavity and the pulmonary artery. The area of the pulmonary valve orifice is normally 2 cm^2/m^2; it is about 0.5 cm^2 at birth and increases in size with body growth. In general, the effective valve area must be decreased about 60 percent before there is a hemodynamically significant obstruction to flow. PSPG may reach 150 to 240 mmHg in severe cases. The degree of obstruction is assessed by the peak and mean systolic pressure gradients and the amount of flow across the valve. In neonates, severe stenosis can be associated with a relatively small pressure difference if the flow is very low as a result of right ventricular failure. If pulmonary flow is normal, patients with PSPG at rest <40 mmHg have mild stenosis and patients with PSPG >75 mmHg have severe stenosis.

When the pulmonary stenosis is severe, the right ventricle may fail and the cardiac output may be decreased at rest; this is associated with elevation of both the right ventricular end-diastolic pressure and the right atrial mean pressure. This may cause the foramen ovale to open and allow shunting of blood from the right atrium to the left atrium, resulting in arterial oxygen desaturation and cyanosis. In most adolescent or adult patients with significant pulmonary stenosis, the resting cardiac output is within normal limits but usually does not increase normally during exercise. In contrast, younger children may be able to increase cardiac output during exercise, even with significant obstruction.[119,150]

CLINICAL MANIFESTATIONS

Pulmonary stenosis is one of the most common congenital heart defects and accounts for about 10 percent of patients in most large study populations (Table 63-1). The stenosis is at the level of the pulmonary valve in most instances, but it can occur within the right ventricle, in the pulmonary arteries, or in a combination of the two. Infants with severe stenosis with patency of the foramen ovale may have right-to-left shunting.

History Most infants and children are asymptomatic, but a small percentage with very severe obstruction manifest symptoms, usually mild fatigue or shortness of breath with exertion. Young infants with critical obstruction present with cyanosis if there is a patent foramen ovale or ASD. Squatting and syncope are rare in childhood.[151]

Physical Examination Patients with a dysplastic valve and occasional supravalvular stenosis have consistent noncardiac abnormalities in a familial syndrome described by Noonan,[149] with short stature, hypertelorism, ptosis, low-set ears, and mental retardation.

In older patients with valvular pulmonary stenosis, cyanosis is uncommon, except with severe obstruction and an atrial communication. Hepatomegaly and the murmur of tricuspid regurgitation may be present with severe obstruction. With at least moderate obstruction, a prominent a wave is seen on examination of the jugular venous pulse. A systolic thrill in the suprasternal notch and at the left upper sternal border is present with significant obstruction unless there is isolated subvalvular stenosis. The right ventricular parasternal impulse becomes increasingly forceful with more severe obstruction. *An early systolic click with expiration that disappears with inspiration heard at the left upper sternal border is the hallmark of valvular stenosis unless the obstruction is severe or the valve is dysplastic.* A click is not present with isolated stenosis at other levels. As the obstruction increases in severity, the pulmonary component of the second heart sound becomes progressively softer and more delayed, becoming inaudible when the right ventricular pressure reaches systemic levels or greater. The second heart sound is normal or accentuated with supravalvular stenosis. A fourth heart sound is heard if the obstruction is severe. The characteristic systolic murmur is harsh, crescendo-decrescendo in shape, and best heard at the left upper sternal border with radiation toward the left clavicle. The murmur radiates more to the axilla and back with supravalvular stenosis. The duration of the murmur and the timing of peak intensity correlate well with the severity of obstruction. With mild to moderate stenosis, the murmur peaks in midsystole and ends at or before the aortic component of the second heart sound. In patients with severe stenosis, the murmur peaks late in systole and extends beyond the aortic component of the second heart sound (see Chaps. 10 and 59).[151]

Chest Roentgenogram Most patients have a normal or only slightly increased heart size, primarily of the right ventricle. Significant enlargement is seen with critical obstruction and is an ominous sign. Characteristically, the main and proximal left pulmonary arteries are prominent as a result of poststenotic dilatation when the stenosis is valvular. This finding may be absent with very severe obstructions, with a dysplastic valve, in very young infants, or with stenosis above or below the valve. The pulmonary vascular pattern is normal in most of these patients, but the vascularity is diminished in those with a right-to-left shunt at the atrial level.

Electrocardiogram Right ventricular forces in the anterior precordial leads correlate reasonably well with the degree of obstruction.[151] They are normal or demonstrate mild hypertrophy with an rsR′ pattern if there is mild obstruction. With severe stenosis, there is right axis deviation, right atrial hypertrophy, and very tall pure R waves in the anterior precordial leads. The presence of a qR pattern in these leads is almost always a sign of very severe obstruction. Those with a dysplastic valve frequently have a superior QRS axis.

Echocardiogram Two-dimensional imaging allows identification of the level of obstruction, and Doppler studies provide an excellent measure of severity. Shunting at the atrial level also can be evaluated.[152]

Cardiac Catheterization Diagnostic catheterizations are rarely necessary, but data obtained before balloon dilation demonstrate an elevated right ventricular systolic pressure with a distinct systolic pressure difference across the narrowed segment, as demonstrated by slow withdrawal of the catheter from the distal pulmonary arterial branches to the proximal right ventricle. Simultaneous measurement of systemic arterial and right ventricular pressures with measurement of flow is necessary to assess severity accurately. The right ventricular end-

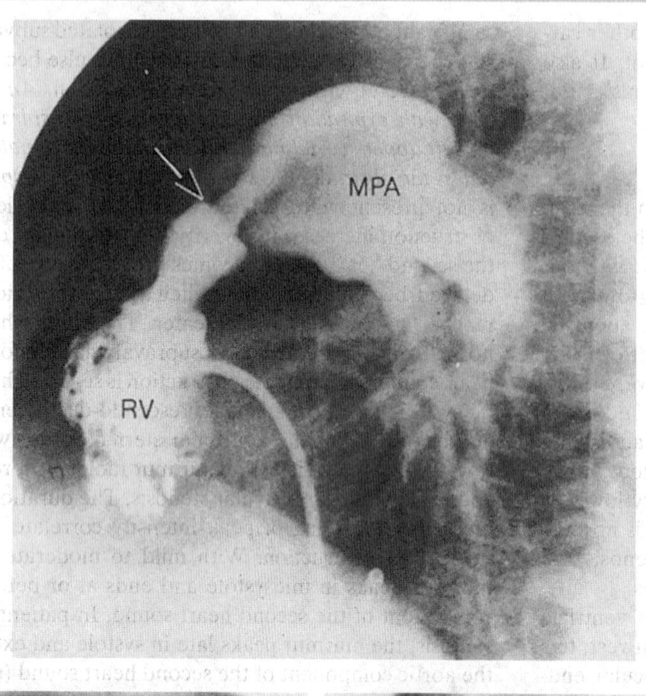

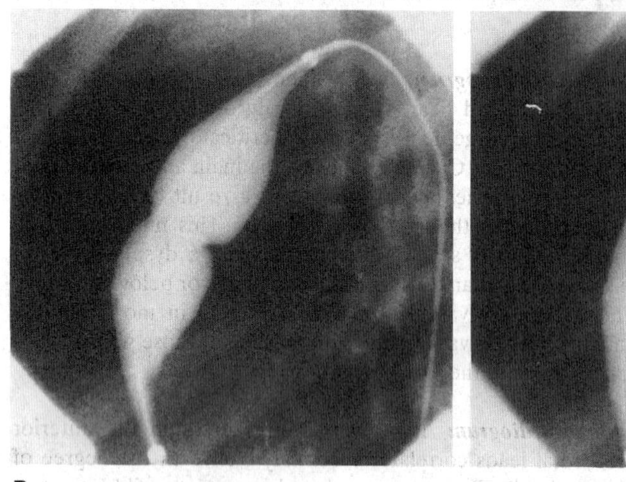

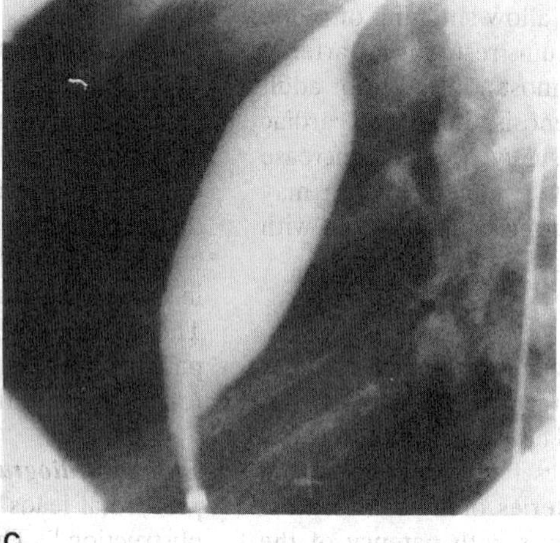

FIGURE 63-28 *A*. Lateral view of a right ventricular (RV) angiogram demonstrating the typical features of valvular pulmonary stenosis with doming of the pulmonary valve (*arrow*) and a narrow jet of contrast entering the dilated main pulmonary artery (MPA). *B*. An 18-mm balloon is inflated across the 14-mm annulus. A moderate waist is seen at 1 atmosphere of pressure. *C*. The waist is eliminated at 4 atmospheres of pressure. (From Lock JE, Keane JF, Perry SB. *Diagnostic and Interventional Catheterization in Congenital Heart Disease*. 2d ed. Boston: Kluwer; 2000.)

diastolic pressure and right atrial *a* wave may be elevated. Systemic oxygen saturation is diminished only in those with more severe obstruction and a patent foramen ovale or, less commonly, a true ASD. A left-to-right shunt at the atrial level is detected in some patients with mild to moderate obstruction. With valvular stenosis, right ventricular angiography demonstrates thickened and doming valve leaflets and a jet of contrast material entering the dilated pulmonary artery (Fig. 63-28*A*). Doming is not characteristic of the dysplastic valve. Infundibular subvalvular narrowing caused by muscular hypertrophy may occur secondary to the valvular stenosis or rarely as an isolated anomaly. Isolated anomalous muscle bundles in the right ventricle also may be seen. Pulmonary arterial angiography best demonstrates the sites of obstruction with supravalvular stenoses. Ventricular volume studies have demonstrated depressed ventricular function in patients with right-to-left shunts. Balloon dilation is discussed below under "Management."

NATURAL HISTORY AND PROGNOSIS

The clinical course of valvular stenosis is favorable in most patients with mild to moderate obstruction. In a national cooperative study,[153] 86 percent of patients had no significant increase in their pressure gradients over a 4- to 8-year interval. Those with a significant increase were less than 4 years of age and had at least moderate stenosis initially. Progression during the period of growth seems to be the likely explanation for most of the increases, but a few patients developed subvalvular muscular hypertrophy, which increased the obstruction. Even mild obstruction may progress significantly in some infants during the first year of life. The prognosis of those with severe obstruction without intervention is poor, especially in infants with critical obstruction. With severe obstruction, right ventricular damage and dysfunction can ensue over the years, and heart failure or arrhythmias can cause premature death in adults.[154] Tricuspid regurgitation also may result. Obstruction of the subvalvular type frequently increases with time, while supravalvular stenosis usually does not progress. Brain abscess can occur if a right-to-left shunt is present. Infective endocarditis with vegetations on the valve, pulmonary arterial wall, or infundibular region is also a risk. The children originally followed and treated as part of the national cooperative study cited above[151,153] were reevaluated 15 to 25 years later.[155] Among the 580 patients alive at the completion of the previous study, new data were available on 464 (78.4 percent). The probability of 25-year survival was 95.7 percent compared with an expected age- and sex-matched control group survival of 96.6 percent. Ninety-seven percent were asymptomatic. Although cardiac catheterization studies were not repeated, clinical examination and echocardiography at follow-up suggested no pulmonary stenosis in 2 percent, mild stenosis in 93 percent, moderate stenosis in 3 percent, and severe stenosis in only 1 percent. Pulmonary regurgitation was present in 40 percent, usually secondary to surgical valvotomy. Endocarditis was uncommon, as were ventricular arrhythmias.

MANAGEMENT

Management obviously depends on the severity of obstruction. For those with mild to moderate valvular pulmonary stenosis, periodic reexamination is indicated to detect any evidence of progression, with more frequent evaluation for those under 1 year of age. Measures to treat heart failure should be instituted in an infant with critical stenosis, but prompt intervention is mandatory. Cyanosis or a right ventricular systolic pressure well above systemic levels also is an indication for prompt intervention. Intervention is warranted in older children when the gradient exceeds 75 mmHg and is clearly not indicated when the gradient is less than 25 mmHg. *In the intermediate group, there is still some controversy, but general practice suggests valvuloplasty when the gradient exceeds 40 mmHg, although objective data to support therapy at this level are lacking.*

Balloon valvuloplasty has replaced surgical therapy as a first approach. Through the femoral vein, a balloon catheter is advanced across the valve and inflated to about 120 percent of the size of the pulmonary annulus, ripping the domed valve and thus relieving the obstruction (Fig. 63-28*B*).

The Valvuloplasty and Angioplasty of Congenital Anomalies Registry has published the combined results on 822 children.[156] Valvuloplasty resulted in improvement in most children with valvular obstruction, reducing the gradient from 71 ± 33 mmHg to 28 ± 24 mmHg. Valvuloplasty is, not surprisingly, less effective in children with a dysplastic pulmonary valve.[156,157] Complications were uncommon (5 in 822, or 0.6 percent), including two deaths. Valvuloplasty also has been performed in critical neonatal pulmonary stenosis with cyanosis caused by right-to-left shunting at the atrial level with a high success rate.[158,159] Subvalvular obstruction is less amenable to dilatation.

Peripheral pulmonary stenosis also has been occasionally amenable to dilatation, although the results are frequently less dramatic because of the multiple areas of stenosis and the fact that the complications, including pulmonary artery rupture, are more common.[160,161] Recently, stents have been used, with promising results,[161] in those with peripheral pulmonary artery stenosis in an attempt to keep open vessels that recoil back to normal size after the balloon is deflated. For those in whom there is isolated subvalvular stenosis or associated defects or in whom balloon dilatation has failed, surgical intervention is recommended.

The risk of death after pulmonary artery dilation is higher than that after dilation of the valve.[160] In the large collaborative study cited above, the death rate was 3 percent, although a more recent study from the author's institution found a mortality rate less than 1 percent among 400 cases.[162]

SURGICAL MANAGEMENT

Operation rarely is indicated for isolated pulmonary valvular stenosis; balloon valvuloplasty is virtually always successful in eliminating a clinically significant obstruction. A thickened, immobile, dysplastic pulmonary valve, however, is best treated by complete surgical excision (valvectomy). A small annulus is augmented with a pericardial or Dacron gusset.[163]

Subvalvular pulmonary stenosis is relieved through a right ventriculotomy, a main pulmonary arteriotomy, or a right atriotomy. Hypertrophic parietal and septal muscle bands constituting the fibrous orifice of the os infundibulum and obstructing moderator bands or muscle bundles within the body of the right ventricle are excised. Care is exercised to avoid injury to major coronary arterial branches. The right ventriculotomy usually can be closed by direct suturing, but a small oval patch of pericardium or Dacron can be used to prevent constriction of the outflow tract. Right ventricular function is compromised minimally by a small patch that does not extend across the annulus; larger patches to the pulmonary arterial bifurcation probably impair ventricular performance but may be necessary when there is associated annular or main pulmonary arterial hypoplasia. When possible, excision from the pulmonary artery or the right atrium is preferred to avoid ventricular injury. Excellent relief of right ventricular outflow tract obstruction can be expected after resection. Mortality and significant morbidity are rare.

Stenoses of main or extraparenchymal branch pulmonary arteries can be relieved by pericardial, synthetic, or homograft aortic or pulmonary arterial patches if the obstruction is proximal. Proximal coarctations in the larger portion of the arterial tree are more readily corrected than are those in small distal branches beyond the bifurcation of either the right or the left pulmonary artery, where results are poor.[164] In these instances, catheter balloon angioplasty, although certainly not without risk, offers nonsurgical relief of obstruction even in the small pulmonary arterial branches and should be considered the procedure of choice for distal pulmonary arterial stenoses.[160,161]

Prophylaxis against infective endocarditis is recommended for all patients whether or not surgery is performed, although the risks seem to be lower than they are with many other congenital anomalies.

Tetralogy of Fallot

PATHOLOGY

Tetralogy of Fallot is characterized by biventricular origin of the aorta above a large VSD (Fig. 63-29), obstruction to pulmonary blood flow, and right ventricular hypertrophy. Fibrous continuity of the aortic origin and the anterior mitral valve is maintained.[66]

The right ventricular infundibulum lies anterior to the position of the VSD and is bounded by the anterior and septal walls anteriorly and medially; the posterior wall is said to be a vertical crista supraventricularis or displaced conus septum.[165] The right ventricular infundibulum is a distinctive channel, but the caliber varies widely from only mild obstruction to atresia. Usually, it exhibits a significant degree of stenosis and is the dominant site of the obstruction to pulmonary flow that is characteristic of tetralogy.

The pulmonary valve is often malformed, usually being either bicuspid or unicuspid. That valve may contribute to pulmonary stenosis, but only uncommonly is it the only site of significant obstruction to pulmonary flow. Characteristically, the pulmonary trunk is thin-walled and its lumen is more narrow than normal, but usually it is wider than either the right ventricular infundibulum or the orifice of the pulmonary valve. The aorta is wider than normal, its change in caliber being roughly opposite to that of the pulmonary trunk. The foramen ovale is frequently patent in patients of all ages. In all cases of tetralogy with significant pulmonary obstruction, collateral branches to the lungs arise from the aorta.

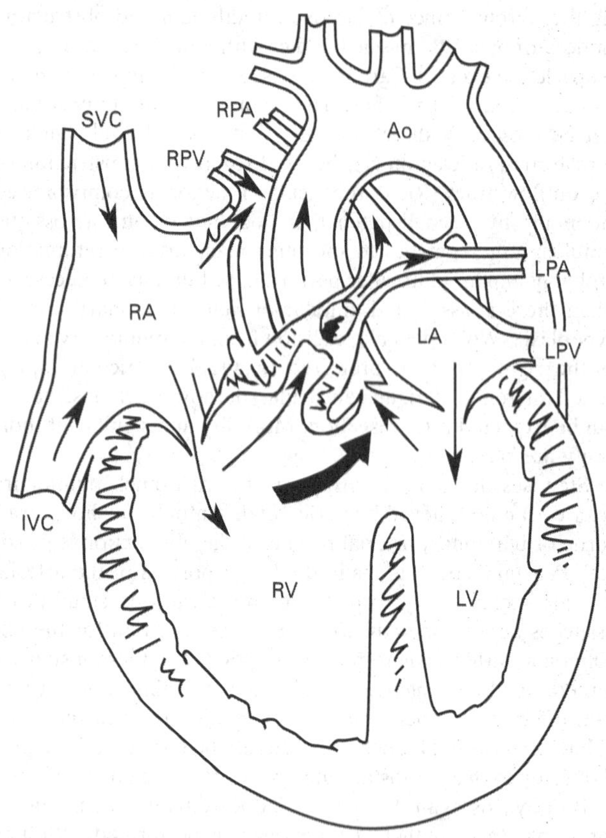

FIGURE 63-29 Classic tetralogy of Fallot. There are infundibular and pulmonary valvular stenoses. There is also right-to-left shunting at the atrial level. SVC = superior vena cava; IVC = inferior vena cava; RA = right atrium; RV = right ventricle; RPA = right pulmonary artery; LPA = left pulmonary artery; RPV = right pulmonary vein; LPV = left pulmonary vein; LA = left atrium; LV = left ventricle; Ao = aorta. (From Edwards.[66] Reproduced with permission from the publisher and author.)

There is invariably a large malalignment VSD. Anterior, middle, or apical muscular defects are also present in up to 5 percent of children seen as infants. Many close spontaneously, but if corrective surgery is to be performed successfully, they must be evaluated.

Coronary artery abnormalities are not uncommon. The anterior descending coronary artery in the interventricular septum may arise from the right instead of the left coronary artery. Although physiologically unimportant preoperatively, the course across the right ventricular outflow tract makes the usual site of right ventriculotomy and outflow patch unavailable during reparative surgery, frequently necessitating a conduit to "jump over" the vessel. The anatomy of the coronary circulation used to require angiography to establish, but more recently echocardiography with Doppler color flow has been sufficient to detail the distribution of the proximal coronary circulation in most cases.

ASSOCIATED CONDITIONS

The condition most commonly associated with tetralogy of Fallot is right aortic arch (about 30 percent).[166] A persistent left superior vena cava has been described in 10.6 percent of cases. When an associated ASD exists, this anomaly is referred to as *pentalogy of Fallot.* The ductus arteriosus may be absent, present unilaterally on either the right or the left side, or bilateral.

ABNORMAL PHYSIOLOGY

Since the VSD is usually large, with an area about as great as that of the aortic valve, both ventricles and the aorta have essentially the same systolic pressures. The most important hemodynamic factor is the ratio between the resistance to flow into the aorta and the resistance to flow across the stenotic right ventricular infundibulum. If the stenosis is not severe, the resistance to right ventricular outflow is not large, the pulmonary flow may be twice the systemic flow, and the arterial oxygen saturation may be normal (acyanotic tetralogy of Fallot). However, the resistance to the pulmonary flow may be increased markedly, causing right-to-left shunting, arterial desaturation, and subsequent polycythemia. When the pulmonary stenosis is very severe, the pulmonary blood flow may be by way of collateral vessels from the systemic arteries to the distal pulmonary arteries beyond the stenosis. The infundibular obstruction, which may be in part dynamic, is increased by drugs, heart rate maneuvers, and activities that increase myocardial contractility or decrease right ventricular volume. In addition, the infundibular hypertrophy may increase gradually over time. Since the systolic pressure in the right ventricle cannot exceed that in the left ventricle because of the large VSD, the right ventricle is "protected" from excessive pressure and work, and so congestive heart failure is uncommon.

Hypercyanotic episodes (spells) in patients with tetralogy are of uncertain origin. It is likely that some episodes are caused by unusual hyperactivity of muscular fibers in the right ventricular outflow tract that produce or exaggerate the infundibular stenosis, increasing pulmonary resistance and thus increasing the right-to-left shunting. Some spells may be caused by a decrease in peripheral resistance and systemic arterial pressure, which also may cause the right-to-left shunt to increase and pulmonary blood flow to decrease.

CLINICAL MANIFESTATIONS

Tetralogy of Fallot is the most common congenital cardiac defect that causes cyanosis. Tetralogy with an associated ASD, or pentalogy of Fallot, is not distinguishable clinically. For a discussion on the hypoxemia and the consequences in tetralogy, see the section on cyanosis and its complications earlier in this chapter.

History Most of these patients now are diagnosed prenatally by ultrasound or present in the first days or weeks of life with a heart murmur. If the right ventricular obstruction is severe, cyanosis is present at birth and is exacerbated when the ductus closes. If the obstruction is milder, the infant may be acyanotic with left-to-right flow through the VSD and occasionally may develop congestive heart failure. In this group, gradually increasing right ventricular obstruction may reduce the left-to-right shunt, and eventually, when infundibular resistance and pulmonary resistance exceed systemic resistance, right-to-left shunting develops, resulting in cyanosis.

Dyspnea with exertion occurs commonly in toddlers and older children with unrepaired defects. Attacks of suddenly increasing cyanosis associated with hyperpnea, or hypoxic spells,[167] are common between ages 2 months and 2 years. There are many precipitating events, including infection, exertion, and summer heat. They occur most often in the morning, with increasing irritability. The frequency and duration vary widely, but prolonged episodes can lead to syncope, seizures, and death. Squatting with exercise is common from 1.5 to 10 years of age in those not previously repaired. These problems are becoming uncommon as more and more children undergo early repair.

Physical Examination Growth is usually normal unless cyanosis is extreme. Clubbing of the fingers and toes occurs after 3 months of age and is proportional to the level of cyanosis. Signs of congestive heart failure do not appear in tetralogy of Fallot during childhood unless there is a superimposed illness such as anemia or infective endocarditis.

Increased right ventricular activity is observed. A systolic thrill may be palpable at the left midsternal border, with a harsh midsystolic murmur in that location. Softer murmurs signal more severe obstruction and are common when presentation is in the newborn period or during hypoxic spells. The murmur ends before the second heart sound, which is characteristically single. A continuous murmur is heard if a PDA or large collateral vessels are present. An early systolic ejection sound at the left sternal border and apex is uncommon; its presence suggests primarily valvular pulmonary stenosis.

Chest Roentgenogram The total heart size is usually normal on chest roentgenography, but right ventricular enlargement is present in the lateral view. The aorta arches to the right in many cases. Pulmonary flow is diminished. The pulmonary segment is concave and the apex is elevated, giving the *coeur en sabot* (boot-shaped) contour. A very young infant may have only diminished pulmonary flow.

Electrocardiogram In tetralogy of Fallot, the mean QRS axis of the ECG is usually to the right, between +90° and +210°. There is right ventricular hypertrophy, with a tall R wave in the right precordial leads and a deep S wave in the left leads. Some of these patients have right atrial hypertrophy.

Echocardiogram Two-dimensional echocardiography can delineate the anatomic components of tetralogy.[168] Anomalies of the coronary arteries can be demonstrated, and associated defects can be excluded.

Hematologic and Other Laboratory Studies Before surgical repair, the hemoglobin and hematocrit should be measured and pulse oximetry should be performed in all patients at initial evaluation and periodically thereafter for determination of the degree of polycythemia and the early detection of anemia relative to the degree of cyanosis. The latter is common, especially in those under 2 years of age, and may predispose a patient to cerebrovascular accidents. Platelet counts and clotting studies may be advisable in older unrepaired patients with marked polycythemia, particularly if a surgical procedure is planned. Serum uric acid levels should be measured if polycythemia is severe and long-standing.

Cardiac Catheterization In an increasing number of centers, the quality of echocardiography (especially when done in neonates or infants) is sufficiently diagnostic to outline the right ventricular and proximal pulmonary artery anatomy, rule out additional muscular VSDs, and establish the proximal coronary circulation. As a consequence, diagnostic cardiac catheterization and angiography are less commonly performed preoperatively than they were in the past in children with tetralogy of Fallot.

In those in whom the study is performed, the right ventricular systolic pressure is equal to the pressure in the left ventricle and aorta. If the pulmonary artery can be entered, the pressure will be normal or low. The level or levels of obstruction can be evaluated by careful pullback to the right ventricle. Caution should be observed if the pulmonary artery is entered, as the catheter may critically reduce the pulmonary flow and cause a hypoxic episode. Systemic arterial oxygen saturation is reduced because of right-to-left shunting from the right ventricle to the left ventricle. If a patent foramen ovale or ASD is present, there may be an additional right-to-left or bidirectional shunt at the atrial level. Selective biplane right ventricular angiography will demonstrate levels of obstruction, continuity and size of the pulmonary arteries, and size and position of the ventricular defect. If this is not demonstrated by echocardiography or aortography, selective coronary arteriography should be performed on all patients preoperatively to demonstrate the coronary arterial pattern.[169]

MEDICAL MANAGEMENT

Although the definitive treatment of tetralogy of Fallot is surgical, medical management plays a role before surgery and in the postoperative period. For a severely cyanotic newborn, prostaglandin administration is of benefit[91] to keep the ductus open until surgery can be done. Before surgery, the hematocrit and hemoglobin should be monitored and iron-deficiency anemia should be treated promptly to prevent strokes. Fever or other illness that would lead to dehydration and possible thrombotic complications should be treated promptly.

Hypoxic spells in an infant should be treated initially by placing the infant in the knee-chest position and administering a high concentration of oxygen and morphine sulfate. If acidosis is present and does not correct spontaneously and promptly, intravenous sodium bicarbonate and an alpha-adrenergic agonist should be given. Propranalol may be useful in preventing hypoxic spells.[170]

Bacterial endocarditis is a serious complication, especially in those who have had a systemic-to-pulmonary artery shunt. Meticulous care should be taken to maintain good dental hygiene, and prophylactic antibiotics at times of predictable risk are mandatory (see Chap. 73).

SURGICAL MANAGEMENT

Historically, the approach to tetralogy of Fallot has been either palliation or corrective surgery. The introduction of an aorta-to-pulmonary-artery shunt for the treatment of tetralogy of Fallot[171] truly can be called the beginning of effective treatment for pediatric cardiovascular disease. When open heart surgery was initiated in the 1950s, tetralogy of Fallot was among the first lesions to be corrected.[172] Over the years, the age at which corrective surgery can be performed has dropped so that in many centers primary repair is the procedure of choice at any age. Palliation, when it is now performed, almost inevitably involves a modified Blalock-Taussig shunt that interposes a graft between the subclavian artery and the ipsolateral pulmonary artery, usually on the side opposite the aortic arch.[173] Even in the perinatal period, the placement of a 4-mm tube will result in satisfactory palliation for a year in more than 90 percent of infants.

Surgical correction for those with pulmonary stenosis involves closing the VSD, usually through a right ventriculotomy, resecting infundibular muscle, and, if the infundibulum, pulmonary valve, and main pulmonary artery are hypoplastic, using a pericardial patch to open the narrowed area. Care must be taken to avoid heart block while closing the VSD and avoid cutting a major branch of the coronary artery. If a patent foramen ovale is present, it usually is left open to allow decompression in the perioperative period. If a true ASD is present (pentology of Fallot), it should be closed to avoid left-to-right shunting once the right ventricle has recovered from the perioperative insult.[174]

Children with tetralogy of Fallot and pulmonary atresia with good-sized pulmonary arteries usually are repaired by closing the VSD and interposing a conduit, frequently an aortic homograft, between the right ventricle and the pulmonary artery.[175] If this is done in children under 7 or 8 years of age, replacement of the conduit is to be expected secondary to somatic growth. Children with tetralogy of Fallot and hypoplastic and/or discontinuous pulmonary arteries require an individualized approach that frequently involves balloon dilation of hypoplastic vessels, unifocalization of discontinuous vessels, and, it is hoped, eventual repair with a conduit closing the VSD.[176] Operative and early mortality rates for repair of tetralogy of Fallot are now quite low in most centers. Kirklin and coworkers[173] in the early 1980s reported mortality rates of 1.6 percent with operations at 5 years of age to 4.1 percent at 1 year of age. At Children's Hospital in Boston, there was a 4.2 percent mortality rate among 330 children under 1 year of age operated on between 1973 and 1990, with a mortality rate of only 2.5 percent in the past 6 years of the study (1984–1990).[174] Late complications have included residual peripheral pulmonary stenosis, a small incidence of residual VSDs, and, rarely, aortic regurgitation. The long-term survivors have had atrial or, more commonly, ventricular arrhythmias and continue to be at risk for infective endocarditis.

Physicians at the Mayo Clinic, the first center to use the pump oxygenator to repair tetralogy of Fallot in the 1950s, have reported a minimum 30-year follow-up of the 162 30-day survivors of surgery.[177] The 32-year actuarial survival rate was 86 percent, with subgroup survival rates of those less then 5 years old, 5 to 7 years old, and 8 to 11 years old at the time of surgical repair being 90, 93, and 91 percent, respectively. Late sudden death from cardiac causes occurred in 10 patients during the 32-year period. The performance of some previous palliative operation (Waterston or Pott's shunts) but not a palliative Blalock-Taussig shunt was associated with higher mortality. With earlier surgery and less utilization of palliative procedures, it is hoped that the surgical results will be even better for children born in the 1980s and 1990s and beyond.

Ebstein's Anomaly

PATHOLOGY

In Ebstein's anomaly, the anterior leaflet of the tricuspid valve is attached normally to the annulus, but varying portions of the posterior and septal leaflets are displaced downward, being attached to the ventricular wall below the annulus. The proximal part of the right ventricle is thin-walled and continuous with the right atrium. The functional right ventricle is small and is made up of the apical and infundibular portions of the right ventricle. An additional common finding is that the papillary muscles and chordae are highly malformed, with great variation in the manner of attachment of the two involved leaflets to the right ventricular wall. Commonly, multiple direct attachments of valvular tissue to the right ventricular mural endocardium occur.[178,179]

An interatrial communication is present in most cases, usually taking the form of a patent foramen ovale. Continuity of right atrial and right ventricular myocardial tissues, in addition to the usual connections by way of the main conduction pathways, has been observed. *The presence of Ebstein's anomaly has been associated with maternal lithium use during pregnancy, although the risk ratio remains unclear.*[180]

ABNORMAL PHYSIOLOGY

Ebstein's anomaly results in obstruction to right ventricular filling because of a decrease in the size of the right ventricle, part of which is incorporated into the huge right atrium. The deformed tricuspid valve also frequently is associated with tricuspid regurgitation with a right-to-left shunt through the foramen ovale. In the perinatal period, when the pulmonary vascular resistance is high, the tricuspid regurgitation may be severe. This results in increased right atrial pressure and, when the patent foramen ovale is open, severe cyanosis. As the pulmonary vascular resistance falls, the right-to-left shunting is decreased and hypoxemia improves. In older children, right-sided congestive heart failure with edema and/or ascites may develop.

CLINICAL MANIFESTATIONS

History Approximately one-half of reported patients develop symptoms of cyanosis and right-sided heart failure in early infancy. The remainder present with a murmur or abnormal chest roentgenogram, but with no symptoms, in early childhood or because of gradual progression of symptoms through late childhood or adult life.[181] The most common symptom is dyspnea on exertion. The spectrum of exercise intolerance has been described.[182] Palpitations resulting from supraventricular tachyarrhythmias occur in 20 to 30 percent of these children. Occasionally, syncope occurs as a result of arrhythmia or low cardiac output if the atrial septum is intact.

Physical Examination A newborn with elevated pulmonary vascular resistance has severe cyanosis. In older infants and children, cyanosis and clubbing are mild. Only a small percentage do not have an ASD or patent foramen ovale and thus are not cyanotic. The precordium is generally quiet even in those with striking cardiomegaly. The liver is enlarged, and the jugular venous pulse may be elevated. The holosystolic murmur of tricuspid regurgitation is heard at the lower left sternal border and may be accompanied by a "scratchy" diastolic murmur of tricuspid stenosis. The first heart sound is split and loud, and the second heart sound is widely and persistently split. Loud third and fourth heart sounds are usual, especially in older patients.

Chest Roentgenogram Heart size, as shown by chest roentgenography, varies, but the heart is ordinarily very large because of the very dilated right atrium. In those with cyanosis, pulmonary blood flow is diminished correspondingly.

Electrocardiogram Giant, peaked P waves are common, along with a prolonged PQ interval and right ventricular conduction delay or complete right bundle branch block. In approximately 10 percent of these patients, the pattern of Wolff-Parkinson-White syndrome (with a short PQ interval and slurring of the initial QRS forces or a delta wave) is seen.[181]

Echocardiogram Two-dimensional echocardiography is very helpful in the diagnosis (Fig. 63-30), identifying the lesion, depicting the degree of displacement of the tricuspid valve into the right ventricle, and assessing the severity of the tricuspid regurgitation. In neonates, evaluation of the pulmonary valve usually allows a distinction between anatomic pulmonary atresia from absence of opening of the valve caused by severe tricuspid regurgitation and high pulmonary vascular resistance.[183]

Cardiac Catheterization There is a higher than usual risk associated with cardiac catheterization because of the frequency of rhythm disturbances. Proper precautions and prompt use of cardioversion when necessary minimize this risk. In most cases, echocardiography and color Doppler evaluation are sufficient, and catheterization is performed less commonly than it was previously.

There is usually right-to-left shunting at the atrial level. Right atrial hypertension is present. The characteristic right ventricular pressure recording is not obtained until the catheter is advanced to the apex or outflow tract. An intracardiac ECG demonstrates, on pullback from the right ventricle, an area where the ECG is ventricular but the pressure is atrial in contour.[184] This method is not infallible, but it provides good evidence of tricuspid displacement with an "atrialized" portion of the right ventricle.

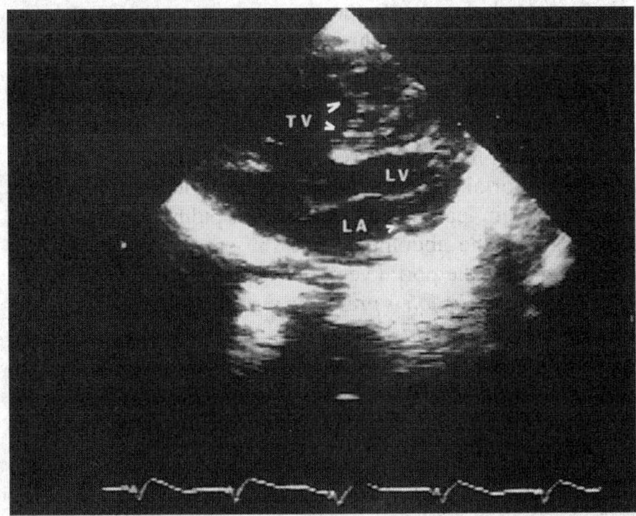

FIGURE 63-30 Two-dimensional echocardiogram in parasternal view in a patient with Ebstein's anomaly of the tricuspid valve (TV). Numerous attachments of the tricuspid valve (*arrowheads*) to the interventricular septum and right ventricular apex are seen. LV = left ventricle; LA = left atrium.

NATURAL HISTORY AND PROGNOSIS

The natural history varies greatly with the severity of the abnormality. In a study of 50 patients who presented in the neonatal period, 9 (18 percent) died in the perinatal period, with late deaths in another 15 (9 from hemodynamic deterioration, 5 sudden, and 1 noncardiac), for a 10-year actuarial survival of 61 percent.[185] In a study that included more children who presented after the perinatal period, the probability of survival was 50 percent at 47 years of age.[186] Predictors of poor outcome were New York Heart Association class III or IV, cardiothoracic ratio >65 percent, and atrial fibrillation.

For women who survive into adulthood without significant arrhythmias or cyanosis, successful pregnancy with good fetal outcome is possible.[187]

MEDICAL MANAGEMENT

Medical therapy varies depending on the severity of disease and the age at presentation. For those presenting with cyanosis in the perinatal period, procrastination until the pulmonary vascular resistance has decreased may be the best strategy. For those who are severely hypoxemic, maintaining the patency of the ductus with PGE_1 may be lifesaving. Reducing the pulmonary vascular resistance with nitric oxide may reduce right-to-left shunting and improve oxygenation.[188] Persistence of severe cyanosis beyond 1 week of age suggests pulmonary stenosis or pulmonary atresia in addition to Ebstein's deformity of the tricuspid valve.

For children with arrhythmias, an electrophysiologic study may be indicated. For those with disabling or life-threatening arrhythmias, radiofrequency ablation may be performed with initial success rates of about 80 percent but recurrences in 30 percent of patients.[189]

In older children who develop right-sided congestive heart failure, anticongestive measures with digoxin and diuretics may be tried, although this level of deterioration is usually an indication for surgical intervention.

SURGICAL MANAGEMENT

The surgical management of Ebstein's disease remains problematic. In the perinatal period, when the pulmonary vascular resistance is high, watchful waiting is probably the best approach. If the child remains severely hypoxemic (saturations <75 percent) after the pulmonary vascular resistance falls, palliation with a Blalock-Taussig shunt to improve pulmonary blood flow may be sufficient to relieve hypoxemia, and this should allow growth to an age at which other procedures can be considered.[190] For children in whom hypoxemia remains a significant problem, three approaches have been used. The first is a Glenn anastomosis connecting the superior vena cava to the right pulmonary artery, allowing inferior vena cava blood to go through the right atrium and ventricle to the pulmonary artery.[191] A more definitive procedure that eliminates hypoxemia that is used primarily for children with single ventricle but now is applied in this situation as well is the modified Fontan. In this approach, the tricuspid valve is oversewn and the patent foramen ovale is closed, diverting all systemic venous return to the pulmonary arteries by passing the right heart.[192] In a small group of patients, this has been done with success.

The more common approach has been tricuspid valve reconstruction or replacement, usually with a bioprosthesis. Among 189 patients operated on at the Mayo Clinic over a period of

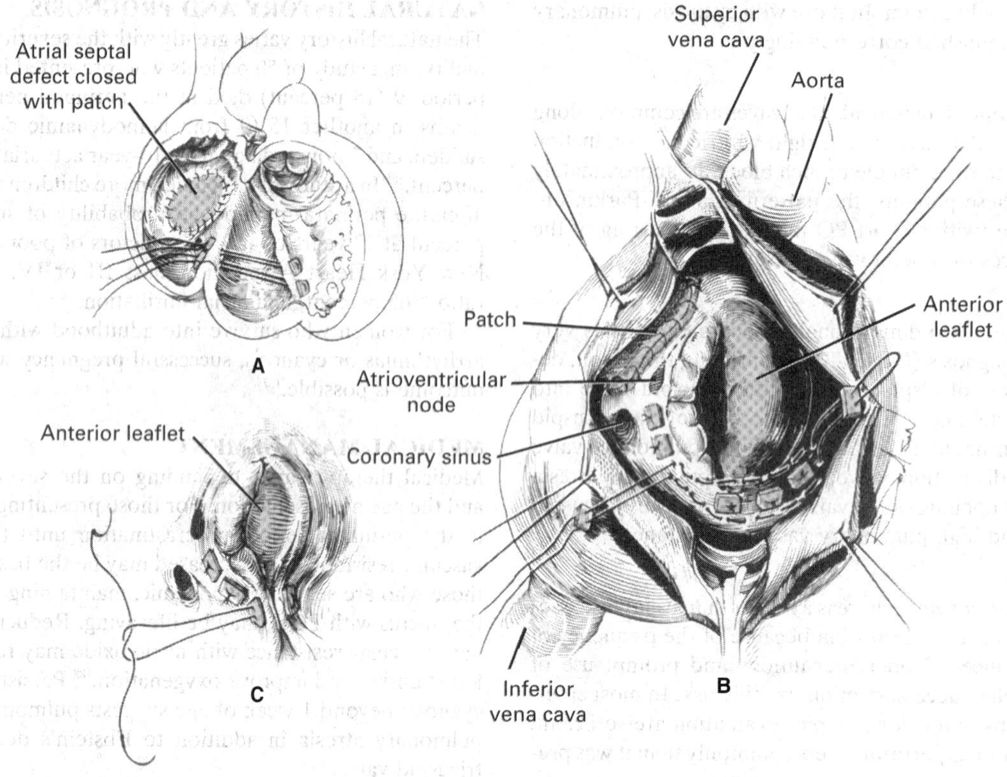

FIGURE 63-31 Danielson repair of Ebstein's malformation. *A.* Anterior cutaway drawing. The atrial septal defect is closed securely with a patch. Pledgeted sutures are placed to position the posterior leaflet at the annulus and imbricate the "atrialized" right ventricular chamber. *B* and *C.* Drawing of the right atrium showing the annuloplasty suture passed through two pledgets. Tying of this suture reduces dilation of the tricuspid valve so that the large anterior leaflet can meet the two smaller cusps and constitute a functional, essentially monocusp valve.

almost 20 years, there were 12 hospital deaths (6.3 percent) and an additional 10 late deaths. Among those followed more than 1 year after operation, more than 90 percent were in New York Heart Association class I or II.[193] More recently, other approaches have been suggested, including reconstruction of the normally shaped right ventricle with repositioning of the displaced leaflet of the tricuspid valve at the normal level[194] and reimplantation of the tricuspid valve leaflets with a vertical plication of the atrialized portion of the right ventricle to reduce its size (Fig. 63-31).[195] *Although the newer approaches seem promising in small numbers of patients in the short run, many patients with the milder form of the disease can live well into adulthood,*[196] *and so indications for the newer operations in patients who are asymptomatic or only mildly limited remain problematic.*

ABNORMALITIES OF THE PULMONARY VENOUS CONNECTIONS

Total Anomalous Pulmonary Venous Connection

PATHOLOGY

When all pulmonary veins terminate in a systemic vein or the right atrium, the term *total anomalous pulmonary venous connection* or *return* is applied (Fig. 63-32). Usually the pulmonary veins leave the lung and then join a chamber-like confluence posterior to the left atrium. From the confluence of veins, one primitive embryologic vessel persists and leads to the anomalous termination. Less commonly, two or more vessels lead to multiple sites of termination.

If the left cardinal vein persists, drainage flows superiorly into the innominate vein and then to the superior vena cava and right atrium or inferiorly into a persistent left superior vena cava and coronary sinus to the right atrium. If the right cardinal vein persists, drainage is to the superior vena cava, the azygous vein, or the right atrium directly. These types are sometimes referred to collectively as supracardiac or supradiaphragmatic drainage and almost never are associated with pulmonary venous obstruction.[197]

If the site of termination is infradiaphragmatic, with connection to the portal venous system or the inferior vena cava, the anomalous vein leaves the confluence of pulmonary veins and descends into the abdomen along the esophagus to join the ductus venosus, the portal vein, or the left gastric vein. *Pulmonary venous obstruction is present in virtually all cases of infradiaphragmatic connection.*[197]

In all cases of total anomalous pulmonary venous connection, there is a patent foramen ovale. The atrium and ventricle of the left side are small in comparison with the right-sided chambers but are within normal limits in regard to absolute size. In the absence of asplenia or polysplenia syndromes, associated anomalies are not common.

ABNORMAL PHYSIOLOGY

In this anomaly, all the blood from both the pulmonary and systemic circulations eventually returns to the right atrium. In neonates with the connection below the diaphragm, the increase

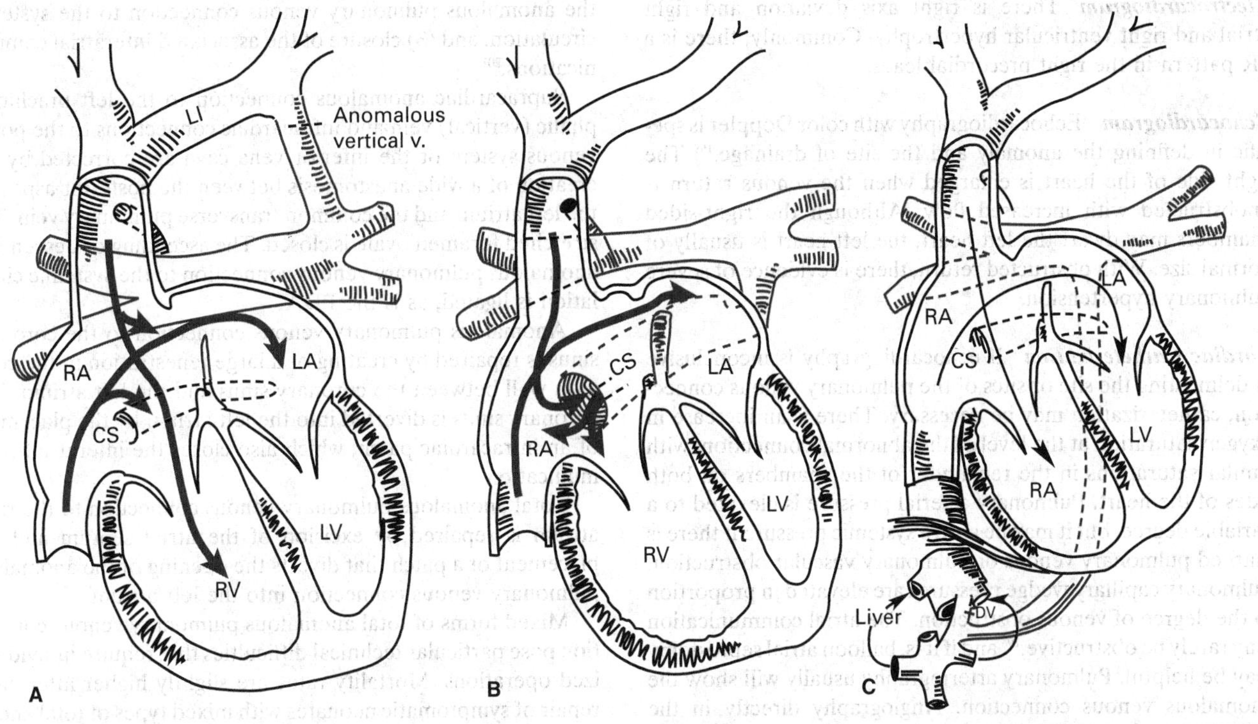

FIGURE 63-32 Three common types of total anomalous pulmonary venous connection. *A.* Total anomalous pulmonary venous connection to the left brachiocephalic (innominate) vein (LI). *B.* Total anomalous pulmonary venous connection to the coronary sinus (CS). *C.* Total anomalous pulmonary venous connection of the infradiaphragmatic type to the ductus venosus (DV). RA = right atrium; RV = right ventricle; LA = left atrium; LV = left ventricle.

in pulmonary flow as the pulmonary resistance decreases after birth cannot be accommodated and the obstruction to flow causes a marked increase in pulmonary venous pressure, resulting in a very high pulmonary vascular resistance. If the ductus arteriosus is still open, the pulmonary vascular resistance exceeds systemic vascular resistance with a right-to-left shunt at the ductal level. When the ductus closes, the increased pulmonary resistance results in increased right ventricular pressure. If the right ventricle fails, the right atrial pressure will increase, and right-to-left shunting at the atrial level may be present, often with profound hypoxemia.

In older children with unobstructed damage above the diaphragm (supracardiac), the pulmonary resistance is usually low. This low resistance facilitates a high pulmonary flow. With mixing of all pulmonary and systemic flow in the right atrium, the oxygen saturation is usually relatively high, resulting in physiology similar to that of an ASD and mild cyanosis.[198]

CLINICAL MANIFESTATIONS

Total Anomalous Pulmonary Venous Connection with Pulmonary Venous Obstruction Neonates with total anomalous pulmonary venous connection below the diaphragm who have pulmonary venous obstruction present with cyanosis, which may be severe, and dyspnea. Symptoms frequently develop beyond 12 h of age, allowing differentiation from respiratory distress syndrome. In addition to dyspnea, feeding difficulties and cardiac failure are seen.

The physical findings are usually unimpressive. The heart is not hyperactive, and thrills are absent. The second heart sound may be split, with an increased pulmonary component. Significant murmurs are uncommon.

Total Anomalous Pulmonary Venous Connection without Pulmonary Venous Obstruction These patients are usually asymptomatic at birth, although some may develop transient tachypnea. Presentation typically occurs during the first year of life. Some of these children have tachypnea and feeding difficulties, with frequent respiratory infections. Cyanosis often is mild and may not be clinically apparent. Other children may be asymptomatic and present with a heart murmur.

The cardiac examination is similar to that of an ASD with increased right-sided flow. The right ventricular impulse is usually hyperactive. The jugular venous pulse is elevated, and hepatomegaly appears early. There is a diffuse and hyperdynamic right ventricular impulse. The second heart sound is split and relatively fixed; the loudness of the pulmonary component may be increased. There is usually a grade 2 or 3 midsystolic flow murmur at the left sternal border. At the lower sternal border, there are a middiastolic rumble and prominent third and fourth heart sounds. Rales may be heard over the lung fields, and periorbital edema is common. A continuous murmur rarely may be heard over the common venous channel.

Chest Roentgenogram With the unobstructed types, the heart is enlarged with increased pulmonary flow. Pulmonary edema is uncommon. In patients with return to the left innominate vein, there may be a characteristic bulging of the superior mediastinum bilaterally, producing a "snowman," or figure-of-eight, contour. With obstructed types, the heart size is nearly normal; there is very marked pulmonary edema, which may give a granular appearance to the lungs, making differentiation from respiratory distress syndrome difficult in a newborn.

Electrocardiogram There is right axis deviation and right atrial and right ventricular hypertrophy. Commonly, there is a qR pattern in the right precordial leads.

Echocardiogram Echocardiography with color Doppler is specific in defining the anomaly and the site of drainage.[199] The right side of the heart is enlarged when the venous return is unobstructed with increased flow. Although the right-sided chambers may dwarf the left heart, the left heart is usually of normal size. With obstructed return, there is evidence of severe pulmonary hypertension.

Cardiac Catheterization If echocardiography is inconclusive in delineating the site or sites of the pulmonary venous connection, catheterization may be necessary. There is an increase in oxygen saturation at the level of the abnormal connection, with similar saturations in the remainder of the chambers on both sides of the heart. Pulmonary arterial pressure is elevated to a variable degree, but it may be above systemic pressure if there is marked pulmonary venous or pulmonary vascular obstruction. Pulmonary capillary wedge pressures are elevated in proportion to the degree of venous obstruction. The atrial communication may rarely be obstructive,[198] and if it is, balloon atrial septostomy may be helpful. Pulmonary arteriography usually will show the anomalous venous connection. Angiography directly in the common venous channel, if it is entered, will outline its course and any sites of obstruction optimally.

NATURAL HISTORY AND PROGNOSIS

The natural history varies depending on the degree of obstruction of egress of blood from the pulmonary veins.[198] Those who present in the perinatal period with severe cyanosis and respiratory distress, usually with pulmonary venous drainage below the diaghram, represent a medical emergency and will die without early surgery.

Those with supracardiac drainage and some degree of obstruction and therefore pulmonary hypertension are frequently sufficiently tachypneic that feeding is problematic, and they fail to gain weight at a normal rate. They tolerate respiratory infections poorly and occasionally need emergency surgery for respiratory failure.

Those with no pulmonary venous obstruction have large left-to-right shunts and mild cyanosis but may have no or minimal symptoms at rest or exercise. If corrective surgery is not performed, they are at risk for pulmonary vascular disease.[200]

MEDICAL MANAGEMENT

For neonates with severe cyanosis and respiratory disease, oxygen, a respirator, and PGE_1 can be used to temporize but survival is dependent on early surgery. For those with mild pulmonary hypertension and failure to thrive, surgery usually is performed semielectively. For those with no pulmonary hypertension, who usually present with murmurs and findings similar to those of an atrial septal defect, surgery is more elective but little is gained by waiting, and more centers are advocating early repair in this group as well.[201]

SURGICAL MANAGEMENT

Correction of total anomalous pulmonary venous connection requires (1) creation of a large communication between the left atrium and the pulmonary venous system, (2) obliteration of the anomalous pulmonary venous connection to the systemic circulation, and (3) closure of the associated interatrial communications.[201]

Supracardiac anomalous connection to the left brachiocephalic (vertical) vein and infracardiac connections to the portal venous system or the inferior vena cava are corrected by the creation of a wide anastomosis between the posterior aspect of the left atrium and the common transverse pulmonary vein. The stretched foramen ovale is closed. The ascending or descending anomalous pulmonary venous connection to the systemic circulation is ligated, as is the PDA.

Anomalous pulmonary venous connection to the coronary sinus is repaired by creating of a large fenestration in the common wall between the coronary sinus and the left atrium. The coronary sinus is diverted into the left atrium by the placement of an intracardiac patch, which also closes the interatrial communication.

Total anomalous pulmonary venous connection to the right atrium is repaired by excision of the atrial septum and the placement of a patch that diverts the opening of the anomalous pulmonary venous connection into the left atrium.

Mixed forms of total anomalous pulmonary venous connection pose particular technical difficulties that require individualized operations. Mortality rates are slightly higher after early repair of symptomatic neonates with mixed types of total anomalous pulmonary venous connections.

Although the results of repair of total anomalous pulmonary venous connection without obstruction in an older child have always been quite good, until recently neonates with obstructed total venous return have been problematic. In the 1960s and early 1970s, the surgical mortality rate exceeded 50 percent.[202] Between 1970 and 1980, surgical techniques improved and the mortality rate was reduced to 10 to 20 percent.[203] More recently, surgical results have continued to improve, with no mortality among 27 infants who underwent reparative surgery at Children's Hospital in Boston in the late 1980s.[204] Late survival has been quite good, with 98 percent surviving a median of 87 months in one study.[205]

After a satisfactory operative course, the prognosis has been excellent in those in whom a large common pulmonary vein can be attached to the back wall of the left atrium with a relatively large anastomosis. For those initially with obstructed total anomalous pulmonary venous return, the left atrium may be small and the anastomosis may be more difficult. Late obstruction of one or more pulmonary veins has been seen. When present, the obstruction can be approached by balloon dilation, stent placement, or repeat surgery.[206]

MALPOSITION OF THE CARDIAC STRUCTURES

Definition and Terminology

The *segmental approach* to the diagnosis of complex congenital heart disease[207] provides an orderly, effective method for determining the anatomic and hemodynamic interrelationships of the cardiac chambers, valves, and great vessels. For this approach to be better understood, certain definitions are helpful. Positioning of viscera is described as situs solitus, inversus, or ambiguous. In *situs solitus* (S), the distribution of all the organs is recognized as normal, for example, a left-sided stomach and spleen, a predominantly right-sided liver, a trilobed right lung, and a bilobed left lung. In *situs inversus* (*totalis*) (I), the organs show a perfect mirror image in regard to left and right to that of situs solitus. Anteroposterior relations are not disturbed. When neither situs solitus nor situs inversus can be identified, *situs ambiguous* (A) is said to be present. This usually applies in cases of asplenia or polysplenia.

With the rarest of exceptions, the *atria follow the body situs* and are so designated (morphologic right atrium to the right of the left atrium in atrial situs solitus and to the left of the left atrium in atrial situs inversus). The AV canal consists of the tricuspid valve, the mitral valve, and the septum of the AV canal and connects the atrial portion with the ventricular portion of the heart. As a rule, *each AV valve is part of the specific ventricle into which it leads*. The valve situs may be solitus, inversus, or ambiguous.

The alignment or type of AV or ventriculoarterial (VA) connection addresses the issue of what flows into what. The connection may be described at the AV or VA level as concordant (e.g., right atrium to right ventricle, left ventricle to aorta) or discordant (e.g., right atrium to left ventricle, left ventricle to pulmonary artery) or may be considered an arrangement that requires a special description. In the case of AV alignment in which the atria are not lateralized, the alignment would be ambiguous. In the univentricular heart, the designation would be double-inlet, absent right, or absent left AV connection. Special descriptions in the case of VA alignment or type of VA connection include double-outlet and single-outlet VA connection. The mode of connections, either AV or VA, addresses the structural makeup of the connecting segments: the AV canal and the infundibulum or conus. The mode of AV connection may be normal, common, stenotic, imperforate, atretic, double-orifice, overriding, straddling, or unguarded. The mode of VA connection may be expressed in terms of the position and development of the conus or infundibulum, which, although normally incorporated into the right ventricle, is not an intrinsic part of the true right ventricle. It may be described as subpulmonary, subaortic, very deficient, or bilaterally present or absent.[208]

The position of the ventricles may be described by the terms *d loop* and *l loop*. When the morphologic right ventricle lies to the right of the morphologic left ventricle, the ventricular portion of the heart is said to exhibit a d loop (D). The ventricles are said to be noninverted or in the solitus position. When the ventricular relations are reversed, l loop (L) is said to be present. The ventricles are inverted or in the inversus position. *These relationships are independent of the visceral or atrial situs as well as the position of the heart or its chambers within the chest.*

The great arteries may deviate from the usual with respect to both their anteroposterior and lateral (left-to-right) relationships. In solitus (S) or *normally related great arteries* (NRGA), the aortic origin lies to the right of and posterior to the position of the pulmonary valve. In the inversus (I) relationship, the anteroposterior relationships are not disturbed but the aortic origin lies to the left of the pulmonary arterial origin. In *transposition of the great arteries* (TGA), the aorta arises from the anatomic right ventricle, the pulmonary artery arises from the anatomic left ventricle, and usually the aortic origin is more anterior than that of the pulmonary artery.

When the aortic origin lies to the right of the pulmonary origin, the transposition is called *dextro* or *d transposition* (D-TGA) (see the discussion of complete transposition of the great arteries, below). When the aortic origin lies to the left of the pulmonary origin, *levo transposition* (L-TGA) is said to be present (see the section on congenitally corrected transposition, below).

When the abnormal relationship of the great arteries is neither complete nor corrected transposition, the term *malposition of the great arteries* (MGA) may be used. Malpositions are designated as D-MGA or L-MGA, depending on the laterality in the relation between the origins of the two great arteries.[208] Within this group are found examples of the abnormal VA alignment, where one great artery arises from the appropriate ventricle and the other great artery also arises from the same (or inappropriate) ventricle. These are examples of *double-outlet right ventricle* (DORV) or *double-outlet left ventricle* (DOLV). Also included is the arterial malposition termed *anatomically corrected malposition* (ACM). This is characterized by the great arteries having a normal VA alignment (concordant), but with the aorta anterior to the pulmonary artery by virtue of an abnormal mode of VA connection: the presence of a well-developed conus lying beneath both the aorta and the pulmonary artery or only beneath the aorta. The route for the flow of blood in ACMs may be normal or abnormal, depending on the AV alignment.[208]

The Segmental Approach to Diagnosis

The segmental, or step-by-step, approach is a valuable tool for arriving at the correct diagnosis in patients with complex congenital heart disease and is independent of cardiac position. In order, one determines (1) the locations of the right and left atria and their venous connections, (2) the location of the right and left ventricles and their alignment with the atria, (3) the mode of connection of the AV valves to the ventricles, (4) the position of the great arteries and their alignment with the ventricles, and (5) the location and status of the infundibulum. In addition, one must search for associated malformations between and within each of these segments.

Determining atrial situs can be accomplished in most instances by taking advantage of the high degree of abdominal visceroatrial concordance. With abdominal situs solitus (S), the liver is on the right and the right atrium almost invariably is on the right as well; with abdominal situs inversus (I), the liver is on the left and the right atrium almost invariably is on the left. With abdominal situs ambiguous (A), the liver may be placed almost symmetrically across the midline and the atria may be located normally or inverted or both atria may have morphologic characteristics of either the right atrium or the left atrium (Fig. 12-4). A symmetric liver is found in approximately 60 percent of patients with situs ambiguous. Lateralization of the liver, which is evident in the remainder, may simulate either situs solitus or situs inversus.

When both atria have characteristics of a right atrium,[209] *dextroisomerism*, or "bilateral right-sidedness," is said to be present. This situation is usually, though not invariably, accompanied by asplenia. When both atria have characteristics of a left atrium, *levoisomerism*, or "bilateral left-sidedness," is said to exist. This usually, but again not invariably, is accompanied by polysplenia.

Bronchial situs, as determined by overpenetrated chest roentgenogram or bronchial tomography, is an excellent predictor of atrial situs, but the most accurate technique appears to be two-dimensional echocardiography with Doppler color flow mapping. The hepatic portion of the inferior vena cava, which almost always enters the morphologic right atrium, usually can be identified easily, as can the connections and structural details of the superior vena cava, coronary sinus, pulmonary veins, atrial septum, and atrial appendages.

Additional clinical clues to atrial situs may be obtained from the ECG, where a superior and leftward orientation of the P-wave vector suggests levoisomerism and polysplenia. Howell-Heinz and Howell-Jolly bodies in the peripheral blood smear are characteristic of dextroisomerism or asplenia.

For determination of the AV, ventricular, and VA relationships, high-quality selective biplane angiography, supplemented by equally high-quality two-dimensional echocardiography with Doppler color flow mapping, is essential.[209] Symbols used to designate the combination or sequence of segments are arranged in order as follows: (1) the visceroatrial or bronchoatrial situs, (2) the ventricular loop, and (3) the relations of the great arteries. These may be included within parentheses and preceded by abbreviations that indicate the VA alignment, for example, TGA, DORV, or single ventricle (SV). Associated malformations such as VSD, pulmonary stenosis, and straddling tricuspid valve may be listed after the parentheses. Thus, the typical or usual transposition of the great arteries with situs solitus, d-ventricular loop, and aorta arising from the right ventricle and to the right of the pulmonary artery, with an intact ventricular septum (IVS), would be designated TGA (SDD) IVS. The designation for typical corrected transposition (TGA) with situs solitus (S), l-ventricular loop (L), aorta arising from the morphologic right ventricle and lying to the left of the pulmonary artery (L), with VSD and pulmonary stenosis (PS), would be TGA (SLL), VSD, PS. This designation would apply to transposition with situs solitus, whether the heart lay in the right or left chest (dextrocardia or levocardia, respectively). It should be noted that the description of the position of the heart within the chest would offer no additional information referable to the intracardiac anatomy or great vessel alignment.[207]

Levocardia, Dextrocardia, and Mesocardia

The position of the cardiac apex indicates a condition of levocardia, dextrocardia, or mesocardia.

The trend today is to discard the terms *dextroposition, dextroversion, mirror-image dextrocardia,* and *isolated dextrocardia* because they do not provide any significant information beyond what is already known—that the cardiac apex is in the right chest—and to use the broad term *dextrocardia* for all right-sided hearts, followed by a description of the visceroatrial situs. In the case of patients in whom the heart appears to have been pulled or pushed into the right chest by massive atelectasis or hypoplasia of the right lung, diaphragmatic hernia, eventration of the diaphragm, pleural effusion, obstructive emphysema, or pneumothorax, an appropriate descriptive phrase should be added. The term *isolated levocardia* is applied to all left-sided hearts with situs inversus or situs ambiguous, and a description of the visceroatrial situs should follow.

Dextrocardia with complete situs inversus occurs in approximately 2 per 10,000 live births. *The incidence of congenital heart disease is relatively low among these individuals and is estimated to be about 3 percent.* Dextrocardia with situs solitus or situs ambiguous is considerably less common and occurs in perhaps 1 in 20,000 live births. The incidence of congenital heart disease is extremely high in this situation, however, probably in the range of 90 percent or greater. From these figures, one could project that approximately 12 percent of individuals found to have dextrocardia and congenital heart disease would have complete situs inversus. This estimate compares favorably with the figure of 18 percent observed in large autopsy series. About 50 percent of patients with dextrocardia and heart disease have situs solitus, and the remainder, perhaps 30 percent, have situs ambiguous.[207] An l-ventricular loop is found in the majority of patients with dextrocardia regardless of situs but is most common, as one might expect, among patients with situs inversus, in whom it approaches 80 percent. Cardiac malformations usually, although not invariably, are severe and complex. The most common lesions and their approximate frequency are as follows: transposition of the great arteries, 50 to 75 percent; double-outlet right ventricle, 10 to 18 percent; VSD, 60 to 80 percent; single ventricle, 15 to 40 percent; and pulmonary stenosis or atresia, 70 to 80 percent.[207] Approximately three-quarters of transposed great arteries have the segmental arrangement of corrected transposition. Tetralogy of Fallot is distinctly uncommon. Polysplenia or asplenia is found in about one-third of patients with dextrocardia and almost invariably with situs ambiguous. Kartagener's syndrome, the triad of situs inversus, sinusitis, and bronchiectasis, results from impaired ciliary movement. It is present in approximately 20 percent of patients with dextrocardia and situs inversus totalis.[210] The incidence of isolated levocardia has been estimated at approximately 0.6 per 10,000 live births. It is estimated that over 90 percent of affected individuals have associated heart disease. Situs inversus is present in approximately 15 percent, and the remainder have situs ambiguous, with the ratio of asplenia to polysplenia or accessory spleens being from 2.5:1 to 1.5:1. The associated defects are comparable in complexity and severity to those associated with dextrocardia. *Mesocardia* may exist as a variant position of the normal heart or a variant position of dextrocardia or isolated levocardia.

MEDICAL AND SURGICAL MANAGEMENT

Medical management of patients with cardiac malposition is similar to that of patients with normally located hearts, with the exceptions of continuous daily antibiotic coverage and pneumococcal vaccine for patients with asplenia and the particular attention to detail that is necessary to establish the correct diagnosis in individuals with unusual and complex malformations. Surgical management differs in the technical considerations imposed by the malposition of the heart itself, the frequency of occurrence of the l-ventricular loop, and the variability of the intracardiac conduction system.

Dextro Transposition of the Great Arteries

DEFINITION

In this condition, the aorta and the pulmonary artery are misplaced in relation to the ventricular septum, with the aorta arising from the right ventricle and the pulmonary artery arising from the left ventricle (discordant VA connection).

PATHOLOGY

In the majority of cases, there are situs solitus of the atria and viscera (S) and concordance of the AV connection and the right

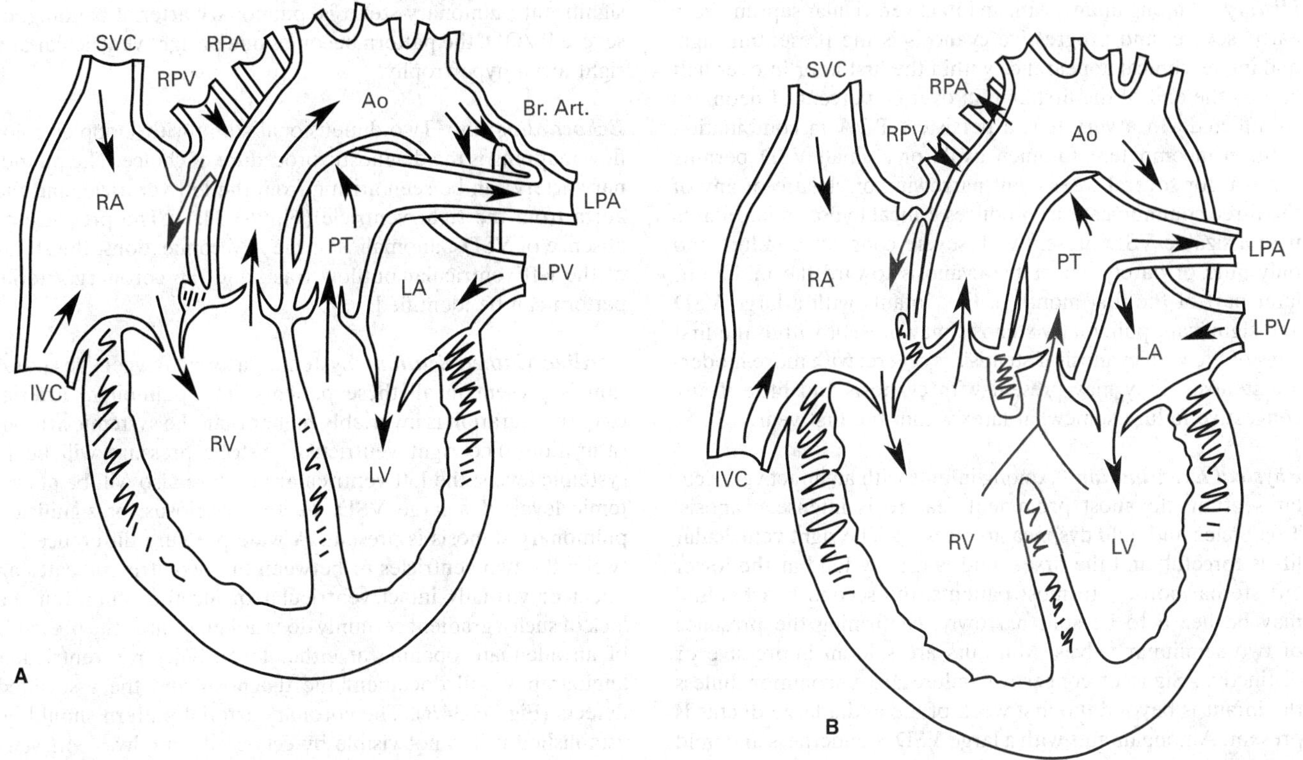

FIGURE 63-33 Complete D transposition of the great arteries. *A.* With intact ventricular septum. A patent foramen ovale and enlarged bronchial arteries (Br. Art.) are present. *B.* With ventricular septal defect and without pulmonary stenosis. SVC = superior vena cava; IVC = inferior vena cava; RA = right atrium; RV = right ventricle; Ao = aorta; LA = left atrium; LV = left ventricle.

ventricle lies to the right of the left ventricle (d loop, D) (Fig. 63-33). The aorta lies to the right of the pulmonary arterial origin (d transposition, D) and is anterior. Of the communications between the two sides of the circulation, a narrow patent foramen and PDA are common in very young infants. The ventricular septum is intact in approximately half these patients, and another 10 percent have only a very small VSD. The remainder have a large VSD or multiple VSDs.[211]

Pulmonary stenosis of significance is very uncommon among neonates with an intact ventricular septum but develops with the passage of time in approximately one-third of patients in whom the right ventricle continues to be the systemic ventricle. In most cases it is mild and usually, though not invariably, is the result of a bulging of the ventricular septum into the left ventricular outflow area. Approximately one-third of patients with a large VSD have significant left ventricular outflow tract obstruction (pulmonary stenosis). Causes of this obstruction include leftward malalignment of the infundibular septum, the presence of a membranous collar or ridge encircling the left ventricular outflow tract, anomalous adhesion of the anterior mitral leaflet to the ventricular septum, stenotic deformity of the pulmonary valve, and, rarely, an aneurysm of endocardial tissue related to the VSD.[212]

The coronary arteries usually arise from the two aortic sinuses adjacent to the pulmonary trunk—the "facing sinuses"—with the most common arrangement being the right coronary artery arising from the rightward sinus and the left coronary artery, with its anterior descending and circumflex branches, arising from the leftward sinus.

Hypertensive pulmonary vascular disease may occur at an inordinately early age and may occur even in patients with an intact ventricular septum and initially low left ventricular pressures. Three-quarters or more of patients with d transposition, situs solitus, and d loop [TGA (SDD)] either have no significant associated cardiac defects or have relatively simple malformations in the form of VSD, ASD, PDA, or pulmonary stenosis. The remainder have more complicated lesions and will not be discussed in this section.

ABNORMAL PHYSIOLOGY

The systemic and pulmonary circulations are arranged so that the systemic venous return is conducted back to the systemic arterial system and the pulmonary venous return is conducted back to the pulmonary arterial system, with no obligatory mixing or interchange. For survival, there must be communication between the two circulations in the form of a patent foramen ovale, a PDA, or a VSD. The hemodynamics are dependent on the combination of defects present and particularly on the amount of mixing between the systemic and pulmonary circulations. The right ventricle is the systemic ventricle, and its systolic pressure is the same as systemic arterial pressure.

CLINICAL MANIFESTATIONS

Approximately 3 to 4 percent of children with recognized congenital heart disease have transposition of the great arteries (Table 63-1). Males are more commonly afflicted than are females in a ratio between 2:1 and 3:1.

History Among infants with an intact ventricular septum, very early, severe, and progressive cyanosis is the presenting sign, making its clinical appearance within the first hour in over half and by the end of the first 24 h in over 60 percent of neonates so afflicted.[3] In a very few, a persistent PDA in combination with an incompetent foramen ovale or a small VSD permits survival for several weeks, but narrowing or closure of any of the three communications produces critical hypoxemia. Infants with a sizable VSD present with severe congestive failure and only mild or barely detectable cyanosis toward the middle or later part of the first month of life. Infants with a large VSD and significant pulmonary stenosis may present within the first days of life with cyanosis if stenosis is severe; with more moderate stenosis, they may present with cyanosis and little if any congestive failure somewhat later within the first year.

Physical Examination Among infants with an intact ventricular septum, the most prominent feature is intense cyanosis. Tachypnea and mild dyspnea are present. The right ventricular lift is forceful, and the first sound is usually loud at the lower left sternal border. In most patients, the second heart sound may be heard to be split narrowly, confirming the presence of two semilunar valves. Murmurs are seldom impressive or distinctive. Signs of congestive failure are uncommon unless the infant is beyond the first week of life and a large ductus is present. Among infants with a large VSD, slenderness and mild cyanosis or a grayish pallor are apparent. Breathing is labored, and both the right and left ventricular impulses are hyperactive. A thrill is uncommon. A systolic murmur at the lower left sternal border is usually present but is seldom loud or completely holosystolic. A gallop rhythm and a diastolic flow rumble at the apex are typical. Infants and children with VSD and significant pulmonary stenosis generally are severely cyanotic.

Chest Roentgenogram With an intact ventricular septum, the heart size and pulmonary vascularity appear normal or at the upper limits of normal during the first week. Later, a narrow base caused by the displaced pulmonary artery may give rise to the characteristic "egg-on-side" contour. Impressive cardiomegaly, pulmonary plethora, and this characteristic contour are more common during the second week and beyond. With a large VSD, marked cardiac enlargement involving all chambers, impressive pulmonary plethora, and the egg-on-side contour are present. With significant pulmonary stenosis, the heart resembles that of a patient with tetralogy of Fallot, but it is usually slightly larger and the pulmonary vascularity is less diminished than one would expect for a comparable degree of clinical cyanosis. A right aortic arch is present in 4 to 16 percent of those patients.

Electrocardiogram If the ventricular septum is intact, the ECG may reveal tall or peaked P waves by the second or third day of life; however, clearly abnormal right ventricular forces usually are not apparent until the latter part of the first week. The persistence of an upright T wave in leads V_1 and V_{3R} beyond 4 days of age provides an early clue that the right ventricular systolic pressure is at systemic levels. An older infant will have abnormal right axis deviation and marked right ventricular hypertrophy. A large VSD with a large pulmonary blood flow usually will produce biatrial and biventricular hypertrophy. If pulmonary blood flow is reduced toward normal, whether by significant pulmonary stenosis, pulmonary arterial banding, or severe PVOD, the pattern becomes one of right ventricular and right atrial hypertrophy.

Echocardiogram Two-dimensional study with Doppler color flow mapping is the diagnostic procedure of choice. The pulmonary artery can be seen arising from the left ventricle, and the aorta from the right ventricle (Fig. 63-34*A*). The presence or absence of VSDs, anomalies of the AV connections, the status of the left ventricular outflow tract, and the coronary arterial pattern can be identified.

Cardiac Catheterization Systemic arterial oxygen desaturation is present in all these patients. The pulmonary arterial oxygen saturation is invariably higher than the systemic arterial saturation. The right ventricular systolic pressure will be at systemic levels; the left ventricular pressure also will be at systemic levels if a large VSD, ductus arteriosus, or significant pulmonary stenosis is present. A wide pressure difference between the two ventricles or between the two atria indicates an intact or virtually intact ventricular or atrial septum, but the lack of such a gradient certainly does not guarantee the presence of an adequate opening at either level. Selective ventricular angiography will document the diagnosis and the associated defects (Fig. 63-34*B*). The coronary arterial pattern should be established if it is not visible by echocardiography.[213] *All newborns with transposition can benefit from balloon atrial septostomy at catheterization by virtue of the increased mixing of the pulmonary and systemic venous circulations and the decompression of the left atrium.*

NATURAL HISTORY AND PROGNOSIS

Without balloon septostomy or surgical intervention, 50 percent of infants with transposition die within the first month and 90 percent die within the first year of life.[214] Those with an intact ventricular septum die very early from hypoxemia. Those with a large VSD usually live somewhat longer, but the majority die in the first months of congestive failure; the few survivors have severe PVOD. Those with a large VSD and pulmonary stenosis have the best outlook, but the average life expectancy is barely 5 years even with this combination of defects. With an adequate interatrial opening, whether natural, balloon-induced, or surgically created, infants with an intact ventricular septum do relatively well during the first year. Increasing cyanosis during the first year in these patients may be due to a gradual diminution of the size of the atrial septal opening, narrowing or closure of a persistent PDA or small VSD, the gradual development of subvalvular pulmonary stenosis, or the development of PVOD. Before age 2 years, cerebrovascular accidents are a hazard to these hypoxemic infants and occur almost invariably in a setting of relative anemia rather than extreme polycythemia. The appearance of PVOD is unusual but can occur within the first 12 months of life. It becomes more common, approaching 40 percent, in the second year of life and thereafter. Infants with a large VSD and no significant pulmonary stenosis will develop PVOD and become prohibitive risks for corrective surgery by the end of the first year of life. Those with a VSD and severe pulmonary stenosis usually become progressively more cyanotic.

Palliative and subsequent corrective operations have enabled a relatively large group of patients to survive beyond infancy and early childhood. Among the survivors of the atrial switch operations, such as the Mustard and Senning procedures, are found residual abnormalities such as pulmonary stenosis and PVOD as well as complications that result from surgery. These complications include residual intraatrial baffle leaks, systemic and/or pulmonary venous obstruction, and arrhythmias. Late sudden death has been described in about 3 percent of survivors and very possibly results from arrhythmias. Finally, right ventricular dysfunction with or without progressive tricuspid regurgitation has been documented in many of the somewhat older survivors of atrial inversion operations and raises the question of whether the right ventricle can function adequately as the systemic arterial ventricle beyond adolescence and early adult life.

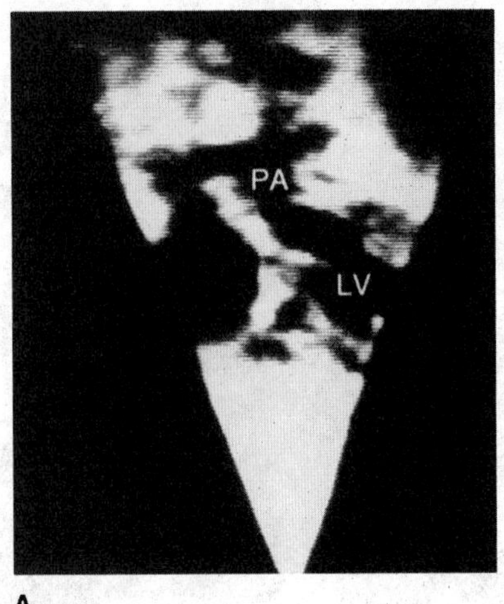

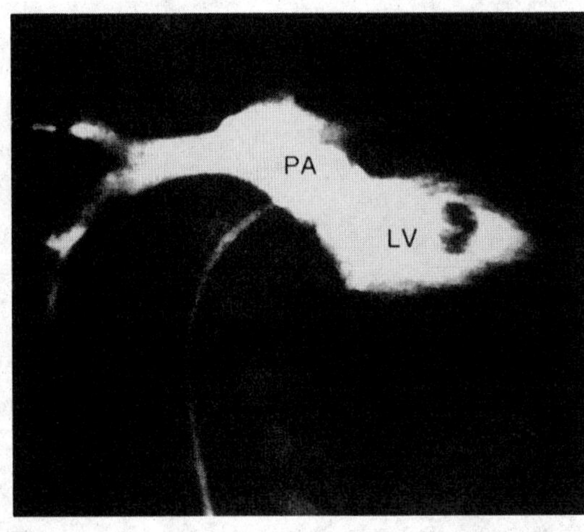

FIGURE 63-34 *A.* Two-dimensional echocardiogram. The left ventricle leads to a bifurcating great vessel (pulmonary artery, PA), confirming transposition. *B.* Anterolateral projection of an angiogram in the smooth-walled left ventricle (LV). The dye is ejected into the pulmonary artery.

While complications have been problematic for some, long-term follow-up of the group as a whole has been good. The Toronto experience is the oldest and largest. Among 534 children who underwent a "Mustard" procedure since 1962, there were 52 early deaths (9.7 percent). Survival at 5 years was 89 percent, and it was 76 percent at 20 years.[215] In a study from New Zealand of 113 hospital survivors of surgery performed between 1964 and 1982, survival at 10, 20, and 28 years was 90 80, and 80 percent, respectively, with 76 percent of survivors being New York Heart Association class I.[216] There has been less long-term follow-up of survivors of the "Senning" type of atrial repair. In a recent study of 100 patients, the actuarial survival at 13 years was 90 percent for those with simple transposition and 78 percent survival for those with complex disease.[217]

MEDICAL MANAGEMENT

The first step in the treatment of infants with an intact ventricular septum is to provide without delay an adequate systemic arterial oxygen saturation. This can be achieved in almost all instances by establishing an adequate interatrial opening with balloon atrial septostomy and providing adequate systemic arterial-to-pulmonary arterial shunting via the ductus with the use of intravenous PGE_1 infusion;[91] the latter procedure frequently is supplemented by endotracheal intubation to compensate for prostaglandin-related apnea. The adequacy of the atrial septostomy opening can be determined by a sustained increase in the systemic arterial oxygen saturation to above 60 percent and verified by direct visualization with two-dimensional echocardiography. If the relief of hypoxemia is unsatisfactory with PGE_1 alone and if the interatrial opening is judged by echocardiography to be small, the alternatives are to perform a balloon atrial septectomy without delay or to proceed directly with corrective surgery in the form of the arterial switch operation.

SURGICAL MANAGEMENT

Arterial switch repair is now the preferred surgical alternative to the atrial inversion procedures for a neonate with an intact ventricular septum and for a slightly older infant with a large VSD and without significant structural pulmonary stenosis (Fig. 63-35). Arterial switching should be performed within the first 2 to 3 weeks of life, before left ventricular systolic pressure falls significantly below that of the right ventricle. For infants beyond 3 weeks of age, if the ratio of left ventricular to right ventricular pressure has fallen below 0.60, a pulmonary arterial band may be applied with or without a systemic-to-pulmonary arterial shunt and the arterial switch operation may be performed approximately 1 week later. Most patterns of coronary arterial origin and course appear to be amenable to the operation, and infants as small as 2.0 kg may be repaired successfully.

In some centers, the surgical risks have been reduced to about 5 to 10 percent,[218] although in other centers, the surgical mortality continues to be higher.[219] Short- and medium-term prognosis is good,[220] but longer-term studies are awaited. The most common problem has been stenosis at the pulmonary artery anastomotic site.[221] When severe, this usually has been amenable to balloon dilation or stenting.[222]

For infants with transposition, a large VSD, and pulmonary hypertension, the arterial switch technique with VSD closure must be carried out within the first 2 months of life to prevent severe PVOD. Infants with a large VSD and severe pulmonary stenosis usually may be palliated with a systemic-to-pulmonary arterial shunt and repaired in later infancy or as young children,[175] although some centers are doing reparative surgery in infancy.[223] Finally, the severe hypoxemia present in children with a large VSD and severe PVOD may be reduced by an intraatrial repair performed as a palliative procedure, with no attempt at closure of the VSD.[224]

Double-Outlet Right Ventricle

PATHOLOGY

In this malformation, more than 50 percent of the semilunar valve orifices of both great arteries arise from the morphologic right ventricle. In most cases, the ventricles display a d loop, and the pulmonary arterial origin is normally positioned, arising from a conus above the right ventricle. The aorta also arises

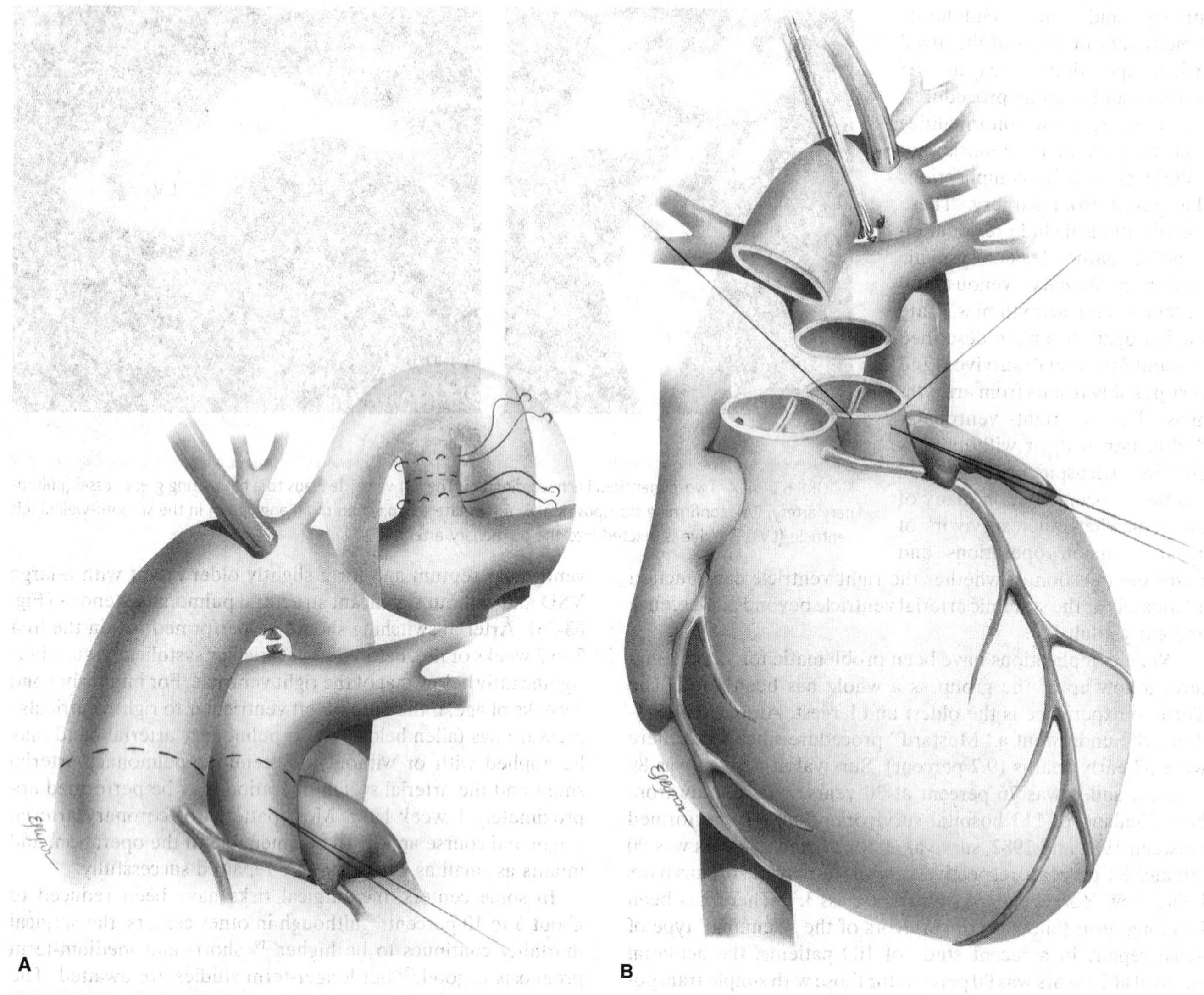

FIGURE 63-35 Surgical technique of the arterial switch operation. *A.* Aortic cannula is positioned distally in the ascending aorta, the ductus arteriosus is divided between suture ligatures, and the branch pulmonary arteries are dissected out to the hilum to provide adequate mobility for anterior translocation. The broken lines represent the levels of transection of the aorta and the main pulmonary artery. Marking sutures are placed in the anticipated sites of coronary transfer. *B.* Transection of the great arteries. The left ventricular outflow tract, neoaortic valve, and coronary arteries are inspected thoroughly. *C.* The coronary arterial buttons are excised from the free edge of the aorta to the base of the sinus of Valsalva. *D.* The coronary buttons are anastomosed to V-shaped excisions made in the neoaorta. *E.* The pulmonary artery is brought anterior to the aorta (Lecompte maneuver). Anastomosis of the proximal neoaorta is shown. *F* and *G.* The coronary donor sites are filled with autologous pericardial patches. A single U-shaped patch (*F*) or two separate patches (*G*) may be used. *H.* Completed anastomosis of the proximal neopulmonary artery and the distal pulmonary artery. (Modified from Castaneda AR. Anatomic correction of transposition of the great arteries at the arterial level. In: Sabiston DC Jr, Spencer FC, eds. *Surgery of the Chest.* 5th ed. Philadelphia: Saunders; 1990. Reproduced with permission from the authors and publisher.)

from the right ventricle above conal tissue. The two semilunar valves are at about the same level, and there is no fibrous continuity between the semilunar and mitral valves (Fig. 63-36).

In most cases, the aortic origin is to the right (d malposition) of the pulmonary arterial origin, with the two vessels usually displaying a side-by-side relationship. Uncommonly, the aortic origin is distinctly anterior to the pulmonary origin or the aorta arises to the left (l malposition) of the pulmonary artery.[225]

With rare exceptions, there is a VSD. The condition may be subdivided further on the basis of the relation of the VSD to the origin of the great arteries. The VSD is subaortic in approximately two-thirds of patients, subpulmonary (*Taussig-Bing heart*) in 18 percent, related to both great arteries (*doubly committed*) in 3 percent, and remote or unrelated to either great artery in about 7 percent.[225]

ASSOCIATED CONDITIONS

Pulmonary stenosis occurs in over half these cases, with the condition usually resulting from a narrow subpulmonary conus. ASD, subaortic stenosis, and coarctation of the aorta are also relatively common, with the latter particularly associated with the subpulmonary defect. Obstruction at the mitral valve may be observed in about one-fifth of cases of double-outlet right ventricle. Mitral valve straddling of the VSD and varying degrees of left ventricular hypoplasia also are encountered.

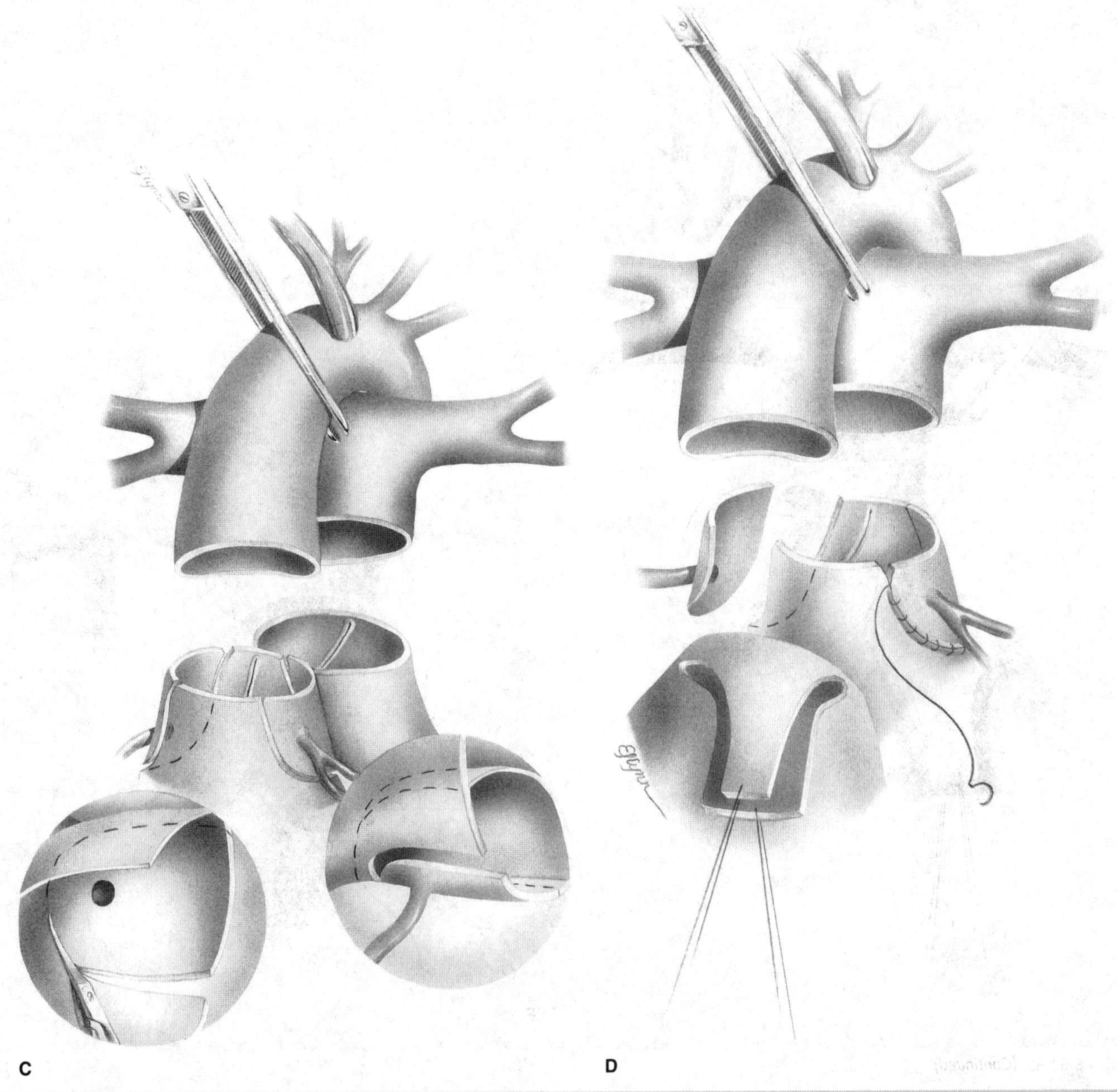

FIGURE 63-35 (*Continued*)

CLINICAL MANIFESTATIONS

Double-outlet right ventricle, or origin of both great arteries from the right ventricle, is a relatively rare malformation that is found in only 0.8 percent of patients with congenital heart disease. It is of considerable importance, however, because its clinical and laboratory features frequently resemble those of more common and more easily correctable malformations. Double-outlet right ventricle reflects the relationship of the great vessels to the ventricular septum; the presentation and treatment of children with this condition depend on the associated anomalies.

History and Physical Examination Patients with a subaortic VSD without pulmonary stenosis (Fig. 63-36*A*) have the same findings on examination as do patients with a large isolated VSD. Congestive failure appears within a few weeks of birth, and cyanosis is seldom described. Those with a subaortic VSD and pulmonary stenosis (Fig. 63-36*B*) usually present after the newborn period and follow a course similar to that of patients with tetralogy of Fallot. Patients with a subpulmonary defect without pulmonary stenosis (Fig. 63-36*C*), the Taussig-Bing malformation, resemble patients with transposition of the great arteries and a large VSD without pulmonary stenosis. The findings are those of severe congestive failure and cyanosis.

Chest Roentgenogram Cardiomegaly with pulmonary overperfusion is characteristic of all types of this anomaly without pulmonary stenosis. Double-outlet right ventricle with subaortic VSD and pulmonary stenosis resembles tetralogy of Fallot. In the case of subpulmonary VSD without pulmonary stenosis,

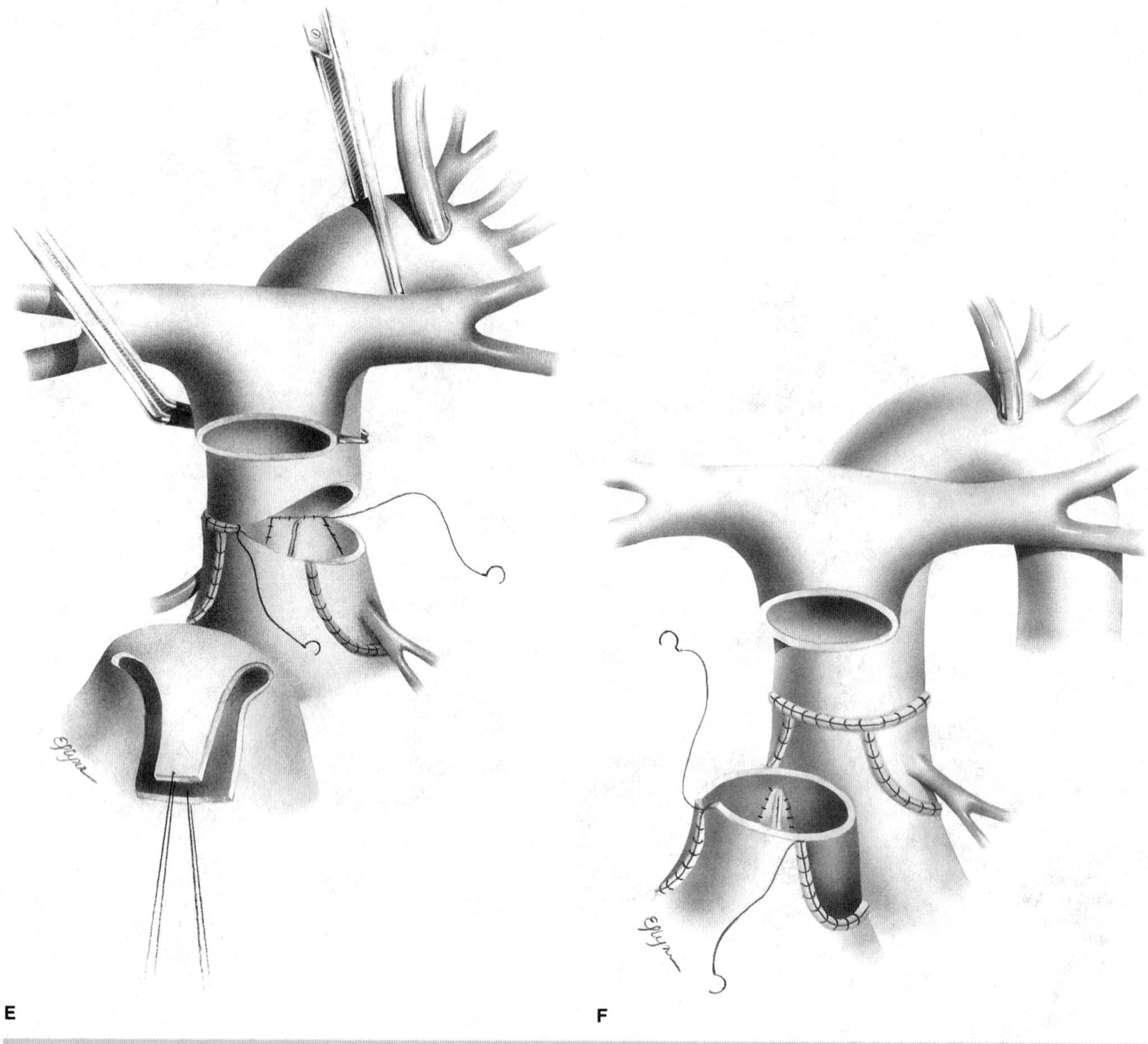

FIGURE 63-35 (*Continued*)

the pulmonary artery usually lies beside rather than posterior to the aorta; this clearly visible, dilated main pulmonary artery may permit distinction of this malformation from transposition, which it mimics so closely.

Electrocardiogram Right axis deviation and right atrial and right ventricular hypertrophy are characteristic of double-outlet right ventricle.

Echocardiogram Two-dimensional echocardiography is very useful in demonstrating the anatomic components and associated defects.[225,226]

Cardiac Catheterization There is an increase in oxygen saturation at the right ventricular level. The pulmonary arterial saturation is lower than that of the aorta in patients with a subaortic VSD and is invariably higher than that of the aorta in those with a subpulmonary septal defect and transposition physiology. Left ventricular systolic pressure may be higher than right pressure if the VSD is small and restrictive. Selective right and left ventricular biplane angiography and an aortogram are recommended.

NATURAL HISTORY AND PROGNOSIS

The clinical course of each variety of double-outlet right ventricle is determined by the associated defects. Without surgical intervention, those with an unguarded pulmonary artery either die in infancy with congestive failure or develop PVOD. Spontaneous narrowing or closure of the VSD may occur and is life-threatening. Increasing dyspnea, increasing intensity of the systolic murmur, and progressive left ventricular hypertrophy suggest this complication. Patients with pulmonary stenosis tend to have progressive obstruction and cyanosis.

MEDICAL MANAGEMENT

Vigorous treatment of heart failure is required for those without pulmonary stenosis. Almost all cases are best treated with surgical palliation or correction in infancy. If there is pulmonary

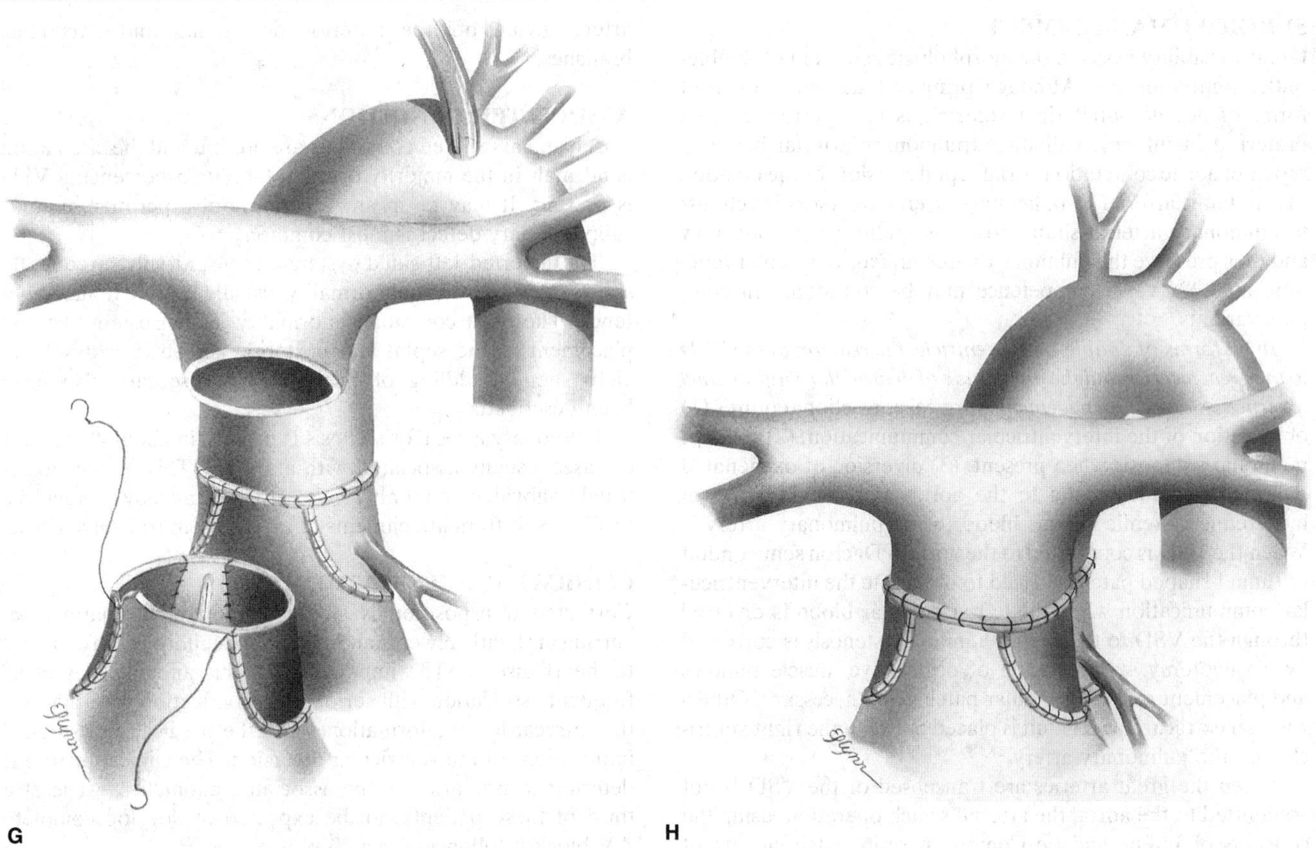

G

H

FIGURE 63-35 (*Continued*)

hypertension, banding or correction should be done by 2 to 3 months of age. Patients with ventricular hypoplasia, mitral stenoses, straddling AV valves, or a remote VSD are usually not candidates for biventricular repair, and initial palliation should prepare the child for a modification of the Fontan operation. Whether or not corrective surgery has been performed, all patients in whom the left ventricular output must pass through the VSD should be observed continuously for the possibility of spontaneous narrowing and obstruction at that site.

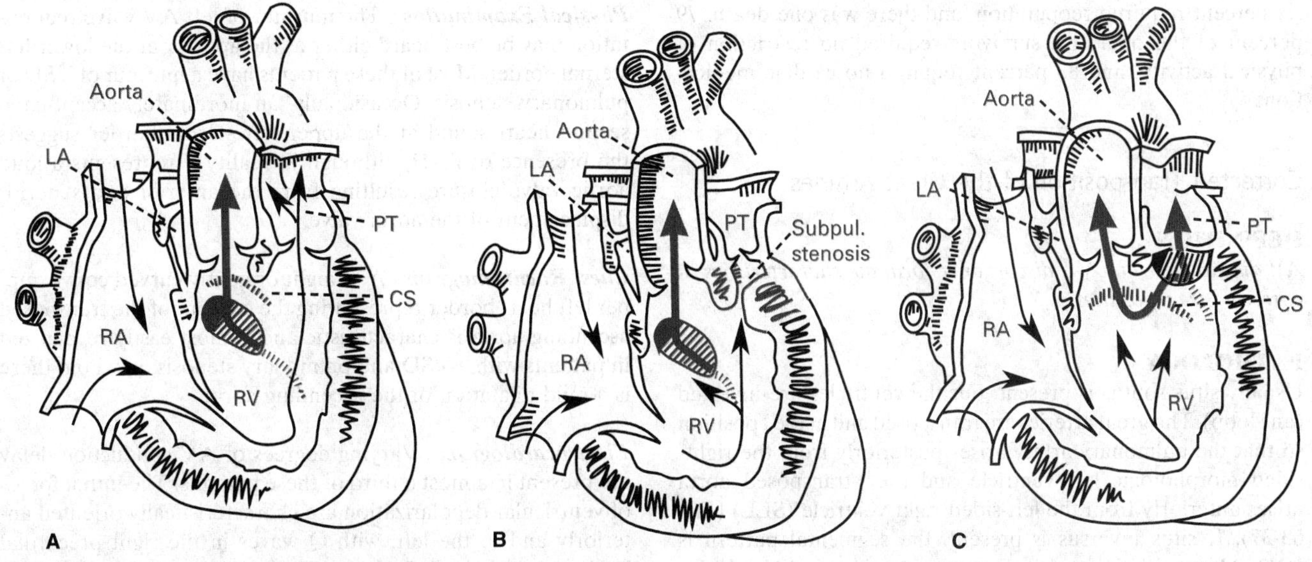

FIGURE 63-36 Double-outlet right ventricle. *A.* With subaortic ventricular septal defect without pulmonary stenosis. *B.* With subaortic ventricular septal defect and subpulmonary stenosis (Subpul. stenosis). *C.* With subpulmonary, supracristal ventricular septal defect. The so-called Taussig-Bing complex. RA = right atrium; RV = right ventricle; CS = crista supraventricularis; LA = left atrium; PT = main pulmonary arterial trunk.

SURGICAL MANAGEMENT

Great variability exists in the morphologic spectrum of double-outlet right ventricle. Although primary total repair of most forms of double-outlet right ventricle is now performed and preferred in infancy, palliation (pulmonary arterial banding, repair of aortic coarctation, atrial septal excision, or the creation of a systemic arterial-to-pulmonary arterial or systemic venous-to-pulmonary arterial shunt) to adjust pulmonary blood flow and thus preserve the pulmonary vascular bed, ventricular function, and AV valve competence may be considered in complex variants.

In all forms of double-outlet ventricle, the relation of the VSD to the great arteries and the magnitude of ventricular outflow tract obstruction dictate management. Surgical correction requires (1) obliteration of the interventricular communication, (2) relief of pulmonary stenosis when present, (3) diversion of oxygenated pulmonary venous blood to the aorta, and (4) diversion of hypoxemic systemic venous blood to the pulmonary artery.[227] When the VSD is committed to the aorta, a Dacron semiconduit or tunnel-shaped patch is placed to obliterate the interventricular communication while the left ventricular blood is diverted through the VSD to the aorta. Pulmonary stenosis is corrected by a valvotomy, with excision of obstructive muscle bundles and placement of a transannular patch when necessary. Otherwise, an extracardiac conduit is placed between the right ventricle and the pulmonary artery.[228,229]

When the great arteries are transposed or the VSD is not committed to the aorta, the arterial switch operation, using the concepts of Jatene and Le Compte, permits patch closure of the VSD, directing left ventricular blood into the neoaorta.[230] Further consideration of repair of double-outlet right ventricle associated with more complex defects is beyond the scope of this discussion. For a patient who is not a candidate for biventricular repair because of hypoplasia of a ventricle or a straddling AV valve, initial palliation should prepare the child for a modification of the Fontan operation.

In a 10-year review of repair of double-outlet right ventricle in 73 patients,[228] early mortality was 11 percent, with an overall actuarial survival estimate at 8 years of 81 percent. Twenty-six percent required reoperation, and there was one death; 79 percent of the operative survivors required no restriction of physical activity, and 83 percent required no cardiac medications.

Corrected Transposition of the Great Arteries

DEFINITION

AV discordance and VA discordance form the characteristics of corrected transposition.

PATHOLOGY

Usually situs solitus is present, but the ventricles are inverted (an l loop). The great arteries are transposed and in the l position so that the pulmonary artery arises posteriorly from the right-sided morphologic left ventricle and the l-transposed aorta arises anteriorly from the left-sided right ventricle (SLL) (Fig. 63-37). If situs inversus is present, the segmental pattern is IDD. Along with the ventricular inversion, there is AV valvular inversion. The two coronary arteries arise from the right and left (posteriorly facing) sinuses, with the right-sided coronary artery giving off the anterior descending and circumflex branches.[231]

ASSOCIATED CONDITIONS

Rarely, no associated conditions are present and the circulation is normal. In the majority of cases (about 75 percent), a VSD is present. It may be in any location, but a perimembranous subpulmonary defect is most common.

The inverted left-sided systemic tricuspid valve frequently shows some degree of abnormality, usually leading to incompetence. The most common abnormality is an Ebstein-like displacement of the septal and posterior leaflets, but dysplasia, clefts, and straddling of the ventricular septum also have been described.

Pulmonary atresia or stenosis is present in about 40 percent of cases, usually associated with a VSD.[231] This obstruction is usually subvalvular, is only rarely valvular, and may characteristically result from attachments of accessory mitral valve tissue.

CLINICAL MANIFESTATIONS

Corrected transposition is an uncommon malformation, occurring in slightly fewer than 1 percent of children with congenital heart disease. The importance of this anomaly lies in its frequent association with serious AV conduction disturbances, the intracardiac malformations, and the medical and surgical implications of the ventricular inversion. The clinical picture is determined primarily by the associated anomalies. At least a third of these patients can be expected to develop complete AV block if followed for a 20-year period.[232]

History A slow, irregular heart rate often is detected in utero, and 10 percent of patients with congenital complete block prove to have corrected transposition. Patients with a large VSD without pulmonary stenosis usually present within the first month or so of life with symptoms indistinguishable from those of infants with a large VSD alone. Patients with VSD and pulmonary stenosis may present with symptoms of cyanosis and resemble patients with tetralogy of Fallot.

Physical Examination The murmur of left AV valve regurgitation may be best heard either at the apex or at the lower left sternal border. Most of these patients have a murmur of VSD or pulmonary stenosis. Occasionally, an inordinately accentuated second heart sound at the upper left sternal border suggests the presence of PAH, although in reality it represents a loud aortic valve closure resulting from the anterior and superior displacement of the aorta valve.

Chest Roentgenogram A straight or gently curved convex upper left heart border representing the contour of the transposed ascending aorta is characteristic and is most easily recognized in patients with a VSD and pulmonary stenosis, in whom there is a mild dilatation of the ascending aorta.

Electrocardiogram Varying degrees of AV conduction delay are present in almost a third of these patients. The initial forces of ventricular depolarization are characteristically oriented anteriorly and to the left, with Q waves in the right precordial leads and not in leads I, V_5, and V_6 resulting from depolarization of the septum from the left side (right ventricle) to the right side (left ventricle). With normal or nearly normal pressure in

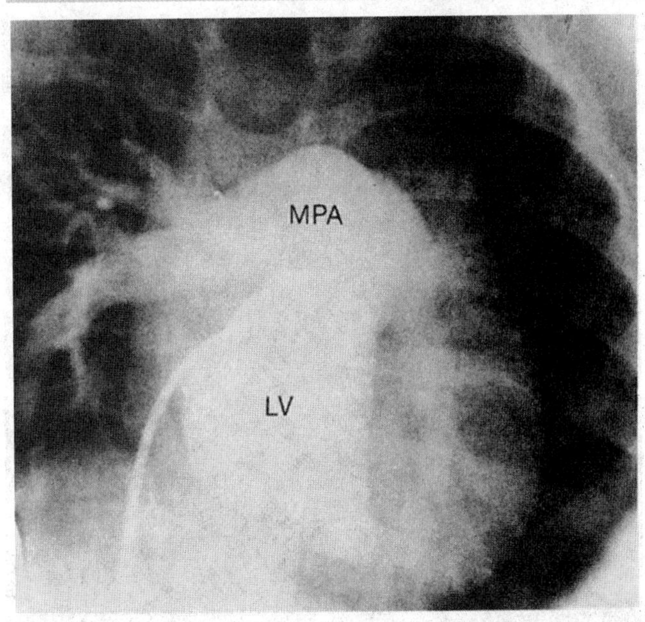

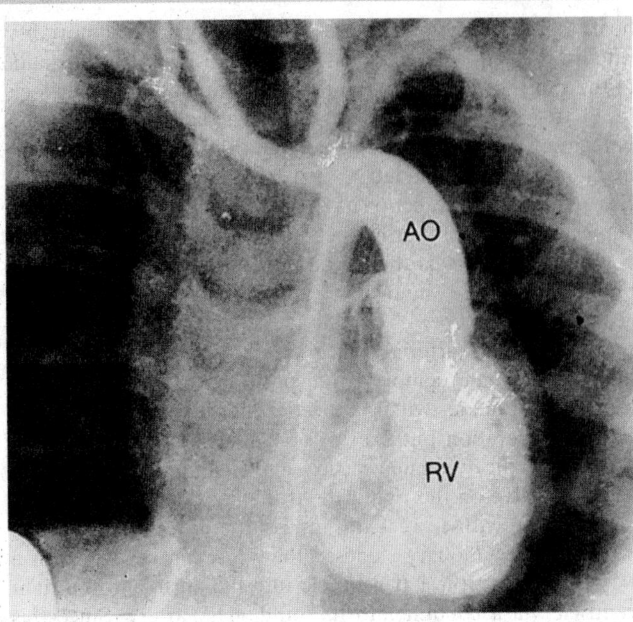

FIGURE 63-37 *A.* Posteroanterior view of the left ventricular (LV) angiogram in a child with corrected transposition of the great arteries. The main pulmonary artery (MPA) arises from the smooth-walled left ventricle, which receives the systemic venous blood. *B.* Posteroanterior view of the right ventricular angiogram (RV). The ascending aorta (AO) arises to the left of the pulmonary artery from the more heavily trabeculated right ventricle, which receives the pulmonary venous blood. The ventricular septum, seen here perpendicular to the frontal plane, is intact.

the systemic venous or morphologic left ventricle, a QS pattern in the right and an RS pattern in the left precordial leads are usual.

Echocardiogram Using a segmental approach, two-dimensional echocardiography permits identification of the anatomic components and associated defects.[233]

Cardiac Catheterization When diagnostic catheterization is performed, the morphologic left ventricle is entered from the right atrium, and in the presence of a VSD, the catheter may cross the defect, traverse the morphologic right ventricle, and enter the ascending aorta in the position normally occupied by the pulmonary artery. Entry into the medially placed pulmonary artery may be much more difficult, but the use of flow-guided catheters permits successful entry for the measurement of pressure. Selective angiography in both ventricles will outline the defects. The ventricular septum usually lies in the anteroposterior plane, and frequently a VSD may be imaged best angiographically in the frontal view (Fig. 63-37). Gentle manipulation of the catheter within the heart is indicated, since the production of varying degrees of transient AV block is not uncommon, and in rare instances, the block may prove permanent.

NATURAL HISTORY AND PROGNOSIS

The clinical course is determined primarily by the severity of the associated defects. It is estimated that only about 1 percent of individuals with corrected transposition have an otherwise normal heart. Even with complicating anomalies, survival to adulthood is possible.[234] Congestive heart failure associated with a large VSD has been the most common cause of death, with most fatalities occurring within the first year of life. AV conduction abnormalities tend to be progressive, and complete AV block may appear at any age. Similarly, left AV valve regurgitation may present at any age and significantly alters the long-term outcome.[235] Finally, the morphologic right ventricle may not be capable of sustaining adequate cardiac output over a normal life span.[236]

MEDICAL MANAGEMENT

Management of corrected transposition includes the treatment of congestive failure, cyanosis, and AV block and the prevention of infective endocarditis. Patients with severe pulmonary hypertension or congestive heart failure should undergo early banding of the pulmonary artery or repair of the defect. Similarly, patients with a VSD, severe pulmonary stenosis, and cyanosis benefit from systemic-to-pulmonary artery shunting procedures or total correction. Those with a congenital block require prompt pacemaker therapy. Patients with significant left AV valve regurgitation require valve replacement. Regularly scheduled follow-up examinations are recommended for all these patients to detect progressive AV conduction disorders and the progression or late appearance of left AV valve incompetence. Antibiotic coverage as protection against infective endocarditis is recommended, as is the introduction of an afterload reducer at the first appearance of AV valve regurgitation.[237]

SURGICAL MANAGEMENT

The conventional approach has been correction of the underlying lesion, closure of the ventricular septal defect in those with an isolated VSD, and closure of the VSD and a conduit from the left (pulmonary) ventricle to the pulmonary artery in those with L-TGA, VSD, and PS.[238] Unfortunately, this approach frequently has led to suboptimal results because of a very high incidence of complete heart block, increasing left AV valve regurgitation, and right systemic ventricular dysfunction and heart failure.[235] Despite recent advances, operative mortality rates for VSD or VSD and pulmonary stenosis or atresia remain in the range of 4 to 15 percent with postoperative heart block in 14 to 33 percent.[239,240] The 10-year actual survival was 83 percent in one study[239] and 55 percent in the other.[240] Replacement of the regurgitant left AV valve at the first sign of progressive ventricular dysfunction has been recommended to preserve ventricular function but has been of limited utility.[241]

In view of the less than optimum results with the standard procedures, more innovative approaches have been suggested.[242] For those with a VSD in association with corrected transposition, an arterial switch can be performed and, since this would create complete transposition, an atrial switch as well. This "double-switch" procedure is clearly a much more complex operation but has the advantage of leaving the left ventricle as the systemic ventricle and leaving the problematic tricuspid valve on the right side of the heart.

For those with corrected transposition, a ventricular septal defect, and pulmonary stenosis, the VSD can be closed in a way that diverts the left ventricle into the aorta and the right ventricle via a conduit into the pulmonary artery. Since this also would create transposition physiology, one needs to do an atrial switch by Mustard's or Senning's technique. Although the early mortality for this approach is about 10 percent,[243,244] it is hoped and expected that the long-term results will be superior to those of the more conventional approach.

Single Ventricle

DEFINITION

The univentricular heart, or single ventricle, is characterized by the entire flow from the two atria being carried directly through the left and/or right AV valves into the single ventricular chamber. The double-inlet type of AV connection may take the form of either one common or two separate AV valves; straddling of one AV valve sometimes is included. The VA connections may be concordant (pulmonary artery from right ventricle and aorta from left ventricle), discordant (pulmonary artery from left ventricle and aorta from right ventricle), double-outlet (both great arteries from either the left or the right ventricle), or single-outlet (atresia of one great artery). Alternatively, one of the AV valves may be atretic. This is associated with normally related great vessels or transposition of the great arteries.

PATHOLOGY

A common type of single ventricle is associated with triscupid atresia in which the ventricle has the morphology of a left ventricle. There may be normally related great vessels (type I), D transposition of the great arteries (type II), or L transposition (type III). Depending on the size of the ventricular communication with the hypoplastic right ventricle, there may be pulmonary atresia (A), pulmonary stenosis (B), or no pulmonary stenosis (C).

In a large series,[245] about two-thirds were type I, and of these about two-thirds had pulmonary stenosis (I B). Among the one-third with transposition, the most common variety is without pulmonary outflow obstruction (II C). L transposition accounts for less than 5 percent in almost all series of children with tricuspid valve atresia.

When the mitral valve is severly stenotic or atretic, the left ventricle and aorta are usually hypoplastic or atretic (hypoplastic left heart syndrome). In this situation, it is the right ventricle that is the predominant ventricle. Depending on the severity of the left-sided hypoplasia, the ascending aorta and aortic arch are usually hypoplastic as well.

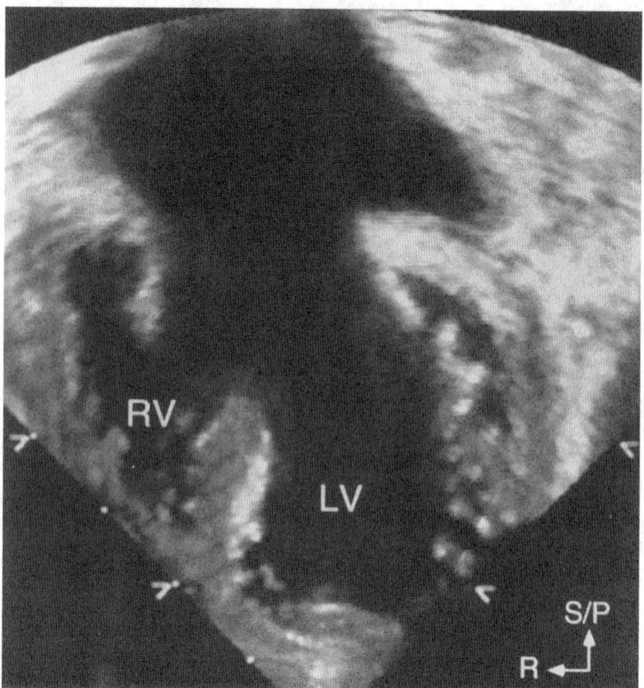

FIGURE 63-38 A malaligned atrioventricular canal with a large left ventricle (LV) and small right ventricle (RV). This would be repaired by a single ventricle approach (Fontan). (From Levine J and Geva T.[85] Reprinted with permission of the author and publisher.)

When there is one large atrioventricular valve or when both AV valves are present, the valve may straddle the ventricular septum, producing one large ventricle and one small ventricle (Fig. 63-38). The most common situation (65 to 70 percent of cases) is that in which the dominant ventricular chamber has the trabecular pattern of a left ventricle and communicates through an opening, the bulboventricular foramen, with a rudimentary right ventricle.[246] The VA connection is discordant (transposition of the great arteries) in about 90 percent of these patients. In about 20 percent of cases, the dominant ventricle shows the trabecular features of a right ventricle and the rudimentary chamber shows those of a left ventricle. The majority of these patients have a double-outlet VA connection from the main chamber, and a smaller number have a single-outlet connection with pulmonary atresia.[246] In 10 to 14 percent, neither ventricular sinus can be identified; this is the so-called primitive ventricle.

The term *Holmes' heart,* which is of historical interest, refers to a double-inlet left ventricle with situs solitus, normally related great arteries (SDS), an absent right ventricular sinus, and a subpulmonary infundibular outlet chamber communicating with the left ventricle via a restrictive bulboventricular foramen.[247]

ASSOCIATED CONDITIONS

Pulmonary stenosis or atresia is common. Subaortic stenosis and coarctation of the aorta occurs in association with L transposition and may result from a narrow bulboventricular foramen. In those with tricuspid or mitral atresia, an atrial communication is present.

CLINICAL MANIFESTATIONS

This complex and challenging malformation is relatively rare. The clinical picture is determined largely by the associated defects, among which pulmonary stenosis or atresia, which is present in a little over half of the patients, and obstruction to aortic flow are the most important.

All these patients have some degree of systemic hypoxemia because of mixing of the two sides of the circulation. If pulmonary stenosis or atresia is present, the presenting symptom is usually cyanosis. Without pulmonary stenosis, the presentation is usually congestive heart failure at 2 to 6 weeks of age as the pulmonary resistance falls. For those with subaortic stenosis and/or coarctation of the aorta, failure can occur within the first days of life as the ductus arteriosus closes. Physical examination depends on the combination of lesions present, but systolic ejection murmurs and a single second heart sound are very common.

Chest Roentgenogram Almost all these patients have at least some degree of cardiac enlargement. Those with little or no pulmonary stenosis generally have very large hearts with marked pulmonary plethora. Only patients with very severe pulmonary stenosis or atresia show a nearly normal heart size and diminished pulmonary arterial blood flow.

Electrocardiogram Evidence of right or left ventricular hypertrophy is common depending on which ventricle predominates.

Echocardiography Two-dimensional echocardiography with Doppler color flow studies can identify the morphologic and functional features of this malformation that are necessary to establish the diagnosis and formulate a plan for clinical management.[248]

Cardiac Catheterization A degree of systemic arterial oxygen desaturation is present in all these patients, although the severity appears to be related mainly to the volume of pulmonary blood flow. Careful recording of intracardiac and arterial pressures is essential to detect significant or potentially significant obstruction to blood flow across either AV valve, across the atrial septum, or between the ventricle and the aorta or pulmonary artery. The morphologic features of the ventricle, the relation of the aorta and the pulmonary artery, and other features can be established with high-quality selective ventricular angiography, using specially angled views to supplement conventional views.[249]

NATURAL HISTORY AND PROGNOSIS

Since by definition only one ventricle is "usable," treatment must be aimed at preserving the anatomy, physiology, and function to allow this single ventricle to support the circulation and establishing a method for systemic venous return to go to the lungs without a second pumping chamber.

These patients usually present as newborns with cyanosis, congestive failure, or a combination of both. Those in whom pulmonary arterial pressure and blood flow are increased require surgery to prevent death from congestive heart failure or progressive PVOD. Patients with severe pulmonary stenosis or atresia require systemic-to-pulmonary arterial shunting procedures. Among patients with univentricular heart, there is a propensity for the development of subaortic obstruction[250] and AV valve regurgitation.[251] Both threaten ventricular compliance and diminish the likelihood of successful long-term palliation.[252] Survivors are subject to the threats of infective endocarditis, brain abscess, and progressive PVOD.

MEDICAL MANAGEMENT

Early recognition and identification of patients with these complex defects are important so that successful palliative surgical procedures can be carried out for the relief of congestive failure or cyanosis. PGE_1 is useful in neonates with ductal-dependent defects.[91] An adequate interatrial communication is essential for those with mitral or tricuspid atresia. For those with pulmonary stenosis or atresia, a Blalock-Taussig shunt can be livesaving. Ventricular function and AV valvular competence are preserved by early creation of a bidirectional modified Glenn anastomosis (superior vena cava to undivided pulmonary artery).[253] Subaortic stenosis or obstruction at the bulboventricular foramen can be bypassed by anastomosis of the proximal pulmonary artery to the lateral aspect of the ascending aorta while pulmonary blood flow is delivered to the distal pulmonary arterial tree through a systemic arterial or systemic venous shunt.[254,255] Digitalis and diuretics may be necessary for patients with continuing heart failure. Care should be taken that anemia or severe polycythemia does not develop and that these patients are protected adequately against infective endocarditis. The pulmonary vascular bed must be protected and ventricular function and compliance must be preserved carefully if more definitive procedures are to be considered.

SURGICAL MANAGEMENT

Long-term palliation of children with a single ventricle is usually a three-stage approach: (1) initial palliation in the perinatal period, (2) a bidirectional Glenn at 6 to 18 months of age, and (3) a modified Fontan at 1 to 3 years of age. For complex problems, a heart transplant soon after birth has been suggested.[256]

Initial palliation for patients with univentricular AV connections requires adjustment of pulmonary blood flow with a pulmonary arterial band when it is excessive or the creation of a shunt when it is diminished. The modified Blalock-Taussig shunt is preferred in neonates. Relief of aortic stenosis and the creation of an adequate atrial communication frequently are necessary as well. The prognosis is affected adversely by a single ventricle of the right ventricular type[257] and the evolution of AV valvular regurgitation[258] or subaortic obstruction.[259]

Ventricular function and AV valvular competence are preserved by early creation of a bidirectional modified Glenn anastomosis, in which the superior vena cava is divided with the caudad portion patched closed; the cephalad portion is sutured to the top of the right pulmonary artery. If pulmonary atresia is not present, the main pulmonary artery is closed.[260] Subaortic stenosis or obstruction at the bulboventricular foramen can be palliated by anastomosis of the proximal pulmonary artery to the lateral aspect of the ascending aorta, while pulmonary blood flow is delivered to the distal pulmonary arterial tree through a systemic arterial or systemic venous shunt (the Damus-Kaye-Stansel operation). Other surgical options for the relief of subaortic obstruction are direct enlargement of the bulboventricular foramen (VSD), the modified Norwood operation,[255] and the arterial switch operation.[261]

Although initially some types of single ventricle were repaired by dividing the common chamber into the right and left ventricles, this has largely been abandoned because of unacceptably high initial mortality resulting from problems in connecting the ventricles to the appropriate great vessels without interfering with the atrioventricular valves and the high incidence of complete heart block.

The current approach is a modification of the principal suggested by Fontan and Baudet[262] to bypass the right side of the heart, directing systemic venous blood directly to the pulmonary arteries and allowing the single functioning ventricular chamber to pump blood to the systemic circulation. First, if it has not been done already, a bidirectional Glenn anastomosis is constructed (see above), and then an intraatrial tunnel is constructed to divert the inferior vena caval blood to the caudad portion of the superior vena cava, which then is connected to the underside of the right pulmonary artery (Fig. 63-39). A fenestration in the baffle sometimes is used to decompress the right side in the perioperative period. Recently, instead of tunnelling within the atrium, an external conduit has been used between the inferior vena cava (IVC) and the right pulmonary artery ligating the IVC–right atrial junction. The single ventricle is thus relieved of the burden of the volume overload and ventricular hypertrophy required to maintain the pulmonary circulation and is asked only to deliver systemic cardiac output.[262]

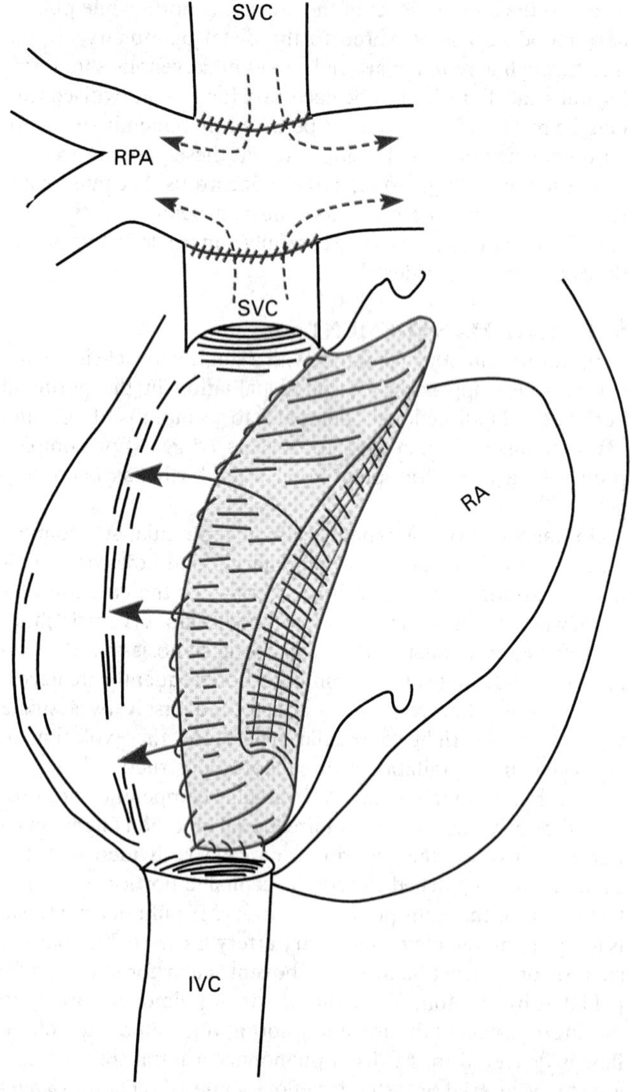

FIGURE 63-39 The modified Fontan operation. The superior vena cava (SVC) is divided. The cephalad portion is anastomosed to the superior aspect of the right pulmonary artery (RPA), and an intraatrial baffle is constructed from the inferior vena cava (IVC) to the superior vena cava along the lateral wall of the right atrium (RA). The caudad portion of the SVC then is connected to the inferior aspect of the right pulmonary artery.

The surgical risks depend on patient selection. For those with complex forms of single ventricle and those with elevated pulmonary pressure or resistance, ventricular dysfunction, or atrioventricular valve regurgitation, the risks are increased. For those without risk factors and with tricuspid atresia or double-inlet left ventricle, the risks are less than 5 percent.[263] Even for those with some risk factors or with more complex disease, at some centers the mortality is under 10 percent.[263,264]

For children with hypoplastic left heart syndrome, the survival from the three-stage procedure (initial Norwood, bidirectional Glenn, and Fontan) is approximately 50 percent,[265] although some centers are reporting a survival rate as high as 76 percent.[266] There does not seem to be any significant difference in survival in centers that use the three-stage anatomic "repair" from primary heart transplantation in the perinatal period at 36 months of age.[265]

Quality and length of life are clearly improved, but persistent problems (AV valvular regurgitation, systemic embolization, limitation of exercise tolerance, protein-losing enteropathy, atrial arrhythmias, and deterioration of ventricular function) occur with a frequency of about 1 percent per year.[263] For patients with progressive deterioration, cardiac transplantation is recommended.

CONGENITAL ABNORMALITIES OF THE CORONARY ARTERIAL CIRCULATION

Coronary Arteriovenous Fistula

PATHOLOGY

A coronary arteriovenous fistula is a fistulous communication between a coronary artery and a cardiac chamber, the coronary sinus, or the pulmonary trunk (Fig. 63-40).

The site of origin may involve any of the epicardial coronary arteries. *The right coronary artery is the site of origin in somewhat over half the cases, and the two most common sites into which the fistula feeds are a cardiac vein (usually the coronary sinus) and the right ventricle.* Although solitary communication is the rule, there may be multiple sites of termination. A fistula into the pulmonary trunk usually is characterized by one or more vessels opening into the pulmonary trunk and connecting with branches of each of the two main coronary arteries. The artery or arteries feeding the fistula are grossly enlarged and tortuous. Saccular aneurysms may develop in segments of dilated vessels; such aneurysms usually are observed in adults and frequently show calcification of the wall.

CLINICAL MANIFESTATIONS

Many patients with a coronary arteriovenous fistula are asymptomatic.[267,268] In some, the magnitude of the shunt into the right side of the heart is great enough to cause congestive heart

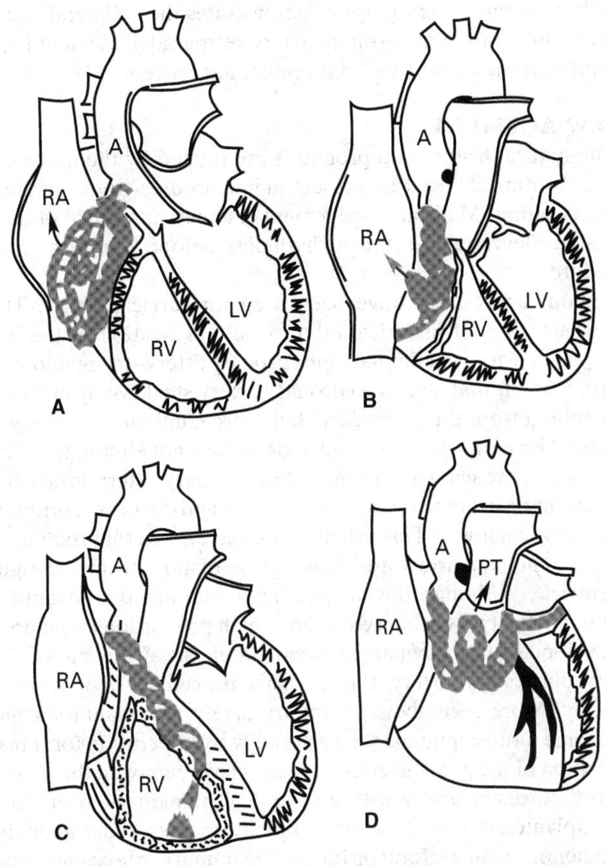

FIGURE 63-40 Anomalous communications of coronary arteries. *A.* Right coronary artery communicates with coronary sinus. *B.* Right coronary artery communicates with right atrium (RA). *C.* Anomalous communication of right coronary artery with right ventricle (RV). *D.* Two coronary arteries arise from the aorta (A) and make collateral communication with accessory coronary artery arising from pulmonary trunk (PT). LV = left ventricle.

failure, with a tendency for this to occur in early infancy or after 40 years of age. The classic finding is that of a continuous murmur with an unusual location, since it is loudest over the fistula. It may have a louder diastolic component, especially if communication is with the right ventricle. In those with large shunts, there may be cardiomegaly and increased pulmonary flow shown by chest roentgenography and right ventricular hypertrophy shown by ECG. Transthoracic echocardiography is usually diagnostic in children;[269] transesophageal studies may be necessary in adults. At cardiac catheterization, an increase in oxygen saturation may be encountered, usually in the right atrium or right ventricle, if the shunt is large enough. Selective coronary arteriography will demonstrate the involved coronary artery and the site of entry of the fistula. The most common complication is infective endocarditis, but thrombosis, myocardial ischemia, and rupture may occur.

SURGICAL MANAGEMENT

Except for very small fistulas, closure is recommended, since the flow tends to increase with age and these patients are at risk for infective endocarditis, congestive heart failure, and myocardial ischemia. Until relatively recently, closure was invariably surgical. Occasionally, closure was done without a coronary bypass by placing obliterating mattress sutures across the fistula beneath the coronary artery as it passes over the surface of the heart.[270] More commonly, cardiopulmonary bypass is preferred for safe exposure of large or multiple fistulas, such as those entering the right atrium near the junction of the superior vena cava and the right atrium, those arising from the artery to the sinoatrial node, and those between the left coronary artery and the left ventricle.[271] The orifice of the fistula is obliterated by direct suture or the placement of a Dacron or pericardial patch. Fistulas have been closed from within the open coronary artery; the artery then is repaired by direct suturing. Surgical mortality should be minimal;[271] the long-term results have been favorable.[272]

Fistulas have been closed by interventional catheterization techniques. Perry and associates[273] attempted to close fistulas in nine patients: four from the left circumflex artery, three from the left anterior descending artery, and two from the right coronary artery. Gianturco coils were used in six patients and a double-umbrella in two, with coils and an umbrella used in one. All were completely occluded. In three patients with multiple fistulas, no attempt was made in the catheterization laboratory and the patients were referred for surgery. This "noninvasive" technique seems to be applicable to some children and adults with coronary AV fistulas, although long-term follow-up is necessary to be certain that the fistulas do not recur.

Origin of the Left Coronary Artery from the Pulmonary Artery

PATHOLOGY AND PATHOPHYSIOLOGY

In this anomaly, the left coronary artery arises from the pulmonary artery rather than from the aorta (Fig. 63-41). In the perina-

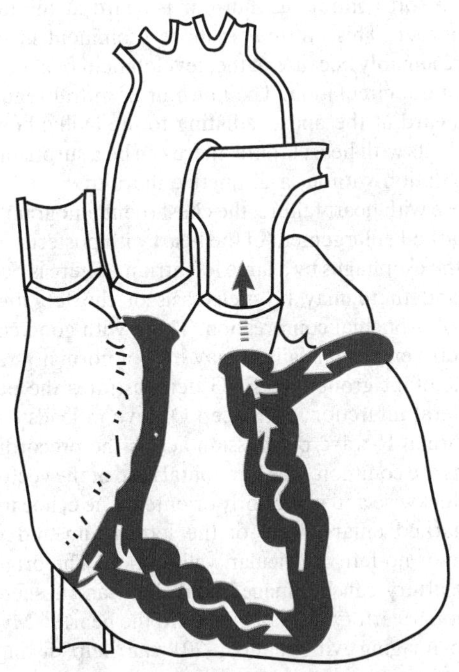

FIGURE 63-41 Anomalous origin of the left coronary artery from the pulmonary trunk. With time, wide collaterals develop between the two coronary systems so that right coronary arterial blood is shunted into the left coronary system and thence into the pulmonary trunk.

tal period, the pulmonary artery pressure is high and the left coronary is perfused with venous blood. Problems arise when the pulmonary resistance and pulmonary artery pressure fall and the diastolic pressure is insufficient to perfuse the left ventricular myocardium. In the absence of collateral vessels from the right coronary, left ventricular ischemia and eventually infarction of the left ventricular wall and papillary muscles occur. This in turn leads to congestive heart failure, usually by 3 to 8 weeks of age.

In a small group of children, extensive collaterals between the right coronary (arising normally from the aorta) and the left system develop. Perfusion via the right may be sufficient to oxygenate the left ventricular myocardium so that no ischemia develops. Over time, the higher perfusion pressure in the aorta may allow a left-to-right shunt into the pulmonary artery through the right and then the left coronary system. Eventually this may lead to a "steal" of blood from the myocardium into the lower-resistance pulmonary circuit.

CLINICAL MANIFESTATIONS

The clinical spectrum and mode of presentation in patients with this abnormality vary.[274,275] The majority of these patients present at 6 to 12 weeks of age. Acute episodes of irritability, profuse cold sweating, pallor (? angina), and respiratory distress occur, with evidence of heart failure. Less often, these patients present at an older age with mitral regurgitation and heart failure. A few reach adolescence or adulthood with no or relatively few symptoms other than occasional exertional angina or palpitations. Sudden death may be the first and only sign of this condition.

On physical examination, the heart is enlarged, with an abnormal left ventricular apex impulse. Other signs of failure are usually present. Pallor and clammy skin are common. In some patients, a soft continuous murmur is heard at the upper left sternal border. This murmur is more prominent in older patients, presumably because of the development of a more extensive collateral circulation. The murmur of mitral regurgitation may be heard at the apex, radiating to the axilla; however, in young infants with heart failure, there can be a surprising degree of regurgitation without a distinctive murmur.

In those with heart failure, the chest roentgenogram typically shows marked enlargement of the heart with posterior displacement of the esophagus by a large left atrium. There is pulmonary edema, and there may be atelectasis of the left lower lobe because of bronchial compression. Those with good collaterals and no left ventricular failure may have a normal x-ray.

In the infant group, the ECG demonstrates the pattern of anterolateral infarction, with deep Q wave in leads I and aVL and abnormal R-wave progression across the precordium. Arrhythmias are common. The horizontal loop of the vectorcardiogram is clockwise and posteriorly oriented. The echocardiogram shows marked enlargement of the left atrium and ventricle with little or no left ventricular wall motion. The origin of the coronary artery can be imaged, and flow can be seen toward the pulmonary artery instead of toward the heart.[276] Myocardial perfusion imaging with thallium-201 can help distinguish an anomalous coronary artery from congestive cardiomyopathy.[277]

At cardiac catheterization, there may be an increase in saturation in the pulmonary artery if there is enough retrograde flow. There is usually some pulmonary hypertension, with very elevated pulmonary wedge pressure. Aortography or selective right coronary arteriography demonstrates the collateral circulation filling the left coronary artery retrogradely, with at least faint opacification of the main pulmonary artery.

MANAGEMENT

The natural history and prognosis are related by the modes of presentation. Those who present in infancy die without surgical intervention. Medical management is aimed at control of congestive heart failure and arrhythmias before a surgical procedure.

Four approaches have been used for surgical repair. The first, which is of historical interest only, is ligation of the left coronary artery to eliminate the coronary artery–to–pulmonary artery shunt that acts as a coronary artery steal. Many children benefited from this procedure, but there continued to be myocardial ischemia and late sudden death was not eliminated. The second approach was to tunnel the coronary artery inside the pulmonary artery to the wall of the aorta and create an aortopulmonary window.[278] This usually required an external roofing of the pulmonary artery to allow egress of flow from the right ventricle. Although this surgical approach has the advantage of making a two-coronary system, a high proportion of children developed supravalvular pulmonary stenosis at the site of the intrapulmonary artery tunnel. This procedure is now used rarely. More recently, as coronary artery reimplantation has become more common in the arterial switch operation for transposition of the great arteries, surgeons have removed the anomalous coronary artery with a button of pulmonary artery and reimplanted it onto the aorta.[279] Finally, in a few older patients, saphenous vein grafting or internal mammary artery implantation has been used.[280]

The late results after surgery have been quite good.[279,281] The congestive heart failure frequently improves, the heart becomes smaller, the left ventricular shortening fraction improves, and mitral regurgitation tends to regress. Interestingly, the infarction pattern on ECG with deep anterolateral Q waves frequently disappears, suggesting that the poor function is due to extreme ischemia rather than infarction (hybernating myocardium).[282]

References

1. Mitchell SC, Korones SB, Berendes HW. Congenital heart disease in 56,109 births: Incidence and natural history. *Circulation* 1971; 43:323–332.
2. Hoffman JIE, Christianson R. Congenital heart disease in a cohort of 19,502 births with long-term follow-up. *Am J Cardiol* 1978; 42:641–647.
3. Fyler DC. Report of the New England Regional Infant Cardiac Program. *Pediatrics* 1980; 65:II375–II461.
4. Perry LW, Neill CA, Ferencz C, et al. Infants with congenital heart disease: The cases. In: Ferencz C, Rubin JD, Loffredo CA, Magee CA, eds. *Epidemiology of Congenital Heart Disease: The Baltimore-Washington Infant Heart Study 1981–1989.* Mount Kisco, NY: Futura; 1993:33–61.
5. Fyler DC, ed. *Nadas' Pediatric Cardiology.* Philadelphia: Hanley & Belfus; 1992:273.
6. Keith JD. Prevalence, incidence and epidemiology. In: Keith JD, Rowe RD, Vlad P, eds. *Heart Disease in Infancy and Childhood,* 3d ed. New York: Macmillan; 1978:3.
7. Nora JJ. Causes of CHD—old and new modes, mechanisms and models. *Am Heart J* 1993; 125:1409–1418.
8. Belmont JW. Recent progress in the molecular genetics of congenital heart defects. *Clin Genet* 1998; 54:11–9.

9. Hall JG. Catch 22. *J Med Genet* 1993; 30:801–802.
10. Dawes GS. *Foetal and Neonatal Physiology: A Comparative Study of the Changes at Birth.* Chicago: Year Book; 1968:90.
11. Lind J, Wegelius C. Human fetal circulation: Changes in the cardiovascular system at birth and disturbances in the postnatal closure of the foramen ovale and ductus arteriosus: Cold Spring Harbor Symposium. *Quant Biol* 1954; 19:109–125.
12. Rudolph AM, Heymann MA. The circulation of the fetus in utero. *Circ Res* 1967; 21:163–184.
13. Rudolph AM, Heymann MA. Circulatory changes with growth in the fetal lamb. *Circ Res* 1970; 26:289–299.
14. Rudolph AM, Heymann MA. Cardiac output in the fetal lamb: The effects of spontaneous and induced changes of heart rate on right and left ventricular output. *J Obstet Gynecol* 1976; 124:183–192.
15. Teitel DF, Iwamoto HS, Rudolph AM. Effects of birth-related events on central flow patterns. *Pediatr Res* 1987; 22:557–566.
16. Coceani F, Olley PM. Role of prostaglandins, prostacyclin, and thromboxanes in the control of prenatal patency and postnatal closure of the ductus arteriosus. In: Heymmann MA, ed. *Prostaglandins in the Perinatal Period.* New York: Grune & Stratton; 1980:109.
17. Rudolph AM. Fetal and neonatal pulmonary circulation. *Annu Rev Physiol* 1979; 41:383–395.
18. Fineman JR, Soifer SJ, Heymann MA. Regulation of vascular tone in the perinatal period. *Annu Rev Physiol* 1995; 57:115–134.
19. Heymann MA, Rudolph AM. Effects of congenital heart disease on fetal and neonatal circulations. *Prog Cardiovasc Dis* 1972; 15:115–143.
20. Levin DL, Heymann MA, Kitterman JA, et al. Persistent pulmonary hypertension in the newborn infant. *J Pediatr* 1976; 89: 626–630.
21. Fox WW, Duara S. Persistent pulmonary hypertension in the neonate: Diagnosis and management. *J Pediatr* 1983; 103: 505–514.
22. Kinsella JP, Abman SH. Recent developments in inhaled nitric oxide therapy of the newborn. *Curr Opini Pediatr* 1999: 11:121–125.
23. UK Collaborative randomized trial of neonatal extracorporeal membrane oxygenation: UK Collaborative ECMO Trial Group. *Lancet* 1996: 348:75–82.
24. Talner NS. Heart failure. In: Emmanouilides GC, Riemenschneider TA, Gutgesell HP, eds. *Moss and Adams Heart Disease in Infants, Children, and Adolescents Including the Fetus and Young Adult,* 5th ed. Baltimore: Williams & Wilkins; 1995:1746.
25. Seguchi M, Nakazawa M, Momma K. Effect of enalapril on infants and children with congestive heart failure. *Cardiol Young* 1992; 2:14–19.
26. Fischbein CA, Rosenthal A, Fischer EG, et al. Risk factors of brain abscess in patients with congenital heart disease. *Am J Cardiol* 1974; 34:97–102.
27. Phornphutkul C, Rosenthal A, Nadas AS, Berenberg W. Cerebrovascular accidents in infants and children with cyanotic congenital heart disease. *Am J Cardiol* 1973; 32:329–334.
28. Beekman RH, Tuuri DT. Acute hemodynamic effects of increasing hemoglobin concentration in children with a right to left ventricular shunt and relative anemia. *J Am Coll Cardiol* 1985; 5:357–362.
29. Gidding SS, Stockman JA III. Effect of iron deficiency on tissue oxygen delivery in cyanotic congenital heart disease. *Am J Cardiol* 1988; 61:605–607.
30. Ross EA, Perloff JK, Danovitch GM, et al. Renal function and urate metabolism in late survivors with cyanotic congenital heart disease. *Circulation* 1986; 73:396–400.
31. Henriksson P, Varendh G, Lundstrom NR. Haemostatic defects in cyanotic congenital heart disease. *Br Heart J* 1979; 41:23–27.
32. Waldman JD, Czapek EE, Paul MH, et al. Shortened platelet survival in cyanotic heart disease. *J Pediatr* 1975; 87:77–79.
33. Territo MC, Rosove MH, Perloff JK. Cyanotic congenital heart disease: Hematologic management, renal function, and urate metabolism. In: Perloff JK, Child JS, eds. *Congenital Heart Disease in Adults.* Philadelphia: Saunders; 1991:93.
34. Aram DM, Ekelman BL, Ben Shachar G, Levinsohn MW. Intelligence and hypoxemia in children with congenital heart disease: Fact or artifact? *Am J Coll Cardiol* 1985; 6:889–893.
35. Cameron JW, Rosenthal A, Olson AD. Malnutrition in hospitalized children with congenital heart disease. *Arch Pediatr Adolesc Med* 1995; 149:1098–1102.
36. Schuurmans FM, Pulles-Heintzberger CF, Gerver WJ, et al. Longterm growth of children with congenital heart disease: A retrospect study. *Acta Paediatr* 1998; 87:1250–1255.
37. Rabinovitch M. Pathophysiology of pulmonary hypertension. In: Emmanouilides GC, Riemenschneider TA, Allen HD, Gutgesell HP, eds. *Moss and Adams Heart Disease in Infants, Children, and Adolescents,* 5th ed. Baltimore: Williams & Wilkins; 1995: 1659.
38. Heath D, Edwards JE. The pathology of hypertensive pulmonary vascular disease: A description of six grades of structural changes in the pulmonary arteries with special reference to congenital cardiac septal defects. *Circulation* 1958; 18:533.
39. Turanlahti MI, Laitinen PO, Sarna SJ, Pesonen E. Nitric oxide, oxygen and prostacyclin in children with pulmonary hypertension. *Heart* 1998; 79:169–174.
40. Nihill MR. Clinical management of patients with pulmonary hypertension. In: Emmanouilides GC, Riemenschneider TA, Allen HD, Gutgesell HP, eds. *Moss and Adams Heart Disease in Infants, Children, and Adolescents,* 5th ed. Baltimore: Williams & Wilkins; 1995:1695.
41. Gersony WM. Long-term follow-up of operated congenital heart disease. *Cardiol Clin* 1989; 7:915–923.
42. Freed MD. Infective endocarditis in the adult with congenital heart disease. *Cardiol Clin* 1993; 11:589–602.
43. Morris CD, Reller MD, Menashe VD. Thirty year incidence of infective endocarditis after surgery for congenital heart defect. *JAMA* 1998; 279:599–603.
44. Keane JF, Driscoll DJ, Gersony WM. Second Natural History Study of Congenital Heart Defects: Results of treatment of patients with aortic valvar stenosis. *Circulation* 1993; 87 (suppl):I16–I27.
45. Hart EM, Garson A Jr. Psychosocial concerns of adults with congenital heart disease: Employability and insurability. *Cardiac Clin* 1993; 11:711–715.
46. Schmaltz AA, Neudorf U, Winkler UH. Outcome of pregnancy in women with congenital heart disease. *Cardiol Young* 1999; 9:88–96.
47. Strong WB. Introduction: Pediatric cardiology exercise testing. *Pediatri Cardiol* 1999; 20:1–3.
48. Chandar JS, Wolff GS, Garson A Jr, et al. Ventricular arrhythmias in postoperative tetralogy of Fallot. *Am J Cardiol* 1990; 65:655–661.
49. Gelatt M, Hamilton RM, McCrindle BW, et al. Arrhythmia and mortality after the Mustard procedure: A 30-year single-center experience. *J Am Coll Cardiol* 1997; 29:194–201.
50. Fishberger SB, Wernovsky G, Gentiles TL, et al. Factors that influence the development of atrial flutter after the Fontan operation. *J Thorac Cardiovasc Surg* 1997; 113:80–86.
51. Moreau GA, Graham TP Jr. Clinical assessment of ventricular function after surgical treatment of congenital heart defects. *Cardiol Clin* 1989; 7:439–452.
52. Turina MI, Siebenmann R, von Segesser L, et al. Late functional deterioration after atrial correction for transposition of the great arteries. *Circulation* 1989; 80:I162–I167.
53. Mertens L, Hagler DJ, Sauer U, et al. Protein-losing enteropathy

after the Fontan operation: An international multicenter study: PLE study group. *J Thorac Cardiovasc Surg* 1998; 115:1063–1073.

54. Graham TP, Gutgesell HP. Ventricular septal defects. In: Emmanouilides GC, Riemenschneider TA, Allen HD, Gutgesell HP, eds. *Moss and Adams Heart Disease in Infants, Children, and Adolescents,* 5th ed. Baltimore: Williams & Wilkins; 1995:724.
55. Alpert BS, Cook DH, Varghese PJ, Rowe RD. Spontaneous closure of small ventricular septal defects: Ten-year follow-up. *Pediatrics* 1979; 63:204–206.
56. Trowitzsch E, Braun W, Stute M, Pielmeier W. Diagnosis, therapy, and outcome of ventricular septal defects in the 1st year of life: A two-dimensional colour-Doppler echocardiography study. *Eur J Pediatr* 1990; 149:758–761.
57. Weidman WH, Blount SG Jr, DuShane JW, et al. Clinical course in ventricular septal defect. *Circulation* 1977; 56:I156–I169.
58. Rhodes L, Keane JF, Keane JP, et al. Long follow-up (to 43 years) of ventricular septal defect with audible aortic regurgitation. *Am J Cardiol* 1990; 66:340–345.
59. Gersony WM, Hayes CJ. Bacterial endocarditis in patients with pulmonary stenosis, aortic stenosis or ventricular septal defect. *Circulation* 1977; 56:I84–I87.
60. Gersony WM, Hayes CJ, Driscoll DJ, et al. Bacterial endocarditis in patients with aortic stenosis, pulmonary stenosis or ventricular septal defect. *Circulation* 1993; 87(suppl I):I121–I126.
61. Driscoll DJ, Michels VV, Gersony WM, et al. Occurrence risk for congenital heart defects in relatives of patients with aortic stenosis, pulmonary stenosis, or ventricular septal defect. *Circulation* 1993; 87(suppl I):I114–I120.
62. Casteneda AR, Jonas RA, Mayer JE, Hanley FL. *Cardiac Surgery of the Neonate and Infant.* Philadelphia: Saunders; 1994:187–203.
63. Moller JH, Patton C, Varco RL, Lillchei CW. Late results (30–35 years) after operative closure of isolated ventricular septal defect from 1954–1960. *Am J Cardiol* 1991; 68:1491–1497.
64. Rocchini A, Lock JE. Defect closure: Umbrella devices. In: Lock JE, Keane JF, Perry SB, eds. *Diagnostic and Interventional Catheterization in Congenital Heart Disease.* Boston: Kluwer; 2000:179.
65. Lewis FJ, Winchell P, Bashour FA. Open repair of atrial septal defects: Results in sixty-three patients. *JAMA* 1957; 165:922.
66. Edwards JE. Classification of congenital heart disease in the adult. In: Roberts WC, ed. *Congenital Heart Disease in Adults.* Philadelphia: Davis; 1979:1.
67. Mahoney LT, Truesdell SC, Krzmarzick TR, Lauer RM. Atrial septal defects that present in infancy. *Am J Dis Child* 1986; 140:1115–1118.
68. Benson DW, Sharkey A, Fatkin D, et al. Reduced penetrance, variable expressivity, and genetic heterogeneity of familial atrial septal defects. *Circulation* 1998; 97:2043–2048.
69. Murphy JG, Gersh BJ, McGoon MD, et al. Long-term outcome after surgical repair of isolated atrial septal defect: Follow-up at 27–32 years. *N Engl J Med* 1990; 323:1645–1650.
70. Seward JB, Tajik AJ. Transesophageal echocardiography in congenital heart disease. *Am J Cardiol Imaging* 1990; 4:215–222.
71. Dall'Agata A, McGhie J, Taams MA, et al. Secundum atrial septal defect is a dynamic three dimensional entity. *Am Heart J* 1999; 137:1075–1086
72. Hamilton WT, Hattajee CE, Dalen JE, et al. Atrial septal defect secundum: Clinical profile with physiologic correlates. In: Roberts WC, ed. *Adult Congenital Heart Disease.* Philadelphia: Davis; 1987:395.
73. Steele PM, Fuster V, Cohen M, et al. Isolated atrial septal defect with pulmonary vascular obstructive disease, long-term follow-up and prediction of outcome after surgical correction. *Circulation* 1987; 76:1037–1042.
74. Prieto LR, Foreman CK, Cheatham JP, Latson LA. Intermediate-term outcome of transcatheter secundum atrial septal defect closure using the Bard Clamshell Septal Umbrella. *Am J Cardiol* 1996; 78:1310–1312.
75. Masura J, Lange PE, Wilkinson JL, et al. US/International multicenter trial of atrial septal catheter closure using the Amplatzer Septal Occluder: Initial results (abstract). *Am J Card* 1998; 31(supplement A):57A.
76. Zamora R, Rao PS, Lloyd TR, et al. Intermediate-term results of Phase I Food and Drug Administration Trials of buttoned device occlusion of secundum atrial septal defects. *J Am Coll Cardiol* 1998; 31:674–676.
77. St. John-Sutton MG, Tajik AJ, McGoon DC. Atrial septal defect in patients ages 60 years or older: Operative results and long-term postoperative follow-up. *Circulation* 1981; 64:402–409.
78. Healy JE Jr. An anatomic survey of anomalous pulmonary veins: Their clinical significance. *J Thorac Cardiovasc Surg* 1952; 23:433–444.
79. Silverman NH. Anomalous pulmonary venous connections. In: Silverman NH, ed. *Pediatric Echocardiography.* New York: Williams & Wilkins; 1993:179.
80. Saalouke MG, Shapiro SR, Perry LW, Scott LP III. Isolated partial anomalous pulmonary venous drainage associated with pulmonary vascular obstructive disease. *Am J Cardiol* 1977; 39:439–444.
81. Rogers HM, Edwards JE. Incomplete division of the atrioventricular canal with patent interatrial foramen primum (persistent common cardioventricular ostium): Report of five cases and review of the literature. *Am Heart J* 1948; 36:28.
82. Rastelli GC, Ongley PA, Kirklin JW, McGoon DC. Surgical repair of the complete form of persistent common atrioventricular canal. *J Thorac Cardiovasc Surg* 1968; 55:299–308.
83. Rose V, Izukawa T, Moes CA. Syndromes of asplenia and polysplenia: A review of cardiac and non-cardiac malformations in 60 cases with special reference to diagnosis and prognosis. *Br Heart J* 1975; 37:840–852.
84. Lacro RV. Dysmorphology. In: Fyler DC, ed. *Nadas' Pediatric Cardiology.* Philadelphia: Hanley & Belfus; 1992:37.
85. Levine J, Geva T. Echocardiographic assessment of common atrioventricular canal. *Prog Pediatr Cardiol* 1999; 10:137–151.
86. Nora JJ, Nora AH. Maternal transmission of congenital heart diseases: New recurrence risk figures and the questions of cytoplasmic inheritance and vulnerability to teratogens. *Am J Cardiol* 1987; 59:459–463.
87. Kirklin JW, Barratt-Boyes BG. Atrioventricular canal defect. In: Kirklin JW, Barratt-Boyes BG, eds. *Cardiac Surgery,* 2d ed. New York: Churchill Livingstone; 1993:693.
88. Hanley FL, Fenton KN, Jonas RA, et al. Surgical repair of complete atrioventricular canal defects in infancy: Twenty-year trends. *J Thorac Cardiovasc Surg* 1993; 106:387–397.
89. Alexi-Meskishvili V, Ishino K, Dahnert I, et al. Correction of complete atrioventricular septal defects with the double-patch technique and cleft closure. *Ann Thorac Surg* 1996; 62:519–525.
90. Daebritz S, del Nido PJ. Surgical management of common atrioventricular canal. *Prog Pediatri Cardiol* 1999; 10:161–171.
91. Freed MD, Heymann MA, Lewis AB, et al. Prostaglandin E-1 in infants with ductus arteriosus-dependent congenital heart disease. *Circulation* 1981; 64:899–905.
92. Gersony WM, Peckham GJ, Ellison RC, et al. Effects of indomethacin in premature infants with patent ductus arteriosus: Results of a national collaborative study. *J Pediatr* 1983; 102: 895–906.
93. Siassi B, Blanco C, Cabal LA, Coran AG. Incidence and clinical features of patent ductus arteriosus in low-birthweight infants: A prospective analysis of 150 consecutively born infants. *Pediatrics* 1976; 57:347–351.
94. Varvarigou A, Bardin CL, Beharry K, et al. Early ibuprofen administration to prevent patent ductus arteriosus in premature newborn infants. *JAMA* 1996; 275:539–544.
95. Castaneda AR, Jonas RA, Mayer JE, Hanley FL. *Cardiac Surgery of the Neonate and Infant.* Philadelphia: Saunders; 1994:203.

96. Satur CR, Walker DR, Dickinson DF. Day case ligation of patent ductus arteriosus in preterm infants: A 10-year review. *Arch Dis Child* 1991; 66:477–480.
97. Bell Thomson J, Jewell E, Ellis FH Jr, Schwaber JR. Surgical technique in the management of patent ductus arteriosus in the elderly patient. *Ann Thorac Surg* 1990; 30:80–83.
98. Laborde F, Folligvet T, Batisse A, et al. Video-assisted thorascopic surgical interruption: The technique of choice for patent ductus arteriosus. *J Thorac Cardiovasc Surg* 1995; 110:1681–1685.
99. Burke RP, Wernovsky G, van der Velde M, et al. Video-assisted thorascopic surgery for congenital heart disease. *J Thorac Cardiovasc Surg* 1995; 109:499–507.
100. Portsmann W, Wierny L. Percutaneous transfemoral closure of the patent ductus arteriosus: An alternative to surgery. *Semin Roentgenol* 1981; 16:95–102.
101. Rashkind WJ, Cuaso CC. Transcatheter closure of patent ductus arteriosus. *Pediatr Cardiol* 1979; 1:3–7.
102. Shim D, Fedderly RT, Beekman RH III, et al. Follow-up of coil occlusion of patent ductus arteriosis. *J Am Coll Cardio* 1996; 28:207–211.
103. Sakakibara S, Konno S. Congenital aneurysm of the sinus of Valsalva: Anatomy and classification. *Am Heart J* 1962; 63: 405–424.
104. Takach TJ, Reul GJ, Duncan JM, et al. Sinus of Valsalva aneurysm or fistula: Management and outcome. *Ann Thorac Surg* 1999; 68:1573–1577.
105. Shaffer EM, Snider AR, Beekman RH, et al. Sinus of Valsalva aneurysm complicating bacterial endocarditis in an infant: Diagnosis with two-dimensional and Doppler echocardiography. *J Am Coll Cardiol* 1987; 9:588–591.
106. Clagett OT, Kirklin JW, Edwards JE. Anatomic variations and pathologic changes in 124 cases of coarctation of the aorta. *Surg Gynecol Obstet* 1954; 98:103.
107. Bharati S, Lev M. The surgical anatomy of the heart in tubular hypoplasia of the transverse aorta (preductal coarctation). *J Thorac Cardiovasc Surg* 1986; 91:79–85.
108. Gardiner HM, Celermajer DS, Sorensen KE, et al. Arterial reactivity is significantly impaired in normotensive young adults after successful repair of aortic coarctation in childhood. *Circulation* 1994; 89:1745–1750.
109. Beekman RH. Coarctation of the aorta. In: Emmanouilides GC, Riemenschneider TA, Allen HD, Gutgesell HP, eds. *Moss and Adams Heart Disease in Infants, Children, and Adolescents,* 5th ed. Baltimore: Williams & Wilkins; 1995:1111.
110. Ing FF, Starc TJ, Griffiths SP, Gersony WM. Early diagnosis of coarctation of the aorta in children: A continuing dilemma. *Pediatrics* 1996; 98:378–382.
111. Campbell M. Natural history of coarctation of the aorta. *Br Heart J* 1970; 32:633–640.
112. Fletcher SE, Nihill MR, Grifka RG, et al. Balloon angioplasty of native coarctation of the aorta: Mid-term follow-up and prognostic factors. *J Am Coll Cardio* 1995; 25:730–734.
113. Zehr KJ, Gillinov AM, Redmond JM, et al. Repair of coarctation of the aorta in neonates and infants: A thirty-year experience. *Ann Thorac Surg* 1995; 59:33–41.
114. Kreutzer J, Perry SB. Stents. In Lock JE, Keane JF, Perry SB, eds. *Diagnostic and Interventional Catheterization in Congenital Heart Disease*, 2d ed. Boston, Kluwer; 2000:221.
115. Parks WJ, Ngo TD, Plauth WH, et al. Incidence of aneurysm formation after Dacron patch aortoplasty repair for coarctation of the aorta: Long-term results and assessment utilizing magnetic resonance angiography with three-dimensional surface rendering. *J Am Coll Cardiol* 1995; 26:266–271.
116. Kirklin JW, Barratt-Boyes BG. Coarctation of the aorta and interrupted aortic arch. In: Kirklin JW, Barratt Boyes BJ, eds. *Cardiac Surgery,* 2d ed. New York: Churchill Livingstone; 1993:1263.
117. Quaegebeur JM, Jonas RA, Weinberg AD, et al. Outcomes in seriously ill neonates with coarctation of the aorta: A multi-institutional study. *J Thorac Cardiovasc Surg* 1994; 108:841–854.
118. Pollock JC, Jamieson MP, McWilliam R. Somatosensory evoked potentials in the detection of spinal cord ischemia in aortic coarctation repair. *Ann Thorac Surg* 1986; 41:251–254.
119. Driscoll DJ, Wolfe RR, Gersony WM, et al. Cardiorespiratory responses to exercise of patients with aortic stenosis, pulmonary stenosis, and ventricular septal defect. *Circulation* 1993; 87(suppl I):I102–I113.
120. Silverman NH. *Pediatric Echocardiography.* New York: Williams & Wilkins; 1993:386.
121. Rhodes LA, Colan SD, Perry SB, et al. Predictors of survival in neonates with critical aortic stenosis. *Circulation* 1991; 84:2325–2335.
122. Keane JF, Driscoll DJ, Gersony WM, et al. Second Natural History Study of Congenital Heart Defects: Results of treatment of patients, with aortic valvular stenosis. *Circulation* 1993; 87(suppl I):I16–I27.
123. Yetman AT, Rosenberg HC, Joubert GI. Progression of asymptomatic aortic stenosis identified in the neonatal period. *Am J Cardiol* 1995; 75:636–637.
124. McCrindle BW, for the Valvuloplasty and Angioplasty of Congenital Anomalies (VACA) Registry investigators. Independent predictors of immediate results of percutaneous balloon aortic valvotomy in childhood. *Am J Cardiol* 1996; 77:286–293.
125. Moore P, Egito E, Mowrey H, et al. Midterm results of balloon dilatation of congenital aortic stenosis: Predictors of success. *J Am Coll Cardiol* 1996; 27:1257–1263.
126. Egito ES, Moore P, O'Sullivan J, et al. Transvascular balloon dilation for neonatal critical aortic stenosis: Early and midterm results. *J Am Coll Cardiol* 1997; 442–447.
127. Kirklin JW, Barratt-Boyes BG. Congenital aortic stenosis. In: Kirklin JW, Barratt-Boyes BH, eds. *Cardiac Surgery,* 2d ed. New York: Churchill Livingstone; 1993:1195.
128. Elkins RC, Knott-Craig CJ, Ward KE, Lane MM. The Ross operation in children: 10-year experience. *Ann Thorac Surg* 1998; 65:496–502.
129. Hawkins JA, Minich LL, Tani LY, et al. Late results and reintervention after aortic valvotomy for critical aortic stenosis in neonates and infants. *Ann Thorac Surg* 1998; 1758–1762.
130. Najm HK, Coles JG, Black MD, et al. Extended aortic root replacement with aortic allografts or pulmonary autografts in children. *J Thorac Cardiovasc Surg* 1999; 118:503–509.
131. Graham TP Jr, Bricker JT, James FW, Strong WB. 26th Bethesda conference: Recommedations for determining eligibility for competition in athletes with cardiovascular abnormalities: Task Force 1: Congenital heart disease. *J Am Coll Cardiol* 1994; 24:867–873.
132. Fyler DC. Aortic outflow abnormalities. In: Fyler DC, ed. *Nadas' Pediatric Cardiology.* Philadelphia: Hanley & Belfus; 1992:506.
133. Van Son JA, Edwards WD, Danielson GK. Pathology of coronary arteries, myocardium, and great arteries in supravalvular aortic stenosis. *J Thorac Cardiovasc Surg* 1994; 108:21–28.
134. Ensing GJ, Schmidt MA, Hagler DF, et al. Spectrum of findings in a family with nonsyndromic autosomal dominant supravalvular aortic stenosis: A Doppler echocardiographic study. *J Am Coll Cardiol* 1989; 13:413–419.
135. Zalzstein E, Moes CA, Musewe NN, Freedom RM. Spectrum of cardiovascular anomalies in Williams-Beuren syndrome. *Pediatr Cardiol* 1991; 12:219–223.
136. French JW, Guntheroth WG. An explanation of asymmetric upper extremity blood pressure in supravalvular aortic stenosis: The Coanda effect. *Circulation* 1970; 42:31–36.
137. Van Son JA, Danielson GK, Puga FJ, et al. Supravalvular aortic stenosis: Long term results of surgical treatment. *J Thorac Cardiovasc Surg* 1994; 107:103–114.
138. Wright GB, Keane JF, Nadas AS, et al. Fixed subaortic stenosis

in the young: Medical and surgical course in 83 patients. *Am J Cardiol* 1983; 52:830–835.
139. Choi JY, Sullivan ID. Fixed subaortic stenosis: Anatomic spectrum and nature of progression. *Br Heart J* 1991; 65:280–286.
140. Freedom RM, Pelech A, Brand A, et al. The progressive nature of subaortic stenosis in congenital heart disease. *Int J Cardiol* 1985; 8:137–148.
141. Cape EG, Vanauker MD, Sigfusson G, et al. Potential role of mechanical stress in the etiology of pediatric heart disease: Septal shear stress in subaortic stenosis. *J Am Coll Cardiol* 1997; 30:247–254.
142. Drinkwater DC, Laks H. Surgery for subvalvular aortic stenosis. *Prog Pediatr Cardiol* 1994; 3:189–201.
143. Maginot KR, Williams RG. Fixed subaortic stenosis. *Prog Pediatr Cardiol* 1994; 3:141–149.
144. Kirklin JW, Ellis FH Jr. Surgical relief of diffuse subvalvular aortic stenosis. *Circulation* 1961; 24:739.
145. DeVries AG, Hess J, Witsenburg M, et al. Management of fixed subaortic stenosis: A retrospective study of 57 cases. *J Am Coll Cardiol* 1992; 19:1013–1017.
146. Braverman AC. Bicuspid aortic valve and associated aortic wall abnormalities. *Curr Opin Cardiol* 1996; 11:501–503.
147. Koretzky ED, Moller JH, Korns ME, et al. Congenital pulmonary stenosis resulting from dysplasia of valve. *Circulation* 1969; 40:43–53.
148. Li MD, Coles JC, McDonald AC. Anomalous muscle bundle of the right ventricle: Its recognition and surgical treatment. *Br Heart J* 1978; 40:1040–1045.
149. Noonan JA. Hypertelorism with Turner phenotype, a new syndrome associated with congenital heart disease. *Am J Dis Child* 1968; 116:373–380.
150. Stone FM, Bessinger FB Jr, Lucas RV Jr, Moller JH. Pre- and postoperative rest and exercise hemodynamics in children with pulmonary stenosis. *Circulation* 1974; 49:1102–1106.
151. Ellison RC, Freedom RM, Keane JF, et al. Indirect assessment of severity in pulmonary stenosis. *Circulation* 1977; 56(suppl I):I14–I20.
152. Lima CO, Sahn DJ, Valdez-Cruz LM, et al. Noninvasive prediction of transvalvular pressure gradient in patients with pulmonary stenosis by quantitative two-dimensional echocardiographic Doppler studies. *Circulation* 1983; 67:866–871.
153. Nugent EW, Freedom RM, Nora JJ, et al. Clinical course in pulmonary stenosis. *Circulation* 1977; 56(suppl I):I38–I47.
154. Mody MR. The natural history of uncomplicated valvular pulmonic stenosis. *Am Heart J* 1975; 90:317–321.
155. Hayes CJ, Gersony WM, Driscoll DJ, et al. Second natural history of congenital heart defects: Results of treatment of patients with pulmonary valvular stenosis. *Circulation* 1993; 87(suppl I): I28–I37.
156. Stanger P, Cassidy SC, Girod DA, et al. Balloon pulmonary valvuloplasty: Results of the Valvuloplasty and Angioplasty of Congenital Anomalies Registry. *Am J Cardiol* 1990; 65:775–783.
157. Marantz PM, Huhta JC, Mullins CE, et al. Results of balloon valvuloplasty in typical and dysplastic pulmonary valve stenosis: Doppler echocardiographic follow-up. *J Am Coll Cardiol* 1988; 12:476–479.
158. Ali Khan MA, al-Yousef S, Huhta JC, et al. Critical pulmonary valve stenosis in patients less than 1 year of age: Treatment with percutaneous gradational balloon pulmonary valvuloplasty. *Am Heart J* 1989; 117:1008–1014.
159. Ladysans EJ, Qureshi SA, Parsons JM, et al. Balloon dilation of critical stenosis of the pulmonary valve in neonates. *Br Heart J* 1990; 63:362–367.
160. Kan JS, Marvin WJ Jr, Bass JL, et al. Balloon angioplasty—branch pulmonary artery stenosis: Results from the Valvuloplasty and Angioplasy of Congenital Anomalies Registry. *Am J Cardiol* 1990; 65:798–801.
161. O'Laughlin MP. Catheterization treatment of stenosis and hypoplasia of pulmonary arteries. *Pediatr Cardiol* 1998; 19:48–56.
162. Baker CM, McGowen FX, Lock JE, Keane JF. Management of pulmonary artery trauma due to balloon dilation. *J Am Coll Cardiol* 1998; 31(suppl A):57A.
163. Vancini M, Roberts KD, Silove ED, Singh SP. Surgical treatment of congenital pulmonary stenosis due to dysplastic leaflets and small valve annulus. *J Thorac Cardiovasc Surg* 1980; 79:464–468.
164. McGoon MD, Fulton RE, Davis GD, et al. Systemic collateral and pulmonary artery stenosis in patients with congenital pulmonary valve atresia and ventricular septal defect. *Circulation* 1977; 56:473–479.
165. Becker AE, Connor M, Anderson RH. Tetralogy of Fallot: A morphometric and geometric study. *Am J Cardiol* 1975; 35:402–412.
166. Rao BN, Anderson RC, Edwards JE. Anatomic variations in the tetralogy of Fallot. *Am Heart J* 1971; 81:361–371.
167. Morgan BC, Guntheroth WG, Bloom RS, Fyler DC. A clinical profile of paroxysmal hyperpnea in cyanotic congenital heart disease. *Circulation* 1965; 31:66–69.
168. Hagler DJ, Tajik AJ, Seward JB, et al. Wide-angle two-dimensional echocardiographic profiles of conotruncal abnormalities. *Mayo Clin Proc* 1980; 55:73–82.
169. Formanek A, Nath PH, Zollikofer C, Moller JH. Selective coronary arteriography in children. *Circulation* 1980; 61:84–95.
170. Ponce FE, Williams LC, Webb HM, et al. Propanolol palliation of tetralogy of Fallot: Experience with long-term drug treatment in pediatric patient. *Pediatrics* 1973; 52:100–108.
171. Blalock A, Taussig HB. The surgical treatment of malformations of the heart in which there is pulmonary stenosis or pulmonary atresia. *JAMA* 1945; 128:129.
172. Lillehei CW, Cohen M, Warden HE, et al. Direct vision intracardiac surgical correction of the tetralogy of Fallot, pentalogy of Fallot, and pulmonary atresia defects: Report of the first 10 cases. *Ann Surg* 1955; 142:418–442.
173. Kirklin JW, Blackstone EH, Kirklin JK, et al. Surgical results and protocols in the spectrum of tetralogy of Fallot. *Ann Surg* 1983; 198:251–265.
174. Castaneda AR, Jonas RA, Mayer JE, Hanley FL. Tetralogy of Fallot. In: *Cardiac Surgery of the Neonate and Infant.* Philadelphia: Saunders; 1994:215.
175. Rastelli GC, Wallace RB, Ongley PA. Complete repair of transposition of the great arteries with pulmonary stenosis: A review and report of a case corrected by using a new surgical technique. *Circulation* 1969; 39:83–95.
176. Kreutzer J, Perry SB, Jonas RA, et al. Tetralogy of Fallot with diminutive pulmonary arteries: Preoperative pulmonary valve dilation and transcatheter rehabilitation of pulmonary arteries. *J Am Coll Cardiol* 1996; 27:1741–1747.
177. Murphy JG, Gersh BJ, Mair DD, et al. Long-term outcome in patients undergoing surgical repair of tetralogy of Fallot. *N Engl J Med* 1993; 329:593–599.
178. Lev M, Liberthson RR, Joseph RH, et al. The pathologic anatomy of Ebstein's disease. *Arch Pathol* 1970; 90:334–343.
179. Schreiber C, Cook A., Ho SY, et al. Morphologic spectrum of Ebstein's malformation: Revisitation relative to surgical repair. *J Thorac Cardiovasc Surg* 1999; 117:148–155.
180. Cohen LS, Friedman JM, Jefferson JW, et al. A reevaluation of risk of in utero exposure to lithium. *JAMA* 1994; 271:146–150.
181. Watson H. Natural history of Ebstein's anomaly of tricuspid valve in childhood and adolescence: An international co-operative study of 505 cases. *Br Heart J* 1974; 36:417–427.
182. Driscoll DJ, Mottram CD, Danielson GK. Spectrum of exercise intolerance in 45 patients with Ebstein's anomaly and observations on exercise tolerance in 11 patients after surgical repair. *J Am Coll Cardiol* 1988; 11:831–836.

183. Roberson DA, Silverman NH. Ebstein's anomaly: Echocardiographic and clinical features in the fetus and neonate. *J Am Coll Cardiol* 1989; 14:1300–1307.
184. Hernandez FA, Richkind R, Cooper HR. The intracavitary electrocardiogram in the diagnosis of Ebstein's anomaly. *Am J Cardiol* 1958; 1:181–190.
185. Celermajer DS, Cullen S, Sullivan ID, et al. Outcome in neonates with Ebstein's anomaly. *J Am Coll Cardiol* 1992; 19:1041–1046.
186. Gentles TL, Calder AL, Clarkson PM, Neutze JM. Predictors of long-term survival with Ebstein's anomaly of the tricuspid valve. *Am J Cardiol* 1992; 69:377–381.
187. Donnelly JE, Brown JM, Radford DJ. Pregnancy outcome and Ebstein's anomaly. *Br Heart J* 1991; 66:368–371.
188. Kulik TJ. Inhaled nitric oxide in the management of congenital heart disease. *Curr Opin Cardiol* 1996; 11:75–80.
189. Reich JD, Auld D, Hulse E, et al. The Pediatric Radiofrequency Ablation Registry's experience with Ebstein's anomaly: Pediatric Electrophysiology Society. *J Cardiovasc Electrophysiol* 1998; 9:1370–1377.
190. Starnes VA, Pitlick PT, Bernstein D, et al. Ebstein's anomaly appearing in the neonate: A new surgical approach. *J Thorac Cardiovasc Surg* 1991; 101:1082–1087.
191. Marianeschi SM, McElhinney DB, Reddy VM, et al. Alternative approach to the repair of Ebstein's malformation: Intracardiac repair with ventricular unloading. *Ann Thorac Surg* 1998; 66:1546–1550.
192. Van Son JA, Falk V, Black MD, et al. Conversion of complex neonatal Ebstein's anomaly into functional tricuspid or pulmonary atresia. *Eur J Cardiothorac Surg* 1998; 13:280–284.
193. Danielson GK, Driscoll DJ, Mair DD, et al. Operative treatment of Ebstein's anomaly. *J Thorac Cardiovasc Surg* 1992; 104:1195–1202.
194. Carpentier A, Chauvaud S, Mace L, et al. A new reconstructive operation for Ebstein's anomaly of the tricuspid valve. *J Thorac Cardioasc Surg* 1988; 96:92–101.
195. Quaegebeur JM, Sreeram H, Fraser AG, et al. Surgery for Ebstein's anomaly: The clinical and echocardiographic evaluation of a new technique. *J Am Coll Cardiol* 1991; 17:722–728.
196. Radford DJ, Graff RF, Neilson GH. Diagnosis and natural history of Ebstein's anomaly. *Br Heart J* 1985; 54:517–522.
197. Lucas RV Jr, Lock JE, Tandon R, Edwards JE. Gross and histologic anatomy of total anomalous pulmonary venous connections. *Am J Cardiol* 1988; 62:292–300.
198. Gathman GE, Nadas AS. Total anomalous pulmonary venous connection: Clinical and physiologic observations of 75 pediatric patients. *Circulation* 1970; 42:143–154.
199. Chin AJ, Sanders S, Sherman F, et al. Accuracy of subcostal two-dimensional echocardiography in prospective diagnosis of total anomalous pulmonary venous connection. *Am Heart J* 1987; 113:1153–1159.
200. Newfeld EA, Wilson A, Paul MH, Reisch JS. Pulmonary vascular disease in total anomalous pulmonary venous drainage. *Circulation* 1980; 61:103–109.
201. Castaneda AR, Jonas RA, Mayer JE, Hanley FL. *Cardiac Surgery in the Neonate and Infant.* Philadelphia: Saunders; 1994:157.
202. Behrendt DM, Aberdeen E, Waterson DJ, Bonham-Carter RE. Total anomalous pulmonary venous drainage in infants: I. Clinical and hemodynamic findings, methods, and results of operation in 37 cases. *Circulation* 1972; 46:347–356.
203. Norwood WI, Hougen TJ, Castaneda AR. Total anomalous pulmonary venous connection: Surgical considerations. *Cardiovasc Clin* 1981; 11:353–364.
204. VanderVelde M, Parness IA, Colan SD, et al. Two-dimensional echocardiography in the pre- and postoperative management of total anomalous pulmonary venous connection. *J Am Coll Cardiol* 1991; 18:1746.
205. Bando K, Turrentine MW, Ensing GJ, et al. Surgical management of total anomalous pulmonary venous connection: Thirty-year trends. *Circulation* 1996; 94(suppl):II12–II26.
206. Lacour-Gayet F, Zoghbi J, Serraf AE, et al. Surgical management of progressive pulmonary venous obstruction after repair of total anomalous pulmonary venous connection. *J Thorac Cardiovasc Surg* 1999; 117:679–687.
207. Van Praagh R, Weinberg PM, Smith SD, et al. Malpositions of the heart. In: Adams FH, Emmanouilides GC, Riemenschneider TA, eds. *Moss' Heart Disease in Infants, Children, and Adolescents,* 4th ed. Baltimore: Williams & Wilkins; 1989:530.
208. Van Praagh R. Segmental approach to diagnosis. In: Fyler DC, ed. *Nadas' Pediatric Cardiology.* Philadelphia: Hanley & Belfus; 1992:27.
209. Van Praagh S, Santini F, Sanders SP. Cardiac malpositions with special emphasis on visceral heterotaxy (asplenia and polysplenia syndromes). In: Fyler DC, ed. *Nadas' Pediatric Cardiology.* Philadelphia: Hanley & Belfus; 1992:589.
210. Rooklin AR, McGeady SJ, Mikaelian DO, et al. The immotile cilia syndrome: A cause of recurrent pulmonary disease in children. *Pediatrics* 1980; 66:526–538.
211. Fyler DC. D-transposition of the great arteries. In: Fyler DC, ed. *Nadas' Pediatric Cardiology.* Philadelphia: Hanley & Belfus; 1992:557.
212. Paul MH, Wernovsky G. Transposition of the great arteries. In: Emmanouilides GC, Riemenschneider TA, Allen HD, Gutgesell HD, eds. *Moss and Adams Heart Disease in Infants, Children, and Adolescents,* 5th ed. Baltimore: Williams and Wilkins; 1995:1154.
213. Yoo S, Burrows PE, Moes CAF, et al. Evaluation of coronary arterial patterns in complete transposition by laidback aortography. *Cardiol Young* 1996; 6:149–155.
214. Liebman J, Cullum L, Belloc NB. Natural history of transposition of the great arteries: Anatomy and birth and death characteristics. *Circulation* 1969; 40:237–262.
215. Gelatt M, Hamilton RM, McCrindle BW, et al. Arrhythmia and mortality after the Mustard procedure: A 30-year single-center experience. *J Am Coll Cardiol* 1997; 29:194–201.
216. Wilson NJ, Clarkson PM, Barratt-Boyes BG, et al. Long-term outcome after the Mustard repair for simple transposition of the great arteries: 28-year follow-up. *J Am Coll Cardiol* 1998; 32:758–765.
217. Kirjavainen M, Happonen JM, Louhimo I. Late results of Senning operation. *J Thorac Cardiovasc Surg* 1999; 117:488–495.
218. Wernovsky G, Mayer JE Jr, Jonas RA, et al. Factors influencing early and late outcome of the arterial switch operation for transposition of the great arteries. *J Thorac Cardiovasc Surg* 1995; 109:289–301.
219. Gutgesell HP, Massaro TA, Kron IL. The arterial switch operation for transposition of the great arteries in a consortium of University Hospitals. *Am J Cardiol* 1994; 74:959–960.
220. Wernovsky G, Freed MD. Transposition of the great arteries: Results and outcome of the arterial switch operation. In: Freedom RM, ed. *Atlas of Heart Diseases,* vol XII, *Congenital Heart Disease.* Philadelphia: Current Medicine; 1997:16.1.
221. Williams WG, Quaegebeur JM, Kirklin JW, Blackstone EH. Outflow obstruction after the arterial switch operation: A multiinstitutional study: Congenital Heart Surgeons Society. *J Thorac Cardiovasc Surg* 1997; 114:975–987.
222. Nakanishi T, Matsumoto Y, Seguchi M, et al. Balloon angioplasty for postoperative pulmonary artery stenosis in transposition of the great arteries. *J Am Coll Cardiol* 1993; 22:859–866.
223. Castaneda AR, Jonas RA, Mayer JE, Hanley FL. *Cardiac Surgery of the Neonate and Infant.* Philadelphia: Saunders; 1994:444.
224. Sagin-Saylam G, Somerville J. Palliative Mustard operation for transposition of the great arteries: Late results after 15–20 years. *Heart* 1996; 75:72–77.
225. Hagler DJ. Double-outlet right ventricle. In: Emmanouilides TA, Riemenschneider TA, Allen HD, Gutgesell HP, eds. *Moss and*

Adams Heart Disease in Infants, Children, and Adolescents, 5th ed. Baltimore: Williams & Wilkins; 1995:1246–1270.

226. Snider AR, Serwer GA. *Echocardiography in Pediatric Heart Disease.* Chicago: Year Book; 1990:190–195.
227. Kirklin JW, Barratt-Boyes BG. Double outlet right ventricle. In: Kirklin JW, Barratt-Boyes BG, eds. *Cardiac Surgery,* 2d ed. New York: Churchill Livingstone; 1993:1469.
228. Aoki M, Forbess JM, Jonas RA, et al. Result of biventricular repair for double-outlet right ventricle. *J Thorac Cardiovasc Surg* 1994; 107:338–349.
229. Belli E, Serraf A, Lacour-Gayet F, et al. Surgical treatment of subaortic stenosis after biventricular repair of double-outlet right ventricle. *J Thorac Cardiovasc Surg* 1996; 112:1570–1580.
230. Mavroudis C, Backer CL, Muster AJ, et al. Taussig-Bing anomaly: Arterial switch versus Kawashima intraventricular repair. *Ann Thorac Surg* 1996; 61:1330–1338.
231. Freedom RM. Congenitally corrected transposition of the great arteries: Definitions and pathologic anatomy. *Pediatr Cardiol* 1999; 10:3–16.
232. Fischbach PS, Law IH, Serwer GS. Congenitally corrected I-transposition of the great arteries: Abnormalities of atrioventricular conduction. *Prog Pediatr Cardiol* 1999; 10:37–43.
233. Snider AR, Serwer GA, Ritter SB. Abnormalities in ventricular connection. In: Snider AR, Serwer GA, Ritter SB, eds. *Echocardiography in Pediatric Heart Disease.* St. Louis: Mosby; 1990: 317–323.
234. Connelly MS, Liu PP, Williams WG, et al. Congenitally corrected transposition of the great arteries in the adult: Functional status and complications. *J Am Coll Cardiol* 1996; 27:1238–1243.
235. Lundstrom U, Bull C, Wyse RK, Somerville J. The natural and "unnatural" history of congenitally corrected transposition. *Am J Cardiol* 1990; 65:1222–1229.
236. Cowley CG, Rosenthal A. Congenitally corrected transposition of the great arteries: The systemic right ventricle. *Prog Pediatr Cardiol* 1999; 10:31–35.
237. Warnes CA. Congenitally corrected transposition: The uncorrected misnomer (editorial comment). *J Am Coll Cardiol* 1996; 27:1244.
238. Kirklin JW, Barratt-Boyes BG. Congenitally corrected transposition of the great arteries. In: Kirklin JW, Barratt-Boyes BG, eds. *Cardiac Surgery,* 2d ed. New York: Churchill Livingstone; 1993:1511.
239. Sano T, Riesenfeld T, Karl TR, Wilkinson JL. Intermediate term outcome after intracardiac repair of associated cardiac defects in patients with atrioventricular and ventriculoarterial discordance. *Circulation* 1995; 92(suppl II):II272–II278.
240. Termignon JL, Leca F, Vouhe PR, et al. "Classic" repair of congenitally corrected transposition and ventricular septal defect. *Ann Thorac Surg* 1996; 62:199–206.
241. Van Son JA, Danielson GK, Huhta JC, et al. Late results of systemic atrioventricular valve replacement in corrected transposition. *J Thorac Cardiovasc Surg* 1995; 109:642–653.
242. Ilbawi MN, DeLeon SY, Backer CL, et al. An alternative approach to the surgical management of physiologically corrected transposition with ventricular septal defect and pulmonary stenosis or atresia. *J Thorac Cardiovasc Surg* 1990; 100:410–415.
243. Imai Y. Double-switch operation for congenitally corrected transposition. *Adv Cardiac Surg* 1997; 9:65–86.
244. Reddy VM, McElhinney DB, Silverman NH, Hanley FL. The double switch procedure for anatomical repair of congenitally corrected transposition of the great arteries in infants and children. *Euro Heart J* 1997; 18:1470–1477.
245. Rosenthal A, Dick M. Tricuspid atresia. In: Emmanouilides GC, Riemenschneider TA, Allen HD, Gutgesell HD, eds. *Moss and Adams Heart Disease in Infants, Children, and Adolescents,* 5th ed. Baltimore: Williams & Wilkins; 1995:902.
246. Hagler DJ, Edwards WD. Univentricular atrioventricular connection. In: Emmanouilides GC, Riemenschneider TA, Allen HD, Gutgesell HD, eds. *Moss and Adams Heart Disease in Infants, Children, and Adolescents,* 5th ed. Baltimore: Williams & Wilkins; 1995:1278.
247. Dobell ARC, Van Praagh R. The Holmes heart: Historic associations and pathologic anatomy. *Am Heart J* 1996; 132:437–445.
248. Silverman NH. *Pediatric Echocardiography.* New York: Williams & Wilkins: 1993:279.
249. Freedom RM, Culham JAG, Moes CAF. *Angiocardiography of Congenital Heart Disease.* New York: Macmillan; 1989.
250. George BL, Kaplan S. Single ventricle and subaortic obstruction. *Prog Pediatr Cardiol* 1994; 3:167–176.
251. Moak JP, Gersony WM. Progressive atrioventricular valvular regurgitation in single ventricle. *Am J Cardiol* 1987; 59:656–658.
252. Donofrio MT, Jacobs ML, Norwood WI, Rychik J. Early changes in ventricular septal defect size and ventricular geometry in the single left ventricle after volume-unloading surgery. *J Am Coll Cardiol* 1995; 26:1008–1015.
253. Mainwaring RD, Lamberti JJ, Moore JW. The bidirectional Glenn and Fontan procedures—integrated management of the patient with a functionally single ventricle. *Cardiol Young* 1996; 6:198–207.
254. Van Son JA, Reddy VM, Haas GS, Hanley FL. Modified surgical techniques for relief of aortic obstruction in (SLL) hearts with rudimentary right ventricle and restrictive bulboventricular foramen. *J Thorac Cardiovasc Surg* 1995; 110:909–915.
255. Norwood WI, Lang P, Hansen DD. Physiologic repair of aortic atresia-hypoplastic left heart syndrome. *N Engl J Med* 1983; 308:23–26.
256. Bailey LL, Nehlsen-Cannarella SL, Doroshow RW, et al. Cardiac allotransplantation in newborns as therapy for hypoplastic left heart syndrome. *N Engl J Med* 1986; 315:949–951.
257. Mayer JE, Bridges ND, Lock JE, et al. Factors associated with marked reduction in mortality for Fontan operation in patients with single ventricle. *J Thorac Cardiovasc Surg* 1992; 103:444–452.
258. Moak JP, Gersony WM. Progressive atrioventricular valvular regurgitation in single ventricle. *Am J Cardiol* 1987; 59:656–658.
259. Matitiau A, Geva T, Colan SD, et al. Bulboventricular foramen size in infants with double-inlet left ventricle or tricuspid atresia with transposed great arteries: Influence on initial palliative operation and rate of growth. *J Am Coll Cardiol* 1992; 19:142–148.
260. Jacobs ML, Rychik J, Rome JJ, et al. Early reduction of the volume work of the single ventricle: The hemi-Fontan operation. *Ann Thorac Surg* 1996; 62:456–462.
261. Van Son JA, Reddy VM, Haas GS, Hanley FL. Modified surgical techniques for relief of aortic obstruction in (SLL) hearts with rudimentary right ventricle and restrictive bulboventricular foramen. *J Thorac Cardiovasc Surg* 1995; 110:909–915.
262. Fontan F, Baudet E. Surgical repair of tricuspid atresia. *Thorax* 1971; 26:240–248.
263. Cetta F, Feldt RH, O'Leary PW, et al. Improved early morbidity and mortality after Fontan operation: The Mayo Clinic experience, 1987 to 1992. *J Am Coll Cardiol* 1996; 28:480–486.
264. Petrossian E, Reddy VM, McElhinney DB, et al. Early results of the extracardiac conduit Fontan operation. *J Thorac Cardiovasc Surg* 1999; 117:688–696.
265. Jacobs ML, Blackstone EH, Bailey LL. Intermediate survival in neonates with aortic atresia: A multi-institutional study: The Congenital Heart Surgeons Society. *J Thorac Cardiovasc Surg* 1998; 116; 417–434.
266. Bove EL. Surgical treatment for hypoplastic left heart syndrome. *Jpn J Thorac Cardiovasc Surg* 1999; 47:47–56.
267. Tkebuchava T, Von Segesser LK, Vogt PR, et al. Congenital coronary fistulas in children and adults: Diagnosis, surgical technique and results. *J Cardiovasc Surg* 1996; 37:29–34.
268. Vavuranakis M, Bush CA, Boudoulas H. Coronary artery fistulas

in adults: Incidence, angiographic characteristics, natural history. *Cathet Cardiovasc Diagn* 1995; 35:116–120.

269. Velvis H, Schmidt KG, Silverman NH, Turley K. Diagnosis of coronary artery fistula by two-dimensional echocardiography, pulsed Doppler ultrasound and color flow imaging. *J Am Coll Cardiol* 1989; 14:968–976.
270. Urruita SCO, Falashci G, Ott DA, Cooley DA. Surgical management of 56 patients with congenital coronary artery fistulas: Report of three cases. *Ann Thorac Surg* 1983; 35:300–307.
271. Mavroudis C, Backer CL, Rocchini AP, et al. Coronary artery fistulas in infants and children: A surgical review and discussion of coil embolization. *Ann Thorac Surg* 1997; 63:1235–1242.
272. Blanche C, Chaux A. Long-term results of surgery for coronary artery fistulas. *Int Surg* 1990; 75:238–239.
273. Perry SB, Rome J, Keane JF, et al. Transcatheter closure of coronary artery fistulas. *J Am Coll Cardiol* 1992; 20:205–209.
274. Hurwitz RA, Caldwell RL, Girod DA, et al. Clinical and hemodynamic course of infants and children with anomalous left coronary artery. *Am Heart J* 1989; 118:1176–1181.
275. Wesselhoeft H, Fawcett JS, Johnson AL. Anomalous origin of the left coronary artery from the pulmonary trunk: Its clinical spectrum, pathology, and pathophysiology, based on a review of 140 cases with seven further cases. *Circulation* 1968; 38:403–425.
276. Schmidt KG, Cooper MJ, Silverman NH, Stanger P. Pulmonary artery origin of the left coronary artery: Diagnosis by two-dimensional echocardiography, pulsed Doppler ultrasound and color flow mapping. *J Am Coll Cardiol* 1988; 11:396–402.
277. Gutgesell HP, Pinsky WW, DePuey EG. Thallium-201 myocardial perfusion imaging in infants and children: Value in distinguishing anomalous left coronary artery from congestive cardiomyopathy. *Circulation* 1980; 61:596–599.
278. Takeuchi S, Imamura H, Katsumoto K, et al. New surgical method for repair of anomalous left coronary artery from pulmonary artery. *J Thorac Cardiovasc Surg* 1979; 78:7–11.
279. Cochrane AD, Coleman DM, Davis AM, et al. Excellent long-term functional outcome after an operation for anomalous left coronary artery from the pulmonary artery. *J Thorac Cardiovasc Surg* 1999; 117:332–342.
280. El-Said GM, Ruzyllo W, Williams RL, et al. Early and late results of saphenous vein graft for anomalous origin of left coronary artery from pulmonary artery. *Circulation* 1973; 48(suppl III):2–6.
281. Rein AJ, Colan SD, Parness IA, Sanders SP. Regional and global left ventricular function in infants with anomalous origin of the left coronary artery from the pulmonary trunk: Preoperative and postoperative assessment. *Circulation* 1987; 75:115–123.
282. Rahimtoola SH. Concept and evaluation of hibernating myocardium. *Annu Rev Med* 1999; 50:75–86.

CHAPTER 64

CONGENITAL HEART DISEASE IN ADULTS

Carole A. Warnes / John E. Deanfield

Congenital heart disease occurs in 5 to 10 per 1000 live births.[1] Without early treatment, the majority of patients would die in infancy or childhood, with only 5 to 15 percent surviving until puberty.[2] The advent of surgical procedures, from ligation of a patent arterial duct[3] in 1939 to the innovations of the 1990s, as well as advances in medical treatment, has transformed the outlook for children with even complex defects. The majority now survive into adolescence and adult life (Chap. 63). This success story has radically altered both the size and complexity of the population of young adults with congenital heart disease. In the United States alone, well over a half-million patients with functionally important congenital cardiac malformations have reached adulthood in the past three decades.[4] Despite the fact that most patients now surviving to adult life will have undergone surgery during childhood, "total correction" is not the rule.[5] The term *total correction* is itself a misnomer, perhaps with the exception of the successfully ligated ductus arteriosus without residua. The misperception of "cure" leads adults not to seek understanding of their anomaly, to fail to follow endocarditis prophylaxis, and to fail in pursuing continued cardiac care. The majority, if not all, require long-term surveillance, and many need reoperation. Other adults may require their first operation for congenital heart lesions that were well tolerated during childhood.

Both the "natural" survivors and the postoperative patients require specialized medical care. Arrhythmia is common, as are residual or deteriorating hemodynamic problems and endocarditis. Although cardiologists specializing in the care of adults may be expert in one or more of these areas, the critical relationship between rhythm and hemodynamic status in hearts with complex circulations (as after a Fontan operation or after intra-atrial repair for transposition) may lead to treatment errors by those inexperienced in the treatment of congenital heart defects. Patients with cyanosis require special care because of erythrocytosis, bleeding, renal problems, and arthropathy; moreover, they require specific counseling and management regarding pregnancy. In addition to the medical problems, psychosocial problems such as the search for employment, life and health insurance, participation in sports, sexual activity, and contraception are of great importance to adolescents and young adults with congenital heart disease. Many of the "normal" ordeals of growing up are more difficult for this group, in whom chronic illness, embarrassing scars, and/or exercise limitation may inhibit normal social intercourse and maturation.

Over the last few years, the specialist needs of this growing population have begun to be appreciated. In addition to the challenge of continuing the expert care of their complex cardiac problems from the pediatric environment into the much wider adult medical community, knowledge of the long-term fate of patients with congenital heart disease is essential for pediatric cardiologists in order to refine initial management strategy. A rather short-term view of "success" or "failure" has been encouraged by rapid changes in medical and surgical policies over the last three decades. Nevertheless, there are clear examples, such as the management of transposition of the great arteries, where awareness of long-term problems has altered the primary surgical approach. The Mustard or Senning procedures (see below) provide a physiologic repair at acceptably low risk but may result in long-term systemic ventricular dysfunction, arrhythmias, and sudden death. This has enabled the introduction of anatomic repair by the arterial-switch procedure, despite high surgical mortality in the early series, with the expectation of a more satisfactory long-term outcome. Other debates, over such issues as the place of Fontan operations, cavopulmonary anastomosis, and systemic-to-pulmonary shunts, are not yet resolved and will be strongly influenced by the accumulation of rigorously collected outcome data, not merely for survival but also for morbidity and quality of life.

The optimal solutions for delivery of care to the adult with congenital heart disease will depend on the different medical systems in operation around the world. The common requirements include collaboration between pediatric and adult cardiologists; the establishment of a few specialist centers with appropriate medical, surgical, anesthetic, and nonmedical staff together with investigational facilities; the establishment of treatment guidelines, and centralization of accumulating knowledge.[6] The report of a consensus conference on adult congenital heart disease commissioned by the Canadian Cardiovascular Society represents an important step forward.[7] This includes recommendations for training and a hierarchy of care from the community to the specialist center. Similar training guidelines have been published in the United States.[8]

MEDICAL CONSIDERATIONS

Many young adults with congenital heart disease have mild lesions that have not required and may not ever require surgery. The commonest defects in this category are small ventricular septal defect, mild pulmonary valve stenosis, mild aortic valve stenosis, and mitral valve prolapse (Table 64-1). Such patients need infrequent follow-up (e.g., biannual) to assess any progression in severity of the lesion, to reinforce the need for antibiotic prophylaxis against infective endocarditis (Chap. 73), and to obtain psychosocial advice. Other patients reach adult life with more complex defects that are still unrepaired. Some may still be candidates for palliative or definitive surgery, whereas in others surgery may no longer be possible, often because of the presence of irreversible pulmonary vascular disease. More and more survivors of surgery in childhood are now reaching adult life; they now form the largest group of patients (Table 64-2). The majority need continuing medical surveillance, since late cardiovascular problems may result from hemodynamic disturbances, arrhythmia, and endocarditis. Such patients can also develop noncardiac problems as a consequence of their heart disease (e.g., secondary to cyanosis) and are, of course, susceptible to all the potential acquired "medical problems" of adulthood.

TABLE 64-1 Common Congenital Heart Defects Compatible with Survival to Adult Life without Surgery or Interventional Catheterization

Mild pulmonary valve stenosis
Peripheral pulmonary stenosis
Bicuspid aortic valve
Mild subaortic stenosis
Mild supravalvar aortic stenosis
Small atrial septal defect
Small ventricular septal defect
Small patent ductus arteriosus
Mitral valve prolapse
Ostium primum atrial septal defect (atrioventricular septal defect)
Marfan's syndrome
Ebstein's anomaly
Corrected transposition (atrioventricular-ventriculo-arterial discordance)
Balanced complex lesions (e.g, double-inlet ventricle with pulmonary stensosis)
Defects with pulmonary vascular obstructive disease (Eisenmenger's syndrome)

Hemodynamics

Study of the hemodynamic consequences of repaired and unrepaired congenital heart disease is a crucial aspect of long-term follow-up. Progressive congestive cardiac failure secondary to myocardial deterioration is the most common cause of disability and death in patients whose ventricles may have been subjected to many years of volume and pressure loading, often with chronic hypoxia. A significant number of the adult postoperative patients with congenital heart disease have been repaired at older ages than is the current practice. This may result in greater preoperative damage and pulmonary vascular disease, which may persist postoperatively. In the early era of open-heart surgery, myocardial protection was sometimes less than optimal, resulting in myocardial damage.

It should also be appreciated that postoperative circulations created by the repair of many congenital heart defects result in an adequate physiologic repair (e.g., deoxygenated blood to lungs and oxygenated blood to the body) but often have far from normal anatomy. For example, after the Mustard and Senning operation for transposition of the great arteries, the right ventricle remains on the systemic side of the circulation. Some of these patients have evidence of deteriorating right ventricular function, and there is increasing concern that this will become a major life-threatening problem with longer follow-up.[9] Similar concerns have been expressed for systemic ventricular function after the Fontan operation.[10] The different morphologic characteristics and loading conditions for these ventricles suggest that standard indices of ventricular function,

TABLE 64-2 Common Congenital Heart Defects Surviving to Adult Life after Surgery/Interventional Catheterization

Aortic valve disease, valvotomy or replacement
Pulmonary stenosis, valvotomy
Tetralogy of Fallot
Atrial septal defect
Ventricular septal defect
Atrioventricular septal defect
Transposition of the great arteries, atrial redirection
Complex transposition of the great arteries
Total anomalous pulmonary venous connection
Pulmonary atresia/ventricular septal defect
Fontan operation for complex congenital heart disease
Ebstein's anomaly
Coarctation of the aorta
Mitral valve disease

derived from studies of structurally normal hearts, may be inappropriate for such patients (see also Chap. 20).[11] Prospective serial studies are beginning to define "normal ranges" for congenital heart defects and to examine their "natural" and "unnatural" history.[12]

Residual hemodynamic defects are often present in repaired patients and may cause problems even many years after surgery. These may be amenable to further surgery (see below) or require long-term medical treatment. Medical management of cardiac failure in patients with congenital heart disease is adopting therapies shown to be of benefit in large-scale clinical trials of patients with heart failure from predominantly cardiomyopathy or ischemic heart disease.[13–15] Appreciation of ventricular "remodeling" and the effect of neurohumeral responses on symptoms and disease progression has led to increasing and earlier use of angiotensin-converting enzyme inhibitors and, in some cases, beta blockers and long-acting calcium antagonists in addition to standard therapy with digoxin and diuretics (see Chap. 21). These agents may also slow the rate of progressive deterioration in ventricular function reported in certain congenital heart diseases even when they have been adequately "corrected."

Cyanosis

Adults with congenital heart disease may have central cyanosis from right-to-left shunting secondary to their unrepaired cardiac defect or to pulmonary vascular disease (Eisenmenger's syndrome; see Chap. 63). The latter complication should be seen less frequently in years ahead as a result of the trend toward early recognition and repair of congenital heart disease in infancy. Currently, however, a significant number of patients reach adult life with pulmonary vascular disease as a result of lesions such as large ventricular septal defect, atrioventricular (AV) septal defect, truncus arteriosus, and double-outlet right ventricle. Their pulmonary vascular resistance may already have been too high for surgical repair at the time of diagnosis; in others, pulmonary vascular disease may have progressed despite repair of the congenital heart defect.

Chronic cyanosis may lead to erythrocytosis and hyperviscosity. Many patients with cyanotic congenital heart disease establish a stable high hematocrit but few symptoms of hyperviscosity.[16] They have a low risk of stroke and do not require venesection.[17] In others, the hemoglobin concentration may rise progressively. Once it exceeds 20 g/dL, they are at risk from thromboembolic complications and may suffer from headache, dizziness, and fatigue. Symptoms may be improved with judicious venesection by the removal of 500 mL of blood and volume replacement with normal saline or dextrose solution.[17,18] Overzealous venesection, however, may result in both acute and chronic problems, including cardiovascular collapse in patients with Eisenmenger's syndrome, iron depletion, microcytosis, and hyperviscosity in its own right.[19] The paradoxical anemia of erythrocytotic patients with iron deficiency due to repeated phlebotomy may be missed and indeed has been shown to increase the risk of stroke.[20] It has been demonstrated that phlebotomies and microcytosis were strongly associated with stroke, perhaps due to the fact that iron-deficient red blood cells are less deformable than are normal red blood cells and do not pass through the microcirculation as readily as do iron-replete cells.

Patients with chronic cyanosis also develop defective hemostasis from abnormalities in platelet function and in the coagulation and fibrinolytic systems,[19,20] especially patients with marked erythrocytosis. The risk of hemorrhage, especially at surgery, is well recognized and may be fatal. Hyperuricemia is common because of increased red cell turnover and renal dysfunction. Arthralgia is well recognized, but gouty arthritis is rare and may be misdiagnosed. Renal impairment can deteriorate to renal failure as a result of relatively minor interventions, such as injection of contrast medium at angiography or the injudicious use of nonsteroidal anti-inflammatory agents.[21,22] Patients with right-to-left shunts are at risk of paradoxic embolus, which may cause a cerebrovascular accident or renal infarction. Air filters must be utilized with all intravenous lines. A cerebral abscess is a well-known complication of a septic embolus and must always be considered in the cyanotic patient with any neurologic symptoms, however transient, or low-grade fever. Facial and truncal acne is common, and is not only a cosmetic problem but a potential source of sepsis. A specific concern has been the safety of air travel in adults with cyanotic congenital heart disease, since in-flight atmospheric conditions on commercial jets approach altitude equivalents of 6000 to 8000 ft (1829 to 2438 m). In a recent report, however, only modest (approximately 6 percent) decreases in systemic arterial oxygen saturation were found, with no adverse effects.[23]

Progressive kyphoscoliosis has been recognized for many years as a complication of congenital heart disease.[24] It is common in cyanotic patients and those with previous thoracotomy. The degree of deformity, if left untreated, may become profound and compromise pulmonary function. Treatment with bracing or insertion of a Harrington rod may be indicated, since the kyphoscoliosis may significantly reduce both the quality and quantity of life. Surgical repair is not possible, however, in those with Eisenmenger's syndrome, since the surgical risk is too high.

The prognosis for patients with Eisenmenger's syndrome depends on the site of the lesion and the medical and cardiac care they receive.[25–27] Death may result from right-sided heart failure, pulmonary hemorrhage, or arrhythmia. It can also occur prematurely due to potentially avoidable complication, such as inappropriate drug therapy or injudicious general anesthesia. Special care must be employed during noncardiac surgery, utilizing cardiac anesthesia, maintenance of preload, and cardiac monitoring.[28] Recent data suggest promise for chronic prostacyclin therapy in reducing pulmonary artery pressure, but this is preliminary.[29]

Infective Endocarditis

Patients with both unoperated and operated congenital heart disease are at risk from infective endocarditis. Lifelong antibiotic prophylaxis is recommended, but the specific indications and optimal regimens are still debated.[30,31] The American Heart Association Special Report on Prevention of Infective Endocarditis has stratified risk groups for the various lesions.[31] Prophylaxis is advocated for all lesions except isolated secundum atrial septal defect and repaired secundum atrial septal defect, ventricular septal defect, or patent ductus arteriosus without residua beyond 6 months (see Chap. 73). The wide variety of portals of entry includes dental work, skin sepsis, obstetric and gynecologic procedures, genitourinary and gastrointestinal interventions, and surgery.[32,33] There is also a risk of bacteremia and infective endocarditis in young adults who have their ears pierced or acquire a tattoo.[34] Patients must be educated and preferably should carry an information card with them. The symptoms of endocarditis may be subtle, and the diagnosis must be considered in any patient who experiences unexplained malaise or fever. Injudicious prescription of antibiotics without previous blood culture may mask the problem and make bacteriologic diagnosis and appropriate treatment difficult. Both general measures, such as oral hygiene as well as skin and nail care, and appropriate antibiotic treatment are important. Among 102 patients with congenital heart disease who filled in a questionnaire, there was a disturbing lack of knowledge about endocarditis prevention measures and indeed about their cardiac lesion in general.[35]

Electrophysiologic Problems

Arrhythmias and conduction defects have a major impact on the prognosis and management of both unoperated and operated patients and have been linked to sudden death in a number of conditions.[36,37] The principles of diagnosis and treatment are similar to those employed in patients with arrhythmia due to other causes (see Chap. 24), with some important exceptions. Rhythm disturbances that may be benign in a structurally normal heart may be life-threatening in congenital heart disease. Restoration of sinus rhythm is usually much more important, and rate control of atrial arrhythmias is usually not a good treatment option. Special consideration must be given before the use of therapies that may have negative inotropic properties. In unoperated patients, chamber dilatation, myocardial hypertrophy, and fibrosis may all contribute to the genesis of arrhythmia. In operated patients, additional sinus or AV node damage and atrial and/or ventricular scarring may cause electrophysiologic problems. The etiology is multifactorial, and the clinical significance of arrhythmia depends very much on the hemodynamic context in which it occurs.

Supraventricular arrhythmia and sinus node injury, not surprisingly, occur most often in conditions with "atrial defects" or those requiring atrial surgery.[38,39] Abnormalities of sinus node function are common in patients with atrial septal defect, particularly the sinus venosus type,[40] and are often seen after Mustard or Senning operation for transposition of the great arteries.[41] Sinus node dysfunction has also been reported after surgery for tetralogy of Fallot, the Fontan procedure, and many other operations for congenital heart lesions.[42] Clinical manifestations include sinus bradycardia, sinoatrial block, sinus arrest, and occasionally the tachybradycardia syndrome with paroxysmal atrial flutter and fibrillation. Although bradycardia has been postulated as the cause of sudden death in some conditions, current evidence indicates that tachyarrhythmia is usually a more likely explanation (see below).[41]

In sinus node disease, insertion of a pacemaker is indicated for patients with symptoms resulting from a slow heart rate, such as tiredness, dizziness, and syncope or for an extremely low heart rate (see Chap. 31). Indications in asymptomatic individuals are still controversial, since the arrhythmia is benign in many cases. It should be noted that pacing may be difficult because of the complex underlying anatomy and lack of a suitable site for endocardial lead fixation.[43] The choice of pacemaker will depend on the precise indication. The simplest VVI pacemaker may be adequate prophylaxis against bradycardia-related sudden death. In general, however, rate-responsive pacemakers are preferable, and dual-chamber pacing may provide the best hemodynamics (see also Chap. 31).[44,45]

Injury to the AV node and proximal conduction tissue may result from surgery for lesions such as ventricular septal defect, AV septal defect, or tetralogy of Fallot. Transient complete AV block in the postoperative period has been shown to have prognostic significance in some reports, particularly if the site of damage is below the bundle of His. In a 30-year follow-up of ventricular septal defect repair at the Mayo Clinic, the development of transient complete heart block for over 72 h followed by resumption of sinus rhythm was a strong independent predictor of late mortality.[46] Whether transient perioperative AV block warrants permanent pacing and whether an invasive electrophysiologic study can help stratify risk are unresolved.[38] Postoperative right bundle-branch block is frequent after ventriculotomy and may be due to injury related to closure of a ventricular septal defect or to interruption of distal Purkinje fibers by ventriculotomy or muscle resection.[37,38] Occasionally, the electrocardiographic (ECG) pattern of right bundle-branch block with left-axis deviation occurs (bifascicular block), and there may also be PR-interval prolongation (trifascicular block).[47,48] Early reports suggested that these findings were harbingers of sudden cardiac death due to complete heart block.[49] More recent studies, however, have not substantiated this adverse prognosis.[50]

Tachyarrhythmias can be life threatening. Late sudden death has been reported in several lesions, both before and after repair. In general, the worse the disease (i.e., more complex anatomy and/or more extensive surgery), the greater the incidence of sudden death, although aortic stenosis and coarctation are also represented in this group. Studies suggest that the risk increases incrementally 20 years after surgical repair.[51] The identification of patients at risk and their management are important but controversial issues. After the Mustard and Senning operation, atrial flutter with a rapid ventricular response is dangerous, especially when it occurs in association with right ventricular dysfunction or venous pathway obstruction.[52] Medical or electrical cardioversion should be promptly used to restore sinus rhythm, and drug therapy may need to be accompanied by pacemaker insertion. Recently, ablation (surgical or catheter) has been advocated for certain cases of atrial flutter (see Chap. 28). Atrial tachyarrhythmias are also common after the Fontan operation; sinus node injury, atrial suturing, and a dilated hypertensive right atrium probably contribute.[42,51] Modification of the operation to exclude the right atrium from the Fontan circuit, the total cavopulmonary connection, may reduce the incidence of potentially serious early and late rhythm disturbances.[53,54]

Ventricular arrhythmias are known to occur after open-heart surgery, particularly repair of tetralogy of Fallot.[48,55] Studies using ambulatory ECG monitoring in postoperative patients have documented asymptomatic complex ectopy and nonsustained ventricular tachycardia in up to 50 percent of patients,[55–57] and more than 20 percent have inducible ventricular tachycardia at electrophysiologic study.[58,59] Experimental and clinical studies have shown that the electrical substrate for reentry arrhythmia is present in the right ventricle.[60] In several reports, older age at surgery is a predisposing factor,[57,61] an observation that suggests factors present at the time of repair may be involved in the genesis of postoperative arrhythmia, in addition to the myocardial damage occurring at the time of surgery or during postoperative follow-up.[62] This is consistent with morphologic studies that have documented increasing fibrosis of the right ventricle as part of the natural history of defects such as tetralogy of Fallot.[63] The current practice of early surgical repair for tetralogy of Fallot may reduce the incidence of such postoperative ventricular arrhythmia, and encouraging preliminary data support this view.[62,64] Other postulated risk factors include elevated right ventricular systolic pressure, reduced right ventricular ejection fraction, pulmonary regurgitation, and a ventriculotomy scar.[65] The clinical significance of nonsustained ventricular tachycardia and especially the indications for prophylactic antiarrhythmic therapy remain unclear.[52] There is a disparity between the high frequency of ventricular arrhythmia and the much lower incidence of sudden death.[66,67] The predictive value of an abnormal ambulatory ECG or of electrophysiologic study has not been established. Furthermore, prophylactic antiarrhythmic therapy has not been shown to be of value in asymptomatic patients with congenital heart defects. Such therapy may have proarrhythmic potential, be negatively inotropic, or have serious extracardiac side effects. As a result, there is insufficient evidence to advocate prophylactic treatment for asymptomatic individuals with nonsustained arrhythmia. On the other hand, there are a few cases of sudden death, out-of-hospital ventricular fibrillation, and/or sustained ventricular tachycardia in almost all large series of patients after repair of tetralogy of Fallot. Identification of at-risk individuals and appropriate treatment remain a challenge. Recent reports have indicated a link between the electrical and mechanical properties of the right ventricle, which may have clinical relevance.[68] The QRS duration on the surface ECG correlates with cardiothoracic ratio and, in a retrospective review, a QRS greater than 180 ms was a sensitive and specific marker for sudden death or out-of-hospital cardiac arrest.[69] Others have not confirmed this.[70] Further refinements in risk stratification in adults with tetralogy of Fallot or other congenital heart lesions are necessary and probably will involve hemodynamic and electrophysiologic testing both at rest and after exercise, evaluation of ventricular late potentials (Chap. 26), and heart rate variability.[71] It should be remembered, however, that, despite the attention given to ventricular arrhythmia after repair of tetralogy of Fallot, a major source of morbidity in such patients is from atrial arrhythmia.[72]

Radiofrequency ablation, so successfully used to treat arrhythmia in patients with structurally normal hearts (Chap. 28), is being applied to patients with congenital heart disease. These applications represent some of the most challenging electrophysiologic procedures because of the complex cardiac anatomy, enlarged chamber size, and abnormal localization of the underlying conduction system. Nevertheless, ablation may have a role, not merely in subjects with accessory pathways or AV reentry tachycardia, but also in intraatrial reentry arrhythmias that may be present after operations such as Fontan and Mustard or Senning procedures.[73,74]

Pregnancy

An increasing number of women with complex and postoperative congenital heart defects are reaching childbearing age. Advice is sought on both maternal and fetal risk as well as on the incidence of congenital heart disease in the offspring. In the United States, most maternal cardiac disease is congenital in origin. Data are accumulating regarding outcomes of pregnancy in many complex anomalies.[75–80] Prepregnancy counseling is mandatory for all patients whether operated or unoperated. The evaluation should include a detailed history, physical examination, ECG, and chest x-ray along with a comprehensive echocardiogram to evaluate ventricular function, all valve lesions and defects, and pulmonary artery pressure. If pulmonary artery pressure and resistance is in doubt following noninvasive testing, a cardiac catheterization may be necessary. An exercise test may facilitate a detailed assessment of functional capacity.

There are profound changes in the maternal cardiovascular system during pregnancy, including a large (30 to 40 percent) increase in blood volume, a fall in peripheral vascular resistance, and an increase in cardiac output (approximately 40 percent; see also Chap. 82). In general, women with left-to-right shunts or valvular regurgitation tolerate pregnancy well, whereas those with right-to-left shunts or valvular stenosis do less well.[81,82] Asymptomatic young women with small or moderate left-to-right shunts and normal pulmonary artery pressures can expect an uncomplicated pregnancy and labor. In the presence of a large left-to-right shunt, however, heart failure may be provoked or aggravated by pregnancy. Patients with cyanosis have the most problems in carrying a fetus to term and have a high incidence of early spontaneous abortion. Early studies showed that, with higher degrees of cyanosis (as reflected by the maternal hemoglobin), the incidence of spontaneous abortion increased and the handicap to fetal growth became more pronounced. Infants are unlikely to survive if the maternal hemoglobin level is above 18 g/dL.[83] A study from Presbitero et al. demonstrated a clear relationship between the degree of hypoxia and fetal loss (Table 64-3).[84] When the maternal oxygen saturation was 85 percent, only 2 out of 17 pregnancies (12 percent) resulted in live-born infants. Only 41 of 96 pregnancies (43 percent) produced a live birth in 45 cyanosed mothers. There were 49 spontaneous abortions and 6 stillbirths in this series, again reflecting the high risk that maternal cyanotic congenital heart disease poses for the fetus. Meticulous care during pregnancy and delivery lessened the maternal complication rate,

TABLE 64-3 Fetal Outcome in Cynotic Congenital Heart Disease and Its Relation with Maternal Cyanosis

Hemoglobin, g/dL[a]	Pregnancy, no.	Live Births, no.	Live Born, %
≤16	28	20	71
17–19	40	18	45
≥20	26	2	8
Arterial Oxygen Saturation, %[b]	**Pregnancy, no.**	**Live Births, no.**	**Live Born, %**
≤85	17	2	12
85–89	22	10	45
≥90	13	12	92

[a]Hemoglobin level unknown in two pregnancies.
[b]Arterial oxygen saturation unknown in 44 pregnancies.
SOURCE: From Presbitero P, Somerville J, Stone S, et al. Pregnancy in cyanotic congenital heart disease: Outcome of mother and fetus. *Circulation* 1994; 89:2673–2676. Reproduced with permission from the publisher and authors.

but this was still considerable. Such patients require rest and a short labor as well as avoidance of dehydration and sepsis. In such situations, the decision as to whether to continue with the pregnancy depends on an assessment of the risk to the mother and fetus as compared with the patient's desire to have children.

An elevated pulmonary vascular resistance, from either Eisenmenger's syndrome or primary pulmonary hypertension, is a clear contraindication to pregnancy. Pregnancy for women with Eisenmenger's syndrome carries approximately a 50 percent mortality rate.[85] Termination of pregnancy is always preferable; ideally, this should be done with cardiac anesthesia. If such patients are seen late in pregnancy and termination is not feasible, management should concentrate on maintenance of adequate preload and avoidance of vasodilation. The ideal management around the time of delivery for these patients is controversial because individual experience is small. Vaginal delivery is usually associated with less blood loss than is cesarean section. The latter, however, can be done quickly with all medical personnel in attendance. One report has suggested an approach of elective delivery by cesarean section under general anesthesia.[86] The use of prophylactic heparin before and after delivery is also controversial, and there is no established consensus.[86,87] Even after successful delivery, however, death frequently occurs within the few days following from deteriorating hemodynamics or pulmonary infarction.[85] Patients with Marfan's syndrome and aortic root dilation (greater than 40 mm) are at greater risk of aortic dissection and rupture, and while those without preexisting cardiovascular disease whose aortic root is smaller often tolerate pregnancy well, the risk is unpredictable.[88,89] Patients with severe aortic stenosis are also at increased risk because of the fall in afterload that accompanies pregnancy and exaggerates the valve gradient.[90,91] While early reports suggested a high risk of aortic rupture and cerebral hemorrhage in patients with aortic coarctation,[92] recent data have been more encouraging.[93] Fetal risk is increased, however, presumably as a result of compromised placental blood supply.

The management of pregnant women with mechanical prosthetic cardiac valves is a special problem because of the risk to the mother of thromboembolism and the risk to the fetus of anticoagulants (warfarin crosses the placenta and is teratogenic).[94,95] Depending on the condition involved and the mother's motivation and compliance, the use of subcutaneous heparin in the first and third trimesters and warfarin in the midtrimester is one treatment option. Heparin, however, is a poor anticoagulant during pregnancy; even with meticulous control of anticoagulation, there is still an increased risk of valve thrombosis.[96] In addition, there is also an increased risk of fetal loss with this approach. Because of the poor results with heparin, some authors have advocated the use of warfarin throughout pregnancy despite the risk of fetal teratogenicity.[97] This risk may be less if the dose of warfarin is less than 5 mg/day.[98] Nonetheless, this approach is still very controversial, despite the fact that fetal teratogenicity with warfarin may have been overemphasized (see Chap. 44).[99] Before prescribing any cardiovascular drug during pregnancy, the effects on both mother and fetus must be considered.

Management of labor should be specifically directed toward avoidance of rapid changes in circulatory volume, blood pressure, or cardiac output. In most cases, vaginal delivery is recommended, with careful attention to maternal position and analgesic agents. The American Heart Association no longer recommends endocarditis prophylaxis for vaginal delivery.[31] This recommendation, however, is not based on controlled data, and most cardiologists recommend antibiotics under these circumstances for almost all congenital heart defects.

Genetic Counseling

The risk of recurrence is an increasingly important issue as more males and females with congenital heart disease reach reproductive age, and genetic counseling should be provided for all potential parents. Recent genetic advances are clarifying the etiology of a number of congenital heart diseases. It has been estimated that the cause of congenital heart disease is genetic in approximately 8 percent of cases (e.g., velocardiofacial syndrome and Holt-Oram syndrome with autosomal dominant transmission) and environmental in 2 percent (e.g., congenital rubella syndrome).[100] In the remainder, genetic and environmental factors are thought to interact.[101] The greater the number of affected first-degree relatives within the family, the greater the recurrence risk. Recurrence risks in siblings of patients with congenital heart disease are well documented and range between 1 and 8 percent.[102] For the affected potential parents, however, the risk of recurrence in offspring is the key information, and fewer data exist. Early reports suggested that recurrence risks were considerably higher in offspring compared to siblings. Studies, such as the Second Natural History of Congenital Heart Defects, have suggested a low risk (1.2 percent for aortic stenosis, 2.8 percent for pulmonary stenosis, and 2.9 percent for ventricular septal defects).[103] There is considerable variation in recurrence risks in reported series, and factors inherent in study design, ascertainment bias, and follow-up account for many of the differences. In addition, certain forms of congenital heart disease recur more frequently than others (e.g., left ventricular outflow tract obstruction), and the recurrence risk appears to be higher in pregnancies with affected mothers rather than fathers. Accumulation of further information will be invaluable for counseling of patients. Fetal cardiac ultrasound at approximately 18 weeks of pregnancy facilitates early diagnosis.

Investigation and Imaging

Transthoracic echocardiography and cardiac catheterization with angiocardiography are the principal investigations in pediatric cardiology. Transthoracic echocardiography is an invaluable tool in adults also, although image acquisition is more challenging because of body habitus and chest wall abnormalities as a result of previous surgeries.[104] Transesophageal echocardiography is becoming increasingly important for the definition of cardiac structure and function,[104–106] and multiplane probes with color-flow Doppler imaging allow simultaneous assessment of anatomy and physiology. Specific areas and lesions of the heart that are well imaged in this way include systemic and pulmonary venous drainage, atrial lesions (including baffle function), AV valve morphology and function, left ventricular outflow tract lesions (including the ascending aorta in Marfan's syndrome), and intracavity thrombus or vegetations (Fig. 64-1).[106,107]

Magnetic resonance imaging (MRI) can also provide valuable anatomic information, which in some cases is superior to that from ultrasound, even via a transesophageal approach. Rapid technologic advances—including three-dimensional image reconstruction; software to study hemodynamics, such as velocity mapping; and cine-MRI—may reduce the need for invasive investigation (Fig. 64-2).[108–110] The expertise required both to acquire and to interpret MRI information is likely to be confined to specialized regional centers, but access to the MRI facility should be available to all units managing adult patients with congenital heart disease.

In parallel with the decreasing need for diagnostic cardiac catheterization, there has been a dramatic rise in the indications for and scope of interventional procedures in adult patients with congenital heart disease.[111] Residual defects after repair that are amenable to treatment in the catheterization laboratory include coronary fistulas, paravalvular leaks, and pulmonary artery stenoses. Optimum management of patients with complex congenital heart disease can often be achieved by planned collaboration between surgeon and interventional cardiologist. In other patients with a range of relatively simple lesions—including patent ductus arteriosus, pulmonary valve stenosis, atrial septal defect/patent foramen ovale, and certain forms of ventricular septal defect—definitive treatment avoiding surgery may be achieved by interventional catheterization.

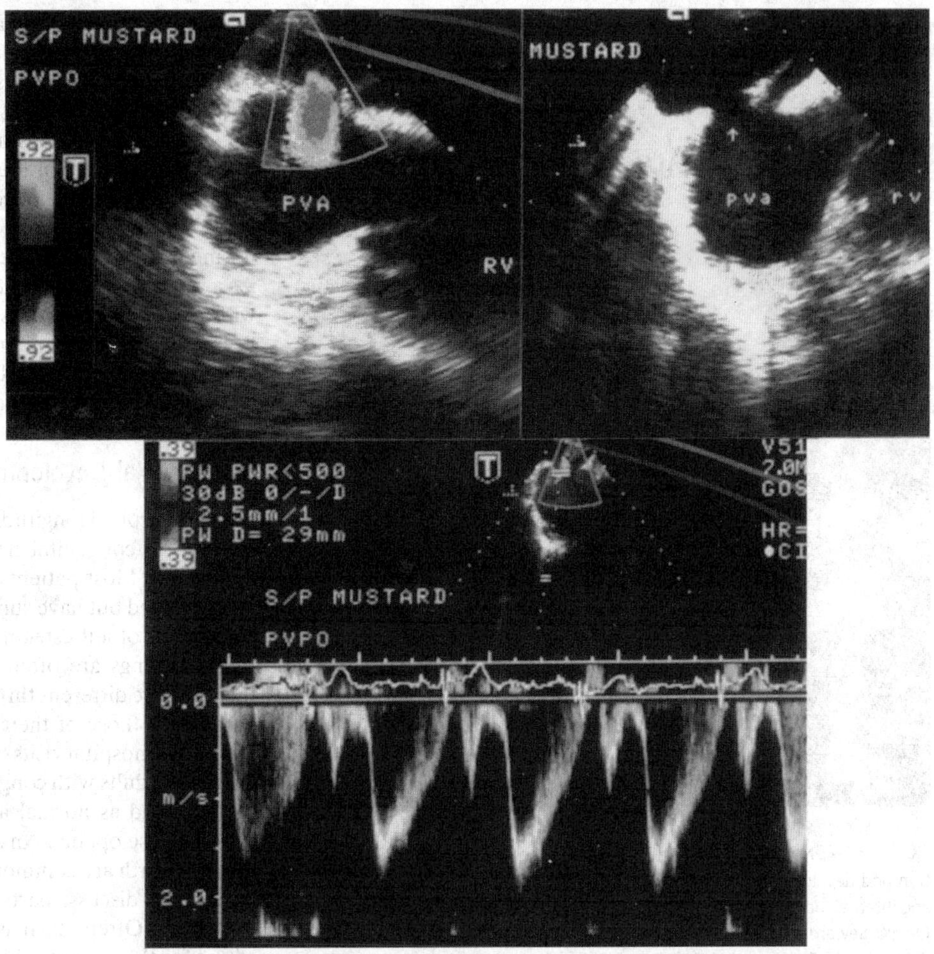

FIGURE 64-1 Transesophageal echocardiogram and Doppler evaluation after a Mustard operation for transposition of the great arteries. There is moderate pulmonary venous obstruction, indicated by the accelerated flow through the narrowing indicated by the arrow. PVA, pulmonary venous atrium; RV, right ventricle. (Courtesy of Dr. I. D. Sullivan, Great Ormond Street Hospital for Children, London.)

PSYCHOSOCIAL ASPECTS

During adolescence, a crucial transition occurs for the patient with congenital heart disease. By the end of the teenage years, the young adult must understand the nature and implications of his or her heart problem. Sensible advice and guidance must be available regarding employment, insurance, socialization, contraception, exercise, and sports.

Employment

Most patients can work and should have access to employment appropriate to their physical and intellectual capabilities. The report of the Natural History Study of Congenital Heart Defects suggested that, among patients with ventricular septal defect, pulmonary stenosis, and aortic stenosis, in comparison with national normal standards, a greater percentage achieved higher levels of education (college and beyond).[112] No similar data are yet available for large groups of patients with more complex defects, although their situation will undoubtedly prove worse.

Despite the excellent potential of many adults with congenital heart disease, job discrimination is frequently encountered, even when a patient has been cleared by a cardiologist. In the United States, the National Rehabilitation Act of 1973 seeks to prevent job discrimination by employers with 10 or more employees by obliging them to consider only the present capacity of applicants to perform a given job and not projections of future deterioration. In other countries, employers frequently take into account future prospects for absenteeism or premature career curtailment. In these circumstances, young adults with congenital heart defects are often at a disadvantage, particularly if they apply for jobs with long training periods.

Restrictions for employment exist for jobs in which the safety of others is the direct responsibility of an individual, such as driving a bus or truck. Most armed services exclude applicants with a cardiac history. The regulations for commercial airline pilots are clearer and subject to regular review. In Europe, a risk of sudden cardiac death or acute disability below 1 percent per annum is the maximum considered acceptable for multicrew flights and below 0.1 percent per annum for solo flights. The number of congenital heart defects in which low risk rates are clearly defined remains small.[113]

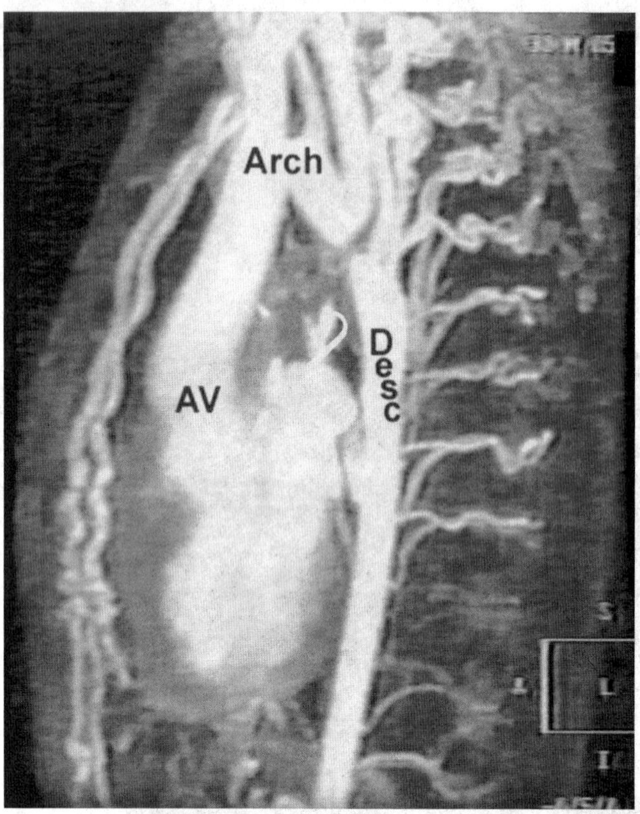

FIGURE 64-2 MRI angiogram of a 33-year-old man showing a severe coarctation and development of extensive collateralization involving the intercostal and internal mammary arteries. AV, aortic valve; Desc, descending aorta. (From Oh JK, Seward JB, Tajik AJ. Congenital heart disease. In: Oh JK, Seward JB, Tajik AJ, eds: *The Echo Manual*, 2d ed. Philadelphia: Lippincott-Raven, 1999: 233. Reproduced with permission from the publisher and authors.)

Insurance

Possession of adequate life insurance is often a prerequisite for a home mortgage. Insurance companies are of necessity fiscally conservative. As a result, life insurance is difficult to obtain for many young adults in the absence of adequate long-term survival data for their congenital heart lesions. Most of the data used to assess risk are either incorrect or out of date and do not apply to currently performed medical or surgical procedures. In 1986, a survey in the United States recorded that only patients with very simple lesions were insured at regular rates.[114] These included mild pulmonary valve stenosis, uncomplicated repaired atrial septal defect, ventricular septal defect, and patent ductus arteriosus. A similar survey in the United Kingdom in 1993 evaluated both employment status and insurability of young adults with congenital heart disease.[115] In general, policies were as restrictive as those in the earlier survey, with mitral valve prolapse (without regurgitation), postoperative patent ductus arteriosus, and coarctation insurable at standard rates and all other lesions being either insurable at higher rates or not insurable at all. Marked inconsistencies were found, making "shopping around" mandatory. This situation is likely to improve when health care professionals are able to provide high-quality follow-up data on morbidity and mortality rates relevant to current treatment protocols (see Chap. 104).

Despite surgical repair, long-term cardiac care into adult life is usually required for patients with congenital heart disease. In many countries, health care provision and financing are changing rapidly, with costs spiraling dramatically.[116] There are particular problems in systems that rely on private health insurance. Medical expenses incurred during childhood are usually reimbursed as part of the parents' policy. This coverage often ceases to be available once the patient reaches the age of majority. A new policy sought at this stage at best excludes benefits for medical or surgical treatment of the cardiac condition itself. As a result, the level of medical surveillance of the adult patient with congenital heart disease drops dramatically after age 21 years. This is a major problem, since, with adequate regular follow-up, costs for adults with congenital heart disease are considerably lower than those for other chronic diseases.

Psychosocial Development

Large controlled longitudinal studies of the psychosocial consequences of congenital heart disease are rare and difficult to interpret.[117] Most patients with congenital heart disease appear well adjusted but have subtle feelings of "difference" from their peers. Lack of self-esteem and fear of isolation are common.[118–120] These feelings are often compounded by frequent reminders that they are different through limitation of their activities compared with those of their peers, the presence of scars, cardiac symptoms, hospital visits, and family anxiety. As a result, adolescents and adults with congenital heart disease should be encouraged to lead as normal a life as possible and to discuss their heart disease openly. Anxieties about sexual activity, marriage, and childbirth are common, but patients often find these aspects difficult to discuss, particularly with the doctor in a regular clinic.[120–122] Often, such issues are best handled by the team caring for the patient, which may include a nurse, social worker, and psychologist. As the child with congenital heart disease matures, one of the most potent effects on his or her life is parental overprotection. In adolescents and young adults, this may result in enormous resentment and rebellion against all adult authority figures, including the doctor. Compliance with medical treatment and advice can be affected.

The impact of congenital heart disease on intellectual development is controversial. Interpretation of testing must take into account the very abnormal childhood experienced by many patients, with absences from school for medical reasons as well as decreased social interaction. In addition, patients have often had an overprotected childhood, and their attitude to testing procedures may be different from those of their peers. All studies of intellect exclude patients with genetic syndromes and other dysmorphic, somatic, or neurologic defects, but subtle abnormalities are easily missed.[123] Certain aspects of development appear to be more specifically affected by congenital heart disease. For example, walking is delayed in cyanotic children, but speech is not. This will affect the relevance of early IQ testing to later performance. Currently, data suggest that cyanosis is associated with mild intellectual impairment.[124–126] This association is reduced by early corrective surgery, even involving cardiopulmonary bypass.

Contraception

Sexually active adolescents and young adults should be given appropriate advice about contraception.[127,128] In general, the low-dose estrogen oral contraceptive pill is safe for young women with congenital heart disease.[129] Exceptions include women with hypertension (e.g., associated with coarctation of the aorta) and those with pulmonary vascular disease or cyanosis with associated erythrocytosis. Progesterone preparations are alternatives, although they have a lower contraceptive efficacy.[130] They are, however, inappropriate for patients with cardiac failure because of the tendency for fluid retention; moreover, progesterone-only pills can cause depression in adolescents. Barrier methods, either using condom or diaphragm, are safe and effective, but intrauterine devices should probably not be used because of the risk of endocarditis and of increased bleeding, particularly in cyanotic women.[131] In women with severe pulmonary vascular disease or with lesions in which pregnancy would result in high maternal risk, laparoscopic sterilization should be considered.

Exercise and Sports

Exercise is of both physical and psychological benefit. It leads to improved cardiovascular fitness and decreased likelihood of obesity, hypertension, and ischemic heart disease.[132,133] Furthermore, participation in exercise and sports is part of normal socialization in adolescent and adult life. In many adults with congenital heart disease, exercise capacity is diminished, even after surgery. Reduced performance may also reflect lack of regular exercise in protected individuals with congenital heart defects. This is often reinforced by doctors who, if in doubt, tend to limit exercise.

The Twenty-sixth Bethesda Conference provided recommendations for competition in athletics by patients with cardiovascular abnormalities.[134] Sports are broadly categorized into those involving dynamic exercise and those involving static exercise, although these two types of exercise are at two extremes of a continuum. Another important consideration is the danger of bodily injury from collision or the consequences of syncope. Significant disease or death precipitated by exercise in patients with congenital heart disease is rare, but the other consideration is whether prolonged long-term exercise might contribute to progressive hemodynamic deterioration (e.g., left ventricular hypertrophy and aortic stenosis). In some cases, exercise capacity is clearly normal and the risk is minimal, as after closure of a small patent ductus arteriosus. In others, exercise capacity is limited and the risk is high, as in severe pulmonary hypertension. Between these extremes is a gray area in which recommendations must take into account the individual, the underlying cardiac defect, hemodynamic status, and the type of sport and form of exercise contemplated (e.g., social or competitive, or contact or noncontact). Formal testing should be performed (preferably including measurement of oxygen uptake), both as a measure of the effects of submaximal and maximal exercise and also as a reassurance to the patient. A 12-min walking test provides a good guide to functional capacity, whereas a treadmill protocol with more strenuous effort is employed to assess risk by revealing occult arrhythmia, ischemia, or fall in blood pressure (Chap. 14). Subjective estimates of exercise capacity are often inaccurate.

In general, volume overload, valve regurgitation, and left-to-right shunts are associated with good exercise tolerance, while pressure overload, valve stenosis, and right-to-left shunt are not. The recommendations provided by the Bethesda Conference should be considered guidelines only. The physician with knowledge of the severity of the patient's lesion and physiologic and psychologic response to training and competition may choose to modify these recommendations.[134] Those patients with a history of symptomatic arrhythmia, syncope, pulmonary hypertension, or myocardial dysfunction deserve special attention, since they are probably at higher risk. Patients with fixed, elevated pulmonary vascular resistance have limited exercise capacity, and for them exercise has considerable risk. Walking should be encouraged but strenuous exercise avoided. The most controversial recommendations are those for aortic stenosis and Marfan's syndrome. It could be argued that exercise may increase the risk of sudden death or progression of left ventricular hypertrophy in the former (see Chap. 56) and of progressive aortic dilatation in the latter (see Chap. 76). Thus, patients with more than mild aortic stenosis should be counseled against moderate to strenuous activities. Patients with Marfan's syndrome, particularly those with aortic root dilatation, should be counseled against isometric exercise and activities with the potential for bodily collision. Supervised training programs for adults with congenital heart disease can improve aerobic fitness and increase the safe level at which they can participate in sports. Such programs also improve psychological adjustment and self-esteem.

SURGICAL CONSIDERATIONS

Reoperations

Reoperations in adults with congenital heart disease provide a particular challenge.[135,136] The risks are often higher than for primary procedures. Careful preoperative planning should include complete understanding of the cardiac anatomy and its relationships to neighboring structures, and study of previous operative reports. Sternal reentry is particularly risky when the ventricle immediately beneath the sternum is a high-pressure chamber or when an extracardiac conduit lies in this position. The use of Gore-Tex membranes under the sternum may reduce the difficulties of future repeat procedures. Postoperative hemodynamic and respiratory problems are particularly common after reoperation because of the increased duration of surgery, previously scarred myocardium and/or lung disease, and greater use of blood products. The need for reoperation may come as a shock to patients and relatives who may have believed that childhood surgery was curative. As a result, resentment is frequent, and tact is required. Indications for reoperation are shown in Table 64-4.

Inevitable Reoperation

Early repair of congenital heart defects that have involved insertion of a prosthetic valve or extracardiac conduit commonly results in a need for reoperation to replace prostheses that are either too small or have undergone degeneration. Extracardiac conduits are commonly used for repair of pulmonary atresia with ventricular septal defect, truncus arteriosus, transposition with left ventricular outflow tract obstruction and/or ventricular septal defect, congenitally corrected transposition with left ventricular outflow tract obstruction, and/or ventricular septal defect and were used in early Fontan operations. Development

TABLE 64-4 Indications for Reoperation in Adults with Congenital Heart Disease

1. Inevitable reoperation after definitive repair prosthetic valves, extracardiac conduits placed at an early age that become of inadequate size because of body growth
2. Residual defects after definitive repair: ventricular septal defect after tetralogy of Fallot and left AV valve regurgitation after AV septal defect repair
3. New/recurrent defects after definitive repair: subaortic stenosis, restenosis of aortic valve, pulmonary regurgitation in tetralogy of Fallot
4. Staged repair of complex defects: pulmonary atresia with ventricular septal defect
5. Unexpected complications: infective endocarditis
6. Heart/heart-lung transplantation for uncorrectable congenital heart disease
7. Patient operated on for congenital heart disease with new acquired heart disease: coronary disease

of obstruction is influenced by the type and size of conduit, technique of insertion, and timing of the original operation. In one series of 143 survivors of heterograft conduit insertion, all had to be replaced by 10 years.[137] A homograft aorta or pulmonary artery and valve have also been used for the repair of pulmonary atresia with ventricular septal defect.[138] Fresh or frozen homografts in childhood have not performed as well as initially hoped.[139] Calcification and obstruction remain significant complications. However, because of their favorable handling characteristics, homografts remain the conduits of choice for many reconstructions.[140,141] Besides the conduit itself, improved operative technique and the use of a large conduit have clear beneficial influence on the need for early replacement. This may be facilitated by utilizing a prosthetic roof of pericardium placed over the fibrous tissue bed of the explanted conduit, thus permitting a large tissue valve to be inserted.[142] Patients with right-sided conduits need careful follow-up, particularly toward the end of the expected life of the conduit. Although conduit obstruction may be suspected from clinical examination, the signs of severe obstruction may be subtle and may be missed. As a result, replacement may be performed too late. The consequent major deleterious effects on right ventricular function increase the risk of surgery and may not be fully reversible. Regular, noninvasive evaluation by transthoracic or transesophageal echocardiography or MRI is indicated in selected patients and may provide the information usually obtained by cardiac catheterization and angiography. Reoperation is usually indicated if the right ventricular pressure is 75 percent of the systemic or if there is evidence of deteriorating ventricular function.[143]

Residual and Recurrent Defects

Residual and recurrent defects may be difficult to distinguish unless careful assessment after the original repair has been performed. They may have a major impact on morbidity and mortality rates, as when major left AV valve regurgitation persists after repair of AV septal defect.[144] Much more long-term follow-up data are needed before guidelines for reoperation for relatively minor residual abnormalities, such as mild left AV valve regurgitation, in this situation can be established.

The reported need for reoperation after the commonly performed reparative operation for tetralogy of Fallot varies between 1.8 and 13 percent over a follow-up of up to 31 years.[145,146] Ventricular septal defect and right ventricular outflow tract obstruction are the commonest residual abnormalities. Pulmonary regurgitation is extremely common and inevitable after transannular patching as part of the original repair. The hemodynamic consequences of pulmonary regurgitation for the right ventricle are greater in the presence of other defects, such as residual obstruction and/or ventricular septal defect. Pulmonary valve replacement has not been frequently required in the first two decades after repair but may become increasingly performed because of the late deleterious effects of pulmonary regurgitation on the right ventricle.[147] Current indications include progressive right ventricular dilatation and a decrease in exercise tolerance.[148] This is often accompanied by progressive tricuspid regurgitation and atrial arrhythmias. When surgery is performed before the development of right ventricular failure, both clinical status and right ventricular function improve.[149] The optimal method for assessing pulmonary regurgitation in serial follow-up has not been determined; therefore, appropriate guidelines for intervention are still not established.

Several studies have emphasized the palliative nature of aortic valvotomy in childhood.[150-152] Isolated aortic stenosis most frequently results from a bicuspid aortic valve, although in neonates and infants the structural abnormality of the aortic valve is more severe and the results of surgery even worse (see Chap. 63). In a series of 59 patients who underwent open aortic valvotomy at over 1 year of age, the actuarial survival rate was 94 percent at 5 years but only 77 percent at 22 years. Reoperation was carried out in 36 percent, and the actuarial probability of reoperation was 44 percent at 22 years. When serious events, comprising death, reoperation, and endocarditis, were grouped together, 92 percent were free of events at 5 years but only 39 percent at 22 years. Others have reported a similar long-term outcome.[150] The causes of restenosis have not been studied in detail but appear to be related to the degree of residual obstruction.

Staged Repair

For complex congenital heart disease, definitive repair may not be possible until the anatomy and physiology of the circulation have been improved by one or more palliative procedures as part of a staged approach to "correction." This course is often necessary for patients with pulmonary atresia and ventricular septal defect, hypoplastic pulmonary arteries, and multifocal pulmonary blood supply. Palliative procedures to increase flow to the central pulmonary arteries and unifocalization of pulmonary flow by anastomosis (direct or indirect) of collateral vessels to the pulmonary arteries may eventually result in the ability to perform a repair (conduit insertion between the right ventricle and pulmonary artery and ventricular septal defect closure) with an acceptable postoperative right ventricular/left ventricular pressure ratio.[153,154] Good surgical results have been reported from such an approach, but the long-term outcome is not yet known.[155]

Other situations in which definitive repair may be indicated in the young adult include complex congenital heart defects with one functioning ventricle palliated by a systemic-pulmonary shunt or pulmonary artery banding in childhood. In selected patients who fulfill the stringent criteria for a Fontan operation, it is likely that long-term results will be better after a Fontan operation than when the ventricle is left with a chronically increased load resulting from a systemic pulmonary shunt.[12] The Fontan operation, however, should be considered palliative rather than curative: long-term problems are frequent.

Unexpected Reoperations

Indications for unexpected reoperation include thrombosis in a low-flow circulation such as the Fontan, prosthetic valve failure or thrombosis, and infective endocarditis. The latter may be particularly difficult to diagnose in complex congenital heart disease where the site of vegetations may not be easy to image (e.g., in a Blalock-Taussig shunt). Reoperation in the patient with uncontrolled endocarditis carries a particularly high risk.

Heart and Heart-Lung Transplantation

Despite the major successes of the last three decades, an increasing number of patients survive to adult life with deteriorating clinical status. Their only remaining prospect may be a heart or heart-and-lung transplant (see Chap. 22). These patients often present specific surgical problems of multiple previous chest incisions, complex venous anatomy, and borderline pulmonary vascular resistance. In addition, the young adult with end-stage heart disease may not have the ideal social milieu to cope with the demands of transplantation and may require considerable psychological support. Nonetheless, the results in this group of patients may be excellent.[156] The shortage of donors and the ability to monitor rejection in a single organ have stimulated great interest in single-lung transplantation for patients with primary pulmonary hypertension and Eisenmenger's syndrome (in conjunction with closure of the shunt).[157]

First Operations for Congenital Heart Disease in Adults

The first surgical repair of a congenital heart defect may be required in a teenager or an adult because the lesion was mild and of little hemodynamic significance in childhood but progressed in severity with time. Examples of such lesions include a bicuspid aortic valve with progressive stenosis (see Chap. 56), Marfan's syndrome with aortic root dilatation (see Chap. 76), and Ebstein's anomaly with worsening symptoms. Alternatively, lesions such as small to moderate atrial septal defects may have been missed or misdiagnosed until adult life. In certain complex congenital heart defects, the combination of lesions produces a balanced hemodynamic state compatible with prolonged survival without intervention. Patients with double-inlet ventricle and pulmonary stenosis, complex pulmonary atresia, and tetralogy of Fallot may remain well until the second and even third decades of life before deteriorating.[158] The contemplation of heart surgery in an adolescent or young adult is often terrifying, implying the acceptance of the presence of a serious heart problem by the patient and his or her immediate friends and family. The scar on the chest may cause embarrassment, and the patient may be discriminated against both socially and at work. All these issues need to be dealt with sympathetically by the physician.

Noncardiac Surgery

When performed without adequate preparation, noncardiac surgery in adults with congenital heart disease is a major cause of avoidable morbidity and death. All the anesthetic risks encountered for cardiac reoperation apply equally to noncardiac surgery, but in the latter the patient may be managed by medical staff who may be unfamiliar with the significance of the congenital heart disease. Many patients with congenital heart defects are at increased risk for arrhythmia and from agents that depress ventricular function. The surgeon must be aware of the presence of a pacemaker or pacing leads that may affect the safe use of diathermy. Prophylaxis against infective endocarditis is usually indicated, and the choice of antibiotic regimen is dictated by the surgical procedure or intervention being undertaken (see Chap. 73). In patients with pulmonary vascular disease, general anesthesia may have disastrous consequences, with a sudden fall in systemic vascular resistance.[28] Similar hemodynamic changes may induce a severe hypercyanotic spell in a patient with uncorrected tetralogy of Fallot, and meticulous pre-, intra-, and postoperative hemodynamic monitoring is mandatory, together with the avoidance of vasodilating anesthetic agents, hypoxia, hypoventilation, and blood or volume loss. Cyanotic patients also have impaired hemostasis, and some patients may be taking anticoagulants. Intravenous lines, drugs, and infusions must be managed carefully in patients with intracardiac shunts, since air or emboli may reach the systemic circulation. The safety of noncardiac surgery in adults with congenital heart disease is greatly increased when physicians, anesthesiologists, and surgeons familiarize themselves with these issues, seek specialized advice, and, if necessary, refer the patient to a team with more experience.

SPECIFIC LESIONS

General Considerations

Some lesions that are commonly seen in adult congenital heart disease, as a result of both natural and unnatural survival, are listed in Tables 64-1 and 64-2.

Interpretation of the literature on long-term outcome of congenital heart defects is hampered by a number of difficulties. First, follow-up is still short, and numbers of survivors are small for many defects. The era of open-heart surgery for congenital heart defects only began in the 1950s, and "correction" has only been attempted much more recently for many categories of patients now beginning to reach adult life (e.g., the Fontan operation). Second, surgical practice has undergone a process of evolution during this time, with new operations for some lesions (e.g., transposition of the great arteries) or major change in operative technique for others (e.g., the Fontan operation). Third, major advances in cardiopulmonary bypass and myocardial protection have accompanied improved preoperative diagnosis and recognition of intracardiac anatomy, particularly of the disposition of the conduction tissues. Finally, for almost all lesions, the management philosophy has changed, with a trend to early primary repair as opposed to initial palliation. For many defects, therefore, long-term outcome data relevant to current practice are not available.

Correct application of survival analysis is essential for interpretation of follow-up data. In particular, the use of hazard functions providing an estimate of *instantaneous risk* is particularly valuable. The following section deals with some specific defects seen in adults with congenital heart disease.

Atrial Septal Defect

Atrial septal defects are among the commonest congenital anomalies in adolescents and adults, accounting for up to 30 percent of congenital heart disease in this age group.[159,160] Approximately 75 percent of defects are ostium secundum defects, 20 percent ostium primum defects (discussed below), and 5 percent sinus venosus defects; defects at other sites are rare (see Chap. 63).[161,162] Associated lesions include pulmonary stenosis, mitral valve prolapse, and mitral regurgitation. Atrial septal defects may be associated with other syndromes, including the Holt-Oram syndrome (see Fig. 10-2)[163] and may be familial.[164] In the latter, conduction disease manifesting as prolongation of the PR interval and, rarely, heart block have been described.[164] Lutembacher syndrome (atrial septal defect coexisting with mitral stenosis) is now very uncommon.

NATURAL HISTORY

Survival into adulthood is the rule, and patients living into their eighties and nineties have been reported.[159] Life expectancy, however, is not normal. Death during the first 20 years of life is infrequent, but after the age of 40 years, the mortality rate increases to about 6 percent per year.[165,166] Defects may go unrecognized for many years because symptoms are rare until later life and physical signs may be subtle. Later, the natural history is characterized by progressive symptoms and cardiomegaly, the development of atrial arrhythmias, right ventricular hypertrophy, and pulmonary hypertension. The mechanisms for the development of symptoms are multifactorial[159] and include the following:

1. Change in left ventricular compliance from superimposed hypertension or coronary artery disease may increase the shunt with age. Long-standing right ventricular volume overload, although relatively well tolerated, ultimately leads to right ventricular dysfunction and progression of tricuspid regurgitation.
2. Supraventricular arrhythmias, particularly atrial fibrillation and flutter, increase with time and may cause symptoms and cardiac failure (Fig. 64-3).
3. Progressive pulmonary hypertension may become symptomatic after the third decade of life.
4. Rarer complications may occur, including systemic and pulmonary emboli, recurrent chest infections, and infective endocarditis (in patients with coexisting mitral valve disease).

MANAGEMENT

Surgical closure either by direct suture or use of a patch has been performed for more than 40 years (see Chap. 63). Surgery carries a low risk (less than 1 percent operative mortality rate),

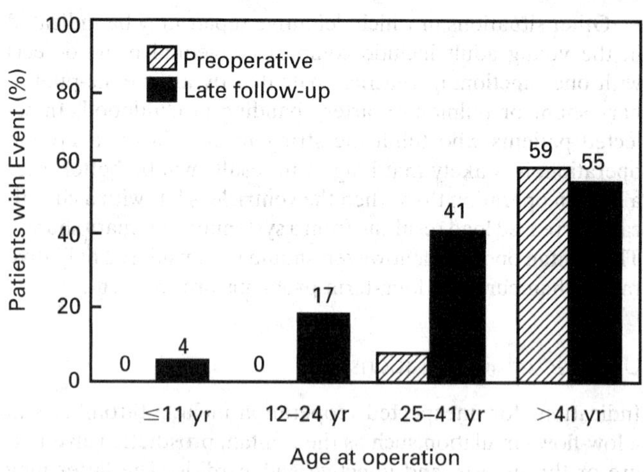

FIGURE 64-3 Incidence of atrial flutter or atrial fibrillation preoperatively and at late follow-up according to the age at operation after repair of atrial septal defect. (From Murphy JG, Gersh BJ, McGoon MD, et al. Long-term outcome after surgical repair of isolated atrial septal defects: Follow-up at 27–32 years. *N Engl J Med* 1990; 323:1645. Reproduced with permission from the publisher and authors.)

provided that the pulmonary vascular resistance is not significantly elevated.[162] In older patients, the indication for closure is a little more controversial. Shah et al. compared the outcome of patients treated medically and surgically when diagnosed after the age of 25 years.[167] This unrandomized study followed patients for more than 20 years and concluded that there was no difference in survival or symptoms between the two groups and no difference in the incidence of new arrhythmia, stroke, or other embolic phenomena in the follow-up period. Notably, however, more than 70 percent of patients in both the medical and surgical groups were asymptomatic at presentation, which may partly explain the favorable outcome of the medically treated group, who had a 91 percent survival. Konstantinides et al. evaluated 179 patients with secundum atrial septal defect 40 years of age or older and compared the outcome of medically and surgically treated groups.[168] They demonstrated a reduced mortality rate after surgical closure, with a 95 percent surgical survival versus an 84 percent medical survival at 10 years. Nonfatal cardiovascular complications, however, were similar, with atrial fibrillation and flutter occurring with a similar incidence in both groups. The functional status of the medically treated group deteriorated in 34 percent of patients and improved in many of the surgical patients, particularly those in class III or IV. It thus seems reasonable to conclude that symptomatic adult patients will improve after surgical repair, and the only real contraindication is severe pulmonary vascular disease. When surgery is delayed, symptoms are likely to be progressive, and surgical repair is less likely to prevent problems with atrial fibrillation and thromboembolic events. For those with preexisting atrial fibrillation, a concomitant right-sided maze procedure may facilitate restoration and maintenance of sinus rhythm.[169] The management of the asymptomatic adult patient is less clear, but certainly closure of the defect halts progression of right ventricular volume overload, tricuspid regurgitation, and progression of pulmonary vascular disease, and it can be accomplished with low surgical risk. The standard surgical approach remains a midline sternotomy, but patients should be made aware of the alternatives of thoracotomy or inframammary incision. Although morbidity rates may be higher, the resulting scar may be less offensive, especially to young women.

Closure of atrial septal defect has been achieved in selected patients by use of a variety of occlusion devices inserted at cardiac catheterization.[170–174] Several alternatives have been evaluated, but no large series with adequate follow-up are yet available for comparison with surgery. The attractions of closing defects without open-heart surgery are obvious. Eventually, the transcatheter technique may supplant surgery as the method of closure for atrial septal defects of appropriate size, morphologic characteristics, and location. In addition, the presence of a patent foramen ovale has been suggested as a risk factor for cerebral embolus. Determining the risk of clinical events in asymptomatic subjects with patent foramen ovale and indications for treatment are highly controversial areas. Catheter treatment may become the method of choice for patients who have a clear indication for intervention.

LATE RESULTS

In a recent study of patients undergoing surgical repair of an atrial septal defect between 1956 and 1960, late survival of patients undergoing operation at below 24 years of age was not significantly different from that of an age- and sex-matched control population. Late survival in patients aged 25 to 41 years was good but less than that of the control population, while repair after age 41 years was associated with significantly poorer late survival (see Fig. 64-3). The combination of older age at operation and pulmonary hypertension had an additive effect on late mortality rates.[175] In this and other series, the propensity for atrial fibrillation and flutter increased as a function of age both before and after operation (Fig. 64-4).[175,176] Twenty-two percent of late deaths were due to stroke, and all occurred in patients with postoperative atrial fibrillation or flutter. These data support the current policy of repair at a preschool age (Chap. 63). A separate study of 66 patients who underwent closure of atrial septal defect between 60 and 78 years of age implied a benefit in survival in patients discharged from the hospital compared with unoperated historical age- and sex-matched controls.[177] A study of patients over 70 years of age showed improved survival of patients in New York Heart Association (NYHA) class II and III when treated surgically compared to medical treatment. Patients in NYHA class IV did poorly with medical or surgical treatment.

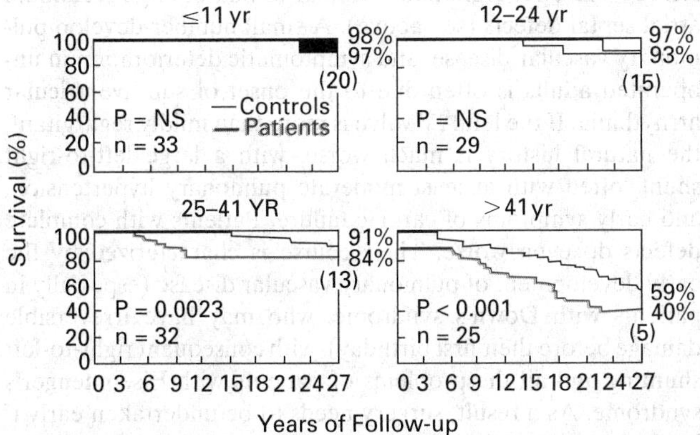

FIGURE 64-4 Long-term survival of perioperative survivors of atrial septal defect repair by age at time of operation. Controls are survival in an age- and sex-matched population. (From Murphy JG, Gersh BJ, McGoon MD, et al. Long-term outcome after surgical repair of isolated atrial septal defects: Follow-up at 27–32 years. *N Engl J Med* 1990; 323:1645. Reproduced with permission from the publisher and authors.)

The near-normal survival and low morbidity rates in patients undergoing repair within the first two decades of life have important implications for employment and insurance recommendations. Such patients should be encouraged to lead a normal life, and competitive sports should not be restricted in the absence of hemodynamic or electrophysiologic sequelae. Patients who have undergone repair in the third decade of life or later require careful regular surveillance. Although late survival is good, the development of supraventricular arrhythmia and risk of cerebrovascular accident are of concern. Anticoagulation is indicated in patients with atrial fibrillation and should be considered in those with supraventricular tachycardia or atrial flutter in the absence of other contraindications (see also Chaps. 24 and 44). Long-term follow-up is recommended for patients repaired in adult life who have increased pulmonary artery pressure at the end of operation, pre- and postoperative arrhythmia, ventricular dysfunction, or coexisting heart disease.

Ventricular Septal Defect

Isolated ventricular septal defect, although one of the commonest congenital abnormalities in infants and children, is far less frequent in the adolescent and adult for several reasons.[159] First, most patients with a hemodynamically significant defect will have undergone repair in childhood; second, spontaneous decrease in size and closure are common for small or moderate perimembranous or muscular defects (this decreases in frequency with increasing age); finally, patients with large, unoperated defects may die earlier in life.[178] The spectrum of isolated ventricular septal defects in the adult is thus limited to the following four groups of patients: (1) those with small, restrictive defects that were either small to begin with or have partially closed; (2) those with Eisenmenger's syndrome and a predominant right-to-left shunt with cyanosis,[179] who need to be distinguished from those who develop secondary infundibular pulmonary stenosis, which can also decrease the left-to-right shunt and may result in cyanosis with shunt reversal (see Chap. 63);[180] (3) the occasional patient with a moderately restrictive defect in whom the diagnosis has been overlooked or who has not had closure in childhood; and (4) those who have had their defects closed in childhood.

NATURAL HISTORY

The natural history of small, restrictive ventricular septal defects is very favorable. Nevertheless, the risk of infective endocarditis persists (developing in almost 4 percent of patients with ventricular septal defect), and lifelong prophylaxis is required. Spontaneous closure may occasionally still occur in adult life. A subset of patients with perimembranous defects or defects in the outlet septum may develop aortic cusp prolapse and aortic regurgitation. This may be progressive and is often severe by the end of the second decade of life. As incompetence increases, the ventricular septal defect may become "closed" by the prolapsing cusp; if it is left to develop, however, aortic valve replacement may be necessary.[181] Such defects are associated with a high risk of infective endocarditis. Severe and progressive pulmonary vascular disease is a feature of older patients with nonrestrictive large defects. Eisenmenger's syndrome is compatible with survival into young adult life, but the complications of right-sided heart failure, paradoxical emboli, and erythrocytosis usually result in death by the third decade (see Chap. 63). Occasionally, patients with moderate-sized ventricular septal defects and left-to-right shunts who did not develop pulmonary vascular disease present in adolescence and young adult life with symptoms of fatigue, effort intolerance, and respiratory infections.

MANAGEMENT

Patients with small ventricular septal defects are asymptomatic and should be managed conservatively. Continued medical follow-up is, however, helpful to remind patients about the need for prophylaxis against infective endocarditis and to minimize inappropriate discrimination during the search for employment and insurance. Ventricular septal defects associated with aortic cusp prolapse and aortic regurgitation should be repaired even when the shunt is small in an effort to prevent progressive deterioration of the aortic valve. Surgical repair is indicated in the rare adult with a significant left-to-right shunt (pulmonary/systemic flow ratio exceeding 2:1) and a low pulmonary vascular resistance. The management of patients with large defects and infundibular narrowing causing right-to-left shunting and cyanosis is similar to that for tetralogy of Fallot (see below).

Unfortunately, adults are still seen with a large ventricular septal defect and pulmonary vascular disease. In those with borderline pulmonary vascular resistance (7 to 10 U/m^2), surgery may be attempted, but the benefits are unpredictable, since the pulmonary vascular disease may progress despite closure of the defect (see Chap. 63).[182] Medical management and consideration for heart-lung or single-lung transplantation are the only realistic options for patients with established severe pulmonary vascular disease, although prostacyclin may hold some promise.[29]

LATE RESULTS

Late results of surgery are good, but the life expectancy for the whole group is not normal. In a study of 179 operative survivors between 1956 and 1959, 30-year survival was 82 percent, compared with 97 percent in age- and sex-matched controls.[180] Only 25 percent of patients in the series were over 10 years of age at surgery, and their 30-year survival of 70 percent was substantially lower than the 88 percent in patients under 2 years of age at operation. Thirty-year survival was 83 percent for patients aged 3 to 10 years at surgery. Older age at repair and preoperative pulmonary vascular disease are important predictors of late outcome. Postoperative conduction defects, especially right bundle-branch block, are common, but complete heart block, which was seen in the early surgical experience, is now rare. Late ventricular arrhythmia has been reported, as after repair of tetralogy of Fallot.[183] The incidence of late sudden death, however, is extremely low, and prophylactic antiarrhythmic therapy in asymptomatic patients is not indicated.

Certain selected ventricular septal defects may be closed with transcatheter devices. One report described closure of 21 muscular ventricular septal defects in 12 patients, half of whom had complex heart defects.[184] All the defects were closed successfully, and subsequent cardiac surgery for associated lesions was performed in 11 of 12 patients.

In postoperative patients, the risk of late infective endocarditis is very small, provided that the defect is isolated and is completely closed. Antibiotic prophylaxis, however, is often advised, particularly for 6 months postoperatively. Recommendations regarding physical activity and competitive sports require detailed evaluation, which may include exercise testing, cross-sectional echocardiography, and ambulatory ECG monitoring. The presence of abnormal left ventricular function, a more than trivial residual shunt, arrhythmia, or any degree of pulmonary hypertension mandates some restriction of physical activity.

Atrioventricular Septal Defect

The term *atrioventricular septal defect* describes the spectrum of lesions that involve a defect at the site of the normal AV septum, resulting in an abnormality involving the AV valves, ventricular architecture, and left ventricular outflow tract. A variety of classifications have been used (see Chap. 63), but the defects are usefully divided into "partial" and "complete" forms. In the former, there is a defect in the primum or inferior part of the atrial septum but no direct intraventricular communication (ostium primum defect). In the latter, there is a large ventricular component beneath either or both the superior or inferior bridging leaflets of the AV valve. The deficiency of ventricular septum together with the abnormal AV valve or valves produces an elongated left ventricular outflow tract characteristically described as having a "gooseneck" appearance at angiography. The morphologic and functional features, together with the associated cardiac and noncardiac abnormalities, determine the natural history. Subaortic stenosis is a common association and may occur de novo even after surgical repair.[185]

NATURAL HISTORY

In the New England Regional Cardiac Registry, 5 percent of newborns with cardiac disease had AV septal defects, with two-thirds being the "complete" form.[186] Down's syndrome is very frequently associated, especially with complete defects. The noncardiac features, especially mental retardation, have a major influence on management in adolescence and adult life.

The natural history of partial AV septal defects with little left AV valve regurgitation is similar to that of large secundum atrial septal defects (see above). A small number develop pulmonary vascular disease, and symptomatic deterioration in unoperated adults is often due to the onset of supraventricular arrhythmia. If the left AV valve is more than mildly regurgitant, the natural history is much worse, with a large left-to-right shunt, often with at least moderate pulmonary hypertension, and early symptoms of cardiac failure. Patients with complete defects do even worse. Their course is characterized by the early development of pulmonary vascular disease (especially in patients with Down's syndrome, who may have irreversible damage before their first birthday), with consequent right-to-left shunting and all the problems of patients with Eisenmenger's syndrome. As a result, surgery needs to be undertaken early if it is to be successful, and most uncorrected patients seen by the adolescent or adult cardiologist will have a pulmonary vascular resistance that is too high for repair (greater than 8 to 10 U/m^2; see Chaps. 15 and 63). Their outcome is poor, but survival into their thirties is possible. Uncorrected patients with partial AV septal defects may present to the adult cardiologist for consideration of surgery, which should be recommended for those with a significant left-to-right shunt in the absence of other contraindications.

MANAGEMENT

Surgical repair involves closure of the atrial and ventricular septal defects and restoration of a competent left AV valve as far as is possible (see Chap. 63).[187] The surgical mortality rate in experienced centers is approximately 10 percent for complete defects and less than 5 percent for partial defects.[162]

LATE RESULTS

Patients with repair of both partial and complete forms of AV septal defect have now been followed for more than 20 years. Late results are good in the absence of pulmonary vascular disease and significant residual left AV valve regurgitation. Some patients with complete defects who were corrected later in childhood, before the need for correction in early infancy was appreciated, have developed progressive pulmonary vascular disease. This late complication should be greatly reduced in patients undergoing repair in the first 6 months of life, as is now technically feasible (see Chap. 63). Even patients who are repaired late in adult life (at 40 years of age or more) can have excellent results, with an early mortality rate of only 6 percent and a good chance of left AV valve repair in experienced hands.[188]

During long-term follow-up, careful attention must be paid to the status of the left AV valve. If the regurgitation increases in severity, reoperation and mitral valve replacement may be necessary.[144] Monitoring for arrhythmia at intervals is also currently recommended; in general, little intervention is usually required, apart from lifelong infective endocarditis prophylaxis. Surgically repaired non-Down's patients without pulmonary vascular disease can often enjoy life without cardiovascular disability and should not be discouraged from competitive sports, pregnancy, or employment. Restrictions are clearly required for those with pulmonary vascular disease, left AV valve regurgitation, or mitral valve replacement on anticoagulants. Patients with Down's syndrome, both operated and unoperated, are demanding, and their families require considerable support from the physician as well as from educational and social services. The recurrence risk of congenital heart disease in offspring of mothers with AV septal defect is higher than average, and potential parents should be counseled.

Tetralogy of Fallot

Tetralogy of Fallot is the commonest form of cyanotic congenital heart disease seen in the adult. Nonetheless, in the developed world the unoperated patient with tetralogy of Fallot has, fortunately, become a rarity, since the overwhelming majority of patients will have undergone palliation or, more often, repair in childhood. From an anatomic and pathophysiologic standpoint, the manifestations of tetralogy of Fallot are similar in all age groups, although hypercyanotic spells, which are often seen in infants and young children, are rare in adults. The development of systemic hypertension with age is a problem, since it increases the afterload to both ventricles.[159,189] Although pulmonary blood flow may improve, this occurs at the expense of right ventricular failure. Acquired calcific aortic stenosis has similar effects. Aortic regurgitation may occur as a result of cusp prolapse into the subaortic ventricular septal defect, and the aorta itself may be dilated. The aortic regurgitation may also be exacerbated by infective endocarditis. Since the volume overload is transmitted to both ventricles, patients may present with right ventricular failure as a consequence of aortic regurgitation. The development of chronic obstructive lung disease is another manifestation of an acquired cardiopulmonary disease that may place the adult patient with tetralogy of Fallot at particular risk.

NATURAL HISTORY

Survival into the seventh decade is described,[190] but the natural history in the unoperated patient, which is determined by the severity of obstruction of the right ventricular outflow tract and pulmonary vasculature, is poor. Only 25 percent of patients reach the age of 10 years; 11 percent are alive at 20 years, 6 percent at age 30 years, and only 3 percent at age 40 years.[159,162,191] Complications of right-to-left shunting and erythrocytosis, which include stroke and cerebral abscess, are common and, in many instances, fatal. Patients are at continuing risk of infective endocarditis; the development of congestive heart failure in adolescence or early adult life is a major cause of death, as is arrhythmia. Myocardial fibrosis resulting from long-standing right ventricular pressure overload and hypoxemia are postulated mechanisms.[192] Prior palliative surgery with a Cooley or Waterston shunt (between the ascending aorta and right pulmonary artery) or a Potts shunt (between the descending aorta and the left pulmonary artery) can lead to the late development of pulmonary vascular disease.[193]

MANAGEMENT

The focus of medical treatment in unoperated patients is on the elevated hematocrit, bleeding disorders, and abnormal uric acid metabolism and the complications of pregnancy. Repair is indicated in all suitable patients, and the principles and techniques are not significantly different in adults than in children (see Chap. 63).[161] Most adults are suitable candidates for repair, but occasionally a patient with an underdeveloped pulmonary vascular bed may require a palliative shunt procedure. Intracardiac repair consists of closure of the ventricular septal defect and relief of right ventricular outflow tract obstruction. In some patients, this may require excision of the pulmonary valve and patch reconstruction of the anulus and outflow tract. In the occasional patient with an anomalous origin of the left coronary artery from the right coronary artery, a conduit between the right ventricle and pulmonary artery may be required.[162]

LATE RESULTS

Late survival is excellent, even in patients who underwent repair during the very early years of open heart surgery.[162] At the Mayo Clinic, the cumulative 30-year survival for patients undergoing successful surgery between 1956 and 1960 was 86 percent compared to 95 percent in age- and sex-matched controls (Fig. 64-4).[194] In a previous series of 396 hospital survivors of repair between 1955 and 1962 at the same institution, 91 percent were alive at 20 years. At 30 years, 77 percent of the initial cohort of 106 patients undergoing surgery between 1954 and 1960 by Lillehei and associates were alive, including 1 patient who was 45 years of age at the time of operation.[195] Surgery cannot be considered "curative," since survival, even in excellent series, is slightly but significantly worse than for a matched control population. The risk factors for an adverse late outcome include older age at surgery, preoperative congestive heart failure, a previous Potts shunt, persistent right ventricular systolic hypertension, and a residual ventricular septal defect.[175,193] Late death may be sudden, due to tachyarrhythmia or, very rarely in the current era, to conduction disease (see above).[50] Left and right ventricular failure due to right ventricular pressure overload or left ventricular volume overload is another important cause of late death in older patients.[159]

The late functional outcome is excellent for the majority of patients. Most lead normal lives, but the results appear to be better in those undergoing surgery at a younger age.[196] Persistent or recurrent symptoms are usually the result of incomplete relief of right ventricular systolic hypertension or recurrent or residual ventricular septal defects. These problems are often manifest within the first few years after surgery and may require reoperation. Progressive aortic dilatation and aortic regurgitation may also occur, requiring aortic valve replacement.[197] Pulmonary regurgitation may be well tolerated for decades but may be associated with late impairment of exercise capacity and, frequently, atrial arrhythmias. Right ventricular volume overload may also be well tolerated for years but ultimately results in right ventricular failure and progressive tricuspid regurgitation. Pulmonary valve replacement can be accomplished with a low risk.[149] In some patients, isolated right ventricular restrictive physiology may paradoxically improve exercise performance and reduce cardiac enlargement, due possibly to shortening of the duration of pulmonary regurgitation.[68]

Recent information links pulmonary regurgitation, cardiomegaly, QRS duration, and potentially life-threatening ventricular arrhythmia.[68,69] This may be important for identification of risk of late sudden death, which has been a rare event in most long-term follow-up series. Asymptomatic ventricular arrhythmia is very common during long-term follow-up. It is again related to older age at repair, but the link between nonsustained ventricular arrhythmia and adverse clinical outcome is uncertain (see above).[61,62] Objective testing has emphasized the effects of older age at operation on subsequent exercise performance. This is essentially normal for children repaired at below 5 years of age but is usually impaired when surgery is undertaken in adolescence or adulthood.[198]

Before unrestricted physical activity after repair of tetralogy of Fallot can be recommended, careful evaluation—including echocardiography, ECG monitoring, and exercise testing—should be undertaken. Normal activity, including competitive sports, seems reasonable if surgery has been performed at a young age, right and left ventricular function and size are normal, and there are no residual ventricular septal defect, significant right ventricular outflow tract obstruction, or worrisome arrhythmia. In those who do not fulfill these stringent criteria, the degree to which physical activity should be restricted must be individualized. Currently, long-term follow-up of all patients with tetralogy of Fallot is recommended.

Pulmonary Stenosis

Isolated pulmonary valve stenosis is a common form of adult congenital heart disease and is characterized typically by a trileaflet valve with fused commissures. A dysplastic valve without commissural fusion occurs infrequently in otherwise normal children but more commonly in patients with Noonan's syndrome (see Fig. 10-13).[159] Subvalvar stenosis due to infundibular hypertrophy is usually a secondary phenomenon in response to obstruction to right ventricular outflow but may occur as a rare isolated entity. Supravalvar or peripheral pulmonary artery stenosis is also extremely uncommon as an isolated entity but is associated with tetralogy of Fallot and supravalvar aortic stenosis in Williams' syndrome (see Fig. 10-25).

NATURAL HISTORY

Prolonged survival into adult life is common and depends upon the severity of obstruction. In patients with severe pulmonary stenosis, symptoms of right-sided failure increase with time because of progressive obstruction and alterations in right ventricular compliance.[199] In the Joint Study of the Natural History of Congenital Heart Disease, 19 percent of patients with severe stenosis aged 2 to 11 years and 37 percent aged 12 to 21 years were symptomatic. The natural history of moderate pulmonary stenosis in older patients is more favorable, with less tendency to progression.

MANAGEMENT

Patients with mild stenosis are asymptomatic and require no intervention other than antibiotic prophylaxis against infective endocarditis. In patients with more severe stenosis (>140-mm gradient between the right ventricle and pulmonary artery), intervention to reduce severity should be considered even if there are no symptoms.

Surgical valvotomy for isolated pulmonary stenosis has been successfully performed for more than 40 years. Perioperative morbidity and mortality rates are minimal beyond the neonatal period in patients without severe congestive cardiac failure or right ventricular dysplasia.[162] Late results are also excellent. In a study from the Mayo Clinic of patients undergoing surgery between 1956 and 1957, late survival for those undergoing valvotomy who are over 21 years of age was similar but not identical to that of an age- and sex-matched control population (Fig. 64-5). Among patients undergoing surgery at an older age, late survival, although still good, was less than that of the control population (Fig. 64-6).[200] This effect of age on late outcome, which was independent of the use of ventriculotomy and outflow patches and of pulmonary regurgitation, is likely the result of long-standing pressure overload on the right ventricle. Late functional results are excellent, and pulmonary regurgitation is well tolerated in the short and medium term. More severe pulmonary regurgitation may result when a pulmonary valvectomy or transanular patch is required, as may be the case for a small or dysplastic valve; the long-term consequences on the right ventricle and functional capacity are not yet well documented (see "Tetralogy of Fallot," above).

Surgical valvotomy is now rarely required after infancy because of the advent of catheter balloon pulmonary valvotomy. In most institutions, balloon valvotomy is the initial procedure of choice at all ages. In the series of 822 patients in the Valvuloplasty and Angioplasty of Congenital Heart Abnormalities registry, gradient reduction was substantially worse in patients with dysplastic valves.[201] Interventional catheter procedures should be confined to centers with experienced operators.

Long-term follow-up data are not yet available. It appears that the excellent early results are maintained for at least 5 years. The late effects of pulmonary regurgitation resulting from the use of large balloons need to be determined. The risk of infective endocarditis in patients with mild pulmonary stenosis

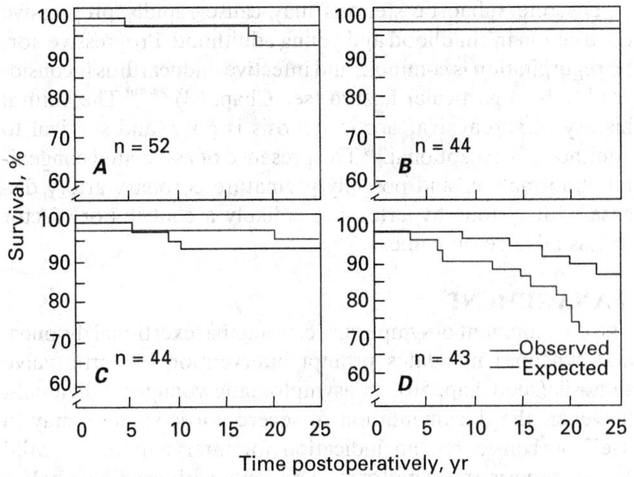

FIGURE 64-5 Long-term survival of perioperative survivors of surgical repair of pulmonary valve stenosis by age at time of operation. *A*. Ages 0 to 4 years. *B*. Ages 5 to 10 years. *C*. Ages 11 to 20 years. *D*. Ages 21 to 68 years. Expected is survival in an age- and sex-matched population. Values of p for comparison between the expected and observed survivals: .07, .34, .16, and <.002 for panels *A*, *B*, *C*, and *D*, respectively. (From Kopecky SL, Gersh BJ, McGoon MD, et al. Long-term outcome of patients undergoing surgical repair of isolated pulmonary valve stenosis: Follow-up at 20–30 years. *Circulation* 1988; 78:1150. Reproduced with permission from the publisher and authors.)

or in those with mild gradients after surgical or balloon valvotomy is low. Long-term follow-up is recommended to evaluate not only the right ventricular outflow tract gradient but also pulmonary regurgitation, right ventricular function, and exercise performance. In patients with good relief of pulmonary stenosis, no restriction of physical activities, including competitive sports, is required. In those with moderate residual obstruction or right ventricular dysfunction, exercise intensity should be reduced (see also Chap. 77).

Left Ventricular Outflow Tract Obstruction

Congenital left ventricular outflow tract obstruction may occur at valvar, subvalvar, and supravalvar levels (see Chap. 85). Aortic valve stenosis is a common abnormality in adults with congenital heart disease. It may either be an isolated defect or be associated with other lesions, such as coarctation or ventricular septal defect. It is usually due to a bicuspid aortic valve, which may be present in 1 to 2 percent of the total adult population and is three to four times more common in males than in females.[202] Unicuspid and tricuspid stenotic valves are less common.[162] Subvalvar stenosis encompasses a morphologic spectrum of fibrous or fibromuscular obstructions; it can be a discrete "membrane" below the aortic valve, a discrete fibromuscular ridge, or a diffuse narrowing extending well into the left ventricular cavity forming a "tunnel."[203] The condition occurs more commonly in patients with long and narrow left ventricular outflow tracts,[204] and perhaps this morphologic feature promotes turbulence and shear stresses that stimulate cellular proliferation.[205] Abnormal ventricular bands or chords may also contribute to obstruction, along with abnormal chordal attachments of the anterior mitral valve leaflet. A dynamic component of obstruction may also occur as left ventricular hypertrophy progresses. Common associated anomalies include ventricular septal defect and coarctation of the aorta. Supravalvar stenosis is the least common variety of left ventricular outflow tract obstruction in adolescents and adults, except in the context of Williams' syndrome.[206]

NATURAL HISTORY

The natural history of congenital valvar aortic stenosis in adults is variable but is characterized by progressive stenosis with time (Fig. 64-7; see Chap. 56).[159] By the age of 45 years, approximately half of all bicuspid aortic valves have some degree of narrowing. The severity of obstruction at the time of diagnosis correlates

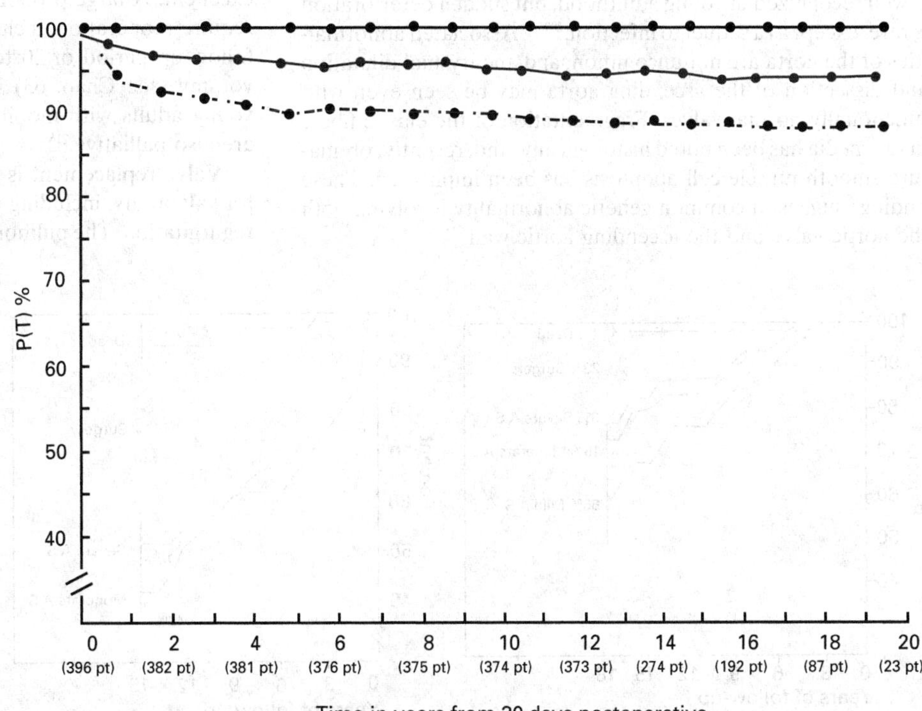

FIGURE 64-6 Probability of deterioration in operative survivors after repair of tetralogy of Fallot plotted against time in years. Time of deterioration is defined as the postoperative year in which late death (*middle curve*) or in which death, reoperation, or symptoms occurred (*bottom curve*). The top curve represents the controlled expected survival on the basis of an age- and sex-matched distribution. The number of patients at each follow-up interval is denoted in parentheses. (From Fuster V, McGoon DC, Kennedy M, et al. Long-term evaluation (12–22 years) of open-heart surgery for tetralogy of Fallot. *Am J Cardiol* 1980; 46:635. Reproduced with permission from the publisher and authors.)

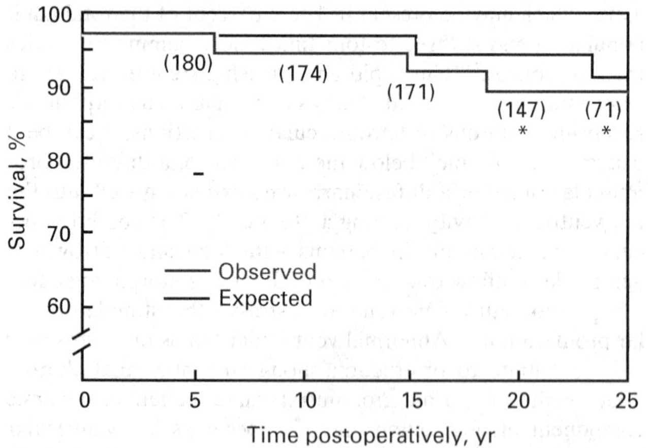

FIGURE 64-7 Long-term survival of perioperative survivors following surgical repair of isolated pulmonary stenosis and expected survival of age- and sex-matched control populations. Difference between expected and observed $p < .002$. (From Kopecky SL, Gersh BJ, McGoon MD, et al. Long-term outcome of patients undergoing surgical repair of isolated pulmonary valve stenosis: Follow-up at 20–30 years. *Circulation* 1988; 78:1150. Reproduced with permission from the American Heart Association and authors.)

with the pattern of progression (Fig. 64-8).[207] Bacterial endocarditis is relatively uncommon (1.8 to 2.7 cases per 100 patient-years),[208] but antibiotic prophylaxis is necessary, even for functionally normal valves. Slowly progressive aortic regurgitation is well recognized in young adulthood, but sudden deterioration is rare, except as a sequel to infection.[209,210] Associated abnormalities of the aorta are not uncommon, and aneurysmal dilatation and dissection of the ascending aorta may be seen even with functionally normal valves. Fragmentation of the elastic fibers in the media has been noted histologically, and, recently, premature smooth muscle cell apoptosis has been implicated. These findings suggest a common genetic abnormality involving both the aortic valve and the ascending aortic wall.[211]

Discrete subaortic stenosis may cause rapidly progressive obstruction in childhood and young adulthood. Progressive aortic regurgitation is common, and infective endocarditis is considered to be a particular hazard (see Chap. 63).[209,210] The natural history of supravalvar aortic stenosis is poor, and survival to adulthood is exceptional.[159] The presence of associated congenital abnormalities and possibly premature coronary artery disease with systolic hypertension is likely a contributory factor to this adverse outcome.

MANAGEMENT

The development of symptoms (e.g., angina, exertional dyspnea, and syncope) mandates prompt intervention in aortic valve stenosis (see Chap. 56). In asymptomatic younger individuals, however, the documentation of severe aortic stenosis may in itself be considered an indication for intervention.[212,213] Mild aortic stenosis in asymptomatic patients with gradients below 50 mmHg warrants careful surveillance. The management of patients in the intermediate group (gradients 50 to 75 mmHg) is more controversial, but evidence argues in favor of elective intervention. Calculation of aortic valve area is important, since left ventricular–aortic gradients may be misleading if there is reduced cardiac output.

Surgery in the young adult with congenital aortic stenosis must be considered palliative.[152,214] In the absence of calcification, young patients may be candidates for aortic valvotomy (see also Chaps. 56 and 63). Perioperative mortality rates in adolescents and adults are extremely low, and late survival is excellent. A large proportion (35 to 45 percent), however, will require reoperation, including aortic valve replacement, over a follow-up period of 20 to 25 years.[150,152] Catheter balloon valvotomy (see Chap. 63) has been utilized in adolescents and young adults with mobile noncalcified valves, but the results are also palliative.[215]

Valve replacement is the only option for valves unsuitable for valvotomy, including those with significant calcification and regurgitation. The pulmonary autograft (Ross) operation represents an attractive surgical alternative to prosthetic or homograft aortic valve replacement. The choice of operation is discussed elsewhere (see Chap. 56), but the age and size of the patient are major considerations, as are individual characteristics that determine the safety of anticoagulation, such as the desire for future pregnancies.

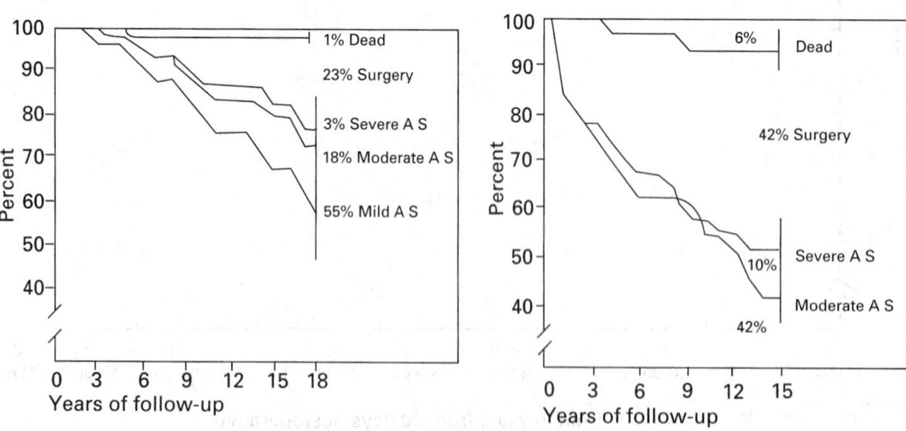

FIGURE 64-8 (*Left*) Cumulative actuarial curves of 153 patients presenting with *mild* aortic stenosis. Bars show ±1 standard error in age at presentation 6.5 years (range 1 to 25 years); mean follow-up was 8.8 years (range 1 to 26 years). (*Right*) Cumulative actuarial curves of 54 patients presenting with *moderate* aortic stenosis. Conventions are as in the left-hand figure. Mean age at presentation was 11.8 years (range 1 to 25 years). Mean follow-up was 8.5 years (range 1 to 24 years). (From Hossack KF, Neutze JM, Lowe JB, Barratt-Boyes BG. Congenital valvar aortic stenosis: Natural history and assessment for operation. *Br Heart J* 1980; 43:561. Reproduced with permission from the publisher and authors.)

Subaortic stenosis is usually amenable to more definitive surgical repair. This fact, in conjunction with the potential for progressive aortic regurgitation, justifies a more aggressive approach even in asymptomatic patients with lesser gradients.[216,217] Excision of the obstructive membrane, together with a myectomy or myotomy, is usually required. Subaortic stenosis occasionally recurs, and persistent or progressive aortic regurgitation may develop. Operative mortality rates are low, but the risks are greater in patients with "tunnel" forms of obstruction and in patients with obstruction at several levels. Such situations usually require a more aggressive surgical intervention with extensive myectomy, a Konno procedure, or modification thereof.[218]

Hospital mortality rates for repair of supravalvular aortic stenosis are low, and late morbidity and mortality rates are also excellent. Nevertheless, residual abnormality, such as aortic regurgitation or stenosis, may persist after aortoplasty.

Medical follow-up of patients who have undergone surgical or balloon valvotomy should focus on the development of restenosis, the severity and progression of aortic regurgitation, and the constant hazard of infective endocarditis. Echocardiography has facilitated serial evaluation of gradients, valve areas, ventricular dimensions, function, and mass. The acceptable level of physical activity in patients with left ventricular outflow tract obstruction remains very controversial. It is debatable whether any patient who has had significant obstruction should be allowed to participate in competitive sports. We consider a residual gradient greater than 20 mmHg or persistent left ventricular hypertrophy to be contraindications to vigorous physical activity. Before one approves strenuous activity in others, evaluation should include ECG monitoring and maximal exercise testing (see Chap. 14).

Coarctation of the Aorta

Although coarctation of the aorta is a congenital malformation, nearly 20 percent of the cases presenting at the Mayo Clinic over a 20-year period were diagnosed initially in adolescence or adulthood. Most commonly, coarctation diagnosed at ages beyond childhood was discovered in asymptomatic patients in whom a routine physical examination for athletic participation or employment disclosed upper limb hypertension with diminished or absent femoral pulses. Coarctation of the aorta may occur anywhere along the descending aorta, even below the diaphragm, but in more than 95 percent of cases it is located below the origin of the left subclavian artery, and may involve the origin of this vessel. Usually, there is a discrete infolding of the aortic wall, causing eccentric narrowing of the lumen. Frequently, there is secondary aortic dilatation proximal and distal to the coarcted area.

NATURAL HISTORY

Isolated, severe aortic coarctation may cause congestive heart failure as early as the neonatal period. More frequently, however, coarctation producing symptoms during early infancy is associated with other congenital cardiovascular abnormalities, such as ventricular septal defect, left ventricular outflow tract obstruction, or mitral valve abnormality. Many patients with undetected coarctation will remain symptom-free until adolescence or early adulthood, when symptoms such as headaches related to hypertension, leg fatigue, or leg cramps may develop. Occasionally, a major catastrophic event, such as a cerebrovascular accident, infective endocarditis, or even rupture of the aorta, is the first recognized symptom. A bicuspid aortic valve is found in approximately 25 to 50 percent of patients with coarctation, and these abnormal valves have a tendency to calcify in early or middle adult life, producing aortic stenosis. Aortic stenosis may be the presenting condition, and subsequent investigation may disclose an additional coarctation of the aorta. In the era before surgical intervention, approximately 50 percent of patients with coarctation died within the first three decades, and 75 percent were dead by age 50.[219] Death was most frequently caused by a complication of hypertension, such as stroke or aortic dissection, but other causes included endocarditis, endarteritis, and congestive heart failure.

MANAGEMENT

Infrequently, a mild degree of coarctation may be present that would not justify intervention. In the great majority of cases, however, symptoms or the presence of significant upper-body hypertension mandate surgical repair. On occasion, an asymptomatic adolescent or adult patient with a severe coarctation will be normotensive at rest because of well-developed collaterals around the coarctation site. Such patients have inappropriate hypertension with exercise, however, and should be repaired. There is evidence that residual hypertension and late complications are directly related to age at the time of repair.[220]

Surgery for coarctation has been available since 1945.[221] Various techniques have been used, including end-to-end anastomosis, patch grafting, and the use of the subclavian flap technique.[222] Aneurysmal or atherosclerotic changes in the aorta found in adolescents or adults may occasionally mandate the use of an interposition prosthetic graft. Surgery is performed without cardiopulmonary bypass, and the risk of death from operation is small, although it is higher in adults than in children. Serious morbidity is rare, but occasionally paraplegia secondary to spinal cord ischemia and bowel ischemia or infarction occur.[223] For patients who require concomitant surgical procedures, such as aortic valve replacement, an ascending-to-descending aortic bypass may be utilized through a median sternotomy.[224] Some patients require antihypertensive medication because of transient postoperative hypertension for a short period, whereas in others hypertension may persist, requiring long-term treatment.

Balloon angioplasty of native coarctation has been utilized, but the role of this technique remains controversial.[225] Immediate reduction of the degree of obstruction and gradient is usually possible but is achieved at the price of tearing both the aortic intima and media. Late aneurysm formation, presumably secondary to the disruption of the media, has been observed.[226] Currently, most centers do not perform catheter balloon angioplasty as the primary procedure for coarctation, reserving it for recoarctation, where it appears to have a much greater role.[227] Balloon-expandable stents have also been utilized recently with good results, although long-term follow-up data are not available.[228–231]

LATE RESULTS

The Mayo Clinic has published late results in 646 patients with coarctation operated upon between 1946 and 1981.[220] The median age at operation was 16 years (range 1 week to 72 years) with 72 patients (11 percent) over age 35 years of age. Although survival was good (91 percent at 10 years and 72 percent at 30 years), the mean age of death was 38 years, confirming the previous finding that life expectancy is reduced, even after repair. In this and other series reporting long-term follow-up, the most common cause of death was premature coronary artery disease with secondary myocardial infarction.[232,233] Other causes included congestive heart failure, stroke, and ruptured aortic aneurysm. Age at operation was a powerful prognostic factor.

The older the patient at the time of repair, the greater the probability of premature death, making it highly likely that the duration of preoperative obstruction and hypertension is important in the etiology of arterial disease and subsequent cardiovascular events.

The incidence of recoarctation with all surgical techniques is low for repairs performed after infancy, but surgery in later years for associated abnormalities, such as aortic and mitral valve disease, may be required. The majority of survivors are asymptomatic, but there is a high incidence of late hypertension, despite satisfactory early fall in blood pressure after surgery and good relief of obstruction. In one series, only 32 percent of patients were normotensive 30 years after repair, and 25 percent were significantly hypertensive.[233] Long-term blood pressure surveillance, including blood pressures with exercise, is therefore mandatory, since hypertension is directly related to many of the late vascular complications.[220,232,233] This incidence may decline significantly as more patients are diagnosed and repaired during infancy or early childhood. Long-term regular follow-up should also include surveillance of the repaired aorta (MRI imaging is very suitable), assessment of the aortic valve, and endocarditis prophylaxis.

Transposition of the Great Arteries

In complete transposition of the great arteries, the aorta arises from the right ventricle and the pulmonary artery from the left ventricle (discordant ventriculoarterial connection). As a result, the systemic and arterial circulations run "in parallel" rather than "in series," and predominantly desaturated blood enters the aorta. Oxygenation and survival depend on mixing between the systemic and pulmonary circulations at the atrial level in simple transposition (via a patent foramen ovale or atrial septal defect; see Chap. 63). In approximately half the cases, there are associated anomalies: ventricular septal defect (30 percent), left ventricular outflow tract obstruction (5 to 10 percent), ventricular septal defect with left ventricular outflow tract obstruction (10 percent), patent ductus arteriosus, and, more rarely, coarctation of the aorta or AV valve anomalies.[234] These associated conditions affect both the natural history and surgical management.

NATURAL HISTORY

Transposition of the great arteries is relatively common, but the natural history is so poor that very few patients survive past childhood without intervention. Death is usually due to profound hypoxia and its hematologic consequences. In transposition of the great arteries with large ventricular septal defect, severe hypoxia is rare, but patients do badly as a result of heart failure from excessive pulmonary flow and early pulmonary vascular disease.[129] Transposition with ventricular septal defect and left ventricular outflow tract obstruction presents with early hypoxia. Occasionally, prolonged survival into adult life may occur with a large atrial septal defect, ventricular septal defect, and/or patent ductus arteriosus, with the development of pulmonary vascular disease (Eisenmenger's syndrome) or with associated ventricular septal defect and left ventricular outflow tract obstruction.

MANAGEMENT

The outlook has been transformed by the use of catheter balloon atrial septostomy.[235] In the late 1950s and early 1960s, the Senning[236] and Mustard[237] operations, involving atrial redirection of the systemic and pulmonary venous returns, were introduced. These operations are usually performed between 3 and 12 months of age, with a trend over the years to earlier surgery. Both procedures have been undertaken with excellent early mortality rates (approximately 2 percent operative mortality rate and less than 10 percent for the whole early-management protocol). Long-term follow-up for both procedures is now available, with comparable late results, apart from a lower incidence of baffle obstruction after the Senning operation.[238] Follow-up now extends to 30 years in some patients.[239] A recent study reported actuarial survival rates of 90 percent, 80 percent, and 80 percent at 10, 20, and 28 years, respectively, after the Mustard repair.[240,241] Seventy-six percent of the survivors were in NYHA class I. Thus, cardiologists are likely to see patients who have undergone these types of atrial redirection. Late problems, however, are now recognized, with sudden death, arrhythmia, tricuspid regurgitation, and right (systemic) ventricular dysfunction being the major concerns.[240] These late complications have led to the increasing acceptance of the arterial switch operation as the operation of choice.[242] This procedure involves transection and reanastomosis of the great arteries (aorta to left ventricle and pulmonary artery to right ventricle) with coronary artery transfer. The mortality rate for this procedure has decreased, but the long-term results into adult life are not yet available. For transposition with ventricular septal defect, the mortality rate for atrial repair with ventricular septal defect closure has always been higher than for simple transposition, and arterial switch is the operation of choice. Transposition with ventricular septal defect and left ventricular outflow tract obstruction is usually palliated in infancy with a systemic-to-pulmonary shunt followed by repair by the Rastelli procedure in later childhood.[243] This operation involves closure of the ventricular septal defect to connect the left ventricle to the aorta and insertion of a valved conduit from the right ventricle to the pulmonary artery. Long-term results are good, but further surgery to replace the extracardiac conduit in adolescent and adult life is inevitable (see "Surgical Considerations," above).

LATE RESULTS

Two specific problems after atrial redirection have caused concern during long-term follow-up: arrhythmia and systemic ventricular dysfunction. Loss of sinus rhythm is progressive and has not been prevented by modification of surgical technique for either the Mustard or the Senning operation.[41,244] In most cases, it is asymptomatic, but occasionally profound bradycardia may necessitate pacemaker insertion. There appears, however, to be no relationship between loss of sinus rhythm and risk of sudden death. More worrisome is the development of atrial tachyarrhythmias, including atrial flutter. This arrhythmia has profound hemodynamic consequences after intraatrial repair and is a risk factor for sudden death, especially in the presence of right ventricular dysfunction. Deteriorating performance of the right ventricle supporting the systemic circulation has been reported in some patients, but the precise basis for this problem remains unclear.[9] Although a major concern, it is not yet known whether or not ventricular performance will inevitably deteriorate in the majority of patients and, if so, over what period.[9]

Risk stratification for sudden death remains a clinical challenge. Late death cannot be predicted merely from serial ECGs or ambulatory monitoring.[41] This difficulty underscores the need for a more sophisticated approach involving both electrophysiologic and hemodynamic measurements. Assessment should include evaluation of cardiac performance at rest and exercise, and evaluation of systemic and venous pathways. Transesophageal echocardiography is particularly useful in this situation. Heart transplantation should be considered in the patient who has severe right ventricular failure or disabling arrhythmias. An alternative approach is to perform pulmonary artery banding as preparation for conversion of the atrial repair to an arterial switch. Published results have indicated a significant surgical mortality rate for this approach. As a result, case selection and timing, as well as optimal surgical strategy, remain unclear.[245] The rather limited information after arterial switch operation suggests that electrophysiologic problems are much less prevalent.[246] More recent studies confirm the theoretical advantages of anatomic repair over atrial repair with respect to preservation of sinus node function and lower prevalence of clinically relevant tachyarrhythmias.[247] The systemic left ventricle after the switch is at risk from the surgical procedure itself, potential myocardial ischemia from coronary distortion, and aortic regurgitation. Early results, however, are encouraging, but few patients have yet reached adult life.[248] Because of the high incidence of observed and potential medical problems, all patients who have had both atrial and arterial repair of transposition of the great arteries should have lifelong follow-up by a cardiologist at a center specializing in adult congenital heart disease.

Congenitally Corrected Transposition (Atrioventricular and Ventriculoarterial Discordance)

In congenitally corrected transposition of the great arteries, there is a discordant AV connection (right atrium to left ventricle and left atrium to right ventricle) and a discordant ventriculoarterial connection (left ventricle to pulmonary artery and right ventricle to aorta). As a result of this "double discordance," the systemic and pulmonary venous returns flow to the appropriate great arteries, giving rise to the potentially confusing term *corrected transposition*.[249]

NATURAL HISTORY

In a small proportion of cases (approximately 10 percent in reported series, but this is probably an underestimate), there are no associated cardiac defects.[250,251] Such individuals are pink and asymptomatic, and survival to the ninth decade has been reported.[76] The only specific difference from normal hearts is the tendency to develop AV conduction problems and complete heart block. Complete heart block may be present from birth (approximately 10 percent of patients)[252] and is said to develop in about 2 percent of patients per year.[253] It is not clear whether the systemic right ventricle in patients with corrected transposition can maintain function over extended periods or whether this has an impact on outcome, since few studies have examined enough patients without associated defects over a long enough period. The majority of patients have a ventricular septal defect (90 percent) and/or pulmonary stenosis (80 percent).[250] The combination of these lesions may cause cyanosis. Abnormalities of the tricuspid valve (systemic AV valve) are common and may be due to an intrinsic tricuspid valve abnormality, such as Ebstein's malformation. These defects influence the natural history and surgical strategy required.

MANAGEMENT

Strategies and indications for surgery differ from those in patients with normal connections because of the potential for the operation to aggravate systemic ventricular dysfunction, systemic AV valve incompetence, or conduction problems. Palliative surgery in childhood is sometimes performed, since definitive repair may involve insertion of an extracardiac conduit. In a large retrospective study of 111 patients managed over a 20-year period, it was concluded that patients with symptomatic heart failure should be repaired before the systemic ventricle dilates and the tricuspid regurgitation becomes severe.[251] Patients with more than mild tricuspid regurgitation whose valves were not replaced did very poorly. In contrast, the patients with cyanosis did much better, and the timing of intracardiac surgery can be delayed and be determined by the patient's symptoms. In one recent series of surgical repair of 127 patients, 56 percent required reoperation within 20 years for AV valve regurgitation, pulmonary stenosis, or both.[254] Left AV valve regurgitation is common in adults with congenitally corrected transposition[255] and tends to be progressive.[256] It may be related to an Ebstein-like malformation of the left AV valve, but these valves, in contrast to Ebstein's anomaly of the right AV valve, cannot be repaired adequately and always need to be replaced. Left AV valve replacement should always be performed before there is compromise of systemic (morphologic right) ventricular function. In one series of 40 patients, left AV valve replacement was accomplished without surgically induced complete heart block, with an early mortality rate of 10 percent (n = 4) and 8 late deaths.[257] The principal cause of death in all 12 patients was systemic ventricular failure. Survival correlated with preoperative systemic ventricular ejection fraction of 44 percent or greater. It thus seems appropriate to refer these patients for valve replacement at the earliest signs of ventricular dysfunction.

Recently, alternative surgical strategies involving a "double switch" have been adopted by some units. These involve an atrial repair by a Mustard or Senning operation together with connection of the left ventricle to the aorta (via a patch through the ventricular septal defect) or an arterial switch.[258,259] The advantage of these approaches is that the morphologic left ventricle (with mitral valve) supports the systemic circulation. While this is an attractive option, it should be stressed that few patients who have received double-switch procedures have reached adolescence, and long-term follow-up data are not yet available for comparison with the conventional surgical approach.

LATE RESULTS

The long-term outcome for well-repaired patients is good, but those with severe symptomatic heart failure preoperatively do badly. Atrial arrhythmias are common in long-term follow-up and in one recent series occurred in 36 percent of survivors.[260] Since repairs may involve insertion of an extracardiac conduit, prosthetic AV valve, and pacemaker, careful long-term follow-up is mandatory.

Complex Lesions

A number of complex congenital heart defects involve structural abnormalities that preclude the creation of a biventricular circulation. The changing nomenclature and classification that have been applied to these defects over the years are a major source of confusion (see Chap. 63). This group of patients includes those with double-inlet ventricle (single ventricle), absent right or left AV connection (tricuspid or mitral atresia), some cases of pulmonary atresia/intact ventricular septum, and cases with straddling of an AV valve and hypoplastic left or right ventricles. The natural history of these defects is highly variable and depends to a large extent on the impact of the associated defects. In a recent report of 191 patients with double-inlet ventricle presenting in the first year of life, the actuarial survival rate before definitive repair for the whole group was 57 percent at 1 year and 42 percent at 10 years.[158] On multivariate analysis, pulmonary stenosis, balanced pulmonary flow, and older age at presentation were factors favoring survival, while right atrial isomerism, common AV orifice, pulmonary atresia, obstruction to systemic output, and anomalous pulmonary venous return were detrimental. Despite the complex morphologic defects, prolonged natural survival is possible, particularly if the physiology is well balanced.[261] The patients with double-inlet left ventricle with discordant ventriculoarterial connection and pulmonary stenosis with balanced pulmonary flow do best, with predicted actuarial survivals of 96 percent at 1 year and 91 percent at 10 years.

MANAGEMENT

For most patients with complex congenital heart disease, prolonged survival into adult life is possible only with one or more palliative operations (e.g., systemic to pulmonary shunt, Glenn shunt, pulmonary artery banding, and relief of systemic outflow obstruction) or after a Fontan-type procedure. With palliative surgery alone, clinical deterioration usually begins in the second decade of life and is often due to progressive ventricular dysfunction and/or AV valve regurgitation.[262–264]

TABLE 64-5 Indications for Hospitalizations after Fontan Procedure for 215 Surviving Patients Who Returned a Questionnaire

Indication	Patients Hospitalized (No.)[a]
Cardiac operation	62
Other	57
Arrhythmia	52
Pacemaker insertion or replacement	22
Heart failure	14
Abdominal swelling	10
Leg edema	9
Endocarditis	7
Protein-losing enteropathy	6
Hypoproteinemia	4
Stroke	4
Liver problems	1
Brain abscess	1

[a]A patient may have provided multiple indications for one hospitalization.

SOURCE: Driscoll DJ, Offord KP, Feldt RH, et al. Five- to fifteen-year follow-up after Fontan operation. *Circulation* 1992; 85:469–496. Reproduced with permission from the publisher and authors.

The goals of management during childhood have been to maintain suitable anatomy and physiology for the Fontan circulation. A number of modifications of Fontan's original operation have been introduced (Fig. 64-9).[265–268] The basic principle is to separate the systemic and pulmonary circuits by returning systemic venous blood to the pulmonary artery without incorporating a subpulmonary ventricle. This circulation is less "flexible" than one with two functioning ventricles; the operative risk and postoperative status are largely dependent on the patient's suitability. Most important are a low pulmonary vascular resistance and adequate ventricular function (both systolic and diastolic), allowing the circulation to operate with an acceptably low systemic venous pressure. Careful preoperative hemodynamic assessment is vital to optimize patient selection. The operative risk varies considerably among institutions.

LONG-TERM RESULTS

The early and medium-term results of the successful Fontan operation are excellent when compared to the preoperative status of the patients. Improvements in arterial saturation and exercise tolerance have been confirmed by objective testing.[268] The patients with the best hemodynamics can perform well at submaximal levels of exercise equivalent to most normal daily activities.[269] With longer follow-up, however, increasing problems develop (Table 64-5).[270,271] Fontan's own analysis of 334 patients revealed a premature decline in survival and functional status and a late rise in hazard for which no risk factors could be identified other than the Fontan state per se.[271] Arrhythmia

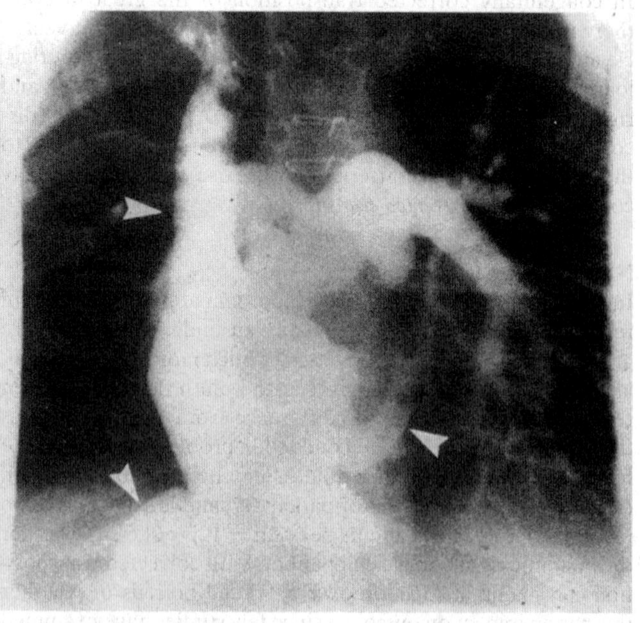

A

FIGURE 64-9 Angiograms. *A.* Fontan conduit from right atrium to pulmonary artery. There is dilatation of the right atrium with filling of the inferior vena cava, superior vena cava, and coronary sinus. *B.* Total cavopulmonary connection. The superior vena cava is connected to the right pulmonary artery ("bidirectional Glenn"), and the inferior vena cava is baffled to the pulmonary artery. (Courtesy of Dr. I. D. Sullivan, Great Ormond Street Hospital for Children, London.)

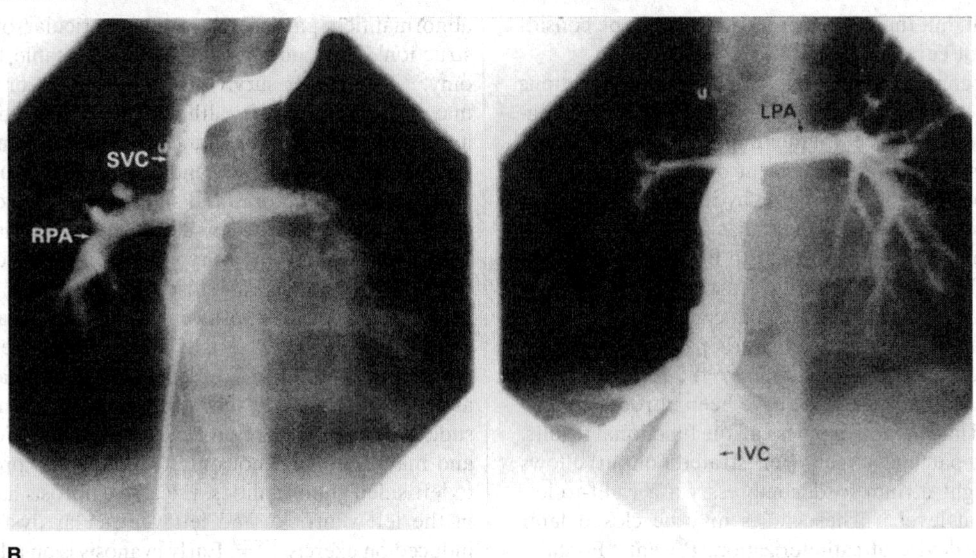

FIGURE 64-9 (*Continued*)

is a particularly common problem and occurs in approximately 20 percent at 10-year follow-up (Table 64-6).[270] Other problems include thrombus in the atria and declining ventricular function.[270–272] Anticoagulation policy differs widely even among specialist centers. The increasing concerns regarding stasis of blood in the right atrium and thrombus formation have led to wider routine use of long-term anticoagulants, but this is not standard practice. Patients with a history of documented atrial arrhythmias, a fenestration in the Fontan connection, and "smoke" in the right atrium on echocardiography have the strongest indications for anticoagulation.

Protein-losing enteropathy (PLE) is another important complication and probably results from elevated systemic venous pressure, which subsequently causes lymphangiectasia. PLE is associated with fluid accumulation, such as pleural effusion, ascites, and peripheral edema. The diagnosis can be confirmed by quantifying gastrointestinal protein loss utilizing alpha$_1$ antitrypsin clearance. The cumulative risk for the development of PLE by 10 years in one reported large series was approximately 13 percent;[273] once this complication had developed, the 5-year survival rate was approximately 50 percent. Therapy includes sodium restriction, dietary modification, and anticongestive measures such as diuretics and afterload-reducing agents. Many patients require periodic albumin infusion, but medical management of PLE is usually only partially successful. Obstruction in the Fontan circuit should always be ruled out as a potential cause, since reoperation may result in resolution of the PLE. Chronic subcutaneous heparin therapy may also resolve the PLE,[274,275] as may percutaneous atrial fenestration.[265,276] Occasional reports suggest improvement with steroid therapy.[277] Cardiac transplantation appears to pose a high risk and does not always resolve the protein loss.[274] Other concerns are the effects of nonpulsatile pulmonary flow, favoring the development of pulmonary arteriovenous malformations, as seen after the Glenn anastomosis.[278] Extrapolation of these data to current

TABLE 64-6 Arrhythmias in 215 Survivors of the Fontan Operation

Results from Follow-up Questionnaire	5 Years Postop Patients		Current Patients	
	No.	%	No.	%
Syncope	18	8	17	8
Rapid heart rate (tachycardia)	44	20	45	21
Slow heart rate (bradycardia)	17	8	15	7
Palpitations	51	24	60	28
Atrial flutter or fibrillation	26	12	41	19
Premature ventricular contractions	13	6	15	7
Ventricular tachycardia	9	4	13	6
Pacemaker	[b]	[b]	22	10
Number of antiarrhythmic medications[a]				
0	179	83	167	78
1	31	13	40	19
2	5	2	8	4

[a]Excluding digitalis.
[b]"Presence of a pacemaker" asked only for patient's current status.
SOURCE: From Driscoll DJ, Offord KP, Feldt RH, et al. Five-to-fifteen-year follow-up after Fontan operation. *Circulation* 1992; 85:469–496. Reproduced with permission from the publisher and authors.

practice is difficult, but the Fontan procedure should be considered palliative, not curative.

Despite these complications, more and more modifications of the Fontan operation are being performed, and more long-term data are necessary to see whether important complications can be reduced in this way. Much recent interest has involved conversion of the Fontan to a more "hydrodynamically efficient" circuit to improve atrial arrhythmias and PLE.[279] A high mortality rate, however, is associated with PLE surgery, and in one series only 50 percent of the survivors were cured.[274] Atrial arrhythmias may also persist after Fontan conversion[279,280] even though hydrodynamics are improved. Perhaps concomitant arrhythmia circuit cryoablation may improve the results.[281]

Some surgical modifications that have been introduced may improve early and late hemodynamics and the functional results. Perforation of the patch at surgery (fenestrated Fontan) allows a hypertensive right atrium to decompress via a right-to-left shunt at the atrial level.[282] These holes may be closed later with an occlusion device at catheterization. Recent "Fontan" operations have excluded the right atrium from the circulation, creating a total cavopulmonary connection (superior vena cava to right pulmonary artery via a bidirectional Glenn anastomosis and inferior vena cava blood channeled to the pulmonary artery).[283] Data suggest improved flow and energy characteristics compared to the standard atriopulmonary connection and fewer early supraventricular arrhythmias.[46] Other modifications have created an extracardiac Fontan connection using a tube graft in the hope of preventing atrial distention and atrial arrhythmias.[284,285]

All patients who have complex congenital heart defects palliated by systemic-to-pulmonary shunt, cavopulmonary anastomosis (bidirectional Glenn), or Fontan should have lifelong regular cardiac follow-up at a specialist center. Particular attention should be paid to ventricular function, detection of thrombus in the right atrium, residual shunts, systemic AV valve regurgitation, AV malformations in the lung, obstruction at the Fontan anastomosis (especially in early operations involving a right atrium-to-pulmonary artery conduit), and PLE (see above).

Ebstein's Anomaly of the Tricuspid Valve

Ebstein's anomaly is characterized by displacement of the proximal attachments of the tricuspid valve from the AV ring into the right ventricle (see Chap. 63). This structural abnormality divides the right ventricle into an "atrialized" portion and a distal "ventricularized" portion. The severity is variable and accounts for the broad clinical spectrum, from severe disease causing fetal or neonatal death to mild disease compatible with natural survival as late as the eighth decade of life.[286] Ebstein's anomaly is an uncommon defect occurring in less than 1 percent of patients with congenital heart disease, but it is disproportionately represented in the adult congenital heart disease population because of its favorable natural history.

The diagnosis of Ebstein's anomaly is now much easier with echocardiography, which has altered our understanding of the natural history. In a large collaborative study of Ebstein's anomaly reported in 1974, only 7 percent of patients were under 1 year of age.[286] It is not surprising that neonates presenting with Ebstein's anomaly represent the worst end of the spectrum, with a severe anatomic defect and a high incidence of associated abnormalities, particularly right ventricular outflow tract obstruction. Their poor outcome is predictable from their anatomy.[287] Those who survive this period with or without surgery may live into adult life, although there is continued morbidity and death throughout childhood. Many patients are minimally symptomatic in childhood and do not present until adolescence or adult life. Symptoms and signs, when they develop, include cyanosis due to right-to-left shunting at the atrial level, dyspnea and fatigue secondary to hypoxia and low cardiac output, and palpitation due to supraventricular arrhythmia. Ebstein's anomaly is often associated with ventricular preexcitation, which may involve one or more, usually right-sided, accessory pathways. Approximately 25 to 30 percent of adults will have symptomatic arrhythmias that may be difficult to treat and can result in sudden death.[288] Progressive heart failure may develop with time and may be related not only to right-sided problems but also to left-sided abnormalities. Excessive fibrosis has been reported in the left ventricle, and left ventricular dysfunction may be induced on exercise.[287,289] Early cyanosis is an adverse risk factor for survival, as is congestive cardiac failure.[290]

MANAGEMENT

Surgery may consist of repair or replacement of the tricuspid valve together with closure of the atrial septal defect to prevent cyanosis (Fig. 64-10).[291] In 189 patients aged 11 months to 64 years (mean 19.1 years), a tricuspid valve reconstruction was possible in 58.2 percent, and in 36.5 percent a prosthetic valve, usually a bioprosthesis, was inserted. In the occasional patient, the atrial septal defect may be responsible for a left-to-right shunt and can be closed as the sole procedure. In others, the functioning right ventricle is too small for a biventricular circulation, and a Fontan procedure may be the only option. Cross-sectional echocardiography is very useful in determining whether the tricuspid valve is amenable to repair, delineating the mobility or tethering of the elongated anterior leaflet and the presence or absence of fenestration. The results of surgery are affected by the presence of arrhythmia. Uncontrolled preoperative supraventricular arrhythmia is a risk factor for early postoperative rhythm problems that may have serious hemodynamic consequences.[288] It is usually recommended that division of an accessory pathway be performed at the time of tricuspid valve surgery. The pathways are usually in the posteroseptal or right free-wall position and may be multiple. An alternative approach is to perform catheter radiofrequency ablation of the accessory pathway (see Chap. 28) before surgery. Thus far, few such procedures have been performed in patients with Ebstein's anomaly. In hearts with marked enlargement of the right atrium, catheter ablation is challenging and, in the setting of an atrial communication, poses the additional risk of a paradoxical embolus and stroke. If there are no accessory pathways, a right-sided maze procedure at the time of tricuspid valve surgery may successfully control supraventricular arrhythmia.[169]

LATE RESULTS

The long-term outlook for well-repaired patients is good; reduction in heart size is usual (see Fig. 64-10), and atrial arrhythmias are reduced. Exercise capacity improves postoperatively, particularly in those who are cyanotic before surgery.[292] Of 149 patients receiving a porcine bioprosthesis in the Mayo Clinic series, the 10-year survival was 92.5 percent, and 92 percent of the survivors were NYHA class I or II. Bioprosthesis durability in the tricuspid position performs favorably, with freedom from bioprosthesis replacement being 80.6 percent at 10 and 15 years.[293]

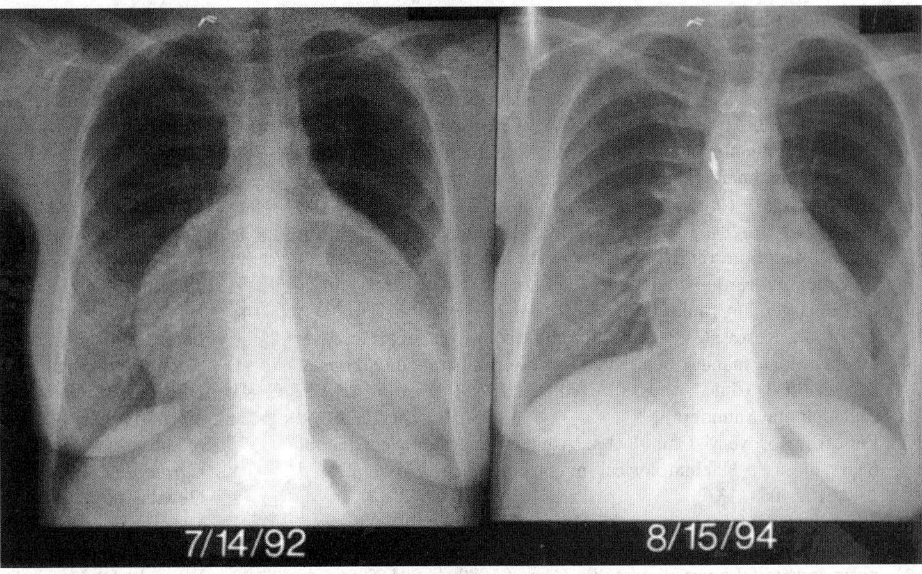

FIGURE 64-10 (*Left*). The chest radiograph shows severe cardiac enlargement associated with Ebstein's anomaly in a 32-year-old woman. She had had a right Blalock-Taussig shunt at age 12. (*Right*). Following tricuspid valve repair and closure of a secundum atrial septal defect, there has been dramatic reduction in the size of the heart.

Marfan's Syndrome

Although the autosomally dominant Marfan's syndrome is congenital in the sense that the patient is born with an abnormal gene or genes, the heart defect is usually acquired. Mutations of fibrillin 1, the main constituent of extracellular microfibrils, are the cause of the pleiotropic manifestations of Marfan's syndrome.[294] The typical phenotypic features—tall, thin stature; pectus deformities; arachnodactyly; and high-arched palate—by which the condition is currently diagnosed, may be obvious, subtle, or absent (see Fig. 10-7). Cardiovascular complications occur in 30 to 60 percent of patients and are the cause of a decreased life expectancy.[295] Mitral valve prolapse is the commonest finding in the pediatric population,[296] but aortic root dilation with a potential for aortic dissection or severe aortic valve regurgitation is the most serious later complication.[297] In a review of 257 patients seen between 1939 and 1972, the median age of death was reported to be about 45 years, with aortic root problems accounting for three-fourths of the deaths (see also Chap. 76).[295] By 1995, a multicenter study reported that the median survival had improved to 72 years.[298]

MANAGEMENT

The risk of dissection is broadly related to the degree of dilation of the aortic root. Dilation can be followed serially by regular cross-sectional echocardiography, which should be performed at least annually. Particularly close monitoring is necessary during puberty and the rapid-growth phase of adolescence. Treatment with beta blockade has been advocated for patients with evidence of aortic root enlargement. Elective aortic root replacement has a low operative mortality rate, but, in contrast, emergency repair, usually for acute aortic dissection, carries a much higher early mortality rate. In a recent multicenter study of 675 patients having aortic root replacement, the 30-day mortality rate was 1.5 percent for those having elective repair, 2.6 percent for those having urgent repair (within 7 days of a surgical consultation), and 11.7 percent for those having emergency repair (within 24 h of a surgical consultation).[297] Forty-six percent of the 158 patients with aortic dissection had an aneurysm with a diameter of 6.5 cm or less. Elective aortic root surgery, therefore, is generally recommended when the aorta exceeds 5.5 cm in diameter.[299] The aortic valve itself may also need to be replaced, although preliminary results from valve-sparing procedures, which eliminate the need for long-term anticoagulants necessary for conventional mechanical valve replacements, suggest cautious optimism.[297,300] It is important to note that more than 10 percent of patients in the multicenter study had problems with the residual aorta, emphasizing the need for continued vigilance of the aorta with MRI or computed tomographic scanning and meticulous control of blood pressure. Since regular, long-term follow-up visits are required, patients with Marfan's syndrome are not uncommon in adult congenital heart clinics. In addition to cardiac care, such patients need expert help with skeletal and ocular problems, genetic counseling, advice on physical activity (see above), and general psychosocial support.

References

1. Ferencz C, Rubin J, McCarter R, et al. Congenital heart disease: Prevalence at live birth. *Am J Epidemiol* 1985; 121:31–36.
2. MacMahon B, McKeown T, Record R. The incidence and life expectation of children with congenital heart disease. *Br Heart Jr* 1953; 15:121–129.
3. Gross R, Hubbard J. Surgical ligation of a persistent ductus arteriosus. *JAMA* 1939; 112:729–731.
4. Perloff J. Congenital heart disease in adults. In: Kelly W, ed. *Textbook of Internal Medicine*. Philadelphia: Lippincott; 1989:223.
5. Stark J. Do we really correct congenital heart defects? *J Thorac Cardiovasc Surg* 1989; 97:(1)1–9.
6. Warnes C. Establishing an adult congenital heart disease clinic. *Am J Card Imaging* 1995; 9:11–14.
7. *1996 Consensus Conference on Adult Congenital Heart Disease*. Montreal: Canadian Cardiovascular Society; 1996.
8. Skorton D, Cheitlin M, Freed M, et al. Training in the care of adult patients with congenital heart disease. *J Am Coll Cardiol* 1995; 25:1–34.
9. Graham T, Arwood G, Boucek R, et al. Abnormalities of right ventricular function following Mustard's operation for transposition of the great arteries. *Circulation* 1975; 52:678–684.
10. Penny D, Redington A. Angiographic demonstration of incoordinate motion of the ventricular wall after the Fontan operation. *Br Heart J* 1991; 66:456–459.
11. Redington A. Functional assessment of the heart after corrective surgery for complete transposition. *Cardio Young* 1991; 1:84–90.
12. Gewillig M, Lundstrom U, Deanfield J, et al. Impact of the Fontan

operation on left ventricular size and contractility. *Circulation* 1990; 81:118–127.
13. Packer M, O'Connor C, Ghali J, et al. Effect of amlodipine on morbidity and mortality in severe chronic heart failure. *N Engl J Med* 1996; 335:1107–1114.
14. CIBIS Investigators and Committees. A randomized trial of beta-blockade in heart failure: The Cardiac Insufficiency Bisprolol Study (CIBIS). *Circulation* 1994; 90:1765–1773.
15. Pfeffer M, Braunwald E, Moye L, et al. Effect of captopril on mortality and morbidity in patients with left ventricular dysfunction after myocardial infarction: Results of the survival and ventricular enlargement trial. *N Engl J Med* 1992; 327:669–677.
16. Territo M, Rosove M, Perloff J. Cyanotic congenital heart disease: Haematologic management, renal function, and urate metabolism. In: Perloff J, Child J, eds. *Congenital Heart Disease in Adults*. Philadelphia: Saunders; 1991:94.
17. Perloff J, Rosove M, Child J, et al. Adults with cyanotic congenital heart disease: Haematological management. *Ann Intern Med* 1988; 109:406–413.
18. Oldershaw P, St. John Sutton, M. Haemodynamic effects of haematocrit reduction in patients with polycythaemia secondary to cyanotic congenital heart disease. *Br Heart J* 1980; 44:584–588.
19. Rosove M, Hocking W, Canobbio M, et al. Chronic hypoxaemia and decompensated erythrocytosis in cyanotic congenital heart disease. *Lancet* 1986; 2:313–315.
20. Ammash N, Warnes CA. Cerebrovascular events in adult patients with cyanotic congenital heart disease. *J Am Coll Cardiol* 1996; 28:768–772.
21. Ross E, Perloff J, Danovitch G, et al. Renal function and urate metabolism in late survivors with cyanotic congenital heart disease. *Circulation* 1986; 73:396–400.
22. Dittrich S, Haas NA, Buhrer C, et al. Renal impairment in patients with long-standing cyanotic congenital heart disease. *Acta Paediatr* 1998; 87:949–954.
23. Harinck E, Hutter P, Hoorntje T, et al. Air travel and adults with cyanotic heart disease. *Circulation* 1996; 93:272–276.
24. Jordan C, White R Jr, Fischer K, et al. The scoliosis of congenital heart disease. *Am Heart J* 1972; 84:463–469.
25. Niwa K, Perloff J, Kaplan S, et al. Eisenmenger syndrome in adults: Ventricular septal defect, truncus arteriosus, univentricular heart. *J Am Coll Cardiol* 1999; 34:223–232.
26. Daliento L, Somerville J, Presbitero P, et al. Eisenmenger syndrome: Factors relating to deterioration and death. *Eur Heart J* 1998; 19:1845–1855.
27. Somerville J. How to manage the Eisenmenger syndrome. *Int J Card* 1997; 63:1–8.
28. Ammash N, Connolly H, Abel M, et al. Noncardiac surgery in Eisenmenger syndrome. *J Am Coll Cardiol* 1999; 33:222–227.
29. Rosenzweig EB, Kerstein D, Barst RJ. Long-term prostacyclin for pulmonary hypertension with associated congenital heart defects. *Circulation* 1999; 99:1858–1865.
30. Working Party of the British Society for Antimicrobial Chemo. The antibiotic prophylaxis of infective endocarditis. *Lancet* 1982; 2:1323–1326.
31. Dajani A, Talbert K, Wilson W, et al. Prevention of bacterial endocarditis. *JAMA* 1997; 277:1794–1801.
32. Sullivan N, Sutter V, Mims M, et al. Clinical aspects of bacteremia after manipulation of the genitourinary tract. *J Infect Dis* 1973; 127:49–55.
33. DeSwiet M, Ramsey I, Rees G. Bacterial endocarditis after insertion of intrauterine contraceptive device. *Br Med J* 1975; 2:76–77.
34. Cetta F, Graham LC, Lichtenberg RC, et al. Piercing and tattooing in patients with congenital heart disease: Patient and physician perspectives. *J Adolesc Health* 1999; 24:160–162.
35. Cetta F, Warnes CA. Adults with congenital heart disease: patient knowledge of endocarditis prophylaxis. *Mayo Clin Proc* 1995; 70:50–54.
36. Godman M, Roberts N, Izukawa T. Late postoperative conduction disturbances after repair of ventricular septal defect and tetralogy of Fallot. *Circulation* 1974; 49:214–221.
37. Vetter V, Horowitz L. Electrophysiologic residua and sequelae of surgery for congenital heart defects. *Am J Cardiol* 1982; 50:588–604.
38. Garson A Jr. Chronic postoperative arrhythmia. In: Gillette P, Garson A Jr, eds. *Pediatric Arrhythmia: Electrophysiology and Pacing*. Philadelphia: Saunders; 1990:667.
39. Dodo H, Gow R, Hamilton R, et al. Chaotic atrial rhythm in children. *Am Heart J* 1995; 129:990–995.
40. Boelens M, Friedli B. Sinus node function and conduction system before and after surgery for secundum atrial septal defect: An electrophysiologic study. *Am J Cardiol* 1984; 53:1415–1420.
41. Deanfield J, Camm J, Macartney F, et al. Arrhythmia and late mortality after Mustard and Senning operation for transposition of the great arteries: An eight year prospective study. *J Thorac Cardiovasc Surg* 1988; 96:569–576.
42. Gewillig M, Wyse R, de Leval M, et al. Early and late arrhythmia after the Fontan operation: Predisposing factors and clinical consequences. *Br Heart J* 1992; 67:72–79.
43. Warfield D, Hayes D, Hyberger L, et al. Permanent pacing in patients with univentricular heart. *PACE* 1999; 22:1193–1201.
44. Ward D, Clarke B, Schofield P, et al. Long-term transvenous ventricular pacing in adults with congenital abnormalities of the heart and great arteries. *Br Heart J* 1983; 50:325–329.
45. Stewart W, DiCola V, Hawthorne J. Doppler ultrasound measurement of cardiac output in patients with physiologic pacemakers: Effects of left ventricular function and retrograde ventriculoatrial conduction. *Am J Cardiol* 1984; 54:308–312.
46. Murphy J, Gersh B, Warnes C, et al. The late survival after surgical repair of isolated ventricular septal defect [abstract]. *Circulation* 1989; 80(suppl II):490.
47. Kulbertus H, Coyne J, Hallidie-Smith K. Conduction disturbances before and after surgical closure of ventricular septal defect. *Am Heart J* 1969; 77:123–131.
48. Deanfield J, McKenna W, Hallidie-Smith K. Detection of late arrhythmia and conduction disturbance after correction of tetralogy of Fallot. *Br Heart J* 1980; 44:577–583.
49. Wolff G, Rowland T, Ellison R. Surgically induced right bundle branch block with left anterior hemiblock. *Circulation* 1972; 46:587–594.
50. Deanfield J. Late ventricular arrhythmias occurring after tetralogy of Fallot: Do they matter? *Int J Cardiol* 1991; 30:143–150.
51. Silka MJ, Hardy BG, Menashe VD, et al. A population-based prospective evaluation of risk of sudden cardiac death after operation for common congenital heart defects. *J Am Coll Cardiol* 1998; 32:245–251.
52. Gewillig M, Cullen S, Mertens B, et al. Risk factors for arrhythmia and death after Mustard operation for simple transposition of the great arteries. *Circulation* 1991; 84(suppl IV):187–192.
53. Balaji S, Gewillig M, Bull C, et al. Arrhythmias after the Fontan procedure: Comparision of total cavopulmonary connection and atriopulmonary connection. *Circulation* 1991; 84(suppl IV): 162–167.
54. Gardiner H, Dhillon R, Bull C, et al. Prospective study of the incidence and determinants of arrhythmia after total cavopulmonary connection. *Circulation* 1996; 94(suppl II):II-17–II-21.
55. Garson A, Nihill M, McNamara D, et al. Status of the adult and adolescent after repair of tetralogy of Fallot. *Circulation* 1979; 59:1232–1240.
56. Kavey R, Blackman M, Sondheimer H. Incidence and severity of chronic ventricular dysrhythmia after repair of tetralogy of Fallot. *Am Heart J* 1982; 342–350.
57. Vaksmann G, Fournier A, Davignon A, et al. Frequency and prognosis of arrhythmias after operative "correction" of tetralogy of Fallot. *Am J Cardiol* 1990; 66:346–349.

58. Lucron H, Marcon F, Bosser G, et al. Induction of sustained ventricular tachycardia after surgical repair of tetralogy of Fallot. *Am J Cardiol* 1999; 83:1369–1373.
59. Marie P, Marcon F, Brunotte F, et al. Right ventricular overload and induced sustained ventricular tachycardia in operatively "repaired" tetralogy of Fallot. *Am J Cardiol* 1992; 69:785–789.
60. Deanfield J, McKenna W, Rowland E. Local abnormalities of right ventricular depolarization after repair of tetralogy of Fallot: A basis for ventricular arrhythmia. *Am J Cardiol* 1985; 55:522–526.
61. Deanfield J, McKenna W, Presbitero P, et al. Ventricular arrhythmia in unrepaired and repaired tetralogy of Fallot: Relation to age, timing of repair and haemodynamic status. *Br Heart J* 1984; 52:77–86.
62. Sullivan I, Presbitero P, Gooch V, et al. Is ventricular arrhythmia in repaired tetralogy of Fallot an effect of operation or a consequence of the course of the disease? *Br Heart J* 1987; 58:40–44.
63. Jones M, Ferrans V. Myocardial degeneration in congenital heart disease: Comparison of morphologic findings in young and old patients with congenital heart disease associated with muscular obstruction to right ventricular outflow. *Am J Cardiol* 1977; 39:1051–1063.
64. Walsh E, Rockenmacher S, Keane J, et al. Late results in patients with tetralogy of Fallot repaired during infancy. *Circulation* 1988; 77:1062–1067.
65. Kobayashi J, Hirose H, Nakano S, et al. Ambulatory electrocardiographic study of the frequency and cause of ventricular arrhythmia after correction of tetralogy of Fallot. *Am J Cardiol* 1984; 54:1310–1313.
66. Quattlebaum T, Varghese J, Neill C, et al. Sudden death among postoperative patients with tetralogy of Fallot: A follow-up study of 243 patients for an average of twelve years. *Circulation* 1976; 54:289–293.
67. Dunnigan A, Pritzker M, Benditt D, et al. Life-threatening ventricular tachycardias in later survivors of surgically corrected tetralogy of Fallot. *Br Heart J* 1984; 52:198–206.
68. Gatzoulis M, Clark A, Newman C, et al. Right ventricular diastolic function 15–35 years after repair of tetralogy of Fallot: Restrictive physiology predicts superior exercise performance. *Circulation* 1995; 91:1775–1781.
69. Gatzoulis M, Till J, Somerville J, et al. Mechanoelectrical interaction in tetralogy of Fallot: QRS prolongation relates to right ventricular size and predicts malignant ventricular arrhythmias and sudden death. *Circulation* 1995; 92:231–237.
70. Larson M, Warnes C. Repaired tetralogy of Fallot: ECG predictors of death and ventricular tachycardia [abstract]. *J Am Coll Cardiol* 1998; 31(suppl A):355A.
71. McLeod K, Hillis W, Houston A, et al. Reduced heart rate variability following repair of tetralogy of Fallot. *Heart* 1999; 81:656–660.
72. Roos-Hesselink J, Perlroth J, McGhie J, et al. Atrial arrhythmias in adults after repair of tetralogy of Fallot: Correlations with clinical, exercise, and echocardiographic findings. *Circulation* 1995; 91:2214–2219.
73. Rodefeld M, Gandhi S, Huddleston C, et al. Anatomically based ablation of atrial flutter in an acute canine model of the modified Fontan operation. *J Thorac Cardiovasc Surg* 1996; 112:898–907.
74. Kalman J, VanHare G, Olgin J, et al. Ablation of "incisional" reentrant atrial tachycardia complicating surgery for congenital heart disease: Use of entrainment to define a critical isthmus of conduction. *Circulation* 1996; 93:502–512.
75. Canobbio MM, Mair DD, van der Velde M, et al. Pregnancy outcomes after the Fontan repair. *J Am Coll Cardiol* 1996; 28:763–767.
76. Connolly HM, Grogan M, Warnes CA. Pregnancy among women with congenitally corrected transposition of the great arteries. *J Am Coll Cardiol* 1999; 33:1692–1695.
77. Connolly HM, Warnes CA. Outcome of pregnancy in patients with complex pulmonic valve atresia. *Am J Cardiol* 1997; 79:519–521.
78. Zuber M, Gautschi N, Oechslin E, et al. Outcome of pregnancy in women with congenital shunt lesions. *Heart* 1999; 81:271–275.
79. Genoni M, Jenni R, Hoerstrup SP, et al. Pregnancy after atrial repair for transposition of the great arteries. *Heart* 1999; 81:276–277.
80. Connolly HM, Warnes CA. Ebstein's anomaly: Outcome of pregnancy. *J Am Coll Cardiol* 1994; 23:1194–1198.
81. Warnes C. Cyanotic congenital heart disease, . In: Oakley C, eds. *Heart Disease in Pregnancy*. London: BMJ Publishing Group; 1997:83–96.
82. Warnes C, Elkayam U. Congenital heart disease and pregnancy. In: Elkayam U, Gleicher N, eds. *Cardiac Problems in Pregnancy*. New York: John Wiley and Associates; 1998; 39–53.
83. Neill C, Swanson S. Outcome of pregnancy in congenital heart disease [abstract]. *Circulation* 1961; 24:1003.
84. Presbitero P, Somerville J, Stone S, et al. Pregnancy in cyanotic congenital heart disease: Outcome of mother and fetus. *Circulation* 1994; 89:2673–2676.
85. Gleicher N, Midwall J, Hochberger D, et al. Eisenmenger's syndrome and pregnancy. *Obst Gynecol* 1975; 34:721–741.
86. Avila W, Grinberg M, Snitcowsky R, et al. Maternal and fetal outcome in pregnant women with Eisenmenger's syndrome. *Eur Heart J* 1995; 16:460–464.
87. Pitts J, Crosby W, Basta L. Eisenmenger's syndrome in pregnancy: Does heparin prophylaxis improve the maternal mortality rate? *Am Heart J* 1977; 93:321–326.
88. Rossiter J, Repke J, Morales A, et al. A prospective longitudinal evaluation of pregnancy in the Marfan syndrome. *Am J Obstet Gynecol* 1995; 173:1599–1606.
89. Elkayam U, Ostrzega E, Shotan A, et al. Cardiovascular problems in pregnant women with the Marfan syndrome. *Ann Intern Med* 1995; 123:117–122.
90. Siu SC, Sermer M, Harrison DA, et al. Risk and predictors for pregnancy-related complications in women with heart disease. *Circulation* 1997; 96:2789–2794.
91. Lao T, Sermer M, Magee L, et al. Congenital aortic stenosis and pregnancy: A reappraisal. *Am J Obstet Gynecol* 1993; 169:540–545.
92. Mendelson C. Pregnancy and coarctation of the aorta. *Am J Obstet Gynecol* 1940; 39:1014–1021.
93. Connolly H, Ammash N, Warnes C. Pregnancy in women with coarctation of the aorta [abstract]. *J Am Coll Cardiol* 1996; 27(suppl A):43A.
94. Hall J, Pauli R, Wilson K. Maternal and fetal sequelae of anticoagulation during pregnancy. *Am J Med*, 1980; 68:122–140.
95. Iturbe-Alessio I, Del Carmen Fonseca M, Mutchinik O, et al. Risks of anticoagulant therapy in pregnant women with artificial heart valves. *N Eng J Med* 1986; 315:1390–1393.
96. Salazar E, Izaguirre R, Verdejo J, et al. Failure of adjusted doses of subcutaneous heparin to prevent thromboembolic phenomena in pregnant patients with mechanical cardiac valve prostheses. *J Am Coll Cardiol* 1996; 27:1698–1703.
97. Sbarouni E, Oakley C. Pregnancy and prosthetic heart valves. *Br Heart J* 1994; 71:196–201.
98. Cotrufo M, deLuca T, Calabro R, et al. Coumadin anticoagulation during pregnancy in patients with mechanical valve prostheses. *Eur J Cardiothorac Surg* 1991; 5:300–305.
99. Elkayam U. Anticoagulation in pregnant women with prosthetic heart valves. *J Am Coll Cardiol* 1996; 27:1704–1706.
100. Nora J, Nora A. The evolution of specific genetic and environmental counseling in congenital heart disease. *Circulation* 1978; 57:205–213.
101. Burn J. The aetiology of congenital heart disease. In: Anderson R, Macartney F, Shinebourne E, et al., eds. *Paediatric Cardiology*. Edinburgh: Churchill Livingstone; 1987:15.
102. Allan L, Crawford D, Chita S, et al. Familial recurrence of congenital heart disease in a prospective series of mothers referred for fetal echocardiography. *Am J Cardiol* 1986; 58:334–337.

103. Driscoll D, Michels V, Gersony W, et al. Occurrence risk for congenital heart defects in relatives of patients with aortic stenosis, pulmonary stenosis, or ventricular septal defect. *Circulation* 1993; 87(suppl I):I-114–I-120.
104. Houston A, Hillis S, Lilley S, et al. Echocardiography in adult congenital heart disease. *Heart* 1998; 80 (suppl 1):12–26.
105. Tworetzky W, McElhinney DB, Brook MM, et al. Echocardiographic diagnosis alone for the complete repair of major congenital heart defects. *J Am Coll Cardiol* 1999; 33:228–33.
106. Stumper O. Imaging the heart in adult congenital heart disease [editorial]. *Heart* 1998; 80:535–536.
107. Ammash NM, Seward JB, Warnes CA, et al. Partial anomalous pulmonary venous connection: diagnosis by transesophageal echocardiography. *J Am Coll Cardiol* 1997; 29:1351–1358.
108. Choe YH, Ko JK, Lee HJ, et al. MR imaging of non-visualized pulmonary arteries at angiography in patients with congenital heart disease. *J Korean Med Sci* 1998; 13:597–602.
109. Hartnell GG, Notarianni M. MRI and echocardiography: How do they compare in adults? *Semin Roentgenol* 1998; 33:252–261.
110. Wimpfheimer O, Boxt LM. MR imaging of adult patients with congenital heart disease. *Radiol Clin North Am* 1999; 37:421–438.
111. Harrison D, McLaughlin P. Interventional cardiology for the adult patient with congenital heart disease: The Toronto Hospital experience. *Can J Cardiol* 1996; 12:965–971.
112. Gersony WM, Hayes CJ, Driscoll DJ, et al. Second natural history study of congenital heart defects. Quality of life of patients with aortic stenosis, pulmonary stenosis, or ventricular septal defect. *Circulation* 1993;87(suppl I): I-52–I-65.
113. Deanfield J. Adult congenital heart disease with special reference to the data on long-term follow-up of patients surviving to adulthood with or without surgical correction. *Eur Heart J* 1992; 13(suppl H):111–116.
114. Truesdell S, Skorton DJ, Lauer RM. Life insurance for children with cardiovascular disease. *Pediatrics* 1986; 77:687–691.
115. Celermajer D, Deanfield J. Employment and insurance for young adults with congenital heart disease. *Br Heart J* 1993; 69:539–543.
116. Garson A, Allen H, Gersony W, et al. Cost of congenital heart disease in children and adults: Sources of variation assessed by multicenter study [abstract]. *Circulation* 1991; 84(suppl II):II-385.
117. Mahoney L, Truesdell S, Hamburgen M, et al. Insurability, employability, and psychosocial considerations. In: Perloff J, Child J, eds. *Congenital Heart Disease in Adults*. Philadelphia: Saunders; 1991: 178.
118. Kellerman J, Zeltzer L, Ellenberg L, et al. Psychological effects of illness in adolescence: Anxiety, self-esteem, and perception of control. *J Pediatr* 1980; 97:126–131.
119. Brandhagen D, Feldt R, Williams D. Long-term psychologic implications of congenital heart disease: A 25-year follow-up. *Mayo Clin Proc* 1991; 66:474–479.
120. Utens EM, Bieman HJ, Verhulst FC, et al. Psychopathology in young adults with congenital heart disease. Follow-up results. *Eur Heart J* 1998; 19:647–651.
121. Zeltzer L, Kellerman J, Ellenberg L, et al. Psychologic effects of illness in adolescence: Impact of illness in adolescents—crucial issues and coping styles. *J Pediatr* 1980; 97:132–138.
122. Gupta S, Giuffre RM, Crawford S, et al. Covert fears, anxiety and depression in congenital heart disease. *Cardiol Young* 1998; 8:491–499.
123. Myers-Vando R, Steward M, Folkins C, et al. The effects of congenital heart disease on cognitive development, illness causality concepts, and vulnerability. *Am J Orthopsychiatr* 1979; 49:617–625.
124. Silbert A, Wolff P, Mayer B, et al. Cyanotic heart disease and psychological development. *Pediatrics* 1969; 43:192–200.
125. Aram D, Ekelman B, Ben-Shachae G, et al. Intelligence and hypoxemia in children with congenital heart disease. *J Am Coll Cardiol* 1985; 6:889–893.
126. Newburger J, Silbert A, Buckley L, et al. Cognitive function and age at repair of transposition of the great arteries in children. *N Engl J Med* 1984; 310:1495–1499.
127. Huffman J. Sex and the teenager. In: Huffman J, Dewhurst J, Capuaro V, eds. *The Gynecology of Childhood and Adolescence*. Philadelphia: Saunders; 1981:527.
128. Swan L, Hillis WS, Cameron A. Family planning requirements of adults with congenital heart disease [editorial]. *Heart* 1997; 78:9–11.
129. Bonnar J. Coagulation effects of oral contraception. *Am J Obstet Gynecol* 1987; 157:1042–1048.
130. Fraser I. Progestogens for contraception. *Austr Fam Phys* 1988; 17:882–885.
131. Whittemore R. Pregnancy and congenital heart disease. In: Adams F, Emmanoulides G, Riemenschneider T, eds. *Heart Disease in Infants, Children, and Adults*. Baltimore: Williams & Wilkins; 1989:684.
132. Rocchini A, Katch V, Anderson J, et al. Blood pressure in obese adolescents: Effects of weight loss. *Pediatrics* 1988; 82:16–23.
133. Powell K, Thompson P, Casperen C, et al. Physical activity and the incidence of coronary heart disease. *Annu Rev Public Health* 1987; 8:281–287.
134. 26th Bethesda Conference. Recommendations for determining eligibility for competition in athletes with cardiovascular abnormalities. *J Am Coll Cardiol* 1994; 24:845–899.
135. Stark J, Pacifico A, eds. *Reoperations in Cardiac Surgery*. Berlin: Springer-Verlag; 1989.
136. Dore A, Glancy DL, Stone S, et al. Cardiac surgery for grown-up congenital heart patients: Survey of 307 consecutive operations from 1991 to 1994. *Am J Cardiol* 1997; 80:906–913.
137. Jonas R, Freed M, Mayer J Jr, et al. Long-term follow-up of patients with synthetic right heart conduits. *Circulation* 1985; 72(suppl II):77–83.
138. Ross D, Somerville J. Correction of pulmonary atresia with a homograft aortic valve. *Lancet* 1966; 2:1446–1447.
139. Merin G, McGoon D. Reoperation after insertion of aortic homograft as a right ventricular outflow tract. *Ann Thorac Surg* 1973; 16:122–126.
140. Shabbo F, Wain W, Ross D. Right ventricular outflow reconstruction with aortic homograft conduit: Analysis of the long-term results. *Thorac Cardiovasc Surg* 1980; 28:21–25.
141. Di Carlo D, de Leval M, Stark J. "Fresh" antibiotic sterilized aortic homografts in extracardiac valved conduits. *Thorac Cardiovasc Surg* 1984; 32:10–14.
142. Cerfolio R, Danielson G, Warnes C, et al. Results of an autologous tissue reconstruction for replacement of obstructed extracardiac conduits. *J Thorac Cardiovasc Surg* 1995; 110:1359–1366.
143. Stark J. Reoperations in patients with extracardiac valved conduits. In: Stark J, Pacifico A, eds. *Reoperations in Cardiac Surgery*. Berlin: Springer-Verlag; 1989:271.
144. Studer M, Blackstone E, Kirklin J, et al. Determinants of early and late results of repair of atrioventricular septal (canal) defects. *J Thorac Cardiovasc Surg* 1982; 84:523–542.
145. Poirier R, McGoon D, Danielson G, et al. Late results after repair of tetralogy of Fallot. *J Thorac Cardiovasc Surg* 1977; 73: 900–908.
146. Zhao H, Miller D, Reitz B, et al. Surgical repair of tetralogy of Fallot: Long-term follow-up with particular emphasis on late death and reoperation. *J Thorac Cardiovasc Surg* 1985; 89:204–220.
147. Ebert P. Second operation for pulmonary stenosis or insufficiency after repair of tetralogy of Fallot. *Am J Cardiol* 1982; 50:637–640.
148. Wessel H, Cunningham W, Paul M, et al. Exercise performance in tetralogy of Fallot after intracardiac repair. *J Thorac Cardiovasc Surg* 1980; 80:582–593.
149. Yemets I, Williams W, Webb G, et al. Pulmonary valve replacement late after repair of tetralogy of Fallot. *Ann Thorac Surg* 1997; 64:526–530.
150. Presbitero P, Somerville J, Revel-Chion R, et al. Open aortic

valvotomy for congenital aortic stenosis: Late results. *Br Heart J* 1982; 47:26–34.
151. Stewart J, Paton B, Blunt S Jr, et al. Congenital aortic stenosis: Ten to twenty years after valvulotomy. *Arch Surg* 1978; 113:1248–1252.
152. Hsieh K, Keane J, Nadas A, et al. Long-term follow-up of valvulotomy before 1968 for congenital aortic stenosis. *Am J Cardiol* 1986; 58:338–341.
153. Puga F, Leoni F, Julsrud P, et al. Complete repair of pulmonary atresia, ventricular septal defect, and severe peripheral arborization abnormalities of the central pulmonary arteries: Experience with preliminary unifocalization procedures in 38 patients. *J Thorac Cardiovasc Surg* 1989; 6:1018–1029.
154. Sullivan I, Wren C, Stark J, et al. Surgical unifocalisation in pulmonary atresia and ventricular septal defect: A realistic goal? *Circulation* 1988; 78(suppl III):5–13.
155. Watterson K, Wilkinson J, Kari T, et al. Very small pulmonary arteries: The central end-to-side shunt. *Ann Thorac Surg* 1991; 52:1132–1137.
156. Speziali G, Driscoll DJ, Danielson GK, et al. Cardiac transplantation for end-stage congenital heart defects: The Mayo Clinic experience, Mayo Cardiothoracic Transplant Team [comments]. *Mayo Clin Proc* 1998; 73:923–928.
157. Mendeloff EN, Huddleston CB. Lung transplantation and repair of complex congenital heart lesions in patients with pulmonary hypertension. *Semin Thorac Cardiovasc Surg* 1998; 10:144–151.
158. Franklin R, Spiegelhalter D, Anderson R, et al. Double inlet ventricle presenting in infancy: Survival without definitive repair. *J Thorac Cardiovasc Surg* 1991; 101:767–776.
159. Child J, Perloff J. Natural survival patterns: A narrowing base. In: Child J, Perloff J, eds., *Congenital Heart Disease in Adults*. Philadelphia: Saunders; 1991:21.
160. Borow K, Braunwald E. Congenital heart disease in the adult. In: Braunwald E, eds. *Heart Disease*. Philadelphia: Saunders; 1988:976.
161. Warnes C, Fuster V, Driscoll D, et al. Atrial septal defect. In: Giuliani E, Fuster V, Gersh B, et al., eds. *Cardiology Fundamentals and Practice*. St. Louis: Mosby-Year Book; 1991:1622.
162. Kirklin J, Barratt-Boyes BG, eds. *Cardiac Surgery*. New York: Wiley; 1986.
163. Massumi R, Nutter D. The syndrome of familial defects of the heart and upper extremities (Holt-Oram syndrome). *Circulation* 1966; 34:65–76.
164. Nora J, McNamara D, Fraser F. Hereditary factors in atrial septal defect. *Circulation* 1967; 35:448–456.
165. Perloff J. Ostium secundum atrial septal defect: Survival for 87–94 years. *Am J Cardiol* 1984; 53:388–389.
166. Campbell M. Natural history of atrial septal defect. *Br Heart J* 1970; 32:820–826.
167. Shah D, Azhar M, Oakley C, et al. Natural history of secundum atrial septal defect in adults after medical or surgical treatment: A historical prospective study. *Br Heart* 1994; 71:224–228.
168. Konstantinides S, Geibel A, Olschewski M, et al. A comparison of surgical and medical therapy for atrial septal defects in adults. *N Engl J Med* 1995; 333:469–473.
169. Theodoro D, Danielson G, Porter C, et al. Right-sided maze procedure for right atrial arrhythmias in congenital heart disease. *Ann Thorac Surg* 1998; 65:149–154.
170. Lock J. The adult with congenital heart disease: Cardiac catheterization as a therapeutic intervention. *J Am Coll Cardiol* 1991; 18:330–331.
171. Hellenbrand W, Fahey J, McGowan F, et al. Transesophageal echocardiographic guidance of transcatheter closure of atrial septal defect. *Am J Cardiol* 1990; 66:207–213.
172. Banerjee A, Bengur AR, Li JS, et al. Echocardiographic characteristics of successful deployment of the Das AngelWings atrial septal defect closure device: Initial multicenter experience in the United States. *Am J Cardiol* 1999; 83:1236–1241.
173. Thanopoulos BD, Laskari CV, Tsaousis GS, et al. Closure of atrial septal defects with the Amplatzer occlusion device: Preliminary results [comments]. *J Am Coll Cardiol* 1998; 31:1110–1116.
174. Walsh KP, Tofeig M, Kitchiner DJ, et al. Comparison of the Sideris and Amplatzer septal occlusion devices. *Am J Cardiol* 1999; 83:933–936.
175. Murphy J, Gersh B, McGoon M, et al. Long-term outcome after surgical repair of isolated atrial septal defect. *N Engl J Med* 1990; 323:1645–1697.
176. Brandenburg R Jr, Holmes D Jr, Brandenburg R, et al. Clinical follow-up study of paroxysmal supraventricular arrhythmias after operative repair of a secundum type atrial septal defect in adults. *Am J Cardiol* 1983; 51:273–276.
177. St. John Sutton M, Tajik A, McGoon D. Atrial septal defect in patients aged 60 or older: Operative results and long-term postoperative follow-up. *Circulation* 1981; 64:402–409.
178. Engle M, Kline S, Borer J. Ventricular septal defect. In: Roberts W, ed. *Adult Congenital Heart Disease*. Philadelphia: Davis; 1987:409.
179. Wood P. The Eisenmenger syndrome or pulmonary hypertension with reversed central shunt. *Br Med J* 1958; 2:701–709.
180. Warnes C, Fuster V, Driscoll D, et al. Ventricular septal defect. In: Guiliani E, Fuster V, Gersh B, et al., eds. *Cardiology: Fundamentals and Practice*. St. Louis: Mosby-Year Book; 1991:1639.
181. Tatsuno K, Konno S, Sakakibara S. Ventricular septal defect with aortic insufficiency: Angiocardiographic aspects and a new classification. *Am Heart J* 1973; 85:13–21.
182. Cartmill T, DuShane J, McGoon D, et al. Results of repair of ventricular septal defect. *J Thorac Cardiovasc Surg* 1966; 52:486–499.
183. Blake R, Chung E, Wesley H, et al. Conduction defects, ventricular arrhythmias and late death after surgical closure of ventricular septal defect. *Br Heart J* 1982; 47:305–315.
184. Bridges N, Perry S, Keane J, et al. Preoperative transcatheter closure of congenital muscular ventricular septal defects. *N Engl J Med* 1991; 324:1312–1317.
185. Reeder G, Danielson G, Seward J, et al. Fixed subaortic stenosis in atrioventricular canal defect: A Doppler echocardiographic study. *J Am Coll Cardiol* 1992; 20:386–394.
186. Report of the New England Regional Infant Cardiac Program. *Pediatrics* 1980; 65(suppl):441–444.
187. Rastelli G, Ongley P, Kirklin J, et al. Surgical repair of the complete form of persistent common atrioventricular canal. *J Thorac Cardiovasc Surg* 1968; 55:299–308.
188. Bergin M, Warnes C, Tajik A, et al. Partial atrioventricular canal defect: Long-term follow-up after initial repair in patients greater than or equal to 40 years old. *J Am Coll Cardiol* 1995; 25:1189–1194.
189. Abraham K, Cherian G, Rao V, et al. Tetralogy of Fallot in adults: A report on 147 patients. *Am J Med* 1979; 66:811–816.
190. Phadke A, Phadke S, Handy M, et al. Acyanotic Fallot's tetralogy with survival to the age of 70 years: Case report. *Indian Heart J* 1977; 29:46–49.
191. Bertranou E, Blackstone E, Hazelrig J, et al. Life expectancy without surgery in tetralogy of Fallot. *Am J Cardiol* 1978; 42:458–466.
192. Deanfield J, Ho S, Anderson R, et al. Late sudden death after repair of tetralogy of Fallot: A clinicopathological study. *Circulation* 1983; 67:636–641.
193. Katz N, Blackstone E, Kirklin J, et al. Late survival and symptoms after repair of tetralogy of Fallot. *Circulation* 1982; 65:403–410.
194. Murphy J, Gersh B, Mair D, et al. Long-term outcome in patients undergoing surgical repair of tetralogy of Fallot. *N Engl J Med* 1993; 329:593–599.
195. Lillehei C, Varco R, Cohen M, et al. The first open heart corrections of tetralogy of Fallot: A 26–31 year follow-up of 106 patients. *Ann Surg* 1986; 204:490–501.
196. Wennevold A, Rygg I, Lauridsen P, et al. Fourteen- to nineteen-

year follow-up after corrective repair of tetralogy of Fallot. *Scand J Thorac Cardiovasc Surg* 1982; 16:41–45.
197. Dodds GA 3d, Warnes CA, Danielson GK. Aortic valve replacement after repair of pulmonary atresia and ventricular septal defect or tetralogy of Fallot. *Thorac Cardiovasc Surg* 1997; 113: 736–741.
198. Bjarke B. Oxygen uptake and cardiac output during submaximal and maximal exercise in adult subjects with totally corrected tetralogy of Fallot. *Acta Med Scand* 1975; 197:177–186.
199. Nugent E, Freedom R, Nora J, et al. Clinical course in pulmonary stenosis. *Circulation* 1977; 56(suppl I):I-38–I-47.
200. Kopecky S, Gersh B, McGoon M, et al. Long-term outcome of patients undergoing surgical repair of isolated pulmonary valve stenosis: Follow-up at 20 to 30 years. *Circulation* 1988; 78:1150–1156.
201. Mullins C, Latson L, Neches W, et al. Balloon dilatation of miscellaneous lesions: Results of Valvuloplasty and Angioplasty of Congenital Anomalies Registry. *Am J Cardiol* 1990; 65:802–803.
202. Friedman W, Johnson A. Congenital aortic stenosis. In: Roberts W, ed. *Adult Congenital Heart Disease.* Philadelphia: Davis; 1987:357.
203. Kelly D, Wulfsberg B, Rowe R. Discrete subaortic stenosis. *Circulation* 1972; 46:309–322.
204. Kleinert S, Geva T. Echocardiographic morphometry and geometry of the left ventricular outflow tract in fixed subaortic stenosis. *J Am Coll Cardiol* 1993; 22:1501–1508.
205. Freedom R. The long and short of it: Some thoughts about the fixed forms of left ventricular outflow tract obstruction. *J Am Coll Cardiol* 1997; 30:1843–1846.
206. Williams J, Barratt-Boyes B, Lowe J. Supravalvular aortic stenosis. *Circulation* 1961; 24:1311–1318.
207. Mills P, Leech G, Davies M, et al. The natural history of a nonstenotic bicuspid aortic valve. *Br Heart J* 1978; 40:951–957.
208. Gersony W, Hayes C. Bacterial endocarditis in patients with pulmonary stenosis, aortic stenosis, or ventricular septal defect. *Circulation* 1977; 56(suppl I):I-84–I-87.
209. Fontana R, Edwards J. *Congenital Cardiac Disease: A Review of 357 Cases Studied Pathologically.* Philadelphia: Saunders; 1962.
210. Muna W, Ferrans V, Pierce J, et al. Discrete subaortic stenosis in Newfoundland dogs: Association of infective endocarditis. *Am J Cardiol* 1978; 41:746–754.
211. Bonderman D, Gharehbaghi-Schnell E, Wollenek G, et al. Mechanisms underlying aortic dilatation in congenital aortic valve malformation. *Circulation* 1999; 99:2138–2143.
212. Cohen L, Friedman W, Braunwald E, et al. Natural history of mild congenital aortic stenosis elucidated by serial hemodynamic studies. *Am J Cardiol* 1972; 30:1–5.
213. Wagner H, Ellison R, Keane J, et al. Long-term follow-up of valvotomy before 1968 for congenital aortic stenosis. *Am J Cardiol* 1986; 58:338–341.
214. Kugelmeier J, Egloff L, Real F, et al. Congenital aortic stenosis: Early and late results of aortic valvotomy. *Thorac Cardiovasc Surg* 1982; 30:91–95.
215. Sandhu S, Lloyd T, Crowley D, et al. Effectiveness of balloon valvuloplasty in the young adult with congenital aortic stenosis. *Cathet Cardiovasc Diagn* 1995; 36:122–127.
216. Somerville J, Stone S, Ross D. Fate of patients with fixed subaortic stenosis after surgical removal. *Br Heart J* 1980; 43:629–647.
217. Brauner R, Laks H, Drinkwater D Jr, et al. Benefits of early surgical repair in fixed subaortic stenosis. *J Am Coll Cardiol* 1997; 30:1835–1842.
218. van Son J, Schaff H, Danielson G, et al. Surgical treatment of discrete and tunnel subaortic stenosis: Late survival and risk of reoperation. *Circulation* 1993; 88:II59–II69.
219. Campbell M. Natural history of coarctation of the aorta. *Br Heart J* 1970; 32:633–640.
220. Cohen M, Fuster V, Steele P. Coarctation of the aorta: Long-term follow-up and prediction of outcome after surgical correction. *Circulation* 1989; 80:840–845.
221. Gross R, Hufnagel C. Coarctation of the aorta: Experimental studies regarding its surgical correction. *N Engl J Med* 1945; 233:287–293.
222. Waldhausen J, Shitman V, Werner J, et al. Surgical intervention in infants with coarctation of the aorta. *J Thorac Cardiovasc Surg* 1981; 81:323–325.
223. Keen G. Spinal cord damage and operations for coarctation of the aorta: Aetiology, practice, and prospects. *Thorax* 1987; 42:11–18.
224. Morris R, Samuels L, Brockman S. Total simultaneous repair of coarctation and intracardiac pathology in adult patients. *Ann Thorac Surg* 1998; 65:1698–1702.
225. Sperling D, Dorsey T, Rowen M, et al. Percutaneous transluminal angioplasty of congenital coarctation of the aorta. *Am J Cardiol* 1983; 51:562–564.
226. Ritter S. Coarctation and balloons: Inflated or realistic? *J Am Coll Cardiol* 1989; 13:696–699.
227. Yetman AT, Nykanen D, McCrindle BW, et al. Balloon angioplasty of recurrent coarctation: A 12-year review. *J Am Coll Cardiol* 1997; 30:811–816.
228. Ebeid M, Prieto L, Latson L. Use of balloon-expandable stents for coarctation of the aorta: Initial results and intermediate-term follow-up. *J Am Coll Cardiol* 1997; 30:1847–1852.
229. Rao P, Thapar M, Wilson A, et al. Intermediate-term follow-up results of balloon aortic valvuloplasty in infants and children with special reference to causes of restenosis. *Am J Cardiol* 1989; 64:1356–1360.
230. Magee A, Brzezinska-Rajszys G, Qureshi S, et al. Stent implantation for aortic coarctation and recoarctation. *Heart* 1999; 82:600–606.
231. de Lezo J, Pan M, Romero M, et al. Immediate follow-up findings after stent treatment for severe coarctation of aorta. *Am J Cardiol* 1999; 83:400–406.
232. Maron B, Humphries J, Rowe R, et al. Prognosis of surgically corrected coarctation of the aorta: A 20-year postoperative appraisal. *Circulation* 1973; 47:119–126.
233. Presbitero P, Demarie D, Villani M, et al. Long-term results (15–30 years) of surgical repair of aortic coarctation. *Br Heart J* 1987; 57:462–467.
234. Fyler D. Report of the New England regional cardiac infant program. *Pediatrics* 1980; 65:375–460.
235. Rashkind W, Mille W. Creation of an atrial septal defect without thoracotomy: A palliative approach to complete transposition of the great arteries. *JAMA* 1966; 196:991–992.
236. Senning A. Surgical correction of transposition of the great vessels. *Surgery* 1959; 45:966–980.
237. Mustard W. Successful two-stage correction of transposition of the great vessels. *Surgery* 1964; 55:469–472.
238. Turina M, Seibenmann R, Segesser L, et al. Late functional deterioration after atrial correction for transposition of the great arteries. *Circulation* 1989; 80(suppl I):162–167.
239. Gelatt M, Hamilton R, McCrindle B, et al. Arrhythmia and mortality after the Mustard procedure: a 30-year single-center experience. *J Am Coll Cardiol* 1997; 29:194–201.
240. Wilson NJ, Clarkson PM, Barratt-Boyes BG, et al. Long-term outcome after the Mustard repair for simple transposition of the great arteries. 28-year follow-up. *J Am Coll Cardiol* 1998; 32:758–765.
241. Puley G, Siu S, Connelly M, et al. Arrhythmia and survival in patients 18 years of age after the Mustard procedure for complete transposition of the great arteries. *Am J Cardiol* 1999; 83:1080–1084.
242. Jatene A, Fontes V, Paulista P, et al. Successful anatomic correction of transposition of the great vessels: A preliminary report. *Arg Braz Cardiol* 1975; 28:461–464.
243. Rastelli G, Wallace R, Ongley P. Complete repair of transposition

of the great arteries with pulmonary stenosis: A review and report of a case corrected by using a new surgical technique. *Circulation* 1969; 39:83–95.
244. Flinn C, Wolff G, Dick M, et al. Cardiac rhythm after the Mustard operation for complete transposition of the great arteries. *N Engl J Med* 1984; 310:1635–1638.
245. Mee R. Two-stage repair: Pulmonary artery banding and switch. *J Thorac Cardiovasc Surg* 1986; 92:385–390.
246. Wernovsky G, Hougen T, Walsh E, et al. Mid-term results after the arterial switch operation for transposition of the great arteries with intact ventricular septum: Clinical, hemodynamic, echocardiographic, and electrophysiologic data. *Circulation* 1988; 77:1333–1344.
247. Rhodes L, Wernovsky C, Keane J, et al. Arrhythmias and intracardiac conduction after the arterial switch operation. *J Thorac Cardiovasc Surg* 1995; 19:303–310.
248. Colan S, Trowitzsch E, Wernovsky G, et al. Myocardial performance after arterial switch operation for transposition of the great arteries with intact ventricular septum. *Circulation* 1988; 78:132–141.
249. Warnes G. Congenitally corrected transposition: The uncorrected misnomer. *J Am Coll Cardiol* 1996; 27:1244–1245.
250. Allwork S, Bentall H, Becker A, et al. Congenitally corrected transposition of the great arteries: Morphologic study of 32 cases. *Am J Cardiol* 1976; 38:910–923.
251. Lundstrom U, Bull C, Wyse R, et al. The natural and "unnatural" history of congenitally corrected transposition. *Am J Cardiol* 1990; 65:1222–1229.
252. Friedberg D, Nadas A. Clinical profile with congenitally corrected transposition of the great arteries: A study of 60 cases. *N Engl J Med* 1970; 282:1053–1059.
253. Huhta J, Maloney J, Ritter D, et al. Complete atrioventricular block in patients with atrioventricular discordance. *Circulation* 1983; 67:1374–1377.
254. Yeh T, Connelly M, Coles J, et al. Atrioventricular discordance: Results of repair in 127 patients. *J Thorac Cardiovasc Surg* 1999; 117:1190–1203.
255. Prieto LR, Hordof AJ, Secic M, et al. Progressive tricuspid valve disease in patients with congenitally corrected transposition of the great arteries. *Circulation* 1998; 98:997–1005.
256. Voskuil M, Hazekamp MG, Kroft LJ, et al. Postsurgical course of patients with congenitally corrected transposition of the great arteries. *Am J Cardiol* 1999; 83:558–562.
257. van Son J, Danielson G, Huhta J, et al. Late results of systemic atrioventricular valve replacement in corrected transposition. *J Thorac Cardiovasc Surg* 1995; 109:642–653.
258. Yagihari T, Kishimoto H, Isobe F, et al. Double switch operation in cardiac anomalies with atrioventricular and ventriculoarterial discordance. *J Thorac Cardiovasc Surg* 1994; 107:351–358.
259. Ilbawi M, DeLeon S, Backer C, et al. An alternative approach to the surgical management of physiologically corrected transposition with ventricular septal defect and pulmonary stenosis or atresia. *J Thorac Cardiovasc Surg* 1990; 100:410–415.
260. Connelly M, Piu P, Williams W, et al. Congenitally corrected transposition in the adult: Functional status and complications. *J Am Coll Cardiol* 1996; 27:1238–1243.
261. Ammash N, Warnes C. Survival into adulthood of patients with unoperated single ventricle. *Am J Cardiol* 1996; 77:542–544.
262. LaCorte M, Dick M, Scheer G, et al. Left ventricular function in tricuspid atresia: Angiographic analysis in 28 patients. *Circulation* 1975; 52:996–1000.
263. Moodie D, Ritter D, Tajik A, et al. Long-term follow-up in the unoperated univentricular heart. *Am J Cardiol* 1984; 53:1124–1128.
264. Moodie D, Ritter D, Tajik A, et al. Long-term follow-up after palliative operation for univentricular heart. *Am J Cardiol* 1984; 53:1648–1651.
265. Warnes C, Feldt R, Hagler D. Protein-losing enteropathy after the Fontan operation: Successful treatment by percutaneous fenestration of the atrial septum. *Mayo Clin Proc* 1996; 71:378–379.
266. Fontan F, Baudet E. Surgical repair of tricuspid atresia. *Thorax* 1971; 26:240–248.
267. Choussat A, Fontan E, Besse P, et al. Selection criteria for Fontan's procedure. In: Anderson R, Shinebourne E, eds. *Paediatric Cardiology*. Edinburgh: Churchill Livingstone; 1977:559–566.
268. Fontan F, Deville C, Quagebeur J, et al. Repair of tricuspid atresia in 100 patients. *J Thorac Cardiovasc Surg* 1983; 85:647–660.
269. Gewillig M, Lundstrom U, Bull C, et al. Exercise responses in patients after Fontan repair: Patterns and determinants of performance. *J Am Coll Cardiol* 1990; 15:1424–1432.
270. Driscoll D, Offord K, Felot R, et al. Five to fifteen year follow-up after Fontan operation. *Circulation* 1992; 81:1520–1536.
271. Fontan F, Kirklin J, Fernandez G, et al. Outcome after a "perfect" Fontan operation. *Circulation* 1990; 81:152–1536.
272. Matsuda H, Kawashima Y, Kishimoto H, et al. Problems with the modified Fontan operation for univentricular heart of the right ventricular type. *Circulation* 1987; 76(suppl II):II-45–II-52.
273. Feldt R, Driscoll D, Offord K, et al. Protein-losing enteropathy after the Fontan operation. *J Thorac Cardiovasc Surg* 1991; 112:672–680.
274. Mertens L, Hagler DJ, Sauer U, et al. Protein-losing enteropathy after the Fontan operation: an international multicenter study: PLE study group. *J Thorac Cardiovasc Surg* 1998; 115:1063–1073.
275. Kelly AM, Feldt RH, Driscoll DJ, et al. Use of heparin in the treatment of protein-losing enteropathy after Fontan operation for complex congenital heart disease. *Mayo Clin Proc* 1998; 73:777–779.
276. Mertens L, Dumoulin M, Gewillig M. Effective percutaneous fenestration of the atrial septum in protein-losing enteropathy after the Fontan operation. *Br Heart J* 1994; 72:591–592.
277. Zellers T, Brown K. Protein-losing enteropathy after the modified Fontan operation: Oral prednisone treatment with biopsy and laboratory proved improvement. *Pediatr Cardiol* 1996; 17:115–117.
278. Mathur M, Glenn W. Long-term evaluation of cavopulmonary artery anastomosis. *Surgery* 1973; 74:889–916.
279. Kreutzer J, Keane J, Lock J, et al. Conversion of modified Fontan procedure to lateral atrial tunnel cavopulmonary anastomosis. *J Thorac Cardiovasc Surg* 1996; 111:1169–1176.
280. van Son J, Mohr F, Hambsch J, et al. Conversion of atriopulmonary or lateral atrial tunnel cavopulmonary anastomosis to extracardiac conduit Fontan modification. *European J C-T Surg* 1999; 15:150–157.
281. Deal B, Mavrousid C, Backer C, et al. Impact of arrhythmia circuit cryoablation during Fontan conversion for refractory atrial tachycardia. *Am J Cardiol* 1999; 83:563–568.
282. Bridges N, Lock J, Castaneda A. Baffle fenestration with subsequent transcatheter closure: Modifications of the Fontan operation for patients at higher risk. *Circulation* 1990; 82:1681–1689.
283. de Leval M, Kilner P, Gewillig M, et al. Total cavopulmonary connection: A logical alternative to atriopulmonary connection for complex Fontan operations. *J Thorac Cardiovasc Surg* 1988; 96:682–695.
284. Laschinger J, Redmond J, Cameron D, et al. Intermediate results of the extracardiac Fontan procedure. *Ann Thorac Surg* 1996; 62:1261–1267.
285. Petrossian E, Reddy V, McElhinney D, et al. Early results of the extracardiac conduit Fontan operation. *J Thorac Cardiovasc Surg* 1999; 117:688–696.
286. Watson H. Natural history of Ebstein's anomaly of the tricuspid valve in childhood and adolescence: An internation cooperative study of 505 cases. *Br Heart J* 1974; 36:417–427.
287. Celermajer D, Dodd S, Greenwald S, et al. Morbid anatomy in neonates with Ebstein's anomaly of the tricuspid valve: Pathophysiologic and clinical implications. *J Am Coll Cardiol* 1992; 19:1049–1053.

288. Till J, Celermajer D, Deanfield J. The natural history of arrhythmias in Ebstein's anomaly [abstract]. *J Am Coll Cardiol* 1992, 19(suppl A):273A.
289. Saxena A, Fong L, Tristram M, et al. Late noninvasive evaluation of cardiac performance in mildly symptomatic older patients with Ebstein's anomaly of the tricuspid valve: Role of radionuclide imaging. *J Am Coll Cardiol* 1991; 17:182–186.
290. Kumar A, Fyler D, Miettinen O, et al. Ebstein's anomaly: Clinical profile and natural history. *Am J Cardiol* 1981; 28:84–95.
291. Danielson G, Driscoll D, Mair D, et al. Operative treatment of Ebstein's anomaly. *J Thorac Cardiovasc Surg* 1992; 104:1195–1202.
292. MacLellan-Tobert S, Driscoll D, Mottram C, et al. Exercise tolerance in patients with Ebstein's anomaly. *J Am Coll Cardiol* 1997; 29:1615–1622.
293. Kiziltan H, Theodoro D, Warnes C, et al. Late results of bioprosthetic tricuspid valve replacement in Ebstein's anomaly. *Ann Thorac Surg* 1998; 66:1539–1545.
294. Ramirez F, Gayraud B, Pereira L. Marfan syndrome: New clues to genotype-phenotype correlations. *Ann Med* 1999; 31:202–207.
295. Murdoch J, Walker B, Halpern B, et al. Life expectancy and causes of death in the Marfan syndrome. *N Engl J Med* 1972; 286:804–808.
296. Pyeritz R, Wappel M. Mitral valve dysfunction in the Marfan syndrome. *Am J Med* 1983; 74:797–807.
297. Gott VL, Greene PS, Alejo DE, et al. Replacement of the aortic root in patients with Marfan's syndrome. *N Engl J Med* 1999; 340:1307–1313.
298. Silverman D, Burton K, Gray J, et al. Life expectancy in the Marfan syndrome. *Am J Cardiol* 1995; 75:157–160.
299. Coady M, Rizzo J, Hammond G, et al. What is the appropriate size criterion for resection of thoracic aortic aneurysms? *J Thorac Cardiovasc Surg* 1997; 113:476–491.
300. Yacoub M, Gehle P, Chandrasekaran V, et al. Late results of a valve-preserving operation in patients with aneurysms of the ascending aorta and root. *J Thorac Cardiovasc Surg* 1998; 115:1080–1090.

PART ELEVEN

CARDIOMYOPATHY AND SPECIFIC HEART MUSCLE DISEASES

CHAPTER 65

CLASSIFICATION OF CARDIOMYOPATHIES

Jay W. Mason

Despite controversy in classifying the cardiomyopathies, there is general agreement on the definition. Cardiomyopathy is a primary disorder of the heart muscle that causes abnormal myocardial performance and is not the result of disease or dysfunction of other cardiac structures. Thus, the term *cardiomyopathy* excludes cases of myocardial failure due to myocardial infarction (so-called ischemic cardiomyopathy, a misnomer), systemic arterial hypertension, and valvular stenosis or regurgitation. Although cardiomyopathy is easily defined, classification of its various forms is difficult. This difficulty results because the great majority of cases of cardiomyopathy are associated with generalized cardiac dilatation and ventricular systolic dysfunction, in which the etiology is unknown.

CLASSIFICATION SCIENCE

Physicians and biomedical scientists use classification schemes to draw relations and distinctions between diseases. This process promotes understanding and aids recollection. Even disorders we know little about can be understood if appropriately placed in a class with other disorders we do know about.

The science of classification requires that all items within the classified domain be included and that each item appear in only one class. Inability to make clear distinctions between biologic systems makes this latter requirement the most demanding. Classification must be based on those features of the individual units within the domain that are understood or recognizable and that permit a useful distinction between groups.

Thus, the classification of cardiomyopathies should be based on an extensive, current category of knowledge about heart diseases and should be as useful as possible to physicians and scientists.

CATEGORIES OF KNOWLEDGE ABOUT CARDIOMYOPATHIES

Knowledge about cardiomyopathies falls into several categories: Etiology, gross anatomy, histology, genetics, biochemistry, immunology, hemodynamic function, prognosis, treatment, and others. No single classification scheme can utilize all of these areas of knowledge because there is so much overlap between them.[1]

The best classifications use a single category of knowledge with which to separate items in the domain. However, the most useful knowledge category differs among users of the classification. A histologic classification will be useful to the pathologist, while a functional categorization is more valuable to the treating physician. If only one classification is to be used by both clinicians and scientists, etiologic categorization seems to be most successful. It must be recognized, however, that no single classification can serve all users and all purposes.

Several commonly employed classifications of cardiomyopathy are discussed below. For clarity, the primary categories of each classification are displayed in Tables 65-1 to 65-6, but only a few representative diseases are mentioned within each category. The exceptions are the etiologic classification (Table 65-3) and the *International Classification of Disease,* Ninth Revision (ICD-9) classification (Table 65-5), in which more nearly complete listings are provided.

THE WORLD HEALTH ORGANIZATION CLASSIFICATION

The only currently used clinical classification of cardiomyopathy that was developed by consensus is that of the *World Health Organization* (WHO) and the International Society and Federation of Cardiology.[2,3] This scheme is outlined in Table 65-1. Because it was developed by a panel of experts and has the implied backing of the WHO, it is widely recognized and frequently used. Although it has been in existence since 1980, it has not gained general acceptance.

The 1980 WHO committee[2] reserved the term *cardiomyopathy* for myocardial disease of unknown cause. This somewhat restricted usage has not been adopted widely and is not fully adhered to in this text. The more common usage includes all

TABLE 65-1 World Health Organization Classifications of Cardiomyopathies

- I. Former WHO classification[a]
  - A. Heart muscle diseases of unknown cause
    1. Dilated cardiomyopathy
    2. Hypertrophic cardiomyopathy
    3. Restrictive cardiomyopathy
    4. Unclassified cardiomyopathy
  - B. Specific heart muscle disease
    1. Infective
    2. Metabolic
       a. Endocrine
       b. Familial storage diseases and infiltrations
       c. Deficiency
       d. Amyloid
    3. General system disease
       a. Connective tissue disorders
       b. Infiltrations and granulomas
    4. Heredofamilial
       a. Muscular dystrophies
       b. Neuromuscular disorders
    5. Sensitivity and toxic reactions
- II. New WHO classification[b]
  - A. Functional classification of cardiomyopathy
    1. Dilated cardiomyopathy
    2. Hypertrophic cardiomyopathy
    3. Restrictive cardiomyopathy
    4. Arrhythmogenic right ventricular cardiomyopathy
    5. Unclassified cardiomyopathies
  - B. Specific cardiomyopathies
    1. Ischemic cardiomyopathy
    2. Valvular cardiomyopathy
    3. Hypertensive cardiomyopathy
    4. Inflammatory cardiomyopathy
       a. Idiopathic
       b. Autoimmune
       c. Infectious
    5. Metabolic cardiomyopathy
       a. Endocrine
       b. Familial storage diseases and infiltrations
       c. Deficiency
       d. Amyloid
    6. General system disease
       a. Connective tissue disorders
       b. Infiltrations and granulomas
    7. Muscular dystrophies
    8. Neuromuscular disorders
    9. Sensitivity and toxic reactions
    10. Peripartal cardiomyopathy

[a]This dates from 1980; see reference 2.
[b]This dates from 1995; see reference 3.
NOTE: These are listings of major categories only; specific disorders are not listed.

TABLE 65-2 Functional Classification of Cardiomyopathies

- I. Cardiac dilatation
  - A. With systolic failure
    1. Idiopathic dilated cardiomyopathy
    2. Late cardiac amyloidosis
    3. Tachycardia-induced congestive failure
  - B. Without systolic failure
    1. High cardiac output state
    2. Bradycardia-induced congestive failure
- II. Cardiac hypertrophy
  - A. With obstruction
    1. Hypertrophic obstructive cardiomyopathy
  - B. Without obstruction
    1. Hypertrophic cardiomyopathy
    2. Left ventricular hypertrophy due to systemic hypertension
- III. Cardiac restriction
  - A. Early cardiac amyloidosis
  - B. Endomyocardial fibrosis

NOTE: This is a complete listing of primary categories, but only a few specific examples are provided for illustration.

forms of heart disease in which the myocardium is primarily involved, as defined at the start of this chapter, but excludes valvular heart disease, systemic arterial hypertension, and coronary atherosclerosis. In its 1995 classification, the WHO committee (entirely new except for one member) moved toward this more common usage, stating, "With increasing understanding of etiology and pathogenesis, the difference between cardiomyopathy and specific heart muscle disease has become indistinct."[3]

Examination of the 1980 and 1995 WHO classifications reveals that they are, in fact, somewhat awkward schemes that employ two separate categorizations in series, one based primarily on left ventricular morphology and function and the other based on etiology. A resultant disadvantage is that diseases are placed in two schema that overlap.

FUNCTIONAL CLASSIFICATION OF CARDIOMYOPATHIES

The most widely used functional classification of cardiomyopathy recognizes three disturbances of function: dilatation, hypertrophy, and restriction (Table 65-2). *Dilatation* is dominated by left ventricular cavity enlargement and systolic failure. *Hypertrophy* includes both obstructive and nonobstructive forms. *Restriction* is characterized by inadequate compliance causing restriction of diastolic filling. The value of this scheme is that virtually all cardiomyopathies are readily placed in one of the three categories, and the therapeutic approaches to each category are distinctly different. For example, left ventricular afterload reduction is a cornerstone of therapy for dilated cardiomyopathies with systolic failure, but is of little benefit in the restrictive forms. There are some shortcomings of the functional classification however. Many diseases are physiologically heterogeneous. Almost all hypertrophic conditions have an element of diastolic restriction. Most dilated ventricles display

TABLE 65-3 Etiologic Classification of Cardiomyopathies

- I. Infective/inflammatory
  - Idiopathic lymphocytic myocarditis
  - Peripartum myocarditis
  - Eosinophilic myocarditis
  - Giant-cell myocarditis
  - Viral myocarditis
  - Rickettsial myocarditis
  - Bacterial myocarditis
  - Mycobacterial heart disease
  - Spirochetal heart disease
  - Fungal myocarditis
  - Protozoal myocarditis
  - Metazoal myocarditis
  - Helminthic myocarditis
  - Chemical or drug hypersensitivity
  - Autoimmune myocarditis
- II. Metabolic
  - A. Endocrine
    - 1. Thyroid disease
      - Thyrotoxicosis
      - Hypothyroidism
    - 2. Pheochromocytoma
    - 3. Acromegaly
    - 4. Diabetes mellitus
    - 5. Carcinoid heart disease
  - B. Uremia
  - C. Hyperoxaluria
  - D. Gout
  - E. Storage diseases and infiltrative processes
    - 1. Lysosomal storage diseases
      - GM1 gangliosidosis
      - Tay-Sachs disease and variants
      - Sandhoff's disease
      - Niemann-Pick disease
      - Gaucher's disease
      - Fabry's disease
      - Farber's disease
      - Fucosidosis
      - Hurler's syndrome
      - Scheie's syndrome
      - Hunter's syndrome
      - Sanfilippo
      - Morquio
      - Moroteaux-Lamy
    - 2. Glycogen storage diseases
      - Pompe's disease
      - Cori's disease
      - Andersen's disease
      - Dominantly inherited cardioskeletal myopathy with lysosomal glycogen storage and normal acid maltase levels
    - 3. Refsum's syndrome
    - 4. Hand-Schüller-Christian
    - 5. Adipositos cordis
    - 6. Hemochromatosis
  - F. Deficiencies
    - 1. Electrolyte
      - Hypocalcemia
      - Hypophosphatemia
    - 2. Nutritional
      - Kwashiorkor
      - Beriberi
      - Pellagra
      - Scurvy
      - Selenium
      - Carnitine
- III. Amyloid
  - AL (primary amyloid, myeloma-associated amyloid)
  - AA (secondary amyloid, familial Mediterraneanfever-associated amyloid)
  - AF (familial amyloid)
  - SSA (senile cardiac amyloid, senile systemic amyloid)
  - IAA (atrial amyloid)
- IV. General system disorders
  - A. Collagen vascular (connective tissue)
    - Systemic lupus erythematosus
    - Polyarteritis nodosa
    - Rheumatoid arthritis
    - Scleroderma
    - Dermatomyositis
    - Whipple's disease
    - Kawasaki's disease
  - B. Sarcoidosis
  - C. Neoplastic
- V. Muscular dystrophies, myopathies, and neuromuscular disorders
  - A. Muscular dystrophies
    - Duchenne's muscular dystrophy
    - Becker's muscular dystrophy
    - Myotonic dystrophy
    - Facioscapulohumeral muscular dystrophy
    - Limb girdle dystrophy
    - Scapuloperoneal dystrophy, including Emery-Dreifuss
    - Congenital muscular dystrophy
    - Distal muscular dystrophy
  - B. Congential myopathies
    - Central-core disease
    - Nemaline myopathy
    - Myotubular myopathy (centronuclear)
    - Congenital fiber-type disproportion
  - C. Mitochondrial myopathies, including Kearns-Sayre syndrome
  - D. Neuromuscular disorders, Friedreich's ataxia
- VI. Toxicity, hypersensitivity, and physical agent effects
  - A. Toxic effects
    - 1. Caused by drugs, heavy metals, and chemical agents
      - Alcohol (ethyl)
      - Amphetamine/methamphetamine
      - Anthracyclines
      - Antidepressants
      - Antimony
      - Arsenic
      - Arsine gas
      - Carbon monoxide
      - Catecholamines
      - Chloroquine
      - Cobalt
      - Cocaine
      - Cyclophosphamide
      - Emetine
      - 5-Fluorouracil
      - Hydrocarbons
      - Interferon
      - Lead
      - Lithium
      - Mercury
      - Methysergide
      - Paracetamol
      - Phenothiazines
      - Phosphorus
      - Reserpine
    - 2. Caused by scorpions, spiders, arthropods, and snakes
      - Scorpions
      - Arthropods
      - Black widow spider
      - Snakes
  - B. Hypersensitivity reactions
    - Acetazolamide
    - Amitriptyline
    - Amphotericin B
    - Ampicillin
    - Carbamazepine
    - Chlorthalidone
    - Hydrochlorothiazide
    - Indomethacin
    - Isoniazid
    - Methyldopa
    - Oxyphenbutazone
    - Para-aminosalicylic acid
    - Penicillin
    - Phenindione
    - Phenylbutazone
    - Phenytoin
    - Streptomycin
    - Sulfadiazine
    - Sulfisoxazole
    - Sulfonylureas
    - Tetracycline
  - C. Physical agents
    - Heat
    - Hypothermia
    - Radiation
- VII. Miscellaneous
  - Peripartum heart disease
  - Tachycardia-induced cardiomyopathy
  - Ectodermal dysplasia-associated cardiomyopathy
  - Idiopathic endocardial fibrosis
  - Endocardial fibroelastosis
  - Infantile cardiomyopathy
  - Arrhythmogenic right ventricular dysplasia

NOTE: This is an essentially complete listing of cardiomyopathies of known cause.

myocyte hypertrophy. Some diseases change from one category to another during their course; the best example is cardiac amyloidosis, which initially exhibits diastolic stiffness, with complete preservation of systolic performance, followed years later by dilatation and systolic failure.

The functional scheme also associates diseases that have vastly different causes, some of which require special therapeutic interventions. For example, the primary therapy for cardiac hemochromatosis, often an initially restrictive disease, is removal of excessive iron stores; this would not, of course, be

TABLE 65-4 Endomyocardial Biopsy Histology Classification of Cardiomyopathies

I. Inflammatory/immune cardiomyopathy
- Lymphocytic myocarditis
- Rheumatic carditis
- Sarcoidosis
- Giant cell myocarditis
- Cardiac allograft rejection
- Chagas' cardiomyopathy
- Hypersensitivity myocarditis

II. Infectious cardiomyopathy
- Toxoplasmosis
- Lyme carditis
- Cytomegalovirus

III. Infiltrative cardiomyopathy
- Glycogen storage
- Hemochromatosis
- Right ventricular lipomatosis
- Amyloidosis

IV. Cardiac tumors
- Cardiac origin
- Noncardiac origin

V. Miscellaneous specific cardiomyopathies
- Anthracycline cardiotoxicity
- Endocardial fibrosis
- Endocardial fibroelastosis
- Fabry's disease
- Carcinoid disease
- Irradiation injury
- Kearns-Sayre syndrome
- Henoch-Schönlein purpura
- Chloroquine cardiomyopathy
- Carnitine deficiency
- Hypereosinophilic syndrome

VI. Nonspecific abnormalities
- Idiopathic dilated cardiomyopathy
- Other cardiomyopathies of unknown cause

VII. No histologic abnormality

NOTE: This represents a relatively complete listing of diagnoses that have been made by endomyocardial biopsy and reported in the literature.

effective treatment for other diseases similarly classified. Despite its shortcomings, the functional classification of cardiomyopathy remains the most popular among clinicians because it is based on easily understood physiology and is relevant to therapy.

ETIOLOGIC CLASSIFICATION

This scheme utilizes knowledge about cardiomyopathies more extensively than all the others. It has the most primary categories because there are numerous known causes that are not interrelated. Table 65-3 categorizes the diseases covered in Chaps. 69, 73 to 80, 85, 86, and 91 to 94. The general outline established by WHO in 1980 is followed roughly. In many cases the etiologic agent is poorly understood (e.g., uremic "cardiomyopathy"), or the cardiomyopathy is associated with another disease, but the mechanism responsible for heart failure is not known (e.g., cardiomyopathy of systemic neoplasia).

While this classification has the advantage of being inclusive, it has the disadvantage of being awkwardly long. It has 7 primary and 42 secondary categories. In addition, most similarly classified disorders are anatomically, physiologically, and therapeutically unrelated. Thus, this classification is not used routinely by clinicians. It has been used most frequently as an organizational scheme in textbooks and reviews concerning heart muscle disease and cardiomyopathy.

TABLE 65-5 ICD-9 Classification of Heart Disease

ICD-9 Code	Description
402.00	Hypertensive heart disease, malignant, w/o CHF
402.01	Hypertensive heart disease, malignant, w CHF
402.10	Hypertensive heart disease, benign, w/o CHF
402.11	Hypertensive heart disease, benign, w CHF
402.90	Hypertensive heart disease, unspecified, w/o CHF
402.91	Hypertensive heart disease, unspecified, w CHF
422.90	Acute myocarditis, unspecified
422.91	Idiopathic myocarditis
425.0	Endomyocardial fibrosis
425.1	Hypertrophic obstructive cardiomyopathy
425.2	Obscure cardiomyopathy of Africa
425.3	Endomyocardial fibroelastosis
425.4	Idiopathic cardiomyopathy
425.5	Alcoholic cardiomyopathy
425.7	Nutritional and metabolic cardiomyopathy
425.8	Cardiomyopathy in other diseases classified elsewhere
425.9	Secondary cardiomyopathy, unspecified
428.0	Congestive heart failure
428.1	Left heart failure
428.9	Heart failure, unspecified
429.0	Myocarditis, unspecified
429.1	Myocardial degeneration
429.3	Cardiomegaly
429.82	Hyperkinetic heart disease
674.84	Postpartum cardiomyopathy

CHF = congestive heart failure.

ENDOMYOCARDIAL BIOPSY CLASSIFICATION

Because the heart can be safely biopsied, antemortem histologic diagnosis can be used to classify cardiomyopathies. Dozens of specific myocardial diseases can be detected by biopsy (Table 65-4). The great strength of histologic diagnosis is that it is definitive and unequivocal when a specific disease is observed. In contrast, numerous deficiencies make this method of classification relatively restricted in use. The foremost problem is that, although the number of specific histologic diagnoses is large, they represent a small proportion of all cases—certainly fewer

TABLE 65-6 Therapeutic Classification of Cardiomyopathies

I. Reduce ventricular afterload
  Idiopathic dilated cardiomyopathy
  Late cardiac amyloidosis
II. Reduce ventricular preload
  Endocardial fibrosis
  Early cardiac amyloidosis
III. Increase ventricular compliance
  Hypertrophic cardiomyopathy
IV. Relieve ventricular obstruction
  Hypertrophic obstructive cardiomyopathy
V. Improve cardiac rhythm
  Cardiomyopathy of persistent tachycardia
VI. Specific therapy
  A. Replace deficiency
    Carnitine deficiency cardiomyopathy
  B. Remove toxic agent
    Hemochromatosis
    Hypersensitivity
  C. Immunosuppression
    Giant cell myocarditis
    Lymphocyte myocarditis(?)
  D. Correct systemic disease
    Uremic cardiomyopathy
    Cardiomyopathy of cancer
    Systemic lupus erythematosus

NOTE: This is a complete listing of primary categories with a few specific examples for illustration.

than 15 percent. The histology in most patients with cardiomyopathy is nonspecific and nondiagnostic. Hypertrophy, or fiber attenuation, and fibrosis may be seen in varying degrees in almost any disorder and are the only findings in most cases of idiopathic dilated cardiomyopathy and hypertrophic cardiomyopathy (as well as in many instances of heart failure due to myocardial infarction and valvular dysfunction). Furthermore, completely normal histology may occasionally be seen on biopsy in cases of severe dilatation and systolic failure.

Myocardial biopsy samples can be subjected to several additional analytic techniques that expand the potential for classification using endomyocardial biopsy. While at present these analyses are only investigational and none can be generally applied, it is likely that one or more of them will become clinically useful in the future and could form the basis of a classification with wide appeal.

ICD-9 CLASSIFICATION

ICD-9-CM stands for *International Classification of Disease*, Ninth Revision, Clinical Modification. This system was developed by WHO in 1948 for registering disease incidences. In 1977, the United States National Center for Health Statistics modified the ICD-9 code to allow coding of medical records. That modification is the current ICD-9-CM. In 1989 it became mandatory for physicians in the United States to include an ICD-9-CM code on their Medicare claims. It is fascinating to see how utterly different a classification system intended for governmental statistics and claims payment is in comparison to those intended for scientific or clinical purposes. The code is a remarkable hodgepodge, combining multiple categories of knowledge into one classification system. Diseases are variously defined according to one or more features such as etiology, anatomy, physiology, comorbidity, symptoms, and even method and extent of diagnosis. It is no wonder that this code is impossible to remember and notoriously ambiguous and difficult to use. In Table 65-5, the codes describing cardiomyopathies have been extracted from the 1999 version of the ICD-9-CM, where they appear in several groups scattered throughout the listing. Relatively few—25—cardiomyopathy diagnoses are coded, and these represent only 9 specific entities. Some well-recognized myocardial diseases are completely ignored, such as arrhythmogenic right ventricular dysplasia. This classification system and the method of classification it represents are certainly not recommended to physicians and scientists. ICD-9-CM should remain in the bailiwick of bureaucrats and serve as a paragon of classification chaos.

THERAPEUTIC CLASSIFICATION

A classification based on specific therapies borrows heavily from the functional and the etiologic classifications of cardiomyopathy. This classification adds information regarding treatment that is not available in other schemes and therefore may be useful to clinicians.

Nevertheless, this classification has several shortcomings. First, often more than one class of therapy is appropriate for a disease. Therefore, the classification must categorize diseases on the basis of their *primary* therapy. This introduces some instability to the classification, since therapeutic preferences are subject to variance in opinion and to change with new research. The greatest fault of therapeutic categorization is that when new therapies are introduced, the existing classification becomes obsolete. The therapeutic classification shown in Table 65-6 illustrates the sensitivity of this approach to opinion. Some might argue, for example, that diuretic therapy remains the primary treatment for dilated cardiomyopathy.

Note that some commonly employed therapies, such as inotropic agents and cardiac transplantation, do not appear in Table 65-6 because they are often not the initial or primary therapies.

GENE-BASED CLASSIFICATION

Aside from traumatic, iatrogenic, infectious, and certain other secondary cardiac disorders, most heart diseases result from an abnormality of gene function. Many diseases caused by adverse gene behavior are due to inherited or acquired genetic mutations. Several diseases are now defined genetically, including hypertrophic cardiomyopathy, long QT syndrome, forms of dilated cardiomyopathy, muscular dystrophies involving the heart, and arrhythmogenic right ventricular dysplasia. A genetic classification of cardiomyopathies would specify the type of genetic disorder (chromosomal, single genic, polygenic, mitochondrial, or somatic cellular) and the mode of inheritance (autosomal or X-linked, and dominant or recessive), the chromosomes or chromosomal locations involved, and the genes involved. A complete genetic classification might also specify the specific mutation or the regional location of the mutation within the gene, since phenotype does and therapy might vary with each specific mutation or region of mutation. A classification system based upon genetic mutations is diagnostically and therapeutically useless unless the biochemical and resultant physiologic aberrations are understood. Thus, the classification should specify the affected protein products of the mutations, as well as the affected functions provided by the proteins.

In the future, many cardiac diseases will be shown to be due to genes functioning at the extremes of normal behavior, and these behavior abnormalities could be classified in much the same way as inherited mutations. Gene-based classification will become the best classification system for cardiomyopathies, because it will at once precisely and uniquely define the disease, and make evident the necessary diagnostic and therapeutic actions.[4]

SUMMARY

No single classification of cardiomyopathy is generally accepted within the biomedical community. An attempt to gain a consensus for one of the many classifications in current use is not likely to succeed because we are unable to subdivide meaningfully cases of idiopathic dilated cardiomyopathy, which constitute the large majority of all cases. At present, it seems best for the individual health practitioner or scientist to use the classification scheme that best serves his or her purpose. For clinicians, this will often be the functional classification.

In the future, a widely acceptable classification may develop that is based on the molecular genetics of myocardial disease. Although this field is only beginning to develop, it is the discipline most likely to contribute to the understanding of causes and the development of new treatments for myocardial disease.

References

1. Abelmann WH. Classification and natural history of primary myocardial disease. *Prog Cardiovasc Dis* 1984; 27:73–94.
2. Report of the WHO/ISFC task force on the definition and classification of cardiomyopathies. *Br Heart J* 1980; 44:672–673.
3. Richardson P, McKenna W, Bristow M, et al. Report of the 1995 World Health Organization/International Society and Federation of Cardiology task force on the definition and classification of cardiomyopathies. *Circulation* 1996; 93:841–842.
4. Keating MT, Sanguinetti MC. Molecular genetic insights into cardiovascular disease. *Science* 1996; 272:681–685.

CHAPTER 66

DILATED CARDIOMYOPATHIES

Michael R. Bristow / Luisa Mestroni / Teresa J. Bohlmeyer / Edward M. Gilbert

This chapter describes the phenotypic and clinical characteristics of the primary and secondary dilated cardiomyopathies, the most common cause of the clinical syndrome of chronic heart failure.[1] Heart failure is an enormously important clinical problem that, if not contained or solved, ultimately may overwhelm health care resources.[2] The clinical syndrome of heart failure is a complex process where the primary pathophysiology is quickly obscured by a variety of superimposed secondary adaptive, maladaptive, and counterregulatory processes (see also Chap. 20). Heart failure is best understood and approached from the vantage point of *myocardial failure,* most commonly associated with a dilated cardiomyopathy phenotype.[3] As an indication of the importance of the problems of cardiomyopathy and heart failure, the cardiomyopathies have been reclassified recently by a World Health Organization/International Society and Federation of Cardiology (WHO/ISFC) task force[3] (and elaborated on further below).

IMPORTANCE OF HEART FAILURE

Due to its high prevalence (1–1.5 percent of the adult population) and high morbidity, including frequent hospitalizations, the clinical syndrome of heart failure is among the most costly medical problems in the United States.[2] Despite improvements in the treatment of heart failure introduced in the last 10 years, including the general availability of cardiac transplantation and better medical treatment, clinical outcome following the onset of symptoms has not changed substantially.[1] That is, mortality remains high (median survival of 1.7 years for men and 3.2 years for women),[1] the natural history remains progressive,[1] the cost is excessive,[2] and disability[2] and morbidity[2,4] are among the highest of any disease or disease syndrome.

RELATIONSHIP OF MYOCARDIAL FAILURE AND DILATED CARDIOMYOPATHIES TO THE CLINICAL SYNDROME OF HEART FAILURE

The vast majority of the cases of heart failure are caused by heart muscle disease (cardiomyopathy). Within the WHO categorization[3] of cardiomyopathy (Table 66-1), the most common cause of the clinical syndrome of heart failure is a secondary (ischemic, valvular, hypertensive, etc.) or a primary (e.g., idiopathic or familial) *dilated cardiomyopathy,* defined as a ventricular chamber exhibiting increased diastolic and systolic volumes

TABLE 66-1 The World Health Organization/International Society and Federation of Cardiology Classification of the Cardiomyopathies[3]

Category	Definition
I. Dilated (DCM) 1. Primary 2. Secondary	↑ EDV, ↑ ESV; low EF
II. Restrictive (RCM) 1. Primary 2. Secondary	↓ EDV, ↔ ESV; ↑ FP, ↔ EF
III. Hypertrophic (HCM)	↑ ↑ Septal and ↑ posterior wall thickness, myofibrillar disarray Mutation in sarcomeric protein, autosomal dominant inheritance
IV. Arrhythmogenic RV Dysplasia (ARVC)	Fibrofatty replacement of RV myocardium Autosomal dominant (most) and recessive inheritance
V. Unclassified 1. Primary 2. Secondary	Not meeting criteria for other categories Features of > one category

ABBREVIATIONS: EDV = end-diastolic volume; ESV = end systolic volume; EF = LV ejection fraction; FP = LV filling pressure; CM = cardiomyopathy.

and a low (<40 percent) ejection fraction. The natural history of the clinical syndrome of heart failure depends on the course of myocardial failure, since (1) the most powerful single predictor of outcome is the degree of left ventricular (LV) dysfunction, as assessed by the LV ejection fraction,[5] (2) treatment that improves intrinsic ventricular function improves heart failure natural history,[6] and (3) treatment that ultimately worsens intrinsic function, such as many types of positive inotropic agents, is associated with an adverse effect on outcome.[6]

THE WHO/ISFC CLASSIFICATION OF CARDIOMYOPATHIES

The WHO/ISFC classification of cardiomyopathies was revised recently[3] to accommodate several rapidly emerging realities. The first was that the molecular genetic basis of previously unknown types of heart muscle disease is rapidly being elucidated, and so it really makes no sense to reserve the classification for "unknown etiologies" of cardiomyopathy.[7] The second consideration was that many of the mechanisms responsible for the natural history of myocardial dysfunction are qualitatively similar in primary versus secondary dilated cardiomyopathies,[8] which accurately predicted a qualitatively similar response to treatment targeted at these mechanisms.[9,10] This made the exclusion of secondary or "known cause"[7] cardiomyopathies gratuitous, and their inclusion in the new classification allows all cardiomyopathies to be classified under one scheme.

As shown in Table 66-1, the WHO/ISFC cardiomyopathy classification uses two separate methods to define the individual categories. The first is based on the global anatomic description of chamber dimensions in systole and diastole. Thus the dilated and restrictive categories have definitions based on LV dimensions or volume, which also define function via calculated ejection fraction (see Table 66-1). The justification for this is that these two groups have distinct natural histories and respond distinctly differently to medical treatment. The second method of creating individual categories within the WHO/ISFC classification is for cardiomyopathies that are genetically based, have unique myocardial phenotypic features, and do not exhibit extracardiac phenotypes. Thus hypertrophic cardiomyopathy (HCM), caused by mutations in contractile proteins manifesting as a unique phenotype, merits a separate category. The same is true for arrhythmogenic right ventricular dysplasia (ARVC), which also has a unique phenotype and likely will turn out to be completely genetic in basis, as has HCM. On the other hand, genetic cardiomyopathies without unique phenotypes, such as the dilated cardiomyopathy of Becker-Duchenne, are included as one form of the anatomic/chamber dimension category (category I).

The WHO/ISFC classification includes another assignment of nomenclature in "secondary" cardiomyopathies, i.e., those associated with known cardiac or systemic processes.[3] These are referred to as *specific cardiomyopathies,* named for the disease process with which they are associated. Thus an ischemic cardiomyopathy would be a specific cardiomyopathy related to previous myocardial infarction (MI) and the subsequent remodeling process, which usually would fall within the dilated class. On the other hand, a hypertensive cardiomyopathy might be classified as either dilated or restrictive depending on the chamber dimensions. Therefore, the correct term for these cardiomyopathies would be *ischemic dilated cardiomyopathy* and *hypertensive dilated* (or *restrictive*) *cardiomyopathy.*

MOLECULAR MECHANISMS IN CARDIOMYOPATHIES AND MYOCARDIAL FAILURE: DISEASE PHENOTYPE PRODUCED BY ALTERATIONS IN GENE EXPRESSION

As shown in Table 66-2, there are three general categories of mechanisms whereby altered gene expression can lead to a phenotypic change in cardiac myocytes.[11] These are (1) a single-gene defect, e.g., as present in β-myosin heavy-chain codon 403 in familial HCM[12] and in an analogous region of the α-myosin heavy chain in HCM transgenic mouse models,[13,14] (2) polymorphic variation in modifier genes, such as is present in many components of the renin-angiotensin system,[15–19] and (3) maladaptive regulated expression of completely normal genes, such as for the mechanisms responsible for progressive myocardial dysfunction and remodeling in secondary dilated cardiomyopathies.[6,11]

Genetic Causes of Cardiomyopathies in Humans and Animal Models

The ability to genetically manipulate the cardiovascular system has made it possible to investigate the role of a number of genes in the developing and adult mouse heart (for a review, see Robbins[20]). The discovery that mutations in sarcomeric proteins lead to HCM has made it possible to generate animal models for this disease.[13,14] In the case of myosin mutations, a single genetic defect initiates a pathway that ultimately leads to hypertrophy and then in males results in late decompensation and ventricular dilatation.[14] Multiple gene mutations have now been associated causally with familial dilated cardiomyopathies, as discussed later in this chapter.

TABLE 66-2 Three General Mechanisms by Which Alterations in Gene Expression Can Influence the Development or Progression of a Dilated Cardiomyopathy

Type of Process	Examples
Gene mutation	Cardiac α-actin,[34] desmin,[35] dystrophin,[36,37] lamin[38,39]
Polymorphic variation in modifier genes	Angiotensin converting enzyme (ACE),[16,43,44] β_2-adrenergic receptor[46]
Altered expression of a completely normal, wild type gene	Decreased expression: β_1-adrenergic receptors,[8] α-MHC,[47,48] SERCA-2[49] Increased expression: ANP,[50] β-MHC,[47] ACE,[51,52] TNF-α,[53] endothelin,[54] βARK[55]

ABBREVIATIONS: MHC = myosin heavy chain; TNF = tumor necrosis factor; βARK = β-adrenergic receptor kinase; SERCA = sarcoplasmic reticulum calcium ATPase; ANP = atrial natriuretic peptide.

A serendipitous genetic model of dilated cardiomyopathy and heart failure (*myf*5 mice) has been generated by activation of a skeletal muscle genetic program in the heart.[21] These mice have a dilated cardiomyopathy phenotype characterized by progressive myocardial dysfunction and dilatation. They develop the clinical syndrome of heart failure, and they have an extraordinarily high (>90 percent at 260 days) heart failure–related mortality.[21] Another serendipitous genetic model of dilated cardiomyopathy is the muscle LIM protein (MLP) knockout mouse.[22] MLP is a positive regulator of muscle differentiation that is ordinarily expressed at high levels in the heart and which may be involved in myofibrillar protein assembly along the actin-based cytoskeleton.[22] MLP knockout mice exhibit typical features of dilated cardiomyopathy, including decreased systolic and diastolic function and β-adrenergic receptor pathway desensitization.[22]

These characteristics make this model very useful in assessing the mechanisms that lead to the development and progression of myocardial failure. Thus, in transgenic mouse models, both altered expression of contractile proteins and perturbation of myocyte cytoarchitecture can lead to the dilated cardiomyopathy phenotype.

There are several additional transgenic mouse models of cardiomyopathy that may be more relevant to the production of a dilated phenotype in humans. Three of them involve overexpression of components of the adrenergic receptor pathway, the heterodimeric G-protein α_s subunit ($G\alpha_s$)[23,24] and the β_1-[25,26] and β_2-adrenergic receptors.[27] These β-adrenergic pathway transgenic mouse models exhibit similar histopathology consisting of myocyte hypertrophy and increased fibrosis, evidence of apoptosis, systolic and diastolic dysfunction, and ultimately, development of LV dilatation.[23–28]

Several transgenic models of concentric or symmetrical LV hypertrophy have now been reported, including overexpression of the protooncogenes *ras*[29] and *myc*,[30] α_1-adrenergic receptors,[31] the heterodimeric G-protein α subunit ($G\alpha_q$),[32] and protein kinase C (PKC).[33] The mechanisms for the induction of increased ventricular wall thickness are diverse, inasmuch as the *ras*, α_1-receptor, $G\alpha_q$, and PKC overexpressors exhibit true cellular hypertrophy with an increase in cell size,[29,31–33] whereas the *myc* animal exhibits cardiac myocyte hyperplasia.[30] The HCM phenotypes discussed earlier illustrate the principle that apparently diverse signals can culminate in the same phenotype, presumably by converging on final common pathways.

Multiple gene defects have been identified that can produce a dilated cardiomyopathy in humans, as discussed in more detail in the section on familial forms of dilated cardiomyopathy. As listed in Table 66-2, these include mutations in the cardiac α-actin,[34] desmin,[35] dystrophin,[36,37] and lamin[38,39] genes.

Polymorphic Variation in Modifier Genes

Genes exhibit polymorphic variation; i.e., normal variants of genes exist in the population that are of slightly different size or sequence.[40] Some gene polymorphisms are associated with differences in function of the expressed protein gene product, and some of these differences in function likely account for "biologic variation" routinely encountered in population studies of disease susceptibility or clinical response to treatment.

Examples of "modifier" genes that may have an impact on the natural history of a dilated cardiomyopathy (see Table 66-2) include the angiotensin-converting enzyme (ACE) *DD* genotype, where individuals are homozygous for the "deletion" variant, which is associated with increased circulating[15] and cardiac tissue[41] ACE activity. The *DD* genotype appears to increase the extent of hypertrophy in HCM[42] and may be a risk factor for early remodeling after MI[43] and for the development of end-stage ischemic or idiopathic dilated cardiomyopathy.[16,44] Other potentially important polymorphic variants that may influence the natural history of a cardiomyopathy involve the angiotensin AT_1 receptor[18,45] and β_2-adrenergic receptors.[46]

Altered, Maladaptive Expression of a Completely Normal Gene

The third way in which altered gene expression can contribute to the development of a cardiomyopathy is altered, maladaptive expression of a completely normal "wild type" gene.[11] This occurs most commonly in the context of progression of heart muscle disease and myocardial failure, which is the natural history of virtually all cardiomyopathies once they are established. Examples in this category (see Table 66-2) include downregulation of β_1-adrenergic receptors,[8] α-myosin heavy chain (α-MHC),[47,48] and sarcoplasmic reticulum Ca^{2+} ATPase[49] genes and upregulation in the atrial natriuretic peptide (ANP),[50] β-myosin heavy chain (β-MHC),[47] ACE,[51,52] tumor necrosis factor (TNF-α),[53] endothelin,[54] β-adrenergic receptor kinase (βARK)[55] genes. These concepts are discussed further below.

PATHOPHYSIOLOGIC PROCESSES INVOLVED IN MYOCARDIAL DYSFUNCTION, REMODELING, AND THEIR PROGRESSION

Tissue preparations and myocytes isolated from failing human hearts exhibit evidence of decreased contractile function.[56] Assuming that loading conditions and ischemia are not adversely affecting cardiac myocyte function, in the setting of chronic systolic dysfunction from a dilated cardiomyopathy, progressive myocardial failure is most likely caused by myocardial cell loss or changes in the gene expression of proteins that regulate or produce muscle contraction. Figures 66-1 and 66-2 summarize these general points and emphasize the central roles of the renin-angiotensin system (RAS) and the adrenergic nervous system (ANS) in promoting cell loss, growth and remodeling, and altered gene expression.[6]

Myocardial Dysfunction and Remodeling due to Altered Expression of Contractility Regulating Genes and Changes in Sarcomeric Assembly

Gene expression can be defined, broadly, as the expression of a fully or normally functioning protein gene product or, more narrowly (and commonly), as the steady-state abundance of a gene's mRNA transcript. Using either definition, numerous abnormalities of gene expression of normal, wild-type genes have been demonstrated in the failing human heart, as discussed earlier, with examples listed in Table 66-2. In order to characterize the abnormalities that may account for progressive myocardial dysfunction and remodeling, it is useful to subdivide them into two general categories,[57] as shown in Table 66-3. The first category encompasses mechanisms that subserve *intrinsic* function, or the mechanisms responsible for contraction and relaxation of the heart in the basal or resting state. *Intrinsic function* is defined as myocardial contraction and relaxation in the absence of extrinsic influences, such as neurotransmitters or hormones. The second general category is *modulated* function, which comprises the mechanisms responsible for the remarkable ability of the heart to increase or decrease its performance dramatically (by 2- to 10-fold) and rapidly in response to various physiologic or physical stimuli. Other critical organs such as the brain, kidney, and liver do not exhibit this quality. *Modulated function* is defined as stimulation or inhibition of myocardial contraction or relaxation by endogenous bioactive compounds, including neurotransmitters, cytokines, autocrine/paracrine substances, and hormones.

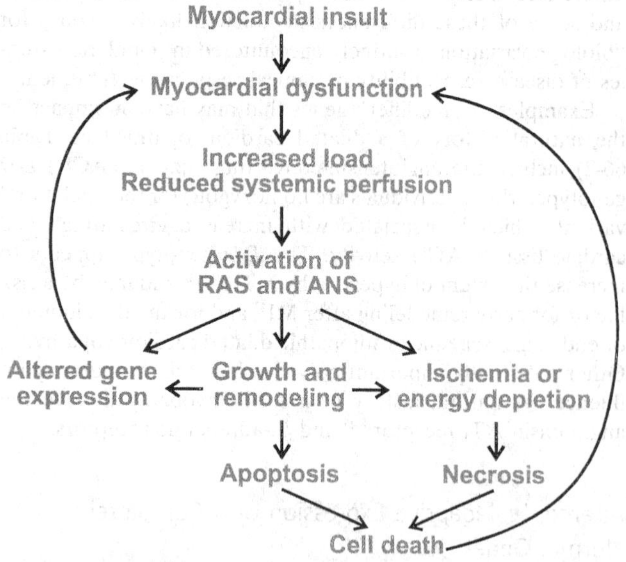

FIGURE 66-1 Relationship of neurohormonal activation and production of cardiac myocyte loss due to apoptosis and necrosis and altered gene expression. Cell loss and altered gene expression result in more myocardial dysfunction, and a vicious cycle is established. RAS = renin angiotensin system; ANS = adrenergic nervous system.

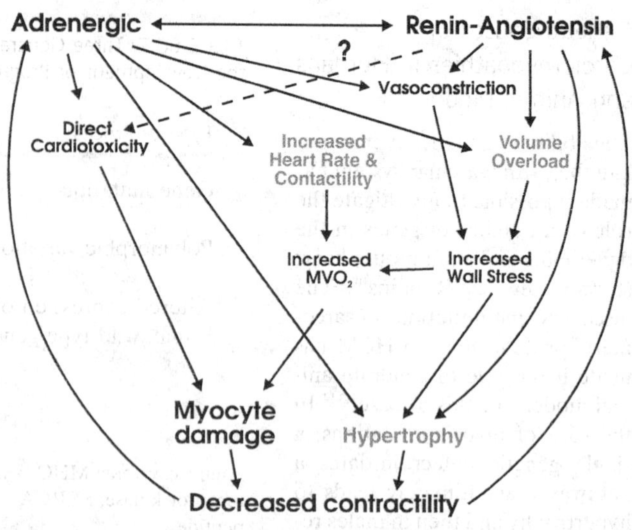

FIGURE 66-2 Heart failure compensatory mechanisms that are activated to support the failing heart. Light-colored areas indicate physiologic mechanisms that stabilize pump function.

In the failing human heart, changes are present in the expression of genes potentially responsible for both general types of myocardial function depicted in Table 66-2.[6,57] Abnormalities of intrinsic function include the factors responsible for an altered length-tension relation,[58–60] a blunted force-frequency response,[61,62] and/or the signals responsible for abnormal cellular and chamber remodeling.[63,64] In the case of the abnormal force-frequency and length-tension responses, the evidence favors abnormal contractile function of individual cardiac myocytes.[56] As shown in Table 66-3, these abnormalities likely reside in the contractile proteins or their regulatory elements,[47,48,65–67] mechanisms involved in excitation-contraction coupling,[49] or the cytoskeleton.[22,68–70] However, within these possibilities for altered intrinsic function, there is not currently a consensus as to which specific abnormalities are present in idiopathic dilated cardiomyopathy (IDC), the most common form of heart failure studied in humans. For cellular remodeling, in both human ventricles[71,72] and animal models,[64,73] the assembly of sarcomeres in series leads to a myocyte that is markedly increased in length but not in diameter, which contributes to remodeling at the chamber level. Such remodeling places the chamber and the myocyte at an energetic disadvantage because of the attendant increase in wall stress,[74] which is one of the major determinants of myocardial oxygen consumption. Inadequate myocyte energy production, particularly associated with key subcellular ion flux mechanisms or the myosin ATPase cycle,[75] in turn would contribute to myocyte contractile dysfunction. Moreover, the hypertrophy process itself leads to a qualitative change in contractile protein gene expression (induction of a "fetal" gene program) that reduces contractile function.[11,47,48,65] On the other hand, cardiac myocyte contractile dysfunction likely plays a role in the remodeling process, inasmuch as medical treatment that improves intrinsic myocardial function can reverse remodeling.[6] Thus contractile dysfunction and remodeling at the cellular level are intimately related to the progressive contractile dysfunction and chamber enlargement that define the natural history of myocardial failure.[76] These concepts are summarized in Fig. 66-3.

TABLE 66-3 General Categorization of Myocardial Function

Intrinsic (Function in the Absence of Neural or Hormonal Influence)	Modulated (Function that May Be Stimulated or Inhibited by Extrinsic Factors Including Neurotransmitters, Cytokines, or Hormone)
• Contractile proteins	• R-G-adenylyl cyclase pathways
• E-C coupling mechanisms	• R-G-phospholipase C pathways
• R-G-adenylyl cyclase pathways	
• Bioenergetics	
• Cytoskeleton	
• Sarcomere and cell remodeling	

ABBREVIATIONS: E-C = excitation-contraction; R-G = receptor–G-protein.

In contrast to abnormalities of intrinsic function, a consensus has been reached on several specific abnormalities in the stimulation component of modulated function. Most of these changes concern β-adrenergic signal transduction.[8,11,57] The ability of β-adrenergic stimulation to increase heart rate and contractility is markedly attenuated in the failing heart due to multiple changes at the level of receptors, G-proteins, and adenylyl cyclase. This produces a major abnormality in the stimulation component of modulated function. In addition, the inhibition component of modulated function is also abnormal in the failing heart, due to a reduction in parasympathetic drive.[77]

There is obviously overlap between the two major subdivisions of myocardial function. Recent data indicate that even in the absence of adrenergic stimulation, β-adrenergic receptors have intrinsic activity.[78–81] That is, a small number of receptors are in an activated state without agonist occupancy and as such can support intrinsic myocardial function.[79,80] Thus overexpression of human β_2-adrenergic receptors is able to markedly increase intrinsic myocardial function,[80] as is enhancement of sarcoplasmic reticulum calcium uptake and release by genetic ablation of the phospholamban gene.[82] The recent realization that active state, agonist-unoccupied β-adrenergic receptors can modulate intrinsic myocardial function is the reason why the "R-G-adenylyl cyclase" mechanism appears in both categories in Table 66-3.

Progressive Myocardial Dysfunction and Remodeling due to Loss of Cardiac Myocytes

The second general mechanism by which myocardial function may be adversely affected is by loss of cardiac myocytes, which also may play a role in the progression of ventricular dysfunction in dilated cardiomyopathies. Cardiac myocyte loss can occur via toxic mechanisms producing necrosis or by "programmed cell death" producing apoptosis. Apoptosis, which is likely due to a combination of growth signaling and cell cycle dysregulation, has been described in end-stage IDC,[83] as well as in the β_1-adrenergic receptor,[25] the $G\alpha_s$ overexpressor transgenic mice,[28] and in models of hypertrophy.[84] However, the human hearts with IDC or ischemic cardiomyopathy were taken from very late stage, literally dying patients maintained on multiple powerful intravenous inotropic medications,[83] and it is not clear if apoptosis plays a significant role in remodeling and/or chamber systolic dysfunction until this point in the natural history of the dilated cardiomyopathies.

IMPORTANCE OF "COMPENSATORY" MECHANISMS IN THE PROGRESSION OF MYOCARDIAL FAILURE

As depicted in Figs. 66-1 and 66-2, there is now a large body of information supporting the idea that *activation of the ANS and RAS compensatory mechanisms contributes to, or is responsible for, the progressive nature of both myocardial failure and the natural history of the heart failure clinical syndrome.*[6] This evidence includes the observations that activation of both these systems is associated with progression of myocardial dysfunction and the heart failure syndrome and clinical trial data that consistently demonstrate that inhibition of these systems can prevent deterioration in or improve myocardial function as well as reduce mortality.[6,10] Despite the fact that in human heart failure

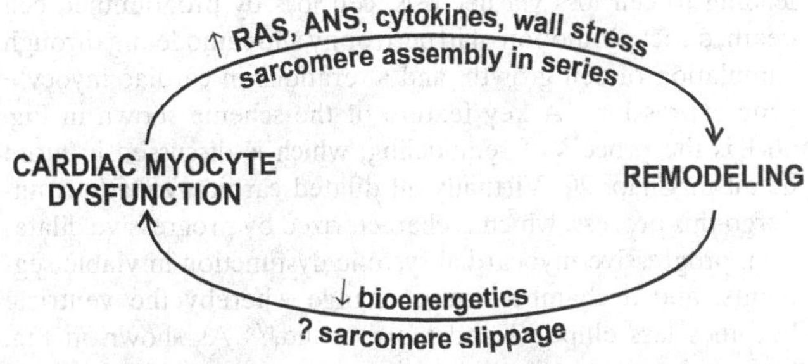

FIGURE 66-3 Relationship between progressive myocardial dysfunction and remodeling. RAS = renin angiotensin system; ANS = adrenergic nervous system.

we now know that chronic activation of the ANS and RAS contributes to the progressive nature of myocardial dysfunction, we know virtually nothing about how these systems adversely affect the biology of the cardiac myocyte. What we do know is that mechanisms within both general categories outlined in Table 66-3 must be involved in the adverse myocardial effects mediated by the ANS and RAS. This is so because modulated function may be improved by treatment with ACE inhibitors or β-blocking agents. Progressive myocardial dysfunction and remodeling are attenuated by both β-blocking agents and ACE inhibitors, and in cardiomyopathies, intrinsic myocardial function is improved and remodeling is reversed by chronic treatment with β-blocking agents.[6] Additionally, mortality in chronic heart failure is directly related to activation of the ANS[85,86] and RAS[87] and may be related to activation of other neurohormonal or autocrine/paracrine systems as well.

Regardless of the type or cause of dilated cardiomyopathy, an initial myocardial insult resulting in this phenotype exhibits common pathophysiologic features that are summarized in Fig. 66-1. That is, a myocardial insult that produces systolic dysfunction will be followed by the initiation of processes designed to temporarily stabilize pump function. The possible mechanisms available for such stabilization are in fact limited. As shown in Fig. 66-2, in chronological order of their action, they are an increase in heart rate and contractility mediated by an increase in cardiac β-adrenergic signaling (produced within seconds of the onset of pump dysfunction), volume expansion in order to use the Frank-Starling mechanism to increase stroke volume (evident within hours of the onset of pump dysfunction), and cardiac myocyte hypertrophy to increase the number of contractile elements (evident within days to weeks of the onset of pump dysfunction). As shown in Fig. 66-2, these compensatory adjustments are largely accomplished by activation of the RAS and ANS. However, despite the short-term (days to months) stability achieved via these mechanisms, they ultimately prove harmful.[6] The best evidence that chronic, continued activation of the RAS and ANS contributes to progressive myocardial dysfunction and remodeling comes from clinical trials where both inhibitors of the RAS (ACE inhibitors) and ANS (β-adrenergic receptor–blocking agents) prevent these two phenomena, and β-blocking agents actually may reverse remodeling and progressive systolic dysfunction,[6] as alluded to.

Much current work is focused on the precise pathophysiologic mechanisms by which activation of the RAS and ANS produces remodeling and adverse effects on myocardial function. Some of the possibilities are given in Fig. 66-1, and they include an exacerbation of ischemia and/or energy depletion leading to cell loss via necrosis, cell loss by programmed cell death, direct promotion of hypertrophy and remodeling through stimulation of cell growth, and alterations in cardiac myocyte gene expression.[6] A key feature of the schema shown in Fig. 66-1 is the process of remodeling, which is discussed in more detail in Chap. 20. Virtually all dilated cardiomyopathies undergo this process, which is characterized by progressive dilatation, progressive myocardial systolic dysfunction in viable segments, and a chamber shape change whereby the ventricle becomes less elliptical and more round.[6,63] As shown in Fig. 66-3, this places the ventricle at an energetic disadvantage,[6,63,74] which likely contributes to further myocardial dysfunction, which then contributes to progressive remodeling. The latter observation is based on data obtained with β-adrenergic blocking agents, which produce an improvement in systolic dysfunction that can be detected prior to a reversal in remodeling.[6] As emphasized by Fig. 66-3, each myocardial degenerative process likely begets the other, leading to an inexorably progressive deterioration in myocardial performance and clinical condition.

SCOPE OF DILATED CARDIOMYOPATHIES

The number of cardiac or systemic processes that can produce or are associated with a dilated cardiomyopathy are plentiful and remarkably varied, as shown in Table 66-4. The dilated phenotype is by far the most common form of cardiomyopathy, comprising over 90 percent of subjects referred to specialized centers.[88] In the United States, the most common dilated cardiomyopathy is ischemic dilated cardiomyopathy,[1] or the cardiomyopathy that follows MI. Other common secondary dilated cardiomyopathies are hypertensive and valvular dilated cardiomyopathies, both produced in part by chronically increased wall stress. The primary cardiomyopathy, IDC, is another relatively common dilated phenotype,[89,90] as discussed below.

SELECTED, COMMON TYPES OF DILATED CARDIOMYOPATHIES

Ischemic Cardiomyopathy

DEFINITION/DIAGNOSIS

Ischemic cardiomyopathy is defined as a dilated cardiomyopathy in a subject with a history of MI or evidence of clinically significant (i.e., ≥70 percent narrowing of a major epicardial artery) coronary artery disease, in whom the degree of myocardial dysfunction and ventricular dilatation is not explained solely by the extent of previous infarction or the degree of ongoing ischemia.[3] In other words, *an ischemic dilated cardiomyopathy is present when a post-MI left ventricle experiences remodeling and a drop in ejection fraction.*

DISTINCT PATHOPHYSIOLOGY

Dilatation of the left ventricle and a decrease in ejection fraction occurs in 15 to 40 percent of subjects within 12 to 24 months following an anterior MI[91,92] and in a smaller percentage of subjects following an inferior MI.[92] Based on limited data,[43] it is tempting to speculate that the subjects who undergo the remodeling process and develop an ischemic dilated cardiomyopathy are individuals with particularly heightened compensatory mechanisms (see Figs. 66-1 and 66-2), perhaps as a result in polymorphic variation in these systems.[16] As discussed earlier, the remodeling process is an attempt by the compromised ventricle to increase its performance by increasing stroke volume, but ultimately, it correlates with an adverse outcome[6,63] in the long term.

The gross pathology of ischemic cardiomyopathy includes transmural or subendocardial scarring, representing old MIs, that may comprise up to 50 percent of the LV chamber. The histopathology of the noninfarcted regions is similar to changes that occur in IDC,[71] as discussed below.

PROGNOSIS

Several studies have concluded that ischemic cardiomyopathy patients have a worse prognosis than subjects with a "non-

TABLE 66-4 Types of Dilated Cardiomyopathies

- Ischemic insult (ischemic cardiomyopathy)
- Valvular disease (mitral regurgitation, aortic regurgitation, aortic stenosis) (valvular cardiomyopathy)
- Chronic hypertension (hypertensive cardiomyopathy)
- Tachyarrhythmias (supraventricular, ventricular, atrial flutter)
- Familial (autosomal dominant, X-linked)
- Idiopathic
- Toxins
  - Ethanol
  - Chemotherapeutic agents (anthracyclines such as doxorubicin and daunorubicin)
  - Cobalt
  - Antiretroviral agents (zidovudine, didanosine, zalcitabine)
  - Phenothiazines
  - Carbon monoxide
  - Lithium
  - Lead
  - Cocaine
  - Mercury
- Metabolic abnormalities
  - Nutritional deficiencies (thiamine, selenium, carnitine, protein)
  - Endocrinologic disorders (hypothyroidism, acromegaly, thyrotoxicosis, Cushing's disease, pheochromocytoma, catecholamines, diabetes mellitus)
  - Electrolyte disturbances (hypocalcemia, hypophosphatemia)
- Infectious
  - Viral (coxsackie virus, cytomegalovirus, HIV)
  - Rickettsial
  - Bacterial
  - Mycobacterial
  - Spirochetal
  - Fungal
  - Parasitic (toxoplasmosis, trichinosis, Chagas' disease)
- Systemic disorders
  - Systemic lupus erythematosis
  - Juvenile rheumatoid arthritis
  - Polyarteritis nodosa
  - Kawasaki disease
  - Collagen vascular disorders (scleroderma, lupus erythematosus, dermatomyositis)
  - Hemochromatosis
  - Amyloidosis
  - Sarcoidosis
  - Pseudoxanthoma elasticum
  - Hypereosinophilic syndrome
- Hypersensitivity myocarditis
- Peri/postpartum dysfunction
- Arrhythmogenic right ventricular dysplasia or cardiomyopathy
- Infantile histiocytoid
- Neuromuscular dystrophies
  - Becker or Duchenne's muscular dystrophy, X-linked cardioskeletal myopathy
- Facioscapulohumoral muscular dystrophy
- Erb's limb-girdle dystrophy
- Myotonic dystrophy
- Friedreich's ataxia
- Emery-Dreifuss muscular dystrophy
- Inborn errors of metabolism
- Mitochondrial cardiomyopathies
- Keshan cardiomyopathy

ischemic" dilated cardiomyopathy,[93,94] probably because the risk of ischemic events is added to the risk of having a dilated cardiomyopathy.

TREATMENT

The treatment of ischemic dilated cardiomyopathy and chronic heart failure is covered in detail in Chap. 21. In general, treatment consists of the use of ACE inhibitors in asymptomatic or symptomatic patients, the use of diuretics in volume-overloaded subjects, and the use of digoxin in subjects who remain symptomatic on the former medications. An emerging treatment strategy is the use of β-adrenergic blocking agents in mild to moderately symptomatic subjects,[6,10] whereas in both ischemic and nonischemic dilated cardiomyopathies,[9,10,95–97] second- and third-generation compounds improve LV function,[6,9–11] reduce hospitalizations,[9,10,95–97] and lower mortality.[9,10] Additionally, adjunctive therapy includes anticoagulation in subjects with lower LV ejection fractions to prevent thromboembolic complications, amiodarone to treat symptomatic arrhythmias, maintaining potassium levels in the high normal (4.3–5.0 meq/L) range to prevent sudden death, frequent clinic visits to adjust medications, and an aggressive approach to treating ischemia, including revascularization.

Hypertensive Cardiomyopathy

DEFINITION/DIAGNOSIS

A *hypertensive dilated cardiomyopathy* is diagnosed when myocardial systolic function is depressed out of proportion to the increase in wall stress. In other words, a subject presenting in heart failure with a hypertensive crisis would not carry this diagnosis unless ventricular dilatation and depressed systolic function remained after correction of the hypertension. In addition to producing a "pure" form of hypertensive cardiomyopathy, hypertension is a major risk factor for heart failure from any cause.[98] Within the WHO/ISFC classification, "hypertensive heart disease" may present in the "dilated," "restrictive," or "unclassified" categories.

DISTINCT PATHOPHYSIOLOGY

The most important pathophysiologic element in hypertension in dilated cardiomyopathy is sustained increased systolic wall stress. Interestingly, in both systolic pressure overloaded right and left ventricles, phenotypic expression is qualitatively variable[99,100] and can include dilatation and systolic dysfunction without increased wall thickness, increased wall thickness, concentric hypertrophy with or without systolic dysfunction, and systolic dysfunction without concentric hypertrophy. Other contributors to the pathophysiology of hypertensive cardiomyopathies are local neurohormonal mechanisms.[101]

PROGNOSIS

The prognosis depends on the presence of other comorbid conditions such as diabetes mellitus and coronary artery disease, as well as the extent of control of afterload. Compared with other forms of cardiomyopathy, in the absence of comorbid conditions, the prognosis of hypertensive cardiomyopathy in subjects whose afterload is controlled is probably better than for most other types of dilated cardiomyopathy.[102]

TREATMENT

The treatment is as for ischemic dilated cardiomyopathy, except that afterload must be vigorously controlled.[101] This consists of the addition of pure antihypertensive vasodilators such as amlodipine or α-blocking agents to standard heart failure therapy.

Valvular Cardiomyopathy

DEFINITION/DIAGNOSIS

A *valvular cardiomyopathy* occurs when a valvular abnormality is present and myocardial systolic function is depressed out of proportion to the increase in wall stress. This most commonly occurs with left-sided regurgitant lesions (mitral regurgitation and aortic regurgitation), less commonly occurs with aortic stenosis, and never occurs as a consequence of pure mitral stenosis.

DISTINCT PATHOPHYSIOLOGY

The classic explanation for the typical phenotypes observed in valvular cardiomyopathies relates to exposure to different types of wall stress.[103] Within this construct, the pattern of eccentric hypertrophy derives from increased diastolic wall stress.[103] Thus long-standing mitral regurgitation most commonly results in compensated eccentric hypertrophy that can progress to a dilated failing phenotype. Aortic regurgitation is a particularly poorly tolerated hemodynamic insult because wall stress is increased in both systole and diastole,[103] and when decompensation occurs, ventricular volume will be increased with or without increased wall thickness. Aortic stenosis classically results in compensated concentric hypertrophy, but when decompensation occurs, a variety of phenotypes can be observed that are similar to hypertensive cardiomyopathies. A disturbing and fairly commonly observed phenomenon is the development of a dilated cardiomyopathy after surgical correction of mitral and sometimes aortic valve disease in subjects who preoperatively had only mild LV dysfunction. These cases are likely due to the superimposition of myocardial damage resulting from open heart surgery and/or underlying dysfunction that was likely greater than appreciated preoperatively.

PROGNOSIS

The prognosis is variable and depends on the number of associated conditions, the nature and extent of the valvular abnormality, and most important, the severity of the cardiomyopathy at the time of surgical correction (see below). In general, *severely depressed myocardial function will not improve much with surgical repair of aortic regurgitation or mitral regurgitation, but the prognosis is likely to be improved because of elimination of some of the hemodynamic insult.* Replacement of the mitral valve should not be attempted in the majority of subjects with severe mitral regurgitation and LV ejection fractions less than 25 percent because of prohibitively high operative/perioperative mortality rates. On the other hand, there is no impairment of LV systolic function severe enough to preclude valve replacement of severe aortic stenosis, since function invariably will improve on relief of the hemodynamic insult, and the prognosis is relatively good.

TREATMENT

The treatment of a valvular dilated cardiomyopathy is surgical valve replacement or repair as soon as the cardiomyopathy is detected. Catheter valvuloplasty may be an option for severe aortic stenosis (AS) patients who are not good surgical candidates for reasons other than heart failure.[104] Medical treatment may be the only option in subjects with aortic insufficiency or mitral regurgitation whose LV function is severely impaired. The medical treatment of either disorder should be as mentioned earlier for ischemic cardiomyopathy plus aggressive afterload reduction, usually hydralazine/nitrates on top of ACE inhibitors. The calcium channel blocker amlodipine is another option for afterload reduction,[105] particularly for aortic insufficiency, where calcium channel blocker therapy has been shown to improve survival.[106]

Idiopathic Dilated Cardiomyopathy, Including Familial Forms

DEFINITION/DIAGNOSIS

IDC is diagnosed by excluding significant coronary artery disease, valvular abnormalities, and other causes. IDC is a relatively common cause of heart failure, with an estimated prevalence rate of 0.04 percent[89] and incidence rates varying from 0.005 to 0.006 percent.[89,90] The true incidence of IDC is undoubtedly higher, owing to the fact that subjects may remain asymptomatic until marked ventricular dysfunction has occurred. The incidence of IDC increases with age, and males are afflicted at a higher rate than are females.[89] As discussed below, histologic features are nonspecific and consist of myocardial cell hypertrophy and varying amounts of increased interstitial fibrosis. Although the diagnosis is not difficult, problems arise when an apparent IDC presents in someone with a history of hypertension or excessive alcohol intake. In such cases, it is best to reassign the etiology to alcohol only when the intake has exceeded 80 g/day for males and 40 g/day for females for more than 5 years and to hypertensive heart disease when blood pressure has been uncontrolled and high (>160/100 mmHg), as well as sustained (for years). All subjects with an unexplained dilated cardiomyopathy need a thyroid-stimulating hormone (TSH) determination done to exclude hypo- or hyperthyroidism, and subjects with diastolic dysfunction need to have an infiltrative process excluded. As discussed below, this is best done by performing an endomyocardial biopsy.

DISTINCT PATHOPHYSIOLOGY

IDC may be familial in as many as 35 to 50 percent of the patients when first-degree relatives are carefully screened.[107,108] The analysis of the phenotype identifies a wide range of clinical and pathologic forms indicating genetic heterogeneity. Accordingly, several chromosomal assignments for gene location have been made, and recently, as shown in Table 66-2, several genes have been identified.[34–39,109–118] The majority of familial patients present with autosomal dominant inheritance and a phenotype characterized by low and age-related penetrance (which is the proportion of carriers who manifest the disease). It is estimated that only 20 percent of gene carriers under the age of 20 display the disease phenotype.[119] Autosomal dominant dilated cardiomyopathy can be due to mutations of the cardiac actin[34] or desmin gene,[35] but in the majority of cases the disease gene is still unknown. The detection of an altered creatine kinase level can indicate the existence of a subclinical skeletal muscle disease. In these patients, an X-linked inheritance suggests mutations in the dystrophin gene,[36,37,120–122] whereas an autosomal dominant transmission and the presence of conduction defects and arrhythmia suggests mutations in the lamin A/C gene.[38,39] In *laminopathy,* the phenotype of the affected relatives can be very variable, from a pure IDC to a mild Emery-Dreifuss-like or limb-girdle-like muscle dystrophy[39] (see Chap. 62). Skeletal muscle and endomyocardial biopsy are diagnostic in X-linked dilated cardiomyopathy, showing abnormalities of dystrophin protein expression by immunocytochemistry.[123,124] Finally, autosomal recessive transmission of dilated cardiomyopathy occurs in mutations of sarcoglycan genes, which encode for dystrophin complex–associated proteins.[125]

Dystrophin, sarcoglycans, desmin, and lamin are cytoskeletal proteins. The contractile protein cardiac α-actin also has a force-transmission or cytoskeletal role.[34] Other data support the hypothesis that IDC could represent, in the majority of cases, a disease of the cytoskeleton; absence of the protein metavinculin in the myocardium was reported in one IDC patient,[70] and as discussed earlier, a dilated cardiomyopathy can be created in mice[22] or is present in a hamster line[126] related to mutations in cytoskeletal genes. However, as discussed earlier, it appears that other genetic abnormalities such as mutations in contractile proteins[14,21,34,127,128] and overexpression of β-adrenergic receptors[25–27] or $G\alpha_s$[24] also can produce a dilated phenotype.

In children, X-linked familial IDC suggests mutation in the G4.5 or tafazzin gene, particularly if associated with certain other signs (such as endocardial fibroelastosis, neutropenia, short stature, or skeletal muscle abnormalities).[116] The function of tafazzin is still unknown. In mitochondrial DNA (mtDNA) mutations, myocardial dysfunction usually is associated with multiorgan involvement (encephalopathy, lactic acidosis, skeletal muscle abnormalities, retinitis pigmentosa, etc.).[129] It is still unclear whether a mtDNA mutation can lead to an isolated IDC phenotype in adults.

Although still incomplete, new knowledge on the genetics of IDC has important clinical implications. The frequency of familial forms indicates the need of family screening in IDC, which can allow genetic counseling, an early detection of the disease, and early therapeutic interventions in affected relatives. The complexity of the phenotype requires an accurate skeletal muscle investigation, which can direct the diagnosis toward a specific type of familial myopathy. Finally, family investigations require more sensitive diagnostic criteria[130] that are able to detect minor cardiac abnormalities as initial signs of the disease. These include initial dilatation without marked systolic dysfunction, arrhythmia, and isolated wall and other abnormalities.[39,108,131]

The major morphologic feature of IDC on postmortem examination is dilatation of the cardiac chambers.[130,131] One ventricle (usually the left) may be more dilated than the other ventricle. The weight of the heart is increased in IDC, with a mean cardiac weight of 551 g for women and 632 g for men.[131] Although there is an increase in muscle mass and myocyte cell volume in IDC, LV wall thickness is usually not increased because of the marked dilatation of the ventricular cavities. Grossly visible scars may be present in either ventricle, and while most scars are small, some may be large and transmural. Scarring occurs in the absence of significant narrowing of the epicardial coronary arteries. In most cases, the degree of fibrosis does not appear to be extensive enough to cause changes in systolic or diastolic function. Intracardiac thrombi and mural endocardial plaques (from the organization of thrombi) are present at necropsy in more than 50 percent of patients with IDC.[132,133] The effect of anticoagulation on the incidence of thrombi has not been studied carefully, but systemic and pulmonary emboli are more frequent in patients with ventricular thrombi or plaques.[134]

The characteristic findings of IDC on microscopy are marked myocyte hypertrophy, very large, bizarrely shaped nuclei[135–137] (Fig. 66-4), increased interstitial fibrosis (see Fig. 66-4), myocyte atrophy, and myofilament loss.[133,138] In isolated cardiac myocytes, the major cellular phenotypic change is marked increase in cell length without a concomitant increase in diameter.[72] As described earlier, this cellular lengthening or remodeling contributes to the chamber remodeling/dilatation that characterizes IDC and other cardiomyopathies. These morphologic changes in IDC are not specific and are generally found in secondary cardiomyopathies such as in the noninfarcted regions of ischemic dilated cardiomyopathy.[71] Also, the morphometric changes in IDC do not correlate with the severity of illness.[137,138] Ultrastructural abnormalities such as mitochondrial changes, T-tubular dilatation, and intracellular lipid droplets may be observed in IDC but also can be observed in other forms of heart disease.[137] There may be interstitial parenchymal and perivascular focal infiltrates of small lymphocytes.[136–140] The lymphocytic infiltrates that are present on histologic examination in IDC are not associated with adjacent myocyte damage, in contrast to myocarditis where adjacent myocyte necrosis is observed. Fibrosis is nearly always present in IDC,[136–140] and its pattern is quite variable from a fine perimyocytic distribution to coarse scars indistinguishable from those present in chronic ischemia. However, small intramural arteries and capillaries are structurally normal in IDC.[137]

A number of immune regulatory abnormalities have been identified in IDC, including humoral and cellular autoimmune reactivity against myocytes,[141] decreased natural killer cell activity,[142] and abnormal suppressor cell activity.[143,144] These abnormalities suggest that immune defects may be important etiologic factors in the development of IDC. These findings, however, are not universally present in patients with IDC, and some abnormalities are also present in other types of heart muscle disease. For example, an increase in the cardioselective M7 antimitochondrial antibodies is found in both IDC and hypertrophic cardiomyopathy but not in heart failure from coronary artery disease.[145] The incidence of some autoreactive antibodies, such as antinuclear and antifibrillary antibodies, increases with the severity of heart failure.[146] It is likely that many of the antibodies detected in IDC and other myocardial diseases do not have pathogenic relevance, but rather are secondary to the primary degenerative process. However, it is possible that certain antibodies present in IDC may have important functional implications. For example, anti-β_1-adrenergic receptor antibodies[147,148] could modify β-adrenergic receptor activity[149] and produce chronic increases in signal transduction that are harmful to the failing heart. Disturbed energy metabolism from antibodies to the ADP/ATP carrier of the inner mitochondrial membrane is another potential pathogenetic autoimmune mechanism[150,151]; these antibodies are present in some individuals with IDC[150] and have been shown to impair metabolism and myocardial function.[151]

There has been great interest in histocompatibility locus antigens (HLAs) in IDC because these antigens are known to be associated with immune regulatory functions, and many autoimmune diseases are found to have positive HLA antigenic associations. HLA associations also have been identified in IDC; the frequency of HLA-B27, HLA-A2, HLA-DR4, and HLA-DQ4 is increased compared with controls, and the frequency of HLA-DRw6 is decreased compared with controls.[152] Genetic abnormalities in the HLA region potentially could alter immune response and thereby increase disease susceptibility to infectious agents such as enteroviruses. Thus the association in IDC with specific HLAs suggest a possible immunologic etiology for this disease. However, these specific HLAs are present in less than 50 percent of patients with IDC, and the heterogeneity of these antigens does not point to a unique site for a putative disease-associated gene. Thus, while the autoimmune hypothesis is an attractive candidate for the etiology of some cases of IDC, it remains unproved.

A clinical and pathologic syndrome that is similar to IDC may develop after resolution of viral myocarditis in animal models and biopsy-proven myocarditis in human subjects.[153] This has led to speculation that IDC may develop in some individuals as a result of subclinical viral myocarditis. Theoretically, an episode of myocarditis could initiate a number of autoimmune reactions that injure the myocardium and ultimately result in the development of IDC. The

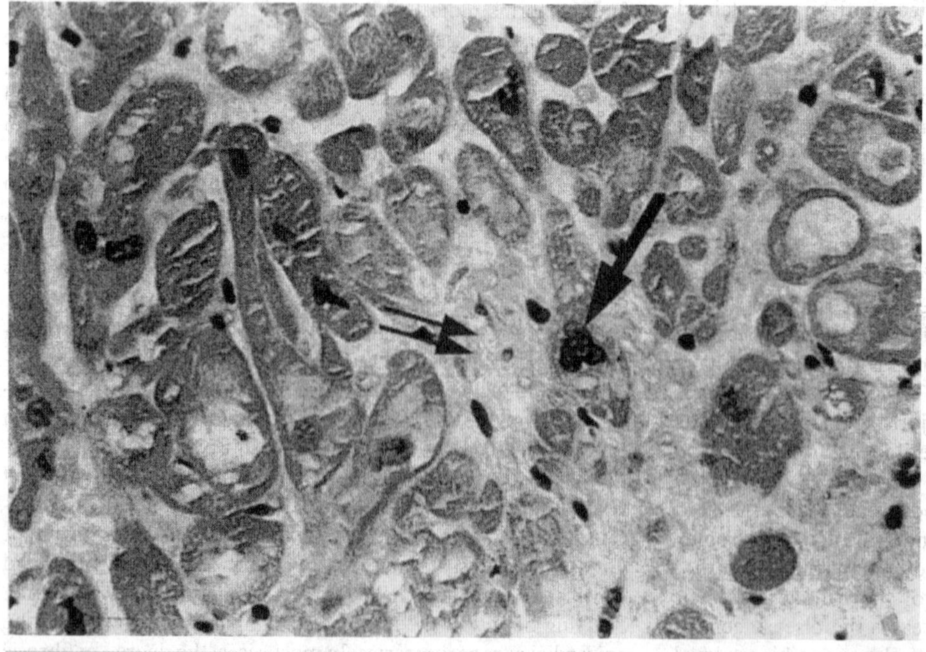

FIGURE 66-4 Right ventricular endomyocardial biopsy from a subject with IDC. Note the increased nuclear size (*arrow*) and the increased interstitial fibrosis.

abnormalities in immune regulation and the variety of antimyocardial antibodies present in IDC are consistent with this hypothesis. However, it is generally not possible to isolate an infectious virus or to demonstrate the presence of viral antigens in the myocardium of patients with IDC.[153,154] Enteroviral RNA sequences are found in heart biopsy samples in IDC, but only in approximately one-third of patients.[154–156] Furthermore, active myocardial inflammation is usually not detected in IDC.[139,140] However, in controlled trials, corticosteroid therapy of patients with IDC does not result in significant clinical improvements.[157] Importantly, recent experimental data have shown in vitro and in vivo that the enteroviral protease 2A is able to cleave dystrophin and disrupt the cytoskeleton in cardiac myocytes, providing a potential link between viral infection and a genetic model of the disease.[158] Furthermore, analysis of human viruses other than enteroviruses suggests that adenoviruses, herpesvirus, and cytomegalovirus also can cause myocarditis and potentially IDC, particularly in children and young subjects.[159,160] Further investigation will be necessary to understand the significance of these findings, particularly in the adult population.

As also discussed in Chap. 22, endomyocardial biopsy of the right or left ventricle may be a valuable diagnostic adjunct for diagnosing specific myocardial processes that can produce a dilated phenotype, such as myocarditis and infiltrative cardiomyopathies. Since several of these other dilated cardiomyopathies may have specific treatments and/or a different prognosis than IDC, endomyocardial biopsy may be warranted in many individuals presenting with a dilated cardiomyopathy. In the future, biopsy may be used more frequently to identify genetic disorders resulting in abnormal gene or protein expression,[50] such as now can be done to diagnose Becker-Duchenne cardiomyopathy.[123,124] Since special staining, electron microscopy, or molecular analysis of the biopsy material may be necessary, endomyocardial biopsy is best performed in specialized cardiomyopathy/heart failure centers.

PROGNOSIS

Several studies of the natural history of IDC have been conducted.[159,160] The prognosis is generally better than for ischemic cardiomyopathy,[93,94] and prior to the routine use of ACE inhibitors, survival was approximately 50 percent in 5 years.[161] The prognosis has been improved substantially since then,[162] inasmuch as ACE inhibition,[163] cardiac transplantation[164] and β-adrenergic blockade[10] are all effective treatments in this cardiomyopathy.

TREATMENT

The treatment of IDC is similar to that discussed earlier for ischemic cardiomyopathy, except that there is no issue of revascularization. The risk of thromboembolic complications may be higher than in ischemic cardiomyopathy, resulting in a lower threshhold for anticoagulation. β-Adrenergic blockade produces a quantitatively greater degree of improvement in LV function compared with ischemic cardiomyopathy[165,166] either because there is a greater degree of adrenergic activation[8] or there is more viable myocardium to work with in IDC. Approximately 10 percent of IDC subjects treated with β-adrenergic blockade will normalize their myocardial function, and this form of treatment should be offered to all IDC patients who do not have a contraindication before considering cardiac transplantation.[167]

SELECTED SPECIFIC DILATED CARDIOMYOPATHIES WITH UNIQUE MANAGEMENT ISSUES

Anthracycline Cardiomyopathy

DEFINITION/DIAGNOSIS

The commonly used and highly efficacious anthracycline antibiotic anticancer agents doxorubicin and daunorubicin produce a dose-related cardiomyopathy[168–173] that may limit their clinical application. Within the WHO/ISFC classification, an anthracycline cardiomyopathy would most likely be in the "dilated" category, but because the extent of dilatation initially may be minimal (see below), it also could be in the "unclassified" category. The cardiomyopathy produced by these agents depends on the total cumulative dose, and for the more widely used compound doxorubicin (Adriamycin), the incidence of heart failure due to cardiomyopathy dramatically increases above total cumulative doses of 450 mg/m^2 in subjects without underlying cardiac problems or other risk factors.[169] *Prior mediastinal radiation involving the heart is a powerful risk factor for anthracycline cardiomyopathy,*[170] *and the risk is also evident if radiation treatment follows chemotherapy.*[172,173] In subjects with risk factors, anthracycline cardiomyopathy can present at lower cumulative doses than 450 mg/m^2.[170–172]

Although the diagnosis of anthracycline cardiomyopathy can be made clinically, the definitive diagnosis depends on the demonstration of a substantial number of cardiac myocytes exhibiting the characteristic anthracycline effect.[168,170–173] Tissue sampling is best done by endomyocardial biopsy, which allows for "thin section" electron microscopic processing of the sample and more definitive resolution of the anthracycline effect with light microscopy.[168,170–173]

DISTINCT PATHOPHYSIOLOGY

In the absence of a tissue diagnosis, anthracycline cardiomyopathy may be diagnosed clinically by exclusion of other causes of cardiomyopathy in a subject who has had at least 350 mg/m^2 of doxorubicin or the equivalent amount of another anthracycline. As shown in Fig. 66-5, the anthracycline cardiac myocytic lesion consists of cell vacuolization progressing to cell dropout, and when 16 to 25 percent of the total number of sampled cells exhibit this morphology, myocardial dysfunction results.[170]

There are some distinguishing clinical features of anthracycline cardiomyopathy that may relate to its pathophysiology. These include a relative absence of hypertrophy and dilatation and a higher heart rate (110–130 beats per minute) than is usually encountered in ambulatory heart failure. The reasons for these features are that the onset of symptoms may be relatively acute (remodeling takes time to develop), and the anthracycline inhibits contractile protein synthesis,[174] reducing the amount of compensatory dilatation and remodeling. In this situation, the only option available for stabilizing cardiac output is increasing the heart rate, since increasing stroke volume via a larger end-diastolic volume has been precluded. The increased heart rate is produced by a greater than expected hyperadrener-

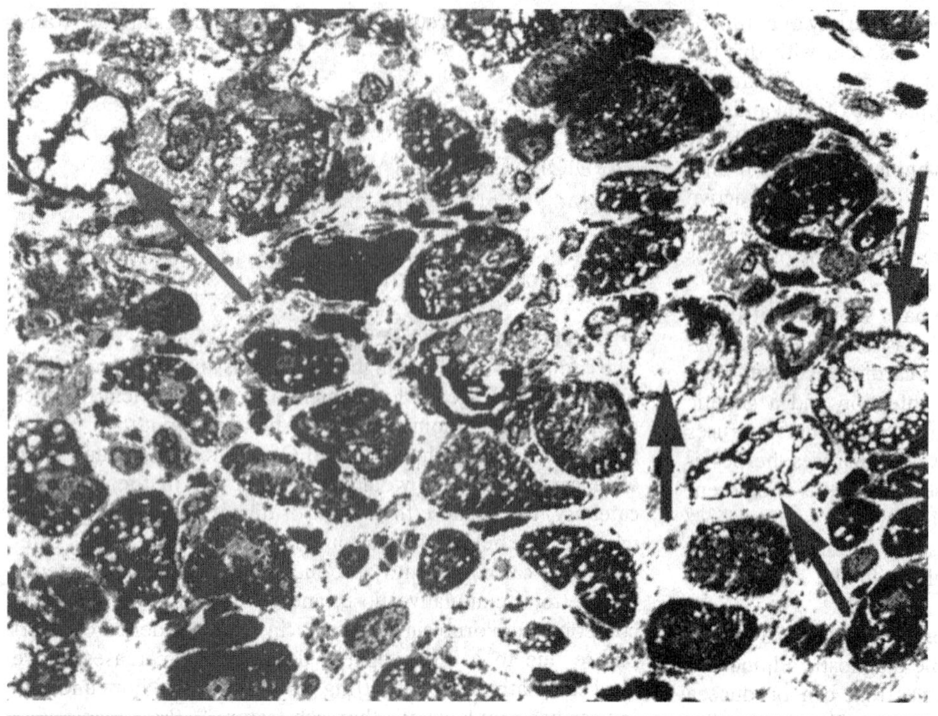

FIGURE 66-5 Cardiac myocyte vacuolization in cases of Adriamycin cardiomyopathy classified on endomyocardial biopsy as grade 3 by the Billingham classification.[170,171,178]

gic state, and so these subjects may be exceptionally dependent on adrenergic support.

PROGNOSIS

The prognosis of anthracycline cardiomyopathy is variable and depends on numerous factors, including the age and underlying prechemotherapy cardiac status of the patient and the time of presentation relative to the last dose of drug. Subjects who present late (several months) or very late (years) after the last dose have a better prognosis because the anthracycline myocardial effect takes at least 60 days to become fully manifest.[175] That is, subjects who develop heart failure within a few days of the last dose of drug have an additional cardiomyopathic burden to face, since the last one to two doses produce their full morphologic effect over the next 1 to 2 months.

TREATMENT/PREVENTION

Subjects who develop anthracycline cardiomyopathy should be treated aggressively with conventional heart failure treatment, since some degree of reversibility is likely. Conventional treatment consists of ACE inhibitors, digoxin, and diuretics. β-Adrenergic blockade has been used successfully in some subjects,[176,177] but because of the high adrenergic drive, it may be difficult to administer. On the other hand, the heightened adrenergic mechanism may be producing a commensurate amount of adverse effect on the myocardium, and so the potential for a favorable response may be even greater than in other kinds of cardiomyopathy. In severe refractory cases, cardiac transplantation may be performed provided that the patient's cancer is in complete remission and is not likely to recur ($\approx$70 percent chance of cure).

Several strategies have been shown to lower the risk of developing anthracycline cardiomyopathy without compromising the chemotherapy response rate. These include using endomyocardial biopsy and right-sided heart catheterization with exercise to assess risk, which virtually eliminates clinical cardiomyopathy and allows more anthracycline to be administered to less susceptible subjects[178]; using serial radionuclide angiography with[179] or without[180] exercise as a monitoring strategy, which may be somewhat helpful but because of a low specificity reduces the total amount of chemotherapy that can be administered safely to some subjects[178,179]; giving the agents as low-dose weekly[181] or as 48- to 72-h infusions[182] rather than as every 3- to 4-week boluses; using a liposomal formulation[183]; or concomitantly administering a second agent that reduces toxicity.[184] Unfortunately, none of these strategies completely eliminates the risk of developing a clinical cardiomyopathy.

Postpartum Cardiomyopathy

DEFINITION/DIAGNOSIS

Postpartum or *peripartum cardiomyopathy* is defined as the presentation of systolic dysfunction and clinical heart failure during the last trimester of pregnancy or within 6 months of delivery.[185] Given the extreme hemodynamic load produced by pregnancy, it is perhaps surprising that postpartum cardiomyopathy is not more common.

DISTINCT PATHOPHYSIOLOGY

Postpartum cardiomyopathy most likely will be classified within the "dilated" WHO/ISFC category but occasionally will be "unclassified" because dilatation and remodeling have not had time to occur. Postpartum cardiomyopathy is likely a heterogeneous group of disorders consisting of the addition of the hemodynamic load of pregnancy to a variety of underlying myocardial processes, including hypertensive heart disease, familial or idiopathic dilated cardiomyopathy, and myocarditis.[185,186]

PROGNOSIS

Approximately half of subjects who develop postpartum cardiomyopathy will recover completely,[187] and the majority of the rest will improve. Subjects who have developed a postpartum cardiomyopathy should never become pregnant again, even if myocardial function has recovered fully.

TREATMENT

Treatment should be aggressive and as for IDC. Cardiac transplantation may be required in severely compromised patients who do not improve.

Amyloid Cardiomyopathy

DEFINITION/DIAGNOSIS

As discussed in Chap. 68, amyloidosis is a group of diseases characterized by extracellular deposition of proteins characterized by their unique β-pleated sheet conformation and recognized electron microscopically as randomly arranged nonbranching fibers ranging from 8 to 14 nm in length. Amyloidosis is classified according to the type of amyloid protein involved.[188] Amyloidosis involving the heart is not rare and accounts for up to 10 percent of all nonischemic cardiomyopathies in autopsy studies.[189,190]

Amyloid cardiomyopathy may present in the WHO/ISFC "restrictive," "dilated," or "unclassified" categories. Most commonly it presents as a restrictive cardiomyopathy with conduction system abnormalities. In the setting of systemic amyloidosis (secondary or primary forms), the presence of increased wall thickness on echocardiogram plus low electrocardiographic voltage is highly suggestive of cardiac involvement.[191] In primary systemic amyloidosis, a monoclonal immunoglobulin spike is detectable in urine or serum in approximately 80 percent of subjects.[192] The definitive diagnosis of amyloid cardiomyopathy is made by tissue examination, ideally premortem by endomyocardial biopsy.[191] In systemic forms, the tissue diagnosis may be made by rectal, skin, or tongue biopsy of any abnormal tissue in these locations coupled with an unexplained myocardial process. As shown in Fig. 66-6, the characteristic histologic signature of amyloid is extracellular deposition of a fibrillar protein with a characteristic periodicity on electron microscopy.[193] Although a Congo Red stain can identify most cases, electron microscopy is more sensitive and specific and should be used routinely when amyloid is suspected.

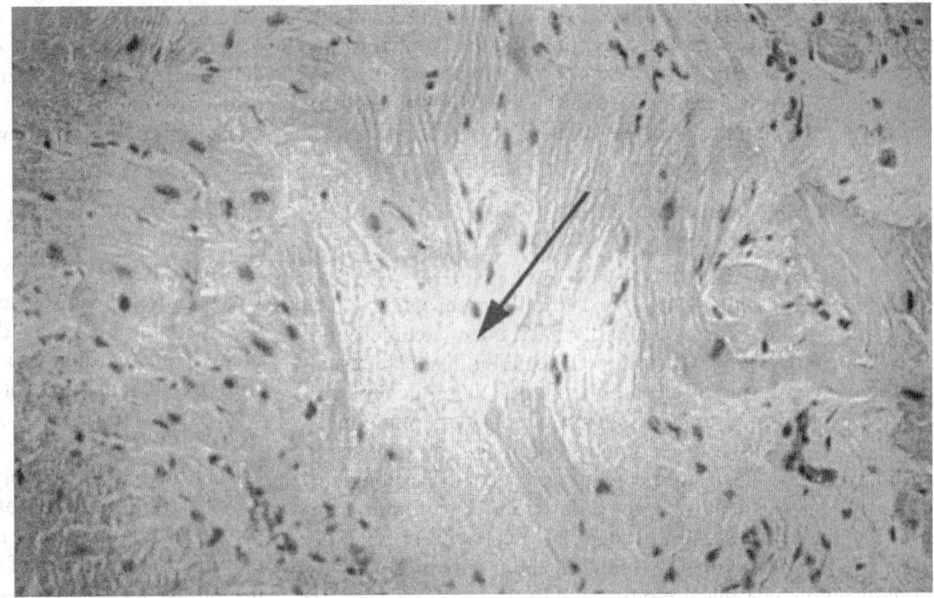

A

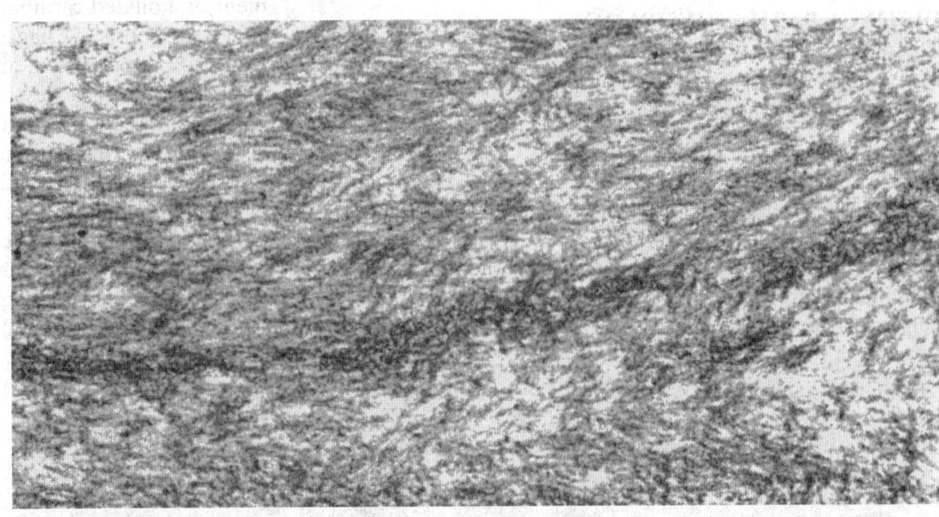

B

FIGURE 66-6 *A.* Right ventricular biopsy demonstrating interstitial amyloid deposition (H&E stain, ×100). *B.* Electron micrograph of the same biopsy specimen illustrating the characteristic 8- to 14-nm, nonbranching, randomly oriented amyloid fibrils.

DISTINCT PATHOPHYSIOLOGY

Although the source and chemical nature of amyloid protein differs among the various types of amyloidosis, the tissue/organ pathophysiology is the same, i.e., the slow destruction of the heart by the inexorable deposition of a β-pleated sheet fibril that is insoluble and impervious to proteolytic digestion.[190]

PROGNOSIS

The prognosis is uniformly bad regardless of the type of amyloidosis, and the majority of patients with amyloid cardiomyopathy are dead within 2 years of diagnosis.

TREATMENT

There is no definitive treatment of amyloid cardiomyopathy. Treatment is completely empirical and consists of diuretics when needed, pacemaker treatment of bradyarrhythmias, and the avoidance of digoxin, which may be arrhythmogenic in any infiltrative cardiomyopathy. There is limited evidence that chemotherapy directed at amyloid secretion by abnormal β-lymphocytes can produce favorable effects in some patients.[194] Cardiac transplantation should be avoided even in primary localized amyloid cardiomyopathy because it will invariably recur in the heart or in other organs. The exception may be familial forms of amyloidosis, where the abnormal protein is a transthyretin or prealbumin variant synthesized in the liver. Combined liver and heart transplantation can be curative in this situation.[195]

Alcohol Cardiomyopathy

DEFINITION/DIAGNOSIS

An *alcohol cardiomyopathy* is said to be present when other causes of a dilated cardiomyopathy have been excluded and there is a history of heavy, sustained alcohol intake. The usual requirement in terms of alcohol amount is 100 g alcohol per day, typically over several years. However, in susceptible individuals it is likely that lower amounts of intake can produce a cardiomyopathy. The histologic features of alcohol cardiomyopathy are nonspecific and do not differ from IDC. Other than history, the only potentially distinguishing feature between IDC and alcohol cardiomyopathy is that the latter may present with a relatively high cardiac output.

DISTINCT PATHOPHYSIOLOGY

The pathophysiology of alcohol cardiomyopathy is thought to be related to the toxic effects of alcohol, plus in some subjects nutritional components such as thiamine deficiency.

PROGNOSIS

The prognosis depends on the degree of impairment of myocardial function and the extent of abstinence from alcohol and, in an extremely compromised patient, the administration of thiamine. There is evidence that the prognosis is somewhat better for alcohol cardiomyopathy than for IDC.[196]

TREATMENT

The treatment of alcohol cardiomyopathy does not differ from IDC, except the inclusion of total abstinence from alcohol. Obviously, these subjects are not good candidates for cardiac transplantation because of the high relapse rate to alcoholism.

Chagas' Cardiomyopathy

DEFINITION/DIAGNOSIS

Chagas' disease is discussed in Chap. 69 as a cause of myocarditis. In addition, Chagas' disease is the most common cause of nonischemic cardiomyopathy in South and Central America, with over 10 million people afflicted.[197] It is caused by a parasite, the leishmanial or tissue form of the protozoan *Trypanosoma cruzi*. Although in the United States the vector (*Triatoma*, or kissing bug) is found only in the Southwest, Chagas' disease may be transmitted by blood transfusions, and as a result, it could become relatively more important in this country. The natural history consists of an initial myocarditis most commonly presenting in childhood, associated with acute myocardial infection followed by recovery and in some individuals the development of a dilated cardiomyopathy 10 to 30 years later.

The diagnosis of Chagas' cardiomyopathy is based on clinical (history, LV functional, and electrocardiographic) criteria and a positive serologic test for *T. cruzi*.[198] Electrocardiographic abnormalities consist of bundle-branch or hemiblocks (indeed, hemiblocks were first described by Rosenbaum et al.[199] in Chagas' afflicted hearts with discrete foci of involvement), LV hypertrophy, and first- or second-degree atrioventricular (AV) block.[200] The histologic lesion of chronic Chagas' consists of mononuclear infiltrates, fibrosis, and as shown in Fig. 66-7, foci of the leishmanial form of *T. cruzi* in myocardial fibers. The LV functional abnormalities initially may be segmental and may include an apical aneurysm but later become more global.[198,200]

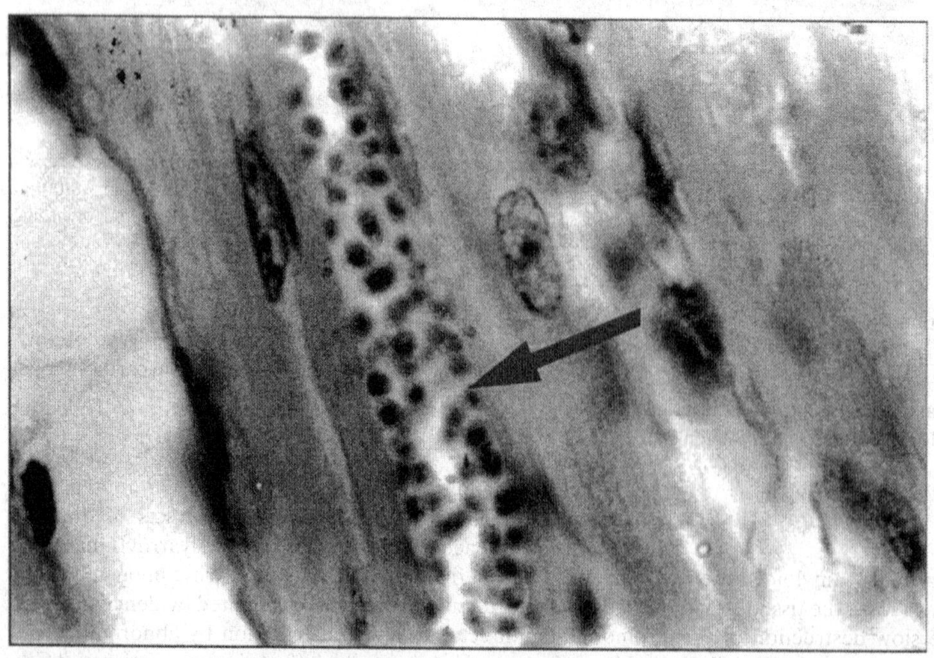

FIGURE 66-7 Leishmanial forms of *T. cruzi* within the swollen cytoplasm of a cardiac myocyte (Chagas' cardiomyopathy) (H&E stain, ×250). (Courtesy Dr. Elmer Koneman.)

DISTINCT PATHOPHYSIOLOGY

The basis for Chagas' cardiomyopathy is unknown but may be immunologic, whereby antibodies generated against *T. cruzi* cross-react with cardiac myocyte antigens including myosin.[201]

PROGNOSIS

The prognosis is relatively good for a dilated cardiomyopathy and similar to IDC; the 5-year survival in Chagas' cardiomyopathy with heart failure is around 50 percent.[198] Compared with IDC, death likely occurs more commonly due to an arrhythmic mechanism.[198] However, as for IDC and most other dilated cardiomyopathies, mortality risk depends directly on the degrees of ventricular dysfunction and exercise intolerance.[198]

TREATMENT

There is no definitive treatment for Chagas' cardiomyopathy, and nonspecific treatment includes pacemaker implantation for heart block and heart failure treatment as for IDC. The one exception may be the more frequent use of amiodarone, which appears to be particularly effective in treating arrhythmias associated with Chagas' cardiomyopathy and in one study reduced mortality compared with standard treatment.[202] The role of cardiac transplantation is still somewhat uncertain, but it can be done at acceptable risk,[203] especially when coupled with trypanocidal agents.[204]

SUMMARY

Dilated cardiomyopathies are important because they are the most common cause of heart failure, which is the single most costly medical problem in the adult U.S. population. Cardiomyopathies in general are a heterogeneous group of diseases, but they can be classified under a newly modified WHO/ISFC classification system, which, although imperfect, should be of great value in standardizing the terminology and encouraging systematic investigative and clinical approaches to diagnosis and treatment. Within this classification system, primary and secondary dilated cardiomyopathies comprise the single largest and most important group. Current diagnosis and treatment of dilated cardiomyopathies vary somewhat among the various types, but the cornerstones of medical management are similar in most cases.

Genetic causes and influences on the natural history of dilated cardiomyopathies are the new frontier in this field, and their elucidation is almost certain to lead to new therapeutic and diagnostic approaches. In the near future, molecular genetic testing will be done routinely for many cardiomyopathies that may have a single gene defect as the cause. As we learn more about the influence of polymorphic genetic variation on the natural history and selection of specific medical therapy, genetic testing will be performed in most patients with cardiomyopathies.

References

1. Ho KKL, Anderson KM, Kannel WB, et al. Survival after the onset of congestive heart failure in Framingham Heart Study subjects. *Circulation* 1993; 88:107–115.
2. O'Connell JB, Bristow MR. Economic impact of heart failure in the United States: Time for a different approach. *J Heart Lung Transplant* 1994; 13:S107–S112.
3. Richardson P, McKenna W, Bristow MR, et al. Report of the 1995 World Health Organization/International Society and Federation of Cardiology Task Force on the definition and classification of cardiomyopathies. *Circulation* 1996; 93:841–842.
4. Guccione AA, Felson DT, Anderson JJ, et al. The effects of specific medical conditions on the functional limitations of elders in the Framingham Study. *Am J Public Health* 1994; 84:351–358.
5. Cohn JN, Johnson GR, Shabetai R, et al, for the V-HeFT VA Cooperative Studies Group. Ejection fraction, peak exercise oxygen consumption, cardiothoracic ratio, ventricular arrhythmias, and plasma norepinephrine as determinants of prognosis in heart failure. *Circulation* 1993; 87(suppl VI):VI-5–VI-16.
6. Eichhorn EJ, Bristow MR. Medical therapy can improve the biologic properties of the chronically failing heart: A new era in the treatment of heart failure. *Circulation* 1996; 94:2285–2296.
7. WHO/ISFC Task Force on Cardiomyopathies. Report of the WHO/ISFC Task Force on the definition and classification of cardiomyopathies. *Br Heart J* 1980; 44:672–673.
8. Bristow MR, Anderson FL, Port JD, et al. Differences in β-adrenergic neuroeffector mechanisms in ischemic vs idiopathic dilated cardiomyopathy. *Circulation* 1991; 84:1024–1039.
9. Packer M, Bristow MR, Cohn JN, et al. Effect of carvedilol on morbidity and mortality in patients with chronic heart failure. *N Engl J Med* 1996; 334:1349–1355.
10. Bristow MR. β-Adrenergic receptor blockade in chronic heart failure. *Circulation* 2000; 101:558–569.
11. Bristow MR. Why does the myocardium fail? New insights from basic science. *Lancet* 1998; 352(suppl):8–14.
12. Geisterfer-Lawrence AA, Kass S, Tanigawa G, et al. A molecular basis for familial hypertrophic cardiomyopathy: A beta-cardiac myosin heavy chain missense mutation. *Cell* 1990; 62:999–1006.
13. Geisterfer-Lawrence AA, Christe M, Conner DA, et al. A mouse model of familial hypertrophic cardiomyopathy. *Science* 1996; 272:731–735.
14. Vikstrom KL, Factor SM, Leinwand LA. Mice expressing mutant myosin heavy chains are a model for familial hypertrophic cardiomyopathy. *Mol Med* 1996; 2:556–567.
15. Tiret L, Rigat B, Visvikis S, et al. Evidence, from combined segregation and linkage analysis, that a variant of the angiotensin I-converting enzyme (ACE) gene controls plasma ACE levels. *Am J Hum Genet* 1992; 51(1):197–205.
16. Raynolds MV, Bristow MR, Bush E, et al. Angiotensin-converting enzyme DD genotype in patients with ischæmic or idiopathic dilated cardiomyopathy. *Lancet* 1993; 342:1073–1075.
17. Jeunemaitre X, Charru A, Rigat B, et al. Sib-pair linkage analysis of renin gene haplotypes in human essential hypertension. *Hum Genet* 1992; 88:301–306.
18. Bonnardeaux A, Davies E, Jeunemaitre X, et al. Angiotensin II type 1 receptor gene polymorphisms in human essential hypertension. *Hypertension* 1994; 24:63–69.
19. Jeunemaitre X, Soubrier F, Kotelevtsev Y, et al. Molecular basis of human hypertension: Role of angiotensinogen. *Cell* 1992; 71:169–180.
20. Robbins, J. Gene targeting and animal models of cardiovascular disease. *Circ Res* 1993; 73:3–9.
21. Edwards JG, Lyons GE, Micales BK, et al. Cardiomyopathy in transgenic *myf*5 mice. *Circ Res* 1996; 78:379–387.
22. Arber S, Hunter JJ, Ross J Jr, et al. MLP-deficient mice exhibit a disruption of cardiac cytoarchitectural organization, dilated cardiomyopathy, and heart failure. *Cell* 1997; 88:393–403.
23. Iwase M, Bishop SP, Uechi M, et al. Adverse effects of chronic endogenous sympathetic drive induced by cardiac $G_{s\alpha}$ overexpression. *Circ Res* 1996; 78:517–524.
24. Iwase M, Uechi M, Vatner DE, et al. Dilated cardiomyopathy induced by cardiac Gs-alpha overexpression (abstract). *Circulation* 1996; 94:I-16.
25. Bisognano JD, Wenberger HD, Bohlmeyer TJ, et al. Myocardial-directed overexpression of the human beta1-adrenergic receptor in transgenic mice. *J Mol Cell Cardiol* 2000; 32:817–830.
26. Engelhardt S, Hein L, Wiesman F, Lohse MJ. Progressive hypertrophy and heart failure in β_1-adrenergic receptor transgenic mice. *Proc Natl Acad Sci USA* 1999; 96:7059–7064.
27. Liggett SB, Tepe NM, Lorenz JN, et al. Early and delayed consequences of β_2-adrenergic receptor overexpression in mouse hearts: Critical role for expression level. *Circulation* 2000; 101:1707–1714.
28. Geng Y-J, Ishikawa Y, Vatner DE, et al. Apoptosis of cardiac myocytes in $G_{s\alpha}$ transgenic mice. *Circ Res* 1999; 84(1):34–42.
29. Hunter JJ, Tanaka N, Rockman HA, et al. Ventricular expression of a MLC-2v-*ras* fusion gene induces cardiac hypertrophy and selective diastolic dysfunction in transgenic mice. *J Biol Chem* 1995; 270:23173–23178.
30. Robbins RJ, Swain JL. C-*myc* protooncogene modulates cardiac

hypertrophic growth in transgenic mice. *Am J Physiol* 1992; 62:H590–H597.

31. Milano CA, Dolber PC, Rockman HA, et al. Myocardial expression of a constitutively active α_{1B}-adrenergic receptor in transgenic mice induces cardiac hypertrophy. *Proc Natl Acad Sci USA* 1994; 91:10109–10113.
32. D'Angelo DD, Sakatra Y, Lorenz JN, et al. Transgenic Gαq overexpression induces cardiac contractile failure in mice. *Proc Natl Acad Sci USA* 1997; 94:8121–8126.
33. Wakasaki H, Koya D, Schoen FJ, et al. Targeted overexpression of protein kinase Cβ2 isoform in myocardium causes cardiomyopathy. *Proc Natl Acad Sci USA* 1997; 94(17):9320–9325.
34. Olson TM, Michels VV, Thibodeau SN, et al. Actin mutation in dilated cardiomyopathy, a heritable form of heart failure. *Science* 1998; 280:750–752.
35. Li D, Tapscoft T, Gonzalez O, et al. Desmin mutation responsible for idiopathic dilated cardiomyopathy. *Circulation* 1999; 100: 461–464.
36. Towbin JA, Hejtmancik F, Brink P, et al. X-linked cardiomyopathy (XLCM): Molecular genetic evidence of linkage to the Duchenne muscular dystrophy (dystrophin) gene at the Xp21 locus. *Circulation* 1993; 87:1854–1865.
37. Muntoni F, Cau M, Ganau A, et al. Deletion of the dystrophin muscle-promoter region associated with X-linked dilated cardiomyopathy. *N Engl J Med* 1993; 329:921–925.
38. Fatkin D. Missense mutations in the rod domain of the lamin A/C gene as causes of dilated cardiomyopathy and conduction system disease. *N Engl J Med* 1999; 341:1715–1724.
39. Brodsky GL, Muntoni F, Miocic S, et al. A lamin a/c gene mutation associated with dilated cardiomyopathy with skeletal muscle involvement. *Circulation* 2000; 101:1394–1399.
40. Lander ES, Schork NJ. Genetic dissection of complex traits. *Science* 1994; 265:2037–2048.
41. Jan Danser AH, Maarten ADH, Schalekamp MD, et al. Angiotensin-converting enzyme in the human heart: Effect of the deletion/insertion polymorphism. *Circulation* 1995; 92:1387–1388.
42. Lechin M, Quinones MA, Omran A, et al. Angiotensin I converting enzyme genotypes and left ventricular hypertrophy in patients with hypertrophic cardiomyopathy. *Circulation* 1995; 92:1808–1812.
43. Pinto YM, van Gilst WH, Kingma JH, Schunkert H, for the Captopril and Thrombolysis Study Investigators. Deletion-type allele of the angiotensin-converting enzyme gene is associated with progressive ventricular dilatation after anterior myocardial infarction. *J Am Coll Cardiol* 1995; 25:1622–1626.
44. Andersson B, Sylven C. The DD genotype of the angiotensin-converting enzyme gene is associated with increased mortality in idiopathic dilated cardiomyopathy. *J Am Coll Cardiol* 1996; 28:162–167.
45. Raynolds MV, Roden RL, Blain-Nelson P, et al. Association of genetic variants in the angiotensin II type 1 receptor and angiotensinogen with end-stage heart muscle disease. *J Am Coll Cardiol* 1996; 27A.
46. Liggett SB, Wagoner LE, Craft LL, et al. The Ile164 β_2-adrenergic receptor polymorphism adversely affects the outcome of congestive heart failure. *J Clin Invest* 1998; 102(8):1534–1539.
47. Lowes BD, Minobe WA, Abraham WT, et al. Changes in gene expression in the intact human heart: downregulation of α-myosin heavy chain in hypertrophied, failing ventricular myocardium. *J Clin Invest* 1997; 100:2315–2324.
48. Miyata S, Minobe WA, Bristow MR, Leinwand LA. Myosin isoform expression in the failing and non-failing human heart. *Circ Res* 2000; 86:386–390.
49. Mercadier JJ, Lompre AM, Duc P, et al. Altered sarcoplasmic reticulum Ca-ATPase gene expression in the human ventricle during end-stage heart failure. *J Clin Invest* 1990; 85:305–309.
50. Feldman AM, Ray PE, Silan CM, et al. Selective gene expression in failing human heart: Quantification of steady-state levels of messenger RNA in endomyocardial biopsies using the polymerase chain reaction. *Circulation* 1991; 83:1866–1872.
51. Studer R, Reinecke H, Muler B, et al. Increased angiotensin I converting enzyme gene expression in the failing human heart: Quantification by competitive RNA polymerase chain reaction. *J Clin Invest* 1994; 94:301–310.
52. Zisman LS, Asano K, Dutcher DL, et al. Differential regulation of cardiac angiotensin converting enzyme binding sites and AT1 receptor density in the failing human heart. *Circulation* 1998; 98:1735–1741.
53. Torre-Amione G, Kapadia S, Lee J, et al. Tumor necrosis factor-α and tumor necrosis factor receptors in the failing human heart. *Circulation* 1996; 93:704–711.
54. Zolk O, Quattek J, Sitzler G, et al. Expression of endothelin-1, endothelin-converting enzyme, and endothelin receptors in chronic heart failure. *Circulation* 1999; 99:2118–2123.
55. Ungerer M, Böhm M, Elce JS, et al. Altered expression of β-adrenergic receptor kinase and β_1-adrenergic receptors in the failing human heart. *Circulation* 1993; 87:454–463.
56. Davies CH, Davia K, Bennett JG, et al. Reduced contraction and altered frequency response of isolated ventricular myocytes from patients with heart failure. *Circulation* 1995; 92:2540–2549.
57. Bristow MR, Gilbert EM. Improvement in cardiac myocyte function by biologic effects of medical therapy: A new concept in the treatment of heart failure. *Eur Heart J* 1995; 16(suppl. F):20–31.
58. Ross J, Braunwald E. Studies on Starling's law of the heart: IX. The effects of impeding venous return on performance of the normal and failing ventricle. *Circulation* 1964; 30:719–727.
59. Schwinger RHG, Böhm M, Koch A, et al. The failing human heart is unable to use the Frank-Starling mechanism. *Circ Res* 1994; 74:959–969.
60. Holubarsch C, Thorsten R, Goldstein DJ, et al. Existence of the Frank-Starling mechanism in the failing human heart: Investigations on the organ, tissue, and sarcomere levels. *Circulation* 1996; 94:683–689.
61. Feldman MD, Gwathmey JK, Phillips P, et al. Reversal of the force-frequency relationship in working myocardium from patients with end-stage heart failure. *J Appl Cardiol* 1988; 3:273–283.
62. Muleiri LA, Hasenfuss G, Leavitt B, et al. Altered myocardial force-frequency relationship in the human heart failure. *Circulation* 1992; 85:1743–1750.
63. Cohn JN. Structural basis for heart failure: Ventricular remodeling and its pharmacological inhibition. *Circulation* 1995; 91:2504–2507.
64. Gerdes AM, Capasso JM. Structural remodeling and mechanical dysfunction of cardiac myocytes in heart failure. *J Mol Cell Cardiol* 1995; 27:849–856.
65. Nadal-Ginard B, Mahdavi V. Molecular basis of cardiac performance. *J Clin Invest* 1989; 84:1693–1700.
66. Hirzel HO, Tuchschmid CR, Schneider J, et al. Relationship between myosin isoenzyme composition, hemodynamics, and myocardial structure in various forms of human cardiac hypertrophy. *Circ Res* 1985; 57:729–740.
67. Anderson PAW, Malouf NN, Oakley A, et al. Troponin T isoform expression in humans: A comparison among normal and failing adult heart, fetal heart, and adult and fetal skeletal muscle. *Circ Res* 1991; 69:1226–1233.
68. Tsutsui H, Ishihara K, Cooper G IV. Cytoskeletal role in the contractile dysfunction of hypertrophied myocardium. *Science* 1993; 260:682–687.
69. Yoshida K, Ikeda S, Nakamura A, et al. Molecular analysis of the Duchenne muscular dystrophy gene in patients with Becker muscular dystrophy presenting with dilated cardiomyopathy. *Muscle Nerve* 1993; 16:1161–1166.
70. Maeda M, Holder E, Lowes B, et al. Dilated cardiomyopathy

associated with deficiency of the cytoskeletal protein metavinculin. *Circulation* 1997; 95(1):17–20.
71. Gerdes AM, Kellerman SE, Moore JA, et al. Structural remodeling of cardiac myocytes from patients with chronic ischemic heart disease. *Circulation* 1992; 86:426-430.
72. Gerdes AM, Kellerman SE, Schocken DD. Implications of cardiomyocyte remodeling in heart dysfunction. In: Dhalla NS, Beamish RE, Takeda N, Nagano N, eds. *The Failing Heart.* New York: Raven Press; 1995:197–205.
73. Gerdes AM, Odera T, Wang X, McCune SA. Myocyte remodeling during progression to failure in rats with hypertension. *Hypertension* 1996; 28(4):609–614.
74. Zhang J, McDonald KM. Bioenergetic consequences of left ventricular remodeling. *Circulation* 1995; 92:1011–1019.
75. Sata M, Sugiura S, Yamashita H, et al. Coupling between myosin ATPase cycle and creatine kinase cycle facilitates cardiac actomyosin sliding in vitro: A clue to mechanical dysfunction during myocardial ischemia. *Circulation* 1996; 93:310–317.
76. Cintron C, Johnson G, Francis G, et al. Prognostic significance of serial changes in left ventricular ejection fraction in patients with congestive heart failure. *Circulation* 1993; 87(suppl VI):VI-17–VI-23.
77. Binkley PF, Nunziata E, Haas GH, et al. Parasympathetic withdrawal is an integral component of autonomic imbalance in congestive heart failure: Demonstration in human subjects and verification in a paced canine model of ventricular failure. *J Am Coll Cardiol* 1991; 18:464–472.
78. Chidiac P, Hebert TE, Valiquette M, et al. Inverse agonist activity of β-adrenergic antagonists. *Mol Pharmacol* 1994; 45:490–499.
79. Mewes T, Dutz S, Ravens U, Jakobs KH. Activation of calcium currents in cardiac myocytes by empty β-adrenoceptors. *Circulation* 1993; 88:2916–2922.
80. Milano CA, Allen LF, Rockman HA, et al. Enhanced myocardial function in transgenic mice overexpressing the β_2-adrenergic receptor. *Science* 1994; 264:562–566.
81. Bond RA, Leff P, Johnson TD, et al. Physiological effects of inverse agonists in transgenic mice with myocardial overexpression of the β_2-adrenoceptor. *Nature* 1995; 374:272–276.
82. Luo W, Grupp IL, Harrer J, et al. Targeted ablation of the phospholamban gene is associated with markedly enhanced myocardial contractility and loss of β-agonist stimulation. *Circ Res* 1994; 75:401–409.
83. Narula J, Haider N, Virmani R, et al. Apoptosis in myocytes in end-stage heart failure. *N Engl J Med* 1996; 335:1182–1189.
84. Teiger E, Than VD, Richard L, et al. Apoptosis in pressure overload-induced heart hypertrophy in the rat. *J Clin Invest* 1996; 97:2891–2897.
85. Cohn JN, Levine TB, Olivari MT, et al. Plasma norepinephrine as a guide to prognosis in patients with chronic congestive heart failure. *N Engl J Med* 1984; 311:819–823.
86. Kaye DM, Lefkovits J, Jennings GL, et al. Adverse consequences of high sympathetic nervous activity in the failing human heart. *J Am Coll Cardiol* 1995; 26:1257–1263.
87. Swedberg K, Eneroth P, Kjekshus J, Wilhelmsen L. Hormones regulating cardiovascular function in patients with severe congestive heart failure and their relation to mortality. *Circulation* 1990; 82:1730–1736.
88. Bristow MR, O'Connell JB. Myocardial diseases. In: Kelley WN, ed. *Textbook of Internal Medicine,* 3d ed. Philadelphia: Lippincott; 1997:398–405.
89. Codd MB, Sugrue DD, Gersh BJ, Melton LJ. Epidemiology of idiopathic dilated and hypertrophic cardiomyopathy: A population based study in Olmstead County, MN, 1975–1984. *Circulation* 1989; 80:564–572.
90. Rakar S, Sinagra G, Di Lenarda A, et al. Epidemiology of dilated cardiomyopathy: A prospective post-mortem study of 5252 necropsies. *Eur Heart J* 1997; 18:117–123.
91. McKay RG, Pfeffer MA, Pasternak RC, et al. Left ventricular remodeling after myocardial infarction: A corollary to infarct expansion. *Circulation* 1986; 74:693–702.
92. Mitchell GF, Lamas GA, Vaughan DE, Pfeffer MA. Left ventricular remodeling in the year after myocardial infarction: A quantitative analysis of contractile segment lengths and ventricular shape. *J Am Coll Cardiol* 1992; 19:1136–1144.
93. Franciosa JA, Willen M, Ziesche S, Cohn JN. Survival in men with severe chronic left ventricular failure due to either coronary heart disease or idiopathic dilated cardiomyopathy. *Am J Cardiol* 1983; 51:831–836.
94. Likoff MJ, Chandler SL, Kay HR. Clinical determinants of mortality in chronic congestive heart failure secondary to idiopathic dilated or to ischemic cardiomyopathy. *Am J Cardiol* 1987; 59(6):634–638.
95. Bristow MR, Gilbert EM, Abraham WT, et al. Carvedilol produces dose-related improvements in left ventricular function and survival in subjects with chronic heart failure. *Circulation* 1996; 94:2807–2816.
96. MERIT-HF Study Group. Effect of metoprolol CR/XL in chronic heart failure: Metoprolol CR/XL Randomized Intervention Trial in Congestive Heart Failure (MERIT-HF). *Lancet* 1999; 353:2001–2006.
97. CIBIS-II Investigators and Committees. The cardiac insufficiency bisoprolol study II (CIBIS-II): A randomised trial. *Lancet* 1999; 353:9–13.
98. Levy D, Larson MG, Vasan RS, et al. The progression from hypertension to congestive heart failure. *JAMA* 1996; 275:1557–1562.
99. Quaife RA, Lynch D, Badesch DB, et al. Right ventricular phenotypic characteristics is subjects with primary pulmonary hypertension or idiopathic dilated cardiomyopathy. *J Cardiac Failure* 1999; 5:46–54.
100. Devereux RB, Roman MJ. Left ventricular hypertrophy in hypertension: Stimuli, patterns, and consequences. *Hypertens Res* 1999; 22(1):1–9.
101. Bristow MR. Mechanisms of development of heart failure in the hypertensive patient. *Cardiology* 1999; 92:3–6.
102. Nielsen I. The natural history of hypertensive heart disease as suggested by echocardiography. *Acta Med Scand Suppl* 1986; 714:165–169.
103. Grossman W. Cardiac hypertrophy: Useful adaptation or pathologic process? *Am J Med* 1980; 69:576–584.
104. Moreno PR, Jang IK, Block PC, Palacios IF. The role of percutaneous balloon valvuloplasty in patients with cardiogenic shock. *J Am Coll Cardiol* 1994; 23:1071–1075.
105. Packer M, O'Conner CM, Ghali JK, et al. Effect of Amlodipine on morbidity and mortality in severe chronic heart failure. *N Engl J Med* 1996; 335:1107–1114.
106. Scognamiglio R, Rahimtoola SH, Fasoli G, et al. Nifedipine in asymptomatic patients with severe aortic regurgitation and normal left ventricular function. *N Engl J Med* 1994; 331(11): 689–694.
107. Grunig E, Tasman JA, Kucherer H, et al. Frequency and phenotypes of familial dilated cardiomyopathy. *J Am Coll Cardiol* 1998; 31:186–194.
108. Baig MK, Goldman JH, Caforio ALP, et al. Familial dilated cardiomyopathy: Cardiac abnormalities are common in asymptomatic relatives and may represent early disease. *J Am Coll Cardiol* 1998; 31:195–201.
109. Krajinovic M, Pinamonti B, Sinagra GF, et al. Linkage of familial idiopathic dilated cardiomyopathy to chromosome 9. *Am J Hum Genet* 1995; 57:846–852.
110. Durand J-B, Bachinski LL, Bieling LC, et al. Localization of a gene responsible for familial dilated cardiomyopathy to chromosome 1q32. *Circulation* 1995; 92:3387–3389.
111. Siu B, Niimura H, Osborne JA, et al. Familial dilated cardio-

myopathy locus maps to chromosome 2q31. *Circulation* 1999; 99:1022–1026.

112. Jung M, Poepping I, Perrot A, et al. Investigation of a family with autosomal dominant dilated cardiomyopathy defines a novel locus on chromosome 2q14-q22. *Am J Hum Genet* 1999; 65:1068–1077.

113. Bowles KL, Gajarski R, Porter P, et al. Gene mapping of familial autosomal dominant dilated cardiomyopathy to chromosome 10q21-23. *J Clin Invest* 1996; 98:1355–1360.

114. Kass S, MacRae C, Graber HL, et al. A gene defect that causes conduction system disease and dilated cardiomyopathy maps to chromosome 1p1-1q1. *Nature Genet* 1994; 7:546–551.

115. Olson TM, Keating MT. Mapping a cardiomyopathy locus to chromosome 3p22-p25. *J Clin Invest* 1996; 97:528–532.

116. D'Adamo P, Fassone L, Gedeon A, et al. The X-linked gene G4.5 is responsible for different infantile dilated cardiomyopathies. *Am J Hum Genet* 1997; 61:862–867.

117. van der Kooi AJ, van Meegen M, Ledderhof TM, et al. Genetic localization of a newly recognized autosomal dominat limb-girdle muscular dystrophy with cardiac involvement (LGMD1B) to chromosome 1q11-21. *Am J Hum Genet* 1997; 60:891–895.

118. Messina DN, Speer MC, Pericak-Vance MA, McNally EM. Linkage of familial dilated cardiomyopathy with conduction defect and muscular dystrophy to chromosome 6q23. *Am J Hum Genet* 1997; 61:909–917.

119. Mestroni L, Rocco C, Gregori D, et al. Familial dilated cardiomyopathy: Evidence for genetic and phenotypic heterogeneity. *J Am Coll Cardiol* 1999; 34:181–190.

120. Ortiz-Lopez R, Li M, Su J, et al. Evidence for a dystrophin missense mutation as a cause of X-linked dilated cardiomyopathy. *Circulation* 1997; 95:2434–2440.

121. Muntoni F, Di Lenarda A, Porcu M, et al. Dystrophin gene abnormalities in two patients with idiopathic dilated cardiomyopathy. *Heart* 1997; 78:608–612.

122. Milasin J, Muntoni F, Severini GM, et al. A point mutation in the 5′ splice site of the dystrophin gene first intron responsible for X-linked dilated cardiomyopathy. *Hum Mol Genet* 1996; 5:73–79.

123. Bies RD, Maeda M, Roberds SL, et al. A 5′ dystrophin duplication mutation causes membrane deficiency of alpha-dystroglyean in a family with X-linked cardiomyopathy. *J Mol Cell Cardiol* 1997; 29 (12):31175–31188.

124. Maeda M, Nakao S, Miyazato H, et al. Cardiac dystrophin abnormalities in Becker muscular dystrophy assessed by endomyocardial biopsy. *Am Heart J* 1995; 129:702–707.

125. Melacini P, Fanin M, Duggan DJ, et al. Heart involvement in muscular dystrophies due to sarcoglycan gene mutations. *Muscle Nerve* 1999; 22:473–479.

126. Nigro V, Okazaki Y, Belsito A, et al. Identification of the Syrian hamster cardiomyopathy gene. *Hum Mol Genet* 1997; 6:601–607.

127. Fatkin D, Christe ME, Aristizabal O, et al. Neonatal cardiomyopathy in mice homozygous for the Arg403Gln mutation in the alpha cardiac myosin heavy chain gene. *J Clin Invest* 1999; 103:147–153.

128. McConnell BK, Jones KA, Fatkin D, et al. Dilated cardiomyopathy in homozygous myosin-binding protein-C mutant mice. *J Clin Invest* 1999; 104:1235–1244.

129. Tiranti V, Jaksch M, Hofmann S, et al. Loss-of-function mutations of SURF-1 are specifically associated with Leigh syndrome with cytochrome c oxidase deficiency. *Ann Neurol* 1999; 46: 161–166.

130. Mestroni L, Maisch B, McKenna WJ, et al. Guidelines for the study of familial dilated cardiomyopathies. *Eur Heart J* 1999; 20:93–102.

131. Crispell KA, Wray A, Ni H, et al. Clinical profiles of four large pedigrees with familial dilated cardiomyopathy: Preliminary recommendations for clinical practice. *J Am Coll Cardiol* 1999; 34:837–847.

132. Silver MA. Anatomy of the failing heart in dilated cardiomyopathy. In: Engelmeier RS, O'Connell JB, eds. *Drug Therapy in Dilated Cardiomyopathy and Myocarditis*. New York: Marcel Dekker; 1988:1–12.

133. Roberts WC, Siegel RJ, McManus BM. Idiopathic dilated cardiomyopathy: Analysis of 152 necropsy patients. *Am J Cardiol* 1987; 60:1340–1355.

134. Falk RH, Foster E, Coats MH. Ventricular thrombi and thromboembolism in dilated cardiomyopathy: A prospective follow-up. *Am Heart J* 1992; 123:136–142.

135. Rowan R, Maesk MA, Billingham ME. Ultrastructural morphometric analysis of endomyocardial biopsies. *Am J Cardiovasc Pathol* 1988; 2:137–144.

136. Baandrup U, Olsen EG. Critical analysis of endomyocardial biopsies from patients suspected of having cardiomyopathy. *Br Heart J* 1981; 45:475–486.

137. Arbustini E, Pucci R, Pozzi R, et al. Ultrastructural changes in myocarditis and dilated cardiomyopathy. In: Baroldi G, Camerini F, Goodwin JF, eds. *Advances in Cardiomyopathies*. Berlin: Springer-Verlag; 1990:274–289.

138. Schwarz F, Mall G, Zebe H, et al. Determinants of survival in patients with congestive cardiomyopathy: Quantitative morphologic findings and left ventricular hemodynamics. *Circulation* 1984; 70:923–928.

139. Tazelaar HD, Billingham ME. Leukocytic infiltrates in idiopathic dilated cardiomyopathy. *Am J Surg Pathol* 1986; 10:405–412.

140. Hammond EH, Anderson JL, Menlove RL. Diagnostic and prognostic value of immunofluorescence and electron-microscopic findings in idiopathic dilated cardiomyopathy. In: Bavoldi G, Camerini F, Goodwin JF, eds. *Advances in Cardiomyopathies*, 1st ed. Berlin: Springer-Verlag; 1990:290–301.

141. Kawai C, Takatsu T. Clinical and experimental studies on cardiomyopathy. *N Engl J Med* 1975; 293:592–597.

142. Anderson JL, Carlquist JF, Hammond EH. Deficient natural killer cell activity in patients with idiopathic dilated cardiomyopathy. *Lancet* 1982; 2:1124–1127.

143. Fowles RE, Bieker CP, Stinson EB. Defective in vitro suppressor cell function in idiopathic congestive cardiomyopathy. *Circulation* 1979; 59:483–491.

144. Gerli R, Rambotti P, Spinozzi F, et al. Immunologic studies of peripheral blood from patients with idiopathic dilated cardiomyopathy. *Am Heart J* 1986; 112:350–355.

145. Klein R, Maisch B, Kochsiek K, Berg PA. Demonstration of organ specific antibodies against heart mitochondria (anti-M) in sera from patients with some forms of heart disease. *Clin Exp Immunol* 1984; 58:283–292.

146. Maisch B, Deeg P, Liebau G, Kichsiek K. Diagnostic relevance of humoral and cytotoxic immune reactions in primary and secondary dilated cardiomyopathy. *Am J Cardiol* 1983; 52:1071–1078.

147. Limas CJ, Goldenberg IF, Limas C. Autoantibodies against β-adrenoreceptors in human idiopathic dilated cardiomyopathy. *Circ Res* 1989; 64:97–103.

148. Magnusson Y, Marullo S, Hoyer S, et al. Mapping of a functional autoimmune epitope on the β_1-adrenergic receptor in patients with idiopathic dilated cardiomyopathy. *J Clin Invest* 1990; 86:1658–1663.

149. Magnusson Y, Wallukat G, Waagstein F, et al. Autoimmunity in idiopathic dilatated cardiomyopathy: Characterization of antibodies against the β_1-adrenoceptor with a positive chronotropic effect. *Circulation* 1994; 89:2760–2767.

150. Schultheiss H-P, Bolte HD. Immunological analysis of autoantibodies against the adenine nucleotide translocator in dilated cardiomyopathy. *J Mol Cell Cardiol* 1985; 17:603–617.

151. Schultheiss H-P. Disturbance of the myocardial energy metabolism in dilated cardiomyopathy due to autoimmunological mechanisms. *Circulation* 1993; 87(suppl IV):IV-43–IV-48.

152. Anderson JL, Carlquist JF, Lutz JR, et al. HLA A, B, and DR

typing in idiopathic dilated cardiomyopathy: A search for immune response function. *Am J Cardiol* 1984; 33:1326–1330.
153. Gilbert EM, Mason JW. Immunosuppressive therapy of myocarditis. In: Engelmeier RS, O'Connell JB, eds. *Drug Therapy in Dilated Cardiomyopathy and Myocarditis*. New York: Marcel Dekker; 1987:233–263.
154. Archard LC, Freeke CA, Richardson PJ, Olsen EGJ. Persistence of enterovirus RNA in dilated cardiomyopathy: A progression from myocarditis. In: Shultheiss H-P, ed. *New Concepts in Viral Heart Disease*. Berlin: Springer-Verlag; 1989:347–359.
155. Giacca M, Severini GM, Mestroni L, et al. Low frequency of detection by nested polymerase chain reaction of enterovirus ribonucleic acid in endomyocardial tissue of patients with idiopathic dilated cardiomyopathy. *J Am Coll Cardiol* 1994; 24:1033–1040.
156. Bowles NE, Richardson PJ, Olsen ECJ, Archard LC. Detection of Coxsackie-B virus specific RNA sequences in myocardial biopsy samples from patients with myocarditis and dilated cardiomyopathy. *Lancet* 1986; 1:1120–1128.
157. Parrillo JE, Cunnion RE, Epstein SE, et al. A prospective, randomized, controlled trial of prednisone for dilated cardiomyopathy. *N Engl J Med* 1989; 321:1061–1067.
158. Badorff C, Lee GH, Lamphear BJ, et al. Enteroviral protease 2A cleaves dystrophin: Evidence of cytoskeletal disruption in an acquired cardiomyopathy. *Nature Med* 1999; 5:320–326.
159. Pauschinger M, Doerner A, Kuehl U, et al. Enteroviral RNA replication in the myocardium of patients with left ventricular dysfunction and clinically suspected myocarditis. *Circulation* 1999; 99(7):889–895.
160. Martin AB, Webber S, Fricker FJ, et al. Acute myocarditis: Rapid diagnosis by PCR in children. *Circulation* 1994; 90(1):330–339.
161. Fuster V, Gersh BJ, Giuliani ER, et al. The natural history of idiopathic dilated cardiomyopathy. *Am J Cardiol* 1981; 47: 525–531.
162. Redfield MM, Gersh BJ, Bailey KR, et al. Natural history of idiopathic dilated cardiomyopathy: Effect of referral bias and secular trend. *J Am Coll Cardiol* 1993; 22:1921–1926.
163. The SOLVD Investigators. Effect of angiotensin converting enzyme inhibition with enalapril on survival in patients with reduced left ventricular ejection fraction and congestive heart failure: Results of the Treatment Trial of the Studies of Left Ventricular Dysfunction (SOLVD), a randomized double blind trial. *N Engl J Med* 1991; 325:293–302.
164. Hosenpud JD, Novick RJ, Bennett LE, et al. The Registry of the International Society for Heart and Lung Transplantation: Thirteenth official report (1996). *J Heart Lung Transplant* 1996; 15:655–674.
165. Woodley SL, Gilbert EM, Anderson JL, et al. β-Blockade with bucindolol in heart failure due to ischemic vs idiopathic dilated cardiomyopathy. *Circulation* 1991; 84:2426–2441.
166. Bristow MR, Colucci WS, Fowler MB, et al. Effect of carvedilol on survival and hospitalization in patients with ischemic or nonischemic cardiomyopathy (abstract). *Circulation* 1996; 94:I-338.
167. Waagstein F, Bristow MR, Swedberg K, et al. Beneficial effects of metoprolol in idiopathic dilated cardiomyopathy. *Lancet* 1993; 342:1441–1446.
168. Bristow MR, Mason JW, Billingham ME, Daniels JR. Doxorubicin cardiomyopathy: Evaluation by phonocardiography, endomyocardial biopsy, and cardiac catheterization. *Ann Intern Med* 1978; 88:168–175.
169. Von Hoff DD, Layard MW, Basa P, et al. Risk factors for doxorubicin-induced congestive heart failure. *Ann Intern Med* 1979; 91:710–717.
170. Bristow MR, Mason JW, Billingham ME, Daniels JR. Dose-effect and structure function relationships in doxorubicin cardiomyopathy. *Am Heart J* 1981; 102:709–718.
171. Bristow MR, Billingham ME, Mason JW, Daniels JR. The clinical spectrum of anthracycline antibiotic cardiotoxicity. *Cancer Treat Rep* 1978; 62:873–879.
172. Billingham ME, Bristow MR, Glatstein J, et al. Adriamycin cardiotoxicity: Endomyocardial biopsy evidence of enhancement by irradiation. *Am J Surg Pathol* 1977; 1:17–23.
173. Kantrowitz NE, Bristow MR. Cardiotoxicity of antitumor agents. *Prog Cardiovasc Dis* 1984; 27:195–200.
174. Lewis W, Kleinerman J, Puszkin S. Interaction of adriamycin in vitro with myofibrillar proteins. *Circ Res* 1982; 50:547–553.
175. Jaenke RS. Delayed and progressive myocardial lesions after Adriamycin administration in rabbits. *Cancer Res* 1976; 36:2958–2966.
176. Eiswirth CC, Bowden RE, Kazamias T, et al. Treatment of Adriamycin cardiomyopathy with metoprolol. *Circulation* 1986; 74(supp II):1236.
177. Shaddy RE, Olsen SL, Bristow MR, et al. Efficacy and safety of metoprolol in the treatment of doxorubicin-induced cardiomyopathy in pediatric patients. *Am Heart J* 1995; 129:197–199.
178. Bristow MR, Lopez MB, Mason JW, et al. Efficacy and cost of cardiac monitoring in patients receiving doxorubicin. *Cancer* 1982; 50(1):32–41.
179. McKillop JH, Bristow MR, Goris ML, et al. Sensitivity and specificity of radionuclide ejection fractions in doxorubicin cardiotoxicity. *Am Heart J* 1983; 105:1048–1056.
180. Alexander J, Dainiak N, Berger HJ, et al. Serial assessment of doxorubicin cardiotoxicity with quantitative radionuclide angiocardiography. *N Engl J Med* 1979; 300:278–283.
181. Torti FM, Bristow MR, Howes AE, et al. Endomyocardial biopsy evidence of reduced cardiotoxicity of doxorubicin delivered on a weekly schedule. *Ann Intern Med* 1983; 99:745–749.
182. Legha SS, Benjamin RS, Mackay B, et al. Reduction of doxorubicin cardiotoxicity by prolonged continuous intravenous infusion. *Ann Intern Med* 1982; 96:133–139.
183. Rahman A, More N, Schein PS. Doxorubicin-induced chronic cardiotoxicity and its prevention by liposomal administration. *Cancer Res* 1982; 42:1817–1825.
184. Speyer JL, Green MD, Kramer E, et al. Protective effect of the bispiperazinedione ICRF-187 against doxorubicin-induced cardiac toxicity in women with advanced breast cancer. *N Engl J Med* 1988; 319(12):745–752.
185. Julian DG, Szekely P. Peripartum cardiomyopathy. *Prog Cardiovasc Dis* 1985; 27:223–240.
186. Midei MG, DeMent SH, Feldman AM, et al. Peripartum myocarditis and cardiomyopathy. *Circulation* 1990; 81:922–928.
187. O'Connell JB, Costanzo-Nordin MR, Subramanian R, et al. Peripartum cardiomyopathy: Clinical, hemodynamic histologic and prognostic characteristics. *J Am Coll Cardiol* 1986; 8:52–56.
188. Jacobson DR, Busbaum JN. Genetic aspects of amyloidosis. *Adv Hum Genet* 1991; 20:69–75.
189. Kyle RA, Griepp PR. Amyloidosis (AL): Clinical and laboratory feature in 229 cases. *Mayo Clin Proc* 1983; 58:665–672.
190. Glenner GG. Amyloid deposits and amyloidosis. *N Engl J Med* 1980; 302:1283–1292.
191. Hamer JP, Janssen S, van Rijswik MH, Lie KI. Amyloid cardiomyopathy in systemic non-hereditary amyloidosis: Clinical, echocardiographic and electrocardiographic findings in 30 patients with AA and 24 patients with AL amyloidosis. *Eur Heart J* 1992; 13:623–627.
192. Stone MJ. Amyloidosis: A final common pathway for protein deposition in tissues. *Blood* 1990; 75:531–545.
193. Schroeder JS, Billingham ME, Rider AK. Cardiac amyloidosis: Diagnosis by transvenous endomyocardial biopsy. *Am J Med* 1975; 59:269–273.
194. Kyle RA, Gertz MA, Greipp PR, et al. A trial of three regimens for primary amyloidosis: Colchicine alone, melphalan and prednisone, and melphalan, prednisone, and colchicine. *N Engl J Med* 1997:336(17)1202–1207.

195. Holmgren G, Ericzon B-G, Groth C-G. Clinical improvement and amyloid regression after liver transplantation in hereditary transthyretin amyloidosis. *Lancet* 1993; 341:1113–1116.
196. Prazak P, Pfisterer M, Osswald S, et al. Differences of disease progression in congestive heart failure due to alcoholic as compared to idiopathic dilated cardiomyopathy. *Eur Heart J* 1996; 17(2):251–257.
197. World Health Organization Expert Committee Chagas' disease. *World Health Organ Tech Rep Ser* 1984; 697:50–55.
198. Mady C, Cardoso RHA, Barretto ACP, et al. Survival and predictors of survival in patients with congestive heart failure due to Chagas' cardiomyopathy. *Circulation* 1994; 90:3098–3102.
199. Rosenbaum MB. The hemiblocks: Diagnostic criteria and clinical significance. *Mod Concepts Cardiovasc Dis* 1970; 39:141–146.
200. Laranja FS, Dias E, Nobrega G, Miranda A. Chagas' disease: A clinical, epidemiological, and pathological study. *Circulation* 1956; 14:1035–1060.
201. Tibbetts RS, McCormick TS, Rowland EC, et al. Cardiac antigen-specific autoantibody production is associated with cardiomyopathy in *Trypanosoma cruzi*-infected mice. *J Immunol* 1994; 152(3):1493–1499.
202. Nul DR, Grancelli HO, Perrone SV, et al. Randomised trial of low-dose amiodarone in severe congestive heart failure. *Lancet* 1994; 344:493–498.
203. Bocchi EA, Bellotti G, Mocelin AO, et al. Heart Transplantation for chronic Chagas' heart disease. *Ann Thorac Surg* 1996; 61:1727–1733.
204. Blanche C, Aleksic I, Takkenberg JJM, et al. Heart transplantation for Chagas' cardiomyopathy. *Ann Thorac Surg* 1995; 60:1406–1409.

CHAPTER 67

HYPERTROPHIC CARDIOMYOPATHY

Barry J. Maron

Hypertrophic cardiomyopathy (HCM) is a genetically transmitted primary cardiac disease that has been of great interest to clinicians and laboratory scientists because of its particularly diverse clinical, morphologic, pathophysiologic, and molecular genetic manifestations.[1–22] Because of the broad and heterogeneous HCM disease spectrum as well as the relatively low prevalence in cardiologic practice, a measure of confusion and uncertainty has persisted regarding this condition.

HISTORICAL CONSIDERATIONS

There is some uncertainty regarding the first gross anatomic description of HCM. About 1900, French and German authors reported four patients at autopsy in whom striking hypertrophy involving the ventricular septum appeared to be responsible for obstruction to left ventricular ejection.[23,24] The first unequivocal description of HCM was the detailed pathologic report of Teare,[25] which stimulated widespread interest in this disease among cardiologists, pathologists, and surgeons. Teare described a condition in eight patients (seven of whom died suddenly) characterized by an asymmetric pattern of left ventricular wall thickening and nondilated ventricular cavities. The striking ventricular septal hypertrophy and bizarre arrangement of muscle bundles observed in these patients was initially thought to represent a benign tumor of the heart.

NOMENCLATURE AND PREVALENCE

Over the past 40 years, numerous studies have led to a dramatic evolution of our concepts concerning the clinical and pathologic spectrum of HCM; in the process, the disease has acquired a myriad of names[7] (Fig. 67-1). This multiplicity of descriptive terms largely reflects the enormous clinical, functional, and morphologic diversity of this disease. However, many of the terms that have been used to describe HCM are somewhat misleading by emphasizing the presence of left ventricular outflow obstruction at rest, a clinical feature that occurs in only a minority of HCM patients (about 20 to 25 percent).[1,3,5] The prevalence of HCM appears to be about 0.2 percent in the general population[26] and 1 percent in primary medical practice[27] based on identification of the disease phenotype with two-dimensional (2D) echocardiography. It is possible, however, that many individuals with HCM go undetected in the community because they manifest no or only mild symptoms and are not referred for echocardiographic studies.[28–31] Reports from a large number of diverse geographic areas suggest that HCM has extensive if not worldwide occurrence; there is also some evidence that the morphologic expression of the disease may differ in certain ethnic or racial groups (such as Japanese).[32–34]

DEFINITION AND CRITERIA FOR DIAGNOSIS

The clinical diagnosis of HCM is based on definition of the most characteristic morphologic feature of the disease—i.e., thickening of the left ventricular wall associated with a nondilated cavity in the absence of another cardiac or systemic disease capable of producing the magnitude of hypertrophy evident (e.g., systemic hypertension or aortic stenosis)[7] (Fig. 67-2). Because the nonobstructive form of HCM is predominant, the well-described clinical features of dynamic obstruction to left

Asymmetrical hypertrophic cardiomyopathy
Asymmetrical hypertrophy of the heart
Asymmetrical septal hypertrophy
Brock's disease
Diffuse muscular subaortic stenosis
Diffuse subvalvular aortic stenosis
Dynamic hypertrophic subaortic stenosis
Dynamic muscular subaortic stenosis
Familial hypertrophic cardiomyopathy
Familial hypertrophic subaortic stenosis
Familial muscular subaortic stenosis
Familial myocardial disease
Functional aortic stenosis
Functional hypertrophic subaortic stenosis
Functional obstructive cardiomyopathy
Functional obstruction of the left ventricle
Functional obstructive subvalvular aortic stenosis
Functional subaortic stenosis
Hereditary cardiovascular dysplasia
HYPERTROPHIC CARDIOMYOPATHY
Hypertrophic constrictive cardiomyopathy
Hypertrophic hyperkinetic cardiomyopathy
Hypertrophic infundibular aortic stenosis
Hypertrophic nonobstructive cardiomyopathy
Hypertrophic obstructive cardiomyopathy
Hypertrophic stenosing cardiomyopathy
Hypertrophic subaortic stenosis
Idiopathic hypertrophic cardiomyopathy
Idiopathic hypertrophic obstructive cardiomyopathy
Idiopathic hypertrophic subaortic stenosis
Idiopathic hypertrophic subvalvular stenosis
Idiopathic muscular hypertrophic subaortic stenosis
Idiopathic muscular stenosis of the left ventricle
Idiopathic myocardial hypertrophy
Idiopathic stenosis of the flushing chamber of the left ventricle
Idiopathic ventricular septal hypertrophy
Irregular hypertrophic cardiomyopathy
Left ventrical muscular stenosis
Low subvalvular aortic stenosis
Muscular aortic stenosis
Muscular hypertrophic stenosis of the left ventricle
Muscular stenosis of the left ventricle
Muscular subaortic stenosis
Muscular subvalvular aortic stenosis
Non-dilated cardiomyopathy
Nonobstructive hypertrophic cardiomyopathy
Obstructive cardiomyopathy
Obstructive hypertrophic aortic stenosis
Obstructive hypertrophic cardiomyopathy
Obstructive hypertrophic myocardiopathy
Obstructive myocardiopathy
Pseudoaortic stenosis
Stenosing hypertrophy of the left ventricle
Stenosis of the ejection chamber of the left ventricle
Subaortic hypertrophic stenosis
Subaortic idiopathic stenosis
Subaortic muscular stenosis
Subvalvular aortic stenosis of the muscular type
Teare's disease

FIGURE 67-1 The multitude of terms used to describe HCM.

ventricular outflow—such as systolic anterior motion of the mitral valve, partial premature closure of the aortic valve, and a loud systolic ejection murmur—are not required for diagnosis.[1] Also, not all individuals harboring a genetic abnormality capable of producing the clinical and morphologic abnormalities of HCM show left ventricular hypertrophy at all phases of life.[10,22,31,35–37] For example, some children with HCM will not have left ventricular wall thickening identifiable by 2D echocardiogram prior to about age 16[35] and a few adults with incomplete penetrance may also show little or no hypertrophy.[10,36,38–40]

MORPHOLOGIC CHARACTERISTICS

Gross Features

Left ventricular hypertrophy is the gross anatomic marker of HCM and the likely determinant of many of the clinical features identifiable in most patients with this disease[1–7,16–18] (Figs. 67-3 and 67-4). Since the left ventricular cavity is usually small or normal in size, the increased left ventricular mass is due almost entirely to an increase in wall thickness. Although a symmetric (concentric) pattern of left ventricular hypertrophy can be observed,[12,18,41] the distribution of hypertrophy is almost always asymmetric; i.e., with segments of the left ventricular wall thickened to a dissimilar degree, and with the ventricular septum showing disproportionate magnitude of hypertrophy.[12,18] Examination of the heart at necropsy also typically shows dilatation of the atria, enlargement and elongation of the mitral valve leaflets, and areas of replacement fibrosis (scarring) in the left ventricular wall.[16,17,20,42,43] In addition, most hearts show a characteristic fibrous plaque on the mural endocardium of the left ventricular outflow tract in apposition to the thickened anterior mitral leaflet, presumably resulting from systolic (or diastolic) contact between mitral valve and septum[16] (Fig. 67-3).

Based on both echocardiographic and necropsy analyses of large numbers of patients, it is apparent that the HCM disease spectrum is characterized by vast structural diversity with regard to the patterns and extent of left ventricular hypertrophy [12,18,41,43] (Figs. 67-5 and 67-6). Indeed, no single phenotypic expression can be considered "classic" or particularly typical of this disease. While maximal thickness of the left ventricular wall varies greatly, the average value in a population is usually 21 to 22 mm. Wall thickness is markedly increased in many patients, with some showing the most severe hypertrophy observed in any cardiac disease (60 mm is the most extreme dimension).[44,45] On the other hand, the HCM phenotype is not always expressed as a particularly thickened left ventricle;

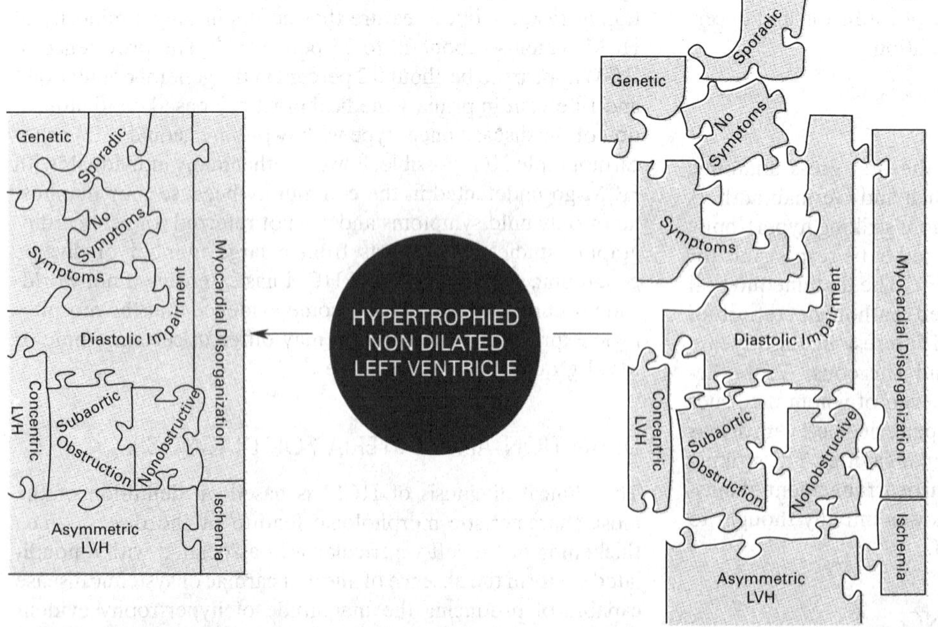

FIGURE 67-2 Diagrammatic representation of the basic morphologic definition of HCM (*dark circle*) as it unifies the clinical and morphologic diversity characteristic of the disease spectrum.

some patients may show only a mild increase of 15 to 18 mm, and a few genotyped affected individuals have been observed with normal thicknesses (≤12 mm).[10,36,40,46] Often the pattern of wall thickening is strikingly heterogeneous, involving noncontiguous segments of left ventricle (i.e., with areas of normal thickness evident in between), or with marked differences in wall thickness in adjacent segments of the wall. Transitions between thickened areas and regions of normal thickness are often sharp and abrupt, not infrequently creating right-angled contours of the wall.

In most patients the pattern of hypertrophy is diffuse, involving both septum and substantial portions of the lateral free wall, while the posterior segment of free wall is usually least affected by the hypertrophic process.[12,18] In others, hypertrophy involves only the ventricular septum while sparing the free wall. Of note, in an important proportion of patients (about one-third), wall thickening may be relatively mild and confined to a single segment of left ventricle.[12,13,18] Such segmental hypertrophy is usually localized to the anterior septum but may also be limited to the posterior septum,[12,18] anterolateral free wall,[12,18] posterior free wall,[47] or even the most apical portion of the left ventricle.[14,15,32,48–50] Therefore, the ventricular septum is usually, but not always, prominently involved in the hypertrophic process. Infiltrative and myocardial storage diseases such as cardiac amyloid and Fabry's disease may occasionally mimic HCM morphologically (Chap. 10).

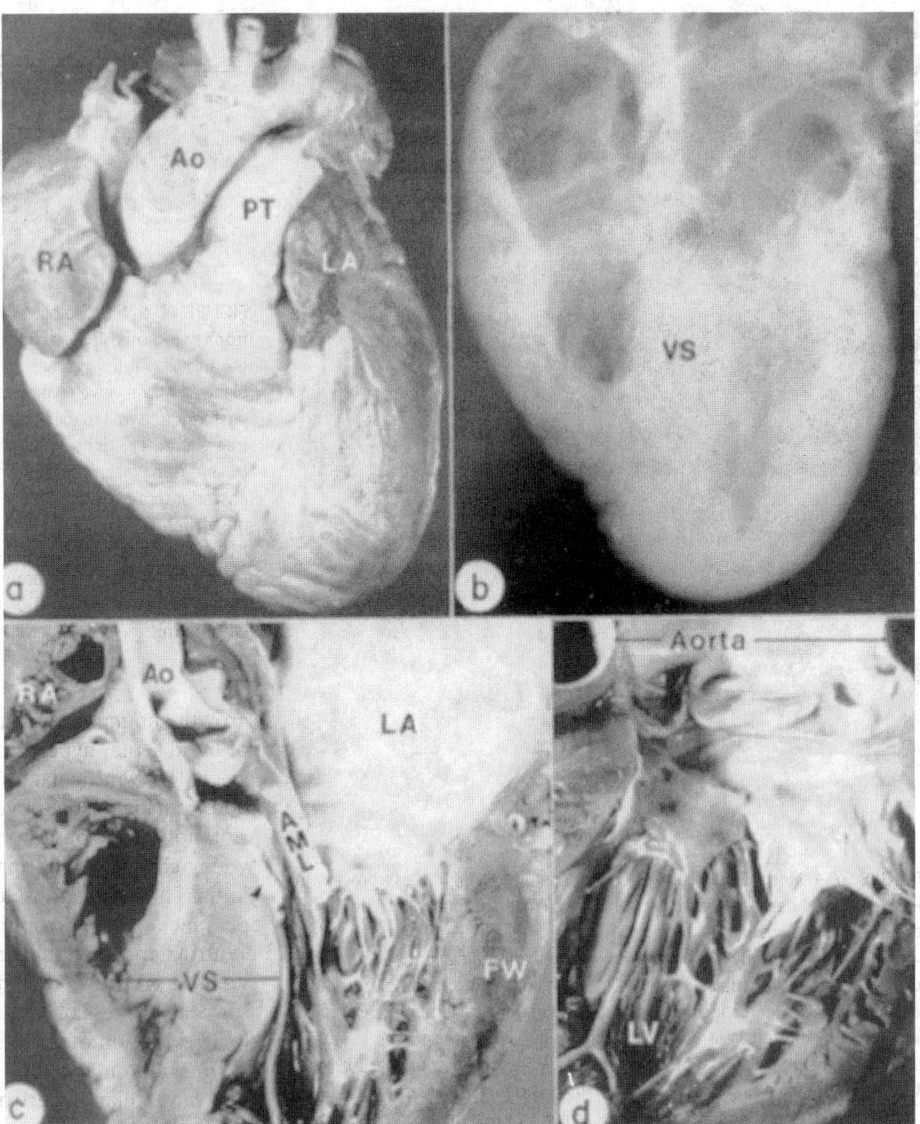

FIGURE 67-3 Anatomic features of HCM are demonstrated in the heart of a 26-year-old man. *A.* Exterior view; both right atrium (RA) and left atrium (LA) are dilated. Ao = aorta; PT = pulmonary trunk. *B.* Radiography of specimen showing asymmetric thickening of ventricular septum (VS). *C.* Coronal section; the septum is clearly thicker than left ventricular free wall (F); an endocardial mural contact plaque (*arrowhead*) is present in the left ventricular outflow tract in apposition to the anterior mitral leaflet (AML). *D.* Closer view of plaque and thickened anterior leaflet. (From Roberts WC et al.[16] with permission from the authors and publisher.)

Hypertrophy confined to the left ventricular apex ("apical HCM") has been reported most commonly by Japanese investigators,[32,34,49] who have described this subgroup of HCM patients to be clinically benign and with a "spade" deformity of the left ventricular cavity on angiography and a distinctive electrocardiographic (ECG) pattern of deep ("giant") T-wave inversion. Reports from outside Asia would suggest, however, that apical hypertrophy is uncommonly accompanied by marked T-wave inversion and associated with adverse outcome in some patients.[14,15,48,50] This heterogeneous morphologic expression described for HCM is underlined by the fact that even first-degree relatives with the disease usually show great dissimilarity in the pattern of left ventricular wall thickening.[11]

In some young athletes, segmental hypertrophy of the anterior ventricular septum (wall thicknesses of 13 to 15 mm), consistent with a relatively mild morphologic expression of HCM, may often be difficult to distinguish from the physiologic left ventricular hypertrophy that can represent an adaptation to intense forms of athletic training.[51,52] In asymptomatic individuals within this morphologic "gray zone," the differential diagnosis between athlete's heart and nonobstructive HCM can often be resolved by clinical assessment and noninvasive testing[52] (Fig. 67-7).

HCM can represent a congenital heart malformation in which phenotypic expression in the form of left ventricular wall thickening begins during fetal development[53] and is evident at or shortly after birth.[54–56] Indeed, HCM has been reported in a small number of very young children, including a few infants under 6 months of age.[54–56] When HCM presents in infancy, the

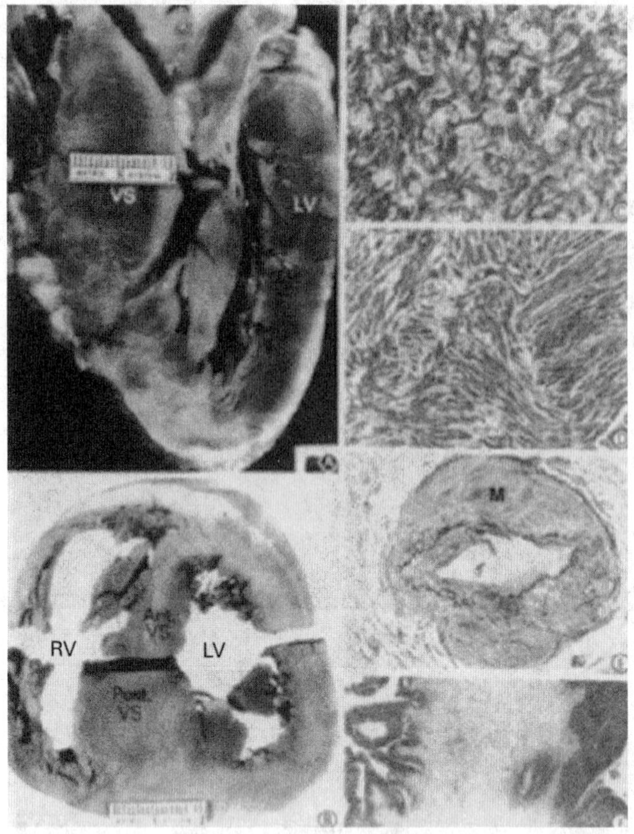

FIGURE 67-4 Morphologic components of the underlying disease process in HCM. *A.* Gross heart specimen sectioned in a cross-sectional plane similar to that of the echocardiographic (parasternal) long axis. The pattern of left ventricular hypertrophy is asymmetric, with wall thickening confined primarily to the anterior ventricular septum (VS), which bulges into the left ventricular outflow tract. *B.* Heart specimen illustrating a different pattern of hypertrophy, in which marked left ventricular wall thickening is localized to the posterior portion of the ventricular septum (Post. VS), while the anterior septum (Ant. VS) is only mildly thickened. *C* and *D.* Histopathology characteristic of the left ventricle in HCM. *C.* Septal myocardium shows markedly disordered architecture, with adjacent hypertrophied cardiac muscle cells arranged at perpendicular and oblique angles to each other. *D.* Bundles of hypertrophied cells show a disorganized, "interwoven" arrangement. *E.* Intramural coronary artery with apparently narrowed lumen and thickened wall due primarily to medial (M) hypertrophy. *F.* Extensive scarring of ventricular septum, which is transmural in distribution. LV = left ventricular free wall. (From Maron BJ et al.[3] with permission from the authors and publisher.)

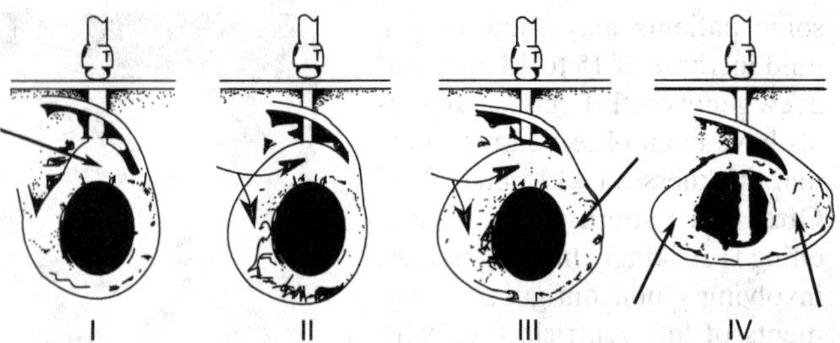

FIGURE 67-5 Morphologic variability in HCM, based on observations made from two-dimensional echocardiography; areas of hypertrophy are indicated by arrows. All images are drawn in the standard short-axis cross-sectional plane at mitral valve level with anterior chest wall and transducer to the top, posterior free wall to the bottom, posterior septum to the left, and anterolateral free wall to the right. *I.* Relatively mild left ventricular hypertrophy confined to anterior portion of ventricular septum. *II.* Hypertrophy of anterior and posterior septum in the absence of free wall thickening. *III.* Diffuse hypertrophy of substantial portions of both ventricular septum and anterolateral free wall. *IV.* Included are more unusual patterns of hypertrophy in which the thickened portions of left ventricle are present in the posterior septum or anterolateral free wall (as shown here) or at the left ventricular apex. (From Maron BJ[12] with permission from the author and publisher.)

disease is usually associated with marked septal hypertrophy as well as severe progressive congestive heart failure and biventricular outflow obstruction.[54,55,57] However, most cases of idiopathic left ventricular hypertrophy presenting in the first 2 years are not true HCM due to sarcomere protein mutations, but are often associated with other conditions such as Noonan syndrome.[57]

Later in childhood, serial echocardiographic investigations have shown prominent left ventricular remodeling. The morphologic expression of HCM is not usually complete until adulthood,[35,58] and during adolescence children often show striking spontaneous increases in wall thicknesses (i.e., of about 100 percent) and more widespread distribution of hypertrophy, including de novo development of wall thickening, when body growth and maturation are accelerated (Fig. 67-8). Progression of basal septal hypertrophy associated with a developmentally small left ventricular outflow tract appears to be the major determinant for the development of mitral valve systolic anterior motion and outflow obstruction during childhood.[59] In some young children, abnormalities on the 12-lead ECG may be the initial clinical manifestation of HCM, even preceding the appearance of hypertrophy on the echocardiogram.[31,60] Such left ventricular remodeling is usually not associated with development or progression of symptoms or sudden death and appears to be an expression of the genetically predetermined morphologic evolution of the disease.[35,61]

In symptomatic adult patients with HCM, the magnitude of left ventricular hypertrophy may *decrease* with aging.[62] Very marked degrees of hypertrophy (e.g., maximum wall thickness ≥30 mm) are largely limited to patients under age 40, while older patients over age 60 generally have more modest hypertrophy and rarely show wall thicknesses >25 mm. The explanation for this inverse relation between age and magnitude of hypertrophy could be a higher rate of premature death in younger patients with severe morphologic forms or, alternatively, to a process of wall thinning and remodeling occurring very gradually over long periods of time in many patients.[61]

Histologic Features

Several histologic features of left ventricular myocardium represent components of the primary cardiomyopathic disease process in HCM[1,3,42,63–73]: (1) disarray of cardiac muscle cells (myocytes) (Fig. 67-4*C* and *D*); (2) replacement fibrosis (Fig. 67-4*F*); (3) expansion of the interstitial (matrix) collagen compartment; and (4) abnormally small intramural coronary arteries (Fig. 67-4*E*). Marked distortion of cellular architecture with myocyte disarray, described prominently by Teare in his initial report of HCM,[25] is a characteristic feature of the left ventricle.[64–68,71] Many cardiac muscle cells in both the ventricular septum and left ventricular free wall show increased transverse diameter and

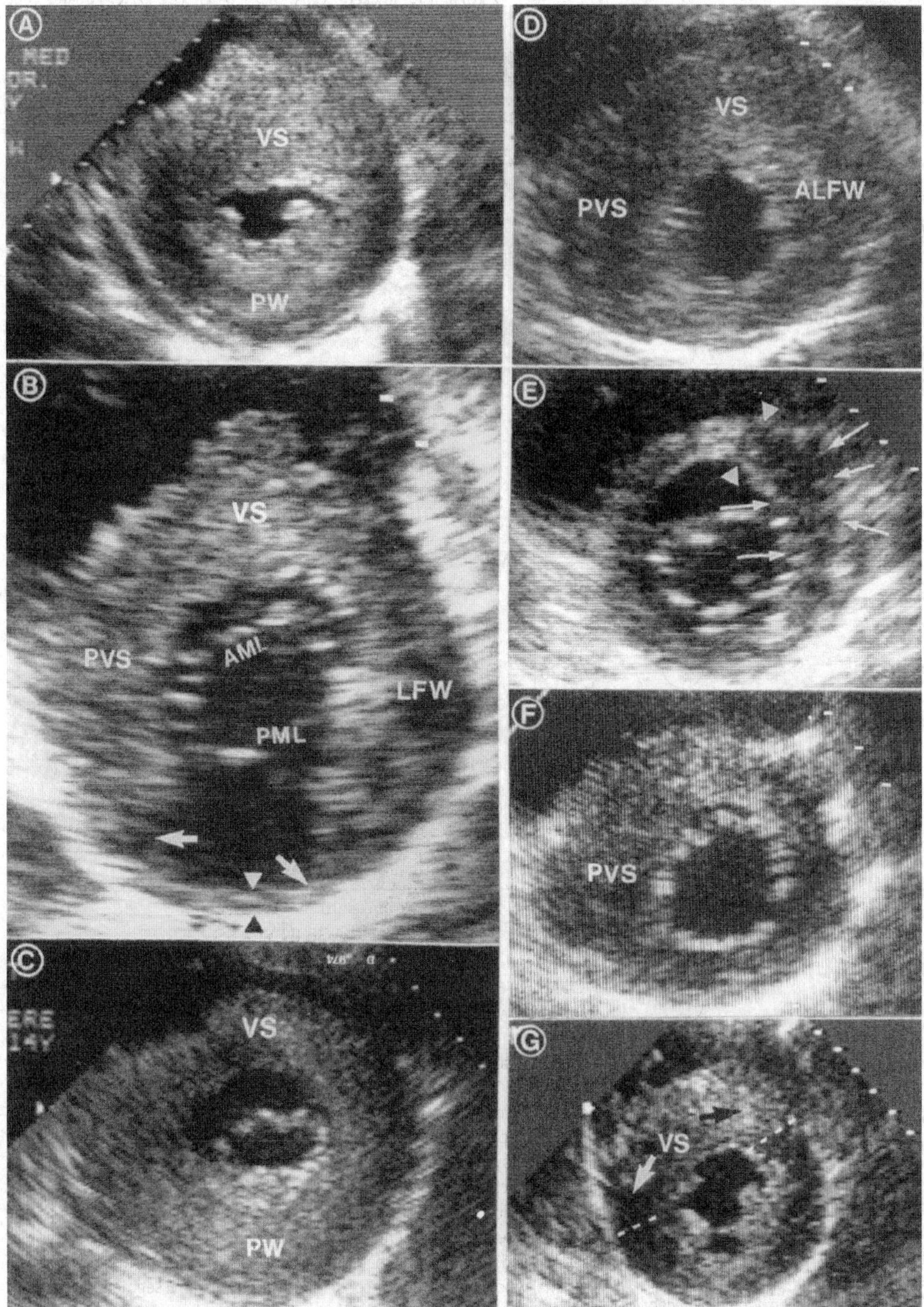

FIGURE 67-6 Variability of patterns of left ventricular hypertrophy in patients with hypertrophic cardiomyopathy, shown in a composite of diastolic stop-frame images in the parasternal short-axis plane. *A, B,* and *D.* Wall thickening is diffuse, involving substantial portions of ventricular septum and free wall. At the papillary muscle level (*A*), all segments of the left ventricular wall are hypertrophied, including the posterior free wall (PW), but the pattern of thickening is asymmetric, with the anterior portion of ventricular septum (VS) massive (i.e., 50 mm). *B.* Hypertrophy is diffuse, involving three segments of the left ventricle but with the posterior wall spared and thin (<10 mm) (*arrowheads*) and with particularly abrupt changes in wall thickness evident (*arrows*). *C.* Marked hypertrophy in a pattern distinctly different from that in *A, B,* and *D,* in which the thickening of the posterior wall is predominant and the ventricular septum is of nearly normal thickness. *D.* Diffuse distribution of hypertrophy involving three segments of the left ventricle similar to that in *B* but without sharp changes in the contour of the wall. *E.* Hypertrophy predominantly of lateral free wall (*arrows*) and only a small portion of the contiguous anterior septum (*arrowheads*). *F.* Hypertrophy predominantly of posterior ventricular septum (PVS) and, to a lesser extent, the contiguous portion of the anterior septum. *G.* Thickening of anterior and posterior septum to a similar degree but with sparing of the free wall. Calibration dots are 1 cm apart. AML = anterior mitral leaflet; LVW = lateral free wall; PML = posterior mitral leaflet. (From Klues HG et al.[18] with permission from the authors and publisher.)

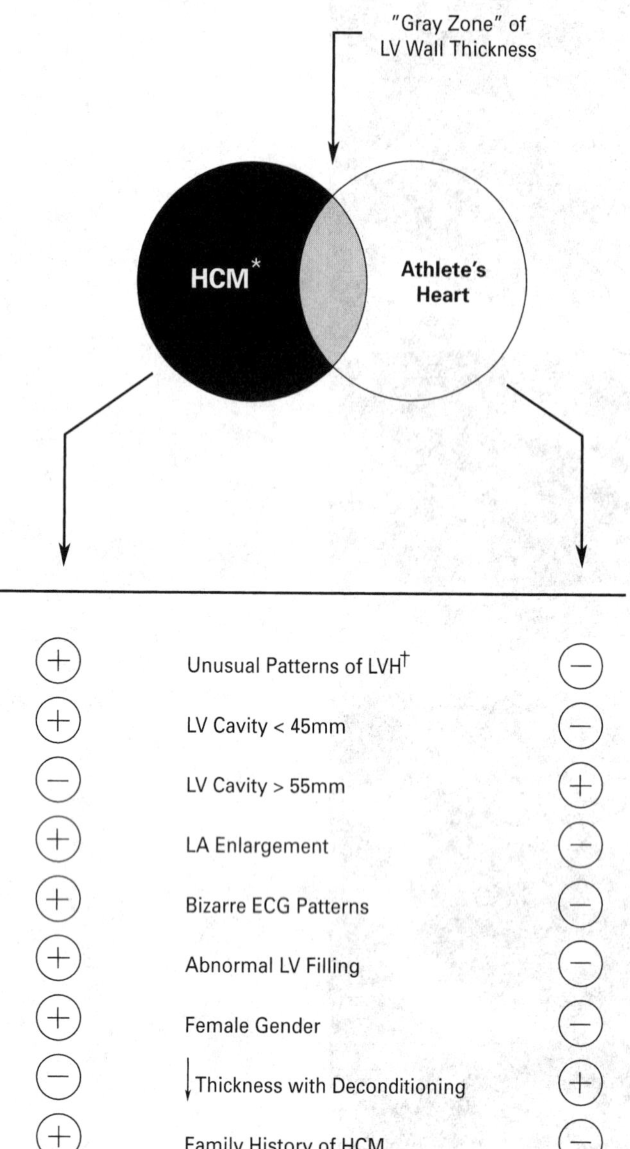

FIGURE 67-7 Criteria used to distinguish HCM from athlete's heart when left ventricular (LV) wall thickness is within the shaded gray zone of overlap, consistent with both diagnoses. *Assumed to be the nonobstructive form, since substantial mitral valve systolic anterior motion would confirm, per se, the diagnosis of HCM in an athlete. †May involve a variety of abnormalities, including heterogeneous distribution of LV hypertrophy in which adjacent regions may be of greatly different thicknesses, with sharp transitions evident between segments; also, asymmetric patterns in which anterior ventricular septum is spared from the hypertrophic process and the region of predominant thickening may be in the posterior septum or anterolateral or posterior free wall. ↓ = decreased; LA = left atrial. (From Maron BJ et al.[52] with permission from the authors and Williams & Wilkins.)

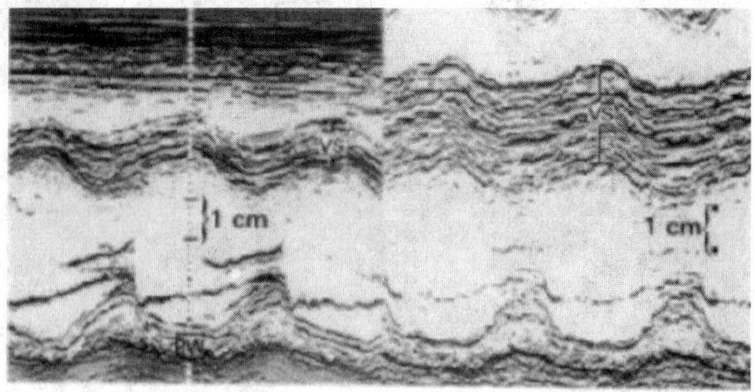

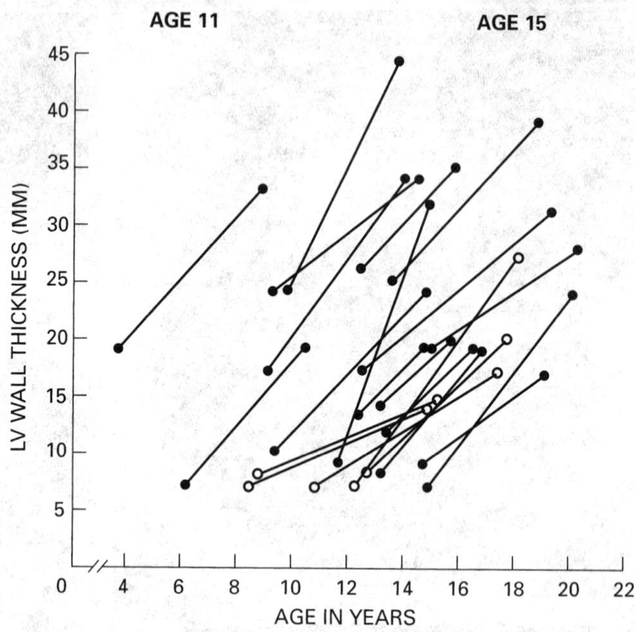

FIGURE 67-8 Development and progression of left ventricular hypertrophy in children with HCM. *Upper panel:* Development of marked hypertrophy of the anterior basal ventricular septum (VS). M-mode echocardiograms shown here were obtained at the same cross-sectional level in a girl with a family history of HCM. At age 11, ventricular septal thickness was at upper limit of normal (10 mm); at age 15, septal thickness had increased markedly (to 33 mm), and appearance of the echocardiogram is typical of HCM. The patient remained asymptomatic throughout this period of time but died suddenly and unexpectedly at age 17. PW = posterior left ventricular free wall. *Lower panel:* Dynamic, striking changes in left ventricular wall thickness with age in 22 children; each patient is represented by the left ventricular segment that showed the greatest change in wall thickness. Open symbols denote 5 patients who had no evidence of hypertrophy in any segment of the left ventricle at the initial evaluation but subsequently developed de novo hypertrophy typical of HCM. (From Maron BJ et al.[35] with permission of the authors and the Massachusetts Medical Society.)

bizarre shapes, maintain intercellular connections with several adjacent cells, and are arranged in a disorganized pattern at oblique and perpendicular angles to each other. This myocyte disarray is present in about 95 percent of patients dying of HCM and usually occupies substantial portions of both septum (i.e., about 33 percent) and left ventricular free wall (i.e., 25 percent) (see Fig. 74-4*C* and *D*). However, there is little correlation between absolute wall thickness and amount of disorganized myocardium in segments of the left ventricular wall.[71] Therefore areas of normal or only mildly increased left ventricular wall thickness may also show evidence of the cardiomyopathic process in HCM, in the form of cellular disarray.[71]

Dispersion of disorganized cardiac muscle cells throughout the left ventricular myocardium may impair intercellular transmission of normal electrophysiologic impulses, predispose to electrical instability, and thereby serve as an arrhythmogenic

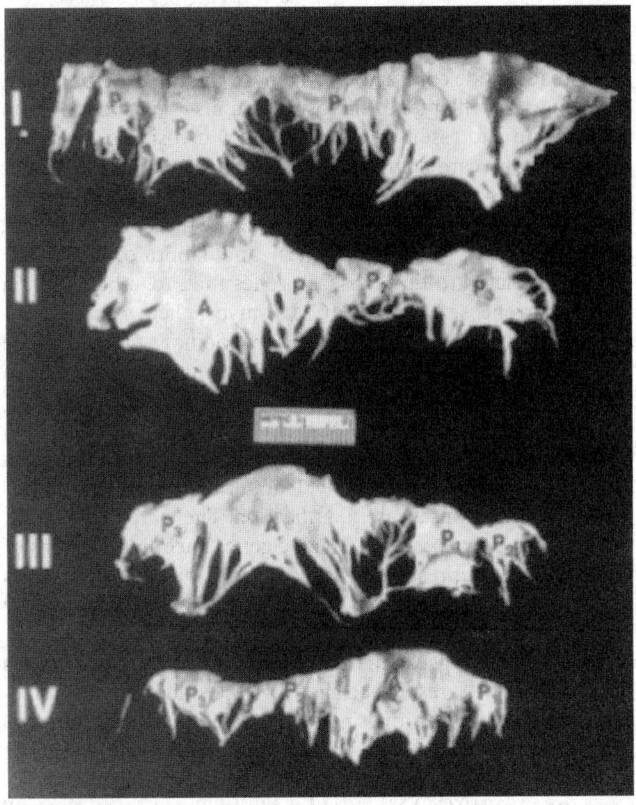

FIGURE 67-9 Mitral valves from three patients with obstructive HCM, aged 31, 29, and 60 years (I, II, and III), and from a normal control patient without cardiovascular disease (IV), showing variation in valvular size and structure present in HCM. Valves are opened with the circumference displayed in a horizontal orientation, exposing the atrial surface, with annular margin to top and chordal attachments to bottom. *I.* Large valve (area 22 cm^2) in which both the anterior (A) and posterior (P) leaflets are greatly elongated and increased in area. *II.* Large valve in which increased valve size (area 18 cm^2) is due primarily to elongation and enlargement of the anterior leaflet (A). *III.* Segmental elongation and increased area confined to a scallop of posterior leaflet. (From Klues HG et al.[20] with permission of the authors and Lippincott Williams & Wilkins.)

substrate responsible for the genesis of primary ventricular tachycardia/fibrillation.[74]

Patients with HCM (and without atherosclerotic coronary artery disease) often exhibit myocyte necrosis and replacement fibrosis in the left ventricle at necropsy.[42,63,69,72] A spectrum of severity and distribution is observed ranging from isolated small

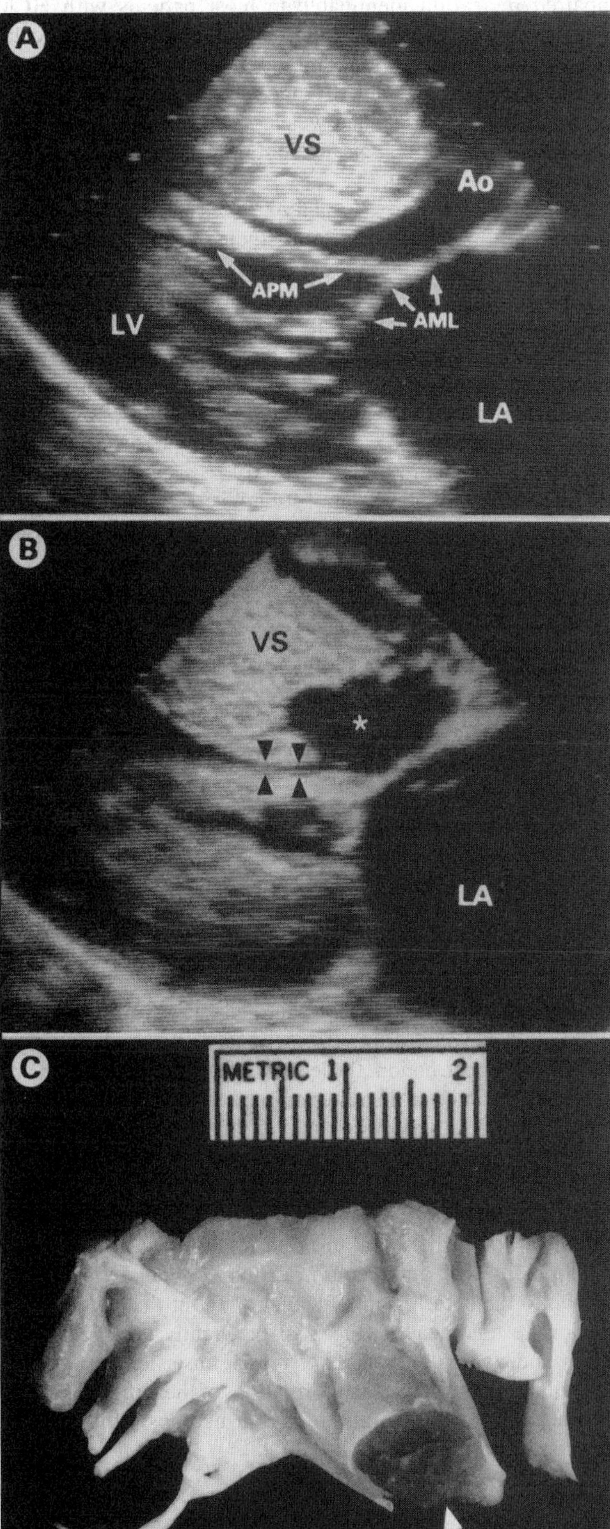

FIGURE IT Anomalous papillary muscle insertion directly into anterior mitral leaflet (*AML*) in patient with obstructive HCM. *A. Before myotomy-myectomy:* parasternal long-axis echocardiogram shows AML in direct continuity with the hypertrophied anomalous anterolateral papillary muscle (*APM*), which displaced anteriorly within the left ventricular cavity, producing a long area of midcavity muscular contact with the ventricular septum (VS) and outflow obstruction (*arrows*); tips of the mitral leaflets coapt in the usual position, and typical systolic anterior motion is absent (*small arrows*). *B. After myotomy-myectomy:* Long-axis echocardiogram shows extensive muscular resection (*), extending from base of the septum to beyond the distal margins of the anterior mitral leaflet; nevertheless, a large area of direct muscular contact remains after operation between papillary muscle and ventricular septum (*arrowheads*), which is responsible for persistent and marked obstruction to left ventricular outflow. *C.* Mitral valve specimen excised at operation; a massively hypertrophied anterolateral anomalous papillary muscle (*arrow*) inserted directly into the body of the anterior leaflet. Ao = aorta; LA = left atrial; LV = left ventricle. (From Klues HG et al.[19] with permission of the authors and Lippincott Williams & Wilkins.)

scars to extensive, grossly visible replacement scarring that may even be transmural[42] (Fig. 67-4*F*). These areas of fibrosis, which likely result from repetitive bursts of myocardial ischemia or are related in some other way to the underlying cardiomyopathic disease process, can be identifiable during life as irreversible thallium-201 myocardial perfusion abnormalities[75] and may well contribute to the increased ventricular chamber stiffness and impaired relaxation identifiable in most patients with HCM as well as representing a nidus for the genesis of ventricular arrhythmias.[1,3,5,74] In addition, the interstitial collagen matrix of the left ventricle is substantially increased in size; its components (perimysial coils, pericellular weaves, and struts) are increased in number and morphologically abnormal, often showing a disorganized arrangement.[73]

Abnormal intramural coronary arteries are present in about 80 percent of patients with HCM studied at necropsy and are most commonly evident in the ventricular septum.[69,70] The walls of these arterioles are thickened (because of increased smooth muscle cells, collagen, elastic fibers, and mucoid deposits in the media and intima), and frequently the lumen appears narrowed and compromised (Fig. 67-4*E*). Increased numbers or clusters of abnormal intramural arteries are often observed within or at the margins of sizable areas of fibrosis.[42,69] This association between abnormal intramural coronary arteries and myocardial scarring suggests that a form of "small-vessel disease" present in patients with HCM may be responsible for myocardial ischemia and necrosis.[69]

Mitral Valve Abnormalities

Morphometric analysis of mitral valves removed at operation or necropsy from patients with outflow obstruction supports the concept that primary structural abnormalities of the mitral valve are also characteristic of many patients with HCM[20,43] (Fig. 67-9). About two-thirds of patients show alterations in mitral valve size and shape, with an increased mitral valve tissue area (up to twice normal) due primarily to leaflet elongation (but without evidence of myxomatous degeneration). These enlarged valves demonstrate considerable structural heterogeneity, either with both the anterior and posterior leaflets increased in size or asymmetric and segmental enlargement of one leaflet.[20] Mitral valve systolic anterior motion and outflow obstruction may occur both with normal or enlarged mitral valves but show age-related morphologic and functional features. In younger patients with obstruction, the leaflets are usually elongated and the valve is situated more posterior in the left ventricular outflow tract (at end-diastole), in contrast to elderly patients in whom the mitral valve is often normal-sized and situated much closer to the ventricular septum.[43]

In addition, other HCM patients show a congenital malformation of the mitral apparatus due to an arrest in embryonic development, with anomalous insertion of papillary muscle directly into the anterior mitral leaflet (without the interposition of chordae tendineae)[19] (Fig. 67-10). Greatly enlarged mitral valves and anomalous papillary muscle insertion represent a constellation of structural malformations of the mitral apparatus (in >50 percent of patients studied at necropsy) that expand the morphologic definition of HCM.[19,20,43]

ETIOLOGY AND GENETICS

HCM is a mendelian trait with an autosomal dominant pattern of familial inheritance.[1–5,8–11,22,38–40,76–83] Based on 10 years of molecular genetic studies, it is now known that HCM is genetically heterogeneous and caused by mutations in any one of nine genes that encode contractile proteins of the cardiac sarcomere, involving thick filaments (myosin subunits—i.e., beta-myosin heavy chain and essential and regulatory myosin light chains), thin filaments (cardiac troponin T, cardiac troponin I, α-tropomyosin, and α-actin), and—in the case of titin cardiac myosin-binding protein C—the structural network that joins thick and thin filaments.[5,8–11,22,38–40,76–83] Clinical and laboratory data are largely restricted to three disease genes that, together, explain most occurrences of familial HCM: β-myosin heavy chain, myosin-binding protein C, and cardiac troponin T. Overall, more than 100 individual disease-causing HCM mutations have been reported, either of the missense type (with the replacement of one amino acid by another) or mutations leading to truncated proteins. Indeed, most genotyped pedigrees show a mutation apparently unique to that family. Undoubtedly, numerous other genes and mutations await identification. The fact that all mutations known to cause HCM involve genes encoding proteins of the sarcomere represents a unifying principle that permits us to regard this heterogeneous condition as a single disease entity (and as a disease of the sarcomere).[5,8–10,84]

It has been suggested that the prognosis of HCM varies considerably with respect to many of the mutations reported. For example, some β-myosin heavy chain point mutations appear benign (e.g., Val606Met), whereas others are more virulent and associated with reduced survival (e.g., Arg403Gln, Arg453-Cys, and Arg719Trp).[8,9,22,76,82] In addition, cardiac troponin-T mutations may have malignant forms associated with reduced survival even though cardiac hypertrophy is often relatively mild.[5,22,38,39] Although, collectively, these observations suggest that genetic data may ultimately predict prognosis and influence clinical management, at present such a risk stratification strategy should be regarded as preliminary considering the relatively small number of genotyped families and the aforementioned genetic heterogeneity.

Occurrence of premature sudden cardiac death in a family should dictate a genetic and/or echocardiographic evaluation in surviving relatives, since the clinical expression of HCM may be particularly virulent in certain families (e.g., "malignant" HCM).[85] Also, because HCM is the most common cause of sudden unexpected death in young competitive athletes,[86] youthful family members should be screened for HCM prior to participation in intense athletic training. Because phenotypic (i.e., morphologic) expression of HCM may not be complete until 17 to 18 years of age,[35] a single screening echocardiogram during early childhood may not definitively exclude HCM. Therefore, children in families with HCM in whom left ventricular hypertrophy is absent on 2D echocardiography should continue to have examinations periodically until they achieve full growth and maturation. There now appears to be one clear exception to the tenet that development or progression of left ventricular hypertrophy does not occur in adulthood—i.e., myosin-binding protein-C mutations[10,46] (Fig. 67-11), which are associated with age-related penetrance; in some young adults, the HCM phenotype may not be evident on echocardiography, and is delayed until much later in life[10,46] (Fig. 67-12).

Routine echocardiographic screening at ≤12 years of age is usually unproductive, since phenotypic expression of the mutant gene is rarely present at that age.[31,35,59,77] Family screening can usually be deferred in young children until adolescence unless they are involved in intense sports programs (such as swimming

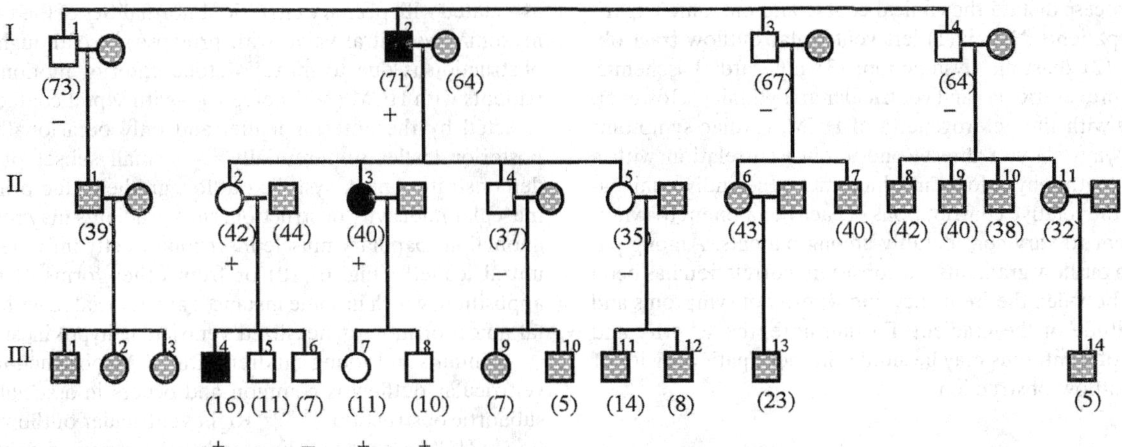

FIGURE 67-11 Pedigree of HCM family with a myosin-binding protein C mutation and variable penetrance. The genetically affected 42-year-old woman (II.2) is both the offspring of an affected parent (I.2), the mother of a 16-year-old affected child (III.4), and the sister of an affected 40-year-old sibling (II.3). In contrast to her father, child, and sister, this woman (II.2) showed no evidence of left ventricular hypertrophy and the HCM phenotype by two-dimensional echocardiography (or 12-lead ECG).

and tennis) or are members of families with HCM-related sudden deaths.[85]

With the advent of preclinical genetic diagnosis of HCM, a number of asymptomatic youthful family members have been identified as affected on the basis of a DNA diagnosis in the absence of typical phenotypic features of their disease (as assessed with echocardiography and electrocardiography).[5,10,22,31,36,37,40] The increasing availability of gene-based diagnosis will lead to the identification of greater numbers of children and adults with a preclinical diagnosis of HCM (i.e., who have a gene defect but no phenotypic manifestations of

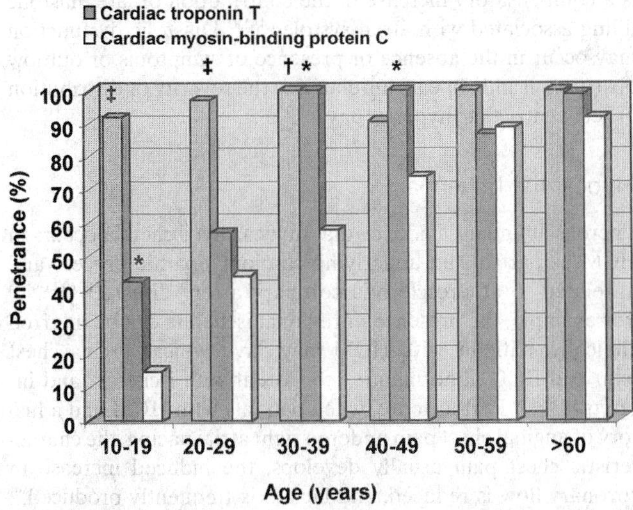

FIGURE 67-12 Age-related penetrance of familial HCM caused by mutations in the genes for cardiac myosin-binding protein C, cardiac troponin T, and cardiac β-myosin heavy chain. Solid bars denote the percentage of persons with both cardiac myosin-binding protein C mutations and left ventricular hypertrophy. Comparable clinical data for cardiac troponin T and β-myosin heavy chain are shown. Significant differences in the penetrance of familial HCM caused by cardiac myosin-binding protein C mutations and by mutations in cardiac troponin T or cardiac β-myosin heavy chain are indicated as follows: * = $p < 0.05$; ≁ = $p < 0.005$; ≠ = $p < 0.001$. (From Niimura H et al.[10] with permission of the authors and the Massachusetts Medical Society.)

HCM).[5,10,22,31,36,37,40] At present, the clinical implications of such gene abnormalities and the appropriate management are largely unresolved issues, although—of note—very few such patients have been reported with adverse outcome.[87,88] Therefore there is not sufficient evidence available at present to preclude such individuals from competitive athletics in the absence of cardiac symptoms or risk factors such as family history of sudden cardiac death.[89] It should be emphasized that, at present, due to the substantial genetic heterogeneity of HCM and the complex, time-consuming, and expensive techniques required for genetic screening, DNA diagnosis is quite demanding, permits only research-oriented genotyping of selected pedigrees, and is not routinely available for clinical practice.[22]

Although the reported sarcomeric protein mutations are regarded as disease-causing for HCM, many of the abnormal and primary structural features of this disease are not confined to protein abnormalities of the sarcomere but extend to alterations in connective tissue elements—e.g., mitral valve enlargement and elongation as well as other anomalies of the mitral apparatus,[19,20,43] abnormal small intramural coronary arteries,[69,70] and an expanded collagen matrix.[72,73] This fact, together with the observations that the patterns of left ventricular hypertrophy in closely related family members are usually dissimilar[11] and that hypertrophy is frequently confined to only a portion of the wall,[11–13,18] suggests that phenotypic expression is importantly influenced by genetic factors other than the causal mutation (e.g., by modifier genes)[90] or by undefined environmental influences.

PATHOPHYSIOLOGY

The symptoms of HCM are varied and include those of pulmonary congestion—such as exertional dyspnea, orthopnea, and paroxysmal nocturnal dyspnea—as well as fatigue, chest pain (which may be atypical of angina pectoris), palpitations, and impaired consciousness, including dizziness, near syncope, and syncope. The onset of symptoms is often in early adulthood between 20 and 40 years of age, although they can become evident at any age.

A number of pathophysiologic components of the HCM

disease process dictate the clinical course and outcome experienced by patients[1,3–5,91–101]: (1) left ventricular outflow tract obstruction; (2) diastolic dysfunction; (3) myocardial ischemia; and (4) supraventricular and ventricular arrhythmias. However, consistent with the heterogeneity of HCM, cardiac symptoms do not always show a direct (one-to-one) correlation with a particular pathophysiologic mechanism in the individual patient, and the relative contributions of each component to symptoms appear to vary considerably among patients. Among patients with outflow gradients, no consistent correlation has been identified between the frequency and severity of symptoms and the magnitude of the gradient. Furthermore, the severity and character of symptoms may be similar in those patients with or without outflow obstruction.

Outflow Obstruction

Obstruction to left ventricular outflow exhibited by patients with HCM (due to systolic anterior motion of the mitral valve and midsystolic contact with the ventricular septum)[4,6,94–97,102,104] is characteristically dynamic, showing spontaneous variability.[2] Interventions or circumstances that decrease myocardial contractility (e.g., beta-blocking drugs) or increase ventricular volume or arterial pressure (squatting or vasoconstrictor agents) have the effect of reducing or abolishing subaortic obstruction. Interventions or circumstances that increase contractility (exercise or infusion of isoproterenol) or decrease arterial pressure or ventricular volume (Valsalva maneuver or a hypotension-producing agent) will increase or provoke obstruction. Not uncommonly, patients with little or no obstruction to left ventricular outflow under basal conditions are capable of generating substantial labile gradients with physiologic or pharmacologic provocations[2–4] or just after the cessation of exercise.[98]

The increase in systolic intraventricular pressure associated with outflow obstruction may increase myocardial wall stress and oxygen demand. It is generally conceded that outflow obstruction in HCM can, in some patients, have long-term detrimental consequences on left ventricular function and be responsible for the genesis of symptoms.[1–6,95] The magnitude of the systolic pressure gradient can be reliably estimated noninvasively by the magnitude and duration of mitral valve systolic anterior motion on M-mode echocardiogram[4,6,94,95] or, more easily and quantitatively, by continuous-wave Doppler interrogation, obviating the necessity of performing serial cardiac catheterizations.[105] The combined use of color-coded, pulsed, and continuous-wave Doppler echocardiography allows assessment of the site and severity of outflow obstruction[104] (Chap. 13).

For the subaortic gradient to occur in HCM, several of the following morphologic and hemodynamic factors will be present: (1) reduced outflow tract dimension at end-diastole; (2) substantial hypertrophy involving the basal anterior ventricular septum; (3) displacement of mitral valve and papillary muscles anteriorly within the ventricular cavity; (4) increased length of the mitral leaflets; and (5) hyperdynamic left ventricular ejection, creating a high-velocity jet which streams through the narrowed outflow tract, pulling the mitral leaflets forward toward the septum (i.e., Venturi effect), or perhaps more likely due to drag (the hydrodynamic pushing force of flow) on the leaflets as they protrude into the outflow tract.[90] While mitral regurgitation due to outflow obstruction is usually mild-to-moderate in HCM, it may occasionally be much more severe when associated with primary intrinsic abnormalities of the valve (e.g., myxomatous mitral valve with prolapse).[106] Although outflow obstruction is due to mitral systolic anterior motion in most patients with HCM (>95 percent)—with septal contact usually effected by the anterior leaflet and only occasionally by the posterior leaflet preferentially[103]—a small subset of patients demonstrate a peak systolic outflow gradient due primarily to muscular midcavity obstruction; such gradients may result from anomalous papillary muscle insertion directly into the anterior mitral leaflet[19] (Fig. 67-10) or from other forms of muscular apposition, which in some instances are associated with segmental apical or more generalized ventricular hypokinesia.[107]

In infants and young children with HCM, obstruction to right ventricular outflow is common and occurs in association with subaortic obstruction.[54,55,95,108] Right ventricular outflow obstruction in HCM is produced by greatly hypertrophied right ventricular musculature (crista supraventricularis, moderator band, or trabeculae), reflecting an excessive hypertrophic process, and projecting into the relatively small outflow tract.[109]

Diastolic Dysfunction

Echocardiographic, Doppler, contrast, or radionuclide angiographic and hemodynamic studies of left ventricular diastolic function have identified characteristic abnormalities in relaxation and filling that are present in about 80 percent of patients with HCM[1,3,4,6,92,93,99,110–113] and are presumed to have an important role in the genesis of fatigue, exertional dyspnea, and angina pectoris. Therefore, considering the overall HCM disease spectrum, diastolic dysfunction is probably the single most important pathophysiologic mechanism responsible for symptoms. Prior studies have shown that the early filling phase of diastole is significantly prolonged and associated with a decreased rate and volume of rapid filling.[1,4,92,93] Associated with this alteration is a compensatory increase in the contribution of late diastolic filling associated with atrial systole.[1,4,92,93] Diastolic dysfunction may occur in the absence or presence of symptoms or outflow obstruction and appears unrelated to the severity or distribution of left ventricular hypertrophy.[92,113]

Myocardial Ischemia

There is abundant evidence that myocardial ischemia occurs in HCM as part of the underlying cardiomyopathic process and unrelated to atherosclerotic coronary artery disease.[1,3,69,70,91,114] For example, the presence of regional ischemia can be inferred clinically; patients with HCM may have typical angina chest pain and ECG abnormalities consistent with ischemia and infarction.[115,116] Furthermore, when patients with HCM and a history of anginal chest pain undergo right atrial pacing, the characteristic chest pain usually develops, the induced increase in coronary flow is reduced, and lactate is frequently produced.[91] Also, such patients may have fixed or exercise-induced reversible thallium-201 defects indistinguishable from those of patients with myocardial ischemia secondary to coronary artery disease.[75] Nevertheless, it has proven exceedingly difficult to measure or quantitate precisely the extent and location of such ischemia or to consistently derive clinical correlations or prognostic information for this finding.[110]

Myocardial ischemia and impaired vasodilator reserve in HCM may be due to several potential mechanisms: (1) compromised coronary blood flow to the left ventricular myocardium because of abnormal intramural coronary arteries (i.e., "small vessel disease"); (2) excessive myocardial oxygen demand that exceeds the capacity of the coronary system to deliver oxygen; or (3) prolonged diastolic relaxation, resulting in elevated myocardial wall tension.

ELECTROCARDIOGRAPHIC FEATURES

The 12-lead ECG is abnormal in about 90 percent of patients with HCM and shows a wide variety of patterns, often bizarre in appearance.[2,4,48–50,116] However, no particular ECG alteration is characteristic of most patients with HCM; common abnormalities are increased precordial voltages consistent with left ventricular hypertrophy, ST-segment changes and T-wave inversion, left atrial enlargement, abnormally deep Q waves, and diminished or absent R waves in the right precordial leads. Infants and young children often have the paradoxic finding of right ventricular hypertrophy on ECG, which may reflect obstruction to right ventricular outflow.

PREPARTICIPATION SCREENING FOR HCM IN ATHLETIC POPULATIONS

Detection of preexisting cardiovascular abnormalities (such as HCM) with the potential for significant morbidity or sudden death during intense physical activity is an important objective of the widespread practice of preparticipation screening of high school[117,118] and college-aged athletes.[119] In the United States, customary screening practice dictates a personal and family history and physical examination.[117–119] However, under the conditions of standard screening, it is difficult to identify or raise the suspicion of HCM, given that the vast majority of patients have the nonobstructive form of the disease with either no or only a soft systolic heart murmur, and that historical clues such as syncope or family history of sudden death are also uncommon.[1,118] Ideally, the detection of HCM would be enhanced by the incorporation of noninvasive testing during screening, such as 12-lead ECG[120] or echocardiography.[118] However, cost-efficacy and other considerations make the routine application of such tests impractical throughout the United States.[118] Echocardiographic screening for HCM is also limited by the frequency of borderline wall-thickness measurements (and the uncertainty and anxiety created by such findings), as well as the fact that the HCM phenotype may not always be detectable with echocardiography prior to about age 16.[35]

NATURAL HISTORY INCLUDING SUDDEN CARDIAC DEATH

HCM may be identified clinically at virtually any age, from infancy to old age (with even a few patients >90 years of age). Understanding the clinical course of HCM, particularly when viewed in the context of predicting outcome for individual patients, has for 40 years been constrained by three obstacles: (1) uncommon occurrence of the disease (i.e., 0.2 percent in the general population)[26]; (2) heterogeneity of disease expression[1–22,29,32–34,37–46,58–62,77–83,121]; and (3) tertiary center referral bias.[28,122,123]

Indeed, because much of the considerable published literature on HCM is based on studies performed at tertiary referral centers,[28,124–130] the overall clinical picture of HCM that has emerged is profoundly influenced by the biases created by highly selective patient referral patterns,[28,122,123] which has led to an overestimation of the overall risk for premature death and morbidity. This concept is substantiated by the fact that annual mortality figures from such referral centers are considerably higher (3 to 4 percent and up to 6 percent in children)[108,125,126,128,129] than those more recently reported in relatively unselected regional populations (about 1 percent per year).[122,131–136] Indeed, patient referral patterns are probably the strongest determinants of our prevailing perceptions regarding the clinical expression and impact of HCM.[122,123]

In general terms, it is reasonable to characterize HCM as a complex disorder capable of important clinical consequences, including causing premature death in some patients. However, the disease has a more favorable overall clinical course than previously thought, as many patients achieve normal life expectancy with little or no disability and often without the aid of therapeutic interventions. These observations emphasize the need to provide many HCM patients, including many children, with reassurance regarding their clinical outlook, as well as prudence concerning possible adverse consequences.

On the other hand, when HCM is viewed in terms of patient subgroups (rather than the overall disease), some individuals are clearly at much higher risk and may be subject to three modes of death: (1) sudden and unexpected, often in the young; (2) progressive heart failure in midlife; and (3) stroke associated with atrial fibrillation, largely in the elderly.

While frequent in children and young adults, sudden death is not confined to these age groups and may also occur in midlife and beyond, without a statistically significant predilection for any particular age group. Therefore the potential risk period in HCM is particularly long. However, reports of sudden death in infants and very young children are exceedingly rare. Sudden death in HCM usually occurs in previously asymptomatic (or only mildly symptomatic) patients, and such catastrophes are often the first clinical manifestation of the disease.[124] Although most patients die in the morning hours[137] while engaged in sedentary pursuits or during mild exertion, a substantial proportion collapse during or just after vigorous physical activity.[86,124] The latter observation—as well as the fact that HCM is the most common cause of sudden death among young competitive athletes[86] (Fig. 67-13)—supports the view that intense physical activity can act as a trigger for sudden death in the presence of underlying cardiovascular disease.[138] Therefore it is prudent to recommend the disqualification of young athletes with HCM from intense competitive sports, in accord with the standards of the 26th Bethesda Conference,[89] in an effort to decrease the risk of exercise-related sudden death.

Based on stored electrogram data from HCM patients experiencing appropriate implantable cardioverter-defibrillator discharges, ventricular tachycardia/fibrillation appears to be the primary mechanism most commonly responsible for sudden death in HCM,[74] although a number of other mechanisms may also be involved.[139–146] No particular symptom complex has been shown to be reliably associated with subsequent sudden death in HCM with the exception of recurrent or exertional syncope, particularly in the young.[5] Furthermore, patients with or without subaortic obstruction may die suddenly, and some patients appear to tolerate marked outflow obstruction for virtually their

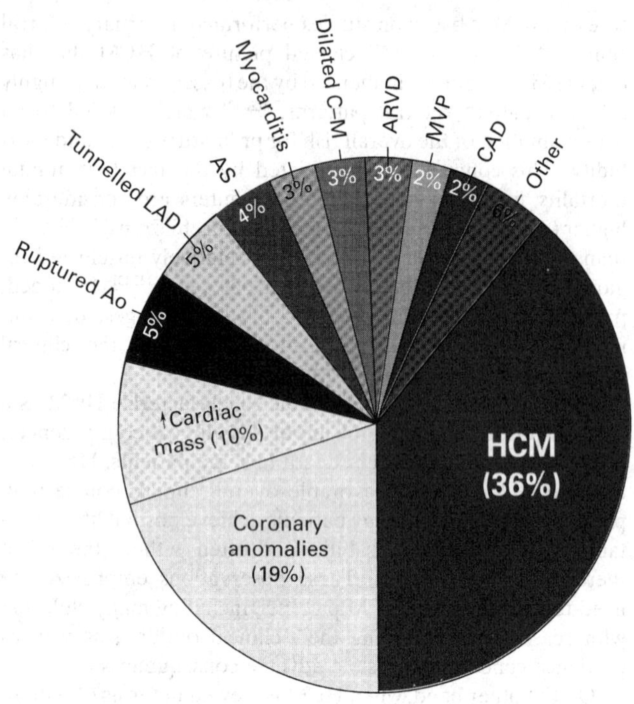

FIGURE 67-13 Causes of sudden cardiac death in young competitive athletes (median age, 17), based on systematic tracking of 158 athletes in the United States, 1985 to 1995. In an additional 2 percent, no evidence of cardiovascular disease sufficient to explain death was found at necropsy; ↑ (increased) cardiac mass = hearts with increased weight and some morphologic features consistent with (but not diagnostic of) HCM. Ao = aorta; LAD = left anterior descending coronary artery; AS = aortic stenosis; C-M = cardiomyopathy; ARVD = arrhythmogenic right ventricular dysplasia; MVP = mitral valve prolapse; CAD = coronary artery disease; HCM = hypertrophic cardiomyopathy. (Adapted from Maron BJ et al.[86] with permission of Lippincott Williams & Wilkins.)

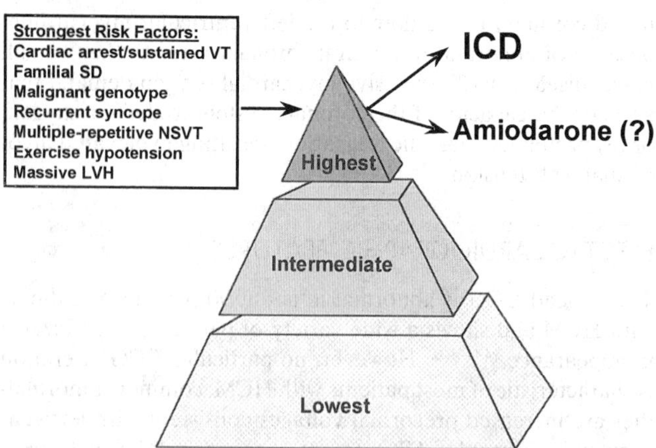

FIGURE 67-14 Assessment of risk for sudden cardiac death in HCM population. Treatment for the prevention for sudden death is limited to that small subset perceived to be at highest risk compared to all other patients with HCM, based on the presence of ≥1 of the risk factors shown. Patients regarded as low risk are asymptomatic with mild left ventricular hypertrophy and *without* either ventricular tachycardia on ambulatory Holter ECG, hypotensive blood pressure response to exercise, and family history of premature HCM-related death. ICD = implantable cardioverter-defibrillator; LVH = left ventricular hypertrophy; NSVT = nonsustained ventricular tachycardia; SD = sudden death; VT = ventricular tachycardia. (From Maron,[1] with permission of the author and *Lancet*.)

entire lives without adverse consequences.[122] Indeed, the presence or magnitude of the outflow gradient has not been independently associated with increased risk for sudden death, although an association with heart failure–related or total cardiovascular mortality has been cited.[122,136,148]

However, other disease variables have been associated with an increased likelihood of sudden death. The most important of these proposed risk factors include[1,5,8,9,22,38,74,82,85,145,147–149] (Fig. 67-14) the following: prior cardiac arrest or sustained ventricular tachycardia, "malignant" genotype or family history of premature HCM death, multiple-repetitive (or prolonged) bursts of nonsustained ventricular tachycardia on ambulatory ECGs, massive degree of left ventricular hypertrophy (wall thickness, ≥30 mm). A hypotensive blood pressure response to exercise may also be informative regarding risk but is encumbered by a low positive predictive accuracy and is much more powerful as a negative predictor of outcome.[139,140]

A recent retrospective analysis of children with HCM suggested that an intramural course of a segment of the proximal left anterior descending coronary artery (i.e., myocardial bridging) constitutes a risk factor for sudden cardiac arrest.[145] It was proposed that such muscular bridges could produce systolic coronary arterial narrowing, residual diastolic compression, and myocardial ischemia, thereby justifying surgical unroofing when detected.

The data available at this time do not provide convincing evidence that programmed electrical stimulation has a major role in risk stratification in HCM. Particularly aggressive programmed stimulation protocols with triple ventricular premature depolarizations seldom induce monomorphic ventricular tachycardia but frequently trigger polymorphic ventricular tachycardia or ventricular fibrillation in patients with HCM.[5,150] Based on experience in HCM as well as in coronary artery disease and dilated cardiomyopathy, these latter arrhythmias are generally regarded as nonspecific responses.[5]

END-STAGE PHASE

A final phase of disease evolution occurring in about 10 percent of symptomatic patients in a referral-based population has been variously referred to as the "end-stage," "burned-out," or "dilated" phase of HCM[61] (Fig. 67-15). This distinctive clinical course is characterized by progressive congestive symptoms with marked exercise limitation and atrial arrhythmias, associated with substantial left ventricular remodeling—i.e., enlarging left ventricular cavity size (occasionally with marked absolute dilatation), thinning of portions of the wall, systolic dysfunction, and—in a few patients—spontaneous reduction of the subaortic gradient. Therefore, the disease in end-stage patients is transformed from the typical morphologic and functional appearance of HCM (hyperdynamic, hypertrophied, and nondilated left ventricle) to a clinical state that is more suggestive of a dilated form of cardiomyopathy (Chap. 66) in which the thickness of the left ventricular wall may be virtually normal. Many such patients exhibit irreversible myocardial perfusion abnormalities, which undoubtedly represent areas of extensive myocardial scarring.[42,63,69,75]

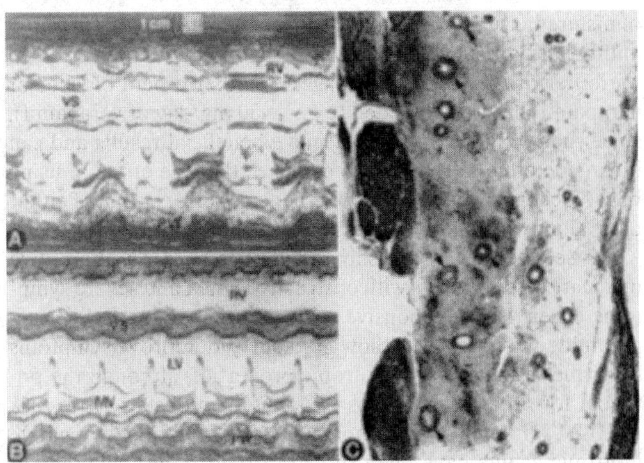

FIGURE 67-15 Studies in patients with HCM and normal extramural coronary arteries showing changes occurring in association with progressive congestive cardiac failure and transmural myocardial infarction (end-stage phase). *A.* Echocardiographic study from a 26-year-old patient with exertional chest pain and dyspnea. Ventricular septum (VS) is markedly thickened (23 mm) and pattern of hypertrophy is asymmetric. Left ventricular end-diastolic dimension is reduced (38 mm), and there is a trivial degree of mitral systolic anterior motion (*arrow*). PW = posterior wall; RV = right ventricle. *B.* From same patient at 30 years of age (9 months before death) after clinical deterioration with progressive cardiac failure, pulmonary edema associated with chronic atrial fibrillation, and cardiopulmonary collapse. Appearance of left ventricle has changed dramatically. Septum has thinned considerably (to 13 mm) and is about as thick as the posterior wall; left ventricular (LV) and right ventricular cavities have enlarged substantially. MV = mitral valve. *C.* Low-power photomicrograph of a specimen from a patient with a clinical course similar to that of the patient in *A* and *B* showing transmural scarring of the septum and numerous abnormal intramural coronary arteries, some with thickened walls and narrowed lumen (*arrows*) (Magnification ×6). (From Maron BJ et al.[3] with permission of the authors and the Massachusetts Medical Society.)

It is possible that the morphologic and functional changes that result in end-stage depression of left ventricular contractile function are due to impaired coronary blood flow and myocardial ischemia resulting from small-vessel coronary artery disease. Patients evolving into the end-stage phase of HCM or experiencing sudden and unexpected cardiac death may coexist in the same family (and share the identical disease-causing mutation).[151] Also, a few patients with aborted episodes of cardiac arrest have themselves died many years later in the end-stage phase.[152]

HYPERTROPHIC CARDIOMYOPATHY IN THE ELDERLY

Older patients (over age 60 to 65) with morphologic and clinical features consistent with HCM have been reported.[1,21,153,154] In certain of these patients, HCM may be well tolerated to particularly advanced ages (i.e., 80 to 90 years) and therefore should be regarded as a disease compatible with normal longevity. In an unselected HCM population, about 20 percent of patients had achieved the age of ≥75 years.[122] In other elderly patients, symptoms are not present early in life, but severe functional limitation and heart failure may intervene abruptly for the first time after age 60 to 65.[21,153,155] This prolonged period of symptomatic latency is notable for a disease usually expressed morphologically by age 20 and in which symptoms are usually evident by age 40 to 50.

Older patients with HCM differ in many respects from many younger patients with regard to certain morphologic features.[21,153–155,156] Older patients characteristically have relatively small hearts with only modestly increased left ventricular wall thickness (usually 20 mm)[21,62,122,155] and severely distorted outflow tract morphology, with greatly reduced size, and exaggerated anterior displacement of a normal-sized mitral valve. Substantial deposits of calcium in the mitral annular region are frequently present and may contribute to anterior displacement of the valve in some patients. Outflow obstruction often occurs in the presence of restricted mitral valve systolic anterior motion, with contact between ventricular septum and anterior mitral leaflet produced by a combination of anterior excursion of the mitral valve toward the septum and posterior movement of septum toward the mitral valve.[43] It is uncertain whether the HCM phenotype in such older patients always conveys the same genetic etiology as in younger patients; however, some older patients have been documented to carry the same mutant genes encoding sarcomeric proteins characteristic of other (younger) HCM patients.

MEDICAL TREATMENT

Asymptomatic Patients and Prevention of Sudden Cardiac Death

Those patients with clear evidence of high risk should be offered treatment for the prevention of sudden cardiac death.[1,5] The implantable cardioverter-defibrillator (ICD) has proved effective and reliable in relatively young and high-risk HCM patients by virtue of sensing ventricular tachycardia/fibrillation and restoring sinus rhythm by appropriate defibrillation shocks or antitachycardia pacing at an overall rate of 7 percent per year.[74] The ICD may be lifesaving,[74,157] both in the context of secondary prevention after cardiac arrest or in sustained ventricular tachycardia (11 percent per year) or for primary (prophylactic) prevention due to the perception of high risk based on ≥1 sudden death risk factors.[74] Alternatively, long-term prophylactic treatment with amiodarone[158] would seem less realistic in relatively young HCM patients, given the potential side effects and the long risk period in HCM as well as the paucity of data substantiating amiodarone as affording effective protection against sudden cardiac death specifically in this disease. Prophylactic and empiric administration of beta blockers or verapamil to asymptomatic patients for the primary purpose of reducing the risk for sudden death, for which there are no or little data, now seems outdated in view of the availability of more definitive therapeutic measures such as the ICD. Drug treatment to prevent or delay progression of congestive symptoms is empiric, with a complete lack of any controlled data.

Alleviation of Symptoms

Therapeutic strategies for symptomatic patients with HCM are summarized in Fig. 67-16. Responses of HCM patients to medical treatment are highly variable; consequently, therapy must often be tailored to the individual requirements of symptomatic patients.[1,5,159] Historically, beta-adrenergic blocking drugs (pro-

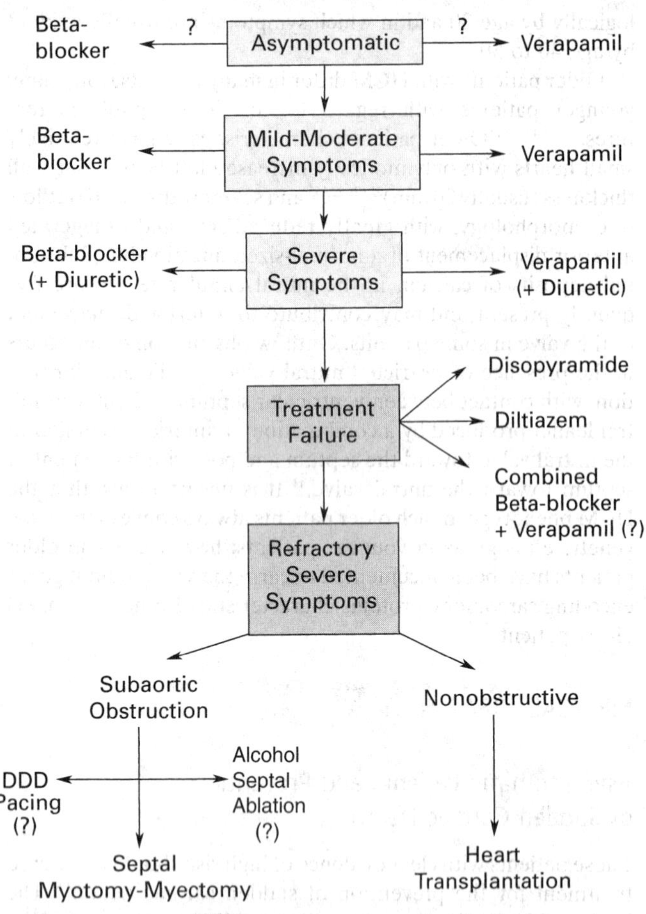

FIGURE 67-16 Therapeutic strategies for patients with HCM. Question marks indicate treatment recommendations that are largely unresolved.

pranolol or more cardioselective agents such as atenolol, metoprolol, or nadolol) have been utilized extensively to relieve symptoms in patients with either the obstructive or nonobstructive form of HCM.[1,3–6,159] The beneficial effects of beta blockers on symptoms (principally exertional dyspnea and chest pain) and exercise capacity appear to be due largely to decreased heart rate, with consequent prolongation of diastole, increased passive left ventricular filling, and decreased filling pressures. By reducing inotropic state, beta blockers may also lessen myocardial oxygen demand and decrease the left ventricular outflow gradient during exercise when sympathetic tone is increased.

Calcium channel blockers (principally verapamil) are also important therapeutic agents in the management of symptomatic patients with HCM.[1,160,161] Orally administered verapamil provides improvement in cardiac symptoms and exercise tolerance for many patients with HCM, including those who have failed to benefit from beta blockers. This symptomatic improvement with verapamil appears to be due largely to normalization of left ventricular filling parameters.[1,5]

Beta blockers and verapamil are usually administered empirically at the onset of symptoms by titrating drug dosage to the historical assessment of functional disability, although some investigators utilize exercise testing with or without measurement of oxygen consumption to gauge the effect of medications on symptoms. Furthermore, there is no consensus on the sequence with which beta blockers and verapamil should be administered; usually a trial with one or the other drug is initiated and should a benefit fail to result, the patient is converted to the other drug. Excessive dosages of either a beta blocker or verapamil should be avoided (e.g., >480 mg/day of verapamil), since such drug levels rarely achieve beneficial results and can incur side effects. There is no evidence that the effect of using beta blockers and verapamil together is superior to that of either drug alone, and this combination should be avoided.

At selected centers, disopyramide has been an alternative medication for patients with obstructive HCM and severe symptoms otherwise unresponsive to standard therapy.[6,162–164] Disopyramide may reduce outflow gradient and improve symptoms by virtue of its negative inotropic properties, although the potential for proarrhythmia has constituted an obstacle to its use in HCM for some investigators. The aforementioned negative inotropic agents have been shown to reduce outflow gradient in HCM by slowing left ventricular ejection acceleration.[164]

Some patients with particularly severe symptoms of heart failure despite treatment with beta blockers or verapamil may show symptomatic improvement with the judicious addition of diuretic agents.[3] The aforementioned therapeutic considerations apply to those patients with HCM in whom symptoms of congestive failure typically occur in the presence of normal or hyperdynamic systolic performance. Conversely, in the subgroup of patients experiencing congestive symptoms secondary to systolic dysfunction (i.e., end-stage HCM)[1,4–6,61,159] therapeutic strategy is similar to that employed for heart failure in other diseases with impaired systolic function, including the use of diuretics, angiotensin-converting enzyme inhibitors, and digitalis; ultimately, heart transplantation should be considered in this subgroup of patients[61,165] (see Chap. 22).

Prevention of Infective Endocarditis

Bacterial endocarditis, a recognized complication of HCM, is virtually confined to patients with the obstructive form of the disease (and mitral valve systolic anterior motion) with a prevalence of about 0.5 percent.[166] Vegetations most commonly involve the anterior mitral leaflet or septal endocardium at the site of mitral valve contact (likely a consequence of the high-velocity outflow jet) and less commonly the aortic valve.[166,167]

Atrial Fibrillation

Atrial fibrillation is a particularly important arrhythmia in HCM,[134,168,169] reportedly occurring in up to about 20 percent of patients followed longitudinally with this disease.[122,134] Atrial fibrillation is associated with an increased risk for systemic thromboembolism, heart failure, and death.[1,3–6] Of note, HCM patients with atrial fibrillation usually show substantial left atrial enlargement but, paradoxically, usually only relatively mild left ventricular hypertrophy.[168] Onset of atrial fibrillation may importantly impair the clinical course in HCM, probably because absence of the atrial systolic contribution to ventricular filling is critical to cardiac function in patients with such poorly compliant ventricles. In many patients, however, chronic atrial fibrillation appears to be reasonably well tolerated as long as ventricular rate is controlled.[169] Beta-adrenergic blocking agents or verapamil are usually efficacious in controlling heart rate in patients with chronic atrial fibrillation. Recurrent atrial fibrillation is managed by restoring sinus rhythm with electrical cardioversion, if necessary, or alternatively by drugs—with amiodarone probably the most effective antiarrhythmic agent for the prevention of recurrent atrial fibrillation. Because of the risk of peripheral embolism and stroke, anticoagulant therapy should be administered (and continued indefinitely) in most patients once atrial fibrillation has been documented.

SURGICAL TREATMENT

Operation is regarded as the standard treatment for those HCM patients with obstruction to left ventricular outflow under basal conditions (gradient ≥50 mmHg), and severe drug-refractory symptoms.[1,3–6,159,170–186] Therefore surgery is performed to relieve incapacitating symptoms and subaortic obstruction by normalizing the markedly increased systolic intraventricular pressures.[1,3–6,159,170–186] General agreement is lacking, however, as to whether symptomatic patients with marked outflow gradients—which are present solely or predominantly under provokable conditions such as exercise or with maneuvers in the catheterization laboratory (e.g., isoproterenol infusion, amyl nitrite inhalation, or Valsalva maneuver)—are appropriate operative candidates.[2,4,6,171,179]

Ventricular septal myotomy-myectomy (Morrow operation)[170] (Fig. 67-17) is the surgical procedure of choice; a small amount of muscle is removed from the basal anterior septum (usually about 2 to 6 g) through an aortotomy. However, mitral valve replacement has been employed[177,179,184] in selected patients when the operative site for muscular resection in the basal anterior portion of the septum is relatively thin (i.e., ≤18 mm) or when the distribution of septal hypertrophy is atypical.[179]

Occasionally, patients have outflow obstruction from a mechanism other than mitral valve systolic anterior motion. For example, anomalous papillary muscle insertion directly into anterior mitral leaflet without the interposition of the chordae tendineae (Fig. 67-10) producing muscular mid-ventricular obstruction[19] should always be contemplated prior to surgery, since the operative strategy may require a more extensive myectomy[186] or possibly mitral valve replacement.[19] Suture plication of the anterior mitral leaflet (in combination with myotomy-myectomy) has also been introduced in patients judged to have a greatly enlarged mitral valve, so as to reduce the likelihood that mitral valve systolic anterior motion will persist postoperatively.[185]

Intraoperative 2D echocardiography is an important guide to mapping the distribution and magnitude of septal hypertrophy [179,187,188] and determining how the muscle resection should be tailored to the distribution of septal hypertrophy in the individual patient to achieve the desired hemodynamic result and avoid iatrogenic complications such as ventricular septal defect. Transesophageal echocardiography (Chap. 13) may also be useful in assessing morphologic and functional abnormalities during surgery, particularly of the mitral valve.[187,188]

Results from a number of North American and European centers employing septal myotomy-myectomy over the past 40 years, in about 2000 patients, have demonstrated salutary hemodynamic as well as symptomatic effects.[1,3–6,159,170–183,189] Operative mortality at the most experienced centers has improved over the past several years and is presently less than 1 to 2 percent.[1,5] Older patients with associated cardiac lesions, such as coronary artery disease requiring bypass grafting, may be at greater operative risk.[190]

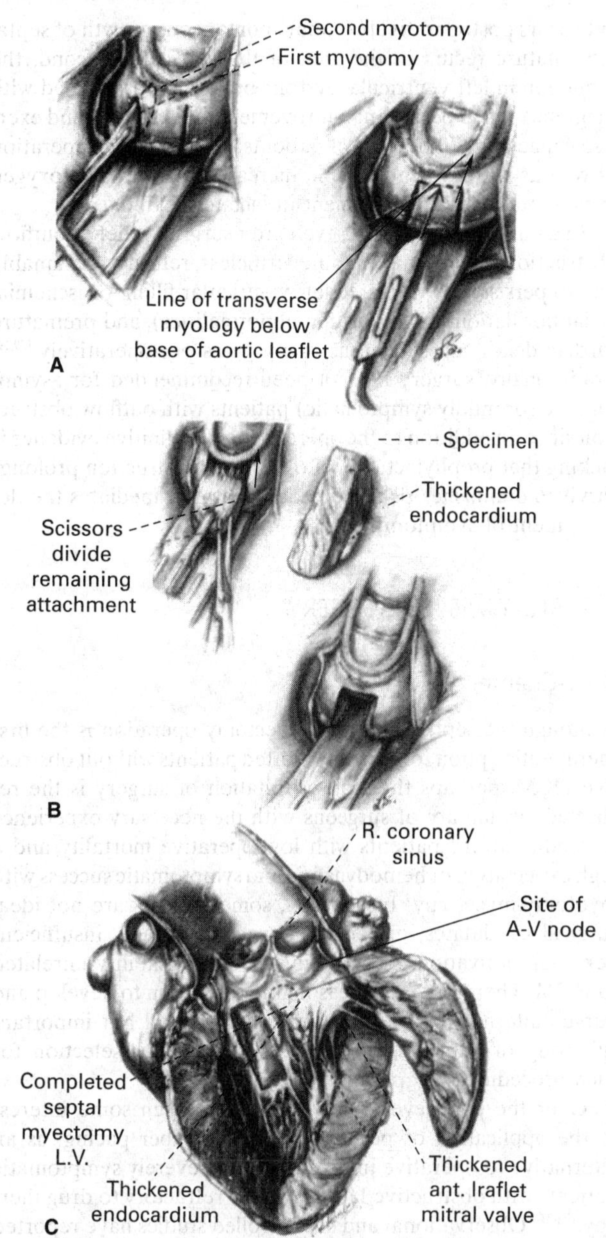

FIGURE 67-17 Illustration of ventricular septal myotomy-myectomy operation (Morrow procedure). *A.* Two vertical, parallel myotomies are made in the cephalad portion of the septum about 1 cm apart. Transverse incision is then made, connecting the two parallel myotomies. *B.* Attachments of the muscle bar to the septum are divided; this segment of muscle is isolated and then excised. *C.* After completion of the myotomy-myectomy, a rectangular channel about 4 cm long and 2 cm wide is evident extending from the aortic annulus to a point just distal to the caudal margins of the mitral leaflets. (From Maron BJ et al.[176] with permission from the authors and the *European Heart Journal.*)

Several important effects of operation have been defined in patients with HCM.[1,3–6,159,170–183,189] First, in more than 90 percent of patients, myotomy-myectomy (or mitral valve replacement) abolishes or substantially reduces the basal subaortic gradient and mitral valve systolic anterior motion without importantly compromising left ventricular function; this consequence of surgery appears to be permanent, with no evidence that the gradient recurs postoperatively or that spontaneous growth of septal musculature recurs in the area of the resection. Second, the reduction in left ventricular systolic pressure is associated with a significant and persistent improvement in symptoms and exercise capacity in 70 percent of patients ≥5 years after operation as well as with a demonstrable increase in myocardial oxygen consumption and improvement in lactate metabolism.[191]

In a minority of patients, even after surgical relief of outflow obstruction, symptoms may nevertheless return (presumably due to persistently impaired left ventricular filling or ischemia, atrial fibrillation, or conduction abnormalities), and premature cardiac death can still ensue many years postoperatively.[189,191] Traditionally, surgery has not been recommended for asymptomatic (or mildly symptomatic) patients with outflow obstruction since, in addition to the operative risk, definitive evidence is lacking that prophylactic relief of outflow obstruction prolongs survival, diminishes risk for sudden death, or mediates the development of symptoms.

ALTERNATIVES TO SURGERY

Dual-Chamber Pacing

Although the septal myotomy-myectomy operation is the first therapeutic option for severely limited patients without obstructive HCM, perhaps the major limitation of surgery is the restricted availability of surgeons with the necessary experience to readily afford patients with low operative mortality and a high expectation of hemodynamic and symptomatic success with myotomy-myectomy. In addition, some patients are not ideal surgical candidates, either due to advanced age, insufficient personal motivation, or a limiting medical disability unrelated to HCM. Therefore it is a reasonable aspiration to develop and pursue alternatives to operation for this small but important subgroup of patients. However, proper patient selection for such procedures is a paramount consideration.

Over the past several years there has been some interest in the application of permanent dual-chamber pacing, as an alternative to operative intervention, for severely symptomatic patients with obstructive HCM who are refractory to drug therapy.[192–194] Observational and uncontrolled studies have reported pacing to be associated with reduction in outflow gradient and amelioration of symptoms in many patients over relatively short time periods.[172–174] However, this reported symptomatic benefit has not been consistently accompanied by improved exercise tolerance documented by objective parameters (e.g., treadmill exercise duration and measured oxygen consumption). Randomized, double-blind, crossover pacing studies have shown that the subjectively perceived symptomatic improvement reported by patients is largely due to a placebo effect.[195–197] In addition, the effect of pacing on outflow gradient and symptoms is variable and reduction in obstruction is often much more modest than that achieved with surgery.[196,198] Other laboratory catheterization studies report dual-chamber pacing to have deleterious effects on left ventricular systolic and diastolic function.[199–201] For these reasons and because the underlying HCM disease process and the risk for sudden death do not appear to be altered by permanent dual-chamber pacing, this potential treatment modality cannot be regarded as a primary treatment for the diverse clinical and functional spectrum of HCM.[196] However, there may well be a therapeutic role for certain subsets of patients with this disease.[196,201] In one randomized study, those patients ≥65 years old showed the most convincing benefit from pacing.[196]

Alcohol Septal Ablation

A second, recently introduced potential alternative to surgery is alcohol septal ablation, in which about 2 mL of alcohol is injected directly into the first septal perforator coronary artery for the purpose of producing an MI, septal thinning, and reduced mitral valve systolic anterior motion.[202–205] This procedure is intended to mimic the morphologic and functional consequences of ventricular septal myotomy-myectomy. At present the septal ablation technique is associated with a risk similar to that of surgery but is capable of producing a substantial reduction in the basal gradient. As yet, there is little objective substantiation for the improvement in symptoms reported by many patients over short-term follow-up. This is of particular importance in assessing symptomatic and functional changes for a disease in which pathophysiology is complex and symptoms are variable, often difficult to assess by history, and subject to a placebo effect.[196] As is the case with pacing, alcohol ablation should not be regarded as a primary treatment for the disease or one capable of reducing the risk of sudden death. Indeed, there is concern[206,207] that this intervention could paradoxically increase the future long-term risk for life-threatening ventricular tachyarrhythmias and sudden death—a risk directly attributable to the intramyocardial scar produced by alcohol ablation (which is not present following myotomy-myectomy) in a patient population that already harbors an arrhythmogenic substrate and often a particularly long period of risk.

References

1. Maron BJ. Hypertrophic cardiomyopathy. *Lancet* 1997; 350: 127–133.
2. Braunwald E, Lambrew CT, Rockoff D, et al. Idiopathic hypertrophic subaortic stenosis: I. A description of the disease based upon an analysis of 64 patients. *Circulation* 1964; 30(suppl IV):3–217.
3. Maron BJ, Bonow RO, Cannon RO, et al. Hypertrophic cardiomyopathy: Interrelation of clinical manifestations, pathophysiology, and therapy. *N Engl J Med* 1987; 316:780–789, 844–852.
4. Wigle ED, Sasson Z, Henderson MA, et al. Hypertrophic cardiomyopathy: The importance of the site and extent of hypertrophy—A review. *Prog Cardiovasc Dis* 1985; 28:1–83.
5. Spirito P, Seidman CE, McKenna WJ, Maron BJ. Management of hypertrophic cardiomyopathy. *N Engl J Med* 1997; 30:775–785.
6. Wigle ED, Rakowski H, Kimball BP, et al. Hypertrophic cardiomyopathy: Clinical spectrum and treatment. *Circulation* 1995; 92:1680–1692.
7. Maron BJ, Epstein SE: Hypertrophic cardiomyopathy: A discussion of nomenclature. *Am J Cardiol* 1979; 43:1242–1244.
8. Marian AJ, Roberts R. Recent advances in the molecular genetics of hypertrophic cardiomyopathy. *Circulation* 1995; 92:1336–1347.
9. Schwartz K, Carrier L, Guicheney P, et al. Molecular basis of familial cardiomyopathies. *Circulation* 1995; 91:532–540.
10. Niimura H, Bachinski LL, Sangwatanaroj S, et al. Mutations in the gene for human cardiac myosin-binding protein C and late-onset familial hypertrophic cardiomyopathy. *N Engl J Med* 1998; 338:1248–1257.
11. Ciró E, Nichols PF, Maron BJ. Heterogeneous morphologic ex-

pression of genetically transmitted hypertrophic cardiomyopathy: Two-dimensional echocardiographic analysis. *Circulation* 1983; 67:1227–1233.
12. Maron BJ, Gottdiener JS, Epstein SE. Patterns and significance of distribution of left ventricular hypertrophy in hypertrophic cardiomyopathy: A wide-angle, two-dimensional echocardiographic study of 125 patients. *Am J Cardiol* 1981; 48:418–428.
13. Spirito P, Maron BJ, Bonow RO, et al. Severe functional limitation in patients with hypertrophic cardiomyopathy and only mild localized left ventricular hypertrophy. *J Am Coll Cardiol* 1979; 44:401–412.
14. Webb JG, Sasson Z, Rakowski H, et al. Apical hypertrophic cardiomyopathy: Clinical follow-up and diagnostic correlates. *J Am Coll Cardiol* 1990; 15:83–90.
15. Louie EK, Maron BJ. Apical hypertrophic cardiomyopathy: Clinical and two-dimensional echocardiographic assessment. *Ann Intern Med* 1987; 106:663–670.
16. Roberts CS, Roberts WC. Morphologic features. In: Zipes DP, Rowlands DJ, eds. *Progress in Cardiology 2/2.* Philadelphia: Lea & Febiger; 1989:3.
17. Olsen EG. Anatomic and light microscopic characterization of hypertrophic obstructive and non-obstructive cardiomyopathy. *Eur Heart J* 1983; 4 (suppl F):1–8.
18. Klues HG, Schiffers A, Maron BJ. Phenotypic spectrum and patterns of left ventricular hypertrophy in hypertrophic cardiomyopathy: Morphologic observations and significance as assessed by two-dimensional echocardiography in 600 patients. *J Am Coll Cardiol* 1995; 26:1699–1708.
19. Klues HG, Roberts WC, Maron BJ. Anomalous insertion of papillary muscle directly into anterior mitral leaflet in hypertrophic cardiomyopathy: Significance in producing left ventricular outflow obstruction. *Circulation* 1991; 84:1188–1197.
20. Klues HG, Maron BJ, Dollar AL, et al. Diversity of structural mitral valve alterations in hypertrophic cardiomyopathy. *Circulation* 1992; 85:1651–1660.
21. Lewis JF, Maron BJ. Elderly patients with hypertrophic cardiomyopathy: A subset with distinctive left ventricular morphology and progressive clinical course late in life. *J Am Coll Cardiol* 1989; 13:36–45.
22. Maron BJ, Moller JH, Seidman CE, et al. Impact of laboratory molecular diagnosis on contemporary diagnostic criteria for genetically transmitted cardiovascular diseases: Hypertrophic cardiomyopathy, long-QT syndrome, and Marfan syndrome. *Circulation* 1998; 98:1460–1471.
23. Liouville H. Rétrécissement ventriculo-aortique. *Gazette Med Paris* 1869; 24:161–163.
24. Schmincke A. Über linseitige muskulöse Conusstenosen. *Dtsch Med Wochenschr* 1907; 33:2082.
25. Teare D. Asymmetrical hypertrophy of the heart in young adults. *Br Heart J* 1958; 20:1–18.
26. Maron BJ, Gardin JM, Flack JM, et al. Prevalence of hypertrophic cardiomyopathy in a general population of young adults: Echocardiographic analysis of 4111 subjects in the CARDIA study. *Circulation* 1995; 92:785–789.
27. Maron BJ, Peterson EE, Maron MS, et al. Prevalence of hypertrophic cardiomyopathy in an outpatient population referred for echocardiographic study. *Am J Cardiol* 1994; 73:577–580.
28. Spirito P, Chiarella F, Carratino L, et al. Clinical course and prognosis of hypertrophic cardiomyopathy in an outpatient population. *N Engl J Med* 1989; 320:749–755.
29. Shapiro LM, Zezulka A. Hypertrophic cardiomyopathy: A common disease with a good prognosis: Five year experience of a district general hospital. *Br Heart J* 1983; 50:530–533.
30. Maron BJ, Mathenge R, Casey SA, et al. Clinical profile of hypertrophic cardiomyopathy identified de novo in rural communities. *J Am Coll Cardiol* 1999; 33:1590–1595.
31. Rosenzweig A, Watkins H, Hwang D-S, et al. Preclinical diagnosis of familial hypertrophic cardiomyopathy by genetic analysis of blood lymphocytes. *N Engl J Med* 1991; 325:1753–1760.
32. Yamaguchi H, Ishimura T, Nishiyama S, et al. Hypertrophic nonobstructive cardiomyopathy with giant negative T waves (apical hypertrophy): Ventriculographic and echocardiographic features in 30 patients. *Am J Cardiol* 1979; 44:401–412.
33. Ando H, Imaizumi T, Urabe Y, et al. Apical segmental dysfunction in hypertrophic cardiomyopathy: Subgroup with unique clinical features. *J Am Coll Cardiol* 1990; 16:1579–1588.
34. Koga Y, Itaya K-I, Toshima H. Prognosis of hypertrophic cardiomyopathy. *Am Heart J* 1984; 108:351–359.
35. Maron BJ, Spirito P, Wesley Y, et al. Development and progression of left ventricular hypertrophy in children with hypertrophic cardiomyopathy. *N Engl J Med* 1986; 315:610–614.
36. Charron P, Dubourg O, Desnos M, et al. Diagnostic value of electrocardiography and echocardiography for familial hypertrophic cardiomyopathy in a genotyped adult population. *Circulation* 1997; 96:214–219.
37. Charron P, Dubourg O, Desnos M, et al. Diagnostic value of electrocardiography and echocardiography for familial hypertrophic cardiomyopathy in genotyped children. *Eur Heart J* 1998; 19:1377–1382.
38. Watkins H, McKenna WJ, Thierfelder L, et al. The role of cardiac troponin T and α tropomyosin mutations in hypertrophic cardiomyopathy. *N Engl J Med* 1995; 332:1058–1064.
39. Moolman JC, Corfield VA, Posen B, et al. Sudden death due to troponin T mutations. *J Am Coll Cardiol* 1997; 29:549–555.
40. Maron BJ, Niimura H, Casey SA, et al. Hypertrophic cardiomyopathy in adult patients without left ventricular hypertrophy: Genotype–phenotype correlations for cardiac myosin binding protein-C mutations (abstr). *Circulation* 1998; 98(suppl I): I-596–I-597.
41. Shapiro LM, McKenna WJ. Distribution of left ventricular hypertrophy in hypertrophic cardiomyopathy: A two-dimensional echocardiographic study. *J Am Coll Cardiol* 1983; 2:437–444.
42. Maron BJ, Epstein SE, Roberts WC. Hypertrophic cardiomyopathy and transmural myocardial infarction without significant atherosclerosis of the extramural coronary arteries. *Am J Cardiol* 1979; 43:1086–1102.
43. Klues HG, Roberts WC, Maron BJ. Morphologic determinants of echocardiographic patterns of mitral valve systolic anterior motion in obstructive hypertrophic cardiomyopathy. *Circulation* 1993; 87:1570–1579.
44. Louie EK, Maron BJ. Hypertrophic cardiomyopathy with extreme increase in left ventricular wall thickness: Functional and morphologic features and clinical significance. *J Am Coll Cardiol* 1986; 8:57–65.
45. Maron BJ, Gross BJ, Stark SI. Extreme left ventricular hypertrophy. *Circulation* 1995; 92:2748.
46. Charron P, Dubourg O, Desnos M, et al. Clinical features and prognostic implications of familial hypertrophic cardiomyopathy related to the cardiac myosin-binding protein C gene. *Circulation* 1998; 97:2230–2236.
47. Lewis JF, Maron BJ. Hypertrophic cardiomyopathy characterized by marked hypertrophy of the posterior left ventricular free wall: Significance and clinical implications. *J Am Coll Cardiol* 1991; 18:421–428.
48. Alfonso F, Nihoyannopoulos P, Steward J, et al. Clinical significance of giant negative T waves in hypertrophic cardiomyopathy. *J Am Coll Cardiol* 1990; 15:965–971.
49. Sakamoto T, Tei C, Murayama M, et al. Giant T wave inversion as a manifestation of asymmetrical apical hypertrophy (AAH) of the left ventricle: Echocardiographic and ultrasono-cardiotomographic study. *Jpn Heart J* 1976; 17:611–616.
50. Maron BJ, Bonow RO, Seshagiri TN, et al. Hypertrophic cardiomyopathy with ventricular septal hypertrophy localized to the

apical region of the left ventricle (apical hypertrophic cardiomyopathy). *Am J Cardiol* 1982; 49:1838–1848.

51. Pelliccia A, Maron BJ, Spataro A, et al. The upper limit of physiologic cardiac hypertrophy in highly trained elite athletes. *N Engl J Med* 1991; 324:295–301.
52. Maron BJ, Pelliccia A, Spirito P. Cardiac disease in young trained athletes: Insights into methods for distinguishing athlete's heart from structural heart disease with particular emphasis on hypertrophic cardiomyopathy. *Circulation* 1995; 91:1596–1601.
53. Maron BJ, Verter J, Kapur S. Disproportionate ventricular septal thickening in the developing normal human heart. *Circulation* 1978; 57:520–526.
54. Skinner JR, Manzoor A, Hayes AM, et al. A regional study of presentation and outcome of hypertrophic cardiomyopathy in infants. *Heart* 1997; 77:229–223.
55. Maron BJ, Tajik AJ, Ruttenberg HD, et al. Hypertrophic cardiomyopathy in infants. Clinical features and natural history. *Circulation* 1982; 65:7–17.
56. Schaffer MS, Freedom RM, Rowe RD. Hypertrophic cardiomyopathy presenting before 2 years of age in 13 patients. *Ped Cardiol* 1983; 4:113–119.
57. Maron BJ. Hypertrophic cardiomyopathy. In: Allen HD, Gutgesell HP, Clark EB, Driscoll DJ, eds. *Moss and Adam's Heart Disease in Infants, Children and Adolescents,* 6th ed. Baltimore, MD: Lippincott Williams & Wilkins; in press.
58. Spirito P, Maron BJ. Absence of progression of left ventricular hypertrophy in adult patients with hypertrophic cardiomyopathy. *J Am Coll Cardiol* 1987; 9:1013–1017.
59. Panza JA, Maris TJ, Maron BJ. Development and determinants of dynamic obstruction to left ventricular outflow in young patients with hypertrophic cardiomyopathy. *Circulation* 1992; 85:1398–1405.
60. Panza JA, Maron BJ. Relation of electrocardiographic abnormalities to evolving left ventricular hypertrophy in hypertrophic cardiomyopathy. *Am J Cardiol* 1989; 63:1258–1265.
61. Maron BJ, Spirito P. Implications of left ventricular remodeling in hypertrophic cardiomyopathy. *Am J Cardiol* 1998; 81:1339–1344.
62. Spirito P, Maron BJ. Relation between extent of left ventricular hypertrophy and age in patients with hypertrophic cardiomyopathy. *J Am Coll Cardiol* 1989; 13:820–823.
63. Tanaka M, Fujiwara H, Onodera T, et al. Quantitative analysis of myocardial fibrosis in normals, hypertensive hearts, and hypertrophic cardiomyopathy. *Br Heart J* 1986; 55:575–581.
64. Ferrans VJ, Morrow AG, Roberts WC. Myocardial ultrastructure in idiopathic hypertrophic subaortic stenosis. A study of operatively excised left ventricular outflow tract muscle in 14 patients. *Circulation* 1972; 45:769–792.
65. Maron BJ, Roberts WC. Quantitative analysis of cardiac muscle cell disorganization in the ventricular septum of patients with hypertrophic cardiomyopathy. *Circulation* 1979; 59:689–706.
66. Maron BJ, Anan TJ, Roberts WC. Quantitative analysis of the distribution of cardiac muscle cell disorganization in the left ventricular wall of patients with hypertrophic cardiomyopathy. *Circulation* 1981; 63:882–894.
67. St. John Sutton MG, Lie JT, Anderson KR, et al. Histopathological specificity of hypertrophic obstructive cardiomyopathy. *Br Heart J* 1980; 44:433–443.
68. Fujiwara H, Kawai C, Hamashima Y. Myocardial fascicle and fiber disarray in 25 μ-thick sections. *Circulation* 1979; 59:1293–1298.
69. Maron BJ, Wolfson JK, Epstein SE, et al. Intramural ("small vessel") coronary artery disease in hypertrophic cardiomyopathy. *J Am Coll Cardiol* 1986; 8:545–557.
70. Tanaka M, Fujiwara H, Onodera T, et al. Quantitative analysis of narrowings of intramyocardial small arteries in normal hearts, hypertensive hearts, and hearts with hypertrophic cardiomyopathy. *Circulation* 1987; 75:1130–1139.
71. Maron BJ, Wolfson JK, Roberts WC. Relation between extent of cardiac muscle cell disorganization and left ventricular wall thickness in hypertrophic cardiomyopathy. *Am J Cardiol* 1992; 70:785–790.
72. Factor SM, Butany J, Sole MJ, et al. Pathologic fibrosis and matrix connective tissue in the subaortic myocardium of patients with hypertrophic cardiomyopathy. *J Am Coll Cardiol* 1991; 17:1343–1351.
73. Shirani J, Pick R, Roberts WC, et al. Morphology and significance of the left ventricular collagen network in young patients with hypertrophic cardiomyopathy and sudden cardiac death. *J Am Coll Cardiol.* 2000; 35:36–44.
74. Maron BJ, Shen W-K, Link MS, et al. Efficacy of implantable cardioverter-defibrillators for the prevention of sudden death in patients with hypertrophic cardiomyopathy. *N Engl J Med.* 2000; 342:365–373.
75. O'Gara PT, Bonow RO, Maron BJ, et al. Myocardial perfusion abnormalities in patients with hypertrophic cardiomyopathy: Assessment with thallium-201 emission computed tomography. *Circulation* 1987; 76:1214–1223.
76. Watkins H, Rosenzweig A, Hwang D-S, et al. Characteristics and prognostic implications of myosin missense mutations in familial hypertrophic cardiomyopathy. *N Engl J Med* 1992; 326:1108–1114.
77. Maron BJ, Nichols PF, Pickle LW, et al. Patterns of inheritance in hypertrophic cardiomyopathy: Assessment of M-mode and two-dimensional echocardiography. *Am J Cardiol* 1984; 53:1087–1094.
78. Coviello DA, Maron BJ, Spirito P, et al. Clinical features of hypertrophic cardiomyopathy caused by mutation of a "hot spot" in the alpha-tropomyosin gene. *J Am Coll Cardiol* 1997; 29:635–640.
79. Morgensen J, Klausen IbC, Pedersen AK, et al. α-Cardiac actin is a novel disease gene in familial hypertrophic cardiomyopathy. *J Clin Invest* 1999; 103:R39–R43.
80. Kimura A, Harada H, Park J-E, et al. Mutations in the cardiac troponin I gene associated with hypertrophic cardiomyopathy. *Nature Genet* 1997; 16:379–382.
81. Yamauchi-Takihara K, Nakajima-Taniguchi C, Matsui H, et al. Cardiomyopathy associated with mutations in the α-tropomyosin gene. *Heart* 1996; 76:63–65.
82. Anan R, Greve G, Thierfelder L, et al. Prognostic implications of novel β cardiac myosin heavy chain gene mutations that cause familial hypertrophic cardiomyopathy. *J Clin Invest* 1994; 93:280–285.
83. Flavigny J, Richard P, Isnard R, et al. Identification of two novel mutations in the ventricular regulatory myosin light chain gene (MYL2) associated with familial and classical forms of hypertrophic cardiomyopathy. *J Mol Med* 1998; 76:208–214.
84. Thierfelder L, Watkins H, MacRae C, et al. α-Tropomyosin and cardiac troponin T mutations cause familial hypertrophic cardiomyopathy: A disease of the sarcomere. *Cell* 1994; 77:701–712.
85. Maron BJ, Lipson LC, Roberts WC, et al. "Malignant" hypertrophic cardiomyopathy: Identification of a subgroup of families with unusually frequent premature death. *Am J Cardiol* 1978; 41:1133–1140.
86. Maron BJ, Shirani J, Poliac LC, et al. Sudden death in young competitive athletes: Clinical, demographic and pathological profiles. *JAMA* 1996; 276:199–204.
87. McKenna WJ, Stewart JT, Nihoyannopoulos P, et al. Hypertrophic cardiomyopathy without hypertrophy: Two families with myocardial disarray in the absence of increased myocardial mass. *Br Heart J* 1990; 63:287–290.
88. Maron BJ, Kragel AH, Roberts WC. Sudden death due to hypertrophic cardiomyopathy in the absence of increased left ventricular mass. *Br Heart J* 1990; 63:308–310.
89. Maron BJ, Isner JM, McKenna WJ. Hypertrophic cardiomyopa-

thy, myocarditis and other myopericardial disease, and mitral valve prolapse. Task Force 3. In: 26th Bethesda Conference. Recommendations for determining eligibility for competition in athletes with cardiovascular abnormalities. *J Am Coll Cardiol* 1994; 24:880–885.
90. Lechin M, Quiñones MA, Omran A, et al. Angiotensin-I converting enzyme genotypes and left ventricular hypertrophy in patients with hypertrophic cardiomyopathy. *Circulation* 1995; 92:1808–1812.
91. Cannon RO, Rosing DR, Maron BJ, et al. Myocardial ischemia in hypertrophic cardiomyopathy: Contribution of inadequate vasodilator reserve and elevated left ventricular filling pressures. *Circulation* 1985; 71:234–243.
92. Maron BJ, Spirito P, Green KJ, et al. Noninvasive assessment of left ventricular diastolic function by pulsed Doppler echocardiography in patients with hypertrophic cardiomyopathy. *J Am Coll Cardiol* 1987; 10:733–742.
93. Bonow RO, Fredrick TM, Bacharach SL, et al. Atrial systole and left ventricular filling in patients with hypertrophic cardiomyopathy: Effect of verapamil. *Am J Cardiol* 1983; 51:1386–1391.
94. Pollick C, Rakowski H, Wigle ED. Muscular subaortic stenosis: The quantitative relationship between systolic anterior motion and pressure gradient. *Circulation* 1984; 69:43–49.
95. Maron BJ, Epstein SE. Clinical significance and therapeutic implications of the left ventricular outflow tract pressure gradient in hypertrophic cardiomyopathy. *Am J Cardiol* 1986; 11:752–756.
96. Sherrid MV, Chu CK, Delia E, et al. An echocardiographic study of the fluid mechanics of obstruction in hypertrophic cardiomyopathy. *J Am Coll Cardiol* 1993; 22:816–825.
97. Cape EG, Simons D, Jimoh A, et al. Chordal geometry determines the shape and extent of systolic anterior motion. *J Am Coll Cardiol* 1989; 13:1438–1448.
98. Klues HG, Leuner C, Kuhn H. Hypertrophic obstructive cardiomyopathy: No increase of the gradient during exercise. *J Am Coll Cardiol* 1991; 19:527–533.
99. Briguori C, Betocchi S, Romano M, et al. Exercise capacity in hypertrophic cardiomyopathy depends on left ventricular diastolic function. *Am J Cardiol* 1999; 84:309–315.
100. Lazzeroni E, Picano E, Morozzi L, et al. Dipyridamole-induced ischemia as a prognostic marker of future adverse cardiac events in adult patients with hypertrophic cardiomypathy. *Circulation* 1997; 96:4268–4272.
101. Yamada M, Elliott PM, Kaski JC, et al. Dipyradimole stress thallium-201 perfusion abnormalities in patients with hypertrophic cardiomyopathy: Relationship to clinical presentation and outcome. *Eur Heart J* 1998; 19:500–507.
102. Spirito P, Maron BJ. Patterns of systolic anterior motin of the mitral valve in hypertrophic cardiomyopathy: Assessment by two-dimensional echocardiography. *Am J Cardiol* 1984; 54:1039–1046.
103. Maron BJ, Harding AM, Spirito P, et al. Systolic anterior motion of the posterior mitral leaflet: A previously unrecognized cause of dynamic subaortic obstruction in hypertrophic cardiomyopathy. *Circulation* 1983; 68:282–293.
104. Schwammenthal E, Block M, Schwartzkopff B, et al. Prediction of the site and severity of obstruction in hypertrophic cardiomyopathy by color flow mapping and continuous wave Doppler echocardiography. *J Am Coll Cardiol* 1992; 20:964–972.
105. Panza JA, Petrone RK, Fananapazir L, et al. Utility of continuous wave Doppler in noninvasive assessment of the left ventricular outflow tract reassure gradient in patients with hypertrophic cardiomyopathy. *J Am Coll Cardiol* 1992; 19:91–99.
106. Petrone RK, Klues HG, Panza JA, et al. Significance of the occurrence of mitral valve prolapse in patients with hypertrophic cardiomyopathy. *J Am Coll Cardiol* 1992; 20:55–61.
107. Fighali S, Krajcer Z, Edelman S, et al. Progression of hypertrophic cardiomyopathy into a hypokinetic left ventricle: Higher incidence in patients with midventricular obstruction. *J Am Coll Cardiol* 1987; 9:288–294.
108. Fiddler GI, Tajik AJ, Weidman WH, et al. Idiopathic hypertrophic subaortic stenosis in the young. *Am J Cardiol* 1978; 42:793–799.
109. Maron BJ, McIntosh CL, Klues HG, et al. Morphologic basis for obstruction to right ventricular outflow in hypertrophic cardiomyopathy. *Am J Cardiol* 1993; 71:1089–1094.
110. Lele SS, Thomson HL, Seo H, et al. Exercise capacity in hypertrophic cardiomyopathy: Role of stroke volume limitation, heart rate and diastolic filling characteristics. *Circulation* 1995; 92:2886–2894.
111. Frenneaux MP, Porter A, Caforio ALP, et al. Determinants of exercise capacity in hypertrophic cardiomyopathy. *J Am Coll Cardiol* 1992; 19:1521–1526.
112. Chikamori T, Counihan PJ, Doi YL, et al. Mechanisms of exercise limitations in hypertrophic cardiomyopathy. *J Am Coll Cardiol* 1992; 19:507–512.
113. Spirito P, Maron BJ. Relation between extent of left ventricular hypertrophy and diastolic filling abnormalities in hypertrophic cardiomyopathy. *J Am Coll Cardiol* 1990; 15:808–813.
114. Pasternac A, Noble J, Streulens Y, et al. Pathophysiology of chest pain in patients with cardiomyopathies and normal coronary arteries. *Circulation* 1982; 65:778–789.
115. Elliott PM, Kaski JC, Prasad K, et al. Chest pain during daily life in patients with hypertrophic cardiomyopathy: An ambulatory electrocardiographic study. *Eur Heart J* 1996; 17:1056–1064.
116. Maron BJ, Wolfson JK, Ciró E, et al. Relation of electrocardiographic abnormalities and patterns of left ventricular hypertrophy identified by two-dimensional echocardiography in patients with hypertrophic cardiomyopathy. *Am J Cardiol* 1983; 51:189–194.
117. Glover DW, Maron BJ. Profile of preparticipation cardiovascular screening for high school athletes. *JAMA* 1998; 279:1817–1819.
118. Maron BJ, Thompson PD, Puffer JC, et al. Cardiovascular preparticipation screening of competitive athletes. *Circulation* 1996; 94:850–856.
119. Pfister GC, Puffer JC, Maron BJ. Preparticipation cardiovascular screening for U.S. collegiate student-athletes. *JAMA* 2000; 283:1597–1599.
120. Corrado D, Basso C, Schiavon M, et al. Screening for hypertrophic cardiomyopathy in young athletes. *N Engl J Med* 1998; 339:364–369.
121. Kyriakidis M, Triposkiadis F, Anastassakis A, et al. Hypertrophic cardiomyopathy in Greece: Clinical course and outcome. *Chest* 1998; 114:1091–1096.
122. Maron BJ, Casey SA, Poliac LC, et al. Clinical course of hypertrophic cardiomyopathy in a regional United States cohort. *JAMA* 1999; 281:650–655.
123. Maron BJ, Spirito P. Impact of patient selection biases on the perception of hypertrophic cardiomyopathy and its natural history. *Am J Cardiol* 1993; 72:970–972.
124. Maron BJ, Roberts WC, Epstein SE. Sudden death in hypertrophic cardiomyopathy: A profile of 78 patients. *Circulation* 1982; 67:1388–1394.
125. McKenna WJ, Deanfield JE. Hypertrophic cardiomyopathy: An important cause of sudden death. *Arch Dis Child* 1984; 59:971–975.
126. Hecht GM, Panza JA, Maron BJ. Clinical course of middle-aged asymptomatic patients with hypertrophic cardiomyopathy. *Am J Cardiol* 1992; 69:935–940.
127. Adelman AG, Wigle ED, Ranganathan N, et al. The clinical course in muscular subaortic stenosis: A retrospective and prospective study of 60 hemodynamically proved cases. *Ann Intern Med* 1972; 77:515–525.
128. McKenna WJ, Deanfield JE, Faroqui A, et al. Prognosis in hypertrophic cardiomyopathy: Role of age and clinical electrocardio-

graphic and hemodynamic features. *Am J Cardiol* 1981; 47:532–538.
129. Shah PM, Adelman AG, Wigle ED, et al. The natural (and unnatural) history of hypertrophic obstructive cardiomyopathy. *Circ Res* 1973; 34,35 (suppl II):II-179–II-195.
130. Frank S, Braunwald E. Idiopathic hypertrophic subaortic stenosis: Clinical analysis of 126 patients with emphasis on the natural history. *Circulation* 1968; 37:759–788.
131. Kofflard MJ, Waldstein DJ, Vos J, et al. Prognosis in hypertrophic cardiomyopathy: A retrospective study. *Am J Cardiol* 1993; 72:939–943.
132. Spirito P, Rapezzi C, Autore C, et al. Prognosis in asymptomatic patients with hypertrophic cardiomyopathy and nonsustained ventricular tachycardia. *Circulation* 1994; 90:2743–2747.
133. Cannan CR, Reeder GS, Bailey KR, et al. Natural history of hypertrophic cardiomyopathy: A population-based study, 1976 through 1990. *Circulation* 1995; 92:2488–2499.
134. Cecchi F, Olivotto I, Montereggi A, et al. Hypertrophic cardiomyopathy in Tuscany: Clinical course and outcome in an unselected regional population. *J Am Coll Cardiol* 1995; 26:1529–1536.
135. Takagi E, Yamakado T, Nakano T. Prognosis of completely asymptomatic adult patients with hypertrophic cardiomyopathy. *J Am Coll Cardiol* 1999; 33:206–211.
136. Maki S, Ikeda H, Muro A, et al. Predictors of sudden cardiac death in hypertrophic cardiomyopathy. *Am J Cardiol* 1998; 82:774–778.
137. Maron BJ, Kogan J, Proschan MA, et al. Circadian variability in the occurrence of sudden cardiac death in patients with hypertrophic cardiomyopathy. *J Am Coll Cardiol* 1994; 23:1405–1409.
138. Maron BJ. Cardiovascular risks to young persons on the athletic field. *Ann Intern Med* 1998; 129:379–386.
139. Olivotto I, Maron BJ, Montereggi A, et al. Prognostic value of systemic blood pressure response during exercise in a community-based patient population with hypertrophic cardiomyopathy. *J Am Coll Cardiol* 1999; 33:2044–2051.
140. Sadoul N, Prasas L, Elliott PM, et al. Prospective diagnostic assessment of blood pressure response during exercise in patients with hypertrophic cardiomyopathy. *Circulation* 1997; 96:2987–2991.
141. Nicod P, Polikar R, Peterson KL. Hypertrophic cardiomyopathy and sudden death. *N Engl J Med* 1988; 318:1255–1257.
142. Stafford WJ, Trohman RG, Bilsker M, et al. Cardiac arrest in an adolescent with atrial fibrillation and hypertrophic cardiomyopathy. *J Am Coll Cardiol* 1985; 7:701–704.
143. Krikler DM, Davies MJ, Rowland E, et al. Sudden death in hypertrophic cardiomyopathy: Associated accessory atrioventricular pathways. *Br Heart J* 1980; 43:245–251.
144. Elliott PM, Sharma S, Varnava A, et al. Survival after cardiac arrest in patients with hypertrophic cardiomyopathy. *J Am Coll Cardiol* 1999; 33:1596–1601.
145. Yetman AT, McCrindle BW, MacDonald LC, et al. Myocardial bridging in children with hypertrophic cardiomyopathy—A risk factor for sudden death. *N Engl J Med* 1998; 339:1201–1209.
146. Maron BJ, Fananapazir L. Sudden cardiac death in hypertrophic cardiomyopathy. *Circulation* 1992; 85(suppl I):I-57–I-63.
147. Spirito P, Bellone P, Harris KM, et al. Magnitude of left ventricular hypertrophy predicts sudden death in hypertrophic cardiomyopathy. *N Engl J Med* 2000; 342:1778–1785.
148. Spirito P, Maron BJ. Relation between extent of left ventricular hypertrophy and occurrence of sudden cardiac death in hypertrophic cardiomyopathy. *J Am Coll Cardiol* 1990; 15:1521–2526.
149. Cecchi F, Maron BJ, Epstein SE. Long-term outcome of patients with hypertrophic cardiomyopathy successfully resuscitated after cardiac arrest. *J Am Coll Cardiol* 1989; 13:1283–1288.
150. Kuck K-H, Kunze KP, Schlueter M, et al. Programmed electrical stimulation in hypertrophic cardiomyopathy: Results in patients with and without cardiac arrest or syncope. *Eur Heart J* 1988; 9:177–185.
151. Hecht GM, Klues HG, Roberts WC, et al. Coexistence of sudden cardiac death and end-stage heart failure in familial hypertrophic cardiomyopathy. *J Am Coll Cardiol* 1993; 22:489–497.
152. Maron BJ, Hecht G, Klues HG, et al. Both aborted sudden cardiac death and end-stage phase in hypertrophic cardiomyopathy. *Am J Cardiol* 1993; 72:363–365.
153. Fay WP, Taliercio CP, Ilstrup DM, et al. Natural history of hypertrophic cardiomyopathy in the elderly. *J Am Coll Cardiol* 1990; 16:821–826.
154. Lever HM, Kuram RF, Currie PH, et al. Hypertrophic cardiomyopathy in the elderly: Distinctions from the young based on cardiac shape. *Circulation* 1989; 79:580–589.
155. Lewis JF, Maron BJ. Clinical and morphologic expression of hypertrophic cardiomyopathy in patients ≥65 years of age. *Am J Cardiol* 1994; 73:1105–1111.
156. Chikamori T, Doi YL, Yonezawa Y, et al. Comparison of clinical features in patients ≥60 years of age to those 40 years of age with hypertrophic cardiomyopathy. *Am J Cardiol* 1990; 66:875–877.
157. Silka MJ, Kron J, Dunnigan A, et al. Sudden cardiac death and the use of implantable cardioverter-defibrillators in pediatric patients. *Circulation* 1993; 87:800–807.
158. McKenna WJ, Oakley CM, Krikler DM, et al. Improved survival with amiodarone in patients with hypertrophic cardiomyopathy and ventricular tachycardia. *Br Heart J* 1985; 53:412–416.
159. Louie EK, Edwards LC. Hypertrophic cardiomyopathy. *Prog Cardiovasc Dis* 1994; 36:275–308.
160. Kaltenbach M, Hopf R, Kober G, et al. Treatment of hypertrophic obstructive cardiomyopathy with verapamil. *Br Heart J* 1979; 42:35–42.
161. Rosing DR, Condit JR, Maron BJ, et al. Verapamil therapy: A new approach to the pharmacologic treatment of hypertrophic cardiomyopathy: III. Effects of long-term administration. *Am J Cardiol* 1981; 48:545–553.
162. Sherrid M, Delia E, Dwyer E. Oral disopyramide therapy for obstructive hypertrophic cardiomyopathy. *Am J Cardiol* 1988; 62:1085–1088.
163. Pollick C. Muscular subaortic stenosis: Hemodynamic and clinical improvement after disopyramide. *N Engl J Med* 1982; 307: 997–999.
164. Sherrid MV, Pearle G, Gunsburg DZ. Mechanism of benefit of negative inotropes in obstructive hypertrophic cardiomyopathy. *Circulation* 1998; 97:41–47.
165. Shirani J, Maron BJ, Cannon RO, et al. Clinicopathologic features of hypertrophic cardiomyopathy managed by cardiac transplantation. *Am J Cardiol* 1993; 72:434–440.
166. Spirito P, Rapezzi C, Bellone P, et al. Infective endocarditis in hypertrophic cardiomyopathy: Prevalence, incidence and indications for antibiotic prophylaxis. *Circulation* 1999; 99:2132–2137.
167. Roberts WC, Kishel JC, McIntosh CL, et al. Severe mitral or aortic valve regurgitation, or both, requiring valve replacement for infective endocarditis complicating hypertrophic cardiomyopathy. *J Am Coll Cardiol* 1992; 19:365–377.
168. Spirito P, Lakatos E, Maron BJ. Degree of left ventricular hypertrophy in chronic atrial fibrillation in hypertrophic cardiomyopathy. *Am J Cardiol* 1992; 69:1217–1222.
169. Robinson KC, Frenneaux MP, Stockins B, et al. Atrial fibrillation in hypertrophic cardiomyopathy: A longitudinal study. *J Am Coll Cardiol* 1990; 15:1279–1285.
170. Morrow AG, Reitz BA, Epstein SE, et al. Operative treatment in hypertrophic subaortic stenosis: Techniques and the results of pre- and postoperative assessments in 83 patients. *Circulation* 1975; 52:88–102.
171. Williams WG, Wigle ED, Rakowski H, et al. Results of surgery for hypertrophic obstructive cardiomyopathy. *Circulation* 1987; 76(suppl V):104–108.

172. McCully RB, Nishimura RA, Tajik AJ, et al. Extent of clinical improvement after surgical treatment of hypertrophic obstructive cardiomyopathy. *Circulation* 1996; 94:467–471.
173. Robbins RC, Stinson EB. Long-term results of left ventricular myotomy and myectomy for obstructive hypertrophic cardiomyopathy. *J Thorac Cardiovasc Surg* 1996; 111:586–594.
174. Schoendube FA, Klues HG, Reigh S, et al. Long-term clinical and echocardiographic follow-up after surgical correction of hypertrophic obstructive cardiomyopathy with extended myectomy and reconstruction of the subvalvular mitral apparatus. *Circulation* 1995; 92(suppl II):II-122–II-127.
175. Schulte HD, Bircks WH, Loesse B, et al. Prognosis of patients with hypertrophic obstructive cardiomyopathy after transaortic myectomy: Late results up to twenty-five years. *J Thorac Cardiovasc Surg* 1993; 106:709–717.
176. Maron BJ, Epstein SE, Morrow AG. Symptomatic status and prognosis of patients after operation for hypertrophic obstructive cardiomyopathy: Efficacy of ventricular septal myotomy and myectomy. *Eur Heart J* 1983; 4(suppl F):175–185.
177. Krajcer Z, Leachman RD, Cooley DA, et al. Septal myotomy-myectomy versus mitral valve replacement in hypertrophic cardiomyopathy: Ten-year follow-up in 185 patients. *Circulation* 1989; 80(suppl I):I-57–I-64.
178. Mohr R, Schaff HV, Danielson GK, et al. The outcome of surgical treatment of hypertrophic obstructive cardiomyopathy: Experience over 15 years. *J Thorac Cardiovasc Surg* 1989; 97:666–674.
179. McIntosh CL, Maron BJ. Current operative treatment of obstructive hypertrophic cardiomyopathy. *Circulation* 1988; 78:487–495.
180. Cohn LH, Trehan H, Collin JJ. Long-term follow-up of patients undergoing myotomy-myectomy for obstructive hypertrophic cardiomyopathy. *Am J Cardiol* 1992; 70:657–660.
181. ten Berg JM, Maarten JS, Knaepen PJ, et al. Hypertrophic obstructive cardiomyopathy: Initial results and long-term follow-up after Morrow septal myectomy. *Circulation* 1994; 90:1781–1785.
182. Heric B, Lytle BW, Miller DP, et al. Surgical management of hypertrophic obstructive cardiomyopathy: Early and late results. *J Thorac Cardiovasc Surg* 1995; 110:195–208.
183. Theodoro DA, Danielson GK, Feldt RH, et al. Hypertrophic cardiomyopathy in pediatric patients: Results of surgical treatment. *J Thorac Cardiovasc Surg* 1996; 112:1589–1599.
184. McIntosh CL, Greenberg CJ, Maron BJ, et al. Clinical and hemodynamic results after mitral valve replacement in patients with obstructive hypertrophic cardiomyopathy. *Ann Thorac Surg* 1989; 47:236–246.
185. McIntosh CL, Maron BJ, Cannon RO, et al. Initial results of combined anterior mitral leaflet plication and ventricular septal myotomy-myectomy for relief of left ventricular outflow tract obstruction in patients with hypertrophic cardiomyopathy. *Circulation* 1992; 86:II-60–II-67.
186. Maron BJ, Nishimura RA, Danielson GK. Pitfalls in clinical recognition and a novel operative approach for hypertrophic cardiomyopathy with severe outflow obstruction due to anomalous papillary muscle. *Circulation* 1998; 98:2505–2508.
187. Marwick TH, Stewart WJ, Lever HM, et al. Benefits of intraoperative echocardiography in the surgical management of hypertrophic cardiomyopathy. *J Am Coll Cardiol* 1992; 20:1066–1072.
188. Grigg LE, Wigle ED, Williams WG, et al. Transesophageal Doppler echocardiography in obstructive hypertrophic cardiomyopathy: Clarification of pathophysiology and importance in intraoperative decision making. *J Am Coll Cardiol* 1992; 20:41–52.
189. Maron BJ, Merrill WH, Freier PA, et al. Long-term clinical course and symptomatic status of patients after operation for hypertrophic subaortic stenosis. *Circulation* 1978; 57:1205–1213.
190. Siegman IL, Maron BJ, Permut LC, et al. Results of operation for coexistent obstructive hypertrophic cardiomyopathy and coronary artery disease. *J Am Coll Cardiol* 1989; 13:1527–1533.
191. Cannon RO, McIntosh CL, Schenke WH, et al. Effect of surgical reduction of left ventricular outflow obstruction on hemodynamics, coronary flow, and myocardial metabolism in hypertrophic cardiomyopathy. *Circulation* 1989; 79:766–775.
192. Jeanrenaud X, Goy J-J, Kappenberger L. Effects of dual-chamber pacing in hypertrophic obstructive cardiomyopathy. *Lancet* 1992; 339:1318–1323.
193. Fananapazir L, Epstein ND, Curiel RV, et al. Long-term results of dual-chamber (DDD) pacing in obstructive hypertrophic cardiomyopathy: Evidence for progressive, symptomatic and hemodynamic improvement and reduction of left ventricular hypertrophy. *Circulation* 1994; 90:2731–2742.
194. Slade AKB, Sadoul N, Shapiro L, et al. DDD pacing in hypertrophic cardiomyopathy. A multicentre clinical experience. *Heart* 1996; 75:44–49.
195. Nishimura RA, Trusty JM, Hayes DL, et al. Dual-chamber pacing for hypertrophic cardiomyopathy: A randomized, double-blind, crossover trial. *J Am Coll Cardiol* 1997; 29:435–441.
196. Maron BJ, Nishimura RA, McKenna WJ, et al. Assessment of permanent dual-chamber pacing as a treatment for drug-refractory symptomatic patients with obstructive hypertrophic cardiomyopathy: A randomized, double-blind cross-over study (M-PATHY). *Circulation* 1999; 99:2927–2933.
197. Linde C, Gadler F, Kappenberger L, et al. Placebo effect of pacemaker implantation in obstructive hypertrophic cardiomyopathy. *Am J Cardiol* 1999; 83:903–907.
198. Ommen SR, Nishimura RA, Squires RW, et al. Comparison of dual-chamber pacing versus septal myectomy for the treatment of patients with hypertrophic obstructive cardiomyopathy: Early and late results. *J Thorac Cardiovasc Surg* 1995; 110:195–208.
199. Nishimura RA, Hayes DL, Holmes DR, et al. Effects of dual-chamber pacing on systolic and diastolic function in patients with hypertrophic cardiomyopathy: Acute Doppler echocardiographic and catheterization hemodynamic study. *J Am Coll Cardiol* 1996; 27:427–430.
200. Betocchi S, Losi M-A, Piscione F, et al. Effects of dual-chamber pacing in hypertrophic cardiomyopathy on left ventricular outflow tract obstruction and on diastolic function. *Am J Cardiol* 1996; 77:498–502.
201. Kappenberger L, Linde C, Daubert C, et al. Pacing in hypertrophic obstructive cardiomyopathy: A randomized crossover study. *Eur Heart J* 1997; 18:1249–1256.
202. Seggewiss H, Gleichman U, Faber L, et al. Percutaneous transluminal septal myocardial ablation in hypertrophic obstructive cardiomyopathy: Acute results and 3-month follow-up on 25 patients. *J Am Coll Cardiol* 1998; 31:252–258.
203. Knight C, Kurbaan AS, Seggwiss H, et al. Nonsurgical septal reduction for hypertrophic obstructive cardiomyopathy: Outcome in the first series of patients. *Circulation* 1997; 95:2075–2081.
204. Lakkis NM, Nagueh SF, Kleiman NS, et al. Echocardiography-guided ethanol septal reduction for hypertrophic obstructive cardiomyopathy. *Circulation* 1998; 98:1750–1755.
205. Geitzen FH, Leuner ChJ, Raute-Kreinsen U, et al. Acute and long-term results after transcoronary ablation of septal hypertrophy (TASH): Catheter interventional treatment for hypertrophic cardiomyopathy. *Eur Heart J* 1999; 20:1342–1354.
206. Maron BJ. New interventions for obstructive hypertrophic cardiomyopathy: Promise and prudence (editorial). *Eur Heart J* 1999; 20:1292–1294.
207. Spirito P, Maron BJ. Perspectives on the role of new treatment strategies in hypertrophic obstructive cardiomyopathy (editorial). *J Am Coll Cardiol* 1999; 33:1071–1075.

CHAPTER 68

RESTRICTIVE, OBLITERATIVE, AND INFILTRATIVE CARDIOMYOPATHIES

Brian D. Hoit

RESTRICTIVE CARDIOMYOPATHY

Definition of Restrictive Cardiomyopathy

The World Health Organization (WHO) and World Heart Foundation define cardiomyopathies as heart muscle diseases of unknown etiology and classify them according to hemodynamic and pathophysiologic criteria.[1] Although this definition differentiates primary cardiomyopathies from other pathologic processes that disturb myocardial function—such as ischemic, hypertensive, valvular, and congenital heart diseases—the WHO classification, despite recent modifications, remains controversial. The clinicopathologic classification scheme initially proposed by Goodwin is similar and includes dilated or congestive, hypertrophic, and restrictive forms.[2] *Restrictive cardiomyopathy* refers to either an idiopathic or systemic myocardial disorder characterized by restrictive filling, normal or reduced left ventricular (LV) and right ventricular (RV) volumes, and normal or nearly normal systolic (LV and RV) function. Thus, the clinical and hemodynamic picture thus simulates constrictive pericarditis and is characterized by elevated venous pressure with prominent X and Y descents, a small or normal sized LV, and pulmonary congestion. Restrictive cardiomyopathy may be noninfiltrative or infiltrative and occurs with or without obliteration; infiltration may be interstitial (e.g., amyloid, sarcoid) or cellular (e.g., hemochromatosis).

Restrictive cardiomyopathy has assumed importance in clinical cardiology for several reasons. First, these myocardial disorders epitomize diastolic heart failure; thus, abnormal ventricular diastolic compliance and impaired ventricular filling constitute their central pathophysiologic components and congestion and elevated diastolic pressure are their major clinical and hemodynamic manifestations. Second, the hemodynamic and clinical manifestations may mimic those produced by constrictive pericarditis, which, in contrast to restrictive cardiomyopathy, is a surgically curable disorder. Accordingly, its lack of recognition may have dire consequences. Third, restrictive cardiomyopathy may present with interventricular conduction delays, heart block, or skeletal muscle disease, often making the diagnosis difficult. Fourth, diagnostic criteria for restriction are not universally accepted, and the morphologic spectrum overlaps with hypertrophic cardiomyopathy challenges our traditional concepts of classification.[3] Finally, a comprehensive echo Doppler assessment has become an important, noninvasive means of detecting the pathophysiology, morphology, and prognosis of the restrictive cardiomyopathies.[4,5]

Clinical Features of Restrictive Cardiomyopathy

Involvement of the myocardium (or endomyocardium), and ventricular obliteration, may occur either in isolation or in the setting of systemic or iatrogenic disease (Table 68-1). Thus, in the strictest sense, restrictive cardiomyopathy is not necessarily a primary disease of heart muscle. Irrespective of the etiology, terminology, or the nature of myocardial process, the ventricles are small (generally <110 mL/m^2), and stiff, restricting ventricular filling. Despite normal (or near normal) systolic function, ventricular diastolic, jugular, and pulmonary venous pressures are increased. Typically, LV filling pressures exceed RV filling pressures by more than 5 mmHg, but equalization of the diastolic pressures and a "square root" dip and plateau of early diastolic pressures of the RV and LV may be seen if the compliances of these chambers are similarly affected. Importantly, the hemodynamics of constrictive pericarditis may be simulated. Moreover, elevated atrial pressures produce symptoms of systemic and pulmonary venous congestion (dyspnea, orthopnea, edema, abdominal discomfort), and relatively underfilled ventricles are responsible for reduced cardiac output and fatigue. In patients with restrictive cardiomyopathy as part of a systemic disorder, cardiac symptoms may dominate or overshadow symptoms referable to other organ systems. Patients with constrictive cardiomyopathy generally have lower RV systolic pressures (<40 mmHg) and an RV end-diastolic pressure greater than one-third of the pressure RV systolic pressure as opposed to patients with restrictive cardiomyopathy but these differences are far from absolute.

Physical Findings

Physical examination reflects the elevated systemic and pulmonary venous pressure. Striking elevation of the jugular venous

TABLE 68-1 Classification of the Restrictive Cardiomyopathies

Myocardial
1. Noninfiltrative cardiomyopathies
   - Idiopathic
   - Familial
   - Pseudoxanthoma elasticum
   - Scleroderma
2. Infiltrative cardiomyopathies
   - Amyloidosis
   - Sarcoidosis
   - Gaucher's disease
3. Storage disease
   - Hemochromatosis
   - Fabry's disease
   - Glycogen storage diseases

Endomyocardial
1. Obliterative
   - Endomyocardial fibrosis
   - Hypereosinophilic syndrome
2. Nonobliterative
   - Carcinoid
   - Malignant infiltration
   - Iatrogenic (radiation, drugs)

pulse and prominent X and especially Y descents are characteristic (see Chap. 10). A *diastolic* arterial pulse, owing to a reduced stroke volume and tachycardia, may be seen in severe cases. The apical impulse is not displaced and systolic murmurs of atrioventricular regurgitation and filling sounds marking the abrupt cessation of rapid early diastolic filling may be present.

Diagnostic/Imaging Studies

Electrocardiographic (ECG) abnormalities such as abnormal voltage, atrial and ventricular arrhythmias, and conduction disturbances are frequent; when restrictive cardiomyopathy is due to amyloid infiltration, low voltage is usual (Fig. 68-1). The chest radiograph usually reveals normal-sized ventricles, although atrial enlargement and pericardial effusion may produce an enlarged cardiac silhouette. Pleural effusions and signs of pulmonary congestion may also be present. Echocardiographic findings are nonspecific but in many cases are useful to exculpate other, more common causes of heart failure.

DIFFERENTIATION FROM CONSTRICTIVE PERICARDITIS

Although several clinical, imaging, and hemodynamic features are helpful in distinguishing restrictive cardiomyopathy from constrictive pericarditis (Table 68-2), considerable overlap and diagnostic confusion exist. The pathophysiologic basis for this distinction includes (1) transmission of intrathoracic pressure to the ventricles (limited by the stiff pericardium in constrictive pericarditis but not in restrictive cardiomyopathy); (2) the principal determinant of the diastolic ventricular pressure-volume relation (ventricular versus pericardial compliance in restrictive cardiomyopathy as compared to constrictive pericarditis, itself); and (3) involvement of the ventricular septum in restrictive cardiomyopathy versus the capacity for ventricular interdependence in constrictive pericarditis.

Recently, Doppler techniques (spectral Doppler, color M-mode, and Doppler tissue imaging) have assumed an important role in characterizing the nature of transvalvular filling and in clinically distinguishing between constrictive pericarditis and restrictive cardiomyopathy (see also Chap. 13).[5–7] These Doppler flow patterns and the associated respiratory changes are illustrated in Fig. 68-2. In the *normal subject,* the early filling wave (E) of mitral flow is greater than the late, atrial systolic wave (A), and neither change significantly with respiration. In contrast, the E and A velocities of tricuspid valve flow increase slightly with inspiration. The deceleration time of the LV early diastolic wave ranges from 150 to 240 ms, and the LV isovolumic relaxation time ranges from 70 to 110 ms. Pulmonary venous flow is generally biphasic, with a dominant wave during systole (S) and a smaller wave during diastole (D); respiratory changes are minimal and atrial systolic reversals are generally small. Hepatic vein flow consists of a larger S and smaller D wave with small reversals (V_r and A_r) after each wave, respectively. With expiration, S and D waves decrease and V_r and A_r increase. Doppler tissue imaging (DTI) shows a prominent longitudinal axis velocity in early diastole (E_a >8 cm/s) and a smaller velocity after atrial contraction (A_a). The slope of early diastolic LV filling on color M-mode (Vp) is >45 cm/s. In the patient with *restrictive cardiomyopathy*, mitral valve flow shows an increased E/A ratio (≥2) with a short (<150 ms) deceleration time and a short (<70 ms) isovolumic relaxation time (a "restrictive" pattern of filling) without respiratory variation. The tricuspid valve flow shows an increased E/A ratio without respiratory variation, a shortened deceleration time, and a short isovolumic relaxation time that shortens further with inspiration. The S/D ratio of pulmonary venous flow is <1, atrial reversals are increased (not shown in Fig. 68-1), and there is little respiratory variation. The S/D ratio of hepatic venous flow is <1 and prominent reversals are seen during inspiration. Doppler tissue imaging shows a striking decrease in E_a (<8 cm/s) and the propagation velocity on color M-mode is <45 cm/s.

In *constrictive pericarditis*, mitral and tricuspid valve flows are also "restrictive," but unlike those in restrictive cardiomyopathy, they display marked respiratory variation. The isovolumic relaxation time shortens during expiration. The S/D of pulmonary venous flow is <1, with increased velocities (especially diastolic) in expiration, resulting in a further decrease in the S/D ratio. In contrast to restrictive cardiomyopathy, hepatic venous flow reversals occur in expiration, early diastolic tissue velocities (E_a) are normal on DTI, and the transmitral propagation velocity is >45 cm/s.

Despite the considerable interest and potential clinical value in the ability to discriminate restrictive cardiomyopathy from constrictive pericarditis, there is no uniform agreement regarding the characteristic features of the Doppler indices, especially those of venous flows. Moreover, rigorous studies of the sensitivity and specificity of these Doppler findings are lacking and relatively few patients have been examined. Thus, the diagnostic certainty is related to the number of "pathognomonic" findings in concert with clinical information and additional imaging studies.

One report suggested that radionuclide ventriculographic indices of LV diastolic function could differentiate constrictive pericarditis and restrictive cardiomyopathy.[8] However, measurements of LV filling—such as the peak filling rate, time to peak filling, and various filling fractions—require careful attention to technical detail. The need for stable heart rates, the lack of venous flows, and the inability to observe the influence of respiration on cardiac blood flows are important limitations of the radionuclide ventriculographic technique.

Magnetic resonance imaging (MRI) and computed tomography (CT) are useful for accurately assessing pericardial thickness (Fig. 68-3); a pericardium >4.0 mm thick can distinguish the two entities (see also Chap. 18A).[9] Recent preliminary data suggest that constrictive pericarditis is associated with severe autonomic dysfunction that involves all segments of the autonomic nervous system, whereas in restrictive cardiomyopathy the autonomic dysfunction is localized to the parasympathetic efferent pathway.[10] Invasive hemodynamics may be helpful (below), and occasionally a histologic diagnosis is necessary.

It is important to remember that clinical and laboratory testing, including imaging and pathologic studies, may produce results consistent with mixed constrictive pericarditis and restrictive cardiomyopathy; indeed, the two entities may coexist [for example, after mediastinal irradiation or after coronary artery bypass grafting (CABG)]. In these cases, a decision to treat conservatively or surgically explore a patient requires experienced clinical judgment.

Cardiac Catheterization

Most patients in whom restrictive cardiomyopathy is a serious consideration should undergo right- and left-sided heart catheterization to document the diagnosis, assess severity, and, in some patients, establish the etiology by means of endomyocardial biopsy. As in patients with constrictive pericarditis, extra care must be taken to obtain high-quality pressure recordings with appropriate gain and optimal damping conditions, and to attend to details such

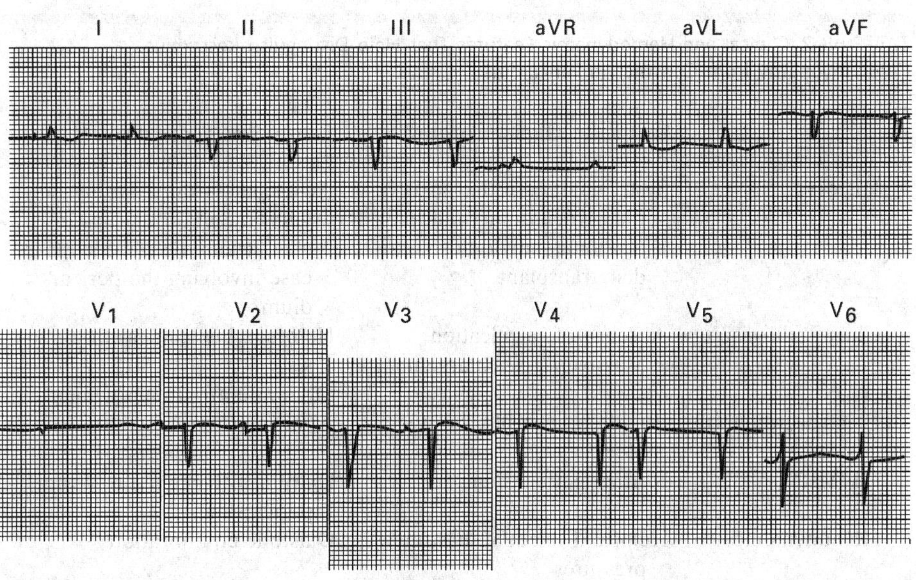

FIGURE 68-1 Electrocardiogram of a patient with amyloidosis. Note the low voltage, which is in striking contrast to the increased left ventricular wall thickness shown echocardiographically. (From Shabetai R. Restrictive, obliterative, and infiltrative cardiomyopathies. In: Alexander WA, Schlant R, Fuster V, et al., eds. *Hurst's The Heart*, 9th ed. New York: McGraw-Hill; 1998:2077. Reproduced with permission.)

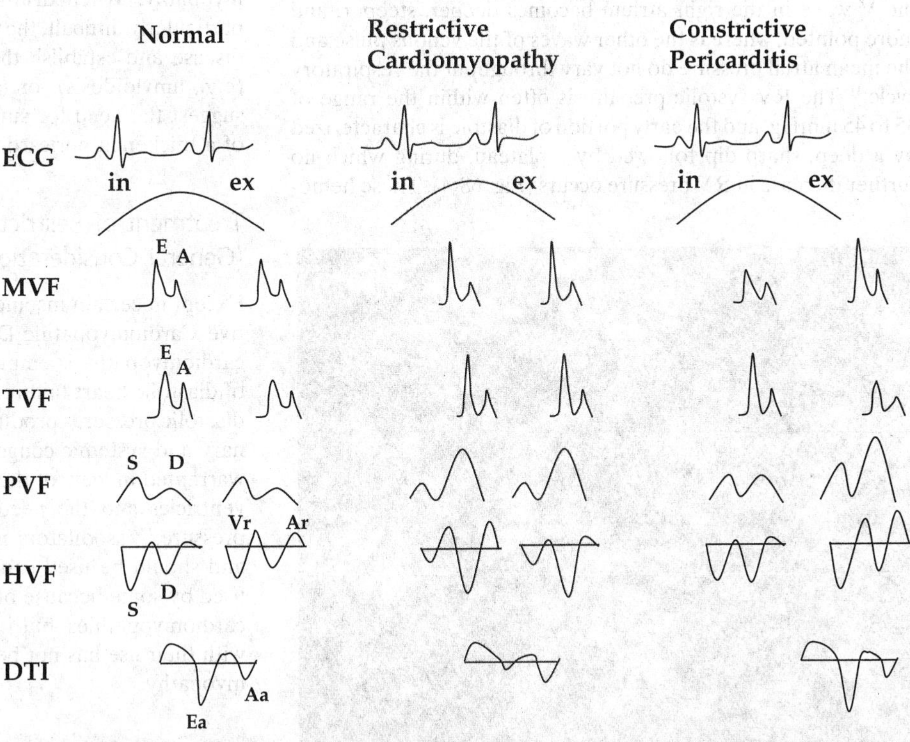

FIGURE 68-2 Schematic of Doppler flows during inspiration (in) and expiration (ex) in normals, restrictive cardiomyopathy, and constrictive pericarditis. See text for details. E, early diastolic filling; A, atrial systolic filling; S, systolic flow; D, diastolic flow; Vr, V-wave reversals; Ar, atrial systolic reversals; Ea, early diastolic tissue velocities; Aa, late diastolic tissue velocites; MVF, mitral valve flow; TVF, tricuspid valve flow; PVF, pulmonary venous flow; HVF, hepatic venous flow; DTI, Doppler tissue imaging. (From Hoit BD. Restrictive cardiomyopathy. In: Pohost G, O'Rourke R, Shah P, Berman D, eds. *Imaging in Cardiovascular Disease*. New York: Lippincott Williams & Wilkins; in press. Reproduced with permission.)

TABLE 68-2 Clinical and Hemodynamic Features That Help Distinguish Restrictive Cardiomyopathy from Constrictive Pericarditis

	Restrictive Cardiomyopathy	Constrictive Pericarditis
History	Systemic disease that involves the myocardium, multiple myeloma, amyloidosis, cardiac transplant	Acute pericarditis, cardiac surgery, radiation therapy, chest trauma, systemic disease involving the pericardium
Chest radiograph	Absence of calcification Massive atrial enlargement	Helpful when calcification persists Moderate atrial enlargement
Electrocardiogram	Bundle branch blocks, AV block	Abnormal repolarization
CT/MRI	Normal pericardium	Helpful if thickened (>4 mm) pericardium
Hemodynamics	Helpful if unequal diastolic pressures Concordant effect of respiration on diastolic pressures	Diastolic equilibration Dip and plateau
Biopsy	Fibrosis, hypertrophy, infiltration	Normal

as the transducer height and system calibration. The venous pressure is elevated and the deep and rapid fall of the right atrial Y descent is striking. During inspiration, the descent of the V wave in the right atrium becomes deeper, steeper, and more pointed, whereas the other waves of the venous pulse and the mean atrial pressure do not vary throughout the respiratory cycle.[11] The RV systolic pressure is often within the range of 35 to 45 mmHg, and the early portion of diastole is characterized by a deep, sharp dip followed by a plateau, during which no further increase in RV pressure occurs (Fig. 68-4). These hemodynamic features are identical to those of constrictive pericarditis and may cause diagnostic confusion. There is usually only modest pulmonary hypertension and the pulmonary arterial diastolic pressure is a few millimeters higher than the pulmonary wedge pressure, which is often quite elevated. It is not uncommon for the pulmonary wedge and the right atrial pressures to be identical and to simulate further the hemodynamics of constrictive pericarditis; however, a higher LV than RV filling pressure strongly favors the diagnosis of restrictive cardiomyopathy rather than constrictive pericarditis. LV systolic pressure is normal, while the LV diastolic pressure tracing shows the same abnormalities as those of the RV (Fig. 68-4).

Left ventriculography usually shows a normal ejection fraction and the absence of major regional wall motion abnormalities. Endomyocardial biopsy is an integral part of the workup of many patients with restrictive cardiomyopathy. When distinction from constrictive pericarditis is particularly difficult, the biopsy may furnish proof of myocardial disease and establish the cause of restrictive cardiomyopathy (e.g., amyloidosis), or (by virtue of unremarkable histology) suggest the need for surgical exploration, even in the absence of a thickened pericardium.

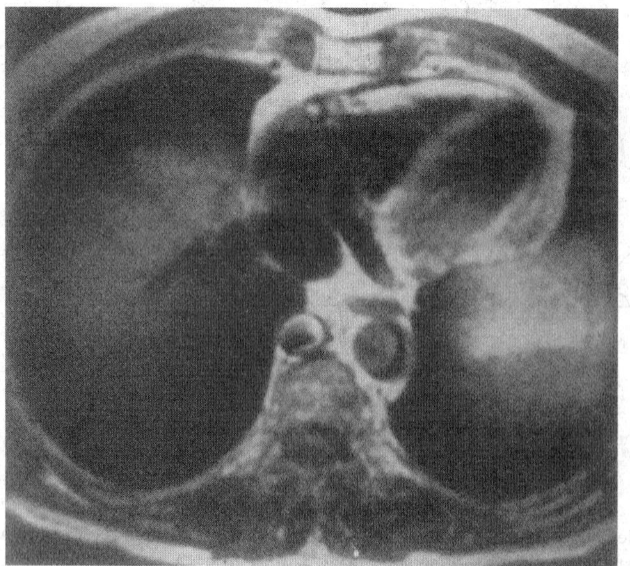

FIGURE 68-3 Magnetic resonance image showing normal pericardium as a low-intensity (*black*) line anterior to the right ventricle between high-intensity (*white*) epicardial and mediastinal fat. (From Hoit BD. Imaging the pericardium. *Cardiol Clin* 1990; 8:588. Reproduced with permission.)

Treatment of Restrictive Cardiomyopathy (General Considerations)

Except in certain instances described below ("Specific Restrictive Cardiomyopathic Diseases"), the treatment of restrictive cardiomyopathy is empiric and directed toward the treatment of diastolic heart failure. Reduction in the elevated ventricular diastolic pressures produces substantial improvement in pulmonary and systemic congestion, but judicious use of diuretics is warranted in view of the steep pressure-volume relation of the ventricles and the need to maintain a relatively high filling pressure. Vasodilators may also jeopardize ventricular filling and should be used cautiously. Calcium channel blockers are used by some because of their beneficial effect in hypertrophic cardiomyopathies, but improvement in ventricular compliance with their use has not been demonstrated in restrictive cardiomyopathy.

SPECIFIC RESTRICTIVE CARDIOMYOPATHIC DISEASES

A useful classification of the restrictive cardiopathies is shown in Table 68-1. This scheme is based upon the cardiac compartment predominantly involved (i.e., myocardial versus endomyocardial) and subdivides the myocardial diseases into the noninfil-

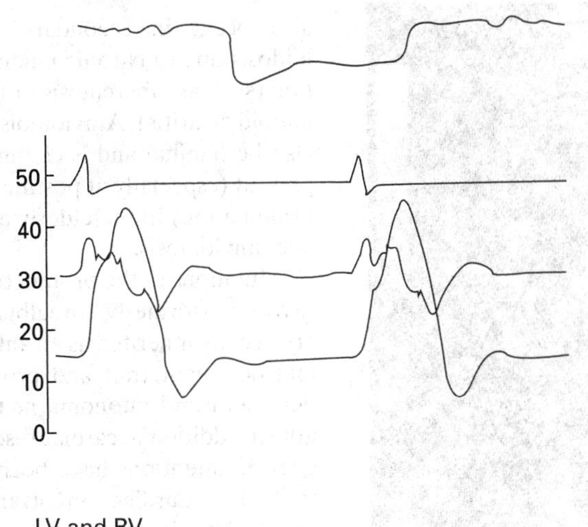

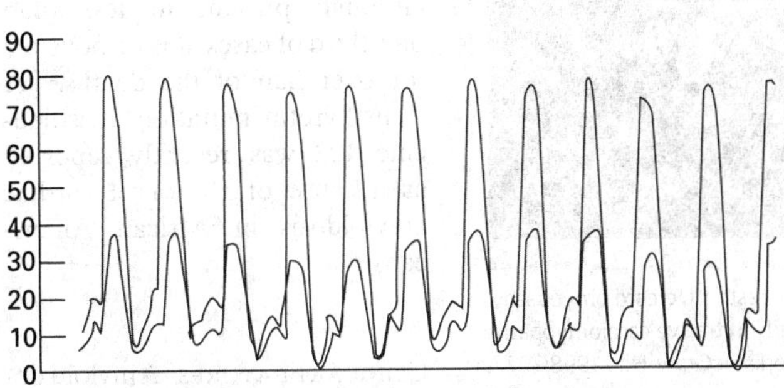

FIGURE 68-4 *Top:* Right-sided heart hemodynamic data from a patient with amyloidosis recorded with a high-fidelity catheter. From the top tracing down is a respirometer, electrocardiogram, right ventricular (RV) dP/dt, and RV pressure. Note the characteristic dip-and-plateau configuration. *Bottom:* Simultaneous RV and LV pressure tracings from another patient with cardiac amyloidosis. In this patient, the typical dip-and-plateau pattern was not present, but during inspiration LV and RV diastolic pressures equilibrated. (From Shabetai R. Restrictive, obliterative, and infiltrative cardiomyopathies. In: Alexander WA, Schlant R, Fuster V, et al., eds. *Hurst's The Heart*, 9th ed. New York: McGraw-Hill; 1998:2079. Reproduced with permission.)

trative, infiltrative, and storage and the endomyocardial diseases into obliterative (i.e., endomyocardial fibrosis and the hypereosinophilic syndrome), carcinoid, infiltrative, and iatrogenic.

Myocardial Diseases

NONINFILTRATIVE CARDIOMYOPATHIES

Idiopathic and Familial Restrictive Cardiomyopathy Recent data suggest that idiopathic restrictive cardiomyopathy may be an autosomal dominant disorder involving myocardium, conduction tissue, and skeletal muscle, with resultant restrictive ventricular filling and heart failure, AV block, and distal skeletal myopathy. Deposition of the intermediate filament desmin has been linked to this syndrome and may represent a distinct pathologic entity; accumulation of desmin immunoreactive material on heart biopsy may be confirmed ultrastructurally.[12,13] Changes in collagen subtypes and matrix metalloproteinase activity may play an important role in the genesis of increased LV stiffness.[14]

Myocyte hypertrophy and fibrosis on endomyocardial biopsy characterize idiopathic restrictive cardiomyopathy, and the absence of myocyte disarray is an important pathologic distinction from hypertrophic cardiomyopathy. However, overlap syndromes characterized by physiologic evidence of restriction and myocyte hypertrophy but without myocyte disarray or LV hypertrophy on echocardiography are reported.[15] Moreover, it was recently postulated that primary restrictive and hypertrophic cardiomyopathies may represent different phenotypic expressions of the same genetic disease.[16] An echocardiographic feature distinguishing primary restrictive cardiomyopathy from cardiac amyloidosis (in addition to the associated clinical features) is the increased LV wall thickness in the latter. In both disorders (and restrictive cardiomyopathies in general), ventricular dimensions are normal or reduced, systolic function is variable, and atrial dimensions are increased.

Two-dimensional and Doppler echocardiography are reliable, noninvasive techniques for diagnosing primary restrictive cardiomyopathy (see Chap. 13).[17] A dominant mitral early diastolic "E" velocity, an increased pulmonary venous atrial systolic "A" reversal velocity and duration, and shortened mitral deceleration time are present in both children and adults with primary restrictive cardiomyopathy (Fig. 68-5). On CT or MRI scans, evidence of restrictive filling (e.g., right atrial and caval enlargement) are common in both restrictive cardiomyopathy and constrictive pericarditis. MRI may differentiate primary restrictive cardiomyopathy from amyloidosis on the basis of tissue characterization.[18]

Pseudoxanthoma Elasticum Pseudoxanthoma elasticum is a rare, genetically heterogeneous disorder characterized by fragmentation and calcification of elastic fibers involving the skin, eyes, and gastrointestinal and cardiovascular systems. Although endocardial fibroelastosis uncommonly causes restrictive cardiomyopathy (Fig. 68-6), coronary artery disease with premature death is a major problem in these patients.[19]

Progressive Systmic Sclerosis Myocardial fibrosis, which may have a patchy distribution and be present in both ventricles, is found in the majority of patients with scleroderma at autopsy. On echocardiography, LV wall thickening in the absence of hypertension and evidence of LV dysfunction may be seen, but heart failure due to either restrictive or dilated cardiomyopathy is rare.[20] Pericardial involvement and electrocardiographic abnormalites (heart block, supraventricular and ventricular tachycardia, and pseudoinfarction patterns) are common. Pulmonary hypertension is a leading cause of morbidity and mortality in patients with scleroderma.

INFILTRATIVE CARDIOMYOPATHIES

Amyloidosis Amyloidosis is a systemic disorder characterized by interstitial deposition of linear, rigid, nonbranching amyloid protein fibrils in multiple organs (e.g., heart, kidney, liver, nerve). Although there are several types of amyloidosis, cardiac involvement is most common in primary amyloidosis (AL type), which is caused by plasma cell production of immunoglobulin light chains; the latter occurs often in association with multiple myeloma. Multiple myeloma is also reported to cause diastolic heart failure in the absence of amyloidosis.[18,21] Cardiac deposition of amyloid protein (protein A, a nonimmunoglobin) may

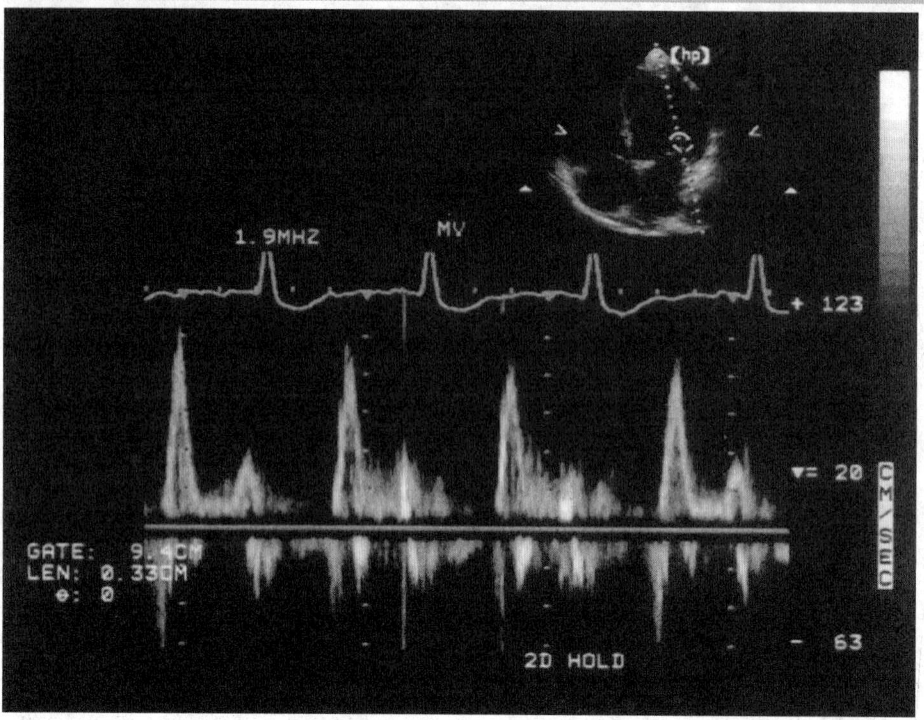

FIGURE 68-5 Doppler record of mitral inflow velocity from a patient with idiopathic restrictive cardiomyopathy. Note the dominant early diastolic wave. (From Shabetai R. Restrictive, obliterative, and infiltrative cardiomyopathies. In: Alexander WA, Schlant R, Fuster V, et al., eds. *Hurst's The Heart*, 9th ed. New York: McGraw-Hill; 1998:2077. Reproduced with permission.)

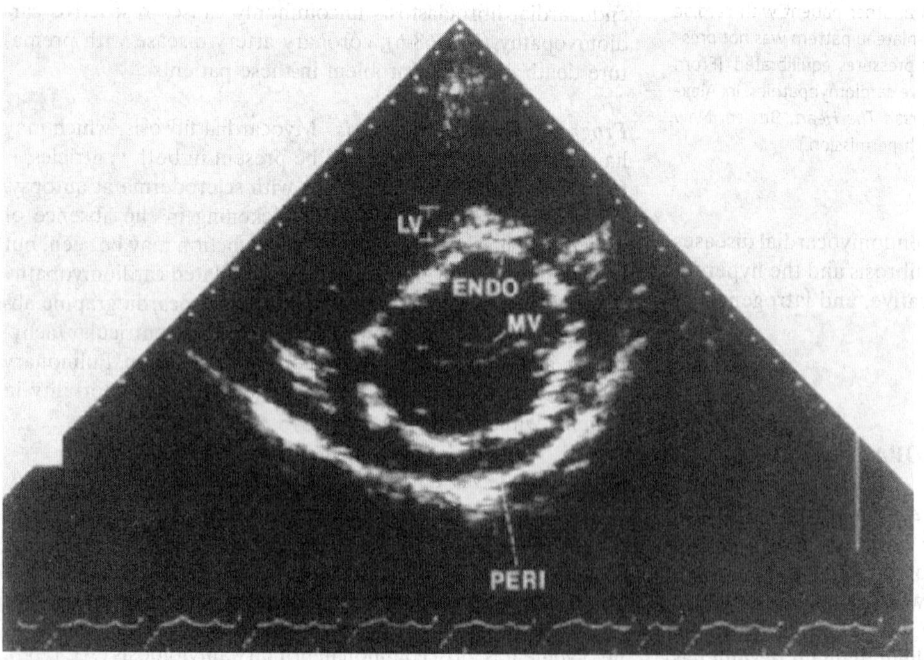

FIGURE 68-6 Short-axis view of the left ventricle (LV) at the mitral valve (MV) level in a patient with pseudoxanthoma elasticum. Note the calcified endomyocardium (ENDO) and echodense pericardium (PERI). The endocardial calcification was clearly visible by fluoroscopy. (From Shabetai R. Restrictive, obliterative, and infiltrative cardiomyopathies. In: Alexander WA, Schlant R, Fuster V, et al., eds. *Hurst's The Heart*, 9th ed. New York: McGraw-Hill; 1998:2085. Reproduced with permission.)

also occur in secondary amyloidosis due to chronic inflammation (such as tuberculosis or rheumatoid arthritis). Amyloidois may also be familial and is commonly present (especially at postmortem examination) in the elderly as senile amyloidosis.

Mutations of the protein transthyretin (formerly prealbumin) are usually inherited as an autosomal dominant trait and produce peripheral and autonomic neuropathy in addition to cardiac disease; over 50 mutations have been described.[22] Cardiac involvement occurs late in the disease and, although present in less than one-third of cases, it is responsible for over half of the deaths.[23] A transthyretin mutation at isoleucine 122 was recently reported as a cause of late-onset cardiac amyloidosis in African Americans.[24]

Clinical Features Amyloid deposits may be interstitial and widespread, resulting in restrictive cardiomyopathy, or localized to (1) conduction tissue, resulting in heart block and ventricular arrhythmias (especially familial amyloid); (2) the cardiac valves, causing valvular regurgitation; (3) the pericardium, producing constriction; and (4) the coronary arteries, resulting in ischemia. Amyloid may be isolated to the subendocardium in senile amyloid and amyloid secondary to chronic disease. Deposition of amyloid and atrial natriuretic factor (ANF) in the atria is frequent in aged hearts.[25] Despite sinus rhythm, atrial mechanical failure and thrombus formation may result due to electromechanical dissociation.[26] Atrial and brain natriuretic peptide are expressed in ventricular myocytes in patients with cardiac amyloidosis.[27] In some cases, the clinical picture is dominated by autonomic neuropathy (orthostatic hypotension, syncope, diarrhea, lack of sweating, and impotence) and nephropathy and cardiac involvement are unrecognized. Cardiac manifestations define a spectrum, often progressive through stages of severity, from the asymptomatic to biventricular failure.

DIAGNOSTIC/IMAGING STUDIES The cardiac silhouette on the chest radiograph may be normal or moderately enlarged. The ECG typically shows decreased voltage, a pseudoinfarction pattern, left axis deviation; arrhythmias and conduction disturbances may predominate the clinical course.

The M-mode echocardiogram may reveal symmetrical wall thickness involving the right and left ventricles, a small or normal LV cavity, variable (but often depressed) systolic function, left atrial enlargement, and a small pericardial effusion (Fig. 68-7). Digitized M-mode tracings may reveal decreased rates of systolic wall thickening and diastolic wall thinning and increased isovolumic relaxation time,[28] especially in the early stages.

Two-dimensional echo findings include thickening of the ventricular myocardium, the interatrial septum and valves (especially the AV valves), enlarged papillary muscles, and dilated atria and inferior vena cava (Fig. 68-8). LV wall thickness is an important prognostic variable; in one study, patients with biopsy-proven amyloidosis having a mean wall thickness ≥15 mm had a median survival of 0.4 years, whereas patients with a mean wall thickness ≤12 mm had a median survival of 2.4 years.[29] Highly reflective echoes producing a granular or sparkling appearance and occurring in a patchy distribution are characteristic echocardiographic findings but are neither sensitive nor specific; concentric hypertrophy, as occurs in hypertension or aortic stenosis, may produce a uniformly speckled or echolucent appearance of the myocardium; and idiopathic hypertrophic cardiomyopathy may display a patchy, granular sparkling. Although they correlate with wall thickness, granular echoes may not be seen. Importantly, their recognition is subjective and is affected by ultrasound instrument settings. Thus, granular sparkling alone is an unreliable finding. The infiltrative pathology associated with amyloidosis may be detected by tissue characterization using MRI.[18] Amyloid cardiomyopathy may exist despite the absence of echocardiographic evidence of infiltration.[30]

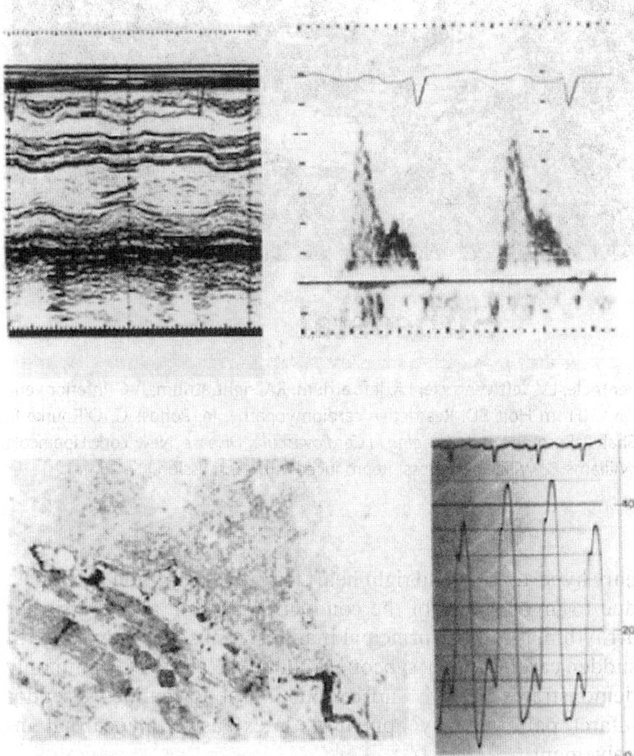

FIGURE 68-7 Amyloidosis. *Top left:* M-mode echocardiogram showing increased thickness of the left ventricular myocardium (calibration mark = 1 cm). *Top right:* Doppler tracing of mitral inflow velocity. Note that the atrial contribution to mitral blood flow velocity is markedly reduced (calibration mark = 20 cm/s). *Bottom left:* electromicrograph showing extensive replacement of myocardium by amyloid. *Bottom right:* Right ventricular pressure tracing. A diastolic dip-plateau pattern is absent because of tachycardia. (From Shabetai R. Restrictive, obliterative, and infiltrative cardiomyopathies. In: Alexander WA, Schlant R, Fuster V, et al., eds. *Hurst's The Heart*, 9th ed. New York: McGraw-Hill; 1998:2083. Reproduced with permission.)

Doppler studies may show the restrictive pattern of LV filling—i.e., a transmitral E/A ratio ≥2 without respiratory variation, transmitral diastolic deceleration time <150 ms, and an isovolumic relaxation time ≤70 ms (Fig. 68-7). The RV filling pattern is often abnormal. The systolic-to-diastolic pulmonary venous flow ratio is <1 and atrial reversals increase with inspiration in the pulmonary and hepatic veins. However, the *earliest sign* of amyloid cardiomyopathy is impaired LV relaxation, manifest by an E/A ratio <1, and increased isovolumic relaxation and transmitral diastolic deceleration times. The severity of combined systolic and diastolic abnormalities can be determined with an echo Doppler index using isovolumic contraction and relaxation and ejection times.[31] In addition, Doppler has shown utility in prognosis; a deceleration time <150 ms and an increased E/A transmitral ratio are strong predictors of cardiac death.[32]

Abnormalities of LV filling are also demonstrated with the LV time-activity curve from radionuclide ventriculography.[33] Moreover, radionuclide imaging using technetium-99m pyrophosphate or Indium-111 antimyosin may be useful in diagnosis. The variable clinical, diagnostic, and prognostic features reflect the location, nature, and extent of amyloid deposition and the temporal course of the disease. Serum and urine protein electrophoresis is diagnostic in most cases of primarily amyloidosis, but monoclonal protein is not secreted in 10 percent of cases.[23] Endomyocardial biopsy of the RV (most helpful if an abdominal fat aspirate is negative) provides the diagnosis, establishes the histochemistry, and quantifies myocardial damage and atrophy.[34]

TREATMENT OF AMYLOIDOSIS The treatment of amyloidosis is unrewarding and symptomatic therapy is fraught with hazard; patients are sensitive to digoxin and calcium channel blockers, and hypotension with vasodilators and diuretics is a threat due to the steep LV pressure-volume relation. Immunosuppressive therapy with melphalan and prednisone is the established treatment regimen for primary (AL) amyloidosis. In a recent study, multiple alkylating agents failed to increase the response rate or survival time over this conventional regimen.[35] Orthotopic cardiac transplantation is generally not recommended because of the systemic nature of amyloidosis and the possibility of recurrence in the transplant, but successful cases have been reported.[36] Liver transplantation may be lifesaving in patients with familial amyloidosis,[37] since the liver is the site of transthyretin production.

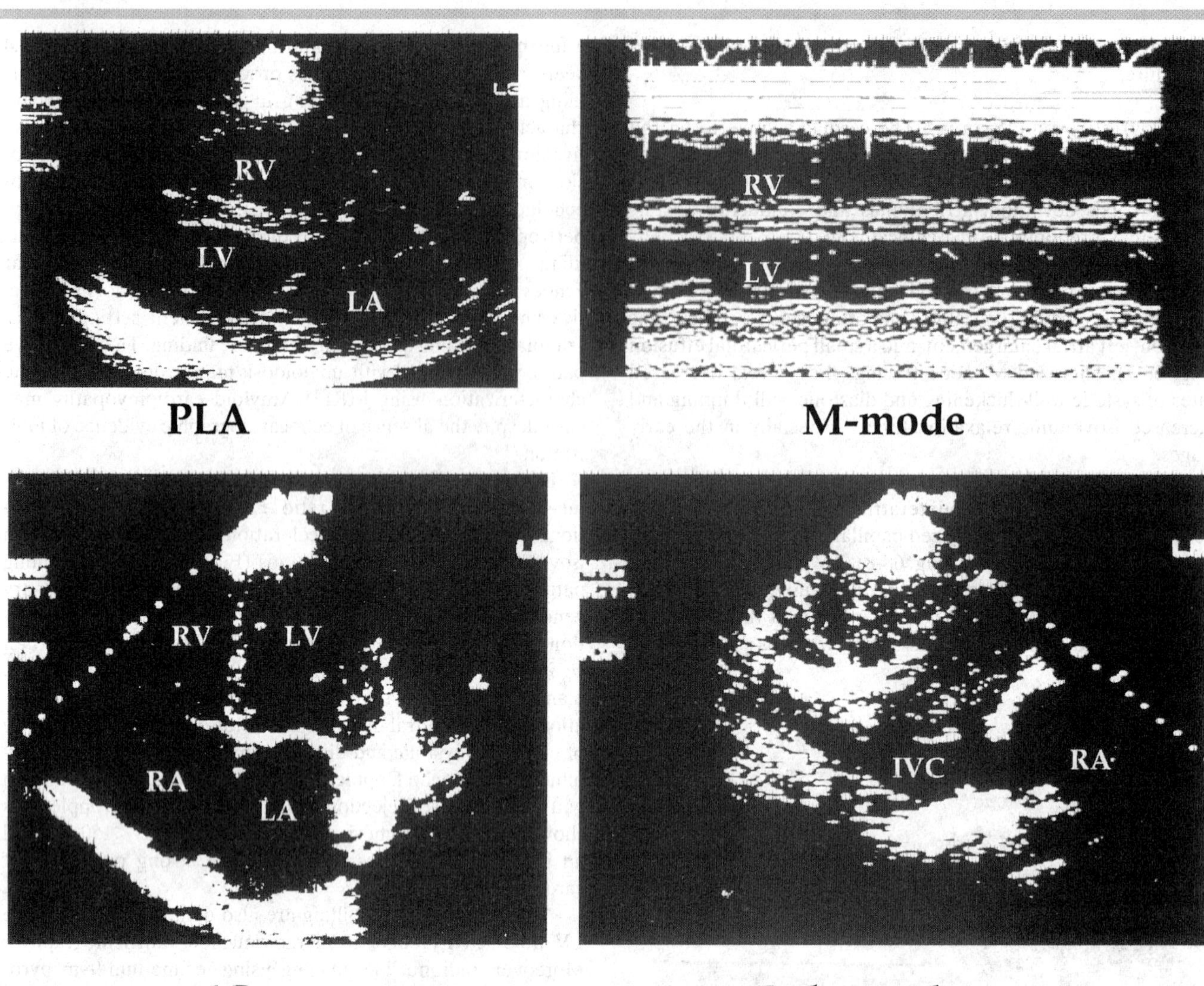

FIGURE 68-8 M-mode and two-dimensional echocardiogram from a patient with biopsy-proven amyloidosis causing hemodynamic restriction. The left ventricular systolic function is mildly impaired, and there is biatrial enlargement and vena cava plethora. Left ventricular hypertrophy is best seen in the M-mode study. PLA, parasternal long axis; 4C, four chamber view; RV, right ventricle; LV, left ventricle; LA, left atrium; RA, right atrium; IVC, inferior vena cava. (From Hoit BD. Restrictive cardiomyopathy. In: Pohost G, O'Rourke R, Shah P, Berman D, eds. *Imaging in Cardiovascular Disease*. New York: Lippincott Williams & Wilkins; in press. Reproduced with permission.)

Sarcoidosis Sarcoidosis is a disorder of unknown etiology characterized by the presence of noncaseating granulomas that involve many organs (e.g., lung, skin, lymph nodes, liver, spleen). Granulomas involve the heart in sarcoidosis in as many as 25 percent of patients but are frequently subclinical.[38] Nevertheless, in approximately half of the fatalities, cardiac involvement is responsible.[39] Rarely, sarcoid is confined to the heart. The combination of extracardiac manifestations and cardiac abnormalities favors a presumptive diagnosis of sarcoidosis without biopsy.

Interstitial granulomatous inflammation initially produces diastolic dysfunction, but later, when the disease is more extensive, it may produce systolic (at times focal) abnormalities. Localized thinning and dilatation of the basilar LV resembling ischemic heart disease are characteristic. Restrictive cardiomyopathy is uncommon. However, sarcoid pulmonary involvement is frequent and produces echo and Doppler findings of pulmonary hypertension and right heart failure. High-grade AV block, due to involvement of the conduction system, and ventricular arrhythmias are the principal manifestations and may result in sudden cardiac death; syncope is common. The ECG commonly demonstrates T-wave and conduction abnormalities. Pseudoinfarct patterns may appear with extensive myocardial involvement.

Echocardiographic findings include evidence of systolic and diastolic LV dysfunction, LV aneurysm formation, abnormal ventricular wall thickness, pericardial effusion, regional wall motion abnormalities in the basal septum with apical sparing, and evidence of cor pulmonale. Thallium 201 and gallium 67 have been used to indicate areas of myocardial involvement and serve to predict the response to corticosteroids. MRI may detect mass lesions due to sarcoid granuloma or scar.[40] Endomyocardial biopsy is useful but may be falsely negative. An important entity in the differential diagnosis is giant-cell myocarditis, which is characterized by a more aggressive and fatal course than cardiac sarcoid.[41]

Treatment with prednisone is warranted in highly suspicious or proven cases because the cardiac granuloma may be sensitive. In patients at high risk for sudden cardiac death, an automatic implantable cardioverter defibrillator (AICD) may be appropriate,[42] and cardiac transplantation is an appropriate consideration in some cases.[43]

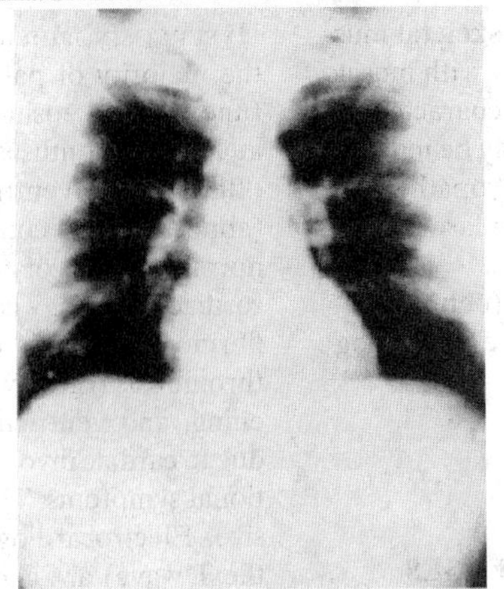

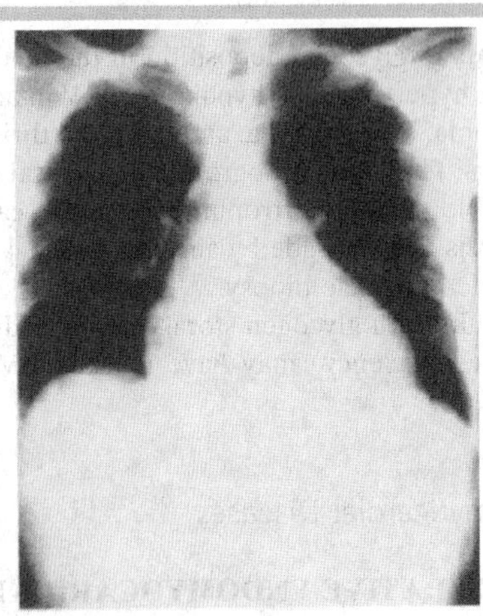

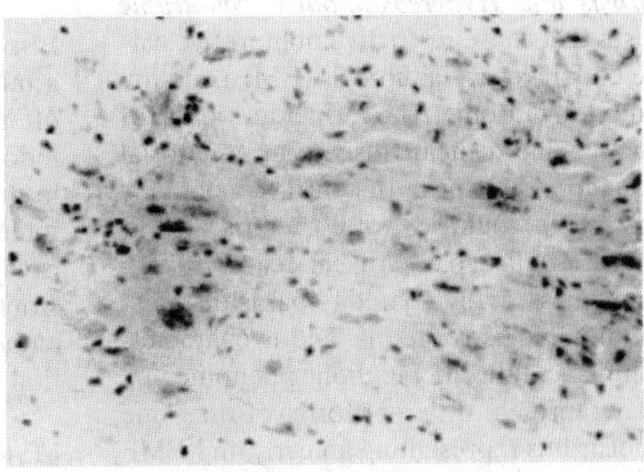

FIGURE 68-9 Chest radiograph of a patient with cardiac hemochromatosis before (*top right*) and after (*top left*) several months of treatment with phlebotomy. *Bottom:* Endomyocardial biopsy that established the diagnosis. (From Shabetai R. Restrictive, obliterative, and infiltrative cardiomyopathies. In: Alexander WA, Schlant R, Fuster V, et al., eds. *Hurst's The Heart*, 9th ed. New York: McGraw-Hill; 1998:2084. Reproduced with permission.)

Gaucher's Disease Gaucher's disease is due to an inherited deficiency of the enzyme β-glucocerebroside, which results in accumulation of cerebroside in the reticuloendothelial system, brain, and heart. Diffuse interstitial infiltration of the left ventricle occurs, with reduced LV wall compliance and cardiac output, but is often subclinical. LV and left-sided valvular thickening and pericardial effusion are seen on echo.[44]

STORAGE DISEASES

Hemochromatosis Primary hemochromatosis is an autosomal recessive iron-storage disease that involves the heart, pancreas, skin, liver, and gonads. Myocardial iron deposition in hemochromatosis, either primary or secondary (e.g., resulting from multiple transfusions, ineffective erythropoeisis), usually produces dilated cardiomyopathy but may cause restrictive cardiomyopathy. Arrhythmia and conduction disturbances are common; indeed, congestive heart failure, conduction abnormalities, and supraventricular and ventricular arrhythmias occur in one-third of patients.[45] Interstitial fibrosis is variable and unrelated to the extent of iron deposition, which occurs in the myocyte; secondarily, myocardial fibrosis may develop. Bronze diabetes and hepatic dysfunction, reflecting iron deposition in the skin, pancreas and liver are frequent associated manifestations.

One report suggests that cardiac involvement progresses temporally from a small, concentrically hypertrophied LV with diastolic dysfunction to a dilated LV with systolic dysfunction.[46] However, this sequence of events is not universally accepted, and systolic abnormalities may require provocation.[47] Findings consistent with either dilated or restrictive cardiomyopathy may be seen; the presence of systolic dysfunction indicates a poor prognosis (Fig. 68-9). Granular sparkling and atrial enlargement may be observed, but these are nonspecific signs. Quantitative ultrasonic analysis of integrated backscatter has been used experimentally to detect changes in the echo reflectivity of the myocardium due to iron deposition in thalassemia major.[48] Computed tomography and magnetic resonance imaging may demonstrate subclinical cardiac involvement, and tissue characterization may be possible with MRI. Endomyocardial biopsy is confirmatory; in selected instances, it may be useful in excluding the diagnosis.

Repeated phlebotomy is recommended for primary hemochromatosis, and the chelating agent desferrioxamine is often beneficial in secondary hemochromatosis. Cardiac transplantation (with or without liver transplantation) may be considered in selected cases.

Fabry's Disease Fabry's disease is an X-linked, genetically heterogeneous disorder of glycosphingolipid metabolism caused by lysosomal ceramide (α-galactosidase) deficiency that leads to accumulation of glycolipid in the heart, skin, and kidneys. Glycolipid accumulation in the myocardium and vascular and valvular endothelium may present with either a restrictive, hypertrophic, or dilated cardiomyopathy, mitral regurgitation, ischemic heart disease, or aortic degeneration. Echocardiographic findings in restrictive cardiomyopathy mimic those seen in amyloid, and LV mass correlates with the severity of disease.[49] Hypertension, mitral valve prolapse, and heart failure are common clinical presentations. Definitive diagnosis may require endomyocardial biopsy.

Pompe's Disease Pompe's disease (glycogen storage type II) is due to an inherited (autosomal recessive) metabolic abnormality due to acid maltase deficiency that causes massive amounts of glycogen deposition in the heart and skeletal muscles. A hypertrophied, hypokinetic LV in an infant with muscle hypotonia, hyperreflexia, and failure to thrive are characteristic findings. The echocardiographic manifestations may be indistinguishable from hypertrophic obstructive cardiomyopathy. The diagnosis can be made by absence of α-1,4-glucosidase activity on skeletal muscle biopsy.

Adults with glycogen storage type III disease (debranching enzyme deficiency) may have marked LVH on echocardiography.[50]

Endomyocardial Diseases

OBLITERATIVE ENDOMYOCARDIAL DISEASES

Endomyocardial Fibrosis and Hypereosinophilic Syndrome Endomyocardial diseases that cause restrictive obliterative cardiomyopathies include endomyocardial fibrosis (EMF) and hypereosinophilic (Loeffler's) syndrome. The former accounts for 10 to 20 percent of deaths due to heart disease in equatorial Africa but is seen throughout the world. In contrast, Loeffler's endocarditis is seen mainly in countries with a temperate climate. Although it shares similar pathological features with EMF, it affects mainly men; is usually related to parasitic infections, leukemia, and immunologic reactions; and is characterized by intense eosinophila and thromboembolic phenomena.[51] The two conditions may represent different forms of the same disease (Loeffler's endocarditis representing an early and EMF an advanced stage), but considerable differences exist. Moreover, the endemic variety EMF may be related to high levels of cerium and low levels of magnesium; it may be pathophysiologically distinct from Loeffler's.[52]

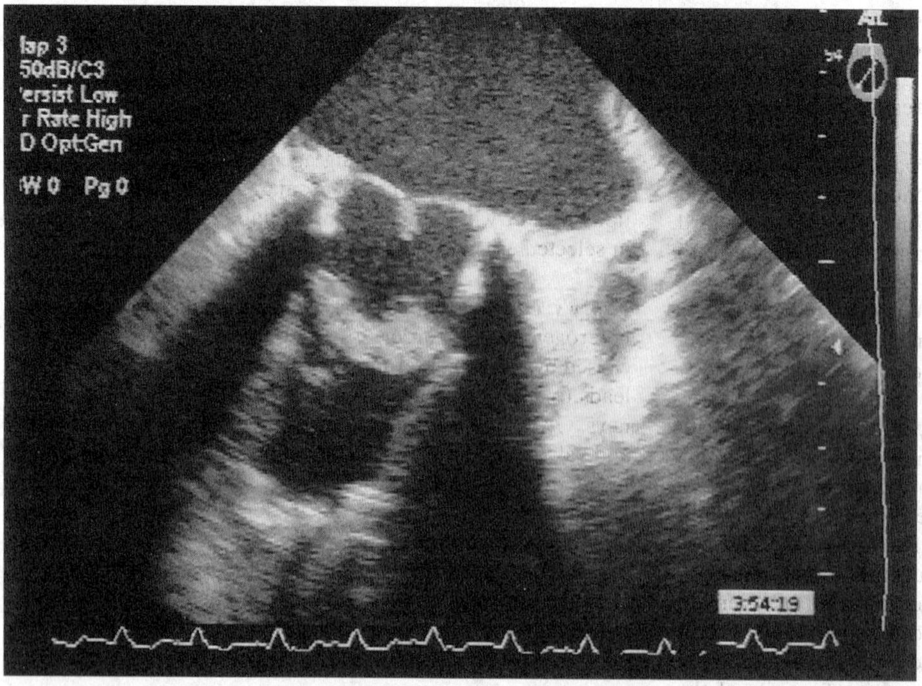

HYPEREOSINOPHILIC SYNDROME Cardiac involvement occurs in the majority of patients with the hypereosinophilic syndrome (unexplained eosinophilia exceeding 1500 eosinophils/mm^3 for at least 6 months and symptoms of organ involvement) and often has a biventricular distribution. Cardiotoxic eosinophils (abnormal cells containing vacuoles and having fewer than the normal number of granules) are central to the pathogenesis. The cardiac pathology consists of an acute eosinophilic myocarditis, fibrinoid vasculitis of the intramural coronary arteries, mural thrombosis (often with eosinophils), fibrotic endocardial thickening, and ventricular obliteration. In addition to symptoms due to cardiac involvement, patients have skin rash and constitutional symptoms. The disease is aggressive and rapidly progressive. Electrocardiographic abnormalities (especially involving the T wave) are common but nonspecific. Hemodynamic findings are typical of restrictive cardiomyopathy.

ENDOMYOCARDIAL FIBROSIS In contrast to Loeffler's, EMF has a more insidious onset, has no gender predilection, and most often affects children and young adults. The disease is more indolent than Loeffler's, and biventricular involvement occurs in only about half the cases. LV involvement produces symptoms due to pulmonary congestion, whereas the less common isolated RV involvement (about 10 percent) may simulate constrictive pericarditis. Atrioventricular valve regurgitation and embolic episodes are frequent complications, and atrial fibrillation is common.

ECHOCARDIOGRAPHIC FEATURES Endomyocardial disease is characterized by endocardial fibrosis of the apex and subvalvular regions of one or both ventricles, resulting in restriction to inflow to the affected ventricle. Although their clinical presentations differ, the pathology, and therefore the cardiac imaging studies, are generally similar in the endomyocardial diseases. M-mode echo findings are nonspecific and digitized M-mode studies reveal a decreased peak filling rate and a decreased duration of the peak filling.[53] On two-dimensional echo, apical obliteration of the right and/or left ventricle, apical thrombus, preservation of ventricular systolic function with thickening of the posterior atrioventricular valve apparatus and posterobasilar LV wall, echo densities in the endocardium, and small ventricular and large atrial cavities are noted (Fig. 68-10).[54] Involvement of the posterior mitral and tricuspid valve leaflets results in mitral and tricuspid regurgitation; less commonly, restricted motion may produce stenosis. Sparing of the outflow tracts is characteristic. Doppler interrogation yields typical patterns of restriction (increased E/A, decreased IVRT, decreased deceleration time), mitral and tricuspid regurgitation, and, less often, stenosis. Not sur-

FIGURE 68-10 Transesophageal echocardiogram from a patient with eosinophilic endocarditis and prosthetic mitral valve replacement. Thrombus is noted below the valve struts, which at the the time of surgery was found to be adherent to the posterior LV wall. Note the apical obliteration and the apical endocardial thickening and calcification.

prisingly, the location, extent, and severity of involvement determine the clinical picture.

TREATMENT OF THE OBLITERATIVE RESTRICTIVE CARDIOMYOPATHIES

Medical therapy of Loeffler's is often ineffective and frustrating. Treatment consists of symptomatic relief, anticoagulants, corticosteroids, and hydroxyurea for myocarditis (interferon α has had some success[55]), and palliative surgery in the late, fibrotic stage. Surgical excision of fibrotic endocardium and valve replacement may offer symptomatic improvement, but at the expense of high (15 to 25 percent) operative mortality. The prognosis of advanced disease is grim (50 percent 2-year mortality), but it is considerably better in those with milder disease.

NONOBLITERATIVE ENDOMYOCARDIAL DISEASES

Carcinoid Syndrome Carcinoid syndrome results from metastatic carcinoid tumors (most commonly arising in the small bowel and appendix, but also the bronchus and other sites) and consists of cutaneous flushing, diarrhea, and bronchoconstriction; involvement of the heart occurs as a late complication of carcinoid syndrome in approximately 50 percent of patients. (see also Chaps. 59 and 77). Hepatic metastases produce serotonin, bradykinin, and other substances that affect right heart structures but are inactivated in the lungs. Thus, LV involvement is distinctly uncommon and its presence suggests a right-to-left intracardiac shunt.[56] Fibrous endocardial plaques comprising smooth muscle cells in a stroma of collagen and acid mucopolysaccharide on the tricuspid and pulmonic valves and right heart endocardium are characteristic. Although tricuspid and pulmonic stenosis and regurgitation dominate the clinical picture, restrictive cardiomyopathy may occur.

The chest radiograph is often normal, but cardiomegaly, pleural effusions, and nodules may be evident; unlike the case with congenital pulmonic stenosis, poststenotic dilatation of the pulmonary artery trunk does not occur.[57] Electrocardiographic abnormalities are common, but nonspecific. Two-dimensional echocardiography reveals thickened, retracted tricuspid and pulmonic valves and right atrial and ventricular enlargement; right atrial wall thickening may be seen on transesophageal echo. Low-velocity tricuspid and pulmonic regurgitation on Doppler indicates normal pulmonary arterial pressures, which is typical of carcinoid heart disease. In one series, echocardiographic findings were detected in two-thirds of patients with carcinoid.[58] In another study, cardiac involvement was associated with a reduced 3-year survival as compared with those without cardiac involvement.[57] Catheterization findings are usually those of tricuspid regurgitation and/or pulmonic stenosis. Therapy is symptomatic, and valvular replacement (mechanical) or repair is warranted in patients with severe valve dysfunction.

Malignant Infiltration Infiltrating tumors of the heart are generally metastatic (lung, breast, melanoma, lymphoma, leukemia) and rarely produce restriction to ventricular filling unless the pericardium is involved (see Chap. 77). Infiltration on echocardiography is suggested by a localized increase in wall thickness, often associated with abnormal wall motion and pericardial effusion. CT and MRI scans are also useful.

Iatrogenic Disease Pericardial disease frequently complicates radiation therapy to the chest and may produce constrictive pericarditis; however, endo- and myocardial involvement may produce restrictive cardiomyopathy, at times presenting years after radiation therapy has been completed.[59] Anthracyclines and methysergide can cause endomyocardial fibrosis. Oils containing L-tryptophan were withdrawn from the market when they were implicated in the genesis of the eosinophilia-myalgia syndrome; this syndrome was associated with restrictive cardiomyopathy.[60] Finally, a restrictive pattern of LV filling is common soon after orthotopic cardiac transplantation and may persist for at least 1 year in as many as 15 percent.[61]

References

1. WHO/ISFC Task Force. Definition and classification of cardiomyopathies. *Br Heart J* 1980; 44:672–673.
2. Goodwin J, Oakley C. The cardiomyopathies. *Br Heart J* 1972; 44:672–673.
3. Angelini A, Calzolari V, Thiene G, et al. Morphologic spectrum of primary restrictive cardiomyopathy. *Am J Cardiol* 1997; 80:1046–1050.
4. Appleton C, Hatle L, Popp R. Demonstration of restrictive ventricular physiology by Doppler echocardiography. *J Am Coll Cardiol* 1988; 11:757–768.
5. Klein A, Cohen G, Pietrolungo J, et al. Differentiation of constrictive pericarditis from restrictive cardiomyopathy by Doppler transesophageal echocardiographic measurements of respiratory variations in pulmonary venous flow. *J Am Coll Cardiol* 1993; 22:1935–1943.
6. Garcia M, Rodriguez L, Ares M, et al. Differentiation of constrictive pericarditis from restrictive cardiomyopathy: Assessment of left ventricular diastolic velocities in longitudinal axis by doppler tissue imaging. *J Am Coll Cardiol* 1996; 27:108–114.
7. Akasaka T, Yoshida K, Yamamuro A, et al. Phasic coronary flow characteristics in patients with constrictive pericarditis: Comparison with restrictive cardiomyopathy. *Circulation* 1997; 96:1874–1881.
8. Gerson M, Fowler N. Differentiation of constrictive pericarditis and restrictive cardiomyopathy by radionuclide ventriculography. *Am Heart J* 1989; 118:114–120.
9. Masui T, Finck S, Higgins C. Constrictive pericarditis and restrictive cardiomyopathy: Evaluation with MR imaging. *Radiology* 1992; 182:369–373.
10. Singh M, Juneja R, Bali HK, et al. Autonomic functions in restrictive cardiomyopathy and constrictive pericarditis: A comparison. *Am Heart J* 1998; 136:443–448.
11. Shabetai R, Fowler NO, Guntheroth WG. The hemodynamics of cardiac tamponade and constrictive pericarditis. *Am J Cardiol* 1970; 26:480–489.
12. Arbustini E, Morbini P, Grasso M, et al. Restrictive cardiomyopathy, atrioventricular block and mild to subclinical myopathy in patients with desmin-immunoreactive material deposits. *J Am Coll Cardiol* 1998; 31:645–653.
13. Zachara E, Bertini E, Lioy E, et al. Restrictive cardiomyopathy due to desmin accumulation in a family with evidence of autosomal dominant inheritance. *G Ital Cardiol* 1997; 27:436–442.
14. Hayashi T, Shimomura H, Terasaki F, et al. Collagen subtypes and matrix metalloproteinase in idiopathic restrictive cardiomyopathy. *Int J Cardiol* 1998; 64:109–116.
15. Cooke R, Chambers J, Curry P. Noonan's cardiomyopathy: A non-hypertrophic variant. *Br Heart J* 1994; 71:561–565.
16. Angelini A, Calzolari V, Thiene G, et al. Morphologic spectrum of primary restrictive cardiomyopathy. *Am J Cardiol* 1997; 80:1046–1050.
17. Cetta F, O'Leary P, Seward J, et al. Idiopathic restrictive cardiomyopathy in childhood: Diagnostic features and clinic course. *Mayo Clin Proc* 1995; 70:634–640.
18. Celetti F, Fattori R, Napoli G, et al. Assessment of restrictive

cardiomyopathy of amyloid or idiopathic etiology by magnetic resonance imaging. *Am J Cardiol* 1999; 83:798–801.
19. Navarro-Lopez F, Llorian A, Ferrer-Roca O, et al. Restrictive cardiomyopathy in psuedoxanthoma elasticum. *Chest* 1980; 78:113–115.
20. Botstein G, LeRoy E. Primary heart disease in systemic sclerosis (scleroderma): Advances in clinical and pathologic features, pathogenesis, and new therapeutic approaches. *Am Heart J* 1981; 102:913–919.
21. Schattner A, Epstein M, Berrebi A, et al. Case report: Multiple myeloma presenting as a diastolic heart failure with no evidence of amyloidosis. *Am J Med Sci* 1995; 310:256–257.
22. Saraiva MJ. Transthyretin mutations in health and disease. *Hum Mutat* 1995; 5:191–196.
23. Kyle RA. Amyloidosis. *Circulation* 1995; 91:1269–1271.
24. Jacobson DR, Pastore RD, Yaghoubian R, et al. Variant-sequence transthyretic (isoleucine 122) in late-onset cardiac amyloidosis in black Americans. *N Engl J Med* 1997; 336:466–473.
25. Kawamura S, Takahashi M, Ishihara T, et al. Incidence and distribution of isolated atrial amyloid: Histologic and immunohistochemical studies of 100 aging hearts. *Pathol Int* 1995; 45:335–342.
26. Dubrey S, Pollak A, Skinner M, et al. Atrial thrombi occurring during sinus rhythm in cardiac amyloidosis: Evidence for atrial electromechanical dissociation. *Br Heart J* 1995; 74:541–544.
27. Takemura G, Takatsu Y, Doyama K, et al. Expression of atrial and brain natriuretic peptides and their genes in hearts of patients with cardiac amyloidosis. *J Am Coll Cardiol* 1998; 4:754–765.
28. Sutton MSJ, Reichek N, Kastor J, et al. Computerized M-mode echocardiographic analysis of left ventricular dysfunction in cardiac amyloid. *Circulation* 1982; 66:790–799.
29. Cueto-Garcia L, Reeder G, Kyle R, et al. Echocardiographic findings in systemic amyloidosis: Spectrum of cardiac involvement and relation to survival. *J Am Coll Cardiol* 1985; 6:737–743.
30. Gertz MA, Grogan M, Kyle RA, et al. Endomyocardial biopsy-proven light chain amyloidosis (AL) without echocardiographic features of infiltrative cardiomyopathy. *Am J Cardiol* 1997; 80:93–95.
31. Tei C, Dujardin KS, Hodge DO, et al. Doppler index combining systolic and diastolic myocardial performance: Clinical value in cardiac amyloidosis. *J Am Coll Cardiol* 1996; 28:658–664.
32. Klein AL, Hatle LK, Taliercio CP, et al. Prognostic significance of Doppler measures of diastolic function in cardiac amyloidosis: A Doppler echocardiography study. *Circulation* 1991; 83: 808–816.
33. Lenihan DJ, Gerson MC, Hoit BD, et al. Mechanisms, diagnosis, and treatment of diastolic heart failure. *Am Heart J* 1995; 130:153–166.
34. Arbustini E, Merlini G, Gavazzi A, et al. Cardiac immunocyte-derived (AL) amyloidosis: An endomyocardial biopsy study in 11 patients. *Am Heart J* 1995; 130:528–536.
35. Gertz MA, Lacy MQ, Lust JA, et al. Prospective randomized trial of melphalan and prednisone versus vincristine, carmustine, melphalan, cyclophosphamide, and prednisone in the treatment of primary systemic amyloidosis. *J Clin Oncol* 1999; 17:262–267.
36. Pelosi F Jr, Capehart J, Roberts WC. Effectiveness of cardiac transplantation for primary (AL) cardiac amyloidosis. *Am J Cardiol* 1997; 79:532–535.
37. Skinner M, Lewis WD, Jones LA, et al. Liver transplantation as a treatment for familial amyloidotic polyneuropathy. *Ann Intern Med* 1994; 15:133–134.
38. Gibbons W, Levy R, Nava S, et al. Subclinical cardiac dysfunction in sarcoidosis. *Chest* 1991; 100:44–50.
39. Perry A, Vuitch F. Causes of death in patients with sarcoidosis: A morphologic study of 38 autopsies with clinicopathologic correlations. *Arch Pathol Lab Med* 1995; 119:167–172.
40. Chandra M, Silverman ME, Oshinski J, et al. Diagnosis of cardiac sarcoidosis aided by MRI. *Chest* 1996; 110:562–565.
41. Cooper LH, Berry G, Rizeq M, et al. Giant cell myocarditis. *J Heart Lung Transplant* 1995; 14:394–401.
42. Okayama K, Kurata C, Tawarchara K, et al. Diagnostic and prognostic value of myocardial scintigraphy with thallium-201 and gallium-67 in cardiac sarcoidosis. *Chest* 1995; 107:330–334.
43. Valantine HA, Tazelaar H, Macoviak J, et al. Cardiac sarcoidosis: Response to steroids and transplantation. *J Heart Transplant* 1987; 5:244–250.
44. Saraclar M, Atalay S, Kocak N, et al. Gaucher's disease with mitral and aortic involvement: Echocardiographic findings. *Pediatr Cardiol* 1991; 13:56–58.
45. Hauser SC. Hemochromatosis and the heart. *Heart Dis Stroke* 1993; 2:487–491.
46. Arnett E, Nienhius A, Henry W, et al. Massive myocardial hemochromatosis: A structure-function conference at the National Heart and Lung Institute. *Am Heart J* 1975; 90:777–787.
47. Dabestani A, Child J, Henze E, et al. Primary hemochromatosis: Anatomic and physiologic characteristics of the cardiac ventricles and their response to phlebotomy. *Am J Cardiol* 1984; 54: 153–159.
48. Lattanzi F, Bellotti P, Picano E, et al. Quantitative ultrasonic analysis of myocardium in patients with thalassemia major and iron overload. *Circulation* 1993; 87:748–754.
49. Goldman M, Cantor R, Schwartz M, et al. Echocardiographic abnormalities and disease severity in Fabry's disease. *J Am Coll Cardiol* 1986; 7:1157–1161.
50. Coleman R, Winter H, Wolf B, et al. Glycogen storage disease type III (glycogen debranching enzyme deficiency): Correlation of biochemical defects with myopathy and cardiomyopathy. *Ann Intern Med* 1992; 116:896–900.
51. Olsen E, Spry C. Relation between eosinophilia and endomyocardial disease. *Prog Cardiovasc Dis* 1985; 27:241–254.
52. Shaper A. What's new in endomyocardial fibrosis? *Lancet* 1993; 342:255–256.
53. Davies J, Gibson D, Foale R, et al. Echocardiographic features of eosinophilic endomyocardial disease. *Br Heart J* 1982; 48:434–440.
54. Gottdiener J, Maron B, Schooley R, et al. Two-dimensional echocardiographic assessment of the idiopathic hypereosinophilic syndrome: Anatomic basis of mitral regurgitation and peripheral embolization. *Circulation* 1983; 67:572–578.
55. Butterfield JH, Gleich GJ. Interferon-alpha treatment of six patients with the idiopathic hypereosinophilic syndrome. *Ann Intern Med* 1994; 121:648–653.
56. Lundin L, Norheim I, Landelius J, et al. Carcinoid heart disease: Relationship of circulating vasoactive substances to ultrasound-detectable cardiac abnormalities. *Circulation* 1988; 77:264–269.
57. Pellikka P, Tajik A, Khandheria B, et al. Carcinoid heart disease: Clinical and echocardiographic spectrum in 74 patients. *Circulation* 1993; 87:1188–1196.
58. Lundin L, Norheim I, Landelius J, et al. Carcinoid heart disease: Relation of circulating vasoactive substances to ultrasound-detectable cardiac abnormalities. *Circulation* 1988; 77:264–269.
59. Brosius FC III, Waller BF, Roberts WC, et al. Radiation heart disease: Analysis of 16 young (aged 15 to 33 years) necropsy patients who received over 3,500 rads to the heart. *Am J Med* 1981; 70:519–530.
60. Berger PB, Duffy J, Reeder GS, et al. Restrictive cardiomyopathy associated with eosinophilia-myalgia syndrome. *Mayo Clin Proc* 1994; 69:162–165.
61. Valantine HA, Fowler MB, Hunt SA, et al. Changes in Doppler echocardiographic indexes of left ventricular function as potential markers of acute cardiac rejection. *Circulation* 1987; 76:V86–V92.

CHAPTER 69

MYOCARDITIS AND SPECIFIC CARDIOMYOPATHIES—ENDOCRINE DISEASE AND ALCOHOL

Donna M. Mancini / Ainat Beniaminovitz

The diagnosis of cardiomyopathy encompasses a wide spectrum of diseases with widely divergent pathogenic mechanisms, that have as their final common pathway the syndrome of congestive heart failure. These heart muscle diseases may be primary or secondary—i.e., resulting from specific cardiac or systemic disorders. A list of etiologies associated with the development of cardiomyopathy is presented in Fig. 69-1.

Coronary artery disease, hypertension, valvular heart disease, and cardiomyopathy are the most common causes of heart failure for both sexes. Comparison of the Framingham[1] and SOLVD[2] (Study of Left Ventricular Dysfunction) registries demonstrates a shift in the predominant etiology of heart failure from hypertension to ischemic heart disease. This probably reflects recent intensified efforts to control high blood pressure.

Inflammatory cardiomyopathies, particularly viral myocarditis, have served as a model to understand the development of heart failure. More than 70 different specific cardiomyopathies associated with general systemic disease, neuromuscular disorders, sensitivity and toxic reactions, and the peripartum state have been described. When considered as a group, these disorders are infrequent; when considered individually, they are rare.

This chapter reviews the inflammatory cardiomyopathies and specific cardiomyopathies with an emphasis on endocrine and infiltrative disorders. Cardiac disorders caused by pulmonary hypertension and congenital cardiac anomalies are not addressed.

ISCHEMIC

Ischemic cardiomyopathy is defined as a dilated cardiomyopathy in a patient with known coronary disease, specifically a patient with a prior history of infarct or a greater than 70 percent narrowing of a major epicardial artery.

Compensatory mechanisms to improve stroke volume result in myocyte hypertrophy, ventricular dilatation, and activation of the sympathetic nervous system. Remodeling of the left ventricle and a decrease in ejection fraction occur in 15 to 40 percent of patients within 12 to 24 months following an anterior wall infarct[3] and in a smaller percentage following an inferior infarction.[4] In the Framingham study, 14 percent of men developed *congestive heart failure* (CHF) within 5 years of a first myocardial infarction[4] and half were dead within 5 years.[5] Prognosis in ischemic heart failure is known to be worse than in other forms of cardiomyopathy,[6,7] presumably due to the superimposed risk of ongoing ischemic events. Aggressive coronary revascularization in instances of significant heart failure may be justified and may achieve a survival benefit without necessarily affecting functional improvement[8] (see also Chaps. 40 and 48).

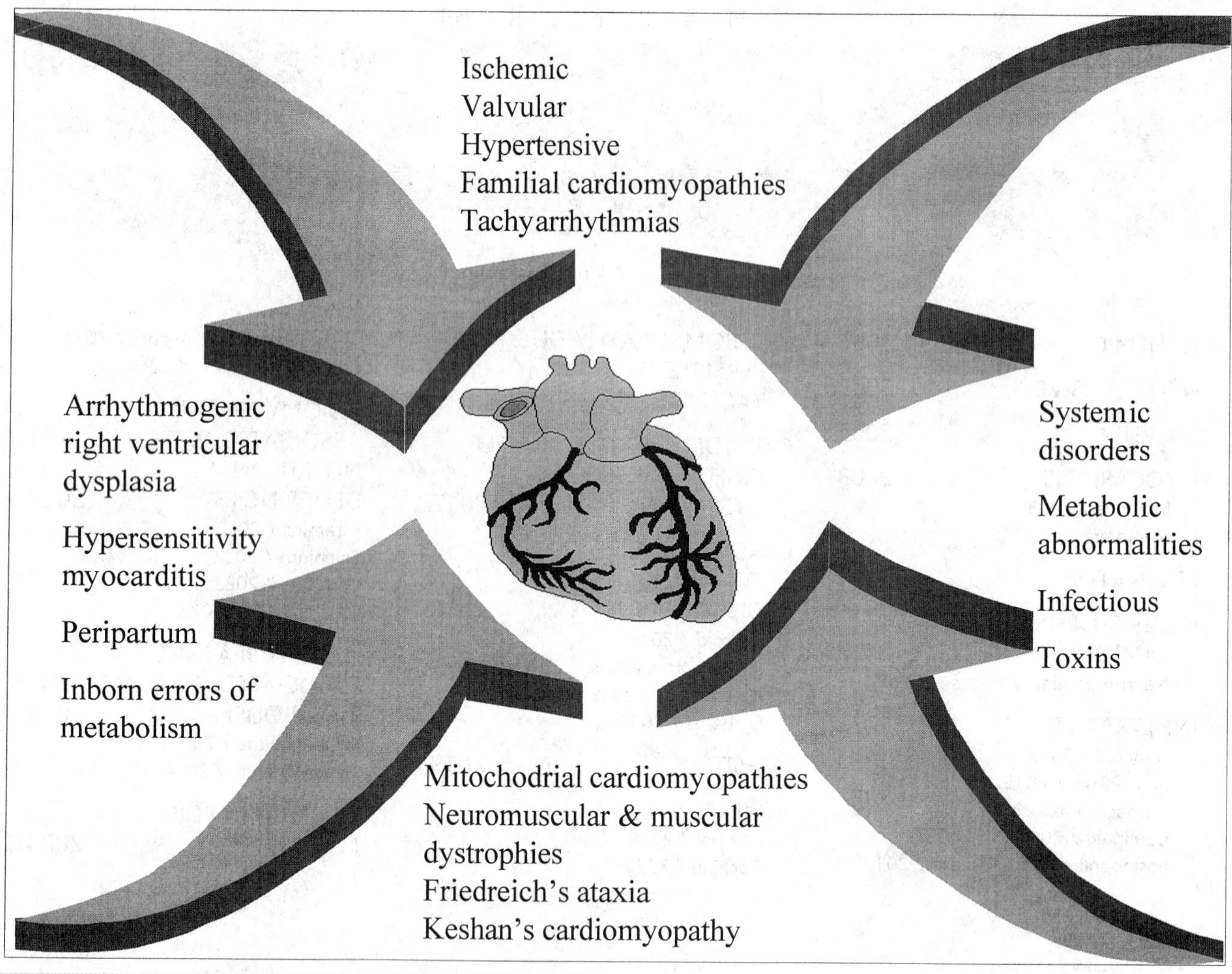

FIGURE 69-1 Various etiologies that can lead to cardiomyopathy.

HYPERTENSIVE

Cardiac hypertrophy due to long-standing arterial hypertension is associated with a high incidence of heart failure.[9] Initially, myocyte hypertrophy occurs to reduce wall stress and to accommodate the increased pressure load imposed on the heart.[10] This increase in myocyte wall thickness is accompanied by biochemical and molecular changes, such as a shift to fetal phenotype gene expression[11] and alterations in the intracellular handling of calcium.[12] Alterations in the nonmyocyte compartment—such as excessive myocardial fibrosis—also ensue.[13] In concert these changes lead to an altered contractile performance of the heart.[14]

Although the precise mechanisms that accelerate the progression from compensated hypertrophy to failure are not known, activation of the renin-angiotensin system has been postulated to play a major role.[15] In vivo, angiotensin II has been shown to increase left ventricular mass[16] and contributes to cardiac phenotype modulation independently from its effect on arterial pressure.[17] In vitro, studies have demonstrated that angiotensin II causes myocyte hypertrophy and promotes interstitial fibrosis.[18] A current clinical trial with the angiotensin-converting enzyme (ACE) inhibitor ramapril has demonstrated that blockade of the renin-angiotensin system in patients with normal left ventricular function but at high risk for cardiovascular events leads to a decrease in the combined end point of death from cardiovascular causes, myocardial infarction, and stroke.[19] This clinical prevention trial further confirms the deleterious effects of the renin-angiotensin axis on cardiac function.

The patient with hypertensive cardiomyopathy typically presents with left ventricular hypertrophy in association with features of dilated or restrictive cardiomyopathy. The prognosis is generally better than that of other forms of cardiomyopathy[20]; however, the prognosis is significantly worsened by the presence of comorbid conditions such as diabetes mellitus, coronary artery disease, and persistent hypertension[21] (see also Chap. 58).

Hypertensive cardiomyopathies are common in the elderly and may be related to an increased prevalence of hypertension due to central arterial stiffness and inherent myocardial changes that occur with normal aging. Recent advances in molecular biology and in echocardiographic and Doppler techniques have led to an improved understanding of the various distinct causes of hypertrophic heart disease in the elderly[22] and the realization that the process is not solely due to the changes associated with aging. Hypertrophic obstructive cardiomyopathy, once thought to be a familial disorder affecting primarily younger individuals, has been diagnosed in older individuals with increasing frequency.[23,24] As shown in Table 69-1, the clinical syndrome, prognosis, and echocardiographic/electrocardiographic findings are somewhat different in the elderly form of the disease.[25]

Similarly, hypertensive hypertrophic cardiomyopathy is another significantly unappreciated cause of hypertensive cardiomyopathy in the elderly.[26] In contrast to the hypertrophic obstructive form, there is a higher female predominance,[26] which is thought to be due to gender-specific differences in the degree of myocyte hypertrophy to intraventricular pressure-overload previously described in women with aortic stenosis.[27] There is no apparent familial component, and patients give a long history of isolated systolic hypertension. In comparison to the prevalence of hypertension in patients over age 65, which varies from 50 to 70 percent, hypertensive hypertrophic cardiomyopathy remains relatively rare, suggesting a unique and currently poorly understood pathophysiology.[28] Many postulate that in hypertensive hypertrophic cardiomyopathy, as in the hypertrophic obstructive form, the development of senescent hypertension may act influentially on an already genetically altered substrate to lead to the respective phenotypes.[29]

TABLE 69-1 Differences between Old and Young Patients with Hypertrophic Cardiomyopathy

Findings	Old	Young
Echocardiographic	Ovoid ventricle	Crescentic ventricle
	Large left atrium	Small left atrium
	LVH diffuse	LVH anterior septum
	Proximal septal bulge	No septal bulge
Mutations	Gene for cardiac myosin-binding protein C	β-myosin heavy chain and cardiac troponin genes
Etiology	Sporadic, 40%	Primarily inherited
Symptoms	More severe	Less severe
Progression	Slower	Rapid
Prognosis	Better	Worse
Sudden death	Uncommon	Common

VALVULAR

Valvular cardiomyopathy is defined as systolic dysfunction out of proportion to the wall stress imposed by the initial valvular lesion.[30] It occurs most commonly with left-sided regurgitant (mitral and aortic insufficiency) rather than stenotic lesions (aortic and mitral stenosis). The prognosis depends on the nature and extent of the valvular abnormality but more importantly on the degree of left ventricular dysfunction at the time of the proposed surgical repair. Generally even severe left ventricular dysfunction due purely to aortic stenosis will have a favorable prognosis after surgical repair. This is in marked contrast to a surgical approach for similar degrees of left ventricular dysfunction due to mitral[31] or aortic regurgitation. Owing to high surgical risks, medical therapy with afterload reduction—and, if indicated, cardiac transplantation—are acceptable modes of therapy in these instances. Cardiac reduction surgery with valve repair has become an increasingly popular modality for treatment of these high-risk patients. No large-center randomized trial is currently available to evaluate the efficacy and safety of this approach.

MYOCARDITIS

Infective

VIRAL

As early as 1806, a relationship between infection and chronic heart disease (diphtheria) was postulated, but it was not until the 1970s, with the advent of endomyocardial biopsies, that diagnosis of myocarditis could be established during life. Multiple infectious etiologies (Table 69-2)[32] have been implicated as the cause of myocarditis, with the most common being viral, specifically, Coxsackie B.[33] In the majority of patients, active myocarditis remains unsuspected because the cardiac dysfunction is subclinical, asymptomatic, and self-limited. Histologic evidence of myocarditis following traumatic death is identified in 1 to 3 percent of autopsies,[34,35] suggesting that the frequency of myocarditis is underestimated by analyzing data only from symptomatic patients.

Pathogenesis Infection by cardiotropic viruses prompted the initial hypothesis that the viral infection was responsible for myocardial injury. However, several investigators noted that cardiac dysfunction increased after the eradication of the infective agent and speculated that the pathogenesis may be due to the immunologic responses initiated by the virus (Fig. 69-2). Support for this theory comes initially from the work of Woodruff, who noted that the histologic evidence of cardiac injury in Coxsackie B infection occurred only after the virus was no longer detectable in the myocardium.[36] Subsequently, demonstration of T-lymphocyte and macrophage infiltration,[37] perforin granules,[38] and a variety of cytokines known to depress myocardial contractility[39] in endomyocardial biopsies of patients with active carditis strengthened the concept of immune-mediated injury. Furthermore, immunosuppressive therapy in animal models attenuated inflammation—with improved survival, less cellular infiltrate, and less necrosis.

The specific immune responses that lead to the myocardial injury are incompletely defined. A murine model of myocarditis induced by coxsackie B3 has provided some insight into immunologic sequence of events. Following infection with coxsackie B3 virus, macrophages are present in the infiltrate until day 8.[40] After macrophage activity decreases, both effector (CD8) and helper (CD4) T cells are identified within myocardial lesions. At peak infiltration, some murine strains showed a predominance of CD8-positive cells while in others CD4 cells predominate, suggesting participation of both humoral- and cell-mediated immune responses.[41] In human subjects, T-lymphocyte and macrophage infiltration characterizes the immunohistochemical picture, whereas B lymphocytes and natural killer cells are absent.[37] T-lymphocyte subset analysis of human serum does not demonstrate consistency in dominance of CD4 or CD8 cells.

TABLE 69-2 Causes of Myocarditis

- Infectious
  - Viruses
    - Coxsackievirus, echovirus, HIV, Epstein-Barr virus, influenza, cytomegalovirus, adenovirus, hepatitis (A and B), mumps, poliovirus, rabies, respiratory synctial virus, rubella, vaccinia, varicella zoster, arbovirus
  - Bacteria
    - *Cornyebacterium diptheriae, Streptococcus pyogenes, Staphylococcus aureus, Haemophilus pneumoniae, Salmonella* spp., *Neisseria gonorrhoeae, Leptospira, Borrelia burgdorferi, Treponema pallidum, Brucella, Mycobacterium tuberculosis,* Actinomyces, *Chlamydia* spp., *Coxiella burnetti, Mycoplasma pneumoniae, Rickettsia* spp.
  - Fungi
    - *Candida* spp., *Aspergillus* spp., *Histoplasma, Blastomyces, Cryptococcus, Coccidioidomyces*
  - Parasites
    - *Trypanosoma cruzii, Toxoplasma, Schistosoma, Trichina*
- Noninfectious
  - Drugs causing hypersensitivity reactions
    - Antibiotics: sulfonamides, penicillins, chloramphenicol, amphotericin B, tetracycline, streptomycin
    - Antituberculous: isoniazid, para-aminosalicylic acid
    - Anticonvulsants: phenindione, phenytoin, carbemazepine
    - Anti-inflammatories: indomethacin, phenylbutazone
    - Diuretics: acetazolamide, chlorthalidone, hydrochlorothiazide, spironolactone
    - Others: amitriptyline, methyldopa, sulfonylureas
  - Drugs not causing hypersensitivity reactions
    - Cocaine, cyclophosphamide, lithium, interferon alpha
  - Nondrug causes
    - Radiation, giant-cell myocarditis

The mechanisms of injury when lymphocytes infiltrate the myocardium are unknown. In the murine model, messenger ribonucleic acid (m-RNA) of perforin, the pore-forming protein mediating cytotoxicity, was identified in cytoplasmic granules of infiltrating cells by in situ hybridization.[42] Similarly, biopsy samples from patients with active myocarditis contain perforin granules in infiltrating cells,[38] implying that direct cytotoxicity can occur. Alternatively, release of cytokines such as interleukin-1, interleukin-6, interleukin-8, and tumor necrosis factor alpha may cause reversible depression of myocardial contractility without resulting in cell death.[39] Therefore, the effect of T cell–mediated immune injury may be either irreversible as a result of cell death through cytotoxicity (perforin) or reversible as a result of injury mediated by cytokines. A marked reduction in myocardial cell damage is noted in T cell–depleted mice inoculated with encephalomyocarditis virus.

Antiheart antibodies in the serum of patients with myocarditis have been reported but may reflect nonspecific myocardial damage.[43] When serum from patients with myocarditis was screened for autoantibodies, high-titer immunoglobulin G (IgG) with cardiac specificity was detected in 59 percent of patients with myocarditis and in none of the normal samples.[44] Antibodies with specificity for contractile and energy-transport proteins have been identified. In sera from patients with active myocarditis, Western immunoblotting demonstrated reactivity of a fraction that includes antibody to the heavy chain of cardiac myosin.[44] In a murine myocarditis model, cardiac myosin antibodies are observed following coxsackie B virus infection.[45] Moreover, injection of cardiac antimyosin antibodies without infection results in myocarditis that is histologically similar to that seen following coxsackie B3 virus infection.[46,47]

The role of viral infection has been deemphasized following the popularization of the immune injury hypothesis. Viral infection is the trigger for the immune response that is deleterious. Attempts to culture virus from human myocardial tissue generally have been unsuccessful. Only a single case report of Coxsackievirus identified in a myocardial biopsy specimen in an adult has been described.[48] However, identification of viral genomic fragments in myocardial samples by in situ hybridization and polymerase chain reaction from patients with myocarditis and dilated cardiomyopathy have been reported.[49–66] These genomic fragments may not be capable of replicating as intact cardiotropic virus but probably serve as a persistent source of antigen to drive the deleterious immune responses.[67]

In addition to the tropism of the virus, host immune responses play an important role in determining the severity of the clinical disease. When quantitative peripheral T- and B-lymphocyte populations were analyzed in patients with dilated cardiomyopathy and myocarditis, no consistent changes were detected.[68,69] However, immunologic assays demonstrate a reduction in the function of natural killer cells, antibody-dependent cellular cytotoxic cells, and suppressor cells and an increase in circulating levels of interleukin-1 and tumor necrosis factor alpha.[69–72] These immunoregulatory defects may predispose the host with a high antigenic load to develop immune responses that are not modulated by the natural inhibitory immunoregulatory mechanisms.

In addition to chronic inflammatory immune mechanism or persistent viral infection, apoptotic cell death may be another mechanism by which myocarditis can result in cardiomyopathy. Several different viruses have been reported to be triggers for apoptosis.

The association between acute myocarditis and dilated cardiomyopathy has been recognized for the past two centuries. However, the link between these two diseases remains circumstantial. Autoreactive antibodies and interleukin-2 receptors are identified commonly in both patients with myocarditis and those with dilated cardiomyopathy. Serologic titers to cardiotropic viruses are more common in patients with cardiomyopathy than in normal subjects. Viral genomic material can be detected more frequently by polymerase chain reaction (PCR) in patients with dilated cardiomyopathy versus other cardiac diseases. Animal models of myocarditis can progress to dilated cardiomyopathy, as can patients with clinically suspected or biopsy-proven myocarditis. However, the percentage of patients with idiopathic dilated cardiomyopathy that represent the end stage of an active myocarditis is unknown.

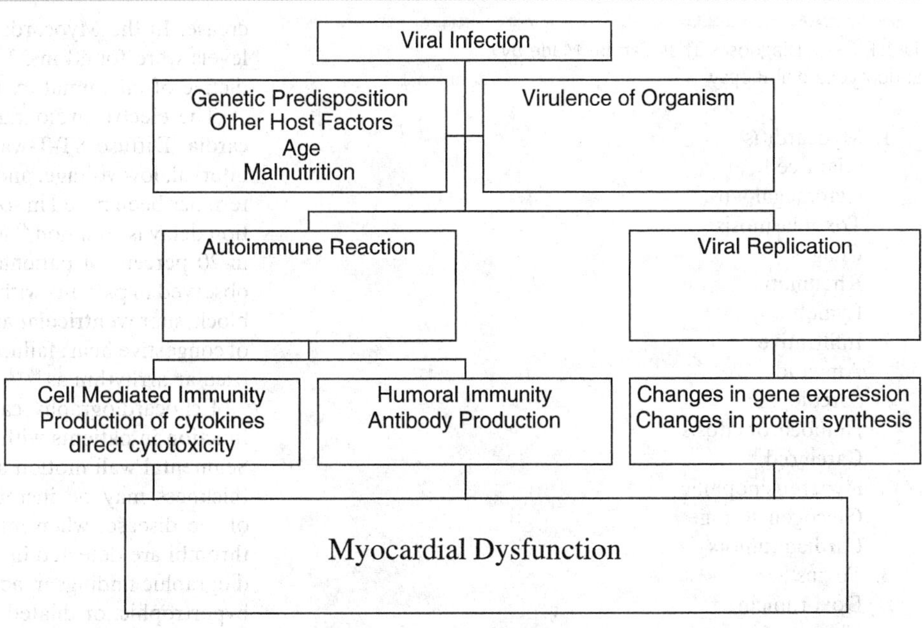

FIGURE 69-2 Flow diagram illustrating various factors that contribute to the development of myocardial dysfunction after viral infection.

Clinical Presentation The clinical manifestations of myocarditis are variable. Most patients have a self-limited disease, whereas others present in profound cardiogenic shock. The most obvious symptom suggesting myocarditis is an antecedent viral syndrome. Flu-like symptoms occur in approximately 60 percent of patients.[73] Chest pain may occur in up to 35 percent of patients and may be typically ischemic, somewhat atypical, or pericardial in character. Occasionally patients will present with a clinical syndrome identical to an acute myocardial infarction, with left ventricular asynergy, electrocardiographic evidence of injury or Q waves, and ischemic cardiac pain[74] (Fig. 69-3). In this syndrome, at autopsy, the coronary arteries are widely patent, although viral coronary arteritis has been reported.[75,76] Coronary vasospasm has also been associated with acute myocarditis.[77]

Patients may present with syncope or palpitations with atrioventricular (AV) block or ventricular arrhythmia. Complete AV block is common with some patients presenting with Stokes-Adams attacks. The complete heart block is generally transient and rarely requires a permanent pacemaker.[78] Sudden cardiac death can be the initial presentation of myocarditis in some patients, presumably from complete heart block or ventricular tachycardia. In a 20-year review of sudden death among Air Force recruits, 20 percent had myocarditis documented at autopsy.[79] In some patients with refractory ventricular arrhythmias, endomyocardial biopsy or autopsy has revealed myocarditis. Systemic or pulmonary thromboembolic disease is also associated with myocarditis.[80,81]

A familial tendency for the development of myocarditis may be present. In one report, a suppressor cell defect was detected, predisposing to development of active myocarditis.[82] Patients with peripartum cardiomyopathy have a high frequency of myocarditis on endomyocardial biopsy.[83] The immunoregulatory changes during and following pregnancy may heighten susceptibility to viral myocarditis, and exposure to trophoblastic antigens may predispose to immune-mediated myocardial injury.

Patients with new-onset left ventricular dysfunction given the diagnosis of idiopathic dilated cardiomyopathy may actually have active myocarditis despite the absence of clinical signs and symptoms of acute infection.[84]

Diagnosis Laboratory findings are generally not diagnostic. Sixty percent of patients will have an elevated erythrocyte sedimentation rate and 25 percent an elevated white blood cell count.[73] Elevated titers to cardiotropic viruses may be present. However, a fourfold rise in IgG titer over a 4- to 6-week period is required to document acute infection. Elevated IgM antibody titer may denote an acute infection more specifically than a rise in IgG antibody titer. Unfortunately, a rise in antibody titer documents only the response to a recent viral infection and does not indicate active myocarditis.

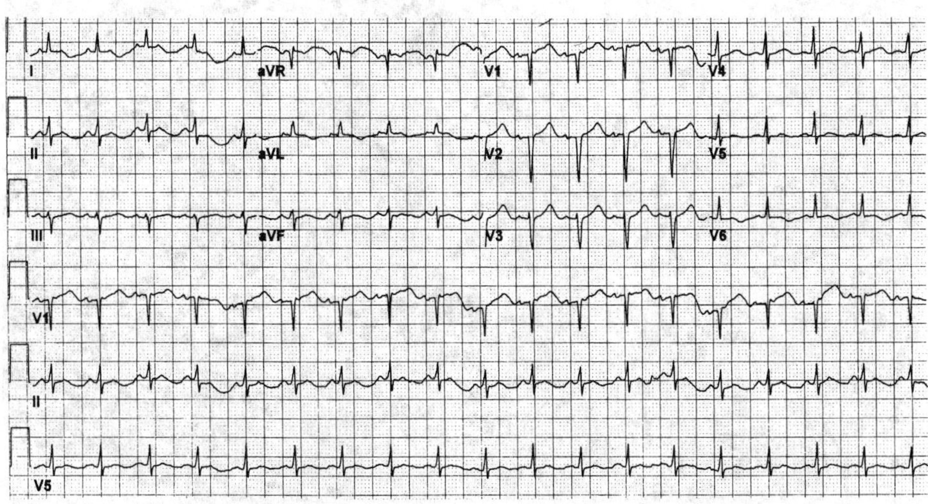

FIGURE 69-3 Electrocardiographic tracing consistent with an anteroseptal myocardial infarction and lateral ischemia in a patient with acute myocarditis and normal coronary arteries.

TABLE 69-3 Diagnoses That Can Be Made by Endomyocardial Biopsy

1. Myocarditis
   - Giant cell
   - Cytomegalovirus
   - Toxoplasmosis
   - Chagas
   - Rheumatic
   - Lyme
2. Infiltrative
   - Amyloid
   - Sarcoid
   - Hemochromatosis
   - Carcinoid
   - Hypereosinophilic
   - Glycogen storage
   - Cardiac tumors
3. Toxins
   - Doxorubicin
   - Chloroquine
   - Radiation injury
4. Genetic
   - Fabry
   - Kearns-Sayre syndrome
   - Right ventricular dysplasia

Abnormalities in peripheral T- and B-lymphocyte counts have been reported, but these findings have not been consistent and cannot be used as diagnostic adjuncts.

Increase in the MB band of CPK is observed in approximately 12 percent of patients.[73] Troponin levels may also increase. In the Myocarditis Treatment Trial, elevated troponin levels were found in 32 percent of the patients and were predictive of inflammatory involvement.

The electrocardiogram most frequently shows sinus tachycardia. Diffuse ST-T-wave changes, prolongation of the QTc interval, low voltage, and even an acute myocardial infarct pattern has been noted in some patients with myocarditis. Conduction delay is common,[85] with left bundle branch block identified in 20 percent of patients. Cardiac arrhythmias are frequently observed in patients with myocarditis, including complete heart block, supraventricular arrhythmias—especially in the presence of congestive heart failure or pericardial inflammation, and ventricular arrhythmias.[86]

Echocardiography can reveal left ventricular systolic dysfunction in patients with a normal-sized left ventricular cavity. Segmental wall motion abnormalities may be observed.[87] Wall thickness may be increased, particularly early in the course of the disease, when inflammation is fulminant.[88] Ventricular thrombi are detected in 15 percent of those studies.[89] Echocardiographic findings in active myocarditis can mimic restrictive, hypertrophic, or dilated cardiomyopathy.

Endomyocardial biopsy is the critical test to confirm the diagnosis. Endomyocardial biopsy techniques enable the repetitive sampling of the human myocardium with minimal discomfort and minor morbidity.[84,90,91] Right ventricular myocardial specimens can be obtained by accessing the right internal jugular or femoral vein. Intravascular biopsy of the left ventricle is infrequently performed due to the higher morbidity associated with this approach. The right ventricular bioptome is positioned under fluoroscopy or echocardiography to sample the interventricular septum.[90] As the myocarditis can be focal, a minimum of four to six fragments are obtained. Sampling error is reduced by less than 5 percent. Using the Stanford bioptome, typical samples are 2 to 3 mm in maximal diameter and 5 mg in wet weight. Samples are processed, paraffin-imbedded, sectioned, and stained with hematoxylin-eosin and trichrome. Special stains are employed if other diagnoses are considered. Diagnoses that can be made or confirmed by endomyocardial biopsy are listed in Table 69-3.

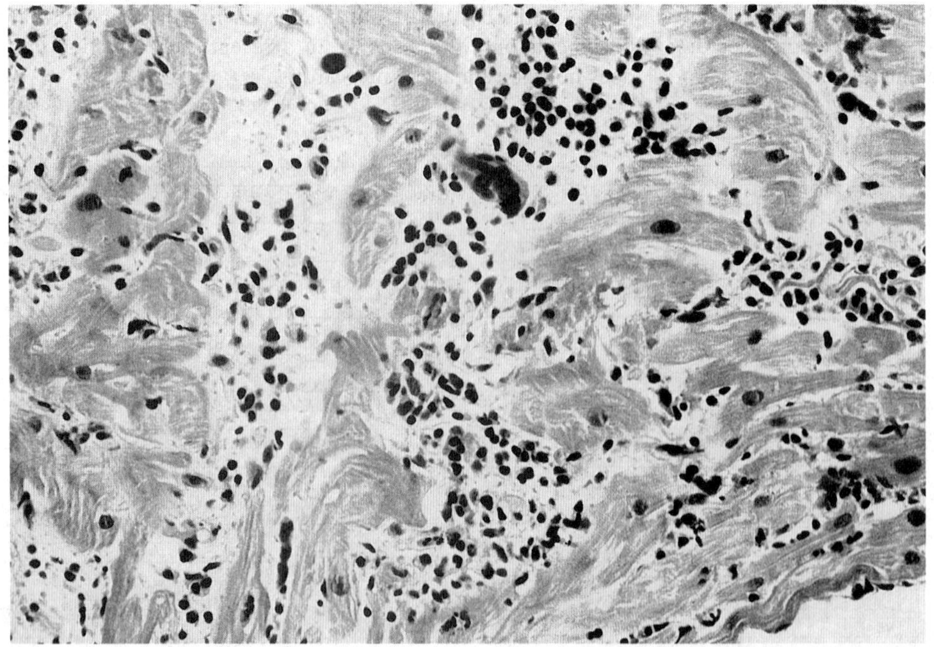

FIGURE 69-4 Photomicrograph showing extensive interstitial infiltrates of lymphocytes and myocytes with focal myocyte necrosis. (H&E, ×40.)

Several investigators have performed endomyocardial biopsies in patients with unexplained congestive heart failure and/or ventricular arrhythmia.[84,92–122] The percentage of patients with biopsies interpreted as myocarditis varied widely, primarily owing to the different diagnostic criteria for active myocarditis used by the investigators. This variability of endomyocardial biopsy criteria prompted a meeting of cardiac pathologists to reach a consensus on the pathologic definition of myocarditis, now known as "the Dallas criteria." Active myocarditis was defined as "an inflammatory infiltrate of the myocardium with necrosis and/or degeneration of adjacent myocytes not typical of the ischemic damage associated with coronary artery disease."[123] Examination of a minimum of four to six fragments from each patient is required for interpretation. The term *borderline* myocarditis is applied when the inflammatory infiltrate is too sparse or myocyte injury is not demonstrated. Repeat biopsy is then suggested. A high frequency of active myocarditis is confirmed by repeat biopsy in patients whose initial histologic samples demonstrated borderline myocarditis.[124] When right ventricular endomyocardial biopsy has failed to establish the diagnosis, sampling the left ventricle may improve diagnostic yield (Fig. 69-4).

Endomyocardial biopsy must be applied as quickly as possible to maximize the diagnostic yield. Biopsies in patients with peripartum cardiomyopathy have the highest yield when performed early after onset of symptoms.[83] Resolution of active myocarditis has been documented within 4 days of initial biopsy, with progressive clearing over several weeks on serial biopsy.[125] Progression of active myocarditis to dilated cardiomyopathy has been documented when serial biopsies are performed.[126]

Newer molecular biology techniques are being applied to the analysis of endomyocardial tissue for the detection of viral nucleic acid. The usefulness of PCR amplification of viral genomic material from endomyocardial tissue in children with suspected myocarditis was shown in a study that found PCR-amplified viral product in 67 percent of the children studied.

Noninvasive Studies Although technetium-99m-pyrophosphate scintigraphy has proved useful in the detection of myocarditis in a murine model, it has not been effective in diagnosing myocarditis in humans. Imaging with gallium 67, an inflammation-avid radioisotope, has shown promise as a screening method for active myocarditis, with a specificity and sensitivity of 83 percent and a negative predictive value of 98 percent in biopsy-proven myocarditis.[100] Indium 111–labeled antimyosin antibody scans can be used to detect myocyte necrosis. Application of this technique in patients with myocarditis has demonstrated a sensitivity of 83 percent, a specificity of 53 percent, and a positive predictive value of a normal scan of 92 percent.[124] In those patients who were antimyosin antibody–positive and biopsy-negative, the possibility of inflammation undetected by biopsy has been considered. Antimyosin imaging, however, detects myocyte injury independent of etiology, and noninflammatory causes of heart muscle injury in young patients may cause false-positive scans. The usefulness of scintigraphy in diagnosing myocarditis is limited by low specificiy, radiation exposure, and expense (see also Chap. 16).

Tissue alterations associated with myocarditis may be identifiable using magnetic resonance imaging (MRI).[127] Preliminary results suggest that myocardial inflammation may induce abnormal signal intensity of the myocardial walls. Use of T2-weighted images to visualize tissue edema has been described in several case reports of patients with active myocarditis. More recently, contrast media–enhanced MRI has been used to characterize myocardial changes in myocarditis. The MRI imaging contrast agent gadopentetate dimeglumine accumulates in inflammatory lesions (see Chap. 18A). It is a hydrophilic agent that accumulates in the extracellular space of water-containing tissues. Gadolinium increases the signal of T1-weighted images. A total of 19 patients with clinically suspected myocarditis and 18 normal subjects underwent contrast-enhanced MRI. Global relative enhancement was higher in patients than controls. Contrast MRI also visualized the area of inflammation and the extent of inflammation and may prove to be a valuable technique in both the diagnosis and monitoring of disease activity.

Despite the promise of noninvasive techniques, endomyocardial biopsy remains the diagnostic standard.

Treatment The immune injury hypothesis generated application of potential therapies, including immunosuppression. Anecdotal success with immunosuppression in active viral myocarditis[101,106] led to the large Multicenter Myocarditis Treatment Trial.[128] In this study, 111 patients with biopsy-proven myocarditis were randomized between conventional medical therapy versus steroid/azathioprine or steroid/cyclosporine immunosuppression. The primary end point of the study was change in ejection fraction over 28 weeks. For all patients, the average increase in ejection fraction over baseline was 9 percent. Treatment assignment was not predictive of improvement in left ventricular ejection fraction, attenuation of clinical disease, or mortality[129] (Fig. 69-5).

Recently, immune modulatory therapy with immune globulin has been shown to be an effective treatment for Kawasaki's disease and new-onset cardiomyopathy in pediatric patients.[130] Subsequently, a small open-label study was performed in 10 adult patients with new-onset heart failure.[131] Significant improvement in left ventricular function was observed in 9 of 10 patients. These findings formed the basis for a multicenter study investigating the use of this treatment modality. The IMAC trial (Intervention in Myocarditis and Acute Cardiomyopathy with immune globulin) used a single infusion of high-dose immunoglobulin (2 g/kg) to treat presumed inflammatory cardio-

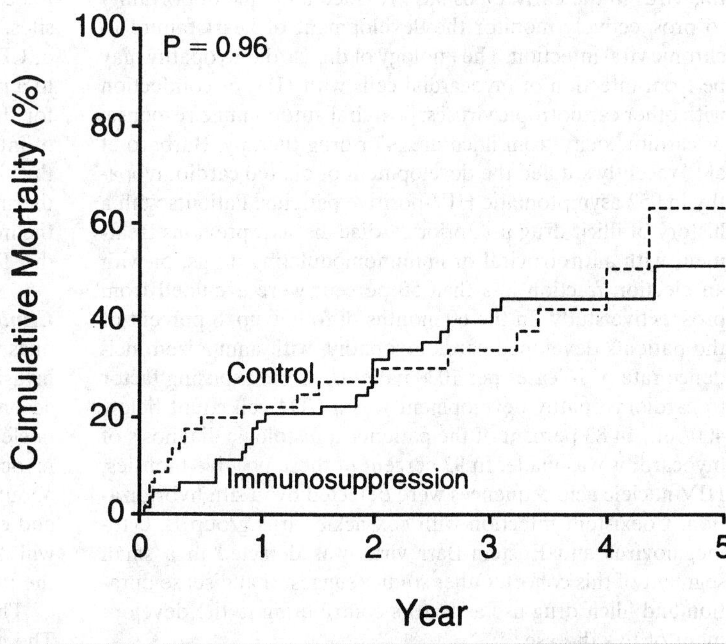

FIGURE 69-5 Actuarial mortality curves from the Myocarditis Treatment Trial illustrating no difference in survival between the treatment groups. (From Mason et al.,[129] with permission.)

myopathies. In this placebo-controlled 6-month trial, the improvement in left ventricular ejection fraction and symptoms was similar in both groups. Thus no benefit of immunomodulation could be demonstrated.

Despite the experimental data supporting the immune injury hypothesis, no randomized study has yet demonstrated the efficacy of immunosuppressive therapy in myocarditis. Immunosuppressive therapy is therefore not routinely recommended for infective myocarditis. Standard heart failure treatment remains the mainstay of therapy.

Prognosis About one-third of those who present with clinical carditis and recover will be left with some cardiac abnormality ranging from mild changes on electrocardiography (ECG) to significant heart failure. The multicenter myocarditis trial provided insight into the natural history of myocarditis with current treatment. The degree of left ventricular dysfunction at initial presentation was most predictive of recovery. Approximately 40 percent of patients fully recovered.[104] Other predictors of recovery included shorter duration of disease and less intensive conventional drug therapy. One-year survival in this study was 80 percent, with a 4-year survival of only 44 percent.

The prognosis of myocarditis depends to some extent on the causative agent, but if clinical heart failure develops, 5-year mortality rates are in the 50 to 60 percent range, comparable with figures seen in idiopathic cardiomyopathy.[132] Chronic inflammation, viral persistence, or both may affect disease progression and prognosis. Future therapies will need to identify the predominant factor to target treatment and hopefully improve survival.

Human Immunodeficiency Virus Human immunodeficiency virus (HIV) is increasingly recognized as a cause of dilated cardiomyopathy. In some inner-city hospitals, it may represent a very common diagnosis. The relatively recent emergence of this virus in the early 1980s has provided a unique opportunity to prospectively monitor the development of heart failure to chronic viral infection. The etiology of this cardiomyopathy may be from infection of myocardial cells with HIV or coinfection with other cardiotropic viruses, postviral autoimmune response, or cardiotoxicity from illicit drugs or drug therapy. Barbaro et al.[133] recently studied the development of dilated cardiomyopathy in 952 asymptomatic HIV-positive patients. Patients with a history of illicit drug use, prior cardiac disease, previous treatment with antiretroviral or immunomodulating drugs, or with an ejection fraction less than 50 percent were excluded from prospective study. In the 60 months of follow up, 8 percent of the patients developed cardiomyopathy, with annualized incidence rate of 16 cases per 1000 patients. A predisposing factor to cardiomyopathy development was a CD4 cell count below 400/mL. In 83 percent of the patients, a histologic diagnosis of myocarditis was made. In 92 percent of these positive biopsies, HIV nucleic acid sequences were detected by in situ hybridization. Coexistent infection with coxsackie virus group B, cytomegalovirus and Epstein-Barr virus was detected in a small segment of this cohort. Other studies suggest that disease duration and illicit drug use as factors contributing to the development of this disease.[134]

As the symptoms of heart failure and HIV can be very similar (i.e., fatigue, wasting, etc.), careful cardiologic follow-up of these patients is probably indicated to detect early development of left ventricular dysfunction. Conventional heart failure management can then be instituted to alleviate cardiac-related symptoms.

Cytomegalovirus Cytomegalovirus may lead to myocarditis in the general population, but ordinarily the myocarditis is self-limited and asymptomatic. In the cardiac transplant recipient, however, cytomegalovirus myocarditis may become a more serious disease resulting in cardiac dysfunction.[135] The treatment of cytomegalovirus myocarditis is intravenous ganciclovir, which effectively eradicates the virus. Early cytomegalovirus infection correlates with the development of allograft coronary artery disease, the major cause of death beyond the first year after cardiac transplantation. It is proposed that infection of either subintimal fibroblasts or endothelial cells results in immunologic injury that predisposes to this potentially fatal condition.

NONVIRAL

Chagas' Disease American trypanosomiasis, or Chagas' disease, is the most common cause of congestive heart failure in the world.[136] This condition results from the bite of the reduviid bug, leading to infection with *Trypanosoma cruzi,* and is endemic to rural South and Central America.

Pathogenesis The pathogenesis of chronic, chagasic cardiomyopathy is controversial because the parasite is rarely present in the myocardium. As in the viral cardiomyopathy model, the cardiac injury is thus thought to be immunologically mediated.[137] Both cellular and humoral immune responses have been implemented in the myocardial injury.[137] Myocardial biopsies demonstrate that the inflammatory infiltrate in chronic Chagas' disease consists mainly of CD8+ T cells, with a low number of CD4+ T cells.[138–140] This suggests some degree of immunologic depression in the host, since the activation of T-helper cells is known to be the most effective mechanism of defense against the parasites.[141] Some have postulated that the diminished expression of CD4+ T cells during acute *T. cruzi* infection may be related to a mechanism of tolerance induced by the parasite. Evidence for this comes from studies that have shown that the addition of interleukin-1 (IL-1) in vitro restores helper T-cell function, thus implementing a macrophage defect in this process.[142] Furthermore, IL-2 and the IL-2 receptor are absent or scarce in the inflammatory infiltrate,[143] attesting to the attenuated role of the T-helper subset in this disease.

Clinical Presentation This parasitic disease has an acute phase, where hematogenous spread of the parasite leads to invasion of various tissues and organ systems. The invasion is accompanied by an intense inflammatory reaction with mononuclear cells and is characterized by fever, sweating, myalgias, myocarditis, hepatosplenomegaly, and a case fatality rate of about 5 percent. Most patients recover from the acute illness and enter an asymptomatic latent phase, but 20 to 30 percent will develop a chronic form of the disease up to 20 years after the initial infection.

The chronic stage is a result of gradual tissue destruction. The gastrointestinal tract and the heart are the most common sites of involvement, with the primary cause of death being cardiac failure. In the gut, the destruction of the myenteric plexus is responsible for the development of megaesophagus and megacolon. In the heart, the myofibrils and the Purkinje fibers are replaced by fibrous tissue, leading to cardiomegaly, congestive heart failure, heart block, and arrhythmia. The microscopic findings are those of extensive fibrosis, but a chronic cellular infiltrate composed of lymphocytes, plasma cells, and macrophages is often present and parasites are found in about a quarter of the patients.

The diagnosis of the acute disease depends on the discovery of trypomastigotes in the blood of the infected individual. In chronic infection, direct diagnosis is less useful due to less circulating trypomastigotes. Xenodiagnosis (where the patient is bitten by reduviid bugs bred in the laboratory and subsequent identification of the parasites in the intestine of the insect) is the most useful test, which will detect infection in about half the patients. The complement-fixation test (Machado-Guerreiro test) also has high sensitivity and specificity for identification of chronic Chagas' disease. In the other lab tests, it is necessary to rely on positive serologic tests (such as the indirect immunofluorescent antibody, the enzyme-linked immunosorbent assay, and the hemagglutination tests) together with symptoms and signs compatible with Chagas' disease.

Endomyocardial biopsy may show active myocarditis using the Dallas criteria.[144] Noninvasive assessment commonly shows segmental wall motion abnormalities, specifically apical aneurysms. Electrocardiographic findings include complete heart block, atrioventricular block, or right bundle branch block with or without fascicular block in 11 percent of infected individuals.[145] Ventricular arrhythmias may require antiarrhythmic drugs, including amiodarone.[146]

The treatment of chronic Chagas' disease is symptomatic and includes a pacemaker for complete heart block, an implantable cardioverter-defibrillator for recurrent ventricular arrhythmia, and standard therapy for congestive heart failure as outlined for other forms of myocarditis. Antiparasitic agents such as Nifurtimox and benzimidazole eradicate parasitemia during the acute phase and are typically curative. They should be administered if the disease has not previously been treated and may be used as prophylaxis if there is a high likelihood of recurrence, such as following immunosuppressive therapy. The role of immunosuppression therapy for chagasic myocarditis is controversial, and heart transplantation is effective for end-stage refractory cardiac disease.

Lyme Carditis Lyme disease may result from infection with the spirochete *Borrelia burgdorferi,* introduced by a tick bite. The initial presenting symptom in patients with the disease who progress to cardiac involvement is frequently complete heart block. Left ventricular dysfunction may be seen but is unusual.[147] Endomyocardial biopsy may show active myocarditis. Rarely are spirochetes seen on biopsy. Corticosteroid administration is helpful in treating Lyme carditis following therapy with tetracycline.[148]

Among other infectious etiologies is *Toxoplasma gondii,* which is curable by pyrimethamine and sulfadiazine[149] and occurs most commonly in the immune-deficient host. Leptospirosis is yet another common cause in fatal cases of myocarditis. Fifty percent of cases have ST- and T-wave changes on electrocardiography.

Rheumatic Carditis One form of myocarditis that has declined dramatically in the latter half of the twentieth century is rheumatic carditis.[150] The availability of antibiotics and changes in the virulence and serotypes of group A streptococcus may explain the decreasing frequency of this disease.[151]

Acute rheumatic fever can occur in children and young adults. It generally follows a group A streptococcal pharyngitis, but only indirect evidence linking the two has been found. Rheumatic carditis may result from a direct toxic effect of some streptococcal product versus an immunologic mechanism.[152–154] Group A streptococci have a number of structural components similar to those of human tissue. Antibodies to streptococci cross-react with the glycoproteins of heart valves. The serum of patients with rheumatic fever contains autoantibodies to myosin and sarcolemma. The Aschoff body, pathognomic for this disorder, represents persistent focal inflammatory lesions in the myocardium. These nodules can persist for years after an acute attack. Macrophages containing myosin have been identified in these nodules.

Clinical diagnosis is made using the Jones criteria[155] (see also Chap. 55). The major manifestations are carditis, polyarthritis, chorea, erythema marginatum, subcutaneous nodules, and evidence of preceding streptococcal infection (i.e., positive throat culture, history of scarlet fever, elevated antistreptolysin titers). Minor criteria are nonspecific findings such as fever, arthralgia, previous rheumatic fever or rheumatic heart disease, elevated ESR or reactive protein, and prolonged PR interval. Diagnosis is made by the presence of two major criteria or one major and two minor criteria. Debate into whether the Jones criteria should be modified to incorporate Doppler-Echo indices are ongoing.[156,157]

Two-thirds of patients present with an antecedent pharyngitis, followed by the symptoms of rheumatic fever in 1 to 5 weeks, with a mean presentation of 18.6 days. Severe carditis resulting in death can occur but is unusual. CHF is observed in only 5 to 10 percent of cases. Usually the carditis is mild, with the predominant effect being scarring of the heart valves. Physical exam is notable for fever and heart murmurs reflecting the acute valvulitis. The mitral valve is involved three times as frequently as the aortic valve; therefore mitral murmurs are more common. Mitral regurgitation is the most common finding. A mid diastolic murmur over the apical area can frequently be heard. This

TABLE 69-4 Drug Causes of Eosinophilic Myocarditis

Drug	
Acetazolamide	Oxyphenylbutazone
Amitriptyline	Para-aminosalicylic acid
Amphotericin B	Penicillin
Ampicillin	Phenindione
Carbamazepine	Phenobarbital
Cefaclor	Phenylbutazone
Chloramphenicol	Phenytoin
Chlorthalidone	Spironolactone
Desipramine	Streptomycin
Hydrochlorothiazide	Sulfadiazine
Indomethacin	Sulfisoxazole
Interleukin-4	Sulfononylureas
Isoniazid	Tetanus toxoid
Methyldopa	Tetracycline

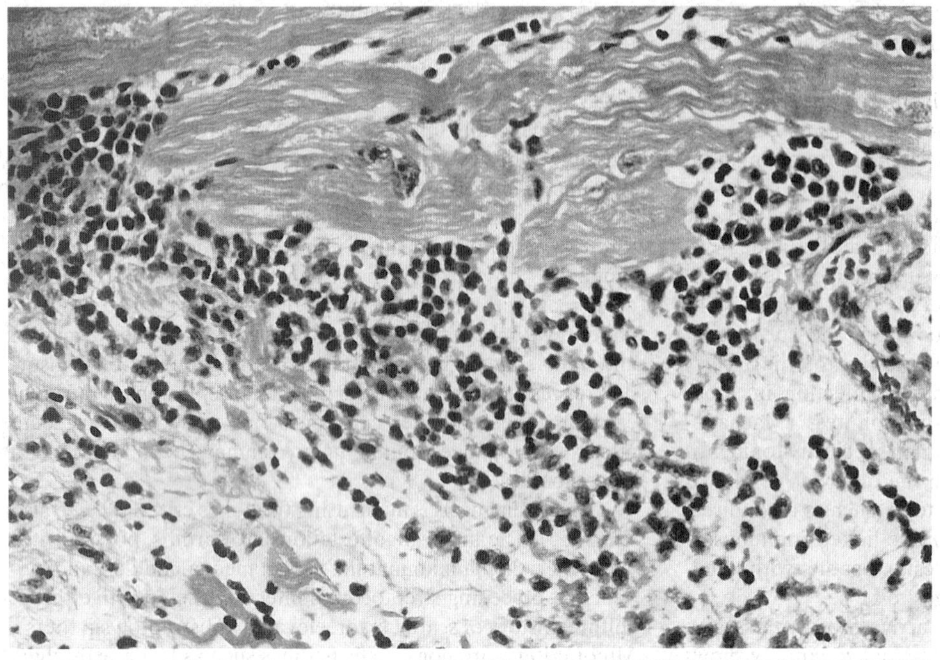

FIGURE 69-6 Photomicrograph showing interstitial infiltrates rich in eosinophils. (H&E, ×40.)

Laboratory tests suggestive of rheumatic fever include antibodies to antistreptolysin O and anti-DNAase B, an elevated sedimentation rate, and elevated C-reactive protein. Extracardiac manifestations generally predominant with an acute migratory polyarthritis of the large joints. Aspirin and penicillin are the mainstays of therapy. Corticosteroids can also provide symptomatic relief. Once rheumatic fever is diagnosed, antibiotic prophylaxis is required to prevent recurrent episodes. The most effective method is a single monthly intramuscular injection of 1.2 million units of benzathine Penicillin G until age 21.

is called the Carey Coombs murmur, and its presence almost certainly confirms mitral valvulitis. Aortic insufficiency can be auscultated with aortic valvulitis.

There are no characteristic ECG findings through PR prolongation, and nonspecific ST-T-wave changes are frequently described. Endomyocardial biopsy demonstrates the Aschoff nodules as well as a diffuse cellular interstitial infiltrate including lymphocytes, polymorphonuclear cells, histiocytes, and eosinophils.

Noninfective

HYPERSENSITIVITY

Hypersensitivity myocarditis is an example of the early phase of eosinophilic myocarditis and is thought to be due to an allergic reaction to a variety drugs (Table 69-4). Methyldopa, the penicillins, sulfonamides, tetracycline, and the antituberculous drugs are the pharmaceuticals most commonly associated with this entity. It is characterized by peripheral eosinophilia and infiltration into the myocardium by eosinophils, multinucleated giant cells, and leukocytes (Fig. 69-6).[158] The major basic protein of the eosinophil granule may be detected in the presence of acute necrotizing myocarditis, suggesting toxicity of the granule contents.[159] Good success has been reported with stopping the offending agent and treatment with corticosteroids.[160] Unfortunately, the presence of this condition often goes unnoticed and the first manifestation of cardiac involvement is sudden death due to arrhythmia.

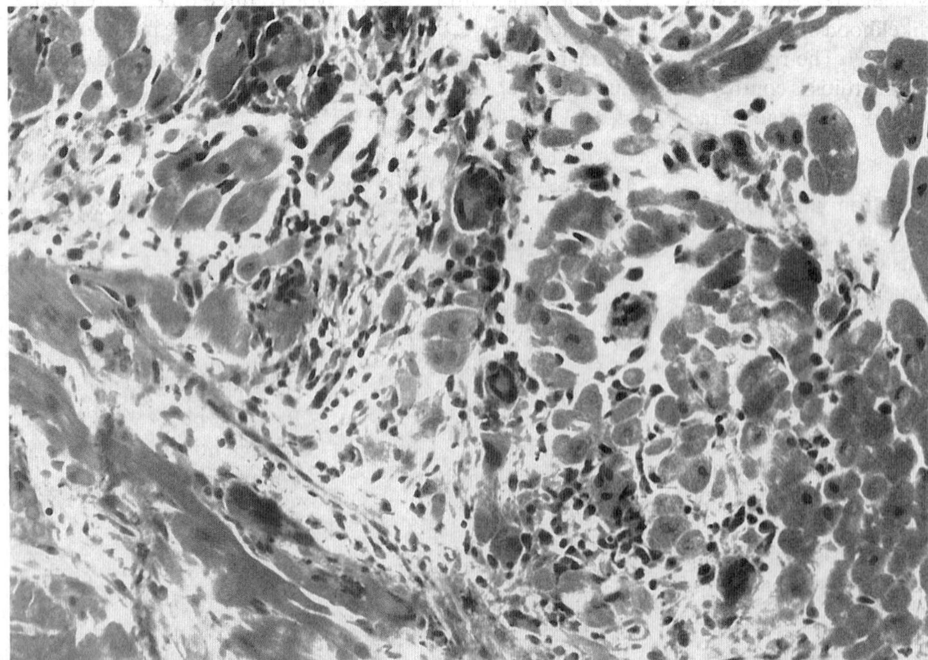

FIGURE 69-7 Photomicrograph showing extensive myocyte damage and infiltrates of mononuclear cells and numerous multinucleated giant cells. (H&E, ×60.)

GIANT-CELL MYOCARDITIS

Giant-cell myocarditis is an extremely rare but aggressive form of myocarditis, typically progressive and unresponsive to medical therapy.[161] This disease is most prevalent in young adults, with a mean age at onset of 42 years (and a range of 16 to 69 years). Association with other autoimmune disorders is reported in approximately 20 percent of cases. Diagnosis is made by endomyocardial biopsy. Widespread or multifocal necrosis with a mixed inflammatory infiltrate including lymphocytes and

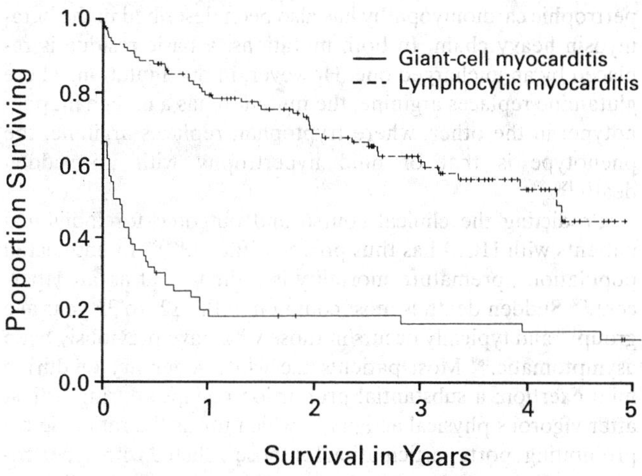

FIGURE 69-8 Kaplan Meier survival curves for patients with giant-cell myocarditis versus lymphocytic myocarditis. (From Cooper et al.,[161] with permission.)

histiocytes is required for histologic diagnosis. Eosinophils are frequently noted, as are multinucleated giant cells in the absence of granuloma (Fig. 69-7). Immunophenotyping of the cellular infiltrate has shown lymphocyte populations composed of T-helper or in some cases T-suppressor cells.

The clinical course is usually characterized by progressive CHF and is frequently associated with refractory ventricular arrhythmia.[162] It is almost uniformly and rapidly fatal. Comparison of survival of patients with giant-cell myocarditis with that of patients with lymphocytic myocarditis demonstrates significantly worse survival in those patients with giant-cell disease (Fig. 69-8). There have been rare reports of response to aggressive immunosuppressive regimens that include cyclosporine and azathioprine in addition to corticosteroids.[162,163] Use of immunosuppressive therapy in these patients appears to prolong survival. Cardiac transplantation represents the best treatment option, though most patients expire prior to identification of a suitable donor. Giant-cell myocarditis may recur following cardiac transplantation, but the frequency of recurrence is unknown. Giant cells can be detected on routine surveillance biopsies up to 9 years posttransplant. This cellular infiltrate may respond to an increase in immunosuppressive therapy.

PERIPARTUM

Peripartum cardiomyopathy is an uncommon form of CHF first described by Virchow in 1870.[164] Estimates of its incidence vary from 1 to 1300 to 1 in 15,000 pregnancies.[165] The disease occurs more commonly in obese multiparous black females over age 30.[166] Cesarean delivery, multiple gestations, preeclampsia, and chronic hypertension are other predisposing factors. Patients present with heart failure in the last trimester of pregnancy or in the first 5 months postpartum. Absence of a demonstrable cause of heart failure and structural heart disease is required to make the diagnosis. Indeed, the hemodynamic stress of pregnancy can frequently unmask previously unknown cardiac disease (see also Chap. 82).

PATHOGENESIS

The etiology of this disorder is unclear. Proposed mechanisms include nutritional deficiencies, genetic disorders, viral or autoimmune etiologies, hormonal problems, volume overload, alcohol, physiologic stress of pregnancy, or unmasking of latent idiopathic dilated cardiomyopathy. Several lines of evidence suggest that peripartum cardiomyopathy may be the result of myocarditis due to a viral illness or an autoimmune etiology.[167–172] Given the relatively immunosuppressed state of pregnancy, susceptibility to cardiotropic viruses is higher,[167] as is the viral load during infection.[168] Furthermore, studies have demonstrated that when cardiac output rises, as is the case in pregnancy, myocardial viral lesions worsen.[169] Additionally, several studies have demonstrated histologic evidence of myocarditis on endomyocardial biopsy samples obtained from patients with peripartum cardiomyopathy.[170–172] Other investigators have postulated an autoimmune etiology to peripartum cardiomyopathy, specifically immunologic responses to fetal and endometrial antigens that cross-react with the patient's myocytes. In one case report, a patient with peripartum cardiomyopathy had antibodies to smooth muscle and actin produced in response to actin and myosin released during uterine degeneration after delivery. These antibodies later cross-reacted with the myocardium and induced cardiomyopathy.[173]

CLINICAL PRESENTATION

The presentation is that of heart failure. Presenting symptoms include shortness of breath, dyspnea on exertion, edema, palpitations, syncope, sudden death, and thromboembolic phenomena. The incidence of thromboembolism is high due to the hypercoagulability of pregnancy. Physical findings are notable for S3, S4, tricuspid or mitral insufficiency murmurs, edema, rales, ascites, hepatomegaly, jugular venous distension. The ECG frequently shows left ventricular hypertrophy. Echocardiographic findings can range from single-chamber left ventricular enlargement to four-chamber dilatation. In a small percentage of patients, endomyocardial biopsy may reveal myocarditis, but generally the findings are nonspecific.

PROGNOSIS AND TREATMENT

Too few patients with peripartum cardiomyopathy have been studied to fully analyze the natural history of the disease. In a small series of 27 patients, left ventricular size was analyzed at 6 months; 14 patients (50 percent) had normal dimensions. None of these patients died of CHF—compared with 85 percent of those patients with persistent cardiomegaly, who died from CHF within 5 years.[174] The authors concluded, therefore, that if the congestive cardiomyopathy persists for more than 6 months, it is likely to be irreversible and to be associated with a worse prognosis. Similar findings were published in another series by O'Connell et al.[83] These authors also noted that those patients with higher ejection fractions and smaller ventricular diastolic dimensions at the time of diagnosis have a better long-term prognosis. Other prognostic studies suggest that those patients with persistent symptoms more than 2 weeks postpartum have a worse prognosis, raising the question as to whether this disorder has different etiologies.[175] The role of corticosteroids in the treatment of this disorder is controversial.[170,171] The incidence of thromboembolism is high due to the hypercoagulabilty of pregnancy; therefore anticoagulation is recommended.[175]

Patients with refractory heart failure referred for transplant have a survival posttransplant comparable with that of patients with idiopathic dilated cardiomyopathy, though higher early rejection rates are noted.

In patients with stable heart failure or recovery of left ventricular function, the possibility of subsequent pregnancy must be addressed. There are several case reports of patients with this diagnosis who went on to subsequent pregnancies. The outcomes of these patients are variable, with a few having uneventful pregnancies and others developing an exacerbation or recurrence of fulminant heart failure. Subsequent pregnancy should be viewed as high risk and all patients with this disorder should be counseled on birth control and even sterilization.

HYPERTROPHIC AND FAMILIAL

Hypertrophic cardiomyopathy is characterized by disproportionate hypertrophy primarily of the left ventricle (Fig. 69-9) and occasionally the right ventricle. It most typically involves the septum but can also be concentric[176] and occurs in the absence of a recognizable stimulus to hypertrophy. This has led many to postulate and subsequently demonstrate a genetic basis to this disease.[177] Inheritance is of an autosomal dominant pattern; however, the phenotypic expression of this disease as measured by echocardiography is highly variable and reflects the different genetic mutations and incomplete penetrance.[178–180] The identification of certain well-characterized genetic abnormalities offers some measure of prognostication. Several familial hypertrophic cardiomyopathy–causing mutations have been characterized in the genes encoding sarcomeric contractile proteins—namely, the beta-myosin heavy chain,[181] cardiac troponin T,[178] alpha tropomyosin,[178] and cardiac myosin–binding protein C.[182,183] Previous theories suggested that variations resulting in a change in charge of the substituted amino acid were associated with a poor survival index.[184,185] However, the genotypic-phenotypic correlation is not always preserved. For example, a cytosine-for-guanine mutation hot spot responsible for familial hypertrophic cardiomyopathy has also been described in the beta-myosin heavy chain. In both mutations, a basic residue is replaced by an uncharged one. However, in one mutation, where glutamine replaces arginine, the mutation has a malignant phenotype; in the other, where tryptophan replaces arginine, the phenotype is that of mild hypertrophy with no sudden death.[186,187]

Predicting the clinical course and outcome for individual patients with HCM has thus proved difficult.[188,189] In unselected populations, premature mortality is estimated at about 1 percent.[186] Sudden death is most common in the 12- to 35-year age group[190] and typically occurs in those who have previously been asymptomatic.[189] Most patients die while sedentary or during mild exertion; a substantial proportion collapse during or just after vigorous physical activity,[190] which forms the rationale for prohibiting sports participation for those afflicted with hypertrophic cardiomyopathy.

The mechanism of sudden death in hypertrophic cardiomyopathy is complex and probably multifactorial.[191] Recurrent syncope is the only symptom that has been shown to be reliably associated with subsequent sudden death.[192] Other proposed risk factors include prior cardiac arrest, sustained ventricular tachycardia, massive left ventricular hypertrophy, a malignant genotype or a previous family history of sudden premature death, repetitive salvos of nonsustained ventricular tachycardia on Holter monitoring, and early onset of symptoms in childhood.[193–196] The main forms of therapy have been primarily beta blockade, calcium channel blockers, amiodarone, and implantable cardioverter-defibrillators, with conflicting data on their impact on mortality.[197] Cardiac transplantation is pursued when significant symptomatic systolic dysfunction develops.[198]

As in the case of the myosin mutations noted in the hypertrophic cardiomyopathies, single genetic defects are presumed to underlie the dilated cardiomyopathies that have been described in several large families. There has been recent evidence that dilated cardiomyopathy is more frequently familial than generally realized.[199] In a single-center study of 96 patients with a diagnosis of idiopathic cardiomyopathy, approximately 20 percent had a familial basis.[200] Other studies have estimated a familial role in up to 50 percent of cases when first-degree relatives are carefully screened.[201] The influence of a preceding viral infection,[202] alcohol use,[203] or pregnancy[204] on the clinical manifestation of cardiomyopathy in familial situations remain unclear.

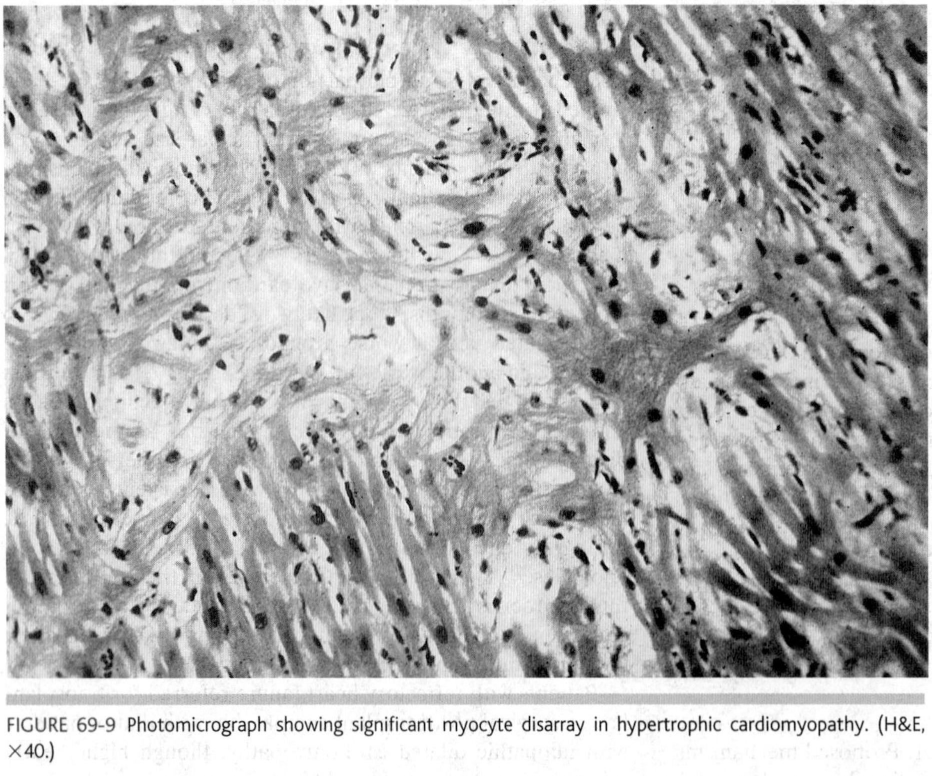

FIGURE 69-9 Photomicrograph showing significant myocyte disarray in hypertrophic cardiomyopathy. (H&E, ×40.)

Neuromuscular Diseases

Several heritable neuromuscular dystrophies may be associated with cardiomyopathy. Included in this category are diseases such as Beckel's, Duchenne's, and X-linked cardioskeletal myopathy, myotonic dystrophy (Stingert's disease), congenital myotonic dystrophy, limb-girdle muscular dystrophy (Erb's disease), familial centronuclear myopathy, Dugelberg-Welander syndrome, Friedreich's ataxia and Barth's syndrome. The myocardial involvement, natural history, and prognosis of each of these disorders are variable.

Duchenne's dystrophy is an X-linked disease with proximal muscle weakness and cardiomyopathy. A dystrophin gene mutation is responsible. Death usually results from respiratory and/or cardiorespiratory failure. Patients with myotonic dystrophy present between age 20 and 50 years, usually with arrhythmias.

Several mitochondrial myopathies have also been described.[177,205] Mitochondria are essential cellular organelles that convert oxygen to biochemically useful energy. Additionally, mitochondria function as calcium storage sites and modulators of cellular pH. As such, mitochondrial function affects muscle and ventricular function. Mitochondria are unique organelles with their own maternally inherited DNA, which encodes several respiratory chain proteins. Genetic defects in the mitochondrial respiratory chain enzymes—specifically complexes I, III, and IV—have been recognized as the cause in some cardiomyopathies. The presentation in mitochondrial myopathies is extremely heterogeneous, as each cell will contain a mixture of normal and mutant DNAs. Deletion mutations in DNA can occur and are frequently observed in these myopathies.

Mitochondrial myopathies include such disorders as Kearns-Sayre syndrome, chronic ophthalmoplegia, myoclonic epilepsy, ragged-red-fiber disease, and mitochondrial encephalomyopathy. The MELAS syndrome—mitochondrial encephalopathy, lactic acidosis, and stroke-like episodes—is associated with cardiomyopathy and generalized microangiopathy. Kearns-Sayre syndrome results from a deletion mutation in mitochondrial DNA. This ocular myopathic disease is associated with dilated or hypertrophic cardiomyopathy with cardiac conduction defects.

Defects in transport of molecules from the cytoplasm into the mitochondria have also been associated with cardiac and skeletal myopathy. One example is that of carnitine deficiency, discussed later in this chapter.

INFILTRATIVE

The infiltrative cardiomyopathies comprise several acquired and heritable conditions; these include amyloidosis, hemochromatosis, carcinoid, sarcoidosis, glycogen storage disease, endocardial fibroelastosis, and endomyocardial fibrosis due to hypereosinophilic syndromes or other collagen vascular disorders such as scleroderma or Churg-Strauss syndrome.

Amyloid

CLASSIFICATION AND PATHOGENESIS

The most commonly encountered of the infiltrative cardiomyopathies is amyloidosis, leading to an overproduction of a monoclonal immunoglobulin protein that is deposited throughout the body. Secondary amyloidosis results from the deposition of a protein other than immunoglobulin. Whereas primary amyloid has no associated systemic diseases, other chronic diseases are present in the secondary form. Secondary amyloidosis may result from familial, senile, or chronic inflammatory processes (rheumatoid arthritis, juvenile rheumatoid arthritis, ankylosing spondylitis, Crohn's disease, tuberculous paraplegia associated with decubitus ulcers, cystic fibrosis, and heroin use with chronically infected cutaneous injection sites). Familial Mediterranean fever is an autosomal recessive inherited disease of Sephardic Jews, Armenians, and other Mediterranean peoples associated with amyloid deposition. In the familial diseases, more than 40 different genetic mutations of the plasma protein transthyretin (prealbumin) have been associated with amyloid deposition. Inheritance is autosomal dominant, with the genetic defect being confined to a single amino acid substitution in the mature protein.[206,207]

The frequency of cardiac involvement varies with the different etiologies. Of patients with primary amyloid, one-third to one-half have cardiac involvement and more than one-fourth have symptomatic heart failure. Cardiac involvement in patients with secondary amyloidosis is much less frequent. Indeed, in amyloid due to chronic inflammatory processes, amyloid protein deposition is usually limited to the intima and media of arterioles and not the heart. Familial amyloidosis is the rarest form of systemic amyloidosis, affecting only about 4 percent of cases; however, cardiomyopathy is present in 68 percent of those affected. Familial amyloidosis can manifest initially with progressive neuropathy, cardiomyopathy, or renal involvement. In some of the families, cardiac amyloidosis is not even symptomatic, while in others cardiac symptoms predominate. Senile cardiac amyloidosis is common in the elderly but often does not lead to a clinical cardiac syndrome and is only detected postmortem.[208]

CLINICAL PRESENTATION

Amyloid fibrils are rigid and as such lead primarily to relaxation abnormalities and diastolic dysfunction; however, when myocardial replacement occurs, systolic dysfunction becomes a prominent feature.[209] The cardiomyopathy may be restrictive or congestive in nature. Systolic left ventricular function deteriorates late in the disease process only after marked amyloid deposition.[210-217] The clinical presentation is that of congestive heart failure, with a more frequent occurrence of right-sided symptoms. Sudden death and myocardial infarction may result from vascular involvement. Atrial arrhythmias, from infiltration of atrial tissue with amyloid, are not uncommon.

DIAGNOSIS

Diagnosis is made by characteristic echocardiographic features and endomyocardial biopsy.[218] Echocardiography can demonstrate symmetric thickening of the left ventricular wall with a diffuse hyper-refractile, granular sparkling appearance of the myocardium (Fig. 69-10*A*) (see also Chap. 13). Abnormal left ventricular diastolic filling manifested by reduction in the rate, in the volume of rapid diastolic filling with enhanced atrial contraction can be seen very early in cardiac amyloidosis.[219] The ECG typically demonstrates low voltage despite marked hypertrophy on echo (Fig. 69-10*B*). A pseudoinfarct or postinfarct anterior wall pattern is often present.[220] Cardiac involvement is generally present when mean left ventricular wall thickness on echocardiogram is greater than 11 mm in the absence of a history of hypertension or valvular heart disease, with unexplained low voltage (<0.5 mV) on the ECG. The majority of patients presenting with cardiac involvement have a mono-

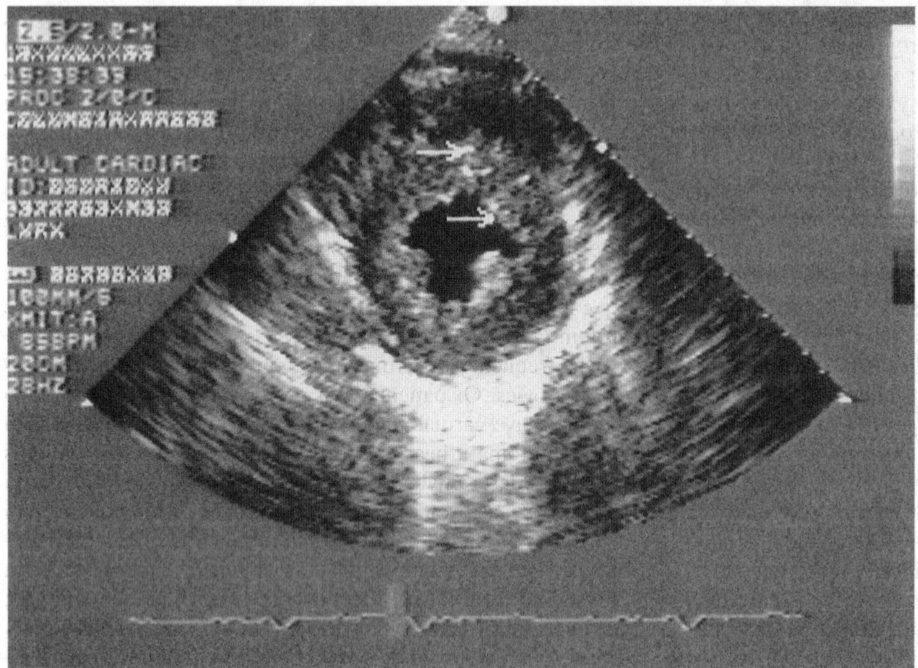

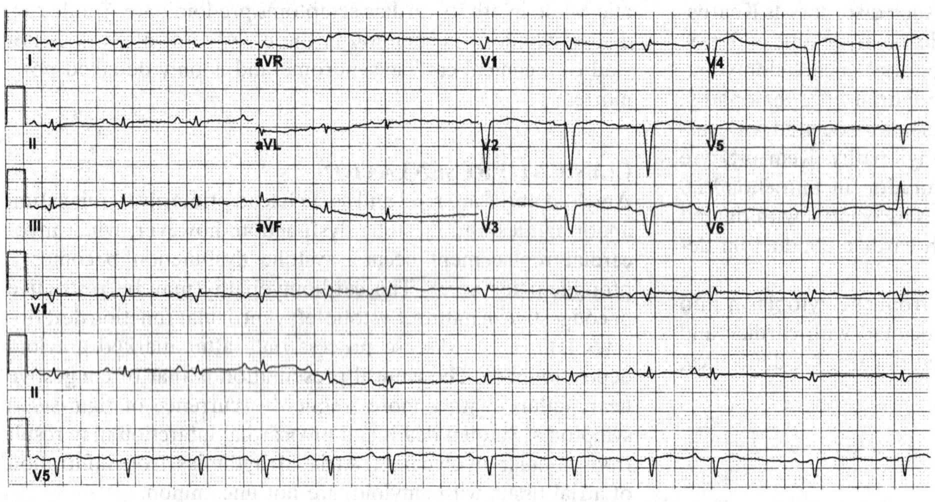

FIGURE 69-10 Cardiac amyloidosis. *A*. Two-dimensional echocardiographic parasternal short-axis view demonstrating symmetrical thickening of the left ventricular wall and granular sparkling appearance of the myocardium. *B*. 12-lead electrocardiogram demonstrating low voltage and a pseudoinfarct pattern. *C*. Photomicrograph showing diffuse interstitial accumulations of waxy homogeneous material. (H&E, ×60.) *D*. Electron microscopy of an amyloid deposit (asterisk) in a cardiac biopsy.

clonal protein spike in the serum or urine reflecting the primary nature of the disease.[210]

Amyloid is detected easily in endomyocardial biopsy specimens using Congo red staining and is seen in the interstitium in a pericellular or nodular pattern, in the endocardium, or in myocardial blood vessels. Sulfated alcian blue, methyl violet, and thioflavine T are other histochemical stains used to detect cardiac amyloid (Fig. 69-10*C*). Immunoperoxidase stains for kappa and lambda light chains and for prealbumin may categorize the type of cardiac amyloid. Electron microscopic examination of biopsy specimens is likely the most sensitive method of recognizing amyloidosis (Fig. 69-10*D*).

Radionuclide imaging using technetium-99m pyrophosphate and indium-111 antimyosin showing increased diffuse uptake can also be used to diagnose cardiac amyloidosis.

TREATMENT

Prognosis is typically poor and treatment ineffective.[221] Increased myocardial concentrations of digoxin may occur from binding of the drug to amyloid fibrils, thus increasing the propensity for digoxin toxicity. Digoxin should therefore be used with caution in these patients. Prognosis depends on the extent of myocardial involvement, but once heart failure is present, the prognosis is poor, with a 5-year survival less than 5 percent. Indeed, patients with primary amyloidosis who fall into New York Heart Association (NYHA) class 3 or have recurrent cardiac syncope rarely survive for more than 6 months. Echocardiography with Doppler assessment can provide prognostic information. A shortened deceleration time and an increased ratio of early diastolic filling velocity to the atrial filling velocity were more powerful predictors of mortality from cardiac causes than left ventricular wall thickness or fractional shortening.[222–224]

A recent clinical trial comparing colchicine to the combination of melphalan, prednisone, and colchicine failed to demonstrate any survival benefit in cases of cardiac amyloid. Stem-cell transplant as treatment for primary amyloidosis is now being investigated.

Because of recurrence in the transplanted heart, results following heart transplantation have proved disappointing.[225] The immediate and early postoperative outcomes are similar to those in patients undergoing transplantation for other cardiac diseases; however, late survival is reduced (39 percent at 48 months) owing to recurrence of the disease in the transplanted organ and progressive disease in other organ systems. With the continuing donor shortage, the outcome associated with primary amyloidosis is unacceptable to the majority of cardiac transplant centers. In the future, combined cardiac and bone marrow transplant may provide successful treatment.

Sarcoidosis

PATHOGENESIS

Sarcoidosis is a systemic granulomatous disease of unknown etiology characterized by enhanced cellular immune responses. The pathologic hallmark of this disease is the noncaseating granuloma (Fig. 69-11). The initial lesion is an inflammatory infiltrate consisting of activated helper-inducer T lymphocytes and abundant macrophages that secrete cytokines. The macrophages aggregate and differentiate into epithelioid and multinucleated giant cells. Fibroblasts, mast cells, collagen fibers, and proteoglycans encase the inflammatory cells into a ball-like cluster. The fibrotic response results in end-organ damage.

Clusters of cases have been observed, suggesting spread by person-to-person exposure or environmental agents/pathogens. Genetic factors may also play a role in the development of the disease, as an exaggerated cellular immune response and the formation of granulomas may develop in genetically predisposed hosts after exposure to the offending antigen.

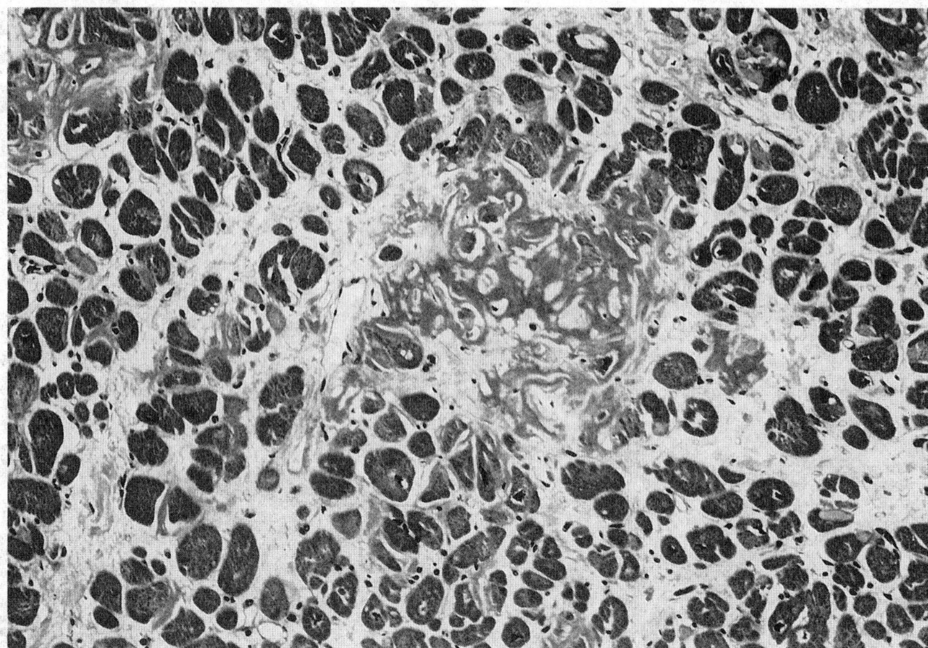

C

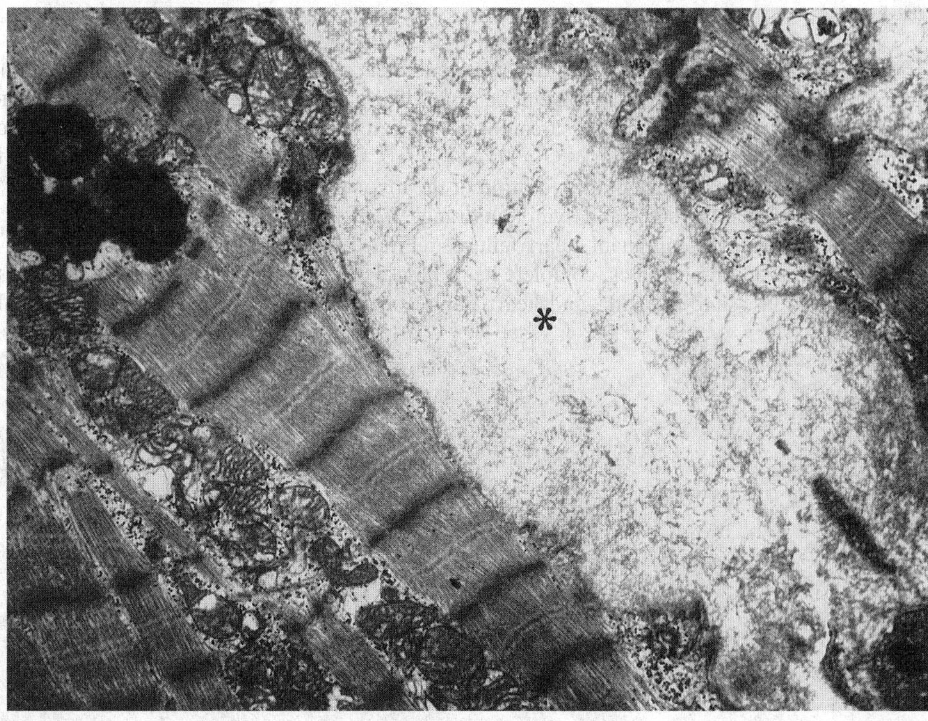

D

FIGURE 69-10 (*Continued*)

CLINICAL PRESENTATION

The clinical manifestations of sarcoidosis are protean. The disease may be widespread or limited to a single organ. Virtually any organ except the adrenal gland may be involved. The lymphoid, pulmonary, cardiovascular, hepatobiliary, and hematologic systems are the most commonly involved, with the lungs being affected in over 90 percent of patients.[226–228]

Cardiac sarcoid is more common than previously recognized. In a recent autopsy study of 38 patients with sarcoidosis, 76 percent had cardiac involvement, accounting for 50 percent of the deaths. In other series, sarcoidosis affected the heart in 25 to 50 percent of autopsy cases with fatality in 50 percent of the cases with cardiac involvement.[229] Cardiac sarcoid is more likely fatal and less likely to be diagnosed antemortem than pulmonary sarcoid. Frequently the initial presentation is that of sudden death. Myocardial involvement peaks between the third and sixth decades of life. Less than 10 percent of patients with sarcoid have symptoms referable to the cardiovascular system.

In myocardial sarcoid, portions of the myocardial wall are replaced by sarcoid granulomas, which preferentially involve the cephalad portion of the ventricular septum or the left ven-

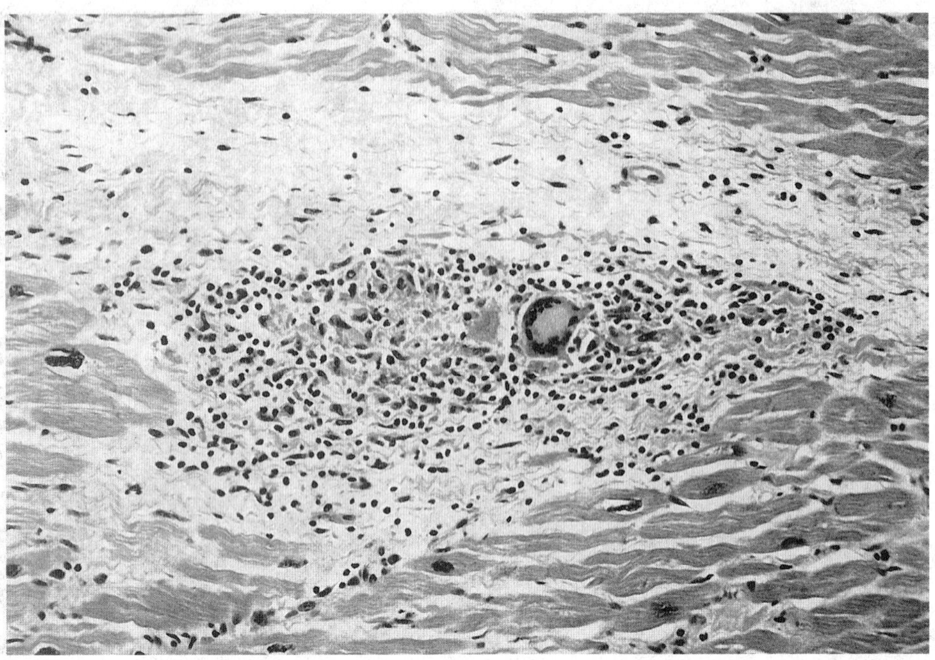

FIGURE 69-11 Photomicrograph showing interstitial noncaseating granulomas with a multinucleated giant cell. (H&E, ×40.)

tricular papillary muscles.[230] Myocardial involvement is much more common than pericardial involvement.[226,231–234] Cor pulmonale due to extensive pulmonary sarcoidosis with interstitial fibrosis may occur.

Because of the varied extent and location of the myocardial granulomas, presenting signs and symptoms range from first-degree heart block to fulminant heart failure.[235] First-degree AV block, bundle-branch block, complete heart block, ventricular arrhythmias, sudden death, and heart failure occur with a frequency of 10 to 20 percent.[235] Heart failure can present as a cardiomyopathy with restrictive hemodynamics or systolic dysfunction. Some 25 percent of the deaths due to cardiac sarcoid are from heart failure, while sudden death accounts for one-third to one-half of the deaths.

DIAGNOSIS

In diagnosing cardiac sarcoid, evidence of other organ system involvement including lymphadenopathy, hepatomegaly, splenomegaly, or pulmonary findings should be sought. In cases where the heart is involved to a much greater degree than are other organs, little or no evidence of extracardiac sarcoidosis may be found. Chest x-ray, ECG, and echocardiography findings will depend on the extent and location of involvement. Due to the scattered nature of the granulomas, endomyocardial biopsy lacks sensitivity and seldom makes the diagnosis despite high specificity. Magnetic resonance imaging has been useful in diagnosing scars or lesions in the myocardium due to sarcoid.[236]

TREATMENT

Although no controlled trials have been performed, high-dose corticosteroids are usually given in the hope that the course of disease may be altered. Administration of corticosteroids can improve cardiac symptoms and reverse ECG changes in over half of the treated patients.[237] Antiarrhythmic drugs should be used as necessary, although drug therapy of ventricular tachycardia in patients with sarcoidosis, even when guided with programmed ventricular stimulation, is associated with a high rate of arrhythmia recurrence or sudden death.[238] Automatic internal cardioverter-defibrillators have been advocated. Prognosis after the diagnosis of cardiac sarcoid is variable but can be poor.[227] In one series of 247 patients, survival was 41 percent at 5 years and 15 percent at 10 years.[226,239] Transplantation is also a successful treatment, as the recurrence of sarcoid in the allograft is low, possibly due to posttransplant steroid therapy.[240]

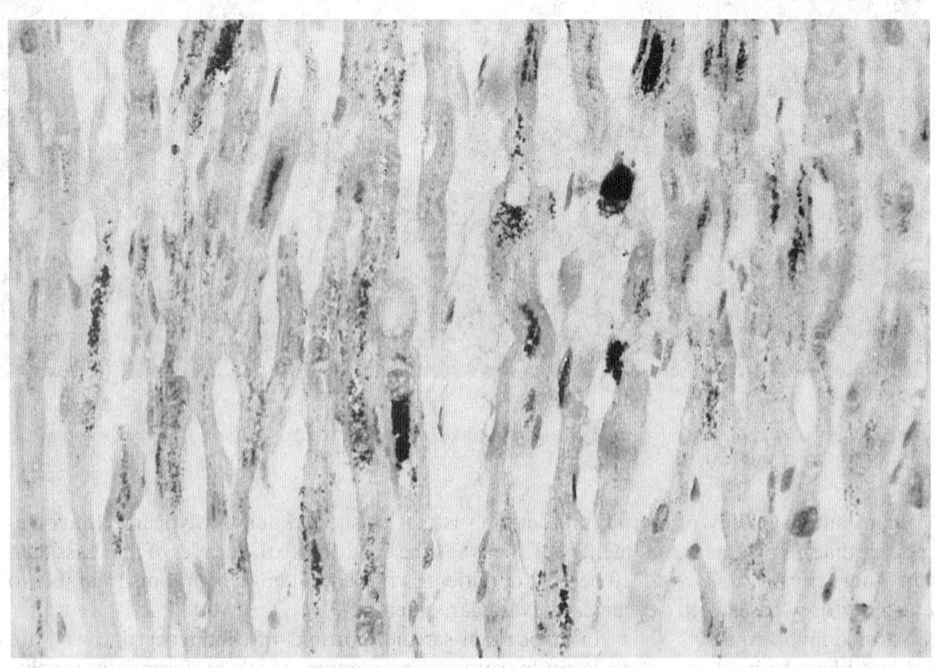

FIGURE 69-12 Photomicrograph showing Perls' stain of hemachromatosis with deposits scattered throughout the myocyte. (×100.)

Hemachromatosis

Primary hemachromatosis is an inborn error of metabolism leading to iron deposition in a variety of organs, including the heart, and resultant secondary myocardial fibrosis. Both restrictive and dilated presentations can occur.[241,242] In contrast to amyloidosis, treatment with phlebotomy[243] is highly effective. In the secondary forms of hemachromatosis due to multiple blood transfusions for blood dyscrasias, chelation therapy is highly effective. Diagnosis is made by symptom constellation in the presence of an elevated serum iron and ferritin. Endomyocardial biopsy is diagnostic (Fig. 69-12).

Carcinoid

Carcinoid heart disease typically leads to a restrictive pattern and often has asymmetrical involvement due to the predilection of the carcinoid for the tricuspid valve apparatus.[244,245] Diagnosis is generally made with right-sided heart findings in the setting of systemic features of carcinoid syndrome. Cardiac involvement responds favorably to control of the primary tumor with chemotherapy or catheter embolization.[244] Tricuspid valve replacement and/or pulmonary valvulotomy and outflow tract enlargement have been recommended when hemodynamically indicated.[244] Alternatively, balloon valvuloplasty for tricuspid or pulmonary stenoses has been used successfully[246] (see also Chaps. 59 and 77).

There are other heritable lesions leading to infiltrative cardiomyopathy. Pseudoxanthoma elasticum (also known as endocardial fibroelastosis) is an inherited disorder of elastic tissue metabolism that leads to a thickening and calcification of the endocardium.[247] Similarly, a number of metabolic inherited disorders cause massive infiltration of the myocardium in infancy and childhood. The best known is Pompe's disease, which is an autosomal recessive disorder caused by a deficiency of the enzyme α-glucosidase, leading to massive glycogen deposition in the cardiac and skeletal musculature. Interestingly, the pathophysiology resembles that of hypertrophic rather than restrictive cardiomyopathy.[248] Prognosis is poor, with no known therapy. Death typically ensues within the first year of life.

Eosinophilic Heart Disease

Eosinophilic heart disease was originally described several decades ago by Löffler,[249] who reported the observation of endocardial lesions, termed "endocarditis parietalis fibroplastica," in association with blood eosinophilia. Although initially thought to represent an isolated disease, Löffler's syndrome is now recognized to be only one manifestation of a spectrum of hypereosinophilic syndromes. Recently cases of isolated eosinophilic myocarditis without signs of endocardial involvement, with or without vasculitis, have been described.[250] Hypereosinophilic syndromes are characterized by peripheral eosinophilia and endocardial disease consisting of eosinophilic infiltration, fibrosis, and eventual occlusion of the ventricular cavity by scar and thrombus.[251] This leads to a very severe form of restrictive myocardial disease referred to as *obliterative myocardial disease*.[252]

PATHOGENESIS

Löffler's endomyocardial disease is considered to be an immunologic disorder caused by clones of abnormal eosinophils infiltrating both sides of the heart. This group of diseases may begin with myocarditis due to the direct toxic effects of the eosinophils and their granules.[253] Indeed, hypersensitivity myocarditis, discussed earlier in this chapter, may be an early variant of this disease. Chronic disease culminates in endomyocardial fibrosis after the disappearance of the initial eosinophilia.[254] The eosinophilic endocardial disease has since been well described[255,256] and is characterized by intense endocardial fibrotic thickening of the apex and subvalvular regions of one or both ventricles. These changes lead to inflow obstruction and restrictive physiology.

CLINICAL PRESENTATION

Löffler's syndrome was initially described primarily in men from temperate climates in their fourth decade of life with a hypereosinophilic syndrome. Diffuse organ involvement may be observed (lungs, bone marrow, brain), with cardiac involvement in more than 75 percent of patients. The typical clinical presentation includes weight loss, fever, cough, skin rash, and congestive heart failure. Overt cardiac dysfunction occurs in about half the patients and is the leading cause of death. Chest x-ray reveals cardiomegaly. ECG findings most commonly include nonspecific ST- and T-wave changes, atrial fibrillation, and right bundle-branch block. Echocardiography commonly demonstrates localized thickening of the left ventricle with valvular leaflet abnormalities[257] and atrial enlargement due to atrioventricular valvular regurgitation and restrictive physiology. In cases of advanced endomyocardial fibrosis, there may be apical obliteration by thrombus[253] but normal systolic function.

Diagnosis is easily established in the acute phase by endomyocardial biopsy and typical ECG images.[252] Variable degrees of acute inflammatory eosinophilic myocarditis are observed. Marked changes can be seen histologically in the coronary vessels, including inflammatory, fibrotic, and thrombotic changes typically containing eosinophils. Fibrotic thickening of up to several millimeters[253] can be observed. Mural thrombosis is common.

Medical therapy with corticosteroids and cytotoxic drugs[159,257,258] in the early stages of disease may substantially improve survival. Routine therapy for heart failure with digitalis, diuretics, afterload reduction, and anticoagulation are adjuncts in the management of these patients. Surgical therapy offers palliation once the later fibrotic stages have been reached.[259]

CARDIOMYOPATHY DUE TO PERSISTENT TACHYCARDIA

Incessant supraventricular or ventricular tachycardia can lead to severe dilated cardiomyopathy in both animals and humans.[260] Successful medical or surgical treatment of the tachyarrhythmia can lead to resolution of the myopathy. The mechanism between the sustained tachycardia and the development of cardiomyopathy is unknown but may be related to depletion of high-energy substrates.

CARDIOMYOPATHY DUE TO RIGHT VENTRICULAR DYSPLASIA

Right ventricular dysplasia is a cardiomyopathy predominantly of the right ventricle. Left ventricle involvement is usually of a lesser and variable degree. Several anomalies may be included under this general heading: Uhl's anomaly,[261] arrhythmogenic right ventricular dysplasia,[262] and right ventricular cardiomyopathy.[263] It is currently recognized as an important inherited cardiomyopathy and a cause of sudden death, especially in youth.[264] Its cause is unknown, although an autosomal dominant pattern with variable expression and penetrance has been suggested, since many cases show a strong familial tendency.[265]

Clinically patients typically present with recurrent ventricular tachycardia of left-bundle-branch-block morphology and, less commonly, CHF. Standard electrocardiography discloses incomplete or complete right-bundle-branch block in most patients or T-wave inversions in leads V_1-V_3 (Fig. 69-13*A*). These conduction or repolarization abnormalities are thought to be due to adipose infiltration of the myocardium. Clinical diagnosis is based on detection of predominantly right ventricular morphologic changes on imaging studies. Echocardiography is an effective tool to demonstrate the characteristic abnormal structure[266] of the right ventricle, including hypokinesis, massive dilatation, and a "parchment-thin" wall[267] (Fig. 69-13*B*). In addition, tricuspid regurgitation and paradoxic ventricular septal wall motion are common. Pathologically, there is variable infiltration or replacement of the right ventricular myocardium by adipose and fibrous tissue.[268]

The importance of right ventricular dysplasia is its association with sudden death, with an incidence of up to 20 percent in some series.[264] Therapy therefore is focused on the prevention of sudden death with implantation of automatic internal cardioverter-defibrillators.

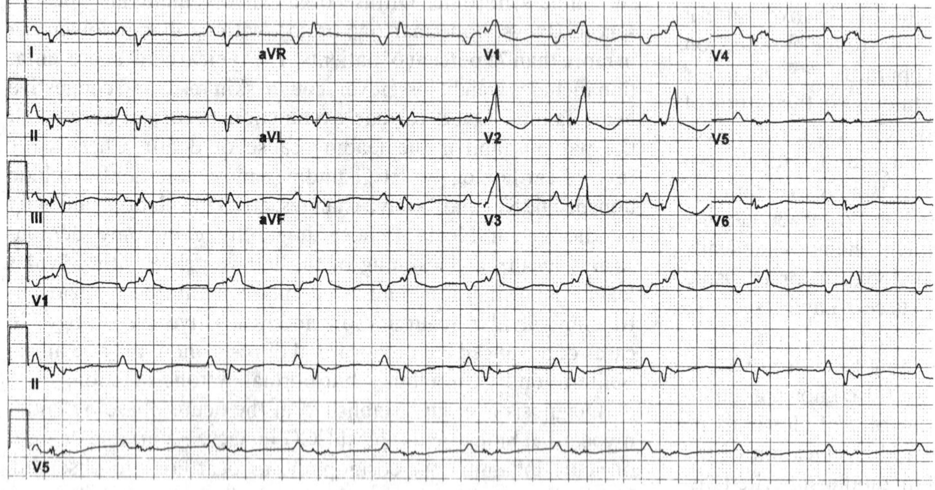

B

FIGURE 69-13 Uhls' anomaly. *A*. Twelve-lead electrocardiogram demonstrating characteristic right bundle branch block with T-wave inversions in leads V_1–V_3. *B*. Two-dimensional echocardiographic four-chamber view demonstrating massive right ventricular dilation with a "parchment-thin" wall.

CARDIOMYOPATHY DUE TO ENDOCRINE DISORDERS

Thyroid

Thyroid hormone has long been recognized to affect the heart and the peripheral vasculature.[269] Changes in cardiac function are mediated by T3 regulation of cardiac-specific genes.[270] Thyroid hormone metabolism is frequently abnormal in patients with CHF. In a study of 84 patients with advanced heart failure, T3 levels were found to be low.[271] Furthermore, a low T3/reverse T3 ratio was the only independent predictor of prognosis when a multivariate regression analysis was performed with known predictors of poor outcome such as ejection fraction, serum sodium, or hemodynamic variables. The low conversion to T3 was postulated to be an adaptive mechanism to decreased catabolism. In a subsequent study, Hamilton et al. studied the effects of intravenous T3 infusion to patients with class III or IV heart failure.[272] Cardiac output increased without a change in left ventricular ejection fraction or filling pressures. This was thought to be secondary to the effects of T3, causing vascular smooth muscle dilatation and therefore peripheral vasodilation. In another study of thyroid hormone replacement in heart failure, 20 patients with class II and III idiopathic dilated cardiomyopathy were given L-thyroxine orally.[273] Cardiac output improved, peripheral vascular resistance decreased, and exercise performance increased. The improved exercise performance was explained by a higher oxygen consumption at peak exercise due to improved oxygen uptake by skeletal muscle, increased perfusion of the musculature, or improved muscle metabolism by local action of L-thyroxine occurring during training. Similar results were obtained in a study by Moruzzi and colleagues.[274] In this series of 20 patients, ejection fraction, cardiac output, and left ventricular diastolic dimensions all increased. Functional capacity and peak exercise cardiac output also improved. The beneficial effects were sustained with the longer therapy regimen.

Like thyroid deficiency, thyroid toxicity can lead to the development of both high-output and low-output cardiac failure. A prolonged tachycardia and high-output state caused by thyrotoxicosis is thought eventually to produce left ventricular dilatation. A consequent progressive decline in systolic function leads to low-output heart failure. This process can often be reversed by reduction of excess hormone levels. In a study of 7 patients with a dilated cardiomyopathy and hyperthyroidism, Umpierrez et al. demonstrated echocardiographic normalization of left ventricular function after treatment with propylthiouracil or methimazole.[275]

Pheochromocytoma

Hypertension and its sequelae are the major cardiovascular manifestations of pheochromocytoma. However, there have been reports of a specific catecholamine-induced myocarditis[276] and/or cardiomyopathy.[277–279] Degenerative and fibrotic myocardial changes have been described in autopsy specimens of patients dying of suprarenal tumors.[276] Although progression to cardiac involvement is unusual, when the presentation of the tumor is aggressive, pheochromocytoma patients typically die of cardiovascular causes, most commonly congestive heart failure or malignant ventricular arrhythmias.[276,277] In the largest series, 15 of the 26 patients with proven pheochromocytomas had a pathologic diagnosis of myocarditis at autopsy.[276] Hemodynamic stabilization is generally obtained with alpha and beta blockers, and prompt adrenalectomy is required to eliminate catecholamine-induced cardiotoxicity. The cardiac abnormalities can be reversed with tumor resection[280,281] (see also Chap. 51).

Acromegaly

It is not clear whether acromegalic cardiomyopathy is a specific entity or is secondary to the hypertension or atherosclerosis associated with this condition. However, 10 to 20 percent of patients with acromegaly develop congestive heart failure.[282] The congestive heart failure that develops in these patients is particularly resistant to conventional therapy[283] owing to higher collagen content in the acromegalic heart.[282] Histopathologically, the myocytes display cellular hypertrophy, patchy fibrosis, and myofibrillar degeneration. Inflammatory and degenerative damage to the sinoatrial and AV nodes can lead to sudden death.[283] Surgery and irradiation remain the mainstays of therapy, but often the cardiopathic manifestations persist despite a fall in growth hormone levels.[284]

Diabetes

Analysis of the Framingham data showed that the risk of developing heart failure was substantially increased among diabetic patients. Even after exclusion of patients with prior coronary or rheumatic disease and controlling for age, hypertension, obesity, and hypercholesterolemia, the diabetic patients have a fivefold increased risk of developing congestive heart failure.[285] This increased incidence suggested that the metabolic abnormalities associated with diabetes may contribute to myocyte dysfunction and produce a diabetes-induced cardiomyopathy. Histologically, this cardiomyopathy shows no evidence of epicardial atherosclerotic disease or abnormalities in myocardial capillary basal lamina.[286,287] Typically, interstitial fibrosis and arteriolar hyalinization are present. Clinically both systolic and diastolic dysfunction can occur, and the severity of the dysfunction is related to the degree of metabolic control.[288]

OBESITY

Heart failure in the markedly obese is usually chronic. It often occurs due to reduction in left ventricular compliance due to the increases in left ventricular mass and resultant elevations of filling pressures. The chronic increases in cardiac work due to an increased myocardial output and arterial hypertension ultimately lead to systolic dysfunction. With exercise and weight reduction, left ventricular mass decreases[289] and function improves.[290] The improvement in function, however, seems limited to those patients whose obesity was of relatively short duration.[291]

TOXINS

Alcohol

Congestive cardiomyopathy as a result of chronic alcohol abuse accounts for up to 45 percent of all dilated cardiomyopathies.[292] The untoward effects of alcohol on cardiac function were initially described more than 100 years ago. As an estimated 10 percent of the adult population are heavy alcohol users, cardiac toxicity from alcohol is a major problem.

PATHOGENESIS

The cardiodepressant effects of alcohol have been demonstrated following acute and chronic ingestion in animal models and in normal and alcoholic human subjects. Chronic excessive alcohol use can result in congestive heart failure, hypertension, and arrhythmias. Cardiac damage results from direct toxic effects of alcohol or one of its metabolites. Nutritional deficiencies, toxic cofactors, sympathetic stimulation, or coexistent hypertension may also contribute to disease development.[293]

Orally ingested alcohol is converted in the liver to acetaldehyde by the alcohol dehydrogenase enzyme system. Acetaldehyde is then converted into acetic acid by oxidation via acetaldehyde dehydrogenase. The activity of these enzyme systems varies greatly between individuals and in particular between races. Thus, depending on individual enzyme system activity, there are varying levels of alcohol and acetaldehyde concentrations after ingestion of an alcoholic beverage. Alcohol and acetaldehyde are both potent vasodilators. Additionally, acetaldehyde results in marked catecholamine release. Both alcohol and acetaldehyde interfere with a variety of cellular metabolic functions, including calcium transport and binding, lipid metabolism and fatty acid composition of the sarcolemma, protein synthesis, myofibrillar ATPase, and mitochondrial respiration.[292,294] Though ethanol can interfere with a number of myocardial metabolic steps, no predominant factor has been identified. Recently a nonoxidative pathway for the metabolism of alcohol in several organ systems including the heart has been described.[295] Nonesterified fatty acids are esterified with ethanol to produce fatty acid ethyl esters (FAEE). These molecules can accumulate in mitochondria and impair cellular function. Fatty acid ethyl esters are synthesized at high rates in the heart owing to the lack of oxidative ethanol metabolism in this organ. Other studies have demonstrated interference with lipid metabolism leading to triglyceride accumulation and alteration of the fatty acid composition of the sarcolemma.[292] Increased levels of acyl-CoA from enhanced glycerol acyltransferase activity may lead to triglyceride accumulation. The cellular membrane shows reduced changes results in decreased calcium uptake by the sarcolemma. Alcohol also is found to be an inhibitor of the sodium-potassium ATPase.

For many years, alcoholic cardiomyopathy was believed to be due to nutritional deficiencies. The stereotypical malnourished skid-row derelict could have a variety of nutritional deficiencies. Indeed, those subjects with heavy beer consumption could develop thiamine deficiency. As beer contains no thiamine, the consumption of this high-calorie, high-carbohydrate beverage can exhaust existing thiamine stores, particularly in the presence of a deficient diet. Thus, a small percentage of patients with alcohol cardiomyopathy may have coexistent thiamine deficiency. However, the majority of patients develop this disease despite adequate diets.[293]

Contamination of alcoholic beverages with heavy metals has resulted in heart failure. In the nineteenth century, an epidemic of heart failure occurred in Manchester, England, following accidental contamination of the beer with arsenic. More recently, in the 1960s, a new variant of alcoholic cardiomyopathy was described.[296] Patients presented with massive pericardial effusion, low cardiac output, elevated venous pressure, and polycythemia. After considerable medical detective work, the syndrome was linked to cobaltous chloride that was added to the beer as a foaming agent to increase and stabilize the beer head. Removal of the additive resulted in the resolution of this miniepidemic.

CLINICAL PRESENTATION

Although approximately 10 percent of the adult population are heavy drinkers, the prevalence of cardiac disease in this group is low—significantly lower than the prevalence of liver disease in the same population. Although patients with alcoholic cirrhosis may have evidence of asymptomatic myocardial disease, the simultaneous presentation of overt alcoholic liver and cardiac disease is extremely rare.[297]

The disease is observed most frequently in males age 30 to 55 years with a greater than 10-year history of heavy alcohol use. The disease is extremely rare in premenopausal women. The amount and duration of alcohol use is frequently difficult to establish. Criteria used to define heavy chronic alcohol use have included such estimates as the use of 125 mL/day of alcohol and/or 30 to 50 percent of daily calories derived from alcohol for a minimum of 10 years. In a study of 50 asymptomatic alcoholic men, Rubin et al. demonstrated that cardiomyopathy, as well as abnormalities of skeletal muscle, are common among persons with chronic alcoholism, and that alcohol is toxic to striated muscle in a dose-dependent manner.[203]

Presenting symptoms include dyspnea on exertion, orthopnea, paroxysmal nocturnal dyspnea, fatigue, weakness, arrhythmias, or embolic phenomena. Atrial fibrillation is extremely common, followed by atrial flutter and ventricular premature contractions. Sudden death can be the initial presentation. ECG findings include first-degree heart block, left ventricular hypertrophy, nonspecific interventricular conduction defects, bundle-branch blocks and prolongation of the QT interval. The echocardiogram frequently shows left ventricular hypertrophy, single- to four-chamber enlargement, and mural thrombi.

In animal studies, left ventricular biopsies from dogs that developed alcoholic cardiomyopathy showed an accumulation of glucoprotein-like material in the interstitium on light microscopy as well as a dilatation of the intercalated discs on electron microscopic evaluation. These studies also demonstrated abnormalities of the sarcoplasmic reticulum and swelling of subsarcolemma regions.[298,299] The severity of these changes related to the duration and extent of alcohol use. Several histologic changes have been described on endomyocardial biopsies in alcoholic cardiomyopathy, but none of these changes are pathognomonic. Changes include myocyte loss, increased fibrosis, loss of sarcolemmal integrity, myofibrillar degeneration, mitochondrial swelling, intercellular edema and accumulation of fatty acids in particular triglycerides, and diminished levels of arachidonate in the cellular membrane.[300] Electron microscopy shows mitochondrial swelling with dense intramitochondrial inclusions, swollen vesiculated sarcoplasmic reticulum, and myofibrillar disruption.

TREATMENT

The mainstay of treatment is abstinence from alcohol. Alcohol withdrawal may have a remarkable impact on disease manifestation and progression, especially in the milder forms of the disease.[301–303] In animal models, following cessation of alcohol use, the hearts recover. In humans, the duration and extent of abuse is correlated with outcome.[304] Prognosis is extremely poor in those patients who continue to drink compared with patients who become abstinent. Ninety-one percent of patients who abstain from alcohol after the initial diagnosis are alive at 42 months, versus 43 percent of those who continue to drink.

Although early in the disease process abstinence can result in recovery, there is a point at which cessation of alcohol is no longer effective,[305] and this correlates with the development of structural histologic abnormalities.[301] Survival of patients with alcoholic dilated cardiomyopathy who are abstinent appears to be significantly better than the long-term survival of patients with a comparable class of CHF due to idiopathic cardiomyopathy.[301,306] In a series of 75 patients with CHF, 23 had alcoholic cardiomyopathy compared with 52 with an idiopathic etiology.[306] Mean left ventricular ejection fraction, diastolic volumes, and NYHA class were similar. Overall survival was measured at 1, 5, and 10 years, and was 100, 81, and 81 percent for patients with alcoholic cardiomyopathy, and 89, 48, and 30 percent for patients with idiopathic cardiomyopathy, respectively. In another series however, no mortality difference was found,[307] but this may be due to persistent alcohol use in that cohort despite the onset of CHF.

Cocaine

Myocardial ischemia, infarction, coronary spasm, cardiac arrhythmias, sudden death, myocarditis, and dilated cardiomyopathy are all reported cardiovascular complications of cocaine abuse.[308] Clinical and experimental evidence suggests a variety of theories for the cardiotoxic effects of cocaine (see also Chap. 71).

The pharmacologic effects of cocaine on the heart partly explain its toxic effects.[309] By blocking the reuptake of norepinephrine, cocaine induces tachycardia, vasoconstriction, hypertension, cardiomyopathy, and ventricular arrhythmias. Cardiomyopathy may then result from secondary changes in the heart due to tachycardia or sustained increased ventricular afterload.

Cocaine has also been shown to exert a direct toxic effect on the heart. In vitro studies with isolated rabbit ventricular tissue[310] or isolated blood-perfused dog preparations[311] showed that high-dose cocaine depressed myocardial contractile force. Acute ventricular dilatation and reversible systolic dysfunction after intravenous cocaine administration have been documented in vivo in dogs.[312]

The risks and manifestations of toxic effects of cocaine in any given individual are unpredictable. The duration or amount of cocaine use is not predictable of disease. For example, among Andean Indians, heart failure rarely occurs from the chewing of coca even though plasma levels of cocaine are comparable to those of intranasal cocaine abusers.[313] This raises the possibility of a genetic susceptibility or that a metabolite or contaminant and not cocaine itself may be the inciting factor for development of cardiac damage.

Dilated cardiomyopathy in the absence of coronary abnormalities and myocarditis has been reported.[314,315] In these cases, myocardial depression is global and is generally reversible; it is attributed to a direct myocardial depressant effect of cocaine.[316]

There are no clinical or histologic features specific for cocaine-induced myocardial damage. Endomyocardial biopsy[308] and autopsy studies[317] confirm the presence of myocyte necrosis and a diffuse inflammatory cellular infiltrate in cocaine users. "Contraction-band necrosis" has been seen in a patient presenting with a clinical course similar to that of catecholamine cardiomyopathy,[318] but this is not characteristic. Although eosinophilic infiltrates can be seen, cocaine is not included in the list of typical drugs associated with a hypersensitivity syndrome. Thus the diagnosis is usually presumptive and is one of exclusion. The treatment of cocaine-related myocarditis and cardiomyopathy is nonspecific and focuses on abstinence and heart failure therapy.

Chemotherapeutic Agents

Several chemotherapeutic agents can cause an acute and/or chronic cardiomyopathy. Among them, the anthracycline group (doxorubicin) and cyclophosphamide are the most common agents associated with heart failure.

Doxorubicin has been used as single or combination therapy for treatment of many different tumors including breast and esophageal tumors as well as sarcomas and lymphomas from the late 1960s. Its use is limited by its cardiotoxicity. The cause of the cardiotoxicity is unknown, but it is suspected to be due to increased oxidative stress from the generation of free radicals by doxorubicin. Moreover, endogenous antioxidants are reduced by treatment with doxorubicin. Increased oxidative stress results in the loss of myofibrils and cellular vacuolization, similar to what is observed with doxorubicin administration.[319]

Doxorubicin can be associated with early or late cardiotoxicity. Risk factors for the development of doxorubicin cardiomyopathy include age greater than 70 years, combination chemotherapy, mediastinal irradiation, prior cardiac disease, hypertension and liver disease. The early or acute cardiotoxicity manifests as a pericarditis-myocarditis syndrome[320] and is not dose-related. Left ventricular dysfunction is rarely seen, but arrhythmias, abnormalities of conduction, decreased QRS voltage, and nonspecific ST-segment and T-wave abnormalities are observed in up to 40 percent of patients.[321] The prognosis is good, with quick resolution of the abnormalities upon discontinuation of therapy.

In contrast, the late or chronic cardiotoxicity is due to the development of a dose-dependent degenerative cardiomyopathy[322] (Fig. 69-14). This syndrome generally occurs at doses above 550 mg/m^2. Serial assessment of nuclear ejection fractions is used clinically to monitor for adverse effects. However, histopathologic grading is most useful in delineating the safety of continued doxorubicin administration.[323] Cardiotoxicity may occur during therapy within a year of the last dose of anthracycline or as late as 6 to 10 years after its cessation. Therefore a course

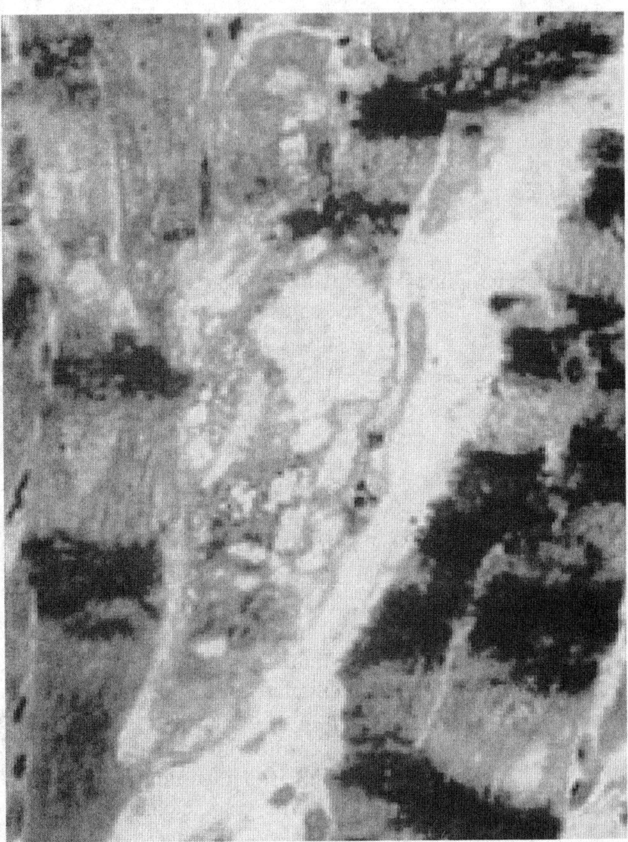

FIGURE 69-14 Loss of myofibrils and vacuolization of cytoplasm (toluidine blue stain, ×40) in a patient with doxorubicin cardiotoxicity. (From Singal et al.,[319] with permission.)

of this chemotherapy commits patients to prolonged cardiac surveillance.

Prognosis depends to some extent on the severity at time of presentation, but the incidence of death even in milder forms remains high.[324] The best management of anthracycline cardiotoxicity is prevention by limiting dosage. Lowering the peak blood levels of the drug by giving a continuous rather than bolus infusion also appears to significantly decrease drug-related damage.[325] Coadministration of doxorubicin with agents that would block free radical formation and not decrease its antineoplastic effects has been studied. Dexrazoxane, an iron chelating agent, has been used in clinical trials of patients with breast cancer or small-cell lung cancer to limit the cardiotoxicity of doxorubicin. The incidence of heart failure and the decrease in ejection fraction is less in those patients receiving combined therapy. Unfortunately, dexrazoxane is a potent myelosuppressive agent potentiating the effects of doxorubicin. It also may interfere with cancer therapy.

Heart failure due to doxorubicin has been very difficult to treat and is typically refractory to conventional therapy. In children with doxorubicin-induced cardiomyopathy, recent reports have described diminished symptoms and improved left ventricular function after treatment with beta blockers. Further studies on the use of these agents are needed.

In contrast to the anthracyclines, cyclophosphamide leads to an acute cardiotoxicity that is not related to cumulative dose.[326]

TABLE 69-5 Major Cardiovascular Complications of Chemical Toxins

Agent	Cardiac Toxicity
Cobalt	Congestive heart failure
Cocaine	Coronary abnormalities, arrhythmias, myocarditis, myocardial depression
Interferon alpha	Arrhythmias, dilated cardiomyopathy, congestive heart failure
Interleukin-2	Myocardial ischemia/infarct, arrhythmias, eosinophilic myocarditis
Phenothiazines	Electrocardiographic, arrhythmias, sudden death
Emetine	Mononuclear and histiocyte infiltration, electrocardiographic abnormalities
Methysergide	Left-sided valvular lesions, fibrotic endocardial and pericardial lesions, restriction and constriction
Chloroquine	Arrhythmias, cardiac dysfunction
Lithium	Arrhythmias, cardiac dilatation with myofibrillar degeneration
Hydrocarbons	Electrocardiographic changes, arrhythmias, and cardiomegaly
Lead	Electrocardiographic changes, arrhythmias, and congestive heart failure
Carbon monoxide	Arrhythmias and transient biventricular dysfunction

Pericarditis, systolic dysfunction, arrhythmias, and myocardial edema make up the spectrum of cardiac abnormalities. Prior left ventricular dysfunction is a risk factor for development of significant cardiomyopathy with cyclophosphamide. Although mortality is not trivial, survivors exhibit no residual cardiac abnormalities.[327]

Chemical Toxins

A variety of compounds can lead to a spectrum of cardiotoxicity, including cardiomyopathy. They include interferon alpha,[328] IL-2,[329] phenothiazines,[330] emetine,[331] methysergide,[332] chloroquine,[333] lithium,[334] hydrocarbons,[335] lead,[336] and carbon monoxide.[337] A summary of the cardiotoxicity seen with each compound is outlined in Table 69-5.

CARDIOMYOPATHIES ASSOCIATED WITH NUTRITIONAL DEFICIENCIES

Vitamins

Thiamine deficiency, or beriberi, causes a high-output state, which leads to left ventricular dilatation and an elevated pulmonary capillary wedge pressure.[338] Vitamin D deficiency, or rickets, and vitamin D excess are associated with cardiovascular morbidity and mortality as well. There are about 25 reported cases of hypocalcemic cardiomyopathy in the adult population caused mostly by idiopathic hypoparathyroidism.[339] Similarly in children, cardiomyopathy has been documented in cases of hypocalcemia caused by vitamin D deficiency rickets.[340] Excess doses of vitamin D in humans have been associated with calcium deposition in the heart and QT shortening but not frank cardiomyopathy. Similarly, vitamin A, vitamin B_6, vitamin C, and niacin deficiency are not directly associated with overt cardiac dysfunction in humans but can be associated with ECG abnormalities.

Selenium

Interest in the role of selenium deficiency in cardiovascular diseases originated from observations of cardiomyopathy and sudden cardiac death in animals with dietary selenium deficiency.[341] Cardiomyopathy associated with inadequate dietary intake of selenium, termed Keshan's disease, has also been described in humans. This syndrome was discovered in regions of China with a low soil content of selenium.[342] Whether the cardiomyopathy results from the actual selenium deficiency or the selenium deficiency increases suspectibility to cardiotropic viruses is unclear. Coxsackievirus B3 (CVB 3/20), which causes no pathology in hearts of selenium-adequate mice, induces extensive myocarditis in selenium-deficient mice.[343] Furthermore, Coxsackievirus B3 recovered from the hearts of selenium-deficient mice and inoculated into selenium-adequate mice induced significant heart damage, suggesting mutation of the virus to a virulent genotype.[344] These findings may underlie the seasonal variation characteristic of Keshan's disease.

This disease is typically seen in children and pregnant women. Both acute and chronic forms of Keshan's disease exist.[345] In the acute form, cardiogenic shock, severe arrhythmias, and pulmonary edema are the manifestations of the systolic impairment. The chronic type shows a moderate to severe heart enlargement with varying degrees of cardiac insufficiency; often patients are asymptomatic. Its incidence is dramatically reduced with supplementation of sodium selenite.

Other than Keshan's disease, circumstantial evidence supports an association between selenium deficiency and cardiomyopathy. Congestive cardiomyopathy with low selenium levels has been reported in patients receiving total parenteral nutrition.[346] Patients with congestive cardiomyopathy have significantly lower serum selenium concentrations than healthy control subjects. Left ventricular ejection fraction is positively correlated with the selenium concentration in patients with cardiomyopathies.[346]

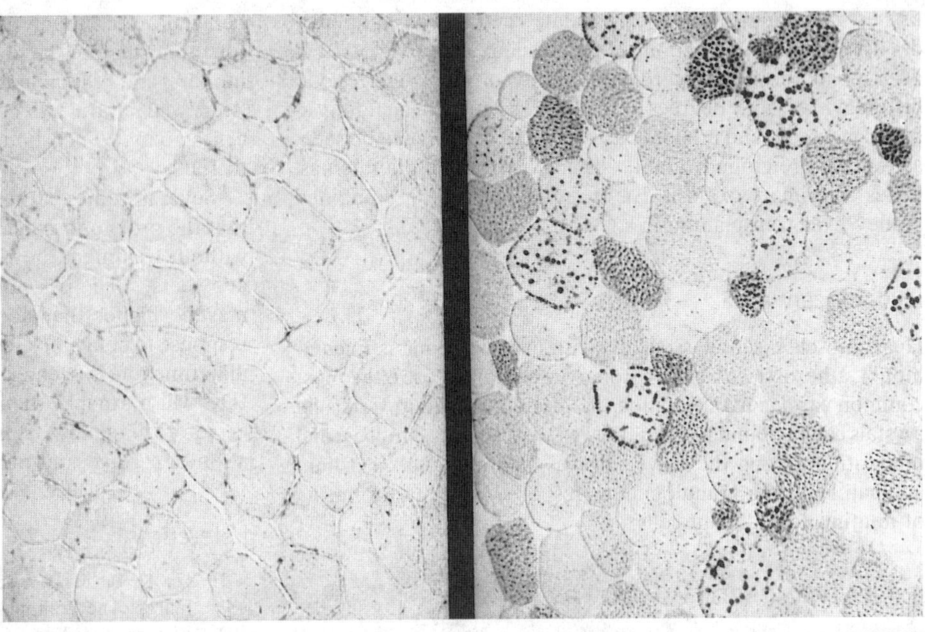

FIGURE 69-15 Photomicrograph of Oil red O stain demonstrating lipid deposits in type I and IIb fibers in normal (*right*) and carnitine-deficient (*left*) skeletal muscle.

Carnitine

L-Carnitine is an essential compound in the transport of long chain fatty acids into mitochondria, where they undergo beta oxidation. Since the normal heart obtains approximately 60 percent of its total energy production from fatty acid oxidation, this function of carnitine is thought to be of major importance.[347] Because of this function of carnitine and numerous case reports that have shown that some patients with carnitine deficiency exhibit cardiomyopathy,[348–350] it is believed that adequate levels of carnitine are required for normal energy metabolism and contractile function of the heart.[351] Interestingly, not all patients with carnitine deficiency exhibit cardiomyopathy. This may be explained perhaps by the degree of carnitine deficiency or by how cardiac performance is assessed.[352]

Deficiencies of carnitine can be either primary or secondary. Primary deficiencies arise from several genetic disorders involving carnitine synthesis or handling. These rare conditions are severe and are associated with muscle and plasma carnitine levels as low as 10 percent of normal (Fig. 69-15). Several case reports have established that primary carnitine deficiency is associated with cardiomyopathy.[353–355] The cardiomyopathy that ensues presents within 3 to 4 years of birth[356] and is profound; clinically, however, it responds to carnitine supplementation.

Secondary carnitine deficiencies are much more common and arise from a large number of genetic diseases associated with defects in acyl-CoA metabolism.[357] In patients with long-chain or short-chain acyl-CoA dehydrogenase deficiency, carnitine levels are reduced to 25 to 50 percent of normal and a depression in cardiac contractile performance has been found.[357,358] Secondary carnitine deficiencies can also be acquired as a result of liver disease, renal disease[359,360] (Fanconi's syndrome, renal tubular acidosis), dietary insufficiencies[361] (chronic total parenteral nutrition, malabsorption), diabetes mellitus, and heart failure.[362] Many of these types of secondary carnitine deficiency are often associated with cardiomyopathy.[355,363] In cases of secondary carnitine deficiency, however, it has been difficult to determine whether the symptoms are due to carnitine deficiency or to the underlying genetic metabolic disorder. Based on this observation and the inconsistent reports of cardiomyopathy with these secondary deficiencies, it appears that a clear and strong association can only be made between cardiomyopathy and primary carnitine deficiency.

Coenzyme Q

Coenzyme Q (2,3-dimethoxy-5 methyl-6-decapreyl-1,4-benzoquinone) is another important factor involved in oxidative phosphorylation in mitochondria of the heart.[364] It has been postulated that its depletion, when found in myocardial biopsies of patients with cardiomyopathy,[365] may contribute to heart failure.[366] Several studies have claimed subjective and objective improvement in patients with heart failure after oral therapy with coenzyme Q.[367–369] These studies were small, unblinded, and uncontrolled trials. Recently a placebo-controlled double-blinded randomized crossover trial of coenzyme Q was performed in 30 patients with heart failure stabilized on conventional vasodilator therapy.[370] In this study, treatment with 3 months of oral coenzyme Q failed to improve resting left ventricular systolic function or quality of life despite an increase in plasma levels of coenzyme Q to more than twice basal values. Thus, given the lack of convincing and consistent data, coenzyme Q supplementation is not included in the basic repertoire of heart failure medications.

CARDIOMYOPATHIES ASSOCIATED WITH ALTERED METABOLISM

Hyperoxaluria

Both primary and secondary oxalosis are characterized by excessive deposition of calcium oxalate crystals in various body tissues, including the heart.[371] Oxalate crystals are frequently deposited in the conduction system, leading to heart block and occasionally in the myocardium and the coronary arteries. On histology, variable degrees of cellular reaction—including fibrosis, necrosis, and mononuclear cell infiltration—can be seen, as well as foreign-body giant cells and myocardial granulomas. Cases of primary oxalosis can be treated with after combined kidney/liver transplantation.[372,373]

Hyperuricemia

Heart muscle disease associated with hyperuricemia is uncommon[374]; atherosclerosis and coronary artery disease are the most common cardiac manifestations associated with gout. Uric acid crystals can be found in the blood vessel walls, in the myocardial interstitium, along the valve surfaces, and in the pericardium and can lead to a granulomatous response with the formation of multinucleated giant cells.[373]

IDIOPATHIC CARDIOMYOPATHY

Idiopathic cardiomyopathy (IDC) is the term used to describe a group of myocardial diseases of unknown cause. Idiopathic dilated cardiomyopathy probably represents the end result of a number of disease processes involving myocyte dysfunction, myocyte loss, myocyte hypertrophy and fibrosis. It is a diagnosis of exclusion. As discussed earlier in this chapter, an idiopathic dilated cardiomyopathy may be the end result of an infectious myocarditis. Endocardial biopsy in patients with dilated cardiomyopathy may reveal an inflammatory infiltrate. Surreptitious alcohol use as well as undiagnosed and untreated hypertension probably represent other etiologies of cardiomyopathy in many of these cases. Familial factors have generally been more predominant in hypertrophic cardiomyopathies than in dilated congestive cardiomyopathy. However more and more data are accumulating to suggest that genetic factors contribute to these cases as well. When one is making the diagnosis of idiopathic dilated cardiomyopathy, it is most important to exclude potentially reversible etiologies (Table 69-6).

The incidence of IDC has been estimated at 0.005 to 0.006 percent,[375] with the incidence increasing with age and males being more commonly afflicted.[376] A number of immune regulatory abnormalities have been characterized in IDC and include humoral and cellular autoimmune reactivity against myocytes,[377] decreased natural killer cell activity,[378] and abnormal suppressor cell activity.[70] Such findings suggest an immunologic etiology to IDC.

Several studies of the natural history of IDC have concluded that the prognosis is better than for ischemic cardiomyopathy[7]; without treatment, however, mortality approaches 50 percent at 5 years.[379] The risk of thromboembolic complications in IDC may be higher than for the ischemic group, but the clinical response to beta blockade as gauged by improvement in ventricular function is greater.[380] About 10 percent of patients with IDC will normalize their ejection fraction on beta blockade[381]; therefore, if tolerated, this therapy is warranted before consideration of cardiac transplantation.

TABLE 69-6 Potentially Reversible Dilated Cardiomyopathies

Ischemic with viable myocardium	Endocrine
Valvular without surgically correctable lesion	Hyperthyroidism
Inflammatory	Pheochromocytoma
CMV	Metabolic
Toxoplasmosis	Hypocalcemia
Mycoplasma	Hypophatemia
Lyme	Uremia
Toxic	Carnitine
Alcohol	Nutritional
Cocaine	Selenium
Cobalt	Thiamine
	Infiltrative
	Hemachromatosis
	Sarcoidosis
	Hypersensitivity

References

1. Ho K, Pinsky J, Kannel W, et al. The epidemiology of heart failure: The Framingham study. *J Am Coll Cardiol.* 1993; 22:6.
2. Limacher M, Yusef G. Gender differences in presentation, morbidity and mortality in the Studies of Left Ventricular Dysfunction (SOLVD): A preliminary report. In: Wenger N, Sperpff L, Packard B, eds. *Cardiovascular Health and Disease in Women.* Greenwich, CT: Le Jacq Communications; 1993.
3. Mckay R, Pfeffer M, Pasternak R, et al. Left ventricular remodeling after myocardial infarction: A corollary to infarct expansion. *Circulation* 1986; 74:693.
4. Mitchell G, Lamas G, Vaughan D, et al. Left ventricular remodeling in the year after myocardial infarction: A quantitative analysis of contractile segment lengths and ventricular shape. *J Am Coll Cardiol* 1992; 19:1136.
5. Mckee P, Catelli W, McNamara P, et al. The natural history of congestive heart failure: The Framingham Study. *N Engl J Med* 1971; 285:1441.
6. Bristow M, Gilbert E, Abraham W, et al. Carvedilol produces dose-related improvements in left ventricular function and survival in subjects with chronic heart failure. *Circulation* 1996; 94:2807.
7. Likoff M, Chandler S, Kay H. Clinical determinants of mortality in chronic congestive heart failure secondary to idiopathic or dilated cardiomyopathy. *Am J Cardiol* 1987; 59:634.
8. Iskander S, Iskandarian A. Prognostic utility of myocardial viability assessment. *Am J Cardiol* 1999; 83(5):696.
9. Kannel W, Castelli W, McNamara P, et al. Role of blood pressure in the development of congestive heart failure in the Framingham study. *N Engl J Med* 1972; 287:781.
10. Grossman W, Jones D, McLaurin, KP. Wall stress and patterns of hypertrophy in the human left ventricle. *J Clin Invest* 1975; 58:56.
11. Lompre A, Schwartz K, d'Albis A, et al. Myosin isoenzyme redistribution in chronic heart overload. *Nature* 1979; 282:105.
12. Arai M, Matsui H, Periasamy M. Sarcoplasmic reticulum gene expression in cardiac hypertrophy and heart failure. *Circ Res* 1994; 74:555.
13. Jalil J, Doering C, Janicki J, et al. Fibrillar collagen and myocardial stiffness in the intact hypertrophied rat left ventricle. *Circ Res* 1989; 64:1041.
14. Lecarpentier Y, Waldenstrom A, Clergue M, et al. Major alterations in relaxation during cardiac hypertrophy induced by aortic stenosis in guinea pig. *Circ Res* 1987; 61:107.
15. Pfeffer J, Pfeffer M, Braunwald E. Influences of chronic captopril therapy on the infarcted left ventricle of the rat. *Circ Res* 1985; 57:84.
16. Khairallah P. Angiotensin and myocardial protein synthesis. In:

Tarazi RC, Dunbar J, Kanabus J, eds. *Perspective in Cardiovascular Research.* New York: Raven Press; 1983.
17. Kim S, Ohta K, Hamaguchi A, et al. Angiotensin II induces cardiac phenotypic modulation and remodeling in vivo in rats. *Hypertension* 1995; 25:1252.
18. Sadoshima JS. I: Molecular characterization of angiotensin II-induced hypertrophy of cardiac myocytes and hyperplasia of cardiac fibroblasts. *Circ Res* 1993; 73:413.
19. Yusuf S, Sleight P, Pogue J, et al. Effects of an angiotensin-converting-enzyme inhibitor, ramapril, on death from cardiovascular causes, myocardial infarction, and stroke in high-risk patients. *N Engl J Med* 2000; 342:145.
20. Nielsen I. The natural history of hypertensive heart disease as suggested by echocardiography. *Acta Med Scand* 1986; 714:165.
21. Levy D, Larson M, Vasan R, et al. The progression from hypertension to congestive heart failure. *JAMA* 1996; 275:1557.
22. Niimura H, Bachinski L, Sangwatanaroj S, et al. Mutations in the gene for cardiac myosin-binding protein C and late-onset familial hypertrophic cardiomyopathy. *N Engl J Med* 1998; 338: 1248.
23. Lewis J, Maron B. Elderly patients with hypertrophic cardiomyopathy: A subset with distinctive left ventricular morphology and progressive clinical course in late life. *J Am Coll Cardiol* 1989; 13:36.
24. Lewis J, Maron B. Clinical and morphological expression of hypertrophic cardiomyopathy in patients >65 years of age. *Am J Cardiol* 1994; 73:1105.
25. Zieman S, Fortuin N. Hypertrophic and restrictive cardiomyopathies in the elderly. *Cardiol Clin* 1999; 17:151.
26. Topol E, Traill T, Fortuin N. Hypertensive hypertrophic cardiomyopathy of the elderly. *N Engl J Med* 1985; 312:277.
27. Aurigemma G, Gaasch W. Gender differences in older patients with pressure-overload hypertrophy of the left ventricle. *Cardiology* 1995; 86:310.
28. Karam R, Lever H, Healy B. Hypertensive hypertrophic cardiomyopathy or hypertrophic cardiomyopathy with hypertension? A study of 78 patients. *J Am Coll Cardiol* 1989; 13:580.
29. Shapiro L. Hypertrophic cardiomyopathy in the elderly. *Br Heart J* 1990; 63:265.
30. Richardson P, McKenna W, Bristow M, et al. Report of the 1995 World Health Organization/International Society and Federation of Cardiology Task Force on the definition and classification of cardiomyopathies. *Circulation* 1996; 93:841.
31. Ramanathan K, Knowles J, Connor M, et al. Natural history of chronic mitral insufficiency: Relation of peak systolic pressure/end-systolic volume ratio to morbidity and mortality. *J Am Coll Cardiol* 1984; 3:1412.
32. Brodison A, Swann J. Myocarditis: A review. *J Infect* 1998; 3:99.
33. Keeling P, Lukaszyk A, Poloniecki J, et al. A prospective case controlled study of antibodies to coxsackie B virus in idiopathic dilated cardiomyopathy. *J Am Coll Cardiol* 1994; 23:593.
34. Stevens P, Underwood Ground K. Occurrence and significance of myocarditis in trauma. *Aerospace Med* 1970; 41:776.
35. Limas C, Goldenberg I, Limas C. Influence of anti-beta-receptor antibodies on cardiac adenylate cyclase in patients with idiopathic dilated cardiomyopathy. *Am Heart J* 1990; 119:1322.
36. Woodruff J. Viral myocarditis: A review. *Am J Pathol* 1980; 101: 427.
37. Chow L, Ye Y, Linder J, et al. Phenotypic analysis of infiltrating cells in human myocarditis. *Arch Pathol Lab Med* 1989; 113:1357.
38. Young L, Joag S, Zheng L-M, et al. Perforin-mediated myocardial damage in acute myocarditis. *Lancet* 1990; 336:1019.
39. Satoh M, Tamura G, Segawa I, et al. Expression of cytokine genes and presence of enteroviral genomic RNA in endomyocardial biopsy tissues of myocarditis and dilated cardiomyopathy. *Virchows Arch* 1996; 427:503.
40. Godeny E, Gauntt C. In situ immune autoradiographic identification of cells in heart tissues of mice with coxsackie virus B3-induced myocarditis. *Am J Pathol* 1987; 129:267.
41. Lodge P, Herzum M, Olszewski J, et al. Coxsackievirus B3 myocarditis. *Am J Pathol* 1987; 128:455.
42. Seko Y, Shinkai Y, Kawasaki A, et al. Expression of perforin in infiltrating cells in murine hearts with acute myocarditis caused by coxsackievirus B3. *Circulation* 1991; 84:788.
43. Camp T, Hess E, Conway G, et al. Immunologic findings in idiopathic cardiomyopathy. *Am Heart J* 1969; 77:610.
44. Neumann D, Burek C, Baughman K, et al. Circulating heart-reactive antibodies in patients with myocarditis or cardiomyopathy. *J Am Coll Cardiol* 1990; 16:839.
45. Neu N, Craig S, Rose N, et al. Coxsackievirus induced myocarditis in mice: Cardiac myosin autoantibodies do not cross-react with the virus. *Clin Exp Immunol* 1987; 69:566.
46. Neu N, Rose N, Beisel K, et al. Cardiac myosin induces myocarditis in genetically predisposed mice. *Immunology* 1987; 139:3630.
47. Pummerer C, Luze K, Grässl G, et al. Identification of cardiac myosin peptides capable of inducing autoimmune myocarditis in BALB/c mice. *J Clin Invest* 1996; 97:2057.
48. Sutton G, Harding H, Truehart L, et al. Coxsackie B4 myocarditis in an adult: Successful isolation of virus from ventricular myocardium. *Aerospace Med* 1967; 38:66.
49. Easton A, Eglin R. The detection of coxsackievirus RNA in cardiac tissue by in situ hybridization. *J Gen Virol* 1988; 69:285.
50. Kandolf R, Hofschneider P. Viral heart disease. *Springer Semin Immunopathol* 1989; 11:1.
51. Bowles N, Rose M, Taylor P, et al. End-stage dilated cardiomyopathy. *Circulation* 1989; 80:1128.
52. Tracy S, Chapman N, McManus B, et al. A molecular and serologic evaluation of enteroviral involvement in human myocarditis. *J Biol Cell Cardiol* 1990; 22:403.
53. Jin O, Sole M, Butany J, et al. Detection of enterovirus RNA in myocardial biopsies from patients with myocarditis and cardiomyopathy using gene amplification by polymerase chain reaction. *Circulation* 1990; 82:8.
54. Grasso M, Arbustini E, Silini E, et al. Search for coxsackievirus B3 RNA in idiopathic dilated cardiomyopathy using gene amplification by polymerase chain reaction. *Am J Cardiol* 1992; 69:658.
55. Weiss L, Movahed L, Billingham M, et al. Detection of coxsackievirus B3 RNA in myocardial tissues by the polymerase chain reaction. *Am J Pathol* 1991; 138:497.
56. Schwaiger A, Umlauft F, Weyrer K, et al. Detection of enteroviral ribonucleic acid in myocardial biopsies from patients with idiopathic dilated cardiomyopathy by polymerase chain reaction. *Am J Heart J* 1993; 126:406.
57. Petitjean J, Kopecka H, Freymuth F, et al. Detection of enteroviruses in endomyocardial biopsy by molecular approach. *J Med Virol* 1992; 37:76.
58. Keeling P, Jeffery S, Caforio A, et al. Similar prevalence of enteroviral genome within the myocardium from patients with idiopathic dilated cardiomyopathy and controls by the polymerase chain reaction. *Br Heart J* 1992; 68:554.
59. Katsuragi M, Yutani C, Mukai T, et al. Detection of enteroviral genome and its significance in cardiomyopathy. *Cardiology* 1993; 83:4.
60. Severini G, Mestroni L, Falaschi A, et al. Nested polymerase chain reaction for high-sensitivity detection of enteroviral RNA in biological samples. *J Clin Microbiol* 1993; 31:1345.
61. Liljeqvist J, Bergström T, Holmström S, et al. Failure to demonstrate enterovirus aetiology in Swedish patients with dilated cardiomyopathy. *J Med Virol* 1993; 39:6.
62. Satoh M, Tamura G, Segawa I. Enteroviral RNA in endomyocardial biopsy tissues of myocarditis and dilated cardiomyopathy. *Pathol Int* 1994; 44:345.
63. Nicholson F, Ajetunmobi J, Li M, et al. Molecular detection and

serotypic analysis of enterovirus RNA in archival specimens from patients with acute myocarditis. *Br Heart J* 1995; 74:522.

64. Ueno H, Yokota Y, Shiotani H, et al. Significance of detection of enterovirus RNA in myocardial tissues by reverse transcription-polymerase chain reaction. *Int J Cardiol* 1995; 51:157.
65. Fujioka S, Koide H, Kitaura Y, et al. Molecular detection and differentiation of enteroviruses in endomyocardial biopsies and pericardial effusions from dilated cardiomyopathy and myocarditis. *Am Heart J* 1996; 131:760.
66. Andreoletti L, Hober D, Decoene C, et al. Detection of enteroviral RNA by polymerase chain reaction in endomyocardial tissue of patients with chronic cardiac diseases. *J Med Virol* 1996; 48:53.
67. Gauntt C, Pallansch M. Coxsackievirus B3 clinical isolates and murine myocarditis. *Virus Res* 1996; 41:89.
68. Gerli R, Rambotti P, Spinozzi F, et al. Immunologic studies of peripheral blood from patients with idiopathic dilated cardiomyopathy. *Am Heart J* 1986; 112:350.
69. Huber K, Gersh B, Sugrue D, et al. T-lymphocyte subsets in patients with idiopathic dilated cardiomyopathy. *Int J Cardiol* 1989; 22:59.
70. Fowles R, Bieber C, Stinson E. Defective in vitro suppressor cell function in idiopathic congestive cardiomyopathy. *Circulation* 1979; 59:483.
71. Anderson J, Fowles R, Bieber C, et al. Idiopathic cardiomyopathy, age, and suppressor-cell dysfunction as risk determinants of lymphoma after cardiac transplantation. *Lancet* 1978; 2:1174.
72. Matumori A, Yamada T, Suzuki H, et al. Increased circulating cytokines in patients with myocarditis and cardiomyopathy. *Br Heart J* 1994; 72:561.
73. Investigators MTT. Incidence and clinical characteristics of myocarditis. *Circulation* 1991; 84:II-2.
74. Costanzo-Nordin M, O'Connell J, Subramanian R, et al. Myocarditis confirmed by biopsy presenting as acute myocardial infarction. *Br Heart J* 1985; 53:25.
75. Saffitz J, Schwartz D, Southworth W, et al. Coxsackie viral myocarditis causing transmural right and left ventricular infarction without coronary narrowing. *Am J Cardiol* 1983; 52:644.
76. Burch G, Shewey L. Viral coronary arteritis and myocardial infarction. *Am Heart J* 1976; 92:11.
77. Ferguson D, Farwell A, Bradley W, et al. Coronary artery vasospasm complicating acute myocarditis. *West J Med* 1988; 148:664.
78. Kimby A, Sodermark T, Volpe U, et al. Stokes-Adams attacks requiring pacemaker treatment in three patients with acute nonspecific myocarditis. *Acta Med Scand* 1980; 207:177.
79. Phillips M, Robinowitz M, Higgins J, et al. Sudden cardiac death in Air Force recruits: A 20-year review. *JAMA* 1986; 256:2696.
80. Tomioka N, Kishimoto C, Matsumori A, et al. Mural thrombus in experimental viral myocarditis in mice: Relation between thrombosis and congestive heart failure. *Cardiovasc Res* 1986; 20:665.
81. Kojima J, Miyazaki S, Fujiwara H, et al. Recurrent left ventricular mural thrombi in a patient with acute myocarditis. *Heart Vessels* 1988; 4:120.
82. O'Connell J, Fowles R, Robinson J, et al. Clinical and pathologic findings of myocarditis in two families with dilated cardiomyopathy. *Am Heart J* 1984; 107:127.
83. O'Connell J, Costanzo-Nordin M, Subramanian R, et al. Peripartum cardiomyopathy: Clinical, hemodynamic, histologic and prognostic characteristics. *J Am Coll Cardiol* 1986; 8:52.
84. Mason J, Billingham M, Ricci D. Treatment of acute inflammatory myocarditis assisted by endomyocardial biopsy. *Am J Cardiol* 1980; 45:1037.
85. Toshima H, Ohkita Y, Shingu M. Clinical features of acute coxsackie B viral myocarditis. *Jpn Circ J* 1979; 43:441.
86. Karjalainen J, Viitasalo M, Kala R, et al. 24-Hour electrocardiographic recordings in mild acute infectious myocarditis. *Ann Clin Res* 1984; 16:34.
87. Chandraratna P, Nimalasuriya A, Reid C, et al. Left ventricular asynergy in acute myocarditis. *JAMA* 1983; 250:1428.
88. Arvan S, Manalo E. Sudden increase in left ventricular mass secondary to acute myocarditis. *Am Heart J* 1988; 116:200.
89. Pinamonti B, Alberti E, Cigalotto A, et al. Echocardiographic findings in myocarditis. *Am J Cardiol* 1988; 62:285.
90. Miller L, Labovitz A, McBride L, et al. Echocardiography-guided endomyocardial biopsy. *Circulation* 1988; 78:III.
91. Caves P, Schultz W, Dong EJ, et al. New instrument for transvenous cardiac biopsy. *Am J Cardiol* 1974; 33:264.
92. Noda S. Histopathology of endomyocardial biopsies from patients with idiopathic cardiomyopathy: Quantitative evaluation based on multivariate statistical analysis. *Jpn Circ J* 1980; 44:95.
93. Baandrup V, Olsen E. Critical analysis of endomyocardial biopsies from patients suspected of having cardiomyopathy: I. Morphological and morphometric aspects. *Br Heart J* 1981; 45:475.
94. Das J, Rath B, Das S, et al. Study of endomyocardial biopsies in cardiomyopathy. *Indian Heart J* 1981; 18:18.
95. Nippoldt T, Edwards W, Holmes DJ, et al. Right ventricular endomyocardial biopsy. *Mayo Clin Proc* 1982; 57:407.
96. Fenoglio JJ, Ursell P, Kellogg C, et al. Diagnosis and classification of myocarditis by endomyocardial biopsy. *N Engl J Med* 1983; 308:12.
97. Unverferth D, Fetters J, Unverferth B, et al. Human myocardial histologic characteristics in congestive heart failure. *Circulation* 1983; 68:1194.
98. Parrillo J, Aretz H, Palacios I, et al. The results of transvenous endomyocardial biopsy can frequently be used to diagnose myocardial diseases in patients with idiopathic heart failure. *Circulation* 1984; 69:93.
99. Zee-Cheng C-S, Tsai C, Palmer D, et al. High incidence of myocarditis by endomyocardial biopsy in patients with idiopathic congestive cardiomyopathy. *J Am Coll Cardiol* 1984; 3:63.
100. O'Connell J, Henkin R, Robinson JA, et al. Gallium-67 imaging in patients with dilated cardiomyopathy and biopsy-proven myocarditis. *Circulation* 1984; 70:58.
101. Daly K, Richardson P, Olsen E, et al. Acute myocarditis: Role of histological and virological examination in the diagnosis and assessment of immunosuppressive treatment. *Br Heart J* 1984; 51:30.
102. Rose A, Fraser R, Beck W. Absence of evidence of myocarditis in endomyocardial biopsy specimens from patients with dilated (congestive) cardiomyopathy. *S Afr Med J* 1984; 66:871.
103. Regitz V, Olsen E, Rudolph W. Histologisch nachweisbare Myokarditis bei Patienten mit eingeschrankter linksventrikularer Funktion. *Herz* 1985; 10:27.
104. Dec G, Palacios I, Fallon J, et al. Active myocarditis in the spectrum of acute dilated cardiomyopathies: Clinical features, histologic correlates, and clinical outcomes. *N Engl J Med* 1985; 312:885.
105. Salvi A, Silvestri F, Gori D, et al. La biopsia endomiocardica: Un'esperienza relativa a 156 pazienti. *G Ital Cardiol* 1985; 15:251.
106. Mortensen S, Baandrup U, Buch J, et al. Immunosuppressive therapy of biopsy proven myocarditis: Experiences with corticosteroids and cyclosporin. *Int J Immunother* 1985; 1:35.
107. Hosenpud J, McAnulty J, Niles N. Lack of objective improvement in ventricular systolic function in patients with myocarditis treated with azathioprine and prednisone. *J Am Coll Cardiol* 1985; 6:797.
108. Cassling R, Linder J, Sears T, et al. Quantitative evaluation of inflammation in biopsy specimens from idiopathically failing or irritable hearts: Experience in 80 pediatric and adult patients. *Am Heart J* 1985; 110:713.
109. French W, Siegel R, Cohen A, et al. Yield of endomyocardial biopsy in patients with biventricular failure. *Chest* 1986; 90:181.
110. Hammond E, Menlove R, Anderson J. Predictive value of immunofluorescence and electron microscopic evaluation of endomyo-

cardial biopsies in the diagnosis and prognosis of myocarditis and idiopathic dilated cardiomyopathy. *Am Heart J* 1987; 114:1055.

111. Maisch B, Bauer E, Hufnagel G, et al. The use of endomyocardial biopsy in heart failure. *Eur Heart J* 1988; 9:59.

112. Chow L, Dittrich H, Shabetai R. Endomyocardial biopsy in patients with unexplained congestive heart failure. *Ann Intern Med* 1988; 109:535.

113. Leatherbury L, Chandra R, Shapiro S, et al. Value of endomyocardial biopsy in infants, children and adolescents with dilated or hypertrophic cardiomyopathy and myocarditis. *J Am Coll Cardiol* 1988; 12:1547.

114. Hobbs R, Pelegrin D, Ratliff N, et al. Lymphocytic myocarditis and dilated cardiomyopathy: Treatment with immunosuppressive agents. *Cleve Clin J Med* 1989; 56:628.

115. Latham R, Mulrow J, Virmani R, et al. Recently diagnosed idiopathic dilated cardiomyopathy: Incidence of myocarditis and efficacy of prednisone therapy. *Am Heart J* 1989; 117:876.

116. Popma J, Cigarroa R, Buja L, et al. Diagnostic and prognostic utility of right-sided catheterization and endomyocardial biopsy in idiopathic dilated cardiomyopathy. *Am J Cardiol* 1989; 63:955.

117. Vasiljevic J, Kanjuh V, Seferovic P, et al. The incidence of myocarditis in endomyocardial biopsy samples from patients with congestive heart failure. *Am Heart J* 1990; 120:1370.

118. Lieberman E, Hutchins G, Herskowitz A, et al. Clinicopathologic description of myocarditis. *J Am Coll Cardiol* 1991; 18:1617.

119. Strain J, Grose R, Factor S, et al. Results of endomyocardial biopsy in patients with spontaneous ventricular tachycardia but without apparent structural heart disease. *Circulation* 1983; 68:1171.

120. Sugrue D, Holmes DJ, Gersh B, et al. Cardiac histologic findings in patients with life-threatening ventricular arrhythmias of unknown origin. *J Am Coll Cardiol* 1984; 4:952.

121. Vignola P, Aonuma K, Swaye P, et al. Lymphocytic myocarditis presenting as unexplained ventricular arrhythmias: Diagnosis with endomyocardial biopsy and response to immunosuppression. *J Am Coll Cardiol* 1984; 4:812.

122. Hosenpud J, McAnulty J, Niles N. Unexpected myocardial disease in patients with life threatening arrhythmias. *Br Heart J* 1986; 56:55.

123. Aretz H, Billingham M, Edwards W, et al. Myocarditis: A histopathological definition. *Am J Cardiovasc Pathol* 1986; 1:3.

124. Dec G, Palacios I, Fallon J, et al. Antimyosin antibody cardiac imaging: Its role in the diagnosis of myocarditis. *J Am Coll Cardiol* 1990; 16:97.

125. Keogh A, Billingham M, Schroeder J. Rapid histological changes in endomyocardial biopsy specimens after myocarditis. *Br Heart J* 1990; 64:406.

126. Billingham M, Tazelaar H. The morphological progression of viral myocarditis. *Postgrad Med J* 1986; 62:581.

127. Gagliardi M, Bevilacqua M, Di Renzi P, et al. Usefulness of magnetic resonance imaging for diagnosis of acute myocarditis in infants and children, and comparison with endomyocardial biopsy. *Am J Cardiol* 1991; 68:1089.

128. Hahn E, Hartz V, Moon R, et al. The Myocarditis Treatment Trial: Design, methods and patient enrollment. *Eur Heart J* 1995; 16:162.

129. Mason J, O'Connell J, Herskowitz A, et al. A clinical trial of immunosuppressive therapy for myocarditis. *N Engl J Med* 1995; 333:269.

130. McNamara D, Rosenblum W, Janosko K, et al. Intravenous immune globulin in the therapy of myocarditis and acute cardiomyopathy. *Circulation* 1997; 95:2476.

131. McNamara D, Starling R, Dec W, et al. Intervention in myocarditis and acute cardiomyopathy with immune globulin: Results from the randomized placebo controlled IMAC trial (abstr). *Circulation* 1999; 100.

132. Grogan M, Redfield M, Baily K, et al. Long term outcome of patients with biopsy proven myocarditis: Comparison with idiopathic dilated cardiomyopathy. *J Am Coll Cardiol* 1995; 26:80.

133. Barbaro G, DiLorenzo G, Grisoris B, Barbarini G. Incidence of dilated cardiomyopathy and detection of HIV in myocardial cells of HIV-positive patients: Gruppo Italiano per lo Studio Cardiologico dei Pazienti Affetti da AIDS. *N Engl J Med* 1998; 339:1093.

134. Flotats A, Domingo P, Carrio I. Dilated Cardiomyopathy in HIV-infected patients. *N Engl J Med* 1999; 340:732.

135. Gonwa T, Capehart J, Pilcher J, et al. Cytomegalovirus myocarditis as a cause of cardiac dysfunction in a heart transplant recipient. *Transplantation* 1989; 47:197.

136. Marsden P. South American trypanosomiasis (Chagas' disease). *Int Rev Trop Med* 1971; 4:97.

137. Sadigursky M, von Kreuter B, Ling P-Y, et al. Association of elevated antisarcolemma, anti-idiotype antibody levels with the clinical and pathologic expression of chronic Chagas myocarditis. *Circulation* 1989; 80:1269.

138. D'Avila Reis D, Jones E, Tostes S, et al. Characterization of inflammatory infiltrate in chronic myocardial lesions: Presence of tumor necrosis factor-alpha+ cells and dominance of granzyme A+, CD8+ lymphocytes. *Am J Trop Med Hyg* 1993; 48:637.

139. Higuchi M, Reis M, Aiello V, et al. Association of an increase in CD8+ T cells with the presence of Trypanosoma cruzi antigens in chronic, human, chagasic myocarditis. *Am J Trop Med Hyg* 1997; 56:485.

140. Araujo F. Development of resistance to Trypanosoma cruzi in mice depends on a viable population of L3zt4+ (CD4+) T lymphocytes. *Infect Immun* 1989; 57:2246.

141. Sher A, Coffman R. Regulation of immunity to parasites by T cells and T cell-derived cytokines. *Annu Rev Immunol* 1992; 10:385.

142. Ribeiro-dos-Santos R, Pirmez A, Savino W. Role of autoreactive immunological mechanisms in chagasic carditis. *Res Immunol* 1991; 142:134.

143. Reis M, Higuchi MdL, Benvenuti L, et al. An in situ quantitative immunohistochemical study of cytokines and IL-2R+ in chronic, human, chagasic myocarditis: Correlation with the presence of myocardial *T. cruzi* antigens. *Clin Immunol Immunopathol* 1997; 83:165.

144. Higuchi M, De Morais C, Barreto A, et al. The role of active myocarditis in the development of heart failure in chronic Chagas' disease: A study based on endomyocardial biopsies. *Clin Cardiol* 1987; 10:665.

145. Maguire J, Mott K, Lehman J, et al. Relationship of electrocardiographic abnormalities and seropositivity to *Trypanosoma cruzi* within a rural community in northeast Brazil. *Am Heart J* 1983; 105:287.

146. Chiale P, Halpern M, Nau G, et al. Efficacy of amiodarone during long-term treatment of malignant ventricular arrhythmias in patients with chronic chagasic myocarditis. *Am Heart J* 1984; 107:656.

147. Steere A, Batsford W, Weinberg M, et al. Lyme carditis: Cardiac abnormalities of Lyme disease. *Ann Intern Med* 1980; 93:8.

148. Olson L, Okafor E, Clements I. Cardiac involvement in Lyme disease: Manifestations and management. *Mayo Clin Proc* 1986; 61:745.

149. Luft B, Billingham M, Remington J. Endomyocardial biopsy in the diagnosis of toxoplasmic myocarditis. *Transplant Proc* 1986; 18:1871.

150. Wallace M, Garst P, Papadimos T, et al. The return of acute rheumatic fever in young adults. *JAMA* 1989; 262:2557.

151. Massell B, Chute C, Walker A, et al. Penicillin and the marked decrease in morbidity and mortality from rheumatic fever in the United States. *N Engl J Med* 1988; 318:280.

152. Stollerman G. Rheumatogenic streptococci and autoimmunity. *Clin Immunol Immunopathol* 1991; 61:131.

153. Bessen D, Jones K, Fischetti V. Evidence for two distinct classes

of streptococcal M protein and their relationship to rheumatic fever. *J Exp Med* 1989; 169:269.
154. Krisher K, Cunningham M. Myosin: A link between streptococci and heart. *Science* 1985; 227:413.
155. Jones T. Diagnosis of rheumatic fever. *JAMA* 1944; 126:481.
156. Vasan R, Shrivastava S, Vijayakumar M, et al. Echocardiographic evaluation of patients with acute rheumatic fever and rheumatic carditis. *Circulation* 1996; 94:73.
157. Narula J, Rahimtoola S. Diagnosis of acute rheumatic carditis: The echoes of change. *Circulation* 1999; 100:1576.
158. Kounis N, Zavras G, Soufas G, et al. Hypersensitivity myocarditis. *Ann Allergy* 1989; 62:71.
159. Spry C, Tai P-C. The eosinophil in myocardial disease. *Eur Heart J* 1987; 8:81.
160. Kim C, Vlietstra R, Edwards W, et al. Steroid-responsive eosinophilic myocarditis: Diagnosis by endomyocardial biopsy. *Am J Cardiol* 1984; 53:1472.
161. Cooper L, Berry G, Shabetai R. Idiopathic giant-cell myocarditis—natural history and treatment. *N Engl J Med* 1997; 336:1860.
162. Zhang S, Kodama M, Hanawa H, et al. Effects of cyclosporine, prednisolone, and aspirin on rat autoimmune giant cell myocarditis. *J Am Coll Cardiol* 1993; 21:1254.
163. Davidoff R, Palacios I, Southern J, et al. Giant cell versus lymphocytic myocarditis: A comparison of their clinical features and long-term outcomes. *Circulation* 1991; 83:953.
164. Brown C, Bertlet B. Peripartum cardiomyopathy: A comprehensive review. *Am J Obstet Gynecol* 1998; 178:409.
165. Cunningham F, Pritchard J, Hankins G, et al. Peripartum heart failure: Idiopathic cardiomyopathy or compounding cardiovascular events? *Obstet Gynecol* 1986; 67:157.
166. Seftel H, Susser M. Maternity and myocardial failure in African women. *Br Heart J* 1961; 43.
167. Farber P, Glasgow L. Factors modulating host resistance to virus infection: II. Enhanced susceptibility of mice to encephalomyocarditis virus infection during pregnancy. *Am J Pathol* 1968; 53:463.
168. Farber P, Glasgow L. Viral myocarditis during pregnancy: Encephalomyocarditis virus infection in mice. *Am Heart J* 1970; 80:96.
169. Takatsu T, Kitamura Y, Morita H, et al. Viral myocarditis and cardiomyopathy. In: Sekigushi M, Olsen E, eds. *Cardiomyopathy.* Tokyo: University of Tokyo Press; 1978.
170. Midei M, Dement S, Feldman A, et al. Peripartum myocarditis and cardiomyopathy. *Circulation* 1990; 81:922.
171. Melvin K, Richardson P, Olson E, et al. Peripartum cardiomyopathy due to myocarditis. *N Engl J Med* 1982; 307:731.
172. Nizeq M, Rickenbocker P, Fowler M, et al. Incidence of myocarditis in peripartum cardiomyopathy. *Am J Cardiol* 1994; 74:74.
173. Knobel B, Melamud E, Kishon Y. Peripartum cardiomyopathy. *Isr J Med Sci* 1984; 20:1061.
174. Demakis J, Rahimtoola S, Sutton G, et al. Natural course of peripartum cardiomyopathy. *Circulation* 1971; 44:1053.
175. Carvalho A, Brandao A, Martinez E, et al. Prognosis in peripartum cardiomyopathy. *Am J Cardiol* 1989; 64:540.
176. Report of the WHO/ISGC Task Force on the Definition and Classification of the Cardiomyopathies. *Br Heart J* 1980; 44:672.
177. Marin-Garcia J, Goldenthal M. Cardiomyopathy and abnormal mitochondrial function. *Cardiovasc Res* 1994; 28:456.
178. Watkins H, McKenna W, Thierfelder L, et al. Mutations in the genes for cardiac troponin T and μ-tropomyosin in hypertrophic cardiomyopathy. *N Engl J Med* 1995; 332:1058.
179. Maron B, Spirito P, Wesley Y, et al. Development and progression of left ventricular hypertrophy in children with hypertrophic cardiomyopathy. *N Engl J Med* 1986; 315:610.
180. Solomon S, Wolff S, Watkins H, et al. Left ventricular hypertrophy and morphology in familial hypertrophic cardiomyopathy with mutations of the b-myosin heavy chain gene. *J Am Coll Cardiol* 1993; 22:498.
181. Schwartz K, Carrier L, Guicheney P, et al. Molecular basis of familial cardiomyopathies. *Circulation* 1995; 91:532.
182. Watkins H, Conner D, Thierfelder L, et al. Mutations in the cardiac myosin binding protein-C gene on chromosome 11 cause familial hypertrophic cardiomyopathy. *Nature Genet* 1995; 11:434.
183. Bonne G, Carrier L, Bercovici J, et al. A splice acceptor site mutation in the cardiac myosin binding protein-C gene causes familial hypertrophic cardiomyopathy. *Nature Genet* 1995; 11:438.
184. Watkins H, Rosenzweig A, Hwang D-S, et al. Characteristics and prognostic implications of myosin missense mutations in familial hypertrophic cardiomyopathy. *N Engl J Med* 1992; 326:1108.
185. Anan R, Greve G, Thierfelder L, et al. Prognostic implications of novel b-cardiac myosin heavy chain gene mutations that cause familial hypertrophic cardiomyopathy. *J Clin Invest* 1994; 93:280.
186. Posen B, Moolman J, Corfield V, et al. Clinical and prognostic evaluation of familial hypertrophic cardiomyopathy in two South African families with different cardiac b-myosin heavy chain gene mutations. *Br Heart J* 1995; 74:40.
187. Dausse E, Komadja M, Fetler L. Familial hypertrophic cardiomyopathy: Microsatellite haplotyping and identification of a hotspot for mutations in the b-myosin heavy chain gene. *J Clin Invest* 1993; 92:2807.
188. Newman H, Sugrue D, Oakley C, et al. Relation of left ventricular function and prognosis in hypertrophic cardiomyopathy: An angiographic study. *J Am Coll Cardiol* 1985; 5:1064.
189. Hecht G, Panza J, Maron B. Clinical course of middle-aged asymptomatic patients with hypertrophic cardiomyopathy. *Am J Cardiol* 1992; 69:935.
190. Maron B, Shirani J, Poliac L, et al. Sudden death in young competitive athletes: Clinical, demographic and pathologic profiles. *JAMA* 1996; 276:199.
191. Maron B, Roberts W, Epstein S. Sudden death in hypertrophic cardiomyopathy: A profile of 78 patients. *Circulation* 1982; 67: 1388.
192. Nicod B, Polikar R, Peterson K. Hypertrophic cardiomyopathy and sudden death. *N Engl J Med* 1988; 318:1255.
193. Mckenna W, Deanfield J, Faroqui A, et al. Prognosis in hypertrophic cardiomyopathy: Role of age and clinical electrocardiographic and hemodynamic features. *Am J Cardiol* 1981; 47:532.
194. Gilligan D, Nihoyannopoulos P, Chan W, et al. Investigation for a hemodynamic basis for syncope in hypertrophic cardiomyopathy: Use of a head-up tilt test. *Circulation* 1992; 85:2140.
195. Maron B, Cecchi F, McKenna W. Risk factors and stratification for sudden cardiac death in hypertrophic cardiomyopathy. *Br Heart J* 1994; 72:S13.
196. Spirito P, Maron B. Relation between extent of left ventricular hypertrophy and occurrence of sudden cardiac death in hypertrophic cardiomyopathy. *J Am Coll Cardiol* 1990; 15:1521.
197. Spirito P, Seidman C, McKenna W, et al. Management of hypertrophic cardiomyopathy. *N Engl J Med* 1997; 30:775.
198. Shirani J, Maron B, Cannon R, et al. Clinicopathologic features of hypertrophic cardiomyopathy managed by cardiac transplantation. *Am J Cardiol* 1993; 73:434.
199. Valentine H, Hunt S, Fowler M, et al. Frequency of familial nature of dilated cardiomyopathy and usefulness of cardiac transplantation in this subset. *Am J Cardiol* 1989; 63:959.
200. Michaels V, Moll P, Miller F, et al. The frequency of familial dilated cardiomyopathy in a series of patients with idiopathic cardiomyopathy. *N Engl J Med* 1992; 326:77.
201. Gregori D, Rocco C, DiLenarda A, et al. Estimating the frequency of familial dilated cardiomyopathy and the risk of misclassification errors (abstr). *Circulation* 1996; 94:I270.
202. Abelmann W, Lorell B. The challenge of cardiomyopathy. *J Am Coll Cardiol* 1989; 13:1219.

203. Rubin E. Alcoholic myopathy in heart and skeletal muscle. *N Engl J Med* 1979; 301:28.
204. Honey M. A case of fatal peripartum cardiomyopathy. *Br Heart J* 1986; 55:114.
205. Anan R, Nakagawa M, Miyata M, et al. Cardiac involvement in mitochondrial diseases. *Circulation* 1995; 91:955.
206. Kushwaha S, Fallon J, Fuster V. Medical progress: Restrictive cardiomyopathy. *N Engl J Med* 1997; 336:267.
207. Carrell R, Lomas D. Conformational disease. *Lancet* 1997; 350:134.
208. Hodkinson H, Pomerance A. The clinical significance of senile cardiac amyloidosis: A prospective clinico-pathological study. *Q J Med* 1977; 46:381.
209. Swanton R, Brooksby I, Davis M, et al. Systolic and diastolic ventricular function in cardiac amyloidosis: Studies in six cases diagnosed with endomyocardial biopsies. *Am J Cardiol* 1977; 39:658.
210. Cohen A. Amyloidosis. In: Wilson J, Braunwald E, Isselbacher K, et al., eds. *Harrison's Principles of Internal Medicine,* 12th ed. New York: McGraw-Hill; 1991.
211. Cohen A. Amyloidosis. *N Engl J Med* 1967; 277:522.
212. Kyle R, Greipp P. Amyloidosis (AL): Clinical and laboratory features in 229 cases. *Mayo Clin Proc* 1983; 58:665.
213. Roberts W, Waller B. Cardiac amyloidosis causing cardiac dysfunction: Analysis of 54 necropsy patients. *Am J Cardiol* 1983; 52:137.
214. Olson L, Gertz M, Edwards W, et al. Senile cardiac amyloidosis with myocardial dysfunction: Diagnosis by endomyocardial biopsy and immunohistochemistry. *N Engl J Med* 1987; 317:738.
215. Nichols W, Liepnieks J, Snyder E, et al. Senile cardiac amyloidosis associated with homozygosity for a transthyretin variant (ILE-122). *J Lab Clin Med* 1990; 117:175.
216. Nordlie M, Sletten K, Husby G, et al. A new prealbumin variant in familial amyloid cardiomyopathy of Danish origin. *Scand J Immunol* 1988; 27:119.
217. Gertz M, Kyle R, Greipp P. Response rates and survival in primary systemic amyloidosis. *Blood* 1991; 77:257.
218. Bhandari A, Nanda N. Myocardial texture characterization by two-dimensional echocardiography. *Am J Cardiol* 1982; 51:817.
219. Click R, Olson L, Edwards W, et al. Echocardiography and systemic diseases. *J Am Soc Echocardiogr* 1994; 7:201.
220. Gertz M, Kyle R. Primary systemic amyloidosis: A diagnostic primer. *Mayo Clin Proc* 1989; 64:1505.
221. Kyle R, Bayrd E. Amyloidosis: Review of 236 cases. *Medicine* 1975; 54:271.
222. Klein A, Hatle L, Taliercio C, et al. Prognostic significance of Doppler measures of diastolic function in cardiac amyloidosis: A Doppler echocardiography study. *Circulation* 1991; 83:808.
223. Klein A, Hatle L, Burstow D, et al. Comprehensive Doppler assessment of right ventricular diastolic function in cardiac amyloidosis. *J Am Coll Cardiol* 1990; 15:99.
224. Klein A, Hatle L, Taliercio C, et al. Serial Doppler echocardiographic follow-up of left ventricular diastolic function in cardiac amyloidosis. *J Am Coll Cardiol* 1990; 16:1135.
225. Hosenpud J, DeMarco T, Frazier O, et al. Progression of systemic disease and reduced long-termed in patients with cardiac amyloidosis undergoing heart transplantation: Follow-up results of a multicenter survey. *Circulation* 1991; 84:III.
226. Bascom R, Johns C. The natural history and management of sarcoidosis. *Adv Intern Med* 1986; 31:213.
227. Roberts W, McAllister H, Ferrans V. Sarcoidosis of the heart: A clinicopathologic study of 35 necropsy patients and review of 78 previously described necropsy patients. *Am J Med* 1977; 63:86.
228. Silverman K, Hutchins G, Bulkley B. Cardiac sarcoid: A clinicopathologic study of 84 unselected patients with systemic sarcoidosis. *Circulation* 1978; 58:1204.
229. Perry A, Vuitch F. Causes of death in patients with sarcoidosis: A morphologic study of 38 autopsies with clinicopathologic correlation. *Arch Pathol Lab Med* 1995; 119:167.
230. Wenger N, Ablemann W, Roberts W. Cardiomyopathy and specific heart muscle disease. In: Hurst J, Schlant R, Rackley C, Sonnenblick E, Wenger N, eds. *The Heart,* 7th ed. New York: McGraw-Hill; 1990.
231. *Tenth International Conference on Sarcoidosis and Other Granulomatous Disorders.* New York: New York Academy of Sciences; 1986.
232. Matsui Y, Iwai K, Tackibana T, et al. Clinicopathologic study of fatal cardiac sarcoidosis. *Ann NY Acad Sci* 1976; 278:455.
233. Stein E, Stimmel B, Siltzbach L. Clinical course of cardiac sarcoidosis. *Ann NY Acad Sci* 1976; 278:470.
234. Burstow D, Tajik J, Bailey K, et al. Two-dimensional echocardiographic findings in systemic sarcoidosis. *Am J Cardiol* 1989; 63:478.
235. Fleming H. Cardiac sarcoidosis. *Semin Respir Med* 1986; 8:65.
236. Fawcett F, Goldberg M. Heartblock resulting from myocardial sarcoidosis. *Br Heart J* 1974; 36:220.
237. Schaedel H, Kirsten D, Schmidt A, et al. Sarcoid heart disease: Results of follow-up investigations. *Eur Heart J* 1991; 12:26.
238. Winters S, Cohen M, Greenberg S, et al. Sustained ventricular tachycardia associated with sarcoidosis: Assessment of the underlying cardiac anatomy and the prospective utility of programmed ventricular stimulation, drug therapy and an implantable antitachycardia device. *J Am Coll Cardiol* 1991; 18:937.
239. Fleming H. Sarcoidosis heart disease. *BMJ* 1986; 292:1095.
240. Valentine H, Tazelaar H, Macoviak J, et al. Cardiac sarcoidosis: Response to steroids and transplantation. *J Heart Transplant* 1987; 5:244.
241. Skinner C, Kenmure C. Hemachromatosis presenting as congestive cardiomyopathy and responding to venesection. *Br Heart J* 1973; 35:466.
242. Short E, Winkle R, Billingham M. Myocardial involvement in idiopathic hemachromatosis, morphological and clinical improvement following venesection. *Am J Med* 1981; 70:1275.
243. Skinner M, Anderson J, Simms R, et al. Treatment of 100 patients with primary amyloidosis: A randomized trial of melphalan, prednisone, and colchicine versus colchicine only. *Am J Med* 1996; 100:290.
244. Strickman N, Hall R. Carcinoid heart disease. In: Kapoor A, Reynolds R, eds. *Cancer and the Heart.* New York: Springer-Verlag; 1986.
245. Pellikka P, Tajik A, Khandheria B, et al. Carcinoid heart disease: Clinical and echocardiographic spectrum in 74 patients. *Circulation* 1993; 87:1188.
246. Onate A, Alsibar J, Inguanzo R, et al. Balloon dilation of tricuspid and pulmonary valve in carcinoid heart disease. *Texas Heart Inst J* 1993; 20:115.
247. Rosenzweig B, Guarneri E, Kronzon I. Echocardiographic manifestations in a patient with pseudoxanthoma elasticum. *Ann Intern Med* 1993; 119:487.
248. Hwang B, Meng C, Lin C, et al. Clinical analysis of 5 infants with glycogen storage disease of the heart-Pompe's disease. *JPN Heart J* 1986; 27:25.
249. Löffler W. Endocarditis parietalis fibroplastica mit Bluteosinophilie, ein eigenartiges Krankheitsbild. *Schweiz Med Wochenschr* 1936; 66:817.
250. Galiuto L, Enriquez-Sarano M, Reeder G, et al. Eosinophilic myocarditis manifesting as myocardial infarction: Early diagnosis and successful treatment. *Mayo Clin Proc* 1997; 72:603.
251. Daves J, Spry C, Sapsford R, et al. Cardiovascular features of 11 patients with eosinophilic endomyocardial disease. *Q J Med* 1983; 52:23.
252. Acquatella H, Schiller N, Puigbo J, et al. Value of two-dimensional echocardiography in endomyocardial disease with and

without eosinophilia: Clinical and pathologic study. *Circulation* 1983; 67:1219.
253. Olsen E, Spry C. Relation between eosinophilia and endomyocardial disease. *Prog Cardiovasc Dis* 1985; 27:241.
254. Moodie D, Baum J, Gill C, et al. Endomyocardial fibrosis: Diagnosis and surgical treatment of two cases occurring in the United States. *Clevel Clin Q* 1986; 53:159.
255. Oakley C, Olsen E. Eosinophilia and heart disease (editorial). *Br Heart J* 1977; 39:233.
256. Solley G, Maldonado J, Gleich G, et al. Endomyocardiopathy with eosinophilia. *Mayo Clin Proc* 1976; 51:697.
257. Hendren W, Jones E, Smith M. Aortic and mitral valve replacement in idiopathic hypereosinophilic syndrome. *Ann Thorac Surg* 1988; 46:570.
258. Arnold M, McGuire L, Lee J. Löffler's fibroplastic endocarditis. *Pathology* 1988; 20:79.
259. Blake D, Palmer I, Olinger G. Mitral valve replacement in idiopathic hypereosinophilic syndrome. *J Thorac Cardiovasc Surg* 1985; 89:630.
260. Packer D, Bardy G, Worley S, et al. Tachycardia-induced cardiomyopathy: A reversible form of left ventricular dysfunction. *Am J Cardiol* 1986; 57:563.
261. Uhl H. A previously undescribed congenital malformation of the heart: Almost total absence of the myocardium of the right ventricle. *Bull Johns Hopkins Hosp* 1972; 91:197.
262. Marcus F, Fontaine G, Guiraudon G, et al. Right ventricular dysplasia: A report of 24 adult cases. *Circulation* 1982; 65:384.
263. Gerlis L, Schmidt-Ott S, Ho S, et al. Dysplastic conditions of the right ventricular myocardium: Uhl's anomaly v arrhythmogenic right ventricular dysplasia. *Br Heart J* 1993; 69:142.
264. Thiene G, Nava A, Corrado D, et al. Right ventricular cardiomyopathy and sudden death in young people. *N Engl J Med* 1988; 318:129.
265. Nava A, Thiene G, Canciani B, et al. Familial occurrence of right ventricular dysplasia: A study involving nine families. *J Am Coll Cardiol* 1988; 12:1222.
266. Kisslo J. Two-dimensional echocardiography in arrhythmogenic right ventricular dysplasia. *Eur Heart J* 1989; 10:22.
267. Segall H. Parchment heart (Osler). *Am Heart J* 1950; 40:948.
268. Hasumi M, Sekiguchi M, Hiroe M, et al. Endomyocardial biopsy approach to patients with ventricular tachycardia with special reference to arrhythmogenic right ventricular dysplasia. *Jpn Circ J* 1987; 51:242.
269. Maitland M, Frishman W. Thyroid hormone and cardiovascular disease. *Am Heart J* 1998; 135:187.
270. Dillman W. Biochemical basis of thyroid hormone action in the heart. *Am J Med* 1990; 88:626.
271. Hamilton M, Stevenson L, Luu M, et al. Altered thyroid hormone metabolism in advanced heart failure. *J Am Coll Cardiol* 1990; 16:91.
272. Hamilton M, Stevenson L. Thyroid hormone abnormalities in heart failure: Possibilities for therapy. *Thyroid* 1996; 6:527.
273. Moruzzi P, Doria E, Agostoni P, et al. Usefulness of L-thyoxine to improve cardiac and exercise performance in idiopathic dilated cardiomyopathy. *Am J Cardiol* 1994; 73:374.
274. Moruzzi P, Doria E, Agostoni P. Medium-term effectiveness of L-thyroxine treatment in idiopathic dilated cardiomyopathy. *Am J Med* 1996; 101:461.
275. Umpierrez G, Challapalli S, Patterson C. Congestive heart failure due to reversible cardiomyopathy in patients with hyperthyroidism. *Am J Med* Sci 1995; 310:99.
276. Van Vliet P, Rarchell H, Titus J. Focal myocarditis associated with pheochromocytoma. *N Engl J Med* 1966; 274:1102.
277. Imperato-McGinley J, Cautier T, Ehlers K, et al. Reversibility of catecholamine-induced dilated cardiomyopathy in a child with a pheochromocytoma. *N Engl J Med* 1987; 316:793.
278. Scott I, Parkes R, Cameron D. Pheochromocytoma and cardiomyopathy. *Med J Aust* 1988; 148:94.
279. Behrana A, Haselton P, Leen C, et al. Multiple extra-adrenal paragangliomas associated with catecholamine cardiomyopathy. *Eur Heart J* 1989; 10:182.
280. Lam J, Shub G, Sheps S. Reversible dilatation of hypertrophied left ventricle in pheochromocytoma: Serial two-dimensional echocardiographic observations. *Am Heart J* 1985; 109:613.
281. Salathe M, Wein P, Ritz R. Rapid reversal of heart failure in a patient with phaeochromocytoma and catecholamine-induced cardiomyopathy who was treated with captopril. *Br Heart J* 1992; 68:527.
282. Lie J, Grossman S. Pathology of the heart in acromegaly: Anatomic findings in 27 autopsied patients. *Am Heart J* 1980; 100:41.
283. Rossi L, Thiene G, Caregaro L, et al. Dysrhythmias and sudden death in acromegalic heart disease. A clinicopathologic study. *Chest* 1977; 72:495.
284. Baldwin A, Cundy T, Butler J, et al. Progression of cardiovascular disease in acromegalic patients treated by external pituitary irradiation. *Acta Endocrinol* 1985; 108:26.
285. Abbott R, Donahue R, Kannel W, et al. The impact of diabetes on survival following myocardial infarction in men vs women. The Framingham Study. *JAMA* 1988; 260:3456.
286. Zoneraich S. *Diabetes and the Heart.* Springfield, IL: Charles C Thomas; 1978.
287. Sutherland C, Fisher B, Frier B, et al. Endomyocardial biopsy pathology in insulin-dependent diabetic patients with abnormal ventricular function. *Histopathology* 1989; 14:593.
288. Hausdorf G, Rieger U, Koepp P. Cardiomyopathy in childhood diabetes mellitus: Incidence, time of onset, and relation to metabolic control. *Int J Cardiol* 1988; 19:225.
289. MacMahon S, Wilcken D, Macdonald G. The effect of weight reduction on left ventricular mass: A randomized controlled trial in young, overweight, hypertensive patients. *N Engl J Med* 1986; 314:334.
290. Alpert M, Terry B, Kelly D. Effect of weight loss on cardiac chamber size, wall thickness, and left ventricular function in morbid obesity. *Am J Cardiol* 1985; 55:783.
291. Backman L, Freyschuss U, Hallberg D, et al. Reversibility of cardiovascular changes in extreme obesity: Effects of weight reduction through jejunoileostomy. *Acta Med Scand* 1979; 205:367.
292. Waldenstrom A. Alcohol and congestive heart failure. *Alcohol Clin Exp Res* 1998; 22:315s.
293. McCall D. Alcohol and the cardiovascular system. *Curr Probl Cardiol* 1987; 12:351.
294. Richardson P, Patel V, Preedy V. Alcohol and the myocardium. *Novartis Foundation Symp* 1998; 216:35.
295. Beckemeier M, Bora P. Fatty acid ethyl esters: Potentially toxic products of myocardial ethanol metabolism. *J Mol Cell Cardiol* 1998; 30:2487.
296. Morin Y, Daniel P. Quebec's beer drinkers cardiomyopathy: Etiologic considerations. *Can Med Assoc J* 1967; 97:926.
297. Krelbrek H, Nielsen B, Eriksen J, et al. Left ventricular performance in alcoholic patients without chronic liver disease. *Br Heart J* 1987; 58:352.
298. Regan T, Khan M, Ettinger P, et al. Myocardial function and lipid metabolism in the chronic alcoholic animal. *J Clin Invest* 1974; 54:740.
299. Regan T, Levinson G, Oldewurtel H, et al. Ventricular function in noncardiacs with alcoholic fatty liver: The role of ethanol in the production of cardiomyopathy. *J Clin Invest* 1969; 48:397.
300. Reitz R, Helsabeck E, Mason D. Effects of chronic alcohol ingestion on the fatty acid composition of the heart. *Lipids* 1973; 8:80.
301. Demakis J, Proskey A, Rahimtoola S, et al. The natural course of alcoholic cardiomyopathy. *Ann Intern Med* 1974; 80:293.
302. Pravin D, Nicolosi G, Lestuzzi C, et al. Normalization of variables of left ventricular function in patients with alcoholic cardiomyop-

athy after cessation of excessive alcohol intake: An echocardiographic study. *Eur Heart J* 1987; 8:535.
303. Milani L, Bagolin E, Sanson A. Improvement of left ventricular function in chronic alcoholics following abstinence of ethanol. *Cardiology* 1989; 76:299.
304. Vecchia L, Bedogni F, Bozzola L, et al. Prediction of recovery after abstinence in alcoholic cardiomyopathy: Role of hemodynamic and morphometric parameters. *Clin Cardiol* 1995; 19:45.
305. Regan T. Alcoholic cardiomyopathy. *Progr Cardiovasc Dis* 1984; 27:141.
306. Prazak P, Pfistere M, Osswald S, et al. Differences of disease progression in congestive heart failure due to alcoholic as compared to idiopathic dilated cardiomyopathy. *Eur Heart J* 1996; 17:251.
307. Ikram H, Williamson H, Won M, et al. The course of idiopathic dilated cardiomyopathy in New Zealand. *Br Heart J* 1987; 57:521.
308. Isner J, Chokshi S. Cardiovascular complications of cocaine. *Curr Probl Cardiol* 1991; 16:538.
309. Waller B. Cocaine and the heart. *Ind Med* 1988; 81:956.
310. Hauge N, Perrault C, Morgan J. Effects of cocaine on intracellular Ca++ handling in mammalian myocardium (abstr). *Circulation* 1988; 78:359.
311. Herman E, Vlck J. A study of direct effect of cocaine on the heart (abstr). *Fed Proc* 1987; 46:1148.
312. Franker T, Temsey-Armos P, Brewster P, et al. Mechanisms of cocaine-induced myocardial depression in dogs. *Circulation* 1990; 81:1012.
313. Van Dyke C, Byck R. Cocaine. *Sci Am* 1982; 246:128.
314. Weiner R, Lockhart J, Schwartz R. Dilated cardiomyopathy and cocaine abuse. *Am J Med* 1986; 81:699.
315. Chakko S, Myerburg R. Cardiac complications of cocaine abuse. *Clin Cardiol* 1995; 18:67.
316. Hale S, Alker K, Rezkalla S, et al. Adverse effects of cocaine in cardiovascular dynamics, myocardial blood flow, and coronary artery diameter in an experimental model. *Am Heart J* 1989; 118:927.
317. Virmani R, Robinowitz M, Smialek J, et al. Cardiovascular effects of cocaine: An autopsy study of 40 patients. *Am Heart J* 1988; 115:1068.
318. Chokshi S, Moore R, Pandian N, et al. Reversible cardiomyopathy associated with cocaine intoxication. *Ann Intern Med* 1989; 111:1039.
319. Singal P, Iliskovic N. Current concepts: Doxorubicin-induced cardiomyopathy. *N Engl J Med* 1998; 339:900.
320. Bristow M, Billingham M, Mason J, et al. Clinical spectrum of anthracycline antibiotic cardiotoxicity. *Cancer Treat Rev* 1978; 873:62.
321. Lena L, Page J. Cardiotoxicity of Adriamycin and related anthracyclines. *Cancer Treat Rev* 1976; 3:111.
322. Lipshultz S, Colan S, Gelber R, et al. Late cardiac effects of doxorubicin therapy for acute lymphoblastic leukemia in childhood. *N Engl J Med* 1991; 324:808.
323. Fowles R. Cardiac catheterization and endomyocardial biopsy. In: Kapoor A, Reynolds R, eds. *Cancer and the Heart*. New York: Springer-Verlag; 1986.
324. Greene H, Reich S, Dalen J. How to minimize doxorubicin toxicity. *J Cardiovasc Med* 1982; 7:306.
325. Legla S, Benjamin R, MacKay B, et al. Reduction of doxorubicin cardiotoxicity by prolonged continuous intravenous infusion. *Ann Intern Med* 1982; 96:133.
326. Goldberg M, Antin J, Guinan E, et al. Cyclophosphamide cardiotoxicity: An analysis of dosing as a risk factor. *Chem Toxins* 1986; 68:1114.
327. Gottdiener J, Applebaum F, Ferrans V, et al. Cardiotoxicity associated with high dose cyclophosphamide therapy. *Arch Intern Med* 1981; 141:758.
328. Deyton L, Walker R, Kovacs J, et al. Reversible cardiac dysfunction associated with interferon alpha therapy in AIDS patients with Kaposi's Sarcoma. *N Engl J Med* 1989; 321:1246.
329. Schuchter L, Hendricks C, Holland K, et al. Eosinophilic myocarditis associated with high-dose interleukin-2 therapy. *Am J Med* 1990; 88:439.
330. Horowitz J. Drugs that induce heart problems: Which agents? What effects? *J Cardiovasc Med* 1983; 8:308.
331. Khan M, Haider B, Thind L. Emetine-induced cardiomyopathy in rabbits. *J Submicrosc Cytol* 1983; 15:495.
332. Harbin A, Gerson M, O'Connell J. Stimulation of acute myopericarditis by constrictive pericardial disease with endomyocardial fibrosis due to methylsergide therapy. *J Am Coll Cardiol* 1984; 4:196.
333. Ratliff N, Estes M, Myles J, et al. Diagnosis of chloroquine cardiomyopathy by endomyocardial biopsy. *N Engl J Med* 1987; 316:191.
334. Brafy H, Horgan J. Lithium and the heart: Unanswered questions. *Chest* 1988; 93:166.
335. Cunningham S, Dalzell G, McGirr P, et al. Myocardial infarction and primary ventricular fibrillation after glue sniffing. *BMJ* 1987; 294:739.
336. Kopp S, Barron J, Tow J. Cardiovascular actions of lead and relationship to hypertension: A review. *Environ Health Perspect* 1988; 78:91.
337. McMeekin J, Finegan B. Reversible myocardial dysfunction following carbon monoxide poisoning. *Can J Cardiol* 1987; 3:118.
338. Watson R. *Nutrition and Heart Disease II*. Boca Raton; FL: CRC Press; 1987.
339. Kudoh C, Tanaka S, Marusaki S, et al. Hypocalcemic cardiomyopathy in a patient with idiopathic hypoparathyroidism. *Intern Med* 1992; 31:561.
340. Mustafa A, Birgas J-L, McCrindle B. Dilated cardiomyopathy as a first sign of nutritional vitamin D deficiency rickets in infancy. *Can J Cardiol* 1999; 15:699.
341. Burk R. Selenium in nutrition. *World Rev Nutr Diet* 1978; 30:88.
342. Yang G. Keshan disease: An endemic selenium-related deficiency disease. In: Chandara R, ed. *Trace Elements in Nutrition of Children*. New York: Raven Press; 1985.
343. Beck M, Kolbeck P, Shi Q, et al. Increased virulence of a human enterovirus (Coxsackievirus B3) in selenium deficient mice. *J Infect Dis* 1994; 170:351.
344. Beck M, Shi Q, Morris V, et al. Rapid genomic evolution of a non-virulent Coxsackievirus B3 in selenium-deficient mice results in selection of identical virulent isolates. *Nature Med* 1995; 1:433.
345. Huttunen J. Selenium and cardiovascular disease—an update. *Biomed Environ Sci* 1997; 10:220.
346. Oster O, Prellwitz W. Selenium and cardiovascular disease. *Biol Trace Elem Res* 1990; 24:91.
347. Neely J, Morgan H. Relationship between carbohydrate metabolism and energy balance of heart muscle. *Annu Rev Physiol* 1974; 36:413.
348. Tripp M, Katcher M, Peters H, et al. Systemic carnitine deficiency presenting as familial endocardial fibroelastosis. *N Engl J Med* 1981; 305:385.
349. Waber L, Valle D, Neill C, et al. Carnitine deficiency presenting as familial cardiomyopathy: A treatable defect in carnitine transport. *J Pediatr* 1982; 101:700.
350. Christensen E, Virke-Jorgensen J. Six years experience with carnitine supplementation in a patient with an inherited defective carnitine transport system. *J Inherit Metab Dis* 1995; 18:233.
351. Rebouche C, Paulson D. Carnitine metabolism and functions in humans. *Ann Rev Nutr* 1986; 6:41.
352. Paulson D. Carnitine deficiency-induced cardiomyopathy. *Mol Cell Biochem* 1998; 180:33.
353. Famularo G, De Simone C. A new era for carnitine. *Immunol Today* 1995; 16:211.
354. Christensen E. Cardiomyopathy and abnormal carnitine metabolism. *J Pediatr* 1989; 114:903.

355. Scholte H, Rodriguez Pereira R, de Jonge P, et al. Primary carnitine deficiency. *J Clin Chem Clin Biochem* 1990; 28:351.
356. Stanley C. Carnitine disorders. *Adv Pediatr* 1993; 42:209.
357. Bennett M, Hale D, Pollitt R, et al. Endocardial fibroelastosis and primary carnitine deficiency due to a defect in the plasma membrane carnitine transport (clinical conference). *Clin Cardiol* 1996; 19:243.
358. Duran M, Loof N, Ketting D, et al. Secondary carnitine deficiencies. *J Clin Chem Clin Biochem* 1990; 28:359.
359. Gahl W, Bernardini I, Dalakas M, et al. Muscle carnitine repletion by long-term carnitine supplementation in nephrotic cystinosis. *Pediatr Res* 1993; 34:115.
360. Ahmad S, Robertson H, Golper T, et al. Multicenter trial of L-carnitine in maintenance hemodialysis patients: II. Clinical and biochemical effects. *Kidney Int* 1990; 38:912.
361. Heinonen O, Takala J. Carnitine status during prolonged total parenteral nutrition. *J Pediatr* 1993; 122:503.
362. Regitz V, Bossaller C, Strasser R, et al. Metabolic alterations in end-stage and less severe heart failure—Myocardial carnitine decrease. *J Clin Chem Clin Biochem* 1990; 28:611.
363. Paulson D, Sanjak M, Shug A. *Carnitine Deficiency and the Diabetic Heart.* Boca Raton; FL: CRC Press; 1992.
364. Crane F. Physiological coenzyme Q function and pharmacological reactions. In: Folkers K, Yamamura Y, eds. *Biomedical and Clinical Aspects of Coenzyme Q.* Amsterdam: Elsevier; 1986.
365. Kitamura N, Yamaguchi A, Otaki M, et al. Myocardial tissue level of coenzyme Q_{10} in patients with cardiac failure. In: Folkers K, Yamamura Y, eds. *Biomedical and Physical Aspects of Coenzyme Q.* Amsterdam, Elsevier; 1984.
366. Folkers K, Vadhanavikit S, Mortensen S. Biochemical rationale and myocardial tissue data on the effective therapy of cardiomyopathy with coenzyme Q_{10}. *Proc Natl Acad Sci USA* 1985; 82:901.
367. Langsjoen P, Langsjoen P, Folkers K. Long-term efficacy and safety of coenzyme Q_{10} therapy for idiopathic dilated cardiomyopathy. *Am J Cardiol* 1990; 65:521.
368. Morisco C, Trimarco B, Condorelli M. Effect of coenzyme Q_{10} therapy in patients with congestive cardiac failure: A long-term muticenter randomized study. *Clin Invest* 1993; 71:S134.
369. Lampertico M, Comis S. Italian muticenter study on the efficacy and safety of coenzyme Q_{10} as adjuvant therapy in heart failure. *Clin Invest* 1993; 71:S129.
370. Waton P, Scalia G, Galbraith A, et al. Lack of effect of coenzyme Q on left ventricular function in patients with congestive heart failure. *J Am Coll Cardiol* 1999; 33:1549.
371. Danpure C. Recent advances in the understanding, diagnosis, and treatment of primary hyperoxaluria type 1. *J Inherit Metab Dis* 1989; 12:210.
372. Rodby R, Tyszka T, Williams J. Reversal of cardiac dysfunction secondary to type 1 primary hyperoxaluria after combined liver-kidney transplantation. *Am J Med* 1991; 90:498.
373. Fyfe B, Israel D, Quish A, et al. Reversal of primary hyperoxaluria cardiomyopathy after combined liver and renal transplantation. *Am J Cardiol* 1995; 75:210.
374. Rosenberg A, Bergstrom L, Troost B, et al. Hyperuricemia and neurologic deficits: A family study. *N Engl J Med* 1970; 282:992.
375. Torp A. Incidence of congestive cardiomyopathy. *Postgrad Med J* 1978; 54:435.
376. Codd M, Sugrue D, Gersh B, et al. Epidemiology of idiopathic dilated and hypertrophic cardiomyopathy: A population based study in Olmstead County, MN 1975–1984. *Circulation* 1989; 80:564.
377. Kawai C, Takatsu T. Clinical and experimental studies on cardiomyopathy. *N Engl J Med* 1975; 293:592.
378. Anderson J, Carliquist J, Hammond E. Deficient natural killer cell activity in patients with idiopoathic dilated cardiomyopathy. *Lancet* 1982; 2:1124.
379. Fuster V, Gersh B, Giuliani E, et al. The natural history of idiopathic dilated cardiomyopathy. *Am J Cardiol* 1981; 47:525.
380. Woodley S, Gilbert E, Anderson J, et al. β-blockade with bucindilol in heart failure due to ischemic vs idiopathic dilated cardiomyopathy. *Circulation* 1991; 84:2426.
381. Waagstein F, Bristow M, Swedberg K, et al. Beneficial effects of metoprolol in idiopathic dilated cardiomyopathy. *Lancet* 1993; 342:1441.

CHAPTER 70

AIDS AND THE CARDIOVASCULAR SYSTEM

Melvin D. Cheitlin

INTRODUCTION

The pandemic of acquired immunodeficiency syndrome (AIDS), after nearly 2 decades, has taken a tragic toll in lives in the United States and threatens a catastrophe in Africa and Southeast Asia. An estimated 10 million people worldwide are infected with the human immunodeficiency virus (HIV), and at least another 12 million have full-blown AIDS.[1] In the United States, over a million people are HIV positive, and about 2 million have been diagnosed with AIDS.[2,3]

In New York City, AIDS has become the most important cause of premature death among patients under age 65. In terms of years of potential life lost, AIDS advanced in rank order from the 8th leading cause of death in 1983 to the leading cause in 1994.[4]

AIDS is caused by infection with a virus of the family Retroviridae. This group of retroviruses comprises enveloped ribonucleic acid (RNA) viruses possessing an RNA-dependent deoxyribonucleic acid (DNA) polymerase (reverse transcriptase). There are two classes of AIDS viruses: HIV-1 and HIV-2.

The most specific definition of infection by HIV is by identification of the HIV organism in the host's tissues. Since isolation of the virus is not easily done and therefore lacks sensitivity, a patient with repeated positive screening test results for antibodies to HIV, as with an enzyme-linked immunosorbent assay (ELISA), confirmed by a supplemental test such as the Western blot immunofluorescence assay, should be considered to be infected by HIV.

The following classification system for the different stages of HIV infection as proposed by the United States Centers for Disease Control (CDC) is helpful[5]:

Group I: Acute infection
Group II: Asymptomatic infection
Group III: Persistent generalized lymphadenopathy (PGL)
Group IV: Chronic disease—AIDS with constitutional disease (such as unexplained diarrhea, weight loss, or fever over 1 month), neurologic disease, secondary infectious diseases, secondary cancers (Kaposi's sarcoma, non-Hodgkin's lymphoma, and primary lymphoma of the brain)

In January 1993, the CDC, together with other state and territorial health departments, broadened the surveillance definition for AIDS in adolescents and adults to add a measure of immunosuppression (a CD4+ T-lymphocyte count <200/μL or a CD4+ percentage <14), as well as three additional clinical conditions: pulmonary tuberculosis, recurrent pneumonia (two or more episodes within a year), or invasive cervical cancer.[6]

Patients with HIV infection have also been divided into three clinical categories. Category A includes asymptomatic patients, those with acute HIV infection or progressive lymphadenopathy. Category B includes symptomatic patients without AIDS-defining conditions. Category C includes patients with 25 AIDS-defining conditions, including opportunistic infections, tumors, central nervous system abnormalities, wasting syndrome, pulmonary tuberculosis, invasive cervical carcinoma, and recurrent pneumonia.[6]

The recognition of human infection by HIV in 1981 represented the startling development of a modern epidemic with many of the aspects of epidemics of the past, such as those of poliomyelitis and the black plague. This infection is due to a retrovirus that invades the nucleus of certain cells containing a specific receptor on their cell membranes and incorporates the DNA copy of HIV in the host's genetic material or genome. After an asymptomatic latent period from infection of 2 to 6 weeks, most patients experience a primary HIV-1 infection that is a self-limited viral syndrome not unlike infectious mononucleosis, characterized by fever, fatigue, pharangitis, lymphadenopathy, and maculopapular rash.[7] Over 95 percent of the patients seroconvert to a positive HIV serology within 6 months, most within 6 to 12 weeks.[8] After an apparent incubation (dormant) period of a mean of 8 to 10 years, the virus can eventually express itself by releasing into the cytoplasm double-stranded DNA copies of the virus, thus killing the cell and invading other immune cells, usually T-helper lymphocytes, to the point that the host's immune defense mechanisms are compromised.[9]

Studies have demonstrated a high rate of viral replication in the lymph nodes during this quiescent period, indicating active progression of the disease, despite the low levels of infectious HIV in the plasma of some patients.[10]

A long-term prospective study showed the actuarial rate of progression from the time of infection to the appearance of AIDS to be 53 percent at 10 years and 68 percent at 14 years after infection, with an increasing progression after 5 years of infection.[11] About 30 percent of patients with PGL will progress to AIDS in 5 years.[12] A minority of patients have an accelerated course and develop full-blown AIDS in 1 or 2 years.[13] Small groups of patients have also been described who have had HIV infection for over 10 years without any symptoms.[14] At some point, there is a breakdown of the body's defense against certain neoplastic changes, resulting in the development of non-Hodgkin's lymphoma and Kaposi's sarcoma. These complications lead inevitably, at least in a very high percentage of cases, to death.

The average length of life after infection in the absence of treatment is approximately 10 years.[11] With the introduction of highly active antiviral therapy (HAART) including nucleocide reverse-transcriptase inhibitors and especially the protease-inhibitor drugs, elimination of the virus from the peripheral blood and prolongation of life have been demonstrated.[15] The impact of the new treatment with multiple drugs is seen in a fall in the rate of AIDS deaths by 12 percent in the United States in 1996 and by 47 percent in 1997.[16]

At the beginning of the epidemic in the United States, the HIV organism struck mainly at the male homosexual population. Later it was found to be transmitted not only through sexual intercourse but also through bloodborne contamination, soon affecting the population using intravenous drugs and other populations receiving blood products and blood transfusions, such as hemophiliacs. The disease is also transmitted perinatally, so that an increasing number of pediatric patients with AIDS are being seen. Although in the U.S. male-to-male sexual activity and intravenous drug users account for 75 percent of cases, in the developing world heterosexual transmission accounts for the majority of cases.[17]

From work with HIV-1, it has been found that the usual way in which the virus attacks cells is through interaction with a receptor on the surface membrane of the cell, the so-called CD4 receptor. This is present in T-helper lymphocytes. Macrophages, microglia, and Langerhans' cells may have specific receptors for HIV other than CD4. Other cells seem to lack an HIV receptor and therefore are much less often found to be sites of infection; the myocardial cell is one such cell.

From the beginning of the epidemic, it was recognized that the heart could be involved but that significant clinical involvement of the heart was unusual. Originally it was believed, through autopsy studies, that the heart was involved mainly because of pericarditis or metastatic Kaposi's sarcoma.[18,19] A few patients with nonbacterial thrombotic endocarditis (NBTE) were reported, but this could be nonspecific, since many of these patients have a wasting disease in which NBTE is not unusual.[20] On further review of autopsy series and clinical series and especially with the study of patients with AIDS who had echocardiography, it was apparent that abnormalities of the heart were seen frequently, even though clinical manifestations of heart disease still remained unusual.

AUTOPSY FINDINGS

The incidence of cardiac involvement at autopsy varies, depending on the definition of cardiac disease. In 15 autopsy series, the incidence of cardiac involvement varies from none to 70 percent of the hearts, depending on whether lymphocytic infiltration with or without myocardial necrosis is included.[18–26] The presence of autopsy-proven cardiac involvement in patients who, during life, had clinically significant cardiac involvement is less impressive, especially if one includes the patients with localized, isolated collections of myocardial lymphocytes.

In evaluating autopsy reports, it is often difficult to discern how many patients had clinically significant abnormalities during life. In the large series of consecutive autopsies of AIDS patients, between 5 and 20 percent appear to have had cardiac lesions of potential clinical importance. These include patients with myocarditis with clinical manifestations, mainly with known pathogens—such as toxoplasmosis, clinically evident pericarditis, or nonbacterial endocarditis—which can cause systemic emboli.[27]

The largest recent autopsy series is by Barbero et al., where 440 AIDS patients had an autopsy. Cardiac involvement was documented in 18.6 percent and dilated cardiomyopathy in 2.7 percent.[28]

More important are the relatively few patients in whom cardiac abnormality was listed as the cause of death. The most common cause of death is respiratory failure and infection.[24,26,29,30] Neoplasm, lymphoma, and encephalopathy are also frequent causes of death.[31] Of 858 autopsied patients with AIDS from 15 series in the literature, only 9 (1 percent) had the cause of death listed as cardiac. If the cases with a recognized etiology for heart disease are removed, only 0.5 percent of deaths were possibly due to HIV "myocarditis."

Right ventricular hypertrophy and/or dilatation was reported in 12 of 71 patients (16.9 percent)[25] and in 18 of 115 patients (15.7 percent).[24] Pericarditis varied in frequency from 3 of 41 (7.3 percent)[20] to 3 of 101 (3 percent).[22]

ECHOCARDIOGRAPHIC FINDINGS

Echocardiography in patients with either AIDS or PGL has been reported in a number of studies.[32–39] The prevalence of echocardiographic abnormalities varies from 15 to 60 percent and would be higher if the finding of mitral valve prolapse, an echocardiographic abnormality that may be related to cachexia, is included. The prevalence of left ventricular hypokinesis also varies from 12.5 to 41 percent in three large series.[33,34,36] In one series,[33] four of the eight patients had congestive heart failure; one died and at autopsy had a dilated cardiomyopathy without evidence of inflammatory myocarditis or cardiac opportunistic infections. Only in this study[33] was clinical congestive heart failure mentioned. Dilated cardiomyopathy was seen only in the hospitalized patients. In a large prospective echocardiographic study in 296 HIV-infected adults that was conducted over 4 years, Currie and colleagues found 13 (4 percent) with dilated cardiomyopathy.[37]

Cecchi and colleagues, from 1398 patients admitted for HIV infection, selected 127 (9 percent) with a clinical suspicion of cardiac disease and did echocardiograms on them: 92 (72 percent) had evidence of cardiac involvement, 6.5 percent of total

HIV patients; 38 (2.7 percent) had pericardial effusion, and 20 (1.4 percent) had dilated cardiomyopathy.[38]

The finding of pericardial effusion was common, varying from 20 to 40 percent.[34,36,38] The incidence of tamponade varies: In one series[34] of 18 patients with pericardial effusion, 5 (28 percent) had tamponade. In this report of 300 patients with AIDS, 16 (5 percent) had clinically apparent heart disease, due in most cases to opportunistic infection or tumor.[34] Over a period of 3 years at the San Francisco General Hospital, Rapaport found that, of 1171 patients hospitalized with AIDS, an echocardiogram was ordered for 88 (7.5 percent) because of suspicion of cardiac disease (personal communication). Of these echocardiograms, 52 (59 percent) showed at least one abnormality. Of the 88 echocardiograms, 16 (18 percent) showed either left ventricular dilatation and/or left ventricular hypokinesis, and 26 (30 percent) showed pericardial effusion. There were no control subjects.

Steffen and colleagues[39] reported the prospectively collected results of echocardiography in 151 HIV-seropositive patients, 92 percent of whom were men with a median age of 37 years, and 73 percent were homosexual men. Of these, 13 percent were intravenous drug users, of whom 74 percent were in Walter Reed stages IV to VI, a classification using counts of T4 helper cells and clinical data.[40] A total of 107 patients (71 percent) had normal echocardiograms. Echocardiographic abnormalities attributed to HIV infection were present in 31 patients (20 percent). There was an association of abnormal echocardiographic findings with advanced clinical stages of the disease. The mortality during follow-up was the same for those with normal echocardiograms (35 of 102) as for those with abnormal echocardiograms (12 of 29) ($p = .48$). Even in those with the most advanced clinical disease, there was no independent prognostic significance of the echocardiographic cardiac involvement, with 44 percent of both echo-normal and echo-abnormal patients dying. This study shows a remarkably low incidence of HIV-associated echocardiographic abnormalities, most often asymptomatic pericardial effusion.

These studies suggest that the prevalence of echocardiographic abnormalities in HIV-positive patients depends on the stage of their clinical illness, with the sickest patients having the most abnormalities.

PERICARDIAL INVOLVEMENT

In general, pericardial effusion and pericarditis constitute the most commonly recognized cardiac involvement in AIDS. At autopsy, Kaposi's sarcoma involvement and lymphoma may be clinically silent, accompanied by asymptomatic pericardial effusion, or they may be clinically important because of pericardial tamponade.[41] Pericarditis due to specific organisms has frequently been reported. These organisms are most commonly *Mycobacterium tuberculosis*[34,42,43] or *Mycobacterium avium–intracellulare*.[35,42,44] One study[34] reported pericardial tamponade in five patients and large pericardial effusions in six. Of the patients with clinical heart disease in this study, 22 percent had echocardiographic evidence of tamponade, and another 33 percent had large pericardial effusions.

In a review of 15 autopsy and echocardiographic studies involving 1139 patients with HIV disease, the incidence of pericardial disease was 21 percent. Most cases were asymptomatic without an identifiable etiology. In those that were symptomatic, about two-thirds were caused by infection or neoplasm and one-third were of undetermined etiology. In the 66 published cases of pericardial tamponade, 26 percent were caused by *M. tuberculosis*.[42]

At San Francisco General Hospital, experience has been similar. In a consecutive series of 88 in-hospital AIDS patients who had echocardiograms, 36 (41 percent) had normal echocardiograms, whereas the most common abnormality, seen in 26 (30 percent), was pericardial effusion. We have recognized a total of 25 patients with AIDS or PGL who have pericardial disease. Ten of these patients had pericardiocentesis, of whom eight (32 percent) presented with tamponade, two had pericardial windows, and one died and was autopsied. Another two patients, who had neither pericardiocentesis nor pericardial windows, died and were autopsied. No etiology was found on examination of either fluid or tissue in any of the 12 patients.

In a prospective echocardiographic study among 231 patients recruited over a 5-year period, the prevalence of pericardial effusion for AIDS patients entering into the study was 5 percent. Over the follow-up time, the incidence of pericardial effusion increased as the stage of the HIV progressed from 0 percent per year in asymptomatic HIV-infected patients to 11 percent per year in patients with AIDS; 80 percent of these effusions were small and asymptomatic.[45] The survival of the AIDS patients who developed pericardial effusion was significantly shorter than the survival of those who did not, 36 percent versus 93 percent at 6 months. This shortened survival period remained significant even after adjustment for lead-time bias and was independent of CD4+ T-cell count.[45] Since death was not due directly to the pericardial effusion, the development of pericardial effusion in the setting of HIV infection probably suggests end-stage HIV disease.

Flum and colleagues also reported that AIDS-associated pericardial effusion was a grave prognostic sign. They reported 29 patients who had surgical windows for large effusions; only in 2 patients did this result in a change in clinical management. The mortality was 69 percent at 8 weeks after pericardial window.[46] They concluded that pericardial biopsy for diagnosis provided little practical therapeutic information and that surgical windows were justified only to relieve tamponade.

The etiology of pericardial effusion or pericarditis is not obvious; it may be HIV infection or other opportunistic viral infections with Coxsackie virus, cytomegalovirus, or neoplastic.[45] Occasionally, pericarditis has been reported to be caused by common organisms such as *Staphylococcus*,[46] *Cryptococcus neoformans*,[47] or herpes simplex virus.[48]

MYOCARDIAL INVOLVEMENT

For a number of years, involvement of the pericardium and myocardium with both common and unusual opportunistic infections and neoplasms, such as Kaposi's sarcoma and lymphoma, has been recognized. At times, this involvement appears to be incidental and associated with the presence of organisms in many tissues, including the heart. Often, this involvement is not accompanied by signs of cell necrosis or even inflammation. At other times, the infection is accompanied by an intense myocarditis. Opportunistic infection has included viruses (herpes simplex, cytomegalovirus, and Coxsackie virus), bacteria, protozoa (*Toxoplasma gondii*), and fungi (*Candida albicans, C. neoformans,* and *Aspergillus fumigatus*).[49–51] These specific infections have been diagnosed at autopsy but also during life with myocardial biopsy. The importance of identifying a specific organism as the cause of the myocarditis rests in the potential for treatment[42,52]; for instance, amphotericin B and flucytosine may be used to treat cryptococcosis. Grange and colleagues[53] reported a case of *T. gondii* myocarditis in a 58-year-old man with AIDS who was treated successfully with pyrimethamine and clindamycin. A similar case was reported by Albrecht and colleagues.[54]

The most common neoplasms are Kaposi's sarcoma and lymphoma of the non-Hodgkin's type.[18,19,24] With Kaposi's sarcoma, the tumor involvement of the myocardium or pericardium is most frequently an incidental finding. On occasion, myocardial involvement by lymphoma is diagnosed by needle biopsy of the myocardium.

One study reported a collection of 21 cases of lymphoma in AIDS patients—3 Hodgkin's and 18 non-Hodgkin's lymphoma of various histologic types—almost all of which were in the high-grade categories.[55] Unfortunately, these tend to be histologically aggressive tumors involving many organs, and they respond poorly to treatment. At times, the patient presents with pericardial tamponade or even superior vena cava syndrome.[56-58] Echocardiography revealing infiltration into the myocardium and/or myocardial or pericardial masses is most helpful in establishing a diagnosis.

CARDIOMYOPATHY

In 1986, Cohen and colleagues reported three patients with AIDS who had clinical, echocardiographic, and morphologic findings of dilated cardiomyopathy.[59] All had a decreased ejection fraction, and two had congestive heart failure. All three died, and two had findings at autopsy compatible with myocarditis resulting in cardiomyopathy. Microscopic examination in both showed focal collections of inflammatory cells together with myofibrillar atrophy and myocardial necrosis. A subsequent report described 58 consecutively autopsied patients.[60] Seven (12 percent) had major clinical cardiovascular abnormalities, including four with congestive heart failure and others with ventricular tachycardia. All were late in the course of their disease. All patients with these major clinical cardiac abnormalities had focal myocarditis at autopsy. The etiology in these cases was not obvious but was believed to be viral myocarditis.

In another study of 71 patients with AIDS, 8 had left ventricular dilatation and decreased contractility and 4 had congestive heart failure.[33] In a similar echocardiographic study, none of 102 AIDS patients had congestive heart failure, although 41 percent had left ventricular hypokinesia.[36]

In autopsy studies reported in the literature, cardiac causes of death have been rare; clinically, the incidence of congestive heart failure has been extremely small, although microscopic focal myocarditis is frequently described. In 14 studies in the literature, 1009 patients with AIDS were reported. A total of eight died of cardiac involvement. One had cryptococcal myocarditis and one had toxoplasmic myocarditis; five came from one institution.[25]

Symptomatic cardiomyopathy in association with HIV-1 infection is uncommon; however, echocardiographic evidence of left ventricular dysfunction is more common, especially in patients who are the furthest along in the course of HIV disease. Individual reports of one to five cases of patients with either dilated left ventricle, hypokinetic left ventricle, or both have been frequent enough to require explanation.[59,61] Furthermore, the occurrence of cardiomyopathy in children, in whom a disease unrelated to HIV infection would be rare, further suggests a relationship between HIV disease and cardiomyopathy.[62]

Lipshultz and colleagues did a prospective study on 196 HIV-infected children, median age 2.1 years. Only two had congestive heart failure at enrollment. An echocardiogram done every 4 months revealed a 2-year accumulative incidence of cardiomyopathy of 4.7 percent (95 percent confidence interval, 1.5–7.9 percent).[63]

Prospective echocardiographic studies have been reported that show a high prevalence of myocardial dysfunction. DeCastro and colleagues did serial echocardiograms prospectively on 136 HIV-positive patients over a mean follow-up time of 415 ± 220 days. Seven AIDS patients developed clinical and echocardiographic findings of global left ventricular dysfunction. Of the six who died, five were autopsied: three had acute lymphocytic myocarditis, one had cryptococcal myocarditis, and one had myocardial fibrosis.[64]

Blanchard and colleagues did serial echocardiograms on 70 HIV-positive outpatients. Of the 50 patients with AIDS, 7 (14 percent) had echocardiographic evidence of left ventricular dysfunction. On repeat echocardiogram, three of the seven had improved left ventricular function, implying a transient problem that caused a transient decrease in left ventricular function.[65]

At San Francisco General Hospital, the cases of 74 AIDS outpatients were prospectively followed using serial quantitative Doppler echocardiography every 4 months. Control populations included HIV-positive patients without disease, HIV-positive patients with AIDS-related complex, and HIV-negative gay men. Over the follow-up period of 16.5 ± 12 months, no differences in left ventricular systolic or diastolic function were detected between the groups and no differences in mean values from the first to the last echocardiogram.[66]

The prospective study by Barbaro and colleagues reported 952 asymptomatic HIV-positive patients whose cases were followed clinically and by echocardiography for 60 ± 5.3 months.[67] By echocardiogram, dilated cardiomyopathy was diagnosed in 76 (8 percent) of patients—an incidence of 1.6 cases per 100 patients per year. A myocardial biopsy was done on all patients with cardiomyopathy, and a histologic diagnosis of myocarditis made in 83 percent. By in situ hybridization HIV nucleic acid sequences were found in 58 patients but only 36 (63 percent) had active myocarditis. Of these 36 patients, 25 percent had other cardiotropic virus infections with Coxsackie B virus in 6 (17 percent), cytomegalovirus in 2 (6 percent), and Epstein-Barr virus in 1 (3 percent). The authors concluded that dilated cardiomyopathy may be related either to direct HIV infection or to an autoimmune process induced by HIV, possibly in association with other cardiotropic viruses.

Possible Reasons for Cardiomyopathy

There are many theories on the etiology of congestive heart failure with a dilated, poorly contracting left ventricle found in the occasional patient. These explanations may well be related also to the more frequently observed echocardiographic reduction in left ventricular function with or without left ventricular dilatation. The most frequently mentioned etiology is that of myocarditis or postmyocarditis cardiomyopathy. There are occasional reports of virus being grown from cardiac muscle. In 1987, Calabrese and colleagues[68] were the first to report the culturing of HIV from a right ventricular myocardial biopsy from a patient with a hypokinetic right ventricle and a normal left ventricle.

There is some evidence that HIV itself invades the myocardial cell. The myocyte has no CD4+ receptors, which are the major way by which the virus enters the cell. Although there are other ways and possibly other receptors by which the virus could invade the cell, no one has convincingly shown the virus or a portion of the viral DNA or RNA within the genome of the myocardial cell.[69] One study reported detecting HIV nucleic acid sequences by in situ hybridization in cardiac tissue sections from 6 of 22 patients examined who had died of AIDS.[61] The hybridization target was thought to be myocytes, but this could not be proved by this technique. Furthermore, the myocardial cells showing the positive hybridization signal were sparse, comprising only one or a few cells per section; the myocardium was normal by light microscopy; and none of the patients had clinical evidence of cardiac disease. Still, the most compelling evidence for the ability of HIV virus to enter the myocardial cell comes from the previously mentioned study by Barbaro and colleagues.[67]

Other Theories for the Development of Cardiomyopathy

OPPORTUNISTIC INFECTIONS

Patients with AIDS are exposed to and susceptible to multiple bacterial, viral, mycotic, and protozoal infections. Epstein-Barr virus and cytomegalovirus are both known to cause myocarditis in AIDS patients.[67,70] *Cryptococcus neoformans* and *T. Gondii* myocarditis have been well described.[29,52,53,71] Myocarditis due to *M. avium–intracellulare* has been reported.[20] *Aspergillus* endocarditis and myocarditis have been reported.[72]

DILATED CARDIOMYOPATHY AS A POSTVIRAL DISORDER

The study of patients with myocarditis without AIDS has shown that the myocarditis can be precipitated by viral infection and that the inflammatory reaction can progress when the virus is no longer recoverable from either the heart or even the patient. The viral infection precipitates an immune reaction either to viral antigen that cross-reacts with a myocardial protein or to altered myocardial protein, which acts as a foreign antigen, thus precipitating the immune reactions that continue the myocardial necrosis and inflammatory cell infiltration[73] (see also Chap. 69).

The evidence that congestive cardiomyopathy is precipitated by a previous viral myocarditis includes the biopsy finding of inflammatory infiltrate in some patients with dilated cardiomyopathy[74,75] and detection of increased elevated viral antibody titers and viral-specific RNA sequences in myocardial biopsies.[76] Thus, the cardiomyopathy can result from a previous infection with a number of organisms that are no longer recoverable from the myocardium.

Herskowitz and colleagues[77] reported the histologic and immunopathologic results of 37 endomyocardial biopsy samples from patients infected with HIV-1 who developed unexplained global left ventricular dysfunction. Twenty-eight patients had New York Heart Association (NYHA) class III and IV congestive heart failure. Four patients had myocarditis secondary to known etiologies. Of the remaining 33 patients, 17 (51 percent) had histologic evidence of idiopathic active or borderline myocarditis. Specific hybridization within myocytes was abnormal in five patients with HIV-1 antisense riboprobe and in 16 of the 33 with cytomegalovirus immediate early (IE-2) antisense riboprobe. This study is compatible with the possibility that cardiotropic virus infection and myocarditis may be important in the pathogenesis of HIV-associated cardiomyopathy.[77]

IMPAIRMENT OF THE IMMUNE MECHANISM LEADING TO CARDIOMYOPATHY

Humorally mediated autoimmune reactions involving antimyosin antibodies may also be implicated in the development of cardiomyopathy.[78] Circulating cardiac autoantibodies have been identified in four of six AIDS patients with cardiomyopathy and in none of the HIV-positive patients without cardiomyopathy. In situ hybridization with genomic probes failed to show evidence of HIV or any other viruses within the heart muscle. Results of ELISA showed a high titer of immunoglobulin G antibody to myosin and to cardiac mitochondrial adenine nucleotide transporter. In this study, it was concluded that the cardiomyopathy may be related not to HIV infection of the heart but rather to autoimmunity. Apparent improvement of left ventricular function in children with AIDS by using intravenously administered immunoglobulin is also suggestive of an immunologic etiology for the left ventricular dysfunction.[79]

ROLE OF CYTOKINES IN MYOCARDITIS

Ho and colleagues[80] proposed a primary role for neuroglial cell damage from the cytolytic effect of release of substances termed *cytokines* from HIV-infected monocytes, the "innocent bystander" destruction mechanism. Cytokines are biologically active mediators and are soluble proteins released by immune cells. Reversible myocardial depression is well documented in human and canine septic shock.[81,82] This was subsequently demonstrated to be due to a "myocardial depressant factor."[83] The exact nature of this myocardial depressant factor is not agreed upon, but it could be related to a variety of mediators of sepsis such as endotoxin and the cytokine tumor necrosis factor (TNF) and interleukin 2.[84]

Other studies showed that the administration of endotoxin-released TNF caused depression of left ventricular function independent of left ventricular volume or loading conditions,[85] and elevated circulating levels of TNF have been noted in patients with severe chronic heart failure.[86] Increased circulating levels of TNF have been noted in patients with advanced HIV-1 infection.[87] This finding is consistent with a finding of increased production of the cytokine TNF by peripheral monocytes of patients with AIDS.[88]

Barbaro and colleagues[89] investigated the myocardial expression of TNF-α and inducible nitric oxide synthase (INOS) in endomyocardial biopsies in patients with HIV dilated cardiomyopathy and compared them with myocardium from patients with idiopathic dilated cardiomyopathy. The mean intensity of both TNF-α and INOS immunostaining was greater in the HIV patients compared with the idiopathic cardiomyopathy patients.

The staining intensity of both TNF-α and INOS was inversely correlated with the CD4 count.

The increased levels of cytokines—including TNF, interleukins 1 and 2, and α-interferon—may lead to myocardial dysfunction either acting locally in a paracrine fashion on adjacent myocardium or systemically causing a decrease in myocardial function.[90,91]

CACHEXIA

Many patients with AIDS have marked weight loss and cachexia. In patients with anorexia nervosa, wall motion as assessed by two-dimensional echo Doppler was found to be abnormal in 8 of 14 patients but not in control subjects; also, lower stroke volume was found in patients compared with controls, possibly because of decreased heart size.[92] Starvation and refeeding studies in animals have demonstrated myofibrillar atrophy and cardiac interstitial edema that are accompanied by a decrease in left ventricular compliance and decreased peak systolic force.[93] These changes are thought to be due to protein-calorie malnutrition. Congestive heart failure may occur, especially during refeeding and recovery.[94]

VITAMIN- AND SELENIUM-DEFICIENCY STATES

Cachectic people can have vitamin-deficiency states; it is doubtful that many patients with cardiomyopathy have this as a prime etiology. Selenium deficiency has been described, together with reduced cardiac selenium levels in AIDS, similar to the Keshan's disease seen in Chinese with selenium deficiency. In one study, 10 patients with AIDS who had decreased left ventricular fractional shortening on echocardiography received sodium selenite for 23 days.[95] Six of eight showed a return toward normal of left ventricular fractional shortening within 21 days. Selenium deficiency has been reported to be common in malnourished pediatric patients with AIDS.[96]

DRUG-INDUCED CARDIOMYOPATHY

The effect of drugs, both recreational and therapeutic, on myocardial function is not well delineated in patients with AIDS. In most patients with AIDS and cardiomyopathy, however, drugs do not seem to be the cause[61,97]; nevertheless, in patients with AIDS, drugs such as doxorubicin, α_2-interferon, and interleukin 2 have been shown to produce cardiomyopathy that is sometimes reversible. Recombinant α_2-interferon-related cardiomyopathy in patients treated for primary renal cancer has been reported.[98] One report described three cases of reversible cardiac dysfunction associated with α-interferon therapy in AIDS patients with Kaposi's sarcoma.[99]

Cocaine use has been associated with myocarditis and dilated cardiomyopathy, which occasionally has been reported to be reversible.[100,101] Pentamidine has been reported to cause ventricular tachycardia.[102] The most common currently used drug in AIDS, zidovudine (AZT), a nucleoside analog, is a drug that inhibits replication of HIV in vitro, probably by inhibiting the reverse-transcriptase enzyme, which is essential to the replication of the retrovirus. No adverse cardiac effects have been reported in phase 1 clinical trials, and one study failed to show cardiotoxicity[103]; however, a toxic mitochondrial myopathy caused by long-term AZT after 12.8 months of therapy has been reported.[104] This myopathy is characterized by abnormal mitochondria with paracrystalloid inclusions. AZT-induced cardiomyopathy in rats has been shown to be related to oxidative damage and activated ADP-ribosylation reactions damaging mitochondrial energy production.[105] Whether this can occur in cardiac muscle in some patients is not clear. Foscarnet therapy for the treatment of cytomegalovirus infection has also been reported to produce a reversible cardiomyopathy.[106]

Conclusions

Clinical heart muscle disease and heart failure in AIDS are unusual. When this condition occurs, there may be explanations other than direct infection with HIV. The exact incidence of heart muscle disease in AIDS is as yet unknown but must be small, and the mechanisms that can cause failure are probably multiple.

METABOLIC CARDIOVASCULAR COMPLICATIONS OF ANTIVIRAL DRUGS

With the introduction of protease inhibitors, a class of drugs that suppresses HIV replication, to the treatment of patients with HIV infection, metabolic abnormalities have been seen that have potential for development of cardiovascular disease. New-onset hyperglycemia similar to type II diabetes mellitus has been described, as well as worsening of preexisting diabetes in 1 to 6 percent of patients. This problem has been described with all of the protease inhibitors.[107] The cause of the hyperglycemia is not known, but it does respond to sulfonylureas, suggesting that the drug causes increased resistance to the peripheral effects of insulin although it is not possible to rule out a reduction in insulin secretion.[108] The treatment of hyperglycemia is similar to that of type II diabetes: diet and oral hypoglycemic drugs.

Lipid metabolic abnormalities have also been seen in patients taking protease inhibitors with extremely high triglyceride levels to over 1000 mg/dL,[109] which can occur within 2 weeks of starting therapy. In a study of ritonavir plus saquinavir, 11 percent of patients developed triglycerides above 1500 mg/dL. There were no instances of pancreatitis. There are also elevations in serum cholesterol.[110]

Although the mechanism by which this drug induces hyperlipidemia is unknown, there is a 60 percent homology of the catalytic region of the HIV-1 protease to which the drugs bind to two proteins regulating lipid metabolism: cytoplasmic retinoic acid-binding protein type I (CRABP-I) and low-density lipoprotein-receptor-related protein (LRP). Binding of the protease inhibitors to LRP would impair hepatic chylomicron uptake and triglyceride clearance.[108] The elevated triglycerides respond to gemfibrozil.

In 45 HIV-infected patients taking protease inhibitors who had abnormally elevated lipids, the National Cholesterol Education Program Guidelines were followed without disrupting the HIV therapy. Mean serum cholesterol prior to initiation of the protease inhibitors was 170 mg/dL. On the protease inhibitor, the mean cholesterol rose to 289 mg/dL, and triglycerides were 879 mg/dL. On diet, gemfibrozil alone, or with atorvastatin, the cholesterol fell to 201 mg/dL ($p = .01$) over a 10-month period.[111]

Finally, an abnormal redistribution of fat from the periphery centrally to the abdomen and thorax has been described. There is a loss of subcutaneous fat from the face and limbs (partial lipodystrophy), and the development of fat deposits in the abdomen ("protease pouch") and dorsocervical fat pad ("buffalo hump").[112–114] The abdominal fat may be either in the subcutaneous tissue or in the intraabdominal visceral fat.[112] The abnormal fat distribution appears to be associated with the use of ritonavir-saquinavir combinations rather than with indinavir and does not respond to dietary restriction or exercise. In patients with a buffalo hump, hypercortosolism has been ruled out as a cause, and half the patients with a buffalo hump had never been on protease inhibitors.[113] The relationship of these abnormalities to protease inhibitors is still not clear.

Since the protease inhibitors are such important drugs in the management of patients with HIV infection, every attempt must be made to control their metabolic side effects without stopping the drug. Diet and oral hypoglycemic drugs can control the hyperglycemia. Gemfibrozil and HMG-CoA reductase inhibitors decrease the elevated triglycerides, cholesterol, and low-density lipoproteins, as noted. A potential problem is that protease inhibitors are metabolized by the hepatic cytochrome P450 CYP4-A system, and these drugs can both induce and/or inhibit the system. Therefore, other drugs metabolized by the cytochrome P450 system can have their plasma levels either decreased or increased when used together with the protease inhibitors, resulting in an extensive list of drug interactions and possibly drug toxicity. The importance of treating the metabolic abnormalities, however, is seen in the increasing number of reports of premature, extensive coronary artery disease in patients taking protease inhibitors.[115]

CLINICAL WORKUP AND THERAPY

The workup of patients with AIDS and suspected cardiac involvement begins with the history and physical examination for symptoms and signs of cardiac disease. Since there is no therapeutic advantage to finding subclinical cardiovascular involvement, there is no justification for screening electrocardiograms or echocardiograms. If there are signs or symptoms suggesting cardiovascular disease—such as a friction rub, an S_3 gallop, or other evidence of congestive heart failure—an echocardiogram is useful in identifying pericardial effusion and in evaluating right and left ventricular function. Invasive diagnostic studies are rarely necessary.

If left ventricular dilatation and hypokinesis are found with or without clinical evidence of heart failure, consideration should be given to stopping all drugs that are not absolutely essential.[116] If, in a 2-week follow-up, echocardiography reveals improvement, the suspected drug should be eliminated.

The question of whether a myocardial biopsy is helpful is controversial. The finding of a treatable cause of biopsy-proved myocarditis is rare. Furthermore, there is no evidence that treating biopsy-proved focal myocarditis with steroids or antimetabolites is effective.[117] Therefore, by available evidence, myocardial biopsy is of little value.

The potential cardiotoxic roles of drugs for opportunistic infection as well as other known etiologies—such as hypertension, hypertrophic cardiomyopathy, and coronary artery disease—should be considered. The treatment of congestive heart failure is similar to that of the treatment of heart failure from other etiologies, e.g., diuretics, digoxin, and angiotensin-converting enzyme inhibitors (see Chap. 21).

CARDIOVASCULAR SURGERY IN AIDS PATIENTS

There has been an increased interest in the danger to AIDS health care workers of becoming infected or of infecting patients and in the possibility of accelerating the disease through surgery. The problem is illustrated by the following questions:

1. Are we performing an expensive procedure that will cause prolonged hospitalization and probably not affect the outcome in AIDS patients?
2. What is the risk of accelerating the disease by surgery?
3. What is the risk of HIV infection to health care workers?
4. What is the risk of getting HIV infection during open-heart surgery?

In general, it is not wise to perform expensive procedures with some degree of morbidity and mortality that result in prolonged hospitalization of patients with a limited life span due to their underlying disease. For this reason, patients with AIDS should not be subjected to surgery that will most probably not significantly affect their survival. Before protease inhibitors were available, probably 70 percent of patients found to have AIDS would die within 3 to 4 years of the diagnosis.[118] Now, with newer drugs, life has been markedly prolonged. Therefore, if patients with AIDS have medically uncontrollable symptoms, invasive procedures that can ameliorate these symptoms are indicated.

With infective endocarditis, the vast majority of HIV-infected patients are intravenous drug users, and the most common valve involved is the tricuspid valve, which almost always can be treated medically. The most frequent problem in which the question of cardiovascular surgery arises in a relatively young subgroup involves the intravenous drug user with infective endocarditis on the aortic and/or mitral valve and congestive heart failure. The presence of HIV disease in these patients, who overall have a high mortality and poor results from surgery, would suggest that they be treated medically for as long as possible.[119] If failure persists, valvular replacement should be done.

HIV-positive patients and patients with PGL who have not had an opportunistic infection or cancer can have a prolonged course over many years and, in general, should be treated like patients without HIV disease. In fact, life span might be prolonged after HIV infection by using combinations of drugs, including reverse-transcriptase inhibitors and the new protease inhibitors. In this subgroup, cardiovascular surgery should be considered for the usual indications.

The question of whether progression of the HIV disease is accelerated by the immunologic challenge that occurs from cardiopulmonary bypass is largely unanswered. Instances of HIV-positive patients who developed AIDS shortly after open-heart surgery have been reported. It is known that cardiopulmonary bypass temporaily depresses phagocytic function and immune globulin production.[120] Cardiopulmonary bypass per se in HIV-negative patients causes prolonged abnormalities in the CD4+/CD8+ T-cell ratio up to 6 days postoperatively.[121] There is, therefore, a basis for concern that cardiopulmonary bypass surgery could accelerate the progression of HIV disease, and this must be taken into consideration.

Whether all patients undergoing cardiovascular surgery or other invasive procedures should have HIV testing is a matter of heated debate. Although the risk to health care personnel is small, HIV infection is usually tantamount to fatal infection; fear is great among both health care workers and the public. On the other hand, AIDS is an emotional subject, and patients who are known to be HIV positive may be subjected to prejudice and discrimination. At present, HIV testing of both health care workers and patients is voluntary; however, there are proposed recommendations requiring disclosure to patients that a health care worker is HIV positive and informed consent from patients before any invasive procedure is done. At present, there is only one instance of transmission of disease by a health care worker, that of an HIV-positive dentist who is believed to have infected five patients, probably from reuse of inadequately sterilized instruments. This matter is still under considerable debate.

Because of this risk, some cardiovascular surgeons and cardiologists are refusing to operate on or catheterize an HIV-positive person or a patient who will not allow an HIV test to be done. In 1989, a survey was done of the attitudes of cardiac surgeons in the United States concerning operating on HIV-positive patients.[122] More than half responded, and two-thirds of these were reportedly willing to perform open-heart surgery on HIV-positive patients no matter how the patients had acquired their HIV infection. One-quarter of the surgeons would not operate no matter how the HIV infection was acquired, and the rest were uncertain. Once the patient has gone from the HIV-carrier state to AIDS, two-thirds of the cardiac surgeons would not operate. Of those responding, 90 percent want to be able to test all their patients for HIV status. Whether these attitudes have changed in the last decade is unknown.

A physician's fear of becoming infected with HIV is understandable, but as in the case of other professions that involved personal dangers, the profession of the physician requires performance. Both the American College of Physicians and the American Medical Association currently have standards stating that physicians may not ethically refuse to treat patients solely because the patients are HIV positive.

As of 1995, the literature has reported 49 health care workers in the United States who had no other risk factors and were known to be HIV negative at exposure who have seroconverted after exposure.[123] The danger to health care personnel is greatest when there is exposure to blood and the chance of accidental needle or knife perforation or blood splash into the eyes or mouth. In one prospective study of 1307 consecutive procedures, accumulated exposure, parenteral or cutaneous, occurred in only 84 procedures (6.4 percent).[124] Parenteral exposure occurred in 1.7 percent. Knowledge of the patient's HIV status or awareness of the patient's high-risk status for such infection did not appear to influence the rate of exposure, suggesting that preoperative testing for HIV infection would not decrease the frequency of accidental exposure to blood.

In combined data from 20 prospective studies of the risk of HIV-1 transmission to health care workers, there were 6498 parenteral exposures among 1948 subjects.[125] The chance of seroconversion was 0.32 percent per exposure (95 percent confidence interval, 0.18 to 0.46 percent); in 2885 mucous membrane exposures, there was one seroconversion (0.03 percent per exposure). The risk of a health care worker developing HIV seroconversion from work-related activities was very low: approximately one infection in 300 documented exposures to HIV-positive blood.

References

1. Chu SY, Berkelman RL, Curran JW. Epidemiology of HIV in the United States. In: De Vita VT, Hellman S, Rosenberg SA, eds. *AIDS: Etiology, Diagnosis, Treatment and Prevention*, 3d ed. Philadelphia: Lippincott; 1992:99–100.
2. Centers for Disease Control and Prevention. HIV/AIDS surveillance report. Atlanta: CDC 1994; 6(2):7.
3. Steele FR. A moving target: CDC still trying to evaluate HIV-1 prevalence. *J NIH Res* 1994; 6:25–26.
4. Obiri GU, Fordyce EJ, Singh TP, et al. Effect of HIV/AIDS versus other causes of death on premature mortality in New York City, 1983–1994. *Am J Epidemol* 1998; 147:840–845.
5. Centers for Disease Control. Classification system for human T-lymphotropic virus type III/lymphadenopathy-associated virus infections. *MMWR* 1986; 35:334–339.
6. Centers for Disease Control. 1993 Revised classification system for HIV infection and expanded surveillance case definition for AIDS among adolescents and adults. *MMWR* 1992; 41(RR-17):1–19.
7. Schacker T, Collier AC, Hughes J, et al. Clinical and epidemiologic features of primary HIV infection. *Ann Intern Med* 1996; 125:257–264.
8. Horsburgh CR Jr, Ou CY, Jason J, et al. Duration of human immunodeficiency virus infection before detection of antibody. *Lancet* 1989; 2:637–640.
9. Bacchetti P, Moss AR. Incubation period of AIDS in San Francisco [letter]. *Nature* 1989; 338:251–253.
10. Feinberg MB, Greene WC. Molecular insights into human immunodeficiency virus type 1 pathogenesis. *Curr Opin Immunol* 1992; 4:466–474.
11. Rutherford GW, Lifson AR, Hessol NA, et al. Course of HIV-1 infection in a cohort of homosexual and bisexual men: An 11 year follow-up study. *BMJ* 1990; 301:1183–1188.
12. Osmond D. Progression to AIDS in persons testing seropositive for antibody to HIV. In: Cohen PT, Sande MA, Volberding PA, eds. *The AIDS Knowledge Base.* Waltham, MA: Medical Publishing Group; 1990:1.1.6.
13. Piatak M Jr, Saag MS, Yang LC, et al. High levels of HIV-1 in plasma during all stages of infection determined by competitive PCR. *Science* 1993; 259:1749–1754.
14. Pantaleo G, Menzo S, Vaccarezza M, et al. Studies in subjects with long-term nonprogressive human immunodeficiency virus infection. *N Engl J Med* 1995; 332:209–216.
15. Deeks SG, Smith M, Holodniy M, et al. HIV-1 protease inhibitors: A review for clinicians. *JAMA* 1997; 277:145–153.
16. Palalla FJ, Delaney KM, Moorman AC, et al. The HIV outpatient study investigators. *N Engl J Med* 1998; 338:853–860.
17. Mann J, Ching , Piot P, et al. The international epidemiology of AIDS. *Sci Am* 1988; 259:82–89.
18. Silver MA, Macher AM, Reichert CM, et al. Cardiac involvement by Kaposi's sarcoma in acquired immune deficiency syndrome (AIDS). *Am J Cardiol* 1984; 53:983–985.
19. Welch K, Finkbeiner W, Alpers CE, et al. Autopsy findings in the acquired immune deficiency syndrome. *JAMA* 1984; 252:1152–1159.
20. Cammarosano C, Lewis W. Cardiac lesions in acquired immune deficiency syndrome (AIDS). *J Am Coll Cardiol* 1985; 5:703–706.
21. Roldan EO, Moskowitz L, Hensly GT. Pathology of the heart in acquired immunodeficiency syndrome. *Arch Pathol Lab Med* 1987; 111:943–946.
22. Wilkes MS, Fortin AH, Felix JC, et al. Value of necropsy in acquired immunodeficiency syndrome. *Lancet* 1988; 2:85–88.
23. Baroldi G, Corallo S, Moroni M, et al. Focal lymphocytic myocarditis in acquired immunodeficiency syndrome (AIDS): A correlative morphologic and clinical study in 26 consecutive fatal cases. *J Am Coll Cardiol* 1988; 12:463–469.

24. Lewis W. AIDS: Cardiac findings from 115 autopsies. *Prog Cardiovasc Dis* 1989; 32:207–215.
25. Anderson DW, Virmani R, Reilly JM, et al. Prevalent myocarditis at necropsy in the acquired immunodeficiency syndrome. *J Am Coll Cardiol* 1988; 11:792–799.
26. Magno J, Margaretten W, Cheitlin M. Myocardial involvement in acquired immunodeficiency syndrome: Incidence in a large autopsy study [abstr]. *Circulation* 1988; 78(suppl II):II-459.
27. Garcia I, Fainstein V, Rios A, et al. Nonbacterial thrombotic endocarditis in a male homosexual with Kaposi's sarcoma. *Arch Internal Med* 1983; 143:1243–1244.
28. Barbaro G, DiLorenzo G, Grisorio B, et al. Cardiac involvement in the acquired immunodeficiency syndrome: A multicenter clinical and pathological study. Gruppo Italiano par lo studio cardiologico dei pazienti affetti da AIDS Investigators. *AIDS Res Hum Retroviruses* 1998; 14:1071–1077.
29. Lanjewar DN, Katdare GA, Jain PP, et al. Pathology of the heart in acquired immunodeficiency syndrome. *Indian Heart J* 1998; 50:321–325.
30. Moskowitz L, Hensley GT, Chan JC, et al. Immediate causes of death in acquired immunodeficiency syndrome. *Arch Pathol Lab Med* 1985; 109:735–738.
31. Murray JF, Garay SM, Hopewell PC, et al. Pulmonary complications of the acquired immunodeficiency syndrome: An update—Report of the second National Heart, Lung and Blood Institute workshop. *Am Rev Respir Dis* 1987; 135:504–509.
32. Kinney EL, Brafman D, Wright RJ II. Echocardiographic findings in patients with acquired immunodeficiency syndrome (AIDS) and AIDS-related complex (ARC). *Cathet Cardiovasc Diagn* 1989; 16:182–185.
33. Himelman RB, Chung WS, Chernoff DN, et al. Cardiac manifestations of human immunodeficiency virus infection: A two-dimensional echocardiographic study. *J Am Coll Cardiol* 1989; 13:1030–1036.
34. Monsuez JJ, Kinney EL, Vittecoq D, et al. Comparison among acquired immune deficiency syndrome patients with and without clinical evidence of cardiac disease. *Am J Cardiol* 1988; 62:1311–1313.
35. Levy WS, Simon GL, Rios JC, et al. Prevalence of cardiac abnormalities in human immunodeficiency virus infection. *Am J Cardiol* 1989; 63:86–89.
36. Corallo S, Mutinelli MR, Moroni M, et al. Echocardiography detects myocardial damage in AIDS: Prospective study in 102 patients. *Eur Heart J* 1988; 9:887–892.
37. Currie PF, Jacob AJ, Foreman AR, et al. Heart muscle disease related to HIV infection: Prognostic implications. *BMJ* 1994; 309:1605–1607.
38. Cecchi E, Parrini I, Chinaglia A, et al. Cardiac complications in HIV infections. *G Ital Cardiol* 1997; 27:917–924.
39. Steffen HM, Muller R, Schrappe-Bächer M, et al. Prevalence of echocardiographic abnormalities in human immunodeficiency virus 1 infection. *Am J Noninvasive Cardiol* 1991; 5:280–284.
40. Redfield RR, Wright DC, Tramont EC. The Walter Reed staging classification for HTLV-III/LAV infection: Special report. *N Engl J Med* 1986; 314:131–132.
41. Chyu KY, Birnbaum Y, Naqvi T, et al. Echocardiographic detection of Kaposi's sarcoma causing cardiac tamponade in a patient with acquired immunodeficiency syndrome. *Clin Cardiol* 1998; 21:131–133.
42. Estok L, Wallach F. Cardiac tamponade in a patient with AIDS: A review of pericardial disease in patients with HIV infection. *Mt Sinai J Med* 1998; 65:33–39.
43. Heidenreich PA, Eisenberg MJ, Kee LL, et al. Pericardial effusion in AIDS: Incidence and survival. *Circulation* 1995; 92:3229–3234.
44. Flum DR, McGinn JT Jr, Tyras DH. The role of the "pericardial window" in AIDS. *Chest* 1995; 107:1522–1525.
45. Azrak EC, Kern MJ, Bach RG. Hemodynamics of cardiac tamponade in a patient with AIDS-related non-Hodgkin's lymphoma. *Cathet Cardiovasc Design* 1998; 45:287–291.
46. Decker CF, Tuazon CU. *Staphylococcus aureus* pericarditis in HIV-infected patients. *Chest* 1994; 105:615–616.
47. Zuger A, Louie E, Holzman RS, et al. Cryptococcal disease in patients with acquired immunodeficiency syndrome: Diagnostic features and outcome of treatment. *Ann Intern Med* 1986; 104:234–240.
48. Freedberg RS, Gindea AJ, Dieterich DT, et al. Herpes simplex pericarditis in AIDS. *NY State J Med* 1987; 87:304–306.
49. Francis CK. Cardiac involvement in AIDS. *Curr Probl Cardiol* 1990; 15:571–639.
50. Zuger A, Louie E, Holzman RS, et al. Cryptococcal disease in patients with the acquired immunodeficiency syndrome: Diagnostic features and outcome of treatment: Clinical review. *Ann Intern Med* 1986; 104:234–240.
51. Hofman P, Drici MD, Gibelin P, et al. Prevalence of toxoplasma myocarditis in patients with the acquired immunodeficiency syndrome. *Br Heart J* 1993; 70:376–381.
52. Kinney EL, Monsuez JJ, Kitzis M, et al. Treatment of AIDS-associated heart disease. *Angiology* 1989; 40:970–976.
53. Grange F, Kinney EL, Monsuez JJ, et al. Successful therapy for *Toxoplasma gondii* myocarditis in acquired immunodeficiency syndrome. *Am Heart J* 1990; 120:443–444.
54. Albrecht H, Stellbrink HJ, Fenske S, et al. Successful treatment of *Toxoplasma gondii* myocarditis in an AIDS patient. *Eur J Clin Microbiol Infect Dis* 1994; 13:500–504.
55. Ioachim HL, Cooper MC, Hellman GC. Lymphomas in men at high risk for acquired immune deficiency syndrome (AIDS): A study of 21 cases. *Cancer* 1985; 56:2831–2842.
56. Montalbetti L, Della Volpe A, Airughi ML, et al. Primary cardiac lymphoma: A case report and review. *Minerva Cardioangiol* 1999; 47:175–182.
57. Levitt LJ, Ault KA, Pinkus GS, et al. Pericarditis and early cardiac tamponade as a primary manifestation of lymphoscarcoma cell leukemia. *Am J Med* 1979; 67:719–723.
58. Golfarb A, King CL, Rosenzweig BP, et al. Cardiac lymphoma in the accquired immunodeficiency syndrome. *Am Heart J* 1989; 118:1340–1344.
59. Cohen IS, Anderson DW, Virmani R, et al. Congestive cardiomyopathy in association with the acquired immunodeficiency syndrome. *N Engl J Med* 1986; 315:628–630.
60. Reilly JM, Cunnion RE, Anderson DW, et al. Frequency of myocarditis, left ventricular dysfunction and ventricular tachycardia in the acquired immune deficiency syndrome. *Am J Cardiol* 1988; 62:789–793.
61. Kaminski HJ, Katzman M, Wiest PM, et al. Cardiomyopathy associated with the acquired immune deficiency syndrome. *J AIDS* 1988; 1:105–110.
62. Lipshultz SE, Orav EJ, Sanders SP, et al. Cardiac structure and function in children with human immunodeficiency virus infection treated with zidovudine. *N Engl J Med* 1992; 327:1260–1265.
63. Lipshultz SE, Easley KA, Orav EJ, et al. Left ventricle structure and function in children with human immunodeficiency virus: The prospective P2 C2 HIV Multicenter Study. Pediatric Pulmonary and Cardiac Complications of Vertically Transmitted HIV Infection (P2 C2 HIV) Study Group. *Circulation* 1998; 97:1246–1256.
64. DeCastro S, d'Amati G, Gallo P, et al. Frequency of development of acute global left ventricular dysfunction in human immunodeficiency virus infection. *J Am Coll Cardiol* 1994; 24:1018–1024.
65. Blanchard DG, Hagenhoff C, Chow LC, et al. Reversibility of cardiac abnormalities in human immunodeficiency virus (HIV)-infected individuals: A serial echocardiographic study. *J Am Coll Cardiol* 1991; 17:1270–1276.
66. Cheitlin MD. Cardiovascular complications of HIV infection. In:

Sande MA, Volberding PA, eds. *The Medical Management of AIDS,* 4th ed. Philadelphia: Saunders; 1995:332.
67. Barbaro G, Di Lorenzo G, Grisorio B, et al. Incidence of dilated cardiomyopathy and detection of HIV in myocardial cells of HIV-positive patients. Gruppo Italiano per lo Studio Cardilogico dei Pazianti Affetti, da AIDS. *N Engl J Med* 1998; 339:1093–1099.
68. Calabrese LH, Proffitt MR, Yen-Lieberman B, et al. Congestive cardiomyopathy and illness related to the acquired immunodeficiency syndrome (AIDS) associated with isolation of retrovirus from myocardium. *Ann Intern Med* 1987; 107:691–692.
69. Grody WW, Cheng L, Lewis W. Infection of the heart by the human immunodeficiency virus. *Am J Cardiol* 1990; 66:203–206.
70. Stewart JM, Kaul A, Gromisch DS, et al. Symptomatic cardiac dysfunction in children with human immunodeficiency virus infection. *Am Heart J* 1989; 117:140–144.
71. Acierno LJ. Cardiac complications in acquired immunodeficiency syndrome (AIDS): A review. *J Am Coll Cardiol* 1989; 13:1144–1154.
72. Cox JN, Di Dio F, Pizzolato GP, et al. *Aspergillus* endocarditis and myocarditis in a patient with the acquired immunodeficiency syndrome (AIDS): A review of the literature—Case report. *Virchows Arch* [*A*] 1990; 417:255–259.
73. Lowry PJ, Thompson RA, Littler WA. Cellular immunity in congestive cardiomyopathy: The normal cellular immune response. *Br Heart J* 1985; 53:394–399.
74. Zee-Cheng CS, Tsai CC, Palmer DC, et al. High incidence of myocarditis by endomyocardial biopsy in patients with idiopathic congestive cardiomyopathy. *J Am Coll Cardiol* 1984; 3:63–70.
75. Parrillo JE, Aretz HT, Palacios I, et al. The results of transvenous endomyocardial biopsy can frequently be used to diagnose myocardial disease in patients with idiopathic heart failure: Endomyocardial biopsy in 100 consecutive patients revealed a substantial incidence of myocarditis. *Circulation* 1984; 69:93–101.
76. Bowles NE, Richardson PJ, Olsen EGJ, et al. Detection of Coxsackie-B-virus-specific RNA sequences in myocardial biopsy samples from patients with myocarditis and dilated cardiomyopathy. *Lancet* 1984; 1:1120–1123.
77. Herskowitz A, WU T-C, Willoughby SB, et al. Myocarditis and cardiotrophic viral infection associated with severe left ventricular dysfunction in late-stage infection with human immunodeficiency virus. *J Am Coll Cardiol* 1994; 24:1025–1032.
78. Herskowitz A, Ansari AA, Neumann DA, et al. Cardiomyopathy in acquired immunodeficiency syndrome: Evidence for autoimmunity [abstr]. *Circulation* 1989; 80(suppl II):II-322.
79. Lipshultz SE, Orav J, Sanders SP, et al. Immunoglobulins and left ventricular structure and function in pediatric HIV infection. *Circulation* 1995; 92:2220–2225.
80. Ho DD, Pomerantz RJ, Kaplan JC. Pathogenesis of infection with human immunodeficiency virus. *N Engl J Med* 1987; 317:278–286.
81. Parker MM, Shelhamer JH, Bacharach SL, et al. Profound but reversible myocardial depression in patients with septic shock. *Ann Intern Med* 1984; 100:483–490.
82. Natanson C, Fink MP, Ballantyne HK, et al. Gram-negative bacteremia produces both severe systolic and diastolic cardiac dysfunction in a canine model that simulates human septic shock. *J Clin Invest* 1986; 78:259–270.
83. Parrillo JE, Burch C, Shelhamer JH, et al. A circulating myocardial depressant substance in humans with septic shock: Septic shock patients with a reduced ejection fraction have a circulating factor that depresses in vitro myocardial cell performance. *J Clin Invest* 1985; 76:1539–1553.
84. Cunnion RE, Parrillo JE. Myocardial dysfunction in sepsis: Recent insights [editorial]. *Chest* 1989; 95:941–945.
85. Suffredini AF, Fromm RE, Parker MM, et al. The cardiovascular response of normal humans to the administration of endotoxin. *N Engl J Med* 1989; 321:280–287.
86. Levine B, Kalman J, Mayer L, et al. Elevated circulating levels of tumor necrosis factor in severe chronic heart failure. *N Engl J Med* 1990; 323:236–241.
87. Lähdevirta J, Maury CPJ, Teppo AM, et al. Elevated levels of circulating cachectin/tumor necrosis factor in patients with acquired immunodeficiency syndrome. *Am J Med* 1988; 85:289–291.
88. Wright SC, Jewett A, Mitsuyasu R, et al. Spontaneous cytotoxicity and tumor necrosis factor production by peripheral blood monocytes from AIDS patients. *J Immunol* 1988; 141:99–104.
89. Barbaro G, Di Lorenzo G, Soldini M, et al. Intensity of myocardial expression of inducible nitric oxide synthase influences the clinical course of human immunodeficiency virus-associated cardiomyopathy. Gruppo Italiano per lo Studio Cardiologico dei pazienti affetti dei AIDS (GISCA). *Circulation* 1999; 100:933–939.
90. Odeh M. The role of tumour necrosis factor-alpha in acquired immunodeficiency syndrome. *J Intern Med* 1990; 228:549–556.
91. Yamamoto N. The role of cytokines in the acquired immunodeficiency syndrome. *Int J Clin Lab Res* 1995; 25:29–34.
92. Goldberg SJ, Comerci GD, Feldman L. Cardiac output and regional myocardial contraction in anorexia nervosa. *J Adolesc Health Care* 1988; 9:15–21.
93. Abel RM, Grimes JB, Alonso D, et al. Adverse hemodynamic and ultrastructural changes in dog hearts subjected to protein-calorie malnutrition. *Am Heart J* 1979; 97:733–744.
94. Schocken DD, Holloway JD, Powers PS. Weight loss and the heart: Effects of anorexia nervosa and starvation. *Arch Intern Med* 1989; 149:877–881.
95. Dworkin BM, Antonecchia PP, Smith F, et al. Reduced cardiac selenium content in the acquired immunodeficiency syndrome. *J Parenter Enteral Nutr* 1989; 13:644–647.
96. Kavanaugh-McHugh AL, Ruff A, Perlman E, et al. Selenium deficiency and cardiomyopathy in acquired immunodeficiency syndrome. *J Parenter Enteral Nutr* 1991; 15:347–349.
97. Kaul S, Fishbein MC, Siegel RJ. Cardiac manifestations of acquired immune deficiency syndrome: A 1991 update. *Am Heart J* 1991; 122:535–544.
98. Cohen MC, Huberman MS, Nesto RW. Recombinant alpha$_2$ interferon-related cardiomyopathy. *Am J Med* 1988; 85:549–551.
99. Deyton LR, Walker RE, Kovacs JA, et al. Reversible cardiac dysfunction associated with interferon alpha therapy in AIDS patients with Kaposi's sarcoma. *N Engl J Med* 1989; 321:1246–1249.
100. Chokshi SK, Moore R, Pandian NG, et al. Reversible cardiomyopathy associated with cocaine intoxication. *Ann Intern Med* 1989; 111:1039–1040.
101. Brown J, Kind A, Francis CK. Cardiovascular effects of alcohol, cocaine, and acquired immune deficiency. *Cardiovasc Clin* 1991; 21:341–376.
102. Wharton JM, Demopulos PA, Goldschlager N. Torsade de pointes during administration of pentamidine isothionate. *Am J Med* 1987; 83:571–576.
103. Richman DD, Fischl MA, Grieco MH, et al. The toxicity of azidothymidine (AZT) in the treatment of patients with AIDS and AIDS-related complex: A double-blind, placebo-controlled trial. *N Engl J Med* 1987; 317:192–197.
104. Dalakas MC, Illa I, Pezeshkpour GH, et al. Mitochondrial myopathy caused by long-term zidovudine therapy. *N Engl J Med* 1990; 322:1098–1105.
105. Szabados E, Fischer GM, Toth K, et al. Role of reactive oxygen species and poly-ADP-ribose polymerase in the development of AZT-induced cardiomyopathy in rats. *Free Radic Biol Med* 1999; 26:302–317.
106. Brown DL, Sather S, Cheitlin MD. Reversible cardiac dysfunction associated with foscarnet therapy for cytomegalovirus esophagitis in an AIDS patient. *Am Heart J* 1993; 125:1439–1441.
107. Eastone JA, Decker CF. New onset diabetes mellitus associated with the use of protease inhibitors. *Ann Intern Med* 1997; 127:948.

108. Carr A, Samaras K, Chisholm DJ, et al. Pathogenesis of HIV-1 protease inhibitor-associated peripheral lipodystrophy, hyperlipidemia, and insulin resistance. *Lancet* 1998; 351:1881–1883.
109. Danner SA, Carr A, Leondard J, et al. Safety, pharmacokinetics and preliminary efficacy of ritonavir, an inhibitor of HIV-1 protease. *N Engl J Med* 1995; 333:1528–1533.
110. Cameron DW, Japour AJ, Xu Y, et al. Ritonavir and saquinavir combination therapy for the treatment of HIV infection. *AIDS* 1999; 13:213–224.
111. Melroe NH, Kopaczewski J, Henry K, et al. Intervention for hyperlipidemia associated with protease inhibitors. *J Assoc Nurses AIDS Care* 1999; 10:55–69.
112. Miller KD, Jones E, Janovsk JA, et al. Visceral abdominal fat accumulation associated with use of indinavir. *Lancet* 1998; 351:871–875.
113. Lo JC, Mullighan K, Tai VW, et al. Buffalo hump in men with HIV-1 infection. *Lancet* 1998; 351:867–870.
114. Carr A, Samaras K, Burton S, et al. A syndrome of peripheral lipodystrophy, hyperlipidemia and insulin resistance in patients receiving HIV protease inhibitors. *AIDS* 1998; 12:F51–F58.
115. Henry K, Melroe IT, Heubsch J, et al. Severe premature coronary artery disease with protease inhibitors [research letter]. *Lancet* 1998; 351:1321–1328.
116. Herskowitz A, Willouby SB, Baughman KL, et al. Cardiomyopathy associated with antiretroviral therapy in patients with HIV infection: A report of six cases. *Ann Intern Med* 1992; 116:311–313.
117. Mason JW, O'Connell JB, Herskowitz A, et al. A clinical trial of immunosuppressive therapy for myocarditis: The Myocarditis Treatment Trial Investigators. *N Engl J Med* 1995; 333:269–275.
118. Centers for Disease Control. Acquired immunodeficiency syndrome: United States—Update. *MMWR* 1986; 35:17–21.
119. Ribera E, Miro JM, Cortes E, et al. Influence of human immunodeficiency virus 1 and degree of immunosuppression in the clinical characteristics and outcome of infective endocarditis in intravenous drug users. *Arch Intern Med* 1998; 158:2043–2050.
120. Utley JR. The immune response. In: *Pathophysiology and Techniques of Cardiopulmonary Bypass I.* Baltimore: Williams and Wilkins; 1982:132–144.
121. Pollock R, Ames F, Rubio P, et al. Protracted severe immune dysregulation induced by cardiopulmonary bypass: A predisposing etiologic factor in blood transfusion-related AIDS? *J Clin Lab Immunol* 1987; 22:1–5.
122. Condit D, Frater RWM. Human immunodeficiency virus and the cardiac surgeon: A survey of attitudes. *Ann Thorac Surg* 1989; 47:182–186.
123. Heptonstall J, Porter K, Gill ON. *Occupational HIV: Summary of published reports.* London: Public Health Laboratory Services. Communicable Disease Surveillance Centre; Dec 1995.
124. Gerberding JL, Littell C, Tarkington A, et al. Risk of exposure of surgical personnel to patients' blood during surgery at San Francisco General Hospital. *N Engl J Med* 1990; 322:1788–1793.
125. Gerberding JL. Management of occupational exposures to bloodborne viruses. *N Engl J Med* 1995; 332:444–451.

CHAPTER 71

EFFECT OF NONCARDIAC DRUGS, ELECTRICITY, POISONS, AND RADIATION ON THE HEART

Andrew L. Smith / Wendy M. Book

This chapter details many deleterious side effects of treatments and environmental agents on the heart. Toxic effects may occur acutely and require emergent intervention or may be chronic and not be manifest until days or years after exposure.

NONCARDIAC DRUGS

Chemotherapeutic Agents

The use of chemotherapeutic agents may result in acute or chronic cardiovascular toxicity. The heart, composed of nonproliferating myocytes, was traditionally thought to be protected from the effects of drugs on rapidly dividing cells. A variety of agents are now recognized to cause cardiovascular complications, including cardiomyopathy, myocarditis, pericarditis, myocardial ischemia, arrhythmias, and peripheral hypotension or vasospasm (see Table 71-1).[1]

Cardiovascular alterations in the patient receiving chemotherapy may be the result of a specific drug or combination of drugs or be related to tumor-associated factors such as hypercoagulability or release of myocardial depressant factors. Correlating a specific therapy with a particular adverse event may be difficult; however, knowledge of side effects of each agent should be considered when prescribing therapy.

ANTHRACYCLINES

The anthracycline antineoplastics—doxorubicin, daunorubicin, and epirubicine—are the leading cause of chemotherapy-related heart disease. These agents may cause cardiac problems during therapy, weeks after completion of therapy, or, unexpectedly, years later.[2] During acute therapy, electrocardiographic (ECG) changes occur in approximately 30 percent of patients and usually regress within weeks. Findings include ST-T changes, decreased QRS voltage, prolongation of the QT interval, and atrial and ventricular ectopy. Sustained atrial or ventricular arrhythmias are rare. The occurrence of early ECG abnormalities does not predict cardiomyopathy and is not an indication to discontinue therapy.[1] The development of persistent sinus tachycardia (although nonspecific) in an otherwise stable oncology patient, however, may raise the suspicion of ventricular dysfunction and impending congestive heart failure.

Congestive heart failure is related to the cumulative dose of the anthracycline administered. The incidences of heart failure at specific doses of doxorubicin include 0.4 percent at 400 mg/m^2 of body surface area, 7 percent at 550 mg/m^2, and 18 percent at 700 mg/m^2 (see Fig. 71-1). Traditionally, the cardiac limiting dose has been described as 550 mg/m^2 because of the acute rise in heart failure seen above this dose. There is great individual variability, however, with reports of heart failure occurring with doses less than 100 mg/m^2 and, conversely, with some patients tolerating greater than 1000 mg/m^2 without cardiac compromise.[3,4] Risk factors for anthracycline-induced cardiomyopathy are debated but include prior chest radiation, age greater than 70, and preexisting heart disease.[3-5] Young women may be at particularly increased risk for late cardiac dysfunction.[5] Rapid infusion schedules associated with higher peak drug concentrations appear to result in greater cardiotoxicity. Combination therapy with cyclophosphamide is an additional risk factor.[1]

The pathogenesis of anthracycline-induced cardiotoxicity is not known. Theories generally implicate free-radical damage. One proposal is that enzymatic reduction of the anthracycline-quinone ring results in lipid peroxidation and cell membrane damage. Another theory involves the formation of an anthracycline-iron complex, which undergoes "redoxcycling" that results

TABLE 71-1 Chemotherapeutic Agents Commonly Associated with Cardiovascular Toxicity

Drug	Associated Toxicity
Anthracyclines	
Doxorubicin	Cardiomyopathy
Daunorubicin	
Epirubicin	
Idarubicin	
Mitoxantrone	
Alkylating agents	
Cyclophosphamide	Reversible systolic dysfunction, hemorrhagic myocarditis
Cisplatin	Raynaud's phenomenon
Antimetabolites	
5-Fluorouracil	Coronary vasospasm
Other	
Amsacrine	Arrhythmias
Paclitaxel	Arrhythmias
Interleukin 2	Hypotension, myocarditis
Interferon alpha	Hypotension, cardiomyopathy

in oxygen radicals and degradation of microsomal, mitochondrial, and membrane lipids. Disturbances of calcium exchange have also been noted.[6]

The average time to clinical development of heart failure symptoms is 1 month from the end of therapy, but it may occur anytime within 1 year. Patient presentation is similar to that for other dilated cardiomyopathies (see Chap. 66). Biventricular systolic dysfunction occurs, and restrictive hemodynamics have been described.[7] The clinical course varies from fulminant heart failure to gradually progressive deterioration. Some patients have reversibility of systolic dysfunction. Therapy, in addition to withholding further anthracycline dosing or other myocardial toxins, is generally considered the same as recommended for patients with heart failure from dilated cardiomyopathy (Chap. 21).

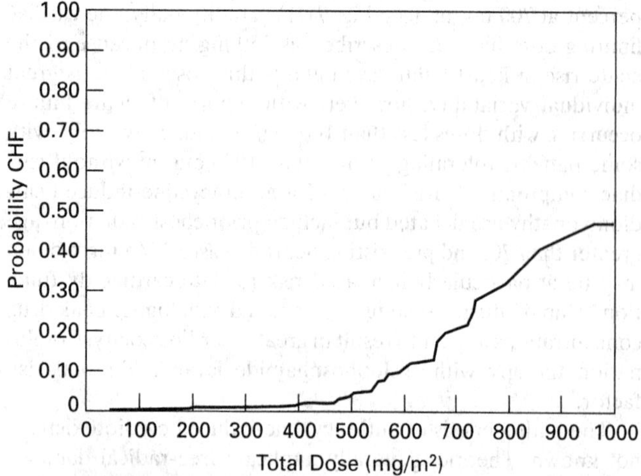

FIGURE 71-1 The development of doxorubicin-induced heart failure is related to cumulative dose. Toxicity may occur at any dose, but at 550 mg/m^2 the probability increases significantly. (From Von Hoff et al.,[3] with permission.)

Noninvasive assessment of left ventricular function has been utilized to guide anthracycline dosing and prevent cardiac toxicity. Serial echocardiography and/or radionuclide angiography (see Chaps. 13 and 16) are most commonly used.[8–10] Improved echocardiographic technologies are likely to increase the use of echocardiography in the adult population. The most commonly used parameter is resting left ventricular ejection fraction. Recognition that resting left ventricular ejection fraction is relatively insensitive for detecting early cardiotoxicity[2] has resulted in investigation of other variables (exercise or dobutamine echocardiography,[9] Doppler velocities, and systolic time intervals) in assessing this problem. These methods have generally been evaluated in small studies and have not gained widespread acceptance in current therapy guidelines. Adult guidelines for serial assessment have been developed. A drop in left ventricular ejection fraction greater than 10 percent (EF units) and to below a normal value of 50 percent is an indication to discontinue therapy. A baseline left ventricular ejection fraction less than 30 percent has generally been considered a contraindication to initiating anthracycline therapy.[10]

Compared with the noninvasive methods, endomyocardial biopsy is considered more specific and provides earlier sensitivity in detection of anthracycline cardiotoxicity. The Billingham score, which quantifies cytoplasmic changes and the percent of myocytes damaged, has been utilized to assess the risk of congestive heart failure.[11] Clinical utility has been limited because of the invasive nature of this procedure and the special expertise required in obtaining and reading the specimens. Additionally, variability of histologic changes and the potential for sampling error have been noted.[12]

There is growing recognition of the occurrence of cardiac dysfunction years after completion of anthracycline therapy. This is particularly of concern in children. One study reported a 23 percent incidence of late cardiac abnormalities (decreased systolic function by noninvasive testing) in survivors of pediatric malignancies treated with anthracycline therapy.[13] The incidence of abnormalities was higher in the patients with the longer elapsed times since therapy, with a 38 percent incidence in patients with a follow-up period greater than 10 years. This study, as well as others,[14] suggests that subclinical myocardial damage may not become clinically evident until years after therapy. Although fewer than 5 percent of these patients had developed clinical heart failure, the potentially progressive nature of systolic dysfunction raises the issue of need for long-term clinical follow-up. There are presently no accepted guidelines, however, in either the pediatric or adult population for chronic monitoring. Early treatment of systolic dysfunction with angiotensin-converting enzyme inhibitors may be warranted in asymptomatic patients.[2] Additionally, patients presenting late after anthracycline therapy with exertional fatigue and normal resting ejection fractions have been noted to have abnormalities on dobutamine echocardiography. This observation suggests abnormalities in cardiac reserve that may lead to symptoms.

Clinical strategies for preventing anthracycline cardiotoxicity have had to balance the need for antineoplastic efficacy. Lower clinical toxicity has been noted with prolonged infusions of doxorubicin over 48 to 96 h in order to avoid high peak concentrations.[15] Several antioxidants have been evaluated, but with inconclusive results.[6,16] *Dexrazoxane,*[17] an iron-chelating agent, reduces free-radical generation by anthracyclines and is approved for use in women with breast cancer after a cumulative dose of doxorubicin of 300 mg/m^2. Studies demonstrate a decrease in cardiotoxicity and most but not all trials have suggested preserved efficacy of antitumor activity. New anthracyclines, including epirubicine and idarubicin, appear to have diminished cardiotoxic effects, although long-term results cannot presently be assessed.[2]

OTHER CHEMOTHERAPEUTIC AGENTS

Mitoxantrone, an anthracendione lacking the amino sugar of anthracyclines, causes cardiotoxicity with features similar to anthracycline-induced cardiomyopathy.[1] This drug appears to have less cardiotoxicity than doxorubicin at equal myelotoxic doses. Cumulative doses above 160 mg/m^2 are associated with an increasing incidence of congestive heart failure.[18]

High-dose *cyclophosphamide* (120 to 240 mg/kg over several days) used in bone marrow transplantation may cause acute cardiac toxicity.[1,19] Symptomatic systolic dysfunction, usually reversible with drug discontinuation, is associated with decreased QRS voltage on the ECG. Pericardial effusions have been noted, and a hemorrhagic myocarditis may result in death. Necropsy data demonstrate endothelial injury with resultant interstitial fibrin deposition and capillary microthrombosis. The cardiotoxicity of cyclophosphamide is likely due to damage from its biologically active metabolites. Rapid metabolizers of cyclophosphamide appear to be prone to cardiotoxicity. The metabolites cause the toxic endothelial damage leading to muscle damage.[19] Cyclophosphamide may also potentiate the cardiotoxic effects of the anthracyclines.[1]

5-*Fluorouracil* may occasionally cause angina, ECG changes, and rarely myocardial infarction.[1,20] The majority of episodes occur during the first cycle of therapy and resolve spontaneously after discontinuation. Arrhythmias and systolic dysfunction have been observed. The understanding of 5-fluorouracil toxicity is complicated because combination chemotherapy is generally utilized, patients may be systemically ill, and many receiving this medication have preexisting coronary artery disease.[20] The incidence of cardiac toxicity is uncertain but ranges from 1 to 8 percent.[21] Patients with known coronary artery disease are at higher risk for serious cardiotoxicity. The mechanism of toxicity remains unclear, although coronary vasospasm has been suspected. Coronary catheterization has generally failed to demonstrate vasomotor hyperreactivity with 5-fluorouracil on ergonovine challenge.

Amsacrine (AMSA) has been associated with prolongation of the QT interval. Malignant ventricular arrhythmias may occur in 1 percent of patients and are exacerbated by hypokalemia.[22]

Paclitaxel (taxol) is being used with increased frequency for breast and ovarian cancer. The most common cardiovascular effect is the development of transient asymptomatic bradycardia, occurring in up to 30 percent of patients. Bradycardia with adverse consequences occurs in only 0.1 percent of patients. A possible relationship of paclitaxel to heart failure has been questioned, but confirmatory data are lacking.[23]

Herceptin (recombinant humanized anti-HER2 antibody) is a relatively new treatment for breast cancer that appears to have favorable antitumor effects when added to standard chemotherapy in selected patients. Unfortunately, cardiac toxicity may limit the use of this drug. In a breast cancer treatment trial, 27 percent of patients receiving doxorubicin, paclitaxel, and Herceptin had cardiac dysfunction compared with 6 percent receiving doxorubicin and paclitaxel without Herceptin. Close cardiac monitoring is warranted.[24]

Immunomodulating Agents

The biological response modifiers *interleukin-2* (IL-2) and *interferon alpha* have been associated with cardiovascular toxicity predominantly secondary to peripheral vasodilatation. IL-2 causes tachycardia, hypotension, and a capillary leak syndrome. Myocarditis has been reported in patients who died soon after initiation of therapy. IL-2 therapy requires pretreatment assessment of cardiovascular risks and close monitoring during drug administration. Interferon alpha may cause supraventricular tachyarrhythmias. A reversible cardiomyopathy has been described.[1,19,25]

Psychotropic Agents

Psychiatric illness, particularly depression, is common in patients with cardiovascular disease[43] (see Chap. 80). Morbidity and mortality following cardiac events are increased in patients with depression, particularly if untreated.[26,27] A variety of psychotropic agents have conduction or vascular effects (see Table 80-11). A thorough understanding of these therapeutic but potentially toxic agents is necessary in the treatment of patients with preexisting cardiac disease. Intentional overdose with these drugs may result in serious cardiac manifestations.

TRICYCLIC ANTIDEPRESSANTS

The tricyclic antidepressants, including the tertiary (amitryptyline, clomipramine, doxepin, imipramine, trimipramine) and secondary (desipramine, nortriptyline, protriptyline) amines, have potentially serious cardiovascular effects. These effects include increased heart rate, orthostatic hypotension, ECG changes, and possible depression of ventricular function. These drugs have electrophysiologic properties similar to the type IA antiarrhythmics. There is the potential for late proarrhythmia in patients with structural heart disease who are taking these agents.[28]

The tricyclic antidepressants have several properties that account for the majority of cardiovascular effects. These drugs inhibit uptake of both norepinephrine and serotonin, resulting in greater toxicity compared to the selective serotonin reuptake inhibitors (SSRIs). A hyperadrenergic state may result in tachycardia. Alpha blockade occurs at higher drug levels and may cause marked hypotension in the setting of overdose. The anticholinergic effects result in tachycardia, dry mouth, and constipation; in overdose they may delay gastrointestinal absorption of the drug. Sodium channel blockade, typical of the type IA antiarrhythmic compounds, results in conduction abnormalities[52] and the potential to suppress ventricular function.[29]

The most frequent side effect of tricyclic antidepressant treatment, orthostatic hypotension, is common in older patients and does not generally improve when doses are reduced to lower levels that will still maintain antidepressant effects. Orthostasis, mediated predominantly by alpha-1 adrenergic receptor blockade, may occur with all of these drugs but is less likely with nortriptyline.[29,30]

The most common ECG changes include nonspecific ST-T changes and prolongation of the QT interval, PR interval, and QRS duration. PR prolongation is due to prolonged infranodal conduction. Patients with preexisting conduction disease, particularly bundle branch block, are at increased risk of toxicity.[31] The type IA antiarrhythmic properties may potentially suppress ventricular ectopy. The results of recent antiarrhythmic studies, however, including those with type I agents, suggest the potential for a proarrhythmic effect for these drugs at therapeutic doses in patients with serious structural heart disease.[28,32] Tricyclic antidepressants are generally contraindicated in the recovery phase following myocardial infarction. Although tricyclic antidepressant therapy may be indicated in the treatment of severely depressed patients, the threshold for use should rise as the severity of heart disease increases or when there is QT prolongation.[28] These issues are discussed in detail in Chap. 80.

Tricyclic antidepressants may impair left ventricular function in patients with severe systolic dysfunction; however, decreases in left ventricular ejection fraction have generally not been noted in patients with moderately impaired function. Tricyclic antidepressant overdose carries a mortality of 2 to 3 percent, which is generally related to cardiac complications. Clinical status at initial presentation and serum drug levels are not predictive of prognosis. QRS prolongation is a sign of toxicity but may be absent in the patient with serious cardiac complications. Rightward deviation of the terminal 40 ms of the frontal plane QRS axis is a more sensitive marker. This finding, manifest by a terminal R wave in lead aV_R, has an 83 percent sensitivity and 63 percent specificity for toxicity.[33]

Aggressive support measures in tricyclic antidepressant overdose should be initiated immediately and include airway maintenance, gastric lavage, and repeated dosing of activated charcoal. Alkalinization with intravenous sodium bicarbonate decreases unbound drug and reverses cardiac and central nervous system conduction defects. Alkalinization is indicated in cardiac arrest, hypotension, arrhythmias, acidosis, and QRS prolongation. Hypotension refractory to volume loading and bicarbonate therapy should be treated with vasopressors, including norepinephrine and phenylephrine, and with vasopressor doses of dopamine. Type I antiarrhythmics (quinidine, procainamide, disopyramide) should not be used. Sodium bicarbonate is the initial therapy for ventricular dysrhythmias.[34]

The duration of monitoring after tricyclic overdose is controversial. Signs of major toxicity generally occur within 6 h of presentation in the emergency department. If clinical or ECG evidence of toxicity is absent and two doses of activated charcoal have been given, patients may not require admission for medical monitoring. Fluoxetine increases tricyclic antidepressant serum levels, and additional monitoring is recommended in patients receiving this medication. Patients with cardiac disease or other serious medical problems may require a longer period of observation.[35]

OTHER ANTIDEPRESSANTS

Selective serotonin reuptake inhibitors (SSRIs) have not been extensively studied in patients with cardiac disease.[36] Case reports of cardiac toxicity are rare, despite the increasing popularity of these agents in the treatment of depression. These agents have rarely been associated with orthostatic hypotension and with bradycardia. Cardiac function does not appear to be depressed by these agents.[37] The SSRIs may affect the cytochrome P450 system and may therefore alter the metabolism of a variety of drugs, including agents used in cardiovascular disease such as antiarrhythmic medications, beta blockers, calcium channel blockers, and warfarin (see Chap. 80).

The monoamine oxidase inhibitors (MAOIs) have little effect on cardiac conduction or myocardial contractility. Orthostatic hypotension is common, particularly in elderly patients. The major concern with these agents is interaction with other drugs or tyramine-containing substances, resulting in hypertensive crisis.[38]

Lithium, used commonly in the treatment of bipolar disorder, is generally well tolerated in patients with cardiac disease. Suppression of sinus node automaticity, resulting in bradycardias, is the most common complication.[39] In patients free of known heart disease, clinically significant sinus node dysfunction occurs in fewer than 1 percent and is reversible with discontinuation of lithium therapy. Preexisting sinus node disease or concomitant therapy with drugs altering sinus node function, however, may result in sinus bradycardia. Lithium-induced hypothyroidism may be a contributing factor.[40] Pacemaker therapy may be required to allow continuation of lithium therapy.

Lithium therapy has been associated with ECG changes simulating hypokalemia. T-wave inversion, prominent U waves, and QT prolongation may occur. PR prolongation, bundle branch block, and complete heart block are rare.[39] Overdose with lithium may result in severe bradycardias requiring temporary pacemaker therapy. A low anion gap may suggest the presence of lithium toxicity.[41]

ANTIPSYCHOTIC AGENTS

The phenothiazine antipsychotic agents have potential cardiac toxicity similar to that of the tricyclic antidepressants. These drugs may cause sinus tachycardia, PR and QT prolongation, and disturbances of intraventricular conduction. Chlorpromazine and thioridazine[42] are the most commonly implicated phenothiazines as causes of torsades de pointes. The butyrophenone haloperidol is also associated with torsades de pointes at high doses given intravenously.[43]

Noncardiac Drugs and Toxic Antidepressants Causing Torsades de Pointes

As discussed above, the tricyclic phenothiazine and other psychotropic agents may prolong the QT interval and induce torsades de pointes. A variety of antiarrhythmic agents, particularly the type I agents, are most strongly associated with this potentially fatal arrhythmia. Other toxic causes of torsades de pointes[44] are listed in Table 71-2.

TABLE 71-2 Noncardiac Drugs and Toxins Known to Cause Torsades de Pointes

Psychotropic agents	Antihistamines
Tricyclic antidepressants	Terfenadine
Tetracyclic antidepressants	Astemizole
Phenothiazines	Other
Haloperidol	Cisapride
Chloral hydrate	Pentamidine
Antibiotics	Probucol
Erythromycin	Arsenic
Trimethoprim-sulfamethoxazole	Organophosphates
	Liquid protein diets

The antibiotics erythromycin and trimethoprim-sulfamethoxazole[45,46] have only rarely been associated with torsades de pointes, the exception being the effect of erythromycin on the metabolism of terfenadine, astemizole, and cisapride. Liquid protein diets and starvation[47] may cause marked electrolyte and chemical disturbances, triggering QT prolongation. Probucol[48] may prolong the QT interval, resulting in torsades de pointes.

The QT prolongation and torsades de pointes reported with the antihistamines terfenadine and astemizole and with cisapride have been associated with high drug levels from excessive dosing or altered metabolism.[49,50] Prolongation of the QT interval induced by terfenadine, astemizole, and cisapride is due to the electrophysiologic activity of blocking HERG, the ion channel that is responsible for the rapid component of the delayed rectifier current for potassium(I_{kr}).[50] These drugs are metabolized by the cytochrome P450 3A isoenzyme.[51] A variety of agents inhibit this isoenzyme, including antifungals (ketoconazole, fluconazole, itraconazole), erythromycin or clarithromycin (not azithromycin), SSRIs (fluvoxamine, nefazodone, fluoxetine, sertaline), quinine, and grapefruit juice. Serious cardiac arrhythmias have been reported in patients taking terfenadine, astemizole, or cisapride with drugs that inhibit the cytochrome P450 3A isoenzyme. Patients with a history of prolonged QT interval or those with serious underlying cardiac disease are at higher risk for this problem. Some women appear to have slow metabolism of these drugs; thus female gender is a risk factor for drug-induced arrhythmias.[50]

Methylxanthines and Beta-Adrenergic Agonists

The methylxanthines caffeine and theophylline have pharmacologic actions of central nervous system stimulation, bronchial smooth muscle relaxation, and cardiac muscle stimulation and have diuretic effects on the kidneys. At therapeutic doses or those consumed in xanthine-containing beverages, these agents competitively inhibit adenosine receptors. At higher doses, they exhibit phosphodiesterase inhibition.[52] The effect of caffeine consumption on the cardiovascular system is variable and depends on chronicity of use, dose exposure, and individual responsiveness. Although elevations of catecholamines may occur with acute administration, this effect resolves with chronic usage. At higher concentrations, caffeine may cause tachycardia and dysrhythmias. Despite the concern that caffeine may be detrimental in patients predisposed to cardiac rhythm disturbances, it appears that moderate amounts of caffeine consumption may be well tolerated in patients with ventricular arrhythmias. The role of coffee, with or without caffeine, as a risk factor for coronary artery disease has been debated. While heavy coffee drinking (>4 cups a day) has been suggested as a potential risk factor for cardiovascular mortality, the data are inconclusive.[53,54]

Theophylline has the potential to cause a slight increase in heart rate with minimal effects on blood pressure. Patients with obstructive lung disease commonly have atrial and ventricular arrhythmias, which can be exacerbated by theophylline therapy. Theophylline toxicity is associated with sinus tachycardia, atrial and ventricular arrhythmias, and hypotension.[55] Hypokalemia, hypercalcemia, hyperglycemia, hypophosphatemia, and metabolic acidosis may occur. Esmolol may be useful in the management of refractory arrhythmias. Dialysis may be helpful in patients with refractory arrhythmias or hypotension.[56,57]

The beta-adrenergic agonists terbutaline and albuterol are commonly used to treat asthma and premature labor. Although adverse reactions are uncommon with aerosol therapy, these agents may cause tachycardia and atrial and ventricular arrhythmias and, rarely, may worsen angina pectoris.[58] Use of oral $beta_2$ agonists has been associated with the development of heart failure.[59] Intravenous therapy may cause hypokalemia and acidosis. Controversy exists over the safety of long-term aerosol therapy with beta-adrenergic agonists in asthma. These concerns, however, relate predominantly to airway hyperresponsiveness and not to direct cardiac toxicity.[60]

Antimigraine Drugs

Ergotamine The ergot alkaloids are commonly used in the treatment of migraine headaches. Ergotamine causes constriction of smooth muscle, and its effect on vascular smooth muscle may result in hypertension and increased peripheral vascular resistance.[61] Ergonovine maleate may be used in the catheterization laboratory to diagnose coronary artery spasm. Chronic use of ergotamine may result in variant angina or myocardial infarction.[61,62] Severe circulatory disturbances of the upper and lower extremities and abdominal arteries have been described.[62] Ergotamine and methysergide have similar chemical structures. Valvular heart disease has been reported with both agents. Either may cause pericardial, pleural, or peritoneal fibrosis or multivalvular heart disease. The occurrence of these side effects is less frequent with ergotamine.[63,64]

Methysergide Methysergide, used in treating vascular headaches, can cause retroperitoneal, pulmonary, and cardiac fibrosis. Cardiac involvement most commonly affects the valves but may affect the endocardium, myocardium, and rarely the aorta. Regurgitant valvular lesions are most common, affecting the mitral and aortic valves more commonly than the tricuspid and pulmonary valves.[65] Patients receiving methysergide therapy should be monitored for the development of murmurs. Therapy should be discontinued if a new murmur is detected. Regression of valvular lesions may occur, although valve replacement is occasionally required. Patients with known valvular disease should not be given methysergide.

Sumatriptan Sumatriptan, a selective serotonin type I agonist, may cause coronary artery vasospasm. Sumatriptan should not be taken within 24 h of treatment with ergotamine-like medications because of the risk of prolonged vasoconstriction.[66]

The antimigraine drugs ergotamine, methysergide, and sumatriptan are generally contraindicated in patients with obstructive coronary artery disease.[67]

Weight-Loss Medications

Dexfenfluramine and the combination of fenfluramine and phentermine may cause valvular heart disease (Chaps. 56, 57, and 59).[68–72] These agents had been prescribed for weight loss in obese patients, but dexfenfluramine and fenfluramine were withdrawn from the market in 1997 when up to 30 percent of users were reported to develop asymptomatic valve regurgitation.[69] Later reports suggested a lower incidence of problems, including reports of valvular regurgitation in approximately

7 percent of dexfenfluramine-treated patients versus 2 to 5 percent of controls.[70] The true incidence of valvular problems is uncertain and differences in reported cases may be secondary to differences in length of therapy, time from therapy to cardiac evaluation, and methods used to determine abnormalities. Mild aortic regurgitation is the most common finding. Abnormalities often improve with cessation of therapy.[71,72]

Histamine H_2-Receptor Antagonists

The histamine H_2-receptor antagonists have rarely been associated with cardiac effects. Episodes of severe bradycardia have been reported as well as hypotension, asystole, and ventricular arrhythmias. These complications have generally occurred with large doses given intravenously.[73] Electrophysiologic studies have not demonstrated any direct effect on sinus node function.[74]

Chloroquine

The antimalarial agent chloroquine is commonly used to treat collagen vascular and dermatologic disorders. Irreversible retinal damage is the primary concern with long-term or high-dose therapy. Skeletal myopathy and less commonly cardiomyopathy may occur. With cardiac involvement, features of restrictive cardiomyopathy are most common. Myocardial biopsy with analysis by electron microscopy showing curvilinear and myeloid bodies is diagnostic. These findings may be seen on skeletal muscle biopsy. The ECG may demonstrate T-wave changes and conduction abnormalities. Acute chloroquine poisoning results in hypotension, tachycardia, and prolongation of the QRS and is often fatal.[75,76]

Oral Contraceptive Agents

Epidemiologic studies prior to the 1980s demonstrated that women using oral contraceptives had an increased risk of cardiovascular disease, including venous thromboembolism, myocardial infarction, hypertension, and stroke.[128] Oral contraceptive formulations used in the 1960s and 1970s consisted of relatively high-dose estrogen. Although rare, the risk of myocardial infarction was increased approximately fourfold. Women smokers, particularly those older than age 35, had a dramatically increased risk of infarction. Coronary angiography done postinfarction not uncommonly demonstrated a discrete lesion in a single vessel or no obstructive lesions, suggesting acute thrombosis as a possible mechanism. The risk of venous thromboembolism was 4 to 10 times that of nonusers during this era.[77,80]

Recent formulations of oral contraceptives consist of less than 50 μg of ethinyl estradiol in combination with a low-dose progestin. Recent studies suggest that these second- and third-generation combined oral contraceptives are much safer in terms of cardiovascular complications.[77] The risks of venous thromboembolism and myocardial infarction are significantly reduced compared with the first-generation agents. Hypertension is rare, and the risk of stroke in otherwise healthy women is only minimally increased.[78]

Third-generation oral contraceptives that contain desogestrol or gestodene are reportedly associated with a 1.5 to 2.5 increased risk of venous thromboembolism compared with the second-generation agents. The significance of this finding has generated controversy, but generally, the cardiovascular risk profile of these agents is considered favorable. However, smokers greater than 35 years of age should use a nonestrogen contraceptive.[77-80]

Anabolic Steroids

Illicit use of androgens has been identified as a problem in competitive athletes and body builders. It is estimated that 300,000 persons in the United States have had recent steroid use and over 1 million have had prior use.[81-83] Anabolic steroids, including testosterone, stanozolol, and nandrolone, are frequently used in combination and at high doses for intermittent periods of several weeks to months. Doses commonly exceed 100 times the doses used for medical purposes.[81] Animal data indicate that these agents can cause abnormal lipids, left ventricular hypertrophy, increased blood volume, and hypertension. Data on human toxicity are limited but suggest similar toxicity.[84] Stanozolol and nandrolone reduce total high-density lipoprotein levels by over 50 percent and increase low-density lipoprotein levels by over 30 percent.[85] Isolated reports of young men (<age 35) developing severe coronary atherosclerosis, myocardial infarctions, or stroke exist in the literature.[81,86] Because of the secrecy surrounding the use of these agents, the full clinical significance of abuse is not known.

Cocaine

Cocaine is a common drug of abuse associated with potentially lethal cardiac toxicity. It is estimated that over 30 million Americans have used cocaine at least once and that 5 million use it regularly.[87] Cocaine may be swallowed, inhaled nasally, smoked, or injected intravenously. Cardiovascular toxicity is broad, ranging from sudden death to chronic cardiomyopathy.[88] A summary of the cardiovascular syndrome associated with illicit cocaine use is shown in Table 71-3. Use of cocaine with other drugs

TABLE 71-3 Cardiovascular Complications of Cocaine

Sudden death
Acute myocardial infarction
Chest pain without myocardial infarction
Accelerated coronary atherosclerosis
Intimal hyperplasia of coronary vessels
Electrocardiographic abnormalities
Sinus tachycardia
Premature ventricular complexes
Ventricular tachycardia
Torsades de pointes
Ventricular fibrillation
Prolongation of QT interval
Early repolarization (ST-segment changes)
Acute reversible myocarditis
Dilated cardiomyopathy
Acute severe hypertension
Acute aortic dissection, rupture
Pneumopericardium
Stroke
Subarachnoid hemorrhage
Endocarditis (intravenous use)

such as ethanol[89] or tobacco[90] may have combined detrimental effects. Cardiovascular susceptibility in an individual is difficult to predict due to the lack of dose-response relationship and the high degree of variability in the individual response to cocaine.[91]

Cocaine has a generalized sympathomimetic effect and has local anesthetic properties.[88] It blocks the reuptake of norepinephrine and dopamine on preganglionic sympathetic nerve terminals. This produces sympathetic stimulation both centrally and peripherally. These catecholamine effects acutely result in tachycardia, hypertension, increased myocardial contractility, and vascular constriction. The local anesthetic effect, occurring through blockade of the fast sodium channel, results in slowed conduction in myocardial tissues. This may result in ECG abnormalities, including prolongation of the PR, QRS, and QT intervals, similar to those seen with toxicity from type I antiarrhythmic agents. These effects increase the vulnerability to reentrant ventricular arrhythmias.[87,88,92]

Use of cocaine may result in increased thrombogenicity.[88,90] Platelet aggregation is enhanced and endothelial function is altered,[94] resulting in the potential for development of coronary thrombosis in the absence of coronary atherosclerosis. Chronic use of cocaine is associated with premature coronary atherosclerosis.[88,93] Cocaine indirectly causes constriction of both diseased and nondiseased coronary artery segments, but its effect is more marked in diseased vessels. Ethanol use and tobacco smoking may worsen the potential for vasospasm.[89,90] In up to one-third of reported cases, patients with cocaine-induced myocardial infarctions have normal coronary arteries.[88] The combined cardiac effects—including early coronary atherosclerosis, coronary vasospasm, increased thrombogenicity, increased myocardial oxygen demands, and proarrhythmic effects—make this drug a lethal threat to users of all ages.

Cocaine may produce direct or indirect myocardial toxicity. Animal studies suggest a direct negative inotropic effect on the heart, possibly related to its local anesthetic properties. Chronic dosing has demonstrated myocardial contraction bands, myofibrillar disorganization, interstitial edema, and mitochondrial swelling. Mononuclear infiltrates have been noted. Myocardial changes may mimic those seen with catecholamine excess, as in pheochromocytoma. Clinical case reports have described transient toxic cardiomyopathy, acute myocarditis, and permanently dilated cardiomyopathy.[88]

Chest pain is the most common reason for cocaine users to seek medical attention. Over 64,000 patients are evaluated annually for cocaine-related chest pain, of whom over half are admitted to the hospital.[95] The evaluation of cocaine-related chest pain is difficult. Prospective studies demonstrate that approximately 6 percent of patients presenting to an emergency department with cocaine-related chest pain have myocardial infarction. These patients are often young men without other risk factors for coronary artery disease except for tobacco smoking. The duration and quality of discomfort does not readily distinguish those eventually noted to have enzyme documentation of infarction. Many young patients have early repolarization patterns with ST elevation in leads V_1 to V_3, a normal variant that may be confused with acute infarction. Infarction has been noted in patients with normal or nonspecific ECGs. Because of the difficulty in excluding myocardial infarctions, patients are often monitored for a period of at least 12 h until enzymes have excluded infarction (Chaps. 40 and 42).[87]

Treatment strategies for cocaine-induced myocardial ischemia have been developed based on the known cardiac and nervous system toxicity of the drug.[87,92] Randomized prospective trials of therapy do not exist. Patients presenting with anxiety, tachycardia, or hypertension may respond well to benzodiazepines. Nitroglycerin may reverse coronary vasoconstriction induced by cocaine. Aspirin may prevent thrombus formation. Patients not responding to these measures may benefit from the alpha-adrenergic antagonist phentolamine or from calcium channel blocker therapy with verapamil.[87] Beta-adrenergic antagonists have been avoided because of the potential of enhanced coronary vasoconstriction and for unopposed alpha-mediated hypertensive crisis. Combined alpha and beta blockade with labetalol has been utilized to treat tachyarrhythmias but is not an accepted therapy for myocardial ischemia.[87] However, the bias against beta blockade is undergoing clinical reevaluation with recognition that beta blockers may block the hyperadrenergic effects that result in thrombosis and vasospasm.[96]

In documented myocardial infarction, thrombolytic therapy is highly effective; however, over 40 percent of patients without infarction will meet accepted ECG criteria for use of lytic therapy.[97] The early repolarization pattern common in young men makes diagnosis difficult, particularly when a prior ECG is not available. Thrombolytic therapy carries increased risk of hemorrhagic stroke in patients with recently uncontrolled hypertension. Therefore emergent coronary angiography may be necessary to document coronary occlusion as well as direct strategies such as primary angioplasty or thrombolysis[147] (see Chap. 42).

Management of supraventricular or ventricular tachyarrhythmias may be facilitated by administration of benzodiazepines. Rhythm disturbances may be exacerbated by acidosis or electrolyte disorders. Intravenous sodium bicarbonate and magnesium may be beneficial. Lidocaine should be used cautiously because of concerns of lowered seizure threshold and potential proarrhythmic effects following recent cocaine use.[92]

Patients with cocaine-associated chest pain not related to myocardial infarction have a favorable 1-year prognosis, particularly if cocaine use is discontinued. Urgent diagnostic cardiac evaluation is not generally recommended. Unfortunately, recurrent cocaine use after cocaine-associated chest pain occurs in over 60 percent of cases.[87]

Methamphetamines

The biologic effects of methamphetamines are similar to those of cocaine, but vasoconstriction is less. Cardiovascular toxicity is common and includes tachycardia, hypertension, and arrhythmias. Chest pain and myocardial infarction are less common than with cocaine.[98] Chronic use may result in a catecholamine-mediated dilated cardiomyopathy.

ELECTRICAL INJURY

Environmental Accidents

Accidental contact with electricity may occur in the home, where young children are particularly vulnerable.[100] Job-related electrical injuries are most common in construction and electrical workers but may also occur on any job in which electrical equipment is used, including the health care setting. Approximately 1200 deaths related to domestic electrical injury occur each year in the United States. There are two to three times as many serious injuries, including burns and neurologic complications.[101] Lightning kills at least 100 people per year in the United States, representing a 30 percent mortality rate in reported cases. Lightning injuries generally occur between May and September in the late afternoon hours, and affect predominantly young people involved in outdoor recreational activities.[102] Death following electrical shock is usually secondary to immediate cardiac rhythm disturbances, although later cardiac complications secondary to internal injury may occur.

PATHOPHYSIOLOGY

The degree of total body injury from electricity is determined by the amount of current delivered, tissue resistance, and duration of contact. Specific organs or tissues injured are in part determined by the path of the current. Electrical injuries are classified as high-voltage (>1000 V) or low-voltage (<1000 V). High-voltage electrical wires and household current (120 or 220 V) are alternating currents (AC) that may result in prolonged exposure due to tetatanic muscle contractions and inability of the victim to "let go." The frequencies of domestically generated AC (50 to 60 cycles per second) result in an increased risk for ventricular fibrillation even at household voltages.[101] Sources of domestic direct current (DC) are usually low-voltage (3 to 24 V), including batteries, appliance transformers, and portable emergency generators and are less likely to cause injury. Lightning is extremely high voltage direct current of brief duration.

Heat injury tissue necrosis is more severe with high-voltage AC. These burns are often internal and may mimic crush injuries. Tissue resistance to current flow is least in nervous and vascular tissues; therefore the heart and neurovascular bundles may serve as conduits for electrical current through the thorax. Arm-to-arm pathway of current is associated with greater risk for cardiac injury, followed by arm-to-leg pathways determined by entry and exit sites. A stride potential, leg to leg, is infrequently associated with cardiac effects.

CARDIOVASCULAR EFFECTS

Cardiac damage in electrical injury may occur as a result of contusion injury or myocardial necrosis or may be in part related to massive release of catecholamines. Typical symptoms or signs of myocardial damage may be absent. Lightning injuries result from brief, high-voltage direct current. Immediate death may be secondary to asystole or ventricular fibrillation or may result from apnea secondary to injury of the central respiratory centers. Lightning strikes may occur by a direct hit, side splash, or ground strike. Direct hits cause mechanical trauma to organs secondary to dissipated energy. Strikes to the chest can result in severe, often reversible global myocardial dysfunction or localized myocardial contusion. ECG abnormalities, including QT_c prolongation and ST-T abnormalities, may be the result of cardiac or neurologic injury. ST elevation has been noted with direct strikes. Conduction abnormalities, including right bundle branch block and complete heart block, have been noted. Pericardial effusions may develop following direct strikes. Elevated levels of CK-MB are generally noted.[102] Splash strikes in which a tree or other object is hit prior to the victim's being hit are associated with CK-MB release in less than two-thirds of patients. Severe myocardial injury is unlikely unless there is a short distance between the directly hit object and the victim. Ground strikes generally do not cause a significant cardiac injury but may be associated with nonspecific ST-T abnormalities.

Domestic alternating current accidents may cause myocardial necrosis and conduction abnormalities. An injury pattern mimicking infarction may be seen on the ECG but is generally related to direct myocardial injury and not from coronary thrombosis.[165] Household voltages (120 to 220 V) may cause sudden death, particularly when they involve arm-to-arm pathways or low skin resistance in a wet victim. Serious myocardial damage is rare.[100]

Treatment for cardiac arrest should be initiated immediately after the patient is disconnected from the current source. Resuscitation efforts should be continued for a prolonged period. In lightning strikes involving multiple victims, attention should be directed first to those who are "apparently dead." This is because there is a higher resuscitation rate for these individuals than for those with medical cardiac arrest. Of note, lightning victims with vital signs generally survive without immediate medical attention.[103]

Patients surviving high-voltage injuries generally require admission, usually for attention to neurologic complications and internal or external burn injuries and less commonly for cardiac monitoring. An initially normal ECG carries a favorable cardiac prognosis, leading some authors to question the need for 24-h ECG monitoring. Patients with arm-to-arm or arm-to-leg passage of current may be at risk for postadmission rhythm disturbances; a higher index of suspicion is required in such patients. Adults and children presenting to the emergency department following low-voltage shocks of less than 240 V have a low incidence of myocardial injury and most do not require further monitoring.[100]

Electroconvulsive Therapy

Electroconvulsive therapy (ECT) is accepted for the treatment of a variety of psychiatric illnesses including depression resistant to pharmacologic therapy, severe suicidal ideation with vegetative signs, acute mania, and depression with intolerance to medication side effects secondary to cardiac problems[104] (see also Chap. 80). ECT involves a brief unilateral or bilateral electrical stimulus to the brain while the patient is under short-acting anesthesia with a hypnotic drug and a muscle depolarizing agent.[105] The shock produces brief, intense stimulation of the central nervous system. Cardiovascular complications may result from this stimulation or from the drugs used to modify the response.[106,107]

Initially, the ECT stimulus activates the vagus nerve and may produce bradycardia, hypotension, and rarely asystole. Sympathetic discharge occurs, which is amplified by a 15-fold rise in epinephrine and 3-fold rise in norepinephrine levels, resulting in tachycardia and hypertension. Transient atrial and ventricular tachyarrhythmias may occur in approximately 10 percent of patients with known or suspected cardiovascular disease. Transient ECG alterations—including ST-T-wave changes, QRS changes, QT prolongation, and peaked T waves—may occur.[104–108]

The mortality rate of ECT is less than 3 in 10,000, and the complication rate is approximately 0.3 percent. Patients with severe heart disease may successfully undergo ECT with acceptable risk. Prior to ECT, electrolyte abnormalities should be

TABLE 71-4 Plants with Cardiac Glycoside Effects

Foxglove (*Digitalis purpurea, D. Lanata*)
Oleander (*Nerium oleander*)
Lily-of-the-valley (*Convallaria majolis*)
Christmas rose (*Helleborus niger*)
Wallflower (*Cheirina cheiri*)
Milkweed (*Asclepias* sp.)

corrected and systemic hypertension should be controlled. Patients with pulmonary disease require special evaluation, because hypoxia and respiratory acidosis may precipitate cardiovascular events.[104]

Following ECT, hypertension and tachycardia may be controlled with adrenergic blockade with intravenous labetalol[109] or esmolol.[107] Other antihypertensive agents such as clonidine or calcium channel blockers may be utilized. Sustained ventricular arrhythmias are treated with lidocaine, but pretreatment with lidocaine is not indicated.[104] Patients with cardiac pacemakers can safely undergo ECT.[110] Currently used pacemakers are not likely to be affected by ECT current. Although these newer devices have not been systematically studied, the 50 to 100 W delivered to the scalp during ECT are probably inadequate to reprogram current pacemakers.

Lithotripsy

Extracorporeal shock wave lithotripsy used to treat renal stones and gallstones has the potential to cause cardiac arrhythmias. Rhythm disturbances may be related to electrical stimulus from the shock wave or from enhanced vagal tone associated with the procedure. Electrocardiographic monitoring is recommended for patients with cardiac disease. Gating of the shock waves to the QRS cycle may be necessary in high-risk patients, although ungated lithotripsy with newer devices is reportedly safe in most patients.[111,112]

POISONS

Plants

A variety of plants contain active cardiac glycosides. Ingestion of these plants may result in a clinical presentation similar to that of digoxin toxicity, including gastrointestinal and visual disturbances as well as dysrhythmias. Plants with cardiac glycoside–like effects[113] are listed (Table 71-4).

Herbal Therapies

The use of herbal treatments and nonprescription remedies is increasing among patients. In one study, 38 percent of congestive heart failure patients questioned were using herbal products.[114] Herbal medicines may contain varying doses and contaminants and are not subject to regulations governing safety and efficacy. Serious adverse effects and drug interactions may therefore occur. The cardiac effects of some herbal remedies are listed in Table 71-5.[115–117]

Snakes and Scorpions

Snake bites cause fewer than 15 deaths per year in the United States but over 40,000 deaths per year worldwide. The majority of lethal snake bites occur in Asia, South America, and Africa. Snake venoms contain a variety of enzymes and toxins that may affect the nervous system, blood vessels, coagulation systems, or heart. The majority of deaths are from the elapids (cobra, mamba, coral snake, taipan), the bites of which cause severe neuromuscular toxicity. Cardiotoxins are present in variable amounts in snake venom. Cobra venoms may cause augmentation of myocardial contraction at low concentration and asystole at high concentration. Rattlesnake venom may affect myocardial sodium channels and depress myocardial contractility. These venoms may cause pulmonary hypertension.[118]

TABLE 71-5 Cardiac Effects of Common Herbal Therapies

Aconite (in Chinese herbal medicines)	Arrhythmias via QT prolongation
Adonis vernalis (pheasant's eye)	Sudden death
Caulophyllum thalictroides (blue cohosh)	Neonatal heart failure, contains cardiac glycosides
Cimicifuga (black cohosh)	Bradycardia
Corydalis racemosa (dl-tetrahydropalmatine)	Hypotension
Corynanthe johimbe (yohimbe)	Hypo- or hypertension, tachycardia
Danshen	Increased bleeding risk with warfarin
Delphinium (larkspur)	Myocardial depression, arrhythmias
Digitalis purpurea (foxglove)	Arrhythmias, heart block
Ephedra (ma huang)	Hypertension, arrhythmias, palpitations, death
Feverfew	Decreased platelet activity
Garlic	Increased bleeding risk with anticoagulants
Ginger	Increased bleeding risk with anticoagulants
Ginkgo	Decreased platelet activity
Hawthorne	Hypotension at high doses
Lingusticum wallichii	Inhibits platelet aggregation, hypotension
Licorice	Hypokalemia, arrhythmias, hypertension
Stephania tetrandra	Interferes with calcium channel blockers, myocardial depressant, hypotension
Tripterygium wilfordii (hook F)	Hypotension, circulatory collapse
Veratrum (hellebore)	Bradycardia, hypotension

SOURCE: From Ernst,[115] Vann,[116] and Yu et al.[117]

Scorpion stings are a common medical problem in areas including India, Southeast Asia, the southwestern United States, Mexico, and Israel. Venoms from different families have different toxicities. The *Buthidae* venoms, primarily neurotoxic, result in spontaneous sympathetic and parasympathetic depolarization. Massive catecholamine release may cause cardiac toxicity, including tachycardia, hypertension, arrhythmias, and myocardial impairment.[119,120]

Arthropods

Direct cardiac effects related to bee, hornet, and wasp stings are difficult to establish. Cardiac complications, including arrhythmias, are generally related to anaphylaxis or epinephrine administration. Animal studies of bee venom toxicity suggest direct cardiac effects.[121,122]

Marine Toxins

Exposure to marine toxins may have serious cardiovascular effects. The venom of scorpion fish can cause sympathetic and parasympathetic discharges. Rhythm disturbances and heart failure may result. Stingray venom contains phosphodiesterases and has rarely been associated with cardiac rhythm disturbances. Ingestion of sea cucumber, which contains holothurin, may result in cardiac glycoside toxicity. Ingestion of pufferfish, which contain tetrodotoxin, may result in vascular collapse and severe bradycardia.[118,123]

Halogenated Hydrocarbons

Halogenated hydrocarbons are used in fire extinguishers, solvents, and refrigerants and in the manufacture of pesticides and plastics. Heavy acute exposure to these compounds may result in cardiac arrhythmias and sudden death.[124] Direct cardiac effects include depression of myocardial contractility and sensitization to the arrhythmogenic effects of catecholamines. Indirect cardiotoxicity may result from hypoxia or central nervous system toxicity.[125]

Organophosphates

Organophosphates, used commercially in pesticides, are powerful inhibitors of acetylcholinesterase, and this inhibition can result in parasympathetic overstimulation. Suicide attempts account for the majority of fatalities associated with ingestion of large doses of organophosphates. Signs and symptoms of ingestion include respiratory depression, bronchospasm and secretion, and pulmonary edema. Deaths are generally related to respiratory failure. Cardiac toxicity is generally associated with QT prolongation. Torsades de pointes, atrioventricular conduction disturbances, and ST-T abnormalities have been noted. Cardiac arrhythmias have been noted up to 15 days after exposure. Direct myocardial toxicity has been postulated, in addition to cholinergic hyperactivity.[126] Treatment includes atropine administration at doses sufficient to dry mucous membranes and to increase heart rate to 100 beats per minute. Obidoxime therapy has also been studied in severe overdoses.[127]

Carbon Monoxide

Toxicity from carbon monoxide is related to tissue hypoxia. Carbon monoxide has a much higher affinity for hemoglobin than does oxygen, preventing adequate oxygen exchange. Carbon monoxide exposure worsens angina pectoris and increases the risk of myocardial infarction. Carbon monoxide poisoning results in ECG abnormalities, including sinus tachycardia, atrial fibrillation, atrioventricular block, and ST-T abnormalities. Cardiac enzyme elevation may occur. Severe exposure can result in myocardial necrosis and cardiomyopathy.[128] Transient evidence of cardiac toxicity, however, is not necessarily associated with long-term sequelae.[129]

RADIATION

Mediastinal radiation—commonly used to treat Hodgkin's disease, lung cancer, breast cancer, and seminoma—may result in acute or late cardiac sequelae. Prior to the 1960s, the heart was thought to be resistant to the effects of clinical radiation. It is now recognized that a variety of cardiac problems may result from radiation, including acute or chronic pericardial disease, coronary atherosclerosis, myocardial dysfunction, conduction defects, and, occasionally, valvular dysfunction (Table 71-6).[130,131]

The incidence of radiation-induced heart disease is influenced by several factors, including total radiation dose, fraction size, volume of heart irradiated, concomitant anthracycline use, and presence of mediastinal tumor.[130] Improved radiation techniques have diminished the occurrence of acute or chronic cardiac toxicity.[132] Cardiac injury has generally been associated with doses above 40 Gy.[130] Increased toxicity is associated with radiation for Hodgkin's disease, where larger volumes of the heart are irradiated, compared to the small cardiac exposure given as adjuvant treatment for breast carcinoma. Large doses per fraction and anterior-weighted fields result in greater toxicity.[133]

Pericardial disease is the most common manifestation of radiation toxicity to the heart. With the current techniques of subcarinal shielding, equal weighting of anterior and posterior ports, and limiting the dose to less than 30 Gy, the incidence of clinical pericarditis is approximately 2.5 percent.[132] Anatomic changes of the pericardium occur in the majority of patients but are clinically silent. Clinically apparent pericarditis is most frequent 4 to 6 months after therapy. Acute pericarditis, asymptomatic pericardial effusion, or pericardial tamponade may occur. Other etiologies of pericarditis should be considered,

TABLE 71-6 Radiation-induced Cardiac Disease

- Pericardial
  - Acute pericarditis
  - Chronic pericarditis
  - Pericardial constriction
- Coronary atherosclerosis
- Restrictive cardiomyopathy
- Dilated cardiomyopathy (concomitant anthracyclines)
- Conduction disease
- Valvular abnormalities

particularly malignant involvement of the pericardium. Pericarditis occurring during treatment of a mediastinal mass contiguous to the heart is generally secondary to tumor effects and does not correlate with late pericardial complications.[134,135]

Radiation may cause an exudative pericarditis. Cellular infiltrate is uncommon. Pericardial fibrosis may follow secondary to fibroblast proliferation and collagen deposition. The majority of patients with pericardial effusion recover spontaneously.[130] Constrictive pericarditis may occur months to years after pericardial effusion or may develop in patients without previously recognized pericardial disease.

The majority of patients with pericardial disease have a relatively benign course. Treatment is based on symptoms, including pericardiocentesis for tamponade and antipyretics for fever. Animal data suggest possible benefit from steroids.[130]

The surgical management of postirradiation constrictive pericarditis is difficult.[134] Extensive mediastinal and pericardial fibrosis make pericardiectomy technically challenging. Surgical morbidity and mortality are significant. Radiation-induced constriction is often associated with coronary atherosclerosis, myocardial dysfunction, or conduction and valvular abnormalities. Comorbid cardiac or general medical conditions should be considered when patients are selected for pericardiectomy.

Clinically important myocardial dysfunction related to radiation generally occurs in combination with pericardial disease. Asymptomatic patients may have varying degrees of myocardial fibrosis. The anterior right ventricle is most susceptible. Areas of fibrosis may be patchy or diffuse. Noninvasive techniques such as echocardiography may show mild impairment of systolic function; however, this is usually not clinically significant.[132] Diastolic abnormalities may occur due to fibrosis.

Restrictive cardiomyopathy has been reported but is rare.[130] Premature coronary artery disease may result from radiation therapy, particularly in patients who were irradiated in an era when cardioprotective techniques were not used. Several series have reported a significantly increased risk of coronary artery disease years following therapeutic radiation involving cardiac exposure.[135] The Stockholm Trial demonstrated increased mortality secondary to coronary artery disease in women receiving high-dose radiation to the heart as adjuvant therapy for carcinoma of the left breast.[135] A review of 635 patients at Stanford treated for Hodgkin's disease before age 21 between the years 1961 and 1991 showed a significantly increased risk for myocardial infarction.[136,137] It is not clear, however, whether present techniques of mediastinal radiation will result in a clinically significant increase in coronary events. Percutaneous angioplasty and coronary bypass surgery have been successful in selected patients. The commonly associated mediastinal and pericardial fibrosis, however, make surgical revascularization more difficult.[130]

Clinically significant valvular heart disease secondary to radiation is rare but, when present, usually involves the aortic or mitral valves.[130,131] Fibrous thickening of the cardiac valves has been noted at autopsy. This thickening often causes asymptomatic aortic or mitral regurgitation.[138] Coexisting pericardial disease is the rule. Symptoms related to valvular dysfunction have been noted to occur 15 to 40 years after radiation treatment. Surgical reports are rare and most commonly are for replacement of the aortic valve due to aortic stenosis.[131]

Radiation may result in fibrosis of the nodal and infranodal pathways. Complete atrioventricular block, right bundle branch block, and, less commonly, left bundle branch block may occur. Progression to complete heart block is rare.

References

1. Frishman WH, Sung HM, Yee HCM, et al. Cardiovascular toxicity with cancer chemotherapy. *Curr Probl Cardiol* 1996; 21: 225–288.
2. Shan K, Lincoff AM, Young JB. Anthracycline-induced cardiomyopathy. *Ann Intern Med* 1996; 125:47–58.
3. Von Hoff DD, Layard MW, Basa P, et al. Risk factors for doxorubicin-induced congestive heart failure. *Ann Intern Med* 1979; 91:710–717.
4. Bristow MR, Mason JW, Billingham ME, Daniels JR. Doxorubicin cardiomyopathy: Evaluation of phonocardiography, endomyocardial biopsy, and cardiac catheterization. *Ann Intern Med* 1978; 88:168–175.
5. Lipschultz SE, Lipsitz SR, Mone SM, et al. Female sex and higher drug dose as risk factors for late cardiotoxic effects of doxorubicin therapy for childhood cancer. *N Engl J Med* 1995; 332:1738–1743.
6. Singal PK, Iliskovic N, Li T, Kumar D. Adriamycin cardiomyopathy: Pathophysiology and prevention. *FASEB J* 1997; 11:931–936.
7. Moreg JS, Oglon DJ. Outcomes of clinical congestive heart failure induced by anthracycline chemotherapy. *Cancer* 1992; 70:2637–2641.
8. Steinherz J, Graham T, Hurwitz R, et al. Guidelines for cardiac monitoring of children during and after anthracycline therapy: Report of the Cardiology Committee of the Children's Cancer Study Group. *Pediatrics* 1992; 89:942–949.
9. Weegner KM, Bledsoe M, Chauvenet A, Wofford M. Exercise echocardiography in the detection of anthracycline cardiotoxicity. *Cancer* 1991; 68:435–438.
10. Schwartz RG, McKenzie WB, Alexander J, et al. Congestive heart failure and left ventricular dysfunction complicating doxorubicin therapy: Seven-year experience using radionuclide angiocardiography. *Am J Med* 1987; 82:1109–1118.
11. McKillop JH, Bristow MR, Goris ML, et al. Sensitivity and specificity of radionuclide ejection fraction in doxorubicin cardiotoxicity. *Am Heart J* 1983; 106:1048–1056.
12. Isner JM, Ferrans VJ, Cohen SR, et al. Clinical and morphologic cardiac findings after anthracycline chemotherapy: Analysis of 64 patients studied at necropsy. *Am J Cardiol* 1983; 51:1167–1174.
13. Steinherz LJ, Steinherz PG, Tan CTC, et al. Cardiac toxicity 4 to 20 years after completing anthracycline therapy. *JAMA* 1991; 266:1672–1677.
14. Leandro J, Dyck J, Poppe D, et al. Cardiac dysfunction late after cardiotoxic therapy for childhood cancer. *Am J Cardiol* 1994; 74:1152–1156.
15. Legha SS, Benjamin RS, MacKay B, et al. Reduction of doxorubicin cardiotoxicity by prolonged continuous intravenous infusion. *Ann Intern Med* 1982; 89:133–139.
16. Siveski-Iliskovic N, Hill M, Chow DA, Signal PK. Probucol protects against adriamycin cardiomyopathy without interfering with its antitumor effect. *Circulation* 1995; 91:10–15.
17. Seifert CF, Nesser ME, Thompson DF. Dexrazoxane in the prevention of doxorubicin-induced cardiotoxicity. *Ann Pharmacother* 1994; 28:1063–1072.
18. Benjamin RS. Rationale for the use of mitoxantrone in the older patient: Cardiac toxicity. *Semin Oncol* 1995; 22:11–13.
19. Feenstra J, Grobbee DE, Remme WJ, Stricker BH. Drug induced heart failure. *J Am Coll Cardiol* 1999; 33:1152–1162.
20. Robben NC, Pippas AW, Moore JO. The syndrome of 5-fluorouracil cardiotoxicity: An elusive cardiopathy. *Cancer* 1993; 71:493–509.
21. Akhtar SS, Salim KP, Bano ZA. Symptomatic cardiotoxicity with

high dose 5-fluorouracil infusion: A prospective study. *Oncology* 1993; 50:441–445.

22. Weiss RB, Grillo-Lopez AJ, Marsoni S, et al. Amsacrine-associated cardiotoxicity: An analysis of 82 cases. *J Clin Oncol* 1986; 4:918–928.
23. Rowinsky EK, Donchower RC. Paclitaxel (taxol). *N Engl J Med* 1995; 332:1004–1014.
24. McNeil C. Herceptin raises its sights beyond advanced breast cancer. *J Natl Cancer Inst* 1998; 90:882–883.
25. DuBois JS, Udelson JE, Atkins B. Severe reversible, global and regional ventricular dysfunction associated with high-dose interleukin-2 immunotherapy. *J Immunother* 1995; 18:119–123.
26. Roose SP, Dalak GW. Treating the depressed patient with cardiovascular problems. *J Clin Psychiatry* 1992; 53(9, suppl):25–31.
27. Fraser-Smith N, Lesperance F, Talajic M. Depression following myocardial infarction: Impact on 6-month survival. *JAMA* 1993; 270:1819–1825.
28. Glassman AH, Roose SP, Bigger JT. The safety of tricyclic antidepressants in cardiac patients—Risk benefit reconsidered. *JAMA* 1993; 269:2673–2675.
29. Franco-Bronson K. The management of treatment-resistant depression in the medically ill. *Psychiatr Clin North Am* 1996; 19:329–348.
30. Glassman AH, Preud'home XA. Review of the cardiovascular effects of heterocyclic antidepressants. *J Clin Psychiatry* 1983; 54(2, suppl):16–22.
31. Roose SP, Glassman AH, Gardina EGV, et al. Tricyclic antidepressants in depressed patients with cardiac conduction disease. *Arch Gen Psychiatry* 1987; 44:273–275.
32. The Cardiac Arrhythmia Suppression Trial II Investigators. Effect of the antiarrhythmic agent moricizine on survival after myocardial infarction. *N Engl J Med* 1992; 327:227–233.
33. Wolfe TR, Caravati EM, Rollin DE. Terminal 40-ms frontal plane QRS axis as a marker for tricyclic antidepressant overdose. *Ann Emerg Med* 1989; 18:348–351.
34. Shanon M. Toxicology reviews: Targeted management strategies for cardiovascular toxicity from tricyclic antidepressant overdose: The pivotal role for alkalinization and sodium loading. *Pediatr Emerg Care* 1998; 14:293–298.
35. Ciraulo DA, Shader RI. Fluoxetine drug-drug interactions: I. Antidepressants and antipsychotics. *J Clin Psychopharmacol* 1990; 10:48–50.
36. Sheline YI, Freedland KE, Carney RM. How safe are serotonin reuptake inhibitors for depression in patients with coronary heart disease? *Am J Med* 1997; 102:54–59.
37. Strik JJMH, Honig A, Lousberg R, et al. Cardiac side effects to two selective serotonin reuptake inhibitors in middle-aged and elderly depressed patients. *Int Clin Psychopharmacol* 1998; 13:263–267.
38. Rudorfer MV, Manji HK, Potter WZ. Comparative tolerability profiles of the newer versus older antidepressants. *Drug Safety* 1994; 10:18–46.
39. Rosenqvist M, Bergfeldt L, Aili H, et al. Sinus node dysfunction during long-term lithium treatment. *Br Heart J* 1993; 70:371–375.
40. Numata T, Abe H, Terao T, et al. Possible involvement of hypothyroidism as a cause of lithium-induced sinus node dysfunction. *PACE* 1999; 22:954–957.
41. Simard M, Gumbiner B, Lee A, et al. Lithium carbonate intoxication: A case report and review of the literature. *Arch Intern Med* 1989; 149:36–46.
42. Kemper AJ, Dunlap R, Pietro DA. Thioridazine-induced torsade de pointes: Successful therapy with isoproterenol. *JAMA* 1983; 249:2931–2934.
43. Di Salvo TG, O'Gara PT. Torsades de pointes caused by high-dose intravenous haloperidol in cardiac patients. *Clin Cardiol* 1995; 18:285–290.
44. Haverkamp W, Shenasa M, Borggrefe M, Breithardt G. Torsades de pointes. In: Zipes DP, Jalife J, eds. *Cardiac Electrophysiology: From Cell to Bedside*, 2nd ed. Philadelphia: Saunders; 1995: 885–899.
45. Orban Z, MacDonald LL, Peters MA, Guslits B. Erythromycin-induced cardiac toxicity. *Am J Cardiol* 1995; 75:859–861.
46. Lopez JA, Harold JG, Rosenthal ML, et al. QT prolongation and torsades de pointes after administration of trimethoprim-sulfamethoxazole. *Am J Cardiol* 1987; 59:376–377.
47. Pringle TH, Scorbie IN, Murray RG, et al. Prolongation of the QT interval during therapeutic starvation: A substrate for malignant arrhythmias. *Int J Obesity* 1983; 7:253–261.
48. Reinoehl J, Frankovich D, Machado C, et al. Probucol-associated tachyarrhythmic events and QT prolongation: Importance of gender. *Am Heart J* 1996; 131:1184–1191.
49. Vitola J, Vukanovic J, Roden D. Cisapride-induced torsades de pointes. *J Cardiovasc Electrophysiol* 1998; 9:1109–1113.
50. Priori SG. Exploring the hidden danger of noncardiac drugs. *J Cardiovasc Electrophysiol* 1998; 9:1114–1116.
51. Nemeroff CB, DeVane CL, Pollack BG. Newer antidepressants and the cytochrome P450 system. *Am J Psychiatry* 1996; 153:311–320.
52. Chen TM, Benowitz NL. Caffeine and coffee: Effects on health and cardiovascular disease. *Comp Biochem Physiol* 1994; 109C:173–189.
53. Grayboys TB, Bedell SE. Caffeine ingestion: Yet another wake-up call? *Am Heart J* 1998; 136:574–575.
54. Swagemakers JJM, Gorgels, APM, Weijenberg MP, et al. Risk indications for out-of-hospital cardiac arrest in patients with coronary artery disease. *J Clin Epidemiol* 1999; 52:601–607.
55. Sessler CN, Cohen MD. Cardiac arrhythmias during theophylline toxicity: A prospective continuous electrocardiographic study. *Chest* 1990; 98:672–678.
56. Seneff M, Scott J, Friedman B, et al. Acute theophylline toxicity and the use of esmolol to reverse cardiovascular instability. *Ann Emerg Med* 1990; 19:671–673.
57. Greenberg A, Piraino BH, Kroboth PD, Weiss J. Severe theophylline toxicity: Role of conservative measures, antiarrhythmic agents and charcoal hemoperfusion. *Am J Med* 1984; 76:854–860.
58. Lee H, Izquierdo R, Evans HE. Cardiac response to oral and aerosol administration of beta agonists. *J Pediatr* 1983; 103:655–658.
59. Martin RM, Dunn NR, Freemantle SH, Mann RD. Risk of non-fatal cardiac failure and ischemic heart disease with long acting B_2 agonists. *Thorax* 1998; 53:558–562.
60. Taylor DR, Sears MR, Cockcroft DW. The beta-agonist controversy. *Med Clin North Am* 1996; 80:719–748.
61. Koh KK, Roe IH, Lee M, et al. Variant angina complicating ergot therapy of migraine. *Chest* 1994; 105:1259–1260.
62. Roithinger FX, Punzengruber C, Gremmel F, et al. Myocardial infarction after chronic ergotamine abuse. *Eur Heart J* 1993; 14:1579–1581.
63. Redfield MM, Nicholson WJ, Edwards WD, Tajik AJ. Valve disease associated with ergot alkaloid: Echocardiographic and pathologic correlations. *Ann Intern Med* 1992; 117:50–52.
64. Allen MB, Tosh G, Walters G, Muers MF. Pleural and pericardial fibrosis after ergotamine therapy. *Respir Med* 1994; 88:67–69.
65. Mason JW, Billingham ME, Friedman JP. Methysergide-induced heart disease: A case of multivalvular and myocardial fibrosis. *Circulation* 1977; 56:889–890.
66. Liston H, Bennett L, Usher B, Nappi, J. The association of the combination of sumtriptan and methysergide in myocardial infarction in a premenopausal woman. *Arch Intern Med* 1999; 159:511–513.
67. VanDenBrink AM, Reekers M, Bax W, et al. Coronary side-effect potential of current and prospective antimigraine drugs. *Circulation* 1998; 98:25–30.
68. Connolly HM, Crary JL, McGoon MD, et al. Valvular heart

disease associated with fenfluramine-phentermine [published correction appears in *N Engl J Med* 1997; 337:1783]. *N Engl J Med* 1997; 337:581–588.

69. Cardiac valvulopathy associated with exposure to fenfluramine or dexfenfluramine: US Department of Health and Human Services interim public health recommendations, Nov 1997. *MMWR* 1997; 46:1061–1066.
70. Weissman NJ, Tighe JF Jr, Gottdiener JS, Gwynne JT. An assessment of heart valve abnormalities in obese patients taking dexfenfluramine, sustained-release dexfenfluramine, or placebo. *N Engl J Med* 1998; 339:725–732.
71. Hensrud DD, Connolly HM, Grogan M, et al. Echocardiographic improvement over time after cessation of use of fenfluramine and phentermine. *Mayo Clin Proc* 1999; 74:1191–1197.
72. Shively BK, Roldan CA, Gill EA, et al. Prevalence and determinants of valvulopathy in patients treated with dexfenfluramine. *Circulation* 1999; 100:2161–2167.
73. MacMahon B, Bakshi M, Walsh MJ. Cardiac arrhythmias after intravenous cimetidine. *N Engl J Med* 1981; 305:832–833.
74. Gould L, Reddy CVR, Singh BK, Zen B. Electrophysiologic properties of cimetidine in man. *Pacing Clin Electrophysiol* 1981; 4:3–7.
75. Cubero GI, Reguero JJ, Ortega JM. Restrictive cardiomyopathy caused by chloroquine. *Br Heart J* 1993; 69:451–452.
76. Ratliff NB, Estes ML, Myles JL, et al. Diagnosis of chloroquine cardiomyopathy by endomyocardial biopsy. *N Engl J Med* 1987; 316:191–193.
77. Rosenberg L, Begaud B, Bergan U, et al. What are the risks of third generation oral contraceptives? *Hum Reprod* 1996; 11:687–693.
78. Jick H, Jick SS, Gurewich V, et al. Risk of idiopathic cardiovascular death and nonfatal venous thromboembolism in women using oral contraceptives with differing progestagen compounds. *Lancet* 1995; 346:1589–1593.
79. Schwingl PJ, Ory HW, Visness CM. Estimates of the risk of cardiovascular death attributable to low-dose oral contraceptives in the United States. *Am J Obstet Gynecol* 1999; 180: 241–249.
80. Consensus Conference on Combination Oral Contraceptives and Cardiovascular Disease. *Fertil Steril* 1999; 71:1S–6S.
81. Bagatell CJ, Brewner WJ. Androgens in men—Uses and abuses: *N Engl J Med* 1996; 334:707–714.
82. Yesalis CE, Kennedy NK, Kopstein AN, Bahrke MS. Anabolic-adrogenic steroid use in the United States. *JAMA* 1993; 270:1217–1221.
83. Nieminen MS, Ramo MP, Viitasalo M, et al. Serious cardiovascular side effects of large doses of anabolic steroids in weight lifters. *Eur Heart J* 1996; 17:1576–1583.
84. Blue JG, Lombardo JA. Steroids and steroid-like compounds. *Clin Sports Med* 1999; 18:667–689.
85. Glazer G. Atherogenic effects of anabolic steroids on serum lipid levels: A literature review. *Arch Intern Med* 1991; 151:1925–1933.
86. Mewis C, Spyridopulous I, Kuhlkamp V, Seipel L. Manifestation of severe coronary heart disease after anabolic drug abuse. *Clin Cardiol* 1996; 19:153–155.
87. Hollander JE. The management of cocaine-associated myocardial ischemia. *N Engl J Med* 1995; 333:1267–1272.
88. Kloner RA, Hale S, Alker Rezkalla S. The effects of acute and chronic cocaine use on the heart. *Circulation* 1992; 85:407–419.
89. Pirwitz MJ, Willard JE, Landau C, et al. Influence of cocaine, ethanol, or their combination on epicardial coronary arterial dimensions in humans. *Arch Intern Med* 1995; 155:1186–1191.
90. Moliterno DJ, Willard JE, Lange RA, et al. Coronary-artery vasoconstriction induced by cocaine, cigarette smoking, or both. *N Engl J Med* 1994; 330:454–459.
91. Knuepfer MM, Mueller PJ. Review of evidence for a novel model of cocaine-induced cardiovascular toxicity. *Pharmacol Biochem Behav* 1999; 63:489–500.
92. Om A, Ellahham S, Disciascio G. Management of cocaine-induced cardiovascular complications. *Am Heart J* 1993; 125: 469–475.
93. Hollander JE, Hoffman RS, Burstein JL, et al. Cocaine-associated myocardial infarction: Mortality and complications. *Arch Intern Med* 1995; 155:1081–1086.
94. Wilbert-Lampe U, Seliger C, Zilker R, et al. Cocaine increases the endothelial release of immunoreactive endothelin and its concentrations in human plasma and urine. *Circulation* 1998; 98:385–390.
95. Hollander JE, Hoffman RS, Gennis P, et al. Prospective multicenter evaluation of cocaine associated chest pain. *Ann Emerg Med* 1994; 1:330–339.
96. Leikin JB. Cocaine and B-adrenergic blockers: A remarriage after a decade-long divorce? *Crit Care Med* 1999; 27:688–689.
97. Gitter MJ, Goldsmith SR, Dunbar DN, Sharkey SW. Cocaine and chest pain: Clinical features and outcome of patients hospitalized to rule out myocardial infarction. *Ann Intern Med* 1991; 115:277–282.
98. Derlet RW, Rice P, Horowitz BZ, Lord RV. Amphetamine toxicity: Experiences with 127 cases. *J Emerg Med* 1989; 7:157–161.
99. Hong R, Matsuyama E, Nur K. Cardiomyopathy associated with the smoking of crystal amphetamine. *JAMA* 1991; 265:1152–1154.
100. Bailey B, Gaudreauh HP, Thivierge RL, et al. Cardiac monitoring of children with household electrical injuries. *Ann Emerg Med* 1995; 25:612–617.
101. Carleton SC. Cardiac problems associated with electrical injury. *Cardiol Clin* 1995; 13:263–277.
102. Lichtenberg R, Dries D, Ward K, et al. Cardiovascular effects of lightning strikes. *J Am Coll Cardiol* 1993; 21:531–536.
103. Jain S, Bandi V. Electrical and lightning injuries. *Crit Care Clin* 1999; 15:319–331.
104. Banazak DA. Electroconvulsive therapy: A guide for family physicians. *Am Fam Physician* 1996; 53:273–278.
105. Sackeim HA, Devanand DP, Prudie J. Stimulus intensity, seizure threshold, and seizure duration: Impact on the efficacy and safety of electroconvulsive therapy. *Psychiatr Clin North Am* 1991; 14:803–843.
106. Rice EH, Sombrotto LB, Markowitz JC, Leon AC. Cardiovascular morbidity in high-risk patients during ECT. *Am J Psychiatry* 1994; 151:1637–1641.
107. O'Connor CJ, Rothenberg DM, Soble JS, et al. The effect of esmolol pretreatment on the incidence of regional wall motion abnormalities during electroconvulsive therapy. *Anesth Analg* 1996; 82:143–147.
108. Graybar G, Goethe J, Levy T, et al. Transient large upright T-wave on the electrocardiogram during multiple monitored electroconvulsive therapy. *Anesthesiology* 1983; 59:467–469.
109. Leslie JB, Kalayjiam RW, Sirgo MA, et al. Intravenous labetolol for the treatment of postoperative hypertension. *Anesthesiology* 1987; 67:413–421.
110. Abiusa P, Dunkelman R, Proper M. Electroconvulsive therapy in patients with pacemakers. *JAMA* 1978; 240:2459–2462.
111. Greenstein A, Kaver I, Lechtman V, et al. Cardiac arrhythmias during nonsynchronized extracorporeal shock wave lithotripsy. *J Urol* 1995; 154:1321–1322.
112. Zeng ZR, Lindstedt E, Roijer A, et al. Arrhythmia during extracorporeal shock wave lithotripsy. *Br J Urol* 1993; 71:10–16.
113. Mashour NH, Lin GI, Frishman WH. Herbal Medicine for the treatment of cardiovascular disease. *Arch Intern Med* 1998; 158:2225–2234.
114. Ackman ML, Campbell JB, Buzak KA, et al. Use of nonprescrip-

tion medications by patients with congestive heart failure. *Ann Pharmacother* 1999; 33:674–679.

115. Ernst E. Harmless herbs? A review of the recent literature. *Am J Med* 1998; 104:170–178.
116. Vann A. The herbal medicine boom: Understanding what patients are taking. *Cleve Clin J Med* 1998; 65:12–13.
117. Yu CM, Chan JCN, Sanderson JE. Chinese herbs and warfarin potentiation by "Danshen." *J Intern Med* 1998; 241:337–339.
118. Karalliedde L. Animal toxins. *Br J Anaesth* 1995; 75:319–327.
119. Gueron M, Ilia R, Sofer S. The cardiovascular system after scorpion envenomation: A review. *Clin Toxicol* 1992; 30:245–258.
120. Blum A, Lubezki A, Sclarovsky S. Black scorpion envenomation: Two cases and review of the literature. *Clin Cardiol* 1992; 15:377–378.
121. Horen WP. Insect and scorpion sting. *JAMA* 1972; 221:894–898.
122. Lefer AM, Curtis MT. Cardiotoxicity of naturally occurring animal peptides. In: Van Stee EW, ed. *Cardiovascular Toxicology*. New York: Raven Press; 1982; 221–258.
123. Brown CK, Shepherd SM. Marine trauma, envenomations and intoxications. *Emerg Med Clin North Am* 1992; 10:385–408.
124. Weill H. Cardiorespiratory effects of inhalant occupational exposures. *Circulation* 1981; 63:250A–252A.
125. Zakhari S, Aviado DM. Cardiovascular toxicology of aerosol propellants, refrigerants, and related solvents. In: Van Stee EW, ed. *Cardiovascular Toxicology*. New York: Raven Press; 1982:281–314.
126. Roth A, Zellinger I, Arad M, Atsmon J. Organophosphates and the heart. *Chest* 1993; 103:576–578.
127. Thiermann H, Mast U, Klimmek R, et al. Cholinesterase status, pharmacokinetics and laboratory findings during obidoxime therapy in organophosphate poisoned patients. *Hum Exp Toxicol* 1997; 16:473–480.
128. Marius-Nunez AL. Myocardial infarction with normal coronary arteries after acute exposure to carbon monoxide. *Chest* 1990; 97:491–494.
129. Roberts JR, Bain M, Klachko MN, et al. Successful heart transplantation from a victim of carbon monoxide poisoning. *Ann Emerg Med* 1995; 26:652–655.
130. Stewart JR, Fajardo LF, Gillette SM, Constine LS. Radiation injury to the heart. *Int J Radiat Oncol Biol Phys* 1995; 31:1205–1211.
131. Mittal S, Berko B, Bavaria J, Herrmann HC. Radiation-induced cardiovascular dysfunction. *Am J Cardiol* 1996; 78:114–115.
132. Arsenian MA. Cardiovascular sequelae of therapeutic thoracic radiation. *Prog Cardiovasc Dis* 1991; 33:299–311.
133. Gustavsson A, Bendahl P, Cwikiel M, et al. No serious late cardiac effects after adjuvant radiotherapy following mastectomy in premenopausal women with early breast cancer. *Int J Radiation Oncol Biol Phys* 1999; 43:745–754.
134. Ni Y, Von Segesser LK, Turina M. Futility of pericardiectomy for postirradiation constrictive pericarditis. *Ann Thorac Surg* 1990; 49:445–448.
135. Shapiro CL, Hardenbergh PH, Gelman R, et al. Cardiac effects of adjuvant doxorubicin and radiation therapy in breast cancer patients. *J Clin Oncol* 1998; 16:3493–3501.
136. Hancock SL, Donaldson SS. Radiation-related heart disease: Risks after treatment of Hodgkin's disease during childhood and adolescence. In: Bricker JT, Green DM, D'Angio GJ, eds. *Cardiac Toxicity After Treatment for Childhood Cancer*. New York: Wiley-Liss; 1993:35–43.
137. Hancock SL, Donaldson SS, Hoppe RT. Heart disease after Hodgkin's treatment in children and adolescents. *J Clin Oncol* 1993; 11:1208–1215.
138. Carlson RG, Mayfield WR, Norman S, Alexander JA. Radiation-associated valvular disease. *Chest* 1991; 99:538–545.

PART TWELVE

PERICARDIAL DISEASES AND ENDOCARDITIS

CHAPTER 72

DISEASES OF THE PERICARDIUM

Brian D. Hoit

INTRODUCTION

Anatomy of the Pericardium

The pericardium is composed of visceral and parietal components. The visceral pericardium is a mesothelial monolayer that adheres firmly to the epicardium, reflects over the origin of the great vessels, and, together with a tough, fibrous coat, envelops the heart as the parietal pericardium (Fig. 72-1). The pericardial space is enclosed between these two serosal layers and normally contains up to 50 mL of a plasma ultrafiltrate, the pericardial fluid. Pericardial reflections around the great vessels tether the pericardium superiorly and result in the formation of two potential spaces: the oblique and transverse sinuses. The left atrium is anterior to the oblique sinus and is therefore largely an extrapericardial chamber; this relationship explains why effusions generally are not seen behind the left atrium. Superior and inferior pericardiosternal and diaphragmatic ligaments limit displacement of the pericardium and its contents within the chest and neutralize the effects of respiration and change of body position. The phrenic nerves are embedded in the parietal pericardium and, for this reason, are vulnerable to injury during pericardial resection.

Histologically, the pericardium is composed predominantly of compact collagen layers interspersed with elastin fibers. The abundance and orientation of the collagen fibers are responsible for the characteristic viscoelastic mechanical properties of the pericardium. For example, the pressure-volume relation of the pericardium is nonlinear; i.e., the relation is initially flat (producing little to no change in pressure for large changes in volume) and develops a "bend" or "knee" at a critical pressure, which terminates in a steep slope (producing large changes in pressure for small changes in volume) (Fig. 72-2). In addition, the pericardium is anisotropic; i.e., it stretches more in the short axis than in the long axis.

Physiology of the Pericardium

The pericardium is not essential for life; no adverse consequences follow congenital absence or surgical removal of the pericardium. However, the pericardium serves many important (although subtle) functions (Table 72-1). The pericardium limits distention of the cardiac chambers and facilitates interaction and coupling of the ventricles and atria.[1] Thus, changes in pressure and volume on one side of the heart can influence pressure and volume on the other side. Limitation of cardiac filling vol-

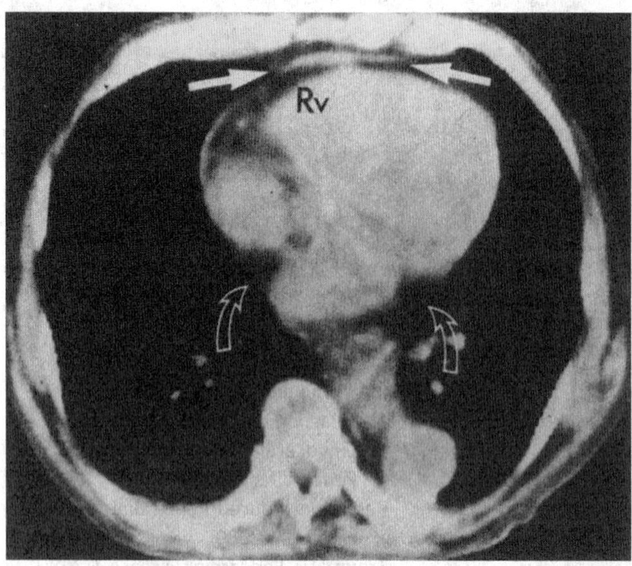

FIGURE 72-1 Computed tomographic (CT) scan shows the normal pericardium as a thin, curvilinear line (*open arrows*). The increased thickening over the anterior surface of the heart (*solid arrows*) is probably an artifact from transmitted right ventricular pulsations. (From Moncada R, Baker M. In: Higgins CB, ed. *CT of the Heart and Great Vessels*. Mt. Kisco, NY: Futura; 1983:292. Reproduced with permission.)

umes by the pericardium also may limit cardiac output and oxygen delivery during exercise.[2] The pericardium also influences quantitative and qualitative aspects of ventricular filling[3]; the thin-walled right ventricle (RV) and atrium are more subject to the influence of the pericardium than is the more resistant, thick-walled left ventricle (LV).[4]

Although the magnitude and importance of pericardial restraint of ventricular filling at physiologic cardiac volumes remain controversial, there is general agreement that pericardial reserve volume (i.e., the difference between unstressed pericardial volume and cardiac volume) is relatively small and that

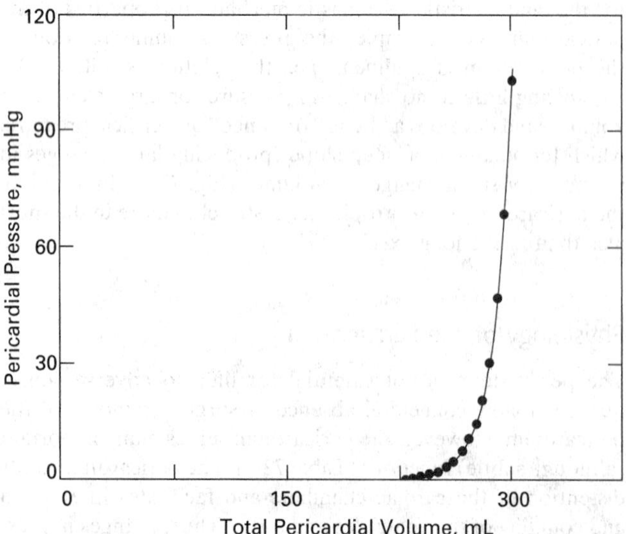

FIGURE 72-2 Pericardial pressure-volume relation in a dog. (From Holt JP. The normal pericardium. *Am J Cardiol* 1970; 26:455. Reproduced with permission.)

TABLE 72-1 Functions of the Pericardium

- Mechanical
  - Effects on chambers
    - Limits short-term cardiac distention
    - Facilitates cardiac chamber coupling and interaction
    - Maintains pressure-volume relation of and output from cardiac chambers
    - Maintains geometry of left ventricle
  - Effects on whole heart
    - Lubricates, minimizes friction
    - Equalizes gravitation, inertial, hydrostatic forces
    - Mechanical barrier to infection
- Immunologic
- Vasomotor
- Fibrinolytic
- Modulation of myocyte structure, function, and gene expression
- Vehicle for drug delivery and gene therapy

pericardial influences become significant when the reserve volume is exceeded. This may occur with rapid increases in blood volume and in disease states characterized by rapid increases in heart size (e.g., acute mitral and tricuspid regurgitation, pulmonary embolism, RV infarction). In contrast, chronic stretching of the pericardium results in "stress relaxation"; this explains why large but slowly developing effusions do not produce tamponade. In addition, the pericardium adapts to cardiac growth by "creep" (i.e., an increase in volume with constant stretch) and cellular hypertrophy. Pericardial thickening, which is characterized by mesothelial cell and matrix rearrangments, and the absence of diastolic abnormalities on echocardiography are features of vibroacoustic disease.[5]

The pericardium serves a variety of other important functions. It prevents excessive torsion and displacement of the heart, minimizes friction with surrounding structures, and is an anatomic barrier to the spread of infection from contiguous structures. The thin layer of pericardial fluid reduces friction on the epicardium and is thought to equalize gravitational forces over the surface of the heart; transmural cardiac pressures therefore do not change during acceleration or differ regionally within cardiac chambers. In addition, pericardial fluid equalizes inertial and hydrostatic forces. The pericardium also has immunologic, vasomotor, and fibrinolytic activity.[6] Epicardial mesothelial cells may modulate myocyte structure and function and gene expression.[7] Finally, the pericardial space has been used as a vehicle for drug delivery in gene therapy; studies using radiolabeled growth factors indicate that substances more consistently and reproducibly gain access to the coronary arteries via pericardial fluid than via endoluminal delivery.[8,9]

PERICARDIAL MICROPHYSIOLOGY

The pericardium is richly innervated; neuroreceptors in the epicardium and fibrosa, sympathetic afferents, stretch-sensitive mechanoreceptors, and phrenic afferents monitor dynamic changes in cardiac volume and tension.[10] Chemo- and mechanoreceptors with sympathetic afferents may be responsible for the transmission of pericardial pain.[11]

The mesothelium of the pericardium is metabolically active

and produces prostaglandin E_2, eicosanoids, and prostacylin; these substances modulate sympathetic neurotransmission and myocardial contractility and may influence epicardial coronary arterial tone. The concentration of angiogenic growth factors bFGF and VEGF increases in unstable angina,[12] suggesting a role for these factors in response to ischemia and injury. The level of brain natriuretic peptide (BNP) in the pericardial fluid is a more sensitive and accurate indicator of ventricular volume and pressure than is either plasma BNP or atrial natriuretic factor and may play an autocrine/paracrine role in heart failure.[13] In addition, levels of pericardial 8-iso-PGF2α (a marker of oxidant stress) increase directly with increasing ventricular dilatation and severity of heart failure, suggesting a role of oxidant stress in ventricular remodeling and the development of heart failure.[14]

Pericardial Pressure

Pericardial pressure measured by a fluid-filled catheter in the pericardial space is subatmospheric and is essentially equal to pleural pressure throughout the respiratory cycle. Small fluctuations related to the events of the cardiac cycle (pericardial pressure is lowest during ventricular ejection) are superimposed on the larger fluctuations related to the events of the respiratory cycle. Although much of the understanding of pericardial physiology is based on fluid pressure, pericardial restraint is a contact force, defined as fluid pressure plus deformational force (much like the force at the knee joint that, although considerable, is negligible when measured with a needle in the joint space). Pericardial contact pressure measured with flat balloons is considerably higher than liquid pressure and varies regionally.[3]

Balloon pressure is similar to the theoretical pericardial pressure that is calculated as the difference in LV diastolic pressure before and after pericardiectomy. This theoretical pressure has important implications for understanding the role of the pericardium in states of altered ventricular loading, such as pulmonary hypertension, aortic stenosis, and congestive heart failure, but does not explain pericardial influences on transmural pressure, for example, during acceleration and deceleration. When liquid versus contact pressure is more relevant is controversial among physiologists but is far less relevant to clinicians, who measure pericardial pressure only when there is a pericardial effusion.

Pathology of the Pericardium

In view of its simple structure, clinicopathologic processes involving the pericardium are understandably few; indeed, pericardial heart disease includes only pericarditis (an acute, subacute, or chronic fibrinous, "noneffusive," or exudative process) and its complications, tamponade and constriction (an acute, subacute, or chronic adhesive, fibrocalcific response), and congenital lesions. However, despite a limited number of clinical syndromes, the pericardium is affected by virtually every cate-

TABLE 72-2 Causes of Pericardial Heart Disease

- Idiopathic
- Infectious
  - Bacterial (pneumococcus, streptococcus, staphlococcus, *Haemophilus influenzae,* gram-negative rods, *B. melitensis, F. tularensis, Legionella pneumophilia, P. gonorrhoeae, N. meningitidis,* Lyme disease, myocoplasma)
  - Viral (coxsackie virus, echovirus, adenovirus, varicella, influenza, cytomegalovirus, HIV, hepatitis B, mumps, infectious mononucleosis)
  - Mycobacterial (*M. tuberculosis, M. avium-intracellulare*)
  - Fungal (histoplasmosis, coccidioidomycosis, blastomycosis, *Candida albicans, Nocardia,* actinomycosis)
  - Protozoal (toxoplasmosis, echinococcosis, amebiasis)
  - AIDS-associated
- Neoplastic
  - Primary (mesothelioma, fibrosarcoma)
  - Secondary (breast, lung, melanoma, lymphoma, leukemia)
- Immune/inflammatory
  - Connective tissue diseases (rheumatoid arthritis, systemic lupus erythematosis, scleroderma, acute rheumatic fever, dermatomyositis, mixed connective tissue disease, Wegener's granulomatosis)
  - Arteritis (temporal arteritis, polyarteritis nodosa, Takayasu's arteritis)
  - Acute myocardial infarction and post-MI (Dressler's syndrome)
  - Postcardiotomy
  - Posttraumatic
- Metabolic
  - Nephrogenic
  - Aortic dissection
  - Myxedema
  - Amyloidosis
- Iatrogenic
  - Radiation injury
  - Instrument/device trauma (implantable defibrillators, pacemakers, catheters)
  - Drugs (hydralazine, procainamide, daunorubicin, isoniazid, anticoagulants, cyclosporine, methysergide, phenytoin, dantrolene, mesalazine)
  - Cardiac resuscitation
- Traumatic
  - Blunt
  - Penetrating
  - Surgical
- Congenital
  - Pericardial cysts
  - Congenital absence of pericardium
  - Mulibrey nanism

gory of disease, including infections, neoplastic, immune/inflammatory, metabolic, iatrogenic, traumatic, and congenital etiologies. Thus, the physician is likely to encounter patients with pericardial disease in a variety of settings, either as an isolated phenomenon or as a complication of a variety of systemic disorders, trauma, or certain drugs.

Pericardial disease often remains clinically silent and may be detected only during the evaluation of unrelated complaints by the electrocardiogram (ECG), chest radiography, or echocardiography. Despite exhaustive etiologic lists (Table 72-2), the cause of pericardial heart disease often is never identified. Recently, an increased prevalence of pericarditis, (owing largely to therapeutic advances such as cardiovascular surgery, hemodialysis, and radiation therapy), pericardial involvement in AIDS, and advances in the recognition, diagnosis, and therapy of pericarditis and its complications have resulted in a resurgence of interest in pericardial heart disease. The remainder of this chapter reviews pericarditis and its sequelae, pericardial effusions, cardiac tamponade and constrictive pericarditis, and congenital diseases of the pericardium.

ACUTE PERICARDITIS

Acute fibrinous or dry pericarditis is a syndrome characterized by typical chest pain, a pathognomonic pericardial friction rub, and specific ECG changes. A variety of conditions are associated with acute pericarditis (Table 72-2). The following description refers to viral and idiopathic pericarditis without significant effusion. Specific forms of pericardial heart disease are reviewed later in the chapter.

History

Acute pericarditis typically produces sharp retrosternal pain that radiates to the trapezius ridge and is aggravated by lying down and relieved by sitting up; its onset frequently is heralded by a prodrome of fever, malaise, and myalgia (Fig. 72-3). The pain of pericarditis is often worse with inspiration and is difficult to distinguish from pleurisy; in some cases, the pain is indistinguishable from that of myocardial infarction. The quality, severity, and location of pain vary greatly, and chest pain may be absent in acute pericarditis, especially in early pericarditis complicating myocardial infarction or cardiac surgery and in uremic pericarditis.

Physical Findings

The hallmark of acute pericarditis is the pericardial friction rub; because of its superficial, creaky, or scratchy character, it often is likened to the sound of walking on dry snow or the squeak of a leather saddle (Fig. 72-3). Rubs are heard anywhere over the precordium but most often between the lower left sternal edge and the cardiac apex; they usually are heard best with the diaphragm of the stethoscope applied firmly and with respiration suspended. Most pericardial friction rubs are independent of the respiratory cycle, but on occasion they are louder during inspiration. The pericardial rub may be confined to ventricular systole but most often includes a component during atrial systole and occasionally during ventricular diastolic filling, resulting in biphasic and triphasic rubs, respectively. Biphasic rubs must be distinguished from murmurs of mixed aortic valve disease, and monophasic rubs often are mistaken for systolic murmurs. Frequent examinations are necessary to detect a rub because of its evanescent nature; pericardial fluid does not prevent a friction rub.

In uncomplicated pericarditis, the jugular venous pressure usually remains normal. Ventricular third and fourth heart sounds indicate coexisting myocardial disease. The history and physical examination are helpful also in recognizing complications and in identifying underlying diseases associated with pericarditis. Depending on the etiology, there may be fever and other signs of inflammation or systemic illness.

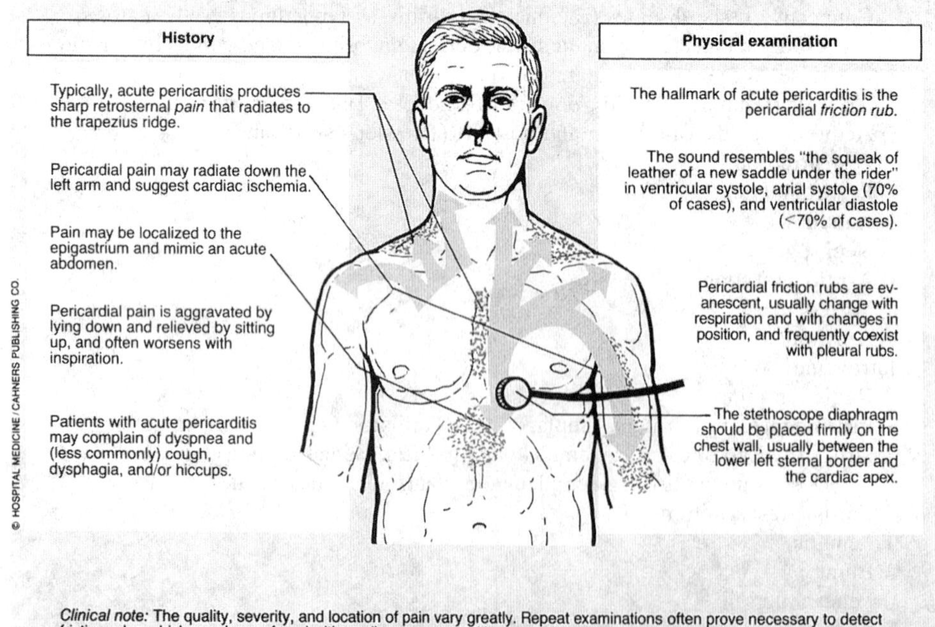

FIGURE 72-3 Clinical features of acute pericarditis: history and physical examination. (From Hoit BD. Acute pericarditis: Diagnosis and differential diagnosis. *Hosp Pract* 1991; 27:23–43. Reproduced with permission.)

Electrocardiography

The ECG may either confirm the clinical suspicion of pericardial disease or first alert the clinician to the presence of pericarditis (Fig. 72-4). Serial tracings may be needed to distinguish the ST-segment elevations caused by acute pericarditis from those caused by acute myocardial infarction

(MI) or normal early repolarization. The ST-T wave changes in acute pericarditis are diffuse and have characteristic evolutionary changes. In the first stage, ST-segment elevations (which differ from ischemic ST elevations by their upward concavity and seldom exceed 5 mm in height) typically occur within a few hours of the onset of chest pain and persist for hours or days. Depression of the PR segment (except in lead aVR) may be seen in this stage and may differentiate acute pericarditis from early repolarization variants.[15] In the second stage, the ST segments return to baseline; at this point, the T waves may appear normal or exhibit a loss of amplitude. In the third stage, tracings show inversion of T waves. T-wave inversions may persist indefinitely, particularly with tuberculous, uremic, or neoplastic pericarditis. The ECG normalizes in the variably present fourth stage. In a typical case of acute pericarditis, the approximate time frame for these ECG changes is 2 weeks. However, only about half of patients with acute pericarditis display all four ECG stages, and variations are very common. Atrial arrhythmias complicate 5 to 10 percent of cases of acute pericarditis.[16]

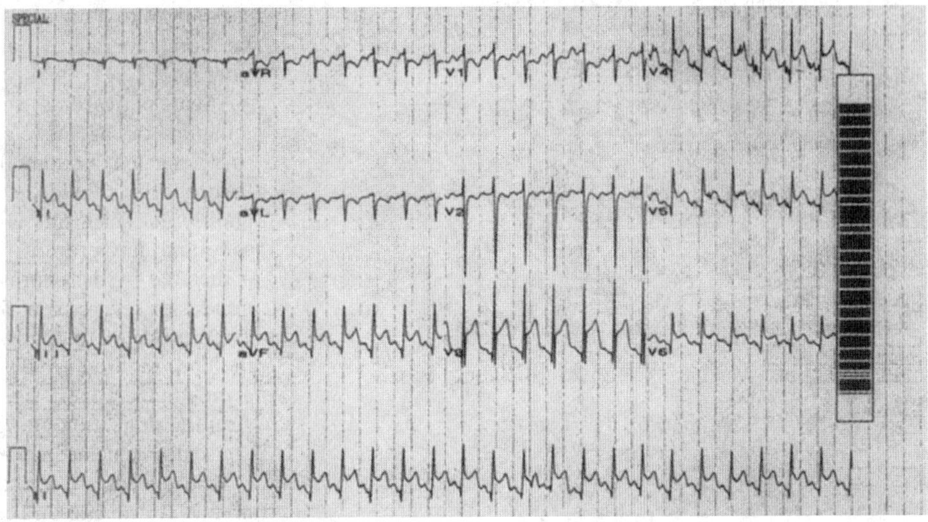

FIGURE 72-4 Twelve-lead electrocardiogram from a patient with acute pericarditis. (From Hoit BD. Pericardial disease and pericardial heart disease. In: O'Rourke RA, ed. *Stein's Internal Medicine*, 5th ed. St. Louis, Missouri: Mosby-Year Book; 1998:273. Reproduced with permission.)

The ST-segment elevation seen in acute pericarditis usually can be distinguished from that of acute MI by the absence of Q waves, the upwardly concave ST segments, and the absence of associated T-wave inversions. The acute ST-segment elevation of Prinzmetal's variant of angina is more transitory and is associated with ischemic pain. Although the ST-segment elevation in the early repolarization variant (common in young individuals, especially blacks, athletes, and psychiatric patients) may simulate the ECG of acute pericarditis, the former is distinguished by the absence of PR-segment depression and evolutionary ST-T wave changes.

Imaging and Laboratory Studies

In uncomplicated acute pericarditis, the chest radiograph is generally normal. However, an enlarged cardiac silhouette may be evident because of a moderate or large pericardial effusion (Fig. 72-5). The chest radiograph may provide evidence of tuberculosis, fungal disease, pneumonia, or neoplasm.

Echocardiographic identification of pericardial effusion confirms the clinical diagnosis of acute pericarditis (Fig. 72-6), but a patient with purely fibrinous acute pericarditis often has a normal echocardiogram. Echocardiography estimates the volume of pericardial fluid, identifies cardiac tamponade, suggests the basis of pericarditis, and documents associated acute myocarditis with congestive heart failure.

Although ^{99}technetium pyrophosphate scans may be positive in patients with pericarditis associated with epicarditis and gallium scans have proved useful in displaying the characteristics of purulent pericarditis, these tests rarely are used to diagnose acute pericarditis.

Nonspecific blood markers of inflammation, such as the erythrocyte sedimentation rate and the white blood cell count, usually increase in cases of acute pericarditis. Patients with extensive epicarditis occasionally have increases in serum cardiac isoenzymes suggestive of acute MI.

Therapy for Acute Pericarditis

Hospitalization is warranted for most patients who present with an initial episode of acute pericarditis to determine the etiology

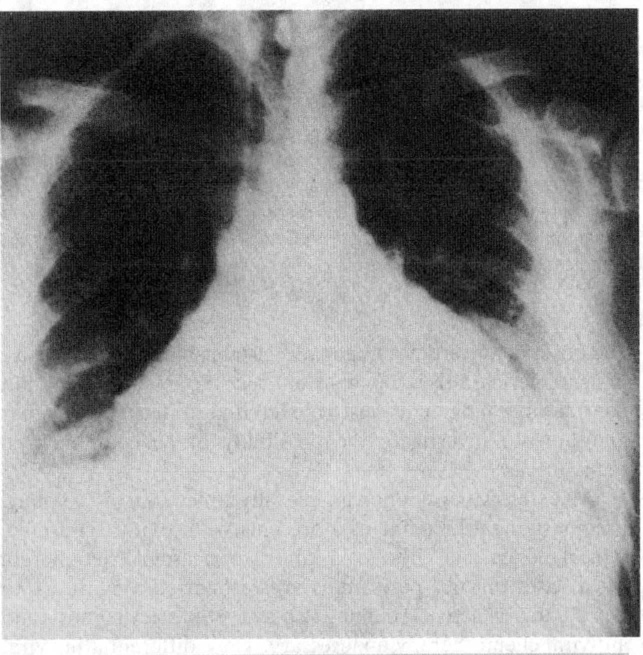

FIGURE 72-5 Chest radiograph from a patient with a large pericardial effusion. Note the "flask-shape" appearance of the cardiac silhouette. (From Hoit BD. Imaging the pericardium. *Cardiol Clin* 1990; 8:588. Reproduced with permission.)

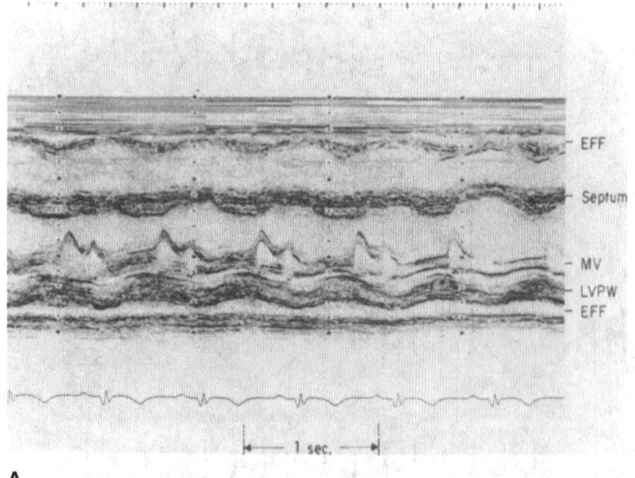

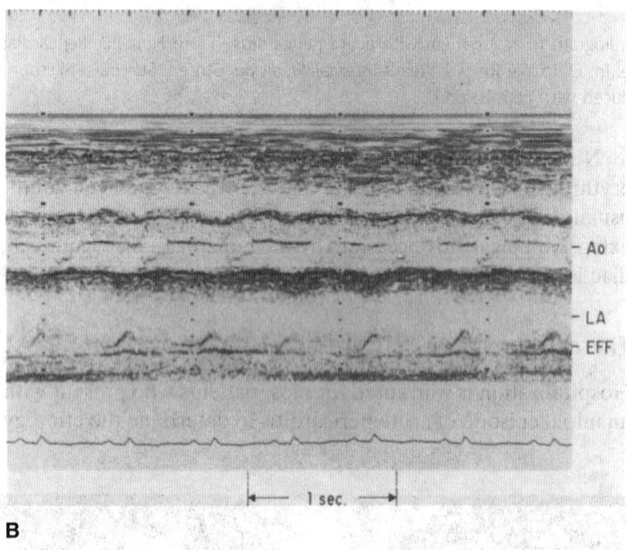

FIGURE 72-6 M-mode echocardiograms of pericardial effusion (EFF). *A.* The effusion appears as an echo-free space posterior to the left ventricular posterior wall (LVPW). Note that parietal pericardium has relatively flat motion throughout the cardiac cycle. MV = mitral valve. *B.* Pericardial effusion behind the left atrium (LA). Note the exaggerated motion of the posterior left atrial wall. (From Hoit BD. Imaging the pericardium. *Cardiol Clin* 1990; 8:588. Reproduced with permission.)

and observe for cardiac tamponade. Establishing the exact cause of acute pericarditis is an important aspect of management, but considerable judgment must be exercised in deciding whether and how to investigate the possibility of concomitant systemic disease.

An extensive evaluation is generally unnecessary in a young, previously healthy adult who presents with a viral syndrome, typical pericardial chest pain, and a pericardial friction rub. Most cases of viral pericarditis are recognized long after the period of viral activity, making a specific etiologic diagnosis and antiviral chemotherapy unnecessary. Thus, differentiating viral from idiopathic pericarditis is difficult, expensive, and generally of little practical importance. Depending on the history and symptoms at presentation, trauma, myocarditis, systemic lupus erythematosus (SLE), and/or purulent pericarditis require consideration in younger patients. In older adults, myocardial infarction, tuberculosis, and neoplastic disease should be considered.

Acute pericarditis usually responds to oral nonsteroidal anti-inflammatory agents (e.g., ASA 650 mg q3–4h or ibuprofen 600 to 800 mg q6h). Indomethacin reduces coronary blood flow and theoretically should be avoided. Some data suggest that the addition of colchicine (1 mg/day) is effective for an acute episode and may prevent recurrences.[17] The intensity of therapy is dictated by the distress of the patient; narcotics may be required for severe pain. Some cases necessitate steroid therapy (prednisone 60 to 80 mg/day) for a week to control pain, with the dose tapered rapidly thereafter. Corticosteroids should be avoided unless there is a specific indication. They may enhance viral multiplication and produce recurrences when the dose is tapered; colchicine may be useful in this situation. Nevertheless, corticosteroids are useful in acute pericarditis associated with uremic pericarditis and connective tissue diseases. Importantly, tuberculous and pyogenic pericarditis should be excluded before steroid therapy is initiated.

Patients in whom pericarditis represents one manifestation of systemic illness (such as sepsis, uremia, connective tissue disease, or neoplasia) should, in addition to palliative and supportive treatment, receive therapy directed toward the primary disorder.

RECURRENT PERICARDITIS

Recurrent or relapsing acute pericarditis is one of the most distressing disorders of the pericardium for both patient and physician; it may occur with or without pericardial effusion and occasionally is associated with pleural effusion or parenchymal pulmonary lesions. Recurrences occur with highly variable frequency over a course of many years. The reasons for relapse are unclear, but the phenomenon suggests that acute pericarditis itself may represent or generate an autoimmune process. Recurrences may be spontaneous but more commonly are associated with discontinuation or tapering doses of anti-inflammatory drugs. When associated with pericardial effusion, relapsing pericarditis can cause cardiac tamponade; however, this is unusual.

Painful recurrences of pericarditis may respond to nonsteroidal anti-inflammatory agents but commonly require corticosteroids. Once steroids are administered, dependency and the development of steroid-induced abnormalities are potential sequelae. Prednisone is begun at a high dose (60 to 80 mg/day), but rapid tapering should be initiated within a few days of clinical resolution. When necessary, the risks of long-term steroids should be minimized by using the lowest possible dose, alternate-day therapy, combinations with nonsteroidal drugs, or colchicine (1 to 2 mg/day).[18] In the most difficult cases, relapse occurs every time the dose of prednisone is reduced below 5 to 20 mg/day. When this occurs, the patient should be maintained for several weeks on the lowest suppressive dose before the next taper commences. Azathioprine (50 to 100 mg/day) also has been used to prevent recurrent episodes.[19] Although encouraging results have been reported in a series of patients who underwent pericardiectomy for recurrent pericarditis, pericardiectomy may simply abbreviate rather than terminate the painful recurrences. Thus, pericardiectomy should be considered only when repeated attempts at medical treatment have clearly failed.

PERICARDIAL EFFUSION

Etiology

Accumulation of transudate, exudate, or blood in the pericardial sac is a common complication of pericardial disease and should be sought in all patients with acute pericarditis.

Pericardial effusions are reported to be associated with heart failure, valvular disease, and myocardial infarction in 14, 21, and 15 percent of cases, respectively.[20] Hydropericardium results from elevated right atrial pressure and limited venous and lymphatic drainage from the pericardium. Although this is the usual explanation for effusions associated with heart failure and LV hypertrophy, recurrent bloody effusions that can be attributed only to congestive heart failure may occur.

Pericardial effusions are very common after cardiac surgery. In 122 consecutive patients studied before and serially after cardiac surgery, effusions were present in 103 patients; the majority appeared by postoperative day 2, reached their maximum size by postoperative day 10, and usually resolved without sequelae within the first postoperative month.[21] Symptoms and physical findings of significant postoperative pericardial effusions are frequently nonspecific, and echo-detection and echo-guided pericardiocentesis, when necessary, are safe and effective; prolonged catheter drainage reduces the recurrence rate.[22] Pericardial effusions in cardiac transplant patients are associated with an increased incidence of acute rejection.[23] Chronic effusive pericarditis is an entity of unknown etiology that may be associated with large, asymptomatic effusions. Many conditions that cause pericarditis (e.g., uremia, tuberculosis, neoplasia, connective tissue disease) produce chronic pericardial effusions.

Nature of the Pericardial Fluid

Characteristics of the pericardial fluid other than culture and cytology are usually too nonspecific to be of diagnostic value. However, in one retrospective series, one-fifth of the patients had a specific etiologic diagnosis that had implications for management and prognosis.[24] Moreover, in certain situations it is mandatory to determine the nature of the pericardial fluid. For example, in patients with neoplastic disease, it is important to determine whether pericardial effusion indicates invasion of the pericardium or a complication of radiation therapy. Cytologic examination of the fluid is also important in cases in which the primary tumor has not been identified clearly. In cases of bacterial or other nonviral infections, it becomes necessary to discover whether the pericardial effusion is exudative and to culture pericardial fluid; this is particularly important when tuberculous or fungal pericarditis is suspected. Transudative effusions (hydropericardium) occur in heart failure and other states associated with chronic salt and water retention (including pregnancy), and exudative effusions occur in a large number of the infectious and inflammatory causes of pericarditis. Although frank hemorrhagic effusions suggest recent intrapericardial bleeding, sanguineous and serosanguineous effusions occur in many infectious and inflammatory disorders. In certain disorders, the nature of the pericardial fluid has greater diagnostic value. For example, chylous pericarditis implies injury or obstruction to the thoracic duct, and cholesterol pericarditis is either idiopathic or associated with hypothyroidism, rheumatoid arthritis, or tuberculosis.

Diagnostic Studies

Specific diagnoses are possible using visual, cytologic, and immunologic analysis of the pericardial effusion and pericardioscopic-guided biopsy of the epicardium and pericardium.[20,25] Observations using these techniques have suggested that (1) fibrin strands and neovascularization are common in inflammatory pericardial diseases, (2) the etiology of viral pericarditis can be established by using a variety of methods, such as in situ hybridization, microneutralization, and polymerase chain reaction, (3) combined analysis of the cytology in the effusion and epicardial biopsy are most important, and pericardial biopsy is often inconclusive, and (4) viral and autoreactive effusions are associated with high titers of antimyolemmal and antisarcolemmal antibodies and in vitro cardiocytolysis of isolated rat heart cells. However, the clinical utility of these diagnostic methods and observations remains to be determined.

There are clinical situations in which it is unnecessary to obtain pericardial fluid for analysis. For example, when pericardial effusion is found in a patient with typical viral or idiopathic pericarditis, pericardiocentesis should not be considered unless the effusion fails to respond to anti-inflammatory treatment or cardiac tamponade develops. Similarly, when a patient undergoing chronic hemodialysis develops pericardial effusion, examination of pericardial fluid is needed only when the clinical course suggests a different etiology or when hemodynamic embarrassment is suspected.

IMAGING STUDIES

Echocardiography is the procedure of choice for the diagnosis of pericardial effusion. Although flask-shaped enlargement of the cardiac silhouette on chest radiography occurs with a moderate or large pericardial effusion (Fig. 72-5), differentiation of large effusions from cardiac dilatation often is difficult or impossible. In contrast, the relative contributions of cardiac enlargement and pericardial effusion to overall cardiac enlargement and the relative roles of tamponade and myocardial dysfunction to altered hemodynamics can be evaluated with echocardiography. Attention to technical detail results in excellent sensitivity and specificity. The diagnostic feature on M-mode echocardiography is the persistence of an echo-free space between parietal and visceral pericardium throughout the cardiac cycle (Fig. 72-6). Separations that are observed only in systole represent clinically insignificant accumulations. Two-dimensional (2-D) echocardiography (Fig. 72-7) has superior spatial orientation and allows delineation of the size and distribution of pericardial effusion as well as detection of loculated fluid. As the amount of pericardial fluid increases, fluid distributes from the posterobasilar LV apically and anteriorly and then laterally and posteriorly to the left atrium. Fluid adjacent to the right atrium is an early sign of pericardial effusion. Frondlike, bandlike, or shaggy intrapericardial echoes should alert one to the possibility of a difficult and potentially less therapeutic pericardiocentesis (Fig. 72-8) but have little value in identifying the cause of the effusion.

Pericardial effusions are easily detected by computed tomography (Fig. 72-9). The size, geometry, and distribution of pericardial effusions can be obtained with this technique, and the attenuation coefficients for blood, exudate, chyle, and serous fluid are generally sufficiently characteristic to identify the nature of the effusion. Computed tomography may be useful in identifying loculated and atypically loculated pericardial effu-

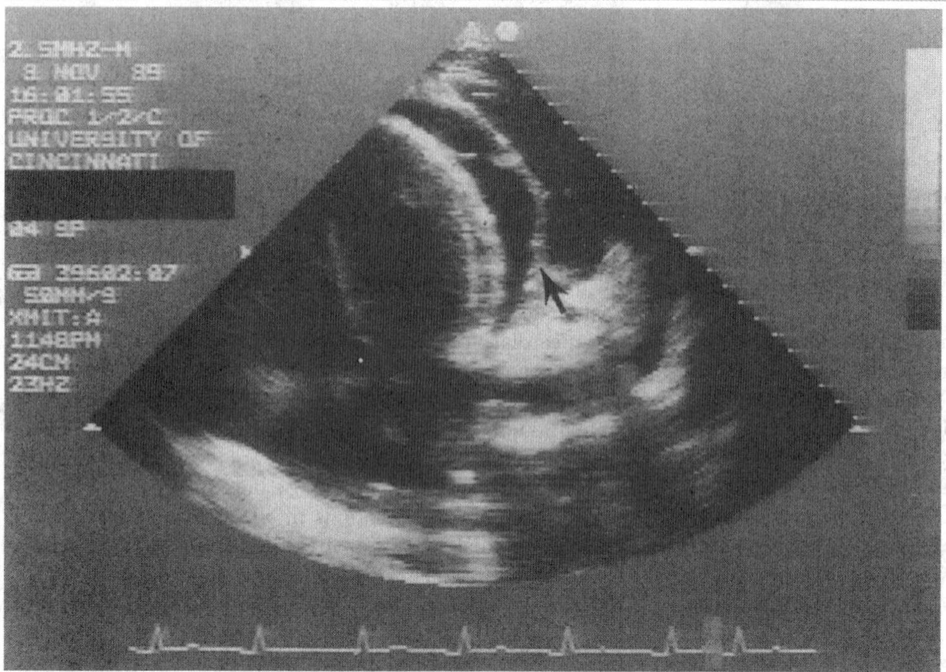

FIGURE 72-7 Two-dimensional echocardiogram from a patient with pleural and pericardial effusions. The thickness of the pericardium (*arrow*) can be appreciated in this patient. (From Hoit BD. Imaging the pericardium. *Cardiol Clin* 1990; 8:596. Reproduced with permission.)

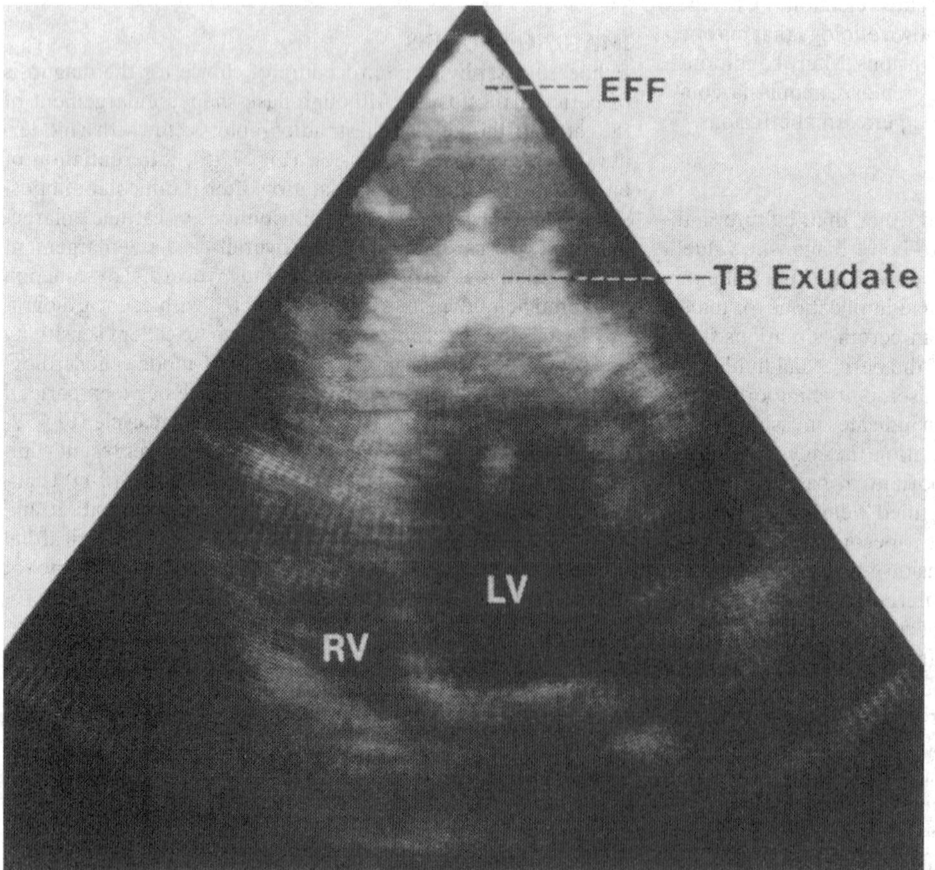

FIGURE 72-8 Two-dimensional echocardiogram from a patient with tuberculous pericarditis. Note the thickened pericardium with shaggy exudate that bridges a large pericardial effusion (EFF). (From Hoit BD. Imaging the pericardium. *Cardiol Clin* 1990; 8:590. Reproduced with permission.)

sions and in guiding pericardiocentesis. Loculated and recurrent pericardial effusions can be treated safely and effectively with video-assisted thoracoscopic pericardial fenestration.[26]

Magnetic resonance imaging (MRI) detects pericardial effusion with high sensitivity and provides an estimate of pericardial fluid volume; in addition, it effectively detects loculated pericardial effusion and pericardial thickening.[27] Inflamed pericardium and adhesions have a high signal intensity relative to pericardial fluid and myocardium, providing a potential means of identifying the nature of the effusion.

Treatment of Pericardial Effusion

Drainage of a pericardial effusion is usually unnecessary unless purulent pericarditis is suspected or cardiac tamponade supervenes, although on occasion, pericardiocentesis is needed to establish the etiology of a hemodynamically insignificant pericardial effusion. Persistent or progressive effusion, particularly when the cause is uncertain, also warrants pericardiocentesis. However, routine drainage of a large pericardial effusion without tamponade or suspected purulent pericarditis has a low diagnostic yield and no clear therapeutic benefit.[28] Anticoagulants should be discontinued temporarily if possible to reduce the risk of cardiac tamponade. In patients on chronic oral anticoagulation, heparin should be used, since its effect can be reversed rapidly. Large effusions may respond to nonsteroidal anti-inflammatory drugs, corticosteroids, or colchicine.[17] Specific treatment for pericardial effusion is considered below.

CARDIAC TAMPONADE

Cardiac tamponade is a hemodynamic condition characterized by equal elevation of atrial and pericardial pressures, an exaggerated inspiratory decrease in arterial systolic pressure (pulsus paradoxus), and arterial hypotension.

Arterial hypotension is generally a late sign in chronic effusions, and occasionally, a heightened sympathoadrenal state produces systemic hypertension. As intrapericardial pressure rises, venous pressures increase to maintain cardiac filling and prevent collapse of the cardiac chambers. Although the absolute intracardiac pressures are elevated, the transmural pressures—i.e., cavitary diastolic pressure minus pericardial pressure—are practically zero or even negative. The greatly reduced preload is responsible for the fall in cardiac output, and when compensatory mechanisms are exhausted, arterial pressure decreases.

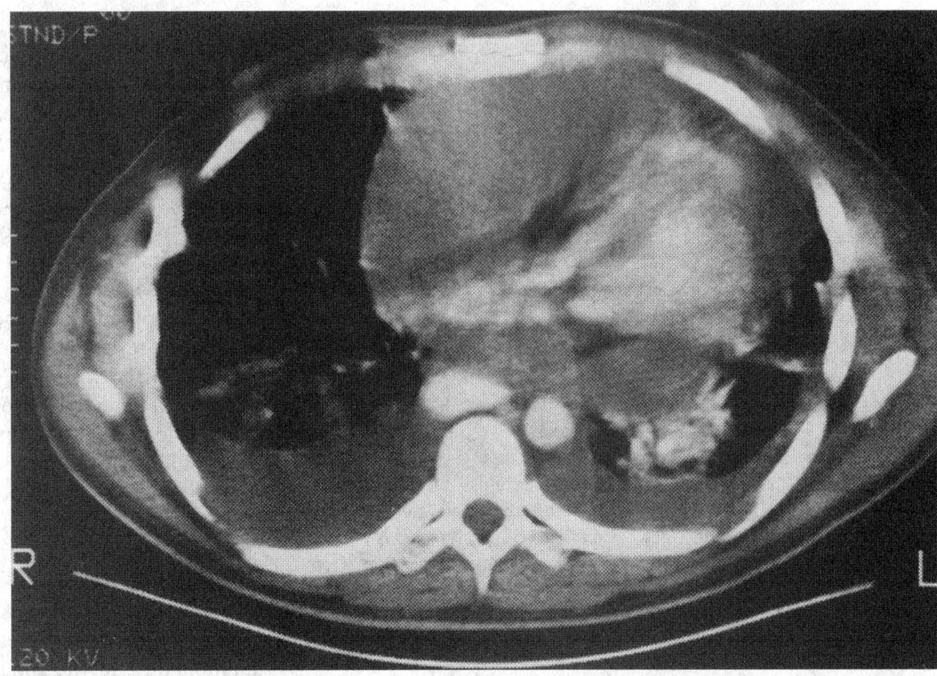

FIGURE 72-9 Computed tomographic scan from a patient with a large pericardial effusion. Note the compression of contrast-filled cardiac chambers. (From Hoit BD. Imaging the pericardium. *Cardiol Clin* 1990; 8:590. Reproduced with permission.)

Clinical Features

Cardiac tamponade may be acute or chronic and should be viewed hemodynamically as a continuum ranging from mild (pericardial pressure lower than 10 mmHg) to severe (pericardial pressure higher than 15 to 20 mmHg). Mild cardiac tamponade is frequently asymptomatic, whereas moderate tamponade and especially severe tamponade produce precordial discomfort and dyspnea.

Tamponade may be so sudden that the patient does not complain of symptoms; in less drastic circumstances, patients with acute cardiac tamponade may complain of severe shortness of breath accompanied by chest tightness and dizziness. The venous pressure is greatly elevated, and the systemic arterial pressure is severely depressed. Pulsus paradoxus usually can be appreciated but may be absent when hypotension is extreme. In striking contrast to the elevation of venous pressure, arterial hypotension, and pulsus paradoxus, cardiac pulsations often are impalpable (Beck's triad). In the most severe cases, consciousness may be impaired, and except for the raised venous pressure, such patients appear to be in hypovolemic shock.

When cardiac tamponade complicates a diagnostic procedure, vague discomfort, generalized uneasiness, and precordial pain are common. Fluoroscopy shows an enlarged cardiac silhouette and diminished pulsations.

Cardiac tamponade should be suspected in a victim of recent chest trauma who appears to be in shock, especially when the venous pressure is elevated. When circumstances are deemed life-threatening, an immediate therapeutic trial of rapid infusion of fluid and diagnostic pericardiocentesis should be attempted. Otherwise, pericardiocentesis should be delayed until the presence of significant pericardial fluid can be demonstrated by prompt echocardiography. An exception to this rule is when tamponade occurs in the diagnostic laboratory; in this instance, when pressures are being monitored and fluoroscopy is available, the diagnosis can be established safely without echocardiographic confirmation.

Other causes of acute tamponade are cardiac rupture complicating acute MI and rupture of a dissecting hematoma of the proximal aorta. Although successful pericardiocentesis may relieve aortic tamponade and increase hemorrhage, a limited pericardiocentesis is reasonable if cardiac tamponade is severe enough to be considered a threat to survival. Finally, after cardiac surgery, dyspnea and fatigue should raise the suspicion of tamponade; in these instances, the effusion is often loculated, and echocardiographic and hemodynamic findings may be unreliable.

A large number of diseases may be associated with more slowly developing cardiac tamponade. In these instances, symptoms may be due to the underlying illness, the culpable pericardial disease, and/or the tamponade itself. Many patients with inflammatory pericarditis give a history of prodromal fever, myalgia, and arthralgia, and patients with neoplastic disease may have symptoms associated with the neoplasm and its treatment. The symptoms of cardiac compression include rapidly progressive dyspnea accompanied by fullness or tightness in the chest, occasionally with dysphagia; pericardial pain is often absent. The course may be less rapid, allowing time for an increase in abdominal girth and the rapid onset and progression of edema.

Pathophysiology

Elevated intrapericardial pressure exerted on the heart throughout the cardiac cycle, with only slight momentary relief when intrapericardial pressure falls (owing to the decrease in cardiac volume during ventricular ejection), is responsible for the pathophysiologic findings of cardiac tamponade. To understand the relation between venous and pericardial pressures in cardiac tamponade, it is useful to review the normal biphasic pattern of venous return. A surge of venous return occurs at the onset

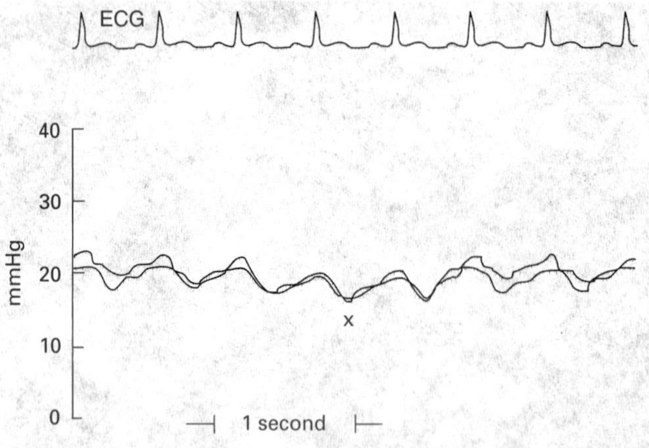

FIGURE 72-10 Simultaneous right atrial and pericardial pressures from a patient with severe cardiac tamponade. The pressures are elevated and equal to one another, and only the X descent on the right atrial tracing is present; the Y descent is absent. The pressures fall normally during inspiration. (From Shabetai R. Diseases of the pericardium. In: Alexander WA, Schlant R, Fuster V, et al., eds. *Hurst's The Heart,* 9th ed. New York: McGraw-Hill; 1998:2179. Reproduced with permission.)

of ventricular ejection and is accompanied by a small reduction in intrapericardial pressure. A second surge of venous return occurs in early diastole, when the tricuspid valve opens and atrial pressure decreases. In contrast, the venous return in cardiac tamponade is unimodal and is confined to ventricular systole, and in severe cardiac tamponade, venous return is halted in diastole, at a time when cardiac volume and intrapericardial pressure are maximal. Pericardial pressure and right atrial pressure are elevated above normal and are equal to each other (Fig. 72-10). The inspiratory fall in intrathoracic pressure is transmitted to the pericardial space and preserves the normal inspiratory increase in systemic venous return (Kussmaul's sign is absent).

Although systolic ventricular function is often supranormal, unrelieved extreme tamponade becomes fatal when venous pressure cannot increase to equal the pericardial pressure and maintain circulation. In severe cases, diminution of myocardial perfusion is aggravated by direct compression of the epicardial coronary arteries, abnormal transmyocardial distribution of blood flow, and, as a result, impaired ventricular systolic function.

PULSUS PARADOXUS

In healthy individuals, systolic blood pressure may decline by as much as 10 mmHg during quiet inspiration. Pulsus paradoxus is an exaggeration of this normal physiologic response. A number of normal and abnormal mechanisms combine to create pulsus paradoxus in cardiac tamponade. Inspiratory augmentation of systemic venous return in cardiac tamponade increases the volume of the right side of the heart at the expense of the left side. The volume of the left side of the heart is decreased, in part by bulging of the intraventricular septum from right to left (changing the size, shape, and compliance of the LV) and in part by increased transmural pericardial pressure (decreasing pulmonary venous return). However, the inspiratory expansion of the volume of the right side of the heart and the transit time of the resulting augmented right heart stroke volume are important in the genesis of pulsus paradoxus. In addition, the negative thoracic pressure produced by inspiration is transmitted to the aorta, increasing LV afterload and reducing stroke volume. LV stroke volume falls more sharply than normal in response to decreased ventricular filling in cardiac tamponade because the small ventricle is operating on the steep ascending limb of the Starling curve. Finally, inspiratory traction by the diaphragm on the taut pericardium, reflex changes in vascular resistance and cardiac contractility, and increased respiratory effort owing to pulmonary congestion contribute to the genesis of pulsus paradoxus.

Pulsus paradoxus appears when both ventricles fill against a common resistance. Therefore, when LV diastolic pressure is elevated by coexisting LV disease, pulsus paradoxus does not develop in cardiac tamponade.[29] Similarly, atrial septal defects and aortic regurgitation prevent reciprocal inspiratory changes in the filling of the two sides of the heart; therefore, in these conditions, cardiac tamponade can occur without pulsus paradoxus.[30]

Physical Findings

Physical findings are dictated by both the severity of cardiac tamponade and the time course of its development. Careful inspection of the jugular venous pulse waveform is essential for the diagnosis, although the venous pressure may be normal in early tamponade, whereas extreme elevations of venous pressure may go unrecognized in a recumbent or semirecumbent patient. Compression of the heart by pericardial fluid results in a characteristic loss of the atrial Y descent, but because of the decrease in intrapericardial pressure that occurs during ventricular ejection, the systolic atrial filling wave and the X descent are maintained. Kussmaul's sign, a failure of venous pressure to decrease during inspiration, is a sign of constriction and generally is not seen in pure cardiac tamponade.

An inspiratory decline of systolic arterial pressure exceeding 10 mmHg (pulsus paradoxus) may be detected with palpation of an arterial pulse, such as the femoral or brachial artery, and quantified by using sphygmomanometry by subtracting the pressure at which Korotkoff's sounds are heard only during expiration from the pressure at which sounds are heard through the respiratory cycle. The origin of the paradoxical pulse is complex and multifactorial, and pulsus paradoxus is neither sensitive nor specific for cardiac tamponade.[30] Nevertheless, in the appropriate clinical setting, pulsus paradoxus is a key finding that signifies cardiac tamponade, and its presence should be sought diligently.

Diagnostic and Imaging Studies

Low voltage on the ECG and/or electrical alternans should suggest cardiac tamponade. However, electrical alternans is insensitive, occurring in only about 20 percent of instances.[31] When effusion is massive, the heart swings freely within the pericardial sac and acquires a pendular, rotary motion that is associated with electrical alternans. When tamponade is suspected, an echocardiogram should be obtained unless even a brief delay might prove life-threatening. During inspiration, a greater than normal increase in RV dimension and a decrease in LV dimension occur in many cases of tamponade. These respiratory changes also accompany other conditions associated with pulsus paradoxus, such as chronic obstructive lung disease and pulmonary embolism.[32] Diastolic collapse of the RV, which is recognized as an abnormal posterior motion of the anterior RV wall during diastole (Fig. 72-11), signifies that pericardial pressure exceeds early diastolic RV pressure, i.e., that transmural RV diastolic pressure is negative (see also Chap. 13). Although this sign is a relatively sensitive and specific marker for tamponade, RV diastolic collapse is sensitive to alterations in ventricular loading conditions and may not be seen in the presence of RV hypertrophy. In addition, right heart chamber collapse occurs with smaller collections of fluid and higher pericardial pressures when there is coexisting LV dysfunction.[29] Late diastolic right atrial collapse is virtually 100 percent sensitive for tamponade but is less specific (Fig. 72-12). A duration of right atrial collapse exceeding one-third of the cardiac cycle increases specificity without sacrificing sensitivity.[33] Posterior loculated effusions after cardiac surgery have been reported to produce left atrial and LV diastolic collapse.[34,35] The value of transesophageal echocardiography has been recognized in the detection and treatment of unusual cases of cardiac tamponade.[36] In patients with unexplained hypotension who are undergoing transesophageal echo, a diagnosis of a nonventricular limitation to cardiac output was associated with improved survival in the intensive care unit compared with a diagnosis of ventricular disease or hypovolemia/low systemic vascular resistance.[37]

During cardiac tamponade, tricuspid and pulmonary flow velocities measured by Doppler echocardiography (Fig. 72-13) increase markedly with inspiration, and mitral and aortic valve flow velocities decrease significantly compared with normal control patients and patients with asymptomatic effusions.[38] Changes in the pattern of venous flow (reflecting the predominance of systolic flow) and exaggerated respiratory variations of venous flow velocities (Fig. 72-14) also are seen in cardiac tamponade.[39] Indeed, abnormal venous flow had a good correlation with clinical tamponade with greater sensitivity than RV diastolic collapse and greater specificity than right atrial collapse.[40]

Cardiac Catheterization

The diagnosis of cardiac tamponade is confirmed by right heart catheterization. The right atrial, pulmonary capillary wedge, and pulmonary artery diastolic pressures are elevated, usually between 10 and 30 mmHg, and are equal within 4 to 5 mmHg (Fig. 72-15). Pericardial pressure is elevated and is equal to right atrial pressure; the degree of elevation is related to both the severity of tamponade and the patient's intravascular volume status (Fig. 72-16). The right atrial and wedge pressure tracings reveal an attenuated or absent Y descent. Cardiac output is reduced, and systemic vascular resistance is elevated. Equal elevation of diastolic pressures also may be seen with dilated cardiomyopathy and with RV infarction. Neither Kussmaul's sign nor the early ventricular diastolic dip and plateau (i.e., the "square root" sign) characteristic of pericardial constriction is seen in tamponade.

Management of Cardiac Tamponade

Removal of small amounts of pericardial fluid (~50 mL) produces considerable symptomatic and hemodynamic improvement because of the steep pericardial pressure-volume relation. Unless there is concomitant cardiac disease or coexisting constriction (i.e., effusive-constrictive pericarditis), removal of all the pericardial fluid normalizes pericardial, atrial, ventricular diastolic, and arterial pressures and cardiac output.

Unless the situation is immediately life-threatening, pericardiocentesis should be performed by experienced staff in a facility equipped for hemodynamic monitoring. The advantages of needle pericardiocentesis include the ability to perform careful

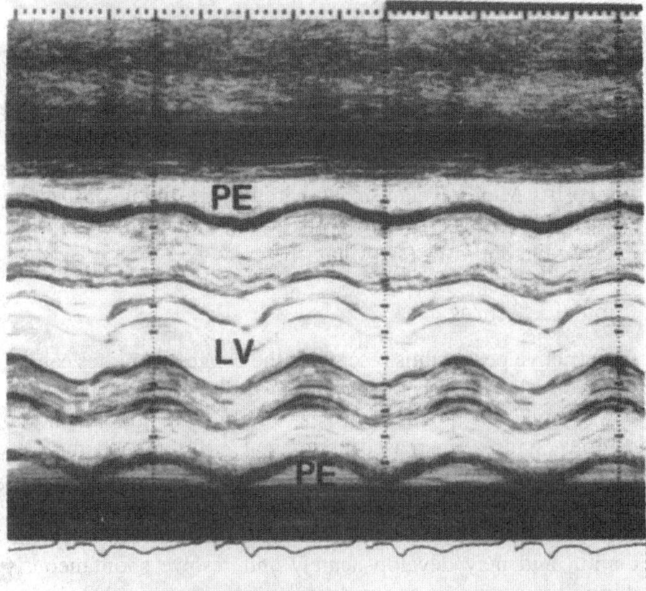

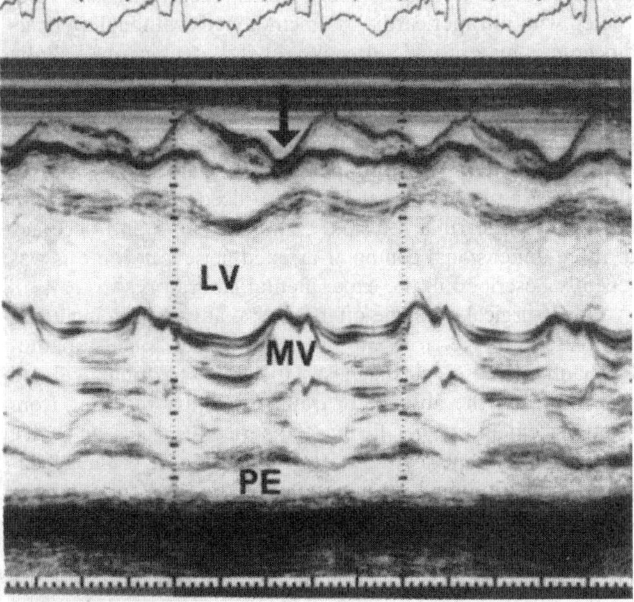

FIGURE 72-11 M-mode echocardiograms of pericardial effusion. The effusion (PE) appears as an echo-free space surrounding the heart. The effusion on the left does not cause cardiac compression. The effusion on the right demonstrates right ventricular diastolic collapse (*arrow*), evident as abnormal motion of the anterior free wall of the right ventricle that occurs after the mitral valve (MV) opens. LV-left ventricle. (From Hoit BD. Pericardial disease and pericardial heart disease. In: O' Rourke RA, ed. *Stein's Internal Medicine*, 5th ed. St. Louis, Missouri: Mosby-Year Book; 1998:273. Reproduced with permission.)

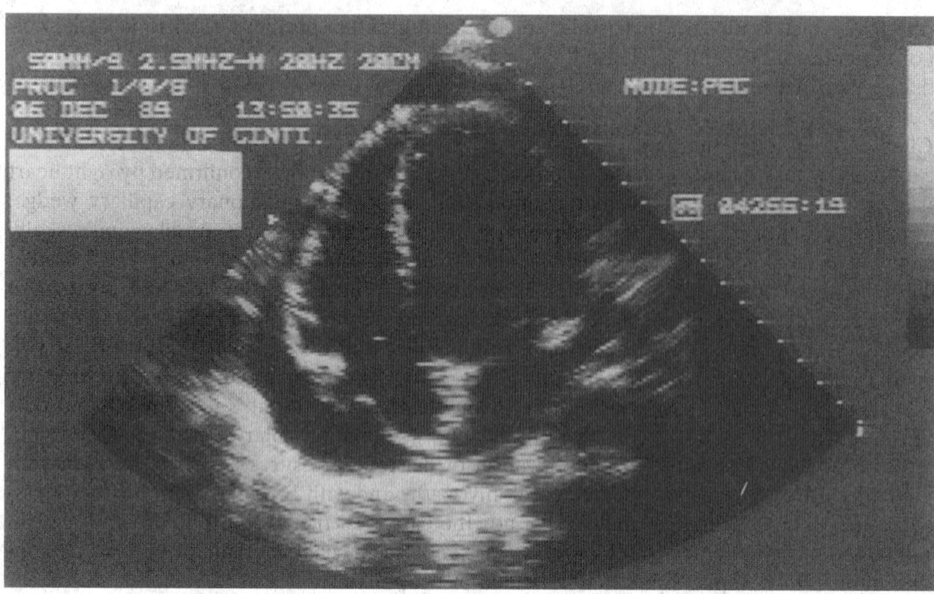

FIGURE 72-12 Two-dimensional echocardiogram in the apical four-chamber view. During late diastole, there is inversion of the lateral wall of the right atrium. (From Hoit BD. Imaging the pericardium. *Cardiol Clin* 1990; 8:593. Reproduced with permission.)

hemodynamic measurements and relatively simple logistic and personnel requirements. The safety of the procedure has been improved by using 2-D echo guidance.[41] A catheter can be advanced over a guidewire into the pericardial space and remain there for several days; sclerosing agents, steroids, urokinase, and specific chemotherapeutic agents may be given through the catheter.[42,43] In a pilot study, intrapericardial instillation of cisplatin for 24 hours prevented recurrence of a hemodynamically significant pericardial effusion after 6 to 12 months in 14 out of 15 patients with a neoplastic effusion; in 12 out of 14 patients with autoreactive pericarditis, recurrence was prevented with intrapericardial triamcinolone.[25] Although pericardiocentesis may provide effective relief, percutaneous balloon pericardiotomy, subxiphoid pericardiotomy, or the surgical creation of a pleuropericardial or peritoneal-pericardial window[44,45] may be required. Nevertheless, in one retrospective review, pericardiocentesis with intrapericardial sclerotherapy was as effective as an open surgical drainage procedure in patients with malignant pericardial effusion.[46] The feasibility and accuracy of three-dimensional computer-assisted pericardiocentesis was recently described in the experimental laboratory.[47]

Open surgical drainage offers several advantages, including complete drainage, access to pericardial tissue for histopathologic and microbiologic diagnoses, the ability to drain loculated effusions, and the absence of traumatic injury resulting from blind placement of a needle into the pericardial sac. The choice between needle pericardiocentesis and surgical drainage depends on institutional resources and physician experience, the etiology of the effusion, the need for diagnostic tissue samples, and the prognosis of the patient. Needle pericardiocentesis is often the best option when the etiology is known and/or the diagnoses of tamponade is in question, and surgical drainage is optimal when the presence of tamponade is certain but the etiology is unclear. It should be recognized that surgical approaches (subxiphoid pericardiotomy and thoracoscopic drainage) can be performed using local anesthesia with little attendant morbidity. Irrespective of the method of retrieval, pericardial fluid should be sent for smear, culture, and cytology.

Fluids should be given to patients with cardiac tamponade who are awaiting pericardial drainage in an effort to expand the intravascular volume. Dobutamine or nitroprusside may be used to increase cardiac output after the blood volume has been expanded, but only as a temporizing measure. Vagal reflexes complicating tamponade and pericardiocentesis are treated with atropine. Positive-pressure breathing should be avoided, and if present, metabolic acidosis should be corrected.

Recurrent effusions may be treated by repeat pericardiocentesis, sclerotherapy with tetracycline, surgical creation of a pericardial window, or pericardiectomy. A pericardial window usually is performed in patients with malignant effusions, and pericardiectomy may be required for recurrent effusions in dialysis patients. In critically ill patients, a pericardial window may be created percutaneously with a balloon catheter.[48,49]

CONSTRICTIVE PERICARDITIS

Constrictive pericarditis is a condition in which a thickened, scarred, and often calcified pericardium limits diastolic filling of the ventricles. Although acute pericarditis from most causes may eventuate in constrictive pericarditis, the most common antecedents are idiopathic conditions, cardiac trauma and surgery, tuberculosis and other infectious diseases, neoplasms (particularly lung and breast), radiation therapy, renal failure, and connective tissue diseases. Rare causes include Dressler's syndrome, sarcoidosis, Whipple's disease, amyloidosis, and dermatomyositis. Mulibrey nanism is a hereditary form of constrictive pericarditis that is associated with abnormalities of the *mu*scle, *li*ver, *br*ain, and *ey*es (see Chap. 10).

Clinical Features

Constrictive pericarditis resembles the congestive states caused by myocardial disease and chronic liver disease. Patients generally complain of fatigue, dyspnea, weight gain, abdominal discomfort, nausea, increased abdominal girth, and edema. Although symptoms usually develop over years, they progress over a period of months in patients with subacute constrictive pericarditis after trauma, cardiac surgery, and mediastinal irradiation and may develop acutely and resolve spontaneously during the course of pericarditis.[50]

Physical Findings

Physical findings include ascites, hepatosplenomegaly, edema, and, in long-standing cases, severe wasting. This general appearance often leads to an erroneous diagnosis of hepatic cirrhosis. However, misdiagnosis is avoided through a careful examination of the neck veins. In constrictive pericarditis, the venous pressure is elevated and displays deep Y and often deep X descents. The venous pressure fails to decrease with inspiration (Kussmaul's sign), but frank inspiratory swelling of the neck veins is uncommon. Kussmaul's sign lacks specificity, as it is seen also in cases of restrictive cardiomyopathy, RV failure and infarction, and tricuspid stenosis.[51] The heart is often normal-sized, and when it is not, enlargement is modest. A pericardial knock that is similar in timing to the third heart sound is pathognomonic but occurs infrequently.[51,52] Pulsus paradoxus may occur with associated pericardial effusion (effusive-constrictive pericarditis). Except in severe cases, the arterial blood pressure is normal.

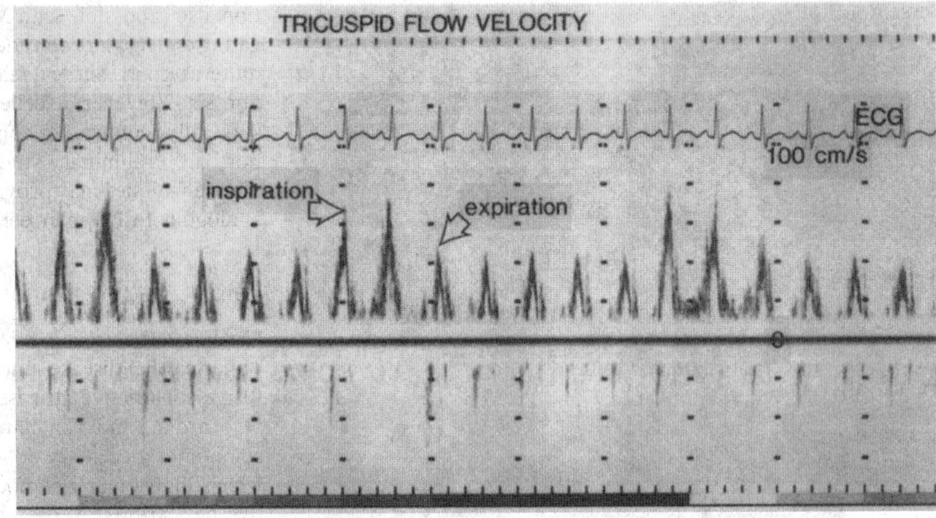

A

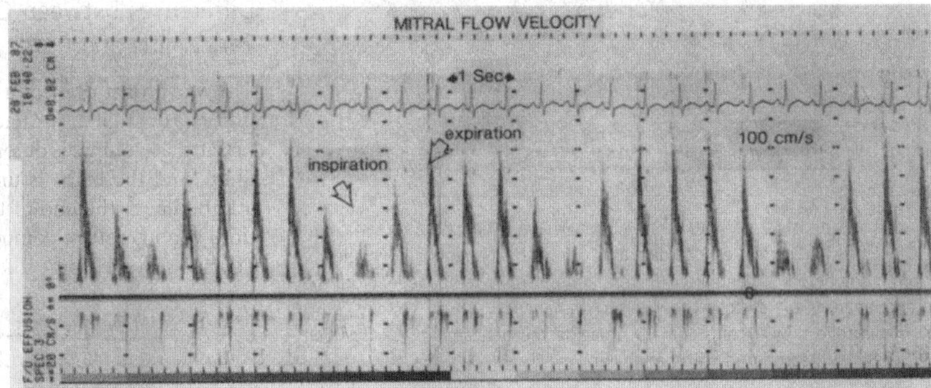

B

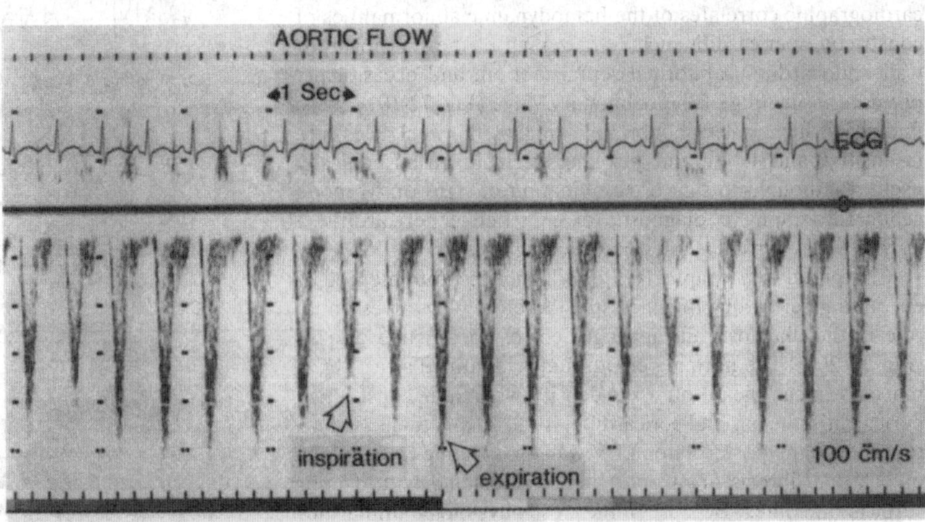

C

FIGURE 72-13 Doppler echocardiogram in a patient with cardiac tamponade. Note the inspiratory increase of tricuspid flow velocities (*A*) and the expiratory increase of mitral (*B*) and aortic (*C*) flow velocities. (From Hoit BD. Imaging the pericardium. *Cardiol Clin* 1990; 8:594. Reproduced with permission.)

Diagnostic and Imaging Studies

Low QRS voltage, nonspecific T-wave changes, and P mitrale are common, but the ECG findings are nonspecific (Fig. 72-17). Atrial fibrillation is seen in approximately one-third of cases, and atrial flutter is seen less often, although the exact percentage of atrial arrhythmias depends on the duration of constriction.

The cardiac silhouette may be normal or enlarged. Pericardial calcification is present in less than half the cases seen in the United States and Europe. Pericardial calcification may be seen with chronic adhesive pericarditis in the absence of constriction, but then it is usually less dense and has a more patchy distribution (Fig. 72-18).

Pericardial thickening and calcification and abnormal ventricular filling produce characteristic changes on the M-mode echocardiogram.[53] Increased pericardial thickness is suggested by parallel motion of the epicardium and parietal pericardium, which are sep-

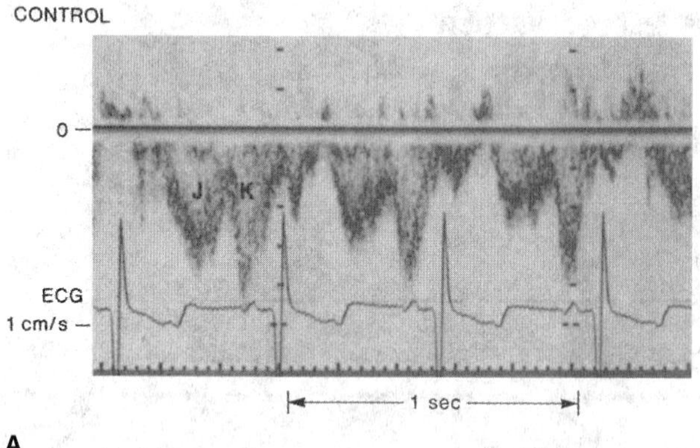

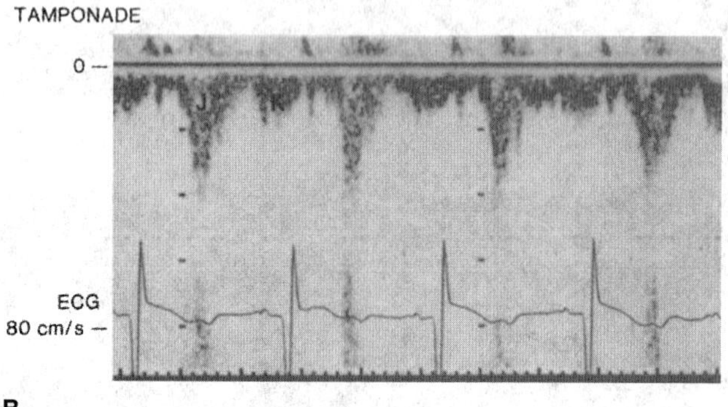

FIGURE 72-14 Doppler echocardiograms of pulmonary venous flow velocity from a dog before (*A*) and after (*B*) creation of cardiac tamponade. Note the predominance of systolic flow after tamponade. J = systolic flow; K = diastolic flow. (From Hoit BD. Imaging the pericardium. *Cardiol Clin* 1990; 8:595. Reproduced with permission.)

arated by a relatively echo-free space at least 1 mm thick. Echocardiographic correlates of the hemodynamic abnormalities of constrictive pericarditis include flattening of the LV posterior wall endocardium, abnormal septal motion, and occasionally premature opening of the pulmonary valve (Fig. 72-19). These findings, which reflect abnormal filling of the ventricles, are insensitive and subtle and lack the specificity to be clinically useful. Although no sign or combination of signs on M-mode echocardiography is diagnostic of constrictive pericarditis, a normal study virtually rules out the diagnosis.[53]

Computed tomography (CT) is a highly accurate method of evaluating pericardial thickness and therefore plays an essential role in the diagnosis and management of constrictive disease (Fig. 72-20).[54] The normal pericardium is identified as a 1- to 2-mm curvilinear line of soft tissue density, whereas in constrictive pericarditis, the parietal pericardium is 4 to 20 mm thick. Failure to visualize the posterolateral LV wall on dynamic CT suggests myocardial fibrosis or atrophy and is associated with a poor surgical outcome.[55] Because of the close physiologic similarities of constrictive pericarditis and restrictive cardiomyopathy, increased pericardial thickness detected by tomographic scanning is the most reliable means of distinguishing between the two disorders, as normal pericardial thickness excludes most cases of constrictive pericarditis. CT also is useful in planning pericardiectomy because of its ability to define the distribution of pericardial thickening.[56]

Accurate definition of pericardial thickness and its distribution also is possible with MRI (Fig. 72-21).[27,57] Unlike CT, ECG gating is necessary for adequate visualization, resolution is not quite as good, and calcification is difficult to distinguish from fibrosis. However, excellent diagnostic accuracy in identifying surgically confirmed constrictive pericarditis has been reported.[58] Preliminary studies suggest that phase velocity mapping techniques may provide additional diagnostic information, analogous to Doppler echo.

Cardiac Catheterization

Cardiac catheterization is used to confirm the clinical suspicion of pericardial disease, uncover occult constriction, diagnose effusive-constrictive disease, and identify associated coronary, myocardial, and valvular disease. Endomyocardial biopsy is sometimes necessary to exclude restrictive cardiomyopathy, which shares many hemodynamic abnormalities with constrictive pericarditis.

Differences between Constrictive Pericarditis and Cardiac Tamponade

The waveform of venous pressure in constrictive pericarditis differs from that in cardiac tamponade. In constrictive pericarditis, cardiac volume is determined by the thickened, rigid pericardium, and the heart is unable to exceed this volume, which is attained near the end of the first third of diastole. During ejection, venous return commences unimpeded, and therefore, the normal systolic surge of venous return is preserved. Cardiac

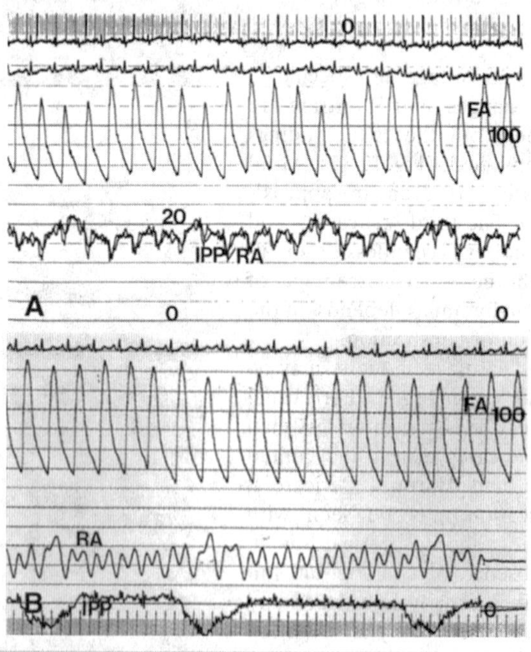

FIGURE 72-15 Hemodynamic record from a patient with cardiac tamponade before (*A*) and after (*B*) pericardiocentesis. *A*. Pulsus paradoxus is evident from the femoral artery (FA) pressure tracing. Note the absent Y descent on the right atrial (RA) tracing and the equal and elevated RA and pericardial (IPP) pressures. *B*. After removal of pericardial fluid, pericardial and right atrial pressures decrease and the pulsus paradoxus disappears. (Courtesy of Noble O Fowler, MD. From Hoit BD. Pericardial disease and pericardial heart disease. In: O'Rourke RA, ed. *Stein's Internal Medicine*, 5th ed. Mosby-Year Book;1998:273. Reproduced with permission.)

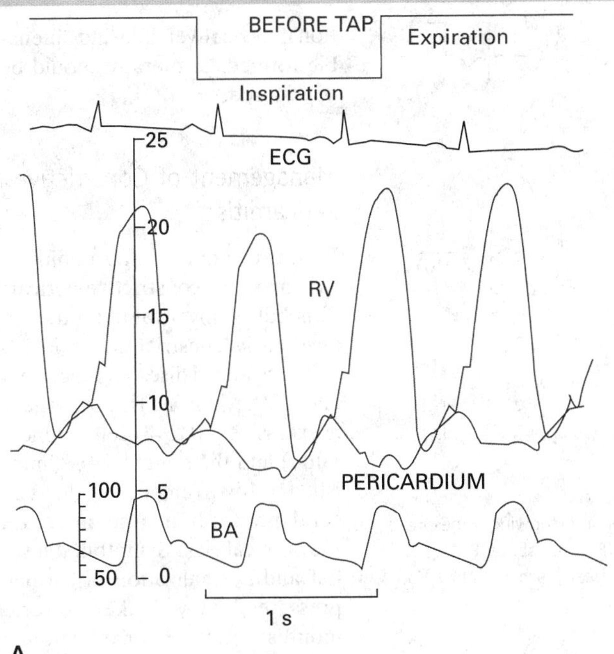

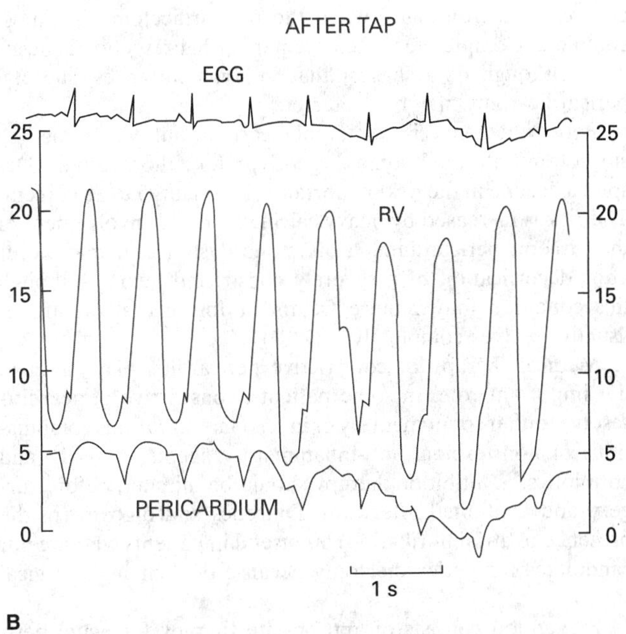

FIGURE 72-16 *A.* Low-pressure cardiac tamponade. Right ventricular (RV) diastolic pressure is only slightly elevated but is equal to pericardial pressure. Hypotension and pulsus paradoxus are absent. *B.* After pericardiocentesis, pericardial pressure is consistently lower than ventricular diastolic pressure. (From Shabetai R. Diseases of the pericardium. In Alexander WA, Schlant R, Fuster V, et al., eds. *Hurst's The Heart,* 9th ed. New York: McGraw-Hill; 1998:2185. Reproduced with permission.)

compression remains insignificant at end systole (unlike cardiac tamponade), so that when the tricuspid valve opens, blood fills the ventricles at a supranormal rate. Thus, in constrictive pericarditis, the venous return is biphasic, but with a diastolic component greater than or equal to the systolic component.

Unlike cardiac tamponade, the intrapericardial space is obliterated in constrictive pericarditis. As a result, during inspiration, the decreased intrathoracic pressure is not transmitted to the heart, venous pressure does not fall, and systemic venous return fails to increase. Another important distinction from cardiac tamponade is that early diastolic filling is faster than normal in constrictive pericarditis, and consequently, the ventricular diastolic pressure is characterized by a dip in early diastole (Fig. 72-22). By the end of the rapid filling phase, the ventricles are completely filled and the ventricular diastolic pressure remains unchanged and elevated for the remainder of diastole. The resultant pattern of ventricular diastolic pressure in constrictive pericarditis is referred to as the "dip-and-plateau pattern" or the "square-root sign."

In contrast to cardiac tamponade, early diastolic filling in constrictive pericarditis is unrestrained, and only at the end of the first third of diastole does the stiff pericardium abruptly restrict ventricular filling. As a result, ventricular pressure falls rapidly in early diastole and subsequently rises abruptly to an elevated level, where it remains until the next ventricular systole. End-diastolic ventricular pressures and mean atrial pressures are elevated and nearly equal (within 5 mmHg), and end-diastolic volumes and, consequently, stroke volume and cardiac output are reduced. These pathophysiologic changes are responsible for the hemodynamic and physical findings that characterize constrictive pericarditis.[51]

Pulsus paradoxus is much less common in constrictive pericarditis than it is in cardiac tamponade because in constrictive pericarditis, inspiratory increases in venous return and in the volume of the right side of the heart seldom occur, and the position of the ventricular septum relative to the two ventricles is not as dramatically altered.

Systolic LV function is usually unimpaired in both constrictive pericarditis and cardiac tamponade. Long-standing calcific constrictive pericarditis may invade the myocardium and coronary vessels, leading to conduction disturbances and impaired ventricular function.

Syndromes of Constrictive Pericarditis

Classic *chronic constrictive pericarditis* is encountered less frequently than it was in the past, whereas *subacute constrictive pericarditis* is becoming more common. In the latter syndrome, pericardial calcification is uncommon and the course may span a matter of weeks to a few years. *Postoperative constrictive pericarditis* is an important cause of constriction, with a reported incidence of 0.2 percent[59]; this incidence is surprisingly low considering that in these operations the pericardium is subject to cellular injury and is exposed to proinflammatory substances such as blood and local hypothermia.

Occult constrictive pericarditis requires a fluid challenge for detection.[60] In the first series reported, the patients complained of nondescript chest pain, for which they underwent cardiac catheterization and coronary arteriography. Although hemodynamic studies revealed normal basal atrial and ventricular pressures, the right atrial pressure waveform assumed the characteristics of constrictive pericarditis and the diastolic pressures in the two ventricles became equal after a rapid infusion (10 min) of approximately 1 L of saline solution. Histologic examination confirmed the surgical findings of a thickened and fibrosed pericardium. Rapid, large fluid challenges at cardiac catheterization should be administered with caution; furthermore, the induction of hemodynamic changes suggesting constrictive pericarditis by

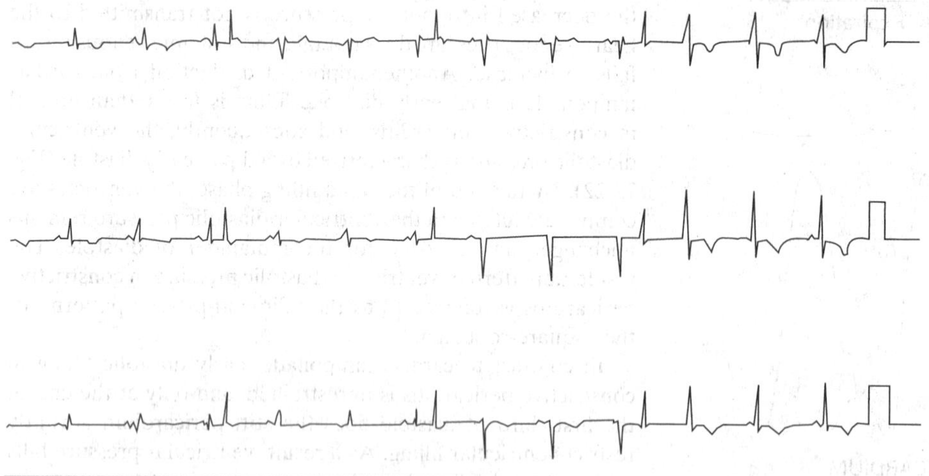

FIGURE 72-17 Electrocardiogram of a patient with tuberculous constrictive pericarditis showing widespread inversed polarity of the T waves. Leads are mounted in the conventional sequence. (From Shabetai R. Diseases of the pericardium. In Alexander WA, Schlant R, Fuster V, et al., eds. *Hurst's The Heart*, 9th ed. New York: McGraw-Hill; 1998:2188. Reproduced with permission.)

this technique should seldom, if ever, be taken alone as an indication for pericardiectomy.

Localized constrictive pericarditis is rare, but occasionally a localized band constricts the inflow or outflow region of one or more of the cardiac chambers. The clinical picture then simulates valve disease or venous obstruction. Evidence of *transient* (*acute*) *constriction* may occur in ~15 percent of patients with acute effusive pericarditis.[61] Therefore, before one proceeds with pericardiectomy, the possibility that pericardial constriction may be reversible and amenable to medical therapy should be considered.

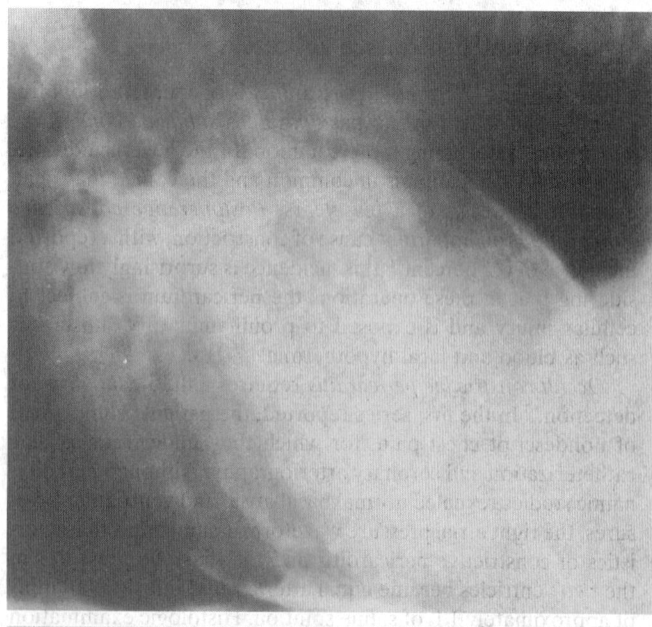

FIGURE 72-18 Calcification of the pericardium seen on a lateral chest radiograph in a patient with chronic constrictive pericarditis. (Courtesy of Ralph Shabetai, MD. From Hoit BD. Imaging the pericardium. *Cardiol Clin* 1990; 8:595. Reproduced with permission.)

Management of Constrictive Pericarditis

Pericardiectomy is the definitive treatment for constrictive pericarditis but is unwarranted either in very early constriction or in severe, advanced disease (functional class IV), when the risk of surgery is excessive (30 to 40 percent mortality) and the benefits are diminished.[62] Involvement of the visceral pericardium also increases the surgical risk. Symptomatic relief and normalization of cardiac pressures may take several months after pericardiectomy; they occur sooner when the operation is carried out before the disease is too chronic and when the pericardiectomy is almost complete. Complete or extensive pericardial resection is desirable, although data suggest that in some instances, subtotal pericardiectomy may be preferred.[63]

Pericardiectomy is commonly carried out via a median sternotomy, although some surgeons prefer a thoracotomy. Despite a decline in the risk of mortality, it remains 5 to 15 percent. The risk is increased by heavy calcification and involvement of the visceral pericardium. LV systolic dysfunction may occur after decortication of a severely constricted heart. Although this condition may require treatment for several months, it usually resolves completely.

Medical therapy of constrictive pericarditis plays a small but important role. In some patients, constrictive pericarditis resolves either spontaneously or in response to various combinations of nonsteroidal anti-inflammatory agents, steroids, and antibiotics.[50] Antibiotic therapy should be initiated before surgery and continued afterward. Diuretics and digoxin (in the presence of atrial fibrillation) are useful in patients who are not candidates for pericardiectomy because of their high surgical risk.

Prevention consists of appropriate therapy for acute pericarditis and adequate pericardial drainage. Although urokinase instillation is promising, corticosteroids are often ineffective.

EFFUSIVE-CONSTRICTIVE PERICARDITIS

Effusive-constrictive pericarditis occurs when pericardial fluid accumulates between the thickened, fibrotic parietal pericardium and visceral pericardium. Neoplasia, chest irradiation, infection, idiopathic pericarditis, and connective tissue diseases are common antecedents. Transient effusive-constrictive pericarditis may complicate chemotherapy.[64] The hemodynamic features are those of cardiac tamponade before, and constrictive pericarditis after, pericardiocentesis. Thus, removal of pericardial fluid fails to lower atrial and ventricular diastolic pressures, but the previously attenuated or absent atrial Y descent becomes prominent (Fig. 72-23).

SPECIFIC FORMS OF PERICARDIAL HEART DISEASE

Idiopathic Pericarditis

Acute pericarditis is most often idiopathic and is typically a self-limited disease lasting 2 to 6 weeks.[65] Recurrence occurs in 25 percent of cases and occasionally proves resistant to therapy. Small pericardial effusions occur commonly, but cardiac tamponade is unusual. Heart failure caused by associated myocarditis and constrictive pericarditis are uncommon. These complications usually can be detected by clinical and echocardiographic evaluation. The clinical course and prognosis of individuals with pericarditis are otherwise determined largely by the presence and nature of any underlying disease.

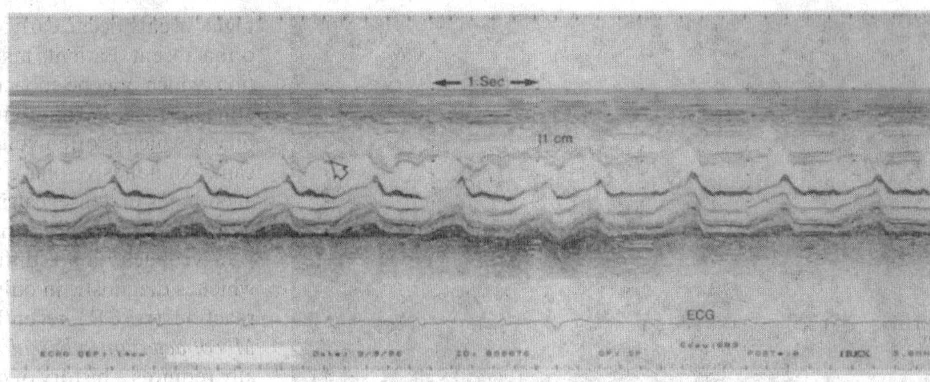

FIGURE 72-19 M-mode echocardiogram from a patient with constrictive pericarditis. An abrupt posterior motion of the septum begins after the onset of atrial systole. This atrial systolic notch is not seen on premature or paced beats. Note also the thickened pericardium and flat posterior wall in middle and late diastole. (From Tei C, Child JS, Tanaka H, et al. Atrial systolic notch on the interventricular septum echogram: An echocardiographic sign of constrictive pericarditis. *J Am Coll Cardiol* 1983; 1:908. Reproduced with permission.)

Infectious Pericarditis

VIRAL PERICARDITIS

Viral pericarditis is the most common infectious type, although a definitive diagnosis from acute and convalescent (3 weeks) viral neutralizing antibodies is generally not helpful in a sporadic case of pericarditis. Viral isolation from pericardial fluid and in situ hybridization techniques have been used to identify a specific etiology.[20,66] However, viral infection often is presumed rather than proved, and many cases are classified as idiopathic. Epicardial biopsy via a pericardioscope is a promising investigative technique for establishing the etiology of acute pericarditis. Common viral infections causing acute pericarditis are those resulting from echovirus and coxsackie virus; however, a great many different viruses may cause pericarditis (Table 72-2).

BACTERIAL PERICARDITIS

Bacterial (purulent) pericarditis most often is caused by streptococci, staphylococci, and gram-negative rods; *Haemophilus influenzae* is an important cause in children.[67] The increasing frequency of cardiac surgery and instrumentation, selection-induced changes in the flora responsible for hospital-acquired infections, and the prolonged survival of immunocompromised hosts (HIV, steroids) have changed the incidence and bacterial spectrum of purulent pericarditis. Pericardial involvement often is unrecognized when it complicates systemic infection; unusually high fever and white blood cell counts are clues to the presence of pericarditis. Children and immunosuppressed patients of all ages are most vulnerable, and the characteristic features of acute pericarditis are frequently absent. The course of bacterial pericarditis is fulminant, often presenting with cardiac tamponade; adhesive and constrictive pericarditis are common sequelae in survivors and may develop suddenly and early.[67,68] However,

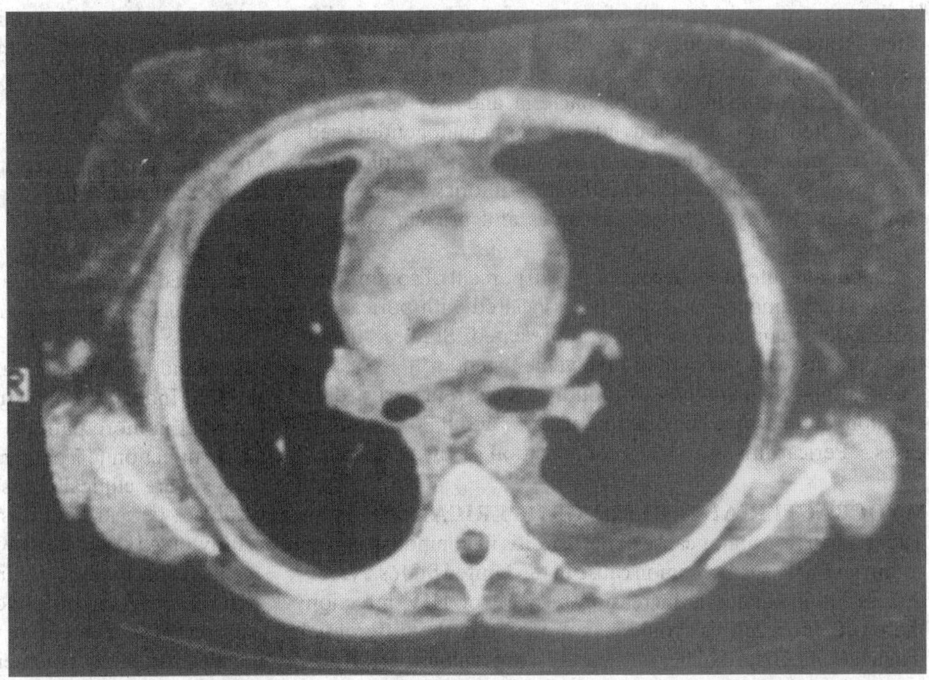

FIGURE 72-20 Computed tomogram from a patient with constrictive pericarditis. The diffusely thickened pericardium is bordered by low-intensity epicardial and mediastinal fat. (Courtesy of Dr. N. O. Fowler. From Hoit BD. Imaging the pericardium. *Cardiol Clin* 1990; 8:597. Reproduced with permission.)

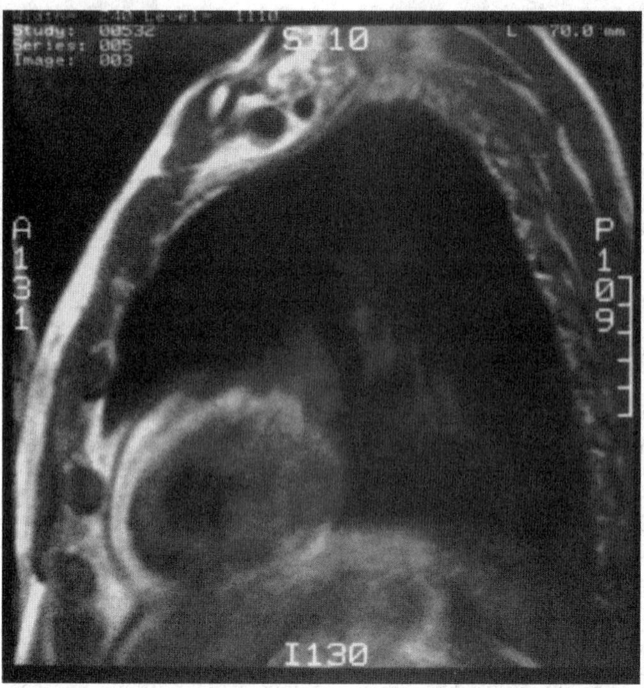

FIGURE 72-21 MRI scan (spin-echo image) from a patient with constrictive pericarditis. The pericardium is viewed as a line of low signal intensity (black) sandwiched between higher-intensity epicardial and pericardial fat (white). Note the regional variation of pericardial thickness, which is normally 1 to 2 mm. (From Hoit BD. Pericardial disease and pericardial heart disease. In: O'Rourke RA, ed. *Stein's Internal Medicine*, 5th ed. St. Louis, Missouri: Mosby-Year Book;1998:273. Reproduced with permission.)

pericarditis complicating systemic infection and sepsis may go unrecognized and misdiagnosed.[69] Many patients lack the typical findings of pericarditis, and the diagnosis of purulent pericarditis often is made either at autopsy or after cardiac tamponade develops; empyema is a common antecedent.[67] Purulent pericarditis rarely is caused by anaerobic bacteria, and the few reported cases resulted from contiguous infection or hematogenous seeding.[70] Bacterial pericarditis is treated with surgical exploration and drainage and appropriate systemic antibiotics. Fibrinolytics may be used to lyse fibrous adhesions and prevent constrictive pericarditis.[71–73]

Legionella infections account for ~10 percent of community-acquired pneumonias and may be associated with pericarditis more often than previously was appreciated. Studies suggest that patients with pericardial involvement tend to be younger and healthier than are those without it.[74] Recurrent pericarditis, effusion, and chronic constriction occur in about 20 percent of cases.[75] Pericarditis is an early complication of Lyme disease.[76]

MYOCBACTERIAL AND FUNGAL PERICARDITIS

Tuberculosis is a major cause of pericarditis in nonindustrialized countries but is an uncommon cause in the United States. Nevertheless, its incidence is increasing because of HIV infection; therefore, tuberculosis should be considered in the differential diagnosis of pericardial heart disease.[77] Tuberculous pericarditis results from hematogenous spread of primary tuberculosis or from the breakdown of infected mediastinal lymph nodes; therefore, affected individuals generally lack the typical symptoms and signs of pulmonary tuberculosis. Fever, weight loss, and night sweats occur early; pericardial pain and friction rubs are often absent. Patients may present with tamponade or constriction, which may be subacute. A fibrinous pericarditis with caseating necrosis and mononuclear infiltrate gives rise to an effusive phase, which is often voluminous and hemodynamically significant. An adhesive phase follows resolution of the effusion and eventuates in dense, calcific adhesions with clinical constriction in nearly 50 percent of patients.

Mycobacteria are difficult to culture from pericardial fluid, which is diagnostic in only one-third of cases; polymerase chain reaction (rtPCR) recently was used to amplify and identify *Mycobacterium tuberculosis.*[78] A presumptive diagnosis generally requires a history of contact and/or purified protein derivative conversion (although the latter lacks sensitivity and specificity). Gadolinium-enhanced MRI may be useful in early diagnosis.[79] Increased adenosine deaminase activity in pericardial fluid is supportive. However, the diagnosis of tuberculous pericarditis is based on (1) histologic identification, (2) culture of *M. tuberculosis,* (3) pericarditis with proven extracardiac tuberculosis, or (4) pericardial effusion responsive to antituberculosis therapy.

Early pericardiectomy has been recommended by some researchers in all cases of tuberculosis pericarditis, but the long-term (16 years) prognosis of patients without cardiac compression during the acute illness who are treated with medical therapy alone is excellent.[80] Multiple-drug therapy and corticosteroids are effective in tuberculous pericarditis, whereas atypical mycobacterial infections (especially *M. avium-intracellulare*) may be resistant to treatment. Patients with tuberculous pericarditis should receive triple-drug therapy (isoniazid, rifampin, and streptomycin or ethambutol) for a minimum of 9 months. Corticosteroids may be useful if pericardial effusion persists or recurs during therapy; pericardiectomy may be necessary for recurrent cardiac tamponade. Patients should be observed for constriction; up to half these patients will require pericardiectomy.[81] In contrast, pericarditis complicating deep fungal infection (histoplasmosis, coccidioidomyocosis) may be immunologic, resolve spontaneously, and not require specific therapy. Surgical decompression and specific antifungal therapy may be necessary for disseminated infection with *Candida, Aspergillus, Actinomycetes,* and *Nocardia.*

AIDS PERICARDITIS

Acquired immunodeficiency syndrome (AIDS) is an important cause of pericardial heart disease. Typically, pericardial effusions are small and asymptomatic in outpatients, but large effusions and tamponade are common in hospitalized patients with AIDS. Indeed, in one study, a moderate or large effusion was present in more patients with symptomatic than asymptomatic HIV infection (17 percent versus 2 percent), and most of these cases were clinically unsuspected.[82] The incidence and prevalence of pericardial effusion in a prospective, 5-year follow-up study of AIDS patients were high (11 percent/year and 5 percent, respectively).[83] A literature review of echocardiographic and autopsy series found an average incidence of pericardial disease of 21 percent.[84]

Pericardial involvement may be due to associated malignancies (e.g., lymphoma and Kaposi's sarcoma), viruses (including HIV) and opportunistic infections (e.g., mycobacteria, cytomegalovirus, *Nocardia,* and cryptococci) and, irrespective of its cause, predicts a poor prognosis in patients with HIV infection.[85]

Large, symptomatic pericardial effusion in patients with HIV infection should be aggressively investigated, as two-thirds of these cases have an identifiable cause.[84] Tamponade in patients with HIV is mycobacterial (*M. tuberculosis* or *avium-intracellulare*) in origin in approximately one-third of patients.[84]

In 68 patients with HIV infection prospectively admitted to the intensive care unit, only 5 had evidence of cardiac disease, but 35 had echocardiographic abnormalities (20 effusions, 2 with tamponade, 15 cases of left ventricular dysfunction, and 4 valvular abnormalities).[86] The presence of an effusion was associated with greater 6-month mortality in patients with AIDS (96 percent versus 36 percent); interestingly, an asymptomatic pericardial effusion may signal end-stage HIV disease, independent of the CD4 count and albumin level.[83]

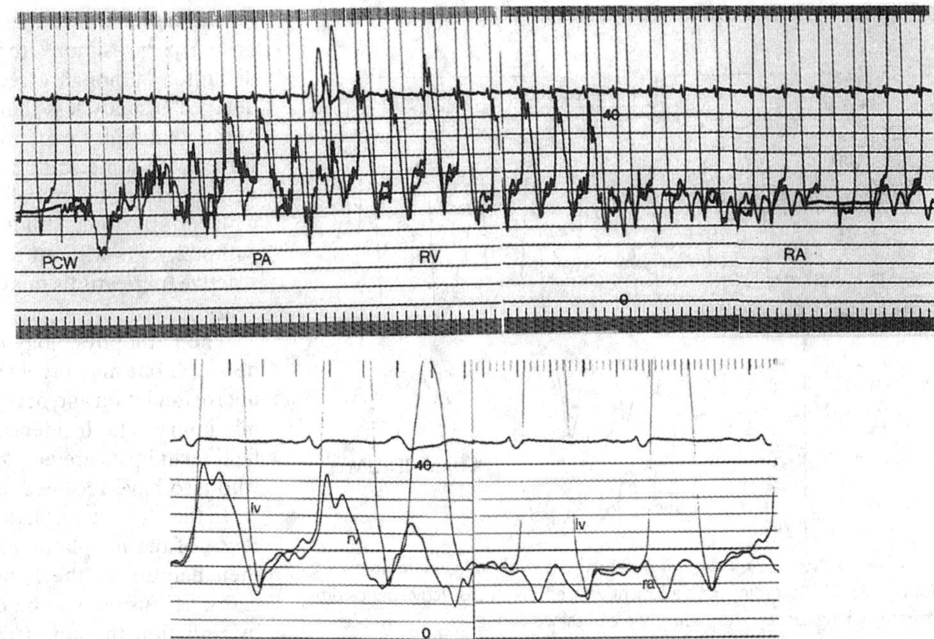

FIGURE 72-22 Hemodynamic record of a patient with surgically proven constrictive pericarditis. *Top*. Slow paper speed recording of high-gain left ventricular (LV) pressure and simultaneous right heart pullback from pulmonary capillary wedge (PCW) to pulmonary artery (PA), right ventricle (RV), and right atrium (RA). *Bottom*. Fast paper speed recording of LV and simultaneous RV and RA pressure tracings. Note the increased and equal atrial and diastolic pressures, the prominent X and Y descents on the RA tracing, and the dip and plateau on the RV and LV tracings during longer diastoles. (Courtesy of Peter J. Engel, MD. From Hoit BD. Pericardial disease and pericardial heart disease. In: O'Rourke RA, ed. *Stein's Internal Medicine*, 5th ed. St. Louis, Missouri: Mosby-Year Book; 1998:273. Reproduced with permission.)

Neoplastic Pericarditis

Metastatic neoplasia remains the leading cause of pericardial disease in hospitalized patients, most often in patients with lung or breast cancer, melanoma, lymphoma, and acute leukemia. Many cases are asymptomatic and are found only incidentally at autopsy, but others cause symptoms and may progress to cardiac tamponade. Primary cardiac tumors may invade the pericardium directly.

Primary mesothelioma of the pericardium is a rare and highly lethal tumor.[87] Signs and symptoms are nonspecific, and chest radiography and echocardiography are insensitive for its detection; CT and MRI are the most promising diagnostic tests. Other primary tumors of the pericardium are quite rare.

In patients with elevated jugular pressure and an intrathoracic mass, an important inclusion in the differential diagnosis is the superior vena cava syndrome. In this disorder, the characteristic pulsations of the jugular veins are not observed and pulsus paradoxus is not present. However, in a patient with respiratory distress, pulsus alternans, arrhythmia, and/or tachycardia, pulsus paradoxus may be obscured.

The pericardium may be thickened and cause constriction; less commonly, effusive-constrictive pericarditis occurs. Echocardiography rapidly and accurately detects pericardial effusion, identifies metastatic lesions, and provides evidence for cardiac compression. MRI is particularly useful in evaluating pericardial mass lesions. Neoplastic cells can be recovered from the pericardial fluid, which is usually bloody, in many cases. However, it is important to remember that more than half of pericardial effusions in cancer patients are due to causes other than metastatic disease, such as infections, radiation, and drug therapy; thus, the presence of pericarditis in cancer patients does not imply imminent death.[88]

Postmyocardial Infarction Pericarditis

Pericarditis is common in the first few days after an MI, occurring in as many as 28 to 43 percent of fatal infarctions, but is clinically apparent in as few as 7 percent of cases.[89] When friction rub is required for diagnosis, there is an underestimation of the incidence of postinfarction pericarditis. On average, pericarditis was diagnosed by rub alone in 14 percent compared with 25 percent when classic symptoms, a rub, or both were used as diagnostic criteria.[90] The detection of atypical T-wave evolution on ECG (i.e., either persistent positivity or temporally late positivity) may be a more sensitive and objective means of diagnosing postinfarction pericarditis.[91]

Pericardial involvement is related to infarct size and is associated with a poor prognosis.[92] An important clinical problem is the extent to which acute pericarditis in myocardial infarction influences management with anticoagulants. A pericardial friction rub occurring in the first 2 or 3 days without an associated pericardial effusion should not influence clinical decisions, but pericarditis occurring later in the course or accompanied by pericardial effusion or tamponade is a contraindication to anticoagulant therapy.

In a prospective, consecutive series of 174 patients with acute myocardial infarction, pericarditis occurred in 24 percent and was associated with anterior infarct location, heparin therapy,

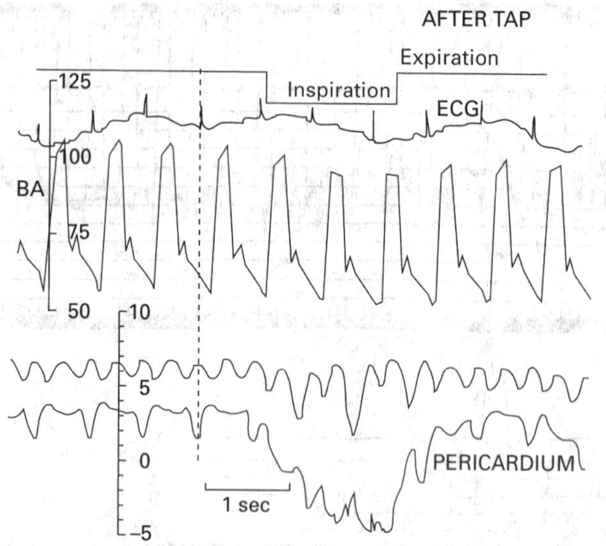

FIGURE 72-23 Recording from a patient with effusive-constrictive pericarditis caused by lung cancer. The tracings were obtained during the pericardiocentesis; right atrial pressure elevation persists, and there are prominent X and Y descents without respiratory variation. (From Shabetai R. *The Pericardium*. New York: Grune & Stratton; 1981:273. Reproduced with permission.)

and pericardial effusion.[93] Cardiac tamponade seldom occurs, except in patients who receive systemic anticoagulants or have cardiac rupture.

Thrombolytic therapy almost invariably precedes the development of pericarditis; therefore, clinical decision making usually is not affected. Surprisingly, thrombolytic therapy reduces the incidence of postinfarction pericarditis by approximately one-half.[94] However, when acute pericarditis is mistaken for acute myocardial infarction, thrombolytic therapy can have calamitous consequences. In patients treated mistakenly for myopericarditis with thrombolytics, the outcome was favorable.[95]

Dressler's syndrome (postmyocardial infarction syndrome) consists of pleuropericardial chest pain, friction rub, fever, leukocytosis, and pulmonary infiltrates. It usually occurs weeks or months (>10 days to 2 weeks) after the causative infarction. Dressler's syndrome may be caused by a combination of viral activation and myocardial antibodies and is clinically and pathogenetically similar to the postpericardiotomy syndrome. Cardiac tamponade of and late constriction may occur. For reasons that are not entirely clear, thrombolytic therapy has helped render post–myocardial infarction pericarditis nearly extinct.[96]

Radiation-Induced Pericardial Disease

Radiation injury to the pericardium is said to occur after exposure in excess of 4000 rads; the incidence also is dependent on the use of subcarinal blocks, the nature of the radiation source, and the duration and fractionation of the radiation regimen. For example, approximately 20 percent of Hodgkin's disease patients receiving ^{60}Co radiation with anterior weighting of the beam develop pericarditis, whereas the incidence of pericarditis after high-dose radiation for breast cancer (which includes less of the heart in the radiation field) is less than 5 percent.

Acute pericarditis occurring early during therapy is uncommon and most likely is a result of the radiation-induced effects on the tumor rather than a direct toxic effect of the radiation on the pericardium.[97] In this instance, therapy should not be disrupted, although a reduction in dose may be necessary. A delayed (usually less than 1 year but highly variable) form of pericardial injury may present as acute pericarditis or effusion (often with some degree of cardiac compression). The reaction of the pericardium to radiation is fibrinous inflammation,[98] often with an effusion. Although the acute lesion usually subsides within 2 years without sequelae, constrictive and effusive-constrictive pericarditis may become manifest only after many years.

The pathophysiology of radiation pericarditis is poorly understood but may involve extensive damage to the pericardial microcirculation and pericardial lymphatics with resultant ischemic injury. The incidence increases when anteriorly weighted field techniques are employed and is more common in patients who also have received adjunctive chemotherapy.

In the effusive stage, the differential diagnosis includes recurrence of the neoplasm, and examination of pericardial fluid is then helpful, as the fluid is positive in about 30 percent of cases.[99] Effusion may be due to the hypothyroid state induced by radiation therapy. Cytology is reliable in breast and lung cancer but less so in lymphoma and leukemia, where pericardial biopsy may be needed. Acute radiation-induced pericarditis can be managed symptomatically as acute idiopathic pericarditis. Hemodynamically insignificant pericardial effusion also can be managed conservatively, as spontaneous resolution is the rule; however, pericardiectomy should be offered to symptomatic patients with large, recurrent pericardial effusions. Constrictive pericarditis requires pericardiectomy unless the biopsy reveals significant endomyocardial fibrosis.

Traumatic Pericardial Disease

Blunt trauma and penetrating trauma are important causes of pericarditis, particularly among young men.[100] Chronic constrictive pericarditis, recurrent pericardial effusion, and recurrent acute pericarditis are well-recognized complications. Traumatic pericarditis may be life-threatening. The application of echocardiography in the trauma unit rapidly and accurately diagnoses hemopericardium in patients with potentially penetrating cardiac wounds.[101] Failure to repair the injury responsible for tamponade is associated with a poor clinical outcome.[102] Constrictive pericarditis occasionally occurs and may be delayed, presenting weeks or years after the injury.[103] Chylous pericardial effusions generally follow traumatic or surgical injury to the thoracic duct but may result from neoplastic obstruction of the thoracic duct or may be idiopathic.

Nephrogenic Pericardial Disease

Pericarditis complicates both uremia and dialytic therapy (hemo- and peritoneal dialysis) and may be clinically silent. The clinical manifestation of nephrogenic pericardial disease may be acute fibrinous pericarditis, pericardial effusion, or cardiac tamponade; classic constrictive pericarditis is rare.

The pathogenesis remains unknown. The etiology of pericarditis in dialyzed patients may be different from that in end-stage renal disease. The theory that uremic pericarditis is a chemical response to retained products of metabolism fails to account for a poor relationship between the blood urea nitrogen

(BUN) or other nitrogenous metabolites and the frequency of pericarditis. Since pericarditis is less common in patients undergoing peritoneal dialysis than in those receiving hemodialysis, there is a possible role for "middle molecules." Moreover, the hemorrhagic diathesis seen in the uremic syndrome may predispose to pericarditis; the resultant pericarditis is highly vascular, and consequently, the uremia or dialysis-related pericardial effusion is generally bloody. Renal insufficiency is associated with increased susceptibility to infection, and therefore, the possibility of viral, tuberculous, or even bacterial pericarditis must be considered. Immunologic abnormalities also have been implicated as a cause of pericardial disease in this setting. A presumptive diagnosis of dialysis-related pericarditis should be made only after other causes of pericardial heart disease (such as neoplasia and post-MI) that are common in this patient population have been excluded.

The clinical manifestations of cardiac tamponade may be atypical and difficult to distinguish from cardiovascular deterioration in patients undergoing hemodialysis. Cardiac tamponade remains one of the principal causes of hemodialysis-associated morbidity and terminates fatally in 20 percent of cases.

Although intensification of dialysis is an accepted treatment modality for hemodynamically insignificant disease, considerable controversy exists regarding the optimal management of large, persistent, or recurrent pericardial effusion and tamponade. Severe tamponade is an indication for pericardial drainage, but a conservative approach—intensification of dialysis and nonsteroidal anti-inflammatory agents—may suffice in less severe cases. The instillation of nonabsorbable steroids directly into the pericardial space has been advocated.[42] Dialysis-associated effusive pericarditis usually responds to an intensification of dialysis and regional heparinization or to a change to peritoneal dialysis. Pericardiectomy may be necessary for intractable effusions.

Myxedema Pericardial Disease

Pericarditis with effusion (sometimes containing cholesterol) occurs in about one-third of patients with myxedema. Effusions develop slowly and may reach a prodigious size; slow resolution usually follows the institution of thyroid replacement therapy. A case of hypothyroidism and viral pericarditis in a patient presenting to the emergency room with abdominal pain and shock was reported recently.[104]

Connective Tissue Disease–Related Pericardial Disease

Pericarditis may accompany virtually any connective tissue disease and may present as either acute or chronic pericarditis with or without an effusion.[105] Although tamponade, effusive-constrictive disease, and constrictive pericarditis are recognized complications, most cases are subclinical and in many instances are recognized only at autopsy.[106]

Rheumatoid pericardial disease is more common in middle-aged men in whom the onset of arthritis is acute. Serologic tests for rheumatoid disease are usually positive, and typical rheumatoid nodules are common. Rheumatoid arthritis is one of the causes of cholesterol pericarditis. Constrictive pericarditis is usually subacute and seldom is calcific. Pericardiectomy may be required within months of the first diagnosis of acute pericarditis and is almost always required within 5 years.[107,108]

Effusions are common in patients with SLE, and recurrent pericarditis, adhesion, and constriction may eventuate[109]; indeed, pericardial disease develops in nearly all patients with SLE when life is prolonged by steroid treatment. The pericardial fluid usually has a high protein content and a normal or slightly reduced glucose content; LE cells may be found. As in rheumatoid arthritis, the complement level is low.

Pericardial involvement may be found in systemic sclerosis (scleroderma), often in association with cardiomyopathy and diffuse scleroderma.[110] Dermatomyositis is not infrequently associated with pericardial involvement, including tamponade. Pericarditis is a rare complication in a wide variety of connective tissue disorders and arteritides (Table 72-2).

Iatrogenic Pericardial Disease

Iatrogenic pericardial disease results from both the calculated complications and the unanticipated misadventures of diagnostic and therapeutic procedures. Radiation pericarditis is one type of iatrogenic pericardial disease and was discussed earlier.

Postcardiotomy syndrome, which complicates 5 to 30 percent of cardiac operations, usually appears in the second or third week to 2 months after cardiac surgery; affected patients frequently have high titers of antiheart and antiviral antibodies and may develop cardiac tamponade.

Cardiac perforation complicating diagnostic cardiac catheterization and pacemaker insertion, complications of endoscopic sclerotherapy of esophageal varices, and automatic defibrillator electrode placement are other causes of iatrogenic pericardial disease. Pericardial abnormalities may develop in response to a number of drugs, of which the more important are hydralazine, procainamide, and daunorubicin, although these abnormalities have been reported with a number of agents (Table 72-2). Cardiac tamponade after thrombolysis with rtPA given for stroke has been reported.[111]

CONGENITAL PERICARDIAL HEART DISEASE

Absence and Partial Absence of the Pericardium

Congenital absence of the pericardium is an uncommon anomaly, usually involving a portion or the whole of the left parietal pericardium. Its presence usually is suspected from the chest radiogram, which shows a leftward shift of the cardiac silhouette, elongation of the left heart border, and radiolucencies between the aortic knob and the pulmonary artery and between the left hemidiaphragm and the base of the heart (Fig. 72-24). This anomaly may be associated with congenital malformations of the heart and lungs.[112]

Although most of these patients are asymptomatic, chest pain may result from torsion of the great vessels, and recurrent pulmonary infections may be a significant feature. Physical findings are not often helpful, but a conspicuous LV heave may be found when the deficiency is substantial. Systolic and diastolic murmurs have been described.

The ECG in patients with complete absence of the left side of the pericardium usually shows an incomplete right bundle branch block. Echocardiographic changes consist of RV enlargement and paradoxical septal motion. Contrast-enhanced CT and MRI detect lesions missed by chest radiography and

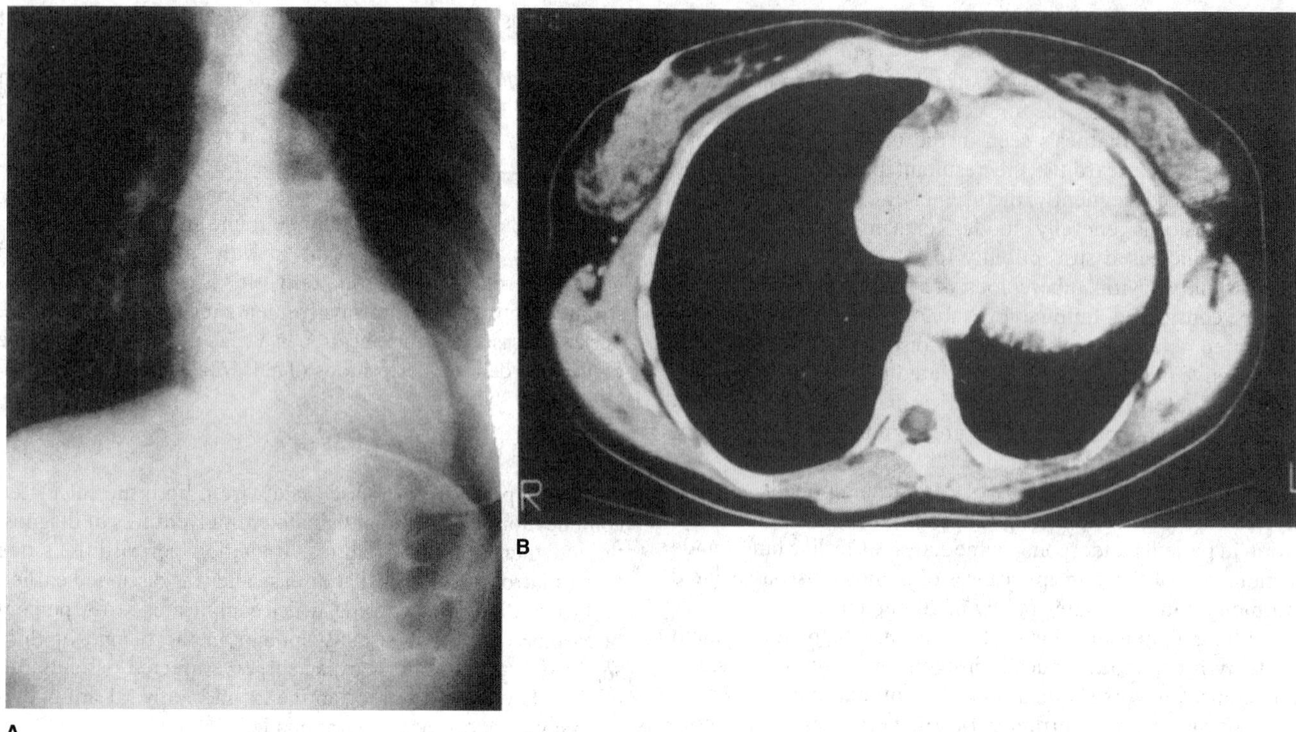

FIGURE 72-24 *A.* Posteroanterior chest radiogram of a patient with congenital absence of the pericardium. *B.* Computed tomography scan of the same patient. (Reproduced with permission from Hoit BD. Imaging the pericardium. *Cardiol Clin* 1990; 8:598.)

echocardiography and reliably establish the anatomy of the defect.[113]

Total and very small defects are not associated with pathophysiologic changes, whereas medium-size defects may allow herniation of the left atrium. Strangulation requires surgical closure or enlargement of the defect to reduce the herniation; this may be accomplished with a thoracoscope.

Pericardial Cysts

Pericardial cysts are rare remnants of defective embryologic development of the pericardium. Cysts usually present as a prominent round, sharply demarcated opacity seen on chest radiography in an asymptomatic patient. They vary greatly in size and most commonly are found in the right cardiophrenic angle, although hilar and mediastinal locations are observed occasionaly. Cysts are benign and produce no local or general symptoms; their importance lies in differentiation from neoplasm. Although they can be demonstrated on echocardiography, the nature of the lesion usually is confirmed by CT. A case of video-assisted surgical excision of a recurrent pericardial cyst has been reported.[114]

References

1. Shabetai R. The pericardium: An essay on some recent developments. *Am J Cardiol* 1978; 42(6):1036–1043.
2. Hammond HK, White FC, Bhargava V, et al. Heart size and maximal cardiac output are limited by the pericardium. *Am J Physiol* 1992; 263(6 part 2):H1675–H1681.
3. Hoit BD, Lew WY, LeWinter M. Regional variation in pericardial contact pressure in the canine ventricle. *Am J Physiol* 1988; 255(6 part 2):H1370–H1377.
4. Ditchey R, Engler RL, LeWinter MM, et al. The role of the right heart in acute cardiac tamponade in dogs. *Circ Res* 1981; 48:701–710.
5. Castelo Branco NA, Aguas AP, Sousa Pereira A, et al. The human pericardium in vibroacoustic disease. *Aviat Space Environ Med.* 1999; 70:A54–A62.
6. Spodick D. Macrophysiology, microphysiology, and anatomy of the pericardium: A synopsis. *Am Heart J* 1992; 124:1046–1051.
7. Eid H, Larson DM, Springhorn JP, et al. Role of epicardial mesothelial cells in the modification of phenotype and function of adult rat ventricular myocytes in primary coculture. *Circ Res* 1992; 71(1):40–50.
8. Laham RJ, Hung D, Simons M. Therapeutic myocardial angiogenesis using percutaneous intrapericardial drug delivery. *Clin Cardiol* 1999; 22:I-6–I-9.
9. Stoll HP, Carlson K, Keefer LK, et al. Pharmacokinetics and consistence of pericardial delivery directed to coronary arteries: Direct comparison with endoluminal delivery. *Clin Cardiol* 1999; 22:I-10–I-16.
10. Spodick DH. *The Pericardium: A Comprehensive Textbook.* New York: Marcel Dekker; 1997.
11. Kostreva DR, Pontus SP. Pericardial mechanoreceptors with phrenic afferents. *Am J Physiol* 1993; 264:H1836–H1846.
12. Fujita M, Ikemoto M, Kishishita M, et al. Elevated basic fibroblast growth factor in pericardial fluid of patients with unstable angina. *Circulation.* 1996; 94:610–613.
13. Tanaka T, Hasegawa K, Fujita M, et al. Marked elevation of brain natriuretic peptide levels in pericardial fluid is closely associated with left ventricular dysfunction. *J Am Coll Cardiol* 1998; 31(2):399–403.
14. Mallat Z, Philip I, Lebret M, et al. Elevated levels of 8-iso-prostaglandin F2alpha in pericardial fluid of patients with heart

failure: A potential role for in vivo oxidant stress in ventricular dilatation and progression to heart failure. *Circulation* 1998; 97(16):1536–1539.
15. Wanner WR, Schaal SF, Bashore TM, et al. Repolarization variant versus acute pericarditis: A prospective electrocardiographic and echocardiographic evaluation. *Chest* 1983; 83:180–184.
16. James JN. Pericarditis and the sinus node. *Arch Intern Med* 1962; 110:305–311.
17. Adler Y, Finkelstein Y, Guindo J, et al. Colchicine treatment for recurrent pericarditis: A decade of experience. *Circulation* 1998; 97(21):2183–2185.
18. Guindo J, Rodriguez de la Serna A, Ramio J, et al. Recurrent pericarditis: Relief with colchicine [see comments]. *Circulation* 1990; 82(4):1117–1120.
19. Marcolongo R, Russo R, Laveder F, et al. Immunosuppressive therapy prevents recurrent pericarditis. *J Am Coll Cardiol* 1995; 26(5):1276–1279.
20. Maisch B. Percardial diseases, with a focus on etiology, pathogenesis, pathophysiology, new diagnostic imaging methods, and treatment. *Curr Opin Cardiol* 1994; 9(3):379–388.
21. Weitzman LB, Tinker WP, Kronzon I, et al. The incidence and natural history of pericardial effusion after cardiac surgery—an echocardiographic study. *Circulation* 1984; 69:506–511.
22. Tsang TS, Barnes ME, Hayes SN, et al. Clinical and echocardiographic characteristics of significant pericardial effusions following cardiothoracic surgery and outcomes of echo-guided pericardiocentesis for management: Mayo Clinic experience, 1979–1998. *Chest* 1999; 116(2):322–331.
23. Ciliberto GR, Anjos MC, Gronda E. Significance of pericardial effusion after heart transplantation. *Am J Cardiol* 1995; 76: 297–300.
24. Mueller XM, Tevaearai HT, Hurni M, et al. Etiologic diagnosis of pericardial disease: The value of routine tests during surgical procedures. *J Am Coll Surg* 1997; 184(6):645–649.
25. Maisch B, Pankuweit S, Brilla C, et al. Intrapericardial treatment of inflammatory and neoplastic pericarditis guided by pericardioscopy and epicardial biopsy—results from a pilot study. *Clin Cardiol* 1999; 22(I suppl 1):I17–I22.
26. Geissbuhler K, Leiser A, Fuhrer J, et al. Video-assisted thoracoscopic pericardial fenestration for loculated or recurrent effusions. *Eur J Cardiothorac Surg* 1998; 14(4):403–408.
27. Sechtem U, Tsholakoff D, Higgins CB. MRI of the abnormal pericardium. *AJR* 1986; 147:245–252.
28. Merce J, Sagrista-Sauleda J, Permanyer-Miralda G, et al. Should pericardial drainage be performed routinely in patients who have a large pericardial effusion without tamponade? *Am J Med* 1998; 105(2):106–109.
29. Hoit BD, Gabel M, Fowler NO. Cardiac tamponade in left ventricular dysfunction. *Circulation* 1990; 82(4):1370–1376.
30. Hoit BD, Shaw D. The paradoxical pulse in tamponade: Mechanisms and echocardiographic correlates. *Echocardiography* 1994; 11:477–487.
31. Spodick DH. Electric alteration of the heart: Its relation to the kinetics and physiology of the heart during cardiac tamponade. *Am J Cardiol* 1962; 10:155–165.
32. Settle HP Jr, Engel PJ, Fowler NO, et al. Echocardiographic study of the paradoxical arterial pulse in chronic obstructive lung disease. *Circulation* 1980; 62(6):1297–1307.
33. Gillam LD, Guyer DE, Gibson TC, et al. Hydrodynamic compression of the right atrium: A new echocardiographic sign of cardiac tamponade. *Circulation* 1983; 68(2):294–301.
34. Chuttani K, Pandian NG, Mohanty PK. Left ventricular diastolic collapse: An echocardiographic sign of regional cardiac tamponade. *Circulation* 1991; 83:1999–2006.
35. Russo AM, O'Connor WH, Waxman HL. Atypical presentations and echocardiographic findings in patients with cardiac tamponade occurring early and late after cardiac surgery. *Chest* 1993; 104(1):71–78.
36. Golub RJ, McNulty CM, McClellan JR, et al. Usefulness of transesophageal Doppler echocardiography in the surgical drainage of a loculated purulent pericardial effusion. *Am Heart J* 1993; 126:724–727.
37. Heidenreich PA, Stainback RF, Redberg RF, et al. Transesophageal echocardiography predicts mortality in critically ill patients with unexplained hypotension. *J Am Coll Cardiol* 1995; 26(1): 152–158.
38. Appleton CP, Hatle LK, Popp RL. Relation of transmitral flow velocity patterns to left ventricular diastolic function: New insights from a combined hemodynamic and Doppler echocardiographic study. *J Am Coll Cardiol* 1988; 12:426–440.
39. Hoit BD, Ramrakhyani K. Pulmonary venous flow in cardiac tamponade: Influence of left ventricular dysfunction and the relation to pulsus paradoxus. *J Am Soc Echocardiogr* 1991; 4(6):559–570.
40. Merce J, Sagrista-Sauleda J, Permanyer-Miralda G, et al. Correlation between clinical and Doppler echocardiographic findings in patients with moderate and large pericardial effusion: Implications for the diagnosis of cardiac tamponade. *Am Heart J* 1999; 138(4):759–764.
41. Callahan JA, Seward JB, Nishimura RA, et al. Two-dimensional echocardiographically guided pericardiocentesis: Experience in 117 consecutive patients. *Am J Cardiol* 1985; 55(4):476–479.
42. Quigg RJ Jr, Idelson BA, Yoburn DC, et al. Local steroids in dialysis-associated pericardial effusion: A single intrapericardial administration of triamcinolone. *Arch Intern Med* 1985; 145(12): 2249–2450.
43. Shepherd FA, Morgan C, Evans WK, et al. Medical management of malignant pericardial effusion by tetracycline sclerosis. *Am J Cardiol* 1987; 60(14):1161–1166.
44. Olson JE, Ryan MB, Blumenstock DA. Eleven years' experience with pericardial-peritoneal window in the management of malignant and benign pericardial effusions. *Ann Surg Oncol* 1995; 2(2):165–169.
45. Allen KB, Faber LP, Warren WH, et al. Pericardial effusion: Subxiphoid pericardiostomy versus percutaneous catheter drainage. *Ann Thorac Surg* 1999; 67(2):437–440.
46. Girardi LN, Ginsberg RJ, Burt ME. Pericardiocentesis and intrapericardial sclerosis: Effective therapy for malignant pericardial effusions. *Ann Thorac Surg* 1997; 64(5):1427–1428.
47. Chavanon O, Barbe C, Troccas J, et al. Accurate guidance for percutaneous access to a specific target in soft tissue: Preclinical study of computer-assisted pericardiocentesis. *J Laparoendosc Adv Surg Tech* 1999; 9(3):259–266.
48. Ziskind AA, Pearce AC, Lemmon CC, et al. Percutaneous balloon pericardiotomy for the treatment of cardiac tamponade and large pericardial effusions: Description of technique and report of the first 50 cases. *J Am Coll Cardiol* 1993; 21(1):1–5.
49. Selig MB. Percutaneous transcatheter pericardial interventions: Aspiration, biopsy, and pericardioplasty. *Am Heart J* 1993; 125: 269–271.
50. Oh JK, Hatle LK, Mulvagh SL, Tajik AJ. Transient constrictive pericarditis: Diagnosis by two-dimensional Doppler echocardiography. *Mayo Clin Proc* 1993; 68(12):1158–1164.
51. Fowler NO. Constrictive pericarditis: Its history and current status. *Clin Cardiol* 1995; 18:341–350.
52. Schiavone WA. The changing etiology of constrictive pericarditis in a large referral center. *Am J Cardiol* 1986; 58:373–375.
53. Engel PJ, Fowler NO, Tei CW, et al. M-mode echocardiography in constrictive pericarditis. *J Am Coll Cardiol* 1985; 6:471–474.
54. Isner JM, Carter BL, Bankoff MS, et al. Differentiation of constrictive pericarditis from restrictive cardiomyopathy by computed tomographic imaging. *Am Heart J* 1983; 105:1019–1025.
55. Rienmuller R, Doppman JL, Lissner J, et al. Constrictive pericar-

dial disease: Prognostic significance of a nonvisualized left ventricular wall. *Radiology* 1985; 156(3):753–755.
56. Oren RM, Grover-McKay M, Stanford W, et al. Accurate preoperative diagnosis of pericardial constriction using cine computed tomography. *J Am Coll Cardiol* 1993; 22(3):832–838.
57. Sayad DE, Clarke GD, Peshock RM. Magnetic resonance imaging of the heart and its role in current cardiology. *Curr Opin Cardiol* 1995; 10(6):640–649.
58. Blackwell GG, Pohost GM. The usefulness of cardiovascular magnetic resonance imaging. *Curr Probl Cardiol* 1994; 19(3): 117–175.
59. Kutcher MA, King SB III, Alimurung BN, et al. Constrictive pericarditis as a complication of cardiac surgery: Recognition of an entity. *Am J Cardiol* 1982; 50:742–748.
60. Bush CA, Stang JM, Wooley CF, et al. Occult constrictive pericardial disease: Diagnosis by rapid volume expansion and correction by pericardiectomy. *Circulation* 1977; 56:924–930.
61. Sagrista-Sauleda J, Permanyer-Miralda G, Candell RJ, et al. Transient cardiac constriction: An unrecognized pattern of evolution in effusive acute idiopathic pericarditis. *Am J Cardiol* 1987; 59:961–966.
62. Seifert FC, Miller DC, Oesterle SN, et al. Surgical treatment of constrictive pericarditis: Analysis of outcome and diagnostic error. *Circulation* 1985; 72(3 part 2):II264–II273.
63. Nataf P, Cacouch P, Dorent R. Results of subtotal pericardiectomy for constrictive pericarditis. *Eur J Cardiothorac Surg* 1993; 7:252–256.
64. Woods T, Vidarsson B, Mosher D, et al. Transient effusive-constrictive pericarditis due to chemotherapy. *Clin Cardiol* 1999; 22(4):316–318.
65. Fowler NO, Harbin AD. Recurrent acute pericarditis: Follow-up study of 31 patients. *J Am Coll Cardiol* 1986; 7:300–305.
66. Maisch B, Drude L. Epi and pericardial biopsy by pericardioscopy. *Circulation* 1990; 82:III-417.
67. Sagrista-Sauleda J, Barrabes JA, Permanyer-Miralda G, et al. Purulent pericarditis: Review of a 20-year experience in a general hospital. *J Am Coll Cardiol* 1993; 22(6):1661–1665.
68. Klacsmann PG, Bulkey BH, Hutchins GM. The changed spectrum of purulent pericarditis: An 86-year autopsy experience in 200 patients. *Am J Med* 1977; 63:666–673.
69. Arsura EL, Kilgore WB, Strategos E. Purulent pericarditis misdiagnosed as septic shock. *South Med J* 1999; 92(3):285–288.
70. Skiest D, Steiner D, Werner M, et al. Anaerobic pericarditis: Case report and review. *Clin Infect Dis* 1994; 19:435–440.
71. Mann-Segal DD. The use of fibrinolytics in purulent pericarditis. *Intensive Care Med* 1999; 25(3):338–339.
72. Defouilloy C, Meyer G, Slama M, et al. Intrapericardial fibrinolysis: A useful treatment in the management of purulent pericarditis. *Intensive Care Med* 1997; 23(1):117–118.
73. Winkler WB, Karnik R, Slany J. Treatment of exudative fibrinous pericarditis with intrapericardial urokinase. *Lancet* 1994; 344: 1541–1542.
74. Puelo J, Matar F, McKeown P, et al. Legionella pericarditis diagnosed by direct fluorescent antibody staining. *Ann Thorac Surg* 1995; 60:444–446.
75. Nelson D, Rensimer E, Raffin T. Legionella pneumophilia pericarditis without pneumonia. *Arch Intern Med* 1985; 145:926.
76. Nagi KS, Joshi R, Thakur RK. Cardiac manifestations of Lyme disease: A review. *Can J Cardiol* 1996; 12(5):503–506.
77. Mastroianni A, Coronado O, Chiodo F. Tuberculous pericarditis and AIDS: Case reports and review. *Eur J Epidemiol* 1997; 13(7):755–759.
78. Rana BS, Jones RA, Simpson IA. Recurrent pericardial effusion: The value of polymerase chain reaction in the diagnosis of tuberculosis. *Heart* 1999; 82(2):246–247.
79. Hayashi H, Kawamata H, Machida M, et al. Tuberculous pericarditis: MRI features with contrast enhancement. *Br J Radiol* 1998; 71(846):680–682.
80. Long R, Younes M, Patton N, et al. Tuberculous pericarditis: Long-term outcome in patients who received medical therapy alone. *Am Heart J* 1989; 117(5):1133–1139.
81. Fowler N. Tuberculous pericarditis. *JAMA* 1991; 266:99–103.
82. Silva-Cardoso J, Moura B, Martins L, et al. Pericardial involvement in human immunodeficiency virus infection. *Chest* 1999; 115(2):418–422.
83. Heidenreich PA, Eisenberg MJ, Kee LL, et al. Pericardial effusion in AIDS: Incidence and survival [see comments]. *Circulation* 1995; 92(11):3229–3234.
84. Estok L, Wallach F. Cardiac tamponade in a patient with AIDS: A review of pericardial disease in patients with HIV infection. *Mt Sinai J Med.* 1998; 65(1):33–39.
85. Chen Y, Brennessel D, Walters J, et al. Human immunodeficiency virus-associated pericardial effusion: Report of 40 cases and review of the literature. *Am Heart J* 1999; 137(3):516–521.
86. Blanc P, Boussuges A, Souk-aloun J, et al. Echocardiography on HIV patients admitted to the ICU. *Intensive Care Med* 1997; 23(12):1279–1281.
87. Thomason R, Schlegel W, Luccam M. Primary malignant mesothelioma of the pericardium. *Tex Heart Inst* 1994; 21:170–174.
88. Wilkes JD, Fidias P, Vaickus L, et al. Malignancy-related pericardial effusion: 127 cases from the Roswell Park Cancer Institute. *Cancer* 1995; 76(8):1377–1387.
89. Widimsky P, Gregor P. Pericardial involvement during the course of myocardial infarction: A long-term clinical and echocardiographic study. *Chest* 1995; 108(1):89–93.
90. Fowler NO. *The Pericardium in Health and Disease.* Mt. Kisco, NY: Futura; 1985.
91. Oliva P, Hammill S, Edwards W. Electrocardiographic diagnosis of postinfarction regional pericarditis: Ancillary observations regarding the effect of reperfusion on the rapidity and amplitude of T wave inversion after acute myocardial infarction. *Circulation.* 1993; 88:896–904.
92. Correale E, Maggioni AP, Romano S, et al. Comparison of frequency, diagnostic and prognostic significance of pericardial involvement in acute myocardial infarction treated with and without thrombolytics: Gruppo Italiano per lo Studio della Sopravvivenza nell'Infarto Miocardico (GISSI). *Am J Cardiol* 1993; 71(16):1377–1381.
93. Madias J, Perdoncin R, Bartoszyk O. Pericarditis and pericardial effusion in patients with acute myocardial infarction. *Am J Noninvas Cardiol* 1994; 8:270–277.
94. Correale E, Maggioni AP, Romano S, et al. Pericardial involvement in acute myocardial infarction in the post-thrombolytic era: Clinical meaning and value. *Clin Cardiol* 1997; 20(4):327–331.
95. Millaire A, de Groote P, Decoulx E, et al. Outcome after thrombolytic therapy of nine cases of myopericarditis misdiagnosed as myocardia infarction. *Eur Heart J* 1995; 16(3):333–338.
96. Shahar A, Hod H, Barabash GM, et al. Disappearance of a syndrome: Dressler's syndrome in the era of thrombolysis. *Cardiology* 1994; 85(3–4):255–258.
97. Stewart J, Fajardo L. Radiation-induced heart disease: An update. *Prog Cardiovasc Dis* 1984; 27:173–194.
98. Benoff LJ, Schweitzer P. Radiation therapy-induced cardiac injury. *Am Heart J* 1995; 129(6):1193–1196.
99. King D, Nieberg R. The use of cytology to evaluate pericardial effusions. *Ann Clin Lab Sci* 1979; 9:18–23.
100. Liedtke JA, DeMuth WE. Nonpenetrating cardiac injuries: A collective review. *Am Heart J* 1973; 86:687–697.
101. Rozycki GS, Feliciano DV, Oshsner MG, et al. The role of ultrasound in patients with possible penetrating cardiac wounds: A prospective multicenter study. *J Trauma* 1999; 46(4):543–551.
102. Thakur RK, Aufderheide TP, Boughner DR. Emergency echo-

cardiographic evaluation of penetrating chest trauma. *Can J Cardiol* 1994; 10(3):374–376.

103. Meleca MJ, Hoit BD. Previously unrecognized intrapericardial hematoma leading to refractory abdominal ascites. *Chest* 1995; 108(6):1747–1748.

104. Gupta R, Munyak J, Haydock T, et al. Hypothyroidism presenting as acute cardiac tamponade with viral pericarditis. *Am J Emerg Med* 1999; 17(2):176–178.

105. Langley RL, Treadwell EL. Cardiac tamponade and pericardial disorders in connective tissue diseases: Case report and literature review. *J Natl Med Assoc* 1994; 86(2):149–153.

106. Spodick DH. Pericarditis in systemic diseases: Diseases of the pericardium. *Cardiol Clin* 1990; 8:709–715.

107. Hakala M, Pettersson T, Tarkka M, et al. Rheumatoid arthritis as a cause of cardiac compression: Favourable long-term outcome of pericardiectomy. *Clin Rheumatol* 1993; 12:199–203.

108. Thould A. Constrictive pericarditis in rheumatoid arthritis. *Ann Rheum Dis* 1986; 45:89–94.

109. Moder KG, Miller TD, Tazelaar HD. Cardiac involvement in systemic lupus erythematosus. *Mayo Clin Proc* 1999; 74(3): 275–284.

110. Thompson AE, Pope JE. A study of the frequency of pericardial and pleural effusions in scleroderma. *Br J Rheumatol* 1998; 37(12):1320–1321.

111. Kasner SE, Villar-Cordova CE, Tong D, et al. Hemopericardium and cardiac tamponade after thrombolysis for acute ischemic stroke. *Neurology* 1998; 50(6):1857–1859.

112. Nasser W. Congenital absence of the left pericardium. *Am J Cardiol* 1970; 26:466–478.

113. Gassner I, Judmaier W, Fink C, et al. Diagnosis of congenital pericardial defects, including a pathognomonic sign for dangerous apical ventricular herniation, on magnetic resonance imaging. *Br Heart J* 1995; 74:60–66.

114. Horita K, Sakao Y, Itoh T. Excision of a recurrent pericardial cyst using video-assisted thoracic surgery. *Chest* 1998; 114(4): 1203–1204.

CHAPTER 73

INFECTIVE ENDOCARDITIS

Merle A. Sande / Mrinka Kartalija / Jeff Anderson

Infective endocarditis is the disease caused by microbial infection of the endothelial lining of the heart. Its characteristic lesion is a *vegetation,* which usually develops on a heart valve but occasionally appears elsewhere on the endocardium. Sometimes a nidus of infection develops on the lining of a large artery, causing *infective endarteritis;* this variant can produce clinical findings that resemble those of infective endocarditis.

DEFINITIONS AND TERMINOLOGY

The following abbreviations for various forms of endocarditis will be used in this chapter:

- IE: Infective endocarditis
- SBE: Subacute bacterial endocarditis
- ABE: Acute bacterial endocarditis
- NVE: Native valve endocarditis
- PVE: Prosthetic valve endocarditis
- NBTE: Nonbacterial thrombotic endocarditis

The terms *subacute* and *acute bacterial endocarditis* (SBE and ABE) have descriptive value when accurately applied. SBE progresses over a period of weeks to months and is usually caused by organisms of low virulence such as viridans streptococci, which possess limited ability to infect other tissues.[1-4]

In contrast, ABE evolves over a period of days to 1 or 2 weeks; the clinical progress is rapidly changing, complications develop earlier, and the diagnosis is usually made in less than 2 weeks.[4-6] ABE is most often caused by primary pathogens such as *Staphylococcus aureus,* which are capable of causing invasive infection at many other sites in the body.

Infection of a heart valve that was either previously normal or damaged by congenital or acquired disease is termed *native valve endocarditis* (NVE). Infection of an artificial heart valve is termed *prosthetic valve endocarditis* (PVE). This infection was first arbitrarily defined as early PVE, when onset is within the first 2 months after surgery, and as late PVE thereafter.[6-11] Some authors have defined infections occurring between 2 months and 1 year of valve replacement as intermediate PVE,[11] while others consider any prosthetic valve infection beginning before 1 year as early PVE.

Sterile vegetations sometimes develop within the heart. The term *noninfective endocarditis* is a misnomer, because the lesions are primarily thrombotic rather than inflammatory.[12] Thus the term *nonbacterial thrombotic endocarditis* (NBTE) is used broadly to describe any sterile vegetation. This category includes a spectrum of lesions ranging from microscopic aggregates of platelets to the large vegetations of marantic endocarditis, which sometimes develop in patients with terminal malignancy or other chronic diseases.[13–15]

Infective endocarditis is designated best by naming the infecting organism, for example, "*Staph. aureus* endocarditis" or "*Candida albicans* PVE." This terminology is specific and informative, allowing useful inferences about the likely natural history, prognosis, and treatment of the case in question.

EARLY STUDIES

Riviere, Lancisi, and Morgagni each described patients who died with endocarditis in the seventeenth and eighteenth centuries.[16] Jean-Baptiste Bouillaud introduced the terms *endocardium* and *endocarditis* between 1824 and 1835. By 1846, Virchow recognized valvular vegetations at autopsy, but the microbial etiology of infective endocarditis was not fully appreciated until Virchow et al. independently demonstrated bacteria in vegetations between 1869 and 1872.[16]

William Osler studied the disease extensively, choosing infective endocarditis as the subject for his Goulstonian lectures of 1885.[17,18] Further major contributions to the knowledge of the natural history, pathogenesis, and pathology of the disease were made by Lenharz, Harbitz, and Schottmuller[16] in Germany; by Horder[19] in England; and by Blumer,[1] Thayer,[2] Allen,[20] Libman and Friedberg,[21] and Beeson et al.[22] in the United States. The technique of blood culture was introduced in Europe and the United States between 1890 and 1910.[3] In 1955, Kerr published a classic monograph summarizing the state of knowledge on subacute bacterial endocarditis to that date.[3]

Attempts to cure endocarditis before the advent of antimicrobial drugs were unsuccessful. In 1939, one patient with infective endarteritis involving a patent ductus arteriosus was cured by surgical closure of the ductus.[23] The first successes in the treatment of endocarditis are closely linked to the history of penicillin.[24] The first patient to receive parenteral penicillin was a young man with streptococcal endocarditis who was treated in 1940 at Columbia University in New York.[25] Although the patient did not receive enough penicillin to effect a cure, his treatment antedated the first administration of penicillin to a patient by Florey's team (Abraham et al.) in Oxford[26] by several months. After initial failures, by 1944 it had been established that penicillin,[27] unlike sulfonamides,[28] could cure most cases of streptococcal endocarditis. Subsequently, the antibiotic treatment of endocarditis was clearly established.[29–33] After antibiotics, the next great advance was cardiac valve replacement for treatment of endocarditis in 1965,[34] which provided an essential intervention to improve survival rates in selected patients.

EPIDEMIOLOGY

Incidence

The incidence of infective endocarditis can only be estimated, because it is not a reportable disease. Various studies in developed countries have estimated the incidence to be 1.6 to 6.0 cases per 100,000 person-years.[35–39] In the United States, this would result in 4000 to 15,000 new cases per year. In a study from the Delaware Valley, where the population includes a large number of intravenous drug users (IDU), the estimated rate was much higher: 11.6 cases per 100,000 per year.[40]

Evolution of the Clinical Syndrome

IE today is a different disease from that seen in the preantibiotic era, when its salient clinical features were exhaustively reported.[1–3] Since 1961, many authors have described the "changing face" of "modern endocarditis,"[41–47] identifying the following trends:

- Increased median age of patients
- Increased ratio of males to females
- Increased proportion of acute cases
- Reduced incidence of some of the classic physical signs of advanced SBE, such as Osler's nodes, finger clubbing, splenomegaly, or Roth's spots
- Decreased proportion of cases due to streptococci, with an increased incidence of staphylococci
- Lengthened list of etiologic organisms, with more reports of cases caused by gram-negative bacilli, fungi, and miscellaneous rare or unusual microbes
- Increased number of cases in IDU
- Increased number of prosthetic valve infections
- Increased incidence of concomitant human immunodeficiency virus (HIV) infection and endocarditis

Susceptible Populations

These striking changes in the clinical features and epidemiology of IE are due to changes in susceptible populations, to earlier diagnosis and treatment of patients with subacute disease and to the impact of antibiotic therapy.[45,48] The prevalence of rheumatic valvular disease, formerly the most common substrate for endocarditis, has steadily decreased; meanwhile, the number of children surviving with congenital heart disease has increased. The number of individuals using illicit drugs intravenously has increased markedly in the United States and Europe since the 1960s, and HIV has spread widely throughout this group as well.[49]

Effect of Antibiotics

Although the advent of antibiotics revolutionized treatment of endocarditis, the overall incidence of the disease has not changed strikingly. The availability of rapidly effective treatments for pneumococcal pneumonia and gonorrhea has probably been responsible for the striking decrease in the incidence of endocarditis caused by *Streptococcus pneumoniae* and *Neisseria gonorrhoeaea* since 1944, while the incidence of reported cases caused by miscellaneous unusual antibiotic-resistant organisms has increased during the antibiotic era.[48,50–53] Apart from these special cases, the widespread use of antimicrobial agents seems to have exerted considerably less influence than have alterations in the populations at risk on the changing epidemiology of endocarditis.[45] Prophylactic use of antibiotics before medical procedures that cause bacteremia has not reduced the incidence of endocarditis significantly; this is not surprising considering

TABLE 73-1 Approximate Frequency of Major Preexisting Cardiac Lesions in Patients with Infective Endocarditis in the United States

Lesion	Children under 2 years, %	Children 2–15 Years, %	Adults 15–50 Years, %	Adults >50 Years, %	Adults Who Are IV Drug Abusers, %
No known heart disease	50–70	10–15	10–20	10	50–60
Congenital heart disease[a]	30–50	70–80	25–35	15–25	10
Rheumatic heart disease	Rare	10	10–15	10–15	10
Degenerative heart disease	0	0	Rare	10–20	Rare
Previous cardiac surgery	5	10–15	10–20	10–20	10–20
Previous endocarditis	Rare	5	5–10	5–10	10–20

[a]Includes mitral valve prolapse.
SOURCE: Adapted from Refs. 35–51, 58–70, 81, 202.

that only a small proportion of all cases can be attributed to such procedures.[54–56] Also, startling studies question the effectiveness of prophylactic antibiotics during dental procedures to prevent endocarditis.[56,57]

Preexisting Heart Disease

Some patients develop endocarditis even though they have no known heart disease. This is most common in cases of ABE,[57] in children less than 2 years of age,[58–64] and in IDUs.[65–70] Most patients who develop IE, however, have a preexisting cardiac condition. Approximate figures for the frequency of the main predisposing factors in children, adults, and IDUs are given in Table 73-1.

The relative propensity of various cardiac lesions to become infected can be estimated by noting their frequency in published series of cases of IE, even though there is wide variation among individual studies (Table 73-2).

Mitral valve prolapse (MVP) can predispose to endocarditis.[71–78] (see Chap. 58). MVP underlies 15 to 30 percent or more of cases.[35,72,75,76,80] However, MVP is common and represents a broad spectrum of valvular and clinical disease. The annual percentage of patients with MVP that develop complications (including IE) is small, and the need for IE prophylaxis is controversial. Hence, American Heart Association recommendations include an algorithm to more clearly define when prophylaxis is recommended in MVP.[79] The risk of IE is primarily increased (five- to eightfold) when MVP is associated with regurgitation.[72,73,78] The use of prophylactic antibiotics is supported by cost-benefit analysis in those with auscultatory or Doppler evidence for mitral insufficiency.[79] In contrast, endocarditis risk is not increased in the absence of regurgitation and prophylaxis is not recommended[2,8,9,79] (see Chap. 58).[72,73] However, this remains controversial. Although commonly used to confirm diagnoses, routine use of echocardiography does not appear to be cost effective.[74]

Children

IE occurs at all ages but is relatively uncommon during childhood and rare during infancy,[58–64,81,82] although the incidence is increasing among smaller infants with cyanotic disease.[83] Males predominate—65 percent in one series.[84] Endocardial infection in children with no predisposing heart disease develops most often in association with infection elsewhere, often in infants and very young children.[85] Endocarditis in these settings is likely to be caused by invasive pathogens and follow an acute course. IE can occur as a rare complication of septicemia caused by staphylococci or group B streptococci or of pneumonia, other respiratory tract infections, osteomyelitis, and severe burns.[58,62]

TABLE 73-2 Estimates of the Relative Risk of Infective Endocarditis Posed by Various Cardiac Lesions

Relatively High Risk	Intermediate Risk	Very Low or Negligible Risk
Prosthetic heart valves	Mitral valve prolapse with regurgitation	Mitral valve prolapse without regurgitation
Previous infective endocarditis	Pure mitral stenosis	Trivial valvular regurgitation by echocardiography without structural abnormality
Cyanotic congenital heart disease	Tricuspid valve disease	Atrial septal defects, secundum type
Aortic valve disease	Pulmonary valve disease	Arteriosclerotic plaques
Mitral regurgitation	Asymmetric septal hypertrophy	Coronary artery disease
Mitral regurgitation and stenosis	Hyperalimentation or pressure-monitoring lines that reach the right atrium	Syphilitic aortitis
Patent ductus arteriosus	Nonvalvular intracardiac prosthetic implants	Cardiac pacemakers
Ventricular septal defect	Degenerative valvular disease in elderly patients	Surgically corrected cardiac lesions (without prosthetic implants, more than 6 months after operation)
Coarctation of the aorta		

SOURCE: Adapted from Refs. 36, 38, 39, 43, 50, 51, 71–81, 86, 116, 370.

Nosocomial cases associated with intravenous catheters are important.[85] Endocarditis complicating congenital or other preexisting heart lesions is more likely to occur in older children and present as a subacute disease without an obvious portal of entry.[85] Children with a systemic pulmonary shunt constructed surgically are most likely to have endocarditis caused by viridans streptococci.[84] *Haemophilus influenzae* type B endocarditis is very rare, even though this organism was a common cause of bacteremia in children prior to the introduction of conjugate vaccines.

The leading underlying cardiac lesions in children are tetralogy of Fallot and other forms of cyanotic congenital heart disease, ventricular septal defects, aortic stenosis, patent ductus arteriosus, pulmonary stenosis, and coarctation of the aorta. A high proportion of cases (77 percent of those with chronic heart disease) occur in children who have undergone palliative or corrective surgery for congenital cardiac defects.[62,84,86] Atrial septal defects of the ostium secundum type very rarely become infected (Chap. 64). Successful repair of ventricular septal defects and closure of patent ductus arteriosus appears to have greatly reduced the risk of endocarditis. In developed countries, preexisting rheumatic heart disease is now much less common than congenital disease. No underlying cardiac disease is found in about 15 percent of children with endocarditis, but the proportion is higher in those less than 2 years of age (Table 73-1).

A firm diagnosis of IE is more difficult to make in infants and small children than it is in adults. Signs and symptoms, however, are similar: fever occurs in 99 percent of pediatric cases, fatigue in 60 percent, arthralgias in 17 percent, petechiae in 21 percent, changing murmur in 21 percent, splenomegaly in 21 percent, and congenative heart failure in 9 percent. Blood cultures are positive in over 90 percent of the cases, which is also similar to adults. Viridans streptococci account for 38 percent of cases, *Staph. aureus* for 32 percent, enterococci for 7 percent, and a mixture of gram-positive cocci and gram-negative organisms for the rest.[84] Once the diagnosis is suspected, improved diagnostic criteria can help determine whether the child has endocarditis.[85] The clinical manifestations of acute rheumatic fever may mimic endocarditis (and vice versa), but fortunately the two conditions rarely coexist.

The choice of antibiotic treatment for children should be governed by the same principles as for adults, with appropriate 0dose adjustment for age. As in adults, valve replacement or other potentially curative surgical treatment should not be delayed if the child has heart failure that does not respond well to medical therapy.[87] Children with *Staph. aureus* endocarditis are most likely to have persistent fever bactermia, and complications, require surgery, and have a higher mortality rate than those who do not have *Staph. aureus*.[84,88]

The Elderly

With the increase in elderly people, endocarditis in this group has become more common.[89–92] The median age of patients with endocarditis has risen steadily for three decades, from about 30 to about 50 years. At present, approximately one-fourth of all patients are over age 60.[35,93] The annual risk for endocarditis is strongly age-related, being about 5 times higher in patients over age 80.[39] Male patients now outnumber females by approximately 1.5 to 1 overall, but by as much as 8 to 1 among patients over age 60.[33,94] Elderly patients are more likely to have underlying degenerative or calcific valve lesions.[90] Older patients (>70 years) had a higher proportion of bacteria from a gastrointestinal source (group D streptococci and enterococci accounted for 50 percent of cases in one series).[92] There is a higher mortality rate (28 versus 13 percent) for patients who are <70 years.[92]

Intravenous Drug Users

Illicit intravenous drug use poses a high risk for IE.[65–70,95] IDUs are 300 times more likely to die suddenly with IE than are nonusers.[96] Bacteremias related to parenteral drug abuse are common and arise either from direct intravenous injection of bacteria or from the skin flora and local infections at injection sites, including cellulitis, abscesses, or suppurative thrombophlebitis. Addicts seldom use sterile injection techniques, sometimes even taking water from toilet bowls to dissolve their drugs. Nevertheless, the organisms that cause drug-related endocarditis most frequently originate from the addict's skin and mucosal bacterial flora.[97] Strains of *Staph. aureus* cause more than 60 percent of cases of endocarditis among parenteral drug abusers, more than all other species combined.[50,70] Infections with gram-negative bacilli, especially *Pseudomonas* species[98,99] or yeasts and other fungi,[100] are notably more common than in nonaddicts (Table 73-3). *Candida parapsilosis* and other *Candida* species are the most common fungi causing drug-related endocarditis, but occasional infections with a wide range of other fungal species have been recorded.[100,101] Polymicrobial and culture-negative cases of endocarditis occur occasionally in IDUs, but together account for less than 5 percent of cases.[65,67,70,102]

Endocarditis in addicts frequently follows an acute course,[5,65,66,101] reflecting the high frequency of *Staph. aureus* infection. This finding partly explains the overall modest increase in the proportion of acute to subacute cases that has been observed over the past 25 years.[45]

The outstanding clinical feature of endocarditis in IDUs is the unusually high incidence of right-sided valvular infection. In various series, the tricuspid valve is involved in 60 to 70 percent of cases.[50,61,103] The aortic and/or mitral valves are involved in 30 to 40 percent.[50,103] More than one valve on either side of the heart may be infected simultaneously. Pulmonary valve infection is unusual even among IDUs, occurring in only some 2 percent of cases.

Tricuspid vegetations commonly embolize to the lungs, causing septic pulmonary infarcts, which result in multiple focal opacities on chest x-ray, sometimes with cavitation. In a drug addict with fever, this radiologic finding is a highly characteristic sign of acute right-sided endocarditis.[5,70] Mortality rates are much lower (4 percent) with endocarditis in IDUs than in other patient populations, even though the most common cause is *Staph. aureus*. This most likely reflects the benign nature of tricuspid valve involvement compared to left-sided disease.

Patients Infected with Human Immunodeficiency Virus

The primary risk factor for IE in HIV-infected people is the continued use of intravenous drugs, although IE is independently associated with HIV infection. Prior endocarditis, female sex, and skin abscesses are independent risk factors.[104] In one study, the adjusted odds ratio for HIV-infected IDUs with CD4 cell levels > 350 who developed endocarditis was 2.31 versus non-HIV-infected IDUs, but increased to an odds ratio of 8.31

TABLE 73-3 Frequency of Various Organisms Causing Infective Endocarditis[a]

Organism	NVE, %	IV Drug Abusers, %	Early PVE, %	Late PVE, %
Streptococci	60	15–25	5	35
Viridans, alpha-hemolytic	35	5–10	<5	25
Streptococcus bovis	10	<5	<5	<5
Enterococcus faecalis	10	10	<5	<5
Other streptococci	<5	<5	<5	<5
Staphylococci	25	50	50	30
Coagulase-positive	23	50	20	10
Coagulase-negative	<5	<5	30	20
Gram-negative aerobic bacilli	<5	5	20	10
Fungi	<5	<5	10	5
Miscellaneous bacteria	<5	5	5	5
Diphtheroids, propionibacteria	<1	<5	5	<5
Other anaerobes	<1	<1	<1	<1
Rickettsiae	<1	<1	<1	<1
Chlamydiae	<1	<1	<1	<1
Polymicrobial infection	<1	1–5	5	5
Culture-negative endocarditis	5–10	<5	<5	<5

[a]These are representative figures collated from the literature; wide local variations in frequency are to be expected. NVE = native valve endocarditis; PVE = prosthetic valve endocarditis; IV = intravenous.
SOURCE: Adapted from Refs. 43, 51, 65–70, 100–110, 115, 159.

when the CD4 cell count fell to < 350.[107] Several cases of *Bartonella* endocarditis have been reported in patients with acquired immunodeficiency syndrome (AIDS);[105] this appears to be a rare instance of true opportunistic infection of the endocardium. Patients in the earlier stages of HIV infection respond well to standard treatment for endocarditis, but mortality due to IE is high after the CD4+ T-cell count falls below 200 cells per cubic millimeter [49,106] (see also Chap. 70).

Post-Cardiac Surgery Patients

Intracardiac operations, especially valve replacements, have created a whole new population at risk for IE. In the 1950s, surgeons first noted that *Staph. epidermidis* endocarditis occurred fairly frequently after mitral valvotomy.[108] Subsequently, *Staph. epidermidis,* which rarely infects native valves, has become a common cause of both early and late PVE (Table 73-3).[8–11,95] Contamination of blood circulating through pump oxygenators with *Staph. epidermidis* or other organisms or from the operating room air can initiate infection at the time of operation, resulting in early PVE. In late PVE, the causative organisms usually originate from the normal flora of the skin or gastrointestinal tract, but their portal of entry largely remains unknown. Gram-negative bacilli and fungi infect prosthetic valves much more frequently than native valves, especially in early postoperative cases.[11,95,109] The spectrum of organisms causing late PVE more nearly resembles that of subacute native valve infection (Table 73-3).

Figure 73-1 shows the curve for incidence of PVE per month after valve replacement. The peak time of onset is 3 to 9 weeks after operation, with the risk falling quickly thereafter.[9] This important time relationship emphasizes that *Staph. epidermidis* and certain other organisms are often inoculated during or immediately after surgery, while streptococci infect the prosthesis during bacteremias that may occur at any time, unrelated to surgery.

The total number of cases of postsurgical endocarditis has increased along with the number of operations, even though the incidence per patient has decreased. This decrease reflects improved operative techniques and possibly the use of prophylactic antibiotics. Currently the rate is about 0.5 percent for early PVE, with a range of 0.3 to 1.2 percent.[8–11]

Patients with prosthetic valves now routinely survive for many years and remain at higher risk for late IE for the rest of their lives.[11,95,109,110] Late PVE occurs at a rate of about 0.3 to 0.5 percent per year.

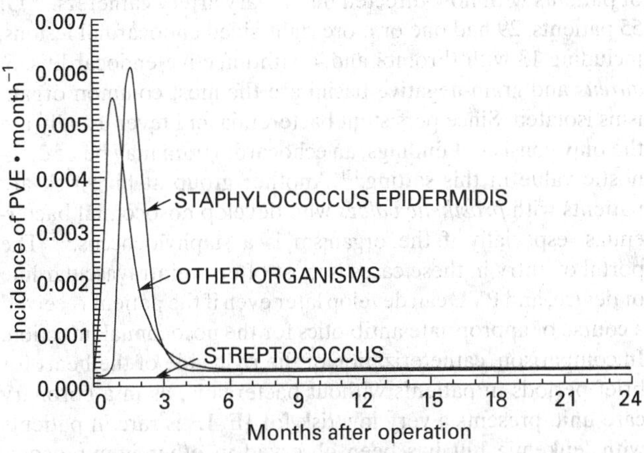

FIGURE 73-1 Incidence of prosthetic valve endocarditis (PVE) over 24 months after valve replacement. The hazard function has been stratified according to the infecting organisms. (From Ivert TSA, Dismukes WE, Cobbs CG, et al. Prosthetic valve endocarditis. *Circulation* 1984; 69:223. Reproduced with permission.)

Obstetric and Gynecologic Patients

Endocarditis occurring as a complication of pregnancy is most likely to develop at the time of delivery or in the puerperium.[111] Normal delivery presents a low risk of endocarditis, even in the presence of preexisting valvular disease,[112] but bacteremias associated with perinatal infective complications such as endometritis, parametritis, septic thrombophlebitis in pelvic veins, or urinary tract infection can seed the mother's endocardium.[111] Septic abortion or pelvic infection related to intrauterine contraceptive devices also can provide the portal of entry for bacteremia resulting in endocarditis.[113] The organisms most often involved are *Enterococcus faecalis,* group B streptococci, *Staph. aureus,* and occasionally gram-negative enteric bacilli or anaerobes.

Nosocomial Endocarditis

Hospital-acquired IE can involve either prosthetic or native valves.[114,115] This serious complication is not rare; one study[116] reported no fewer than 35 examples of probable nosocomial endocarditis among 125 cases (28 percent), and the rate may be rising.[114] Intensive medical care predisposes to endocarditis in several ways. Endocardial damage can be produced by surgery, by intracardiac catheters, and by intravascular devices such as hyperalimentation catheters and cerebrospinal fluid shunts if they reach into the right atrium. Portals of entry for microorganisms are provided by wounds, biopsy sites, pacemakers, intravenous and arterial catheters,[117] urinary catheters, and intratracheal airways. In one study, 75 percent of the suspected sources of infection were vascular access sites.[118] Nosocomial bacteremias arising from local infections are common in seriously ill patients. Up to two-thirds of patients with nosocomial endocarditis had no known predisposing cardiac abnormalities.[118]

Many of the previously mentioned factors coexist in *severely burned* patients. In one study, either NBTE or IE was found at autopsy in all of 6 burned patients who sustained repeated episodes of bacteremia while a pressure-monitoring catheter was maintained in the right side of the heart before death.[119] This observation has been confirmed in another autopsy study of patients with flow-directed pulmonary artery catheters.[120] Of 55 patients, 29 had one or more right-sided endocardial lesions, including 13 with thrombi and 4 with infective endocarditis. *S. aureus* and gram-negative bacilli are the most common organisms isolated. Since persistent bacteremia and fever usually are the only consistent findings, an echocardiogram may be of diagnostic value in this setting.[121] Another group at high risk are patients with *prosthetic valves* who develop nosocomial bacteremias, especially if the organism is a staphylococcus.[115] The portal of entry in these cases is most often an intravascular line or device, and PVE can develop later even if the patient received a course of appropriate antibiotics for the nosocomial infection. In comparison, catheterization of the right side of the heart for brief periods in patients without bacteremia, as in a coronary care unit, presents a very low risk for IE. IE is rare in patients with leukemia but has been observed in other immunocompromised patients—for example, after bone marrow transplantation[122] and heart transplantation.[123] In a report of 46 cases after solid organ transplantation, *Aspergillus fumigatus* and *Staph. aureus* were causative in 50 percent, whereas viridans streptococci were isolated in only 4 percent. Six of 10 cases that occurred within 30 days of transplantation were fungal. No predisposing cardiac abnormality was known to be present in 80 percent. Infected venous access devices and wounds were suspected portals of entry in three-fourths of the cases. The mortality rate was 57 percent, and most infections were not diagnosed prior to death.[124]

Overall, the leading organisms causing nosocomial endocarditis are staphylococci, enterococci, *Candida* species, and gram-negative bacilli. *Staph. aureus* is especially associated with wound infections, cellulitis, and cannula infections; *Staph. epidermidis* with ventriculoatrial shunts; and *C. albicans* with parenteral alimentation.

The prognosis for nosocomial native valve endocarditis is worse than for other forms of native valve infection (up to 50 percent mortality).[114,118] These patients often have serious underlying disease that may delay diagnosis of endocarditis by obscuring the symptoms and signs, while the organisms most commonly involved (staphylococci and enterococci) are more difficult to eradicate than viridans streptococci.

Hemodialysis

Creation of arteriovenous shunts for hemodialysis predisposes patients to develop IE by providing a ready portal of entry for bacteremias. Another possible factor is increased cardiac output. Dogs with high cardiac output due to surgically created arteriovenous fistulas are predisposed to develop not only infective endarteritis at the site of the shunt but endocarditis as well.[125] Therefore, it is not surprising that endocarditis has been reported in 2 to 6 percent of patients on long-term hemodialysis employing either arteriovenous fistulas or cannulas. *Staph. aureus* and *Staph. epidermidis* have been the most common etiologic organisms, followed by viridans streptococci and *E. faecalis.*[126] The diagnosis of endocarditis is difficult in these patients, partly because coexisting intravascular infection at the shunt site often confuses the clinical picture. Mortality is high (53 percent), and a high index of suspicion and use of an echocardiography followed by aggressive treatment of both shunt infections and endocarditis in dialysis patients are necessary to improve outcome.[126] In one study of 20 cases of IE in hemodialysis patients, vegetations were found in 50 percent by transthoracic echocardiogram (TTE) and 81 percent by transesophageal echocardiogram (TEE).[127] In 65 hemodialysis patients with *Staph. aureus* bacteremia, 8 (12 percent) were found to have IE by TEE (6 of whom had normal TTEs).[128]

Pacemaker Infective Endocarditis

The placement of permanent pacemaker leads into the right ventricle may result in endocardial lead infection in 0.2 to 7 percent of patients. These may occur early (6 weeks to 3 months after placement) and are caused by *Staph. epidermidis* in 90 percent, or late, when *Staph. epidermidis* or *Staph. aureus* each account for nearly 50 percent, with gram-negative bacilli causing the remaining few. The definitive diagnosis usually requires TEE, which will detect vegetations in or around the leads in >90 percent of cases. The chest x-ray is predictive in one-third for pulmonary emboli. Cure requires removal of the pacemaker generator and leads, and treatment with antibiotics.[129–132]

Infective Endarteritis

Focal intravascular infection located outside the heart itself can mimic most of the clinical manifestations of endocarditis, including vascular and immunologic phenomena.[50] In the past, about one-quarter of all patients with an uncorrected patent ductus arteriosus developed bacterial endarteritis.[3] Coarctations of the aorta also presented a significant risk, but endocarditis located on an associated bicuspid aortic valve was 3 times more common than was endarteritis with vegetations located in the coarctation. Endarteritis occasionally complicates traumatic arteriovenous fistulas, but arteriosclerotic aneurysms rarely become infected.[50] When bacterial endarteritis does occur within an aneurysm, the organisms usually grow in a multilayered thrombus in the lumen of the aneurysm rather than in vegetations.

The spectrum of organisms causing infective endarteritis is similar to that found in endocarditis except that there is a higher frequency of infection with salmonellae in arteriosclerotic abdominal aneurysms.[50,133] The pattern of embolization observed differs according to the site of infection. Thus, petechiae may occur on the skin of the lower extremities in a patient with an infected abdominal aneurysm, and infarctions may appear in the lungs of a patient with an infected dialysis fistula in the forearm.

Because many of the congenital and acquired vascular lesions that predispose to infective endarteritis can be corrected by modern surgery, endarteritis—except in arteriovenous shunts constructed for the purpose of hemodialysis—is uncommon today in developed countries.

ETIOLOGIC ORGANISMS

The range of microbial species that can cause infective endocarditis is extraordinarily wide, yet only a few species account for the great majority of cases. On native valves, streptococci and staphylococci together cause more than 80 percent of infections.[38,43,51,116] By comparison, NVE caused by *Staph. epidermidis,* enteric bacilli, and fungi are uncommon. Among IDUs and patients with prosthetic valves, the incidence of infection due to these organisms is higher. Table 73-3 offers representative data from the literature on the relative frequency of the major etiologic organisms on native valves, in drug addicts, and on prosthetic valves. It should be emphasized that the relative frequency with which various organisms cause endocarditis can vary widely between countries and between medical centers.

Streptococci

Streptococci cause more cases of endocarditis than any other group of organisms.[38,51,134–136] The alpha-hemolytic or viridans streptococci account for the majority of these cases, but have decreased in frequency when compared with others during the last 30 years. Viridans streptococci are ubiquitous (although outnumbered by anaerobes) in the oropharyngeal and gastrointestinal flora. They are usually low-grade pathogens (except for *Strep. milleri*), often recovered from clinical specimens in mixed culture with other organisms but seldom themselves causing disease. Their strong association with SBE is therefore determined by the frequency with which they enter the bloodstream and by their ability to adhere to endocardium rather than by their innate virulence.

The nomenclature of these organisms is complex and has been subject to repeated revisions.[134,137,138] The following species frequently cause SBE: *Strep. sanguis, Strep. mitis, Strep. oralis,* and *Strep. gordonii.* Many other species occasionally cause SBE; for example, the *Strep. milleri* group: *Strep. anginosus, Strep. intermedius,* and *Strep. constellatus.*[134,136,137] A few cases are caused by strains that require media supplemented with L-cysteine or pyridoxine for growth.[139–142] These strains are more difficult to isolate from blood and seem to be more difficult to eradicate with antibiotic treatment than the other viridans streptococci.

Group D streptococci are next in frequency among the streptococci as a cause of endocarditis.[94,143,144] The nonenterococcal group D species, *Strep. bovis,* accounts for about one-fifth of streptococcal cases. IE caused by *Strep. bovis* tends to occur in older patients, affect multiple valves, and require surgery more commonly than IE caused by other organisms.[145] Gastrointestinal lesions, especially colonic polyps and cancers, are present in > 50 percent of patients who develop *Strep. bovis* bacteremia and/or endocarditis.[146,147] Hence, recovery of this species from blood cultures should prompt investigation for colonic disease, whether or not the patient has gastrointestinal symptoms.

Strains of *E. faecalis* (enterococci) cause about 10 percent of streptococcal cases. In the past it was said that this species caused endocarditis "in young women and old men," because it was found in association with infections of the genital and urinary tract in women of childbearing age and of the urinary tract in old men with prostatic disease. Today, enterococcal endocarditis is also likely to be found in drug addicts, in patients with nosocomial endocarditis, and in those with chronic renal failure.[94] Enterococci commonly cause urinary tract, wound, and intravenous line infections, which often give rise to nosocomial bacteremias.[148,149] Fewer than 2 percent of such patients have endocarditis, but if enterococcal bacteremia is community-acquired without a primary focus of infection, about one-third will have IE.[148] Antibiotic resistance, especially in strains of *E. faecium,* presents major difficulties in treatment of enterococcal endocarditis.[94,150–152]

Many other species and strains of streptococci occasionally cause endocarditis, but they are rare compared with the viridans and group D organisms. *Strep. pneumoniae* endocarditis has become uncommon since the advent of antibiotics. This species causes acute endocarditis,[153] affects primarily the aortic valve in patients without underlying valvular disease (15 of 16 in one series), and often requires immediate valve replacement for aortic insufficiency and cardiac failure (7 of 16).[154,155] In debilitated alcoholics, bacteremic pneumococcal pneumonia is occasionally complicated by the development of pneumococcal endocarditis and meningitis. This triad of simultaneous pneumococcal infections carries an extremely poor prognosis.[153] Beta-hemolytic streptococci rarely cause IE, but in a report of 31 cases, one-third had underlying diabetes mellitis, three-fourths had significant complications, and one-half required cardiac surgery.[156] In children, group A streptococcus may complicate varicella.[157] Group B streptococcal endocarditis is also rare, but may complicate obstetric or other surgical procedures (abortions) or injection drug use, and may involve the tricuspid valve.[158]

Staphylococci

Staph. aureus is the leading cause of acute bacterial endocarditis. Median duration of illness prior to hospitalization was 3 days in one series.[160] It is the predominant etiologic organism in IDUs with endocarditis[70] and frequently causes PVE.[95] *Staph. aureus* endocarditis is also a complication of diabetes mellitis (13 percent in one study), corticosteroid therapy (11 percent), cirrhosis (5 percent), malignancy (4 percent), and chronic renal failure (4 percent).[160] In nosocomial cases, infected intravascular devices were the most common portal of entry. Because it is an invasive primary pathogen, patients with staphylococcal ABE often develop disseminated disease with metastatic infections in skin and soft tissue, bone, joints, eye, or brain.[159–162] More than one-third of patients with *Staph. aureus* endocarditis will have central nervous system involvement.[160]

Only a minority of all patients with *Staph. aureus* bacteremia have endocarditis (6 to 15 percent), and it is often difficult to identify this subgroup clinically. However, use of TEE in this setting is highly effective in establishing the diagnosis of IE. Factors that increase the probability that such a patient has endocarditis are (1) community-acquired bacteremia, (2) absence of a primary focus of infection, and (3) presence of metastatic foci of staphylococcal infection. Up to two-thirds of patients with all 3 of these characteristics have endocarditis.[162] *Staph. epidermidis* is a rare cause of native valve infection (<5 percent), usually associated with an indolent subacute or chronic course.[163] However, serious complications, including systemic embolization, congestive heart failure, myocardial abscess, and valve destruction are common and mortality is high (up to 36 percent).[164] *Staph. lugdunensis,* a recently described species of coagulase negative staphylococcus, appears to be especially virulent and more likely to infect native cardiac valves than *Staph. epidermidis*.[165] In striking contrast, *Staph. epidermidis* is a common cause of PVE (40 to 50 percent), which may follow either an acute or subacute clinical course.[163,166]

Gram-Negative Bacteria

Although most of the species of gram-negative bacteria that colonize and/or infect humans have been reported to cause IE, they account for only a small proportion of cases of native valve infection. A significant subgroup of cases are caused by a group of nutritionally fastidious gram-negative bacilli: *Haemophilus* species, *Actinobacillus actinomycetemcomitans, Cardiobacterium hominis, Eikenella corrodens*, and *Kingella kingae*. These are often referred to by the acronym HACEK, which is derived from their initials,[167,168] and cause approximately 3 percent of cases of IE. In one report, most patients had symptoms between 2 weeks and 3 months and presented with fever, a new or changing murmur, splenomegaly, and emboli.[169] Blood cultures usually took 3 to 4 days to turn positive.[169] Prognosis with medical therapy and surgery, when necessary (one-fourth of patients), was good, with 87 percent overall survival.

Cases caused by *Haemophilus* predominate in this group. Endocarditis caused by this genus is usually due to *H. parainfluenza* (62 percent), *H. aphrophilus* (21 percent), *H. paraphrophilus* (10 percent), and only rarely to *H. influenzae*. *Haemophilus* endocarditis is characterized by large vegetations and arterial emboli (35 to 60 percent).[170]

The common aerobic enteric gram-negative bacilli seldom cause endocarditis. For example, cases of endocarditis caused by *Escherichia coli* and *Klebsiella* are notably rare,[99] even though these species frequently cause gram-negative bacteremia. The reasons for this striking disparity are probably multiple, including low adhesiveness of gram-negative enteric bacilli to heart valves[171] and fibrin[172] and susceptibility of many strains to complement-mediated bacteriolysis.[173] Despite these factors, two special populations are at increased risk of gram-negative endocarditis: IDUs and patients with prosthetic valves. Gram-negative bacilli account for about 5 percent of endocarditis in IDUs,[65,68–70] with *Pseudomonas* species, *Serratia*, and *Enterobacter* species predominating. Gram-negative bacilli cause 15 to 20 percent of early PVE and about 10 percent of late PVE.[11,95] Strains of gram-negative bacilli such as *Stenotrophomonas (Xanthomonas) multophilia,* which are resistant to most antibiotics, are becoming more common. They typically cause nosocomial IE (50 percent), occur on prosthetic heart valves (50 percent), and are associated with IDUs or indwelling vascular catheters (18.8 percent).[174]

Interesting but unusual cases caused by species of *Salmonella, Brucella, Acinetobacter,* and other gram-negative bacilli have been reported.[99] *Brucella* endocarditis is well known in the Mediterranean basin[175–177] but is rare in most other regions. Endocarditis caused by anaerobic bacteria is rare (1 percent or less of cases),[178,179] possibly because the oxygen tension in heart blood is too high to favor growth of these species on the endocardium.

N. gonorrhoeaea causes an acute form of the disease,[2] often involving the right side of the heart. Like the pneumococcus, *N. gonorrhoeaea* has become uncommon as a cause of endocarditis since the introduction of penicillin.[51,52]

Yeasts and Dimorphic Fungi

Although many species of yeasts and other fungi can infect the endocardium, only two genera account for the great majority: *Candida* and *Aspergillus*.[100,101,180,181] *Candida* causes native valve infections in IDUs and in patients receiving parenteral alimentation, while *Aspergillus* species often involve prosthetic valves. Fungal infection of native valves in nonaddicts is rare (Table 73-3).

Miscellaneous Organisms

Many less common organisms occasionally cause endocarditis; for example, *Coxiella burnetii* (Q fever) and *Chlamydia*. Q-fever endocarditis is a chronic, febrile systemic illness with prominent hepatic as well as cardiac valvular involvement.[182–188] Most cases have been reported from Europe, Canada, and Australia and occur in approximately 7 percent of cases of Q fever. Patients typically present with intermittent fever for months to years (91 percent) or with congestive heart failure (77 percent), and almost all have underlying valvular heart disease (97 percent). Diagnosis is difficult and usually based on serology or identification of the organism in cardiac tissue.[183] One report indicates that *Bartonella* may cause up to 3 percent of cases of IE[189]; in the past, most of these cases were listed as culture-negative, while some were misdiagnosed as chlamydial due to false-positive cross-reacting serologic tests.[189] When suspected on clinical and epidemiological grounds (homeless patient: *Bartonella quintana;* close association with cats: *Bartonella henselae*), PCR (polymerase chain reaction)-based genomic detection or antibody determination are considerably more sensitive than culture in identification of the organism.[190] Chlamydial endocarditis is rare; a few cases have been reported in bird fanciers.[191,192] In such cases, the etiologic diagnosis can be established only by specialized culture techniques, serologic studies, or examination of vegetations using immunofluorescent antibodies. More than 50 cases of *Listeria monocytogenes* endocarditis in both native and prosthetic valves have been reported with a high mortality rate (37 percent).[193] Many other unusual species occasionally infect prosthetic valves, including *Mycoplasma hominis,*[194] *Legionella* species,[53] and mycobacteria.[195] Some examples of rare or unusual organisms that have caused one or more cases of endocarditis are listed in Table 73-4.

Culture-Negative Endocarditis

The term, *culture-negative endocarditis*, refers to the active IE whose repeated blood cultures are all negative.[196–198] This syndrome was occasionally observed in the preantibiotic era,[199] usually in subacute cases of long duration (*Endocarditis lenta*). Today, most (but not all) culture-negative cases are caused by antibiotic treatment that is sufficient to suppress the bacteremia but not to sterilize the vegetation. In most such cases, organisms will eventually reappear in the blood after antibiotics are discontinued, usually within a few days. The blood cultures from a few patients with active endocarditis remain persistently culture-negative after antibiotics are stopped.[116]

Negative blood culture results should be expected from about one-fifth of patients with NVE or PVE caused by *Candida* or other yeasts,[101] and from four-fifths of patients with endocarditis caused by *Aspergillus* or other molds.[101,180,200,201]

The reported incidence of culture-negative endocarditis varies widely. Among large unselected series of cases collected from several hospitals, as much as 15 to 20 percent may be culture-negative.[51,196–198] Smaller series of patients studied by a single clinical and laboratory team that is experienced in evaluation of endocarditis usually show only about 5 percent culture-negative cases.[202,203] Thus, in a patient with suspected IE, other diagnoses should be meticulously excluded before a diagnosis of culture-negative endocarditis is accepted. When a patient appears to have IE but blood cultures are negative, the following checklist of possibilities should be considered:

- The patient has received some antibiotic therapy, commonly an oral drug such as ampicillin that was taken at home.
- The etiologic organism is slow-growing, requiring longer incubation of the blood culture for isolation, e.g., some nutritionally variant streptococci, some HACEK species, or mycobacteria.
- The etiologic organism is nutritionally fastidious, requiring special procedures or supplemented media for isolation, e.g., nutritionally variant streptococci, *C. burnetii* (Q fever), *Chlamydia, Mycoplasma, Bartonella,* and *Legionella.*
- The etiologic organism is a strict anaerobe, requiring anaerobic culture conditions.
- The etiologic organism is *Aspergillus* or another mold; these are rarely recovered from blood during the course of endocarditis (although they may be recovered from an arterial embolus removed at surgery).
- The etiologic organism is nonculturable, which is usually diagnosed by PCR on cardiac tissue during surgery for valve insufficiency. Few clinical cases are present as these patients may not have gastrointestinal symptoms, although most will have arthralgias.[200]
- The patient has an alternative diagnosis that simulates IE—e.g., rheumatic fever, tuberculosis, brucellosis, etc.
- The patient has NBTE or marantic endocarditis, associated with a major underlying disease such as malignancy or tuberculosis.
- The patient has Libman-Sacks endocarditis (a variant of NBTE), associated with antiphospholipid antibody syndrome and/or systemic lupus erythematosus.

In some cases, a working diagnosis of endocarditis based on clinical manifestations can be supported by the progress of the disease and good response to empiric antibiotic treatment. If blood culture results always remain negative, a definitive etiologic diagnosis can be made only by detecting organisms in an infected embolus or in vegetations excised during surgery or at autopsy.

TABLE 73-4 Some Unusual or Rare Causes of Infective Endocarditis

Bacteria	Fungi
Bacillus cereus	*Blastoschizomyces capitatus*
Bartonella elizabethae	*Conidiobolus* sp.
Bartonella henselae	*Curvularia lunata*
Corynebacterium diphtheriae biotype *gravis*	*Engyodontium album*
Corynebacterium jeikeium	*Fusarium oxysporum*
Corynebacterium pseudodiphtheriticum	*Histoplasma capsulatum*
Erysipelothrix rhusiopathiae	*Neosartorya fischeri*
Haemophilus influenzae type b	*Phialophora richardsiae*
Lactobacillus species	*Pseudallescheria boydii*
Legionella species	*Scedosporium inflatum*
Mycoplasma hominis	*Scedosporium apiospermum*
Rothia dentocariosa	*Thermomyces lanuginosus tsiklinsky*
Streptobacillus moniliformis	*Trichosporon beigelii*

PATHOGENESIS AND PATHOLOGY

A general concept of the pathogenesis of NBTE and SBE is presented in Fig. 73-2.

Noninfective Endocarditis

Sterile thrombotic lesions may develop on heart valves in a variety of clinical conditions.[204] Small aggregates of platelets can occasionally be found on normal valves, but they occur frequently on the surfaces of valves damaged by congenital, rheumatic, or granlomatous disease[205] or by IE. These could be considered as incipient vegetations or microvegetations.

The common factor leading to platelet deposition is endothelial damage. This exposes subendothelial connective tissue containing collagen, which activates platelets to adhere and aggregate at the site. These microscopic platelet thrombi may embolize away harmlessly, or they may be stabilized and grow by deposition of fibrin and more platelets to form vegetations of NBTE. This process can be duplicated experimentally by

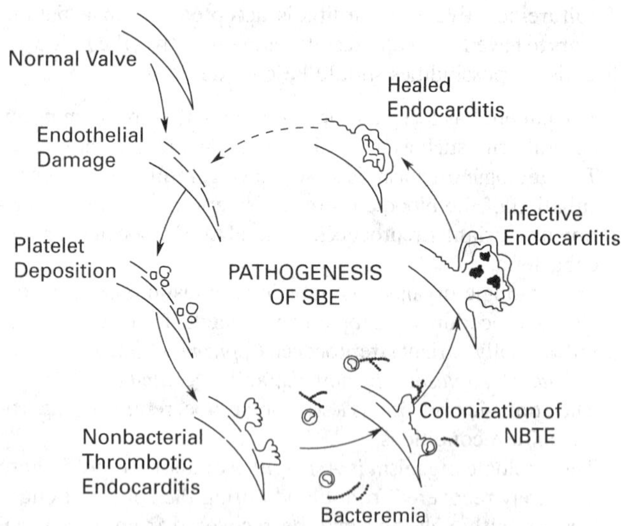

FIGURE 73-2 The main events in the pathogenesis of nonbacterial thrombotic endocarditis (NBTE) and subacute bacterial endocarditis (SBE).

catheter-induced endothelial damage in animals.[206] In humans, intracardiac pressure-monitoring catheters may produce identical lesions.[119,120] Both experimental[207] and human[119,122,204] NBTE can be colonized by circulating bacteria, resulting in IE.

The vegetations of marantic endocarditis occur most often in patients with advanced malignancy[13–15] but may also complicate other chronic wasting diseases, such as tuberculosis or uremia.

Sterile vegetations (termed *Libman-Sacks endocarditis*—see Chap. 76) sometimes develop in patients with systemic lupus erythematosus and/or antiphospholipid antibodies.[208] Typically, Libman-Sacks vegetations are small, sessile masses located on the ventricular surfaces of the mitral valve leaflets.

The vegetations of NBTE are friable white or tan masses, usually situated along the lines of valve closure (Fig. 73-3, Plate 101). These vary greatly in size; from tiny to large and exuberant, with a corresponding tendency to embolize to arteries supplying the myocardium, spleen, kidney, brain, mesentery, or extremities and causing infection. Since there is little inflammatory

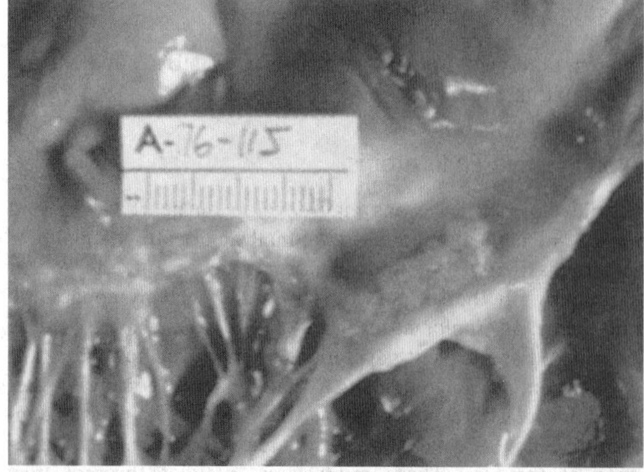

FIGURE 73-3 (Plate 101) Typical vegetation of nonbacterial thrombotic endocarditis found at necropsy in a cachectic patient who died with disseminated lung cancer.

reaction at the site of attachment, fresh vegetations can dislodge and embolize frequently.[204] Histologically, the vegetations of NBTE consist of degenerating platelets interwoven with strands of fibrin, forming a bland, eosinophilic mass, featureless except for a few trapped leukocytes.[204,206]

Pathogenesis of Infective Endocarditis

For IE to develop, two events are essential. First, microbes must attach to an endocardial surface. Second, the microbes must persist and multiply locally, eluding host defense mechanisms. In the case of SBE, which usually develops on previously abnormal valves, bacteria circulating in the bloodstream probably colonize preexisting platelet aggregates or NBTE.[204] It is not known whether ABE, which often affects apparently normal valves, develops in a like manner by colonization of microscopic sterile vegetations, or by direct microbial invasion of normal endothelium.

A critical initial step in the pathogenesis of IE is the attachment or adherence of the circulating microorganism to the disrupted cardiac valve endothelium that has deposits of fibrin and platelets (NBTE). The characteristic that gives the microbe selective adherence advantage to this surface are virulence factors for the development of IE. Early studies identified dextran production in viridans streptococci as an important adherence factor (it had been previously shown to be important in adherence to teeth and production of dental caries).[172] A host of other microbial factors have been described. These include a fibrinectin-binding protein,[377] enterococcal aggregation substance, and enterococcal binding substances (proteins that also mediate formation of mating aggregate between bacteria that cause horizontal transfer of plasmids encoding such things as antibiotic resistance[210] and FimA, a surface-associated protein found on oral streptoccoci and enterococci, that, when used as an antigen (similar to other surface proteins of the Lral family) produce an antibody that reduces adherence to valve surfaces and reduces development of endocarditis in animal model.[209–212] Since FimA is found in 80 percent of streptococci and enterococci strains that produce endocarditis, a protective vaccine strategy is an intriguing probability. Binding to fibronectin appears to be an important property shared by many but not all of the bacterial species that commonly cause endocarditis.[50,209] Clumping factor produced by coagulase-positive staphylococci favors attachment to fibrinogen, adherence to platelet-fibrin clots, and ability to cause endocarditis in rats.[213] Extracellular slime production by coagulase-negative staphylococci may favor localization on prosthetic valves.[214] *Thus, microbial adherence, which can be mediated by a variety of different surface components and receptors, is a key virulance factor for colonization of the endocardium.*[50,209]

The role of the platelet in this postadherance event has been elucidated. First, adherence of *Staph. aureus* to platelets is an important virulance factor for development of experimental IE.[219–225] In addition, acetylsallicylic acid treatment reduces *Staph. aureus*-induced platelet aggregation and adherence to fibrin (with or without platelets) matrices in vitro and reduced vegetation size and embolic events in vivo.[224,225] When *Staph. aureus* (or enterococci) adhere to damaged valves in vivo, tissue thromboplastin is generated, which locally activates the clotting cascade, generating thrombin.[205,220] A vegetation is formed that provides a protected environment for unrestricted bacterial growth. However, thrombin also elicits the secretion from platelets of a low-molecular-weight cationic protein with potent antimicrobial properties (against *Staph. aureus, Staph. epidermidis,* viridans streptococci and *Candida*) termed *thrombin-induced platelet microbiocidal protein* (tPMP).[221] Strains of *Staph. aureus* that are resistant to tPMP are more likely to cause endocarditis in animals and humans.[222] In addition, strains that hypersecrete alpha toxin (a toxin known to lyse platelets and release tPMP) produced a less virulent form of IE, likely due to the antimicrobial action of tPMP.[223]

Therefore, once lodged on NBTE, bacteria must elude local defenses, including platelet microbicidal proteins[215] and leukocytes, if they are to survive. Microbes that cannot do this may die out quickly after adhering to the endocardium.[216] Those that can survive antimicrobial defense mechanisms multiply rapidly in the vegetation, soon reaching high numbers and then entering a stationary growth phase.[207] The vegetation provides an ideal supporting stroma for the growth of microbial colonies, into which essential nutrients can diffuse from the blood. The presence of bacteria is a powerful stimulus for further thrombosis,[217,218] which may be mediated by thromboplastin generated by leukocytes when they are exposed to fibrin.[218] New layers of fibrin are deposited around growing bacteria, causing the vegetations to enlarge.[206] Inflammatory cytokines are produced by monocytes[226] (and presumably other leukocytes) in response to endocardial infection and likely cause some of the patient's symptoms.

The location of vegetations is relevant to understanding and managing endocarditis. Approximate incidence of vegetations at various locations is given in Table 73-5. The frequency of involvement of each valve is directly proportional to the mean blood pressure upon it;[227] thus, the left side of the heart is involved much more often than the right. This rule does not hold true for acute endocarditis in IDUs, in whom tricuspid infection by *Staph. aureus* predominates (Table 73-5).

Vegetations are usually located on the downstream side of anatomic abnormalities in the heart or great vessels. Rodbard[228] developed the unifying concept that vegetations usually arise at a site where blood flows from a high-pressure source (e.g., the left ventricle) through a narrow orifice (e.g., a stenotic aortic valve) into a low-pressure sink (e.g., the aorta). Illustrative examples from human disease include aortic stenosis, ventricular septal defect, coarctation, and mitral regurgitation. Experimentally, Rodbard showed that bacteria carried in an aerosol flowing through a constricted tube into an area of low pressure were deposited on the walls of the tube immediately beyond the constriction due to Venturi pressure effects and turbulence.[228] These observations fit well with the actual location of vegetations found at autopsy in cases of endocarditis (Fig. 73-4). Vegetations also may develop on jet lesions, which are areas of

TABLE 73-5 Approximate Frequency of Anatomic Location of Vegetations in SBE, ABE, and Endocarditis Associated with IV Drug Abuse[a]

Location	SBE, %	ABE, %	Endocarditis in IV Drug Abusers, %
Left-sided valves	85	65	40
Aortic	15–26	18–25	15–20
Mitral	38–45	30–35	15–20
Aortic and mitral	23–30	15–20	13–20
Right-sided valves	5	20	50–70
Tricuspid	1–5	15	45–65
Pulmonary	1	Rare	2
Tricuspid and pulmonary	Rare	Rare	3
Left- and right-sided sites	Rare	5–10	5–10
Other sites (patent ductus, ventricular septal defect, coarctation, jet lesions)	10	5	5

[a]SBE = subacute bacterial endocarditis; ABE = acute bacterial endocarditis.
SOURCE: Adapted from Refs. 51, 65–70, 86, 116, 159, 227, 230.

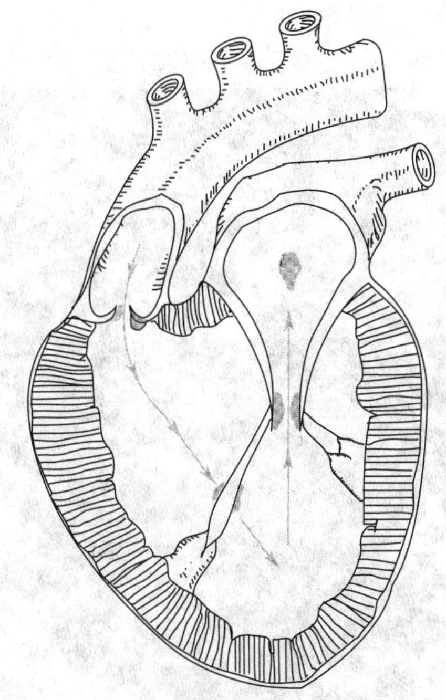

FIGURE 73-4 The sites where endocarditis occurs in aortic and mitral regurgitation. The arrows on the left indicate a high-velocity regurgitant stream passing through the orifice of an incompetent aortic valve into a low-pressure sink (left ventricle in diastole). Vegetations appear on the ventricular surface of the aortic valve. The regurgitant stream may cause a jet lesion on the chordae tendineae of the anterior leaflet of the mitral valve. The arrow on the right shows regurgitation from the high-pressure source of the left ventricle during systole into the left atrium, with vegetations developing on the atrial surface of the mitral valve. Vegetations also can occur on the jet lesion where the regurgitant stream through the mitral valve strikes the atrial endocardium, an area known as *MacCallum's patch*. (From Rodbard S. Blood velocity and endocarditis. *Circulation* 1963; 27:8. Reproduced with permission.)

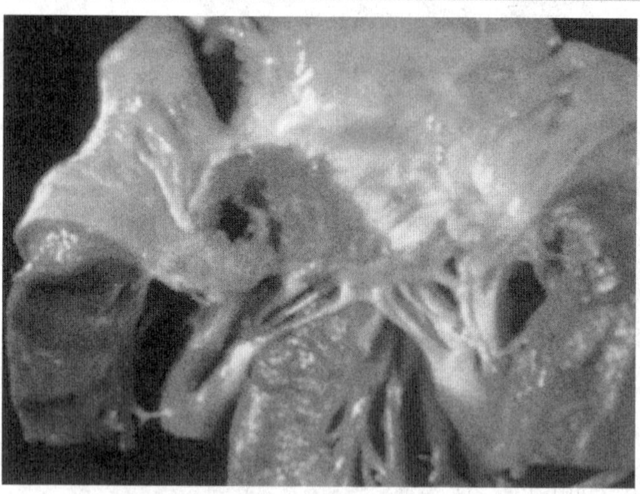

FIGURE 73-5 (Plate 102) Typical vegetation of bacterial endocarditis, complicated by perforation of the anterior mitral valve leaflet. Note that the valve shows preexisting chronic rheumatic disease, with thickening, deformity, and fusion of chordae tendineae.

endothelial roughening and reactive fibrosis at sites where a swift, turbulent regurgitant stream of blood strikes the endothelium.[229] *MacCallum's patch,* on the wall of the left atrium in some patients with mitral regurgitation, is an example of a jet lesion; an infected vegetation occasionally develops at this site (Fig. 73-4).

Vegetations of infective endocarditis vary greatly in size and morphology, from small (<1 mm), warty nodules to large (several centimeters), cauliflower-like polypoid masses. That may cause functional stenosis of valve orifices (Fig. 73-5, Plate 102). Fungal vegetations are often larger than bacterial ones, but otherwise the etiologic species does not correlate reliably with vegetation size. Their color also varies widely, from white to tan to greenish-gray.[67,230] Histologically, colonies of microorganisms are found embedded in a fibrin-platelet matrix.[206,207,231,232] The vegetation characteristically contain relatively few leukocytes that are prevented from reaching bacteria by layers of fibrin, which form protective barriers around colonies (Fig. 73-6).

Development of an abscess is one of the most important complications of valvular infection, and it occurs more frequently with ABE than it does with SBE.[229,231] Abscesses often develop by direct extension of active infection into the fibrous cardiac skeleton—that is, into the rings of supporting connective tissue around the valves. From there, abscesses can extend into the adjacent myocardium and rupture into the pericardium. Hematogenous seeding occasionally leads to development of abscesses elsewhere in the myocardium.

Abscesses are found in the majority of patients who die with active prosthetic valve infection, often spreading around the sewing ring of the prosthesis and causing partial dehiscence of the prosthetic valve.[11,95] Because these valve-ring abscesses are located close to the cardiac conduction system, conduction disturbances commonly result.[233]

FIGURE 73-6 Electron micrograph of a vegetation of experimental streptococcal endocarditis (×7800). Note the very large number of cocci in colonies, the protective layers of fibrin, and the absence of leukocytes—all factors that may impede the efficacy of antimicrobial therapy. (From Durack DT. Experimental bacterial endocarditis: 4. Structure and evolution of very early lesions. *J Pathol* 1975; 115:81. Reproduced with permission.)

Immune Response

Presence of bacteria in endocardial vegetations stimulates the humoral immune system to produce nonspecific antibodies. This can result in a polyclonal increase in gamma globulins, positive rheumatoid factor, and, occasionally, false-positive serologic test results for syphilis.[234] Rheumatoid factor develops in 25 to 50 percent of patients with SBE present for >6 weeks and can provide a useful diagnostic clue; it reverts to negative after eradication of the organisms.[235-237] Antiendocardial and antisarcolemmal antibodies have been detected in 60 to 100 percent of cases;[238] they are more commonly found in SBE than they are in ABE.

Specific antibodies to many of the commensal organisms that cause SBE may be present in low titer before infection. Titers rise during active infection[3] and fall after treatment.

Hemolytic complement levels are low in about 30 percent of patients early in the course of endocarditis, rising later and returning to normal after treatment.[239-245] The lowest levels are found in patients with immune-complex glomerulonephritis.

Circulating immune complexes have been detected in 82 to 97 percent of patients with either ABE or SBE.[244-247] Higher concentrations are correlated with the presence of extracardiac manifestations such as arthritis, splenomegaly, and glomerulonephritis; with longer duration of illness; and with hypocomplementemia. Several studies confirm that glomerulonephritis in patients with endocarditis is mediated by immune complexes.[248,249] It is likely but unproven that arthritis and tenosynovitis—and possibly pericarditis, Osler's nodes, and Roth's spots[244,246,247]—also may represent inflammatory responses involving immune complexes. Antibodies to teichoic acids were found in the serum of 93 percent of patients with *Staph. aureus* endocarditis,[250] but this did not prove to be useful as a routine diagnostic test. Additional relevant information on experimental infective endocarditis is contained in References 251 to 254.

CLINICAL MANIFESTATIONS

Clinical and laboratory manifestations of infective endocarditis can be grouped under three headings (Table 73-6):

- Evidence of a systemic infection
- Evidence of an intravascular lesion
- Evidence of an immunologic reaction to infection

History

The symptoms of subacute endocarditis develop insidiously and with great variability.[3,43,51,116] Fevers, chills, rigors, and night sweats provide evidence of systemic infection. General malaise—with anorexia, fatigue, and weakness—is typical. Weight loss is common, along with headaches and musculoskeletal complaints, including myalgias, arthralgias, and back pains.[255] This symptom complex is often described by the patient or the physician as a "flu-like illness." Evidence of an intravascular lesion is provided by symptoms of left- or right-sided heart failure and by manifestations of embolization, such as focal neurologic injury, chest pain, flank pain, left-upper-quadrant pain, hematuria, or ischemia of an extremity. Symptoms usually persist and worsen intermittently over 4 to 8 weeks before the diagnosis is made.[256,257]

In the acute form of IE, the course is accelerated, and the symptoms are often accentuated in severity. Patients experience hectic fevers, rigors, and prostration, usually leading to hospital admission within a few days.[5,51,103,251,258]

Symptoms of cardiac failure may develop gradually or worsen suddenly in either acute or subacute disease due to mechanical complications such as perforation of a valve leaflet, rupture of one of the chordae tendineae, rupture of a sinus of Valsalva, or development of functional stenosis from obstruction of blood flow by large vegetations.[231,259] Alternatively, heart failure may develop insidiously, or preexisting chronic heart

TABLE 73-6 Summary of the Major Clinical Manifestations of Infective Endocarditis

Manifestation	History	Examination	Investigations
SYSTEMIC INFECTION	Fever, chills, rigors, sweats, malaise, weakness, lethargy, delirium, headache, anorexia, weight loss, backache, arthralgia, myalgia Portal of entry: oropharynx, skin, urinary tract, drug addiction, nosocomial bacteremia	Fever, pallor, weight loss, asthenia, splenomegaly	Anemia, leukocytosis (variable), raised erythrocyte sedimentation rate, positive blood culture, abnormal cerebrospinal fluid
INTRAVASCULAR LESION	Dyspnea, chest pain, focal weakness, stroke, abdominal pain, cold and painful extremities	Murmurs, signs of cardiac failure, petechiae (skin, eye, mucosae), Roth's spots, Osler's nodes, Janeway lesions, splinter hemorrhages, stroke, mycotic aneurysm, ischemia or infarction of viscera or extremities	Blood in urine, chest roentgenogram, echocardiography, arteriography, liver-spleen scan, lung scan, brain scan, CT scan, histology, culture of emboli
IMMUNOLOGIC REACTIONS	Arthralgia, myalgia, tenosynovitis	Arthritis, signs of uremia, vascular phenomena, finger clubbing	Proteinuria, hematuria, casts, uremia, acidosis, polyclonal increases in gamma globulins, rheumatoid factor, decreased complement, immune complexes in serum, antistaphylococcal teichoic acid antibodies

SOURCE: Adapted from Refs. 3–6, 43, 50, 51, 116.

failure may worsen due to progressive damage to the valves or associated structures. Myocarditis or myocardial infarction due to coronary artery embolism may contribute to heart failure.

Physical Examination

The physical exam in IE is a diagnosticians delight since the variety of unique physical findings often allows one to make the diagnosis at the bedside.

Patients with endocarditis may appear acutely or chronically ill. Intermittent chills, rigors, and sweating often provide evidence of a systemic infection. Asthenia and recent weight loss are often notable. Anemia is common,[85] especially in SBE, so many patients are pale. The skin of some patients with long-standing SBE shows the sallow hue of uremia.[3]

VASCULAR PHENOMENA

Patients with endocarditis may exhibit a variety of striking physical findings arising from vascular abnormalities.

Petechiae In both SBE and ABE, petechiae are common; they are rare in NBTE. In a few cases, the petechiae have a pale central spot. Most are due to microembolization to small vessels in the skin or mucous membranes. They are commonly found in crops in the conjunctual sac, on the hard palate, behind the ears and over the chest. But all areas of the trunk and extremities may be affected.

Splinter Hemorrhages Linear subungual hemorrhages, resembling tiny splinters of wood under the nails but not reaching the nail margin, are found in about 20 percent of patients with SBE. They are probably caused by microembolization to linear capillaries under the nail. Because splinter hemorrhages are found in some 5 to 8 percent of patients admitted to the hospital who do not have endocarditis, they are of limited diagnostic value when occuring alone.[260]

Osler's Nodes These are painful, tender, erythematous nodules in the skin of the extremities, usually in the pulp of the fingers[261] (Fig. 10-17, Plate 34; Fig. 10-18). Occasionally, the center of these pea-sized, red lesions is pale, but necrosis does not occur. Osler's nodes occur in 10 to 20 percent of patients with SBE and in fewer than 10 percent of patients with ABE.[261] They are probably caused by inflammation around the site of lodgment of small, infected emboli in distal arterioles, because the etiologic organism can be recovered from some of the lesions.[262] Inflammation due to focal immunologic reactions probably contributes to formation of Osler's nodes, especially in subacute cases.[247]

Janeway Lesions Janeway lesions are small (less than 5 mm), flat, nontender red spots, irregular in outline, found on the palms and soles of a few patients with SBE and ABE. Unlike petechiae, they are not hemorrhagic, and they blanch on pressure.[3,44]

Ocular Lesions Conjunctival petechiae show up as small, bright-red hemorrhages that are easily seen if the upper and lower eyelids are everted. These petechiae are not specific for endocarditis, being found sometimes after cardiac surgery and occasionally in septicemia (Fig. 73-7, Plate 103). Nevertheless, the discovery of conjunctival hemorrhages in a patient with unexplained fever and a heart murmur makes the diagnosis of endocarditis highly likely.

Retinal hemorrhages are found in 10 to 25 percent of cases of both SBE and ABE. They are quite variable in appearance. Some simply represent petechiae in the retina; their round or flame-shaped outline is determined by the layer of the retina in which they develop. Those with a white or yellow center surrounded by a bright-red, irregular halo are known as *Roth's spots,* which probably represent cytoid bodies and associated hemorrhage caused by microinfarction of retinal vessels. Roth's spot are not foci of bacterial infection and are nonspecific to IE.

Loss of vision during the course of endocarditis can occur from embolization to the brain or to the retinal artery, from optic neuritis, or from ophthalmitis. Endophthalmitis may occur in patients with *Candida* endocarditis and/or candidemia. The typical retinal lesions are rounded, white, cotton-like exudates with extension into the vitreous and overlying vitreous haze.[263] Panophthalmitis occurs in some patients with ABE due to hematogenous spread of virulent pathogens.

CLUBBING OF THE FINGERS

Previously common in SBE, finger clubbing is now found in less than 5 percent of cases (Fig. 10-16, Plate 33), presumably because endocarditis is now diagnosed and treated earlier. The pathogenesis of this reaction, which usually resolves after eradication of the infecting organism, is not understood.

SIGNS OF EMBOLIZATION

Decreased or absent arterial pulses in an extremity may signal occlusion of a large artery by a fragment of vegetation. Focal neurologic signs may develop transiently or progress to a completed stroke due to embolization to a cerebral artery (see "Complications," later). Infarctions of the spleen, kidney, or bowel can present with pain and tenderness on palpation of the abdomen, mimicking an acute abdominal event such as bowel obstruction or peritonitis. Myocardial infarction due to obstruction of a coronary artery can cause heart failure or death and is sometimes an unexpected finding at autopsy in patients who

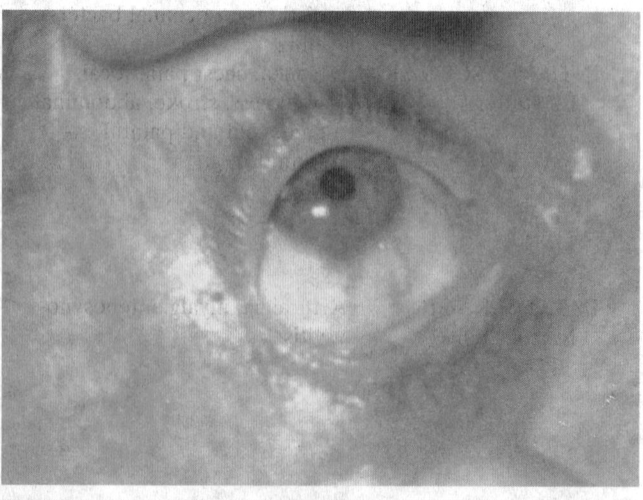

FIGURE 73-7 (Plate 103) Typical conjunctival petechiae in a patient with subacute bacterial endocarditis due to *Streptococcus sanguis*.

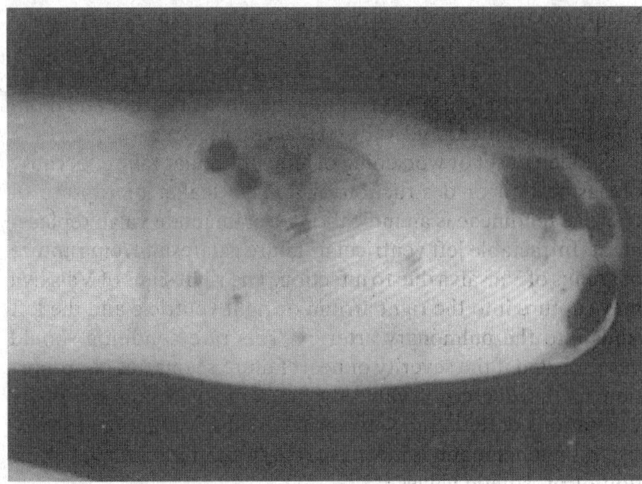

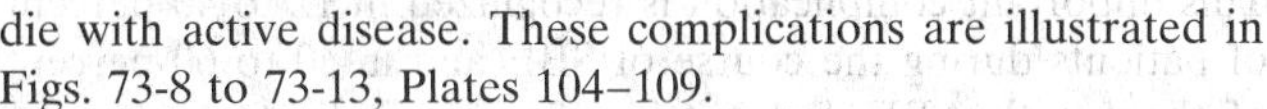

FIGURE 73-8 (Plate 104) Ischemic, hemorrhagic, and pustular lesions on the extremities in acute *Staphylococcus aureus* endocarditis.

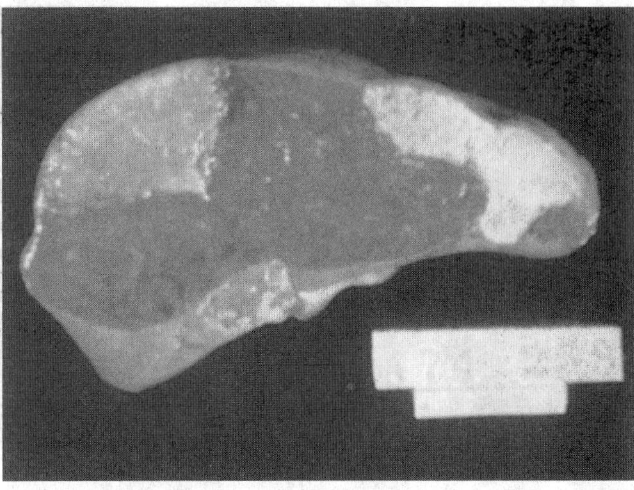

FIGURE 73-10 (Plate 106) Infarctions in the spleen.

die with active disease. These complications are illustrated in Figs. 73-8 to 73-13, Plates 104–109.

SPLENOMEGALY

Development of splenomegaly is common, occurring in about one-quarter of patients with ABE and one-half of those with SBE. The spleen is usually soft and only slightly tender except in the case of recent embolic infarction, when palpation may be very painful. Radionuclide scanning may reveal infarction or a splenic abscess.

CARDIAC EXAMINATION

The pulse is often rapid as a result of fever or congestive failure. Irregularities of conduction may indicate the presence of an abscess near the conducting system. Underlying or newly developed aortic regurgitation associated with IE may result in a collapsing pulse (Chaps. 10 and 56).

One or more murmurs are present in virtually all patients at some stage of the disease. Even though some of the classic findings of IE are less often seen today than they are formerly,

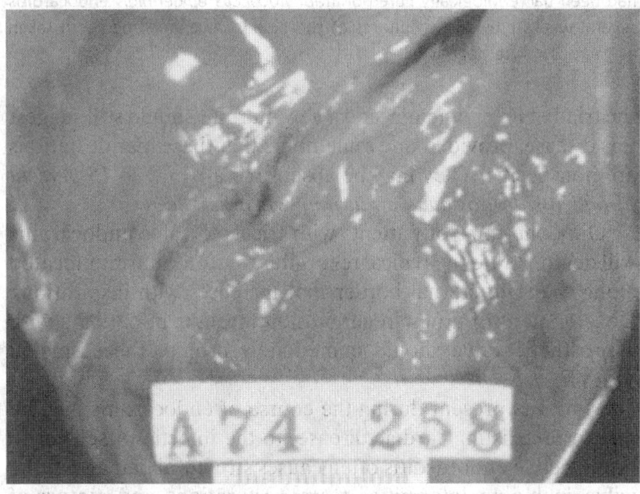

FIGURE 73-11 (Plate 107) An infected embolus in a coronary artery.

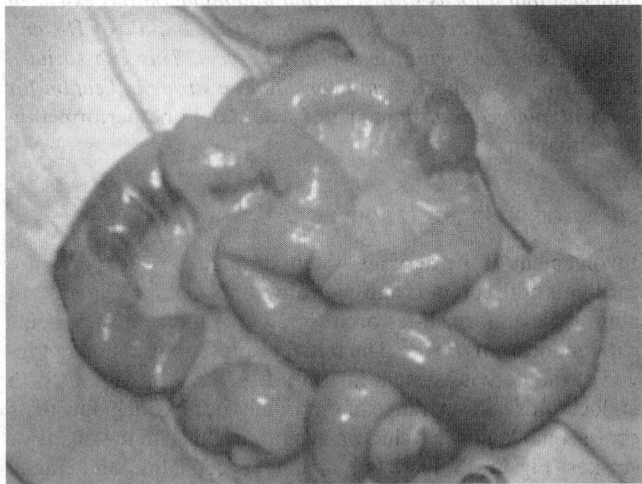

FIGURE 73-9 (Plate 105) Segmental ischemia and necrosis in the gut, presenting as acute abdomen.

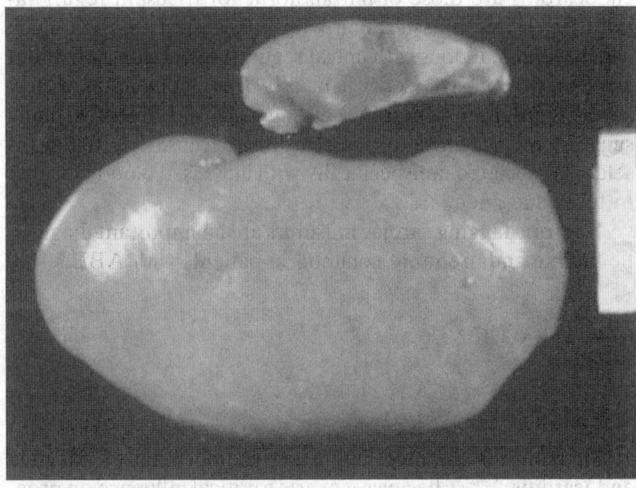

FIGURE 73-12 (Plate 108) Kidney from a patient with subacute bacterial endocarditis, showing two abnormalities: (1) typical ischemic infarctions due to emboli and (2) swelling and petechiae (flea-bitten kidney) due to immune-complex glomerulonephritis.

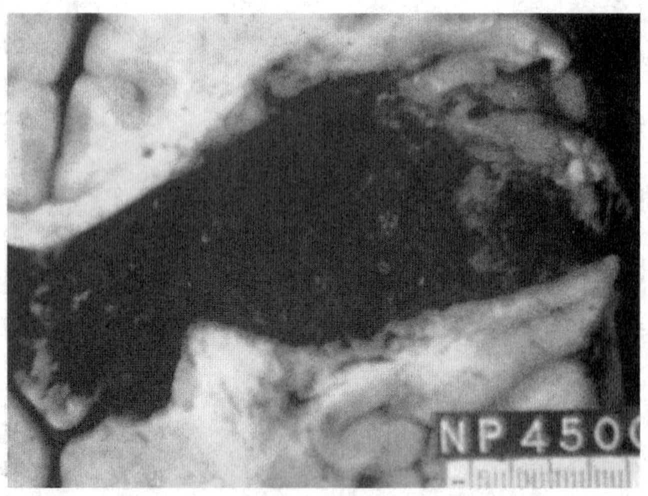

FIGURE 73-13 (Plate 109) Massive cerebral hemorrhage with intraventricular extension due to rupture of a small, peripheral mycotic aneurysm. The patient had been bacteriologically cured of *Staphylococcus epidermidis* endocarditis several weeks previously. Cultures of the blood, valve, and aneurysm taken at necropsy were negative.

the triad of fever, anemia, and a new murmur should still suggest this disease, provided one remembers that these manifestations are nonspecific. They may be absent initially. *Up to 15 percent of patients do not have a murmur when first seen.*

Only one-third of patients with tricuspid valve endocarditis will demonstrate the typical regurgitant systolic murmur located along the right sternal border that increases with inspiration.[5] Development of a new regurgitation murmur in patients with a prosthetic valve should immediately prompt the suspicion of PVE.

Murmurs present during the course of endocarditis may be due to preexisting cardiac disease, to the infection itself, or to both. Active endocarditis often causes structural damage to the valve, including deformities, tears, perforations, and rupture of chordae tendineae. Since these changes often lead to valvular insufficiency, the murmurs most often heard in association with endocarditis are those of mitral, aortic, or tricuspid regurgitation. IE occurs in association with pure mitral stenosis much less often than it does with mitral regurgitation (with or without associated stenosis) (see Chap. 57). Development of a new aortic regurgitation murmur during a febrile illness strongly suggests the diagnosis of endocarditis, because this finding is seldom associated nonspecifically with increased blood flow due to fever and anemia.

New or changing cardiac murmurs are an important diagnostic finding and are more common in patients with ABE.

COMPLICATIONS

Heart Failure

Heart failure is the most important complication of infective endocarditis,[51,264–266] because it exerts a critical influence on prognosis. In 1951, Cates and Christie[215] reported a death rate of 37 percent among 314 patients with SBE who had no heart failure and 85 percent death rate among 94 patients who had moderate or severe failure. In the past, congestive heart failure occurred in up to 55 percent of cases, being more common in patients with aortic valve disease (75 percent) than in those with mitral valve (50 percent) or tricuspid valve disease (19 percent).[265] Today, heart failure is less common because of earlier and more effective treatment and valve replacement surgery.

Sudden onset or worsening of left ventricular failure because of perforation or destruction of a valve leaflet or rupture of chordae tendineae is an indication for immediate valve replacement. Intractable left ventricular failure can result from rupture of a sinus of Valsalva due to infection. The right sinus of Valsalva may rupture into the right atrium or right ventricle and the left sinus into the pulmonary artery.[231] This rare condition should be suspected if the severity of heart failure seems out of proportion to the degree of valve dysfunction. Occasionally, bulky vegetations occlude the valve orifice, causing functional stenosis; this phenomenon is most likely to occur during fungal infection of prosthetic valves.[267,268]

Embolization

This important complication is recognized in 12 to 40 percent of patients during the course of SBE and in 40 to 60 percent of those with ABE, but autopsy findings indicate that many other arterial emboli go undetected. Pelletier and Petersdorf[116] reported a 50 percent incidence of major arterial emboli in 125 cases, affecting brain (25 cases), lung (17 cases), coronary artery (8 cases), spleen (8 cases), extremities (8 cases), gut (4 cases), and eye (3 cases). The presence of infection-related antiphospholipid antibodies has been found to be a major risk factor for embolic events.[269]

Conduction Abnormalities

A conduction abnormality is detected during the course of IE in 4 to 16 percent of patients, especially in association with aortic valve infection.[233,259,270] Types of abnormalities observed include first-degree atrioventricular block (45 percent), third-degree atrioventricular block (20 percent), second-degree atrioventricular block (15 percent), and isolated bundle branch blocks (15 percent).[233] *The development of a new, unstable, or changing conduction abnormality is important because it often indicates that a focus of myocardial inflammation has extended near or into the atrioventricular node or the bundle of His and can be associated with a valve-ring abscess. This is associated with a worse prognosis*[266] *and constitutes a strong indication for surgical intervention.* Immediate TEE should be performed in this situation.

Neurologic Manifestations

Involvement of the nervous system during the course of endocarditis is both common and clinically important.[271–274] Significant neurologic abnormalities occur in 29 to 50 percent of patients with endocarditis.[271,274,275] The initial or presenting complaint involves the nervous system in 10 to 15 percent of patients with endocarditis. A wide range of syndromes occurs, including toxic confusional states, psychiatric symptoms, and minor or major strokes (Fig. 73-13, Plate 00), meningoencephalitis, and cranial or peripheral nerve lesions.[274] (See also Chap. 89.)

Of 55 patients with cerebrovascular complications of endocarditis, four-fifths suffered infarction and one-fifth hemorrhage.[275] Infarction is usually due to embolism, most often to the middle cerebral arteries. In some series, neurologic complications approach or even surpass heart failure as the leading determinant of mortality.[274] Hemorrhage can be a complication of either emboli or mycotic aneurysms.[116,271–273,276,277]

A meningeal reaction cerebritis occurs in 7 to 15 percent of patients, especially those with staphylococcal ABE.[43,271,273–275] This reaction may be mistakenly diagnosed as acute bacterial meningitis because the cerebrospinal fluid contains polymorphonuclear leukocytes and may have a raised protein concentration. In a minority of such cases (up to 20 percent of those with acute staphylococcal infection) cerebrospinal fluid cultures yield the bacteria causing endocarditis. The glucose level, however, is usually normal; the results of cerebrospinal fluid culture are usually negative; and the abnormalities usually resolve without complications during treatment of the endocarditis. Thus, these cerebrospinal fluid abnormalities more often represent a perivascular cerebritis than true bacterial meningitis.

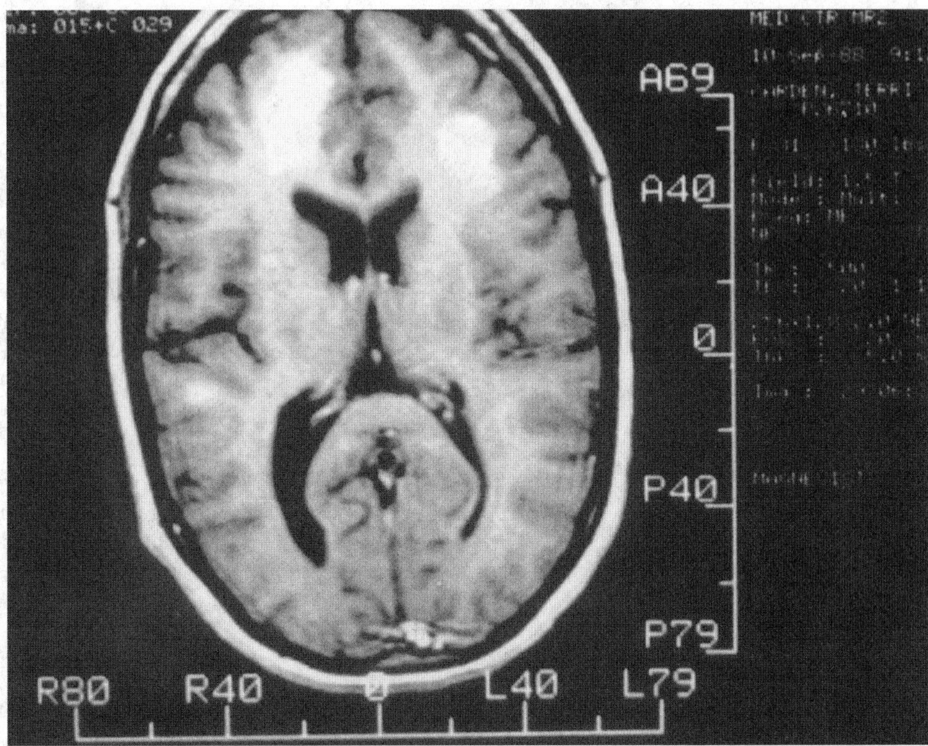

FIGURE 73-14 Magnetic resonance image of the brain in a patient with acute left-sided *Staphylococcus aureus* endocarditis, showing multiple areas of focal cerebritis. This patient had no focal central nervous system signs and recovered fully with antimicrobial therapy. (MRI by courtesy of the Department of Radiology, Duke University, Durham, NC.)

This cerebritis may develop in brain tissue surrounding small infected emboli lodged in cerebral vessels with associated meningoencephalitis.[274] Computed tomography and magnetic resonance imaging often reveal multiple areas of cerebritis, even in patients with no central nervous system symptoms (Fig. 73-14). In patients with ABE, this inflammatory reaction may progress to form a brain abscess, but more often cerebritis will resolve uneventfully during antibiotic treatment of the underlying disease. Brain abscesses are uncommon in patients with SBE.[274] Bacterial meningitis does occur in some patients with pneumococcal endocarditis.[153]

Mycotic Aneurysm

This complication develops in 3 to 15 percent of patients with IE, and the consequences of expansion and rupture of the aneurysm can be very serious, especially in the brain (Fig. 73-13, Plate 109). In order of frequency, the sites most often involved are the proximal aorta, including the sinuses of Valsalva (25 percent of cases), arteries to the viscera (24 percent), arteries to the extremities (22 percent), and arteries to the brain (15 percent).[276–278] Unfortunately, intracerebral aneurysms are often multiple.[277,278]

Mycotic aneurysms develop when the wall of an artery is damaged by the inflammatory response to microbes.[232,243,279,280] These microbes reach the arterial wall via microemboli to the vasa vasorum or by impaction of a larger infected embolus in the lumen. The arterial wall is apparently an unfavorable culture medium for bacteria because the organisms responsible for weakening the vessel often die out spontaneously, even if untreated. The mycotic aneurysm may continue to enlarge even when living organisms are no longer present, due to the physical effects of arterial blood pressure (Fig. 73-9, Plate 105).[276–278,281]

DIFFERENTIAL DIAGNOSIS

Because the clinical manifestations of endocarditis are numerous and often nonspecific, the differential diagnosis of this disease is very wide.[3,43,116,282] Of the many conditions that may be considered, only a few leading examples are listed here.

ABE shares many clinical features with nonendocarditic septicemias due to invasive bacterial pathogens such as *Staph. aureus, Neisseria,* pneumococci, and gram-negative bacilli. The differential diagnosis for a case of ABE might include sepsis, pneumonia, meningitis, brain abscess, stroke, malaria, acute pericarditis, vasculitis, and disseminated intravascular coagulation.

SBE must be considered during the workup of every patient with fever of unknown origin.[202,282,283] Its manifestations can mimic those of rheumatic fever, osteomyelitis, tuberculosis, meningitis, intraabdominal infections, salmonellosis, brucellosis, glomerulonephritis, myocardial infarction, stroke, endocardial thrombi, atrial myxoma, connective tissue diseases; arthrites of unkown etiology, vasculitis, occult malignancies (especially lymphomas), chronic cardiac failure, pericarditis, and even psychoneurosis.

TABLE 73-7 Criteria for Diagnosis of Infective Endocarditis

Definite Infective Endocarditis

PATHOLOGIC CRITERIA

Microorganisms: demonstrated by culture or histology in a vegetation, or in a vegetation that has embolized, or in an intracardiac abscess, *or*

Pathologic lesions: vegetation or intracardiac abscess present, confirmed by histology showing active endocarditis

CLINICAL CRITERIA, USING SPECIFIC DEFINITIONS LISTED IN TABLE 73-8

Two major criteria, *or*

One major and three minor criteria, *or*

Five minor criteria

Possible Infective Endocarditis

Findings consistent with infective endocarditis that fall short of "definite," but not "rejected"

Rejected

Firm alternate diagnosis for manifestations of endocarditis, *or*

Resolution of manifestations of endocarditis, with antibiotic therapy for 4 days or less, *or*

No pathologic evidence of infective endocarditis at surgery or autopsy after antibiotic therapy for 4 days or less

SOURCE: From Durack et al.,[202] with permission.

TABLE 73-8 Definitions of Terminology Used in the Diagnostic Criteria for Endocarditis

Major Criteria

POSITIVE BLOOD CULTURE FOR INFECTIVE ENDOCARDITIS

Typical microorganism for infective endocarditis from two separate blood cultures: viridans streptococci,[a] *Strep. bovis,* HACEK group, or community-acquired *Staph. aureus* or enterococci, in the absence of a primary focus, *or*

Persistently positive blood culture, defined as recovery of a microorganism consistent with infective endocarditis from:

1. Blood cultures drawn more than 12 h apart *or*
2. All of three or a majority of four or more separate blood cultures, with first and last drawn at least 1 h apart

EVIDENCE OF ENDOCARDIAL INVOLVEMENT

Positive echocardiogram for infective endocarditis

1. Oscillating intracardiac mass, on valve or supporting structures, or in the path of regurgitant jet or on implanted material, in the absence of an alternative anatomic explanation, *or*
2. Abscess, *or*
3. New partial dehiscence of prosthetic valve, *or* New valvular regurgitation (increase or change in preexisting murmur not sufficient)

Minor Criteria

- Predisposition: predisposing heart condition *or* intravenous drug use
- Fever: ≥38.0°C (100.4°F)
- Vascular phenomena: major arterial emboli, septic pulmonary infarcts, mycotic aneurysm, intracranial hemorrhage, conjunctival hemorrhages, Janeway lesions
- Immunologic phenomena: glomerulonephritis, Osler's nodes, Roth's spots, rheumatoid factor
- Microbiologic evidence: positive blood culture but not meeting major criterion as previously defined[b] *or* serologic evidence of active infection with oganism consistent with infective endocarditis[c]
- Echocardiogram: consistent with infective endocarditis but not meeting major criterion as previously defined

[a]Including nutritional variant strains.

[b]Excluding single positive cultures for coagulase-negative staphylococci or organisms that do not cause endocarditis.

[c]Positive serologies for *Coxiella* or *Bartonella* may be considered major criteria.[292]

HACEK = *Haemophilus* spp., *Actinobacillus actinomycetemcomitans, Cardiobacterium hominis, Eikenella* spp., and *Kingella kingae*

SOURCE: Adapted from Durack et al.,[202] with pemission.

Diagnostic Criteria

IE can be surprisingly difficult to diagnose with certainty.[202,284] In the course of clinical practice, the diagnosis is suspected much more often than it is confirmed. This is because the presenting symptoms and signs can be highly variable and consistent with many other possible diagnoses. Furthermore, the primary lesion (an endocardial vegetation) is inaccessible to direct inspection except at surgery or autopsy. Major and minor criteria have been defined[202]; they are analogous to the modified Jones criteria[285] (Chap. 55) for diagnosis of acute rheumatic fever[86,202,203] (Tables 73-7 and 73-8). Several diagnostic schemes have been developed to assist the clinician in working through a diagnostic workup, however, it is important to emphasize that while these may be useful guidelines, each patient must be considered on an individual basis. The so-called Duke criteria has received the most attention.[202]

Because the Duke criteria emphasize specificity[203,286] above sensitivity, they should not be used to guide urgent management decisions early in the course of a suspected case. To illustrate: a diagnosis of endocarditis made solely on the basis of presence of fever and a heart murmur would be very sensitive but very nonspecific. These findings alone might make a clinician suspect the diagnosis or begin treatment for endocarditis, but the various diagnostic schemes might guide the clinician to make a final diagnosis, to decide on valve replacement, or to accept the diagnosis for the purpose of epidemiologic studies or clinical trials.

LABORATORY INVESTIGATIONS

Routine Laboratory Tests

Anemia usually develops during the course of SBE.[85,287] It is most often mild or moderate in degree and of the hypoproliferative type, with a normochromic, normocytic smear. Anemia occurs less often in ABE and may be due to hemolysis. Chronic low-grade hemolysis associated with a prosthetic valve may confuse interpretation of the blood picture in a patient with PVE. In addition, blood smear may show schistocytes and other red blood cell fragments. Leukocytosis is not a reliable manifestation of SBE.[85] A low-grade, variable elevation of the polymorphonuclear leukocyte count is characteristic, but in some cases the leukocyte count is normal. A high granulocyte count with an increase in band forms is commonly found in patients with ABE. These neutrophils often show toxic granulations. In a few cases of ABE, staphylococci can be identified inside neutrophils on examination of a gram-stained smear of the buffy coat of the peripheral blood.[288] In addition, abnormal histiocytes may be found in smears of peripheral blood in one-third of patients with SBE,[289] but these tests are not in routine use.

The erythrocyte sedimentation rate (ESR) is elevated in about 90 percent of cases of IE. The median ESR on admission is about 65 mm/h, but the range is wide and 10 percent are in the normal range. The median ESR may rise slightly during treatment and does not fall to normal until 3 to 6 months after diagnosis, so it is not useful as evidence of successful antibiotic therapy. The C-reactive protein is usually elevated (96 percent) and falls to normal more quickly than the ESR during successful treatment.[290] Cryoglobulins have also been reported.[291]

Urinalysis shows microscopic hematuria and/or slight proteinuria in >50 percent of cases, even in the absence of specific renal complications.[3,287] Red blood cell casts and heavy proteinuria are found in those patients who develop immune-complex glomerulonephritis, often in association with decreased total serum complement.[248] Gross hematuria suggests that renal infarction has occurred.

Serologic Tests

Nonspecific serologic abnormalities are common during the course of IE. A positive rheumatoid factor is found in >50 percent of cases of SBE,[235–237] with symptoms for longer than 6 weeks.[202] Rheumatoid factor is rarely positive in patients with ABE. A polyclonal increase in gammaglobulins is characteristic of active endocarditis. Occasional false-positive serologic test results for syphilis occur.[234]

Specific serologic tests are important for the diagnosis of IE caused by *Coxiella* (Q fever) and *Bartonella,* both species that are difficult or slow to grow from culture. In these special cases, positive serology (1:800 antiphase 1 IgG antibody titer for Q fever or positive microimmunofluorescence or PCR test for *Bartonella*) or a single positive blood culture may be added as major criteria for diagnosis of IE.[189,292]

Blood Cultures

Isolation of a typical organism or detection of persistent bacteremia constitutes the most important diagnostic test for endocarditis. Blood cultures should be drawn from all patients with undiagnosed fever and a heart murmur. Cultures should also be taken from patients with other symptoms or signs consistent with endocarditis if no other diagnosis has been made.

Bacteremia in SBE is usually continuous.[22] The number of organisms in venous blood varies widely but is usually between 1 and 200 bacteria per mL in subacute cases. Because most blood cultures in untreated patients will be positive, it is seldom necessary to draw more than 3 separate blood specimens to isolate the organism.[293] In one study, the etiologic organism was recovered from cultures taken on the first day of admission to the hospital in 93 percent of patients with culture-positive endocarditis.[294] In other studies, however, the rate of persistently positive blood cultures was lower, in the range of 62 to 68 percent.[116,202] Additional specimens obtained over a longer period may be needed to isolate the etiologic organism from patients who have received recent antibiotic therapy.

A practical approach for investigation of suspected SBE is to draw 3 separate samples of venous blood, each of 16 to 20 mL, on the first day, with at least 1 h between the first and last venipuncture. Half of each sample should be inoculated into an aerobic broth culture medium, and the other half into another broth (usually anaerobic) medium. These media should be capable of supporting growth of fastidious, nutritionally variant bacteria[139,295] and ideally should contain a resin to remove antibiotics. As soon as a culture turns positive, Gram's stain and subculture should be performed. If all 3 samples (6 bottles) are negative by the second or third day but the diagnosis of endocarditis still seems likely, two more samples of venous blood should be drawn for culture. If the patient had received previous antibiotic therapy, several further venous samples may be taken over the following weeks to identify a possible late recrudescence of bacteremia after partial treatment. For ABE, 3 venous blood samples are drawn for culture and empiric antibiotic therapy is begun at once, because in patients with acute endocarditis, treatment should not be delayed until culture results are available. In cases of *Staph. aureus* endocarditis, greater than 95 percent of blood culture would be positive, usually within 24 hours.[5]

Because *Staph.* epidermidis[251] and diphtheroids[296] can cause endocarditis, special care must be taken during venipuncture to avoid contamination of the specimen with these common skin organisms, which could result in diagnostic confusion. Since endocarditis usually produces continuous bacteremia, all cultures are usually positive; when only 1 of 3 grow a *Staph.* epidermidis or diphtheroid, contamination and not true bacteremia should be suspected! If the diagnosis of endocarditis remains likely, and cultures are negative, cultures should be incubated for 3 weeks and Gram's stains made at 5 days, 2 weeks, and 3 weeks even if no growth is apparent on inspection. The HACEK group of organisms, pyridoxyl requiring viridans streptococci, some fungi, *Bartonella,* and some others may take longer than the standard 3 to 5 days to grow.[297] A number of new seralogic and PCR-based techniques are under development and are desperately needed to clarify diagnosis in these culture-negative cases.[298–300]

Electrocardiography

Electrocardiographic studies should be performed initially and repeated at intervals according to progress during treatment. A disturbance of conduction or onset of myocardial irritability [↑ frequency of ventricular premature complexes (VPCs) or atrial premature complexes (APCs)] that develops during the course of endocarditis suggests extension of infection into the myocardium (see earlier). Such extension may be due to focal myocarditis or to an abscess located close to the conduction system.[110] Thus, development of a prolonged PR interval, if due to an abscess, can have major implications: a probable need for valve replacement and a worse prognosis.[87] Electrocardiograms can reveal evidence of silent myocardial infarction due to embolization of a vegetation to a coronary artery. Continuous electrocardiogram monitoring may be appropriate when conduction or rhythm changes are observed and disease progression is a concern.

Echocardiography

Echocardiographic studies are important in the diagnosis of IE.[301–305] Positive echocardiographic findings, properly defined, constitute an important criteria for the clinical diagnosis of endocarditis and, in the setting of positive blood cultures, essentially establishes the diagnosis of IE.[202] TTE combined with color-flow Doppler imaging (see Chap. 13) provides a wealth of information for both the diagnosis and the management of endocarditis, including the detection of vegetations, valvular perforations[306] and other abnormalities,[307] abscesses, and pericarditis, as well as the assessment of ventricular function (Fig. 73-15*A*–*D*).[302–304] Sensitivity for detection of vegetations, originally in the range of 33 to 63 percent, today is 50 to 75 percent.[307] Sensitivity can be improved to better than 95 percent by use of TEE (see Chap. 14) in selected cases.[270,302] Transesophageal studies also detect abscesses and valve perforation with much greater sensitivity.[304] TEE is markedly better than TTE for evaluation of prosthetic valve endocarditis, especially involving mitral valves.[308,309]

Echocardiography has some limitations.[301] It is not cost-effective as a means of excluding IE in patients with a low pretest probability of having the disease.[310,311] With higher prior probability, a negative study result has useful negative predictive value, especially if transesophageal studies have been performed, but it cannot totally exclude the diagnosis of endocarditis.[170,202,310,311] It is particularly useful in patients with *Staph. aureus* bacteremia. In one study, TTE identified vegetations in 7 of 26 patients with IE, while TEE revealed evidence of vegetations in all (100 percent).[311] These data suggest that a negative TEE allows the clinician to treat for bacteremia alone (usually antibiotic therapy for 2 weeks versus 4 to 6 weeks for IE). Sensitivity for detection of vegetations is somewhat lower on the right side (about 70 percent) than on the left (better than 95 percent).[270,301] The presence of a prosthetic valve sometimes interferes with detection of vegetations, but even in these patients echocardiographic findings are usually informative. Occasionally, the specificity of echocardiography is compromised by false-positive readings for "vegetations" that do not exist. Such readings are particularly common in patients with myxomatous degeneration of valve leaflets or other preexisting disease with focal pathology. This must be considered when surgery is contemplated.

Sequential echocardiograms performed during treatment can guide decisions on the need and timing for surgery by providing objective assessments of cardiac function. For example, premature mitral valve closure due to elevated end-diastolic pressure is a useful echocardiographic sign indicating severe aortic regurgitation, usually requiring urgent valve replacement (see Chap. 56).[270] Echocardiograms may detect development of an abscess, perforation of a valve, or rupture of an infected sinus of Valsalva,[231] all strong indications for surgical intervention. During successful antimicrobial treatment, vegetations may disappear, decrease in size, or even persist unchanged; therefore, serial echocardiograms should not be used as a "test of cure."[301] Significant enlargement of a vegetation during treatment, however, indicates possible treatment failure and constitutes a relative indication for surgical intervention. The valve of echocardiography to determine risk of embolization and/or death is controversial. A large meta-analysis concluded that the odds ratio for embolization was 2.8 ($p < 0.01$) when vegetations >10 mm were detected but did not predict death.[312] In another study of *Staph. aureus*, IE visualization of vegetation by TTE carried a higher risk of embolization or death (68 percent) than identified only by TEE (16 percent, $p < 0.01$).[313] Therefore, the value of echocardiography as a mechanism for predicting outcome remains unclear.[314,315]

Other Imaging Studies

The most important contribution of the chest x-ray in assessment of endocarditis is to provide evidence of early congestive heart failure, because this complication carries such important implications for both prognosis and management (see "Complications," earlier).

Various other x-ray findings can be helpful in assessing patients with endocarditis. The presence of multiple small, patchy infiltrates in the lungs of an IDU with fever strongly suggests the diagnosis of septic emboli arising from right-sided IE.[65–67] Valvular calcification may identify a previously abnormal valve, thus aiding the localization of presumed intravascular infection. Widening of the aorta may be caused by a mycotic aneurysm. Fluoroscopy can demonstrate abnormal motion of a prosthetic valve, indicating presence of a vegetation or partial dehiscence of the valve from the aortic root. This information often helps to decide whether or not valve replacement is needed during management of PVE.

Computed tomography (Chap. 17) and magnetic resonance imaging (Chap. 18)[274] can be helpful in defining the cause of focal neurologic lesions in patients with endocarditis, especially infarction, hemorrhage from a mycotic aneurysm, and brain abscess. The computed tomography scan is very effective for diagnosis of intracranial complications[316] and infected aortic aneurysms.[133] Magnetic resonance imaging adds additional useful information in some cases (Fig. 73-14).[317] In one study, Magnetic resonance imaging provided evidence of cerebral embolization in 12 patients with IE. Angiographic studies are usually used to demonstrate mycotic aneurysms in the brain or elsewhere.[277,278]

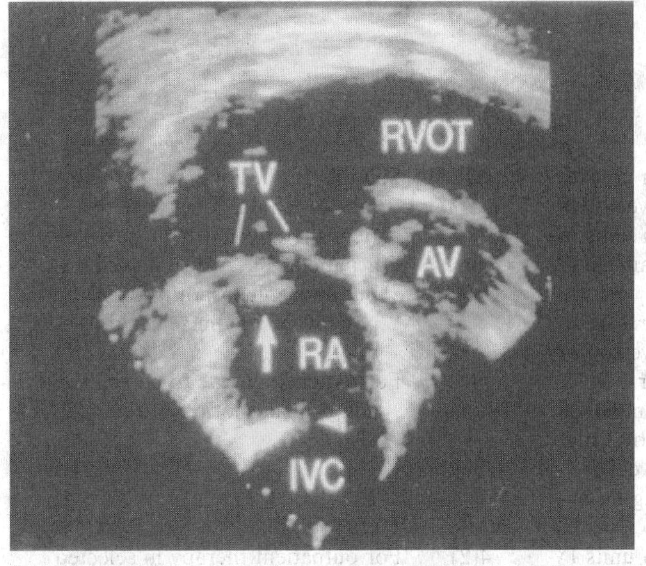

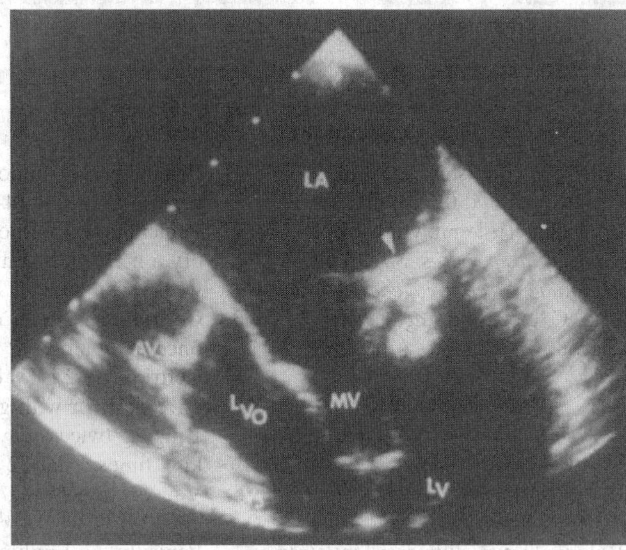

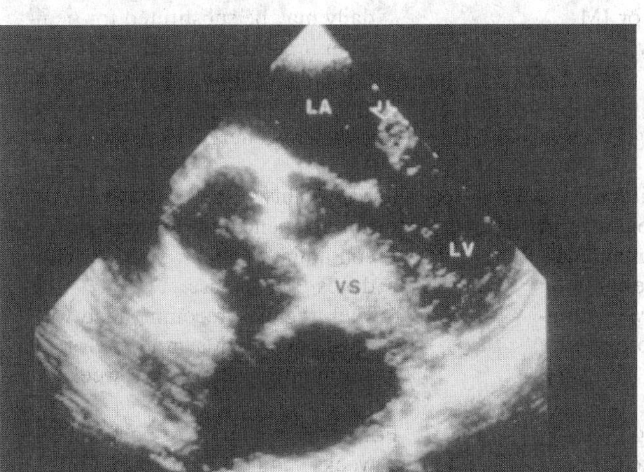

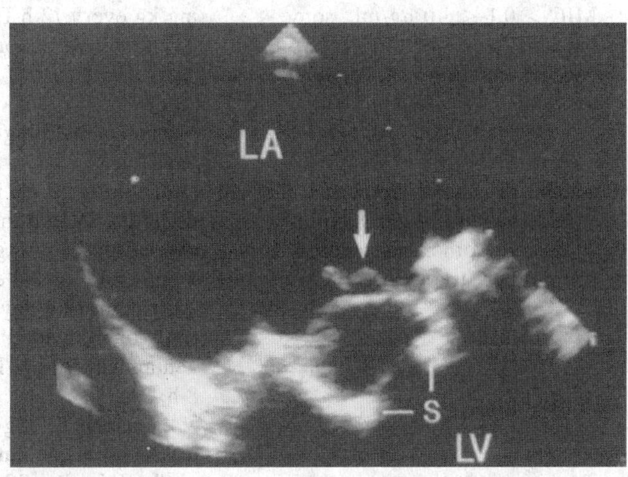

FIGURE 73-15 *A–D.* Echocardiograms from 4 patients with infective endocarditis showing vegetations located at different sites. *A.* Transesophageal echocardiogram (TEE) showing a large vegetation *(arrow)* on the tricuspid valve (TV). IVC = inferior vena cava; RA = right atrium; AV = aortic valve; RVOT = right ventricular outflow tract. *B.* Large vegetation *(arrowhead)* involving both the atrial and ventricular surfaces of the posterior mitral valve leaflet. LA = left atrium; MV = anterior leaflet of the mitral valve; LVO = left ventricular outflow tract; AV = aortic valve. *C.* TEE showing vegetations on both the mitral *(open arrow)* and aortic valve *(arrow)* in a patient with acute *Staphylococcus aureus* endocarditis. LA = left atrium; LV = left ventricle; VS = ventricular septum. *D.* TEE showing a vegetation on the cusp of a bioprosthetic valve *(arrow)*. LA = left atrium; LV = left ventricle; S = artificial valve struts. (Kindly provided by Dr. B. Khanderia and Dr. J. Steckelberg, Mayo Clinic, Rochester, Minn.)

Cardiac Catheterization with Cineangiography

This investigation is usually not necessary for patients who respond well to antimicrobial therapy without developing cardiac failure. When surgical intervention is considered, cardiac catheterization and cineangiography (Chap. 15) can extend and add to information provided by echocardiography. The condition of the coronary arteries should be assessed before valve replacement in adults over 40 years of age, because simultaneous coronary bypass may be indicated if the patient has coronary artery disease. Other relevant anatomic abnormalities such as valvular lesions, congenital defects, asymmetric septal hypertrophy, coarctation of the aorta, or mycotic aneurysm can be better defined. Occasionally, a previously unsuspected diagnosis, such as the presence of a sinus of Valsalva aneurysm, will be made. Physiologic measurements including cardiac output, pressures in the left and right sides of the heart, and the degree of aortic regurgitation may help to decide whether or not valve replacement is indicated and may influence the timing of the operation. Among 35 patients who underwent cardiac catheterization during active endocarditis, the clinical assessment was materially modified by catheterization in 23 patients, the diagnosis of the site of valve involvement was altered in 14, and in 6 valve-ring abscesses were revealed.[318] Surgery was postponed or canceled in 6 patients in whom catheterization revealed only mild hemodynamic abnormalities. There were no serious complications, indicating that catheterization should not be avoided for fear of dislodging emboli when a proper indication exists. In summary,

TABLE 73-9 Treatment Regimens for Infective Endocarditis[a,b]

Organism	Treatment Regimen: Dose and Route	Duration in Weeks	Comments
Fully penicillin-sensitive streptococci: MIC ≤ 0.1 μg/mL viridans (α-hemolytic) streptococci; *Strep. bovis; Strep. pneumoniae; Strep. pyogenes* group A, C, etc.; *Strep. agalactiae* group B	1. Penicillin G 4 million units every 6 h IV alone (4 weeks) *or*	4	Suitable for hospitalized patients but less convenient for outpatient therapy
	2. Penicillin G 4 million units every 6 h IV with gentamicin (2 weeks)	4	For patients allergic to penicillins but not cephalosporins or for outpatient therapy in selected patients
	3. Ceftriaxone 2 g IV or 1 M once daily alone (2 weeks) *or*		
	4. Ceftriaxone 2 g IV or 1 M once daily or with gentamicin 1 mg/kg twice a day or 3 mg/kg 4 times a day (2 weeks)	4	For patients allergic to penicillins and cephalosporins
	5. Vancomycin 15 mg/kg IV every 12 h (4 weeks)[a,b]		
Relatively penicillin-resistant streptococci: MIC > 0.1 < 1.0 μg/mL, some viridans (α-hemolytic) streptococci; some *Strep. pneumoniae;* etc.	1. Penicillin G 4 million units IV every 4 h *plus* gentamicin 1.0 mg/kg every 12 h IV or IM (for first 2 weeks only)[a] *or*	4(2)	For outpatient therapy in selected patients, ceftriaxone 2 g IV once daily may be substituted for penicillin if ceftriaxone MIC ≤ 4 μg/mL, *plus* gentamicin 2.0 mg/kg given once daily
	2. Vancomycin 15 mg/kg IV every 12 h[b]	4	For patients allergic to penicillins
Penicillin-resistant streptococci: MIC ≥ 1.0 μg/mL, *E. faecalis, E. faecium,* other enterococci; some other streptococci	1. Penicillin G 18–30 million units/day IV continuously or in divided doses *plus* gentamicin 1 mg/kg IV or IM every 8 h *or*	4–6	Susceptibility testing needed; do not use penicillin- or ampicillin-containing regimen if strain produces β-lactamase.
	2. Ampicillin 12 g/day IV continuously or in divided doses *plus* gentamicin 1.0 mg/kg IV every 8 h, *or*	4–6	4-week regimen recommended for most cases with symptoms for <3 months, otherwise 6 weeks
	3. Vancomycin 15 mg/kg IV every 12 h *plus* gentamicin 1.0 mg/kg IV every 8 h[a,b]	4–6	For patients allergic to penicillin; 4 weeks should be adequate for most cases; serum levels should be monitored
Staphylococci (in the absence of prosthetic material)	Methicillin-susceptible staphylococci:		
	1. Nafcillin 2 g IV every 4 h IV 4–6 wks *or*	4–6	β-lactam–containing regimens preferred over vancomycin unless patient is definitely hypersensitive to penicillins and cephalosporins; for patients with severe disseminated staphylococcal infection, antimicrobial synergy may be advantageous during early stages of treatment; therefore, gentamicin 1.0 mg/kg IV every 8 h for first 3–5 days only may be added to any of these regimens
	2. Nafcillin 2 g IV every 4 h IV × 4–6 wks plus gentamicin 1.0 mg/kg every 8 h IV × 3–5 days	4–6	
	3. Vancomycin 15 mg/kg IV every 12 h 4–6 wks[b]	4–6	
In right sided uncomplicated tricuspid endocarditis	Nafcillin 2 g IV every 4 h and gentamicin 1 mg/kg twice a day or 3 mg/kg 4 times a day	2	
	Methicillin-resistant staphylococci: Vancomycin 15 mg/kg IV every 12 h[b]	4–6	

TABLE 73-9 Treatment Regimens for Infective Endocarditis (*Continued*)

Organism	Treatment Regimen: Dose and Route	Duration in Weeks	Comments
Staphylococci (associated with prosthetic valve or other prosthetic material)	Methicillin-susceptible staphylococci: Nafcillin 2 g IV every 4 h *plus* gentamicin 1.0 mg/kg IV every 8 h[a] plus rifampin 600 mg orally 4 times a day	≥6	Cefazolin or vancomycin may be substituted for nafcillin if necessary due to drug hypersensitivity
	Methicillin-resistant staphylococci: Vancomycin 15 mg/kg IV every 12 h *plus* gentamicin 1.0 mg/kg IV or IM every 8 h *plus* rifampin 300 mg orally every 8 h[a,b]	≥6	
HACEK group organisms: *Haemophilus* species *Actinobacillus actinomycetemcomitans* *Cardiobacterium hominis* *Eikenella* species *Kingella kingae*	1. Ceftriaxone 2 g IV or IM once daily *or*	4	Other third-generation cephalosporins may be substituted, using appropriate dose adjustment
	2. Ampicillin 12 g/day IV continuously or in divided doses *plus* gentamicin 1.0 mg/kg every 12 h IV or IM[a]	4	Less convenient for outpatient therapy
Pseudomonas aeruginosa, other gram-negative bacilli	Extended-spectrum penicillin *or* third-generation cephalosporin *or* imipenem *plus* aminoglycoside	4–6	Combination therapy recommended; final choice of antibiotic regimen to be made after sensitivity results available
Neisseria species	1. Penicillin G 2 million units IV every 6 h *or*	3–4	Organisms often highly sensitive to penicillin, but must be tested for β-lactamase production; 3 weeks should be adequate for most patients without complications
	2. Ceftriaxone 1 g IV or IM once daily	3–4	

[a]All gentamicin- and vancomycin-containing regimens require monitoring for potential toxicity; monitoring of serum concentrations usually will be required.
[b]Vancomycin dose not to exceed 2.0 g per 24 h.
SOURCE: Adapted from Scheld and Sande[50] and from Wilson et al., and The Sanford Guide 2000.[323]

cardiac catheterization and cineangiography should be performed in most adults with IE who are over 40 years of age and in selected younger patients when surgery is considered.

Radionuclide Imaging

Liver-spleen imaging may reveal defects due to splenic infarction, which confirms embolization. In animals, experimental vegetations have been located by scanning for radiolabeled platelets deposited from the bloodstream onto a growing endocardial lesion.[319] Gallium 67 scans have shown increased uptake in the heart in some patients with endocarditis. Scintigraphic studies following injection of indium 111 labeled leukocytes have detected some intracardiac abscesses,[77,320] but no radionuclide imaging technique has sufficient sensitivity and specificity to justify routine use for detection of vegetations in IE. In selected cases, leukocyte scintigraphy using indium 111 labeled leukocytes can detect mycotic aneurysms and extracardiac foci of infection.[321] Single photon emission computed tomography immunoscintigraphy with antigranulocyte antibody has been described as a nuclear medicine option for diagnosis of IE.

TREATMENT

General Principles

Optimal management aims to eradicate the infecting organism as soon as possible, to operate with correct timing if surgical intervention should be required, and to treat complications. Because IE carries a significant risk of death even when well managed, it is important that treatment be continued long enough to ensure that relapse will not occur. In contrast, patients with the more easily cured forms of endocarditis should not be subjected to unnecessarily long, expensive, and potentially toxic treatment in a hospital.[322] This can happen when physicians treat on the basis of outdated rules, such as the one stating that "endocarditis should be treated for 6 weeks." In fact, many patients can be cured in 2[323–325] or 4 weeks,[326] while some require treatment for 6 weeks or longer.

Microbiologic Tests

To choose and regulate antibiotic therapy correctly, certain basic microbiologic information about the infecting organism is required. For group A streptococcal infection, nothing more than positive identification of the organism is necessary, because these organisms, with only rare exceptions, are still sensitive to low concentrations of penicillin. For other species of streptococci, staphylococci, and most other bacteria, the minimal inhibitory concentration (MIC) of relevant antibiotics should be determined. Some of these organisms are resistant to intermediate or high concentrations of penicillin.[327,328] Many strains are tolerant—that is, inhibited but not killed by antibiotic levels achievable in serum.[329,330] Because there is no definitive evidence that tolerance determines treatment outcome in humans, however, it is not necessary to measure minimal bactericidal concentrations (MBC) in most cases.

The serum bactericidal titer (SBT or Schlichter test) has been used frequently to monitor the treatment of endocarditis.[33,331] In this test, the infecting organism is exposed in vitro to the patient's serum, which is drawn while the patient is receiving antibiotic treatment to determine the maximal dilution of serum that will inhibit and kill the organism. On the basis of empirical clinical experience, it was said that the SBT should be 1:8 or higher at intervals during each day of treatment. For streptococcal endocarditis, this can usually be achieved without difficulty; SBTs are often high, in the range of 1:128 to 1:1024. The SBT is technically difficult to perform and to standardize, however, and after years of use, its clinical utility remains unproven.[331,332] Therefore, SBTs are now regarded as obsolete by most experts. Rarely, measurement of the SBT might be informative: in treating unusual organisms, in using unusual antibiotics, in using unusual regimens (such as oral treatment), or when treatment appears to be failing.

Dosage regimens that result in widely fluctuating antibiotic concentrations in serum are traditionally employed for treatment of endocarditis, and they are usually effective. Whether or not the maintenance of continuous serum antibiotic concentrations offers any therapeutic benefit over intermittent dosing regimens is not known; perhaps continuous infusion of antibiotic would be desirable for treatment of some gram-negative organisms, which regrow more rapidly than most gram-positive organisms when antibiotic levels fall below the minimal inhibitory concentration.

Choice of Antibiotics

Bactericidal antibiotics are generally chosen for treatment of endocarditis whenever possible.[33,326] This is not an absolute rule; some patients have been cured with bacteriostatic drugs such as sulfonamides, tetracycline, or chloramphenicol, but the results of treatment with these agents are unreliable.[28,333,334] Bactericidal action is presumably needed because host defense mechanisms are inadequate in the vegetation; relatively few phagocytes are present, and they are hampered by protective layers of fibrin around the colonies of bacteria (Figs. 73-2 and 73-6). To effect a cure, antibiotic therapy must eradicate organisms completely, without the help of phagocytes to eliminate the subpopulation of microbes that are relatively resistant to antibiotics because they are in the resting phase. In this important respect, IE differs strikingly from bacterial pneumonia in normal hosts, where phagocytes are plentiful and bacteriostatic antibiotics are usually effective. Nevertheless, in treating unusual organisms, it may occasionally be necessary to use a bacteriostatic antibiotic in combination with other drugs to achieve the optimal antibacterial effect. When treatment with unusual combinations of antibiotics is needed, in vitro laboratory tests can be performed to find out whether synergism, indifference, or antagonism exists between them.

For the common forms of bacterial endocarditis caused by gram-positive organisms, specific therapeutic regimens can be recommended with confidence based on extensive published experience.[323,335] Regimens for the more common forms of endocarditis are listed in Table 73-9.

Currently, increasing rates of antibiotic resistance threaten the efficacy of traditional treatment regimens. Penicillin resistance is increasing among viridans streptococci, the majority of which had previously been fully sensitive.[336,337] In 1996, 13 percent of blood culture isolates showed high-level resistance (MIC 4.0 mg/mL or greater) and 42 percent showed intermediate resistance (MIC 0.25 to 2.0 mg/mL).[337] Use of combined antibiotic regimens such as beta-lactam plus aminoglycoside or even vancomycin plus aminoglycoside should be considered for treatment of resistant strains.[336] Synergistic combinations of a beta-lactam and an aminoglycoside have been used successfully to treat enterococci for many years, but increasing resistance among enterococci, especially vancomycin-resistant enterococci, presents new problems for therapy.[338] The most resistant species is *Enterococcus faecium,* which may exhibit high-level resistance to vancomycin as well as intrinsic resistance to beta-lactam antibiotics and imipenem.[94] The optimal treatment for IE caused by these problem strains is not known. Several antibiotic combinations have been tried with some success often with adjunctive surgical valve replacement. These include high-dose ampicillin plus imipenem +/− a fluoroquinolone,[94,339] ampicillin plus imipenem plus vancomycin,[340] ampicillin plus a fluoroquinolone,[341] and quinupristin/dalfopristin plus doxycycline plus rifampin.[342] Since great variability exists between isolates as to sensitivity and whether drugs are cidal or static, in vitro testing with time-kill experiments and testing various drugs alone and in combination will help with selection. An infectious disease consultation is recommended.[94,339–344]

Staph. epidermidis PVE is difficult to eradicate with antibiotics alone.[166] These staphylococci are frequently resistant to semisynthetic penicillins, cephalosporins, and other antibiotics. A regimen combining vancomycin, rifampin, and an aminoglycoside chosen according to sensitivity tests is most likely to succeed. The organism may develop resistance to rifampin during treatment.

Treatment of endocarditis due to less common organisms must be chosen on the basis of more limited published experience,[50,51,108,326] together with the results of tests performed upon the infecting organism in the microbiology laboratory. Treatment must often be individualized. In general, one of the beta-lactam antibiotics should be included in the regimen whenever possible. Combinations of two or more antibiotics are often employed. The list of potentially useful regimens for these rarer forms of infective endocarditis is too long to detail here.

Empiric Therapy

When the etiologic organism is not known, the choice of empiric therapy should depend on whether the patient has acute or subacute disease. ABE requires broad-spectrum therapy that covers *Staph. aureus* as well as many species of streptococci and gram-negative bacilli. SBE requires a regimen that treats most streptococci, including *E. faecalis.* To meet these requirements, the following suggestions are offered:

- For ABE: nafcillin 2.0 g IV q 4 h plus ampicillin 2.0 g IV q 4 h plus gentamicin 1.5 mg/kg IV q 8 h. If methicillin-resistant *Staph. aureus* is considered likely (for example, in a hospital-acquired case), vancomycin 1.0 g IV q 12 h should be substituted for nafcillin in this regimen until the antibiotic sensitivity is known.
- For SBE: ampicillin 2.0 g IV q 4 h plus gentamicin 1.5 mg/kg IV q 8 h.

Treatment should be adjusted as appropriate when the etiologic organism is identified and again when antibiotic sensitivity is known. In those few cases where empiric therapy is administered as a therapeutic trial to help confirm a diagnosis, treatment should be continued without interruption or unnecessary changes for at least 2 weeks; otherwise, no useful diagnostic information will be gained.

Duration of Therapy

Extensive experience with treatment of the common forms of endocarditis provides the basis for recommendations on duration of therapy (Table 73-9). In the case of *Staph. aureus* endocarditis, the response to appropriate treatment can be variable; some patients recover swiftly without complications, especially young IDUs, who can often be cured within 2 weeks.[70,324] In contrast, some patients remain febrile for 10 to 14 days due to complications such as abscesses or other extracardiac manifestations of disseminated staphylococcal disease. Although 4 weeks of therapy is adequate in most cases, this should not be regarded as a rigid rule, because some patients with *Staph. aureus* endocarditis require treatment for 6 weeks or longer to achieve a cure. For *E. faecalis* endocarditis, 4 weeks of treatment is usually adequate. The relapse rate, however, seems to be higher in patients with mitral valve infection and in those who have had symptoms for more than 3 months,[143] where treatment should continue for 6 weeks.

Parenteral treatment can be completed in the patient's home or in the outpatient clinic in carefully selected cases. Availability of antibiotics with long half-lives, such as vancomycin or ceftriaxone, allows once-daily administration. Supervised parenteral treatment outside the hospital should be fully effective in achieving a microbiologic cure and offers obvious benefits: convenience for the patient and cost containment.[344–346] The risks posed by a possible late complication, such as an embolic stroke or the sudden onset of heart failure, must be balanced against these benefits in selecting candidates for home parenteral therapy. Further trials are needed to refine the criteria and proper applications for outpatient therapy for endocarditis, but current experience indicates that more than one-half of endocarditis patients could receive at least some of their treatment as outpatients.

In general, the less extensive the published experience with a particular organism and treatment regimen, the more one should lean toward prolonging treatment in order to provide a reasonable margin of safety. Guidelines for the duration of treatment of the more common etiologic organisms are listed in Table 73-9. For less common organisms, the optimal duration of treatment required may vary according to individual circumstances.

Role of Surgery

Optimal management of IE requires operative intervention during treatment for about one-third of patients.[87,347] Correct selection of this subgroup of patients and optimal timing of surgery are both critically important.[348]

Major indications for surgery are moderate or severe heart failure not responding to medical treatment, valvular obstruction, periannular or myocardial abscess, prosthetic valve dehiscence, persistent bacteremia despite appropriate antibiotics, and fungal infection. In most such cases, surgery should proceed promptly even if the infection is still active.

Relative indications for surgery include recurrent emboli; staphylococcal and gram-negative bacillary infections, especially involving prosthetic valves; persistent fever despite treatment; and vegetations that enlarge during treatment.[11,110,266,348]

Correct timing is the essence of good surgical management of endocarditis.[347] If surgery is undertaken too soon, the risks of operative mortality and the early and late morbidity associated with valve replacement may be inflicted on the patient unnecessarily, because some patients respond well to medical therapy, allowing surgery to be postponed indefinitely. If surgery can be delayed safely, antibiotic therapy should have eradicated or at least greatly reduced the number of organisms in the vegetation and in any sites of metastatic infection, thus increasing the chance of a successful outcome if surgery becomes necessary. If time is available for the effective treatment of complications such as septicemia, renal failure, pneumonia, myocarditis, and neurologic complications[316] before surgery, the operative risk should be lower. In comparison, if surgery is delayed too long, patients may die suddenly, or their hemodynamic status may deteriorate so seriously that surgery is no longer feasible. This would be a tragic error, because many authors have emphasized that both survival and long-term outcome can be improved by earlier operation for selected patients, even if the endocardial infection is still active.[266,349,350]

Careful, frequent reexamination of the patient, together with repeated echocardiographic studies and sometimes cardiac catheterization to confirm the clinical findings, is indicated in every case where operation might be needed. The decision to operate should also be influenced by knowledge of the natural history of the type of endocarditis being treated. For example, penicillin-sensitive streptococcal endocarditis can almost always be cured bacteriologically (Table 73-10), and the immediate prognosis is good provided that cardiac failure or other major complications do not develop. Therefore, surgery should usually be considered only for those patients with cardiac failure that does not respond well to medical treatment. Similarly, because young IDUs with acute staphylococcal endocarditis have a good prognosis,[5,324] surgery should usually be reserved for those who develop intrac-

TABLE 73-10 Estimate of Microbiologic Cure Rates for Various Forms of Endocarditis[a]

Native Valve Endocarditis	Antimicrobial Therapy Alone		Antimicrobial Therapy Plus Surgery	
Viridans streptococci, group A streptococci, *Strep. bovis,* pneumococci, gonococci	98		98	
Enterococcus faecalis	90		>90	
Staph. aureus (in young intravenous drug users)	90		>90	
Staph. aureus (in elderly patients with chronic underlying diseases)	50		70	
Gram-negative aerobic bacilli[b]	40		65	
Fungi	<5		50	
Prosthetic Valve Endocarditis	**Early PVE**	**Late PVE**	**Early PVE**	**Late PVE**
Viridans streptococci, group A streptococci, *Strep. bovis,* pneumococci, gonococci	*c*	80	*c*	90
Enterococcus faecalis	*c*	60	*c*	75
Staph. aureus	25	40	50	60
Staph. epidermidis	20	40	60	70
Gram-negative aerobic bacilli[b]	<10	20	40	50
Fungi	<1	<1	30	40

[a]Morbidity and mortality are significantly greater than these figures for microbiologic cure indicate.
[b]Excluding HACEK species.
[c]Insufficient data to estimate rates.
SOURCE: Adapted from Refs. 9, 11, 32, 33, 110, 116, 259, 323, 324, 350, 365.

table heart failure or definite signs of treatment failure. In contrast, the likelihood that fungal prosthetic valve endocarditis can be eradicated with antifungal drugs alone is negligible (Table 73-10). Such patients should usually undergo valve debridement or replacement early, without waiting to test the remote possibility that antifungal treatment could eradicate the infection.[351] The development of severe aortic regurgitation, especially when accompanied by heart failure, usually requires urgent surgery. Other examples of patients who are highly likely to require operation are those with early-onset PVE, valve-ring abscesses, or gram-negative bacillary infection of prosthetic valves.[11]

Over the past decade, surgical approaches have evolved toward increasingly radical debridement of infected tissue and more extensive use of reconstructive materials.[266,351] For example, an aortic root homograft instead of a standard prosthetic valve is now often inserted after debridement of a valve-ring abscess.[352] The Ross operation, transposing the patient's own pulmonary valve into the aortic position as an autograft after extensive debridement of infected tissue (replacing the pulmonary valve with a homograft) has been advocated as treatment for patients with complicated aortic root infections.[353,354]

In addition to valve replacement, several other surgical procedures may be available for the treatment of endocarditis.[348] Debridement of vegetations ("vegetectomy"), often combined with valvuloplasty, can cure the infection while sparing the native valve in selected patients.[267,268,355] This can be especially beneficial for young patients, women who wish to bear children, and patients who cannot or will not take anticoagulant therapy reliably.

Early consultation with the surgical service should be sought for most patients with endocarditis, so that an appropriate operation can be performed without delay if necessary. The sudden onset of aortic or mitral regurgitation with consequent acute left ventricular failure can occur without warning, even in the most favorable forms of endocarditis.

Anticoagulant Therapy

Even though the infected vegetation is essentially a thrombotic lesion, there is no evidence that anticoagulation has any useful therapeutic effect on the course of the endocarditis itself. On the contrary, early experience showed that simultaneous treatment with penicillin and heparin carried an increased risk of fatal intracerebral hemorrhage.[356] For this reason, anticoagulation was considered to be strongly contraindicated in patients with endocarditis, until further experience showed that warfarin could usually be given safely during the treatment of patients with prosthetic valve infections.[357–359] However in a series of 21 pH with PVE caused by *Staph. aureus,* 12 had CVS events including 6 intracranial hemorrhages and 5 ischemic strokes that had hemorrhagic transformation. All 11 died, and all had been on oral anticoagulants.[359] Currently available information suggests the following guidelines for patients with IE:

- Avoid use of heparin except for urgent indications, such as treatment of massive pulmonary embolism.
- Discontinue or avoid oral anticoagulants if possible, especially in patients with intracranial complications and if *Staph. aureus* is the cause of IE.
- Anticoagulate with warfarin if there is a clear-cut indication, such as a mechanical prosthetic heart valve, taking care to regulate the prothrombin time between International Normalized Ratio (INR) 2.5 and 3.5.

- Choose an antibiotic treatment regimen that does not require intramuscular injections if anticoagulation is instituted.

Thrombolytic agents theoretically could promote lysis or resolution of vegetations. Adjunctive treatment with recombinant tissue plasminogen activator decreased vegetation size and improved the results of short-term penicillin therapy in rabbits with fresh vegetations.[12] Similarly, aspirin therapy can reduce the size of experimental vegetations and improve rate of sterilization by antibiotics.[360] The potential value of antithrombotic agents, however, has not been demonstrated in human beings; thrombolytic therapy might not work on the older vegetations typical of SBE in human beings and could possibly cause serious hemorrhagic complications.

Management of Complications

HEART FAILURE

The development of moderate or severe cardiac failure due to structural valvular damage indicates the need for **prompt surgical intervention** in most patients with endocarditis, even if the intracardiac infection is still active.[347,349] In patients with mild heart failure, the decision should be individualized, always remembering that lives may be lost unnecessarily if cardiac function suddenly worsens, so that surgery becomes either hazardous or unfeasible.

EMBOLI

The occurrence of one or more significant arterial emboli during the treatment of endocarditis is a relative indication for surgery. The predictable early and long-term mortality and morbidity rates of valve replacement must be weighed against the highly unpredictable likelihood of further emboli. For this reason, embolization is a weaker indication for valve replacement than is cardiac failure.[348,349] In the author's opinion, operative intervention during antibiotic treatment should seldom be undertaken solely to prevent further emboli unless the patient has suffered more than one or two proved major emboli. Because the frequency of emboli falls rapidly after 1 to 2 weeks of antibiotic therapy,[361] the most logical time to operate for the purpose of preventing emboli would be early, within 1 week of diagnosis.

RENAL FAILURE

In the preantibiotic era, patients with SBE frequently developed chronic renal failure before they died.[3] Subsequently, both the incidence of renal failure and its importance as a cause of death have greatly diminished. In one series, up to one-third of 204 patients with IE developed evidence of acute renal failure, however. Risk factors for renal failure were increased age, hypertension, thrombocytopenia, IE caused by *Staph. aureus,* and PVE. While the earlier diagnosis and antibiotic treatment have forestalled the development of immune-complex glomerulonephritis, in those (about 5 to 10 percent) who still develop this complication of SBE, timely dialysis can maintain the patient until antibiotic treatment results in disappearance of the bacterial antigens that triggered immune-complex nephritis. Renal function usually normalizes smoothly once infection has been controlled, but recovery may take weeks or months. In a few cases, creatinine clearance worsens for a time despite effective antibacterial treatment, perhaps reflecting persistence of bacterial antigen in vegetations after bacteriologic cure. Corticosteroids may have been of value in a small number of cases.[362] Some patients with septicemia, shock, or disseminated intravascular coagulation associated with ABE develop acute renal failure and require dialysis as part of their intensive care.

MYCOTIC ANEURYSM

This complication is diagnosed in less than 5 percent of patients with IE, but the local consequences of aneurysm expansion and rupture can be very serious, especially in the brain (see Chap. 89).[276,278,279] Small aneurysms will often thrombose or resolve spontaneously during or after antibiotic therapy. Once aneurysms exceed 0.5 to 2 cm in diameter, they are likely to enlarge and eventually rupture despite eradication of the etiologic bacteria by antibiotic therapy.[281] Surgery is indicated for accessible aneurysms before this complication occurs.

Intracranial mycotic aneurysms are especially difficult to manage. They may present with headaches, subarachnoid hemorrhage, or stroke, but many are asymptomatic. Even small aneurysms may bleed at any time; they may be multiple and/or located in inaccessible sites. This presents a therapeutic dilemma: whether to treat conservatively with antibiotics and hope for resolution (risking serious or fatal hemorrhage) or to operate (risking neurologic damage and permanent sequelae). Symptoms or signs consistent with an intracranial aneurysm indicate the need for prompt imaging, using computed tomography and/or magnetic resonance imaging. Cerebral angiography may be needed if the findings are inconclusive. In general, large (over 0.5 cm in diameter) or expanding aneurysms or aneurysms that have already leaked or begun to bleed should be clipped if a surgical approach is feasible. An individualized decision must be made on whether or not to operate for smaller aneurysms that have not leaked or ruptured.

PROGNOSIS

IE is one of the few infectious diseases that are virtually always fatal if untreated. Spontaneous recovery was reported occasionally in the preantibiotic era,[3] but most of these patients probably had illnesses other than IE. The interval between the onset of symptoms and death in patients with untreated subacute disease varied widely, with a median time to death of about 6 months.[3] Almost all patients with acute IE died within less than 4 weeks.

Heart failure is the leading adverse prognostic factor.[264] Other adverse factors include central nervous system complications, renal failure, culture-negative disease, gram-negative bacillary or fungal infection, prosthetic valve infection, and development of abscesses in the valve ring or myocardium.[363] Survival 6 months after PVE in one series was only 54 percent.[364] Six-month survival after early-onset PVE (37 percent) was significantly worse than it was for late-onset PVE (65 percent). Because modern treatment methods, including valve replacement, are effective for treatment of heart failure, central nervous system complications have replaced heart failure as the most important adverse prognostic factor in some case studies.[274]

Favorable prognostic factors include youth, early diagnosis and treatment, infection involving a prolapsing mitral valve, and penicillin-sensitive streptococcal infection. The prognosis is good for young IDUs with *Staph. aureus* infection of the tricuspid valve.[5,335] With earlier diagnosis and appropriate therapy, including surgery, the prognosis for elderly patients can be substantially improved.[90] Eradication of the etiologic organisms (microbiological cure) can be achieved in a high proportion of all patients with bacterial endocarditis.[6,323,344,345] Both early and long-term mortality rates remain significant, however, due to any preexisting disease and added damage caused by endocarditis before the organisms were eradicated. Survival curves after admission with IE show a significant number of late deaths despite microbiologic cure.[9,365]

An analysis of experience over the past 25 years permits a reasonably accurate formulation of the prognosis for microbiologic cure among the various subgroups of patients with IE. Approximate figures are listed in Table 73-10.

RECURRENT ENDOCARDITIS

Recurrent endocarditis is a general term that includes both relapses and reinfections. The term *relapse* refers to recurrence of infection with the same organism because treatment failed. The frequency of relapse can be predicted from published experience for each of the various forms of IE (Table 73-10). Because relapses occasionally occur even after an optimal treatment regimen has been used, follow-up clinical evaluation should be meticulously performed during the first 2 months after treatment. Any clinical suspicion that relapse might have occurred indicates the need to draw blood cultures. Most relapses occur within a few weeks of ending treatment, but living organisms can persist in seemingly healed vegetations for many months and may occasionally cause late relapse.

The term *reinfection* refers to a new episode of endocarditis occurring after the cure of a previous episode.[366] Usually a different etiologic organism is involved, but if the new isolate appears similar to the initial etiologic organism, molecular typing techniques can be used to determine if the case is a relapse or an infection.

Patients remain permanently at risk of reinfection after cure of IE because of residual valve damage superimposed on the original predisposing lesion (see Tables 73-1 and 73-2). Recurrent episodes are fairly common, being recorded in from 2 to 31 percent of cases.[3,46,48,365,366] This wide variation in reported incidence is partly due to variable duration of follow-up. IDUs and patients with severe periodontitis are at highest risk for reinfection. Occasionally, a patient may suffer three or more separate episodes of IE.[366] Patients who have previously had NVE and have required valve replacement, are at high risk to develop prosthetic valve infection (often with a different organism) for reasons that are not yet understood.[9]

THE CHALLENGE OF PROPHYLAXIS

Because various invasive procedures induce bacteremias with bacterial species that often cause IE,[367–369] prophylactic antibiotics are frequently given to susceptible patients in an attempt to prevent bacterial endocarditis. Although antibiotics definitely can prevent endocarditis in experimental animals, its effectiveness in human beings has not been proved in prospective randomized clinical trials and likely never will be. Many relevant questions remain unanswered. These include the following:

- Is antibiotic prophylaxis effective?
- Does the prophylactic effect (benefit) outweigh the potential side effect of the drug cost and influence the emergence of drug-resistant bacteria?
- Which operations and diagnostic procedures should be covered?
- Which patients should receive antibiotics?
- What antibiotic regimens will be most effective?

Although the risk of infection has not been quantitated, it is sufficiently low that most of these questions cannot be answered by clinical trials; the number of susceptible patients required to provide significant results would be too large.[55,349]

Less than 15 percent of SBE cases and even fewer of ABE cases follow identifiable medical procedures that cause transient bacteremias[54,367,368,370]; therefore, the proportion of cases that is potentially preventable by antibiotics is vanishingly small.

Because endocarditis causes serious morbidity and mortality, the American Heart Association and the practicing medical community have accepted the practice of using antibiotic prophylaxis without evidence-based studies. It has been accepted that prevention of even a few cases could be worthwhile. For this reason, currently accepted standards of practice require that an antibiotic regimen be administered before certain dental and surgical procedures in patients with known heart lesions that pose a significant risk of endocarditis.

Because several hundred cases of streptococcal endocarditis following dental and genitourinary tract procedures have been recorded, the potential causative role of these procedures is certainly suggested.[367,368] A rather short "incubation period" for endocarditis is typical, in that most of these patients noticed symptoms within 2 weeks of the procedure.[256] It should be emphasized that the link between a case of endocarditis and a recent procedure causing bacteremia cannot be proved, because the infection could have been caused by one of the transient, asymptomatic, low-grade bacteremias that occur very commonly, induced by everyday events such as chewing and cleaning the teeth. In fact, when 273 cases of endocarditis are examined retrospect from 1, 2, and 3 months prior to endocarditis, no correlation to dental procedures were found.[56,367]

In the absence of prospective controlled trials, empirical recommendations[55,370,371] for prophylaxis of bacterial endocarditis have been made on the basis of indirect information. This information includes the reported frequency of bacteremia after various procedures (Table 73-11); the relative risk posed by the patient's cardiac lesion (Table 73-2); case reports of prophylaxis failures[75]; in vitro susceptibility studies on the relevant organisms, especially streptococci; experimental studies in laboratory animals[254,372]; and retrospective studies in human beings.[373–375]

Information from these sources indicates that experimental endocarditis in animals can be prevented by bactericidal antibiotics; that prevention is probably effective in human beings; that only a small proportion of total cases is potentially preventable by use of antibiotics[370,374]; and that the cost per prevented case would be very high.[76,374] Thus, prevention probably would not be cost-effective as a general strategy, but it might be effective for selected individuals (namely patients with previous IE and patients with prosthetic valves), especially for high-risk procedures such as tooth extractions.[370,376]

For the individual patient, the decision to administer prophylaxis should be made by assessing two main factors: the risk posed by the preexisting cardiac lesion and the risk posed by the procedure that might cause bacteremia. For example, if a patient with a prosthetic valve undergoes prostate resection, antibiotic prophylaxis is recommended because both factors present a significant risk of endocarditis. In contrast, if a patient with mitral valve prolapse is scheduled for gastroscopy, prophylaxis is not necessary because the risk for endocarditis in this setting is very low.[369] Such risk assessments may be difficult or inaccurate; in many situations uncertainties will remain. For these, there is no one "correct" answer; the patient's and the physician's attitudes and preferences may influence the decision to use prophylaxis. Updated consensus recommendations by the AHA may be useful in guiding decision making.[79]

These guidelines emphasize the following points:

1. Most cases are not attributable to an invasive procedure.
2. Cardiac conditions should be stratified into light, moderate, and negligible risk categories; these are primarily based on potential outcomes if endocarditis occurs.
3. There are procedures that may cause high grade bacteremia and for which prophylaxis is most likely to be effective.
4. There is an algorithm to use in deciding on prophylaxis in patients with mitral valve prolapse.
5. The initial dose of amoxicillin is reduced to 2 g for oral and dental procedures and a follow-up dose is no longer recommended; clindamycin (not erythromycin) is recommended as an alternative therapy in penicillin-allergic individuals.
6. Prophylactic recommendations in gastrointestinal and genitourinary procedures have been simplified.[79]

TABLE 73-11 Representative Rates for Frequency of Bacteremia after Various Dental, Diagnostic, and Therapeutic Procedures

Procedure	% Bacteremia	% Range (if available)
None	0	(0–3)
Oral cavity		
Extraction of teeth	60	(18–85)
Periodontal surgery	88	(60–90)
Brushing teeth or irrigation	40	(7–50)
Tonsillectomy	35	(33–38)
Respiratory tract		
Tracheal intubation	<10	(0–16)
Nasotracheal suctioning	16	
Bronchoscopy (rigid bronchoscope)	15	
Bronchoscopy (flexible bronchoscope)	0	
Genitourinary tract		
Catheter insertion and removal	3	(0–26)
Prostatectomy (sterile urine)	12	(11–13)
Prostatectomy (infected urine)	60	(58–82)
Dilatation of strictures	28	(19–86)
Normal delivery	3	(1–5)
Intrauterine device insertion or removal	0	
Gastrointestinal tract		
Upper gastrointestinal endoscopy	4	(0–8)
Transesophageal echocardiography	1	(0–17)
Endoscopic retrograde cholangiopancreatography	5	(0–6)
Barium enema	10	(5–11)
Colonoscopy	5	(0–5)
Sigmoidoscopy (rigid sigmoidoscope)	5	
Sigmoidoscopy (flexible sigmoidoscope)	0	
Proctoscopy	2	
Hemorrhoidectomy	8	
Esophageal dilatation	45	
Vascular system		
Cardiac catheterization	2	(0–5)
Insufficient data		
Insertion and removal of tympanostomy tubes		
Cesarean section		

SOURCE: From Durack,[370] with permission.

Attempted prophylaxis does not always succeed. Of 52 cases of apparent prophylaxis failure in one series, 42 involved patients with heart disease who received oral penicillin or erythromycin, usually to cover dental procedures.[75]

Surprisingly, in one series 12 of 16 patients with known cardiac abnormalities who developed IE with organisms of dental origin and who had a dental procedure within 3 months of onset of IE received prophylactic antibiotics according to AHA guidelines. In fact, only 10 percent of cases of IE in this study would qualify for prophylaxis according to the AHA standards. Even if a prophylaxis was 100 percent effective, it would reduce the incidence of IE by only 2.0 cases per 1,000,000 person-years.

The authors agree with Durack, that on the basis of existing data, it is most reasonable to use prophylaxis prior to dental extractions or gingival surgery including implant placement but not routine dental care, filling of cavities, root canal, cleaning and sealing of teeth, in patients with prosthetic valves or history of prior endocarditis. If any of the four conditions are present, antibiotic prophylaxis seems reasonable.[56]

Common errors in attempted prevention of endocarditis are starting antibiotics too early, continuing for too long, using low doses, covering tooth extractions but not lesser dental procedures, and confusing prevention of rheumatic fever (requiring long-term, low-dose antimicrobial drugs) with prevention of endocarditis (short-term, high-dose).[55]

TABLE 73-12 Suggested Regimens for Prophylaxis of Infective Endocarditis[a]

Standard Regimen	
For dental procedures and oral or upper respiratory tract surgery	Amoxicillin 2.0 g orally 1 h before procedure[b]
Special Regimens	
Parenteral regimen for high-risk patients; also for gastrointestinal (GI) or genitourinary (GU) tract procedures	Ampicillin 2.0 g IM or IV *plus* gentamicin 1.5 mg/kg IM or IV, 0.5 h before procedure,[b] 6 h later, ampicillin 1 g IM or IV or amoxicillin 1 g orally
Parenteral regimen for penicillin-allergic patients	Vancomycin 1.0 g IV *slowly* over 1–2 h; *plus* gentamicin 1.5 mg/kg IM or IV[b]; complete within 30 min of starting the procedure
Oral regimen for penicillin-allergic patients (oral and respiratory tract only)	Clindamycin 600 mg orally 1 h before procedure[b]
Oral regimen for minor GI or GU tract procedures	Amoxicillin 2.0 g orally 1 h before procedure[b]
Parenteral regimen for cardiac surgery including valve replacement	Cefazolin 2.0 g IV on induction of anesthesia, repeated 8 and 16 h later[c] *or* Vancomycin 1.0 g IV *slowly* over 1 h starting on induction of anesthesia, then 0.5 g IV 8 and 16 h later[c]

[a]Note that (1) these regimens are empiric suggestions, no regimen has been proved effective for prevention of endocarditis, and prevention failures may occur with any regimen; (2) these regimens are not intended to cover all clinical situations, and the practitioner should use his or her own judgment on safety and cost-benefit issues in each individual case; (3) one or two additional doses may be given if the period of risk for bacteremia is prolonged.

[b]Pediatric dosages: ampicillin 50 mg/kg; gentamicin 1.5 mg/kg; amoxicillin: for children who weigh more than 60 lb, use same as for adults; for children less than 60 lb, use one-half the adult dose; vancomycin 20 mg/kg; clindamycin 20 mg/kg; cefazolin 30 mg/kg. Do not exceed 2.0 g ampicillin, 120 mg gentamycin.

[c]Vancomycin is preferred if *Staph. epidermidis* is an important cause of postoperative infection in that hospital. Gentamicin 1.5 mg/kg IV or IM may be added to each dose, only if postoperative gram-negative infections have occurred with significant frequency.

SOURCE: Durack DT. Nine controversies in the management of infective endocarditis. In: Petersdorf RG, et al., eds. *Update V: Harrison's Principles of Internal Medicine*. New York: McGraw-Hill; 1984:35; and Dajani, et al. (*JAMA* 1997; 277:1794–1801).[371] Adapted and reproduced with permission of the publisher and author.

In the absence of pelvic infection, prophylaxis for endocarditis in patients with heart lesions is not recommended to cover normal delivery, therapeutic abortion, dilation and curettage, and insertion or removal of intrauterine contraceptive devices. Similarly, antibiotics are not recommended before many common procedures, such as cardiac catheterization, insertion of temporary pacemakers, endotracheal intubation, bronchoscopy, endoscopy, or radiographic contrast studies of the upper and lower gastrointestinal tract. In comparison, some physicians choose to cover even these low-risk procedures in patients with prosthetic valves because they are at higher risk for endocarditis than are patients with native valves. Specific regimens suggested for prophylaxis of endocarditis are listed in Table 73-12.

Cardiac surgeons currently administer antibiotics to virtually all patients undergoing cardiac surgery, attempting to prevent both wound infections and endocarditis, although the efficacy of prophylaxis in prevention of endocarditis has not been proved.[55] Current recommendations call for parenteral administration of an antistaphylococcal antibiotic just prior to operation, followed by 1 or 2 further doses (Table 73-12). The regimen may be modified if local experience shows that cases of early PVE caused by *Staph.* epidermidis or gram-negative bacilli have occurred with significant frequency (Table 73-12).

The paradigms that have been proposed by various expert bodies (including the AHA) for the use of antibiotics to prevent IE have developed over time and have been based on indirect evidence derived from studies in animals that demonstrated that prevention was possible, on case reports tying IE to various procedures known to cause bacteremia, and from a concern about the dire consequences of the disease. These recommendations have been accepted as "standard of care" and failure to follow them has taken on medicolegal implications. Various authors have questioned this practice and new information has emerged calling into question the clinical benefit of prophylactic antibiotics in this setting. This is especially important in an era where overuse of antimicrobials is fueling the dangerous epidemic of antibiotic-resistant bacteria. Therefore, it seems prudent for the various expert committees who write such recommendations to carefully weigh the apparent minimal benefits with the downsides of toxicity, cost, and resistance that has come with excessive use of antibiotics.

NOTE

This chapter is a modification of the original chapter by David Durack in previous editions of this book.

References

1. Blumer G. Subacute bacterial endocarditis. *Medicine* 1923; 2:105–170.

2. Thayer WS. Studies on bacterial (infective) endocarditis. *Johns Hopkins Hosp Rep* 1926; 22:1–185.
3. Kerr A Jr. *Subacute Bacterial Endocarditis.* Springfield, IL: Charles C Thomas; 1955.
4. Hermans PE. The clinical manifestations of infective endocarditis. *Mayo Clin Proc* 1982; 57:15–21.
5. Chambers HF, Korzeniowski OM, Sande MA, National Collaborative Endocarditis Study Group. *Staphylococcus aureus* endocarditis: Clinical manifestations in addicts and nonaddicts. *Medicine* 1983; 62:170–177.
6. Korzeniowski OM, Kaye D. Infective endocarditis. In: Braunwald E, ed. *The Heart: A Textbook of Cardiovascular Medicine,* 4th ed. Philadelphia: Saunders, 1992:1078–1105.
7. Sande MA, Johnson WD Jr, Hook EW, Kay D: Bacteremia associated with cardiac catheterization. *N Engl J Med* 1969; 281:1104–1106.
8. Baumgartner WA, Miller DC, Reitz BA, et al. Surgical treatment of prosthetic valve endocarditis. *Ann Thorac Surg* 1983; 35:87–104.
9. Ivert TSA, Dismukes WE, Cobbs CG, et al. Prosthetic valve endocarditis. *Circulation* 1984; 69:223–232.
10. Braimbridge MV, Eykyn SJ. Prosthetic valve endocarditis. *J Antimicrob Chemother* 1987; 20:173–180.
11. Douglas JL, Cobbs CG. Prosthetic valve endocarditis. In: Kaye D, ed. *Infective Endocarditis,* 2d ed. New York: Raven Press; 1992:375–396.
12. Meyer MW, Witt AR, Krishnan LK, et al. Therapeutic advantage of recombinant human plasminogen activator in endocarditis: Evidence from experiments in rabbits. *Thromb Haemost* 1995; 73:680–682.
13. MacDonald RA, Robbins SL. The significance of nonbacterial thrombotic endocarditis: An autopsy and clinical study of 78 cases. *Ann Intern Med* 1957; 46:255–273.
14. Barry WE, Scarpelli D. Nonbacterial thrombotic endocarditis. *Arch Intern Med* 1962; 109:79–84.
15. Bryan CS. Nonbacterial thrombotic endocarditis in patients with malignant tumors. *Am J Med* 1969; 46:787–793.
16. Major RM. Notes on the history of endocarditis. *Bull Hist Med* 1945; 17:351–359.
17. Osler W. Chronic infectious endocarditis. *Q J Med* 1909; 2:219–230.
18. Osler W. The Goulstonian lectures, on malignant endocarditis. *Br Med J* 1885; 1:467–579.
19. Horder TJ. Infective endocarditis: With an analysis of 150 cases and with special reference to the chronic form of the disease. *Q J Med* 1909; 2:289–329.
20. Allen AC. Nature of vegetations of bacterial endocarditis. *Arch Pathol* 1939; 27:661–671.
21. Libman E, Friedberg CK. *Subacute Bacterial Endocarditis.* New York: Oxford University Press; 1947.
22. Beeson PB, Brannon ES, Warren JV. Observations of the sites of removal of bacteria from the blood in patients with bacterial endocarditis. *J Exp Med* 1945; 81:9–23.
23. Touroff ASW, Vesell H. Subacute streptococcus viridans endocarditis complicating patent ductus arteriosus: Recovery following surgical treatment. *JAMA* 1940; 115:1270–1272.
24. Durack DT. Review of early experience in treatment of bacterial endocarditis, 1940–1955. In: Bisno AL, ed. *Treatment of Infective Endocarditis.* New York: Grune & Stratton; 1981:1–14.
25. Dawson MH, Hunter TH. The treatment of subacute bacterial endocarditis with penicillin: Results in twenty cases. *JAMA* 1945; 127:129–137.
26. Abraham EP, Chain E, Fletcher CM, et al. Further observations on penicillin. *Lancet* 1941; 2:177–189.
27. Loewe L, Rosenblatt P, Greene HJ, Russell M. Combined penicillin and heparin therapy of subacute bacterial endocarditis: Report of seven consecutive successfully treated patients. *JAMA* 1944; 124:144–149.
28. Galbreath WR, Hull E. Sulfonamide therapy of bacterial endocarditis: Results in 42 cases. *Ann Intern Med* 1943; 18:201–203.
29. Bloomfield AL, Armstrong CD, Kirby WMM. The treatment of subacute bacterial endocarditis with penicillin. *J Clin Invest* 1945; 24:251–267.
30. Hunter TH. The treatment of some bacterial infections of the heart and pericardium. *Bull NY Acad Med* 1952; 28:213–228.
31. Finland M. Treatment of bacterial endocarditis (concluded). *N Engl J Med* 1954; 250:419–428.
32. Geraci JE. The antibiotic therapy of infective endocarditis: Therapeutic data on 172 patients seen from 1951 through 1957: Additional observations on short-term therapy (two weeks) for penicillin-sensitive streptococcal endocarditis. *Med Clin North Am* 1958; 42:1101–1148.
33. Weinstein L, Schlesinger J. Treatment of infective endocarditis—1973. *Prog Cardiovasc Dis* 1973; 26:275–296.
34. Wallace AG, Young G Jr, Osterhout S. Treatment of acute bacterial endocarditis by valve excision and replacement. *Circulation* 1965; 31:450–453.
35. Harris SL. Definitions and demographic characteristics. In: Kaye D, ed. *Infective Endocarditis.* 2d ed. New York: Raven Press; 1992:1–18.
36. Steckelberg JM, Wilson WR. Risk factors for infective endocarditis. *Infect Dis Clin North Am* 1993; 7:9–19.
37. Smith RH, Radford DJ, Clark RA, Julian DG. Infective endocarditis: A survey of cases in the southeast of Scotland 1969–72. *Thorax* 1976;31:373–379.
38. Van Der Meer JTM, Thompson J, Valkenburg HA, Michel MF. Epidemiology of bacterial endocarditis in the Netherlands: 1. Patient characteristics. *Arch Intern Med* 1992; 152:1863–1868.
39. Hogevik H, Olaison L, Andersson R, et al. Epidemiologic aspects of infective endocarditis in an urban population: A 5-year prospective study. *Medicine* 1995; 74:324–339.
40. Berlin JA, Abrutyn E, Strom BL, et al. Incidence of infective endocarditis in the Delaware Valley, 1988–1990. *Am J Cardiol* 1995; 76:933–936.
41. Kaye D, McCormack RC, Hook EW. Bacterial endocarditis: The changing pattern since the introduction of penicillin therapy. *Antimicrob Agents Chemother* 1961; 37–46.
42. Uwaydah MM, Weinberg AN. Bacterial endocarditis—A changing pattern. *N Engl J Med* 1965; 273:1231–1235.
43. Lerner PI, Weinstein L. Infective endocarditis in the antibiotic era. *N Engl J Med* 1966; 274:199–206; 259–266; 323–331; 388–393.
44. Finland M, Barnes MW. Changing etiology of bacterial endocarditis in the antibiotic era: Experiences at the Boston City Hospital 1933–1965. *Ann Intern Med* 1970; 72:341–348.
45. Durack DT, Petersdorf RG. Changes in the epidemiology of endocarditis. In: Kaplan EL, Taranta AV, eds. *Infective Endocarditis: An American Heart Association Symposium.* Dallas: American Heart Association; 1977:3–8.
46. Baddour LM. Twelve-year review of recurrent native-valve infective endocarditis: A disease of the modern antibiotic era. *Rev Infect Dis* 1988; 10:1163–1170.
47. Dysson C, Infective endocarditis: An epidemiological review of 128 episodes. *J Infect* 1999; 38(2):87–93.
48. Garvey GJ, Neu HC. Infective endocarditis—An evolving disease: A review of endocarditis at the Columbia-Presbyterian Medical Center, 1968–1973. *Medicine* 1978; 57:105–127.
49. Pulvirenti JJ, Kerns E, Benson C, et al. Infective endocarditis in injection drug users: Importance of human immunodeficiency virus serostatus and degree of immunosuppression. *Clin Infect Dis* 1996; 22:40–45.
50. Scheld WM, Sande MA. Endocarditis and intravascular infections. In: Mandell GL, Douglas RG Jr, Dolin R, eds. *Principles*

and Practice of Infectious Diseases, 4th ed. New York: Churchill Livingstone; 1995:740–783.

51. Weinstein L, Rubin RH. Infective endocarditis—1973. *Prog Cardiovasc Dis* 1973; 16:239–273.
52. Tunkel AR, Mandell GL. Infecting microorganisms. In: Kaye D, ed. *Infective Endocarditis,* 2d ed. New York: Raven Press; 1992:85–97.
53. Tompkins LS, Roessler BJ, Redd SC. Legionella prosthetic-valve endocarditis. *N Engl J Med* 1988; 318:530–534.
54. Bayliss R, Clarke C, Oakley C, et al. The teeth and infective endocarditis. *Br Heart J* 1983; 50:506–512.
55. Durack DT. Prophylaxis of infective endocarditis. In: Mandell GL, Douglas RG Jr, Dolin R, eds. *Principles and Practice of Infectious Diseases,* 4th ed. NewYork: Churchill Livingstone; 1995:793–813.
56. Strom BL, et al. Dental and Cardiac Risk Factors for Infective Endocarditis. *Ann Intern Med* 1998; 129:761–769.
57. Mansur AJ, Grinberg M, da Luz PL, Bellotti G. The complications of infective endocarditis: A reappraisal in the 1980s (see comments). *Arch Intern Med* 1992; 152:2428–2432.
58. Johnson DH, Rosenthal A, Nadas AS. A forty-year review of bacterial endocarditis in infancy and childhood. *Circulation* 1975; 51:581–588.
59. Hansen D, Schmiegelow K, Jacobsen JR. Bacterial endocarditis in children: Trends in its diagnosis, course, and prognosis. *Pediatr Cardiol* 1993; 13:198–203.
60. Saiman L, Prince A, Gersony WM. Pediatric infective endocarditis in the modern era. *J Pediatr* 1993; 122:847–853.
61. Awadallah SM, Kavey RW, Byrum CJ, et al. The changing pattern of infective endocarditis in childhood. *Am J Cardiol* 1991; 68:90–94.
62. Stull TL, LiPuma JJ. Endocarditis in children. In: Kaye D, ed. *Infective Endocarditis,* 2d ed. New York: Raven Press; 1992:313–327.
63. Ifere OAS, Masokano KA. Infective endocarditis in children in the Guinea savannah of Nigeria. *Ann Trop Paediatr* 1991; 11:233–240.
64. Saitoh M, Hishi T, Tamura M, Komoshita S. Forty year review of bacterial endocarditis in infants and children. *Acta Paediatr Jpn* 1991; 33:613–616.
65. El-Khatib MR, Wilson FM, Lerner AM. Characteristics of bacterial endocarditis in heroin addicts in Detroit. *Am J Med Sci* 1976; 271:197–201.
66. Reisberg BE. Infective endocarditis in the narcotic addict. *Prog Cardiovasc Dis* 1979; 22:193–204.
67. Dressler FA, Roberts WC. Infective endocarditis in opiate addicts: Analysis of 80 cases studied at necropsy. *Am J Cardiol* 1989; 63:1240–1257.
68. Weisse AB, Heller DR, Schimenti RJ, et al. The febrile parenteral drug user: A prospective study in 121 patients. *Am J Med* 1993; 94:274–280.
69. Carrel T, Schaffner A, Vogt P, et al. Endocarditis in intravenous drug addicts and HIV infected patients: Possibilities and limitations of surgical treatment. *J Heart Valve Dis* 1993; 2:140–147.
70. Sande MA, Lee BL, Mills J, Chambers HF III. Endocarditis in intravenous drug users. In: Kaye D, ed. *Infective Endocarditis,* 2d ed. New York: Raven Press; 1992:345–359.
71. Corrigall D, Bolen J, Hancock EW, Popp RP. Mitral valve prolapse and infective endocarditis. *Am J Med* 1977; 63:215–222.
72. Clemens JD, Horwitz RI, Jaffe CC, et al. A controlled evaluation of the risk of bacterial endocarditis in persons with mitral-valve prolapse. *N Engl J Med* 1982; 307:776–781.
73. Beton DC, Brear SG, Edwards JD, Leonard JC. Mitral valve prolapse:An assessment of clinical features, associated conditions and prognosis. *Q J Med* 1983; 52:150–164.
74. Heidenreich PA. The clinical impact of echocardiography on antibiotic prophylaxis use in patients with suspected mitral valve prolapse. *Am J Med* 1997; 102(4): 337–343.
75. Durack DT, Kaplan EL, Bisno AL. Apparent failures of endocarditis prophylaxis: Analysis of 52 cases submitted to a national registry. *JAMA* 1983; 250:2318–2322.
76. Clemens JD, Ransohoff DF. A quantitative assessment of predental antibiotic prophylaxis for patients with mitral-valve prolapse. *J Chronic Dis* 1984; 37:531–544.
77. Devereux RB, Hawkins I, Kramer-Fox R, et al. Complications of mitral valve prolapse: Disproportionate occurrence in men and older patients. *Am J Med* 1986; 81:751–758.
78. MacMahon SW, Hickey AJ, Wilcken DEL, et al. Risk of infective endocarditis in mitral valve prolapse with and without precordial systolic murmurs. *Am J Cardiol* 1986; 58:105–108.
79. Dajani AS, Taubert KA, Wilson W, et al. *Prevention of Bacterial Endocarditis.* Dallas: American Heart Association Medical/ Scientific Statement; 1997; 71–0117.
80. MacMahon SW, Roberts K, Kramer-Fox R, et al. Mitral valve prolapse and infective endocarditis. *Am Heart J* 1987; 113:1291–1298.
81. Dhawan A, Grover A, Marwaha RK, et al. Infective endocarditis in children: Profile in a developing country. *Ann Trop Paediatr* 1993; 13:189–194.
82. Elward K, Hruby N, Christy C. Pneumococcal endocarditis in infants and children: Report of a case and review of the literature. *Pediatr Infect Dis J* 1990; 9:652–657.
83. Brook MM, Pediatric bacterial endocarditis: Treatment and prophylaxis. *Pediatr Clin North Am* 1999; 46(2):275–287.
84. Martin JM, Neches WH, Wald ER, et al. Infective endocarditis: 35 years of experience at a children's hospital. *Clin Infect Dis* 1997; 24(4):669–675.
85. Del Pont JM, De Cicco LT, Vartalitis C, et al. Infective endocarditis in children: Clinical analyses and evaluation of two diagnostic criteria. *Pediatr Infect Dis* 1995; 14:1079–1086.
86. Kaplan EL, Rich H, Gersony W, Manning J. A collaborative study of infective endocarditis in the 1970s: Emphasis on infections in patients who have undergone cardiovascular surgery. *Circulation* 1979; 59:327–335.
87. Jung JY, Saab SB, Almond CH. The case for early surgical treatment of left-sided primary infective endocarditis. *J Thorac Cardiovasc Surg* 1975; 70:509–518.
88. Picarelli D, Leone R, Duhagon P, et al. Active infective endocarditis in infants and childhood: Ten-year review of surgical therapy. *J Card Surg* 1997; 12(6):406–411.
89. Bayliss R, Clarke C, Oakley CM, et al. Incidence, mortality and prevention of infective endocarditis. *J R Coll Phys Lond* 1986; 20:15–20.
90. Werner GS, Schulz R, Fuchs FB, et al. Infective endocarditis in the elderly in the era of transesophageal echocardiography: Clinical features and prognosis compared with younger patients. *Am J Med* 1996; 100:90–97.
91. Felder RS, Nardone D, Palac R. Prevalence of predisposing factors for endocarditis among an elderly institutionalized population. *Oral Surg Oral Med Oral Pathol* 1992; 73:30–34.
92. Selton-Suty C, Hoen B, Grentzinger A, et al. Clinical and bacteriological characteristics of infective endocarditis in the elderly. *Heart* 1997; 77(3):260–263.
93. Steckelberg JM, Melton LJ, Ilstrup DM, et al. Influence of referral bias on the apparent clinical spectrum of infective endocarditis. *Am J Med* 1990; 88:582–588.
94. Eliopoulos GM. Enterococcal endocarditis. In: Kaye D, ed. *Infective Endocarditis,* 2d ed. New York: Raven Press; 1992:209–229.
95. Threlkeld MG, Cobbs CG. Infectious disorders of prosthetic valves and intravascular devices. In: Mandell GL, Bennett JE, Dolin R, eds. *Principles and Practice of Infectious Diseases,* 4th ed. New York: Churchill Livingstone; 1995:783–793.
96. Burke AP, Kalra P, Li L et al. Infectious endocarditis and sudden

unexpected death: incidence and morphology of lesions in intravenous addicts and non-drug abusers. *J Heart Valve Dis* 1997; 6(2):198–203.
97. Tuazon CU, Sheagren JN. Increased rate of carriage of *Staphylococcus aureus* among narcotic addicts. *J Infect Dis* 1974; 129:725–727.
98. Reyes MP, Lerner AM. Current problems in the treatment of infective endocarditis due to *Pseudomonas aeruginosa*. *Rev Infect Dis* 1983; 5:314–321.
99. Cohen PS, Maguire JH, Weinstein L. Infective endocarditis caused by gram-negative bacteria: A review of the literature, 1945–1977. *Prog Cardiovasc Dis* 1980; 22:205–242.
100. Rubinstein E, Noriega ER, Simberkoff MS, et al. Fungal endocarditis: Analysis of 24 cases and review of the literature. *Medicine* 1975; 54:331–344.
101. Moyer DV, Edwards JE Jr. Fungal endocarditis. In: Kaye D, ed. *Infective Endocarditis,* 2d ed. New York: Raven Press; 1992:299–312.
102. Baddour LM, Meyer J, Henry B. Polymicrobial infective endocarditis in the 1980s. *Rev Infect Dis* 1991; 13:963–970.
103. Faber M, Frimodt-Moller N, Espersen F, et al. *Staphylococcus aureus* endocarditis in Danish intravenous drug users: High proportion of left-sided endocarditis. *Scand J Infect Dis* 1995; 27:483–487.
104. Spijkerman IJ, van Ameijden EJ, Mientjes GH, et al. Human immunodeficiency virus infection and other risk factors for skin abscesses and endocarditis among injection drug users. *J Clin Epidemiol* 1996; 49(10):1149–1154.
105. Drancourt M, Birtles R, Chaumentin G, et al. New serotype of *Bartonella henselae* in endocarditis and cat-scratch disease. *Lancet* 1996; 347:441–443.
106. Ribera E, et al. Influence of human immunodeficiency virus 1 and degree of immunosuppression in the clinical characteristics and outcome of infective endocarditis in intravenous drug users. *Arch Intern Med* 1998; 158(18):2043–2050.
107. Manoff SB. Human immunodeficiency virus infection and infective endocarditis among injecting drug users. *Epidemiology* 1996; 7(6):566–570.
108. Resnekov L. Staphylococcal endocarditis following mitral valvotomy with special reference to coagulase-negative *Staphylococcus albus*. *Lancet* 1959; 2:597–600.
109. Watanakunakorn C. Prosthetic valve infective endocarditis. *Prog Cardiovasc Dis* 1979; 22:181–192.
110. Karchmer AW, Dismukes WE, Buckley MJ, Austen WG. Late prosthetic valve endocarditis: Clinical features influencing therapy. *Am J Med* 1978; 64:199–206.
111. Seaworth BJ, Durack DT. Infective endocarditis in obstetric and gynecologic practice. *Am J Obstet Gynecol* 1986; 154:180–188.
112. Sugrue D, Blake S, Troy P, MacDonald D. Antibiotic prophylaxis against infective endocarditis after normal delivery—Is it necessary? *Br Heart J* 1980; 44:499–502.
113. Cobbs CG. IUD and endocarditis. *Ann Intern Med* 1973; 78:451.
114. Fernandez-Guerrero ML, Verdejo C, Azofra J, de Gorgolas M. Hospital-acquired infectious endocarditis not associated with cardiac surgery: An emerging problem. *Clin Infect Dis* 1995; 20:16–23.
115. Fang G, Keys TF, Gentry LO, et al. Prosthetic valve endocarditis resulting from nosocomial bacteremia: A prospective, multicenter study. *Ann Intern Med* 1993; 119:560–567.
116. Pelletier LL, Petersdorf RG. Infective endocarditis: A review of 125 cases from the University of Washington Hospitals, 1963–72. *Medicine* 1977; 56:287–313.
117. Raad II, Bodey GP. Infectious complications of indwelling vascular catheters. *Clin Infect Dis* 1992; 15:197–210.
118. Lamas CC. Hospital acquired native valve endocarditis: analysis of 22 cases presenting over 11 years. *Heart* 1998: 79(5):442–447.
119. Ehrie M, Morgan AP, Moore FD, O'Connor NE. Endocarditis with the indwelling balloon-tipped pulmonary artery catheter in burn patients. *J Trauma* 1978; 18:665–666.
120. Rowley KM, Clubb KS, Smith GJW, Cabin HS. Right-sided infective endocarditis as a consequence of flow-directed pulmonary artery catheterization: A clinicopathological study of 55 autopsied patients. *N Engl J Med* 1984; 311:1152–1156.
121. Cartotto RC. Acute bacterial endocarditis following burns: Case report and review. *Burns* 1998; 24(4):369–373.
122. Martino P, Micozzi A, Venditti M, et al. Catheter-related right-sided endocarditis in bone marrow transplant recipients. *Rev Infect Dis* 1990; 12:250–257.
123. Khoo DE, Zebro TJ, English TAH. Bacterial endocarditis in a transplanted heart. *Pathol Res Pract* 1989; 185:445–447.
124. Paterson DL. Infective endocarditis in solid organ transplant recipients. *Clin Infect Dis* 1998; 26(3):689–694.
125. Lillehei CW, Bobb JRR, Visscher MB. The occurrence of endocarditis with valvular deformities in dogs with arteriovenous fistulas. *Ann Surg* 1950; 132:577–590.
126. Cross AS, Steigbigel RT. Infective endocarditis and access site infections in patients on hemodialysis. *Medicine* 1976; 55:453–465.
127. Robinson DL, Bacterial endocarditis in hemodialysis patients, *Am J Kidney Dis* 1997; 30(4):521–524.
128. Marr KA. Incidence and outcome of *Staphylococcus aureus* bacteremia in hemodialysis patients. *Kid Int* 1998; 54(5):1684–1689.
129. Klug D, Lacroix D, Savoye C, et al. Systemic infection related to endocarditis on pacemaker leads: Clinical presentation and management. *Circulation* 1997; 95(8):2098–2107.
130. Cacoub P. Pacemaker infective endocarditis. *Am J Cardiol* 1998; 82(4):480–484.
131. Victor F. Pacemaker lead infection: Echocardiographic features, management, and outcome. *Heart* 1999; 81(1):82–87.
132. Voet JG. Pacemaker lead infection: Report of three cases and review of the literature. *Heart* 1999; 81(1):88–91.
133. Gomes MN, Choyke PL, Wallace RB. Infected aortic aneurysms: A changing entity. *Ann Surg* 1992; 215:435–442.
134. Brennan RO, Durack DT. The viridans streptococci in perspective. In: Remington JS, Swartz MN, eds. *Current Clinical Topics in Infectious Diseases.* New York: McGraw-Hill; 1984:253–289.
135. Sussman JI, Baron EJ, Tenenbaum MJ, et al. Viridans streptococcal endocarditis: Clinical, microbiological, and echocardiographic correlations. *J Infect Dis* 1986; 154:597–603.
136. Watanakunakorn C, Pantelakis J. Alpha-hemolytic streptococcal bacteremia: A review of 203 episodes during 1980–1991. *Scand J Infect Dis* 1993; 25:403–408.
137. Facklam RR. Physiological differentiation of viridans streptococci. *J Clin Microbiol* 1977; 5:184–201.
138. Douglas CWI, Heath J, Hampton KK, Preston FE. Identity of viridans streptococci isolated from cases of infective endocarditis. *J Med Microbiol* 1993; 39:179–182.
139. Carey RB, Gross KC, Roberts RB. Vitamin B6-dependent *Streptococcus mitor (mitis)* isolated from patients with systemic infections. *J Infect Dis* 1975; 131:722–726.
140. Rouff KL. Nutritionally variant streptococci. *Clin Microbiol Rev* 1991; 4:184–190.
141. Bouvet A, Grimont F, Grimont PAD. *Streptococcus defectivus* sp. nov. and *Streptococcus adjacens* sp. nov., nutritionally variant streptococci from human clinical specimens. *Int J Syst Bacteriol* 1989; 39:290–294.
142. Bouvet A. Human endocarditis due to nutritionally variant streptococci: *Streptococcus adjacens* and *Streptococcus defectivus. Eur Heart J* 1995; 16(suppl B):24–27.
143. Wilson WR, Wilkowske CJ, Wright AJ, et al. Treatment of streptomycin-susceptible and streptomycin-resistant enterococcal endocarditis. *Ann Intern Med* 1984; 100:816–823.
144. Moellering RC Jr, Watson BK, Kunz LJ. Endocarditis due to group D streptococci: Comparison of disease caused by *Strepto-*

coccus bovis with that produced by the enterococci. *Am J Med* 1974; 57:239–250.

145. Kupferwasser I. Clinical and morphological characteristics in *Streptococcus bovis* endocarditis: A comparison with other causative microorganisms in 177 cases. *Heart* 1998; 80(3):276–280.
146. Murray HW, Roberts RB. *Streptococcus bovis* bacteremia and underlying gastrointestinal disease. *Arch Intern Med* 1978; 138:1097–1099.
147. Klein RS, Catalano MT, Edberg SC, et al. *Streptococcus bovis* septicemia and carcinoma of the colon. *Ann Intern Med* 1979; 91:560–562.
148. Maki DG, Agger WA. Enterococcal bacteremia: Clinical features, the risk of endocarditis, and management. *Medicine* 1988; 67:248–269.
149. Murray BE. The life and times of the enterococcus. *Clin Microbiol Rev* 1990; 3:46–65.
150. Megran DW. Enterococcal endocarditis. *Clin Infect Dis* 1992; 15:63–71.
151. Eliopoulos GM. Increasing problems in the therapy of enterococcal infections. *Eur J Clin Microbiol Infect Dis* 1993; 12:409–412.
152. Frieden TR, Munsiff SS, Low DE, et al. Emergence of vancomycin-resistant enterococci in New York City. *Lancet* 1993; 342:76–79.
153. Bruyn GAW, Thompson J, Van Der Meer JWM. Pneumococcal endocarditis in adult patients. A report of five cases and review of the literature. *Q J Med* 1990; 74:33–40.
154. Aronin SI. Review of pneumococcal endocarditis in adults in the penicillin era. *Clin Infect Dis* 1998; 26(1):1341–1342.
155. Lindberg J. Pneumococcal endocarditis is not just a disease of the past: An analysis of 16 cases diagnosed in Denmark 1986–1997. *Scand J Infect Dis* 1998; 30(5):469–472.
156. Baddour LM. Infective endocarditis caused by beta-hemolytic streptococci. The Infectious Diseases Society of America's Emerging Infections Network. *Clin Infect Dis* 1998; 26(1):66–71.
157. Winterbotham A. Endocarditis caused by group A beta-hemolytic streptococcus in an infant: Case report and review. *Clin Infect Dis* 1999; 29(1):196–198.
158. Azzam ZS. Group B streptococcal tricuspid valve endocarditis: A case report and review of literature. *Int J Cardiol* 1998; 64(3):259–263.
159. Pankey GA. Acute bacterial endocarditis at the University of Minnesota Hospitals, 1939–1959. *Am Heart J* 1962; 64:583–591.
160. Roder BL. Clinical features of *Staphylococcus aureus* endocarditis: A 10-year experience in Denmark. *Arch Intern Med* 1999; 159(5):462–469.
161. Watanakunakorn C, Tan JS, Phair JP. Some salient features of *Staphylococcus aureus* endocarditis. *Am J Med* 1973; 54:473–481.
162. Bayer AS, Lam K, Gintzon L, et al. *Staphylococcus aureus* bacteremia: Clinical, serologic, and echocardiographic findings in patients with and without endocarditis. *Arch Intern Med* 1987; 147:457–462.
163. Keys TF, Hewitt WL. Endocarditis due to micrococci and *Staphylococcus epidermidis. Arch Intern Med* 1973; 132:216–220.
164. Huebner J. Coagulase-negative staphylococci: Role as pathogens. *Ann Res Med* 1999; 50:223–236.
165. Borgert SJ. Destructive native valve endocarditis caused by *Staphylococcus lugdunensis. South Med J* 1999; 92(8):812–814.
166. Karchmer AW, Archer GL, Dismukes WE. *Staphylococcus epidermidis* causing prosthetic valve endocarditis: Microbiologic and clinical observations as guides to therapy. *Ann Intern Med* 1983; 98:447–455.
167. Chen YC, Chang SC, Luh KT, Hsieh WC. *Actinobacillus actinomycetemcomitans* endocarditis: A report of four cases and review of the literature. *Q J Med* 1992; 81:871–878.
168. Geraci JE, Wilson WR. Endocarditis due to gram-negative bacteria: Report of 56 cases. *Mayo Clin Proc* 1982; 57:145–148.
169. Badley AD. Infective endocarditis caused by HACEK microorganisms. *Ann Rev Med* 1997; 48:25–33.
170. Darras-Joly C. Haemophilus endocarditis: Report of 42 cases in adults and review: Haemophilus Endocarditis Study Group. *Clin Infect Dis* 1997; 24(6):1087–1094.
171. Gould K, Ramirez-Ronda CH, Holmes RK, Sanford JP. Adherence of bacteria to heart valves *in vitro. J Clin Invest* 1975; 56:1364–1370.
172. Scheld WM, Valone JA, Sande MA. Bacterial adherence in the pathogenesis of endocarditis: Interaction of bacterial dextran, platelets, and fibrin. *J Clin Invest* 1978; 61:1394–1404.
173. Durack DT, Beeson PB. Protective role of complement in experimental *E. coli* endocarditis. *Infect Immun* 1977; 16:213–217.
174. Gutierrez RF. Endocarditis caused by *Stenotrophomas maltophilia*: Case report and review. *Clin Infect Dis* 1996; 23(6):1261–1265.
175. Al-Kasab S, Al-Fagih MR, Al-Yousef S, et al. *Brucella* infective endocarditis: Successful combined medical and surgical therapy. *J Thorac Cardiovasc Surg* 1988; 95:862–867.
176. Delvecchio G, Fracassetti O, Lorenzi N. *Brucella* endocarditis. *Int J Cardiol* 1991; 33:328–329.
177. Uddin MJ. The role of aggressive medical therapy along with early surgical intervention in the cure of *Brucella endocarditis. Ann Thorac Cardiovasc Surg.* 1998; 4 (4):209–213.
178. Felner JM, Dowell VR. Anaerobic bacterial endocarditis. *N Engl J Med* 1970; 283:1188–1192.
179. Nastro LJ, Finegold SM. Endocarditis due to anaerobic gram-negative bacilli. *Am J Med* 1973; 54:482–496.
180. Kammer RB, Utz JP. *Aspergillus* species endocarditis: The new face of a not so rare disease. *Am J Med* 1974; 56:506–521.
181. Aspesberro F. Fungal endocarditis in critically ill children. *Eur J Pediatric* 1999; 158(4):275–280.
182. Turck WPG, Howitt G, Turnberg LA, et al. Chronic Q fever. *Q J Med* 1976; 45:193–217.
183. Siegman-Igra Y. Q fever endocarditis in Israel and a worldwide review. *Scand J Infect Dis* 1997; 29(1):41–49.
184. Kimbrough RC, Ormsbee RA, Peacock M, et al. Q fever endocarditis in the United States. *Ann Intern Med* 1979; 91:400–402.
185. Spelman DW. Q fever: A study of 111 consecutive cases. *Med J Aust* 1982; 1:547–553.
186. Falconer H, Terry SI, Spencer H. Cryptococcosis in the West Indies. *West Indian Med J* 1980; 29:142.
187. Raoult D, Marrie T. State of the art clinical article: Q fever. *Clin Infect Dis* 1995; 20:489–496.
188. Raoult D, Brouqui P, Marchou B, Gastaut JA. Acute and chronic Q fever in patients with cancer. *Clin Infect Dis* 1992; 14:127–130.
189. Raoult D, Fournier PE, Drancourt M, et al. Diagnosis of 22 new cases of *Bartonella* endocarditis. *Ann Intern Med* 1996; 125:646–652.
190. La Sacola B. Culture of *Vartonella quintana* and *Bartonella henselae* from human samples: A 5-year experience (1990 to 1998). *J Clin Micorobiol* 1999; 37(6): 1899–1905.
191. Ward C, Ward AM. Acquired valvular heart disease in patients who keep pet birds. *Lancet* 1974; 734–736.
192. van der Bel-Kahn J, Watanakunakorn C, Menefee MG, et al. *Chlamydia trachomatis* endocarditis. *Am Heart J* 1978; 95:627–636.
193. Spyrou N, Anderson M, Foale R. *Listeria* endocarditis: Current management and patient outcome—world literature review. *Heart* 1997; 77(4):380–383.
194. Cohen JI, Sloss LJ, Kundsin R, Golightly L. Prosthetic valve endocarditis caused by *Mycoplasma hominis. Am J Med* 1989; 86:819–821.
195. Malinverni R, Bille J, Glauser MP. Single-dose rifampin prophylaxis for experimental endocarditis induced by high bacterial inocula of *Viridans* streptococci. *J Infect Dis* 1987; 156:151–157.
196. Cannady PB Jr, Sanford JP. Negative blood cultures in infective endocarditis: A review. *South Med J* 1976; 69:1420–1424.

197. Pesanti EL, Smith IM. Infective endocarditis with negative blood cultures: An analysis of 52 cases. *Am J Med* 1979; 66:43–50.
198. Hoen B, Selton-Suty C, Lacassin F, et al. Infective endocarditis in patients with negative blood cultures: Analysis of 88 cases from a one-year nationwide survey in France. *Clin Infect Dis* 1995; 20:501–506.
199. Libman E. The clinical features of cases of subacute bacterial endocarditis that have spontaneously become bacteria-free. *Am J Med Sci* 1913; 146:626–645.
200. Gubler JG. Whipple endocarditis without overt gastrointestinal disease: Report of four cases. *Ann Intern Med* 1999; 131:144–146.
201. Roux JP, Koussa A, Cajot MA, et al. Primary *Aspergillus* endocarditis: Apropos of a case and review of the international literature. *Ann Chir* 1992; 46:110–115.
202. Durack DT, Bright DK, Lukes AS, Duke Endocarditis Service. New criteria for diagnosis of infective endocarditis: Utilization of specific echocardiographic findings. *Am J Med* 1994; 96:200–209.
203. Cecchi E, Parrini I, Chinaglia A, et al. New diagnostic criteria for infective endocarditis. A study of sensitivity and specificity. *Eur Heart J* 1997; 18:1149–1156.
204. Angrist A, Oka M, Nakao K. Vegetative endocarditis. *Pathol Annu* 1967; 2:155–212.
205. Grant RT, Wood JE Jr, Jones TD. Heart valve irregularities in relation to subacute bacterial endocarditis. *Am Heart J* 1928; 14:247–261.
206. Durack DT. Experimental bacterial endocarditis: IV. Structure and evolution of very early lesions. *J Pathol* 1975; 115:81–89.
207. Durack DT, Beeson PB. Experimental bacterial endocarditis: I. Colonization of a sterile vegetation. *Br J Exp Pathol* 1972; 53:44–49.
208. Hojnik M, George J, Ziporen L, Shoenfeld Y. Heart valve involvement (Libman-Sacks endocarditis) in the antiphospholipid syndrome. *Circulation* 1996; 93:1579–1587.
209. Livornese LL Jr, Korzeniowski O. Pathogenesis of infective endocarditis. In: Kaye D, ed. *Infective Endocarditis,* 2d ed. New York: Raven Press; 1992:19–35.
210. Schlievert PM. Aggregation and binding substances enhance pathogenicity in rabbit models of *Enterococcus faecalis* endocarditis. *Infect Immun* 1998; 66(1):218–223.
211. Burnette-Curley D, Wells V, Viscount H, et al. FimA, a major virulence factor associated with *Streptococcus parasanguis* endocarditis. *Infect Immun* 1995; 63:4669–4674.
212. Viscount HB, Munro CL, Burnette-Curley D, et al. Immunization with FimA protects against *Streptococcus parasanguis* endocarditis in rats. *Infect Immun* 1997; 65(3):994–1002.
213. Moreillon P, Entenza JM, Francioli P, et al. Role of *Staphylococcus aureus* coagulase and clumping factor in pathogenesis of experimental endocarditis. *Infect Immun* 1995; 63:4738–4743.
214. Baddour LM, Christensen GD, Hester MG, Bisno AL. Production of experimental endocarditis by coagulase-negative staphylococci: Variability in species virulence. *J Infect Dis* 1984; 150:721–727.
215. Yeaman MR, Puentes SM, Norman DC, Bayer AS. Partial characterization and staphylocidal activity of thrombin-induced platelet microbicidal protein. *Infect Immun* 1992; 60:1202–1209.
216. Dankert J, Hess J, Durack DT. Pathogenesis of viridans streptococcal endocarditis (VSE): Disappearance of adherent streptococci from vegetations. *26th Interscience Conference on Antimicrobial Agents and Chemotherapy* (abstr). 1986.
217. Drake TA, Rogers GM, Sande MA. Tissue factor is a major stimulus for vegetation formation in enterococcal endocarditis in rabbits. *J Clin Invest* 1984; 73:1750–1753.
218. van Ginkel CJW, Thorig L, Thompson J, et al. Enhancement of generation of monocyte tissue thromboplastin by bacterial phagocytosis: Possible pathway for fibrin formation on infected vegetations in bacterial endocarditis. *Infect Immun* 1979; 25:388–395.
219. Sullam PM. Diminished platelet binding in vitro by *Staphylococcus aureus* is associated with reduced virulence in a rabbit model of infective endocarditis. *Infert Immuon* 1996; 64(12):4915–4921.
220. Drake T, Pang M. *Staphylococcus aureus* induces tissue factor expression in cultured human cardiac valve endothelium. *J Infect Dis.* 1988; 66:3476–3479.
221. Dhawan VK, Yeaman MR, Cheung AL, et al. Phenotypic resistance to thrombin-induced platelet microbiocidal protein in vitro is correlated with enhanced virulence in experimental endocarditis due to *Staphylococcus aureus. Infect Immun* 1997; 65(8):3293–3299.
222. Dhawan VK, et al. In vitro resistance to thrombin-induced platelet microbicidal protein is associated with enhanced progression and hematogenous dissemination in experimental *Staphylococcus aureus* infective endocarditis. *Infect Immun* 1998; 66(7):3476–3479.
223. Bayer AS, Ramos MD, Menzies BE, et al. Hyperproduction of alpha-toxin by *Staphylococcus aureus* results in paradoxically reduced virulence in experimental endocarditis: A host defense role for platelet microbicidal proteins. *Infect Immun* 1997; 65(11):4652–4660.
224. Korzeniowski OM, Sande MA. Personal communication.
225. Kupferwasser LI, et al. Acetylsalicylic acid reduces vegetation bacterial density, hematogenous bacterial dissemination, and frequency of embolic events in experimental *Staphylococcus aureus* endocarditis through antiplatelet and antibacterial effects. *Circulation* 1999; 99(21):2791–2797.
226. Capo C, Zugun F, Stein A, et al. Upregulation of tumor necrosis factor alpha and Interleukin-1 beta in Q fever endocarditis. *Infect Immun* 1996; 64:1638–1642.
227. Lepeschkin E. On the relation between the site of valvular involvement in endocarditis and the blood pressure resting on the valve. *Am J Med Sci* 1952; 224:318–319.
228. Rodbard S. Blood velocity and endocarditis. *Circulation* 1963; 27:18–28.
229. Edwards JE, Burchell HB. Endocardial and intimal lesions (jet impact) as possible sites of origin of murmurs. *Circulation* 1958; 18:946–960.
230. Buchbinder NA, Roberts WC. Left-sided valvular active infective endocarditis: A study of forty-five necropsy patients. *Am J Med* 1972; 53:20–35.
231. Scully RE, Mark EJ, McNeely WF, McNeely BU. Case records of the Massachusetts General Hospital. *N Engl J Med* 1996; 334:105–111.
232. McFarland MM. Pathology of infective endocarditis. In: Kaye D, ed. *Infective Endocarditis,* 2d ed. New York: Raven Press; 1992:57–83.
233. DiNubile MJ, Calderwood SB, Steinhaus DM, Karchmer AW. Cardiac conduction abnormalities complicating native valve active endocarditis. *Am J Cardiol* 1986; 58:1213–1217.
234. Phair JP, Clarke J. Immunology of infective endocarditis. *Prog Cardiovasc Dis* 1977; 22:137–144.
235. Williams RC, Kunkel HG. Rheumatoid factor, complement, and conglutinin aberrations in patients with subacute bacterial endocarditis. *J Clin Invest* 1962; 41:666–675.
236. Messner RP, Laxdal T, Quie PG, Williams RC Jr. Rheumatoid factors in subacute bacterial endocarditis—Bacterium, duration of disease or genetic predisposition? *Ann Intern Med* 1968; 68:746–754.
237. Sheagren JN, Tuazon CU, Griffin C, Padmore N. Rheumatoid factor in acute bacterial endocarditis. *Arthritis Rheum* 1976; 19:887–890.
238. Maisch B, Eichstadt H, Kochsick K. Immune reactions in infective endocarditis: I. Clinical data and diagnostic relevance of antimyocardial antibodies. *Am Heart J* 1983; 106:329–337.
239. Weinstein L, Schlesinger JJ. Pathoanatomic, pathophysiologic

and clinical correlations in endocarditis. (First of two parts.) *N Engl J Med* 1974; 291:832–837.

240. Wadsworth AB. A study of the endocardial lesions developing during pneumococcus infection in horses. *J Med Res* 1919; 34:280–291.
241. Mair W. Pneumococcal endocarditis in rabbits. *J Pathol Bacteriol* 1923; 26:426–428.
242. Durack DT, Gilliland BC, Petersdorf RG. Effect of immunization on susceptibility to experimental *Streptococcus mutans* and *Streptococcus sanguis* endocarditis. *Infect Immun* 1978; 22:52–56.
243. Durack DT, Beeson PB. Pathogenesis of infective endocarditis. In: Rahimtoola SH, ed. *Infective Endocarditis.* New York: Grune & Stratton; 1978:1–53.
244. Bayer AS, Theofilopoulos AN, Eisenberg R, et al. Circulating immune complexes in infective endocarditis. *N Engl J Med* 1976; 295:1500–1505.
245. Bayer AS, Theofilopoulos AN, Tillman DB, et al. Use of circulating immune complex levels in the serodifferentiation of endocarditic and nonendocarditic septicemias. *Am J Med* 1979; 66:58–62.
246. Maisch B, Mayer E, Schubert U, et al. Immune reactions in infective endocarditis: II. Relevance of circulating immune complexes, serum inhibition factors, lymphocytotoxic reactions, and antibody-dependent cellular cytotoxicity against cardiac target cells. *Am Heart J* 1983; 106:338–344.
247. Cabane J, Godeau P, Hereeman A, et al. Fate of circulating immune complexes in infective endocarditis. *Am J Med* 1979; 66:277–282.
248. Gutman RA, Striker GE, Gilliland BC, Cutler RE. The immune complex glomerulonephritis of bacterial endocarditis. *Medicine* 1972; 51:1–25.
249. Levy RL, Hong R. The immune nature of subacute bacterial endocarditis (SBE) nephritis. *Am J Med* 1973; 54:645–652.
250. Nagel JG, Tuazon CU, Cardella TA, Sheagren JN. Teichoic acid serologic diagnosis of staphylococcal endocarditis: Use of gel diffusion and counterimmunoelectrophoretic methods. *Ann Intern Med* 1975; 82:13–17.
251. Freedman LR, Valone J Jr. Experimental infective endocarditis. *Prog Cardiovasc Dis* 1979; 22:169–180.
252. Contrepois A. Notes on the history of experimental endocarditis. *Clin Infect Dis* 1995; 20:461–466.
253. Durack DT, Beeson PB. Experimental bacterial endocarditis: II. Survival of bacteria in endocardial vegetations. *Br J Exp Pathol* 1972; 53:50–53.
254. Durack DT. Experience with prevention of experimental endocarditis. In: Kaplan EL, Taranta AV, eds. *Infective Endocarditis: An American Heart Association Symposium.* American Heart Association Monograph No. 52. Dallas: American Heart Association, 1977:28–32.
255. Churchill MA Jr, Geraci JE, Hunder GG. Musculoskeletal manifestations of bacterial endocarditis. *Ann Intern Med* 1977; 87:754–759.
256. Starkebaum MK, Durack DT, Beeson PB. The "incubation period" of subacute bacterial endocarditis. *Yale J Biol Med* 1977; 50:49–58.
257. Karchmer AW. Staphylococcal endocarditis. In: Kaye D, ed. *Infective Endocarditis,* 2d ed. New York: Raven Press; 1992:225–249.
258. Khan MY, Hall WH, Gerding DN. Infective endocarditis in narcotic addicts. *Minn Med* 1975; 83–84.
259. Steckelberg JM, Murphy JG, Wilson WR. Cure rates and long-term prognosis. In: Kaye D, ed. *Infective Endocarditis,* 2d ed. New York: Raven Press, 1992:435–453.
260. Kilpatrick ZM, Greenberg PA, Sanford JP. Splinter hemorrhages—Their clinical significance. *Arch Intern Med* 1965; 115:730–735.
261. Howard EJ. Osler's nodes. *Am Heart J* 1960; 59:633–634.
262. Alpert JS, Krous HF, Dalen JE, et al. Pathogenesis of Osler's nodes. *Ann Intern Med* 1976; 85:471–473.
263. Edwards JE Jr, Foos RY, Montgomerie JZ, Guze LB. Ocular manifestations of *Candida* septicemia: Review of seventy-six cases of hematogenous candida endophthalmitis. *Medicine* 1974; 53:47–75.
264. Cates JE, Christie RV. Subacute bacterial endocarditis: A review of 442 patients treated in 14 centres appointed by the Penicillin Trials Committee of Medical Research Council. *Q J Med* 1951; 20:93–130.
265. Mills J, Utley J, Abbott J. Heart failure in infective endocarditis. *Chest* 1974; 66:151–159.
266. Lytle BW, Priest BP, Taylor PC, et al. Surgical treatment of prosthetic valve endocarditis. *J Thorac Cardiovasc Surg* 1996; 111:198–207.
267. Tanaka M, Abe T, Hosokawa S, et al. Tricuspid valve *Candida* endocarditis cured by valve-sparing debridement. *Ann Thorac Surg* 1989; 48:857–858.
268. Pruett TL, Rotstein OD, Anderson RW, Simmons RL. Tricuspid valve endocarditis: Successful treatment with valve-sparing debridement and antifungal chemotherapy in a multiorgan transplant recipient. *Am J Med* 1986; 80:116–118.
269. Kupferwasser LI, Hafner G, Mohr-Kahaly S, et al. The presence of infection-related antiphospholipid antibodies in infective endocarditis determines a major risk factor for embolic events. *J Am Coll Cardiol* 1999; 33(5):1365–1371.
270. Sokil AB. Cardiac imaging in infective endocarditis. In: Kaye D, ed. *Infective Endocarditis,* 2d ed. New York: Raven Press; 1992:125–150.
271. Ziment I. Nervous system complications in bacterial endocarditis. *Am J Med* 1969; 47:593–607.
272. Pruitt AA, Rubin RH, Karchmer AW, Duncan GW. Neurologic complications of bacterial endocarditis. *Medicine* 1978; 57:329–343.
273. Jones HR Jr, Siekert RG. Neurological manifestations of infective endocarditis: Review of clinical and therapeutic challenges. *Brain* 1989; 112:1295–1315.
274. Francioli P. Central nervous system complications of infective endocarditis. In: Scheld WM, Whitley RJ, Durack DT, eds. *Infections of the Central Nervous System,* 2d ed. New York: Lippincott-Raven, 1997:523–553.
275. Jones HR, Siekert RG, Geraci JE. Neurologic manifestations of bacterial endocarditis. *Ann Intern Med* 1969; 71:21–28.
276. Stengel A, Wolferth CC. Mycotic (bacterial) aneurysms of intravascular origin. *Arch Intern Med* 1923; 31:527–554.
277. Brust JCM, Dickinson PCT, Hughes JEO, Holtzman RNN. The diagnosis and treatment of cerebral mycotic aneurysms. *Ann Neurol* 1990; 27:238–246.
278. Salgado AV, Furlan AJ, Keys TF. Mycotic aneurysm, subarachnoid hemorrhage, and indications for cerebral angiography in infective endocarditis. *Stroke* 1987; 18:1057–1060.
279. Nakata Y, Shionoya S, Kamiya K. Pathogenesis of mycotic aneurysm. *Angiology* 1968; 19:593–601.
280. Masuda J, Yutani C, Waki R, et al. Histopathological analysis of the mechanisms of intracranial hemorrhage complicating infective endocarditis. *Stroke* 1992; 23:843–850.
281. Bamford J, Hodges J, Warlow C. Late rupture of a mycotic aneurysm after "cure" of bacterial endocarditis. *J Neurol* 1986; 233:51–53.
282. Bush LM, Johnson CC. Clinical syndrome and diagnosis. In: Kaye D, ed. *Infective Endocarditis,* 2d ed. New York: Raven Press; 1992:99–115.
283. Durack DT, Street AC. Fever of unknown origin—Reexamined and redefined. *Curr Clin Top Infect Dis* 1991; 11:35–51.
284. von Reyn CF, Levy BS, Arbeit RD, et al. Infective endocarditis: An analysis based on strict case definitions. *Ann Intern Med* 1981; 94:505–517.

285. Dajani AS, Ayoub E, Bierman FZ, et al. Guidelines for the diagnosis of rheumatic fever: Jones criteria, 1992 update. *JAMA* 1992; 268:2069–2073.
286. Dodds GA, Sexton DJ, Durack DT, et al. Negative predictive value of the Duke criteria for infective endocarditis. *Am J Cardiol* 1996; 77:403–407.
287. Kaye MM, Kaye D. Laboratory findings including blood cultures. In: Kaye D, ed. *Infective Endocarditis,* 2d ed. New York: Raven Press; 1992:117–124.
288. Powers DL, Mandell GL. Intraleukocytic bacteria in endocarditis patients. *JAMA* 1974; 227:312–313.
289. Engle RL, Koprowska I. The appearance of histiocytes in blood in subacute bacterial endocarditis. *Am J Med* 1959; 26:965–973.
290. Hogevik H, Olaison L, Andersson R, et al. C-reactive protein is more sensitive than erythrocyte sedimentation rate for diagnosis of infective endocarditis. *Infection* 1997; 25(2):82–85.
291. Agarwal A, Clements J, Sedmak DD, et al. Subacute bacterial endocarditis masquerading as type III essential mixed cryoglobulinemia. *J Am Soc Nephrol,* 1997; 8(12):1971–1976.
292. Fournier PE, Casalta JP, Habib G, et al. Modification of the diagnostic criteria proposed by the Duke Endocarditis Service to permit improved diagnosis of Q fever endocarditis. *Am J Med* 1996; 100:629–633.
293. Belli J, Waisbren BA. The number of blood cultures necessary to diagnose most cases of bacterial endocarditis. *Am J Med Sci* 1956; 232:284–288.
294. Werner AS, Cobbs CG, Kaye D, Hook EW. Studies on the bacteremia of bacterial endocarditis. *JAMA* 1967; 202:127–131.
295. Ellner JJ, Rosenthal MS, Lerner PI, McHenry M. Infective endocarditis caused by slow-growing, fastidious, gram-negative bacteria. *Medicine* 1979; 58:145–158.
296. Gerry JL, Greenough WB. Diphtheroid endocarditis: Report of nine cases and review of the literature. *Johns Hopkins Med J* 1976; 139:61–68.
297. Zbinden R, Hany A, Luthy R, et al. Antibody response in six HACEK endocarditis cases under therapy. *APMIS* 1998; 106(5):547–552.
298. Patel R, Newell J, Procop GW, et al. Use of polymerase chain reaction for citrate synthase gene to diagnose Bartonella quintana endocarditis. *Am J Clin Path* 1999; 112(1):36–40.
299. Goldenberger D, Kunzli A, Vogt P, et al. Molecular diagnosis of bacterial endocarditis by broad-range PCR amplification and direct sequencing. *J Clin Microbiol* 1997; 35(11):2733–2739.
300. Das I, De Giovanni JV, Gray J. Endocarditis caused by *Haemophilus parainfluenzae* identified by 16s ribosomal RNA sequencing. *J Clin Path* 1997; 50(1):72–74.
301. Stewart JA, Silimperi D, Harris P, et al. Echocardiographic documentation of vegetative lesions in infective endocarditis: Clinical implications. *Circulation* 1980; 61:374–380.
302. Mugge A, Daniel WG, Frank G, Lichtlen PR. Echocardiography in infective endocarditis: Reassessment of prognostic implications of vegetation size determined by the transthoracic and transesophageal approach. *J Am Coll Cardiol* 1989; 14:631–638.
303. Pavlides GS, Hauser AM, Stewart JR, et al. Contribution of transesophageal echocardiography to patient diagnosis and treatment: A prospective analysis. *Am Heart J* 1990; 120:910–914.
304. Daniel WG, Mugge A, Martin RP, et al. Improvement in the diagnosis of abscesses associated with endocarditis by transesophageal echocardiography. *N Engl J Med* 1991; 324:795–800.
305. Dodds GAI, Durack DT. Criteria for the diagnosis of endocarditis and the role of echocardiography. *Echocardiography* 1995; 12:663–668.
306. De Castro S, d'Amati G, Cartoni D, et al. Valvular perforation in left-sided infective endocarditis: a prospective echocardiographic evaluation and clinical outcome. *Am Heart J* 1997; 134:656–664.
307. Aly AM, Simpson PM, Humes RA. The role of transthoracic echocardiography in the diagnosis of infective endocarditis in children [in process citation]. *Arch Pediatr Adoles Med* 1999; 153:950–954.
308. Morguet AJ, Werner GS, Andreas S, Kreuzer H. Diagnostic value of transesophageal compared with transthoracic echocardiography in suspected prosthetic valve endocarditis. *Herz* 1995; 20:390–398.
309. Lengyel M. The impact of transesophageal echocardiography on the management of prosthetic valve endocarditis: Experience of 31 cases and review of the literature. *J Heart Valv Dis* 1997; 6:204–211.
310. Lindner JR, Case RA, Dent JM, et al. Diagnostic value of echocardiography in suspected endocarditis: An evaluation based on the pretest probability of disease. *Circulation* 1996; 93:730–736.
311. Fowler VG, Li J, Corey GR, et al. Role of echocardiography in evaluation of patients with *Staphylococcus aureus* bacteremia: experience in 103 patients. *J Am Coll Cardiol* 1997; 30:1072–1078.
312. Tischler MD, Vaitkus PT, et al. The ability of vegetation size on echocardiography to predict clinical complications: A meta-analysis. *J Echocardiog* 1997; 10:562–568.
313. Fowler VG, Sanders LL, Kong LK, et al. Infective endocarditis due to *Staphylococcus aureus*: 59 prospectively identified cases with follow-up. *Clin Infec Dis* 1999; 28(1):106–114.
314. Lancellotti P, Galiuto L, Albert A, et al. Relative value of clinical and transesophageal echocardiographic variables for risk stratification in patients with infective endocarditis. *Clin Cardiol* 1998; 21(8):572–578.
315. De Castro S, Magni G, Beni S, et al. Role of transthoracic and transesophageal echocardiography in predicting embolic events in patients with active infective endocarditis involving native cardiac valves. *Am J Cardiol* 1997; 80(8):1030–1034.
316. Gillinov AM, Shah RV, Curtis WE, et al. Valve replacement in patients with endocarditis and acute neurologic deficit. *Ann Thorac Surg* 1996; 61:1125–1129.
317. Moriarty JA, Edelman RR, Tumeh SS. CT and MRI of mycotic aneurysms of the abdominal aorta. *J Comput Assist Tomogr* 1992; 16:941–943.
318. Welton DE, Young JB, Raizner AE, et al. Value and safety of cardiac catheterization during active infective endocarditis. *Am J Cardiol* 1979; 44:1306–1310.
319. Riba AL, Thakur ML, Gottschalk A, et al. Imaging experimental infective endocarditis with indium-111–labeled blood cellular components. *Circulation* 1979; 59:336–343.
320. Campeau RJ, Ingram C. Perivalvular abscess complicating infective endocarditis: Complementary role of echocardiography and Indium-111–Labeled leukocytes. *J Clin Nucl Med* 1998; 23:582–584.
321. Ben-Haim S, Seabold JE, Hawes DR, Rooholamini SA. Leukocyte scintigraphy in the diagnosis of mycotic aneurysm. *J Nuc Med* 1992; 33:1486–1493.
322. Olaison L, Belin L, Hogevik H, et al. Incidence of beta-lactam-induced delayed hypersensitivity and neutropenia during treatment of infective endocarditis. *Arch Intern Med* 1999; 159(6):607–615.
323. Wilson WR, Karchmer A, Dajani A, et al. Antibiotic treatment of adults with infective endocarditis due to viridans streptococci, enterococci, staphylococci and HACEK microorganisms. *JAMA* 1995; 274:1706–1713.
324. Chambers HF, Miller RT, Newman MD. Right-sided Staphylococcus aureus endocarditis in intravenous drug abusers: Two-week combination therapy. *Ann Intern Med* 1988; 109:619–624.
325. Wilson WR, Geraci JE, Wilkowske CJ, Washington JA. Short-term intramuscular therapy with procaine penicillin plus streptomycin for infective endocarditis due to *Viridans* streptococci. *Circulation* 1978; 57:1158–1161.
326. Baldassare JS, Kaye D. Principles and overview of antibiotic therapy. In: Kaye D, ed. *Infective Endocarditis*. 2d ed. New York: Raven Press; 1992:169–190.

327. Blount JG. Bacterial endocarditis. *Am J Med* 1965; 38:909–922.
328. Pulliam L, Inokuchi S, Hadley WK, Mills J. Penicillin tolerance in experimental streptococcal endocarditis. *Lancet* 1979; 2:957.
329. Denny AE, Peterson LR, Gerding DN, Hall WH. Serious staphylococcal infections with strains tolerant to bactericidal antibiotics. *Arch Intern Med* 1979; 139:1026–1031.
330. Brennan RO, Durack DT. Therapeutic significance of penicillin tolerance in experimental streptococcal endocarditis. *Antimicrob Agents Chemother* 1983; 23:273–277.
331. Reller LB. The serum bactericidal test. *Rev Infect Dis* 1986; 8:803–808.
332. MacGowan A, McMullin C, James P, et al. External quality assessment of the serum bactericidal test: Results of a methodology/interpretation questionnaire. *J Antimicrob Chemother* 1997; 39(2):277–284.
333. Kane LW, Finn JJ. The treatment of subacute bacterial endocarditis with aureomycin and chloromycetin. *N Engl J Med* 1951; 244:623–628.
334. Schein J, Baehr G. Sulfonamide therapy of subacute bacterial endocarditis. *Am J Med* 1948; 4:66–72.
335. Korzeniowski O, Sande MA, National Collaborative Endocarditis Study Group. Combination antimicrobial therapy for *Staphylococcus aureus* endocarditis in patients addicted to parenteral drugs and in nonaddicts: A prospective study. *Ann Intern Med* 1982; 97:496–503.
336. Martinez F, Martin-Luengo F, Garcia A, Valdes M. Treatment with various antibiotics of experimental endocarditis caused by penicillin-resistant *Streptococcus sanguis*. *Eur Heart J* 1995; 16:687–691.
337. Doern GV, Ferraro MJ, Brueggmann AB, Ruoff KL. Emergence of high rates of antimicrobial resistance among viridans group streptococci in the United States. *Antimicrob Agents Chemother* 1996; 40:891–894.
338. Johnson AP, Warner M, Woodford N, et al. Antibiotic resistance among enterococci causing endocarditis in the UK: Analysis of isolates referred to a reference laboratory. *Br Med J* 1998; 317:629–630.
339. Brandt CM, Rouse MS, Laue NW, et al. Effective treatment of multidrug-resistant enterococcal experimental endocarditis with combinations of cell wall-active agents. *J Infect Dis* 1996; 173:909–913.
340. Antony SJ, Ladner J, Stratton CW, et al. High-level aminoglycoside-resistant enterococcus causing endocarditis successfully treated with a combination of ampicillin, imipenem and vancomycin. *Scand J Infec Dis* 1997; 29(6):628–630.
341. Tripodi MF, Locatelli A, Adinolfi LE, et al. Successful treatment with ampicillin and fluoroquinolones of human endocarditis due to high-level gentamicin-resistant enterococci. *Eur J Clin Microbiol Infect Dis* 1998; 17(10):734–736.
342. Matsumura S, Simor AE. Treatment of endocarditis due to vancomycin-resistant Enterococcus faecium with quinupristin/dalfopristin, doxycycline, and rifampin: A synergistic drug combination. *Clin Infect Dis* 1998; 27(6):1554–1556.
343. Landman D, Quale JM; Management of infections due to resistant enterococci: A review of therapeutic options. *J Antimicrob Chemother* 1997; 40(2):161–170.
344. Francioli P, Etienne J, Hoigne R, et al. Treatment of streptococcal endocarditis with a single daily dose of ceftriaxone sodium for 4 weeks: Efficacy and outpatient treatment feasibility. *JAMA* 1992; 267:264–267.
345. Stamboulian D, Bonvehi P, Arevalo C, et al. Antibiotic management of outpatients with endocarditis due to penicillin-susceptible streptococci. *Rev Infect Dis* 1991; 13:S160–S163.
346. Rehm SJ. Outpatient intravenous antibiotic therapy for endocarditis. *Infect Dis Clin N Am* 1998; 12(4):879–901.
347. Aranki SF, Adams DH, Rizzo RJ, et al. Determinants of early mortality and late survival in mitral valve endocarditis. *Circulation* 1995; 92:143–149.
348. Douglas JL, Dismukes WE. Surgical therapy of infective endocarditis on natural valves. In: Kaye D, ed. *Infective Endocarditis*, 2d ed. New York: Raven Press; 1992:397–411.
349. Durack DT. Nine controversies in the management of endocarditis. In: Petersdorf RG, ed. *Update V: Harrison's Principles of Internal Medicine*. New York: McGraw-Hill; 1984:35–45.
350. Vlessis AA, Hovaguimian H, Jaggers J, et al. Infective endocarditis: Ten year review of medical and surgical therapy. *Ann Thorac Surg* 1996; 61:1217–1222.
351. Muehrcke D, Lytle BW, Cosgrove DM III. Surgical and long-term antifungal therapy for fungal prosthetic valve endocarditis. *Ann Thorac Surg* 1996; 60:538–543.
352. Glazier JJ, Verwilghen J, Donaldson RM, Ross DN. Treatment of complicated prosthetic aortic valve endocarditis with annular abscess formation by homograft aortic root replacement. *J Am Coll Cardiol* 1991; 17:1177–1182.
353. Joyce F, Tingleff J, Pettersson G. Expanding indications for the Ross operation. *J Heart Valve Dis* 1995; 4:352–363.
354. Joyce F, Tingleff J, Pettersson G. The Ross operation: Results of early experience including treatment for endocarditis. *Eur J Cardiothorac Surg* 1989; 9:384–392.
355. Hughes CF, Noble N. Vegetectomy: An alternative surgical treatment for infective endocarditis of the atrioventricular valves in drug addicts. *J Thorac Cardiovasc Surg* 1988; 95:857–861.
356. Katz LN, Elek SR. Combined heparin and chemotherapy in subacute bacterial endocarditis. *JAMA* 1944; 124:149–152.
357. Wilson WR, Geraci JE, Danielson GK, et al. Anticoagulant therapy and central nervous system complications in patients with prosthetic valve endocarditis. *Circulation* 1978; 57:1004–1007.
358. Kanis JA. The use of anticoagulants in bacterial endocarditis. *Postgrad Med J* 1974; 50:312–313.
359. Tornos P, Almirante B, Mirabet S, et al. Infective endocarditis due to Staphylococcus aureus: Deleterious effect of anticoagulant therapy. *Arch Intern Med* 1999; 159(5):473–475.
360. Nicolau DP, Marangos MN, Nightingale CH, Quintiliani R. Influence of aspirin on development and treatment of experimental *Staphylococcus aureus* endocarditis. *Antimicrob Agents Chemother* 1995; 39:1748–1751.
361. Steckelberg JM, Murphy JG, Ballard D, et al. Emboli in infective endocarditis: The prognostic value of echocardiography. *Ann Intern Med* 1991; 114:635–640.
362. Conlon PJ, Jefferies F, Krigman HR, et al. Predictors of prognosis and risk of acute renal failure in bacterial endocarditis. *Clin Neph* 1998; 49(2):96–101.
363. Ahern H. Cellular responses to oxidative stress: Extensively studied bacterial systems provide insights into more complex systems and, potentially, human diseases. *ASM News* 1991; 57:627–630.
364. Lu VL, Fang GD, Keys TF, et al. Prosthetic valve endocarditis: Superiority of surgical valve replacement versus medical therapy only. *Ann Thorac Surg* 1994; 58:1073–1077.
365. Ormiston JA, Neutze JM, Agnew TM, et al. Infective endocarditis: A lethal disease. *Aust NZ J Med* 1981; 11:620–629.
366. Welton DE, Young JB, Gentry WO, et al. Recurrent infective endocarditis: Analysis of predisposing factors and clinical features. *Am J Med* 1979; 66:932–938.
367. Everett ED, Hirschmann JV. Transient bacteremia and endocarditis prophylaxis: A review. *Medicine* 1977; 56:61–77.
368. Sullivan NM, Sutter VL, Mims MM, et al. Clinical aspects of bacteremia after manipulation of the genitourinary tract. *J Infect Dis* 1973; 127:49–55.
369. Shorvon PJ, Eykyn SJ, Cotton PB. Gastrointestinal instrumentation, bacteraemia, and endocarditis. *Gut* 1983; 24:1078–1093.
370. Durack DT. Prevention of infective endocarditis. *N Engl J Med* 1995; 332:38–44.
371. Dajani AS, Taubert KA, Wilson WR, et al. Prevention of bacterial

endocarditis: Recommendations by the American Heart Association. *Circulation* 1997; 96:358–366. (*JAMA* 1997; 277:1794–1801)
372. Glauser MP, Francioli P. Relevance of animal models to the prophylaxis of infective endocarditis. *J Antimicrob Chemother* 1987; 20(suppl A):87–93.
373. Horstkotte D, Friedrichs W, Pippert H, Bircks W, Loogen F. Nutzen der Endokarditisprophylaxe bei Patienten mit prothetischen Herzklappen. *Z Kardiol* 1986; 75:8–11.
374. van der Meer JTM, Van Wijk W, Thompson J, et al. Efficacy of antibiotic prophylaxis for prevention of native-valve endocarditis. *Lancet* 1992; 339:135–140.
375. Imperiale TF, Horwitz RI. Does prophylaxis prevent postdental infective endocarditis? A controlled evaluation of protective efficacy. *Am J Med* 1990; 88:131–136.
376. Gould IM, Buckingham JK. Cost effectiveness of prophylaxis in dental practice to prevent infective endocarditis. *Br Heart J* 1993; 70:79–83.

P A R T   T H I R T E E N

THE HEART, ANESTHESIA, AND SURGERY

CHAPTER 74

PERIOPERATIVE EVALUATION AND MANAGEMENT OF PATIENTS WITH KNOWN OR SUSPECTED CARDIOVASCULAR DISEASE WHO UNDERGO NONCARDIAC SURGERY

David S. Bach / Kim A. Eagle

Each year in the United States, approximately 25 million patients undergo noncardiac surgery. Of these, approximately 50,000 patients suffer perioperative myocardial infarction, and more than half of 40,000 perioperative deaths are caused by cardiac events.[1-3] As the population of the United States continues to age over the next several decades, both the total number and the percentage of patients who are over 65 years of age will increase. These patients represent the largest group in whom surgeries are performed, a group in whom approximately a quarter of surgeries are associated with significant risk of cardiac morbidity and death, and a group at increased risk for the presence of cardiac disease. As such, an increasing number of patients with significant perioperative risk can be expected to undergo noncardiac surgery.

Most perioperative cardiac morbidity and deaths are related to myocardial ischemia, congestive heart failure, or arrhythmia. Therefore, preoperative evaluation and perioperative management to reduce morbidity and mortality rates emphasize the detection, characterization, and treatment of coronary artery disease, left ventricular systolic dysfunction, and significant arrhythmias. However, not all patients with underlying cardiac disease are at significantly increased perioperative risk of a morbid cardiac event. The goals of preoperative evaluation are therefore twofold: first, to identify patients at increased risk of an adverse perioperative cardiac event and, second, to identify patients with a poor long-term prognosis due to cardiovascular disease who come to medical attention only because of other disease leading to noncardiac surgery. In this sense, the preoperative evaluation represents an opportunity to identify and treat patients, thereby affecting long-term prognosis, even though their risk at the time of noncardiac surgery may not be prohibitive.

Preoperative evaluation can identify many patients at increased risk of an adverse cardiac event, and perioperative management can affect that risk. The internist and cardiologist, therefore, play a vital role in the evaluation and management of patients before and during noncardiac surgery. This chapter reviews available data and recommendations for the preoperative evaluation and perioperative management of patients with known or suspected cardiovascular disease undergoing noncardiac surgery. However, the nature of preoperative evaluation and perioperative management should be individualized to the patient and the clinical scenario surrounding surgery. Patients presenting with an acute surgical emergency mandate only a rapid preoperative assessment, with subsequent management directed at preventing or minimizing cardiac morbidity and death. Among such patients, a more thorough evaluation can often be performed after surgery. In contrast, patients undergoing an elective procedure with no surgical urgency can undergo a more thorough preoperative evaluation. Among patients presenting for cardiac evaluation prior to "same-day" elective surgery, perioperative risk to the patient must be weighed against the impact of additional testing and cancellation or delay of the surgical procedure.

CLINICAL DETERMINANTS OF PERIOPERATIVE CARDIOVASCULAR RISK

The majority of patients at increased risk of adverse perioperative cardiac events can be identified using simple, clinically assessable features. Specifically, a careful history, physical examination, and review of the resting 12-lead electrocardiogram (ECG) are usually sufficient to allow stratification of most patients into low, intermediate, or high risk for an adverse perioperative cardiac event. A number of investigators have established readily accessible clinical markers that predict increased perioperative risk of myocardial infarction, congestive heart failure, or death.[4–14] Some investigators have used a quantitative scoring system to rank the importance of individual risk factors.[4,12,14] The advantage of such systems rest with the observation that some clinical features are stronger predictors of perioperative risk than are others. At the time of this writing, current recommendations of the American College of Cardiology (ACC) and the American Heart Association (AHA)[15] designate risks factors as belonging to three groups: major, intermediate, and minor (Table 74-1). Using these guidelines, greater weight is given for active than for quiescent disease, and the severity of disease is used to modify its importance.

TABLE 74-1 Clinical Predictors of Increased Perioperative Cardiovascular Risk (Myocardial Infarction, Congestive Heart Failure, Death)

Clinical predictors
MAJOR
Unstable coronary syndromes
Recent myocardial infarction[a] with evidence of important ischemic risk by clinical symptoms or noninvasive study
Unstable or severe[b] angina (Canadian class III or IV)[c]
Decompensated congestive heart failure
Significant arrhythmias
High-grade atrioventricular block
Symptomatic ventricular arrhythmias in the presence of underlying heart disease
Supraventricular arrhythmias with uncontrolled ventricular rate
Severe valvular disease
INTERMEDIATE
Mild angina pectoris (Canadian class I or II)
Prior myocardial infarction by history or pathologic Q waves
Compensated or prior congestive heart failure
Diabetes mellitus
MINOR
Advanced age
Abnormal electrocardiogram (left ventricular hypertrophy, left bundle-branch block, ST-T abnormalities)
Rhythm other than sinus (e.g., atrial fibrillation)
Low functional capacity (e.g., inability to climb one flight of stairs with a bag of groceries)
History of stroke
Uncontrolled systemic hypertension

[a]The American College of Cardiology National Database Library defines recent MI as >7 days but ≤1 month (30 days).
[b]May include "stable" angina in patients who are unusually sedentary.
[c]Campeau L. Grading of angina pectoris. *Circulation* 1976:54:522–523

History

Historical features are important in the identification of patients at increased perioperative cardiac risk. Because most perioperative morbidity and deaths are related to myocardial ischemia, congestive heart failure, and arrhythmias, the assessment of historical risk factors relies heavily on the recognition of coronary artery disease, left ventricular dysfunction, and significant arrhythmias. Risk factors recognized as predictive of increased perioperative risk[15] include advanced age, poor functional capacity, and prior history of coronary artery disease, congestive heart failure, arrhythmia, valvular heart disease, diabetes mellitus, uncontrolled systemic hypertension, and stroke. Coronary artery disease is a major risk factor in the setting of recent myocardial infarction or unstable or severe angina pectoris, and an intermediate risk factor in the setting of mild stable angina pectoris or remote myocardial infarction. Similarly, congestive heart failure is a major risk factor if decompensated and an intermediate risk factor if compensated. A history of arrhythmias may be a major, intermediate, or minor risk factor, depending on the nature and severity of the arrhythmia as well as the presence of underlying heart disease.

A patient's preoperative functional capacity significantly influences the assessment of perioperative cardiac risk. Good functional capacity in an asymptomatic patient predicts low perioperative risk despite the presence of other risk factors. Impaired functional capacity is important in three regards in the assessment of perioperative cardiac risk. First, among patients with chronic coronary artery disease and among those following an acute cardiac event, poor functional capacity is associated with an increased risk of subsequent cardiac morbidity and death.[16] Second, many of the historical features that predict increased perioperative risk assume physical activity. Because most symptoms of cardiac disease are either associated exclusively with or exacerbated by increased physical activity, significant noncardiac limitations in physical capacity are associated with inherent problems in the ability to detect symptoms of and thereby diagnose underlying cardiac diseases. Finally, poor functional capacity is associated with impaired conditioning and therefore a lesser ability to accommodate the cardiovascular stresses that may accompany noncardiac surgery. Because the ability to perform tasks in daily activities correlates well with maximal oxygen uptake on treadmill testing, the assessment of functional capacity on preoperative history is an important feature in the assessment of perioperative risk.

Physical Examination

Features on physical examination may be useful in assessment of perioperative risk. Patients with uncontrolled systemic hypertension should be identified and treated. Because congestive heart failure[4,15,17] and valvular heart disease[4,15,17] are associated with increased risk, physical findings suggestive of these diagnoses should be sought. Elevated jugular venous pressure, pulmonary rales, positive hepatojugular reflux, or a third heart sound on physical examination identify patients with hypervolemia. Patients with aortic stenosis can be identified by a typical murmur with diminished and delayed upstroke of the carotid or brachial pulse. Other cardiac murmurs on physical examination may help identify patients with other forms of valvular heart disease. Patients with mitral stenosis, mitral regurgitation, or aortic regurgitation may be at increased perioperative risk of developing congestive heart failure in the setting of sufficiently severe disease, as well as increased risk of infective endocarditis. Finally, the presence of carotid or other vascular bruits helps identify patients at increased risk of occult coronary artery disease.

Comorbid Diseases

A patient's overall health affects perioperative cardiovascular risk; associated medical conditions may exacerbate risk or complicate perioperative cardiac management. Patients with diabetes mellitus have an increased risk of concomitant coronary artery disease, and the possibility of silent ischemia complicates both the preoperative recognition of coronary artery disease and the perioperative recognition of ischemia. Patients with either restrictive or obstructive pulmonary disease are at increased risk of perioperative respiratory complications, and the associated hypoxemia, hypercapnea, acidosis, and increased work of breathing can exacerbate cardiac stress and precipitate myocardial ischemia. Patients with preexisting renal dysfunction may be predisposed to volume retention in the perioperative period, and hypovolemia may lead to renal hypoperfusion and thereby exacerbate renal dysfunction. Patients with anemia of any cause are at increased risk of myocardial ischemia and congestive heart failure, mediated by increased cardiac stress and increased cardiac work. Optimization of management and control of noncardiac conditions may therefore reduce the risk of cardiac morbidity in the perioperative period.

Surgery-Specific Risks

Perioperative cardiac risk is related in two ways to the type of noncardiac surgery being performed. First, some types of noncardiac surgery identify a group of patients at increased risk for concomitant cardiac disease based on shared risk factors that predispose patients for both noncardiac and cardiac disease. The most notable example of this relationship is seen with peripheral vascular surgery and coronary artery disease. In this case, the same factors that result in clinical peripheral arterial occlusive disease also predispose to the development of coronary artery disease. Among such patients, coronary artery disease may be known or occult, with no symptoms because of the physical limitations associated with surgical peripheral vascular disease. Second, the nature of noncardiac surgery is such that different types of surgery are associated with variable degrees of cardiac stress, mediated by fluctuations in heart rate, blood pressure, intravascular volume, and oxygenation as well as the cardiac stresses associated with duration of the procedure, pain, and neurohumeral activation.[4,5,11,12,18–21] Emergency procedures are associated with a two- to fivefold increase in perioperative cardiac risk compared with elective procedures.[1,17] Other types of noncardiac surgery associated with high perioperative risk include aortic and peripheral vascular surgery, and prolonged abdominal, thoracic, or head and neck procedures with large fluid shifts. The ACC/AHA Task Force Report on Perioperative Cardiac Evaluation[15] stratifies noncardiac surgical procedures as high, intermediate, and low cardiac risk (Table 74-2).

TABLE 74-2 Cardiac Risk[a] Stratification For Noncardiac Surgical Procedures

High (Reported Cardiac Risk Often >5%)
Emergent major operations, particularly in the elderly
Aortic and other major vascular
Peripheral vascular
Anticipated prolonged surgical procedures associated with large fluid shifts and/or blood loss
Intermediate (Reported Cardiac Risk Generally <5%)
Carotid endarterectomy
Head and neck
Intraperitoneal and intrathoracic
Orthopedic
Prostate
Low[b] (Reported Cardiac Risk Generally <1%)
Endoscopic procedures
Superficial procedure
Cataract
Breast

[a] Combined incidence of cardiac death and nonfatal myocardial infarction.
[b] Do not generally require further preoperative cardiac testing.
Source: Eagle et al.,[15] with permission.

The perioperative administration of anesthesia can affect the physiology of cardiac function and therefore may affect perioperative cardiac risk. Although there is no one best myocardial protective anesthetic technique,[22–26] differences in anesthetic techniques may favor the use of one over another for individual patients. Opioid-based general anesthesia generally does not affect cardiovascular function, although the commonly employed inhalational agents cause afterload reduction and decreased myocardial contractility. Spinal anesthesia results in sympathetic blockade, with decreases in both preload and afterload and the potential for shifts in both systemic blood pressure and intravascular volume. In general, hemodynamic affects are minimal when spinal anesthesia is used for infrainguinal procedures, whereas higher dermatomal levels of spinal anesthesia required for abdominal procedures may be associated with significant hemodynamic affects, including hypotension and reflex tachycardia. No study has clearly demonstrated any beneficial change in outcome from the use of pulmonary artery catheters, ST-segment monitoring, or transesophageal echocardiography. Decisions regarding specific anesthetic technique and intraoperative monitoring are therefore best left to the anesthesiologists involved in the patient's care.

Clinical Assessment of Perioperative Risk

Patients at very low risk and those at high risk of an adverse perioperative cardiac event typically can be identified using clinically available features described above. Patients at low risk generally require no additional testing prior to noncardiac surgery. Among patients undergoing elective noncardiac sur-

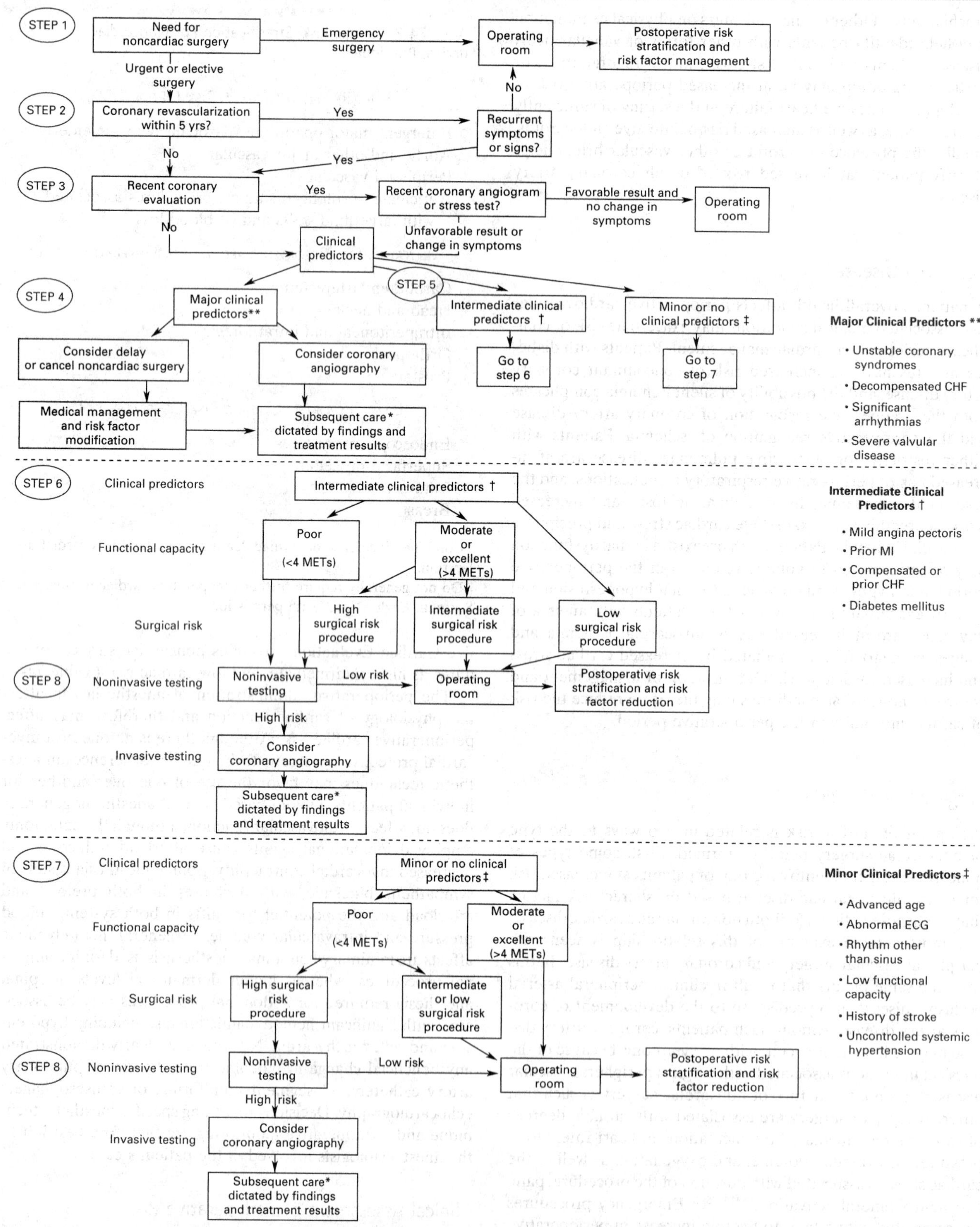

FIGURE 74-1 Stepwise approach to preoperative cardiac assessment. (From Eagle et al.[15] Reproduced with permission from the publisher and authors.)

*Subsequent care may include cancellation or delay of surgery, coronary revascularization followed by noncardiac surgery, or intensified care.

gery in whom risk is determined to be intermediate or high, additional testing may be useful to better define risk.[15] It is useful to employ a stepwise approach to the preoperative assessment of cardiac risk (Fig. 74-1). Using this algorithm, the evaluating clinician first determines the urgency of noncardiac surgery. Then, a history of recent coronary revascularization or recent cardiac testing; clinical features, including the presence of major, intermediate, or minor risk factors; estimation of functional capacity; and the nature of the planned surgical procedure are used to determine whether additional testing may be helpful in further defining perioperative cardiac risk. Such testing may include coronary angiography or noninvasive testing to assess for the presence and significance of coronary artery disease.

PREOPERATIVE TESTING

Factors identifiable on history and physical examination and features inherent to a specific noncardiac surgical procedure are usually sufficient to identify patients at very low or at high risk of morbid perioperative cardiac events. Additional testing is useful to better stratify patients with intermediate cardiac risk and to help guide perioperative management in patients at high risk.

Resting Left Ventricular Function

Impaired left ventricular systolic or diastolic function is predictive of perioperative congestive heart failure. The greatest risk of complications occurs among patients with left ventricular ejection fraction of less than 35 percent; among critically ill patients, severely impaired left ventricular systolic function is associated with a higher risk of death. Preoperative left ventricular systolic function can be assessed noninvasively using radionuclide ventriculography or echocardiography, or invasively using contrast ventriculography. Unless recently defined, preoperative assessment of left ventricular systolic function should be performed among patients with poorly controlled congestive heart failure and should be considered among patients with prior congestive heart failure and among patients with dyspnea of unknown cause.

Functional Testing and Risk of Coronary Artery Disease

EXERCISE TESTING

Preoperative cardiac stress testing is useful in the objective assessment of functional capacity, to help identify patients at risk of perioperative myocardial ischemia or cardiac arrhythmias, and to aid in the assessment of long-term as well as perioperative prognosis. In general, poor functional capacity may be due to advanced age, deconditioning, myocardial ischemia or other causes of reduced cardiac reserve, or poor pulmonary reserve. Reduced functional capacity identifies patients at increased risk of subsequent cardiac morbidity and death.[16] Clinical history can be used to estimate functional capacity. In addition, preoperative exercise testing is a useful tool to objectively assess functional capacity as well as to assess hemodynamic response to stress and the potential for stress-induced myocardial ischemia or cardiac arrhythmias.

In a general population, the mean sensitivity and specificity of exercise electrocardiographic studies for the detection of coronary artery disease are 68 and 77 percent, respectively, with reported ranges of sensitivity from 23 to 100 percent and specificity from 17 to 100 percent.[27] The accuracy of exercise electrocardiographic studies for the detection of coronary artery disease is influenced by the prevalence of disease in the population studied, the degree of exercise achieved, and the number, location, and severity of diseased vessels. The mean sensitivity and specificity for the detection of multivessel disease is 81 and 66 percent, respectively.[28] In addition to assessment for the presence of coronary artery disease, exercise testing is useful for the assessment of prognosis. In a large cohort of 4083 medically treated patients in the Coronary Artery Surgery Study,[29] exercise testing was useful for identifying both high-risk and low-risk subgroups of patients. The mortality rate was 5 percent per year or more among a high-risk subset comprising 12 percent of the total population, who were able to achieve an exercise work load less than Bruce stage I and had an abnormal exercise electrocardiogram. In contrast, mortality was less than 1 percent per year among a low-risk subset comprising 34 percent of the total population, who were able to achieve at least Bruce stage III with a normal exercise electrocardiogram. Preoperative exercise testing has been shown to be useful in the prediction of perioperative cardiac risk among patients undergoing peripheral vascular surgery, abdominal aortic aneurysm repair, or other major noncardiac surgery.[30–40] In these published reports, the negative predictive value for perioperative death or myocardial infarction was 91 to 100 percent, with a positive predictive value of 0 to 81 percent.

NONEXERCISE STRESS TESTING

The ability to perform exercise testing for the assessment of coronary artery disease is limited among many patients undergoing preoperative evaluation for noncardiac surgery. Approximately 30 to 50 percent of patients undergoing noncardiac surgery are unable to achieve an adequate exercise work load for a diagnostic study. This is especially problematic among patients with peripheral vascular occlusive disease, in whom the same factors that cause peripheral disease predispose to coronary atherosclerosis; the surgical peripheral vascular disease severely limits exercise tolerance and therefore the ability to perform diagnostic exercise stress testing. For this reason, pharmacologic stress testing may offer advantages in the preoperative testing of some patients undergoing peripheral vascular surgery as well as other patients who are not able to perform adequate physical exercise due to noncardiac limitations in exercise or functional capacity.

Pharmacologic stress testing for the detection of coronary artery disease can be performed using one of two general methods. Infusion of the adrenergic agonist dobutamine results in increases in heart rate, myocardial contractility, and, to a lesser degree, blood pressure, resulting in increased myocardial oxygen demand. In the setting of a limited oxygen supply, increased demand causes myocardial ischemia. Dobutamine infusion is typically used in conjunction with echocardiographic imaging, whereby inducible ischemia is detected as a regional abnormality in left ventricular wall motion. Alternatively, pharmacological "stress" can be achieved using the coronary vasodilators dipyridamole or adenosine. Nuclear perfusion imaging, such as thallium scintigraphic imaging, is typically used in conjunction with dipyridamole and adenosine. Coronary artery disease is detected as abnormal coronary vasodilator reserve, with heterogeneity of perfusion in response to maximal coronary vasodilation.

Dipyridamole thallium scintigraphy has been extensively studied for the assessment of coronary artery disease and perioperative risk among patients undergoing vascular[11,41–56] and other noncardiac surgery.[57–62] Reports published between 1985 and 1994 found a uniformly high negative predictive value for perioperative morbidity associated with normal dipyridamole thallium scintigraphic results, with values ranging from 95 to 100 percent and an average value of approximately 99 percent. The positive predictive value of dipyridamole thallium redistribution for myocardial infarction or death from cardiac causes has been reported to be from 4 to 20 percent among studies including more than 100 patients. More recent studies have lower positive predictive values. However, this probably reflects changes in clinical practice, with alterations in clinical management made in response to the results of an abnormal scan leading to fewer total perioperative cardiac events. There is also important long-term prognostic value associated with preoperative nuclear perfusion imaging,[46,50,63] suggesting that late postoperative risk after uncomplicated noncardiac surgery can also be predicted by preoperative testing.

Although any abnormality on dipyridamole thallium scintigraphy is suggestive of coronary artery disease and is associated with a higher perioperative cardiac risk compared with patients with a normal scan, perioperative cardiac risk associated with a fixed perfusion defect is substantially lower than that associated with perfusion redistribution. In addition, the size of a perfusion defect is directly related to perioperative cardiac risk.[50,51,53] As such, the ability to predict perioperative cardiac risk is improved with the quantification of abnormalities on nuclear perfusion imaging.

Dobutamine stress echocardiography is well established for the noninvasive detection and characterization of coronary artery disease,[64–69] with an accuracy equivalent to that of dipyridamole thallium scintigraphy. Because the technique has evolved more recently than nuclear perfusion imaging, there are fewer studies that evaluate its utility in the assessment of perioperative cardiac risk. However, six studies published since 1991 have evaluated the utility of dobutamine stress echocardiography for preoperative assessment of patients undergoing vascular or other noncardiac surgery.[70–75] Negative predictive values for perioperative events ranged from 93 to 100 percent. Positive predictive values were 17 to 43 percent for any cardiac event and 7 to 23 percent for predicting myocardial infarction or death. As was seen with later studies using nuclear perfusion imaging, most studies of dobutamine stress echocardiography did not blind treating physicians to stress test results, and subsequent alteration of patient management based on abnormal noninvasive test results presumably contributed to a low event rate despite a positive test result. A meta-analysis of preoperative pharmacologic stress tests[76] demonstrated similar power of

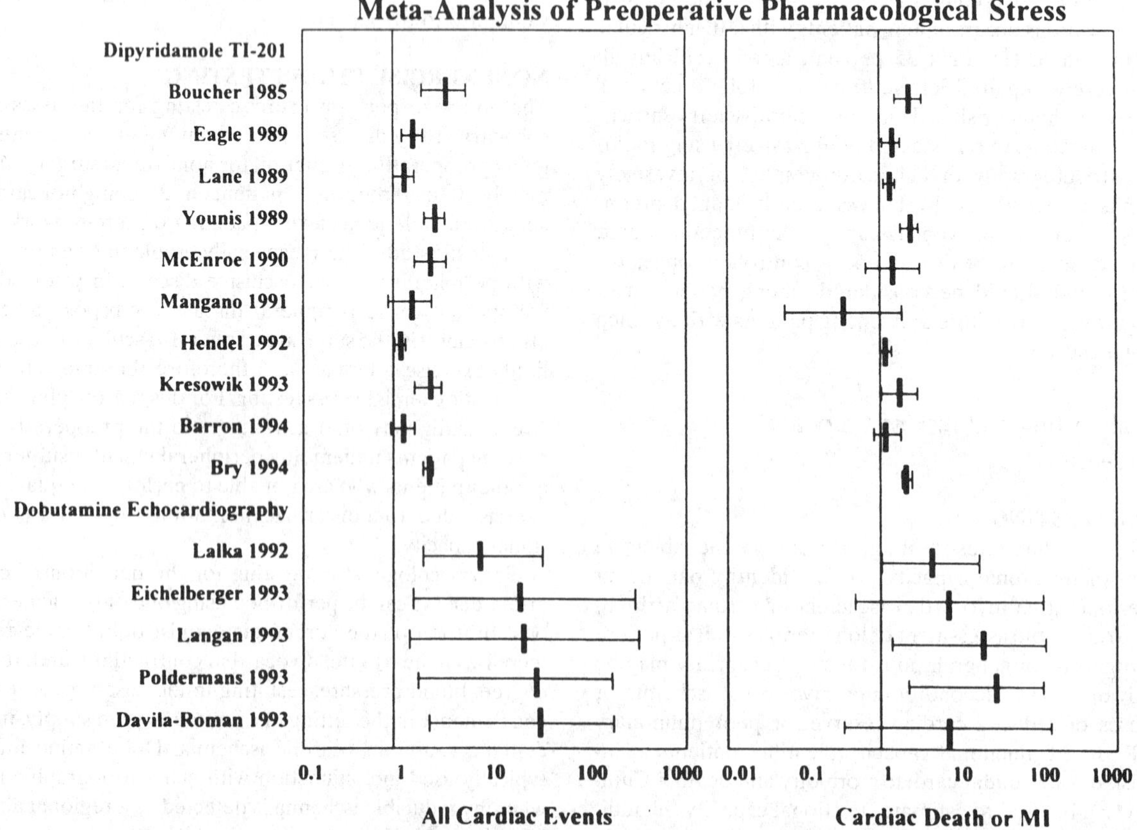

FIGURE 74-2 Univariate odds ratio for intravenous dipyridamole thallium 201 (Tl-201) myocardial perfusion and dobutamine stress echocardiography imaging. The odds ratio for any myocardial ischemic event is depicted on the left and that for cardiac death or nonfatal myocardial infarction on the right. (From Shaw et al.[76] Reproduced with permission from the publisher.)

dobutamine stress echocardiography and dipyridamole thallium scintigraphy in predicting adverse cardiac events after noncardiac surgery (Fig. 74-2).

Because clinical factors are usually able to identify patients at low or at high risk of an adverse cardiac event after noncardiac surgery,[15,21] preoperative stress testing typically has the greatest utility among patients at intermediate risk. Exercise electrocardiographic study allows assessment of functional capacity as well as evaluation for evidence of coronary artery disease based on ST-segment analysis and hemodynamics. Performance of exercise echocardiographic testing or exercise nuclear perfusion imaging should be considered in the presence of significant resting ECG abnormalities that preclude diagnostic testing for coronary artery disease, such as left bundle-branch block, left ventricular hypertrophy with strain, or digitalis effect. Nonexercise stress testing, such as dobutamine stress echocardiographic or dipyridamole thallium scintigraphic studies, should be considered among patients who are unable to perform adequate physical exercise.

FINANCIAL IMPLICATIONS OF NONINVASIVE TESTING

The performance of preoperative noninvasive testing should be based on an assessment of risk and benefit to the patient. In this setting, benefit is defined as the likelihood that testing may alter management and improve outcome because of an adverse perioperative or long-term prognosis. Risk to the patient should include risk associated with additional procedures precipitated by noninvasive testing as well as any risk associated with the noninvasive testing. Although the cost of testing should not play a determining role in the decision, cost must be considered in the present health care environment.

As noted above, clinical features can be used to identify patients at very low risk of an adverse perioperative cardiac event, including asymptomatic patients having undergone coronary revascularization within 5 years as well as those without specific clinical markers for increased risk. Additional testing of selected patients at intermediate or higher risk can potentially reduce the cost of testing without affecting patients' outcomes. Based on a previous study validating the use of selective noninvasive testing before major aortic surgery,[77] the cost implications of selective testing were assessed in the ACC/AHA Task Force report.[15] In the previous study, the application of a clinical algorithm resulted in only 29 percent of 201 patients undergoing noninvasive testing prior to aortic surgery, with an associated 0.5 percent perioperative cardiac mortality rate. Using estimated costs, the use of selected testing was associated with a total cost of $32,886 for 58 patients, compared with an estimated total cost of $113,967 if all 201 had undergone noninvasive screening. The low perioperative mortality rate associated with the use of a clinical algorithm and selected noninvasive testing suggests that substantial cost can be avoided without compromising patients' safety.

PREOPERATIVE THERAPY FOR CORONARY ARTERY DISEASE

Coronary artery disease is responsible for the majority of adverse perioperative cardiac events. Once recognized, specific therapy should be instituted to minimize the risk of perioperative myocardial ischemia, myocardial infarction, or death.

Coronary Revascularization

There are no prospective trials testing the impact of either preoperative coronary artery bypass grafting or percutaneous transluminal coronary angioplasty on perioperative cardiac morbidity and mortality rates. However, several retrospective studies suggest that patients having undergone previous successful surgical coronary revascularization have a low risk of perioperative cardiac events during noncardiac surgery and that the risk of death is comparable to that found among patients with no clinical indications suggestive of coronary artery disease.[78–81]

Although these data support the theory that coronary artery bypass surgery lowers the risk of adverse cardiac events associated with noncardiac surgery, they do not address the overall effect on morbidity and mortality rates associated with the surgical coronary revascularization. However, in the assessment of patients undergoing noncardiac surgery, the well-established long-term benefits of coronary artery bypass surgery should be considered, as should any impact on noncardiac surgical morbidity and mortality rates. There may be some patients for whom coronary artery bypass grafting should be performed prior to noncardiac surgery only because of an otherwise prohibitive perioperative cardiac risk. However, there are many more patients with advanced coronary artery disease who are candidates for surgical coronary revascularization based on long-term prognosis who are identified only during preoperative cardiac assessment. Among such patients, elective noncardiac surgery of intermediate or high risk should generally be postponed for the performance of coronary artery bypass surgery.

There are no prospective studies and few studies of any kind that evaluate the impact of preoperative percutaneous coronary angioplasty on perioperative cardiac morbidity and mortality rates. Three small, retrospective studies[82–84] have suggested that there is a low risk of perioperative myocardial infarction or death following preoperative coronary angioplasty. One study of 1049 noncardiac surgeries performed among 1829 patients enrolled in the Bypass Angioplasty Revascularization Investigation (BARI) trail demonstrated a low incidence of myocardial infarction or death among patients having undergone either coronary artery bypass surgery or percutaneous angioplasty, with events among 1.6 percent of patients in both groups.[85] The absence of any evident difference between groups suggests that previous percutaneous coronary angioplasty confers protection from perioperative cardiac events that is equivalent to that conferred by surgical revascularization. However, based on the limited data available, indications for percutaneous coronary angioplasty among patients undergoing preoperative evaluation should be considered the same as for the general population.[15]

The optimal timing of noncardiac surgery has not been defined for patients who undergo preoperative percutaneous coronary angioplasty. It may be prudent to delay elective noncardiac surgery for a few days following percutaneous coronary angioplasty, due to the early risks of arterial recoil and acute thrombosis. Ideally, elective surgery should be performed within 2 to 3 months of angioplasty, before restenosis can occur. However, patients of more than 6 months following percutaneous coronary angioplasty with no evidence of recurrent ischemia could be considered to have undergone successful revascularization, presumably with a low perioperative risk.

Medical Therapy for Coronary Artery Disease

Several nonrandomized studies have addressed the effect of anti-ischemic medical therapy on perioperative prognosis.[86-93] Although data are lacking to support the empiric use of nitroglycerin or calcium channel blockers, there is increasing evidence that the empiric use of perioperative beta blockers may reduce the risk of an adverse cardiac event. Three small, retrospective studies suggest that perioperative therapy with beta blockers may result in fewer episodes of myocardial ischemia detectable on ECG[91,92] and of acute myocardial infarction.[90] More recently, a randomized study among 112 high-risk patients undergoing vascular surgery demonstrated a reduction in risk of perioperative myocardial infarction or death from 34 to 3 percent with the use of empiric beta blocker therapy.[94] These data support the use of beta blockers therapy among high-risk patients undergoing intermediate or high-risk noncardiac surgery.

MANAGEMENT OF SPECIFIC CONDITIONS

Patients with a variety of medical conditions known to increase cardiovascular risk may require noncardiac surgery. For these patients, appropriate perioperative medical management may prevent the occurrence or minimize the impact of an adverse cardiovascular event. Factors that contribute to increased perioperative risk include interruptions in routine medical therapy as well as physical and mental stresses associated with the surgical procedure and convalescent period. As such, cardiovascular stresses include duress due to the disease for which surgery is planned and alteration in normal medications during the preoperative period; fluctuation in heart rate, blood pressure, intravascular volume, and oxygenation during surgery; dynamic fluid shifts; pain; and limitations in the use of oral medications in the postoperative period. It is important to note that the period of maximum cardiac risk appears to occur in the postoperative period.[95] Because cardiovascular risk is not limited to the intraoperative period, appropriate emphasis should be placed on the treatment of specific conditions throughout all phases of the perioperative period.

Coronary Artery Disease

Among patients with known coronary artery disease undergoing noncardiac surgery, perioperative management should include monitoring for evidence of myocardial ischemia, therapy to prevent and treat ischemia, and postoperative surveillance to ensure that the patient did not experience an ischemic event that could mandate alteration in therapy.

Monitoring can be accomplished with surveillance of ECG ST-segments,[9,95] transesophageal echocardiographic assessment of regional and global left ventricular wall motion,[49] and invasive measurement of pulmonary arterial and pulmonary capillary wedge pressures. Therapy to prevent ischemia should be individualized to the patient and the surgical procedure but in general can include nitroglycerin, beta-adrenergic antagonists, and calcium channel blocking agents alone or in combination. Among many patients with known coronary artery disease, the prevention of ischemia can involve the simple continuation of a routine anti-ischemic regimen or conversion of a regimen to a similar one available for topical or intravenous delivery during periods in which the patient is unable to take medications orally. Nitroglycerin compounds can be administered topically or via intravenous infusion. Several beta-adrenergic antagonists and calcium channel–blocking agents are available for administration via intravenous bolus or infusion. In addition, transdermal clonidine can be substituted for oral beta blockers. In some patients, oral medications can be crushed and delivered through a nasogastric tube that is then clamped for 30 min to allow absorption in the upper intestine. Because of the adverse effects associated with rapid withdrawal of beta-blocking medications as well as the demonstrated benefit associated with their perioperative use,[91,92,94,96-99] every effort should be made to continue these medications during the perioperative period among patients who receive them preoperatively.

At a minimum, an anti-ischemic regimen used prior to surgery should be continued during the perioperative period. Additional anti-ischemic medications can be used empirically and should be used in the event that ischemia is detected during the perioperative period. Intravenous nitroglycerin and/or beta blockers can be titrated to specific end points of heart rate or blood pressure or to resolution of the observed ischemia. In addition, pain relief and correction of any underlying anemia are helpful in reducing tendencies to postoperative ischemia.

Because patients with known coronary artery disease or risk factors for disease are at risk of acute myocardial infarction complicating noncardiac surgery, assessment for change in status is appropriate following a surgical procedure. A simple 12-lead ECG preoperatively, immediately postoperatively, and daily for 2 days is generally sufficient to evaluate for change if there has been no evidence of perioperative ischemia or infarction. Alternative means of assessing for perioperative infarction include assessment of serum creatine kinase (CPK), creatine kinase MB isoenzyme (CPK-MB) fractions, and troponin; echocardiographic assessment of left ventricular wall motion; and nuclear perfusion studies.

At the conclusion of the perioperative period, it is of obvious importance to resume anti-ischemic medications used by the patient prior to undergoing noncardiac surgery. In addition, antiplatelet agents, such as aspirin, which may have been temporarily discontinued prior to surgery, should be reinitiated when no longer contraindicated (see also Chap. 40).

Hypertension

Among patients who are treated for hypertension, preoperative evaluation should include review of present medications and any history of intolerance to previous antihypertensive medications, assessment for adequacy of antihypertensive therapy, and simple measures to evaluate for causes of secondary hypertension and for evidence of target organ damage or associated cardiovascular pathologic conditions. Brief evaluation for rare but potentially treatable causes of secondary hypertension should include assessment for an abdominal bruit, suggestive of renal artery stenosis; for radial-femoral delay, indicative of aortic coarctation; and for hypokalemia in the absence of diuretic use, which could suggest hyperaldosteronism.

Blood pressure should be well controlled prior to elective surgery,[96,97,99,100] and antihypertensive medications should be continued throughout the perioperative period. If there is a period in which the patient is unable to receive oral medications, topical or intravenous equivalents should be substituted. As noted above, rapid withdrawal of beta-blocking medications has associated adverse effects on heart rate and blood pressure, may precipitate myocardial ischemia, and should be avoided.

Mild or moderate preoperative hypertension in the absence of associated cardiovascular or metabolic abnormalities should not necessitate delay of surgery.[101] However, severe hypertension (e.g., diastolic blood pressure of 110 mmHg or greater) should be controlled prior to an elective surgical procedure. If surgery is urgent, then preoperative blood pressure control can usually be achieved rapidly with the use of intravenous beta blockers, calcium blockers, nitroglycerin, or nitroprusside. Finally, patients with preoperative hypertension appear to be predisposed to the development of intraoperative hypotension.[102] A potential for blood pressure lability, with associated ischemia and hypoperfusion, exists among patients with preoperative hypertension; therefore, blood pressure should be carefully monitored and treated if necessary.

Congestive Heart Failure

Congestive heart failure is associated with increased cardiovascular risk during noncardiac surgery.[4,5,9,12,14,103] A careful history and physical examination should include efforts to identify evidence of congestive heart failure, and every effort should be made to treat it prior to surgery.

Congestive heart failure may be the result of a variety of cardiac abnormalities, including left ventricular systolic dysfunction, diastolic dysfunction, and valvular heart disease. Similarly, left ventricular systolic dysfunction may be a harbinger of underlying coronary artery disease. Although congestive heart failure is an independent risk factor for adverse perioperative cardiac outcome, specific underlying causes of congestive heart failure may each be associated with specific independent risks, and the specific nature of the risk may be determined by the nature of the underlying disease. For these reasons, the cause of the underlying process responsible for congestive heart failure should be identified when possible. If left ventricular systolic function is not known, it is generally prudent to establish whether it is normal or abnormal prior to surgery. Similarly, evaluation for left ventricular diastolic dysfunction or valvular heart disease may help in perioperative management. If there are risk factors for coronary artery disease, further evaluation for coronary disease as a cause of left ventricular systolic dysfunction may be appropriate (see also Chap. 21).

Cardiomyopathy

Patients with dilated and hypertrophic cardiomyopathies are predisposed to develop congestive heart failure. Because perioperative management is affected by the nature of the underlying disease, effort should be undertaken to establish the responsible pathologic condition before surgery. Among patients with preoperative signs or symptoms of congestive heart failure, preoperative evaluation should include assessment of left ventricular systolic and diastolic function. Systolic function can be determined noninvasively using either echocardiographic or radionuclide techniques. Echocardiographic imaging offers additional information reflecting diastolic function and valvular function, which could also contribute to congestive heart failure. If not previously performed, preoperative echocardiographic imaging should be strongly considered among patients with congestive heart failure.

Patients with hypertrophic cardiomyopathy require special consideration during the perioperative period. Hypertrophic cardiomyopathy can affect hemodynamics by means of dynamic left ventricular outflow obstruction or may precipitate congestive heart failure mediated by diastolic dysfunction. Left ventricular noncompliance can make patients with hypertrophic cardiomyopathy extremely sensitive to even small amounts of excess intravascular volume, while an underfilled left ventricle can exacerbate dynamic left ventricular outflow obstruction, with a resulting decrease in stroke volume and systemic hypotension. Therefore, perioperative management should be directed at maintaining intravascular volume within a potentially narrow range, avoiding congestive heart failure and minimizing left ventricular outflow obstruction. Catecholamines as a class should be avoided because of their potential to exacerbate dynamic left ventricular outflow obstruction (see also Chap. 51).

Valvular Heart Disease

Most valvular heart disease in an adult population is acquired and therefore increasingly common among older patients undergoing noncardiac surgery. Organic valvular heart disease affects the use of prophylactic antibiotics and can require special consideration for hemodynamic monitoring and medical management in the perioperative period. Although most elective noncardiac surgery need not be delayed, some types of valvular heart disease can pose excessive risk to the patient and should be addressed prior to an elective surgical procedure.

Antibiotic prophylaxis should be used to reduce the risk of infective endocarditis among patients with organic valvular heart disease whenever noncardiac surgery involves a risk of bacteremia. Such procedures include oral, dental, gastrointestinal, and genitourologic procedures, in which normal bacterial flora may gain transient access to the bloodstream. Specific recommendations for prophylactic antibiotic regimens are published for specific types of noncardiac surgery in which there exists an increased risk of infective endocarditis.[104]

AORTIC STENOSIS

Severe aortic stenosis presents the greatest valve-associated cardiovascular risk for patients undergoing noncardiac surgery.[4] The presence of fixed obstruction to left ventricular outflow dramatically limits functional cardiac reserve and may be associated with intracavitary left ventricular pressures in excess of 300 mmHg. Accompanying left ventricular hypertrophy predisposes the patient to diastolic dysfunction and pulmonary congestion. It is important to note that the combination of left ventricular hypertrophy and left ventricular outflow obstruction with high intracavitary pressures predisposes to myocardial ischemia with or without concomitant coronary artery disease. In general, severe or symptomatic aortic stenosis should be addressed prior to the patient's undergoing elective noncardiac surgery. In most cases, aortic valve replacement is indicated as the definitive therapy of choice.[105–107] If cardiac surgery is contraindicated, percutaneous aortic balloon valvotomy can be used to mitigate left ventricular outflow obstruction, even if only as a temporizing measure (see Chap. 56).

MITRAL STENOSIS

The hemodynamic impact associated with mitral stenosis is affected by heart rate. Because increases in heart rate are associated with shortening of the diastolic portion of the cardiac cycle, left ventricular filling is adversely affected by increases in heart rate among patients with even mild or moderate mitral stenosis. As a result, pulmonary congestion can be precipitated by tachycardia of even moderate degree. For this reason, heart rate should be well controlled in the perioperative period among patients with mitral stenosis of any severity. Patients with severe mitral stenosis undergoing high-risk noncardiac surgery may benefit from surgical or percutaneous intervention.[108] The relative risks and benefits and the likelihood of success associated with percutaneous balloon mitral valvotomy, surgical commissurotomy, or mitral valve replacement must be weighed in the context of mitral valve anatomy and other patient-specific factors (see Chap. 57).

AORTIC REGURGITATION AND MITRAL REGURGITATION

Patients with significant aortic regurgitation are predisposed to volume overload in the perioperative period, and volume status should be carefully monitored to prevent pulmonary congestion. In addition, patients with severe aortic regurgitation may benefit from afterload reduction in the form of angiotensin-converting enzyme inhibitors, calcium channel blockers, nitroglycerin, or hydralazine. Just as patients with mitral stenosis are sensitive to tachycardia, patients with significant aortic regurgitation are sensitive to bradycardia. Prolongation of the diastolic interval associated with bradycardia increases the time during which aortic regurgitation occurs and increases total regurgitant volume.

Mitral regurgitation can be due to a variety of underlying causes. As for patients with congestive heart failure, establishing the cause of mitral regurgitation may help define other associated perioperative risks, especially if mitral regurgitation occurs as a manifestation of coronary artery disease. Patients with significant mitral regurgitation may develop volume overload and pulmonary congestion. Diuretics and afterload-reducing therapy should be used to optimize hemodynamic values preoperatively in patients with severe mitral regurgitation undergoing major noncardiac surgery.

Special attention should be paid to left ventricular function in patients with severe mitral regurgitation. The left atrium and pulmonary venous system serve as a low-impedance system that effectively "afterload-reduces" the left ventricle in the setting of significant mitral regurgitation. Because of this, even a mild decrease in left ventricular ejection fraction in the setting of severe mitral regurgitation should be taken as evidence of significant impairment in systolic function and reduced left ventricular functional reserve.

Among patients with mitral valve prolapse, appropriate antibiotic prophylaxis is warranted if there is evidence of regurgitation on either physical examination or echocardiographic Doppler imaging. In addition, antibiotic prophylaxis should be used in patients with mitral valve prolapse and evidence of leaflet thickening and/or leaflet redundancy on echocardiographic imaging[104] (see Chaps. 56 and 57).

PROSTHETIC HEART VALVES

Patients with either tissue or mechanical heart valve prostheses should receive appropriate antibiotic prophylaxis when undergoing noncardiac surgery with an accompanying potential for bacteremia.[104] Patients with mechanical heart valve prostheses also require careful management of anticoagulation in the perioperative period. As a general rule, anticoagulation can be discontinued when necessary for safe performance of noncardiac surgery and should be reinstituted when no longer contraindicated for hemostasis. The risk of valve thrombosis or thromboembolism is related to the location and type of valve prosthesis, the duration in which the patient is not fully anticoagulated, and the level of anticoagulation maintained during that period. A mechanical prosthesis in the mitral position is at greater risk of thrombus formation than is a similar valve in the aortic position, due to the larger cross-sectional area of the mitral prosthesis and associated lower velocities of flow. Similarly, anticoagulation titrated to a subtherapeutic level maintains more protection against thrombus formation than does no anticoagulation. Finally, the risk of thrombus formation is cumulative and increases with the time during which the patient receives less than therapeutic anticoagulation.

Patients who require minimally invasive procedures with a low hemorrhagic risk may be managed by allowing long-term anticoagulation to decrease to a subtherapeutic range and resuming the normal dose of warfarin immediately following the procedure.[109] Among patients with a mechanical heart valve undergoing major noncardiac surgery and in whom anticoagulation is contraindicated at the time of surgery, it is usually prudent to discontinue oral anticoagulation several days prior to surgery and administer intravenous heparin to maintain anticoagulation until the time of surgery. The short half-life of heparin allows the patient to safely undergo surgery within a few hours of its discontinuation. Reestablishing therapeutic anticoagulation usually requires several days after warfarin is initiated, and the patient should again receive heparin in the postoperative period until oral anticoagulation is fully therapeutic. Heparin should be reinitiated when the risk of bleeding is no longer prohibitive and may be started with either a bolus followed by intravenous infusion or with intravenous infusion alone, dictated by the risk of postoperative hemorrhage (see Chap. 60).

Arrhythmia and Conduction Disturbances

Supraventricular and ventricular arrhythmias typically do not represent a serious risk to the patient undergoing noncardiac surgery. However, the arrhythmia may herald the presence of underlying cardiopulmonary disease, and any increased perioperative risk associated with ventricular and supraventricular arrhythmias[4] is most likely due to the underlying disease. The finding of an arrhythmia in the perioperative period should prompt a search for underlying cardiopulmonary disease, drug toxicity, or metabolic derangement that could be both responsible for the arrhythmia and present a risk to the patient.

An otherwise benign arrhythmia can present risk if it unmasks an otherwise silent cardiac disease. For example, a rapid supraventricular tachycardia can provoke myocardial ischemia in the presence of minimal coronary artery disease and similarly can precipitate significant pulmonary congestion in the setting of only mild or moderate mitral stenosis. Ventricular ectopy, including isolated ventricular premature complexes, complex ectopy, and nonsustained ventricular tachycardia, usually do not require specific therapy unless there is evidence of associated hypoperfusion. Thus, hypotension or ongoing myocardial ischemia associated with an arrhythmia warrants therapy directed at the arrhythmia more than would the presence of the arrhythmia alone.

Perioperative atrial fibrillation is common, especially following intrathoracic surgical procedures, where there can be direct atrial irritation, as well as among patients with underlying cardiac or pulmonary diseases. Because of the high-catecholamine state early following major surgery, it may not be possible to establish and maintain normal sinus rhythm in the setting of postoperative atrial fibrillation, and therapy should be directed at rate control and anticoagulation when feasible. Cardioversion of atrial fibrillation in the early postoperative period should be limited to patients with evidence of hemodynamic compromise and hypoperfusion associated with the arrhythmia. For most patients, rate control can be accomplished with the use of beta-adrenergic antagonists or calcium channel–blocking agents administered orally or intravenously. Although digoxin can also be administered, it is typically not as effective for rate control in patients with a high-catecholamine state. Because of the risk of atrial thrombus formation and associated thromboembolic events, patients with atrial fibrillation, including postoperative atrial fibrillation, should be anticoagulated when feasible. Many patients with postoperative atrial fibrillation spontaneously revert to sinus rhythm when perioperative stresses have sufficiently decreased. If a patient does not spontaneously return to sinus rhythm, elective cardioversion should be performed prior to discharge. Any form of cardioversion from atrial fibrillation, whether chemical, electrical, or spontaneous, carries an associated risk of subsequent thromboembolism ascribed to a period of atrial mechanical dysfunction following cardioversion.[110,111] For this reason, patients should receive therapeutic anticoagulation for 3 to 4 weeks following successful cardioversion.

Patients with evidence of intraventricular conduction delay on ECG but without history of symptoms or electrical evidence of advanced heart block do not appear to be at substantial risk of progressing to complete heart block in the perioperative period. If high-grade conduction block develops, treatment can usually be managed in the short term with transthoracic pacing units. Special note should be made of the presence of a left bundle-branch block among patients undergoing right heart catheterization for hemodynamic monitoring. Because of the risk of inducing transient right bundle-branch block during catheter manipulation through the right ventricle, the possibility of complete heart block exists, and measures to provide temporary pacing should be available.

References

1. Mangano DT. Perioperative cardiac morbidity. *Anesthesiology* 1990; 72:153–184.
2. National Center for Health Statistics. *Vital Statistics of the United States: 1980,* vol 2, *Mortality,* part A. DHHS pub no (PHS) 85-1101. Hyattsville, MD: NCHS U.S. Public Health Services; 1985.
3. National Center for Health Statistics. *Vital Statistics of the United States: 1988,* vol 3. DHHS pub no (PHS) 89-1232. Washington, DC: NCHS U.S. Public Health Services; 1989:10–17, 66, 67, 100, 101.
4. Goldman L, Caldera DL, Nussbaum SR, et al. Multifactorial index of cardiac risk in noncardiac surgical procedures. *N Engl J Med* 1977; 297:845–850.
5. Ashton CM, Petersen NJ, Wray NP, et al. The incidence of perioperative myocardial infarction in men undergoing noncardiac surgery. *Ann Intern Med* 1993; 118:504–510.
6. Hollenberg M, Mangano DT, Browner WS, et al. Predictors of postoperative myocardial ischemia in patients undergoing noncardiac surgery: The study of perioperative ischemia research group. *JAMA* 1992; 268:205–209.
7. Hubbard BL, Gibbons RJ, Lapeyre AC III, et al. Identification of severe coronary artery disease using simple clinical parameters. *Arch Intern Med* 1992; 152:309–312.
8. Lette J, Waters D, Bernier H, et al. Preoperative and long-term cardiac risk assessment: Predictive value of 23 clinical descriptors, 7 multivariate scoring systems, and quantitative dipyridamole imaging in 350 patients. *Ann Surg* 1992; 216:192–204.
9. Mangano DT, Browner WS, Hollenberg M, et al. Association of perioperative myocardial ischemia with cardiac morbidity and mortality in men undergoing noncardiac surgery: The study of perioperative ischemia research group. *N Engl J Med* 1990; 323:1781–1788.
10. Michel LA, Jamart J, Bradpiece HA, et al. Prediction of risk in noncardiac operations after cardiac operations. *J Thorac Cardiovasc Surg* 1990; 100:595–605.
11. Eagle KA, Coley CM, Newell JB, et al. Combining clinical and thallium data optimizes preoperative assessment of cardiac risk before major vascular surgery. *Ann Intern Med* 1989; 110:859–866.
12. Detsky AS, Abrams HB, McLaughlin JR, et al. Predicting cardiac complications in patients undergoing non-cardiac surgery. *J Gen Intern Med* 1986; 1:211–219.
13. Foster ED, Davis KB, Carpenter JA, et al. Risk of noncardiac operation in patients with defined coronary disease: The coronary artery surgery study (CASS) registry experience. *Ann Thorac Surg* 1986; 41:42–50.
14. Cooperman M, Pflug B, Martin EW Jr, et al. Cardiovascular risk factors in patients with peripheral vascular disease. *Surgery* 1978; 84:505–509.
15. Eagle KA, Brundage BH, Chaitman BR, et al. Guidelines for perioperative cardiovascular evaluation for noncardiac surgery: Report of the American College of Cardiology/American Heart Association Task Force on Practice Guidelines. *Circulation* 1996; 93:1278–1317.
16. Morris CK, Ueshima K, Kawaguchi T, et al. The prognostic value of exercise capacity: A review of the literature. *Am Heart J* 1991; 122:1423–1431.
17. Detsky AS, Abrams HB, Forbath N, et al. Cardiac assessment for patients undergoing noncardiac surgery: A multifactorial clinical risk index. *Arch Intern Med* 1986; 146:2131–2134.
18. Tarhan S, Moffitt EA, Taylor WF, et al. Myocardial infarction after general anesthesia. *JAMA* 1972; 220:1451–1454.
19. Steen PA, Tinker JH, Tarhan S. Myocardial reinfarction after anesthesia and surgery. *JAMA* 1978; 239:2566–2570.
20. Rao TL, Jacobs KH, El-Etr AA. Reinfarction following anesthesia in patients with myocardial infarction. *Anesthesiology* 1983; 59:499–505.
21. Hertzer NR. Fatal myocardial infarction following peripheral vascular operations: A study of 951 patients followed 6 to 11 years postoperatively. *Cleveland Clin Q* 1982; 49:1–11.
22. Leung JM, Goehner P, O'Kelly BF, et al. Isoflurane anesthesia and myocardial ischemia: Comparative risk versus sufentanil anesthesia in patients undergoing coronary artery bypass graft surgery. The SPI (Study of Perioperative Ischemia) Research Group. *Anesthesiology* 1991; 74:838–847.
23. Baron JF, Bertrand M, Barre E, et al. Combined epidural and general anesthesia versus general anesthesia for abdominal aortic surgery. *Anesthesiology* 1991; 75:611–618.
24. Christopherson R, Beattie C, Frank SM, et al. Perioperative morbidity in patients randomized to epidural or general anesthesia for lower extremity vascular surgery: Perioperative Ischemia

Randomized Anesthesia Trial Study Group. *Anesthesiology* 1993; 79:422–434.

25. Slogoff S, Eeats AS. Randomized trial of primary anesthetic agents on outcome of coronary artery bypass operations. *Anesthesiology* 1989; 70:179–188.
26. Tuman KJ, McCarthy RJ, Spiess BD. Epidural anaesthesia and analgesia decreases postoperative hypercoagulability in high-risk vascular patients. *Anesth Analg* 1990; 70:S414.
27. Gianrossi R, Detrano R, Mulvihill D, et al. Exercise-induced ST depression in the diagnosis of coronary artery disease: A meta-analysis. *Circulation* 1989; 80:87–98.
28. Detrano R, Gianrossi R, Mulvihill D, et al. Exercise-induced ST segment depression in the diagnosis of multivessel coronary disease: A meta analysis. *J Am Coll Cardiol* 1989; 14:1501–1508.
29. Weiner DA, Ryan TJ, McCabe CH, et al. Prognostic importance of a clinical profile and exercise test in medically treated patients with coronary artery disease. *J Am Coll Cardiol* 1984; 3:772–779.
30. McCabe CJ, Reidy NC, Abbott WM, et al. The value of electrocardiogram monitoring during treadmill testing for peripheral vascular disease. *Surgery* 1981; 89:183–186.
31. Cutler BS, Wheeler HB, Paraskos JA, et al. Applicability and interpretation of electrocardiographic stress testing in patients with peripheral vascular disease. *Am J Surg* 1981; 141:501–506.
32. Arous EJ, Baum PL, Cutler BS, et al. The ischemic exercise test in patients with peripheral vascular disease: Implications for management. *Arch Surg* 1984; 119:780–783.
33. Gardine RL, McBride K, Greenberg H, et al. The value of cardiac monitoring during peripheral arterial stress testing in the surgical management of peripheral vascular disease. *J Cardiovasc Surg (Torino)* 1985; 26:258–261.
34. von Knorring J, Lepantalo M. Prediction of perioperative cardiac complications by electrocardiographic monitoring during treadmill exercise testing before peripheral vascular surgery. *Surgery* 1986; 99:610–613.
35. Leppo J, Plaja J, Gionet M, et al. Noninvasive evaluation of cardiac risk before elective vascular surgery. *J Am Coll Cardiol* 1987; 9:269–276.
36. Hanson P, Pease M, Berkoff H, et al. Arm exercise testing for coronary artery disease in patients with peripheral vascular disease. *Clin Cardiol* 1988; 11:70–74.
37. McPhail N, Calvin JE, Shariatmadar A, et al. The use of preoperative exercise testing to predict cardiac complications after arterial reconstruction. *J Vasc Surg* 1988; 7:60–68.
38. Carliner NH, Fisher ML, Plotnick GD, et al. Routine preoperative exercise testing in patients undergoing major noncardiac surgery. *Am J Cardiol* 1985; 56:51–58.
39. Kopecky SL, Gibbons RJ, Hollier LH. Preoperative supine exercise radionuclide angiogram predicts perioperative cardiovascular events in vascular surgery. *J Am Coll Cardiol* 1986; 7:226A.
40. Urbinati S, Di Pasquale G, Andreoli A, et al. Preoperative noninvasive coronary risk stratification in candidates for carotid endarterectomy. *Stroke* 1994; 25:2022–2027.
41. Boucher CA, Brewster DC, Darling RC, et al. Determination of cardiac risk by dipyridamole-thallium imaging before peripheral vascular surgery. *N Engl J Med* 1985; 312:389–394.
42. Cutler BS, Leppo JA. Dipyridamole thallium 201 scintigraphy to detect coronary artery disease before abdominal aortic surgery. *J Vasc Surg* 1987; 5:91–100.
43. Fletcher JP, Antico VF, Gruenewald S, et al. Dipyridamole-thallium scan for screening of coronary artery disease prior to vascular surgery. *J Cardiovasc Surg (Torino)* 1988; 29:666–669.
44. Sachs RN, Tellier P, Larmignat P, et al. Assessment by dipyridamole-thallium-201 myocardial scintigraphy of coronary risk before peripheral vascular surgery. *Surgery* 1988; 103:584–587.
45. McEnroe CS, O'Donnell RF Jr, Yeager A, et al. Comparison of ejection fraction and Goldman risk factor analysis of dipyridamole-thallium 201 studies in the evaluation of cardiac morbidity after aortic aneurysm surgery. *J Vasc Surg* 1990; 11:497–504.
46. Younis LT, Aguirre F, Byers S, et al. Perioperative and long-term prognostic value of intravenous dipyridamole thallium scintigraphy in patients with peripheral vascular disease. *Am Heart J* 1990; 119:1287–1292.
47. Mangano DT, London MJ, Tubau JF, et al. Dipyridamole thallium-201 scintigraphy as a preoperative screening test: A reexamination of its predictive potential. Study of Perioperative Ischemia Research Group. *Circulation* 1991; 84:493–502.
48. Strawn DJ, Guernsey JM. Dipyridamole thallium scanning in the evaluation of coronary artery disease in elective abdominal aortic surgery. *Arch Surg* 1991; 126:880–884.
49. Watters TA, Botvinick EH, Dae MW, et al. Comparison of the findings on preoperative dipyridamole perfusion scintigraphy and intraoperative transesophageal echocardiography: Implications regarding the identification of myocardium at ischemic risk. *J Am Coll Cardiol* 1991; 18:93–100.
50. Hendel RC, Whitfield SS, Villegas BJ, et al. Prediction of late cardiac events by dipyridamole thallium imaging in patients undergoing elective vascular surgery. *Am J Cardiol* 1992; 70:1243–1249.
51. Lette J, Waters D, Cerino M, et al. Preoperative coronary artery disease risk stratification based on dipyridamole imaging and a simple three-step, three-segment model for patients undergoing noncardiac vascular surgery or major general surgery. *Am J Cardiol* 1992; 69:1553–1558.
52. Madsen PV, Vissing M, Munck O, et al. A comparison of dipyridamole thallium 201 scintigraphy and clinical examination: I. The determination of cardiac risk before arterial reconstruction. *Angiology* 1992; 43:306–311.
53. Brown KA, Rowen M. Extent of jeopardized viable myocardium determined by myocardial perfusion imaging best predicts perioperative cardiac events in patients undergoing noncardiac surgery. *J Am Coll Cardiol* 1993; 21:325–330.
54. Kresowik TF, Bower TR, Garner SA, et al. Dipyridamole thallium imaging in patients being considered for vascular procedures. *Arch Surg* 1993; 128:299–302.
55. Baron JF, Mundler O, Bertrand M, et al. Dipyridamole-thallium scintigraphy and gated radionuclide angiography to assess cardiac risk before abdominal aortic surgery. *N Engl J Med* 1994; 330:663–669.
56. Bry JD, Belkin M, O'Donnell TF Jr, et al. An assessment of the positive predictive value and cost-effectiveness of dipyridamole myocardial scintigraphy in patients undergoing vascular surgery. *J Vasc Surg* 1994; 19:112–121.
57. Camp AD, Garvin PJ, Hoff J, et al. Prognostic value of intravenous dipyridamole thallium imaging in patients with diabetes mellitus considered for renal transplantation. *Am J Cardiol* 1990; 65:1459–1463.
58. Iqbal A, Gibbons RJ, McGoon MD, et al. Noninvasive assessment of cardiac risk in insulin dependent diabetic patients being evaluated for pancreatic transplantation using thallium-201 myocardial perfusion scintigraphy. *Transplant Proc* 1991; 23(part 2):1690–1691.
59. Coley CM, Field TS, Abraham SA, et al. Usefulness of dipyridamole-thallium scanning for preoperative evaluation of cardiac risk for nonvascular surgery. *Am J Cardiol* 1992; 69:1280–1285.
60. Shaw L, Miller DD, Kong BA, et al. Determination of perioperative cardiac risk by adenosine thallium-201 myocardial imaging. *Am Heart J* 1992; 124:861–869.
61. Takase B, Younis LT, Byers SL, et al. Comparative prognostic value of clinical risk indexes, resting two-dimensional echocardiography, and dipyridamole stress thallium-201 myocardial imaging for perioperative cardiac events in major nonvascular surgery patients. *Am Heart J* 1993; 126:1099–1106.
62. Younis L, Stratmann H, Takase B, et al. Preoperative clinical

assessment and dipyridamole thallium-201 scintigraphy for prediction and prevention of cardiac events in patients having major noncardiovascular surgery and known or suspected coronary artery disease. *Am J Cardiol* 1994; 47:311–317.

63. Stratmann H, Tamesis B, Wittry M, et al. Dipyridamole sestamibi tomography optimizes perioperative outcome and defines late prognosis in vascular surgery patients. *Circulation* 1993; 88:1–440.
64. Ritchie JL, Bateman TM, Bonow RO, et al. Guidelines for clinical use of cardiac radionuclide imaging: A report of the American College of Cardiology/American Heart Association Task Force on Assessment of Diagnostic and Therapeutic Cardiovascular Procedures (Committee on Radionuclide Imaging), developed in collaboration with the American Society of Nuclear Cardiology. *J Am Coll Cardiol* 1995; 25:521–547.
65. Berthe C, Pierard LA, Hiernaux M. Predicting the extent and location of coronary artery disease in acute myocardial infarction by echocardiography during dobutamine infusion. *Am J Cardiol* 1986; 58:1167–1172.
66. Cohen JL, Green TO, Ottenweller J, et al. Dobutamine digital echocardiography for detecting coronary artery disease. *Am J Cardiol* 1991; 67:1311–1318.
67. Sawada SG, Segar DS, Ryan T, et al. Echocardiographic detection of coronary artery disease during dobutamine infusion. *Circulation* 1991; 83:1605–1614.
68. Martin TW, Seaworth JF, Johns JP, et al. Comparison of adenosine, dipyridamole, and dobutamine in stress echocardiography. *Ann Intern Med* 1992; 116:190–196.
69. Marwick T, Willemart B, D'Hondt AM, et al. Selection of the optimal nonexercise stress for the evaluation of ischemic regional myocardial dysfunction and malperfusion: Comparison of dobutamine and adenosine using echocardiography and 99mTc-MIBI single photon emission computed tomography. *Circulation* 1993; 87:345–354.
70. Lane RT, Sawada SG, Segar DS, et al. Dobutamine stress echocardiography for assessment of cardiac risk before noncardiac surgery. *Am J Cardiol* 1991; 68:976–977.
71. Lalka SG, Sawada SG, Dalsing MC, et al. Dobutamine stress echocardiography as a predictor of cardiac events associated with aortic surgery. *J Vasc Surg* 1992; 15:831–840.
72. Poldermans D, Fioretti PM, Forster T, et al. Dobutamine stress echocardiography for assessment of perioperative cardiac risk in patients undergoing major vascular surgery. *Circulation* 1993; 87:1506–1512.
73. Eichelberger JP, Schwarz KQ, Black ER, et al. Predictive value of dobutamine echocardiography just before noncardiac vascular surgery. *Am J Cardiol* 1993; 72:602–607.
74. Langan EM III, Youkey JR, Franklin DP, et al. Dobutamine stress echocardiography for cardiac risk assessment before aortic surgery. *J Vasc Surg* 1993; 18:905–911.
75. Davila-Roman VG, Waggoner AD, Sicard GA, et al. Dobutamine stress echocardiography predicts surgical outcome in patients with an aortic aneurysm and peripheral vascular disease. *J Am Coll Cardiol* 1993; 21:957–963.
76. Shaw LJ, Eagle KA, Gersh BJ, et al. Meta-analysis of intravenous dipyridamole-thallium-201 imaging (1985 to 1994) and dobutamine echocardiography (1991 to 1994) for risk stratification before vascular surgery. *J Am Coll Cardiol* 1996; 27:787–798.
77. Cambria RP, Brewster DC, Abbott WM, et al. The impact of selective use of dipyridamole-thallium scans and surgical factors on the current morbidity of aortic surgery. *J Vasc Surg* 1992; 15:43–51.
78. Diehl JT, Cali RF, Hertzer NR, et al. Complications of abdominal aortic reconstruction: An analysis of perioperative risk factors in 557 patients. *Ann Surg* 1983; 197:49–56.
79. Crawford ES, Morris GC Jr, Howell JF, et al. Operative risk in patients with previous coronary artery bypass. *Ann Thorac Surg* 1978; 26:215–221.
80. Reul GJ Jr, Cooley DA, Duncan JM, et al. The effect of coronary bypass on the outcome of peripheral vascular operations in 1093 patients. *J Vasc Surg* 1986; 3:788–798.
81. Nielsen JL, Page CP, Mann C, et al. Risk of major elective operation after myocardial revascularization. *Am J Surg* 1992; 164:423–426.
82. Huber KC, Evans MA, Bresnahan JF, et al. Outcome of noncardiac operations in patients with severe coronary artery disease successfully treated preoperatively with coronary angioplasty. *Mayo Clin Proc* 1992; 67:15–21.
83. Elmore JR, Hallett JW Jr, Gibbons RJ, et al. Myocardial revascularization before abdominal aortic aneurysmorrhaphy: Effect of coronary angioplasty. *Mayo Clin Proc* 1993; 68:637–641.
84. Allen JR, Helling TS, Hartzler GO. Operative procedures not involving the heart after percutaneous transluminal coronary angioplasty. *Surg Gynecol Obstet* 1991; 173:285–288.
85. Hassan SA, Hlatky M, Boothroyd D, et al. Impact of prior coronary bypass surgery and angioplasty on peri-operative cardiac outcomes in patients undergoing non-cardiac surgery: Data from Bypass Angioplasty Revascularization Investigation (BARI) study [abstr]. *Circulation* 1999; 100(suppl I):I-529.
86. Coriat P, Daloz M, Bousseau D, et al. Prevention of intraoperative myocardial ischemia during noncardiac surgery with intravenous nitroglycerin. *Anesthesiology* 1984; 61:193–196.
87. Thomson IR, Mutch WA, Culligan JD. Failure of intravenous fentanyl-pancuronium anesthesia. *Anesthesiology* 1984; 61: 385–393.
88. Gallagher JD, Moore RA, Jose AB, et al. Prophylactic nitroglycerin infusions during coronary artery bypass surgery. *Anesthesiology* 1986; 64:785–789.
89. Godet G, Coriat P, Baron JF, et al. Prevention of intraoperative myocardial ischemia during noncardiac surgery with intravenous diltiazem: A randomized trial versus placebo. *Anesthesiology* 1987; 66:241–245.
90. Pasternack PF, Imparato AM, Baumann FG, et al. The hemodynamics of beta-blockade in patients undergoing abdominal aortic aneurysm repair. *Circulation* 1987; 76(suppl 3, pt 2): III-1–III-7.
91. Stone JG, Foex P, Sear JW, et al. Myocardial ischemia in untreated hypertensive patients: Effect of a single small oral dose of a beta-adrenergic blocking agent. *Anesthesiology* 1988; 68:495–500.
92. Pasternack PF, Grossi EA, Baumann FG, et al. Beta blockade to decrease silent myocardial ischemia during peripheral vascular surgery. *Am J Surg* 1989; 158:113–116.
93. Dodds TM, Stone JG, Coromilas J, et al. Prophylactic nitroglycerin infusion during noncardiac surgery does not reduce perioperative ischemia. *Anesth Analg* 1993; 76:705–713.
94. Poldermans D, Boersma E, Bax JJ, et al. The effect of bisoprolol on perioperative mortality and myocardial infarction in high-risk patients undergoing vascular surgery. *N Engl J Med* 1999; 341:1789–1794.
95. Mangano DT, Hollenberg M, Fegert G, et al. Perioperative myocardial ischemia in patients undergoing noncardiac surgery: I. Incidence and severity during the 4 day perioperative period. *J Am Coll Cardiol* 1991; 17:843–850.
96. Stone JG, Foex P, Sear JW, et al. Risk of myocardial ischaemia during anesthesia in treated and untreated hypertensive patients. *Br J Anaesth* 1988; 61:675–679.
97. Prys-Roberts C, Meloche R, Foex P. Studies of anaesthesia in relation to hypertension: I. cardiovascular responses of treated and untreated patients. *Br J Anaesth* 1971; 43:122–137.
98. Cucchiara RF, Benefiel DJ, Matteo RS, et al. Evaluation of esmolol in controlling increases in heart rate and blood pressure during endotracheal intubation in patients undergoing carotid endarterectomy. *Anesthesiology* 1986; 65:528–531.

99. Magnusson J, Thulin T, Werner O, et al. Haemodynamic effects of pretreatment with metoprolol in hypertensive patients undergoing surgery. *Br J Anaesth* 1986; 58:251–260.
100. Goldman L, Caldera DL. Risks of general anesthesia and elective operation in the hypertensive patient. *Anesthesiology* 1979; 50:285–292.
101. Bedford RF, Feinstein B. Hospital admission blood pressure: A predictor for hypertension following endotracheal intubation. *Anesth Analg* 1980; 59:367–370.
102. Slogoff S, Keats AS. Does perioperative myocardial ischemia lead to postoperative myocardial infarction? *Anesthesiology* 1985; 62:107–114.
103. Gerson MC, Hurst JM, Hertzberg VS, et al. Cardiac prognosis in noncardiac geriatric surgery. *Ann Intern Med* 1985; 103:832–837.
104. Dajani AS, Bisno AL, Chung KJ, et al. Prevention of bacterial endocarditis: Recommendations by the American Heart Association. *JAMA* 1990; 264:2919–2922.
105. Bernard Y, Etievent J, Mourand JL, et al. Long-term percutaneous aortic valvuloplasty compared with aortic valve replacement in patients more than 75 years old. *J Am Coll Cardiol* 1992; 20:796–801.
106. Logeais Y, Langanay T, Roussin R, et al. Surgery for aortic stenosis in elderly patients: A study of surgical risk and predictive factors. *Circulation* 1994; 90:2891–2898.
107. Lieberman EB, Bashore TM, Hermiller JB, et al. Balloon aortic valvuloplasty in adults: Failure of procedure to improve long-term survival. *J Am Coll Cardiol* 1995; 26:1522–1528.
108. Reyes VP, Raju BS, Wynne J. Percutaneous balloon valvuloplasty compared with open surgical commissurotomy for mitral stenosis. *N Engl J Med* 1994; 331:961–967.
109. Stein PD, Alpert JS, Copeland J, et al. Antithrombotic therapy in patients with mechanical and biologic prosthetic heart valves. *Chest* 1992; 102(suppl):445S–455S.
110. Black IW, Fatkin D, Sagar KB, et al. Exclusion of atrial thrombus by transesophageal echocardiography does not preclude embolism after cardioversion of atrial fibrillation: A multicenter study. *Circulation* 1994; 89:2509–2513.
111. Fatkin D, Kuchar DL, Thorburn CW, et al. Transesophageal echocardiography before and during direct current cardioversion of atrial fibrillation: Evidence for "atrial stunning" as a mechanism of thromboembolic complications. *J Am Coll Cardiol* 1994; 23:307–316.

CHAPTER 75

ANESTHESIA AND THE PATIENT WITH CARDIOVASCULAR DISEASE

David L. Reich / Joel A. Kaplan

INTRODUCTION

Anesthetizing patients with cardiovascular disease is one of the most difficult challenges facing the anesthesiologist. The constellation of anesthetic drug effects, the physiologic stresses of surgery, and underlying cardiovascular diseases complicate and limit the choice of anesthetic techniques for any particular procedure. Generally speaking, the anesthesiologist's approach to the patient with cardiovascular disease is to select agents and techniques that would optimize the patient's cardiopulmonary function. The perioperative management of a patient with cardiovascular disease requires close cooperation between the cardiologist/internist and the anesthesiologist.[1] Each specialist has a unique knowledge base that complements the others. The approach should emphasize a continuum of care from the preoperative evaluation through the extended postoperative period.

PREOPERATIVE EVALUATION

The assessment of cardiac risk and preoperative optimization of the patient's cardiovascular status are the traditional goals of the preoperative evaluation of patients with cardiovascular disease. In 1977, Goldman et al. introduced the Cardiac Risk Index Score to guide more quantitatively the assignment of cardiac risk in patients undergoing noncardiac surgery.[2] This study had a major impact, because clinicians concluded that improvements in factors such as congestive heart failure symptomatology and general medical condition would decrease cardiac risk. While one major study does not support the predictive value of the Cardiac Risk Index Score or preoperative electrocardiographic ischemic changes in patients with coronary artery disease,[3] the emphasis on preoperative optimization continues and is supported by other studies.[4] This topic is reviewed in Chap. 83. The American College of Cardiology/American Heart Association Task Force on Practice Guidelines published, "Guidelines for Perioperative Cardiovascular Evaluation for Noncardiac Surgery."[5] The algorithmic approach to preoperative evaluation described in these guidelines and that advocated by Mangano and Goldman[6] are valuable in that more consistent clinical approaches should emerge.

The information derived from the cardiac evaluation that is of particular value to the anesthesiologist can be summarized by answers to the following questions:

1. Are further diagnostic studies required prior to elective surgery?
2. Will the patient derive benefit from delaying surgery in order to optimize preoperative medical therapy?
3. Will the patient derive benefit from preoperative myocardial revascularization (angioplasty or surgical revascularization)?
4. Should there be perioperative antithrombotic therapy?
5. What is the regimen of preoperative cardiovascular medications that should be continued through the perioperative period?

The accumulation of historical, clinical, laboratory, echocardiographic, radionuclide, and cardiac catheterization data in a cogent summary form comprises the ideal "medical clearance" consultation for the anesthesiologist. With the benefit of this information, the two specialties can make intelligent decisions regarding the patient's preoperative therapy and the optimal timing of surgery.[7]

PERIOPERATIVE MONITORING

Standards for basic intraoperative monitoring were established by the American Society of Anesthesiologists in 1986.[8] Accordingly, digital pulse oximetry and capnometry have been almost universally applied in the last several years. The indications for the use of more invasive monitors, such as intraarterial and central venous monitoring vary by institution and practitioner (Tables 75-1 and 75-2). The indications for pulmonary arterial catheters (PACs) are especially controversial. There are data from the intensive care setting suggesting that the PAC is harmful,[9] while other data indicate that it may provide prognostic information in the perioperative period.[10] Table 75-3 details specific indications for PAC that many practitioners accept.

The bispectral index is a parameter derived from a proprietary electroencephalographic analysis technology that has been shown to correlate with increasing sedation and loss of con-

TABLE 75-1 Indications for Intraarterial Monitoring

Major surgical procedures involving large fluid shifts and/or blood loss
Surgery requiring cardiopulmonary bypass
Surgery of the aorta
Patients with pulmonary disease requiring frequent arterial blood gases
Patients with recent myocardial infarctions, unstable angina, or severe coronary artery disease
Patients with decreased left ventricular function (congestive heart failure) or significant valvular heart disease
Patients in hypovolemic, cardiogenic, or septic shock, or with multiple organ failure
Procedures involving the use of deliberate hypotension or deliberate hypothermia
Massive trauma
Patients with right heart failure, chronic obstructive pulmonary disease, pulmonary hypertension, or pulmonary embolism
Patients requiring inotropes or intraaortic balloon counterpulsation
Patients undergoing surgery of the aorta requiring cross-clamping
Patients with massive ascites
Patients with electrolyte or metabolic disturbances requiring frequent blood samples
Inability to measure arterial pressure noninvasively (e.g., morbid obesity)

TABLE 75-2 Indications for Central Venous Line Placement

Major operative procedures involving large fluid shifts and/or blood loss in patients with good left ventricular function
Intravascular volume assessment when urine output is not reliable or unavailable (renal failure, urologic surgery)
Patients with tricuspid stenosis
Major trauma
Surgical procedures with a high risk of air embolism, such as sitting position craniotomies
Frequent blood sampling in patients who will not require an arterial line
Venous access for vasoactive or irritating drugs
Chronic drug administration
Inadequate peripheral intravenous access
Rapid infusion of intravenous fluids (using large cannulae)

sciousness.[11] While incomplete amnesia is rare with current anesthetic techniques, bispectral index use has been demonstrated to result in decreased propofol doses and faster recovery from propofol anesthesia.[12]

Transesophageal echocardiography is minimally/moderately invasive and has acquired a much larger role in intraoperative management. The availability of high-frequency transducers and color-flow Doppler mapping has enhanced the ability of anesthesiologists, cardiologists, and surgeons to make intraoperative diagnoses, evaluate hemodynamic aberrations, and assess the quality of cardiac surgical interventions inter alia. Practice guidelines for transesophageal echocardiography have been published by the American Society of Anesthesiologists.[13] Standardized intraoperative examination guidelines for multiplane transesophageal echocardiography have been published[14] and the National Board of Echocardiography has been formed to administer a certifying examination in perioperative transesophageal echocardiography. A list of indications for perioperative transesophageal echocardiography is presented in Table 75-4.

TABLE 75-3 Indications for Pulmonary Artery Catheter Monitoring

Major procedures involving large fluid shifts and/or blood loss in patients with severe coronary artery disease
Patients with recent myocardial infarctions or severely unstable angina
Patients with impaired left ventricular function (congestive heart failure) or significant mitral or aortic valvular pathology
Patients with pericardial tamponade
Patients in hypovolemic, cardiogenic, or septic shock, or with multiple organ failure
Massive trauma
Patients with right-sided heart failure, chronic obstructive pulmonary disease, pulmonary hypertension, or pulmonary embolism
Patients requiring high levels of positive end-expiratory pressure
Hemodynamically unstable patients requiring inotropes or intraaortic balloon counterpulsation
Patients undergoing surgery of the aorta requiring cross-clamping
Patients undergoing hepatic transplantation
Patients with massive ascites

CHOICE OF ANESTHETIC TECHNIQUE

The choice of anesthetic technique is inherently a difficult one because multiple factors must be considered. These include the desires of the patient, the requirements of the surgical procedure, and the patient's underlying medical condition. While a specific anesthetic technique is occasionally desirable for a particular procedure (e.g., spinal anesthesia for transurethral resection of prostate), it is extremely difficult to find scientific evidence that any particular anesthetic approach is superior to reasonable alternatives or that anesthetic technique per se influences patient outcome.[15,16]

There is controversy regarding the effects of regional anesthesia (with postoperative epidural analgesia) on cardiovascular morbidity/mortality in "high-risk" patients. Five prospective randomized trials have addressed this issue. Two reported reduced cardiac morbidity with epidural anesthesia[17,18] and three studies found no difference[19-21] (Table 75-5). *While some studies suggest that regional anesthesia and epidural analgesia have salutary effects in vascular surgical patients, the issue is unresolved due to the limited and conflicting clinical evidence. In addition,*

TABLE 75-4 Practice Guidelines for Perioperative Transesophageal Echocardiography

- Category I indications: Supported by the strongest evidence or expert opinion
  - Intraoperative evaluation of acute, persistent, and life-threatening hemodynamic disturbances in which ventricular function and its determinants are uncertain and have not responded to treatment
  - Intraoperative use in valve repair
  - Intraoperative use in congenital heart surgery for most lesions requiring cardiopulmonary bypass
  - Intraoperative use in repair of hypertrophic obstructive cardiomyopathy
  - Intraoperative use for endocarditis when preoperative testing was inadequate or extension of infection to perivalvular tissue is suspected
  - Preoperative use in unstable patients with suspected thoracic aortic aneurysms, dissection, or disruption who need to be evaluated quickly
  - Intraoperative assessment of aortic valve function in repair of aortic dissections with possible aortic valve involvement
  - Intraoperative evaluation of pericardial window procedures
  - Use in intensive care unit for unstable patients with unexplained hemodynamic disturbances, suspected valve disease, or thromboembolic problems
- Category II indications: Supported by weaker evidence and expert consensus
  - Perioperative use in patients with increased risk of myocardial ischemia or infarction
  - Perioperative use in patients with increased risk of hemodynamic disturbances
  - Intraoperative assessment of valve replacement
  - Intraoperative assessment of repair of cardiac aneurysms
  - Intraoperative evaluation of removal of cardiac tumors
  - Intraoperative detection of foreign bodies
  - Intraoperative detection of air emboli during cardiotomy, heart transplant operations, and upright neurosurgical procedures
  - Intraoperative use during intracardiac thrombectomy
  - Intraoperative use during pulmonary embolectomy
  - Intraoperative use for suspected cardiac trauma
  - Preoperative assessment of patients with suspected acute thoracic aortic dissections, aneurysms, or disruption
  - Intraoperative use during repair of thoracic aortic dissections without suspected aortic valve involvement
  - Intraoperative detection of aortic atheromatous disease or other sources or aortic emboli
  - Intraoperative evaluation of pericardiectomy, pericardial effusions, or evaluation of pericardial surgery
  - Intraoperative evaluation of anastomotic sites during heart and/or lung transplantation
  - Monitoring placement and function of assist devices
- Category III indications: Little current scientific or expert support
  - Intraoperative evaluation of myocardial perfusion, coronary artery anatomy, or graft patency
  - Intraoperative use during repair of cardiomyopathies other than hypertrophic obstructive cardiomyopathy
  - Intraoperative use for uncomplicated endocarditis during noncardiac surgery
  - Intraoperative monitoring for emboli during orthopedic procedures
  - Intraoperative assessment of repair of thoracic aortic injuries
  - Intraoperative use for uncomplicated pericarditis
  - Intraoperative evaluation of pleuropulmonary disease
  - Monitoring placement of intraaortic balloon pumps, automatic implantable cardiac defibrillators, or pulmonary artery catheters
  - Intraoperative monitoring of cardioplegia administration

SOURCE: Modified from American Society of Anesthesiologists. Practice guidelines for perioperative transesophageal echocardiography. *Anesthesiology* 1996; 84:986–1006, with permission.

there are no studies that clearly determine whether or not local anesthesia with intravenous sedation is advantageous compared with general or major regional anesthetic techniques.[5] Therefore, it is essential that the cardiologist/internist does not specifically exclude any anesthetic technique during a preoperative consultation.

Regional anesthetics are not infrequently converted to general anesthetics intraoperatively due to unexpectedly long surgery, patient discomfort, or changes in the surgical plan. No anesthesiologist can be certain that a particular technique will be adequate for the surgical procedure, given the unpredictability of the situation, and the anesthesiologist must have flexibility to alter the technique as needed.

Regional Anesthesia

The term *regional anesthesia* was coined by Cushing for operations where local anesthetics were used on localized areas of the body without loss of consciousness. The advantages of regional anesthesia include simplicity, low cost, and minimal equipment requirements. Many of the adverse effects of general anesthesia are avoided, such as myocardial and respiratory depression.

TABLE 75-5 Clinical Trials Evaluating Effects of Neuraxial Anesthesia on Cardiovascular Morbidity

Study	N	Population	Cardiac Morbidity	Vascular Graft Patency Rate
Yeager et al.[17]	53	Mixed	Reduced with epidural	Not reported
Tuman et al.[18]	80	Vascular surgery	Reduced with epidural	Improved with epidural
Baron et al.[19]	173	Aortic surgery	No difference	Not reported
Christopherson et al.[21]	100	Lower extremity Vascular surgery	No difference	Improved with epidural
Bode et al.[20]	423	Lower extremity Vascular surgery	No difference	Not reported

SOURCE: Modified from Christopherson R, Norris EJ: Regional versus general anesthesia. In: Reich DL, ed. *Anesthesiology Clinics of North America,* Vol. 15. Philadelphia, Saunders; 1997:37, with permission.

The disadvantages include patients' reluctance to be awake in the operating room, anesthetic agents of insufficient duration, and local anesthetic toxicity.

There is little evidence that regional or local anesthesia with intravenous sedation offers improved cardiac morbidity in high-risk patients.

The cardiovascular side effects of regional anesthesia vary depending on the technique chosen. Spinal and epidural anesthesia, for example, may cause major decreases in cardiac preload and afterload, while local anesthetic infiltration and axillary nerve blocks have almost no cardiovascular side effects. Regional anesthetics are contraindicated in anticoagulated patients and those with coagulopathies. Regional anesthesia may also be combined with general anesthesia in adults and children in order to decrease the requirements for the general anesthetic agents and for postoperative analgesia. The institution of analgesia prior to surgical stimulation (preemptive analgesia) may have salutary effects on postoperative pain control.

LOCAL ANESTHESIC AGENTS

The local anesthetics are classified on the basis of their chemical structure as esters or amides. The esters are hydrolyzed by esterases in the plasma, and the amides are metabolized in the liver. The duration of action of local anesthetic agents is affected by the protein-binding characteristics of the molecule and the addition of vasoconstrictors to the local anesthetic solution.[22] Toxic reactions to local anesthetics are generally characterized by central nervous system excitation (seizures), which may be followed by central nervous system depression and cardiovascular collapse.

Cocaine is the original ester local anesthetic. Its clinical use is mainly restricted to topical anesthesia of the nose and airway. It is the only local anesthetic agent that is intrinsically vasoconstrictive, an effect resulting from blockade of catecholamine reuptake at sympathetic nerve terminals. Cocaine's sympathomimetic effects result in central nervous system excitation, which increases requirements for general anesthetics. Cocaine toxicity has resulted in deaths from central nervous system toxicity and arrhythmias.[23] Cocaine can also elicit myocardial ischemia. The tachycardia associated with cocaine contraindicates its use in patients with coronary artery disease, mitral stenosis, or obstructive cardiomyopathy (see also Chap. 71).

Tetracaine is a long-acting ester local anesthetic used in spinal anesthesia. It is also used for topical anesthesia of the eye and airway, but may be toxic in the larger doses required for airway topical anesthesia. Chloroprocaine is a short-acting ester local anesthetic that is used in epidural anesthesia. This agent is rapidly metabolized by serum cholinesterase, leading to a low incidence of toxic reactions.

Compared to the esters, the amide local anesthetics are less rapidly metabolized (in the liver), and the potential for toxic reactions is somewhat greater. Some amide compounds (e.g., lidocaine) also have potent antiarrhythmic actions (see also Chap. 27). Lidocaine and mepivacaine are agents of intermediate duration of action that are commonly used in many types of regional blocks. Etidocaine and bupivacaine are agents of higher potency and longer duration of action that also exhibit more toxicity. Bupivacaine is particularly associated with cardiovascular collapse and arrhythmias upon inadvertent intravascular injection. Ropivacaine is the first new local anesthetic in two decades. It is similar in potency and duration to bupivacaine, but appears to have less cardiovascular toxicity and to cause less motor block.[24]

Epinephrine and phenylephrine may be added to local anesthetic solutions to prolong their duration of action by local vasoconstriction. Epinephrine is typically added in concentrations ranging from 2.5 μg/mL (1:400,000) to 10 μg/mL (1:100,000) for infiltration, nerve blocks, or epidural anesthesia. The systemic absorption of epinephrine occurs slowly and beta-adrenergic effects predominate, resulting in slight tachycardia and diastolic hypotension. In patients whose cardiovascular disease precludes the use of epinephrine, phenylephrine may be substituted at concentrations 10 times higher than that of epinephrine. Epinephrine may induce ventricular arrhythmias in patients anesthetized with halothane (see "Halothane" later).

SPINAL ANESTHESIA

The injection into the subarachnoid space of a relatively small dose of local anesthetic that produces profound motor and sensory blockade is known as spinal anesthesia. Spinal anesthesia also produces blockade of preganglionic sympathetic fibers, which usually results in hypotension. The level of spinal anesthesia is controlled by injection of a hyperbaric or hypobaric solution into the cerebrospinal fluid. The position of the patient is then manipulated to lateralize the blockade or to move the bolus of anesthetic in a more cephalad or caudad direction.

The level of sympathetic blockade is generally two dermatomal segments higher than that of the sensory dermatomal level.

The higher the level of sympathetic blockade, the more profound the arterial and venous vasodilation and postural hypotension. Intravenous hydration with crystalloid solutions is the primary treatment for hypotension. Intravenous boluses of ephedrine (5 to 10 mg) or phenylephrine (20 to 100 μg) are also used to temporarily increase the blood pressure during periods of relative hypovolemia. If the dermatomal level of sympathetic blockade reaches T1, then the patient is effectively sympathectomized. The loss of cardiac accelerator fiber function may lead to bradycardia. Complete sympathectomy always occurs with a "total spinal," which also produces respiratory insufficiency due to intercostal and phrenic nerve root blockade.

Spinal anesthesia must be undertaken cautiously, and with more intensive monitoring, in patients whose cardiovascular stability depends upon the maintenance of a high preload and afterload. Patients with any significant cardiac valvular disease, hypertrophic obstructive cardiomyopathy, or tetralogy of Fallot are prone to hemodynamic decompensation during spinal anesthesia. Patients with coronary artery disease usually tolerate spinal anesthesia well, so long as diastolic arterial pressure is maintained at an appropriate level to preserve coronary perfusion pressure.

EPIDURAL ANESTHESIA

The epidural space, which is filled with loose areolar tissue and a venous plexus, lies immediately external to the dura mater. An indwelling catheter is usually placed percutaneously for intermittent bolus injections or continuous infusions of local anesthetic and/or opioids. The epidural space may be entered by thoracic, lumbar, or caudal approaches. The advantages of epidural anesthesia are similar to those of spinal anesthesia and include moderate hypotension (which tends to decrease intraoperative blood loss) and contracted bowel loops during abdominal surgery. In addition, the ability to administer dilute local anesthetics and opioids through an indwelling epidural catheter is an effective means of postoperative analgesia.

The hemodynamic effects of epidural anesthesia are essentially similar to those of spinal anesthesia except that the onset of sympathetic blockade is more gradual. Thus, with appropriate monitoring, cautious administration of epidural anesthetics has been safely done in patients with mitral valvular disease, aortic stenosis, or hypertrophic obstructive cardiomyopathy. It should be emphasized, though, that intraarterial catheters and PACs may be required to monitor and treat changes in preload and afterload that occur with epidural anesthesia in patients with severe cardiovascular disease.

Generally, 10 to 15 times the volume of local anesthetic is required compared to spinal anesthesia. The potential for inadvertent intravascular injection of a toxic dose of local anesthetic is present. It is also possible inadvertently to inject a large volume into the subarachnoid space and cause a "total spinal" (see "Spinal Anesthesia" earlier).

The hemodynamic consequences of inadvertent intravenous injections of epinephrine-containing solutions may be significant for patients who cannot tolerate tachycardia. Epidural infusions of opioids for postoperative analgesia may be complicated by pruritus, urinary retention, somnolence, and respiratory depression. Thus, appropriate monitoring and nursing care are required.

COMBINED SPINAL-EPIDURAL ANESTHESIA

The injection of intrathecal anesthetic agents via a fine-bore needle through the epidural-introducing trocar followed by epidural catheter placement constitutes combined spinal-epidural anesthesia. The spinal anesthetic provides rapid onset and intense analgesia, while the epidural catheter permits the administration of agents for continued intraoperative anesthesia and postoperative analgesia.[25]

NERVE BLOCKS AND INFILTRATION OF LOCAL ANESTHETIC

Nerve blocks and local anesthetic infiltration may be performed to facilitate surgery of localized areas of the body. The brachial plexus may be blocked by interscalene, supraclavicular, or axillary approaches. The lower extremity may be anesthetized by blocking the femoral, obturator, and sciatic nerves. Local anesthetic infiltration is performed in regions such as the inguinal area to facilitate herniorrhaphies. These blocks, when properly performed, have minimal cardiovascular effects. They do require large volumes of local anesthetic solution, which result in toxic reactions if inadvertent intravascular injection occurs, however. Intercostal blocks are associated with high blood concentrations even without intravascular injection, because the neurovascular bundle enhances absorption of the local anesthetic and multiple blocks are required for clinical efficacy. Epinephrine is occasionally added to prolong the duration of block, but this may be contraindicated in certain patients with cardiovascular disease, such as those with mitral stenosis.

General Anesthesia

General anesthesia is defined as a reversible state consisting of amnesia, analgesia, immobility, and the prevention of undesirable reflexes. The general anesthetics include many drugs, almost all of which have cardiovascular side effects. Intravenous agents are nearly always used for the induction of anesthesia in adults. Anesthesia is maintained using inhalational agents, intravenous agents, or a combination of the two.

Neuromuscular blocking drugs (muscle relaxants) are commonly used to facilitate tracheal intubation and to lower the requirements for anesthetic agents (i.e., the dose of anesthetic that produces adequate amnesia and analgesia may not be sufficient to prevent movement or relax the abdominal musculature). In children, the induction of anesthesia is highly individualized according to patient needs, practitioner, and institution.

The physiologic consequences of general anesthesia have changed dramatically over the last several decades with the development of modern anesthetic agents. Ether and cyclopropane have sympathomimetic properties and were often used with spontaneous ventilation. Modern, nonexplosive inhalational anesthetic agents tend to be cardiac and respiratory depressants. With the exception of brief operations, most general anesthetics include tracheal intubation and mechanical ventilation. As an alternative to tracheal intubation, devices such as the laryngeal mask airway may be used to secure a patient's airway. The loss of consciousness is usually accompanied by a decrease in sympathetic tone. This, as well as the effects of positive pressure ventilation, causes a moderate decrease in cardiac output even when the anesthetic drugs are not myocardial depressants per se.

The patient with cardiovascular disease presents major concerns to the anesthesiologist. General anesthesia masks many of the symptoms of cardiovascular decompensation, such as angina, dyspnea, dizziness, and palpitations. Other signs of cardiovascular disease, such as tachycardia, are nonspecific and may be misinterpreted as hypovolemia or light anesthesia. Fluid shifts, obstructed venous return, and varying levels of noxious stimulation are other variables related to surgery that are unpredictable. It is for these reasons that appropriate monitoring and selection of anesthetic agents are vital to the intraoperative management of the patient with cardiovascular disease.

INTRAVENOUS ANESTHETICS

Intravenous anesthetic induction drugs are composed of lipophilic molecules that have an affinity for neuronal tissue or specific receptors. Their action is generally terminated by redistribution from the vessel-rich tissues (brain, heart, liver, and kidneys) to other tissues (muscle, fat, and skin). Elimination occurs via hepatic metabolism and takes place over several hours. Patients with diminished cardiac output secondary to cardiovascular disease will have prolonged effects from intravenous induction drugs.

Barbiturates Thiopental, an ultra-short-acting thiobarbiturate, is the prototype for agents of its class. It is quick, reliable, and pleasant for patients and does not have excitatory side effects. Its cardiovascular effects are marked by dose-dependent myocardial depression and dilation of venous capacitance vessels. The decrease in cardiac output is usually compensated for by arterial vasoconstriction, so that blood pressure is minimally decreased. Thiopental is a poor analgesic, however, and tachycardia and hypertension are common with tracheal intubation or any painful stimulus.

Standard doses of barbiturate for anesthetic induction are contraindicated in patients with preload-dependent cardiac lesions and/or severely impaired ventricular contractility. This includes patients with pericardial tamponade, mitral regurgitation, aortic regurgitation, mitral stenosis, and dilated cardiomyopathy. Reduced doses and slower injection of the drug will markedly decrease the cardiovascular effects.

Benzodiazepines Benzodiazepines may be used as premedication, to induce anesthesia, or as an adjunct to regional or general anesthesia. Their most useful therapeutic effects include sedation and amnesia. They tend to be unreliable in their rapidity of induction and occasionally fail to induce unconsciousness despite high doses. When used as sole agents, the benzodiazepines have minimal cardiovascular effects. When used in combination with other drugs such as opioids and potent volatile anesthetics, benzodiazepines produce hypotension, which may be due to myocardial depression or decreased systemic vascular resistance.

Opioids Synthetic opioids have assumed a major role in the anesthetic care of patients with cardiovascular disease. They can be used as premedication, as supplements to regional or inhalational anesthesia, as one of the main components of "nitrous-narcotic" anesthesia, or as the primary anesthetic agent (high-dose opioid anesthesia). They are often used as supplements during anesthesia induction to block the hemodynamic response to laryngoscopy and tracheal intubation. While opioids are excellent analgesics, they are unreliable amnesics, provide no muscle relaxation, and are associated with "breakthrough" hypertension and tachycardia intraoperatively.

A further problem with high doses of opioids is that they can produce truncal muscle rigidity, ocular movements, wrist flexion, and shoulder abduction—often referred to as "fentanyl seizures." These events, however, do not produce electroencephalographic changes characteristic of epileptiform activity.[26,27] The truncal rigidity does interfere with ventilation and requires the use of neuromuscular blockers. Ventilatory support is frequently continued postoperatively following high doses of opioids because the elimination half-lives of synthetic opioids are relatively long (1.5 to 4 h). The exception is remifentanil, a new synthetic opioid that is extremely short-acting due to ester hydrolysis. Continuous infusions of remifentanil are notable for the cardiovascular advantages of the synthetic opioids without the prolonged duration of effect.[28] The rapid offset of remifentanil's effect, however, must be counteracted by substituting another method of analgesia so as to avoid acute withdrawal of the opioid effect.

Despite the disadvantages noted earlier, high-dose synthetic (phenylpiperidine) opioid anesthesia does not depress myocardial contractility and is devoid of histamine release. It is therefore associated with markedly stable hemodynamics during anesthetic induction and maintenance in the majority of patients with cardiovascular disease. Nevertheless, patients with high resting sympathetic tone, congestive heart failure, and severe pulmonary hypertension are prone to transient hypotension during anesthetic induction. A mild bradycardia usually occurs on anesthetic induction due to an increase in vagal tone. The bradycardia is often advantageous in patients with diseases such as coronary artery disease or mitral stenosis. The bradycardia effect is reliably antagonized by atropine or pancuronium (see "Neuromuscular Blockade" later) in patients with conditions such as mitral regurgitation, which require faster heart rates. There is a trend to reduce the doses of opioids administered in cardiac anesthesia in order to facilitate more rapid tracheal extubation and discharge from the intensive care unit.[29]

Neither morphine nor meperidine is commonly used intraoperatively. Morphine is often used as premedication and for postoperative analgesia. With higher doses and rapid administration, morphine causes histamine release and is associated with hypotension and increased fluid requirements. It is also a venodilator. Meperidine produces tachycardia and histamine release, and it is a direct myocardial depressant. It has the lowest toxic:therapeutic dose ratio of the clinically relevant opioids.

Anesthesiologists only rarely administer naloxone or other opioid antagonists to reverse the effects of a systemic opioid in patients with cardiovascular disease. In surgical patients, complete reversal of the opioid effect results in the sudden onset of pain and surges in catecholamine levels. Naloxone administration has been complicated by pulmonary edema,[30] arrhythmias,[31] and cardiac arrest.[32] Low doses of intravenous naloxone have been safely used to reverse the pruritus and respiratory depression associated with epidural and intrathecal opioids without reversing the analgesia.[33]

Etomidate Etomidate is an imidazole anesthetic agent that enhances gamma-aminobutyric acid (GABA)-ergic transmission. It is associated with marked hemodynamic stability during bolus administration for anesthetic induction but does not blunt the hemodynamic response to laryngoscopy and tracheal intubation. This is one of the preferred agents for anesthetic induction in patients with valvular or ventricular dysfunction, hypovolemia, or pericardial effusion. Etomidate infusions are not used in the United States because of their association with adrenocortical insufficiency.

Propofol Propofol is a substituted phenol (diisopropylphenol) that may be used for anesthetic induction and maintenance. It is dissolved in a soybean oil and egg lecithin emulsion, which is mildly irritating on injection. Its main advantage is the rapid emergence and psychomotor recovery following termination of the drug infusion. Propofol may also be associated with reduced postoperative nausea and vomiting.[34] Propofol causes dose-dependent hypotension that appears to be due to a combination of myocardial depression and vasodilation. It is prudent to use reduced doses of propofol in patients with aortic or mitral valvular stenosis and cardiomyopathies. Propofol is used increasingly for sedation in intensive care units and to facilitate "fast-track" extubation following cardiac surgery.

Ketamine Ketamine is a cyclohexanone that is chemically related to phencyclidine. Its use as a sole anesthetic is limited by its indirect sympathomimetic effects and emergence delirium. Its sympathomimetic effects are advantageous, however, in certain groups of patients with cardiovascular disease. These include mainly those who are critically dependent on high resting sympathetic tone to maintain an adequate perfusion pressure: patients with pericardial tamponade, hypovolemia, and systemic-to-pulmonary arterial shunts. It is important to reduce the dose of ketamine in those with severe cardiac disease because ketamine is a direct myocardial depressant.[35] In patients who already have maximal sympathetic outflow, hypotension may ensue following ketamine due to an "unmasking" of its myocardial depressant effect. Ketamine is relatively contraindicated in patients who cannot tolerate tachycardia, such as those with coronary artery disease or mitral stenosis.[36]

Alpha$_2$-Adrenergic Agonists Clonidine and dexmedetomidine are alpha$_2$-adrenergic agonists that are sympatholytic, sedative-anxiolytic, antiarrhythmic, analgesic, and reversible.[37,38] Clonidine has also been demonstrated to reduce anesthetic requirements and improve hemodynamic stability during the intraoperative period. Once more convenient and specific compounds are developed, alpha$_2$-adrenergic agents may play a much larger role in the perioperative management of patients with cardiovascular disease.

INHALATIONAL ANESTHETICS

Inhalational anesthetics include nitrous oxide and the potent volatile agents. The study of the uptake and distribution of inhaled drugs with cerebral and cardiovascular effects is practically unique to anesthesiology, and cardiac output is a major determinant of uptake and distribution. The alveolar concentration of a drug is generally equal to the brain concentration. Thus, anything that hastens increases in the alveolar concentration of the drug will speed the onset of anesthesia. Two factors that speed the onset of anesthesia are a diminished cardiac output and an anesthetic agent with low solubility in the blood. Thus, patients with low cardiac output secondary to cardiovascular disease will have a more rapid onset of anesthesia. Intracardiac right-to-left shunting will decrease the onset of anesthesia, whereas left-to-right shunting has negligible effects.

Nitrous Oxide Nitrous oxide is an excellent analgesic but not a very potent anesthetic. Concentrations up to 75 percent may be given safely (so as to maintain an adequate F_{IO_2}), but incomplete amnesia and movement in response to painful stimuli are likely. Thus, nitrous oxide is nearly always administered with other anesthetic agents, such as opioids or potent volatile agents, and neuromuscular blockers. It is also chosen because its relatively low solubility in the blood enhances the rapid onset and termination of its effects.

Nitrous oxide is a weak myocardial depressant, which mildly stimulates the sympathetic nervous system.[39] It does not exacerbate pulmonary hypertension in anesthetized patients with mitral valvular disease,[40] but is nevertheless avoided by most practitioners in patients with severe right ventricular dysfunction. As a sole agent, its cardiovascular effects are minimal, but cardiac output is lowered in the presence of opioids. It also accentuates the negative inotropic effects of potent volatile agents.[41]

Nitrous oxide rapidly diffuses into closed air spaces within the body due to its low blood solubility, high lipid solubility, and high concentrations required. Examples of closed air spaces include bowel gas, pneumothoraces, and air emboli. Once equilibrium is reached, 75% nitrous oxide will quadruple the size of any of these spaces. For this reason, nitrous oxide must be discontinued if a pneumothorax or air embolism is suspected. It is often avoided in cardiothoracic procedures, particularly in children prone to paradoxical embolization, or after cardiopulmonary bypass.

Potent Volatile Agents The use of inhalational anesthesia with potent volatile agents is the most common anesthetic technique because of its relatively low cost, reliable amnesia, and bronchodilation, as well as its low blood solubility and overall safety record. All agents are myocardial depressants and vasodilators and produce some degree of hypotension. The hypotension provides some indication of the depth of anesthesia, as does monitoring of end-tidal gas concentrations and possibly the bispectral index (see "Perioperative Monitoring" earlier).

The effect of these agents is rapidly changed when the inspiratory concentration is adjusted. The ability to titrate inhalational anesthesia is advantageous when compared to intravenous drugs, because the duration of surgical procedures and the degree of surgical stimulation are often unpredictable. For this reason, low doses of volatile anesthetics may be added as supplements to nitrous oxide- or intravenous-based anesthetic techniques for the control of hypertension and the prevention of awareness (incomplete amnesia).

The frequent production of nodal (junctional) rhythm is also common to these agents. The loss of atrial systole may be poorly tolerated, particularly in patients with aortic stenosis, hypertrophic cardiomyopathies, or mitral stenosis. All potent volatile agents have the potential for interactions with calcium channel blockers and beta-adrenergic blockers. Negative inotropic and conduction effects of these drugs may be augmented by the volatile anesthetic agents; however, all cardiac drugs should be continued until the time of surgery.

HALOTHANE Halothane represented a major advance in anesthesia when it was introduced in the 1950s, but its use is restricted by its cardiovascular effects and the small incidence of hepatotoxicity. Halothane depresses the myocardium and the sinoatrial node but is not a potent vasodilator. Thus, cardiac output and heart rate are depressed in a dose-dependent fashion. Blood pressure is not severely decreased, because the decrease in systemic vascular resistance is less than with the other volatile agents at equipotent dosages. This hemodynamic profile is beneficial in situations where myocardial contractility (and oxygen consumption) should be kept low and perfusion pressure maintained high. Examples include ischemic heart disease, hypertrophic obstructive cardiomyopathy, and, especially, tetralogy of Fallot.[42] Halothane is contraindicated in patients with dilated cardiomyopathy, congestive heart failure, aortic stenosis, aortic and mitral regurgitation, and pericardial tamponade.

Halothane lowers the threshold for epinephrine-induced ventricular arrhythmias more than do other volatile agents. As a practical matter, the initial epinephrine dose is restricted to 1.5 μg/kg during infiltration of local anesthetic solutions. If arrhythmias occur due to an inadvertent vascular injection, the halothane should be discontinued. Approximately five times the dose of epinephrine is required to induce ventricular arrhythmias in patients receiving enflurane and isoflurane.

ENFLURANE Enflurane is almost equal to halothane in its negative inotropic effect, but it is more vasodilating and less of a negative chronotrope. Thus, cardiac output is better maintained, but blood pressure is lower than with equipotent dosages of halothane. Enflurane is a reasonable choice as a supplement to intravenous anesthetic techniques when breakthrough hypertension occurs. Enflurane has been used less commonly in recent years for various reasons, including its cardiovascular effects, metabolism to inorganic fluoride, and the emergence of newer agents.

ISOFLURANE Isoflurane is somewhat less negatively inotropic than enflurane or halothane and is a potent arteriolar vasodilator, which tends to maintain cardiac output. Tachycardia frequently occurs at clinical dosages because the baroreceptor reflexes are not impaired. On the basis of its hemodynamic effects, isoflurane would be beneficial in patients with mitral or aortic regurgitation with good ventricular function. It is relatively contraindicated (as a sole agent) in patients with mitral or aortic stenosis, dilated and hypertrophic cardiomyopathies, and pericardial tamponade. Isoflurane is frequently used in patients with coronary artery disease, when it is often combined with opioids or beta-adrenergic blockers to prevent tachycardia and the dose is limited to preserve coronary perfusion pressure. The use of isoflurane remains controversial in patients with coronary artery anatomy that predisposes to coronary "steal."

The coronary steal phenomenon occurs when a zone of myocardium distal to a stenotic coronary artery derives its blood supply from collateral vessels that originate in a zone of myocardium with normal coronary arterial supply. The arterioles in the normal zone are partially constricted, while those in the collateral-dependent zone are maximally dilated due to the "upstream" coronary artery occlusion. This maintains the pressure gradient across the collateral vessels and the perfusion of the collateral-dependent zone. Some arteriolar vasodilators (e.g., adenosine, dipyridamole, and sodium nitroprusside) can dilate the arterioles in the normal myocardial zone, decrease the perfusion pressure across the collateral vessels, and precipitate myocardial ischemia due to coronary steal.

Isoflurane has been shown to induce myocardial ischemia with collateral-dependent myocardial blood flow in canine models[43] and in humans.[44] It remains controversial whether or not isoflurane should be used in patients with coronary artery disease, given the uncertainty regarding coronary artery anatomy in most patients. The tachycardia and hypotension associated with isoflurane, as well as evidence of maldistributed myocardial blood flow, might suggest that it should not be used. Nevertheless, a prospective clinical study in patients with "steal-prone anatomy"[45] and large outcome studies[15,16] have not found intraoperative myocardial ischemia or poorer outcome with isoflurane anesthesia. A reasonable conclusion would be that isoflurane should be used with caution and appropriate monitoring in patients suspected of having "steal-prone" coronary artery anatomy.[46]

DESFLURANE Desflurane is a volatile anesthetic that was introduced into clinical practice in 1992. It is much less soluble in blood than the volatile agents described earlier. Its blood:gas solubility coefficient is similar to that of nitrous oxide. Thus, more rapid induction and emergence would be expected. This is particularly advantageous in ambulatory procedures. Several studies have compared emergence from anesthesia with desflurane with that from other anesthetics and have demonstrated that initial psychomotor recovery is faster,[47] but that hospital discharge criteria occur at about the same time.[48] The coronary vascular effects of desflurane are similar to those of isoflurane, but desflurane is not associated with tachycardia at lower doses.[49] Despite desflurane's similarity to isoflurane with regard to myocardial depression and vasodilation, desflurane has a unique sympathomimetic effect. This effect is seen with rapid increases in end-tidal concentration in the absence of preanesthetic medication. The sympathomimetic action of desflurane can be blocked by fentanyl, esmolol, and clonidine.[50]

SEVOFLURANE The relatively low solubility and minimal airway irritation of sevoflurane make it a very useful anesthetic for the inhalation induction of anesthesia.[51] Its low solubility allows rapid alterations in alveolar concentration during the maintenance period of the anesthetic, thereby improving control of the depth of anesthesia. It is now achieving rapid acceptance in the United States despite initial concerns regarding the potential toxicity of compound A (a breakdown product created in the presence of alkaline carbon dioxide absorbing materials).[52] Biochemical markers of the transient nephrotoxicity of compound A have been measured in healthy volunteers.[53] High fresh gas flow rates are recommended to decrease the concentration of compound A, and it is prudent to avoid its prolonged use in patients with renal dysfunction.

The cardiovascular effects of sevoflurane are similar to those of isoflurane and desflurane except that sevoflurane is not associated with increases in heart rate. Sevoflurane progressively decreases blood pressure in a manner similar to the other volatile anesthetics. In animals, sevoflurane appears to be a slightly less potent coronary vasodilator than isoflurane and has not been associated with coronary steal. Myocardial contractility is depressed in a manner similar to that of equianesthetic concentrations of isoflurane and desflurane, and it does not potentiate epinephrine-induced cardiac arrhythmias. In several prospective, randomized, multicenter studies in which patients with coronary artery disease or risk factors for coronary artery disease received either sevoflurane or isoflurane, the incidence of adverse cardiac outcomes did not differ between treatment groups.[54]

NEUROMUSCULAR BLOCKADE

Benzylisoquinolinium Compounds The benzylisoquinolinium series of nondepolarizing neuromuscular blockers are all derivatives of the curare molecule. Most of these compounds have histamine-releasing properties that are dependent on the dose and rate of administration. *D*-Tubocurarine, metocurine, atracurium, and mivacurium are associated with clinically important histamine release following the administration of bolus doses to facilitate tracheal intubation. The newer agents, doxacurium and cisatracurium, are not associated with histamine release with large ("intubating") doses. While older agents, such as *D*-tubocurarine and metocurine, are mainly dependent upon renal elimination, atracurium and cisatracurium undergo a unique form of spontaneous degradation that is organ-independent (Hofmann elimination). Mivacurium undergoes enzyme-dependent ester hydrolysis.

Aminosteroid Compounds Pancuronium is the classic aminosteroid nondepolarizing neuromuscular blocking drug. The atropine-like molecular structure contains two quaternary nitrogen groups. The tachycardia and hypertension associated with pancuronium have been linked to myocardial ischemia during coronary artery bypass surgery.[55] The anticholinergic effects of pancuronium, however, can be useful (e.g., in patients with mitral regurgitation) for preventing the increase in vagal tone that occurs with high-dose opioid anesthetic inductions. Vecuronium and pipecuronium have minimal cardiovascular effects at usual clinical dosages. Rocuronium has a more rapid onset of action due to its lower potency than the others and has minimal cardiovascular side effects. While pancuronium elimination is almost entirely renal, the newer compounds are also degraded by the liver.

The newest aminosteroid compound is rapacuronium. Following bolus administration, it is characterized by rapid onset of action (due to its low potency) and relatively short duration of action.[56] The side effects include mild histamine release, hypotension, and bronchospasm, but the degree of hypotension did not correlate with histamine levels.[57] Based upon these data, it should be used with caution in patients with preload-dependent lesions and pulmonary hypertension. It is not recommended for infusion use in intensive care, and repeat dosing should be undertaken cautiously due to the presumed accumulation of active metabolites.

Succinylcholine Succinylcholine, essentially di-acetylcholine molecularly, is a depolarizing short-acting neuromuscular blocker that is still used because of its low cost, rapid onset, and short duration of action. Its cardiovascular effects depend on whether nicotinic or muscarinic receptor effects predominate in a given patient. Thus, tachycardia and hypertension or bradycardia and hypotension may occur. Vagal effects tend to predominate with repeated doses or in children. In patients with various disorders (including neuromuscular diseases, recent burns, and massive trauma), hyperkalemic cardiac arrest may occur with succinylcholine administration because of exaggerated release of intracellular potassium from myocytes.

THE POSTOPERATIVE PERIOD AND CARDIAC COMPLICATIONS

Emergence from anesthesia is frequently accompanied by hypertension and tachycardia, which is most often due to incomplete analgesia, but may also be related to withdrawal from antihypertensive drugs, hypoxemia, delirium, or bladder distension. If an underlying modifiable cause is not identified, then intravenous drugs—such as nitroglycerin, labetalol, or esmolol—are frequently used to control hemodynamics in patients with cardiovascular disease. Shivering is another phenomenon that may occur due to hypothermia or emergence from volatile anesthetics. Shivering results in severe increases in oxygen consumption, which may be poorly tolerated by patients with cardiovascular disease. Although the mechanism is unknown, low doses of meperidine decrease or eliminate shivering.[58]

In patients with risk factors, there is a high incidence of postoperative complications, such as myocardial infarction, pulmonary edema, malignant ventricular arrhythmia, and cardiac death.[3] Pain, high catecholamine levels, hypercoagulability, hypovolemia, anemia, intravascular volume shifts, drug effects, and a low level of monitoring all probably contribute to this phenomenon. Prospective trials suggest that prevention of hypothermia[59] and beta-adrenergic blockade during surgery and the postoperative hospitalization[60] may decrease the incidence of these complications in high-risk patients.

Traditionally, the anesthesiologist has not played a major role in postoperative management following discharge from the recovery room/post-anesthesia care unit. This situation has changed with the development of multidisciplinary pain services that administer epidural analgesia and patient-controlled analgesia. As noted earlier, it remains controversial whether or not regional anesthesia and intensive postoperative analgesia are capable of reducing morbidity and mortality. It is conceivable that more effective postoperative analgesia decreases the deleterious effects of the stress response. Future efforts to reduce perioperative risk likely will concentrate on assessing the effects of more intensive postoperative hemodynamic, analgesic, and anticoagulation management.

CONCLUSIONS

The optimal perioperative care of patients with cardiovascular disease is the joint responsibility of anesthesiologists, surgeons, and cardiologists/internists. Any anesthetic agent or technique has the potential for producing adverse effects, and the margin of safety is reduced in patients with cardiovascular disease. It is the anesthesiologist's role to acquire accurate and relevant information from the preoperative evaluation, to apply appropriate monitoring technology, to select an anesthetic technique that is suited to the planned procedure and the condition of the patient, and to manage hemodynamic alterations and analgesic requirements in the perioperative period. As cardiovascular disease continues to become more prevalent in the surgical population and preoperative testing and intraoperative monitoring become more sophisticated, the need for effective communication between the specialties of cardiology and anesthesiology will become even more important.

References

1. Wells PH, Kaplan JA. Optimal management of patients with ischemic heart disease for non-cardiac surgery by complementary anesthesia and cardiology intervention. *Am Heart J* 1981; 102:1030–1040.
2. Goldman L, Caldera DL, Nussbaum SR, et al. Multifactorial index of cardiac risk in noncardiac surgical procedures. *N Engl J Med* 1977; 297:845–850.
3. Mangano DT, Browner WS, Hollenberg M, et al. Association of perioperative myocardial ischemia with cardiac morbidity and mortality in men undergoing noncardiac surgery. *N Engl J Med* 1990; 323:1781–1788.
4. Goldman L. Multifactorial index of cardiac risk in non-cardiac surgery: Ten year status report. *J Cardiothorac Anesth* 1987; 1:237–244.
5. ACC/AHA Task Force on Practice Guidelines. Guidelines for perioperative cardiovascular evaluation for noncardiac surgery. *Circulation* 1996; 93:1278–1317.
6. Mangano DT, Goldman L. Preoperative assessment of patients with known or suspected coronary disease. *N Engl J Med* 1995; 333:1750–1756.
7. Kleinman B, Czinn E, Shah K, et al. The value to the anesthesia-surgical care team of the preoperative cardiac consultation. *J Cardiothorac Anesth* 1989; 3:682–687.
8. American Society of Anesthesiologists. *Standards for Basic Intraoperative Monitoring* (Approved by House of Delegates on October 21, 1986 and last amended on October 21, 1998). Park Ridge, IL: ASA; 1998.
9. Connors AF, Speroff T, Dawson NV, et al. The effectiveness of right heart catheterization in the initial care of critically ill patients. *JAMA* 1996; 276:889–897.
10. Reich DL, Bodian CA, Krol M, et al. Intraoperative hemodynamic predictors of mortality, stroke and myocardial infarction following coronary artery bypass surgery. *Anesth Analg* 1999; 88:814–822.
11. Glass PS, Bloom M, Kearse L, et al. Bispectral analysis measures sedation and memory effects of propofol, midazolam, isoflurane, and alfentanil in healthy volunteers. *Anesthesiology* 1997; 86:836–847.
12. Gan TJ, Glass PS, Windsor A, et al. Bispectral index monitoring allows faster emergence and improved recovery from propofol, alfentanil, and nitrous oxide anesthesia. BIS Utility Study Group. *Anesthesiology* 1997; 87:808–815.
13. American Society of Anesthesiologists. Practice guidelines for perioperative transesophageal echocardiography. *Anesthesiology* 1996; 84:986–1006.
14. Shanewise JS, Cheung AT, Aronson S, et al. ASE/SCA guidelines for performing a comprehensive intraoperative multiplane transesophageal echocardiography examination: Recommendations of the American Society of Echocardiography Council for Intraoperative Echocardiography and the Society of Cardiovascular Anesthesiologists Task Force for Certification in Perioperative Transesophageal Echocardiography. *Anesth Analg* 1999; 89:870–884.
15. Slogoff S, Keats AS. Randomized trial of primary anesthetic agents on outcome of coronary artery bypass operations. *Anesthesiology* 1989; 70:179–188.
16. Tuman KJ, McCarthy RJ, Spiess BD, et al. Does choice of anesthetic agent significantly affect outcome after coronary artery surgery? *Anesthesiology* 1989; 70:189–198.
17. Yeager MP, Glass DD, Neff RK, Brinck-Johnsen T. Epidural anesthesia and analgesia in high-risk surgical procedures. *Anesthesiology* 1987; 66:729–736.
18. Tuman KJ, McCarthy RJ, March RJ, et al. Effects of epidural anesthesia and analgesia on coagulation and outcome after major vascular surgery. *Anesth Analg* 1991; 73:696–704.
19. Baron JF, Bertrand M, Barre E, et al. Combined epidural and general anesthesia versus general anesthesia for abdominal aortic surgery. *Anesthesiology* 1991; 75:611–618.
20. Bode RH Jr, Lewis KP, Zarich SW, et al. Cardiac outcome after peripheral vascular surgery: Comparison of general and regional anesthesia. *Anesthesiology* 1996; 84:3–13.
21. Christopherson R, Beattie C, Frank SM, et al. Perioperative morbidity in patients randomized to epidural or general anesthesia for lower extremity vascular surgery. *Anesthesiology* 1993; 79:422–434.
22. Covino BG. Pharmacology of local anaesthetic agents. *Br J Anaesth* 1986; 58:701–716.
23. Fleming JA, Byck R, Barash PG. Pharmacology and therapeutic applications of cocaine. *Anesthesiology* 1990; 73:518–531.
24. McClure JH. Ropivacaine. *Br J Anaesth* 1996; 76:300–307.
25. Felsby S, Juelsgaard P. Combined spinal and epidural anesthesia. *Anesth Analg* 1995; 80:821–826.
26. Smith NT, Benthuysen JL, Bickford RG, et al. Seizures during opioid anesthetic induction—Are they opioid-induced rigidity? *Anesthesiology* 1989; 71:852–862.
27. Murkin JM, Moldenhauer CC, Hug CC Jr, Epstein CM. Absence of seizures during induction of anesthesia with high-dose fentanyl. *Anesth Analg* 1984; 63:489–494.
28. Dershwitz M, Randel GI, Rosow CE, et al. Initial clinical experience with remifentanil, a new opioid metabolized by esterases. *Anesth Analg* 1995; 81:619–623.
29. Cheng DCH. Fast track cardiac surgery pathways: Early extubation, process of care, and cost containment. *Anesthesiology* 1998; 88:1429–1433.
30. Prough DS, Roy R, Bumgarner J, Shannon G. Acute pulmonary edema in healthy teenagers following conservative doses of intravenous naloxone. *Anesthesiology* 1984; 60:485–486.
31. Azar I, Turndorf H. Severe hypertension and multiple atrial premature contractions following naloxone administration. *Anesth Analg* 1979; 58:524–525.
32. Andree RA. Sudden death following naloxone administration. *Anesth Analg* 1980; 59:782–784.
33. Bell SD, Seltzer JL. Postoperative pain management. In: Kaplan JA, ed. *Vascular Anesthesia.* New York: Churchill-Livingstone; 1991:565.
34. Ewalenko P, Janny S, Dejonckheere M, et al. Antiemetic effect of subhypnotic doses of propofol after thyroidectomy. *Br J Anaesth* 1996; 77:463–467.
35. Kunst G, Martin E, Graf BM, et al. Actions of ketamine and its isomers on contractility and calcium transients in human myocardium. *Anesthesiology* 1999; 90:1363–1371.
36. Reich DL, Silvay G. Ketamine: An update on the first 25 years of clinical experience. *Can J Anaesth* 1989; 36:186–197.
37. Flacke JW. Alpha2-adrenergic agonists in cardiovascular anesthesia. *J Cardiothorac Vasc Anesth* 1992; 6:344–359.
38. Maze M, Tranquilli W. Alpha2-agonists: Defining the role in clinical anesthesia. *Anesthesiology* 1991; 74:581–605.
39. Ebert TJ, Kampine JP. Nitrous oxide augments sympathetic outflow: Direct evidence from human peroneal nerve recordings. *Anesth Analg* 1989; 69:444–449.
40. Konstadt SN, Reich DL, Thys DM. Nitrous oxide does not exacerbate pulmonary hypertension or ventricular dysfunction in patients with mitral valvular disease. *Can J Anaesth* 1990; 37:613–617.
41. Stowe DF, Monroe SM, Marijic J, et al. Comparison of halothane, enflurane, and isoflurane with nitrous oxide on contractility and oxygen supply and demand in isolated hearts. *Anesthesiology* 1991; 75:1062–1074.
42. Samuelson PN, Lell WA. Tetralogy of Fallot. In: Lake CL, ed. *Pediatric Cardiac Anesthesia*, 3d ed. Stamford, CT: Appleton & Lange; 1998:303.

43. Buffington CW, Romson JL, Levine A, et al. Isoflurane induces coronary steal in a canine model of chronic coronary occlusion. *Anesthesiology* 1987; 66:280–292.
44. Reiz S, Balfors E, Sorensen MB, et al. Isoflurane: A powerful coronary vasodilator in patients with coronary artery disease. *Anesthesiology* 1983; 59:91–97.
45. Pulley DD, Kirvassilis GV, Kelermenos N, et al. Regional and global myocardial circulatory and metabolic effects of isoflurane and halothane in patients with steal-prone coronary anatomy. *Anesthesiology* 1991; 75:756–766.
46. Priebe HJ. Isoflurane and coronary hemodynamics. *Anesthesiology* 1989; 71:960–976.
47. Smiley RM, Ornstein E, Matteo RS, et al. Desflurane and isoflurane in surgical patients: Comparison of emergence time. *Anesthesiology* 1991; 74:425–428.
48. Apfelbaum JL, Lichtor JL, Lane BS, et al. Awakening, clinical recovery, and psychomotor effects after desflurane and propofol anesthesia. *Anesth Analg* 1996; 83:721–725.
49. Saidman LJ. The role of desflurane in the practice of anesthesia. *Anesthesiology* 1991; 74:399–401.
50. Weiskopf RB, Eger EI II, Noorani M, Daniel M. Fentanyl, esmolol, and clonidine blunt the transient cardiovascular stimulation induced by desflurane in humans. *Anesthesiology* 1994; 81:1350–1355.
51. Epstein RH, Stein AL, Marr AT, Lessin JB. High concentration versus incremental induction of anesthesia with sevoflurane in children: A comparison of induction times, vital signs, and complications. *J Clin Anesth* 1998; 10:41–45.
52. Smith I, Nathanson MH, White PF. The role of sevoflurane in outpatient anesthesia. *Anesth Analg* 1995; 81(6 suppl):S67–S72.
53. Goldberg ME, Cantillo J, Gratz I, et al. Dose of compound A, not sevoflurane, determines changes in the biochemical markers of renal injury in healthy volunteers. *Anesth Analg* 1999; 88:437–454.
54. Ebert TJ, Harkin CP, Muzi M. Cardiovascular responses to sevoflurane: A review. *Anesth Analg* 1995; 81(6 suppl):S11–S22.
55. Thomson IR, Putnins CL. Adverse effects of pancuronium during high-dose fentanyl anesthesia for coronary artery bypass grafting. *Anesthesiology* 1985; 62:708–713.
56. Wright PM, Brown R, Lau M, Fisher DM. A pharmacodynamic explanation for the rapid onset/offset of rapacuronium bromide. *Anesthesiology* 1999; 90:16–23.
57. Levy JH, Pitts M, Thanopoulos A, et al. The effects of rapacuronium on histamine release and hemodynamics in adult patients undergoing general anesthesia. *Anesth Analg* 1999; 89:290–295.
58. Guffin A, Girard D, Kaplan JA. Shivering following cardiac surgery: Hemodynamic changes and reversal. *J Cardiothorac Anesth* 1987; 1:24–28.
59. Frank SM, Fleisher LA, Breslow MJ, et al. Perioperative maintenance of normothermia reduces the incidence of morbid cardiac events: A randomized clinical trial. *JAMA* 1997; 277:1127–1134.
60. Mangano DT, Layug EL, Wallace A, Tateo I. Effect of atenolol on mortality and cardiovascular morbidity after noncardiac surgery: Multicenter Study of Perioperative Ischemia Research Group. *N Engl J Med* 1996; 335:1713–1720.

PART FOURTEEN

MISCELLANEOUS DISEASES AND CONDITIONS

C H A P T E R 76

THE CONNECTIVE TISSUE DISEASES AND THE CARDIOVASCULAR SYSTEM

Robert C. Schlant / William C. Roberts

The term *connective tissue disease* includes both a group of heritable conditions and a group of nonheritable acquired disorders. The heritable disorders of connective tissue associated with cardiovascular disease include Marfan's syndrome (MS), Ehlers-Danlos syndrome (EDS), pseudoxanthoma elasticum (PXE), osteogenesis imperfecta (OI), annuloaortic ectasia, and familial aneurysms.[1] The nonheritable disorders of connective tissue that may have major cardiovascular involvement include systemic lupus erythematosus (SLE), polyarteritis nodosa (PN), rheumatoid arthritis (RA), ankylosing spondylitis, systemic sclerosis (SS), polymyositis/dermatomyositis, giant-cell arteritis, the Churg-Strauss syndrome, the antiphospholipid syndrome, and possibly syphilis.

HERITABLE CONNECTIVE TISSUE DISEASES

Marfan's Syndrome

EPIDEMIOLOGY

The prevalence of the classic MS is about 5 per 100,000, without gender, racial, or ethnic predilection. Because of the great heterogeneity of the syndrome, the actual prevalence may be considerably greater, probably about 1 per 10,000.[2] MS has an autosomal dominant inheritance with high penetrance. In about 25 to 30 percent of patients, the disorder occurs without a positive family history and appears to be due to a new mutation.

MOLECULAR GENETICS

MS is associated with defects in the fibrillin-1 gene (FBN1) on chromosome 15, where 125 reported and unreported mutations (of several types) have been described[3–12] (see also Chap. 62). Nearly every genotyped family has a unique mutation in the fibrillin genes, with the most common single mutation identified in just four unrelated pedigrees. This intragenic heterogenicity and the large size of the gene have precluded the routine screening of mutations to establish the diagnosis of the MS.[9]

CLINICAL FEATURES

There is considerable variation in the clinical manifestations of MS, even within one family. The ocular, skeletal, and cardiovascular systems are characteristically involved. The four major manifestations include a positive family history, ectopia lentis, aortic root dilatation or dissection, and dural ectasia. Many of the other, relatively mild features of MS occur with a relatively high prevalence in the general population. These features include mitral valve prolapse, early myopia, scoliosis, and joint hypermobility. Other manifestations of MS include anterior chest deformity, especially asymmetric pectus excavatum or carinatum; long, thin extremities (dolichostenomelia) with arachnodactyly; tall stature with increased lower body height (Fig. 10-7); high, narrowly arched palate; myopia; fusiform ascending aortic aneurysm (*anuloaortic ectasia*) with aortic regurgitation (Fig. 76-1); aortic dissection; mitral regurgitation, which can result from a variety of causes, including mitral valve prolapse, dilatation of the mitral annulus, mitral annular calcium, dilatation of the left ventricular cavity, rupture of mitral chordae tendineae, papillary muscle dysfunction, or infective endocarditis; spontaneous pneumothorax; cutaneous striae; and inguinal hernia.[1,2]

In the absence of an unequivocally affected first-degree relative, requirements for the diagnosis include at least one major manifestation with involvement of the skeleton and at least two other systems.[12–14] In the presence of at least one unequivocally affected first-degree relative, there should be involvement of at least two systems; the presence of a major manifestation is still preferred, but this can vary depending on the family's phenotype.[12]

By echocardiogram, mitral valve prolapse occurs in nearly 60 percent of adults and aortic root enlargement in about 70

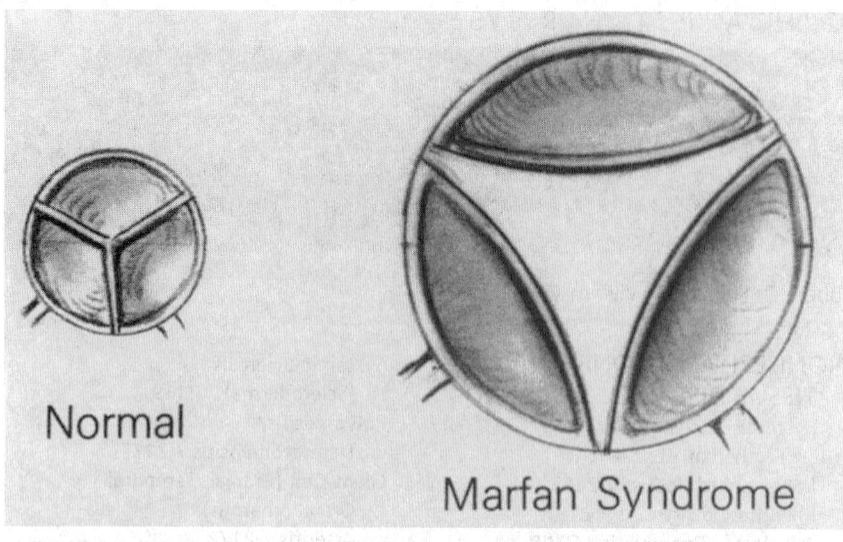

FIGURE 76-1 Mechanism of aortic regurgitation in Marfan's syndrome.

percent of adults with the MS.[15–17] It has been suggested that the MS and mitral valve prolapse are part of a phenotypic continuum.[17]

GENERAL EVALUATION

In addition to carefully recording the personal and family history and physical examination, the patient's height, arm span, and floor-to-pelvis distance should be measured. A slit-lamp ophthalmic examination and an electrocardiogram should be obtained. Patients with MS should be seen at least yearly, and a transthoracic echocardiogram should be obtained annually. Consideration should be given to obtaining a transesophageal echocardiogram or to magnetic resonance imaging (MRI).[18] If the diagnosis is definite or probable, consideration should be given to screening first-degree relatives by echocardiography. Genetic counseling should be offered to all patients. Psychiatric counseling also is often useful. If a patient develops suggestive widening of the proximal aorta, repeat transthoracic or, in some instances, transesophageal echocardiography should be performed more frequently. Patients with possible or definite MS and evidence of mitral valve abnormality should receive antibiotic prophylaxis prior to dental procedures (see Chap. 73).

MANAGEMENT

Patients with MS should avoid isometric, abrupt, or strenuous exertion; contact sports; scuba diving; and trauma. Patients with aortic dilatation and aortic or mitral regurgitation should avoid competitive sports.[19,20] Patients without aortic dilatation and aortic or mitral regurgitation should be allowed to perform low-to-moderate-intensity static and low-intensity dynamic sports, including bowling, golf, and archery.

β-Adrenergic blockade therapy should be used in all patients with MS to retard the rate of dilatation of the aortic root.[2,21,22] Although the optimal dose has not been established, some have suggested giving the largest dose that is clinically tolerated. Selective β_1-adrenergic blocking agents are preferred, although no randomized studies have been performed. Atenolol, which should be administered twice daily, appears to be the most widely used β-adrenergic blocker in this condition.

In asymptomatic patients, repair of aortic aneurysms has been recommended at different degrees of enlargement. Thus, some have advocated repair when the aortic diameter is 55 mm or greater,[23,24] at 60 mm or greater,[21,25–28] or when the aortic diameter increases to twice that of the uninvolved distal aorta.[29–32] Some patients develop aortic dissection with aortic root dimensions less than 50 to 55 mm.[33] Surgical repair is generally recommended when the diameter reaches 55 to 60 mm. Factors that encourage an earlier surgical intervention include a positive family history for aortic dissection or rupture,[34–36] severe aortic or mitral regurgitation, progressive dilatation of the aortic root on serial echocardiograms, the need for other major abdominal aortic or spinal surgical procedures, and planning for a pregnancy. In most patients, the ascending aorta and aortic valve are replaced, and the portion of the aorta containing the coronary ostia is reimplanted,[37] but there are exceptions.[38] Postoperatively annual assessment of the entire aorta by MRI may be useful.

In patients who require a mitral valve procedure, valve repair is usually preferred to replacement, although repair may not always be possible because of a large number of ruptured chordae tendineae, extensive annular calcium, or hugely dilated annuli.[38,39]

PROGNOSIS

While earlier studies indicated that the average lifetime is decreased about 35 percent,[2,40] beta-blocker therapy, antibiotic prophylaxis (against infective endocarditis), and aortic and valvular surgery have probably improved longevity. The most common causes of death of adolescents or adults with the MS are rupture of a fusiform aneurysm of the ascending aorta without longitudinal dissection (Fig. 76-2), ascending aortic dissection with rupture, or congestive heart failure from aortic and/or mitral regurgitation[33] (Fig. 76-3). The major histologic feature in the media of the wall of an aortic aneurysm is a massive loss of elastic fibers[33] (Fig. 76-4). Factors that can predispose to either aortic aneurysm or aortic dissection include systemic arterial hypertension, coarctation of the aorta, pregnancy, and trauma. In children with the MS, the most common cause of death is severe mitral regurgitation (Fig. 76-5).

PREGNANCY

Women with the MS should be counseled regarding the approximately 50 percent risk of transmission of the condition.[41] If the woman has moderate or severe aortic regurgitation or an aortic root diameter exceeding 40 mm, she should be advised that pregnancy greatly increases her risk of premature death. Women with an aortic root diameter of less than 40 mm usually tolerate pregnancy well, but nevertheless the chance of aortic dissection is increased by pregnancy.[42] β-Adrenergic blockers should be administered at least from the midtrimester onward.[43] There may be an advantage to the use of a selective β_1-adrenergic blocker.[44]

During pregnancy, transthoracic echocardiography should be performed every 6 to 10 weeks, depending on the initial findings. Using epidural anesthesia, vaginal delivery in the lat-

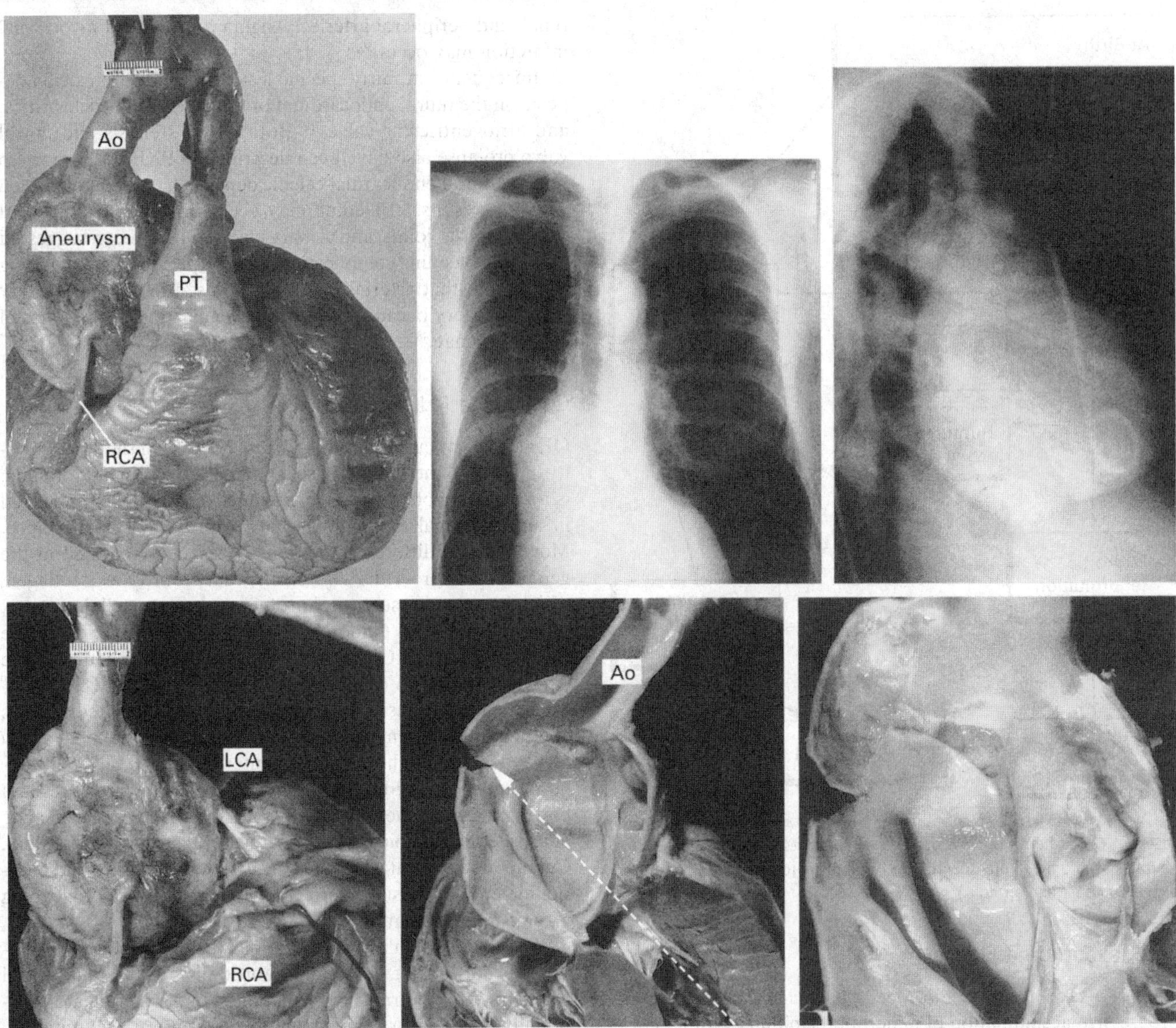

FIGURE 76-2 Heart and aorta of a 38-year-old man who was asymptomatic until exertional dyspnea appeared 5 months before death. *Top left:* Exterior view. Ao, ascending aorta; RCA, right coronary artery; PT, pulmonary trunk. *Bottom left:* Closer view of the massive aortic aneurysm after retracting the pulmonary trunk. LCA, left main coronary artery. The aneurysm does not involve the distal portion of the ascending aorta. *Bottom middle:* View of heart and aorta after removing their anterior half. Death resulted from rupture of the right lateral wall of the aorta at a point where blood ejected from left ventricle contacts the aortic wall (*arrow*). The aneurysmal bulge is mainly to the right. *Bottom right:* Close-up of the multiple healed tears in the ascending aorta. One of the previously incomplete tears ruptured through and through. Posteroanterior chest roentgenogram (*top middle*) and lateral aortogram (*top right*) show massive dilatation of the ascending aorta. (From Roberts and Honig.[33] Reproduced with permission of the publisher and authors.)

eral decubitus position is preferred, and forceps or vacuum delivery is recommended to shorten the second stage of labor. The increases in systemic blood pressure during uterine contractions should be prevented with beta-blocking agents. Postpartum hemorrhage should be anticipated. If fetal maturity can be confirmed in a patient who requires aortic surgery during pregnancy, a Cesarean section can be done before or concomitantly with thoracic surgery.[41,43,44]

Ehlers-Danlos Syndrome

EDS is a heterogeneous group of 14 or more disorders of connective tissue that are characterized primarily by skin fragility, easy bruising, "cigarette paper" scars, skin hyperextensibility, multiple ecchymoses, and joint hypermobility[1,45] (see Fig. 10-5). The numerous types of the EDS have different clinical manifestations, modes of inheritance, and natural history[45] (see also Chap. 62). In several types of the EDS, the heart, heart valves, great vessels, and larger conduit arteries may be involved. Some types of the EDS have spontaneous rupture of the aorta or large arteries, coronary or intracranial aneurysms, and arteriovenous fistulae. Other cardiovascular abnormalities in the EDS include mitral and tricuspid valve prolapse, dilatation of the aortic root, ectasia of the sinuses of Valsalva, aortic regurgitation, renal artery aneurysms, systemic arterial hypertension, and myocardial infarction.[46,47]

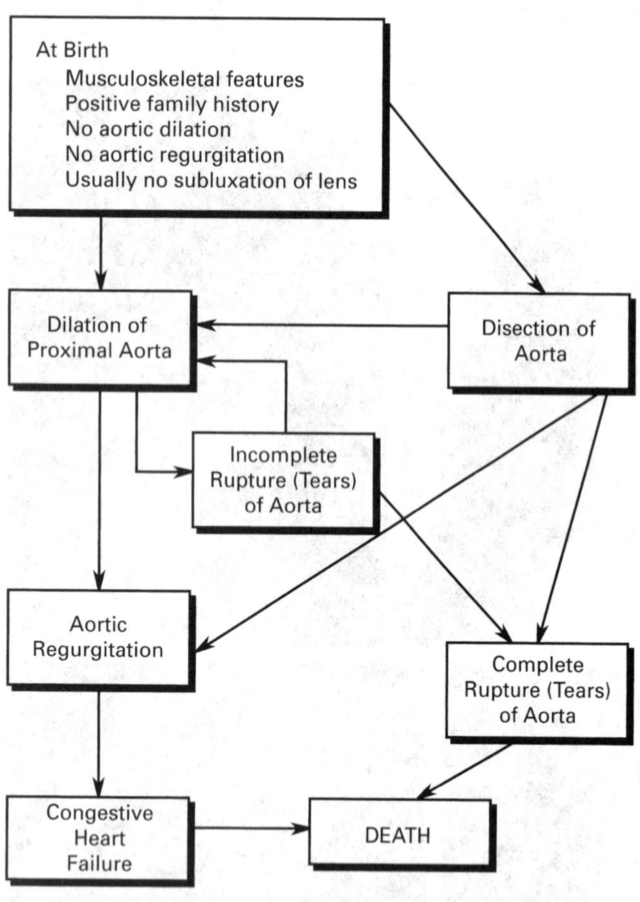

FIGURE 76-3 Scheme of development of cardiovascular complications in Marfan's syndrome. (From Roberts and Honig.[33] Reproduced with permission of the publisher and authors.)

Pseudoxanthoma Elasticum

PXE is a rare heritable disorder that is characterized by the progressive accumulation of mineral precipitants within elastic fibers, particularly those of the skin, Bruch's membrane, and blood vessels. It is transmitted either as an autosomal recessive or as an autosomal dominant trait.[1,48] The estimated prevalence is 1 in 160,000 (see also Chap. 62).

The elastic fiber changes cause skin, eye, gastrointestinal, and cardiovascular manifestations. The skin lesions have been described as resembling a "plucked chicken." Typically, there are yellow macules or papules that produce a rough, cobblestone texture and are maximal in the flexures of the lateral neck, axillae, antecubital fossae, groins, and popliteal spaces. They may form redundant folds of skin[1] (Fig. 10-6). The retinal changes include mottled *peau d'orange* hyperpigmentation, angioid streaks, and an increased incidence of retinal hemorrhage and disk drusen. Angioid streaks, which are breaks in Bruch's membrane behind the retina and are present in 85 percent of patients with PXE, usually develop after the second decade of life. They can be found in numerous other conditions, including MS, EDS, Paget's disease, and sickle cell anemia, although PXE is most common.[49]

There may be calcific deposits in the media of medium-sized arteries. Both vascular deposits similar to Mönckeberg's arteriosclerosis and intimal plaques similar to typical atherosclerotic plaques occur in the coronary, cerebral, gastrointestinal, renal, and peripheral arteries. Angina pectoris and myocardial infarction may occur.[50,51]

Infrequent but fairly specific lesions in PXE are calcific deposits in the mural endocardium of the cardiac ventricles, atria, and atrioventricular valves.[52] Both mitral stenosis and mitral valve prolapse also have been described in PXE.[53,54] Surgery to remove mural endocardial calcific deposits has been performed with fair results.[55] Bleeding may occur in the gastrointestinal system, uterus, joints, and urinary bladder. It has been suggested that some bleeding complications may be prevented by avoiding aspirin and that arterial grafts not be used in coronary artery bypass surgery because of possible calcification of the internal elastic laminae.[48]

Osteogenesis Imperfecta

OI, also known as *brittle bone disease* because of the susceptibility of affected individuals to sustain fractures from mild trauma, is a rare heritable disorder of connective tissue. It is inherited in an autosomal dominant fashion with variable penetrance. More than 80 different mutations have been identified in the genes for either of the two chains that from type I collagen, which is the major structural protein of the extracellular matrix of bone, skin, and tendon.[56] There is a wide variation in the clinical severity of OI, from some forms that are lethal in the perinatal period to other forms that may not be detected.[57–59] Most manifestations of OI are bony, ocular, otologic, cutaneous, and dental. The bony changes manifest themselves in a variety of ways, including short stature, in utero fractures, severe osteoporosis, and severe bone fragility, with repeated fractures and bowing of long bones. The ocular and otologic changes include blue sclerae, angioid streaks in the retina, and hearing loss. Cutaneous and dental changes result in easy bruising and occasional dentinogenesis imperfecta. An increased risk of bleeding may also be present.[59]

The cardiovascular manifestations include aortic regurgitation,[59–63] aortic root dilatation,[59] aortic dissection,[64] and mitral regurgitation.[65] Mitral valve repair and reconstruction are occasionally feasible for patients with severe mitral regurgitation, although most patients require valve replacement. Mitral valve replacement is difficult because of weakness and friability of the tissues and poor wound healing. In addition, some patients have increased bleeding despite normal preoperative coagulation tests and bleeding times.[59,60]

Annuloaortic Ectasia

Annuloaortic ectasia, a pear-shaped enlargement of the sinus and the proximal tubular portions of the ascending aorta, is often part of the MS, where it usually results in aortic regurgitation, partial or complete ascending aortic tears, or both. In some patients, annuloaortic ectasia is familial and no other stigmata of the MS are present.[66] The genetic and molecular changes in these patients are not established. Microscopically, there is severe loss of elastic fibers in the media of the ascending aorta.

Familial Aneurysms

Various types of familial aneurysms involving cardiovascular structures have been reported, including familial aortic dissection,[67] familial aneurysms of the ventricular septum,[68] familial aneurysms of the carotid arteries,[69] and familial intracranial aneurysms.[70] At this time, it is not established that these are heritable disorders of corrective tissue.

Homocystinuria

See Chapter 62.

NONHERITABLE CONNECTIVE TISSUE DISEASES

The acquired or nonheritable autoimmune or connective tissue diseases represent a subset of the arthritides and rheumatic disorders. These disorders are systemic in nature, are commonly linked by a diffuse abnormality of vasculature, and are characterized by inflammatory lesions in skin, joints, muscles, and connective tissue linings such as pleura and pericardium. Involvement of the kidneys, brain, and heart is usually responsible for the fatal and most serious consequences. Specific acquired connective tissue diseases that may have major cardiac involvement include SLE, PN, giant-cell arteritis, RA, ankylosing spondylitis, polymyositis/dermatomyositis, SS, and, possibly, syphilis (Table 76-1). Although certain immunogenetic factors have been identified, their etiology remains uncertain.[71]

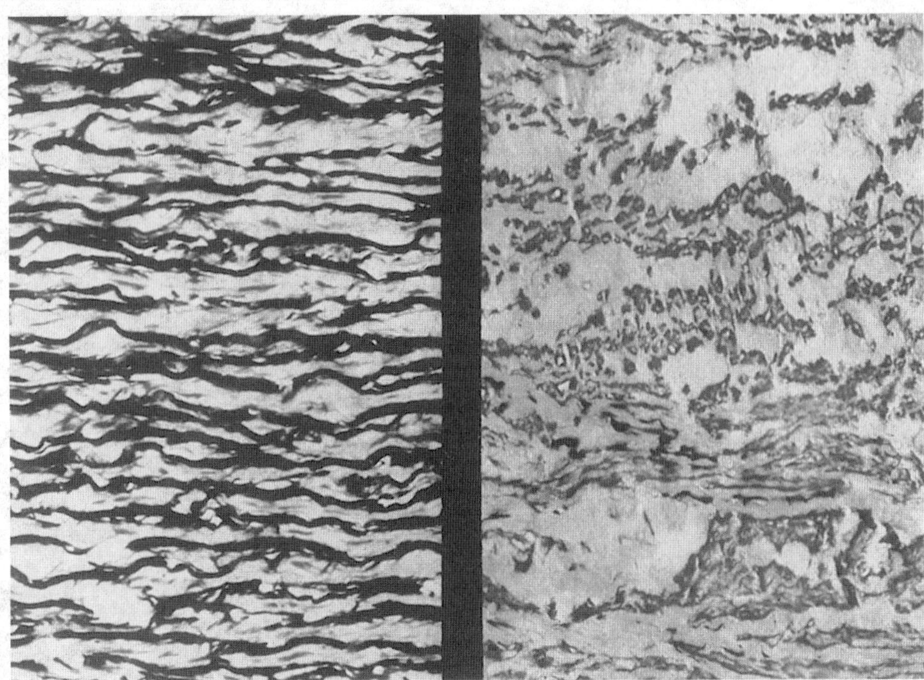

FIGURE 76-4 *Left:* Photomicrograph of the wall of the ascending aorta from a normal subject. *Right:* A similar histologic study (Movat stains) of the wall of an ascending aortic aneurysm in a 35-year-old woman with Marfan's syndrome. Note the virtual absence of elastic fibers. (From Roberts and Honig.[33] Reproduced with permission of the publisher and authors.)

Systemic Lupus Erythematosus

SLE, which is one of the more common autoimmune diseases, is found worldwide and affects all races, is more common among blacks and females of childbearing age, and is usually more severe in blacks than in whites. SLE is much more frequent among females than among males; in patients less than 40 years of age, the female-male ratio is about 8:1. In the United States, the annual incidence of SLE is about 8 per 100,000 and the prevalence is approximately 1 per 2000. The following genes of the human major histocompatibility locus antigens are associated with an increased risk for SLE: HLA-B8, HLA-DR2, HLA-DR3, HLA-DR5, HLA-DR7, HLA-DQ, and null alleles at the C2 and/or C4 loci. Genetic deficiencies of the complement system—i.e., deficiencies of C1q, C2, C4, and C8—predispose individuals to SLE and SLE-like disorders.

The inflammatory process of SLE involves multiple organ systems, including skin, joints, kidneys, brain, heart, and virtually all serous membranes. Its clinical presentation is varied and depends on the organ system(s) involved. Fever, arthritis and arthralgias, skin rashes (Fig. 10-24), and pleuritis are common early signs of SLE.

The immunologic abnormalities of SLE have been well characterized and enable it to be diagnosed despite the diversity of clinical presentations. Typical serologic abnormalities include the presence of antinuclear antibodies (ANAs), positive serum anti-DNA antibodies, positive anti-Smith antibodies, positive anti-ribonucleoprotein (anti-RNP) antibodies, and hypocomplementemia, i.e., low serum C3 and C4. Less specific but frequently identified antibodies include anticytoplasmic antibodies, anticardiolipin (IgGaCL) antibodies, antiphospholipid (aPL) antibodies, and rheumatoid factor. Serum complement is decreased in most patients with SLE, and, insofar as serum complement is usually normal or elevated in other connective tissue disorders (such as RA, PN, SS, and disseminated infections), this serologic test may be useful in the diagnosis of SLE.[72] Certain patients with SLE are more likely to have elevated levels of aPL antibody, particularly those with recurrent venous thrombosis, thrombocytopenia, recurrent fetal loss, hemolytic anemia, livedo reticularis, leg ulcers, arterial occlusions, transverse myelitis, or pulmonary hypertension.[73] Cardiac abnormalities may occur more frequently in patients with increased aPL or anticardiolipin antibody titers compared with patients without increased levels.[71]

Although it may have an acute, fulminating course, SLE most often is characterized by a chronic course marked with exacerbations and remissions; the 10-year survival rate exceeds 80 percent. Nephritis and seizures decrease survival approximately twofold.[74] When patients die of SLE, it is most often in the setting of acute renal failure, central nervous system disease, associated infection, infective endocarditis, or coronary artery disease (see below).

CARDIAC INVOLVEMENT

Probably about 25 percent of patients with SLE have cardiac involvement.[75] In addition to the valvular thickening or verrucae and mitral or aortic valvular regurgitation (or occasional stenosis), there may be pericardial thickening and/or effusion, left ventricular regional or global systolic or diastolic dysfunction, or evidence of pulmonary hypertension.[75] Either valvular regur-

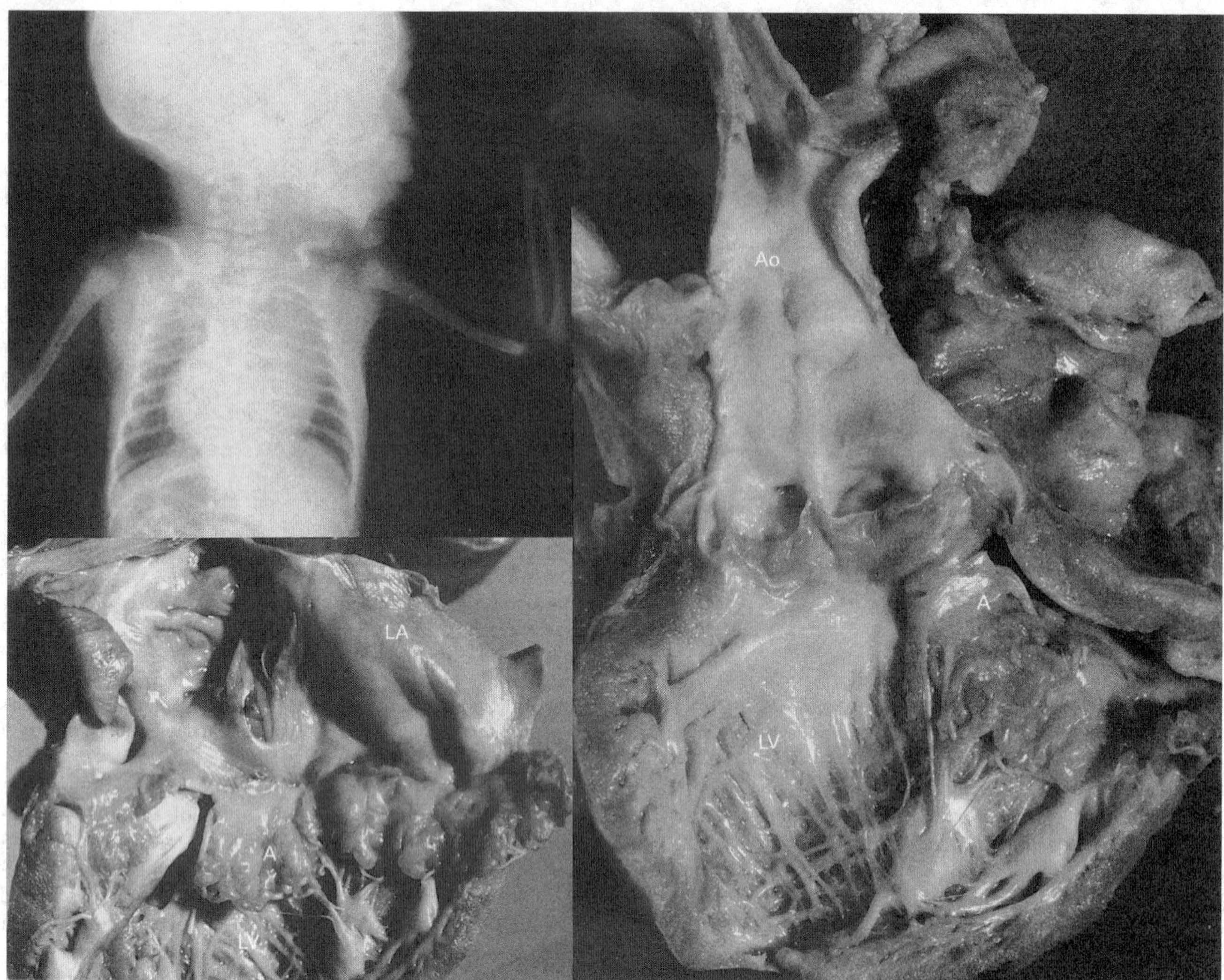

FIGURE 76-5 Congenital floppy mitral valve and floppy tricuspid valve in a 2-day-old boy who had long toes and fingers, a high-arched palate, and a grade 3/6 precordial systolic murmur typical of mitral regurgitation. The heart was enlarged (*top left*), and he died of congestive cardiac failure. At necropsy, the intima of the ascending aorta (Ao) was wrinkled (*right*), suggesting that the underlying media was abnormal at this early stage. Shown here are the opened aorta, aortic valve, and left ventricle (LV). A, anterior mitral leaflet. *Bottom left:* Opened left atrium (LA), mitral valve, and left ventricle (LV). The mitral leaflets are considerably elongated in both longitudinal and transverse dimensions. The left atrium is dilated. (From Roberts and Honig.[33] Reproduced with permission of the publisher and author.)

TABLE 76-1 Primary Cardiac Manifestations of the Nonhereditary Connective Tissue Diseases

Disease	Pericardium	Myocardium	Endocardium (Valves)	Coronary Arteries
Systemic lupus erythematosus	++	+	++	+/−
Systemic sclerosis	+	++	0	++
Polyarteritis nodosa	+/−	+	0	++
Ankylosing spondylitis	0	+/−	++	0
Rheumatoid arthritis	++	+	+	0
Polymyositis/dermatomyositis	++	++	+/−	+/−

NOTE: ++, major site of involvement; +, may be involved, but less frequently; +/−, rarely involved; 0, not involved.

gitation or stenosis due to SLE can require valve replacement.[75] It is unclear whether cardiac abnormalities are significantly more frequent in patients with elevated titers of aPL antibodies.[76-89] In general, valve disease in SLE is frequent but apparently independent of the presence or absence of aPL antibodies.

PERICARDITIS

SLE may cause a pancarditis with abnormalities of pericardium, endocardium, myocardium, and coronary arteries. Pericardial involvement is the most frequent, as observed clinically, by echocardiography, or at autopsy.[75] Pericardial effusions occur at some point in over half of the patients with active SLE. Signs of active or acute pericardial disease may precede (about 5%) the other clinical signs of SLE.[75] In most SLE patients, the pericardial involvement is clinically silent and, if manifest, runs a benign course. Pericardial tamponade may occur and should be considered in patients with unexplained signs of venous congestion.[75] On rare occasions, SLE pericardial disease may lead to pericardial constriction or to acute cardiac tamponade.[75,90] Although the size of the pericardial effusion usually is not sufficiently large to allow aspiration, serologic studies of the pericardial fluid can be useful in diagnosing pericardial effusions due to SLE.

The most common type of pericardial disease in SLE is the presence of diffuse or focal adhesions or fibrinous deposits.[75] The pericardial fluid usually contains mononuclear leukocytes and occasionally lupus erythematosus (LE) cells. In patients with long-standing SLE treated with anti-inflammatory agents, pericardial abnormalities appear to occur with the same frequency as in patients not receiving these agents, but at autopsy the involvement is less extensive and more likely to be fibrous rather than fibrinous. SLE patients with fibrinous pericardial disease, particularly those with severe debilitation or renal failure, are at increased risk for purulent pericarditis, which is usually fatal.[75]

ENDOCARDITIS AND VALVE DISEASE

The cardiovascular lesion of SLE that has received the most attention is the *atypical verrucous endocarditis* first described by Libman and Sacks in 1924,[91] long before SLE was recognized as a systemic disease. The lesions, as they were first described and subsequently attributed to SLE,[92] consist almost entirely of fibrin, and although they may occur on both surfaces of any of the four cardiac valves, they are now most frequently found on the left-sided valves, particularly the ventricular surface of the posterior mitral leaflet (Fig. 76-6).[75] These *verrucae* are similar histologically to those of nonbacterial thrombotic noninfective endocarditis, the valve lesion that occurs most frequently in patients with debilitating illnesses or cancer, except that occasionally hematoxylin bodies, considered the histologic counterpart of LE cells, may be found within Libman-Sacks lesions. While valvular verrucae in SLE (Libman-Sacks lesions) are usually clinically silent, they can be dislodged and embolize and can also become infected, producing infective endocarditis.[75,89] It is prudent to recommend antibiotic prophylaxis against infective endocarditis when patients with SLE undergo procedures that may be associated with bacteremia (see Chap. 73).

Echocardiographically, SLE has a characteristic appearance, with leaflet thickening and valve masses[75,89] (see also Chap. 13). The end-stage or healed form of the verrucous endocarditis of SLE is a fibrous plaque. In some instances, if the thrombotic lesions are extensive enough, their healing may be accompanied by focal scarring and deformity of the underlying valve tissue. This healed form of SLE "endocarditis" may cause valvular dysfunction, particularly mitral and/or aortic regurgitation.[75]

MYOCARDITIS

It is unclear whether infiltration of the myocardial interstitium with acute and/or chronic inflammatory cells and focal myocardial necrosis (i.e., myocarditis) occurs as a natural part of SLE, unassociated with anti-inflammatory drug therapy (glucocorticoid treatment).[75] Several reports have described clinical features consistent with myocarditis, but actual visualization of interstitial myocardial inflammatory cells with associated myofiber necrosis has not been demonstrated histologically. Hemodynamic and echocardiographic studies, however, have shown

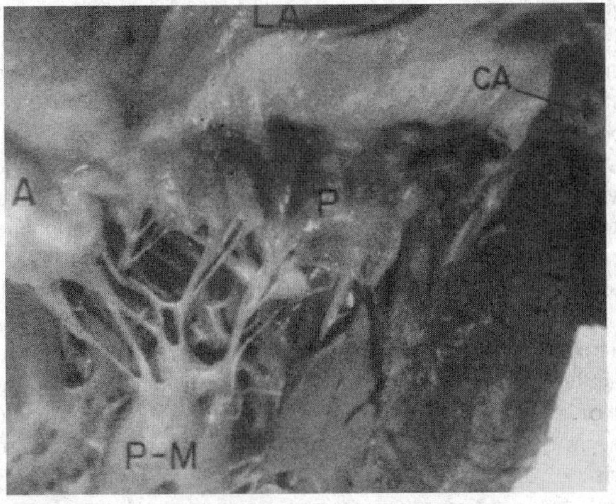

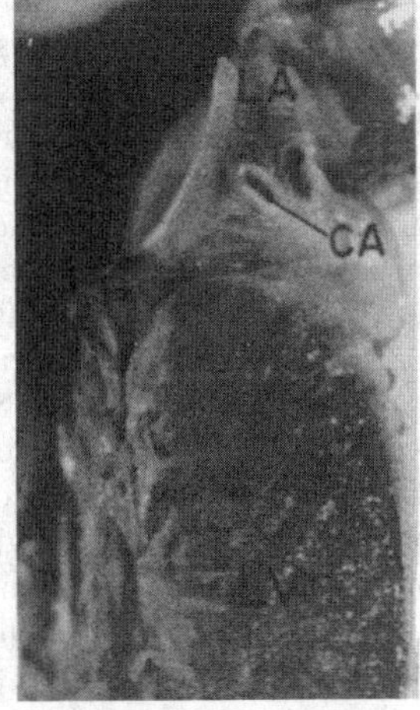

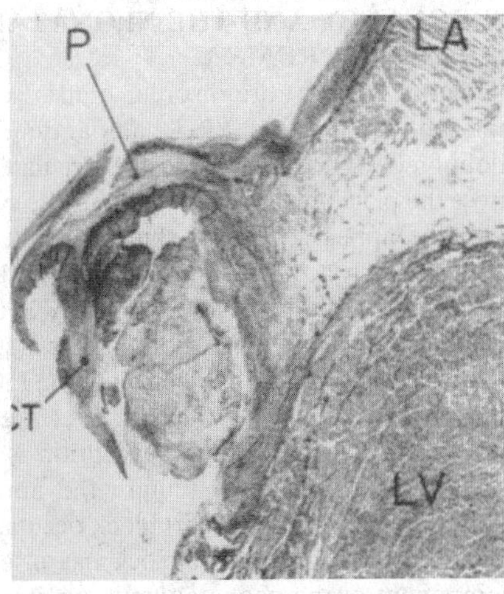

FIGURE 76-6 An example of Libman-Sacks endocarditis in systemic lupus erythematosus. *A* and *B*. The left atrium (LA) and left ventricle (LV) are open. *B* and *C*. Fibrofibrinous verrucae, present on the undersurface of the posterior leaflet (P) of the mitral valve, are often clinically silent. A, anterior leaflet of mitral valve; CA, left circumflex coronary artery; P-M, posteromedial papillary muscle; CT, chorda tendineae. H&E, ×8. (From Bulkley and Roberts.[87] Reproduced with permission from the publisher and author.)

abnormalities in both systolic and diastolic ventricular function in some SLE patients.[75] Whether these abnormalities result from an *autoimmune attack* on the myocardium or from the effects of systemic arterial hypertension, coronary artery disease, or coexisting pericardial disease is unclear (see below).

CORONARY ARTERY DISEASE

Both fatal and nonfatal acute myocardial infarction and sudden coronary death (without demonstrable infarction) from coronary artery disease may occur early in the course of SLE, particularly among young women. Studies of hearts in patients with fatal SLE have demonstrated a high incidence of coronary atherosclerosis in patients who received treatment with glucocorticoids for more than 2 years.[75,93,94] Accelerated coronary atherosclerosis is increasingly recognized as a leading cause of morbidity and mortality among young women patients with SLE who receive long-term glucocorticoid administration.[75,93] Although the causes of this premature coronary atherosclerosis are uncertain, glucocorticoid treatment as well as aPL antibodies have been incriminated. It has been speculated that SLE itself may induce an underlying vasculopathy or arteritis that may facilitate premature atherogenesis from long-term glucocorticoid treatment. Coronary disease in SLE was not described before glucocorticoid therapy was introduced.[75] In one study, the presence of elevated aPL antibodies in patients with SLE correlated with left ventricular (global or segmental) dysfunction, verrucous valvular (aortic or mitral) thickening, and global valvular (mitral or aortic) thickening and dysfunction, as well as mitral regurgitation and aortic regurgitation. Coronary thrombi may occur in patients with active lupus and an acute myocardial infarction in the presence of angiographically normal coronary arteries.[95] SLE also may cause coronary aneurysm;[96,97] aPL antibodies are known to promote platelet aggregation and to be associated with the presence of a clotting tendency, the so-called lupus anticoagulant syndrome.[76]

Inflammation (arteritis) of the wall of the sinus node artery in association with scarring of both sinus and atrioventricular nodes may account for some of the rhythm and conduction disturbances seen in these patients.[98]

PREGNANCY AND THE NEONATAL LUPUS SYNDROME

Neonatal LE is a rare disorder that arises when the so-called anti-Ro, or Sjögren's, (SSA) autoantibodies, mostly immunoglobulin G (IgG), are formed and circulate in pregnant patients, cross the placenta, and cause a lupuslike syndrome in newborns with the appearance of a skin rash and transient cytopenias from passively acquired maternal autoantibodies. Since the half-life of IgG antibodies is approximately 21 to 25 days, the neonatal lupus syndrome in newborn babies is self-limiting; it usually resolves in 3 to 6 months when all of the IgG-containing anti-Ro maternal autoantibodies have been cleared from the neonate's circulation. An unfortunate exception is complete congenital heart block, which may require the implantation of a pacemaker. Once complete heart block occurs, it is usually irreversible. Second-degree heart block has also been reported as a component of the neonatal lupus syndrome. One neonate has been described with first-degree heart block at birth that resolved 6 months later. Antibodies to the Ro (SSA) ribonucleoprotein complexes are present in over 85 percent of sera from mothers of infants with complete congenital heart block. In many patients, antibodies reactive to the La (SSB) antigen as well as the U1RNP protein particle are found in association with anti-Ro (SSA) antibodies.

In most cases, the neonatal lupus syndrome is a benign disorder, and most babies of mothers with anti-Ro (SSA), anti-La (SSB), or anti-U1RNP antibodies do not develop neonatal lupus. *A pregnant woman with SLE with positive anti-Ro, anti-La, or anti-RNP antibodies has a risk of less than 3 percent of having a child with neonatal lupus and congenital heart block. The risk that this patient might have an infant with the neonatal lupus syndrome but without congenital heart block may be as high as 1 in 3.* The neonatal lupus syndrome mediated by the presence of maternal anti-Ro antibodies can occur in babies of mothers who do not have overt SLE, who may or may not meet criteria for a diagnosis of SLE, and who may or may not have a positive test for antinuclear antibodies.

The neonatal lupus syndrome with congenital heart block can be diagnosed by the appearance of fetal bradycardia around week 23 of gestation.[99–101] The cardiac damage with conduction abnormalities in a neonate may result from binding of the passively transferred pathogenic anti-Ro antibodies to Ro (SSA)/La (SSB) antigens present in the fetal heart. It is not known whether these IgG anti-Ro antibodies represent *clinical markers* only or whether they are pathogenic. All mothers of neonates with complete congenital heart block have been HLA-DR3 positive. If a mother is HLA-DR3 positive and has circulating IgG anti-Ro antibodies, her neonate is at risk regardless of the neonate's HLA-DR status.

Other cardiac abnormalities reported in the neonatal lupus syndrome include right bundle branch block, second-degree atrioventricular block, 2:1 atrioventricular block, patent ductus arteriosus, patent foramen ovale, coarctation of the aorta, tetralogy of Fallot, atrial septal defect, hypoplastic right ventricle, ventricular septal defect, dysplastic pulmonic valve, mitral and tricuspid regurgitation, pericarditis, and myocarditis. Most of these patients eventually have a pacemaker inserted.

Pregnant women with SLE should have a serum anti-Ro (SSA) antibody determination as early in pregnancy as possible. Prenatal treatment of established congenital heart block has consisted of the administration of prednisone or dexamethasone and plasmapheresis from week 23 on, although heart block has persisted in most cases. It is unclear whether aggressive anti-inflammatory therapy in an effort to diminish the generalized fetal insult and to lower the titers of circulating anti-Ro (SSA) antibodies makes a difference in fetal cardiac outcome. Fetal echocardiography is useful in following the progression of the disease and also in helping to identify decreased left ventricular contractility, increased cardiac size, tricuspid regurgitation, and pericardial effusion.

Neither dexamethasone nor plasmapheresis has had much success in reversing intrauterine third-degree heart block. Glucocorticoids, however, may be helpful in suppressing an associated inflammatory response producing pleuropericardial effusions or ascites in the fetus. Close monitoring of the clinical course in the prospective mother is also essential because of the risk of exacerbation of the SLE. If fetal bradycardia is present, an *intrauterine therapeutic approach* for as long as possible is recommended to allow for fetal maturation to occur. Ultrasound images can be useful for assessing the degree of cardiac dysfunction present. Following delivery, the neonatologist should be prepared to have a cardiac pacemaker implanted.

Otherwise, all of the other clinical and laboratory features of the neonatal lupus syndrome (with the exception of complete heart block and/or similar severe cardiac fetal disease) should slowly and gradually disappear over the first few months of the baby's life. In one study, one-third of the children with autoantibody-associated congenital heart block died in the early neonatal period;[102] of those who survived, most required a pacemaker.

Women with SLE who are anti-Ro positive should be closely monitored during pregnancy, as should mothers of previous babies born with congenital complete heart block. Pregnant patients who are anti-Ro positive and whose babies have not had fetal bradycardia throughout most of the pregnancy should be reminded that congenital complete heart block is rare and that the neonatal cutaneous lupus syndrome is benign and transient. The long-term prognosis of the mothers of children born with congenital heart block is generally fairly good.[103] In these mothers, the risk of congenital heart block in children of subsequent pregnancies is low.[102] Newborns of mothers with SLE who have a normal pulse rate are unlikely to have significant abnormalities in atrioventricular conduction and do not need screening electrocardiograms at birth.[104]

A higher prevalence of clinical evidence of myocarditis and conduction defects is found in adult anti-Ro-positive patients with SLE than in patients who are anti-Ro negative or in healthy controls.[105] In general, clinical features consistent with myocarditis and conduction defects are relatively common in adults with SLE and seem associated with positive anti-Ro antibodies. Myocarditis at necropsy, however, is rare.[75] In most adults with SLE, positive anti-Ro antibodies have uncommonly been associated with complete heart block.[106] The role of the anti-Ro antibody in inducing heart blocks in adult patients with SLE is unclear.

SECONDARY EFFECTS ON THE HEART

Many, if not most, of the clinically significant cardiac problems occurring in patients with SLE are secondary. Systemic arterial hypertension is common in patients with SLE, particularly those with renal disease and long-standing glucocorticoid therapy, and is a major cause of cardiac enlargement and heart failure.[75] Pulmonary hypertension is also common, approaching 50 percent in a 5-year follow-up study.[107] Uremic pericarditis may occur, of course, in patients with severe renal failure. Premature or accelerated atherosclerosis has been increasingly recognized in young women with SLE receiving long-term glucocorticoid treatment.[75]

THERAPY

Therapy of cardiovascular SLE is the treatment of the underlying disease and includes nonsteroidal anti-inflammatory drugs, glucocorticoids, and, in severe cases, cytotoxic agents such as azathioprine and cyclophosphamide. Systemic arterial hypertension, congestive heart failure, and arrhythmias should be treated with standard therapeutic measures. SLE-induced valve disease can require valve replacement.[75,108,109] Pericardial tamponade may require either high-dose steroids, pericardiocentesis, or placement of a pericardial window, but recurrent effusions or pericardial thickening may develop. Premature cardiovascular events from accelerated atherosclerosis may result in sudden death or myocardial infarction.[75] The antimalarial agent hydroxychloroquine lowers serum cholesterol levels in patients with SLE[110] and may decrease myocardial ischemic damage.[111] An antimalarial such as hydroxychloroquine may be beneficial as a prophylactic agent to prevent premature or accelerated atherosclerosis in young women with SLE receiving long-term treatment with glucocorticoids. Although there are no studies documenting benefit, low-dose aspirin and hydroxychloroquine are often utilized in SLE patients receiving long-term glucocorticoid therapy.

Polyarteritis Nodosa

PN is characterized by segmental necrotizing inflammation of the medium- to small-sized arteries throughout the body, resulting in dysfunction of multiple organ systems. The commonly involved organs are the skin, kidneys, gastrointestinal tract, spleen and lymph nodes, central nervous and musculoskeletal systems, and heart. A variety of cutaneous lesions may be seen: livedo reticularis, palpable purpura, ulcerations, infarcts of distal digits, and nodules. Evidence of glomerulonephritis ranges from low-grade proteinuria to malignant hypertension and acute renal failure.

An association between PN and hepatitis B infection has been recognized for over a decade, and an association with hepatitis C virus infection has also been described;[112] hairy cell leukemia has been described in a few patients with PN. Although the erythrocyte sedimentation rate and serum gamma globulins may be elevated, and rheumatoid factor and antinuclear antibodies may be present, the final clinical diagnosis of PN rests on the combination of multisystem disease and biopsy evidence of active arteritis.[113] In PN, mesenteric vessel angiograms may show aneurysmal dilatation that mimics mycotic aneurysm in infective endocarditis. Since an inflammatory necrotizing arteritis may occur in a variety of disorders, other causes and types of arteritis must be excluded before the diagnosis of PN is made. Classed as separate entities are granulomatous or giant-cell arteritis, hypersensitivity angiitis, temporal arteritis, and arteritis involving the aorta and its major branches. The designation *microscopic polyangiitis* may more appropriately describe patients who have no arteritis, but who have small-vessel vasculitis affecting arterioles, venules, and capillaries. Also, arteritis associated with other connective tissue disorders, for example, rheumatoid vasculitis, is not thought to represent PN when arteritis is the major clinical disease presentation.[113]

CARDIAC INVOLVEMENT

The heart and the coronary arteries are frequent targets of PN. Most often this involvement is a vasculitis of the distal subepicardial coronary arteries just as they penetrate the myocardium (Fig. 76-7). The lesions are characterized by inflammatory infiltrates in the media and adventitia and occasionally by necrosis of the full thickness of the vessel wall, with prominent involvement of the surrounding perivascular connective tissue (Fig. 76-7). The lumens of the involved vessels may contain thrombi, and the walls may be aneurysmal. The latter is responsible for the nodular appearance of the arteries deemed characteristic of this disorder. An even later stage of the vasculitis process is evident as the lesions heal, first showing the formation of granulation tissue and subsequently fibrous tissue replacement of the original components of the artery. In this healing phase, intimal proliferation leading to coronary artery luminal narrowing is evident.[114]

The coronary arterial disease of PN may lead to myocardial

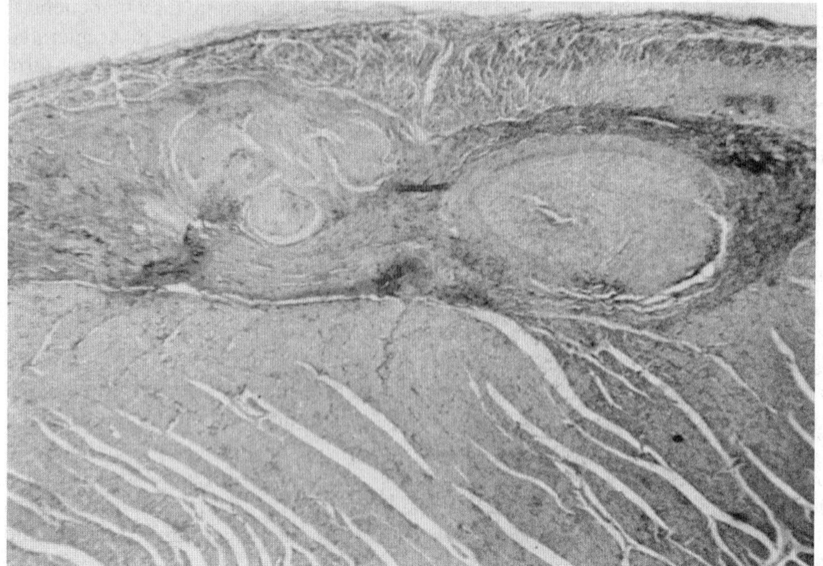

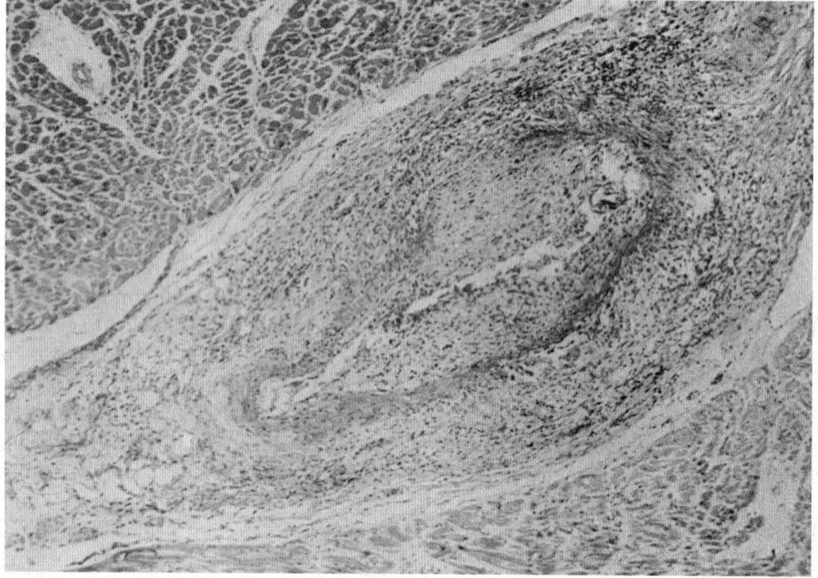

FIGURE 76-7 Polyarteritis nodosa. Examples of the necrotizing vasculitis affecting the extramural and intramural coronary arteries in polyarteritis. *Top:* Extramural coronary arteries. *Bottom:* Intramural coronary arteries. The intramural artery shows a necrotizing arteritis with inflammation involving the full thickness of the vessel. H&E, *top*, ×7; *bottom*, ×22.

infarction.[115] The myocardial necrosis and subsequent replacement fibrosis tend to be focal and patchy throughout the left ventricular wall. This is in contrast to the large areas of grossly visible, regional, subendocardial or transmural necrosis typically seen in the myocardial infarction caused by coronary artherosclerosis (see also Chap. 39).

Conduction system abnormalities have been identified in the heart of patients with PN. The size and location of the sinoatrial node and atrioventricular node arteries make them prime targets for polyarteritis.[116] Atrial and ventricular conduction disturbances may be a primary manifestation of PN, despite minimal involvement of vessels elsewhere in the heart.

Other cardiac abnormalities seen in patients with PN are those that are likely secondary to the underlying systemic arterial hypertension and renal disease. Cardiomegaly and left ventricular hypertrophy most often represent secondary cardiac manifestations of this disease. Similarly, pericardial disease may develop in a patient with PN, but this is most often due to renal insufficiency.

A new autoantibody identified in the serum of patients with systemic vasculitis, especially Wegener's granulomatosis, is the so-called antineutrophil cytoplasmic antibody (ANCA).[117] The ANCA test recognizes antibodies to azurophilic granules present in the cytoplasm of neutrophils. There are two types of ANCA: c-ANCA and p-ANCA. The antigen against which c-ANCA is directed is a 29-kDa serine proteinase. Approximately 90 percent of patients which Wegener's granulomatosis have positive c-ANCA antibodies, the *c* describing the cytoplasmic staining observed under fluorescent microscopy. In contrast, other vasculitides, including PN, tend to have a positive so-called p-ANCA antibody, the *p* describing the perinuclear staining observed in the immunofluorescent assay.

The antigen responsible for the p-ANCA antibody detection appears to be a myeloperoxidase. The detection of serum ANCA levels is a useful laboratory diagnostic marker in the evaluation of the systemic vasculitides, particularly c-ANCA for Wegener's granulomatosis. Serum p-ANCA positivity seems to be nonspecific. For instance, positive p-ANCA may be seen in other chronic inflammatory disorders such as Crohn's enteritis, Felty's syndrome, Kawasaki's vasculitis, leprosy, and tuberculosis. Therefore, the detection of a positive serum p-ANCA in a patient with the clinical picture suggestive of PN should not preclude the need for a biopsy or an angiogram.

CLINICAL MANIFESTATIONS OF CARDIAC DISEASE

Despite the dramatic involvement of coronary arteries that may accompany PN, the most frequent cardiovascular abnormalities seen in patients with PN are unrelated to the coronary arteries per se. Systemic arterial hypertension occurs in approximately 90 percent of these patients and, in combination with chronic renal failure, is the most likely cause of congestive heart failure, which may develop in up to 60 percent of patients.[113] Patients with PN also may develop acute myocardial infarction, which poses the diagnostic question of whether the myocardial injury is due to coronary arteritis with secondary thrombosis or to atherosclerosis, in a population that is typically middle-aged, male, steroid treated, and susceptible to atherosclerotic coronary artery disease as well.[115]

THERAPY

PN has a poor prognosis, especially when systemic arterial hypertension and renal disease are present. Treatment of the heart disease in PN is directed at the specific cardiac dysfunction, and glucocorticoid and other anti-inflammatory agents are administered for the underlying disease. Glucocorticoids are still the initial mainstay of therapy, although they can aggravate coexisting hypertension and even atherosclerosis. Often added to the treatment regimen are glucocorticoid-sparing agents such as cyclophosphamide, azathioprine, or methotrexate. The use of warfarin remains controversial; low-dose aspirin, however, is usually recommended.

Rheumatoid Arthritis

RA, the most common of the connective tissue diseases, is characterized by its deforming erosions of the joints; these erosions result from chronic synovial inflammation and proliferation. It tends to affect women twice as often as men and may run in families. Joint symptoms dominate its course, and symmetric involvement of the hands and wrists is most common. Other joints of the upper and lower extremities and the temporomandibular and sternoclavicular joints also may be affected. The most common systemic or extraarticular manifestations of RA include fever, weight loss, anemia, subcutaneous rheumatoid nodules, and lymphadenopathy. Less frequently, pleuritis and a diffuse, necrotizing vasculitis may occur.

PERICARDIAL INVOLVEMENT

Cardiac involvement is uncommon in RA but may take a variety of forms. A diffuse, nonspecific fibrofibrinous pericarditis occurs in about 50 percent of patients with RA; it is usually clinically silent and is overshadowed by pleuritis or joint pain.[118,119] The pericardial disease tends to be benign, but sizable effusions can occur and require pericardiocentesis, and pericardial constriction can rarely necessitate pericardiectomy. Constrictive pericarditis occurred in 4 of 47 patients with RA whose cases were followed over a 10-year period.[120] The histopathologic findings in all cases after pericardiectomy were consistent with chronic fibrosing pericardial disease. Another study reported on cardiac constriction from rheumatoid pericardial disease. These patients had disease longer, more severe disease, worse functional class, and more extraarticular features when compared with RA patients without cardiac constriction.[121] The presenting clinical features of cardiac constriction included dyspnea, edema, chest pain, and pulsus paradoxus. Chronic, symptomatic pericarditis may require glucocorticoid therapy. RA pericardial disease may shorten survival, especially in the older patients, and be associated with the presence of other cardiac disease, a greater number of extraarticular manifestations, jugular venous distension, and a lower mean systemic blood pressure.[122] Lymphocytic infiltrates of the CD8-positive type may occur in the pericardium of patients with rheumatoid pericardial disease, suggesting that these cells may play a role in the development of the pericardial disease[123] (see also Chap. 72).

MYOCARDIAL AND ENDOCARDIAL INVOLVEMENT

Rarely, rheumatoid nodules focally infiltrate the heart, including the myocardium and the four cardiac valves (Fig. 76-8).[118] These nodules may produce no symptoms, but, if extensive enough or strategically located, they can compromise cardiac function. A rheumatoid nodule may extend from the mural endocardium into a chamber to present as an intracavitary mass.[124] Rheumatoid nodules developing within the valve leaflets may result in mild valvular regurgitation; if the nodule becomes necrotic, perforation of the leaflet can occur and lead to severe valvular regurgitation. The incidence of such valvular infiltration has been estimated at 1 to 2 percent in autopsy studies of patients with RA. Although distinctly uncommon, arrhythmias and conduction disturbances, including complete heart block,[118] and congestive heart failure can also result from RA involvement of the heart. One echocardiographic study of 39 patients with RA detected left ventricular abnormalities in a quarter of the patients.[125] Acute myocardial infarction may be associated with RA.[126]

THERAPY

Since most of the cardiac lesions of RA are clinically silent, it is not certain that the specific therapies used in RA, including nonsteroid anti-inflammatory drugs (NSAIDs), methotrexate, penicillamine, gold, and glucocorticoids, affect the cardiac involvement. Treatment of cardiac constriction from rheuma-

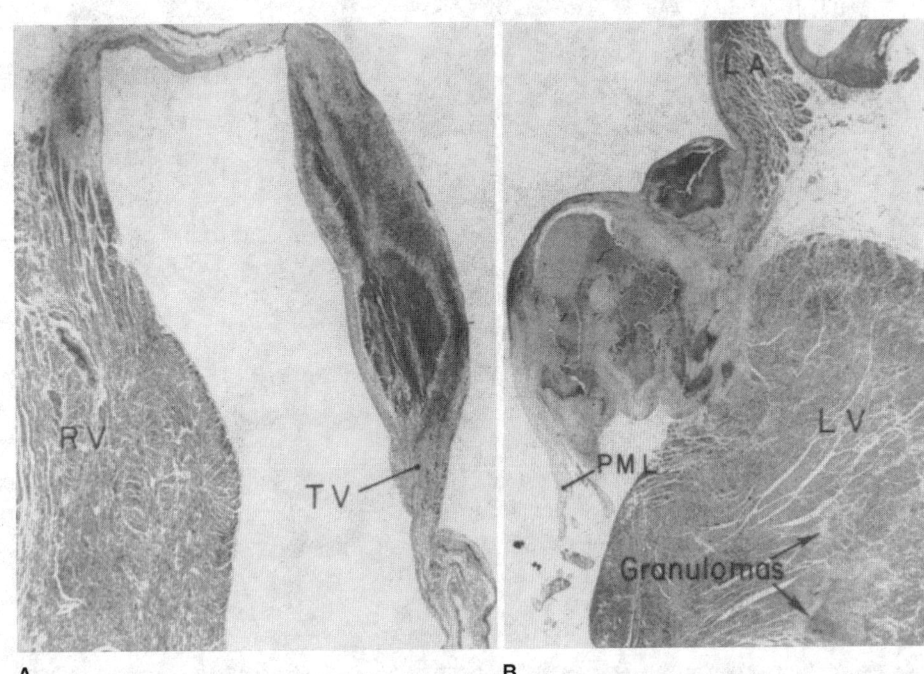

FIGURE 76-8 Rheumatoid arthritis. *A.* A tricuspid valve (TV) infiltrated by rheumatoid nodules. *B.* A mitral valve infiltrated by rheumatoid nodules. In addition, granulomas are present within the left ventricular (LV) wall. LA, left atrium; PML, posterior mitral leaflet; RV, right ventricle. H&E, *A*, ×12; *B*, ×65. (From Roberts WC, Dangel JC, and Bulkley BH.[118] Nonrheumatic valvular cardiac disease: A clinicopathologic survey of 27 different conditions causing valvular dysfunction. In: *Cardiovascular Clinics.* Copyright 1973 by F.A. Davis Company; used by permission of F.A. Davis Company.)

toid pericardial disease may include a trial of high-dose intravenous glucocorticoid (e.g., methylprednisolone) and/or surgical therapy. Pericardiocentesis should be performed only as a lifesaving procedure.[121]

Hydroxychloroquine and NSAIDs are often used. Both have an anticoagulant, antiplatelet effect, which may partially explain why thrombotic events such as deep vein thrombophlebitis as well as acute myocardial infarction are relatively uncommon in patients with RA. Otherwise, conventional treatments of pericarditis, arrhythmias, and conduction disturbances are utilized when these disorders produce clinical symptoms.

Ankylosing Spondylitis

Ankylosing spondylitis is the prototypical example within the group of the seronegative spondyloarthropathies. It is distinctly different from RA. Ankylosing spondylitis is characterized by a progressive inflammatory lesion of the spine, leading to chronic back pain, deforming dorsal kyphosis (Fig. 10-26), and, in its advanced stage, fusion of the costovertebral and sacroiliac joints with immobilization of the spine. This condition is much more frequent in men than in women (9:1), generally first occurring early in life but with a chronic progressive course of 20 to 30 years.[127] The HLA-B27 histocompatibility antigen is found in nearly all patients with ankylosing spondylitis. Other seronegative arthritides that have a high prevalence of this antigen include Reiter's syndrome, psoriatic arthritis, and juvenile arthritis.

CARDIAC INVOLVEMENT

Cardiovascular disease in ankylosing spondylitis takes the form of a sclerosing inflammatory lesion that is generally limited to the aortic root area. The inflammatory process, which extends immediately above and below the aortic valve, typically causes aortic regurgitation[128,129] (Fig. 76-9). As the inflammatory process extends below the aortic valve, it can infiltrate the basal portion of the mitral valve (which is contiguous with the aortic valve) and cause mitral regurgitation.[129] Extension of the inflammatory lesion into the cephalad portion of the ventricular septum, immediately caudal to the aortic valve, accounts for the associated conduction disturbances. Ventricular diastolic dysfunction may also occur.[130]

The major clinical manifestation of ankylosing spondylitis is aortic regurgitation, which occurs in about 5 percent of patients with this condition. Among patients with signs of spondylitis for 10 years, only 2 percent have clinical evidence of aortic regurgitation; by 30 years, that number increases fivefold.[128] Ankylosing spondylitis may be associated with aortic root inflammatory lesions, as may other seronegative spondyloarthropathies such as Reiter's syndrome and psoriatic arthropathy.[128]

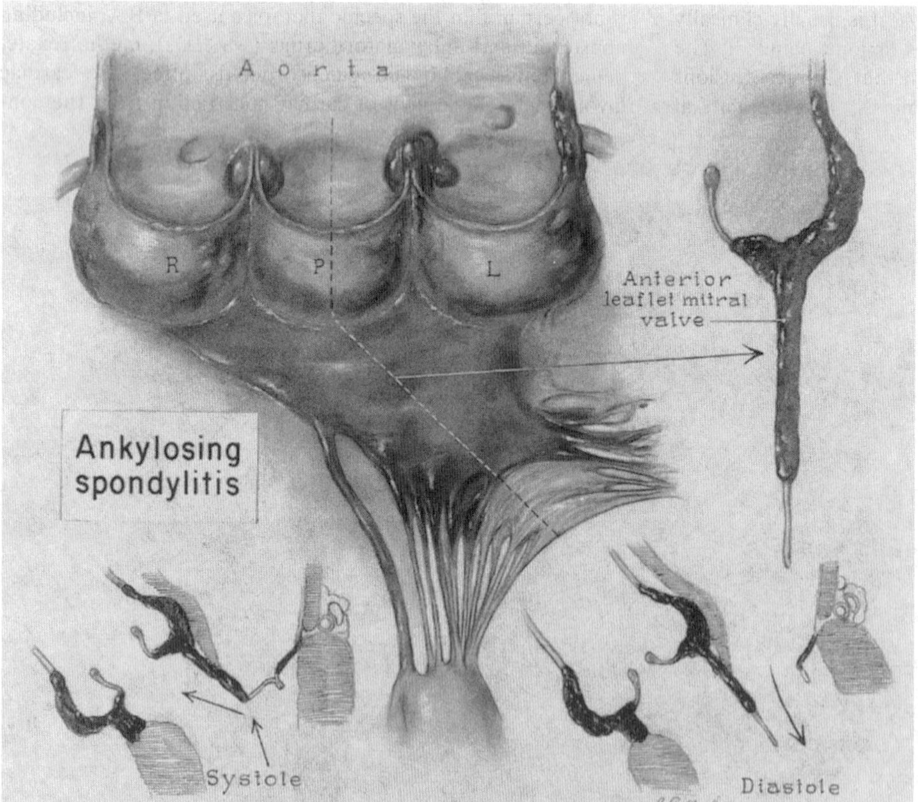

FIGURE 76-9 Diagram showing the characteristic features of ankylosing spondylitis of the heart. The aorta and aortic valve are opened, showing the thickening of the aorta in the vicinity of the aortic valve commissures and the thickening of the anterior mitral leaflet. The small diagrams at the *bottom* of the figure show the thickening in the wall of the aorta behind the sinuses extending below the aortic valve into the membranous ventricular septum and anterior mitral leaflet. In the patient whose heart was portrayed by this diagram, there was also some thickening in posterior mitral leaflet.

THERAPY

Drug therapy for ankylosing spondylitis is primarily directed at relief of the back pain and discomfort. This is accomplished with the use of NSAIDs, methotrexate, and sulfasalazine in addition to physical therapy; phenylbutazone is currently rarely used. Glucocorticoids are not used in this condition except for treatment of iritis. The inflammatory lesion of the heart generally runs a clinically silent course until aortic regurgitation develops. Not infrequently, however, the aortic regurgitation of ankylosing spondylitis may become severe enough to warrant aortic valve replacement[128,129] (see also Chap. 56).

Cardiovascular Syphilis

Although this condition has traditionally not been considered to be a connective tissue disorder, cardiovascular syphilis has histologic features nearly identical to those of ankylosing spondylitis, and spirochetes have never been identified in the aorta of a patient with cardiovascular syphilis. The distribution of the lesions, however, is distinctly different in these two conditions.[118] In cardiovascular syphilis, the process is usually limited to the tubular portion of ascending aorta, i.e., that portion up to the origin of the innominate artery. Because the process as a rule does not extend into the wall of aorta behind the sinuses of Valsalva, aortic regurgitation is infrequent in syphilis. Exactly what percentage of patients with cardiovascular syphilis develop aortic regurgitation is unclear, but it is probably no more than about 15 percent and only those patients in whom the process extends into the wall of aorta behind the sinuses of Valsalva. In syphilis, the process never involves the aortic valve cusps and never extends below (caudal to) the aortic valve. In contrast, in ankylosing spondylitis, the process always involves basal portions of the aortic valve cusps and always extends into the membranous ventricular septum, the basal portion of the anterior mitral leaflet, or both. Thus, because the process in syphilis never extends below the aortic valve, bundle branch or complete heart block and mitral regurgitation never develop in cardiovascular syphilis or, if they do, they are the result of a process other than syphilis. In contrast, heart block and mitral regurgitation are common in ankylosing spondylitis.

Cardiovascular syphilis characteristically involves the entire tubular portion of the aorta, which may become either diffusely or focally dilated. In contrast, in ankylosing spondylitis, the process involves only the proximal 1 cm of the tubular portion of the ascending aorta and then usually in the areas of the aortic valve commissures. Accordingly, aneurysms of the tubular portion of the ascending aorta do not occur in ankylosing spondylitis. Syphilitic aneurysms can become so large that they burrow into the sternum or compress adjacent structures such as the right atrium, superior vena cava, or pulmonary trunk. Rupture into the adjacent structures or into the pericardial sac may also occur.

Histologically, the aortic lesions in both cardiovascular syphilis and ankylosing spondylitis are similar. Both are characterized by extensive thickening by fibrous tissue of the adventitia, with collections of plasma cells and some lymphocytes within these tissues. The vasa vasora are larger than normal, their walls are thickened, and their lumens may be severely narrowed. The inflammatory infiltrates are located primarily in the perivascular locations. The media is thinner than normal and contains scars that are generally located transversely to the long axis of the aorta. Within the scars, elastic fibers may be absent. The overlying intima is thickened, and the intimal process has the "tree bark" appearance of typical atherosclerotic plaques. The intimal thickening is greater in syphilis than in ankylosing spondylitis, probably because the patients with cardiovascular syphilis are generally much older than the patients with ankylosing spondylitis. The average age of death among patients with ankylosing spondylitis and aortic regurgitation is 48 years, whereas the typical patient with cardiovascular syphilis, with or without associated aortic regurgitations, is usually in his or her 70s or 80s.

Systemic Sclerosis (Scleroderma)

SS, which was first identified over two centuries ago, is characterized by its striking skin manifestations; hence the name *scleroderma*. The systemic nature of this disease, and in particular its ability to affect the heart, became apparent much later. In 1943, Weiss and coworkers[131] described a pattern in the cardiac dysfunction of nine patients with scleroderma and correlated these changes with abnormalities in the heart at autopsy in two patients. Moreover, they recognized that the cardiac disease was a manifestation of an underlying primary vascular disorder.

SS is characterized by fibrous thickening of the skin (Fig. 10-22) and fibrous and degenerative alterations of the fingers and of certain target organs, particularly the esophagus, small and large bowels, kidneys, lung, and heart. Central to this degenerative process are diffuse vascular lesions. Functionally, the vascular disorder is characterized by Raynaud's phenomenon, which is a prominent feature of SS. Raynaud's disease of the digits is present in almost all patients with SS and is the first clinical symptom in most. Structurally, the vascular lesions show intimal and adventitial thickening of small- and medium-sized vessels, including arterioles. *The underlying pathophysiology of scleroderma that links structure and function is a Raynaud's-type phenomenon of visceral vasculature that leads to focal vascular lesions and parenchymal necrosis and fibrosis.* This concept is supported by findings in the heart as well as in the lungs and kidneys.[132] The underlying cause of the vascular disease in SS and the role of the immune system in its pathophysiology remain unclear. SS may be related to increased activity of endothelial cells, mast cells, and fibroblasts, perhaps under the influence of immigrant cells, such as T cells, macrophages, or platelets.[131]

Like most connective tissue diseases, SS may have a variable clinical expression. Some patients may have skin involvement predominantly; others have minimal skin abnormalities but severe visceral disease that may therefore evade diagnosis.[132] The CREST (*c*alcinosis, *R*aynaud's phenomenon, *e*sophageal dysmotility, *s*clerodactyly, *t*elangiectasia) syndrome is an SS variant that can be manifest as relatively mild skin changes limited to the face and fingers, but severe lung disease with a primary pulmonary hypertension picture can occur.[133] *Overlap syndromes* are seen when a patient with typical features of SS also has features of SLE or RA. Although SS may run a long and benign course, *malignant* renal, lung, or cardiac disease can occur, with rapid deterioration and death at a young age.

THE CARDIOVASCULAR SYSTEM

Cardiovascular disease in patients with SS can be due to either a primary involvement of the heart by the sclerosing disease or a secondary involvement from disease of the kidney or lungs.

Primary Systemic Sclerosis of the Heart Myocardial involvement is a principal determinant of survival in SS. When the heart is involved directly by scleroderma, a myocardial fibrosis occurs that bears no direct relation to large- or small-vessel occlusions or other anatomic abnormalities. The fibrosis tends to be patchy, involving all levels of the myocardium unpredictably and the right ventricle as often as the left. Focal patchy myocardial cell necrosis may also be evident, and at autopsy over three-quarters of patients with myocardial SS have foci of necrosis.[132] The type of necrosis is myofibrillar degeneration, or contraction-band necrosis (Fig. 76-10). This lesion is characteristic of myocardium that is subjected to transient occlusion followed by reperfusion. This could occur with vascular spasm and also may be induced experimentally by exposing myocardium to high concentrations of catecholamine. Thus, the morphologic characteristics of the myocardial lesions of primary cardiac SS are consistent with a Raynaud's phenomenon of the heart. There is also suggestive evidence that a Raynaud's phenomenon of the pulmonary arterioles may be responsible for the *primary* pulmonary hypertension-type lesion that may occur in CREST

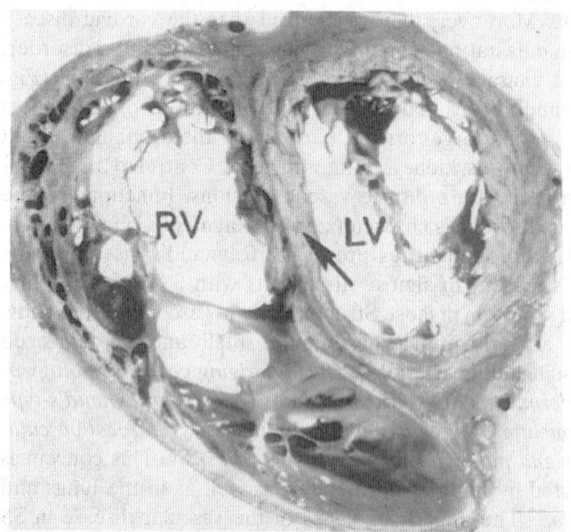

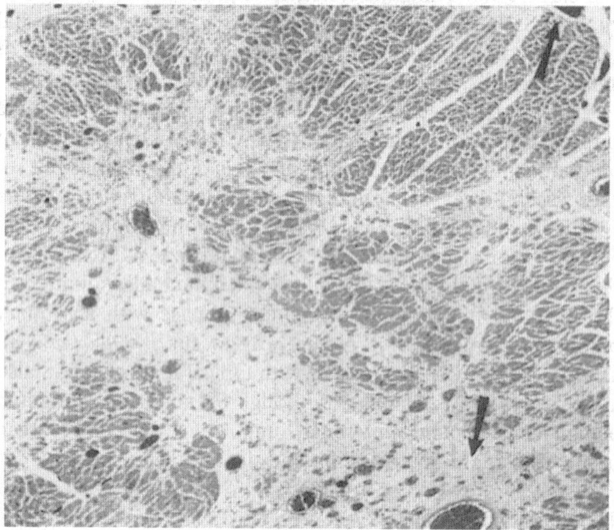

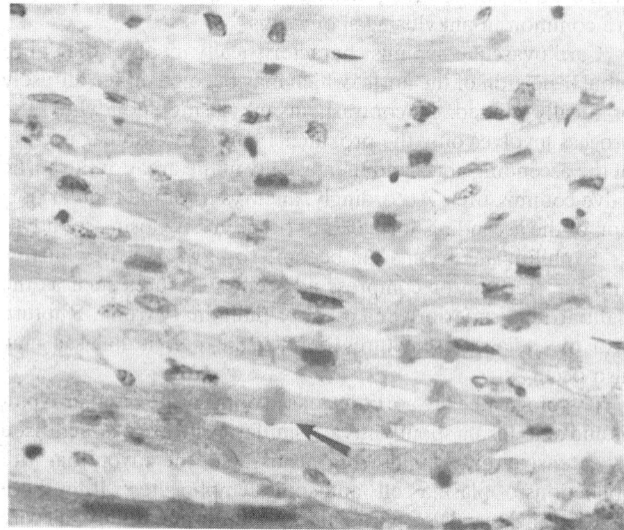

FIGURE 76-10 Systemic sclerosis (SS). *Top:* Cross section through the dilated right (RV) and left (LV) ventricle of a patient with cardiac SS. Marked fibrous scarring of both ventricles is especially evident in the interventricular septum (*arrow*). *Bottom left:* Photomicrograph of myocardium showing replacement fibrosis with patent intramural coronary arteries (*arrows*). *Bottom right:* Higher-power magnification showing contraction-band necrosis of many fibers surrounding the areas of scar. H&E, ×45 and ×60. (From Bulkley.[176] Reproduced with permission form the publisher and author.)

syndrome, and the kidneys in SS can also manifest a Raynaud's-type phenomenon. Some patients with SS have renal Raynaud's phenomenon when digital Raynaud's phenomenon is induced by cold-water immersion.[134] Thus, it is likely that the major visceral manifestations of SS in the heart, lungs, and kidneys are related to the vascular spasm that is evident and readily detectable in the digits. Changes that are comparable to the necrosis and scarring of the fingertips can also develop in the viscera.

The cause of the myocardial necrosis and fibrosis that develop in the setting of patent extramural and intramural vessels is unclear. That the myocardial disease relates in part to immunologic abnormalities or to primary and unrestrained fibrous tissue proliferation remains a possibility. The present evidence, however, suggests that the vascular system—and particularly the smaller arteries and arterioles—is the primary target organ of SS and that the cardiac sclerosis of scleroderma may be a consequence of focal, intermittent, and progressive ischemic injury.

Several functional studies have also suggested that microvascular spasm occurs in patients with cardiac scleroderma. Transient perfusion defects identified by thallium-201 radionuclide imaging in the setting of patent coronary arteries have also been identified in patients with SS and symptomatic cardiac disease.[135] Some patients with SS have reversible cold-induced myocardial perfusion defects as well as cold-induced acute and reversible left ventricular dysfunction.[136]

Clinical Manifestations The clinical features of myocardial SS include biventricular congestive heart failure, atrial and ventricular arrhythmias, myocardial infarction, angina pectoris, and sudden cardiac death.[137,138] These clinical manifestations reflect the underlying conditions of myocardial necrosis and fibrosis and may at times mimic ischemic heart disease due to coronary atherosclerosis. If the myocardial injury is extensive enough, leading to dilated hypodynamic ventricles, a syndrome resembling idiopathic dilated cardiomyopathy (Chap. 66) may be simulated.

Patients with SS may have cardiac involvement but no cardiac symptoms.[137,138] One study[139] examined 18 SS patients by electrocardiography, ambulatory electrocardiography, radionuclide ventriculography, myocardial scintigraphy, and echocardiography and found a high rate of cardiac abnormalities, including ventricular tachycardia in one patient, nonsustained ventricular tachycardia in five, supraventricular tachycardia in six, decreased left ventricular ejection fraction in two, decreased right ventricular ejection fraction in eight, and stress-induced reversible myocardial perfusion abnormalities in six. In other studies of patients with limited scleroderma, noninvasive cardiac techniques such as Doppler echocardiography and thallium-201 perfusion scintigraphy after a cold-stress test or radionuclide ventriculography[140] have found a number of cardiovascular abnormalities, such as mild mitral regurgitation, thickening of papillary muscles, abnormal left and right diastolic function, and systolic pulmonary arterial hypertension. A Japanese study of 13 patients with full-blown SS concluded that patients with SS frequently have deterioration of left ventricular diastolic function, especially those with left ventricular wall thickening out of proportion to left ventricular end-diastolic dimensions.[141]

Other investigators[142] have used electrocardiography and echocardiography to devise a simple *cardiac score* to improve the prediction of prognosis in patients with SS. Skeletal muscle myositis can complicate SS, and such patients may have an increased likelihood of developing myocarditis, heart failure, and symptomatic arrhythmias, and die suddenly.[143] Accordingly, it has been suggested that serum creatine kinase with MB fractionation and studies of left ventricular function be undertaken in patients with SS who have skeletal myositis. Autopsy studies have suggested that up to 50 percent of patients with SS have increased myocardial scar tissue and that up 30 percent of patients have extensive lesions.[144] Some clinical cardiac abnormalities, including symptoms of heart failure or abnormal rhythm with conduction disturbances, may occur in about 40 percent of patients with SS. The cardiac disorder in approximately one-half of patients has been attributed by some researchers to a primary myocardial scleroderma.

Pericardial and Endocardial Disease Pericardial involvement may occur in about 20 percent of patients with SS. Although the pericardial involvement is due to renal failure in as many as two-thirds of patients, some develop a fibrofibrinous or fibrous pericarditis for which no other cause is evident. Exudative pericardial effusions may accompany scleroderma pericardial disease and can be massive.[145] Pericardial tamponade may occur and may precede cutaneous thickening.[146] Rarely, constrictive pericardial disease may result from the pericardial sclerosis. Mitral regurgitation is common in patients with SS.[147] Tricuspid regurgitation occurs in patients with very dilated right ventricular cavities.

Secondary Cardiovascular Disease Since scleroderma most frequently manifests itself as renal and pulmonary parenchymal disease with pulmonary and systemic arterial hypertension, secondary cardiovascular disease is common. Left ventricular hypertrophy and congestive heart failure may be associated with long-standing systemic arterial hypertension and renal disease. Uremic pericarditis may occur. Cor pulmonale with marked right ventricular hypertrophy and right-sided heart failure may result from long-standing severe pulmonary scleroderma.

PULMONARY HYPERTENSIVE DISEASE

Although the pulmonary fibrosis of scleroderma had been known for years, the recognition of a *primary* pulmonary hypertensive lesion independent of parenchymal disease evolved later. Patients with this primary pulmonary vascular lesion tend to develop rapidly progressive dyspnea and right-sided congestive heart failure in the setting of clear lungs. Pulmonary pressures reach the systemic level and are refractory to treatment. Morphologically, the pulmonary arterial lesions show the range of advanced alterations (medial and intimal thickening and plexiform lesions) as seen in Eisenmenger's syndrome and primary pulmonary hypertension. Arterial vasospasm is believed to be a major component of SS primary pulmonary hypertension, and the association is supported by angiographic studies. On occasion, vasodilators such as tolazoline may induce partial lowering of pressure, but the fixed pulmonary lesions and focal thrombotic occlusions of the advanced stages make restoration of normal pressures unlikely. The fact that Raynaud's phenomenon of the digits accompanies idiopathic primary pulmonary hypertension in about one-third of patients[148] suggests that vascular hyperreactivity may be a common link between this disease and scleroderma (see also Chap. 52).

Although uncommon in scleroderma, severe pulmonary hypertension carries a grave prognosis. Sudden unexpected death occurs, and hypotension and death can occur precipitously in the setting of what would appear to be relatively benign procedures such as pericardiocentesis or cardiac catheterization.

TREATMENT

There is no uniformly effective therapy for the cardiovascular disease of SS.[149] Treatment consists of standard therapy for congestive heart failure and arrhythmias. Malignant ventricular arrhythmias in SS have responded seemingly well to insertion of an implantable cardioverter defibrillator[150] (see Chap. 30). Thrombolysis may provide improvement in the Raynaud's phenomenon, cutaneous sclerosis, and digital ulcerations.[151] A pilot study of antithymocyte gamma-globulin (ATGAM) appeared ineffective in improving the skin and pulmonary features of the disease.[152] Nifedipine may improve myocardial perfusion abnormalities as well as systemic and pulmonary hemodynamics in patients with pulmonary hypertension due to SS.[153] Nifedipine and amlodipine may also improve Raynaud's events involving the fingers. Captopril has been shown to improve myocardial perfusion.[154] Potential therapeutic value for SS cardiac disease has been attributed to *D*-penicillamine. No therapy, however, has proved effective for either the systemic disease or its cardiac manifestations.

Polymyositis/Dermatomyositis

These idiopathic autoimmune inflammatory myopathies are rare in the United States, with an estimated annual incidence of about 5 to 10 new patients per million. The clinical features include a typical heliotrope rash in dermatomyositis (DM), with periorbital edema and proximal muscle weakness present in both polymyositis (PM) and DM. PM is basically the same disease except for the absence of a skin rash.[155] Typical laboratory findings include an elevated serum creatine kinase level and elevation of other muscle enzymes such as a serum aldolase, reflecting the presence of muscle breakdown from the inflammatory process. The so-called anti-Jo-1 antibody, detectable in the serum of some patients with PM/DM, has been correlated with inflammatory arthritis, Raynaud's phenomenon, interstitial lung disease, and excess mortality, mostly due to respiratory failure. Typical changes in the electromyogram include short-wave potentials, low-amplitude polyphasic units, and increased spontaneous activity with muscle fibrillation. A positive skeletal muscle biopsy of a proximal muscle such as the deltoid is often confirmatory.[155]

In addition to skeletal muscle involvement, up to 40 percent of patients may have cardiac abnormalities, including atrioventricular conduction defects, tachyarrhythmias, pericarditis with effusion, and a dilated, poorly contracting left ventricle. Myocarditis leading to congestive heart failure has been found in autopsy studies.[156] Rarely, coronary arteritis has been reported in PM/DM. Accordingly, the evaluation of a middle-aged man with known PM/DM who presents with chest pain, or even classic angina with an elevated serum creatine kinase, poses a diagnostic challenge, and the differential diagnosis includes inflammatory myocarditis and coronary arteritis. An increase in cardiac creatine kinase-MB may be "buried" in the marked elevation of skeletal creatine kinase-MB. If coronary angiography is suggestive of coronary vasculitis rather than typical atheromatous plaques, oral high-dose prednisone, 40 to 60 mg daily, is appropriate. This is also the usual initial therapeutic approach in patients with PM/DM even when no cardiac involvement is apparent. There are no clinical studies available comparing the efficacy of glucocorticoid treatment with other immunosuppressive agents such as azathioprine (Imuran), methotrexate, chlorambucil, and cyclophosphamide (Cytoxan).

Most rheumatologists initially use a trial of glucocorticoid therapy in patients with PM/DM. If the response is suboptimal, treatment is instituted with methotrexate, azathioprine (Imuran), chlorambucil, and cyclophosphamide (Cytoxan), in that order. The response to steroids in PM/DM is unpredictable. Some patients do very well on oral prednisone therapy, whereas others fail to respond to any agents. A subset of patients with PM/DM who have the so-called inclusion body myositis are particularly intractable to anti-inflammatory treatment. This is also true for patients who have a rare autoantibody called the anti-signal-recognition-particle (anti-SRP) antibody. Because some patients with PM/DM benefit significantly from an initial trial of high-dose oral or intravenous glucocorticoid therapy, this therapy is usually used first. Intravenous immunoglobulin appears promising in the treatment of PM/DM.[157] Finally, myopathies can arise iatrogenically from commonly used drugs such as cholesterol-lowering agents, statins, and niacin, as well as from colchicine, zidovudine, and methylphenidate hydrochloride (Ritalin).

Giant-Cell (Cranial, Temporal, Granulomatous) Arteritis

Temporal arteritis is a systemic inflammatory vasculitis of unknown etiology that primarily involves extracranial vessels, especially branches of the external carotid artery, but can involve almost any artery in the body, as well as some veins. Giant-cell arteritis occurs almost exclusively in patients over 55 years of age. Common symptoms include headaches, scalp tenderness, jaw claudication, visual disturbances including blindness, diplopia, weight loss, anemia, and, in about 50 percent of patients, musculoskeletal symptoms attributable to polymyalgia rheumatica. Uncommon presentations of giant-cell arteritis include fever of unknown origin, chest pain from aortitis or myocardial infarction, aortic aneurysm,[158,159] coma, peripheral gangrene, peripheral neuropathies, and large-vessel involvement with limb claudication, aortic regurgitation, or stroke. Typical physical findings include tenderness of the temporal or occipital arteries, nodulations of the artery, a pulseless artery, and a tender scalp.

Most giant-cell arteritis patients have a greatly elevated erythrocyte sedimentation rate. The only specific diagnostic test is a temporal artery biopsy that demonstrates granulomatous arterial inflammation with disruption of the internal elastica lamina. Gaint cells need not be present. Unfortunately, the positive yield for giant-cell arteritis in unilateral temporal artery biopsies is no greater than 60 percent, and a contralateral biopsy may be necessary.

Since the occurrence of *skip* lesions in histologic samples is well known in giant-cell arteritis, ideally a 5-cm section of artery should be examined. Angiography is generally not helpful in diagnosis or in selecting a biopsy site. High-dose prednisone therapy is indicated to prevent blindness or to suppress inflammation in the presence of systemic involvement.

Churg-Strauss Vasculitis

Churg-Strauss syndrome, or allergic granulomatosis and angiitis, is a systemic vasculitis that develops in the setting of allergic rhinitis, asthma, and eosinophilia. Sinusitis and pulmonary infiltrates may cause confusion with Wegener's granulomatosis; the absence of cavitating pulmonary nodules or the presence of gastrointestinal involvement is often a helpful distinguishing feature. Peripheral neuropathy, cutaneous involvement, and renal disease are common clinical findings.

Pathologic studies show inflammatory lesions rich in eosinophils with intra- and extravascular granuloma formation. The major morbidity and mortality of Churg-Strauss vasculitis result from cardiac involvement. This may be associated with left ventricular dilatation and a reduced ejection fraction, as well as mitral regurgitation, which may require valve replacement.[158] Left ventricular systolic function may improve significantly with glucocorticoid therapy.[159]

Antiphospholipid Antibody Syndrome

The aPL antibody syndrome has been identified by the presence of aPL antibodies, usually in high titer, or the *lupus anticoagulant,* and any or all of the following clinical events:[160–173] recurrent arterial or venous thromboses, recurrent fetal losses, and thrombocytopenia. Livedo reticularis is also frequently present, and nonhealing leg ulcers and Coombs'-positive hemolytic anemia may be also. Clincally, the terms *anticardiolipin syndrome, antiphospholipid syndrome,* and *lupus anticoagulant syndrome* are usually considered to be equivalent, although some individuals may have one antibody but not the other. A false-positive Venereal Disease Research Laboratory test may also be detected in patients with aPL antibody syndrome; aPL antibodies, however, may be present in asymptomatic individuals. Often, anticardiolipin antibodies cross-react with β_2-glycoprotein 1 (B2GP1) antibodies. The mechanism(s) whereby anticardiolipin or aPL antibodies promote intravascular thrombosis remain(s) uncertain. These antibodies may react with lipid antigens on endothelial cells and/or platelets. The precise nature of the antigen recognized by B2GP1-dependent anticardiolipin antibodies is under active investigation. SLE is frequently present in patients with aPL antibody syndrome. The presence of anticardiolipin antibodies in patients with SLE may be associated with prolonged activated partial thromboplastin time, thrombocytopenia, and positive Coombs' test but not with the lupus anticoagulant (or the aPL) syndrome;[160] the presence of a prolonged activated partial thromboplastin time is strongly associated with venous and arterial thrombosis.

Therapy depends on the clinical setting. Patients with positive aPL antibodies but without evidence of thrombosis or recurrent fetal loss should not be treated. Patients with aPL antibody syndrome who have had thrombotic events or habitual abortions should be treated. Anticoagulation and antithrombotic therapy in these patients has included heparin, warfarin, low-dose aspirin, and the antimalarial agent hydroxychloroquine.[161] Although there is no convincing evidence of benefit, some advocate low-dose aspirin or heparin, with or without low-dose prednisone, alone or in combination to prevent fetal loss. An increased incidence of aortic or mitral regurgitation in association with the *primary* aPL antibody syndrome has been reported as well in patients with SLE who have aPL antibodies. Heart valve involvement, although frequent, appears unrelated to the presence or absence of aPL antibodies. The aPL antibody syndrome is frequently manifest by spontaneous small- and large-vessel arterial thrombosis in the cerebral and ocular circulations.[174] In healthy men, positive anticardiolipin antibody levels are a risk factor for deep venous thrombosis or pulmonary embolus but not for ischemic stroke.[174]

Although there are no controlled trials of therapy to prevent arterial occlusion, low-dose aspirin is often used. Therapy has often included aspirin and warfarin or heparin, as well as low-dose glucocorticoids.[175]

References

1. Beighton P, ed. *McKusick's Heritable Disorders of Connective Tissue,* 5th ed. St Louis: Mosby-Year Book; 1993.
2. Pyeritz PE, McKusick VA. The Marfan syndrome: Diagnosis and management. *N Engl J Med* 1979; 300:772–777.
3. Kainulainen K, Pulkkinen L, Savolainen A, et al. Location of chromosome 15 of the gene defect causing Marfan syndrome. *N Engl J Med* 1990; 323:935–939.
4. Hollister DW, Godfrey M, Sakai LY, Pyeritz RE. Immunohistologic abnormalities of the microfibrillar-fiber system in the Marfan syndrome. *N Engl J Med* 1990; 323:935–939.
5. Lee B, Godfrey M, Vitale E, et al. Linkage of Marfan syndrome and a phenotypically related disorder to two different fibrillin genes. *Nature* 1991; 352:330–334.
6. Maslen CL, Corson GM, Maddox BK, et al. Partial sequence of a candidate gene for the Marfan syndrome. *Nature* 1991; 352: 334–337.
7. Dietz HC, Curring GR, Pyeritz RE, et al. Marfan syndrome caused by a de novo missense mutation in the fibrillin gene. *Nature* 1991; 352:337–339.
8. Dietz HC, Valle D, Francomano CA, et al. The skipping of constitutive exons in vivo induced by nonsense mutations. *Science* 1993; 259:680–683.
9. Dietz HC, McIntosh I, Sakai LY, et al. Four novel FBN1 mutations: Significance for mutant transcript level and EGF-like domain calcium binding in the pathogenesis of Marfan syndrome. *Genomics* 1993; 17:468–475.
10. Dietz HC, Pyeritz RE. Mutations in the human gene for fibrillin-1 (FBN1) in the Marfan syndrome and related disorders. *Hum Mol Genet* 1995; 4:1799–1809.
11. Ramirez F. Fibrillin mutations in Marfan syndrome and related phenotypes. *Curr Opin Genet Dev* 1996; 6:309–315.
12. Burn J, Camm J, Davies MJ, et al. The phenotype/genotype relation and the current status of genetic screening in hypertrophic cardiomyopathy, Marfan syndrome, and the long QT syndrome. *Heart* 1997; 78:110–116.
13. Maron BJ, Moller JH, Seidman CE, et al. Impact of laboratory molecular diagnosis on contemporary diagnostic criteria for genetically transmitted cardiovascular diseases: Hypertrophic cardiomyopathy, long-QT syndrome, and Marfan syndrome. A statement for healthcare professionals from the Councils on Clinical Cardiology, Cardiovascular Disease in the Young, and Basic Science, American Heart Association. *Circulation* 1998; 98:1460–1471.
14. De Paepe A, Devereus RB, Dietz HC, et al. Revised diagnostic criteria for the Marfan syndrome. *Am J Med Genet* 1996; 62: 417–426.
15. Come PC, Fortuin NJ, White RI Jr, McKusick VA. Echocardiographic assessment of cardiovascular abnormalities in the Marfan syndrome: Comparison with clinical findings and with roentgenographic estimation of aortic root size. *Am J Med* 1983; 74:465–474.
16. Roman MJ, Devereus RB, Kramer-Fox R, Spitzer MC. Comparison of cardiovascular and skeletal features of primary valve prolapse and Marfan syndrome. *J Cardiol* 1989; 63:317–321.
17. Glesby MJ, Pyeritz RE. Association of mitral valve prolapse and systemic abnormalities of connective tissue: A phenotypic continuum. *JAMA* 1989; 262:523–518.
18. Wexler L, Higgins CB. The use of magnetic resonance imaging in adult congenital heart disease. *Am J Cardiac Imaging* 1995; 9:15–28.
19. Maron BJ. Heart disease and other causes of sudden death in young athletes. *Curr Probl Cardiol* 1998; 23:477–529.
20. Braverman AC. Exercise and the Marfan syndrome. *Med Sci Sports Exerc* 1998; 30(suppl 10):S387–S395.
21. Salim MA, Alpert BS, Ward JC, Pyeritz RE. Effect of beta-adrenergic blockade on aortic root rate of dilation in the Marfan syndrome. *Am J Cardiol* 1994; 74:629–633.
22. Shores J, Berger KR, Murphy EA, Pyeritz RE. Progression of aortic dilation and the benefit of long-term β-adrenergic blockade in Marfan's syndrome. *N Engl J Med* 1994; 30:1335–1341.
23. Treasure T. Elective replacement of the aortic root in Marfan's syndrome. *Br Heart J* 1993; 69:101–103.
24. Gott VL, Gillinov M, Pyeritz RE, et al. Aortic root replacement: Risk factor analysis of a seventeen-year experience with 270 patients. *J Thorac Cardiovasc Surg* 1995; 109:536–545.
25. Donaldson RM, Emanuel RW, Olsen EG, Ross DN. Management of cardiovascular complications in Marfan syndrome. *Lancet* 1980; 2:1178–1181.
26. Gott VL, Pyeritz RE, McGovern GJ, et al. Surgical treatment of aneurysms of the ascending aorta in the Marfan syndrome: Results of composite-graft repair in 50 patients. *N Engl J Med* 1986; 314:1070–1074.
27. Marsalese DL, Moodie DS, Vacante M, et al. Marfan's syndrome: Natural history and long-term follow-up of cardiovascular involvement. *J Am Coll Cardiol* 1989; 14:422–428.
28. Gott VL, Pyeritz RE, Cameron DE, et al. Composite graft repair in Marfan aneurysm of the ascending aorta: Results in 100 patients. *Ann Thorac Surg* 1991; 52:38–45.
29. Svensson LG, Crawford ES, Coseli JS, et al. Impact of cardiovascular operation on survival in the Marfan patient. *Circulation* 1989; 80(suppl I):I233–I242.
30. Svensson LG, Crawford ES, Hess KR, et al. Dissection of the aorta and dissecting aortic aneurysms: Improving early and long-term surgical results. *Circulation* 1990; 82(suppl IV):IV24–IV38.
31. Pyeritz RE. Marfan syndrome: Current and future clinical and genetic management of cardiovascular manifestations. *Semin Thorac Cardiovasc Surg* 1993; 5:11–16.
32. Smith JA, Fann JI, Miller C, et al. Surgical management of aortic dissection in patients with the Marfan syndrome. *Circulation* 1994; 90(part 2):II235–II242.
33. Roberts WC, Honig HS. The spectrum of cardiovascular disease

in the Marfan syndrome: A clinico-morphologic study of 18 necropsy patients and comparison to 151 previously reported necropsy patients. *Am Heart J* 1982; 104:115–135.
34. Silverman DI, Gray J, Roman MJ, et al. Family history of cardiovascular disease in the Marfan syndrome is associated with increased aortic diameter and decreased survival. *J Am Coll Cardiol* 1995; 26:1062–1067.
35. Hayashi J, Moro H, Namura O, et al. Surgical implication of aortic dissection on long-term outcome in Marfan patients. *Surg Today* 1996; 26:980–984.
36. Bachet J, Goudot B, Dreyfus G, et al. The proper use of glue: A 20-year experience with the GRF glue in acute aortic dissection. *J Card Surg* 1997; 12(suppl 2):243–253.
37. LeMaire SA, Coselli JS. Aortic root surgery in Marfan syndrome: Current practice and evolving techniques. *J Cardvasc Surg* 1997; 12(suppl 2):137–141.
38. David TE. Current practice in Marfan's aortic root surgery: Reconstruction with aortic valve preservation or replacement? What to do with the mitral valve. *J Cardvasc Surg* 1997; 12(suppl 2):147–150.
39. Gillinov AM, Hulyalkar A, Cameron DE, et al. Mitral valve operation in patients with the Marfan syndrome. *J Thorac Cardiovasc Surg* 1994; 107:724–731.
40. Murdoch JL, Walker BA, Halpern BL, et al. Life expectancy and causes of death in the Marfan syndrome. *N Engl J Med* 1972; 286:804–808.
41. Pyeritz RE. Maternal and fetal complications of pregnancy in the Marfan syndrome. *Am J Med* 1981; 71:784–790.
42. Santucci JJ, Katz S, Pogo GJ, Boxer R. Peripartum acute myocardial infarction in Marfan's syndrome, *Am Hear J* 1994; 127:1404–1407.
43. Rossiter JP, Repke JT, Morales AJ, et al. A prospective longitudinal evaluation of pregnancy in the Marfan syndrome. *Am J Obstet Gynecol* 1995; 173:1599–1606.
44. Ulkayan U, Ostrzega E, Shotan A, Mehra A. Cardiovascular problems in pregnant women with Marfan syndrome. *Ann Intern Med* 1995; 123:117–122.
45. Steinmann B, Royce PM, Superti-Furga A. The Ehlers Danlos syndrome. In: Royce PM, Steinmann B, eds. *Connective Tissue and its Heritable Disorders: Molecular, Genetic, and Medical Aspects*. New York: Wiley-Liss; 1993:351.
46. Takahashi T, Koide T, Yamaguchi H, et al. Ehlers-Danlos syndrome *Ann Thorac Surg* 1994; 58:1180–1182.
47. Hamano K, Minami Y, Fujimura Y, et al. Emergency operation for thoracic aortic aneurysm caused by the Ehler-Danlos syndrome. *Ann Thorac Surg* 1994; 58:1180–1182.
48. Lebwohl M, Halperin J, Phelps RG. Occult pseudoxanthoma elasticum in patients with premature cardiovascular disease. *N Engl J Med* 1993; 329:1237–1239.
49. Coleman K, Ross MH, McCabe M, et al. Disk drusen and angioid streaks in pseudoxanthoma elasticum. *Am J Ophthalmol* 1991; 112:166–170.
50. Slade AKB, John RM, Swanton RH. Pseudoxanthoma elasticum presenting with myocardial infarction. *Br Heart J* 1990; 63: 372–373.
51. Kevorkian JP, Masquet C, Kural-Menasche S, et al. New report of severe coronary artery disease in an eighteen-year-old girl with pseudoxanthoma elasticum. *Angiology* 1997; 48:735–741.
52. Rosenzweig BP, Guarneri E, Kronzon I. Echocardiographic manifestations in a patient with pseudoxanthoma elasticum. *Ann Intern Med* 1993; 119:487–491.
53. Lebwohl MG, Distefano D, Prioleau PC, et al. Pseudoxanthoma elasticum and mitral valve prolapse. *N Engl J Med* 1982; 307: 228–231.
54. Fukuda K, Uno K, Fujii T, et al. Mitral stenosis in pseudoxanthoma elasticum. *Chest* 1992; 101:1706–1707.
55. Challenor VF, Conway N, Monro JL. The surgical treatment of restrictive cardiomyopathy in pseudoxanthoma elasticum. *Br Heart J* 1988; 59:266–269.
56. Stover ML, Primorac D, Liu SC, et al. Defective splicing of mRNA from one COL1A1 allele of type I collagen in nondeforming (type I) osteogenesis imperfecta. *J Clin Invest* 1993; 92:1994–2002.
57. Byers PH. Osteogenesis imperfecta. In: Royce PM, Steinmann B, eds. *Connective Tissue and Its Heritable Disorders: Molecular, Genetic and Medical Aspects*. New York: Wiley-Liss; 1993:317.
58. Marini JC, Gerber NL. Osteogenesis imperfecta rehabilitation and prospects for gene therapy. *JAMA* 1997; 277:746–750.
59. Wong RS, Follis FM, Shively BK, Wenly JA. Osteogenesis imperfecta and cardiovascular diseases. *Ann Thorac Surg* 1995; 60: 1439–1443.
60. Hortop J, Tsipouras P, Hanley JA, et al. Cardiovascular involvement in osteogenesis imperfecta *Circulation* 1986; 73:54–61.
61. Almassi GH, Hughes GR, Bartlett J. Combined valve replacement and coronary bypass grafting in osteogenesis imperfecta. *Ann Thorac Surg* 1995; 60:1395–1397.
62. Wood SJ, Thomas J, Braimbridge MV. Mitral valve disease and open heart surgery in osteogenesis imperfecta tarda. *Br Heart J* 1973; 35:103–106.
63. Zegdi R, D'Attellis N, Fornes P, et al. Aortic valve surgery in osteogenesis imperfecta: Report of two cases and review of the literature. *J Heart Valve Dis* 1998; 7:510–514.
64. Moriyama Y, Nishida T, Toyohira H, et al. Acute aortic dissection in a patient with osteogenesis imperfecta. *Ann Thorac Surg* 1995; 60:1397–1399.
65. Fowler NO, Van der Bel-Kahn JM. Indications for surgical replacement of the mitral valve with particular reference to common and uncommon causes of mitral regurgitation. *Am J Cardiol* 1979; 44:148–156.
66. Roman MJ, Devereus RB. Heritable aortic disease. In: Lindsay J, ed. *Diseases of the Aorta*. Philadelphia: Lea & Febiger; 1994:5.
67. Pascal N, Bloor C, Godfrey M, et al. Familial aortic dissecting aneurysm. *J Am Coll Cardiol* 1989; 13:811–819.
68. Chen M, Rigby ML, Redington AN. Familial aneurysms of the interventricular septum. *Br Heart J* 1991; 65:104–106.
69. Jaksche VH. Familiäre Aneurysmen: Vier Karotisaneurysmen aus einer zehnköpfigen Familie. *Zentralbl Neurochir* 1986; 47: 351–353.
70. Elshunnar KS, Whittle IR. Familial intracranial aneurysms: Report of five families. *Br J Neurosurg* 1990; 4:181–186.
71. Boumpas DT, Fessler BJ, Austin HA III, et al. Systemic lupus erythematosus: Emerging concepts. Part 2: Dermatologic and joint disease, the antiphospholipid antibody syndrome, pregnancy and hormonal therapy, morbidity and mortality, and pathogenesis. *Ann Intern Med* 1995; 123:42–53.
72. Wallace DJ, Hahn BH, eds. *Dubois' Lupus Erythematosus*, 4th ed. Philadelphia: Lea and Febiger; 1993.
73. Moder KG, Miller TD, Tazelaar HD. Cardiac involvement in systemic lupus erythematosus. *Mayo Clin Proc* 1999; 74:275–284.
74. Ward MM, Pyun E, Studenski S. Mortality risks associated with specific clinical manifestations of systemic lupus erythematosus. *Arch Intern Med* 1996; 156:1337–1344.
75. Roberts WC, High ST. The heart in systemic lupus erythematosus. *Curr Probl Cardiol* 1999; 24:1–56.
76. Alarcon-Segovia D, Deleze M, Oria CV, et al. Antiphospholipid antibodies and the antiphospholipid syndrome in systemic lupus erythematosus: A prospective analysis of 500 consecutive patients. *Medicine (Baltimore)* 1989; 68:353–365.
77. Leung W-H, Wong K-L, Lau C-P, et al. Association between antiphospholipid antibodies and cardiac abnormalities in patients with systemic lupus erythematosus. *Am J Med* 1990; 89:411–419.
78. Khamashta MA, Cervera R, Asherson RA, et al. Association of antibodies against phospholipids with heart valve disease in systemic lupus erythematosus. *Lancet* 1990; 335:1541–1544.

79. Nihoyannopoulous P, Gomez PM, Joshi J, et al. Cardiac abnormalities in systemic lupus erythematosus. *Circulation* 1990; 82: 369–375.
80. O'Rourke RA. Antiphospholipid antibodies: A marker of lupus carditis? *Circulation* 1990; 82:636–638.
81. Leung WH, Wong KL, Lau C-P, et al. Cardiac abnormalities in systemic lupus erythematosus: A prospective M-mode, cross-sectional and Doppler echocardiographic study. *Int J Cardiol* 1990; 27:367–375.
82. Sturfelt G, Eskilsson J, Nived O, et al. Cardiovascular disease in systemic lupus erythematosus: A study of 75 patients from a defined population. *Medicine (Baltimore)* 1992; 71:216–223.
83. Ong ML, Veerapen K, Chambers JB, et al. Cardiac abnormalities in systemic lupus erythematosus: Prevalence and relationship to disease activity. *Int J Cardiol* 1992; 34:69–74.
84. Kaplan SD, Chartash EK, Pizzarello RA, Furie RA. Cardiac manifestations of the antiphospholipid syndrome. *Am Heart J* 1992; 124:1331–1337.
85. Gleason CB, Stoddard MF, Wagner SG, et al. A comparison of cardiac valvular involvement in the primary antiphospholipid syndrome versus anticardiolipin-negative systemic lupus erythematosus. *Am Heart J* 1993; 125:1123–1129.
86. Khamashta MA, Hughes GRV. Antiphospholipid antibodies and valve disease in patients with systemic lupus erythematosus. *J Am Coll Cardiol* 1993; 22:1268–1271.
87. Bulkley BH, Roberts WC. The heart in systemic lupus erythematosus and the changes induced in it by corticosteroid therapy: A study of 36 necropsy patients. *Am J Med* 1975; 58:243–264.
88. Gabrielli F, Alcini E, Di Prima MA, et al. Cardiac valve involvement in systemic lupus erythematosus and primary antiphospholipid syndrome: Lack of correlation with antiphospholipid antibodies. *Int J Cardiol* 1995; 51:117–126.
89. Roldan CA, Shively BK, Crawford MH. An echocardiographic study of valvular heart disease associated with systemic lupus erythematosus. *N Engl J Med* 1996; 335:1424–1430.
90. Kahl LE. The spectrum of pericardial tamponade in systemic lupus erythematosus: Report of ten patients. *Arthritis Rheum* 1992; 35:1343–1349.
91. Libman E, Sacks B. A hitherto undescribed form of valvular and mural endocarditis. *Arch Intern Med* 1924; 33:701–737.
92. Gross L. The cardiac lesion in Libman-Sacks disease with a consideration of its relationship to acute diffuse lupus erythematosus. *Am J Pathol* 1940; 16:375–407.
93. Sturfelt G, Eskilsson J, Nived O, et al. Cardiovascular disease in systemic disease in systemic lupus erythematosus: A study from a defined population. *Medicine (Baltimore)* 1992; 71:216–223.
94. Petri M, Spence D, Bone LR, Hochberg MC. Coronary risk factors in the Johns Hopkins lupus cohort: Prevalence by patients, and preventive practices. *Medicine (Baltimore)* 1992; 71:291–302.
95. Kutom AH, Gibbs HR. Myocardial infarction due to thrombi without significant coronary artery disease in systemic erythematosus. *Chest* 1991; 100:571–572.
96. Wilson VE, Eck SL, Bates ER. Evaluation and treatment of myocardial infarction complicating systemic lupus erythematosus. *Chest* 1991; 100:571–572.
97. Sumino H, Kanda T, Saski T, et al. Myocardial infarction secondary to coronary aneurysm in systemic lupus erythematosus: An autopsy case. *Angiology* 1995; 46:527–530.
98. James TN, Rupe CE, Monto RW. Pathology of the cardiac conduction system in systemic lupus erythematosus. *Ann Intern Med* 1965; 63:402–410.
99. McCauliffe DP. Neonatal lupus erythematosus: A transplacentally acquired autoimmune disorder. *Sem in Dermol* 1995; 14:47–53.
100. Brucato A, Franceschini F, Buyon JP. Neonatal lupus: Long-term outcomes of mothers and children and recurrence rate. *Clin Exp Rheumatol* 1997; 15:467–473.
101. Rabinerson D, Gruber A, Kaplan B, et al. Isolated persistent fetal bradycardia in complete A-V block: A conservative approach is appropriate—A case report and a review of the literature. *Am J Perinatol* 1997; 14:317–320.
102. Waltuck J, Buyon JP. Autoantibody-associated congenital heart block: Outcome in mothers and children. *Ann Intern Med* 1994; 120:544–551.
103. Press J, Uziel Y, Laxer RM, et al. Long-term outcome of mothers of children with complete congenital heart block. *Am J Med* 1996; 100:328–332.
104. Gobel MM, Dick M II, McCune WJ, et al. Atrioventricular conduction in children of women with systemic lupus erythematosus. *Am J Cardiol* 1993; 71:94–98.
105. Logar D, Kveder T, Rozman B, Pobovisek J. Possible association between anti-Ro antibodies and myocarditis or cardiac conduction defects in adults with systemic lupus erythematosus. *Ann Rheum Dis* 1990; 49:627–629.
106. Martinez-Costa X, Ordi J, Barbera J, et al. High-grade atrioventricular heart block in 2 adults with systemic lupus erythematosus. *J Rheumol* 1991; 18:1926–1928.
107. Winslow TM, Ossipov MA, Fazio GP, et al. Five-year follow up study of the prevalence and progression of pulmonary hypertension in systemic lupus erythematosus. *Am Heart J* 1995; 129:510–515.
108. Kalangos A, Panos A, Sezerman O. Mitral valve repair in lupus valvulitis: Report of a case and review of the literature. *J Heart Valve Dis* 1995; 4:202–207.
109. Morin AM, Boyer JC, Nataf P, Gandjbakhch I. Mitral insufficiency caused by systemic lupus erythematosus requiring valve replacement: Three case reports and a review of the literature. *Thorac Cardiovasc Surg* 1996; 44:313–316.
110. Petri M, Lakatta C, Madger L, Goldman D. Effect of prednisone and hydroxychloroquine on coronary artery disease risk factors in systemic lupus erythematosus: A longitudinal data analysis. *Am J Med* 1994; 96:254–259.
111. Chiariello M, Ambrosio G, Capelli-Bigazzi M, et al. Reduction in infarct size by the phospholipase inhibitor quinacrine in dogs with coronary artery occlusion. *Am Heart J* 1990; 120:801–807.
112. Cacoub P, Lunel-Fabiani F, Le-Thi Huong CLT. Polyarteritis nodosa and hepatitis C virus infection. *Ann Intern Med* 1992; 116:605–606.
113. Alarcon-Segovia D. The necrotizing vasculitides: A new pathogenetic classification. *Symp Rheumatol Dis* 1977; 61:241–260.
114. Schrader ML, Hochman JS, Bulkley BH. The heart in polyarteritis nodosa: A clinicopathologic study. *Am Heart J* 1985; 109:1353–1359.
115. Chu KH, Menapace FU, Blankenship JC, et al. Polyarteritis nodosa presenting as acute myocardial infarction with coronary dissection. *Cathet Cardiovasc Diagn* 1998; 44:320–324.
116. Thiene G, Valente M, Rossi L. Involvement of the cardiac conducting system in panarteritis nodosa. *Am Heart J* 1978; 95:716–724.
117. Charles LA, Jennette JC, Falk RJ. The role of HLGO cells in the detection of antineutrophil cytoplasmic autoantibodies. *J Rheumatol* 1991; 18:491–494.
118. Roberts WC, Dangel JC, Bulkley BH. Nonrheumatic valvular cardiac disease: A clinicopathologic survey of 27 different conditions causing valvular dysfunction. *Cardiovasc Clin* 1973; 4:333–446.
119. Bacon PA, Gibson DG. Cardiac involvement in rheumatoid arthritis: An echocardiographic study. *Ann Rheum Dis* 1974; 33:20–24.
120. Hakala M, Pettersson T, Tarkka M, et al. Rheumatoid arthritis as a cause of cardiac compression: Favourable long-term outcome of pericardiectomy. *Clin Rheumatol* 1993; 12:199–203.
121. Escalante A, Kaufman RL, Quismorio FP Jr, Beardmore TD.

Cardiac compression in rheumatoid pericarditis. *Semin Arthritis Rheum* 1990; 20:148–163.
122. Hara KS, Ballard DJ, Illstrup DM, et al. Rheumatoid pericarditis: Clinical features and survival. *Medicine (Baltimore)* 1990; 69: 81–91.
123. Travaglio-Encinoza A, Anaya JM, Dupuy D, et al. Rheumatoid pericarditis: New immunopathological aspects. *Clin Exp Rheumatol* 1994; 12:313–316.
124. Suriani RJ, Lansman S, Konstadt S. Intracardiac rheumatoid nodule presenting as a left atrial mass. *Am Heart J* 1994; 127: 463–465.
125. Maione S, Valentini G, Giunta A, et al. Cardiac involvement in rheumatoid arthritis: An echocardiographic study. *Cardiology* 1993; 83:234–239.
126. Kotha P, McGreevy MJ, Kotha A, et al. Early deaths with thrombolytic therapy for acute myocardial infarction in corticosteroid-dependent rheumatoid arthritis. *Clin Cardiol* 1998; 21:853–856.
127. Julkunen H. Rheumatoid spondylitis: Clinical and laboratory study of 149 cases compared with 182 cases of rheumatoid arthritis. *Acta Rheumatol Scand* 1962; 172(suppl 4):1–116.
128. Bulkley BH, Roberts WC. Ankylosing spondylitis and aortic regurgitation: Description of the characteristic cardiovascular lesion from study of eight necropsy patients. *Circulation* 1973; 48:1014–1027.
129. Roberts WC, Hollingsworth JR, Bulkley BH, et al. Combined mitral and aortic regurgitation in ankylosing spondylitis: Angiographic and anatomic features. *Am J Med* 1974; 56:237–243.
130. Gould BA, Turner J, Keeling DH, et al. Myocardial dysfunction in ankylosing spondylitis. *Ann Rheum Dis* 1992; 51:227–232.
131. Weiss S, Stead EA, Warren JV, Bailey OT. Scleroderma heart disease: With a consideration of certain other visceral manifestations of scleroderma. *Arch Intern Med* 1943; 71:749–776.
132. Bulkley BH, Klacsmann PG, Hutchins GM. Angina pectoris, myocardial infarction and sudden death with normal coronary arteries: A clinicopathologic study of 9 patients with progressive systemic sclerosis. *Am Heart J* 1978; 95:563–569.
133. Salerni R, Rodnan GP, Leon DR, Shaver JA. Pulmonary hypertension in the CREST syndrome variant of progressive systemic sclerosis (scleroderma). *Ann Intern Med* 1977; 86:394–399.
134. Cannon PJ, Hassar M, Case DB, et al. The relationship of hypertension and renal failure in scleroderma (progressive systemic sclerosis) to structural and functional abnormalities of the renal cortical circulation. *Medicine (Baltimore)* 1974; 53:1–46.
135. Follansbee WP, Curtiss EI, Medsger TA Jr, et al. Physiologic abnormalities of cardiac function in progressive systemic sclerosis with diffuse scleroderma. *N Engl J Med* 1984; 310:142–148.
136. Alexander EL, Firestein GS, Weiss JL, et al. Reversible cold-induced abnormalities in myocardial perfusion and function in systemic sclerosis. *Ann Intern Med* 1986; 105:661–668.
137. Clements PJ, Furst DE. Heart involvement in systemic sclerosis. *Clin Dermatol* 1994; 12:267–275.
138. Deswal A, Follansbee WP. Cardiac involvement in scleroderma. *Rheum Dis Clin North Am* 1996; 22:841–860.
139. Anvari A, Graninger W, Schneider B, et al. Cardiac involvement in systemic sclerosis. *Arthritis Rheum* 1992; 35:1356–1361.
140. Candell-Riera J, Armandans-Gil L, Simeon CP, et al. Comprehensive noninvasive assessment of cardiac involvement in limited systemic sclerosis. *Arthritis Rheum* 1996; 39:1138–1145.
141. Fujimoto S, Kagoshima T, Nakajima T, Dohi K. Doppler echocardiographic assessment of left ventricular diastolic function in patients with progressive systemic sclerosis. *Cardiology* 1993; 83:217–227.
142. Clements PJ, Lachenbruch PA, Furst DE, et al. Cardiac score: A semiquantitative measure of cardiac involvement that improves prediction of prognosis in systemic sclerosis. *Arthritis Rheum* 1991; 34:1371–1380.
143. Follansbee WP, Zerbe TR, Medsger TA Jr. Cardiac and skeletal muscle disease in systemic sclerosis (scleroderma): A high-risk association. *Am Heart J* 1993; 125:194–203.
144. D' Angelo WA, Fries JR, Masi AT, Shulman LE. Pathologic observations in systemic sclerosis (scleroderma): A study of fifty-eight autopsy cases and fifty-eight matched controls. *Am J Med* 1969; 46:428–440.
145. Satoh M, Tokuhira M, Hama N, et al. Massive pericardial effusion in scleroderma: A review of five cases. *Br J Rheumatol* 1995; 34:564–567.
146. Perez-Bocanegra C, Fonollosa V, Simeon CP, et al. Pericardial tamponade preceding cutaneous involvement in systemic sclerosis. *Ann Rheum Dis* 1995; 54:687–688.
147. Kazzam E, Caidahl K, Hallgren R, et al. Mitral regurgitation and diastolic flow profile in systemic sclerosis. *Int J Cardiol* 1990; 29:357–363.
148. Walcott G, Burchell HB, Brown AL. Primary pulmonary hypertension. *Am J Med* 1970; 71:70–79.
149. Pope JE. Treatment of systemic sclerosis. *Rheum Dis Clin North Am* 1996; 22:893–907.
150. Martinez-Taboada V, Olalla J, Blanco R, et al. Malignant ventricular arrhythmia in systemic sclerosis controlled with an implantable cardioverter defibrillator. *J Rheumatol* 1994; 21:2166–2167.
151. Fritzler MJ, Hart DA. Prolonged improvement of Raynaud's phenomenon and scleroderma after recombinant tissue plasminogen activator therapy. *Arthritis Rheum* 1990; 33:274–276.
152. Matteson EL, Shbeeb MI, McCarthy TG, et al. Pilot study of antithymocyte globulin in systemic sclerosis. *Arthritis Rheum* 1996; 39:1132–1137.
153. Alpert MA, Pressly TA, Mukerji V, et al. Acute and long-term effects of infedipine on pulmonary and systemic hemodynamics in patients with pulmonary hypertension associated with diffuse systemic sclerosis, the CREST syndrome and mixed connective tissue disease. *Am J Cardiol* 1991; 68:1687–1690.
154. Kazzam E, Caidahl K, Hällgren R, et al. Noninvasive evaluation of long-term cardiac effects of captopril in system sclerosis. *J Intern Med* 1991; 230:203–212.
155. Plotz PH, Dalakias M, Leff RL, et al. Current concepts in idiopathic inflammatory myopathies: Polymyositis, dermatomyositis, and related disorders. *Ann Intern Med* 1989; 111:143–157.
156. Dalakas MC. Polymyositis, dermatomyositis, and inclusion-body myositis. *N Engl J Med* 1991; 325:1487–1489.
157. Dalakas M, Illa I, Dambrosia JM, et al. A controlled trial of high-dose intravenous immune globulin as treatment for dermatomyositis. *N Engl J Med* 1993; 329:1993–2000.
158. Gonzales EB, Varner WT, Lisse JR, et al. Giant-cell arteritis in the southern United States: An 11-year retrospective study from the Texas Gulf coast. *Arch Intern Med* 1989; 149:1561–1565.
159. Hasley PB, Follansbee WP, Coulehan JL. Cardiac manifestations of Churg-Strauss syndrome: Report of a case and review of the literature. *Am Heart J* 1990; 120:996–999.
160. Abu-Shakra M, Gladman DD, Urowitz MB, Farewell V. Anticardiolipin antibodies in systemic lupus erythematosus: Clinical and laboratory correlations. *Am J Med* 1995; 99:624–628.
161. Khamashta MA, Cudrado MJ, Mujic F, et al. The management of thrombosis in the antiphospholipid-antibody syndrome. *N Engl J Med* 1995; 332:993–997.
162. Brenner B, Blumenfeld Z, Markiewicz W, Reisner SA. Cardiac involvement in patients with primary antiphospholipid syndrome. *J Am Coll Cardiol* 1991; 18:931–936.
163. Beynon HLC, Walport MJ. Antiphospholipid antibodies and cardiovascular disease. *Br Heart J* 1992; 67:281–284.
164. Soler J. Valvular heart disease in the primary antiphospholipid syndrome. *Ann Intern Med* 1992; 116:293–298.
165. Vianna JL, Khamashta MA, Ordi-Ros J, et al. Comparison of the primary and secondary antiphospholipid syndrome: A European multicenter study of 114 patients. *Am J Med* 1994; 96:3–9.

166. Cervera R, Asherson RA, Lie JT. Clinicopathologic correlations of the antiphospholipid syndrome. *Semin Arthritis Rheum* 1995; 24:262–277.
167. Violi F, Ferro D, Quintarelli C. Antiphospholipid antibodies, hypercoagulability and thrombosis. *Haematologica* 1995; 80(suppl 2):131–135.
168. Hojnik M, George J, Ziporen L, Shoenfeld Y. Heart valve involvement (Libman-Sacks endocarditis) in the antiphospholipid syndrome. *Circulation* 1996; 93:1579–1987.
169. Nesher G, Ilany J, Rosenmann D, Abraham AS. Valvular dysfunction in antiphospholipid syndrome: Prevalence, clinical features, and treatment. *Semin Arthritis Rheum* 1997; 27:27–35.
170. Ben-Chetrit E. Anti Ro/La antibodies and their clinical association. *Isr J Med Sci* 1997; 33:251–253.
171. Specker C, Perniok A, Brauckmann U, et al. Detection of cerebral microemboli in APS: Introducing a novel investigation method and implications of analogies with carotid artery disease. *Lupus* 1998; 7(suppl 2):S75–S80.
172. Asherson RA, Cervera R, Piette JC, et al. Catastrophic antiphospholipid syndrome: Clinical and laboratory features of 50 patients. *Medicine (Baltimore)* 1998; 77:195–207.
173. Matsuura E, Kobayashi K, Yasuda T, Koike T. Antiphospholipid antibodies and atherosclerosis. *Lupus* 1998; 7(suppl 2):S135–S139.
174. Ginsburg KS, Liang MH, Newcomer L, et al. Anticardiolipin antibodies and the risk for ischemic stroke and venous thrombosis. *Ann Intern Med* 1992; 117:997–1002.
175. Rosove MH, Brewer PMC. Antiphospholipid thrombosis: Clinical course after the first thrombotic event in 70 patients. *Ann Intern Med* 1992; 117:303–308.
176. Bulkley BH. Progressive systemic sclerosis: Cardiac involvement. *Clin Rheum Dis* 1979; 5–131.

CHAPTER 77

NEOPLASTIC HEART DISEASE

Robert J. Hall / Denton A. Cooley / Hugh A. McAllister, Jr. / O. Howard Frazier / Susan Wilansky

Tumors of the heart, while uncommon, present in protean ways and have challenged the acumen of physicians since the seventeenth century. Antemortem diagnosis, however, was rare. Intracardiac myxoma was first diagnosed, with the aid of angiography, in 1952, with a subsequent attempt to remove the tumor surgically. The first such successful removal with the use of cardiopulmonary bypass was performed in 1954; the patient, then a 40-year-old woman, was still alive 38 years later.[1] Subsequently, increased clinical awareness coupled with angiographic and noninvasive diagnostic techniques led to more frequent correct diagnoses.[2]

The heart may be the site of a primary tumor or may be invaded secondarily by malignancies that arise in adjacent or remote organs. Whether the tumors are primary or secondary, neoplastic heart disease can be expressed in only limited ways (Table 77-1). In the presence of neoplastic disease, pericardial pain, effusion, tamponade, constriction, rapid increase in heart size, new heart murmurs, electrocardiographic changes, atrial or ventricular arrhythmias, atrioventricular (AV) block, and unexplained heart failure are suggestive of secondary invasion of the heart. The triad of obstruction, embolization, and constitutional manifestations characterizes intracavitary tumors, especially myxomas.

PRIMARY TUMORS OF THE HEART

Although less common than other heart tumors, primary tumors of the heart are far more challenging to both the physician and the surgeon. These tumors usually present as intracavitary lesions, and more than 75 percent are benign.[3] Current surgical techniques permit removal and potential "cure" in many patients with primary heart tumors, thus necessitating an awareness of their clinical and hemodynamic presentation.[4]

Primary tumors of the heart and pericardium are rare, with a frequency of 0.001 to 0.28 percent in reported or collected postmortem series.[3] Myxomas constitute nearly 50 percent of all histologically benign tumors of the heart. The frequency of occurrence and classification of 533 primary tumors and cysts of the heart and pericardium collected by the Armed Forces Institute of Pathology are presented in Table 77-2.[5]

Cardiac Myxomas

Intracardiac myxoma is the most frequent benign tumor of the heart. While most (75 percent) are located in the left atrium (LA), myxomas are also found in the right atrium (RA; 18 percent), right ventricle (RV; 4 percent), and left ventricle (LV; 4 percent).[5–7] Cardiac myxomas usually originate from the region of the fossa ovalis but may arise from a variety of locations within the atria.[5] Although myxomas have been reported as originating from the mitral annulus, the mitral valve itself, the aortic valve, and the inferior vena cava, it is likely that true myxomas only arise from the mural endocardium.[6]

PATHOLOGY

Attached to the endocardium by a broad base, myxomas are usually pedunculated, polypoid, and friable, although some may have a smooth surface and be rounded.[8–10] A myxoma appears as a soft, gelatinous, mucoid, usually gray-white mass, often with areas of hemorrhage or thrombosis. They vary from 1 to 15 cm in diameter, with most measuring 5 to 6 cm (Fig. 77-1*A*, *B*, and *C*).[5]

On microscopic examination, the myxoma is composed of an acid mucopolysaccharide myxoid matrix in which polygonal cells and occasional blood vessels are embedded. Channels, often filled with red blood cells, communicate from the surface to deep within the tumor and are lined by endothelial-like cells resembling multipurpose mesenchymal cells, from which the tumor is purported to arise. Similar endothelial cells line the surface of the tumor; however, fibrin, erythrocytes, and organized thrombi also may be present on the surface. Cystic areas; focal or gross hemorrhage; calcification; glandular elements; rarely, bone formation; and even hematopoietic tissue constitute the multiple, although uncommon, variations.[5]

A neoplastic origin of myxomas is supported by the ultrastructural characteristics of the tumor,[14] the results of biochemical analyses,[12] the cultural properties of the tumor cell,[5] and DNA analysis of the tumor.[6] Although myxomas can recur because of their incomplete removal[13] and distant growth of embolic myxomatous material has been observed,[13] the existence of a true malignant cardiac myxoma remains doubtful.[3] The occurrence of multiple tumors within the LA, bilaterally

TABLE 77-1 General Manifestations of Neoplastic Heart Disease

- Pericardial involvement
  - Pericarditis and pain
  - Pericardial effusion
  - Radiographic enlargement
  - Arrhythmia, predominantly atrial
  - Tamponade
  - Constriction
- Myocardial involvement
  - Arrhythmias, ventricular and atrial
  - Electrocardiographic changes
  - Radiographic enlargement
    - Generalized
    - Localized
  - Conduction disturbances and heart block
  - Congestive heart failure
  - Coronary involvement
    - Angina, infarction
- Intracavitary tumor
  - Cavity obliteration
  - Valve obstruction and valve damage
  - Embolic phenomena: systemic, neurologic, and coronary
  - Constitutional manifestations

in each atrium,[14] or simultaneously in the atrium and ventricle[15] raises the possibility of multicentric origin rather than metastasis of the tumor.

AGE, GENDER, AND FAMILIAL OCCURRENCE

Most patients with myxomas are 30 to 60 years of age,[2] although myxomas have been discovered in children, infants, neonates,[16,23] and the elderly.[17] Children have a higher incidence of ventricular myxomas than do adults. A higher incidence in females has characterized most series. Familial occurrence has been reported,[18,19] more frequently in males. Tumors are divided equally on both sides of the heart, and opposite atria are usually involved in afflicted members. Familial cases are associated with a younger age at presentation and a higher recurrence rate.[18,19]

GENERAL OR CONSTITUTIONAL MANIFESTATIONS

While asymptomatic patients with myxoma (Fig. 77-1*C*) have been reported, most present with one or more effects of a triad of constitutional, embolic, and obstructive manifestations.[2] Cardiac myxomas provoke systemic manifestations in 90 percent of the patients, characterized by weight loss, fatigue, fever, anemia (often hemolytic), elevated sedimentation rate, and elevated serum immunoglobulin concentration formed in response to tumor embolization, degenerative changes within the tumor, or overproduction of interleukin-6 by the tumor.[20] The globulin fraction most frequently elevated is immunoglobulin G (IgG), and immunoglobulin A is involved only rarely.[2] Cases involving coexisting cardiac myxoma and IgG multiple myeloma,[21] and systemic AL-amyloidosis have been reported.[22] Less common findings are leukocytosis, thrombocytopenia, clubbing, Raynaud's phenomenon, and breast fibroadenomas.[2] Polycythemia may result from tumor production of erythropoietin.[23] Patients with hemolytic anemia have features of intravascular mechanical destruction. Hemolytic anemia is more likely to occur in patients with calcified myxomas, which are found more commonly in the RA. The protracted multisystemic symptoms produced by myxomas may mimic connective tissue disease and polyarteritis nodosa.[24]

"Syndrome myxoma," or Carney's complex, characterizes a subset of patients with cardiac myxoma, associated with spotty skin pigmentation and peripheral and endocrine neoplasms. These patients, in contrast to those with "sporadic myxoma," are usually younger, have a high frequency of familial myxoma, and more frequently have multiple and recurrent tumors.[25-27]

Infected Myxoma Rarely, an intracavitary myxoma becomes infected, and blood cultures have demonstrated a variety of organisms.[27] Most patients with infected myxomas experience major neurologic embolic events. Thus, surgical resection should be carried out promptly before complications occur.

Embolization Systemic tumor embolization, more commonly from myxomas with irregular, papillary, frondlike surfaces,[8-10]

TABLE 77-2 Tumors and Cysts of the Heart and Pericardium

Type	Number	Percentage
BENIGN		
Myxoma	130	24.4
Lipoma	45	8.4
Papillary fibroelastoma	42	7.9
Rhabdomyoma	36	6.8
Fibroma	17	3.2
Hemangioma	15	2.8
Teratoma	14	2.6
Mesothelioma of the AV node	12	2.3
Granular cell tumor	3	
Neurofibroma	3	
Lymphangioma	2	
Subtotal	319	59.8
Pericardial cyst	82	15.4
Bronchogenic cyst	7	1.3
Subtotal	89	16.7
MALIGNANT		
Angiosarcoma	39	7.3
Rhabdomyosarcoma	26	4.9
Mesothelioma	19	3.6
Fibrosarcoma	14	2.6
Malignant lymphoma	7	1.3
Extraskeletal osteosarcoma	5	
Neurogenic sarcoma	4	
Malignant teratoma	4	
Thymoma	4	
Leiomyosarcoma	1	
Liposarcoma	1	
Synovial sarcoma	1	
Subtotal	125	23.5
Total	533	100.0

SOURCE: McAllister and Fenoglio,[5] with permission.

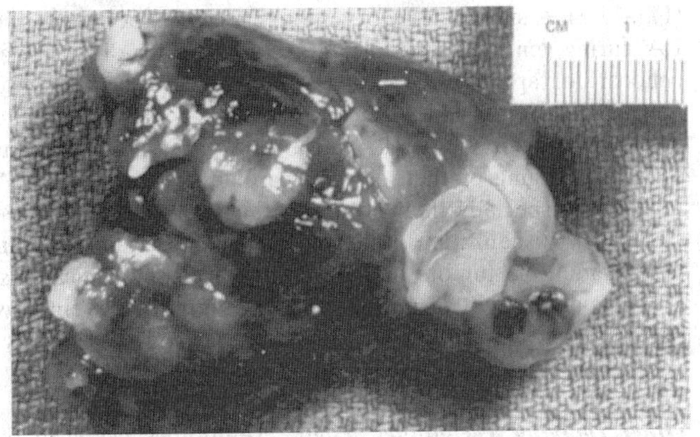

A

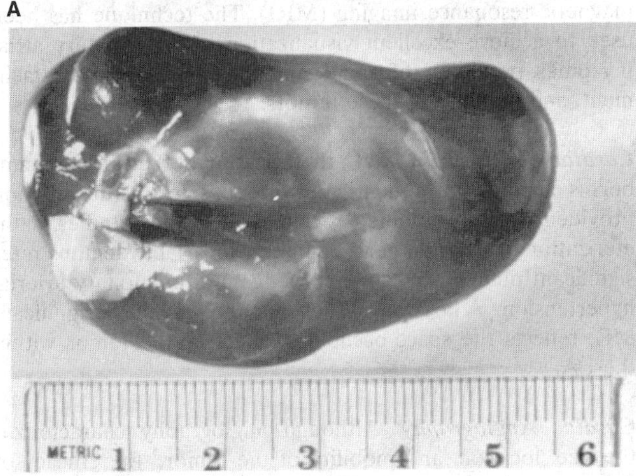

B

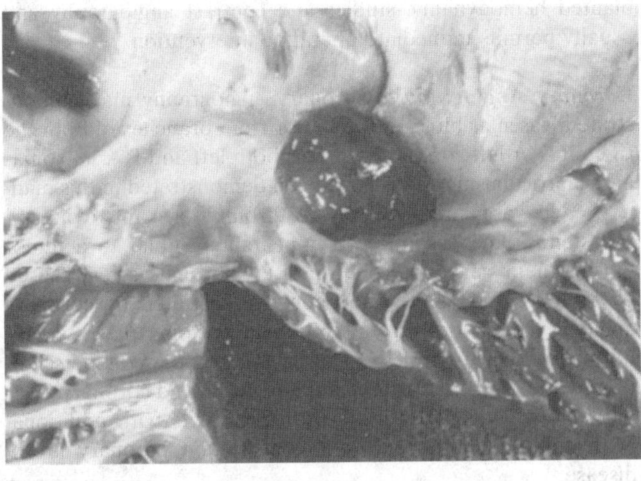

C

FIGURE 77-1 LA myxomas. *A*. More polypoid and irregular. *B*. Smooth-surfaced and rounded. Attachment to a portion of the atrial septum is seen on each tumor. *C*. An asymptomatic sessile myxoma attached above the posterior leaflet of the mitral valve was found coincidentally at necropsy.

occurs in 40 to 50 percent of patients with LA myxoma,[2] with tumor fragments or surface clots embolizing to arteries in the brain, kidneys, and extremities.[28,29] Rarely, a complete LA myxoma becomes detached and lodges in the aortic bifurcation.[30] The size and consistency of such an embolus may require direct exploration of the aortic bifurcation. Histologic examination of emboli recovered at operation from a peripheral artery can aid in diagnosing an otherwise unsuspected intracardiac myxoma.[3] Systemic embolization, especially in a young patient with sinus rhythm, should arouse suspicion of a myxoma once bacterial endocarditis has been ruled out.

Tumor embolization of the central nervous system constitutes about 50 percent of embolic events caused by LA myxomas, may represent the first symptomatic manifestation, is more common in the left hemisphere, and may be multiple and massive.[31] Embolization may be to the extracranial or intracranial cerebral vessels, with the former being amenable to surgical removal. Onset of the neurologic deficit may be gradual or sudden.

Intracranial arterial aneurysms secondary to myxomatous emboli have been demonstrated angiographically. Late rupture with intracranial hemorrhage has been reported. Care must be taken to avoid embolization during surgical removal of an intracardiac myxoma, not only because of the immediate consequences of an embolic phenomenon, but also because viable metastatic foci may cause symptoms years later. As a consequence, the patient who has sustained cerebral emboli is not necessarily "cured" after the primary tumor is surgically removed.[32]

Retinal artery embolism can occur with transient or permanent visual impairment, confirmed by ophthalmoscopic and histopathologic evidence of particulate embolic matter in the retinal artery.[33] Only rarely has occlusion of the retinal artery occurred in the absence of multifocal neurologic manifestations.

Coronary artery embolism associated with myxoma has been documented by both angiography in living patients and histology at postmortem study.[3] Myocardial infarction occasionally is the first manifestation of a myxoma.[34]

General Features Constitutional manifestations and embolic potential are common to varying degrees in patients with myxoma in any intracavitary location. The cardiac manifestations, symptoms, and physical findings are the consequence of the intracavitary mass and the particular location of the tumor. Myxomas of the LA may obstruct either the mitral or pulmonary venous orifices and produce pulmonary venous hypertension, secondary pulmonary hypertension, and right-sided heart failure. The clinical symptoms include dyspnea on exertion, orthopnea, paroxysmal nocturnal dyspnea, acute pulmonary edema, cough, and hemoptysis, along with palpitations, chest pain, fatigue, and peripheral edema. Episodes of syncope or dizziness are frequent, and sudden death may occur. A marked effect of the severity of any symptom caused by a change in position of the patient, especially if recumbency relieves dyspnea,[2] is suggestive of myxoma.

Physical Examination On physical examination, the first heart sound is loud and frequently split, with the second component corresponding to the tumor expulsion from the mitral orifice (see Chap. 10). P_2 is accentuated, and an early diastolic sound, the "tumor plop," is usually heard 80 to 120 ms after the aortic closure sound,[2] resembling an opening snap. The tumor plop may be confused with either an opening snap of the mitral valve or a third heart sound and follows A_2 at an intermediate interval between these events (Fig. 77-2).

An apical diastolic or systolic murmur or both are present in many patients. The auscultatory findings may vary with a change in position of the patient.[2] Features of pulmonary hyper-

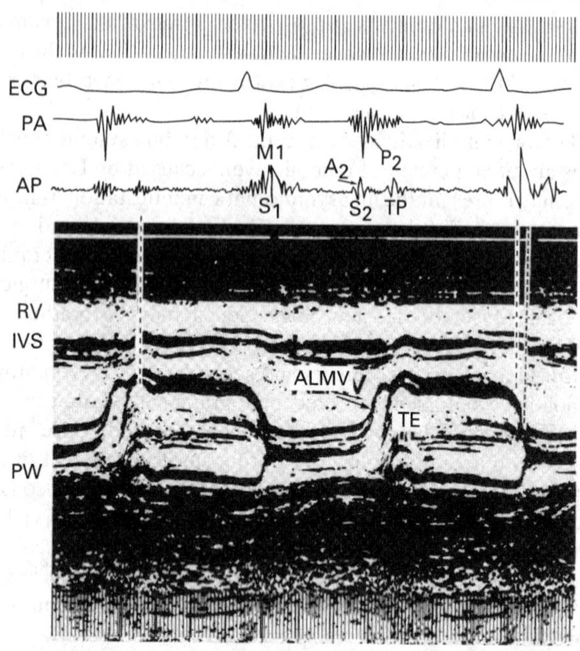

FIGURE 77-2 Recordings of a patient with a cystic LA myxoma, including (*top*) the electrocardiogram, (*middle*) phonocardiograms from the pulmonary area (PA) at high frequency and from the apex (AP) at medium frequency, and (*bottom*) the M-mode echocardiogram at the level of the mitral valve. Time lines equal 0.01-s intervals. The RV, septum (IVS), and posterior wall (PW) of the left ventricle are identified. The loud component of the first sound (M_1) is delayed (Q to M_1 = 0.09 s). The pulmonic second sound (P_2) is accentuated. Multiple linear tumor echoes (TE) are seen behind the anterior leaflet to the mitral valve (ALMV), first appearing at the mitral level 0.04 s after onset of mitral opening and completing the forward movement 0.09 s after onset of mitral opening, at which point the "tumor plop" (TP) is recorded. The A_2–TP interval measures 0.010 s.

tension are frequent and may result in a murmur of tricuspid regurgitation.

Electrocardiogram and Chest X-ray Results of electrocardiographic examination are nonspecific, reflecting hemodynamic alterations similar to those of mitral valvular disease; however, sinus rhythm is generally the rule. The chest roentgenogram reveals LA enlargement and the characteristic changes of pulmonary venous congestion and pulmonary hypertension. The absence of mitral valve calcification and the presence of a LA smaller than might be expected with presumed rheumatic mitral disease are helpful differentiating clues. Calcification may be evident in the tumor even on routine chest film,[35] but this is better visualized and motion is better appreciated on fluoroscopy. The "wrecking-ball" effect of a calcified mobile myxoma may cause destruction of the mitral valve or rupture of the chordae tendineae and may produce severe mitral regurgitation (MR).

Echocardiography The value of ultrasound in the noninvasive diagnosis of intracavitary tumors has been well documented.[2,10] M-mode recordings in patients with a prolapsing LA myxoma typically demonstrate a diminished EF slope of the anterior leaflet of the mitral valve, behind which a dense array of wavy tumor echoes is seen (see Chap. 13). The tumor plop coincides with the completion of this anterior movement of tumor echoes (Fig. 77-2). A similar array of tumor echoes may be seen in the LA during ventricular systole. Transthoracic two-dimensional echocardiography (TTE) and transesophageal echocardiography (TEE) identify the size, shape, point of attachment, and motion characteristics of LA atrial myxomas.[36] TEE permits superior imaging of the posterior cardiac structures and LA myxomas, especially their point of attachment (Fig. 77-3; see Chap. 13). Visualization of all four chambers permits recognition of multiple tumors or tumors in less common locations. Doppler assessment of mitral valve and pulmonary vein flow patterns provides further information regarding the hemodynamic consequences of LA myxomas.

Other Imaging Techniques High resolution is achieved by magnetic resonance imaging (MRI). The technique has been used to achieve excellent visualization of intracavitary atrial myxomas, providing information about the size, shape, attachment, and mobility of these tumors.[37–39]

Cardiac Catheterization Catheterization of the cardiac chambers is currently infrequently performed, since the information provided is readily obtained by echocardiographic studies. Catheterization of the right heart chambers invariably demonstrates significant pulmonary capillary wedge and pulmonary arterial hypertension.[2] A large *v* wave, even in the absence of significant MR, reflects the space-occupying effect of the tumor within the LA.

Cardiac Angiography Although angiography characterizes the size, location, and mobility of the tumor,[2] the efficacy of echocardiography and other imaging techniques has largely supplanted hemodynamic studies and contrast angiography and usually permits immediate operative intervention.

Coronary Angiography Coronary angiography may demonstrate a vascular blush in the tumor from branches of both the right and/or left coronary arteries; both left and RA myxomas and ventricular myxomas have been demonstrated in this manner.[8,55] Neovascularization of a LA thrombus accompanying mitral stenosis may produce an appearance similar to a tumor blush. Aneurysms and occlusion of the coronary artery caused by tumor emboli have also been demonstrated by coronary angiography. Myocardial infarction in myxoma patients with normal coronary arteries has been ascribed to cytokine secretion by the tumor.[40] Cardiac catheterization and coronary angiography are indicated primarily for patients with additional heart disease and to rule out concomitant coronary artery disease.[4]

Differential Diagnosis LA myxomas most often present as, and must be differentiated from, mitral valvular disease.[4] At our institution, intracavitary myxomas were discovered in a ratio of approximately 1 per 100 patients presenting for mitral valve surgery.[2] Characteristically, the clinical course is relatively recent in origin; however, it may occasionally span many years. Fever, constitutional symptoms, and embolic phenomena mimic infective endocarditis[4]; on rare occasions the myxoma itself may be infected. Muscle pain, skin rash, and Raynaud's phenomenon may simulate peripheral vasculitis.[41] Multiple systemic arterial aneurysms secondary to myxomatous embolization have mimicked polyarteritis nodosa.[24] Similarly, coronary artery aneurysmal dilatation and myocardial infarction have been attributed to coronary myxoma embolization. The correct diagnosis will be suspected if the physician maintains a high index of clinical suspicion in patients with diverse and protean features, especially when cardiac, embolic, and constitutional manifestations coexist. Echocardiographic imaging of the heart has greatly facilitated the recognition of intracavitary tumors and results in detection in some patients who are asymptomatic.[15] Intracavitary thrombi may at times mimic intracardiac tumor masses (Fig. 77-4).

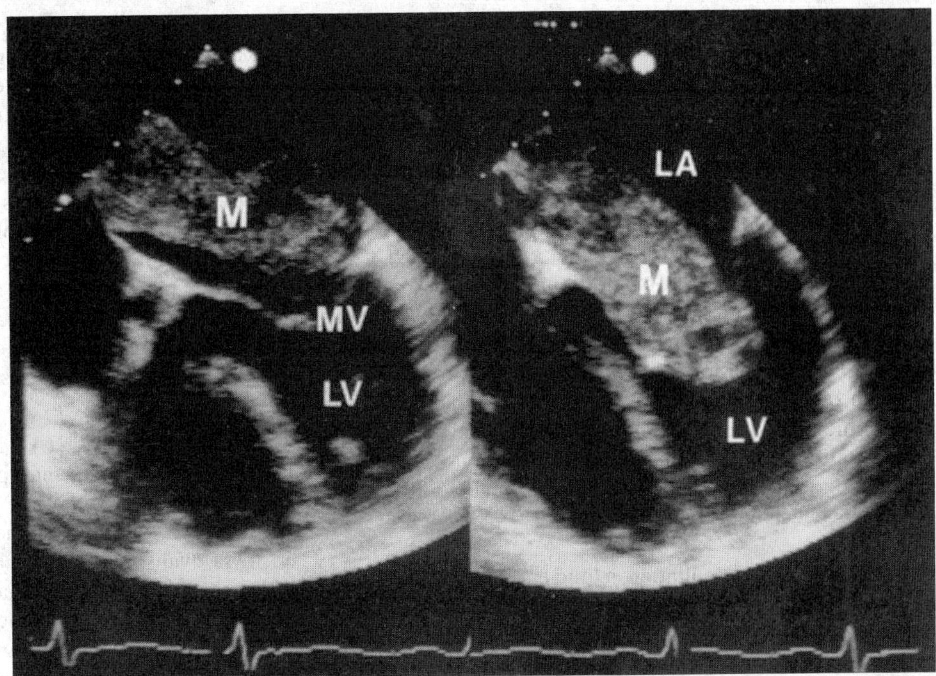

FIGURE 77-3 Transesophageal echocardiogram in the four-chamber view from a 50-year-old man who presented with exertional dyspnea and syncope. A large LA myxoma (M) attached to the interatrial septum is seen prolapsing across the mitral valve (MV) into the LV in diastole (*right panel*). (Courtesy of Susan Wilansky, M.D., Medical Director, Noninvasive Imaging, St. Luke's Episcopal Hospital, Houston, Texas, and Bernardo Triestman, M.D.)

RIGHT ATRIAL MYXOMA

Myxomas in the RA cavity constitute about one-fifth of all myxomas and tend to be more solid, have a wider attachment, and involve a greater amount of the atrial wall or septum than those in the LA. They originate from a variety of locations within the RA, including the inferior margin of the foramen ovale, the tricuspid valve, and the eustachian valve,[6,42,43] and characteristically produce tricuspid valve or vena cava obstruction. A myxoma arising from the inferior vena cava has been reported.[8]

Clinical Manifestations Clinilcaly, symptoms of low cardiac output and manifestations of systemic venous hypertension are present, with a prominent jugular venous *a* wave, hepatomegaly, ascites, edema, and cyanosis,[6] which may be episodic and vary with the position of the patient. Persistence of sinus rhythm is common. Intermittent episodes of syncope and abrupt onset of dyspnea, features never seen with rheumatic tricuspid stenosis, are reported in one-third of these patients.[6] The pendular action of a prolapsing RA myxoma (wrecking-ball effect),[44] especially when it is calcified, may damage or destroy the tricuspid valve and produce severe tricuspid regurgitation.[38]

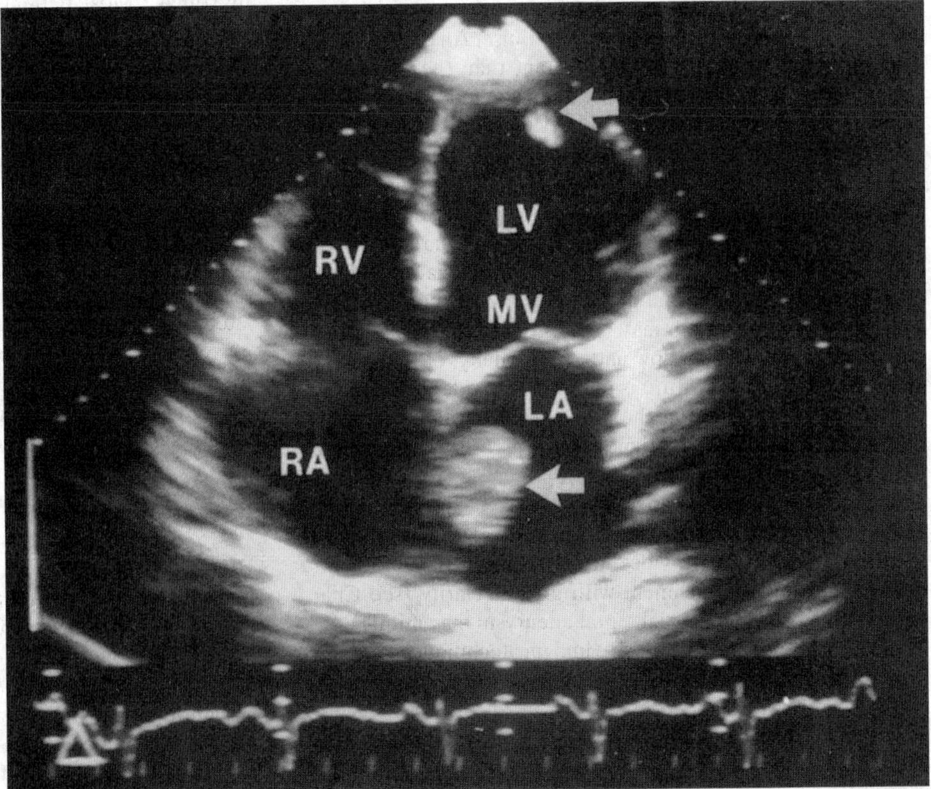

FIGURE 77-4 Two-dimensional echocardiogram, apical four-chamber view, of a patient with advanced congestive cardiomyopathy. Intracavitary masses (arrows), proved at autopsy to be thrombi, are present in the LA attached to the atrial septum (AS) and in the apex of the LV. The latter masses are both sessile and pedunculated. MV, mitral valve. (Courtesy of Carlos de Castro, Department of Cardiology, St. Luke's Episcopal Hospital, Houston, Texas.)

Pulmonary Emboli While embolic tumor phenomena occur less frequently with RA than with LA myxomas, pulmonary emboli have been reported,[6] at times are extensive,[44] and may produce irreversible pulmonary hypertension.[45] RA myxoma has been incorrectly diagnosed as recurrent pulmonary thromboembolism.[46]

Wide dissemination of myxomatous embolization to the pulmonary arteries has been reported, with active infiltration of the media[13] and formation of aneurysms.[6] Paradoxical embolization may occur if an interatrial communication exists.

Systemic Manifestations Constitutional symptoms are less frequent in patients with a RA myxoma.[2] Anemia, polycythemia,[2] and cyanosis have been reported. Polycythemia and cyanosis may be caused by either right-to-left shunting through a patent foramen ovale or atrial septal defect, low cardiac output and hypoxemic stimulation of the bone marrow, intravascular hemoconcentration, or erythropoietin production by the tumor.[23] Mesenteric vasculitis of a nonembolic, probably autoimmune, origin has been reported.[47]

Auscultation On auscultation, a loud early systolic sound may be heard. This sound occurs as late as 80 ms after the mitral component of the first sound and results from expulsion of the tumor from the right ventricle. A palpable tumor shock may coincide with this loud sound.[48] A crescendo murmur with inspiratory augmentation preceding this loud tumor expulsion sound is probably caused by early systolic tricuspid regurgitation (see Chap. 10). There may be a long diastolic murmur or, more commonly, only a late diastolic rumble, augmented by inspiration, accompanying atrial systole. If major injury to the tricuspid valve occurs, the murmur of TR will be present, and large *v* waves will be seen in the jugular venous pulse. An early diastolic sound may be heard but is less constant than the tumor plop that accompanies a LA myxoma. The changing quality of the sound and murmurs may mimic a pericardial rub. Such sounds have been called endocardial friction rubs (see Chap. 10).

Electrocardiogram and Chest X-ray The results of electrocardiography are often normal, although RA enlargement frequently is suggested.[6] Low-voltage, right-axis deviation and varying degrees of right bundle-branch block have been reported.[6] The chest roentgenogram may reveal some prominence or enlargement of the RA shadow and, occasionally, of the RV. An important radiologic feature is the mild or moderate degree of cardiomegaly, considering the severe clinical state of the patients. Calcification in the tumor is more common in patients with myxomas in the right atrium.[2]

Echocardiography TTE and TEE provide excellent images of the RA.[49] The latter provides more detail of the tumor and defines the site of attachment with greater clarity (see Chap. 13). A large prolapsing atrial septal aneurysm may mimic a RA tumor.[50] With current noninvasive imaging techniques, catheterization and angiography of the right-sided heart chambers are rarely necessary.

Differential Diagnosis The clinical features of RA myxoma resemble those of rheumatic tricuspid valvular disease, although the latter is always accompanied by significant mitral and, frequently, aortic valve disease. There are many similarities to constrictive pericarditis and Ebstein's anomaly of the tricuspid valve. Episodic dyspnea, sudden syncope, and variability of symptoms and findings with position of the patient may serve as helpful clues. Changing murmurs, along with fever and anemia, may suggest infective endocarditis. Tricuspid stenosis and regurgitation are prominent in patients with carcinoid syndrome, but involvement of the pulmonary valve and other features of a carcinoid tumor will usually serve to distinguish it from a RA myxoma. Obstruction of the right ventricular (RV) outflow tract may resemble a RA tumor. Pulmonary embolization of other diverse etiologies, with secondary thromboembolic pulmonary hypertension and right-sided heart failure, may be mimicked by RA myxoma. An awareness of the protean manifestations combined with echocardiographic findings usually facilitates a correct diagnosis.

BILATERAL ATRIAL MYXOMA

An atrial myxoma may pass through the foramen ovale and be present in both atria.[51] The tumor is usually shaped like a dumbbell, with the common stalk attached to the margin of the fossa ovalis. Surgery has been successful most often when the correct diagnosis was made preoperatively, emphasizing the importance of echographic exploration of all chambers.[14] Similar echocardiographic findings have been reported in patients with discrete tumors in each atrium. Multichambered cardiac myxomas occasionally involve chambers other than the usual biatrial combination and are more often familial.[6]

LEFT VENTRICULAR MYXOMA

A myxoma originates from the LV in 2.5 to 4 percent of reported myxomas.[3] Most patients are under 30 years of age. Women are affected three times more often than are men, and a short duration of symptoms is also characteristic. Systemic emboli, mostly cerebral,[52] occur in two-thirds of the patients, and constitutional symptoms are usually absent. Attacks of syncope occur in nearly half of the reviewed cases. Symptoms and physical findings are suggestive of aortic or subaortic obstruction. The location and movement of the tumor mass are demonstrated particularly well by TTE and by TEE (Chap. 13).[6] Echoes from an intracavitary LV myxoma must be differentiated from LV thrombi, which are usually apical but occasionally are pedunculated, and from ventricular septal rhabdomyomas. LV and RV myxomas have been identified by MRI (Chap. 18).[53] Planning for surgical excision can be based upon noninvasive imaging without resorting to cardiac catheterization and angiography unless coexistent cardiac or coronary disease is possible.[53,54] The tumor can be removed through a LA approach with mobilization of the anterior leaflet of the mitral valve.[55]

RIGHT VENTRICULAR MYXOMA

Myxomas of the RV are as infrequent as those of the LV. The patient will have symptoms and manifestations of right-sided heart failure, syncope, unexplained fever, and a murmur consistent with pulmonic stenosis. Pulmonary emboli may occur. An "ejection sound" has been reported, as well as delayed closure of the pulmonic valve. A right-sided tumor plop may be heard in diastole.[6] Calcium in the tumor may be recognized on the roentgenogram. Echocardiographic imaging, both TTE and TEE, will detect most RV myxomas.[56] A RV myxoma has been diagnosed in a neonate and has been successfully removed surgically. Other tumors, producing similar outflow tract obstruction, rarely occur within the RV.[6]

SURGERY FOR INTRACAVITARY MYXOMA

Surgical resection of a myxoma is the only acceptable therapy and, in view of the dangers of embolization and sudden death, should be performed promptly.[57] For complete removal of LA myxoma, we use a biatrial approach, excising a full thickness of interatrial septum if the tumor is attached to the region of the fossa ovalis.[58,59] RA myxomas are commonly attached to the fossa ovalis, and, with right-sided tumors, a full thickness of atrial septum also should be resected. If a large portion of the septum is removed, a patch of knitted Dacron cloth should be used for repair to avoid distortion, dysrhythmia, or possible atrial septal defect. We usually induce ventricular standstill with cardioplegia solution before manipulating the heart, to reduce the possibility of fragmentation of the gelatinous tumor. LA myxomas have been removed successfully during pregnancy, utilizing cardiopulmonary bypass, with subsequent uncomplicated completion of a full-term pregnancy. Surgical removal of a RV myxoma in a neonate has been reported.[60]

By its movement within the heart, a myxoma, especially when calcified, may traumatize either AV valve, which may require replacement or repair by annuloplasty.[2] Recurrences of atrial myxomas are rare and usually occur within a 48-month period.[6]

Other Benign Primary Cardiac Tumors

RHABDOMYOMA

The most frequent cardiac tumor in infants and children[3] is a rhabdomyoma, which is probably a hamartoma rather than a true neoplasm.[61] These tumors are usually multiple, usually involve the ventricular myocardium, and project into the cavity or move freely as a pedunculated mass.[62] Associated tuberous sclerosis is present in one-third of the patients.[63] Presenting manifestations may be caused by cardiac obstructive phenomena or by arrhythmias, AV block, pericardial effusion, ventricular preexcitation,[64] and even sudden death. These tumors can mimic pulmonary stenosis and produce hypoxic spells like those seen with tetralogy of Fallot. Ventricular outlet gradients,[64] angiographic abnormalities, echocardiography (Chap. 13), and MRI [65] can lead to demonstration of the tumor and successful surgical resection or heart transplantation.[66] Pedunculated rhabdomyomas that arise from the LA and cause mitral stenosis have been reported. Discrete and multiple myocardial hamartomas and rhabdomyomas have caused incessant ventricular tachycardia in infants and have been successfully removed surgically.[67] Rhabdomyomas are the tumors most frequently found at fetal echocardiography, constituting 17 of 19 fetal tumors found in 14,000 fetal echocardiograms.[68]

FIBROMA

Fibromas are usually ventricular and intramural. Although reported cases have occurred in the age range from newborn to 65 years, most occur in infants and children.[69] Calcification is common. Sudden death, occurring in nearly one-third of the patients, likely is due to involvement of the conduction system, production of arrhythmias, or obstruction of the LV outflow tract.[70] Two-dimensional echocardiography accurately delineates intramural ventricular tumors.[71] Left-axis deviation may occur as an interesting electrocardiographic feature. Total or partial resection of the tumor to relieve obstruction has been reported, with excellent probability of long-term survival. Cardiac transplantation has been used in the management of a young adult with a nonresectable (1030-g) LV fibroma.[72]

PAPILLARY FIBROELASTOMA

Also referred to as papillomas or papillary fibromas, papillary fibroelastomas arise from the cardiac valves[73,74] or occasionally from the ventricular endocardium, are most commonly seen in patients over age 50, and until recently have been a coincidental finding at surgery or postmortem examination. Grossly, these tumors resemble a sea anemone, with multiple papillary fronds attached to the endothelium by a short pedicle. There is a predilection for involvement of the aortic valve,[75] where angina, infarction, or sudden death may result from coronary embolization or ostial occlusion caused by the villous tumor.[3,76,77] Cerebral and ocular emboli from these lesions are being reported with increasing frequency.[103] Origin on right-sided cardiac valves is rare.[78,79] Obstruction of the RV outflow tract has been reported in a patient with a papillary tumor of the tricuspid valve. The tumor is histologically different from Lambl's excrescences, which are degenerative in origin and usually situated on the ventricular aspect of the semilunar valve along the line of closure.[3] Papillary fibroelastomas are being discovered with increasing frequency by echocardiographic (TTE and TEE) imaging of the heart, and because of their potential for cerebral and coronary embolization, surgical excision is recommended for even small papillary fibroelastomas.[80,81] Papillary fibroelastomas may mimic vegetations and bacterial endocarditis.

LIPOMA

Lipomas may occur throughout the heart,[82] including the pericardium. They may be massive. Intrapericardial lipomas may cause pericardial effusion, be mistaken for a pericardial cyst, or present as asymptomatic cardiac or mediastinal enlargement. Intramyocardial lipomas are encapsulated and usually are small.[3] Occasionally, a lipoma arising from the mitral or tricuspid valve may resemble an atrial myxoma on echocardiographic examination[83] and must also be differentiated from a cyst or lymphangioma of the mitral valve.[84] Surgical excision of lipomas yields excellent long-term results. Tissue characterization by MRI permits preoperative identification of these fatty tumors (see Chap. 18).

Lipomatous hypertrophy of the atrial septum is a nonencapsulated hyperplasia of adipose tissue and may not represent a true tumor. Varying in size from 2 to 8 cm, the tumescence may bulge into the atrial cavity or superior vena cava orifice and become a consideration in the differential diagnosis of intracavitary masses.[85] Although often found coincidentally at postmortem study, lipomatous hypertrophy of the atrial septum can be associated with unexplained supraventricular rhythm and conduction disturbances, recurrent pericardial effusion, and sudden death.[3,5] Features of both TTE and TEE are distinctive and include atrial septal thickening with a bilobed appearance due to sparing of the area of the fossa ovalis. Computed tomographic (CT) scanning and MRI provide noninvasive tissue characterization of lipomas that echocardiography does not provide.[86,87] The diagnosis may be confirmed by percutaneous transvenous biopsy.

CYSTIC TUMORS OF THE ATRIOVENTRICULAR NODE

Cystic tumors of the AV node most likely originate from either mesothelial or endodermal rests and are always benign.[6] Patients with these tumors tend to have partial or complete AV block, usually of long duration, and often die of complete heart block or ventricular fibrillation. These tumors are the smallest ones capable of causing sudden death.[6] Reported ages in patients have ranged from the newborn period to the ninth decade of life, with a strong female preponderance. These cystic tumors have also been referred to as mesotheliomas, lymphangioepitheliomas, and congenital polycystic tumors of the AV node.[6] Aside from chance intraoperative finding of this tumor,[88] in vivo recognition has not been reported, although the cystic structure may exceed 3 cm in size. The tumor is usually large enough to be recognized grossly at postmortem examination and should be suspected in all cases of sudden death without apparent cause, especially in children and young adults.[6] Most patients with these cystic tumors of the AV node have demonstrated complete AV block and have recurrent attacks of syncope. Even with complete AV block, a narrow QRS complex is common, and these patients may pursue a stable course for years. Electrophysiologic study discloses a block proximal to the His bundle.[6] Electronic pacing should aid in maintaining an adequate cardiac rate, but examples of electrical instability and sudden death reflect a special hazard in these patients, even during diagnostic electrophysiologic studies and after initiation of effective ventricular pacing. The presence of an accessory bypass tract and intermittent preexcitation has been reported.[89]

VASOFORMATIVE TUMORS

Hemangiomas[90] are rare cardiac tumors usually discovered at postmortem study. Coronary angiography yields a characteristic tumor blush.[6] Spontaneous resolution without treatment of a large cavernous hemangioma of the RV has been reported. Lymphangiomas and vascular hamartomas are rare primary tumors of the heart that usually present as diffuse proliferations rather than as distinct tumors. Therefore, total excision is often not practical.[91] Cardiac transplantation may be considered as an alternative in these cases.

INTRAPERICARDIAL PARAGANGLIOMA

Paragangliomas (pheochromocytomas and chemodectomas) may rarely be localized within the pericardium. Although these tumors may be found overlying or within any cardiac chamber, they most commonly occur over the base of the heart in the major region of vagus nerve distribution.[92] Improved detection and localization to the mediastinum have been provided by iodine-131 metaiodobenzylguanidine nuclear scanning. MRI can further localize cardiac paragangliomas and provide detailed information for guidance of surgical excision.[93] Since these tumors are highly vascular, adherent, and difficult to resect, management with cardiac transplantation may be necessary.[94] Human cardiac explantation and autotransplantation has also been applied to a patient with a large cardiac pheochromocytoma.[95]

MISCELLANEOUS BENIGN TUMORS

The right side of the ventricular septum is rarely the site of a congenital benign thyroid rest. Enlargement results in right ventricular outflow obstruction. Complete resection is indicated, and the condition is curable. Rarely, benign teratomas occur in the ventricular myocardium and may result in sudden death.[96]

Malignant Primary Tumors of the Heart

ANGIOSARCOMA (HEMANGIOSARCOMA)

Almost all primary malignant cardiac tumors are sarcomas,[97] most frequently angiosarcomas, and they usually originate in the RA or pericardium.[98] Intense vascularity may produce a continuous murmur. One-fourth of all angiosarcomas are partially intracavitary, with valvular or vena caval[99] obstruction, and characteristically manifest right-sided heart failure and pericardial tamponade with hemorrhagic fluid. Cardiac rupture due to a RA angiosarcoma has been reported.[6] Atrial angiosarcomas exhibit highly variable histologic patterns, which may overlap those of Kaposi's sarcoma. Echocardiography, angiography, CT, or MRI are helpful in the diagnosis (Fig. 77-5*A*).[100] Coronary angiography may demonstrate angiomatous vessels in the tumor area. The course is rapid, and widespread metastases often make surgery impractical, although tumor excision, radiation, and chemotherapy may offer some relief of symptoms and palliation.[3] An iatrogenic hemangiopericytoma of the right ventricle has been reported following intense radiotherapy to the cardiac area.[101]

RHABDOMYOSARCOMA

Rhabdomyosarcoma is the second most frequent primary sarcoma of the heart and, like angiosarcoma, is prevalent in males. There is no single chamber predilection; multiple sites are common, and significant obstruction of at least one valve is present in half of the patients.[102] Excision of the main tumor mass combined with radiation and chemotherapy has been advocated as the treatment for patients with primary malignant tumor of the heart, but in general the prognosis is poor and survival is short.[3]

OTHER MALIGNANT PRIMARY TUMORS

Fibrosarcoma,[103] liposarcoma,[104] primary malignant lymphoma,[105] and occasionally sarcomas of other basic cell types constitute the remaining but infrequent primary malignant cardiac tumors.[3] The fibrous histiocytoma has a predilection for the LA and rarely involves right-sided cardiac chambers.[106]

Malignant primary cardiac tumors may obstruct cardiac chambers or valves[6] or result in peripheral embolic phenomena.

Surgery for Primary Cardiac Tumors

Effective palliation and local control of the disease can be achieved with extensive resection of malignant primary tumors.[107,108] Echocardiography (see Chap. 13), MRI (see Chap. 18), and CT scanning (see Chap. 52) are all helpful in planning operative resection of cardiac tumors because these tests provide three-dimensional information (Fig. 77-5*B* and *C*).[109] Intraoperative echocardiography may be useful in guiding surgical resection.[110] Adjuvant chemotherapy and radiation therapy are necessary to improve long-term prognosis,[111] and the response to therapy can be assessed by MRI.[6] Cardiac transplantation has been utilized to completely resect an "inoperable" benign tumor and an unresectable malignant primary cardiac neoplasm.[112,113] Cardiac explantation and auto-

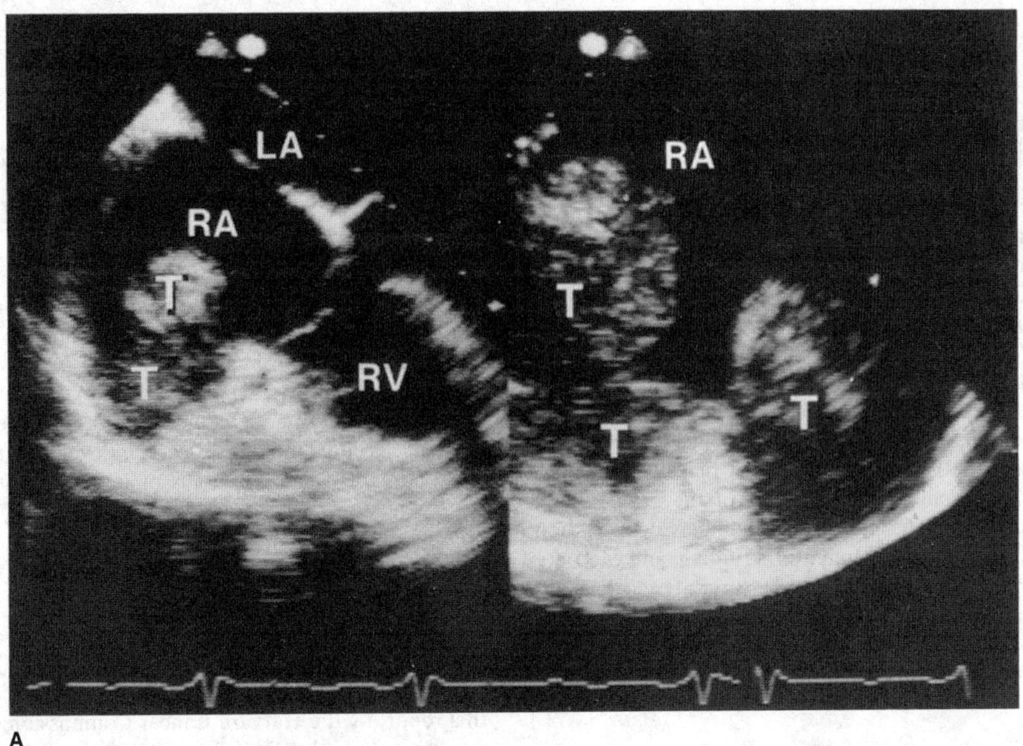

A

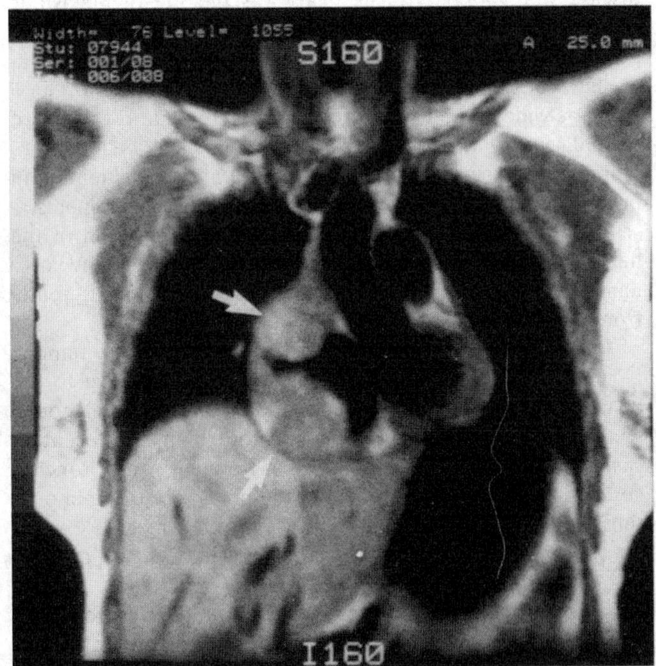

B

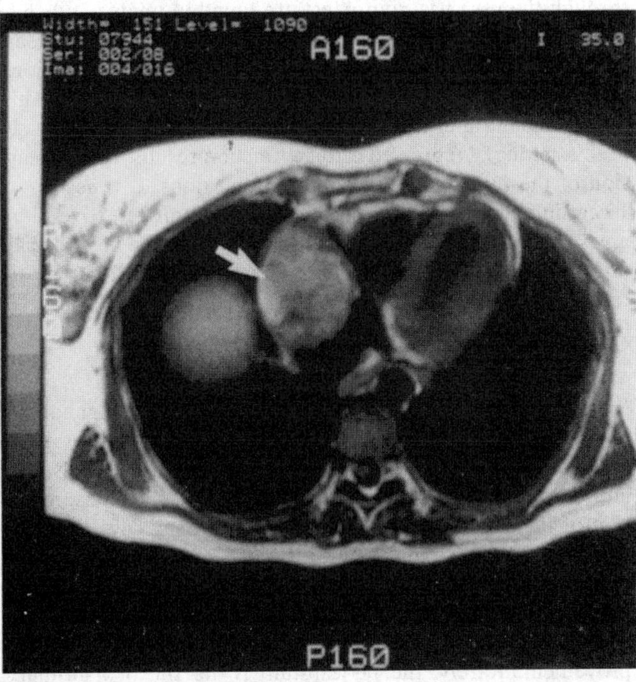

C

FIGURE 77-5 *A*. Biplane transesophageal echocardiogram from a 35-year-old woman who presented with shock of unknown cause. The horizontal plane (*left*) shows a tumor (T) in the RA. The vertical plane (*right*) shows a large, bilobular tumor (T) adherent to the RA wall. Histologic examination proved this to be an angiosarcoma. (Courtesy of Susan Wilansky, M.D., Medical Director, Noninvasive Imaging, St. Luke's Episcopal Hospital, Houston, Texas.) *B* and *C*. Magnetic resonance images. Arrowheads (*B* and *C*) denote a dumbbell-shaped, RA tumor of intermediate signal intensity, which is shown to abut the aorta in the coronal T1-weighted view and the tricuspid valve in the axial T1- weighted view. Note the loss of the usual high–signal-intensity margin (fat) along the right lateral aspect of the aorta in the coronal plane. This raises concern for malignant invasion of the aortic wall. (Courtesy of Clark L. Carrol, M.D., St. Luke's Episcopal Hospital, Texas Children's Hospital, and Texas Heart Institute, Houston, Texas.)

transplantation may facilitate resection of some cardiac tumors (Chap. 22).[114,115]

Tumors of the Pericardium

PERICARDIAL CYSTS

Pericardial, or mesothelial, cysts are the most frequent benign "tumors" of the pericardium. They are usually found coincidentally on a routine roentgenogram. However, 25 to 30 percent of the patients will have chest pain, dyspnea, cough, or paroxysmal tachycardia. Pericardial cysts occur most frequently in the third or fourth decade of life and equally among men and women. The right costophrenic location is the most common, although they may present in the upper mediastinum.[116] Only rarely does the cyst connect with the pericardial cavity. Clinically and radiographically, they resemble other tumors of the pericardium. Hemodynamically significant cardiac-chamber compression rarely results.[117] Echocardiography, CT scanning, and MRI are most helpful in the differential diagnosis. Surgical excision completely relieves symptoms and confirms the diagnosis;[3,6] however, percutaneous aspiration of the cystic contents is an attractive alternative to surgical resection.

TERATOMA

Most teratomas are extracardiac yet intrapericardial and receive their blood supply from the aortic root or pulmonary artery through the vasa vasorum. Most are found in infants and children, with a strong female preponderance.[3] Diagnosis has been established in utero by fetal echocardiography. Recurrent, nonbloody pericardial effusion is common in children with this tumor, and intrapericardial teratoma is the most likely diagnosis in this setting.[6] Depressed cardiac function results from expansion of the tumor to considerable proportions, at times up to 15 cm in diameter. Surgical excision is the only effective therapy[118] and is curative. It is rare for a teratoma to be intracardiac and arise from the interventricular septum, but this type of tumor can be successfully excised.[6]

MESOTHELIOMA

Mesothelioma ranks third in frequency among malignant tumors of the heart and pericardium.[5] The clinical manifestations resemble those of pericarditis, constrictive pericardial disease, and vena cava obstruction. Aspiration and histologic examination of the usually bloody pericardial fluid may be diagnostic. Males outnumber females by a ratio of 2:1, with the peak incidence in the third to fifth decades. The prognosis is poor, surgical excision is usually impossible, and treatment with radiation and chemotherapy generally produces only temporary improvement. Rarely, the pericardium is the site of a primary sarcoma.[119]

Primary Tumors of the Aorta

Primary tumors of the aorta are rare. Most frequently they are malignant sarcomas. Presentation may mimic aortic dissection, coarctation, atherosclerotic occlusive disease, and malignancies in other organs. All portions of the aorta may be involved, and distal metastases are common. Surgical extirpation will relieve the obstructive phenomena, but distant metastases usually lead to disease progression.[120]

SECONDARY TUMORS OF THE HEART

General Considerations

Metastatic tumors involve the heart, the pericardium, or both from a primary origin in some other organ 20 to 40 times more frequently than do primary tumors.[6] These secondary tumors are more frequently carcinomas than sarcomas. Cardiac metastases occur most often in people older than 50 years of age; the incidence is equal in both sexes. The development of otherwise unexplained cardiac symptoms or manifestations, cardiac enlargement, tachycardia, arrhythmias, or heart failure in the presence of neoplastic disease is suggestive of cardiac metastases.

Frequency and Origin of Secondary Tumors

In a report by the Harvard Cancer Commission of 4375 autopsies of patients who died of cancer, myocardial metastases were present in 146 patients (3.4 percent).[121] In a series of 2547 performed at Walter Reed General Hospital, 980 cases of malignant disease were observed. The heart was the site of metastatic tumor in 5.7 percent of the cases and the heart, including the pericardium, in 13.9 percent.[122] In other series, cardiac metastases have been present in patients with malignant tumors in a range as wide as 1.5 to 21 percent. An increased prevalence of secondary cardiac neoplasms in recent years may be related to more vigorous surgical and radiation treatment of patients with primary neoplasms. The relative infrequency of cardiac metastases has been attributed to the strong kneading action of the heart, the metabolic peculiarities of striated muscle, rapid coronary blood flow, and lymphatic connections that drain afferently from the heart.[121]

Cardiac metastases occur with all types of primary tumors. No malignant tumor tends particularly to metastasize to the heart, with the possible exception of malignant melanoma, which involves the myocardium in more than 50 percent of cases.[123] Cardiac metastases are most frequent, with bronchogenic carcinoma and carcinoma of the breast occurring in one-third of the cases.[6] Cardiac infiltration, often macroscopic, is seen in one-half of cases of leukemia and in one-sixth of cases of lymphoma.

Cardiac metastases are encountered with widespread systemic tumor dissemination; only rarely is metastatic tumor limited to the heart or pericardium. Carcinomatous metastases are generally grossly visible, multiple, discrete, small, white, firm nodules; microscopically, they resemble the primary tumor and the metastases in other organs. Diffuse infiltration is characteristic of sarcomatous metastases.

Metastatic tumors are classically thought to reach the heart by embolic hematogenous spread, lymphatic spread, or direct invasion, in descending order of frequency. Lymphatic spread of tumors is particularly frequent with carcinoma of the bronchus and the breast; the proximity of the heart to major mediastinal lymphatic channels seems to explain the high incidence of cardiac metastases from mediastinal tumors.

Manifestations

Secondary tumor involvement of the heart is more often symptomatic, and on rare occasions it may be the first or only expression of a remote primary tumor. At times, as with rapidly developing tamponade, recognition and appropriate therapy must be undertaken promptly. Secondary tumors of the heart may involve the pericardium, myocardium, endocardium, valves, and coronary arteries. Direct invasion of the heart through the venae cavae[124] or pulmonary veins[125] or through an expanding myocardial implant can produce an intracavitary tumor mass and result in obstruction to flow or cause valvular obstruction (Fig. 77-6). Depending on the character and location of the cardiac lesion, a variety of manifestations may serve to identify cardiac involvement.

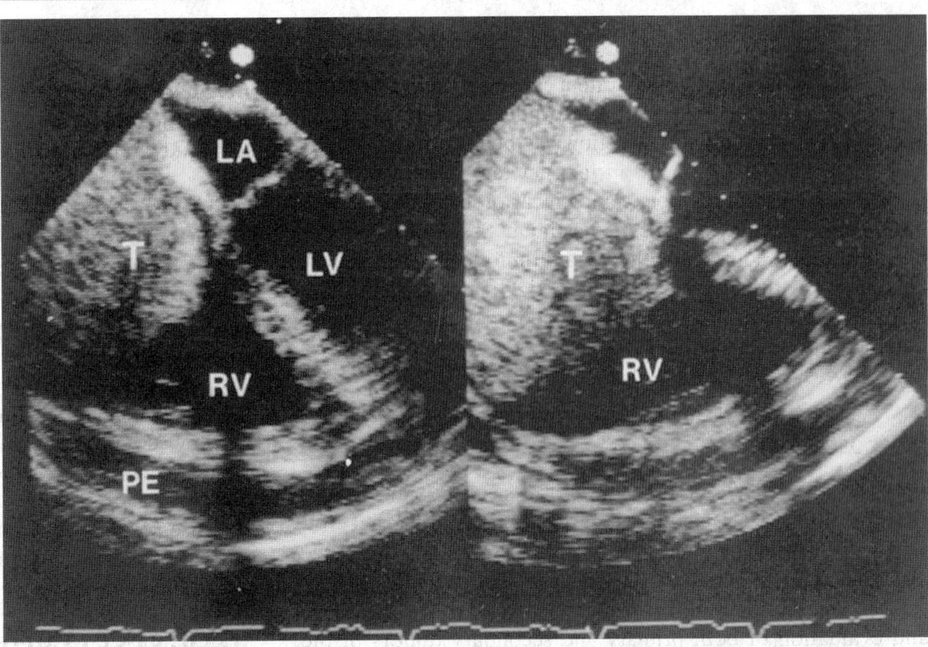

FIGURE 77-6 Transesophageal echocardiogram in a 55-year-old woman who presented with adenocarcinoma of the lung and obstructed superior vena caval syndrome. A large tumor (T) is seen in the RV in systole (*left panel*) and diastole (*right panel*). Subsequent images revealed that it originated from an obstructed superior vena cava. The echo-free space anterior to the RV represented pericardial effusion (PE). (Courtesy of Susan Wilansky, M.D., Medical Director, Noninvasive Imaging, St. Luke's Episcopal Hospital, Houston, Texas.)

PERICARDIAL INVOLVEMENT

Pericardial involvement is often first manifested by chest pain, aggravated by inspiration, and a pericardial friction rub. Accumulation of fluid within the pericardium, often but not always bloody, may result in progressive cardiac enlargement on roentgenogram, with symptoms and signs of cardiac tamponade, and may be the first manifestation of a cardiac malignancy (see Chap. 72). Clinically, the jugular venous pressure is increased, the arterial pressure is reduced, and "pulsus paradoxus" may be present (see Chap. 72). Reduced electrocardiographic QRS voltage can be expected. Electrical alternation, which is generally seen in patients with large effusions and serious tamponade, may indicate the need for prompt pericardiocentesis. The echocardiogram demonstrates pericardial fluid and may demonstrate features of hemodynamic tamponade, diastolic collapse of the RA and RV,[126] inferior vena caval plethora with a blunted inspiratory response, and altered inspiratory intracardiac Doppler flow velocities (see Chap. 72). Pericardial effusion and tamponade may be the first manifestations of cardiac involvement by a malignancy. The association of large quantities of pericardial fluid with tumor encasing the heart frequently results in persistent cardiac constriction, even after pericardiocentesis. Echocardiography and CT imaging are both useful for detecting pericardial metastases. Pericardioscopy performed during surgical drainage procedures has enabled visual diagnoses and guided biopsies of suspicious areas.[127]

MYOCARDIAL INVOLVEMENT

Atrial flutter and fibrillation are frequent, and a patient with either one may be unusually resistant to conventional therapy. Ventricular extrasystoles and serious ventricular arrhythmias[128] may accompany invasion of a tumor into the myocardium. Conduction disturbances and complete AV block also occur. Widespread muscle involvement by tumor invasion or obstruction of the cardiac lymphatic drainage system may cause congestive failure. Rarely, a pedunculated secondary tumor mass may produce a loud murmur and palpable thrill. Myocardial damage and heart failure also may result from some of the chemotherapeutic agents used in the treatment of patients with neoplastic diseases, and combined radiotherapy and chemotherapy may synergistically increase cardiac damage (see Chap. 81). The most frequent electrocardiographic abnormalities seen in patients with neoplastic heart disease are nonspecific changes of the ST segment and the T wave due to myocardial or pericardial involvement by the tumor. Pronounced and prolonged ST-segment elevation in the absence of myocardial infarction may occur with tumor invasion of the heart.[6]

CORONARY ARTERY INVOLVEMENT

In patients with malignant tumor, angina or myocardial infarction may result from concomitant atherosclerosis, coronary occlusion by tumor embolization, or external coronary compression by the tumor as well as from coronary fibrosis or accelerated atherogenesis in patients who have received radiation to the mediastinum.[6,129] The ECG pattern of myocardial infarction also can result from massive invasion of the myocardium by a tumor or from a large pericardial effusion.

INTRACAVITARY TUMOR

Extensions of tumors such as renal cell carcinoma,[130] hepatocellular carcinoma,[131] and uterine leiomyomatosis,[132] along the inferior vena cava and into the RA can present as an intracavitary obstructive mass. Leiomyosarcoma may be primary in the vena cava, most often the inferior, and extend directly into the heart.[133] Intracavitary metastases or an expanding myocardial tumor may progressively obliterate a cardiac chamber or result in a valvular obstruction and, rarely, produce fever of unknown origin. Successful surgical resection has been reported.[134] RA and tricuspid obstruction by an intracavitary mass can mimic pericardial constriction from tumor invasion or from previous intensive radiotherapy to the mediastinum. Systemic or pulmonary emboli, so common with primary tumors of the heart, are uncommon with secondary tumors. Right-sided intracavitary thrombi may mimic primary or secondary tumors on echographic imaging of the heart.[6]

Diagnostic Studies

Echocardiography, TTE and TEE, CT scanning, and, more recently, ultrafast CT facilitate identification of pericardial effusion and intracavitary and pericardial masses (Fig. 77-6)[6] (see also Chaps. 13, 17, and 18A). MRI provides a global view of cardiac anatomy and plays an important role in the diagnosis and evaluation of both primary and secondary tumors of the heart, providing information about the location, extent, and attachment of the tumor.[231] Pericardiocentesis may afford prompt symptomatic relief from pericardial tamponade and often provides a definitive cytologic diagnosis.[135] Ultrasound and fluoroscopic guidance aid in safe pericardial catheter placement (see Chap. 82). The results of endomyocardial biopsy may contribute to the diagnosis in some cases. Bone formation in metastatic osteogenic sarcoma occasionally may be visible radiographically.

Treatment

Malignant pericardial effusion usually recurs rapidly after pericardiocentesis. Depending on the cytologic type and radiosensitivity of the tumor, radiation to the cardiac area with or without systemic chemotherapy is the treatment of choice.[6] The heart can tolerate 20 to 40 Gy, beyond which the risk of radiation-induced pericardial, myocardial, and valvular[136] damage is increased. Patients with malignant pericardial effusions have responded to systemic chemotherapy and to intrapericardial administration of fluorouracil, radioactive gold (nitrogen mustard), and tetracycline.[137] Persistent reaccumulation of fluid may require surgical creation of a pericardial "window."[138] A pericardial-pleural "window" has also been produced with a percutaneous balloon catheter without surgery.[139] Patients with myocardial infiltration by tumor also respond to radiation therapy and systemic chemotherapy. Recurrent ventricular tachycardia has responded to administration of amiodarone.[140] Heart block is treated with temporary or permanent electronic pacing. Surgical removal of intracavitary, obstructing secondary tumors may ameliorate symptoms and prolong survival,[141] as may chemotherapy occasionally. Documentation of tumor regression is possible with echocardiographic imaging. MRI plays an important role in characterizing the three-dimensional extent and attachment of cardiac tumors. This information is of particular importance in planning a surgical approach aimed at either complete removal or palliative debulking of a tumor mass (see Chap. 82).[142]

Special Considerations

LEUKEMIA

Leukemic infiltration of the heart is usually found at postmortem study.[143] Cardiac infiltrates are found in most postmortem studies of patients with acute leukemia, with most having pericardial involvement. Cardiac symptoms are unusual. Chronic lymphocytic leukemia reportedly has caused myocardial infiltration in some patients, as well as mitral valve dysfunction and congestive heart failure.[6] Myocardial rupture has been reported as an early manifestation of acute myeloblastic leukemia.[144] Massive pericardial effusion, often hemorrhagic, and pericardial tamponade have been reported, but overt pericardial effusion is rare.[6] Management consists of pericardiocentesis and chemotherapy; occasionally, surgical decompression of the pericardium is necessitated by recurrent tamponade. Infective endocarditis, commonly fungal, may complicate acute leukemia. Because of advances in treatment and improved long-term remission in patients with acute lymphoblastic leukemia, complicating endocarditis has been managed by valve replacement.

MALIGNANT LYMPHOMA

Involvement of the heart in patients with malignant lymphoma is common, although it is infrequently detected before death. Cardiac or pericardial metastases occur with both Hodgkin's and non-Hodgkin's lymphoma and result from lymphatic and hematogenous spread as well as direct extension from other intrathoracic masses, resulting in predominantly epicardial and pericardial involvement.[3] Cardiac involvement may occasionally be the direct cause of death, but antemortem detection is infrequent.

ACQUIRED IMMUNODEFICIENCY SYNDROME AND HEART NEOPLASMS

Two varieties of malignancies involving the heart have been described in patients with acquired immunodeficiency syndrome (AIDS): Kaposi's sarcoma and, less commonly, malignant lymphoma.[145] Involvement of the heart by Kaposi's sarcoma may be primary or part of a widely disseminated process. The epicardium is a common location, with involvement of the underlying myocardium. Clinical cardiac dysfunction is minimal, although fatal pericardial tamponade has been reported (see Chap. 70).

Lymphomas, usually of high-grade malignant characteristics, occur with increased frequency in patients with AIDS and other immunosuppressed states (Chap. 70). Both primary and, more commonly, secondary lymphomas involve the heart either as a diffuse infiltrative process or as focal nodules in any layer of the heart. Clinical features may be absent in approximately 50 percent of patients. When present, they include cardiomegaly, pericardial effusion and tamponade, congestive failure, atrial arrhythmias, and progressive heart block.[146-149] Echocardiography is useful and demonstrates pericardial effusion, mass lesions, and wall-motion abnormalities. Transvenous biopsy can be useful in making the diagnosis. There is limited experience with heart surgery in this group of patients.

CARCINOID HEART DISEASE

While carcinoid tumors are never primary in the heart and only rarely metastasize to the heart and pericardium, products of the tumor produce a distinctive endocardial and valvular pathologic pattern.[150–153] Tumors producing the carcinoid syndrome most commonly arise in the gastrointestinal tract, but they may also arise in the bronchus, biliary tract, pancreas, and testis.[6,154] Appendiceal carcinoids rarely metastasize or produce the carcinoid syndrome. Ileal carcinoids, containing cytoplasmic granules that take up and reduce silver salts, frequently metastasize to the liver and produce the carcinoid syndrome. These carcinoids contain a high concentration of 5-hydroxytryptamine (5-HT), which is excreted mainly as 5-hydroxyindoleacetic acid (5-HIAA) in the urine. Bronchial, pancreatic, and gastric carcinoid tumors differ morphologically and histochemically, have a worse prognosis, and metastasize more widely than do ileal tumors. They also produce 5-HT and excrete 5-HIAA in the urine; however, the clinical picture may be atypical. Although they bear no morphologic or histochemical relation to the more typical carcinoid tumor, carcinomas of the bronchus, pancreas, or thyroid may occasionally secrete humoral substances that produce the carcinoid syndrome. In gastrointestinal carcinoid disease, the syndrome is produced by secretion of tumor products into the systemic circulation, and its recognition is delayed until after liver metastases. The carcinoid syndrome, which results from the systemic effect of circulating vasoactive amines, consists of cutaneous flushing, intestinal hypermobility, bronchial constriction, edema, and cardiac lesions. Among patients with carcinoid, those with carcinoid heart disease demonstrate strikingly higher plasma serotonin and 5-HIAA levels.[155]

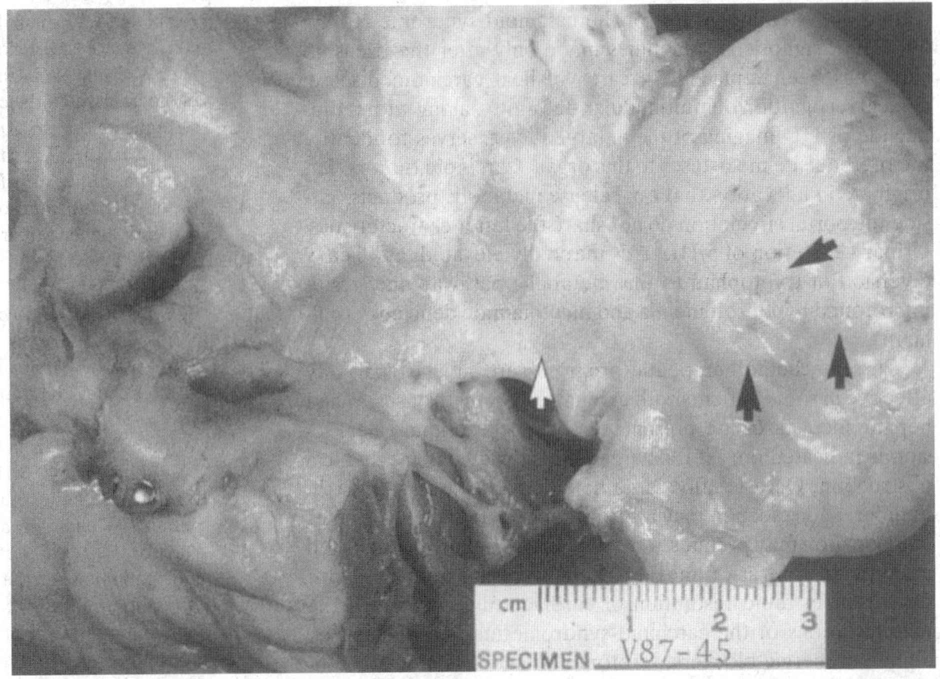

FIGURE 77-7 Carcinoid heart disease. The RA from a patient with carcinoid heart disease and combined tricuspid regurgitation and tricuspid stenosis. Note raised white plaques (black arrow) or the endocardial surface of the dilated RA and tricuspid valve (white arrow). Carcinoid heart disease occurs in 19 to 55 percent of patients with carcinoid.

Cardiac lesions are more commonly found in the right side of the heart than in the left (Fig. 77-6). Left-sided involvement occurs with bronchial tumors, in the presence of an intraatrial communication, or, in the absence of such a communication, when there is extensive right-sided heart involvement. Grossly glistening, white-yellow deposits are found on the pulmonary and tricuspid valves and, to varying degrees, on the RA and RV endocardium (see Chap. 59). Contraction of these deposits leads to tricuspid and pulmonary valve regurgitation and stenosis and occasionally may produce a restrictive type of myopathy.[156] Mitral valve involvement may result in both stenosis and regurgitation. On microscopic examination, the endocardial lesions consist of superficial deposits of fibrous tissue beneath a normal endothelium.[157] Metastatic lesions may be found in the myocardium. Serotonin, 5-HT, and bradykinin have been implicated in the pathogenesis of the cardiac lesions. Transforming growth factor β (TGF-β) has been shown to be produced by the fibroblasts in the carcinoid plaque and may play a critical role in progressive deposition of matrix proteins. The application of antibodies against TGF-β may potentially suppress the plaque progress.

Carcinoid heart disease cannot be recognized clinically until cardiac murmurs and signs of right-sided heart failure develop, especially elevated jugular venous pressure with inspiratory augmentation of the *v* wave, which is characteristic of tricuspid regurgitation (TR). A harsh, holosystolic, lower sternal border murmur with inspiratory accentuation is common, frequently followed by an early diastolic filling sound and diastolic rumble (see Chap. 58). A left upper sternal midsystolic murmur of pulmonic stenosis (PS) may or may not be identified separately. Murmurs of concomitant left-sided heart valvular involvement are rarely identified. There may be a parasternal heave and systolic pulsation of the liver, although enlargement and multinodular irregularity of the liver, ascites, and edema may be features of hepatic metastases without cardiac involvement (Fig. 77-7).

Roentgenographic examination of the chest will show the lung fields to be clear and the pulmonary trunk to be normal in size; the heart may be normal in size or show evidence of RV and RA enlargement. The electrocardiogram may show evidence of RA enlargement, but RV hypertrophy is rare.

Echocardiographic imaging reveals RV volume overload and abnormal right-sided valves. The tricuspid valve is typically thickened, retracted, and fixed in a semiopen position. Doming of the tricuspid valve may be present when the valve is predominantly stenotic. Color-flow Doppler will identify moderate to severe TR in the majority of patients. Pulmonary valve abnormalities are present in one-half of the patients, with pulmonic regurgitation more frequent than PS. Left-sided valvular involvement—mitral more often than aortic—is infrequent (7 percent).

Diagnosis of carcinoid heart disease depends on clinical recognition of the characteristic right-sided heart findings in the setting of systemic features of the carcinoid syndrome (Chap. 59). The diagnosis is sometimes made only after the tricuspid valve has been replaced. In cases of ileal carcinoid disease, clinical recognition of multinodular deformity, along with radionuclide or CT imaging of the enlarged liver, serves to identify the prerequisite metastases to this organ. Carcinoid tumors that originate in a location that can release metabolic products outside the portal circulation do not share the latter characteristics. Urinary excretion of 5-HIAA is markedly elevated, and heavy diversion of tryptophan to this metabolic pathway may result in profound hypoproteinemia and nicotinamide deficiency (pellagra).

Current chemotherapeutic programs are at least partially effective in some patients with extensive liver metastases. When hepatic metastases are present, removing the primary ileal lesion is indicated only if it is large and is producing mechanical obstruction. Occasionally, large hepatic metastases are few in number, and resection may afford symptomatic relief. Catheter embolization may permit segmental hepatic ablation in selected patients. In contrast, removal of an extraportal primary tumor can result in rapid resolution of cardiac failure. Some of the manifestations of the carcinoid syndrome may be blocked by alpha-adrenergic blockers, serotonin antagonists, and somatostatin analogs.[158]

Because heart failure is a frequent cause of disability and death when carcinoid heart disease complicates the carcinoid syndrome, tricuspid valve replacement and pulmonary valvotomy, with outflow tract enlargement if necessary, have been recommended when hemodynamically indicated. Implantation of a bioprosthetic valve[159,160] has generally been discouraged, although a review of reported cases of tricuspid valve replacement showed no significant difference in survival between patients with a bioprosthesis and those with a mechanical valve. Carcinoid plaque extending onto bioprosthetic valves early after surgery has been reported. Surgical mortality rates have been reported from 30 to 60 percent,[161–163] and only a small number of patients have undergone valve surgery. With proper care and planning, general anesthesia can be conducted with minimal risk.[164,165] Balloon valvuloplasty for tricuspid and pulmonary stenoses caused by carcinoid heart disease has been reported.[166]

References

1. Chitwood WR Jr. Clarence Crafoord and the first successful resection of a cardiac myxoma. *Ann Thorac Surg* 1992; 54:997–998.
2. Peters MN, Hall RJ, Cooley DA, et al. The clinical syndrome of atrial myxoma. *JAMA* 1974; 230:695–701.
3. McAllister HA Jr. Primary tumors and cysts of the heart and pericardium. *Curr Probl Cardiol* 1979; 4:1–51.
4. Reynen K. Cardiac myxomas [comments]. *N Engl J Med* 1995; 333:1610–1617.
5. McAllister HA, Fenoglio JJ. *Tumors of the Cardiovascular System*. Washington, DC: Armed Forces; 1978.
6. McAllister H, Hall R, Cooley D. Tumors of the heart and pericardiun. *Curr Probl Cardiol* 1999; 24:57–116.
7. Burke A, Virmani R. Tumors of the heart and great vessels. In: Rosai J, Sobin LH, eds. *Atlas of Tumor Pathology*, Vol 3d ser, fascicle 16. Washington, DC: Armed Forces Institute of Pathology; 1996:231.
8. Shimono T, Makino S, Kanamori Y, et al. Left atrial myxomas: Using gross anatomic tumor types to determine clinical features and coronary angiographic findings. *Chest* 1995; 107:674–679.
9. Burke AP, Virmani R. Cardiac myxoma: A clinicopathologic study. *Am J Clin Pathol* 1993; 100:671–680.
10. Ha JW, Kang WC, Chung N, et al. Echocardiographic and morphologic characteristics of left atrial myxoma and their relation to systemic embolism. *Am J Cardiol* 1999; 83(suppl A8):1579–1582.
11. Wold LE, Lie JT. Scanning electron microscopy of intracardiac myxoma. *Mayo Clin Proc* 1981; 56:198–200.
12. Bashey RI, Nochumson S: Cardiac myxoma. Biochemical analyses and evidence for its neoplastic nature. *NY State J Med* 1979; 79:29–32.
13. Read RC, White HJ, Murphy ML, et al. The malignant potentiality of left atrial myxoma. *J Thorac Cardiovasc Surg* 1974; 68:857–868.
14. Dashkoff N, Boersma RB, Nanda NC, et al. Bilateral atrial myxomas: Echocardiographic considerations. *Am J Med* 1978; 65:361–366.
15. Morgan DL, Palazola J, Reed W, et al. Left heart myxomas. *Am J Cardiol* 1977; 40: 611–614.
16. Balsara RK, Pelias AJ. Myxoma of right ventricle presenting as pulmonic stenosis in a neonate. *Chest* 1983; 83:145–146.
17. Davison ET, et al. Left atrial myxoma in the elderly: Report of four patients over the age of 70 and review of the literature. *J Am Geriatr Soc* 1977; 34:229–233.
18. van Gelder HM, O'Brien DJ, Staples ED, et al. Familial cardiac myxoma. *Ann Thorac Surg* 1992; 53:419–424.
19. Farah MG. Familial cardiac myxoma: A study of relatives of patients with myxoma. *Chest* 1994; 105:65–68.
20. Mochizuki Y, Okamura Y, Iida H, et al. Interleukin-6 and "complex" cardiac myxoma. *Ann Thorac Surg* 1998; 66:931–933.
21. Graham SL, Sellers AL. Atrial myxoma with multiple myeloma. *Arch Intern Med* 1979; 139:116–117.
22. Molstad P, Smith G, Aukrust P. Left atrial myxoma and systemic AL-amyloidosis. *Eur Heart J* 1992; 13:143–144.
23. Burns ER, Schulman IC, Murphy MJ Jr. Hematologic manifestations and etiology of atrial myxoma. *Am J Med Sci* 1982; 284:17–22.
24. Boussen K, Moalla M, Blondeau P, et al. Embolization of cardiac myxomas masquerading as polyarteritis nodosa. *J Rheumatol* 1991; 18:283–285.
25. Carney JA. Carney complex: The complex of myxomas, spotty pigmentation, endocrine overactivity, and schwannomas. *Semin Dermatol* 1995; 14:90–98.
26. Casey M, Mah C, Merliss AD, et al. Identification of a novel genetic locus for familial cardiac myxomas and Carney complex. *Circulation* 1998; 98:2560–2566.
27. Revankar SG, Clark RA. Infected cardiac myxoma: Case report and literature review. *Medicine (Baltimore)* 1998; 77:337–344.
28. Diflo T, Cantelmo NL, Haudenschild CC, et al. Atrial myxoma with remote metastasis: Case report and review of the literature. *Surgery* 1992; 111:352–356.
29. Misago N, Tanaka T, Hoshii T, et al. Erythematous papules in a patient with cardiac myxoma: A case report and review of the literature. *J Dermatol*, 1995. 22:600–605.
30. McMullin GM, Lane R. A rare cause of acute aortic occlusion. *Aust N Z J Surg* 1993; 63:65–68.
31. Browne WT, Wijdicks EF, Parisi JE, et al. Fulminant brain necrosis from atrial myxoma showers. *Stroke* 1993; 24:1090–1102.
32. Furuya K, Sasaki T, Yoshimoto Y, et al. Histologically verified cerebral aneurysm formation secondary to embolism from cardiac myxoma: Case report. *J Neurosurg* 1995; 83:170–173.
33. Rafuse PE, Nicolle DA, Hutnick CM, et al. Left atrial myxoma causing ophthalmic artery occlusion. *Eye* 1997; 11:25–29.
34. Cheitlin MD, McAllister HA, de Castro CM. Myocardial infarction without atherosclerosis. *JAMA* 1975; 231:951–959.
35. Sharratt GP, Grover ML, Monro JL. Calcified left atrial myxoma with floppy mitral valve. *Br Heart J* 1979; 42:608–610.
36. Tighe DA, Rousou JA, Kenia S, et al. Transesophageal echocardi-

ography in the management of mitral valve myxoma. *Am Heart J* 1995; 130:627–629.
37. Matsuoka H, Hamada M, Honda T, et al. Morphologic and histologic characterization of cardiac myxomas by magnetic resonance imaging. *Angiology* 1996; 47:693–698.
38. Kamata J, Yoshioka K, Nasu M, et al. Myxoma of the mitral valve detected by echocardiography and magnetic resonance imaging. *Eur Heart J* 1995; 16:1435–1438.
39. Rittoo D, Cotter L. Detection of a small left atrial myxoma: Value and limitations of four imaging modalities. *J Am Soc Echocardiogr* 1997; 10:874–876.
40. Isobe N, Kanda T, Sakamoto H, et al. Myocardial infarction in myxoma patients with normal coronary arteries: Case reports. *Angiology* 1996; 47:819–823.
41. Huston KA, Combs JJ Jr, Lie JT, et al. Left atrial myxoma simulating peripheral vasculitis. *Mayo Clin Proc* 1978; 53: 752–756.
42. Kuroda H, Nitta K, Ashida Y, et al. Right atrial myxoma originating from the tricuspid valve. *J Thorac Cardiovasc Surg* 1995; 109:1249–1250.
43. Teoh KH, Mulji A, Tomlinson CW, et al. Right atrial myxoma originating from the eustachian valve. *Can J Cardiol* 1993; 9:441–443.
44. Hickie JB, Gibson H, Windsor HM. "The wrecking ball": Right atrial myxoma. *Med J Aust* 1970; 2:82–86.
45. Heck HA Jr, Gross CM, Houghton JL. Long-term severe pulmonary hypertension associated with right atrial myxoma. *Chest* 1992; 102:301–303.
46. Jardine DL, Lamont DL. Right atrial myxoma mistaken for recurrent pulmonary thromboembolism. *Heart* 1997; 78:512–514.
47. Park JM, Garcia RR, Patrick JK, et al. Right atrial myxoma with a nonembolic intestinal manifestation. *Pediatr Cardiol* 1990; 11:164–166.
48. Massumi R. Bedside diagnosis of right heart myxomas through detection of palpable tumor shocks and audible plops. *Am Heart J* 1983; 105:303–310.
49. Lyons SV, McCord J, Smith S. Asymptomatic giant right atrial myxoma: Role of transesophageal echocardiography in management. *Am Heart J* 1991; 121:1555–1558.
50. Angelini P, Wilansky S, Gaos C, et al. Prolapsing large aneurysm of the atrial septum simulating a right atrial mass. *Cathet Cardiovasc Diagn* 1992; 26:122–126.
51. Peachell JL, Mullen JC, Bentley MJ, et al. Biatrial myxoma: A rare cardiac tumor. *Ann Thorac Surg* 1998; 65:1768–1769.
52. Abo-Auda WS, Chidambaram BS, Baker K, et al. Ventricular myxoma presenting as acute visual loss. *Tenn Med* 1998; 91:391–392.
53. Camesas AM, Lichtstein E, Kramer J, et al. Complementary use of two-dimensional echocardiography and magnetic resonance imaging in the diagnosis of ventricular myxoma. *Am Heart J* 1987; 114:440–442.
54. Gulbins H, Reichenspurner H, Wintersperger BJ, et al. Minimally invasive extirpation of a left-ventricular myxoma. *Thorac Cardiovasc Surg* 1999; 47:129–130.
55. Talwalkar NG, Livesay JJ, Treistman B, et al. Mobilization of the anterior mitral leaflet for excision of a left ventricular myxoma. *Ann Thorac Surg* 1999; 67:1476–1478.
56. Nass PC, Niemeyer MG, Brutal de la Riviere A, et al. Left atrial and right ventricular cardiac myxoma: A case report. *Eur J Cardiothorac Surg* 1989; 3:468–470.
57. Jones DR, Warden HE, Murray GF, Hill RC, et al. Biatrial approach to cardiac myxomas: A 30-year clinical experience [comments]. *Ann Thorac Surg* 1995; 59:851–856.
58. Cooley DA. Surgical management of cardiac tumors. In: Kapoor AS, Reynolds RD, eds. Cancer and the Heart. New York: Springer-Verlag; 1977: 126.
59. Massetti M, Babatasi G, Le Page O, et al. Modified biatrial approach for the extensive resection of left atrial myxomas. *Ann Thorac Surg* 1998; 66:275–276.
60. Abushaban L, Denham B, Duff D. 10 year review of cardiac tumours in childhood [comments]. *Br Heart J* 1993; 70:166–169.
61. Fenoglio JJ Jr, McAllister HA, Ferrans VJ. Cardiac rhabdomyoma: A clinicopathologic and electron microscopic study. *Am J Cardiol* 1976; 38:241–251.
62. Howanitz EP, Teske DW, Qualman SJ, et al. Pedunculated left ventricular rhabdomyoma. *Ann Thorac Surg* 1977; 41:443–445.
63. Guereta LG, Burgueros M, Elonza MD, et al. Cardiac rhabdomyoma presenting as fetal hydrops. *Pediatr Cardiol* 1977; 7:171–174.
64. Mehta AV. Rhabdomyoma and ventricular preexcitation syndrome: A report of two cases and review of literature. *Am J Dis Child* 1993; 147:669–671.
65. Boxer RA, La Corte MA, Singh S, et al. Diagnosis of cardiac tumors in infants by magnetic resonance imaging. *Am J Cardiol* 1985; 56:831–832.
66. Demkow M, Sorensen K, Whitehead BF, et al. Heart transplantation in an infant with rhabdomyoma. *Pediatr Cardiol* 1995; 16:204–206.
67. Garson A Jr, Smith RI Jr, Moak JP, et al. Incessant ventricular tachycardia in infants: Myocardial hamartomas and surgical cure. *J Am Coll Cardiol* 1987; 10:619–626.
68. Holley DG, Martin GR, Brenner JI, et al. Diagnosis and management of fetal cardiac tumors: A multicenter experience and review of published reports [comments]. *J Am Coll Cardiol* 1995; 26:516–520.
69. Busch U, Kampmann C, Meyer R, et al. Removal of a giant cardiac fibroma from a 4-year-old child. *Tex Heart Inst J* 1995; 22:261–264.
70. Williams DB, Danielson GK, McGoon DC, et al. Cardiac fibroma: Long-term survival after excision. *J Thorac Cardiovasc Surg* 1982; 84:230–236.
71. Biancaniello TM, Meyer RA, Gaum WE, et al. Primary benign intramural ventricular tumors in children: Pre- and postoperative electrocardiographic, echocardiographic, and angiocardiographic evaluation. *Am Heart J* 1982; 103: 852–857.
72. Jamieson SW, Gaudiani VA, Reitz BA, et al. Operative treatment of an unresectable tumor of the left ventricle. *J Thorac Cardiovasc Surg* 1981; 81:797–799.
73. Ryan PE Jr, Obeid AI, Parker FB Jr. Primary cardiac valve tumors. *J Heart Valve Dis* 1995; 4:222–226.
74. al-Mohammad A, Pambakian H, Young C. Fibroelastoma: Case report and review of the literature. *Heart* 1998; 79:301–304.
75. Grote J, Mugge A, Schafers HJ, et al. Multiplane transoesophageal echocardiography detection of a papillary fibroelastoma of the aortic valve causing myocardial infarction. *Eur Heart J* 1995; 16:426–429.
76. Eckstein FS, Schafers HJ, Grote J, et al. Papillary fibroelastoma of the aortic valve presenting with myocardial infarction. *Ann Thorac Surg* 1995; 60:206–208.
77. Prahlow JA, Barnard JJ. Sudden death due to obstruction of coronary artery ostium by aortic valve papillary fibroelastoma. *Am J Forensic Med Pathol* 1998; 19:162–165.
78. Lee CC, Celik C, Lajos TZ. Excision of papillary fibroelastoma arising from the septal leaflet of the tricuspid valve. *J Card Surg* 1995; 10:589–591.
79. Paelinck B, Vermeersch P, Kockx M. Calcified papillary fibroelastoma of the tricuspid valve. *Acta Cardiol* 1998; 53:165–167.
80. Brown RD Jr, Khandheria BK, Edwards WD. Cardiac papillary fibroelastoma: A treatable cause of transient ischemic attack and ischemic stroke detected by transesophageal echocardiography. *Mayo Clin Proc* 1995; 70:773–778.
81. Grinda JM, Couetil JP, Chauvaud S, et al. Cardiac valve papillary fibroelastoma: Surgical excision for revealed or potential embolization. *J Thorac Cardiovasc Surg* 1999; 117:106–110.
82. Sankar NM, Thiruchelvam T, Thirunavukkaarasu K, et al. Symp-

tomatic lipoma in the right atrial free wall: A case report. *Tex Heart Inst J* 1998; 25:152–154.
83. Barberger-Gateau P, Paquet M, Desaulniers D, et al. Fibrolipoma of the mitral valve in a child: Clinical and echocardiographic features. *Circulation* 1978; 58:955–958.
84. Leatherman L, Leachman RD, Hallman GL, et al. Cyst of the mitral valve. *Am J Cardiol* 1968; 21:428–430.
85. Basu S, Folliguet T, Anselmo M, et al. Lipomatous hypertrophy of the interatrial septum. *Cardiovasc Surg* 1994; 2:229–231.
86. Mortele KJ, Mergo PJ, Williams WF. Lipomatous hypertrophy of the atrial septum: Diagnosis with fat suppressed MR imaging. *J Magn Reson Imaging* 1998; 8:1172–1174.
87. Meaney JF, Kazerooni EA, Jamadar DA, et al. CT appearance of lipomatous hypertrophy of the interatrial septum. *AJR* 1997; 168:1081–1084.
88. Balasundaram S, Halees SA, Duran C. Mesothelioma of the atrioventricular node: First successful follow-up after excision. *Eur Heart J* 1992; 13:718–719.
89. Bharati S, Bauernfeind R, Josephson M. Intermittent preexcitation and mesothelioma of the atrioventricular node: A hitherto undescribed entity. *J Cardiovasc Electrophysiol* 1995; 6:823–831.
90. Pigato JB, Subramanian VA, McCaba JC. Cardiac hemangioma: A case report and discussion. *Tex Heart Inst J* 1998; 25:83–85.
91. Trout HHD, McAllister HA Jr, Giordano JM, et al. Vascular malformations. *Surgery* 1985; 97:36–41.
92. Dresler C, Cremer J, Logemann F, et al. Intrapericardial pheochromocytoma. *Thorac Cardiovasc Surg* 1998; 46:100–102.
93. Hamilton BH, Francis IR, Gross BH, et al. Intrapericardial paragangliomas (pheochromocytomas): Imaging features. *AJR Am J Roentgenol* 1997; 168:109–113.
94. Jeevanandam V, Oz MC, Shapiro B, et al. Surgical management of cardiac pheochromocytoma: Resection versus transplantation. *Ann Surg* 1995; 221:415–419.
95. Cooley DA, Frazier OH, Angelini P. Human cardiac explantation and autotransplantation: Application in a patient with a large cardiac pheochromocytoma. *Tex Heart Inst J* 1985; 12:171–176.
96. Swalwell CI. Benign intracardiac teratoma: A case of sudden death. *Arch Pathol Lab Med* 1993; 117:739–742.
97. Raaf HN, Raaf JH. Sarcomas related to the heart and vasculature. *Semin Surg Oncol* 1994; 10:374–382.
98. Adachi K, Tanaka H, Toshima H, et al. Right atrial angiosarcoma diagnosed by cardiac biopsy. *Am Heart J* 1988; 115: 482–485.
99. Uchita S, Hata T, Sushima Y, et al. Primary cardiac angiosarcoma with superior vena caval syndrome: Review of surgical resection and interventional management of venous inflow obstruction. *Can J Cardiol* 1998; 14:1283–1285.
100. Herrmann MA, Shankerman RA, Edwards WD, et al. Primary cardiac angiosarcoma: A clinicopathologic study of six cases. *J Thorac Cardiovasc Surg* 1992; 103:655–664.
101. Schmid KW, Thurner J Jr, Gruenewald K. Hemangiopericytoma of the heart following treatment of Hodgkin's disease: A case report. *Virchows Arch A Pathol Anat Histopathol* 1987; 411:485–488.
102. Schmaltz AA, and Apitz J. Primary rhabdomyosarcoma of the heart. *Pediatr Cardiol* 1982; 2:73–75.
103. Knobel B, Rosman P, Kishon Y, et al. Intracardiac primary fibrosarcoma: Case report and literature review. *Thorac Cardiovasc Surg* 1992; 40:227–230.
104. Cafferty LL, Epstein JI. Primary liposarcoma of the right atrium. *Hum Pathol* 1987; 18:408–410.
105. Cairns P, Butany J, Fulop J, et al. Cardiac presentation of non-Hodgkin's lymphoma. *Arch Pathol Lab Med* 1987; 111:80–83.
106. Teramoto N, Hayashi K, Miyatani K, et al. Malignant fibrous histiocytoma of the right ventricle of the heart. *Pathol Int* 1995; 45:315–319.
107. Putnam JB Jr, Sweeney MS, Colon R, et al. Primary cardiac sarcomas. *Ann Thorac Surg* 1991; 51:906–910.
108. Turner A, Batrick N. Primary cardiac sarcomas: A report of three cases and a review of the current literature. *Int J Cardiol* 1993; 40:115–119.
109. Rienmuller R, Tiling R. MR and CT for detection of cardiac tumors. *J Thorac Cardiovasc Surg* 1990; 38 (suppl 2):168–172.
110. Mora F, Mindich BP, Guarino T, et al. Improved surgical approach to cardiac tumors with intraoperative two-dimensional echocardiography. *Chest* 1987; 91:142–144.
111. Burke AP, Cowan D, Virmani R. Primary sarcomas of the heart. *Cancer* 1992; 69:387–395.
112. Goldstein DJ, Oz MC, Rose EA, et al. Experience with heart transplantation for cardiac tumors. *J Heart Lung Transplant* 1995; 14:382–386.
113. Harlamert HA, Moulton JS, Lewis W. Images in cardiovascular medicine: Primary malignant fibrous histiocytoma of the heart treated with orthotopic heart transplantation. *Circulation* 1998; 97:703–704.
114. Reardon MJ, DeFelice CA, Sheinbaum R, et al. Cardiac autotransplant for surgical treatment of a malignant neoplasm. *Ann Thorac Surg* 1999; 67:1793–1795.
115. Wagner S, Hutchisson B, Baird MG. Cardiac explantation and autotransplantation. *AORN J* 1999; 70:99–100, 102, 104–112.
116. Stoller JK, Shaw C, Matthay RA. Enlarging, atypically located pericardial cyst: Recent experience and literature review. *Chest* 1977; 89:402–406.
117. Ng AF, Olak J. Pericardial cyst causing right ventricular outflow tract obstruction [comments]. *Ann Thorac Surg* 1997; 63:1147–1148.
118. MacDonald S, Fay JE, Lynn RB. Intrapericardial teratoma: A continuing challenge. *Can J Surg* 1983; 26:81–82.
119. Lazoglu AH, DaSilva MM, Iwahara M, et al. Primary pericardial sarcoma. *Am Heart J* 1994; 127:453–458.
120. Neri E, Miracco C, Luzi P, et al. Intimal-type primary sarcoma of the thoracic aorta presenting as a saccular false aneurysm: Report of a case with evidence of rhabdomyosarcomatous differentiation. *J Thorac Cardiovasc Surg* 1999; 118:371–372.
121. Prichard RW. Tumors of the heart: Review of the subject and report of one hundred and fifty cases. *Arch Pathol* 1951; 51:98–128.
122. DeLoach JF, Haynes JW. Secondary tumors of the heart and pericardium: Review of the subject and report of one hundred thirty-seven cases. *Arch Int Med* 1953; 91:224–249.
123. Emmot WW, Vacek JL, Agee K, et al. Metastatic malignant melanoma presenting clinically as obstruction of the right ventricular inflow and outflow tracts: Characterization by magnetic resonance imaging. *Chest* 1987; 92:362–364.
124. Hayashi J, Ohzeki H, Tsuchida S, et al. Surgery for cavoatrial extension of malignant tumors. *Thorac Cardiovasc Surg* 1995; 43:161–164.
125. Hussain R, Neligan MC. Metastatic malignant schwannoma in the heart. *Ann Thorac Surg* 1993; 56:374–375.
126. Levine MJ, Lorell BH, Diver DJ, et al. Implications of echocardiographically assisted diagnosis of pericardial tamponade in contemporary medical patients: Detection before hemodynamic embarrassment. *J Am Coll Cardiol* 1991; 17:59–65.
127. Millaire A, Wurtz A, de Groote P, et al. Malignant pericardial effusions: Usefulness of pericardioscopy. *Am Heart J* 1992; 124:1030–1034.
128. Sheldon R, Isaac D. Metastatic melanoma to the heart presenting with ventricular tachycardia. *Chest* 1991; 99:1296–1298.
129. Virmani R, Khedekar RR, Robinowitz M, et al. Tumor embolization in coronary artery causing myocardial infarction. *Arch Pathol Lab Med* 1983; 107:243–245.
130. Chatterjee T, Muller MF, Carrel T, et al. Images in cardiovascular medicine: Renal cell carcinoma with tumor thrombus extending through the inferior vena cava into the right cardiac cavities. *Circulation* 1997; 96:2729–2730.

131. Fujisaki M, Kurihara E, Kikuchi K, et al. Hepatocellular carcinoma with tumor thrombus extending into the right atrium: Report of a successful resection with the use of cardiopulmonary bypass. *Surgery* 1991; 109:214–219.
132. Nakayama Y, Kitamura S, Kawachi K, et al. Intravenous leiomyomatosis extending into the right atrium. *Cardiovasc Surg* 1994; 2:642–645.
133. Peh WC, Cheung DL, Ngan H. Smooth muscle tumors of the inferior vena cava and right heart. *Clin Imaging* 1993; 17:117–123.
134. Luck SR, DeLeon S, Shkolnik A, et al. Intracardiac Wilms' tumor: Diagnosis and management. *J Pediatr Surg* 1982; 17:551–554.
135. Salcedo EE, Cohen GI, White RD, et al. Cardiac tumors: Diagnosis and management. *Curr Probl Cardiol* 1992; 17:73–137.
136. McAllister HA, Hall RJ. Iatrogenic heart disease. In: Cheng TO, ed. *The International Textbook of Cardiology*. New York: Pergamon Press; 1977:871.
137. Primrose WR, Clee MD, Johnston RN. Malignant pericardial effusion managed with vinblastine. *Clin Oncol* 1983; 9:67–70.
138. Chan A, Rischin D, Clarke CP, et al. Subxiphoid partial pericardiectomy with or without sclerosant instillation in the treatment of symptomatic pericardial effusions in patients with malignancy. *Cancer* 1991; 68:1021–1025.
139. Palacios IF, Tuzcu EM, Ziskind AA, et al. Percutaneous balloon pericardial window for patients with malignant pericardial effusion and tamponade [comments]. *Cathet Cardiovasc Diagn* 1991; 22:244–249.
140. Leak D. Amiodarone for control of recurrent ventricular tachycardia secondary to cardiac metastasis. *Tex Heart Inst J* 1998; 25:198–200.
141. Chen RH, Gaos CM, Frazier OH. Complete resection of a right atrial intracavitary metastatic melanoma [comments]. *Ann Thorac Surg* 1996; 61:1255–1257.
142. Lynch M, Balk MA, Lee RB, et al. Role of transesophageal echocardiography in the management of patients with bronchogenic carcinoma invading the left atrium. *Am J Cardiol* 1995; 76:1101–1102.
143. Terry LN Jr, Kligerman MM. Pericardial and myocardial involvement by lymphomas and leukemias: The role of radiotherapy. *Cancer* 1970; 25:1003–1008.
144. Bjorkholm M, Ost A, Biberfeld P. Myocardial rupture with cardiac tamponade as a lethal early manifestation of acute myeloblastic leukemia. *Cancer* 1982; 50:1777–1779.
145. Lewis W. AIDS: Cardiac findings from 115 autopsies. *Prog Cardiovasc Dis* 1989; 32:207–215.
146. Aboulafia DM, Bush R, Picozzi VJ. Cardiac tamponade due to primary pericardial lymphoma in a patient with AIDS. *Chest*, 1994; 106:1295–1299.
147. Chyu KY, Birnbaum Y, Naqvi T, et al. Echocardiographic detection of Kaposi's sarcoma causing cardiac tamponade in a patient with acquired immunodeficiency syndrome. *Clin Cardiol* 1998; 21:131–133.
148. Azrak EC, Kern MJ, Bach RG. Hemodynamics of cardiac tamponade in a patient with AIDS-related non-Hodgkin's lymphoma. *Cathet Cardiovasc Diagn* 1998; 45:287–291.
149. Estok L, Wallach F. Cardiac tamponade in a patient with AIDS: A review of pericardial disease in patients with HIV infection. *Mt Sinai J Med* 1998; 65:33–39.
150. Schiller VI, Fishbein MC, Siegel RJ. Unusual cardiac involvement in carcinoid syndrome. *Am Heart J* 1986; 112:1322–1323.
151. Le Metayer P, Constans J, Bernard N, et al. Carcinoid heart disease: Two cases of left heart involvement diagnosed by transthoracic and transoesophageal echocardiography. *Eur Heart J* 1993; 14:1721–1723.
152. Pelikka PA, Tajik AJ, Khandheria BK, et al. Carcinoid heart disease: Clinical and echocardiographic spectrum in 74 patients. *Circulation* 1993; 87:1188–1196.
153. Strickman NE, Hall RJ. Carcinoid heart disease. In: Kapoor AS, Reynolds RD, eds. *Cancer and the Heart*. New York: Springer-Verlag; 1986:135.
154. Koch CA, Azumi N, Furlong MA, et al. Carcinoid syndrome caused by an atypical carcinoid of the uterine cervix. *J Clin Endocrinol Metab* 1999; 84:4209–4213.
155. Robiolio PA, Rigolin VH, Wilson JS, et al. Carcinoid heart disease: Correlation of high serotonin levels with valvular abnormalities detected by cardiac catheterization and echocardiography. *Circulation* 1995; 92:790–795.
156. Johnston SD, Johnston PW, O'Rourke D. Carcinoid constrictive pericarditis. *Heart* 1999; 82:641–643.
157. McAllister HA Jr. Endocrine diseases and the cardiovascular system. In: Silver MD, ed. *Cardiovascular Pathology*, 2d ed. New York: Churchill Livingstone; 1991:1181.
158. Oates JA. The carcinoid syndrome. *N Engl J Med* 1986; 315:702–704.
159. Ridker PM, Chertow GM, Karlson EW, et al. Bioprosthetic tricuspid valve stenosis associated with extensive plaque deposition in carcinoid heart disease. *AM Heart J* 1991; 121:1835–1838.
160. Ohri SK, Schofield JB, Hodgson H, et al. Carcinoid heart disease: Early failure of an allograft valve replacement. *Ann Thorac Surg* 1994; 58:1161–1163.
161. Knott-Craig CJ, Schaff HV, Mullany CJ, et al. Carcinoid disease of the heart: Surgical management of ten patients. *J Thorac Cardiovasc Surg* 1992; 104:475–481.
162. Robiolio PA, Rigolin VH, Harrison JK, et al. Predictors of outcome of tricuspid valve replacement in carcinoid heart disease. *Am J Cardiol* 1995; 75:485–488.
163. Connolly HM, Nishimura RA, Smith HC, et al. Outcome of cardiac surgery for carcinoid heart disease. *J Am Coll Cardiol* 1995; 25:410–416.
164. Propst JW, Siegel LC, Stover EP. Anesthetic considerations for valve replacement surgery in a patient with carcinoid syndrome. *J Cardiothorac Vasc Anesth* 1994; 8:209–212.
165. Neustein SM, Cohen E. Anesthesia for aortic and mitral valve replacement in a patient with carcinoid heart disease. *Anesthesiology* 1995; 82:1067–1070.
166. Onate A, Alcibar J, Inguanzo R, et al. Balloon dilation of tricuspid and pulmonary valves in carcinoid heart disease. *Tex Heart Inst J* 1993; 20:115–119.

CHAPTER 78

DIABETES AND CARDIOVASCULAR DISEASE

Michael E. Farkouh / Elliot J. Rayfield / Valentin Fuster

INTRODUCTION

Diabetes mellitus, whether type 1 or type 2, is a very strong risk factor for the development of coronary artery disease (CAD) and stroke[1,2] (Table 78-1). Eighty percent of all deaths among diabetic patients are due to atherosclerosis, compared with about 30 percent among nondiabetic persons. A large National Institutes of Health (NIH) cohort study revealed that heart disease mortality in the general U.S. population is declining at a much greater rate than it is in diabetic subjects. In fact, diabetic women suffered an increase in heart disease mortality over that period.[3] Among all hospitalizations for diabetic complications, more than 75 percent are due to atherosclerosis. An increase in the prevalence of diabetes has been noted, which in part can be attributed to the aging of the population and an increase in the rate of obesity and the sedentary lifestyle in the United States.

Diabetes accelerates the natural course of atherosclerosis in all groups of patients and involves a greater number of coronary vessels with more diffuse atherosclerotic lesions[4–7] (Fig. 78-1). Cardiac catheterizations in diabetic patients have shown significantly more severe proximal and distal CAD.[8–11] In addition, plaque ulceration and thrombosis have been found to be significantly higher in diabetic patients.[12,13] Cardiovascular complications include CAD, peripheral artery disease, nephropathy, retinopathy, cardiomyopathy, and possible neuropathy (involvement of vasa vasorum). These observations underscore the heightened risks of a diabetic patient to develop vascular disease and compel the physician to correct all the metabolic abnormalities. By understanding the mechanisms underlying all these risks, physicians will be poised to prevent them.

CLINICAL PRESENTATIONS OF DIABETES MELLITUS

The risk factors for the development of diabetes are well established (Table 78-2). About 80 percent of all diabetic patients have type 2 diabetes mellitus, which characteristically occurs after age 40 years. The metabolic mechanisms of type 2 diabetes are the combination of insulin resistance and a genetically programmed defect in the pancreatic beta-cell secretion of insulin. Insulin resistance precedes the onset of type 2 diabetes by about 8 to 10 years and is associated with other cardiovascular risk factors: dyslipidemia, hypertension, and a procoagulant state.[14,15] The combination of these risk factors has been called syndrome X, the metabolic syndrome, and the cardiovascular dysmetabolic syndrome. Many patients with the metabolic syndrome exhibit either impaired fasting glucose (IFG) or impaired glucose tolerance (IGT) for many years before they develop frank diabetes.[16,17]

There are new criteria for the diagnosis of diabetes.[16] The cutoff for the diagnosis of diabetes has been lowered from 140 mg/dL to 126 mg/dL. The upper threshold for normoglycemia has been lowered from 115 mg/dL to 110 mg/dL. A fasting plasma glucose of 110 to 125 mg/dL is now referred to as IFG. These changes eliminate the need for oral glucose tolerance testing for the diagnosis of diabetes, which now rests on an elevation of the fasting plasma glucose level.

In contrast to type 2 diabetes, type 1 diabetes (10 percent of the diabetic population) usually is induced by immunologic destruction of pancreatic beta cells.[18] Type 1 diabetes classically has two peaks (at 4 years and 13 years of age) but can occur at any age. It typically produces microvascular disease (nephropathy, retinopathy) but also results in CAD.

TABLE 78-1 Clinical Evaluation of Risk Factors for the Development of Cardiovascular Disease in Diabetic Patients

Cigarette smoking
  Assess pack-years
Blood pressure
  Duration (if known), current and previous medications, assess presence of orthostatic hypertension.
Serum lipids and lipoproteins
  Dietary habits, alcohol intake, amount of exercise and whether aerobic
  Family history of dyslipidemia, eruptive xanthoma, lipemia, retinalis, xanthelasma, thyroid function tests
  LDL, HDL, cholesterol, fasting triglycerides.
Spot albumin/creatinine ratio (in micro- and macroalbuminuria)
  Serum creatinine
  Don't rely on dipstick protein, since negative results may reflect lack of sensitivity of test
Glycemic status
  Duration of diabetes; family history of diabetes; vascular, renal, and retinal complications
  Laboratory: fasting plasma glucose (FPG), hemoglobin A1c q 3 months: Dx FPG > 126 × 2: impaired fasting glucose 110–126 × 2; when in doubt, have patient undergo 2-h oral glucose tolerance test

TABLE 78-2 Assessment of Predisposing Risk Factors in Diabetic Patients

Body weight and fat distribution
  History
    Age of onset of overweight, family history of obesity
  Physical examination
    Measure body weight (kg), height (m); calculate body mass index (BMI, kg/m^2), BMI of 25–29.9 = overweight, >30.0 = obese, BMI >27 in a diabetic patient should be treated as high risk; measure waist circumference (abdominal obesity is >40 in. in men and >36 in. in women)
  Physical activity
    History: job, activity in sports, walking, aerobics; in women, child care, housework
    Physical examination: assess level of cardiovascular fitness in cardiac rehabilitation facility
  Family history
    History of heart disease, sudden death, elevated cholesterol level, cigarette smoking; hypertension; diabetes, especially in first-degree relatives
  Laboratory
    Measure fasting glucose and lipids in first-degree relatives

Stroke

Compared to nondiabetic subjects, the mortality from stroke in diabetic patients is almost threefold higher.[19] The small paramedial penetrating arteries are the most common site of cerebrovascular disease. In addition, diabetes increases the likelihood of severe carotid atherosclerosis.[20,21] Diabetic patients are likely to suffer increased brain damage with carotid emboli that would result in a transient ischemic attack in a nondiabetic individual.

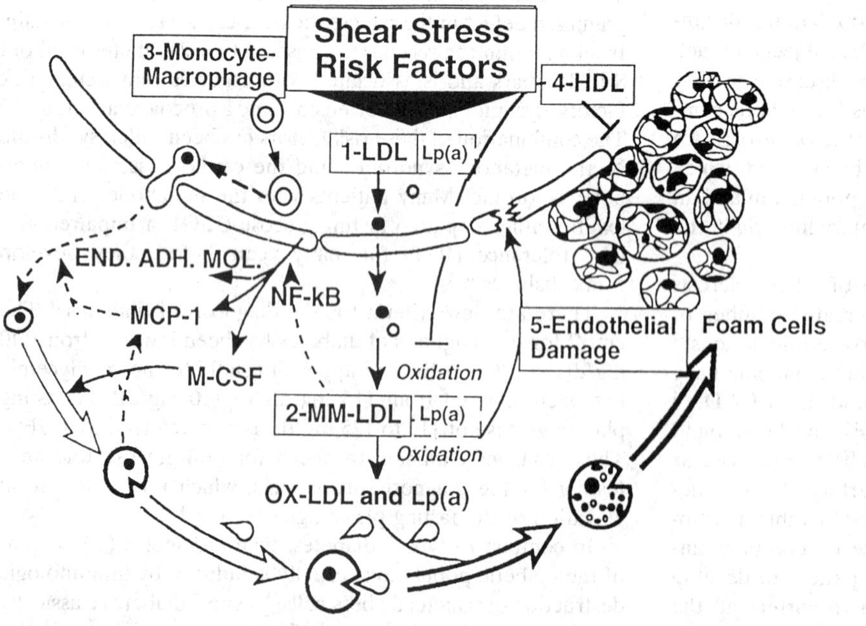

FIGURE 78-1 Schematic of staging (phases and lesion morphology of the progression of coronary atherosclerosis according to the gross pathologic and clinical findings). See text for more details.

Renal Disease

Nephropathy occurs in 40 percent of patients with type 1 and type 2 diabetes. Risk factors include poor glycemic control, hypertension, and ethnicity (blacks, Mexicans, Pima Indians).[22] Table 78-3 summarizes the key points for the assessment of renal status in a diabetic patient. The earliest clinical finding of diabetic kidney disease is microalbuminuria, which may occur at a time when renal histology is essentially normal.[23,24] The Diabetes Control and Complications Trial (DCCT) and the United Kingdom Prospective Diabetes Study group trial (UKPDS) showed that the development and progression of microalbuminuria can be prevented through strict glycemic control. Even once dipstick-positive proteinuria has developed, preliminary data from pancreatic transplant patients show improvement in glomerular pathology at 10 years.[25]

The UKPDS in type 2 diabetics and studies in patients with type 1 diabetes[26] using captopril have shown that control of hypertension slows the progression of nephropathy. The blood pressure should be maintained at <130/85, and angiotensin-converting enzyme (ACE) inhibitors are

TABLE 78-3 Evaluation of Renal Status

Urine albumin and protein
Yearly screen for microalbumin in type 1 and type 2 diabetes; microalbumin/creatinine ratio collected in a spot urine, ideally first morning urine specimen (normal <30 mg/g creatinine); must rule out other diseases that cause proteinuria
If urine albumin/creatinine is >300 mg/g in first morning specimen, macroalbuminuria is present and is usually not reversible with ACE inhibitors; nephrology consult
Nephrotic syndrome: urine protein >3 g/day; nephrology consult
Other reasons to consult nephrologists are diabetic patients with increasing creatinine from 1.4 to over 2.0, elevated creatinine and symptoms of uremia, microalbuminuria not responding to ACE inhibitor
Urinalysis
Red cells, pyuria, casts require nephrology consult
Blood pressure evaluation
If hypertension is present, exclude secondary causes, including with advancing renal insufficiency
Treatment with an ACE inhibitor is preferred first choice even in African-Americans (except if precluded by hyperkalemia or other complications)
Blood urea nitrogen, serum creatinine, and glomerular filtration rate
Yearly creatinine clearance should be obtained with 24-h urine collection and serum creatinine; most accurate way to estimate kidney function without using a radioisotope

the preferred antihypertensive agents.[27,28] The UKPDS, however, showed no difference in blood pressure control with captopril versus atenolol. The benefit of antihypertensive therapy with an ACE inhibitor in type 1 diabetes can be shown early in the course of disease, when microalbuminuria is the only abnormality.[29–31]

There is insufficient evidence to recommend ACE inhibitors in normotensive patients without microalbuminuria.[32] Although screening for microalbuminuria is not as useful in type 2 diabetes patients in predicting the progression to overt nephropathy as it is in type 1 diabetes patients, once microalbuminuria develops, the rate of loss of the glomerular filtration rate (GFR) is equivalent to that in type 1 diabetes.[33,34] Nonetheless, physicians should still recommend screening on at least a yearly basis, since the risk/benefit ratio of diagnosing microalbuminuria justifies treatment with an ACE inhibitor, if not for renal disease alone,[35,36] then for reducing the incidence of myocardial infarction.[37,38]

Patients on ACE inhibitors should be monitored for potassium, since they may develop hyperkalemia in the presence of a type 4 renal tubular acidosis.[27] Sodium restriction will reduce hypertension and therefore is advised. Dietary protein should be adjusted to 0.8 g/kg per day to decrease intraglomerular pressure.[27]

An optimal approach toward diabetic nephropathy combines control of hypertension, preferably with an ACE inhibitor; glycemic control; sodium restriction; and adjustment of protein intake.

Type 2 Diabetes and Coronary Artery Disease

Coronary artery disease is strongly associated with type 2 diabetes mellitus and is the leading cause of death regardless of the duration of disease. There is a twofold to fourfold increase in the relative risk ratio of cardiovascular disease in type 2 diabetes patients compared to the general population.[2,39–43] This increase is particularly disproportionate in diabetic women compared with diabetic men.[39,41,44] The protection that premenopausal women have against CAD is not seen if they suffer from diabetes.[45,46]

The degree and duration of hyperglycemia are a strong risk factor for the development of microvascular complications,[47] but in type 2 diabetes, macrovascular complications have not been documented to be associated with the length or severity of a patient's diabetes.[5,40,43,48] Even impaired glucose tolerance increases cardiovascular risk even though there is minimal hyperglycemia.[41,49–51]

The first detectable sign of a problem in people genetically prone to develop type 2 diabetes is insulin resistance, which can be seen as long as 15 to 25 years before the onset of diabetes.[52] Several atherogenic factors are associated with insulin resistance,[53–59] which can start the atherosclerotic process years before clinical hyperglycemia ensues.[60,61] It is unclear whether the compensatory hyperinsulinemia plays a role in atherosclerosis generation in insulin-resistant patients. A number of prospective studies have shown an association between fasting or postprandial hyperinsulinemia and the future development of CAD.[62–64] However, this association has been demonstrated in middle-aged white men[62–64] but not in women[65] or in other ethnic groups.[66,67]

Hyperglycemia itself plays an important role in enhancing the progression of atherosclerosis in type 2 diabetes. The threshold above which hyperglycemia becomes atherogenic is not known but may be in the range defined as impaired glucose tolerance (i.e., fasting plasma glucose level <126 mg/dL with 30-, 60-, or 90-min plasma glucose concentrations >200 mg/dL and a 2-h plasma glucose level of 140 to 200 mg/dL during an oral glucose tolerance test).[68] Despite the role played by all these factors, population-based studies show that the degree of hyperglycemia increases the risk for CAD and cardiovascular events.[69–71]

Type 1 Diabetes and Coronary Artery Disease

In contrast to type 2 diabetes, cardiovascular risk factors can be examined in relation to hyperglycemia in type 1 diabetes patients. Long-term follow-up of these patients has shown that the incidence of cardiovascular mortality rises after age 30.[72] There is evidence that diabetes accelerates the process of early atherosclerosis that occurs at a young age in the general population. The coronary mortality rate in type 1 diabetes is markedly accelerated, and one-third of these patients will die of CAD by age 55.[72] The protective effect of the premenopausal state is lost for females with type 1 diabetes.

It has been demonstrated that diabetic nephropathy dramatically increases the prevalence of CAD. Diabetic nephropathy is defined by proteinuria, a reduced GFR, and hypertension.

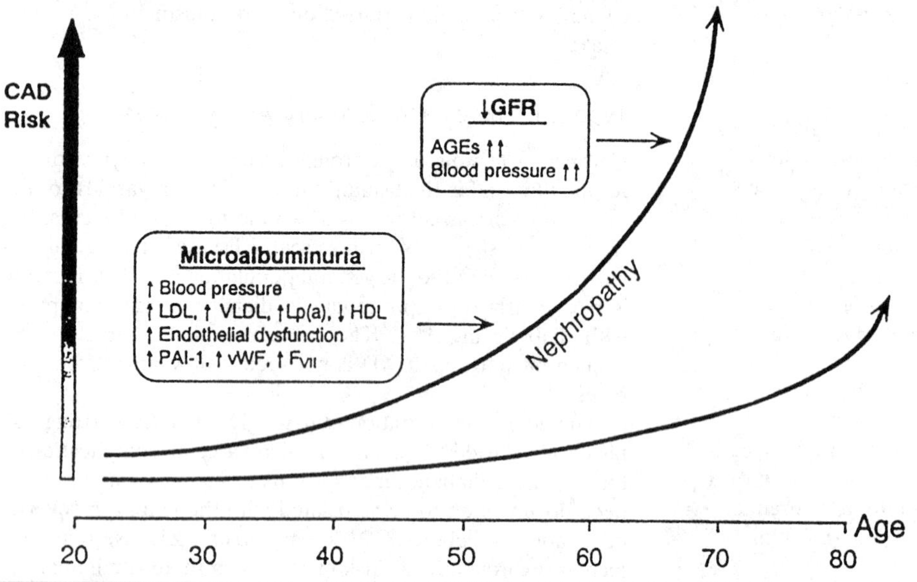

FIGURE 78-2 CAD risk in patients with diabetes mellitus. A subset of genetically predisposed patients develop diabetic nephropathy. In these patients, the risk for CAD increases dramatically. (From Aronson and Rayfield,[138] with permission.)

Patients with proteinuria can be divided into two groups: those with macroalbuminuria (greater than 300 mg/day) and those with microalbuminuria (30 to 300 mg/day). The presence of overt proteinuria increases the risk of cardiovascular mortality almost tenfold compared with the risk in patients without proteinuria.[73] In another cohort, the risk of developing CAD was almost 15 times greater in patients with proteinuria than it was in those without diabetic nephropathy.[72] Since this risk of developing CAD morbidity and mortality has been demonstrated for both macro- and microalbuminuria patients, both must be considered vital in the cardiovascular evaluation of a diabetic patient (Fig. 78-2).

DIABETES AND MECHANISMS OF CARDIOVASCULAR RISKS

Lipoprotein Disorders

Lipid disorders constitute one of the cornerstones in the cardiovascular management of diabetic patients. Many factors influence the lipid profile in these patients, including glycemic control, whether the diabetes is type 1 or type 2, and the presence of diabetic nephropathy.

TYPE OF DIABETES

In type 1 diabetes mellitus, the major determinant in the lipid profile is the level of glycemic control. Low-density lipoprotein (LDL) is moderately increased, triglycerides are markedly increased, and high-density lipoprotein (HDL) is decreased when the level of glycemic control is impaired. For patients with type 2 diabetes, lipid abnormalities are related not only to hyperglycemia but also to the interplay of the insulin-resistant state. Patients with type 2 diabetes may have normal LDL levels but elevated levels of the very low density lipoprotein (VLDL) triglycerides moiety and reduced HDL levels. The expected elevation in VLDL triglyceride is usually no more than 100 percent.

LDL Although LDL levels in patients with controlled type 1 or type 2 diabetes are normal, the atherogenic properties of LDL are increased. There is glycosylation of both apoprotein B[74] and the phospholipid component of LDL,[75] which changes LDL clearance and susceptibility to oxidative modifications. Glycosylation of apoprotein B occurs mainly in the LDL receptor–binding area[74] and is directly related to glucose levels. As a result, there is impairment in the LDL receptor–mediated uptake and therefore clearance of LDL.[76,77] Glycosylation also makes LDL more susceptible to oxidative modification. The product generated by the combined glycosylation and oxidation of LDL is more atherogenic than is either glycosylated or oxidized LDL alone.[78] Such LDL molecules are taken up more easily by the aortic intimal cells and macrophages, resulting in the formation of foam cells.[79–81]

Type 2 diabetic patients with insulin resistance have LDL particles that are small and rich with triglycerides but have little cholesterol in them (small, dense LDL).[82,83] These LDL particles increase the risk of CAD independent of the total LDL level, probably because of their increased susceptibility to oxidative modification. Therefore, even though LDL levels may be normal in these patients, high levels of small, dense LDL may contribute to the increased risk of CAD in such patients.[84]

VLDL Diabetic patients have elevated levels of VLDL as a result of increased free fatty acid mobilization and high glucose levels. There is an increase in triglyceride production by the liver, which results in large, triglyceride-rich VLDL particles.[85] The size of these VLDL particles, which is dependent primarily on the amount of triglycerides available, is an important factor in determining their eventual fate. The conversion of large VLDL particles to LDL is not efficient[86]; therefore, they are cleared from circulation by other pathways. Since the removal of VLDL by lipoprotein lipase also is affected, the level of VLDL triglyceride rises. Furthermore, the abundance of large triglyceride-rich VLDL is associated with an increase in small, dense, atherogenic LDL particles.[87] Numerous studies have shown that elevated triglyceride levels are associated with increased risk for CAD in diabetic patients.[44,88–90] In contrast, elevated triglycerides are not associated with CAD risk in nondiabetic patients.

HDL Low HDL level is a strong risk factor for the development of CAD in both diabetic and nondiabetic patients. There is decreased production and increased catabolism of HDL in diabetes. The decreased HDL production is a result of decreased lipoprotein lipase (LPL) activity. The failure of LPL to efficiently catabolize VLDL results in reduced availability of surface components for HDL production. By contrast, increased catabolism of HDL results from the hypertriglyceridemia of diabetes, producing triglyceride-rich HDL_2 that is prone to catabolism by liver enzymes.[91,92]

MANAGEMENT OF LIPID DISORDERS

Consistent with the National Cholesterol Education Program, the American Diabetes Association has published its consensus document concerning the management of lipid disorders.[93] For the most part, the cornerstone of therapy in diabetes revolves around dietary modifications, weight loss, physical exercise, and maximization of glycemic control.

Type of Diabetes As was previously mentioned, the management of lipid disorders in type 1 diabetes is closely coupled to glycemic control. For type 1 patients, the front-line strategy begins with glycemic control.

In type 1 diabetes, glycemic control can lead to marked reductions in triglyceride levels, but with little or no impact on HDL levels. In type 2, pharmacotherapy is often required sooner than later, given the modest impact of nonpharmacologic strategies.[93]

Medical therapy for hyperlipidemia is similar in diabetic and nondiabetic patients, but diabetic patients require certain considerations.

The hypertriglyceridemia of diabetes can be treated effectively with fibric acid derivatives[94,95] without an adverse effect on glucose metabolism. Type 2 diabetic patients experience a reduction in cardiovascular event rate when treated with gemfibrozil.[96] These drugs cause a 5 to 15 percent drop in LDL levels in patients with normal triglyceride levels, but in patients with hypertriglyceridemia, LDL levels go up. This elevation probably is due to the catabolism of atherogenic LDL particle, resulting in less atherogenic LDL.[97]

Although nicotinic acid lowers both cholesterol and triglyceride levels while raising HDL levels, it generally is not indicated in diabetes. It has an adverse effect on glycemic control[98] that results from the induction of insulin resistance.

Hydroxymethylglutaryl coenzyme A (HMG-CoA) reductase inhibitors are another group of drugs that are useful in lowering cholesterol levels in type 2 diabetes patients without having an adverse effect on glycemic control.[99] In a study assessing the effectiveness of a cholesterol-lowering drug for secondary prevention of morbidity and mortality in patients with angina or prior myocardial infarction, simvastatin was found to be more efficacious in diabetic patients than it was in the overall group.[100]

Bile acid resins can decrease the levels of LDL in diabetic patients,[101] but they can cause a significant rise in triglyceride levels, especially if VLDL levels are already high or if the diabetes is poorly controlled. In patients with high levels of both LDL and VLDL, bile acid resins can be used in low doses in combination with fibric acid derivatives.

Thrombosis and Diabetes

Diabetes mellitus is widely recognized as being perhaps the most significant risk factor for the development of acute coronary syndromes. The relationship between diabetes and acute coronary thrombosis is multifactorial, with the interaction of plaque disruption and the interplay of local and systemic thrombogenic factors playing the primary roles.

PLAQUE DISRUPTION

The inciting role of acute plaque disruption in the development of acute coronary thrombosis is well described. Although the lipid-rich core in plaque is felt to be causative in this process, more aggressive medical management of diabetes can have a favorable impact by decreasing plaque rupture and improving the clinical outcome.[102]

It is well described that not all disruptions of atherosclerotic plaques lead to clinical events. The complex interaction of local and systemic thrombogenic factors is an important determinant of whether clinically significant thrombus formation will occur.

PROTHROMBOSIS

Patients with diabetes demonstrate enhanced platelet aggregation[103,104] that correlates with increased cardiovascular events.[105] Diabetic patients have been shown to have platelets that are hypersensitive to agonists of aggregation.[106,107] The major mechanism is felt to be increased thromboxane production.[108,109] An increased incidence of cardiovascular events in diabetic patients has been shown to be correlated with platelet hyperaggregation.[105]

Diabetic patients have elevated levels of von Willebrand factor that correlate with vascular complications.[110,111] In addition, a relationship has been shown between the insulin resistance syndrome and elevated plasma von Willebrand levels.[112] Similarly, diabetic patients often demonstrate elevated fibrinogen levels, which are also predictive of cardiovascular complications.[113–115] Fibrinogen levels mirror glycemic control.

Factor V, VII, X, XI, and XII levels also are elevated in diabetic patients.[116–118] Factor VII levels correlate directly with fasting plasma glucose levels.[118] Evidence exists linking activation of the coagulation cascade with hyperglycemia. Since antithrombin III activity is decreased with hyperglycemia, glycemic control may play the pivotal role in limiting thrombosis and thrombosis-related complications in diabetic patients.[119]

The insulin resistance syndrome is marked by increased plasminogen-activator inhibitor-1 (PAI-1) levels. Impaired plasma fibrinolytic activity therefore can increase the risk for myocardial infarction.[120] Fasting plasma insulin levels have been shown to be directly correlated to the concentration of PAI-1. Glucose has a direct effect on PAI-1–producing tissues, leading to another explanation for the presence of impaired fibrinolysis in diabetic patients. Even when insulin resistance is adjusted for, serum triglyceride levels have been closely linked to impaired fibrinolysis.[121–123]

Endothelial Dysfunction

Hyperglycemia induces the expression of adhesion molecules such as VCAM-1, ICAM-1, and E-selectin[124] (Fig. 78-3). The binding of advanced glycosylation end products to their receptor results in oxidative stress and the transcription factor NF-κB[125,126] and VCAM-1.[127] These early stages in diabetic atherosclerosis may be the consequence of increased adhesive interactions of monocytes and the endothelial cell surface. Hyperglycemia-induced endothelial dysfunction is believed to result primarily from increased generation of oxygen free radicals that inactivate endothelium-derived relaxing factor (EDRF).[128,129] Enhanced levels of free radicals in the setting of sustained hyperglycemia result in the autooxidation of glucose,[130] the oxidation of lipids,[131] and the metabolism of AGEs.[132] AGEs rapidly inactivate nitric oxide and result in a reduction of endothelium-dependent vaso-

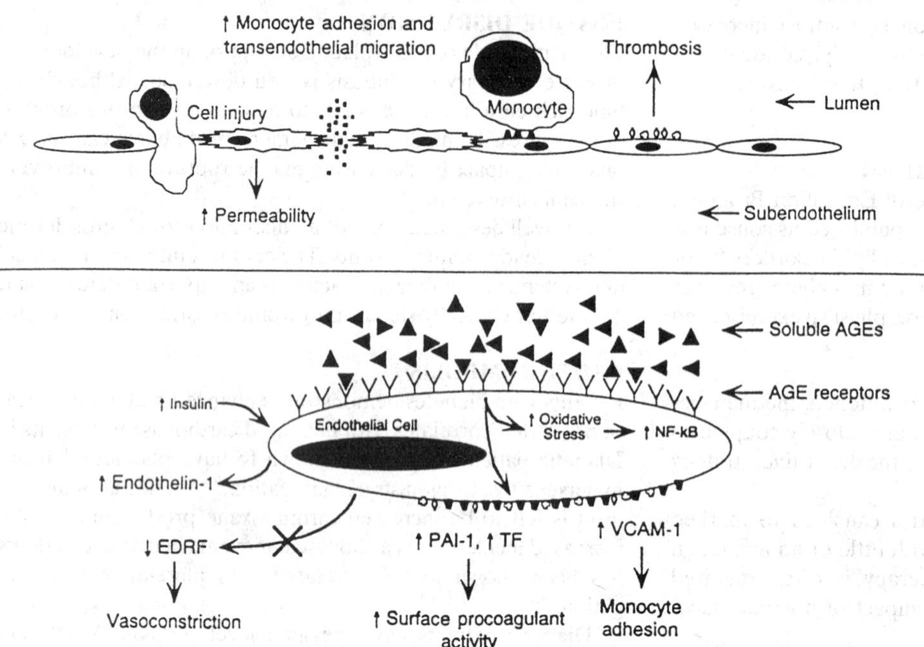

FIGURE 78-3 Generation of a dysfunctional endothelium caused by diabetes. (From Aronson and Rayfield,[138] with permission.)

dilatation.[133] Endothelial dysfunction is measured clinically by the vasodilatory response of forearm resistance vessels to endothelium-dependent agents such as acetylcholine. It recently has been determined that in vivo endothelial dysfunction occurs in subjects whose fasting plasma glucose concentrations fall in the range of IGF = 110 to 126 mg.[134]

Advanced Glycosylation End Products

AGEs are formed by nonenzymatic glucose-protein and lipoprotein interactions, with subsequent cross-linking on vascular tissues.[135,136] In the setting of aging and diabetes, AGEs form at a rate determined by the glucose concentration and the length of exposure.[137] AGEs accelerate atherogenesis by multiple mechanisms that can be classified as receptor-mediated or non-receptor-mediated.[138] AGE deposits have been demonstrated in atherosclerotic plaques and myocardium by immunohistochemistry in patients with diabetes and atherosclerosis.[139] In addition, serum levels of AGEs are significantly increased in type 2 diabetes patients with CAD in contrast to those without CAD.[140] Serum levels of AGEs correlate positively with isovolumetric relaxation time (IVRT) and left ventricular diameter during diastole in type 1 diabetic patients.[141] The systolic parameters did not correlate with serum levels of AGEs.[141]

AGEs can be prevented from forming by pharmacologic means. Aminoguanidines prevent the earlier nonenzymatic Amadori products from progressing to AGEs,[142] and cross-link breakers can break up AGEs in vascular tissues that are already formed.[143]

The cellular interactions for AGE are via a specific receptor for AGE determinants on the cell membrane.[144] Indeed, AGE receptors are present on all cells participating in atherogenesis, such as the monocyte-derieved macrophages, endothelial cells (ECs), and smooth muscle cells (SMCs)[144,145] (Table 78-4). When AGE binds to its receptor, monocytes undergo chemotaxis,[160] followed by mononuclear infiltration through an intact endothelial monolayer.[147,148] Pathologic studies of human atherosclerotic plaques showed infiltration of cells with AGE receptors in a thickened intima.[145] Monocyte-macrophage interactions with AGEs promote several mediators, including interleukin-1 (IL-1), tumor necrosis factor-alpha (TNFα), platelet-derived growth factor (PDGF), and insulin-like growth factor-1 (IGF-1).[146,147,149]

In smooth muscle cells, in the binding of AGE-modified proteins to the AGE receptor by cultured rat SMCs, there is increased cellular proliferation.[161] One can speculate that the response is induced by cytokines or growth factors. In summary, enhanced AGE formation involves receptor-mediated interaction of AGE protein

TABLE 78-4 Atherosclerosis-Promoting Effects of Advanced Glycosylation End Products

Promoting inflammation
*Secretion of cytokines (TNFα, IL-1)[146]
*Chemotactic stimulus for monocytes-macrophages[147,148]
Induction of cellular proliferation
*Stimulation of PDGF[147] and IGF-1[149] secretion from monocyte and (?) SMCs
Endothelial cells
*Increased permeability of EC monolayers[150,151]
*Increased procoagulant activity[150]
*Increased expression of adhesion molecules[152]
*Increased intracellular oxidative stress[153,154]
Extracellular matrix
Collagen cross-linking[155]
Enhanced synthesis of extracellular matrix components[156]
Trapping of LDL in subendothelium[157]
Glycosylated subendothelium matrix quenches NO[158]
Lipoprotein modifications
Glycosylated LDL
Reduced LDL recognition by cellular LDL receptors[76,77]
Increased susceptibility of LDL to oxidative modification[75,78,159]

NOTE: Asterisks indicate receptor-mediated events, whereas lack of an asterisk signifies non-receptor-mediated processes. TNFα: tumor necrosis factor-alpha; IL-1: interleukin-1; PDGF: platelet-derived growth factor; IGF-1: insulin-like growth factor-1; SMC: smooth muscle cells; EC: endothelial cells; LDL: low-density lipoproteins; NO: nitric oxide.

TABLE 78-5 Hyperlipidemia

Trial	Treatment	Outcome	Events Control Group	Events Treatment Group	Relative Risk Reduction, %	Number Needed to Treat	p
4S[162] (secondary prevention) n = 4444 202 DM[a]	Simvastatin	Death, nonfatal MI, revascularization	44/97 (45%)	24/105 (23%)	49	5	<.05
CARE[163] (primary prevention) n = 4159 586 DM	Pravastatin	Death, nonfatal MI, revascularization	112/304 (37%)	81/282 (29%)	21	12	.05
Helsinki Heart Study (primary prevention) n = 4081 135 DM	Gemfibrozil	Death, nonfatal MI, revascularization	8/76 (10.5%)	2/59 (3.4%)	67	14	<.02

[a]n = total number of patients; DM = diabetes mellitus patients.

with vascular wall cells, with subsequent migration of inflammatory cells into the lesion and the elaboration of growth factors and cytokines.

NON-RECEPTOR-MEDIATED MECHANISMS

Glycosylated modification of proteins and lipoproteins can interfere with their normal function (Table 78-4). Glycosylation of matrix components such as type IV collagen, laminen, and vitronectin decreases the binding of anionic heparin sulfate (HS), promoting a greater turnover of HS. The absence of HS may induce a compensatory overproduction of other matrix components by means of altered partitioning of growth factors between matrix-bound proteoglycans and cells.[156] Modification of the cell-binding domain of type IV collagen results in decreased endothelial cell adhesion.[156]

CLINICAL IMPLICATIONS

Lipid Disorders

The management of diabetic patients with lipid abnormalities is a unique challenge to the cardiologist. Important evidence from large randomized trials of lipid-lowering therapies is based on subgroup analyses in which diabetic patients represented less than 10 percent of all the patients enrolled. Two hundred two diabetic patients with a prior history of coronary artery disease were enrolled in the 4S study.[162] Although this number was too small, the comparison of simvastatin with placebo showed almost a 50 percent reduction in coronary events in favor of simvastatin (45 percent versus 23 percent, p = not significant). Similar trends were observed in the CARE trial, which compared pravastatin with placebo in secondary prevention.[163] In the CARE trial, the baseline mean LDL concentration in diabetic patients was 136 mg/dL. LDL was reduced 27 percent in the group receiving pravastatin, which translated into a 25 percent reduction in coronary events over 5 years compared with the control group.[164] Table 78-5 demonstrates the relatively low number needed to treat (NNT) to prevent a major cardiovascular complication in three of the main lipid-lowering trials. These therapies are the cornerstone of diabetic management in the current era.

In the trials of statin therapy in hyperlipidemia, the relative benefit appears similar between diabetic patients and nondiabetic patients. The concern for the clinician is that larger trials focusing on the diabetic population have to be carried out before the magnitude of the benefit of lipid-lowering therapy in reducing cardiovascular events can be determined.

Glycemic Control

The pathophysiology of type 2 diabetes is a consequence of peripheral resistance to insulin action (in muscle and fat cells), increased hepatic glucose production, and decreased secretion of insulin by pancreatic beta cells. About 80 percent of people with type 2 diabetes are obese.

Diet and exercise remain the cornerstone in the management of type 2 diabetes. Pharmacologic agents available to treat type 2 diabetes are insulin, insulin secretagogues (sulfonylureas, repaglinide), alpha glucosidase inhibitors (acarbose, miglitol), and insulin sensitizers (biguanides, thiazolidinediones). Each of these agents targets a different mechanism responsible for the hyperglycemia. Figure 78-4 shows each of these agents and the target organs involved in its mode of action.

The standards of care in patients with diabetes (American Diabetes Associations) are preprandial glucose levels of 80 to

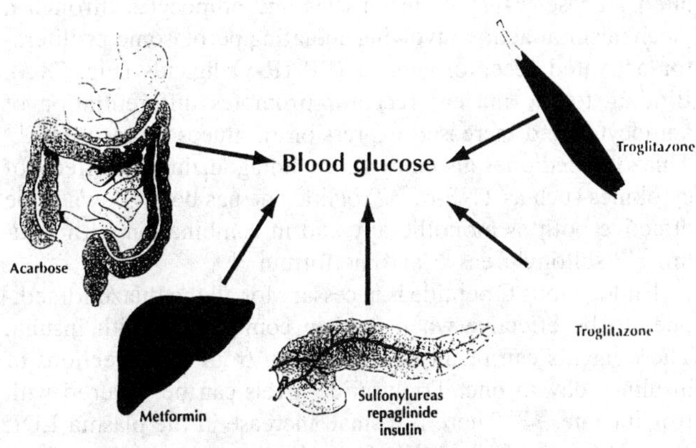

FIGURE 78-4 Mechanism of action of hypoglycemic agents.

120, bedtime glucose levels of 100 to 140, and hemoglobin A1c (Hb-A1c) below 7 percent.[165]

Plasma Hb-A1c reflects the average glucose level of the previous 8 weeks and allows a uniform measure for achieving a target as well as comparing the efficacies of different therapies.

PHARMACOLOGIC MANAGEMENT

Sulfonylureas Sulfonylureas are the typical therapy for lean type 2 diabetics and are used in combinations with other agents in obese type 2 patients. Sulfonylureas bind to a receptor on the beta cells and inhibit the Na-ATP channel; an increase in intracellular calcium results in insulin exocytosis.

Some experts point to a possible risk of increased myocardial damage in patients with known coronary artery disease who use sulfonylureas at the time of an ischemic event.[166] Prevention of protective ischemic preconditioning of the heart by inhibition of the K-ATP channel is the putative mechanism.[167] The UKPDS data do not support this concern. The authors agree and use sulfonylureas in appropriate patients with CAD.

Repaglinide This newer insulin secretagogue binds to a different receptor site than do the sulfonylureas on the K-ATP channel.[168] The half-life of this agent is 3.7 h, which makes it effective for postprandial rather than preprandial hyperglycemia, for use in the elderly, and for diabetic patients with chronic renal failure.[168]

Metformin Metformin is a biguanide drug that has been in use in Europe for over 30 years and was approved in the United States in 1995.[169] The main mode of action of metformin is decreasing hepatic glucose output primarily by inhibiting gluconeogenesis,[170] typically without hypoglycemia.[169]

Metformin is effective alone[171] or in combination with insulin,[172] sulfonylureas,[173] and thiazolidinediones.[174] The drug usually results in weight loss as a result of decreased appetite for up to 1 year after the initiation of therapy.

Significant decreases in LDL cholesterol and triglycerides occur.[173,175] The incidence of lactic acidosis with metformin is 9 per 100,000 person-years.[176] Contraindications to its use include an elevated creatinine (>1.4 in women, >1.5 in men), congestive heart failure, severe pulmonary disease, or any hypoxic state.[177]

Thiazolidinediones This class of drug promotes insulin-stimulated glucose transport in muscles and adipocytes through a mechanism of action involving actuating peroxisome proliferator activated receptor-gamma (PPAR-γ) ligands (Fig. 78-5). Binding to the nuclear receptor promotes differentiation of adipocytes and increased expression of glucose transporter.[178] Thiazolidinediones also may act by antagonizing the effects of cytokines such as TNF-α.[179] Troglitazone has been shown to be effective both as monotherapy and in combination with insulin,[180,181] sulfonylureas,[182] and metformin.[174]

Endogenous C peptide is necessary for all the thiazolidinediones to be effective when used in combination with insulin. These agents can result in a reduction from two injections of insulin a day to one. Triglyceride levels can be lowered with troglitazone.[183,184] There is a small increase in the plasma LDL concentration, along with a favorable increase in the ratio of the buoyant LDL to the more atherogenic small dense LDL.[185]

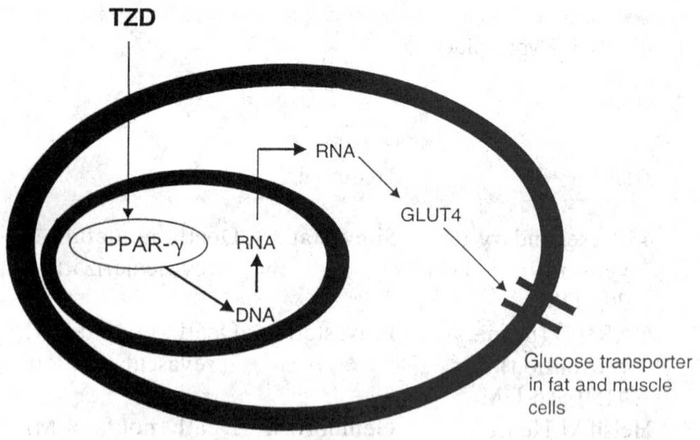

FIGURE 78-5 Mechanism of action of thiazolidinediones.

The thiazolidinediones are associated with weight gain partly resulting from improvement in glycemic control. With troglitazone, monitoring of liver function should be done monthly for the first year and quarterly thereafter.

Troglitazone has resulted in fulminant hepatic failure in about 1 in 60,000 patients on the medication; this is felt to be an idiosyncratic reaction. Patients with a history of liver

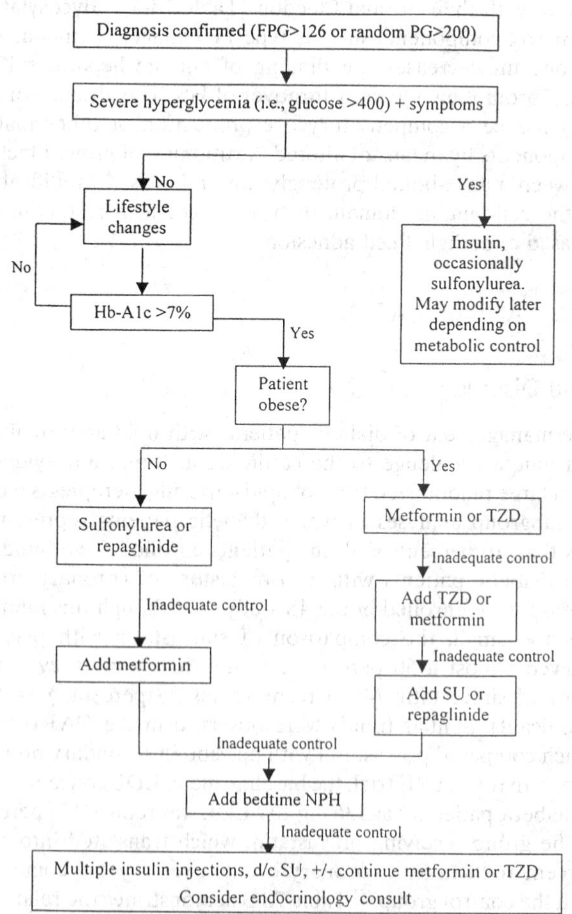

FIGURE 78-6 Algorithm for type 2 diabetes. Note: Acarbose or miglitol can be added anywhere along the treatment pathway. SU = sulfonylurea; TZD = thiazolidinedione.

disease, possibly including hepatitis C (depending on severity), and those who ingest more than a moderate amount of alcohol should not be started on this agent. Because of the potential for liver disease, troglitazone no longer is used as monotherapy unless the patient has been on combination therapy first and has achieved good glycemic control with troglitazone alone.

Two other drugs in this class were approved by the U.S. Food and Drug Administration (FDA) in mid-1999, and the data to date support equal efficacy with less hepatotoxicity. No head-to-head studies of these agents are available. Monitoring of liver function tests with rosiglitazone and pioglitazone is recommended every 2 months for the first year and periodically thereafter, since it has not been determined that serious liver events with troglitazone are a class effect of the thiazolidinediones or are specific to troglitazone.

Rosiglitazone monotherapy results in a decrease of Hgb-A1c of 0.8 to 1.5 percent greater than that seen with placebo, with the greatest reduction seen when it was given in two divided doses.[186,187] Combination studies of rosiglitazone with metformin for 26 weeks resulted in a 1.0 to 1.2 percent placebo-adjusted decrease in Hgb-A1c.[188] Although rosiglitazone is currently approved for use as monotherapy and in combination therapy with metformin, it also is expected to be efficacious with sulfonylureas or insulin. Rosiglitazone has been reported to result in an increase in LDL and HDL cholesterol concentrations between 12 percent and 19 percent, with changes in serum triglycerides similar to those seen with placebo.[189]

Pioglitazone, the newest thiazolidinedione, has been approved for use as monotherapy and in combination with metformins, sulfonylureas, and insulin. In three randomized, double-blind placebo-controlled trials of 16 to 26 weeks' duration, changes in Hgb-A1c were 1.0 to 1.4 percent.[190] Increases in ALT occurred in 0.26 percent of treated patients, a result that was not different from that with placebo.[190] Patients treated with pioglitazone showed a decrease in serum triglyceride (9.3 to 9.6 percent), increases in HDL (12.2 to 19.1 percent), and increases in LDL (5.2 to 6.0 percent) with the 30- to 45-mg doses, respectively.[190]

Alpha-Glucosidase Inhibitors Acarbose and miglitol work in the intestine to reversibly inhibit brush border alpha-glucosidases, resulting in a delay in carbohydrate absorption. Only about 1 percent of the drug is absorbed from the gastrointestinal tract. These drugs cause a 30 percent decrease in postprandial glucose in contrast to a 10 percent decrease in fasting glucose levels. They are adjuncts to other oral agents and rarely are potent enough to be used as monotherapy.

Insulin The natural history of type 2 diabetes is one of progressive beta-cell failure. Therefore, after approximately 10 years of the use of oral hypoglycemic agents, insulin will be required either in combination with oral agents or as the sole therapy. Although endogenous hyperinsulinemia is clearly associated with atherogenesis, there is no compelling evidence of increased risk of cardiovascular disease or increased mortality from exogenous insulin therapy.

Diabetes clinics nationwide have strived to optimize the glycemic control of patients with a view to minimizing the development of coronary and other vascular disease. Figure 78-6 shows an algorithm that is reasonable to use in the management of patients with type 2 diabetes. Table 78-6 shows the clinical trial evidence supporting intensive glycemic control.

TABLE 78-6 Glycemic Control

Trial	Treatment	Outcome	Events Control Group	Events Treatment Group	Relative Risk Reduction, %	Number Needed to Treat	p
Type 1 DM							
DCCT[198] n = 1441 patients[a] free of cardiac disease, HTN, and dyslipidemia	Intensive glycemic control versus conventional therapy	Macrovascular events	40/730 (5.5%)	23/711 (3.2%)	42	43	.08
Type 2 DM							
UKPDS[193–196] In newly diagnosed diabetes mellitus n = 3867	Sulfonylurea or insulin versus conventional therapy	Diabetes-related outcomes	438/1138 (38.4%)	963/2729 (35.2%)	8.3	31	.029
Steno[136] n = 160	Intensive comprehensive (includes hypertension (HTN), dyslipidemia, and glycemic control) therapy versus standard therapy	Macrovascular events Death MI Stroke Vascular ischemia	42/78 (53.8%)	26/77 (33.7%)	37.3	5	.03

[a]n = total number of patients.

TYPE 2 DIABETES: UNITED KINGDOM PROSPECTIVE DIABETES STUDY GROUP TRIAL

A number of important trials have evaluated the effects of glycemic control in cardiac patients with type 2 diabetes. Before the publication of the UKPDS, there was a great deal of controversy about the benefit of intensive glycemic control in type 2 patients. Both the University Group Diabetes Program study and other reports have questioned whether sulfonylureas adversely affect the heart by blocking the ATP-dependent potassium channels.[191,192] Two small, randomized trials suggested that intensive glycemic control with insulin for type 2 diabetics is effective in reducing cardiovascular events. The UKPDS trial is the largest and best conducted study of glycemic control in type 2 diabetic patients. It addresses the issue of the influence of tight glycemic control in reducing micro- and macroangiopathy in newly diagnosed patients with type 2 diabetes mellitus.[193,194] In this multicenter randomized controlled trial, 5102 patients in 23 centers in the United Kingdom were studied between 1977 and 1991. A hypertension study was included to assess whether treating high blood pressure in patients with type 2 diabetes could reduce the risk of diabetic complications.[195]

The first study compared the effects of intensive blood glucose control with either sulfonylurea or insulin and conventional treatment on the risk of micro- and macrovascular complications in type 2 diabetes patients. Intensive glycemic control was defined as a fasting plasma glucose (FPG) level of <108 mg/dL. Over a 10-year period, Hb-A1c was 7.0 percent in the intensive group compared with 7.9 percent in the conventional group. There was a 25 percent risk reduction in microvascular end points in the intensively treated group. No difference existed between the three agents used for intensive glycemic control (chlorpropamide, glibenclimide, and insulin). Patients in the intensive group had more hypoglycemic episodes than did those in the conventional group ($p < .0001$). Finally, none of the individual agents had an adverse effect on cardiovascular outcomes.

UKPDS 34, the second arm of the study, assessed whether intensive glucose control with metformin had any specific advantage or disadvantage. Mean Hb-A1c was 7.4 percent in the metformin group compared with 8.0 percent in the conventional group. Given that intensive glycemic control with metformin appears to decrease the risk of diabetes-related end points in overweight diabetes patients and is associated with less weight gain and fewer hypoglycemic attacks than insulin or sulfonylureas, the authors suggested that metformin may be the first-line pharmacologic therapy of choice in these patients. It should be noted that the UKPDS was conducted before the clinical availability of the thiazolidinediones as well as the statins (although the study did not address the issue of cholesterol reduction in diabetic patients).

A noteworthy finding in the UKPDS was a decrease in the risk of myocardial infarction of 16 percent.[193] The decrease was not statistically significant but demonstrated a trend toward fewer macrovascular events. The approximately 8-year time lag before type 2 diabetes is diagnosed may account for the inability of the UKPDS study to link hyperglycemia with macrovascular events.

UKPDS determined whether intensive blood pressure control prevents micro- and macrovascular complications in patients with type 2 diabetes. Tight blood pressure control was defined as <150/85. The angiotensin-converting enzyme inhibitor (ACE-I) captopril and the beta blocker atenolol were the drugs used to achieve the tight control. Reductions in risk in the group assigned to tight blood pressure control compared with the control group were 24 percent in diabetes-related end points, 32 percent in death from diabetic complications, 44 percent in strokes, and 37 percent in microvascular disease (almost all of which were statistically significant). There was a nonsignificant reduction in all-cause mortality.[193]

UKPDS 39 investigated whether tight blood pressure control with either a beta blocker (atenolol) or an ACE-I (captopril) has a specific advantage in terms of preventing the macro- and microvascular complications of type 2 diabetes. This study involving 1148 hypertensive patients showed that each agent was equally efficacious in reducing blood pressure, the risk of macrovascular end points, and deterioration of retinopathy.[196] Using these two classes of antihypertensive agents, the investigators showed that the blood pressure reduction per se was more important than was the treatment used.

The current strategy for type 2 diabetes mellitus is to optimize Hb-A1c levels with sulfonylureas, insulin-sensitizing agents, or insulin when necessary (see the previous discussion).

TYPE 1 DIABETES: DIABETES CONTROL AND COMPLICATIONS TRIAL

Intensive diabetes control versus standard therapy was evaluated in the DCCT.[197,198] The primary outcome was the development and progression of microvascular disease, but patients were followed for over 6 years so that cardiac events did ensue. There was almost a doubling of the cardiac event rate in patients treated in a conventional manner (40 versus 23 events), but this did not reach statistical significance. Since the patients in this study were between ages 13 and 39 and did not have diabetes for a long enough period, a nearly significant reduction in cardiovascular events is not surprising. Diabetic renal disease is a strong predictor of subsequent cardiovascular events, and therefore, the promising result of reduced proteinuria with intensive therapy in DCCT may translate into a cardioprotective effect in the long term. The current strategy for type 1 diabetes is to optimize glycemic control with multiple injections of insulin or with an insulin pump. Such patients should have a concomitant consultation with an endocrinologist.

Early Detection of Diabetes

Because of the significant increase in major microvascular complications and the risk of premature death, it is important to begin to screen for diabetes at a younger age than 45 years, the current recommendation.[199] Selecting populations at the highest risk for developing diabetes for aggressive screening strategies probably will occur in the next 10 years.

Current measures of cardiovascular surveillance for CAD in asymptomatic diabetic patients focus on routine stress testing in accordance with the American College of Cardiology/American Heart Association (ACC/AHA) guidelines[200] (Table 78-7). Exercise testing in diabetic patients is more likely to be accurate when combined with echocardiography or radionuclide imaging. Diabetic patients are less likely to have an appropriate blood pressure and heart rate response to exercise and less likely to experience any pain corresponding to ST-segment changes caused in part by autonomic dysfunction. The AHA

TABLE 78-7 Detection of Clinical and Subclinical Cardiovascular Disease in Diabetic Patients

A. Stress testing for coronary heart disease
  Consult AHA guidelines for exercise treadmill testing
  Considerations for testing in diabetic patients
    Blunting of heart rate and blood pressure responses
    Painless ST-segment depression common in diabetic patients (autonomic neuropathy)
    Diagnostic specificity of ST-segment depression may be reduced (previous silent myocardial infarction, etc.)
    Exercise or pharmacologic testing (^{99}Tc) perfusion scintography favorable for exercise testing in diabetic patients
    Ambulatory ECG monitoring may be helpful in special instances in diabetic patients to diagnose silent ischemia, but not routinely
B. Noninvasive evaluation of cardiac function
  Echocardiography (Doppler) and radionuclide ventriculography issues in diabetic patients
    Diastolic function common and often precedes systolic dysfunction
    Left ventricular wall motion abnormalities suggest diabetic cardiomyopathy
C. Evaluation of autonomic dysfunction
  In bedside evaluation two or more of these tests are abnormal
    Resting heart rate (supine), 100
    Excess diastolic blood pressure response to handgrip exercise
    Abnormal expiratory/inspiratory RR-interval ratio
    Postural hypotension
  Significance of autonomic dysfunction in diabetic patients
    50% 5-year mortality
    Sudden death common; consider electrophysiologic study
    Greater complications after elective surgery
    Increased danger with general anesthesia
D. Diagnosis of subclinical cardiovascular disease
  History: symptoms of claudication, angina, dyspnea on exertion, cerebrovascular disease
  Physical examination: routine checkup with evaluation of carotid and femoral bruits, peripheral arterial pulses, ratio of ankle to brachial artery systolic blood pressure (marker of subclinical peripheral vascular disease)
  Laboratory: urinary creatinine/albumin ratio (Table 78-1)
  ECG: left ventricular hypertrophy a strong predictor of CAD morbidity and mortality
  Electron beam CT: coronary calcium score highly correlated with total coronary atherosclerosis burden
  Carotid ultrasound: detects subclinical carotid atherosclerosis.

recommends that the finding of subclinical CAD should prompt clinicians to initiate more aggressive preventative measures[201] (Table 78-7).

Hypertension and Nephropathy

To date, there have been no randomized trials primarily evaluating the role of hypertension treatment with nephropathy as the end point in type 1 diabetic patients without microalbuminuria. Hypertensive diabetic patients are treated primarily with ACE inhibitors.

Compared with nondiabetic subjects, diabetic patients in the SHEP (Systolic Hypertension in the Elderly Program cooperative research group) study experienced a more pronounced benefit from treatment with clorthalidone. The 5-year rates of major cardiovascular events are illustrated in Fig. 78-7.[202]

The UKPDS demonstrated no advantage of captopril over atenolol in reducing macrovascular complications.[198] Clearly, this illustrates the significant role lowering of blood pressure plays in reducing adverse events independent of the agent used. The role of further blood pressure reduction even when high-risk patients such as diabetic patients are in the normal range needs to be delineated further. The Hypertension Optimal Treatment (HOT) study showed that the risk of major cardiovascular events in diabetic patients was halved if they had a target diastolic pressure ≤80 mmHg compared with those with a diastolic pressure ≤90 mmHg (p for trend = .005).[203] There was a lower but still significant decrease in the risk of silent myocardial infarction and about a 30 percent risk reduction in

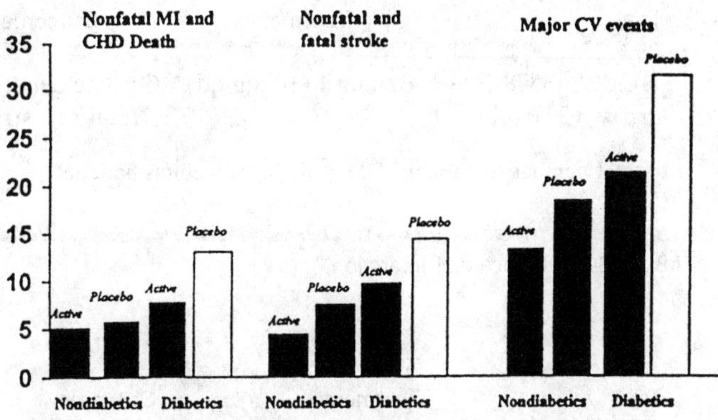

FIGURE 78-7 Five-year rates of nonfatal myocardial infarction (MI) and coronary heart disease (CHD) death, stroke, and major cardiovascular (CV) events by diabetes status and treatment (chlorthalidone vs placebo) in the Systolic Hypertension in the Elderly Program. (Data from Curb et al.[202] and from Furberg CD. Hypertension and diabetes: Current issues. *Am Heart J* 1999; 138:5401, with permission.)

TABLE 78-8 Hypertension

Trial	Treatment	Outcome	Control Group	Treatment Group	Relative Risk Reduction, %	*p*
CAPPP[204] n = 10985 572 DM[a]	Captopril versus conventional therapy	Cardiac death, nonfatal MI, stroke	263	309	33	.03

[a]n = total number of patients; DM = diabetes mellitus patients.

the rate of stroke in the ≤80 mmHg group compared with the ≤90 mmHg group.

The CAPPP trial showed significant lowering of cardiovascular events in hypertensive patients treated with captopril instead of standard therapy with beta blockers or diuretics (Table 78-8).[204] Approximately 5 percent of the patients were diabetic in this trial, and in these patients, similar trends in favor of captopril were observed. The Appropriate Blood pressure Control in Diabetics (ABCD) study also observed a benefit of ACE-I compared with conventional therapy in the treatment of hypertension in diabetic patients.[205]

HOPE

The HOPE trial evaluated over 9000 high-risk patients with evidence of vascular disease or diabetes in a randomized trial comparing ramipril with placebo over a 5-year period. A total of 3578 of these patients were diabetic. This study demonstrated a 22 percent reduction in primary cardiovascular end points of death, myocardial infarction, and stroke in favor of ramipril. The beneficial effect of ramipril was observed over all predefined subgroups. Interestingly, there was a 30 percent reduction in the diagnosis of new diabetic patients in the ramipril-treated arm. This result also was observed in the CAPPP study. Ramipril lowered systolic blood pressure by a mean of only 6 mmHg. This would account for only approximately 40 percent of the reduction in the rate of stroke and about a 25 percent reduction in the rate of myocardial infarction. Therefore, there is some benefit of ramipril independent of the blood pressure–lowering effect that accounts for the impressive cardiovascular protective effect. HOPE provides level 1 evidence supporting the front-line use of ACE-I in the treatment of diabetic patients at risk for cardiovascular events regardless of whether they are hypertensive. In the diabetic subgroup there was even a greater relative risk reduction in primary cardiovascular events (25 percent) (Table 78-9).

Acute Coronary Syndromes

Diabetic patients represent a high-risk group for developing and surviving acute myocardial infarction.[206] In particular, patients with type 1 diabetes have a worse outcome than do patients with type 2 disease, and diabetic women have almost twice the risk of mortality compared with diabetic men.[8,207–209]

Reperfusion therapy is the cornerstone of the management of acute myocardial infarction. In a meta-analysis of all major thrombolytic trials, diabetic patients had a nonsignificant trend toward increased reductions in 35-day mortality rates compared with nondiabetic patients.[210] The potential advantage of angi-

TABLE 78-9 Prevention Study

Trial	Treatment	Outcome	Events Control Group	Events Treatment Group	Relative Risk Reduction, %	Number Needed to Treat	*p*
HOPE[137] 3578 DM n = 9297[a]	Ramipril (10 mg qd)	Cardiac death, nonfatal MI, stroke	351/1769 (19.8%)	277/1808 (15.3%)	25	22	.0004

[a]n = total number of patients; DM = diabetes mellitus patients.

TABLE 78-10 Myocardial Infarction

Trial	Treatment	Outcome	Events Control Group	Events Treatment Group	Relative Risk Reduction, %	Number Needed to Treat	*p*
DIGAMI[211] After MI n = 620[a]	Standard therapy with glucose-insulin infusion versus standard therapy	Long-term (3.4 years) all cause mortality	138/314 (43.9%)	102/306 (33.3%)	24	9	.011

[a]n = total number of patients.

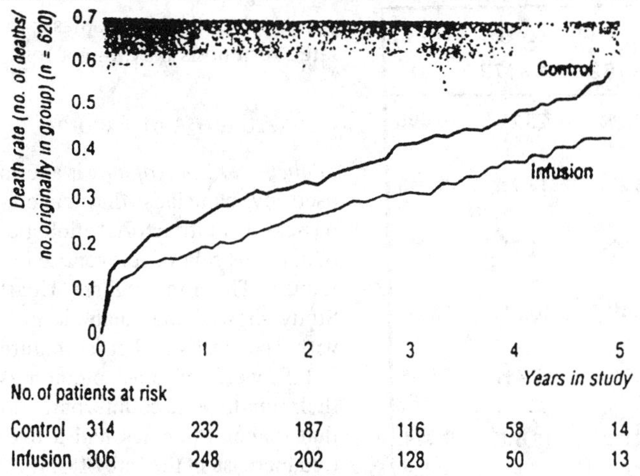

FIGURE 78-8 Actuarial mortality curves during long-term follow-up in patients receiving insulin-glucose infusion and in control group among total DIGAMI cohort. Absolute reduction in risk was 11 percent; relative risk was 0.72 (0.55 to 0.92); $p = .011$. (From Malmberg K for the DIGAMI Study group,[211] with permission.)

oplasty over thrombolytic therapy has not been addressed in the diabetic population.

Besides the use of aspirin and beta blockers, other new treatment strategies are emerging. The utilization of insulin and glucose infusion for at least 24 h after admission followed by intensive long-term insulin, was compared with usual care in the DIGAMI trial (Fig. 78-8 and Table 78-10). A total of 620 diabetic patients were randomized, and the trial demonstrated a 30 percent reduction in mortality at 12 months for the group treated under the intensive program.[211] A new trial is under way to evaluate whether this benefit was the result of acute therapy or the intensive posthospital therapy (Smith and colleagues, unpublished). This new trial also will evaluate the role of changing the diabetic regimen in type 2 diabetes from a sulfonylurea program to a nonsulfonylurea strategy.

Chronic Coronary Artery Disease

The association between CAD and diabetes is strong and has led to screening strategies in diabetic patients even before they are symptomatic. In addition, diabetic patients often are unaware of myocardial ischemic pain, and so silent myocardial infarction and ischemia is markedly increased in this population.[212] There is a heightened concern for the development of sudden cardiac death in diabetics.

Therapeutic modalities in diabetics with CAD revolve around standard therapy with aspirin, beta blockers, calcium channel blockers, and nitrates.

Epidemiologic evidence from the Bezafibrate Infarction Prevention Study registry shows almost a 50 percent reduction in mortality for type 2 patients with chronic CAD who were treated with beta blockers compared with controls.[213] Other randomized trial evidence has demonstrated that diabetes is a strong predictor of death and that diabetic patients may benefit more from beta blocker therapy than do nondiabetics.[214] In general, beta blockers are extremely well tolerated, and masking or prolonging of hypoglycemic symptoms appears to be highly infrequent, particularly with cardioselective beta blockers.

Coronary Revascularization

The high prevalence of CAD in diabetic patients necessitates the frequent use of revascularization procedures in these patients. Both coronary artery bypass grafting and coronary angioplasty are effective in diabetic patients, but the high rate of restenosis diabetic patients experience in the first 6 months after the procedure raises concerns about the long-term benefits of angioplasty.

TABLE 78-11 Coronary Revascularization

Trial	Treatment	Outcome	Events Control Group	Events Treatment Group	Relative Risk Reduction, %	Number Needed to Treat	p
BARI[227] Multivessel CAD n = 1829[a]	CABG vs. PTCA	Mortality from all causes	PTCA 131/915 (14.3%)	CABG 111/914 (12.1%)	15.3	45	.19
Diabetics n = 353 CABG 180 PTCA 173	Same	Same	34.5%	19.4%	43.7	7	.003
EPISTENT[226] n = 2399							
Diabetics (491) n = 335	Stent + abciximab versus Stent + placebo	Death and nonfatal MI at 6 months	Stent + placebo 22/173 (12.7%)	Stent + abciximab 10/162 (6.2%)	51.2	15	.041
n = 318	Stent + abciximab versus PTCA + abciximab	Same	PTCA + abciximab 12/156 (7.8%)	Stent + abciximab 10/162 (6.2%)	20.5	62	.13

[a]n = total number of patients.

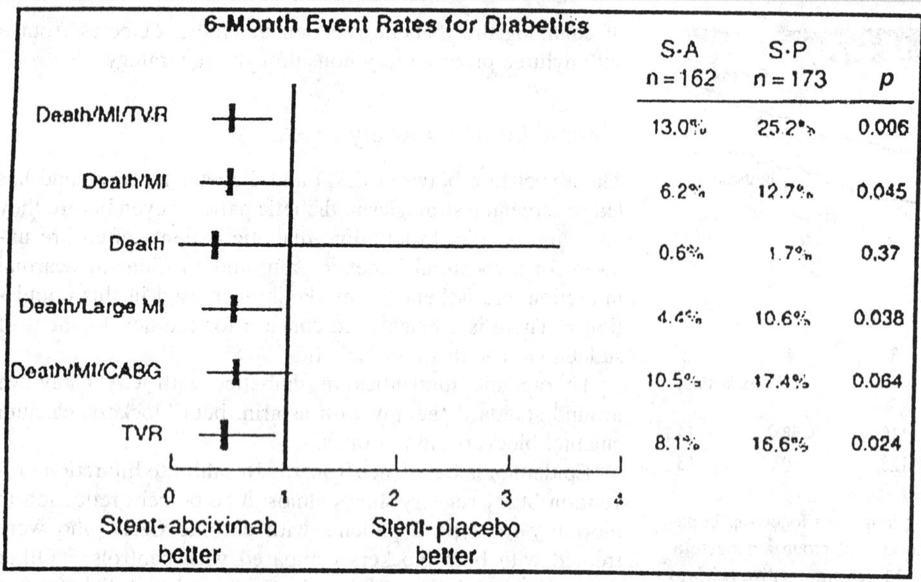

FIGURE 78-9 Absolute percentage of events, 95 percent confidence limits, and point estimates of listed end points for diabetic patients randomized to stenting-abciximab (S-A) or stentin-placebo (S-P). (From Marso SP, Michael A, Lincoff AM, et al. Optimising the percutaneous intervention outcomes for patients with diabetes mellitus. *Circulation* 1999; 100(25):2477, with permission.)

Before the use of stents and IIb-IIIa antagonists, the rate of restenosis after angioplasty in diabetic patients was shown to be as high as 47 to 71 percent.[215–223] The mechanism of restenosis is believed to be related to neointimal hyperplasia, which is tightly linked to the interplay between platelet-thrombus deposition, various growth factors present after injury, and endothelial dysfunction.[224,225]

The best evidence from randomized trials supportive of the utility of stents and abciximab comes from the EPISTENT trial.[226] Among the 2399 patients randomized, 20 percent (491 atients) had diabetes. Patients were assigned to a strategy of stent implantation and placebo, stent implantation and abciximab, or angioplasty and abciximab. For diabetic patients receiving stent and reopro, compared with stent alone, there was a >50 percent reduction in death and nonfatal myocardial infarction at 6 months (Table 78-11). A 6 months, diabetic patients were less likely to require repeat target organ revascularization if they received stent and abciximab (8.1 percent) compared with either stent and placebo (16.6 percent, p = .02) or angioplasty and abciximab (18.4 percent, p = .008). It appears that the effect of abciximab is linked to stent implantation, since elastic recoil and related adverse remodeling are significantly diminished with successful stent deployment, leaving neointimal hyperplasia as the main mode for restenosis. Because of the results of the EPISTENT trial, clinicians are more comfortable recommending percutaneous intervention (Fig. 78-9).

The largest randomized trial comparing angioplasty with bypass surgery in patients with multivessel CAD, the BARI trial, was a landmark study that highlighted the marked benefit of bypass over angioplasty in diabetic patients as opposed to nondiabetic subjects[227] (Fig. 78-10). In the diabetic subgroup, the 5-year mortality was reduced from 34 percent to 19 percent with surgical revascularization, translating into a number needed to treat to prevent one death of only seven (Table 78-11). The most marked difference between the two groups occurred after the first year of follow-up, suggesting that mechanisms other than angioplasty-related restenosis may play a role.

Congestive Heart Failure

Diabetic cardiomyopathy is a term used by clinicians that encompasses the multifactorial etiologies of diabetes-related left ventricular failure. The Framingham Heart Study showed that diabetic men with congestive heart failure (CHF) were twice as common as their nondiabetic counterpart and that diabetic females had a fivefold increase in the rate of CHF.[228] The spectrum of heart failure ranges from asymptomatic to overt systolic failure. Diabetes complicated by hypertension represents a particularly high-risk group for the development of CHF.[229,230] Diastolic dysfunction is exceedingly common (>50 percent prevalence in some studies) and may be linked to diabetes without the presence of concomitant hypertension.[231,232–234]

Given the prominence of the diabetic subgroup in randomized trials of ACE-I in CHF, much emphasis has been placed

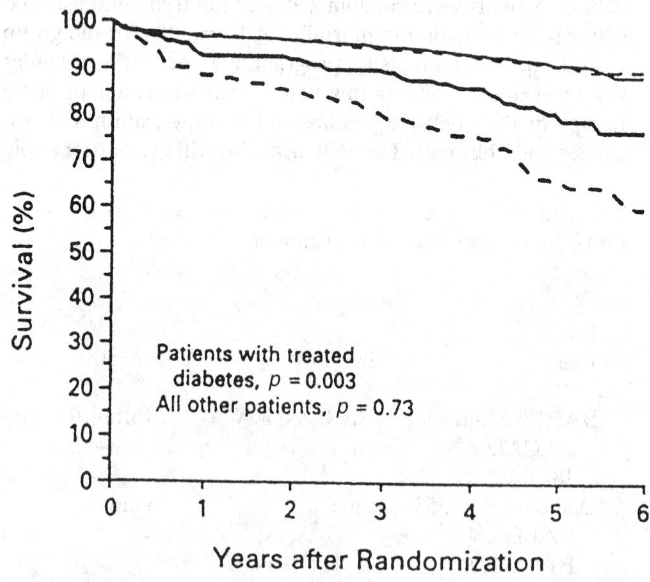

FIGURE 78-10 Survival among patients who were being treated for diabetes at baseline (heavy lines) and all other patients (light lines). Patients assigned to CABG are indicated by solid lines, and those assigned to PTCA by dashed lines. The numbers of patients at risk are shown below the graph at baseline, 3 years, and 5 years. [From the Bypass Angioplasty Revascularization Investigation (BARI) Investigators,[227] with permission.]

TABLE 78-12 Guide to Comprehensive Risk Reduction for Patients with Coronary and Other Vascular Disease who have Diabetes

<table>
<tr><th>Risk Intervention</th><th>Recommendations</th></tr>
<tr><td>Smoking
Goal: complete cessation</td><td>Urge smoking cessation
Try nicoderm patches or xyban; enroll in smoking cessation program</td></tr>
<tr><td>Blood pressure control
Goal: <135/85 mmHg</td><td>Initiate lifestyle modification; weight reduction, increased physical activity; alcohol moderation; sodium restriction in all patients with blood pressure >135/85
Add blood pressure medication if BP not below above goal</td></tr>
<tr><td>Lipid management
Primary goal: LDL≤100 mg/dL
Secondary goals: HDL>35 mg/dL
TG<200 mg/dL</td><td>Start AHA Step II Diet in all patients: ≤30% fat, <7% saturated fat, <200 mg/dL cholesterol
Assess fasting lipid profile. Immediately start cholesterol-lowering drugs when baseline LDL>130 mg/dL
<table>
<tr><td rowspan="3">LDL<100 mg/dL
No drug therapy</td><td>LDL 100–129 mg/dL
Consider adding drug therapy to diet as follows</td><td colspan="2">LDL≥130 mg/dL
Add drug therapy as follows</td><td rowspan="3">HDL<35 mg/dL
Weight management, physical activity, and smoking cessation</td></tr>
<tr><td colspan="3">↘ Suggested drug therapy ↙</td></tr>
<tr><td>TG<200 mg/dL
Statin resin</td><td>TG 200–400 mg/dL
Statin fibrate</td><td>TG>400 mg/dL
Consider combined drug therapy (statin + fibrate)</td></tr>
</table></td></tr>
<tr><td>Glucose control
Goal: nearly normal fasting glucose
Goal: Hb-A 1c ≤1% above normal</td><td>First-step therapy: lifestyle modifications
Second-step therapy: oral hypoglycemic agents (see algorithm)
Third-step therapy: insulin therapy (see algorithm)</td></tr>
<tr><td>Physical activity
Goal: minimum 30 minutes, 3–4 times a week</td><td>Assess risk, preferably with exercise test, to guide prescription
Encourage minimum of 30–60 min of moderate-intensity activity 3–4 times weekly (walking, jogging, cycling, etc.) supplemented by an increase in daily lifestyle activities (e.g., walking breaks at work, using stairs, household work)
Maximum benefit 5 to 6 h a week
Advise medically supervised programs for moderate- to high-risk patients</td></tr>
<tr><td>Weight management</td><td>Start intensive dietary therapy and appropriate physical activity, as outlined above, in patients whose BMI is ≥25 kg/m^2
Particularly emphasize need for weight loss in patients with hypertension, elevated triglycerides, or elevated glucose levels</td></tr>
<tr><td>Antiplatelet agents/ anticoagulants</td><td>Start aspirin 325 mg/day if not contraindicated
Manage warfarin to INR of 2–3.5 for post-MI patients not able to take aspirin</td></tr>
<tr><td>ACE inhibitors in post-MI patients</td><td>Start early post-MI in stable high-risk patients [anterior MI, previous MI, Killip class II (S3 gallop, rales, radiographic congestive heart failure)]
Continue indefinitely for all with LV dysfunction (ejection fraction ≤40%) or symptoms of failure
Use as needed to manage blood pressure or symptoms in all other patients</td></tr>
<tr><td>Beta blockers</td><td>Start in high-risk post-MI patients (arrhythmia, LV dysfunction, inducible ischemia) at 5 to 28 days; continue 6 months minimum; observe usual contraindications; appropriate use of beta-blockers not contraindicated in patients with diabetes; use as needed to manage angina, rhythm, or blood pressure in all other patients</td></tr>
<tr><td>Estrogen</td><td>Observational studies (but not clinical trials) suggest benefit in regard to osteoporosis but not CAD; individualize recommendation consistent with other health risks</td></tr>
</table>

on initiating ACE-I therapy as soon as left ventricular dysfunction is noted, regardless of symptomatology.[235] The results of the HOPE trial probably will translate into even earlier initiation of ACE inhibition in patients without clinical LV dysfunction.

Summary of Clinical Guidelines

Table 78-12 summarizes the AHA recommendations for the indications for risk interventions in diabetic patients with atherosclerotic vascular disease.

FUTURE DIRECTIONS

On the clinical front, there are still many challenges in the prevention and management of diabetic cardiovascular complications. Given the findings of the HOPE trial, the potential for an expanded role for ACE inhibitors in the prevention of cardiovascular and renal disease in all diabetic patients needs to be explored. Glycemic control appears to be the mainstay of long-term diabetes management. Thus, development of better therapies and devices (e.g., closed-loop pumps, islet and pancreatic transplants) for achieving and maintaining Hb-A1c at not only <7 percent but in the normal range of <6 percent will be a primary goal in the next decade. The advent of stenting and the IIb-IIIa antagonist during coronary percutaneous revascularization has led to a reevaluation of the need for coronary bypass surgery in multivessel disease. Confirmation of the results of small trials demonstrating a benefit of intravenous glucose-insulin infusion during acute myocardial infarction is needed before this therapy can be adopted. Finally, the role of gene therapy in the management of diabetic atherosclerotic vascular disease needs to be addressed within the context of all other advances.

References

1. Schwartz CJ, Valente AJ, Sprague EA, et al. Pathogenesis of the atherosclerotic lesion: Implications for diabetes mellitus. *Diabetes Care* 1992; 15:1156–1167.
2. Stamler J, Vaccaro O, Neaton JD, Wentworth D. Diabetes, other risk factors and 12-year cardiovascular mortality for men screened in the multiple risk factor intervention trial. *Diabetes Care* 1993; 16:434–444.
3. Gu K, Cowie CC, Harris MI. Diabetes and decline in heart disease mortality in US adults. *JAMA* 1999; 281:1291–1297.
4. Kawate R, Yamakido M, Nishimoto Y, et al. Diabetes mellitus and its vascular complications in Japanese migrants on the island of Hawaii. *Diabetes Care* 1979; 2:161–170.
5. Head J, Fuller JH. International variations in mortality among diabetic patients: The WHO Multinational Study of Vascular Disease in Diabetics. *Diabetologia* 1990; 33:447–481.
6. Vigorita VJ, Morre GW, Hutchens GM. Absence of correlation between coronary arterial atherosclerosis and severity or duration of diabetes mellitus of adult onset. *Am J Cardiol* 1980; 46:535–542.
7. Waller BF, Palumbo PJ, Lie JT, Roberts WC. Status of the coronary arteries at necropsy in diabetes mellitus after age 30 years: Analysis of 229 diabetic patients with and without evidence of coronary heart disease and comparison to 183 control subjects. *Am J Med* 1980; 69:498–506.
8. Granger CB, Califf RM, Young S, et al. Outcome of patients with diabetes mellitus and acute myocardial infarction treated with thrombolytic agents: The Thrombolysis and Angioplasty in Myocardial Infarction (TAMI) Study Group. *J Am Coll Cardiol* 1993; 21:920–925.
9. Mueller HS, Cohen LS, Braunwald E, et al., for the TIMI investigators. Predictors of early mortality and morbidity after thrombolytic therapy of acute myocardial infarction. *Circulation* 1992; 85:1254–1264.
10. Stein B, Weintraub WS, Gebhart SSP, et al. Influence of diabetes mellitus on early and late outcome after percutaneous transluminal coronary angioplasty. *Circulation* 1995; 91:979–989.
11. Barzilay JI, Kronmal RA, Bittner V, et al. Coronary artery disease and coronary artery bypass grafting in diabetic patients aged >65 years (Report from the coronary artery surgery study [CASS] registry). *Am J Cardiol* 1994; 74:334–339.
12. Davis M, Bland J, Hangartner J, et al. Factors influencing the presence or absence of acute coronary artery thrombi in sudden ischemic death. *Eur Heart J* 1989; 10:203–208.
13. Silva JA, Escobar A, Collins TJ, et al. Unstable angina: A comparison between diabetic and non-diabetic patients. *Circulation* 1995; 92:1731–1736.
14. Hopkins PN, Hunt SC, Wu LL, et al. Hypertension, dyslipidemia, and insulin resistance: Links in a chain or spokes on a wheel? *Curr Opin Lipidol* 1996; 7:241–253.
15. Gray RS, Fabsitz RR, Cowan LD, et al. Risk factor clustering in the insulin resistance syndrome: The Strong Heart Study. *Am J Epidemiol* 1998; 148:869–878.
16. The Expert Committee on the Diagnosis and Classification of Diabetes Mellitus. Report of the Expert Committee on the Diagnosis and Classification of Diabetes Mellitus. *Diabetes Care* 1997; 20:1183–1202.
17. Haffner SM, Stern MP, Hazuda HP, et al. Cardiovascular risk factors in confirmed prediabetic individuals: Does the clock for coronary heart disease start ticking before the onset of clinical diabetes? *JAMA* 1990; 263:2893–2898.
18. Unger RH, Foster DW. Diabetes mellitus. In: Wilson JD, Foster DW, Kronenberg HM, Larsen PR, eds. *Williams Textbook of Endocrinology*. Philadelphia: Saunders; 1998:973.
19. Stamler J, Vaccaro O, Neaton JD, Wentworth D. Diabetes, other risk factors, and 12-year cardiovascular mortality for men screened in the Multiple Risk Factor Intervention Trial (MRFIT). *Diabetes Care* 1993; 16:434–444.
20. Folsom AR, Eckfeldt JH, Weitzman S, et al. Atherosclerosis Risk in Communities Study Investigators. Relation of carotid artery wall thickness in diabetes mellitus, fasting glucose and insulin, body size and physical activity. *Stroke* 1994; 25:66–73.
21. O'Leary DH, Polak JF, Kronmal RA, et al. Distribution and correlates of sonographically detected carotid artery disease in the Cardiovascular Health Study. *Stroke* 1992; 23:1752–1760.
22. Cooper ME. Pathogenesis, prevention, and treatment of diabetic nephropathy. *Lancet* 1998; 352:213–219.
23. Chavers BM, Bilous RW, Ellis EN, et al. Glomerular lesions and urinary albumin excretion in type I diabetes without overt proteinuria. *N Engl J Med* 1989; 320:966–970.
24. Ismail N, Becker B, Strzelczyk P, Ritz E. Renal disease and hypertension in non-insulin-dependent diabetes mellitus. *Kidney Int* 1999; 55:1–28.
25. Lebovitz HE, Wiegmann TB, Cnaan A, et al. Renal protective effects of enalapril in hypertensive NIDDM: Role of baseline albuminuria. *Kidney Int* 1994; 45:S150–S155.
26. Lewis EJ, Hunsicker LG, Bain RP, Rohde RD. The effect of angiotensin-converting-enzyme inhibition on diabetic nephropathy: The Collaborative Study Group. *N Engl J Med* 1993; 329:1456–1462.
27. Grundy SM, Benjamin IJ, Burke GL, et al. Diabetes and cardiovascular disease: A statement for healthcare professionals from the American Heart Association. *Circulation* 1999; 100:1134–1146.

28. Rose BD. Treatment of diabetic nephropathy. Up to Date Computer CD, Feb. 24, 1999.
29. Viberti G, Mogensen CE, Groop LC, Pauls JF. Effect of captopril on progression to clinical proteinuria in patients with insulin-dependent diabetes mellitus and microalbuminuria: European Microalbuminuria Captopril Study Group. *JAMA* 1994; 271:275–279.
30. The Microalbuminuria Captopril Study Group. Captopril reduces the risk of nephropathy in IDDM patients with microalbuminuria. *Diabetologia* 1996; 39:587–593.
31. Ravid M, Savin H, Jutrin I, et al. Long-term stabilizing effect of angiotensin-converting enzyme inhibition on plasma creatinine and on proteinuria in normotensive type II diabetic patients. *Ann Intern Med* 1993; 118:577–581.
32. Golan L, Birkmeyer JD, Welch HG. The cost-effectiveness of treating all patients with type 2 diabetes with angiotensin-converting enzyme inhibitors. *Ann Intern Med* 1999; 131:660–667.
33. Gaber L, Walton C, Brown S, Bakris G. Effects of different antihypertensive treatments on morphologic progression of diabetic nephropathy in uninephrectomized dogs. *Kidney Int* 1994; 46:161–169.
34. Ritz E, Stefanski A. Diabetic nephropathy in type II diabetes. *Am J Kidney Dis* 1996; 27:167–194.
35. Berkman J, Rifkin H. Unilateral nodular diabetic glomerulosclerosis (Kimmelstiel-Wilson): Report of a case. *Metabolism* 1973; 22:715–722.
36. Austin SM, Lieberman JS, Newton LD, et al. Slope of serial glomerular filtration rate and the progression of diabetic glomerular disease. *J Am Soc Nephrol* 1993; 3:1358–1370.
37. Bohlen L, de Courten M, Weidmann P. Comparative study of the effect of ACE-inhibitors and other antihypertensive agents on proteinuria in diabetic patients. *Am J Hypertens* 1994; 7:84S–92S.
38. Tatti P, Pahor M, Byington RP, et al. Outcome results of the Fosinopril versus Amlodipine Cardiovascular Events Randomized Trial (FACET) in patients with hypertension and NIDDM. *Diabetes Care* 1998; 21:597–603.
39. Kannel W, McGee D. Diabetes and glucose tolerance as risk factors for cardiovascular disease: The Framingham Study. *Diabetes Care* 1979; 2:120–126.
40. Jarrett RJ, Shipley MJ. Type 2 (non-insulin dependent) diabetes mellitus and cardiovascular disease—putative association via common antecedents: Further evidence from the Whitehall Study. *Diabetologia* 1988; 31:737–740.
41. Jarrett RJ, McCarthney P, Keen H. The Bedford Study: Ten-year mortality rates in newly diagnosed diabetics, borderline diabetics and normoglycemic controls and the risk indices for coronary heart disease in borderline diabetics. *Diabetologia* 1982; 22:79–84.
42. Fontbonne A, Eschwege E, Cambien F, et al. Hypertriglyceridemia as a risk factor for coronary heart disease mortality in subjects with impaired glucose tolerance or diabetes: Results from the 11-year follow-up of the Paris Prospective Study. *Diabetologia* 1989; 32:300–304.
43. Donahue RP, Orchard TG. Diabetes mellitus and macrovascular complications: An epidemiological perspective. *Diabetes Care* 1992; 15:1141–1155.
44. Barrett-Connor E, Cohn B, Wingard D, Edelstein SL. Why is diabetes mellitus a stronger risk factor for fatal ischemic heart disease in women than in men? The Rancho Bernardo Study. *JAMA* 1991; 256:627–631.
45. Barrett-Connor E, Wingard DL. Sex differential in ischemic heart disease mortality in diabetics: A prospective population-based study. *Am J Epidemiol* 1983; 118:489–496.
46. Nathan DM. Long-term complications of diabetes mellitus. *N Engl J Med* 1993; 328:1676–1685.
47. The Diabetes Control and Complication Trial Research Group. The effect of intensive treatment of diabetes on the development and progression of long-term complications in insulin-dependent diabetes mellitus. *N Engl J Med* 1993; 329:977–986.
48. American Diabetes Association. Consensus statement: Role of cardiovascular risk factors in prevention and treatment of macrovascular disease in diabetes. *Diabetes Care* 1993; 16:72–78.
49. Fuller JH, Shipley MJ, Rose G, et al. Coronary heart disease and impaired glucose tolerance: The Whitehall Study. *Lancet* 1980; 1:1373–1376.
50. Yamasaki Y, Kawamori R, Matsushima H, et al. Asymptomatic hyperglycemia is associated with increased intimal plus medial thickness of the carotid artery. *Diabetologia* 1995; 38:585–591.
51. Crub JD, Rodriguez BL, Burchfiel CM, et al. Sudden death, impaired glucose tolerance and diabetes in Japanese American men. *Circulation* 1995; 91:2591–2595.
52. Kahn CR. Insulin action, diabetogenes and the cause of type II diabetes. *Diabetes* 1994; 43:1066–1084.
53. Ferrannini E, Buzzigoli G, Bonadonna R, et al. Insulin resistance in essential hypertension. *N Engl J Med* 1987; 317:350–357.
54. Zavaroni I, Bonora E, Pagliara M, et al. Risk factors for coronary artery disease in healthy persons with hyperinsulinemia and normal glucose tolerance. *N Engl J Med* 1989; 320:702–706.
55. Larsson B, Savardsudd K, Welin L, et al. Abdominal adipose tissue distribution, obesity and risk of cardiovascular disease and death: 13-year follow-up of participants in the study of men born in 1913. *Br Med J* 1984; 288:1401–1404.
56. Peiris AN, Sothmann MS, Hoffman RG, et al. Adiposity, fat distribution and cardiovascular risk. *Ann Intern Med* 1989; 110:867–872.
57. Laakso M, Barrett-Connor E. Asymptomatic hyperglycemia is associated with lipid and lipoprotein changes favoring atherosclerosis. *Atherosclerosis* 1989; 9:665–672.
58. Modan M, Halkin H, Luskyn A, et al. Hyperinsulinemia is characterized by jointly disturbed plasma VLDL, LDL, and HDL levels. *Arteriosclerosis* 1988; 8:227–236.
59. Laws A, King AC, Haskell WL, Reaven GM. Relation of fasting plasma insulin concentrations to high-density lipoprotein cholesterol and triglyceride concentration in men. *Arterioscler Thromb* 1991; 11:1636–1642.
60. Reaven GM. Role of insulin resistance in human disease (syndrome X): An expanded definition. *Annu Rev Med* 1993; 44:121–131.
61. Reaven GM, Laws A. Insulin resistance, compensatory hyperinsulinemia and coronary heart disease. *Diabetologia* 1994; 37: 948–952.
62. Fontbonne A, Charles MA, Thibult N, et al. Hyperinsulinemia as a predictor of coronary heart disease mortality in a healthy population: The Paris Prospective Study, 15-year follow-up. *Diabetologia* 1991; 34:356–361.
63. Pyorala K, Savolainen E, Kaukola S, Haapakoski J. Plasma insulin as coronary heart disease risk factor: Relationship to other risk factors and predictive value over 9.5 year follow-up of the Helsinki Policeman Study population. *Acta Med Scand* 1985; 701(suppl):38–52.
64. Despres J-P, Lamarche B, Mauriege P, et al. Hyperinsulinemia is an independent risk factor for ischemic heart disease. *N Engl J Med* 1996; 334:952–957.
65. Modan M, Or J, Karasik A, et al. Hyperinsulinemia, sex and risk of atherosclerotic cardiovascular disease. *Circulation* 1991; 84:1165–1175.
66. Liu QZ, Knowler WC, Nelson RG, et al. Insulin treatment, endogenous insulin concentration and ECG abnormalities in diabetic Pima Indians: Cross sectional and prospective analysis. *Diabetes* 1992; 41:1141–1150.
67. Ferrara A, Barrett-Connor E, Edelstein SL. Hyperinsulinemia does not increase the risk of fatal cardiovascular disease in elderly men and women without diabetes: The Rancho Bernardo Study, 1984 to 1991. *Am J Epidemiol* 1994; 140:857–869.

68. Gerstein HC, Yusuf S. Dysglycemia and risk of cardiovascular disease. *Lancet* 1996; 347:949–950.
69. Singer DE, Nathan DM, Anderson KM, et al. Association of HbA1c with prevalent cardiovascular disease in the original cohort of the Framingham Heart Study. *Diabetes* 1992; 41:202–208.
70. Kuusisto J, Makkanen L, Pyorala K, Laakso M. NIDDM and its metabolic control predicts coronary heart disease in elderly subjects. *Diabetes* 1994; 43:960–967.
71. Uusitupa MI, Niskanen LK, Siitonen O, et al. Ten-year cardiovascular mortality in relation to risk factors and abnormalities in lipoprotein composition in type 2 (non-insulin-dependent) diabetic and nondiabetic subjects. *Diabetologia* 1993; 36:1175–1184.
72. Krolewski AS, Kosinki EJ, Warram JH, et al. Magnitude and determinants of coronary artery disease in juvenile-onset, insulin-dependent diabetes mellitus. *Am J Cardiol* 1987; 59:750–755.
73. Borch-Johnsen K, Kreiner S. Proteinuria: Value as predictor of cardiovascular mortality in insulin-dependent diabetes mellitus. *Br Med J* 1987; 294:1651–1654.
74. Bucala R, Mitchell R, Arnold K, et al. Identification of the major site of apolipoprotein B modification by advanced glycosylation end products blocking uptake by the low density lipoprotein receptor. *J Biol Chem* 1995; 270:10828–10832.
75. Bucala R, Makita Z, Koschinsky T, et al. Lipid advanced glycosylation: Pathway for lipid oxidation in vivo. *Proc Natl Acad Sci USA* 1993; 90:6434–6438.
76. Bucala R, Makita Z, Vega G, et al. Modification of low-density lipoprotein by advanced glycosylation end products contributes to the dyslipidemia of diabetes and renal insufficiency. *Proc Natl Acad Sci USA* 1994; 91:9441–9445.
77. Steinbrecher UP, Witztum JL. Glycosylation of low density lipoproteins to an extent comparable to that seen in diabetics slows their catabolism. *Diabetes* 1984; 33:130–134.
78. Lyons TJ. Glycation and oxidation: A role in the pathogenesis of atherosclerosis. *Am J Cardiol* 1993; 71:26B–31B.
79. Sobenin IA, Tertov VV, Koschinsky T, et al. Modified low-density lipoprotein from diabetic patients causes cholesterol accumulation in human intimal aortic cells. *Atherosclerosis* 1993; 100:41–54.
80. Lyons TJ, Klein R, Baynes JW, et al. Stimulation of cholesterol-ester synthesis in human monocyte-derived macrophages by low-density lipoproteins from type I (insulin-dependent) diabetic patients: The influence of nonenzymatic glycosylation of low-density lipoprotein. *Diabetologia* 1987; 30:916–923.
81. Klein RL, Laimins M, Lopes-Varella MF. Isolation, characterization and metabolism of the glycated and nonglycated subfractions of low-density lipoproteins isolated from type I diabetic patients and nondiabetic subjects. *Diabetes* 1995; 44:1093–1098.
82. Fiengold KR, Grunfeld C, Pang M, et al. LDL subclass phenotype and triglyceride metabolism in non-insulin-dependent diabetes. *Arterioscler Throm* 1992; 12:1496–1502.
83. Stewart MW, Laker MF, Dyer RG, et al. Lipoprotein compositional abnormalities and insulin resistance in type II diabetic patients with mild hyperlipidemia. *Arterioscler Throm* 1993; 13:1046–1052.
84. Austin MA, Mykkanen L, Kuusisto J, et al. Prospective study of small LDLs as a risk factor for non-insulin-dependent diabetes mellitus in elderly men and women. *Circulation* 1995; 92:1770–1778.
85. Howard BV, Abbott WF, Beltz WF, et al. The effect of non-insulin-dependent diabetes on very low density lipoprotein and low density lipoprotein metabolism in men. *Metabolism* 1987; 36:870–877.
86. Packard CJ, Munro A, Lorimer AR, et al. Metabolism of apolipoprotein B in large triglyceride-rich very low density lipoproteins of normal and hypertriglyceridemic subjects. *J Clin Invest* 1984; 84:2178–2192.
87. Austin MA, King MC, Vranizan KM, Krauss RM. Atherogenic lipoprotein phenotype: A proposed genetic marker for coronary heart disease risk. *Circulation* 1990; 82:495–506.
88. West KM, Ahuja MMS, Bennett PH, et al. The role of circulation glucose and triglyceride concentration and their interaction with other "risk factors" as determinants of arterial disease in nine diabetic population samples from the WHO multinational study. *Diabetes Care* 1983; 6:361–369.
89. Goldschmid MG, Barrett-Connor E, Edelstein SL, et al. Dyslipidemia and ischemic heart disease mortality among men and women with diabetes. *Circulation* 1994; 89:991–997.
90. Laasko M, Lehto S, Penttila I, Pyorala K. Lipids and lipoproteins predicting coronary heart disease mortality and morbidity in patients with non-insulin-dependent diabetes. *Circulation* 1993; 88:1421–1430.
91. Ginsberg HN. Diabetic dyslipidemia: Basic mechanisms underlying the common hypertriglyceridemia and low HDL cholesterol levels. *Diabetes* 1996; 45(suppl):27S–30S.
92. Patsch JR, Prasad S, Gotto AM, et al. High density lipoprotein 2: Relationship of the plasma levels of this lipoprotein species to its composition, to the magnitude of postprandial lipemia, and to the activities of lipoprotein lipase and hepatic lipase. *J Clin Invest* 1984; 80:341–347.
93. American Diabetes Association, Consensus statement: Detection and management of lipid disorders in diabetes. *Diabetes Care* 1993; 16:828–839.
94. Vinik AI, Colwell JA. Effects of gemfibrozil on triglyceride levels in patients with NIDDM. *Diabetes Care* 1993; 16:37–44.
95. Vega GL, Grundy SM. Gemfibrozil therapy in primary hypertriglyceridemia associated with coronary heart disease: Effect on metabolism of low-density lipoproteins. *JAMA* 1985; 253:2398–2403.
96. Koskinen P, Manttrai M, Manninen V, et al. Coronary heart disease incidence in NIDDM patients in the Helsinki Heart Study. *Diabetes Care* 1992; 15:820–825.
97. Lahdenpera S, Tilly-Kiesi M, Vuorinen-Markkola H, et al. Effects of gemfibrozil on low-density lipoprotein size, density distribution and composition in patients with type II diabetes. *Diabetes Care* 1993; 16:584–592.
98. Garg A, Grundy SM. Nicotinic acid as therapy for dyslipidemia in non-insulin-dependent diabetes mellitus. *JAMA* 1990; 264:723–726.
99. Garg A, Grundy SM. Lovastatin for lowering cholesterol levels in non-insulin dependent diabetes mellitus. *N Engl J Med* 1988; 318:81–86.
100. Scandinavian Simvastatin Survival Study Group. Randomized trial of cholesterol lowering in 4444 patients with coronary heart disease: Scandinavian Simvastatin Survival Study (4S). *Lancet* 1994; 344:1383–1389.
101. Garg A, Grundy SM. Cholestyramine therapy for dyslipidemia in non-insulin-dependent diabetes mellitus. *Ann Intern Med* 1994; 121:416–422.
102. Hope investigators. Effects of an angiotensin converting enzyme inhibitor, ramipril, on cardiovascular events in high-risk patients. *N Engl J Med* 2000; 342:145–153.
103. Winocour PD. Platelet abnormalities in diabetes mellitus. *Diabetes* 1992; 41(suppl 2):26–31.
104. Tschoepe D, Rosen P, Schwippert B, Gries FA. Platelets in diabetes: The role of the hemostatic regulation in atherosclerosis. *Semin Thromb Hemost* 1993; 19:122–128.
105. Breddin H, Krzywanek H, Althoff P, et al. Platelet aggregation as a risk factor in diabetes. *Horm Metab Res Suppl* 1985; 15:63–68.
106. Winocour PD. Platelet abnormalities in diabetes mellitus. *Diabetes* 1992; 41(suppl 2):26–31.
107. Winocour PD. Platelet turnover in advanced diabetes. *Eur J Clin Invest* 1994; 24(suppl 1):34–37.
108. Janero DR. Malondialdehyde and thiobarbituric acid-reactivity

as diagnostic indices of lipid peroxidation and peroxidative tissue injury. *Free Radic Biol Med* 1990; 9:515–540.
109. Davi G, Catalano I, Averna M, et al. Thromboxane biosynthesis and platelet function in type II diabetes mellitus. *N Engl J Med* 1990; 322:1769–1774.
110. Stehouwer CDA, Nauta JJP, Zeldenrust GC, et al. Urinary albumin excretion, cardiovascular disease and endothelial dysfunction in non-insulin-dependent diabetes mellitus. *Lancet* 1992; 340: 319–323.
111. Stehouwer CDA, Donker AJM. Urinary albumin excretion and cardiovascular disease in diabetes mellitus: Is endothelial dysfunction the missing link? *J Nephrol* 1993; 6:72–92.
112. Conlan MG, Folsom AR, Finch A, et al. Associations of factor VII and von-Willebrand factor with age, race, sex and risk factors for atherosclerosis: The atherosclerosis in communities (ARIC) study. *Thromb Haemost* 1993; 70:380–385.
113. Ganda OP, Arkin CF. Hyperfibrinogenemia: An important risk factor for vascular complications in diabetes. *Diabetes Care* 1992; 15:1245–1250.
114. Kannel WB, D'Agostino RB, Wilson RB, et al. Diabetes, fibrinogen and risk of cardiovascular disease: The Framingham experience. *Am Heart J* 1990; 120:672–676.
115. De Feo P, Gaisano GM, Haymond MW. Differential effects of insulin deficiency on albumin and fibrinogen synthesis in humans. *J Clin Invest* 1991; 88:833–840.
116. Garcia Frade LJ, de la Calle H, Alava I, et al. Diabetes mellitus as a hypercoagulable state: Its relationship with fibrin fragments and vascular damage. *Thromb Res* 1987; 47:533–540.
117. Landgraf-Leurs MM, Ladik T, Smolka B, et al. Increased thromboplastic potential in diabetes: A multifactorial phenomenon. *Klin Wochenschr* 1987; 65:600–606.
118. Ceriello A. Coagulation activation in diabetes mellitus: The role of hyperglycaemia and therapeutic prospects. *Diabetologia* 1993; 36:1119–1125.
119. Husted SE, Nielsen HK, Bak JF, Beck-Nielsen H. Antithrombin III activity, von Willebrand factor antigen and platelet function in young diabetic patients treated with multiple insulin injections versus insulin pump treatment. *Eur J Clin Invest* 1989; 19:90–94.
120. Hamsten A, de Faire U, Walldius G, et al. Plasminogen activator inhibitor in plasma: Risk factor for recurrent myocardial infarction. *Lancet* 1987; 2:3–9.
121. Mussoni L, Mannucci L, Sirtori M, et al. Hypertriglyceridemia and regulation of fibrinolytic activity. *Arterioscler Thromb* 1992; 12:19–27.
122. Mehta J, Mehta P, Lawson D, Saldeen T. Plasma tissue plasminogen activator inhibitor levels in coronary artery disease: Correlation with age and serum triglyceride concentrations. *J Am Coll Cardiol* 1987; 9:263–268.
123. Grant PJ, Kruithof EK, Felley CP, et al. Short-term infusions of insulin, triacylglycerol and glucose do not cause acute increases in plasminogen activator inhibitor-1 concentrations in man. *Clin Sci* 1990; 79:513–516.
124. Richardson M, Hadcock SJ, DeReske M, Cybulsky MI. Increased expression in vivo of VCAM-1 and E-selectin by the aortic endothelium of normolipemic and hyperlipemic diabetic rabbits. *Arterioscler Thromb* 1994; 14:760–769.
125. Yan SD, Schmidt AM, Anderson GM, et al. Enhanced cellular oxidant stress by the interaction of advanced glycation end products with their receptors/binding proteins. *J Biol Chem* 1994; 269:9889–9897.
126. Wautier JL, Wautier MP, Schmidt AM, et al. Advanced glycation end products (AGEs) on the surface of diabetic erythrocytes bind to the vessel wall via a specific receptor inducing oxidant stress in the vasculature: A link between surface-associated AGEs and diabetic complications. *Proc Natl Acad Sci USA* 1994; 91:7742–7746.
127. Schmidt AM, Hori O, Chen JX, et al. Advanced glycation end products interacting with their endothelial receptor induce expression of vascular cell adhesion molecule-1 (VCAM-1) in cultured human endothelial cells and in mice. A potential mechanism for the accelerated vasculopathy of diabetes. *J Clin Invest* 1995; 96:1395–1403.
128. Keegan A, Walbank H, Cotter MA, Cameron NE. Chronic vitamin E treatment prevents defective endothelium-dependent relaxation in diabetic rat aorta. *Diabetologia* 1995; 38:1475–1478.
129. Ting HH, Timimi FK, Boles KS, et al. Vitamin C improves endothelium-dependent vasodilation in patients with non-insulin-dependent diabetes mellitus. *J Clin Invest* 1996; 97:22–28.
130. Hunt JV, Dean RT, Wolff SP. Hydroxyl radical production and autoxidative glycosylation: Glucose autoxidation as the cause of protein damage in the experimental glycation model of diabetes mellitus and ageing. *Biochem J* 1988; 256:205–212.
131. Hunt JV, Smith CC, Wolff SP. Autoxidative glycosylation and possible involvement of peroxides and free radicals in LDL modification by glucose. *Diabetes* 1990; 39:1420–1424.
132. Mullarkey CJ, Edelstein D, Brownlee M. Free radical generation by early glycation products: A mechanism for accelerated atherogenesis in diabetes. *Biochem Biophys Res Commun* 1990; 173:932–939.
133. Bucala R, Tracey KJ, Cerami A. Advanced glycosylation products quench nitric oxide and mediate defective endothelium-dependent vasodilation in experimental diabetes. *J Clin Invest* 1991; 87:432–438.
134. Vehkavaara S, Seppala-Lindroos A, Westerbacka J, et al. In vivo endothelial dysfunction characterizes patients with impaired fasting glucose. *Diabetes Care* 1999; 22:2055–2060.
135. Vlassara H. Advanced glycation end-products and atherosclerosis. *Ann Med* 1996; 28:419–426.
136. Stitt AW, Bucala R, Vlassara H. Atherogenesis and advanced glycation: Promotion, progression and prevention. *Ann NY Acad Sci* 1997; 811:115–129.
137. Brownlee M, Cerami A, Vlassara H. Advanced glycation end-products in tissue and the biochemical basis of diabetic complications. *N Engl J Med* 1988; 318:1315–1321.
138. Aronson D, Rayfield EJ. Diabetes. In: Topol E, ed. *Textbook of Cardiovascular Medicine.* Philadelphia: Lippincott-Raven; 1998: 171.
139. Nakamura Y, Horii Y, Nishino T, et al. Immunohistochemical localization of advanced glycosylation end products in coronary atheroma and cardiac tissue in diabetes mellitus. *Am J Pathol* 1993; 143:1649–1656.
140. Kilhovd BK, Berg TJ, Birkeland KI, et al. Serum levels of advanced glycation end products are increased in patients with type 2 diabetes and coronary heart disease. *Diabetes Care* 1999; 22:1543–1548.
141. Berg TJ, Snorgaard O, Faber J, et al. Serum levels of advanced glycation end products are associated with left ventricular diastolic function in patients with type-1 diabetes. *Diabetes Care* 1999; 22:1186–1190.
142. Brownlee M, Vlassara H, Kooney A, et al. Aminoguanidine prevents diabetes-induced arterial wall protein cross-linking. *Science* 1986; 232:1629–1632.
143. Vasan S, Zhang X, Zhang X, et al. An agent cleaving glucose-derived protein crosslinks in vitro and in vivo. *Nature* 1996; 382:275–278.
144. Schmidt AM, Hori O, Brett J, et al. Cellular receptors for advanced glycation end-products: Implications for induction of oxidant stress and cellular dysfunction in the pathogenesis of vascular lesions. *Arterioscler Thromb* 1994; 14:1521–1528.
145. Brett J, Schmidt AM, Yan SD, et al. Survey of the distribution of a newly characterized receptor for advanced glycation end-products in tissues. *Am J Pathol* 1993; 143:1699–1712.
146. Vlassara H, Brownlee M, Manogue KR, et al. Cachetin/TNF and

IL-1 induced by glucose modified proteins: Role in normal tissue remodelling. *Science* 1988; 240:1546–1548.

147. Kirstein M, Brett J, Radoff S, et al. Advanced protein glycosylation induces selective transendothelial human monocyte chemotaxis and secretion of PDGF: Role in vascular diseases of diabetes and aging. *Proc Natl Acad Sci USA* 1990; 87:9010–9014.
148. Vlassara H, Fuh H, Makita Z, et al. Exogenous advanced glycosylation end products induce complex vascular dysfunction in normal animal: A model for diabetic and aging complications. *Proc Natl Acad Sci USA* 1992; 89:12043–12047.
149. Kirstein M, Aston C, Hintz R, Vlassara H. Receptor-specific induction of insulin-like growth factor-1 (IGF-1) in human monocytes by advanced glycosylation end product-modified proteins. *J Clin Invest* 1992; 90:439–446.
150. Esposito C, Gerlach H, Brett J, et al. Endothelial receptor-mediated binding of glucose-modified albumin is associated with increased monolayer permeability and modulation of cell surface procoagulant properties. *J Exp Med* 1989; 170:1378–1407.
151. Wautier JL, Zoukourian C, Chappey O, et al. Receptor-mediated endothelial cell dysfunction in diabetic vasculopathy: Soluble receptor for advance glycation end-products blocks hyperpermeability in diabetic rats. *J Clin Invest* 1996; 97:238–243.
152. Schmidt AM, Osamu H, Chen JX, et al. Advanced glycation end-products interacting with their endothelial receptors induce expression of vascular cell adhesion molecule-1 (VCAM-1) in cultured human endothelial cells in mice. *J Clin Invest* 1995; 96:1395–1403.
153. Yan SD, Schmidt AM, Anderson GM, Zhang J, et al. Enhanced cellular oxidant stress by the interaction of advanced glycation end products with their receptors/binding proteins. *J Biol Chem* 1994; 269:9889–9897.
154. Wautier JL, Wautier MP, Schmidt AM, et al. Advanced glycation end products (AGEs) on the surface of diabetic erythrocytes bind to the vessel wall via a specific receptor inducing oxidant stress in the vasculature: A link between surface-associated AGEs and diabetic complications. *Proc Natl Acad Sci USA* 1994; 91:7742–7746.
155. Brownlee M, Vlassara H, Kooney A, et al. Aminoguanidine prevents diabetes-induced arterial wall protein cross-linking. *Science* 1986; 232:1629–1632.
156. Brownlee M. Glycation and diabetic complications. *Diabetes* 1994; 43:836–841.
157. Brownlee M, Vlassara H, Cerami A. Nonenzymatic glycosylation products on collagen covalently trap low-density lipoprotein. *Diabetes* 1985; 34:938–941.
158. Bucala R, Tracey KJ, Cerami A. Advanced glycosylation products quench nitric oxide and mediate defective endothelium-dependent vasodilatation in experimental diabetes. *J Clin Invest* 1991; 87:432–438.
159. Bowie A, Owens D, Collins P, et al. Glycosylated low density lipoprotein is more sensitive to oxidation: Implications for the diabetic patient? *Atherosclerosis* 1993; 102:63–67.
160. Schmidt AM, Yan SD, Brett J, et al. Regulation of human mononuclear phagocyte migration by cell surface-binding proteins for advanced glycation end-products. *J Clin Invest* 1993; 91:2155–2168.
161. Vlassara H, Bucala R, Striker L. Pathogenic effects of advanced glycosylation: Biochemical, biologic, and clinical implications for diabetes and aging. *Lab Invest* 1994; 70:138–151.
162. Pyorala K, Pedersen DR, Kjekshus J, et al. Cholesterol lowering with simvastatin improves prognosis of diabetic patients with coronary heart disease. *Diabetes Care* 1997; 20:614–620.
163. Sacks FM, Pfeffer MA, Moye LA, et al. The effect of pravastatin on coronary events after myocardial infarction in patients with average cholesterol levels. *N Engl J Med* 1996; 335:1001–1009.
164. CARE Circulation: Goldberg RB, Mellies MJ, Sacks FM, et al. Cardiovascular events and their reduction with pravastatin in diabetic and glucose-intolerant myocardial infarction survivors with average cholesterol levels: Subgroup analyses in the cholesterol and recurrent events (CARE) trial: The Care investigators. *Circulation* 1998; 98:2513–2519.
165. American Diabetes Association: Standard of medical care for patients with diabetes mellitus. *Diabetes Care* 2000; 23(suppl 1): S532–S542.
166. Muhlhauser I, Sawicki PT, Berger M. Possible risk of sulfonylureas in the treatment of non-insulin-dependent diabetes mellitus and coronary artery disease. *Diabetologia* 1997; 40:1492–1496.
167. Cleveland JC, Meldrum DR, Cain BS, et al. Oral sulfonylurea hypoglycemic agents prevent ischemic preconditioning in human myocardium. *Circulation* 1997; 96(1):29–32.
168. Owens DR. Repaglinide—prandial glucose regulator: A new class of oral antidiabetic drugs. *Diabetes Med* 1998; 15(suppl 4): S28–S36.
169. Metformin for non-insulin-dependent diabetes mellitus. *Med Lett Drugs Ther* 1995; 37(948):41–42.
170. Stumvoll M, Nurjhan N, Perriello G, et al. Metabolic effects of metformin in non-insulin-dependent diabetes mellitus. *N Engl J Med* 1995; 333(9):550–554.
171. Garber AJ, Duncan TG, Goodman AM, et al. Efficacy of metformin in type II diabetes: Results of a double-blind, placebo-controlled, dose-response trial. *Am J Med* 1997; 102:491–497.
172. Giugliano D, Quatraro A, Consoli G, et al. Metformin for obese, insulin-treated, diabetic patients: Improvement in glycemic control and reduction of metabolic risk factors. *Eur J Clin Pharmacol* 1993; 44:107–112.
173. DeFronzo RA, Goodman AM, and the Multicenter Metformin Study Group. Efficacy of metformin in patients with non-insulin-dependent diabetes mellitus. *N Engl J Med* 1995; 333:541–549.
174. Inzucchi SE, Maggs DG, Spollett GR, et al. Efficacy and metabolic effects of metformin and troglitazone in type II diabetes mellitus. *N Engl J Med* 1998; 338:867–872.
175. Robinson AC, Burke J, Robinson S, et al. The effects of metformin on glycemic control and serum lipids in insulin-treated NIDDM patients with suboptimal metabolic control. *Diabetes Care* 1998; 21(5):701–705.
176. Stang MR, Wysowski DK, Butler-Jones D. Incidence of lactic acidosis in metformin users. *Diabetes Care* 1999; 22:925–927.
177. *Physician Desk Reference,* ed. 52. Montvale, NJ: Medical Economics Company. 1998; 795–800.
178. Tafuri SR. Troglitazone enhances differentiation, basal-glucose uptake and Glut 1 protein levels in 3T3-L1 adipocytes. *Endocrinology* 1996; 137:4706–4712.
179. Miles PDG, Romeo OM, Higo K, et al. TNF-α-induced insulin resistance in vivo and its prevention by troglitazone. *Diabetes* 1997; 46:1678–1683.
180. Schwartz S, Raskin P, Fonseca V, Graveline JF, for the Troglitazone and Exogenous Insulin Study Group. Effect of troglitazone in insulin-treated patients with type II diabetes mellitus. *N Engl J Med* 1998; 338:861–866.
181. Buse JB, Gumbiner B, Mathias NP, et al. The Troglitazone Insulin Study Group: Troglitazone use in insulin-treated type II diabetic patients. *Diabetes Care* 1998; 21:1455–1461.
182. Horton ES, Whitehouse F, Ghazzi MN, et al. The Troglitazone Study Group: Troglitazone in combination with sulfonylurea restores glycemic control in patients with type II diabetes. *Diabetes Care* 1998; 21:1462–1469.
183. Ghazzi MN, Perez JE, Antonucci TK, et al. The Triglitazone Study Group, Whitcomb RW. Cardiac and glycemic benefits of troglitazone treatment in NIDDM. *Diabetes* 1997; 46:433–439.
184. Maggs DG, Buchanan TA, Burant CF, et al. Metabolic effects of troglitazone monotherapy in type 2 diabetes mellitus. *Ann Intern Med* 1998; 128:176–185.
185. Tack CJJ, Smits P, Demacker PNM, Stalenhoff AFH. Troglitazone decreases the proportion of small, dense LDL and increases

the resistance of LDL to oxidation in obese subjects. *Diabetes Care* 1998; 21:796–797.

186. Patel J, Miller E, Patwardhan R, the Rosiglitazone Study Group. Rosiglitazone improves glycemic control when used as monotherapy in type 2 diabetic patients. *Diabetic Medicine* 1998; 15(suppl 2):S38.
187. Grunberger G, Weston WM, Patwardhan R, Rappaport EB. Rosiglitazone once or twice daily improves the glycemic control in patients with type 2 diabetes. *Diabetes* 1998; 48(suppl 1):A102.
188. Fonesca V, Biswas N, Salzman A. Once-daily rosiglitazone in combination with metformin effectively reduces hyperglycemia in patients with type 2 diabetes. *Diabetes* 1999; 48(suppl 1):A100.
189. Package insert. SmithKline Beecham Pharmaceuticals, Philadelphia.
190. Package insert. Takeda Pharmaceuticals, Lincolnshire, IL.
191. University Group Diabetes Program. A study of the effects of hypoglycemic agents on vascular complications in patients with adult onset diabetes. *Diabetes* 1976; 25:1129–1153.
192. Garratt KN, Hassinger N, Grill DE, et al. Sulfonylurea drug use is associated with increased early mortality during direct coronary angioplasty for acute myocardial infarction among diabetic patients. *J Am Coll Cardiol* 1997; 29:493A (Abstr).
193. UK Prospective Diabetes Study Group. Intensive blood glucose control with sulfonylureas or insulin compared with conventional treatment and risk of complications in patients with type-2 diabetes. UKPDS 33. *Lancet* 1998; 352:837–853.
194. UK Prospective Diabetes Study Group. Effect of intensive blood glucose control with metformin on complications in overweight patients with type-2 diabetes. UKPDS 34. *Lancet* 1998; 352: 854–865.
195. UK Prospective Diabetes Study Group. Tight blood pressure control and risk of macrovascular and microvascular complications in type-2 diabetes. UKPDS 38. *BMJ* 1998; 317:703–713.
196. UK Prospective Diabetes Study Group. Efficacy of atenolol and captopril in reducing risk of macrovascular and microvascular complications in type 2 diabetes. UKPDS 39. *BMJ* 1998; 317: 713–720.
197. The Diabetes Control and Complications Trial Research Group. The effect of intensive treatment of diabetes on the development and progression of long-term complications in insulin-dependent diabetes mellitus. *N Engl J Med* 1993; 329:977–986.
198. The Diabetes Control and Complications Trial Research Group. Effect of intensive diabetes management on macrovascular events and risk factors in the Diabetes Control and Complications Trial. *Am J Cardiol* 1995; 75:894–903.
199. The cost-effectiveness of screening for type 2 diabetes. CDC Diabetes Cost-Effectiveness Study Group, Centers for Disease Control and Prevention. *JAMA* 1998; 280:1757–1763.
200. Gibbons RJ, Balady GJ, Beasley JW, et al. ACC/AHA guidelines for exercise testing: Executive summary: A report of the American College of Cardiology/American Heart Association Task Force on Practice Guidelines (Committee on Exercise Testing). *Circulation* 1997; 96:345–354.
201. Grundy SM, Benjamin IJ, Burke GL, et al. Diabetes and cardiovascular disease: A statement for healthcare professionals from the American Heart Association. *Circulation* 1999; 100:1134–1146.
202. Curb JD, Pressel SL, Cutler JA, et al. Effect of diuretic-based antihypertensive treatment on cardiovascular disease risk in older diabetic patients with isolated systolic hypertension: Systolic Hypertension in the Elderly Program Cooperative Research Group. *JAMA* 1996; 276:1886–1892.
203. Hansson L, Zanchetti A, Carruthers SG, et al., for the HOT Study Group. Effects of intensive blood-pressure lowering and low-dose aspirin in patients with hypertension: Principal results of Hypertension Optimal Treatment (HOT) randomized trial. *Lancet* 1998; 351:1755–1762.
204. Hansson L, Lindholm LH, Niskanen L, et al., for the Captopril Prevention Projects (CAPPP) study group. Effect of angiotensin-converting-enzyme inhibition compared with conventional therapy on cardiovascular morbidity and mortality in hypertension: The Captopril Prevention Project (CAPPP) randomised trial. *Lancet* 1999; 353:611–616.
205. Estacio RO, Jeffers BW, Hiatt WR, et al. The effect of nisoldipine as compared with enalapril on cardiovascular outcomes in patients with non-insulin-dependent diabetes and hypertension. *N Engl J Med* 1998; 338:645–652.
206. Woodfield SL, Lundergan CF, Reiner JS, et al. Angiographic findings and outcome in diabetic patients treated with thrombolytic therapy for acute myocardial infarction: the GUSTO-1 experience. *J Am Coll Cardiol* 1996; 28:1661–1669.
207. Jaffe AS, Spadaro JJ, Schechtman K, et al. Increased congestive heart failure after myocardial infarction of modest extent in patients with diabetes mellitus. *Am Heart J* 1984; 108:31–37.
208. Savage MP, Krolewski AS, Kenien GG, et al. Acute myocardial infarction in diabetes mellitus and significance of congestive heart failure as a prognostic factor. *Am J Cardiol* 1988; 62:665–669.
209. Stone PH, Muller JE, Hartwell T, et al., for the MILIS Study Group. The effect of diabetes mellitus on prognosis and serial left ventricular function after acute myocardial infarction: Contribution of both coronary disease and left ventricular dysfunction to the adverse prognosis. *J Am Coll Cardiol* 1989; 14:49–57.
210. Fibrinolytic Therapy Trialists (FTT) Collaborative Group. Indications for fibrinolytic therapy in suspected acute myocardial infarction: Collaborative overview of early mortality and major morbidity results from all randomized trials of more than 1000 patients. *Lancet* 1994; 343:311–322.
211. Malmberg K, for the DIGAMI Study Group. Prospective randomised study of intensive insulin treatment on long-term survival after acute myocardial infarction in patients with diabetes mellitus. *BMJ* 1997; 314:1512–1515.
212. Zarich S, Waxman S, Freeman RT, et al. Effect of autonomic nervous system dysfunction on the circadian pattern of myocardial ischaemia in diabetes mellitus. *J Am Coll Cardiol* 1994; 24:956–962.
213. Jonas M, Reicher-Reiss H, Boyko V, et al. Usefulness of beta-blocker therapy in patients with non-insulin-dependent diabetes mellitus and coronary heart disease. *Am J Cardiol* 1996; 77:1273–1277.
214. Kendall MJ, Lynch KP, Hjalmarson A, Kjekshus J. Beta-blockers and sudden cardiac death. *Ann Intern Med* 1995; 123:358–367.
215. Holmes DR Jr, Vietstra RE, Smith HC, et al. Restenosis after percutaneous transluminal coronary angioplasty (PTCA): A report from the PTCA Registry of the National Heart, Lung and Blood Institute. *Am J Cardiol* 1984; 53:77C–81C.
216. Weintraub WS, Kosinski AS, Brown CL, King SB. Can restenosis after coronary angioplasty be predicted from clinical variables? *J Am Coll Cardiol* 1993; 21:6–14.
217. Vandormael MG, Deligonul U, Kern MJ, et al. Multilesion coronary angioplasty: Clinical and angiographic outcome. *J Am Coll Cardiol* 1987; 10:246–252.
218. Quigley PJ, Hlatky MA, Hinohara T, et al. Repeat percutaneous transluminal coronary angioplasty and predictors of recurrent restenosis. *Am J Cardiol* 1989; 63:409–413.
219. Lambert M, Bonan R, Cote G, et al. Multiple coronary angioplasty: A model to discriminate systemic and procedural factors related to restenosis. *J Am Coll Cardiol* 1988; 12:310–314.
220. Galan KM, Hollman JL. Recurrence of stenosis after coronary angioplasty. *Heart Lung* 1986; 15:585–587.
221. Rensing BJ, Hermans RM, Vos J, et al. Luminal narrowing after percutaneous transluminal coronary angioplasty. *Circulation* 1993; 88:975–985.
222. Wong SC, Baim DS, Schatz RA, et al. Immediate results and late outcomes after stent implantation in saphenous vein graft

lesions: The multicenter US Palmaz-Schatz stane experience: The Palmaz-Schatz Stent Study Group. *J Am Coll Cardiol* 1995; 26:704–712.

223. Bach R, Jung F, Kohsiek I, et al. Factors affecting the restenosis rate after percutaneous transluminal coronary angioplasty. *Thromb Haemost* 1994; 74(suppl 1):55S–77S.
224. Kornowski R, Mintz GS, Kent KM, et al. Increased restenosis in diabetes mellitus after coronary interventions is due to exaggerated intimal hyperplasia. *Circulation* 1997; 95:1366–1369.
225. Aronson D, Bloomgarden Z, Rayfield EJ. Potential mechanisms promoting restenosis in diabetes mellitus. *J Am Coll Cardiol* 1996; 27:528–535.
226. Lincoff AM, Califf RM, Moliterno DJ, et al., for the Evaluation of Platelet IIb/IIIa Inhibition in Stenting Investigators (EPISTENT). Complementary clinical benefits of coronary artery stenting and blockade of platelet glycoprotein IIb/IIIa receptors. *N Engl J Med* 1999; 341:319–327.
227. The Bypass Angioplasty Revascularization Investigation (BARI) Investigators. Comparison of bypass surgery with angioplasty in patients with multivessel disease. *N Engl J Med* 1996; 335: 217–225.
228. Kannel WB, Hjortland M, Castelli WP. Role of diabetes in congestive heart failure: The Framingham Study. *Am J Cardiol* 1974; 34:29–34.
229. Van Hoeven KH, Factor SM. A comparison of the pathological spectrum of hypertensive, diabetic, and hypertensive-diabetic heart disease. *Circulation* 1990; 82:848–855.
230. Jain A, Avendaro G, Dharamsey S, et al. Left ventricular diastolic dysfunction in hypertension and role of plasma glucose and insulin: Comparison with diabetic heart. *Circulation* 1996; 93:1396–1402.
231. Zarich SW, Arbuckle BE, Cohen LR, et al. Diastolic abnormalities in young asymptomatic diabetic patients assessed by pulse Doppler echocardiography. *J Am Coll Cardiol* 1988; 12:114–120.
232. Raev DC. Which left ventricular function is impaired earlier in the evolution of diabetic cardiomyopathy? An echocardiographic study of young type I diabetic patients. *Diabetes Care* 1994; 17:633–639.
233. Paillole C, Dahan M, Payche F, et al. Prevalence and significance of left ventricular filling abnormalities determined by Doppler echocardiography in young type I (insulin-dependent) diabetic patients. *Am J Cardiol* 1990; 64:1010–1016.
234. Mildenerger RR, Bar-Shlomo B, Druck MN, et al. Clinically unrecognized ventricular dysfunction in young diabetic patients. *J Am Coll Cardiol* 1984; 4:234–238.
235. Shindler DM, Kostis JB, Yusuf S, et al. Diabetes mellitus: A predictor of morbidity and mortality in the Studies of Left Ventricular Dysfunction (SOLVD) trials and registry. *Am J Cardiol* 1996; 77:1017–1020.
236. Gaede P, Vedel P, Parving HH, Pedersen O. Intensified multifactorial intervention in patients with type 2 diabetes mellitus and microalbuminuria: The Steno type 2 randomised study. *Lancet* 1999; 353:617–622.
237. Heart Outcomes Prevention Evaluation Study Investigators. Effects of ramipril on cardiovascular and microvascular outcomes in people with diabetes mellitus: Results of the HOPE study and MICRO-HOPE sub-study. *Lancet* 2000; 355:253–259.

C H A P T E R 79

TRAUMATIC HEART DISEASE

Panagiotis N. Symbas

Accidental or intentional trauma is the leading cause of death, hospitalization, and loss of working days in American society, particularly among young people.[1–3] Cardiac and great vessel injuries are a major contributor to this mortality and morbidity.[4] The heart and/or great vessels may be injured from penetrating and nonpenetrating trauma. Since the diagnostic and therapeutic modalities for the management of heart diseases have become more complex and more invasive, mechanical injuries to the heart caused by iatrogenic trauma have become increasingly important. These injuries result from the complications of various diagnostic, therapeutic, and resuscitative procedures, including cardiac catheterization, percutaneous coronary angioplasty,[5,6] percutaneous aortic or mitral valvuloplasty,[7,8] insertion of pacemaker leads[9] or Swan-Ganz catheters,[10] closed- and open-chest cardiac massage, and electric defibrillation.[11,12] The increasing use of invasive catheters has led to the more frequent migration of these catheters to the heart and the pulmonary vascular beds[13–15] and to nonbacterial thrombotic endocarditis and bacterial endocarditis.

Two other types of cardiac trauma that are not due to mechanical injury warrant separate classification. The first type includes injury to the heart from ionizing radiation, which predominantly causes pericarditis but also may result in myocardial injury.[16–18] The second includes the group of cardiac injuries caused by an electric current,[19,20] which may cause asystole, ventricular fibrillation, other arrhythmias, and myocardial injury (see also Chap. 71).

Many nonpenetrating injuries and an occasional penetrating injury of the heart are well tolerated. Thus, many of these lesions are diagnosed infrequently, since their initial clinical manifestations may be absent or relatively mild, and a lesion may be overlooked unless a high index of suspicion is maintained and specific studies are obtained.[21,22] Frequently, these cardiac injuries are overshadowed by the more overt manifestations of cerebral, abdominal, or musculoskeletal trauma. For these reasons and because only the more severe injuries are reflected in autopsy studies, the actual incidence of traumatic heart disease remains obscure.

PENETRATING INJURIES

Penetrating injuries usually are observed with wounds of the precordium but also may be associated with wounds elsewhere in the chest, neck, or upper abdomen. They usually are due to missile or knife wounds but occasionally are caused by a missile embolus reaching the heart through the venous system or by a needle migrating through the esophagus.

Penetrating Cardiac Trauma

Although penetrating cardiac trauma frequently involves only the free cardiac wall, injury to cardiac valves, chordae tendineae, papillary muscles, the atrial or ventricular septum, coronary arteries, and the conduction system may occur. The multiplicity of heart and great vessel lesions that may be produced by penetrating wounds is indicated in Table 79-1.

The relative frequency of a single penetrating wound of the free cardiac wall is due to its area of exposure on the anterior chest wall. In decreasing order of frequency, the structures affected are the right ventricle, left ventricle, right atrium, and left atrium.[23] Cardiac wounds may be single or multiple; the latter more commonly are caused by missiles.[23,24] Over 50 percent of victims with penetrating cardiac trauma succumb shortly after injury.[25] The remainder survive for varying periods; many can recover completely if treated immediately.

The pathophysiologic consequences and clinical manifestations of penetrating injuries to the heart depend on the size and site of the wound, the mode of injury, and especially the state of the pericardial wound. When the pericardial wound remains open and bleeding occurs freely into the pleural space, there are signs and symptoms of hemothorax and loss of circulating blood volume. When there is intrapericardial hemorrhage with a sealed pericardial wound, cardiac tamponade (see Chap. 72) is the presenting clinical picture. The diagnosis of cardiac injury should be suspected in a patient with chest, lower neck, epigastric, or especially precordial penetrating wounds and with symptoms and signs of cardiac tamponade and/or hemothorax and loss of circulating blood volume. The management of penetrating wounds of the heart consists of immediate thoracotomy and cardiorrhaphy.[23,25–30] When this cannot be done or while appropriate arrangements are being made for thoracotomy, the patient's blood volume should be expanded; pericardiocentesis is performed only to provide time for a safe operation.[23,31]

Although the management of symptomatic patients with a suspected penetrating cardiac wound is clearly defined, the man-

TABLE 79-1 Penetrating Wounds of the Heart

I. Pericardial damage
  A. Laceration or perforation
  B. Hemopericardium with or without cardiac tamponade
  C. Serofibrinous or suppurative pericarditis
  D. Pneumopericardium
  E. Constrictive pericarditis
II. Myocardial damage
  A. Laceration
  B. Penetration or perforation
  C. Retained foreign body
  D. Structural defects
    1. Aneurysm formation
    2. Septal defects
    3. Aorticocardiac fistula
III. Valvular injury
  A. Leaflet or cusp injury
  B. Papillary muscle or chordae tendineae laceration
IV. Coronary artery injury
  A. Laceration or thrombosis with or without myocardial infarction
  B. Arteriovenous fistula
  C. Aneurysm
V. Embolism
  A. Foreign body
  B. Thrombus (septic or sterile)
VI. Infective endocarditis
VII. Rhythm or conduction disturbances

SOURCE: Prepared by Loren F. Parmley, MD, and Thomas W. Mattingly, and modified with permission.

agement of the asymptomatic patients with a penetrating precordial wound presented a considerable dilemma in the past, when the options were either exploratory surgery or observation. Currently, the use of echocardiography by a cardiologist or preferably an immediately available and specially trained trauma surgeon facilitates and makes the treatment of these patients safer by avoiding unnecessary surgery or observation, with its accompanying risk of sudden deterioration and even death.[32]

Residual or Delayed Sequelae of Penetrating Cardiac Trauma

Patients with penetrating cardiac wounds should be observed closely immediately postoperatively and after discharge for the clinical manifestations of residual or delayed sequelae from their penetrating cardiac wounds. Such sequelae may include (1) ventricular or atrial septal defect, (2) injury of the valve cups, leaflets, or chordae tendineae, (3) aortocardiac or aortopulmonary communication, or communication from the coronary artery to the coronary vein or the cardiac chamber, (4) ventricular aneurysms, (5) posttraumatic or postoperative pericarditis, and (6) electrocardiographic abnormalities.[33,34] When symptoms and signs of a structural defect are detected, echocardiography and/or cardiac catheterization should be performed to define the lesion and its hemodynamic significance and determine the proper mode of therapy.[33,35]

Posttraumatic pericarditis, which is similar to the postcardiotomy syndrome seen after cardiac surgery, occurs in approximately 20 percent of all cases of penetrating heart wounds. Symptomatic management is the treatment of choice for this syndrome unless cardiac tamponade or other sequelae, such as purulent or constrictive pericarditis, require surgical intervention.

Missile wounds also may result in the presence of a projectile within the heart after either a direct injury to the heart or an injury to a systemic vein with subsequent migration of the missile to the heart. The missile or the thrombus associated with it may embolize into the systemic or pulmonary arteries.[36–38] Bacterial endocarditis also may occur if the projectile is not completely embedded in the myocardium.[39,40] Rarely, a patient with a projectile in the heart may develop cardiac neurosis, with an almost maniacal desire for removal of the foreign body.[41] In many patients, however, the retained missile in the heart results in no ill effects over a long period of observation.[42,43] Therefore, treatment for missiles in the heart should be individualized according to the patient's clinical course and the location, size, and shape of the missile.[42,43] Missiles that cause symptoms should be removed. Similarly, missiles that are free or partially protruding into a left cardiac chamber should be removed, because their embolization to the systemic arterial system may have serious consequences.[42,43] Missiles in the right side of the heart may be removed or left to embolize to the pulmonary vascular bed, from which they can be retrieved easily.[37] Intramyocardial and intrapericardial bullets and pellets are generally well tolerated and may be left in place.

A missile that has embolized to the systemic arterial bed should be removed surgically without delay unless it has resulted in a significant neurologic deficit.[38] Projectiles adjacent to or embedded within the wall of one of the great or coronary arteries should be extracted to prevent subsequent erosion and bleeding.

Coronary Artery Penetrating Trauma

Coronary artery injuries can result in cardiac tamponade and varying degrees of myocardial ischemia or myocardial infarction. The management of these wounds is dependent on the amount of myocardium at risk. Wounds of major branches of the coronary arterial system are repaired or bypassed, whereas small terminal vessels are ligated. Coronary artery aneurysms and arteriovenous fistulas are rare sequelae of injury, and their treatment should be individualized.[44]

Penetrating Trauma of the Aorta and Great Vessels

The pathophysiology of penetrating wounds to the great vessels is quite similar to that of penetrating wounds to the heart and depends on whether the site of the wound is intra- or extrapericardial.[45,46] In addition to the obvious results of immediate or delayed hemorrhage, a penetrating wound of a great vessel may result in the formation of a false aneurysm, with possible subsequent rupture, or an arteriovenous fistula, producing immediate or latent signs and symptoms of congestive heart failure.[47] Traumatic arteriovenous fistulas occasionally are complicated by the development of bacterial endarteritis and endocarditis.[48] These traumatic vascular lesions should be detected and repaired as soon as possible.

NONPENETRATING INJURIES

The vast majority of blunt injuries to the heart are due to automobile accidents, although other forms of trauma from contact sports, altercations, falls, and so on also may result in this type of injury. The cardiac injury usually is caused by direct compressing or decelerating forces delivered to the chest or rarely by an indirect force delivered to the abdomen or even to the extremities that results in a marked increase in intravascular pressures. A wide variety of injuries are produced by nonpenetrating trauma (Table 79-2).

Cardiac Contusion

Contusion of the heart usually refers to blunt injury to the heart that causes identifiable histopathologic changes within the myocardium. The pathologic lesions of myocardial contusion vary considerably in extent and character, ranging from small areas of petechiae or ecchymosis, which may be either subepicardial or subendocardial, to contusion of the full thickness of the myocardial wall with or without rupture of the heart.[1]

Histologically, various degrees of subepicardial or intramyocardial hemorrhage or disruption of the myocardial fibers and leukocyte infiltration and edema may be present.[1] The forces that produce nonpenetrating lesions of the heart are such that external evidence of chest injury may be meager or undetectable in almost one-third of traumatized patients. This lack of evidence of chest wall injury and the frequent absence of symptoms from the cardiac injury, along with the common presence of other, more obvious injuries to the body, may impede the early diagnosis of cardiac contusion.

TABLE 79-2 Nonpenetrating Trauma of the Heart

1. Pericardial injury
   a. Hemopericardium
   b. Rupture or laceration
   c. Serofibrinous pericarditis
   d. Constrictive pericarditis
2. Myocardial injury
   a. Contusion
   b. Rupture of free cardiac wall, early or delayed
   c. Rupture of septum
   d. Aneurysm
   e. Laceration
3. Disturbances of rhythm or conduction
4. Valve injury
   a. Rupture of valve leaflets, cusp, or chordae tendineae
   b. Contusion of papillary muscle
5. Coronary artery injury
   a. Thrombosis with or without myocardial infarction
   b. Arteriovenous fistula
   c. Laceration with or without myocardial infarction
6. Great vessel injury
   a. Rupture
   b. Aneurysm formation
   c. Aorta-cardiac chamber fistula
   d. Thrombotic occlusion

Patients with contusions of the heart are commonly asymptomatic, but they may complain of pain that is identical in character, location, and radiation to the pain of myocardial ischemia and/or myocardial infarction.[49] The pain is usually transient unless there is concomitant coronary artery injury or occult atherosclerotic coronary heart disease.[50] Coronary thrombosis can result from nonpenetrating trauma, but this is rare and usually is associated with existing atherosclerotic coronary artery disease.[51] In 546 necropsy cases of nonpenetrating cardiac trauma, no instance of coronary thrombosis was found. Dyspnea and hypotension also may be presenting symptoms. In mild or moderate myocardial contusion, these signs may be transient and are usually absent. Cardiac failure is relatively rare; when it is present, the possibility of an associated cardiac injury, such as rupture of the ventricular septum or of one of the cardiac valves, is high. Hemopericardium with or without the signs and symptoms of cardiac tamponade may be associated with myocardial contusion. Laceration of a coronary artery from a nonpenetrating injury also may occur rarely, producing cardiac tamponade or a coronary artery fistula.[52]

The diagnosis of cardiac contusion should be suspected in all patients with significant blunt trauma, particularly to the precordium. Unfortunately, none of the currently available diagnostic tests for myocardial contusion can conclusively establish the diagnosis in all patients. The appropriate use and interpretation of the available tests, however, can assist in the diagnosis of myocardial contusion with reasonable accuracy.

Electrocardiography has been the most widely used test for the diagnosis of contusion of the heart. Various electrocardiographic abnormalities have been considered suggestive of cardiac contusion, such as nonspecific ST-T or Q-wave changes, supraventricular tachyarrhythmias, and ventricular arrhythmias, including fibrillation, which is usually the cause of death at the time of the traumatic impact.[53–55] However, a variety of other clinical conditions[56–59] that are frequently present in traumatized patients (i.e., pain, anxiety, hemorrhage, hypoxia, hypokalemia, head trauma, alcohol or cocaine toxicity) may cause many of these abnormalities. Therefore, the presence of these other causes must be excluded before the electrocardiographic abnormalities are attributed to contusion of the heart.[60–62]

Elevation of the serum level of the MB fraction of creatinine kinase (CK) has been extrapolated from its use in acute myocardial infarction as a diagnostic aid in patients with cardiac contusion. Other clinical conditions that cause elevation in the level of this enzyme—i.e., tachyarrhythmias and skeletal muscle diseases, including trauma (see Chap. 42)—must be excluded before an abnormal level is ascribed to contusion of the heart.[60–62]

Radioisotope imaging of the heart in dogs with experimentally produced cardiac contusion has identified the area of injury only in animals with a full-thickness contusion.[63] Therefore, this is of diagnostic value in only a limited number of patients, since the incidence of full-thickness contusion is low in patients who survive the initial traumatic impact.

Two-dimensional transthoracic and transesophageal echocardiography (TTE and TEE) are useful in the diagnosis of cardiac contusion, particularly of the structural lesions associated with cardiac contusion.[64,65] The sensitivity and specificity of these tests for diagnosing contusion of the heart, however, have not been clearly defined (see Chap. 13).

Circulating cardiac troponin I was measured in a limited number of blunt trauma victims. It was concluded that this test is accurate for diagnosing cardiac contusion.[66] However additional studies are needed to determine its absolute accuracy.

The treatment of myocardial contusion is symptomatic. Appropriate limitation of activity and prevention and early treatment of arrhythmias are the most important therapeutic measures. The possible increased sensitivity of the heart to medications also must be considered when one is deciding what drugs to use in a patient with recent trauma.

Anticoagulants immediately after an injury should be avoided if possible because they may cause bleeding within the myocardium or pericardial space. Congestive heart failure should be treated with angiotensin-converting enzyme (ACE) inhibitors, and antiarrhythmic agents should be used to control ectopic rhythms as appropriate (see Chap. 24). If the myocardial contusion is severe, support with inotropic drugs (see Chap. 23) may be necessary. When all these measures fail, balloon counterpulsation[67] or even a left ventricular assist device[68] may be utilized.

Cardiac Rupture

Although minor, insignificant myocardial contusion of the right ventricle is the most common blunt cardiac injury; the most fatal lesion is rupture of the heart. The rupture may occur in the free cardiac wall or the ventricular septum. Rupture of the free cardiac wall is extremely difficult to diagnose and treat in a timely manner because of the frequently rapid demise of the patient and because traumatic cardiac rupture is often only one of many severe bodily injuries. As a result, rupture of the heart frequently has not been amenable to therapy. Readily available echocardiography in some emergency rooms, however, may increase the number of successfully treated patients.[69] The surgical repair of interventricular septal rupture is accomplished optimally after the patient has been stablized with medical therapy.

Residual or Delayed Sequelae of Blunt Injury to the Heart

Contusion of the heart usually heals with little or no obvious scarring or impairment of cardiac function. Large contusions, however, may cause a decrease in cardiac output, and extensive necrosis may lead to rupture or, rarely, congestive heart failure and the formation of a true or false aneurysm.[70] Cardiac aneurysms may cause arrhythmias, congestive heart failure, rupture, and mural thrombosis with embolism. Because of these complications, surgical repair of a traumatic aneurysm is usually advisable. Localized areas of necrosis and hemorrhage involving the cardiac conduction system may produce varying degrees of atrioventricular block or any of the different types of intraventricular conduction defects.

The most commonly injured valve in surviving patients is the aortic valve, with aortic regurgitation characteristically causing the rapid development of congestive heart failure. Injury of the atrioventricular valves is an uncommon result of nonpenetrating cardiac injury and usually occurs in the presence of severe cardiac trauma, resulting in death. Rupture of the mitral valve leaflet can have hemodynamic consequences somewhat similar to those of aortic valve injury but rarely is encountered clinically. In contrast, tricuspid valve injury may be tolerated for years before surgical correction is required.[71]

Rupture of the papillary muscle or chordae tendineae occurs more frequently than does rupture of valve leaflets. Cardiac contusion also may cause papillary muscle dysfunction with secondary mitral or tricuspid regurgitation.[72] The clinical outcome depends on whether the structures involved are on the right side of the heart, where the lesion may be well tolerated, or the left side, where the high-pressure system can lead to more serious hemodynamic sequelae. The murmurs produced by these lesions are generally typical of valvular regurgitation, but unusual high-pitched systolic and diastolic murmurs of variable loudness also may result (see Chap. 10). Traumatic tricuspid regurgitation may be present despite the absence of detectable murmur.[73] Prompt and correct diagnosis by echocardiographic, hemodynamic, and angiographic studies is important. Patients with hemodynamically significant valvular injury should undergo valvuloplasty or valve replacement.

Pericardial lesions often are overlooked and frequently heal without incident. Hemopericardium may occur but usually is due to the coexisting myocardial injury. When the hemorrhage is severe, cardiac tamponade occurs rapidly. When the oozing of blood or serum into the pericardium is slow, however, dilatation of the pericardial sac can develop over an extended period.

Posttraumatic pericarditis, which is similar to the post–myocardial infarction syndrome, develops less frequently with blunt than with penetrating cardiac injuries. The symptoms and signs of posttraumatic pericarditis are similar to those of pericarditis produced by a wide variety of causes (see Chap. 72). When hemopericardium or hydropericardium is suspected, echocardiography can confirm the diagnosis. Pericardial laceration usually is well tolerated, but herniation of the heart may occur, leading to more serious consequences and death.[74,75]

Aortic Rupture

Rupture of the aorta is the most common blunt injury of the great vessels. Rupture or avulsion of the innominate, carotid, or left subclavian arteries or the venae cavae also has been observed. Because of the variety of mechanical forces produced by blunt trauma (Fig. 79-1), combined with anatomic factors, the most common sites of rupture of the aorta from blunt injury

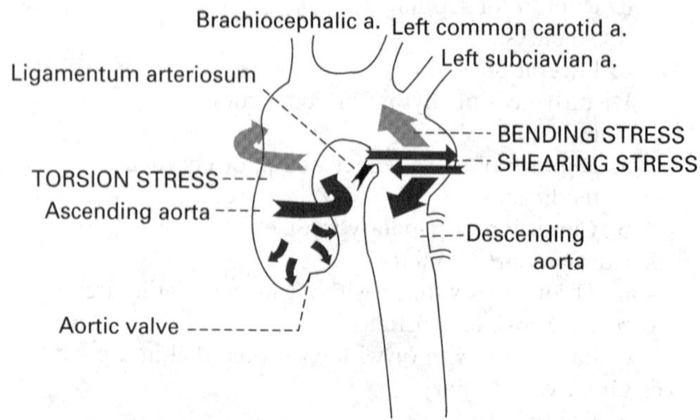

FIGURE 79-1 Diagrammatic illustration of the forces acting on the aortic wall during rupture of the aorta from blunt trauma. (From Symbas PN. *Traumatic Injuries of the Heart and Great Vessels*. Springfield, IL: Charles C Thomas; 1971:153. Courtesy of Charles C Thomas, Publisher, Springfield, Illinois.)

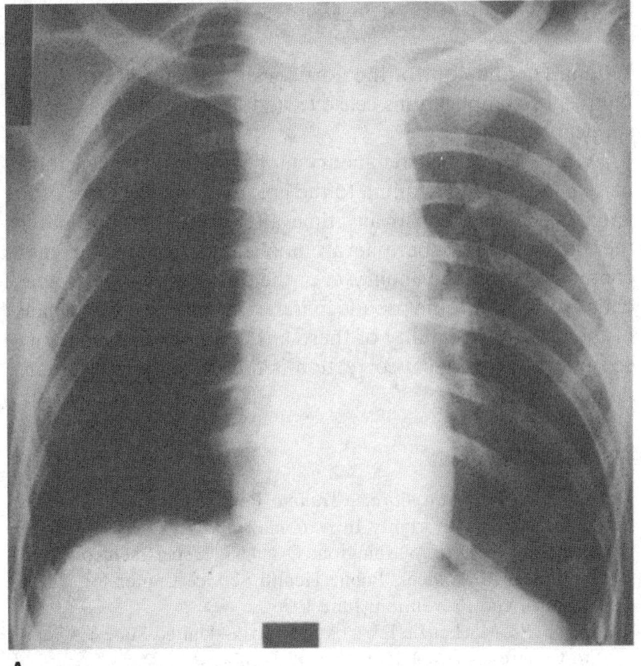

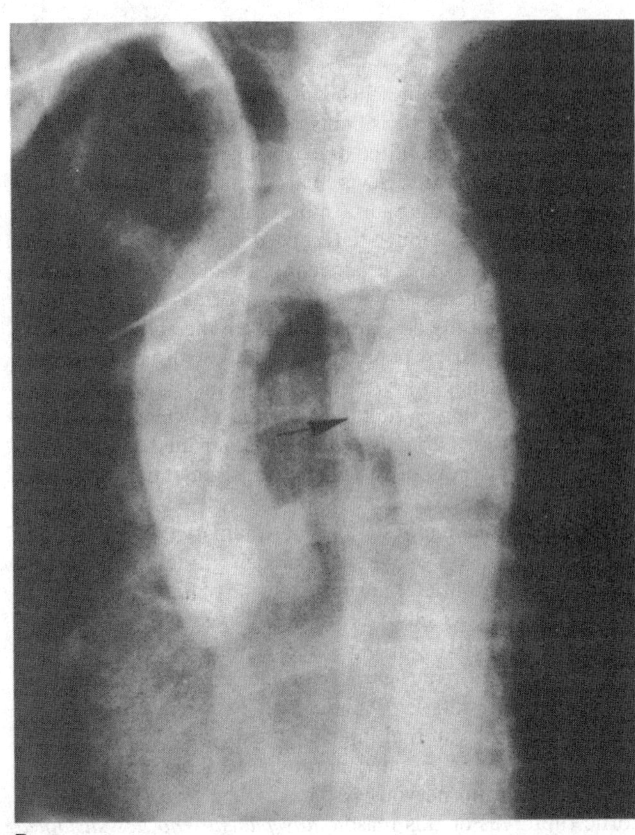

FIGURE 79-2 *A.* Chest roentgenogram of a young man who shortly before admission was involved in an automobile accident. Note the mediastinal widening. *B.* Aortogram the same day showing a false aneurysm distal to the origin of the left subclavian artery and two filling defects, one proximal and one distal to the aneurysm.

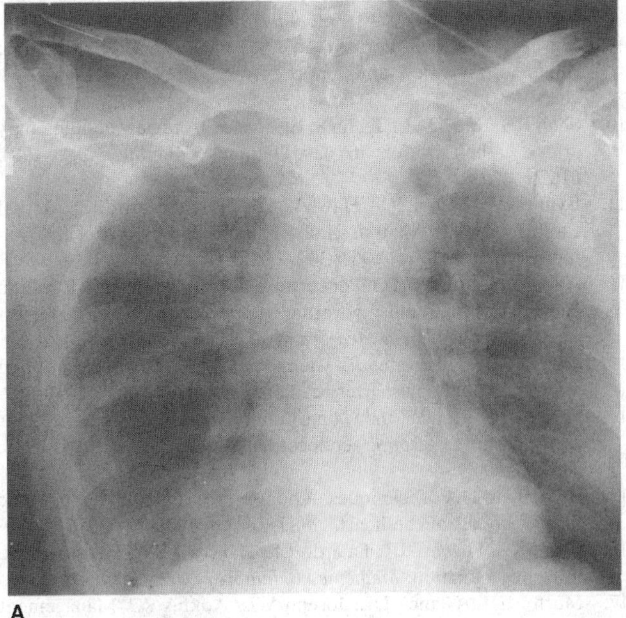

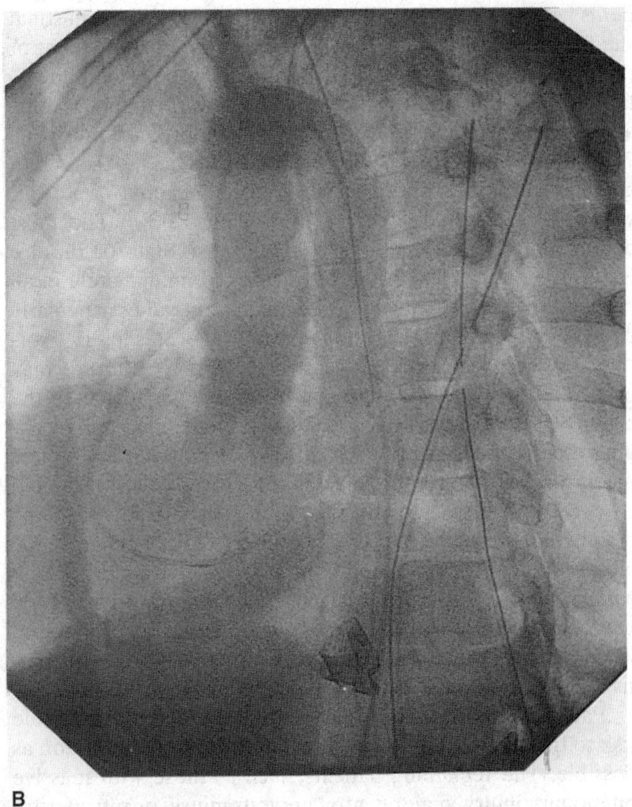

FIGURE 79-3 *A.* Chest roentgenogram of a young man shortly after a vehicular accident. *B.* Aortogram showing rupture of the ascending aorta.

are the descending aorta just distal to the origin of the left subclavian artery (aortic isthmus) and the ascending aorta just proximal to the origin of the brachycephalic artery.[76,77] Because of the high incidence of severe cardiac injury in patients with rupture of the ascending aorta, most of the patients who survive aortic rupture long enough to receive definitive surgical correction are those who have sustained rupture of the aortic isthmus. Occasionally, rupture at the ascending aorta,[78] the aortic arch, and other sites of the descending and even the abdominal aorta may occur. About 20 percent of patients with aortic rupture survive the original injury. A false aneurysm is formed in these patients at the site of rupture, the wall of which consists of adventitia and/or parietal pleura and other mediastinal structures. The intactness of these structures maintains continuity of the circulation.

The common manifestations of traumatic rupture of the aorta are chest and/or midscapular pain, a new murmur, increased pulse amplitude, and hypertension of the upper extremities.[79] Some patients, however, are surprisingly free of any major symptoms or signs from the aortic rupture. Hoarseness, evidence of a superior vena cava syndrome, paraplegia, and anuria are rare manifestations. Although there are occasionally no obvious signs of external injury, patients with rupture of the aorta usually have associated injuries of the skeleton, abdominal viscera, or central nervous system that can mask the signs of aortic rupture. For this reason, *any patient who has sustained severe blunt trauma or has been exposed to major deceleration forces should be suspected of having aortic rupture if there is an increased pulse pressure, upper extremity hypertension, and especially widening of the upper mediastinal silhouette.*

Chest roentgenography is of great diagnostic value in patients with aortic rupture. Widening of the superior mediastinal shadow, depression of the left main bronchus, displacement of the trachea and esophagus to the right, and especially obliteration of the aortic knob shadow are common roentgenographic abnormalities associated with injury at the aortic isthmus (Fig. 79-2). Widening of the mediastinum also has been observed in all cases with rupture of the aortic arch and in about 79 percent with rupture of the ascending aorta (Fig. 79-3).[78] The most definitive procedure to establish the diagnosis of aortic rupture is aortography, which should be performed immediately in all patients whose history, physical examination, and particularly chest roentgenogram suggest the possibility of this injury. Aortography should include the entire aorta, since rupture may occur at sites other than the aortic segment just distal to the origin of the left subclavian artery. Computed tomography scanning also is used widely to evaluate patients with a widened mediastinum.[80] The approximately 55 percent sensitivity and 65 percent sensitivity of this test limit its contribution to the definitive management of these patients.[81] TEE appears to be a useful diagnostic test[66] (see Chap. 13), but there has been no comprehensive study of its diagnostic value for aortic rupture. Until further experience is gained, caution should be exercised when it is used as the sole technique for establishing the diagnosis. Treatment should be undertaken as soon as possible.

Patients with no other organ injuries that add unacceptable risk to the surgical treatment should be operated on as soon as possible. The remaining patients, such as those with massive pulmonary injury, major central nervous injury, or retroperitoneal bleeding, may be treated medically with vasodilators or beta blockers to maintain the systemic blood pressure below 140 mmHg and control the aortic wall tension until the other injuries or complications cease to add unacceptable risk to the surgical treatment.[82]

A chronic false aortic aneurysm may be discovered months or years after blunt trauma to the great vessels. Rupture of the aneurysm may occur at any time after its formation. Rarely, the complications of peripheral embolization from the thrombus contained within the aneurysm or the development of bacterial endaortitis or chronic pseudocoarctation may occur.[83] Because of the relative instability of these aneurysms and the potential complications, surgical correction is the treatment of choice.

References

1. Symbas PN. *Cardiothoracic Trauma.* Philadelphia: Saunders; 1989.
2. James S. Injury mortality. In: *National Summary of Injury Mortality Data, 1987–1993.* Washington, DC: U.S. Department of Health and Human Services, Public Health Service Center for Disease Control and Prevention; June 1996.
3. Price PR, Mackenzie EJ. Cost of injury—United States: A report to Congress. *JAMA* 1989; 262:2803–2804.
4. Kemmerer WT, Eckert WG, Gathwright JB, et al. Patterns of thoracic injuries in fatal traffic accidents. *J Trauma* 1961; 1: 595–599.
5. Bredlau CE, Roubin GS, Leimgruber PP, et al. In-hospital morbidity and mortality in patients undergoing elective coronary angioplasty. *Circulation* 1985; 72:1044–1052.
6. Gaul G, Hollman J, Simpendorfer C, Franco I. Acute occlusion in multiple lesion coronary angioplasty: Frequency and management. *J Am Coll Cardiol* 1989; 13:283–288.
7. Safian RD, Berman AD, Diver DJ, et al. Balloon aortic valvuloplasty in 170 consecutive patients. *N Engl J Med* 1988; 319: 125–130.
8. Nobuyoshi M, Hamasaki N, Kimura T, et al. Indications, complications and short-term clinical outcome of percutaneous transvenous mitral commissurotomy. *Circulation* 1989; 80:782–792.
9. Meyer JA, Millar K. Perforation of the right ventricle by electrode catheters: A review and report of nine cases. *Ann Surg* 1968; 168:1048–1060.
10. Shah KB, Rao TL, Laughlin S, El Etr AA. A review of pulmonary artery catheterization in 6245 patients. *Anesthesiology* 1984; 61:271–275.
11. Bynum WR, Conell RM, Hawk WA. Causes of death after external cardiac massage: Analysis of observations on fifty consecutive autopsies. *Cleve Clin Q* 1963; 30:147–151.
12. Agdal N, Jorgensen TG. Penetrating laceration of the pericardium and myocardium and myocardial rupture following closed chest cardiac massage. *Acta Med Scand* 1973; 194:477–479.
13. Greene JF Jr, Fitzwater JE, Clemmer TP. Septic endocarditis and indwelling pulmonary artery catheters. *JAMA* 1975; 233:891–892.
14. Pace NL, Horton W. Indwelling pulmonary artery catheters: Their relationship to aseptic endocardial vegetation. *JAMA* 1975; 233:893–894.
15. Bloomfield DA. Techniques of nonsurgical retrieval of iatrogenic foreign bodies of the heart. *Am J Cardiol* 1971; 27:538–545.
16. Cohn KE, Stewart JR, Fajardo LF, Hancock EW. Heart disease following radiation. *Medicine* (*Baltimore*) 1967; 46:281–298.
17. Morton DL, Glancy DL, Joseph WL, Adkins PC. Management of patients with radiation-induced pericarditis with effusions: A note on the development of aortic regurgitation in two of them. *Chest* 1973; 64:291–297.
18. De Silva RA, Graboys TB, Podrid PJ, Lown B. Cardioversion and defibrillation. *Am Heart J* 1980; 100:881–895.
19. Bernstein T. Effects of electricity and lightning on man and animals. *J Forensic Sci* 1973; 18:3–11.

20. Jackson SH, Parry DJ. Lightning and the heart. *Br Heart J* 1980; 43:454–527.
21. Moritz AR, Atkins JP. Cardiac contusions: An experimental and pathologic study. *Arch Pathol* 1938; 25:445–462.
22. Samson PC. Battle wounds and injuries of the heart and pericardium: Experiences in forward hospitals. *Ann Surg* 1948; 127:1127–1149.
23. Symbas PN, Harlaftis N, Waldo WJ. Penetrating wounds: A comparison of different therapeutic methods. *Ann Surg* 1976; 183:377–381.
24. Symbas PN. *Cardiothoracic Trauma: Current Problems in Surgery.* St. Louis: Mosby Year Book; 1991:742.
25. Thourani VH, Filiciano DV, Cooper WA, et al. Penetrating cardiac trauma at an urban trauma center: A 22-year experience. *Am Surg* 1999; 65: 811–818.
26. Trinkle JK, Toon RS, Franz JL, et al. Affairs of the wounded heart: Penetrating cardiac wounds. *J Trauma* 1979; 19:467–472.
27. Ivatury RR, Rohman M, Steichen FM, et al. Penetrating cardiac injuries: Twenty-year experience. *Am Surg* 1987; 53:310–317.
28. Attar S, Suter CM, Hankins JR, et al. Penetrating cardiac injuries. *Ann Thorac Surg* 1991; 51:711–716.
29. Knott-Craig CJ, Dalton RP, Rossouw GJ, Barnard PM. Penetrating cardiac trauma: Management strategy based on 129 surgical emergencies over 2 years. *Ann Thorac Surg* 1992; 53:1006–1009.
30. Mitchell ME, Muakkassa FF, Poole GV, et al. Surgical approach of choice for penetrating cardiac wounds. *J Trauma* 1993; 34:17–20.
31. Cooper FW Jr, Stead EA Jr, Warren JV. The beneficial effect of intravenous infusions in acute cardiac tamponade. *Ann Surg* 1944; 120:822–825.
32. Rozycki GS, Feliciano DV, Schmidt JA, et al. The role of surgeon-performed ultrasound in patients with possible cardiac wounds. *Ann Surg* 1996; 224:1–8.
33. Symbas PN, DiOrio DA, Tyras DH, et al. Penetrating cardiac wounds: Significant residual and delayed sequelae. *J Thorac Cardiovasc Surg* 1973; 6:526–532.
34. Symbas PN. *Traumatic Heart Disease: Current Problems in Cardiology.* St Louis: Mosby Year Book; 1991:539.
35. Whisennand HH, Van Pelt SA, Beall AC Jr, et al. Surgical management of traumatic intracardiac injuries. *Ann Thorac Surg* 1979; 28:530–536.
36. Bland EF, Beebe GW. Missles in the heart: A 20-year follow-up report of world war cases. *N Engl J Med* 1966; 274:1039–1046.
37. Symbas PN, Hatcher CR Jr, Mansour KA. Projectile embolus of the lung. *J Thorac Cardiovasc Surg* 1968; 56:97–103.
38. Symbas PN, Harlaftis N. Bullet emboli in the pulmonary and systemic arteries. *Ann Surg* 1977; 185:318–320.
39. Decker HR. Foreign bodies in the heart and pericardium: Should they be removed? *J Thorac Surg* 1939; 9:62.
40. Harken DE. Experiments in intracardiac surgery: I. Bacterial endocarditis. *J Thorac Surg* 1942; 11:656–670.
41. Turner GG. Bullets in the heart for 23 years. *Surgery* 1942; 9:832–852.
42. Symbas PN, Picone AL, Hatcher CR Jr, Vlasis SE. Cardiac missles: A review of the literature and personal experience. *Ann Surg* 1990; 211:639–648.
43. Symbas PN, Vlasis SE, Picone AL, Hatcher CR Jr. Missles in the heart. *Ann Thorac Surg* 1989; 48:192–194.
44. Konecke LL, Spitzer S, Mason D, et al. Traumatic aneurysm of the left coronary artery. *Am J Cardiol* 1971; 27:221–223.
45. Symbas PN, Sehdava JS. Penetrating wounds of the thoracic aorta. *Ann Surg* 1970; 171:441–450.
46. Symbas PN, Kourias E, Tyras DH, Hatcher CR Jr. Penetrating wounds of the great vessels. *Ann Surg* 1974; 179:757–762.
47. Symbas PN, Schlant RC, Logan WD Jr, et al. Traumatic aorticopulmonary fistula complicated by postoperative low cardiac output treated with dopamine. *Ann Surg* 1967; 165:614–619.
48. Parmley LF Jr, Orbison JA, Hughes CW, Mattingly TW. Acquired arteriovenous fistulas complicated by endarteritis and endocarditis lenta due to *Streptococcus faecalis. N Engl J Med* 1954; 250: 305–309.
49. Kissane RW. Traumatic heart diseases, especially myocardial contusion. *Postgrad Med* 1954; 15:114–119.
50. Stern T, Wolf RY, Reichart B, et al. Coronary artery occlusion resulting from blunt trauma. *JAMA* 1974; 230:1308–1309.
51. Levy H. Traumatic coronary thrombosis with myocardial infarction: Postmortem study. *Arch Intern Med* 1949; 84:261–276.
52. Forker AD, Morgan JR. Acquired coronary artery fistula from nonpenetrating chest injury. *JAMA* 1971; 215:289–291.
53. Louhimo I. Heart injury after blunt thoracic trauma: An experimental study on rabbits. *Acta Chir Scand Suppl* 1968; 380:1–60.
54. Dolara A, Morando P, Pampaloni M. Electrocardiographic findings in 98 consecutive nonpenetrating chest injuries. *Dis Chest* 1967; 52:50–56.
55. Jones FL Jr. Transmural myocardial necrosis after nonpenetrating cardiac trauma. *Am J Cardiol* 1970; 26:419–422.
56. Potkin RT, Werner JA, Trobaugh GB, et al. Evaluation of noninvasive tests of cardiac damage in suspected cardiac contusion. *Circulation* 1982; 66:627–631.
57. Hoffman B. The genesis of cardiac arrhythmias. *Prog Cardiovasc Dis* 1966; 8:319–329.
58. Marriott HJ, Nizet PM. Physiologic stimuli simulating ischemic heart disease. *JAMA* 1967; 200:715.
59. Tindall GT, Iwata K, McGraw CP, Vanderveer RW. Cardiorespiratory changes associated with intracranial pressure waves: Evaluation of these changes in 27 patients with head injuries. *South Med J* 1975; 68:407–412.
60. Rapaport E. Serum enzymes and isoenzymes in the diagnosis of acute myocardial infarction. *Mod Concepts Cardiovasc Dis* 1977; 46:43–46.
61. Manor A, Alpan G. Specificity of creatine kinase MB isoenzyme for myocardial injury. *Clin Chem* 1978; 24:2206.
62. Snow N, Richardson JD, Flynt LM Jr. Myocardial contusion: Implication for patients with multiple traumatic injuries. *Surgery* 1982; 92:744–750.
63. Gonzalez AC, Harlaftis N, Gravanis M, Symbas PN. Imaging of experimental myocardial contusion: Observations and pathologic correlations. *AJR* 1977; 128:1039–1040.
64. Miller FA Jr, Seward JB, Gersh BJ, et al. Two-dimensional echocardiographic findings in cardiac trauma. *Am J Cardiol* 1982; 50:1022–1027.
65. Shapiro NG, Yanofsky SD, Trapp I, et al. Cardiovascular evaluation in thoracic blunt trauma using transesophageal echocardiography (TEE). *J Trauma* 1991; 131:835–839.
66. Adams JE III, Davila-Roman VG, Bessey PQ, et al. Improved detection of cardiac contusion with cardiac troponin I. *Am Heart J* 1996; 131:308–312.
67. Snow N, Luca AE, Richardson JD. Intra-aortic balloon counterpulsation for cardiogenic shock from cardiac contusion. *J Trauma* 1982; 22:426–429.
68. Chavanon O, Dutheil V, Hacini R, et al. Treatment of severe cardiac contusion with a left ventricular assist device in a patient with multiple trauma. *J Thorac Cardivasc Surg* 1999; 118:189–190.
69. Symbas NP, Bongiorno PF, Symbas PN. Blunt cardiac rupture: The utility of emergency department ultrasound. *Ann Thorac Surg* 1999; 67:1274–1276.
70. Singh R, Nolan SP, Schrank JP. Traumatic left ventricular aneurysm: Two cases with normal coronary angiograms. *JAMA* 1975; 234:412–414.
71. Liu S, Sako Y, Alexander CS. Traumatic tricuspid insufficiency. *Am J Cardiol* 1970; 26:200–204.
72. Schroeder JS, Stinson EB, Bieber CP, et al. Papillary muscle dysfunction due to nonpenetrating chest trauma, recognition in a potential cardiac donor. *Br Heart J* 1972; 34:645–647.

73. Marvin RF, Schrank JP, Nolan SP. Traumatic tricuspid insufficiency. *Am J Cardiol* 1973; 32:723–726.
74. Munchow OBG, Carter R, Vannix RS, Anderson FS. Cardiac arrest due to ventricular herniation: Report of a case of two successful cardiac resuscitations. *JAMA* 1960; 173:1350–1351.
75. Anderson M, Fredens M, Olesson KH. Traumatic rupture of the pericardium. *Am J Cardiol* 1971; 27:566–569.
76. Feczko JD, Lynch L, Pless JE, et al. An autopsy case review of 142 nonpenetrating (blunt) injuries of the aorta. *J Trauma* 1992; 33:846–849.
77. Symbas PN, Tyras DH, Ware RE, DiOrio DA. Traumatic rupture of the aorta. *Ann Surg* 1973; 178:6–12.
78. Symbas PJ, Horsley SW, Symbas PN. Rupture of the ascending aorta caused by blunt trauma. *Ann Thorac Surg* 1998; 66:113–117.
79. Symbas PN, Tyras DH, Ware RE, Hatcher CR Jr. Rupture of the aorta: A diagnostic triad. *Ann Thorac Surg* 1973; 15:405–410.
80. Fenner MN, Fisher KS, Sergel NL, et al. Evaluation of possible traumatic thoracic aortic injury using aortography and CT. *Am Surg* 1990; 56:497–499.
81. Miller FB, Richardson JD, Thomas HA, et al. Role of CT in diagnosis of major arterial injury after blunt thoracic trauma. *Surgery* 1989; 106:596–603.
82. Galli R, Pacini O, Di Bartolomeo R, et al. Surgical indication and timing of repair of traumatic ruptures of the aorta. *Ann Thorac Surg* 1998; 65:461–464.
83. Kinley CE, Chandler BM. Traumatic aneurysm of thoracic aorta: A case presenting as coarctation. *Can Med Assoc J* 96:279, 1967.

CHAPTER 80

EFFECTS OF MOOD AND ANXIETY DISORDERS ON THE CARDIOVASCULAR SYSTEM

Dominique L. Musselman / William McDonald / Charles B. Nemeroff

And now here's my secret, a very simple secret: It is only with the heart that one can see rightly; what is essential is invisible to the eye. (Antoine de Saint-Exupery, *The Little Prince,* 1943)

INTRODUCTION: DEPRESSION AND COMORBID MEDICAL ILLNESS

The interactions of personality traits, psychiatric symptoms and syndromes, and environmental stressors with the cardiovascular system have long intrigued investigators interested in the factors that contribute to the development and progression of atherosclerotic heart disease. Differences in rates of ischemic heart disease (IHD) remain substantially unexplained even after surveillance of the well-established risk factors. Although the type A personality pattern has been studied intensely as a risk factor for coronary artery disease (CAD),[1] lack of a consistent association between type A behavior and the subsequent development of IHD has stimulated questions about the contributions of the psychological concept of hostility as well as the syndrome of major depression.[2] Increasing evidence is accumulating suggesting that major depression (Table 80-1),[3] a mood disorder, is associated with drastically elevated morbidity and mortality after an index myocardial infarction (MI) and also acts as an independent risk factor in the development of atherosclerotic heart disease.

Depressive syndromes and major depression are exceedingly common. The most recent comprehensive study done in the United States, the National Comorbidity Study, reported lifetime prevalence rates of major depression and dysthymia of 13 percent and 5 percent, respectively.[4] Point prevalence rates of major depression in primary care outpatients range from 2 to 16 percent and 9 to 20 percent for all depressive disorders[5–9] and are even higher among medical inpatients: 8 percent for major depression and 15 to 36 percent for all depressive disorders.[10,11]

Minor depressive disorder (depressive symptoms subthreshold in severity compared with major depression and dysthymia) is also common in the community[12–15] and in primary care clinics.[6,7,16,17] The Epidemiologic Catchment Area Study of over 18,500 individuals reported the lifetime prevalence rate of subthreshold depressive symptoms to be 23 percent in comparison to 6 percent, the sum of the prevalence rates of major depression and dysthymia.[15] Although depression in patients with CAD is diagnosed infrequently by primary care physicians and cardiologists,[18–22] recognition and treatment of major depression is crucial, especially for patients after an MI. Not only do depressed patients experience great difficulties in problem solving and coping with challenges, depression adversely effects compliance with medical therapy[23] and rehabilitation[24,25] and increases medical comorbidity.[24] Minor depressive disorder also is associated with significant functional impairment and substantial increases in health care utilization.[14,15,26,27]

In patients with CAD, depression predicts future cardiac events[20,28,29] and hastens mortality.[22,30,31] Since the 1960s, multiple cross-sectional and longitudinal studies have scrutinized the association of cardiovascular disease (CVD), especially CAD and congestive heart failure (CHF), with depressive symptoms as well as major depression.

TABLE 80-1 DSM-IV Diagnostic Criteria for Depressive Disorders

Major Depressive Disorder

A. Five or more of the following symptoms have been present during the same 2-week period and represent a change from previous functioning; at least one of the symptoms is either (1) depressed mood or (2) loss of interest or pleasure.
   1. Depressed mood
   2. Markedly diminished interest or pleasure
   3. Significant weight loss or weight gain or decrease or increase in appetite
   4. Insomnia or hypersomnia
   5. Psychomotor agitation or retardation (observable by others)
   6. Fatigue or loss of energy nearly every day
   7. Feelings of worthlessness or excessive or inappropriate guilt
   8. Diminished concentration or indecisiveness
   9. Recurrent thoughts of death (not just fear of dying) or suicide

B. The symptoms cause clinically significant distress or impairment in social, occupation, or other important areas of functioning.

C. The symptoms are not due to the direct physiologic effects of a substance or a general medical condition.

D. The symptoms are not better accounted for by bereavement.

Dysthymic Disorder

A. Depressed mood for most of the day, for more days than not, for at least 2 years

B. Presence, while depressed, of two or more of the following:
   1. Poor appetite or overeating
   2. Insomnia or hypersomnia
   3. Low energy or fatigue
   4. Low self-esteem
   5. Poor concentration or difficulty making decisions
   6. Feelings of hopelessness

C. The disturbance is not better accounted for by a chronic major depressive disorder.

SOURCE: Reprinted with permission from the *Diagnostic and Statistical Manual of Mental Disorders*, 4th ed. Copyright 1994, American Psychiatric Association.

EPIDEMIOLOGY

Depression and Cardiovascular Disease

Early studies reported the prevalence of depression to be 18 to 60 percent in patients with CAD.[18,24,31-34] Later studies reported relatively consistent prevalence rates of depression in patients with CVD (patients with CAD) ranging from 16 to 23 percent (mean, 19 percent; median, 18 percent) despite the potential methodologic weaknesses of some of the studies listed in Table 80-2 (such as the use of unmodified psychiatric diagnostic instruments to determine the prevalence of depression, excluding patients because of the severity of CVD, and measuring depressive symptoms at different times after hospital admission) and methodologic differences among the studies (dissimilar patient populations, different diagnostic instruments, different hospitalization status, unspecified type of heart disease).

Although the prevalence of major depressive symptoms in patients hospitalized for CHF has not been as well studied, preliminary evidence indicates that these patients have equally high or even higher rates of major depression.[37,39] However, although severity of physical illness is one of the most important variables associated with depression in patients with other medical illnesses, studies of patients with CVD do not always document a higher prevalence rate of depression in patients with measures of more advanced CVD or a greater level of disability.[20-22,31]

Depression as a Risk Factor for Ischemic Heart Disease

The notion that having a psychiatric illness such as major depression increases one's risk for developing ischemic heart disease remains controversial and often has been "explained" intuitively by the hypothesis that persons with psychiatric disorders generally have other risk factors for the development of CAD.[1] Table 80-3 describes the studies with the most rigorous methods: Those studies have been prospective in design, have used structured clinical interviews or diagnostic instruments, have included other risk factors for CVD in their analyses (such as hypertension, hypercholesterolemia, nicotine and other substance abuse, and physical inactivity), and have been controlled for demographic factors (such as age, sex, and socioeconomic status).

Nearly all the recent studies in Table 80-3 document increased cardiovascular morbidity and mortality in patients with depressive symptoms or major depression, implicating depression *as an independent risk factor* in the pathophysiologic progression of CVD rather than merely as a secondary emotional response to cardiovascular illness. Such large epidemiologic studies may use self-report instruments rather than clinical interviews to evaluate the importance of psychological factors in predicting CVD. Assessments of this type typically are added to large, multiple-risk-factor studies in which population-based samples are followed up prospectively.[1] The advantage of using "dimensional" measures of depression (rather than a categorical diagnosis of major depression) lies in the increased statistical power that allows these studies to detect smaller "effects." However, such epidemiologic data are not equivalent to clinical data. A relatively large clinical study supporting depression as an independent risk factor for CVD observed that patients with major depression experienced elevated mortality rates after an MI. Frasure-Smith and colleagues[22,31] found depression to be a significant predictor of mortality ($p < .001$) in 222 patients 6 months after an MI. Depression remained a significant predictor of mortality ($p = .01$) even after multivariate statistical methodology was used to factor out the effects of left ventricular dysfunction and previous MI. Multiple logistic regression analyses revealed that depression was significantly related to 18-month cardiac mortality even after controlling for other significant multivariate predictors of mortality [previous MI, Killip class,

TABLE 80-2 Prevalence of Major Depression in Patients with Cardiovascular Disease

Study	No./Type of Patients	Diagnostic Method	Prevalence, %
Carney et al., 1988[28]	52 CAD patients undergoing elective cardiac catheterization	DIS[35]	18
Schleifer et al., 1989[21]	283 patients hospitalized with MI	SADS[36]	18
Freedland et al., 1991[37]	60 patients hospitalized for CHF	Modified DIS[35]	17
Frasure-Smith et al., 1993[22]	222 patients hospitalized with MI	DIS[35]	16
Gonzalez et al., 1996[38]	99 hospitalized patients with CAD	DIS[35]	23
Koenig et al., 1998[39]	107 patients hospitalized with primary or secondary diagnosis of CHF	Expanded DIS[35]	37

ABBREVIATIONS: CAD = coronary artery disease; MI = myocardial infarction; DIS = Diagnostic Interview Schedule, Version III; SADS = Schedule for Affective Disorders and Schizophrenia.

SOURCE: Adapted from and reprinted with permission from *Archives of General Psychiatry* 55:580–592, July 1998. Copyrighted 1998, American Medical Association.

frequency of premature ventricular contractions (PVCs)] ($p = .003$).

PATHOPHYSIOLOGY

Hypothalamic-Pituitary-Adrenocortical and Sympathomedullary Hyperactivity

Recent advances in biological psychiatry have included the discovery of numerous neurochemical, neuroendocrine, and neuroanatomic alterations in unipolar depression. Often proposed as important adjuncts in the diagnosis of depressed subjects, some of these biological markers may reflect important pathophysiologic alterations that contribute to the increased vulnerability of depressed patients to CVD. These markers include sympathoadrenal hyperactivity, diminished heart rate variability (HRV), alterations in platelet receptors and/or reactivity, and ventricular instability and myocardial ischemia in reaction to mental stress (Fig. 80-1, Plate 110).

Two primary components that are central to the "fight or flight" stress response observed by Cannon in 1911[62] and the "general adaptation syndrome" described by Selye in 1956[63] are the hypothalamic-pituitary-adrenocortical axis and the sympathoadrenal system. In response to stress, hypothalamic neurons containing corticotropin-releasing factor (CRF) increase the synthesis and release of corticotropin (ACTH), β-endorphin, and other pro-opiomelanocortin (POMC) products from the anterior pituitary gland. Many studies have documented evidence of hypothalamic-pituitary-adrenocortical axis hyperactivity in medication-free patients with major depression, i.e., elevated CRF concentrations in cerebrospinal fluid,[64–69] blunting of the ACTH response to CRF administration, nonsuppression of cortisol secretion after dexamethasone administration, hypercortisolemia, and pituitary and adrenal gland enlargement, as well as direct evidence of increased numbers of hypothalamic CRF neurons in postmortem brain tissue from depressed patients compared with controls.[70,71] Administered corticosteroids have long been known to induce hypercholesterolemia, hypertriglyceridemia, and hypertension. Other atherosclerosis-inducing actions of steroids include injury to vascular endothelial cells[72] and intima[73–75] and the inhibition of normal healing.[76] Indeed, elevated morning plasma cortisol concentrations have been significantly correlated with moderate to severe coronary atherosclerosis in young and middle-aged men.[77]

Many patients with major depression also exhibit dysregulation of the sympathoadrenal system. The adrenal medulla and sympathetic nervous system (SNS) together constitute the sympathoadrenal system. Although central nervous system (CNS) regulation of the sympathoadrenal system has been only partially characterized, hypothalamic CRF-containing neurons provide stimulatory input to several autonomic centers that are involved in regulating sympathetic activity.[78–80] Nerve impulses from regulatory centers in the CNS control catecholamine release from the sympathoadrenal system. Physiologic and pathologic conditions causing sympathoadrenal activation include physical activity, coronary artery ischemia, heart failure, and mental stress. Epinephrine in plasma is derived from the adrenal medulla, whereas plasma norepinephrine (NE) concentrations reflect the secretion of NE largely from sympathetic nerve terminals, with the remaining NE provided by the adrenal medulla and extraadrenal chromaffin cells. Peripheral plasma NE concentrations are determined not only by the rate of release from sympathetic nervous system nerve terminals but also by reuptake into presynaptic terminals, local metabolic degradation, and redistribution into multiple physiologic compartments. Hypersecretion of NE in unipolar depression has been documented by elevated plasma NE and NE metabolite concentrations[81–84] and elevated urinary concentrations of NE and its metabolites. Not only do depressed patients exhibit higher basal plasma concentrations of NE, those with melancholia exhibit even greater elevations in plasma NE concentrations when subjected to orthostatic challenge than do normal control subjects and depressed patients *without* melancholia.[85] Furthermore, depressed patients who are dexamethasone (DST) nonsuppressors exhibit significantly higher basal and cold-stimulated plasma concentrations of NE than do depressed patients who are DST suppressors.[85] After treatment with tricyclic antidepressants (TCAs), urinary excretion of NE and its metabolites diminishes together with plasma NE concentrations,[86–91] although Veith and colleagues[84] reported that chronic treatment with desipramine increased plasma concentrations of NE. Thus, sympathoadrenal hyperactivity seems to represent a state rather than a state or

TABLE 80-3 Antecedent Depression and Subsequent Risk of Cardiovascular Disease

Source	No./Type of Patients	Diagnostic Method	Relative Risk (RR) of Major Depression or Depressive Symptoms for Cardiac Disease or Cardiac Disease–Related Death
Ostfeld et al., 1964[40]	1990 male patients Western Electric Employees	MMPI[41] 16 PF[42]	None
Brozek et al., 1966[43]	258 men	MMPI[41]	None
Goldberg et al., 1979[44]	82 pairs (male and female) of case-control subjects randomly selected from two communities	CES-D Scale[45] and four other depression scales	None
Murphy et al., 1987[46]	1003 male and female subjects from the community	DPAX algorithm[47]	For cardiovascular disease-related death: Men 2.5 Women 1.5
Anda et al., 1993[48]	2832 men and women (age 45–77)	Depression subscale of GWS[49]	For IHD-related death: Depressed affect 1.5 [95% confidence interval (CI): 1.0–2.3] Severe hopelessness 2.1 (95% CI: 1.1–3.9)
Aromaa et al., 1994[29]	5355 men and women (age 40–64)	PSE[50]	For MI: Men 2.62 Women 1.90
Vogt et al., 1994[51]	1187 men and 1386 women (age 18 and older) in an HMO	Depression scale[52]	Depressive symptoms *not* related to incidence of CVD
Simonsick et al., 1995[53]	1063 men and 2398 women (age 65 years and older with hypertension)	CES-D Scale[45]	Elevated rates of CVD-related death in women with high scores on depressive symptoms
Everson et al., 1996[54]	2428 men (age 42–60)	Hopelessness self-report questionnaire	For CVD-related death: RH: 2.52 (95% CI: 1.52–4.17) (moderate hopelessness score) RH: 3.90 (95% CI: 2.14–7.11) (high hopelessness score)
Barefoot and Schroll, 1996[55]	409 men and 321 women (all born in 1914)	MMPI[56]	For MI: 1.7 (95% CI: 1.23–2.34)
Pratt et al., 1996[57]	1551 men and women	DIS	For MI: OR: 2.07 (95% CI: 1.16–3.71) (hx of dysphoria) OR: 4.54 (95% CI: 1.65–12.44) (hx of MDE)
Wassertheil-Smoller et al., 1996[58]	4736 men and women over age 60 with hypertension	CES-D[45]	Baseline CES-D score ≥16 did *not* predict future MI RR of future MI per 5-unit increase in CES-D score: women 1.25 (95% CI: 1.15–1.36)
Callahan et al., 1998[59]	3767 men and women 60 years and older	CES-D[45]	None
Mendes de Leon et al., 1998[60]	2812 men and women 65 years and older	CES-D[45]	None
Ford et al., 1998[61]	1190 men 55 years and older	Depression questionnaire	For MI: RR: 2.12 (95% CI: 1.11–4.06)

ABBREVIATIONS: RH = relative hazard; IHD = ischemic heart disease; MI = myocardial infarction; hx = history; MDE = episode of major depression; OR = odds ratio; CI = confidence interval.

SOURCE: Adapted from and reprinted with permission from *Archives of General Psychiatry* 55:580–592, July 1998. Copyright 1998, American Medical Association.

The Relationship Between Major Depression and Cardiovascular Disease

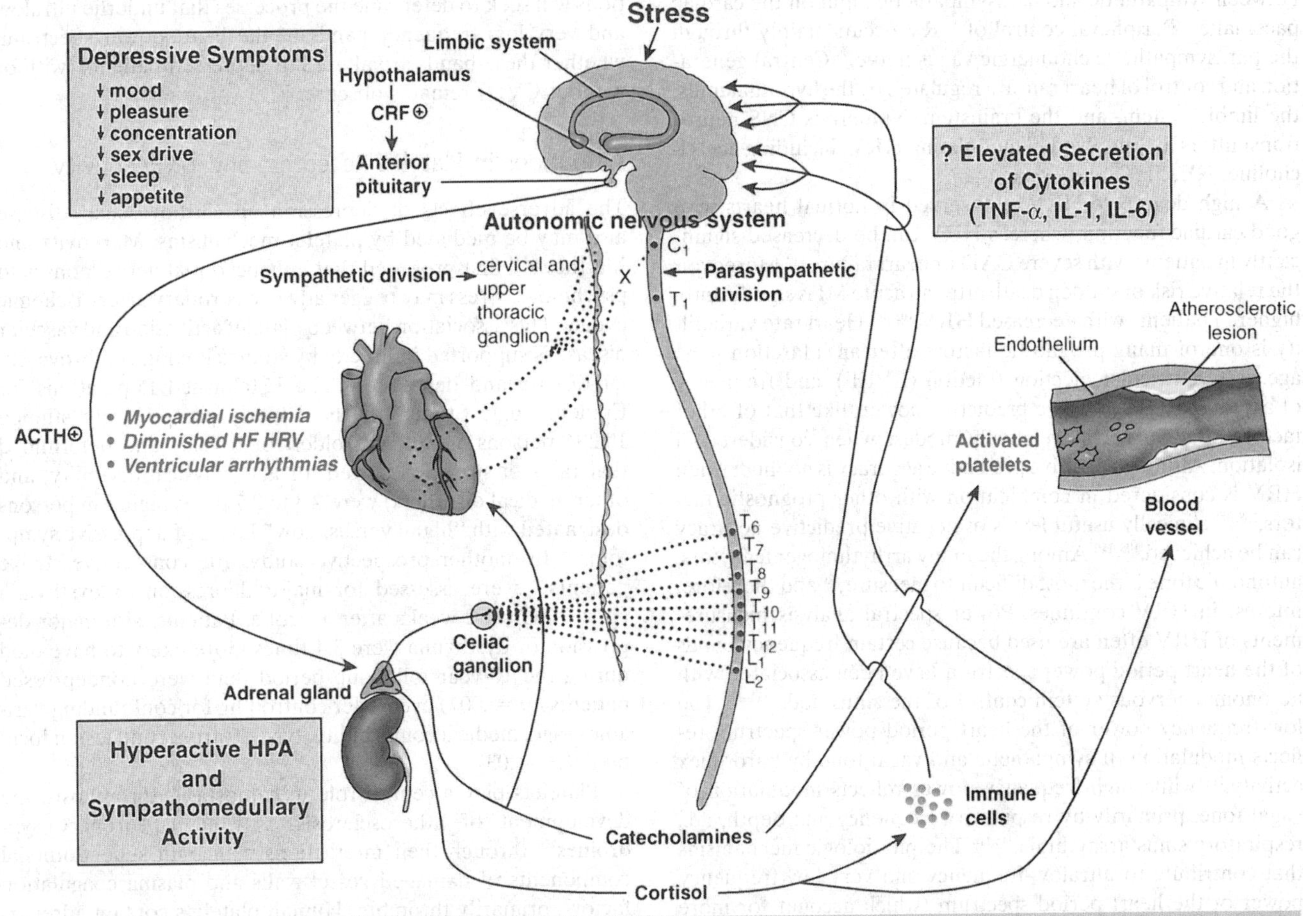

FIGURE 80-1 (Plate 110) Hypothetical schema of pathophysiologic findings associated with depression that probably contribute to increased susceptibility to cardiovascular disease. Autonomic nervous system innervation of the heart via the parasympathetic vagus (X) nerve and sympathetic (postganglionic efferents from the cervical and upper thoracic paravertebral ganglia) nerves is shown. CRF = corticotropin-releasing factor; ACTH = corticotropin; TNF-α = tumor necrosis factor α; IL-1 = interleukin-1; IL-6 = interleukin-6; HRV = heart rate variability; HPA = hypothalamic-pituitary-adrenocortical axis.

trait marker of depression, possibly reflecting increased CRF release within the CNS.

Sympathoadrenal hyperactivity contributes to the development of CVD through effects of catecholamines on the heart, blood vessels, and platelets. Sympathoadrenal activation modifies the function of circulating platelets through direct effects on platelets, catecholamine-induced changes in hemodynamic factors (increased shear stress), circulating lipids, and inhibition of vascular eicosanoid synthesis.[92] Arachidonic acid metabolites such as prostaglandins and leukotrienes contribute to diverse circulatory and hemostatic functions, including inhibition of platelet aggregation, and vascular contractility and permeability.[93] Elevations of plasma NE levels are found most frequently in young hypertensive patients[94] and in subjects with high-cardiac-output borderline hypertension who later proceed to established high-resistance hypertension.[95] Even normotensive depressed patients have been found to exhibit greater heart rates at rest, after orthostasis, and after exercise in comparison with normal controls. These depressed patients also exhibited increased plasma concentrations of NE and serotonin (5HT) at rest.[96] Thus, the sympathoadrenal hyperactivity observed in many patients with major depression may contribute to the development of CVD through the effects of catecholamines on cardiac function and platelets.

Diminished Heart Rate Variability

Alterations in autonomic nervous system activity, as demonstrated by reduced HRV, represent another mechanism that potentially contributes to the diminished survival of depressed patients with CVD. It is believed that the beat-to-beat fluctuations in hemodynamic parameters reflect the dynamic response of cardiovascular control systems to a myriad of naturally occurring physiologic perturbations, such as fluctuations in heart rate associated with respiration. Therefore, HRV may provide a sensitive measure of the functioning of the rapidly reacting sympathetic, parasympathetic, and renin-angiotensin systems. Cardiovascular homeostasis is maintained by the parasympathetic and sympathetic nervous systems through afferent pressor receptors and chemoreceptors and efferents that alter heart rate, atrioventricular conduction, and contractility, and impinge on the peripheral vasculature, altering arterial and venous vasomotor tone.[97] HRV is the standard deviation of successive R–R intervals in sinus rhythm and reflects the interplay and balance between sympathetic and parasympathetic input on the cardiac pacemaker. Peripheral control of HRV occurs mainly through the parasympathetic cholinergic vagus nerve.[98] Central generation and control of heart rate are regulated by the hypothalamus, the limbic system, and the brainstem. Numerous CNS neurotransmitters are involved in modulating HRV, including acetylcholine, NE, 5HT, and dopamine.[99,100]

A high degree of HRV is observed in normal hearts with good cardiac function, whereas HRV can be decreased significantly in patients with severe CAD or heart failure.[101] Moreover, the relative risk of sudden death after an acute MI is significantly higher in patients with decreased HRV.[102–107] Heart rate variability is one of many prognostic factors after an infarction [e.g., age, left ventricular ejection fraction (LVEF), and frequency of arrythmias]. Its positive predictive power, like that of other factors after an MI, is relatively modest when considered in isolation. Although positive predictive accuracy is not high when HRV is considered in combination with other prognostic factors,[108,109] clinically useful levels of negative predictive accuracy can be achieved.[108–110] Among the many arrhythmogenic factors, autonomic tone is the most difficult to measure,[110] and therefore, interest in HRV continues. Power spectral analysis measurements of HRV often are used because certain frequency bands of the heart period power spectrum have been associated with autonomic nervous system control of the sinus node.[111–113] The low-frequency power of the heart period power spectrum reflects modulation of sympathetic and vagal tone by baroreflex activity,[114] while high-frequency power reflects modulation of vagal tone, primarily by respiratory frequency and depth, i.e., respiratory sinus arrhythmia.[115,116] The physiologic mechanisms that contribute to ultralow-frequency and very low frequency power of the heart period spectrum (which account for more than 90 percent of the total power in a 24-h period) remain obscure. In a study of 715 patients after MI, certain frequency bands (total, ultralow, and very low frequencies) of the heart period power spectrum were strongly associated with mortality during 4 years of follow-up even after adjustment for other major risk factors. Indeed, very low frequency power was most strongly associated with death secondary to arrhythmia.[117]

Reduced high-frequency HRV has been observed in depressed patients in comparison with nondepressed groups,[101,118] although discrepant reports exist.[119,120] In patients with angiographically confirmed CAD, diminished HRV during 24-h Holter monitoring was significantly more common in depressed patients than in matched nondepressed patients.[121] Diminished high-frequency HRV is thought to reflect decreased parasympathetic tone, possibly predisposing patients to ventricular arrhythmias and perhaps to the excessive cardiovascular mortality found in CVD patients with a comorbid major depressive disorder.[122] Diminished HRV in patients with major depression also may be contributed to by a deficiency of omega-3 fatty acids[123] in this patient population. Not only have multiple studies documented a deficiency of omega-3 fatty acids in patients with major depression,[124–126] these polyunsaturated lipids possess antiarrhythmic properties and reduce the risk of ventricular arrhythmias.[127–132]

One study (without a placebo control group) revealed normalization of reduced HRV in depressed patients after effective treatment.[133] The prognostic importance of antidepressant-induced improvement in diminished HRV in depressed patients remains an intriguing area of research. Subsequent investigations will seek to determine the processes that underlie ultralow and very low frequency bands of the heart power spectrum; whether these bands are altered in depressed patients (with or without CVD) remains obscure.

Alterations in Platelet Receptors and/or Reactivity

The adverse effects of depression on cardiovascular disease also may be mediated by platelet mechanisms. Markovitz and Matthews[134] first proposed that enhanced platelet responses to psychologic stress may trigger adverse coronary artery ischemic events. This association between platelet activation and vascular disease is supported indirectly by studies linking cerebrovascular disease and depression. The Established Populations for Epidemiologic Studies of the Elderly prospectively studied 10,294 persons age 65 and older for 6 years and determined that rates of stroke (adjusted for age, physical disability, and other medical disorders) were 2.3 to 2.7 times higher in persons designated with "high" versus "low" levels of depressive symptoms.[53] In another prospective study, 103 consecutive stroke patients[135] were assessed for major depression or dysthymia approximately 2 weeks after a stroke. Patients with major depression or dysthymia were 3.4 times more likely to have died during the 10-year follow-up period than were nondepressed patients ($p = .007$) even after controlling for confounding variables (age, medical comorbidity, type of stroke, and lesion location) ($p = .03$).

Platelets play a central role in hemostasis, thrombosis, the development of atherosclerosis, and acute coronary syndromes[136] through their interactions with both subendothelial components of damaged vessel walls and plasma coagulation factors, primarily thrombin. Human platelets contain adrenergic, serotonergic, and dopaminergic receptors. Through activation of platelet alpha$_2$ adrenoceptors, increases in circulating catecholamines (>4 nmol/L) potentiate the effects of other agonists and, at higher concentrations, initiate platelet thrombotic responses, including secretion, aggregation, and activation of the arachidonate pathway. After injury to vessel endothelium, platelets and circulating leukocytes attach to the newly exposed subendothelial layer. Platelets adhere to collagen (and other components of the subendothelial matrix) exposed within a denuded area of the vascular endothelium. Thrombin stimulates platelet activation, converting platelet membrane GPIIb/IIIa complexes into functional receptors for fibrinogen. Activation also is accompanied by extrusion or secretion of platelet storage granule contents into the extracellular environment. Platelets activated at the site of an injury to the vessel wall accelerate the local formation of thrombin and release a variety of products from their storage granules, including chemotactic and mitogenic factors, inducing leukocyte migration from the bloodstream and vascular cell proliferation. These secreted platelet products, e.g., platelet factor 4, β-thromboglobulin (β-TG), and 5HT, stimulate and recruit other platelets and cause irreversible platelet-platelet aggregation, ultimately leading to the formation of a fused platelet thrombus. Platelets also contribute to vascular damage by stimulating lipoprotein uptake by macrophages and mediating vasoconstriction through the production and/or release of substances such as thromboxane A_2, platelet-activating factor, and 5HT.[92] Clinical trials have confirmed the importance of platelets in vascular damage; antiaggregating medications are useful in secondary prevention,[137–139] delay the progression of atherosclerotic lesions,[140] and improve post-MI outcomes.[141,142]

The authors sought to determine whether heightened susceptibility to platelet activation might be a mechanism by which depression in physically healthy young volunteers acts as a significant risk factor for cardiovascular and cerebrovascular disease and/or increased mortality after MI. Utilizing fluorescence-activated flow cytometric analysis, the authors discovered that in comparison with 8 normal controls, 12 depressed patients as a group exhibited enhanced baseline platelet activation as well as increased platelet responsiveness.[143]

In one study, 21 elderly patients suffering from comorbid CVD and major depression exhibited increased platelet activation as measured by markedly elevated plasma concentrations of the platelet secretion products PF4 and β-TG compared with 17 healthy control subjects and 8 *non*depressed age-matched patients with CVD.[144] Although the mechanism or mechanisms responsible remain unknown, the authors believe that heightened susceptibility to platelet activation and secretion underlies, at least in part, the increased vulnerability of depressed patients to CVD and/or mortality after an MI.

Serotonin secreted by platelets induces both platelet aggregation and coronary vasoconstriction, both of which are mediated by $5HT_2$ receptors. Vasoconstriction occurs especially when normal endothelial cell counterregulatory mechanisms of vascular relaxation are defective, as often occurs in patients with CAD.[144–146] Indeed, essential hypertension, elevated plasma cholesterol levels, older age, and smoking, which are well-known predisposing factors for the development of CVD, all contribute to 5HT-mediated platelet activation. Moreover, alterations in platelet 5HT-mediated activation also have been described in affective disorders, most notably major depression. Considerable evidence has accrued in the last two decades that supports the hypothesis that alterations in CNS and platelet serotonergic function occur in depressed patients.[147]

Serotonin-mediated platelet activation can contribute to the development of atherosclerosis, thrombosis, and vasoconstriction. Even though 5HT is a weak platelet agonist, it markedly amplifies platelet reactions to a variety of other agonists such as adenosine diphosphate (ADP), thromboxane A_2, catecholamines, and thrombin. Through an action on $5HT_2$ receptors, serotonin enhances platelet aggregation and the release of intragranular products and arachidonic acid metabolites in response to otherwise ineffective agonist concentrations.[146] This 5HT-induced platelet amplification occurs at the low concentrations attained when indoleamine is released from seeping platelets subjected to shear stresses[148] and from platelet activation by contact with an arterial wall lesion.[149,150] Several investigators have reported *increases* in platelet $5HT_2$ binding density in depressed patients.[151–155] Moreover, the changes appear to be state-dependent in that $5HT_2$ binding-site density returned to control values only in patients who showed clinical improvement. Depressed patients have been found to exhibit significant *reductions* in the number of platelet and brain 5HT transporter sites as detected by [^{3}H] imipramine binding[68,156–158] as well as by the more selective ligand [^{3}H] paroxetine.[147,159] The increased $5HT_2$ receptor binding density and decreased 5HT transporter sites suggest that depressed patients may be particularly susceptible to 5HT-mediated platelet activation and coronary artery vasoconstriction. Decreased numbers of platelet 5HT transporters would potentially hinder the uptake and storage of periplatelet serotonin, exposing the increased numbers of $5HT_2$ receptors to 5HT.[160]

Platelets from depressed patients exhibit significantly increased elevations of intracellular free calcium concentration, $[Ca^{2+}]i$, after 5HT-induced stimulation in comparison to controls.[161–164] Even functionally trivial increases in intraplatelet calcium "prime" the platelet secretion and aggregation response to stimulation by even a "weak" agonist such as 5HT[165] or in response to increased blood flow. Thus, platelets with elevated $[Ca^{2+}]i$, as are observed in depressed patients, probably would exhibit increased activation in comparison with normal comparison subjects under basal conditions or in response to shear-induced aggregation (e.g., after an orthostatic challenge). Future investigations will attempt to confirm and connect the pathophysiologic mechanisms of sympathoadrenal hyperactivity, exaggerated platelet reactivity, and alterations in the platelet 5HT system in depressed patients to the propensity of those patients for the development of CVD.

Myocardial Ischemia and Ventricular Instability in Reaction to Mental Stress

The combination of a vulnerable myocardium after MI, acute ischemia, and negative emotional arousal is thought to trigger fatal ventricular arrythmias.[166] The interplay of these factors in patients with CAD is being scrutinized. Jiang and colleagues[167] longitudinally assessed 126 patients with CAD over a 5-year period. Mental stress–induced myocardial ischemia at baseline in CAD patients was associated with significantly higher rates of subsequent fatal and nonfatal cardiac events independently of age, baseline LVEF, and previous MI. This study proposed that the relation between psychological stress and adverse cardiac events is mediated by myocardial ischemia. Although myocardial ischemia probably is the most significant factor in predisposition to ventricular instability, other factors also contribute. CNS control mechanisms can significantly decrease the threshold for ventricular fibrillation.[168] Ventricular fibrillation is believed to be the mechanism underlying sudden cardiac death, the most common cause of fatality among patients with CAD.[169] Indeed, psychological stress predisposes to abnormal ventricular activity by lowering the ventricular vulnerable-period threshold even to the point of fibrillation. The vagus nerve, however, exerts antiarrthymic activity through a direct action on the ventricular myocardium and interference with sympathetic activity.[170] Increased parasympathetic activity has a protective effect on myocardium electrically destabilized by increased adrenergic tone.[169]

Psychological and physical events can elicit a stress response, which usually is defined as the reaction of an organism to deleterious forces that disturb physiologic homeostasis.[171,172] Psychological stress in humans with CAD increases ventricular ectopic activity and increases the risk of ventricular fibrillation.[173,174] There are several similarities between the stress response and major depression: both can be characterized by increased blood pressure and heart rate as well as increased arousal and increased mobilization of energy stores.[175] Particularly relevant to both the stress response and depression are the critical brain structures the locus coeruleus and the central nucleus of the amygdala, which both are innervated by CRF-containing nerve terminals.[176,177] The stress response and major depression differ in some respects, however. In depression, some aspects of the normal stress response seem to escalate to a pathologic state[178] that fails to respond appropriately to usual counterregulatory responses, resulting in a sustained version of a usually transient phenomenon, i.e., hyperactivity of the hypothalamic-pituitary-adrenocortical (HPA) axis or the sympathoadrenal system. Although many studies have linked stressful life events to the onset of major depression,[179,180] some depressions are clearly endogeneous—i.e., they have no obvious environmental precipitant—although in most of these studies the role of early adverse events that are now known to be of paramount importance was not assessed.

Frasure-Smith and colleagues[31] proposed that depression worsens the prognosis after an MI through another mechanism: PVCs. The risk of sudden cardiac death associated with significant depressive symptoms (Beck Depression Inventory score ≥10) was greatest among patients with 10 or more PVCs per hour (60 percent of these patients died within 18 months), suggesting arrythymia as the link between depression and sudden cardiac death.[31] Depressed patients with CAD are not more likely to have arrhythmias than are nondepressed patients with CAD, but the risk associated with depression is confined largely to patients with PVCs. Patients who were *not* depressed experienced little increase in risk associated with PVCs even in the presence of a low LVEF.[31] Thus, the prognostic impact of PVCs may be related more to depression than to PVCs per se. In the Cardiac Arrhythmia Suppression Trial (CAST),[181] suppression of PVC frequency in post-MI patients did not reduce but actually increased mortality even though PVCs are associated with increased mortality after an MI. Treatment of depression may be necessary to improve survival in depressed patients with PVCs.[182]

ANXIETY DISORDERS AND CARDIOVASCULAR DISEASE

Epidemiology

Anxiety disorders are the most prevalent psychiatric disorders in the United States (Table 80-4), with simple phobias being the most common (9 percent) and social phobia (8 percent) being the most often observed (Tables 80-5 and 80-6). A survey of adult primary care patients (n = 637) enrolled in a health maintenance organization revealed that 10 percent had untreated anxiety disorders.[183]

TABLE 80-4 12-Month Prevalence of DSM-III-R Disorders in the National Comorbidity Survey

Disorder	Percent
Any anxiety disorder	19.3
Any addictive disorder	11.3
Any mood disorder	11.3
Nonaffective psychosis	0.3
Any National Comorbidity Survey disorder	30.9

SOURCE: From Kessler et al.[4]

TABLE 80-5 12-Month Prevalence of Diagnosed Anxiety Disorders in the National Comorbidity Survey

Disorder	Percent
Simple phobia	8.8
Social phobia	7.9
Posttraumatic stress disorder	3.9
Generalized anxiety disorder	3.1
Agoraphobia	2.8
Panic disorder	2.3
Obsessive-compulsive disorder	<1.0
Any anxiety disorder	19.3

SOURCE: From Kessler et al.[4]

Unfortunately, anxiety disorders, though common, remain largely undiagnosed and undertreated.[183,184] Stereotyped as the "worried well," patients with anxiety disorders such as phobias, panic disorder, and generalized anxiety disorder have substantially higher rates of health service utilization, increased social and role disability, diminished quality of life, and poor health outcomes.[183,185–189] Moreover, the comorbidity of anxiety and affective disorders is substantial. Nearly 60 percent of patients with major depression in the National Comorbidity Survey suffered from a comorbid anxiety disorder.[4] Indeed, patients with mixed anxiety and depressive symptoms (or comorbid anxiety and depressive syndromes) suffer increased emotional disability as well as poorer social and role function in comparison to patients with either condition alone.[183,188] *After elective catheterization, the physical disability of patients with CAD at 1 year of follow-up was associated with the severity of these patients' anxiety and depressive symptoms at catheterization,* not *with the number of main coronary vessels stenosed.*[184]

The prevalence of anxiety disorders in patients with CVD has been largely understudied, with most studies focusing on patients with mitral valve prolapse or individuals referred for evaluation of chest pain. Substantial numbers of patients each year who undergo coronary angiography because of symptoms of chest pain (yet have normal coronary arteries) are thought to have anxiety disorders such as panic disorder (Table 80-7). Subsequently categorized as having "atypical chest pain," these patients may suffer chest pain in response to anxiety and/or hyperventilation.[190–193]

However, a large, multicity survey of 875 primary care outpatients revealed that patients with CHF or MI exhibited a point prevalence rate of at least one anxiety disorder (panic disorder, phobia, or generalized anxiety disorder) of 18 percent[189] (Table 80-8). Whether the prevalence of anxiety disorders is elevated in patients who are hospitalized for CAD (e.g., elective coronary catheterization, post-MI, or unstable angina) remains to be determined.

A small number of prospective epidemiologic studies (which control for many of the commonly accepted risk factors for IHD) indicate an increased relative risk of nonfatal and fatal CVD events in patients with anxiety symptoms, even among individuals who have "simple" phobias, e.g., claustrophobia and fear of illness, heights, crowds, or going out alone (Table 80-9).

Moreover, an ancillary study of 348 CAST and CAST II participants who had asymptomatic ventricular arrhythmias

TABLE 80-6 Diagnostic Criteria for the Most Common DSM-IV Anxiety Disorders

DSM-IV Criteria for Simple Phobia

Marked and persistent fear that is excessive or unreasonable, cued by the presence or anticipation of a specific object or situation (e.g., flying, heights, animals, receiving an injection, seeing blood).

Exposure to the phobic stimulus almost invariably provokes an immediate anxiety response, which may take the form of a situationally bound or situationally predisposed panic attack.

The person (adults only) recognizes that the feature is excessive or unreasonable.

The phobic situation is avoided or is endured with intense anxiety or distress.

The avoidance, anxious anticipation, or distress in the feared situations interferes significantly with the person's normal routine, occupational (or academic) functioning or social activities or relationships or there is marked distress about having the phobia.

DSM-IV Diagnostic Criteria for Social Phobia

Marked fear of being focus of attention; avoidance of meeting unfamiliar people and close scrutiny by others

Fear of behaving in embarassing or humiliating way

Extreme anticipatory anxiety which may manifest as a panic attack

DSM-IV Diagnostic Criteria for Posttraumatic Stress Disorder

Experience of a traumatic event

Reexperienced by intrusive and distressing recollection, dreams, flashbacks, distress in similar situations

Persistent avoidance of stimuli associated with trauma

Persistent symptoms of increased arousal

Duration of disturbance of at least 1 month

DSM-IV Diagnostic Criteria for Panic Disorder

Recurrent and unexpected panic attacks plus one or more of the following:
- Persistent concern about having additional attacks (anticipatory anxiety)
- Worry about the consequences of the attacks
- A significant change in behavior related to the attacks (phobic avoidance)

Not due to a substance, medical condition, or mental illness

At least two unexpected panic attacks for diagnosis

Definition of Panic Attack

A period of intense fear or discomfort in which at least four of the following symptoms develop suddenly

—Palpitations or increased heart rate
—Sweating
—Trembling or shaking
—Sensations of shortness of breath or smothering
—Feeling of choking
—Nausea or abdominal distress
—Chest pain or discomfort
—Dizziness, light-headedness, or faintness
—Derealization or depersonalization
—Fear of losing control or going crazy
—Chills or hot flashes
—Paresthesia (numbness or tingling)
—Fear of dying

DSM-IV Criteria for Generalized Anxiety Disorder

Excessive anxiety and worry for more days than not for past 6 months

Difficulty controlling worry

Functional impairment and/or distress

Symptoms not attributable to other causes

Physical symptoms
- Restlessness or feeling keyed up/on edge
- Fatigue
- Muscle tension

Psychological symptoms
- Excessive anxiety or worry
- Difficulty controlling worry
- Irritability
- Difficulty concentrating or mind going blank
- Sleep disturbance

TABLE 80-7 Prevalence of Anxiety Disorders in Patients Referred for Cardiologic Evaluation

Study	No./Type of Patients	Prevalence	Diagnostic Method
Bass and Wade, 1984[194]	99 patients without history of CAD referred for coronary arteriography due to CP	Of 31 patients without CAD: 29% with "anxiety neurosis"	Clinical Interview Schedule[195]
Cormier et al., 1988[196]	98 patients without history of CAD referred for coronary arteriography or ECG exercise tolerance testing due to CP	Of 49 patients without CAD: 47% with panic disorder 39% with major depression 43% with two or more phobias	DIS[35]

ABBREVIATIONS: CAD = coronary artery disease; CP = chest pain; Hx = history.

TABLE 80-8 Prevalence of Comorbid Anxiety Disorders in Primary Care Outpatients*

	Major Depression, %	Hypertension, %	Diabetes, %	Heart Disease, %
Panic disorder	9.4	0.9†	1.1†	1.2†
Phobia	22.7	5.5†	4.8†	9.2†
Generalized anxiety disorder	54.1	10.4†	11.9†	12.4†
Any anxiety disorder	66.3	14.6†	15.5†	17.8†

*Diagnosis of congestive heart failure or myocardial infarction within the previous year, adjusted for patient age, sex, race, education, marital status, income, study site, and each of the other medical or psychiatric conditions.
†Value significantly different from that of patients with current depression ($p \leq .05$), based on regression coefficients.
SOURCE: Sherbourne et al.[189]

TABLE 80-9 Antecedent Anxiety and Subsequent Risk of Cardiovascular Disease

Source	No./Type of Patients	Diagnostic Method	Relative Risk (RR) of Anxiety or Anxiety Symptoms for Cardiac Disease or Cardiac Disease–Related Death
Haines et al., 1987[197]	1457 men (age 40–62)	Crown-Crisp Index	For fatal MI: 3.77 (95% CI: 1.64–8.64)
Eaker et al., 1992[198]	749 women (age 45–64)	Somatic strain scale	For myocardial infarction and fatal CAD: 7.8 (95% CI: 1.9–32.3)
Kawachi et al., 1994[199]	33,999 men (age 42–77)	Crown-Crisp Index	For fatal MI: 2.45 (95% CI: 1.00–5.96) for men with "highest" phobic anxiety
Kawachi et al., 1994[200]	2271 men (age 21–80)	5-item anxiety scale from Cornell Medical Index	For CVD-related sudden death, OR: 4.5 (95% CI: 0.92–21.6)

ABBREVIATIONS: MI = myocardial infarction; CAD = coronary artery disease; CVD = cardiovascular disease; CI = confidence interval; OR = odds ratio.

after MI and were treated with placebo revealed that stressful life events during the initial 4 months of participation in CAST trial and higher anxiety were predictive of mortality independently of the effects of physiologic variables such as diabetes and ejection fraction.[182]

PATHOPHYSIOLOGY OF ANXIETY

The neurocircuitry of anxiety has been postulated to arise from the amygdala, the brain area that registers the emotional significance of environmental stimuli and stores emotional memories. The efferent pathways from the central nucleus of the amygdala travel to a multiplicity of critical brain structures, including the parabrachial nucleus (resulting in dyspnea and hyperventilation), the dorsomedial nucleus of the vagus nerve and nucleus ambiguous (activating the parasympathetic nervous system), and the lateral hypothalamus (resulting in SNS activation).[201] Through reciprocal neuronal pathways connecting the amygdala to the medial prefrontal cortex, cognitive experience of the specific anxiety disorder differs, although fear symptoms may overlap. During panic attacks the fear is of imminent death; in social phobia, the fear is of embarassment; in postraumatic stress disorder, the traumatic memory is remembered or reexperienced; in obsessive-compulsive disorder, obsessional ideas recur and intrude; and in generalized anxiety disorder, anxiety is "free-floating," i.e., not conditioned to specific situations or triggers.[202]

Described in the past with terms such as *cardiac neurosis, irritable heart syndrome, battle fatigue,* and *soldier's heart, panic disorder is the anxiety disorder most often associated with cardiovascular symptoms of chest pain, tachycardia, and dyspnea.* Discrete panic attacks can be induced in the laboratory setting, especially in patients with panic disorder, by a variety of stimuli: sodium lactate, caffeine, isoproterenol, the serotonin receptor agonist m-chlorophenylpiperazine (m-CPP), cholecystokinin tetrapeptide (CCK_4), inhalation of CO_2-enriched air, and voluntary acute hyperventilation of room air. The common element among these disparate inducers may be their ability to stimulate the respiratory rate with the induction of an accompanying subjective sense of breathlessness.[203] Although some researchers have proposed that patients with panic disorder have only a heightened sensitivity to and develop a learned intolerance of tachypnea,[204,205] the higher concordance rate of panic disorder observed in monozygotic compared with dizygotic twins[206] and evidence of altered respiratory rhythym during sleep[207,208] provide evidence of a genetic diathesis and a biological abnormality, respectively, underlying the phenotype of panic disorder.[203]

PATHOPHYSIOLOGY OF ANXIETY DISORDERS: A FOCUS ON THE CARDIOVASCULAR SYSTEM

Although the neurobiology of specific anxiety disorders has not been explored as fully as that of unipolar depression, potential neurochemical, neuroendocrine, and neuroanatomic alterations have not only been identified but increasingly scrutinized. Patients with major depression or anxiety disorders may experience common symptoms, e.g., alterations in psychomotor activity, impairment of sleep, increased appetite, and reduced concentration. Moreover, there are several shared neurobiological findings between patients with certain common syndromal anxiety disorders and those with depression, although differences also exist. The neurobiology of patients with certain anxiety disorders is reviewed below, with attention to mechanisms that contribute to the development of cardiovascular disease and/or cardiac-related mortality: HPA axis activity, sympathomedullary activity, diminished HRV, and alterations in platelet receptor number or function.

The only anxiety disorder in which alterations of HPA axis activity have been documented repeatedly is posttraumatic stress disorder (PTSD). In nearly all controlled studies of PTSD patients, alterations of HPA axis hyperactivity have been documented, including elevations of cerebrospinal fluid (CSF) CRF concentrations[209,210] and blunting of the ACTH response to CRF stimulation.[211] In comparison to control subjects, however, PTSD patients generally exhibit reduced plasma cortisol concentrations, diminished 24-h urinary cortisol concentrations, and a greater suppression of plasma cortisol concentrations in response to low doses (e.g., 0.5 mg) of dexamethasone.[212–216] However the two studies that measured CSF CRF concentrations in PTSD[209,210] found results identical to those repeatedly reported in depression: elevated CSF CRF concentrations. Whether patients with PTSD experience an increased (or decreased) relative risk of CVD is not known. Potential confounds in those studies include the very high rate of comorbid substance abuse and alcoholism as well as tobacco abuse in PTSD patients. Patients with panic disorder do not appear to exhibit alterations in HPA axis function consistently; scrutiny continues of patients with social phobia, generalized anxiety disorder, and obsessive-compulsive disorder.

Sympathomedullary function has been investigated intensively in patients with panic disorder. As was discussed previously, plasma concentrations of catecholamines are determined by the rate of release, local metabolic degradation, synaptic reuptake, and redistribution into other extravascular spaces.[217] To examine systemic as well as regional sympathomedullary kinetics, investigators infuse intravenous trace amounts of radiolabeled NE and epinephrine (EPI). Arterial or "arterialized venous" samples of endogenous catecholamines are then obtained, and a "compartmental analysis" is performed to mathematically fit the data into a two-compartment ("whole-body" versus "cardiac" or "extravascular" versus "vascular"/plasma compartments) model. Whole-body NE "spillover" (the rate of NE appearance in plasma), a sensitive measure of systemic SNS activity, is similar under basal conditions in panic patients and control subjects[218,219] and increases to a similar degree in both groups under laboratory mental stress.[219] Panic patients do, however, exhibit significantly higher cardiac spillover rates of coronary sinus (cardiac-derived) EPI under basal conditions, increased whole-body EPI secretion during laboratory mental stress, and surges of EPI whole-body spillover during panic attacks. Such increases in EPI in panic patients presumably are due to "loading" of sympathetic neuronal stores by uptake from plasma during surges of EPI secretion during panic attacks.[219] Further investigation of cardiac and/or systemic sympathomedullary activation during spontaneous or pharmacologically provoked panic attacks is needed to confirm these findings, along with prospective investigations of the cardiac-related risk of patients with panic disorder.[220,221] However, multiple prospective cohort studies (which control for other accepted risk factors for IHD) report that increasing severity of anxiety is associated with an increased risk for developing elevated systolic blood pressure[222] or hypertension.[223,224] However, given the comorbidity between anxiety and depressive symptoms and syndromes, further studies are required to determine whether the evidence of increased risk for the development of CAD (or hypertension) in anxiety disorder patients is independent of the contribution of depression.[225]

Another area awaiting investigation in patients with anxiety disorders is platelet receptor function, particularly the receptors most integral to thrombovascular repair and disease. Psychobiological studies of patients with panic disorder, in contrast to reports of patients with major depression, have not detected alterations of platelet 5HT transporters and platelet $5HT_2$ receptors. In comparison to control subjects, however, patients with panic attacks have been reported, like those with depression, to exhibit increased plasma concentrations of PF4 and β-TG, providing evidence of increased platelet secretion. Moreover, after treatment of panic patients with alprazolam, plasma concentrations of these alpha granule–specific proteins were reduced significantly.[226] The presence of anxiety disorders has been hypothesized to trigger coronary events through atherosclerotic plaque rupture, coronary vasospasm, ventricular arrhythmias, or atrial arrhthymias.[225] Panic-induced hyperventilation is a well-known precipitant of coronary spasm,[227,228] which in turn may induce ventricular arrhythmias and MI.[200,229,230]

The most compelling evidence regarding the association of anxiety disorders and cardiovascular dysfunction comes from reports of abnormal cardiac autonomic control.[225] Examination of HRV in patients with anxiety disorders has revealed that patients with panic disorder[231–234] and patients with generalized anxiety disorder[235] exhibit reductions in high-frequency HRV.[236] As was noted above, diminished HRV increases the risk of arrhythmias and sudden cardiac death. Indeed, patients with panic disorder or agoraphobia exhibit a higher density of PVCs in comparison to patients with other anxiety disorders[237] and normal comparison subjects.[238,239] Whether patients with panic disorder (or other anxiety disorders) exhibit increased rates of sudden cardiac death remains to be determined.

Although so-called mental disorders may produce effects on cardiovascular function, perhaps less well understood are the cardiovascular contributions to certain anxiety disorders. Whether cardiovascular abnormalities or dysfunction reliably produces symptoms of anxiety is an intriguing area of investigation; e.g., is worsening of CHF associated with an increased incidence of panic attacks? In comparison to gender- and age-matched controls, individuals with cardiac arrhythmias exhibited significantly higher self-reported anxiety scores.[240] Whether a causal biological mechanism exists between PVCs and anxiety symptoms or disorders or there is merely an association remains to be determined.[171,241–243]

Emergency room physicians and cardiologists are well acquainted with the challenges of evaluating patients with an acute onset of chest discomfort, combined with painful and overwhelming anxiety symptoms, which may or may not be associated with clinically significant cardiovascular disease (Table 80-10).

Certainly, the impact of anxiety disorders on the development of and worsening of CVD should be more completely discriminated from the contributions of depressive symptoms or syndromes.[225] Such knowledge carries the promise of anxiety symptom reduction and improved quality of life and the potential for new treatment modalities to enhance cardiovascular function in patients with CVD who have comorbid anxiety disorders.

TABLE 80-10 Medical Conditions Associated with Anxiety Symptoms

Cardiovascular disorders: mitral valve prolapse, coronary artery disease, paroxysmal tachycardia, hypertension, hypotension
Endocrinopathies: hyperthyroidism, hypothyroidism, diabetes, hypoglycemia, hypocalcemia, porphyria, endocrine tumors
Neurologic disorders: migraine headaches, transient ischemic attacks, temporal lobe seizures
Pulmonary disease: asthma, chronic obstructive pulmonary disease, pulmonary embolus
Vestibular dysfunction: Meniere's disease
Infectious diseases: tuberculosis, brucellosis, HIV/AIDS
Drug effects: cocaine abuse, alcohol or sedative withdrawal, sympathomimetics, caffeine, monosodium glutamate, akathesia

Treatment of Major Depression and Anxiety Disorders in Patients with Cardiovascular Disease

As with other medical disorders, effective treatment of major psychiatric illnesses such as major depression and panic disorder and prototype mood and anxiety disorders, respectively, require patient access to informed health care practioners, accurate diagnosis, affordable treatment, and safe, effective treatment modalities. Factors hampering well-conducted psychiatric (psychotherapeutic or psychopharmacologic/somatic) treatment include patient reluctance, social stigma regarding psychiatric treatment, managed care restrictions, and a dearth of psychiatrists and psychologists, particularly in rural areas. However, the evidence of the adverse impact of affective and anxiety disorders on relatively young and physically healthy individuals as well as medically ill patients heralds an opportunity and an accompanying incentive to prevent or limit the personal suffering, economic cost, and social disability associated with mental disorders. Although the safety and efficacy of anxiolytic and antidepressant treatment in patients with cardiovascular disease remain to be truly established in randomized clinical trials, these agents, particularly the newly introduced ones, are prescribed routinely to patients with heart disease. This seems appropriate given the drastic reduction in psychosocial function associated with anxiety or depressive disorders and the extant literature demonstrating the safety, and efficacy of these psychotropic agents in generally healthy populations, some data from psychopharmacologic treatment of medically ill patients, and the paucity of psychiatric practitioners available to patients with severe CVD.

Many heart patients believe that their persistent "worry," "lack of enjoyment of life," or "loss of interest" constitutes an understandable (and untreatable) condition. However, given the prevalence of major depression in patients with heart disease, the astute clinician's index of suspicion should always be heightened. Third-party information (particularly from a spouse or other caregiver) is often more revealing of the true extent of a patient's symptoms (e.g., irritability, social isolation, or listlessness), including attempts to "self-medicate" through abuse of alcohol, prescription medication, or illicit substances. A thorough evaluation of anxiety, panic attacks (if any), and depressive symptoms should be performed, including queries regarding feelings of pessimism, hopelessness, and the wish not to continue living. While the preferences of cardiac patients, as with any medical disorder, should be respected, cardiac patients and their families should always be gently apprised of the risks of untreated depression (CVD-related morbidity and mortality) versus the options of psychotherapeutic and/or psychopharmacologic treatment. Consultation with a knowledgeable mental health provider can assist in the discrimination of depressive disorders from complicated or pathologic grief, delirium, ascertainment of coexisting anxiety disorders (such as generalized anxiety disorder or social phobia), detection of intoxication or withdrawal syndromes, and appropriate emotional reactions.

The efficacy (and safety) of psychotherapeutic treatment of post-MI patients with comorbid major depression or any of the anxiety disorders is not known. However, the Enhancing Recovering in Coronary Heart Disease (ENRICHD) Patients Study, a multicenter, randomized clinical trial sponsored by the National Heart, Lung, and Blood Institute, is under way. ENRICHD is the first large-scale, randomized clinical trial to utilize psychotherapy as an initial intervention targeting post-MI patients with major depression (and/or low social support), proceeding to antidepressant treatment if depressive symptoms do not improve. Psychological interventions with post-MI patients[244–248] targeted to diminish "psychological distress"[246,249] or alter type A personality traits[245] have been studied previously on a more limited scale.

With the introduction of fluoxetine (Prozac) in the United States and citalopram (Celexa) in Europe in 1989, just over a decade of clinical information has been gleaned regarding the selective serotonin reuptake inhibitors (SSRIs) class of antidepressants. Furthermore, during the 1990s, these SSRIs and more recently the 5HT and NE reuptake inhibitor (SSNRI) venlafaxine superseded the benzodiazepines as the first-line treatment of choice for anxiety disorders. These newer antidepressants provide significant reduction of anxiety symptoms in approximately 60 percent of medically healthy patients without having a potential for addiction. SSRIs and SSNRIs have been approved by U.S. Food and Drug Agency for the treatment of panic disorder [paroxetine (Paxil) and sertraline (Zoloft)], social anxiety disorder (social phobia) (paroxetine), obsessive-compulsive disorder [aroxetine, sertraline, fluoxetine and fluvoxamine (Luvox)], and generalized anxiety disorder [venlafaxine (Effexor)] (Table 80-11). It is important to note that the SSRIs, although they all are potent 5HT reuptake inhibitors, also exert unique effects on other neurotransmitter systems. Thus, paroxetine is a very potent inhibitor of NE reuptake, whereas sertraline is a potent inhibitor of dopamine (DA) reuptake. The clinical sequelae of these pharmacologic properties remain obscure.

During the time (often 6 to 8 weeks) before the onset of an antidepressant's anxiolytic effect, benzodiazepines such as lorazepam, alprazolam, and clonazepam may be utilized. These agents are rapidly effective but should be used only for short-term treatment (6- to 8-week duration) of disabling anxiety symptoms. Benzodiazepines are sedating, produce gait instability, impair memory, may induce behavioral disinhibition, are ineffective in the treatment of coexisting depressive syndromes, and place patients at risk of physiologic (and psychological) dependence.

Psychotherapeutic and/or psychopharmacologic treatment of the 15 to 23 percent of post-MI patients who fulfill the criteria for major depression, particularly depressed patients with a comorbid anxiety disorder or subsyndromal anxiety, may have a significant effect (positive or negative) on both medical morbidity and mortality. Because of advances in the medical management of CVD patients, therapeutic trials determining improvement in survival must be quite large[249]; for example, the 22-month CAST trial included 1489 subjects.[181] Such past experience cautions against the raising of hopes for demonstrating improving cardiac outcome through antidepressant treatment of depression and anxiety disorders in patients with CVD. Nevertheless, awaiting the completion of a large-scale mortality trial similar to CAST may not be appropriate in light of the interpersonal, social, and medical burden of depression and early indications of SSRI efficacy in depressed patients with CVD.[250,251]

The use of tricyclic and structurally related antidepressants should be limited in patients with CVD because of the myriad side effects of these drugs on the cardiovascular system, including orthostatic hypotension, tachycardia, reduction in HRV, and slowing of intraventricular conduction (as a result of quinidine-like effects) (Table 80-11). These antidepressants should never be prescribed for patients with bifascicular and left fascicular block.[252,253] Monoamine oxidase inhibitors and trazodone are generally free of effects on cardiac conduction but, like the TCAs, may cause postural hypotension.[254] Because of their fewer potential adverse effects on the cardiovascular system and the lack of lethality from an overdose, pharmacotherapeutic treatment with SSRIs, the SSNRI venlafaxine, or other "atypical" antidepressants (such as bupropion, nefazodone, and mirtazapine) may offer significant advantages in depressed or anxious patients with CVD.

The only known cardiac effect of SSRIs is severe sinus node slowing, which to date has been reported in only a few cases.[262,263] Because 5HT has been implicated in both platelet aggregation and coronary artery vasoconstriction, the SSRIs, which are widely used to treat major depression, may produce effects on platelet function. There have been some reports of alterations of hemostasis[264–266] and platelet aggregation[267] after treatment with fluoxetine.

Because of inhibition of some cytochrome P450 isoenzymes, certain SSRIs may alter the metabolism of medications often used in patients with heart disease. The SSRIs that inhibit the P450 2D6 isoenzyme (fluoxetine, paroxetine, fluvoxamine, and higher doses of sertraline) should be used with caution in patients receiving medications metabolized by the P450 2D6 (e.g., lipophilic beta-blockers and type 1C antiarrhythmics: flecainide, mexiletine, propafenone). SSRIs that inhibit the P450 3A4 isoenzyme (fluoxetine, fluvoxamine, nefazodone) may increase the plasma concentrations of calcium channel blockers and warfarin.[268] Although the antidepressants venlafaxine, bupropion, citalopram, and mirtazapine exhibit minimal hepatic P450 enzyme inhibition, their safety remains to be established in patients with CVD who have comorbid depression or anxiety disorders.

After short-term treatment with buproprion,[269] fluoxetine,[270] paroxetine, fluvoxamine,[120] or paroxetine,[250] depressed patients exhibit no changes in HRV. A recent randomized, double-blind multicenter study compared the efficacy of nortriptyline and

TABLE 80-11 Cardiac-Related Side Effects of Psychotropic Agents Commonly Utilized for Treatment of Anxiety or Depression

Class	Cardiovascular Side Effect(s)	Likely Mechanism of Side Effect	Other Effects/Benefits*
Tricyclic and related cyclic antidepressants Nortriptyline (Pamelor) Imipramine (Tofranil) Amitriptyline (Elavil)	Orthostatic hypotension	Postsynaptic $alpha_1$-receptor blockade	Nortriptyline has lowest incidence of orthostatic hypotension[255,256]
Desipramine (Norpramin) Clomipramine (Anafranil)	Tachycardia	Secondary to hypotension	
Doxepin (Sinequan)	Decreased heart rate variability	Postsynaptic cholinergic receptor blockade	Urinary retention, dry mouth, constipation, confusion, exacerbation of narrow-angle glaucoma
Trimipramine (Surmontil) Protriptyline (Vivactil)	Slowing of intraventricular conduction	Quinidine-like effects	Avoid in patients with: bifascicular block, left bundle branch block, QTc > 44 ms, QRS > 11 ms Fatal in overdose
Monoamine oxidase inhibitors Phenelzine (Nardil) Tranylcypromine (Parnate) Isocarboxizide (Marplan)	Orthostatic hypotension Hypertensive crisis	Inhibition of metabolism of serotonin and catecholamines	Requires adherence to tyramine-free diet and avoidance of other antidepressants, and sympathomimetics Fatal in overdose
Selective serotonin reuptake inhibitors (SSRIs)		Postsynaptic serotonin receptor blockade	Typical SSRI side effects: nausea, insomnia, sexual dysfunction, nervousness
Fluoxetine (Prozac)	Sinus bradycardia[257]	Unknown	Requires 8 weeks for complete washout Inhibitor of CYP-450 IID6 and CYP-450 IIIA4 enzymes Also FDA-approved for treatment of adult obsessive-compulsive disorder (OCD)
Paroxetine (Paxil)	Clinically insignificant decreases in heart rate[250]	Unknown	Inhibitor of CYP-450 IID6 enzyme Also FDA-approved for treatment of social phobia, panic disorder, OCD
Sertraline (Zoloft)	None known		In high doses, inhibitor of CYP-450 IID6 enzyme Also FDA-approved for treatment of panic disorder, adult and pediatric OCD
Fluvoxamine (Luvox)	None known		Potent inhibitor of *multiple* CYP-450 enzymes Also FDA-approved for treatment of adult and pediatric OCD
Citalopram (Celexa)	None known		SSRI with most selective binding to serotonin transporter

TABLE 80-11 Cardiac-Related Side Effects of Psychotropic Agents Commonly Utilized for Treatment of Anxiety or Depression (*Continued*)

Class	Cardiovascular Side Effect(s)	Likely Mechanism of Side Effect	Other Effects/Benefits*
Selective serotonin-norepinephrine reuptake inhibitor (SNRI)			
Venlafaxine (Effexor)	Arrhythmia or cardiac block in overdose[260]	Unknown	No significant inhibition of CYP-450 enzymes
	Increased diastolic blood pressure in doses >300 mg per day[261]	Presynaptic inhibition of norepinephrine reuptake	FDA-approved for treatment of generalized anxiety disorder, major depression Side effect profile similar to SSRIs
Presynaptic $Alpha_2$-Receptor Antagonist			
Mirtazapine (Remeron)	None known	Postsynaptic $histamine_1$ receptor blockade	Very sedating in low doses Weight gain Minimal sexual side effects No significant inhibition of CYP-450 enzymes
Lithium*	Sinus node dysfunction Sinoatrial block T-wave inversion or flattening, particularly in patients >60 years of age Arrythmias and sudden death in patients with cardiac disease	Unknown	Narrow therapeutic index (.6–1.2 mmol/L) Many medications alter lithium plasma levels Fatal in overdose Mood stabilizer for patients with bipolar disorder Yearly ECG in patients over 50
Dopamine and norepinephrine reuptake inhibitor			
Bupropion (Wellbutrin; Zyban)	Significant increases in blood pressure in patients with preexisting hypertension[255]	Presynaptic inhibition of norepinephrine reuptake	No significant inhibition of CYP-450 enzymes Minimal sexual side effects Not proven effective in treatment of anxiety disorders FDA-approved for treatment of nicotine dependence
"Atypical" serotonergic agents			
Trazodone (Desyrel)	Orthostatic hypotension	Postsynaptic $alpha_1$-receptor blockade	Sedation, confusion, dizziness
	Cardiac arrhythmias rare[258]	Unknown	
		Unknown	Rare cases of priapism
Nefazodone (Serzone)	Sinus bradycardia[259]	Unknown	Similar side effect profile as trazodone (except without priapism) Minimal sexual side effects Potent inhibitor of *multiple* CYP-450 enzymes
Psychostimulants			
Dextroamphetamine (Dexedrine) Methylphenidate (Ritalin)	Rarely increases blood pressure or induces tachycardia in therapeutic doses	Release of dopamine and catecholamines	Avoid in patients with hyperthyroidism, severe hypertension, severe angina, tachyarrythmias

TABLE 80-11 Cardiac-Related Side Effects of Psychotropic Agents Commonly Utilized for Treatment of Anxiety or Depression (*Continued*)

Class	Cardiovascular Side Effect(s)	Likely Mechanism of Side Effect	Other Effects/Benefits*
Benzodiazepines Alprazolam (Xanax)		Allosteric alteration of $GABA_A$ receptors	Rapid relief of anxiety symptoms Can cause fatigue, ataxia, drowsiness, amnesia, and behavioral dyscontrol Relatively safe in overdose Physiologic and psychological dependence; withdrawal symptoms without gradual taper of dose
Clonazepam (Klonopin) Lorazepam (Ativan) Oxazepam (Serax)	Hypotension	Muscle relaxation via $GABA_A$ spinal cord receptors	
Partial $5HT_{1A}$-Receptor Agonist Buspirone (Buspar)	None known		FDA-approved for treatment of generalized anxiety disorder Nonaddictive
$Omega_1$ receptor Agonist Zolpidem (Ambien) Zalepelon (Sonata)	None known None known	Potentiation of $GABA_A$ receptor	Sedating Nonaddictive

*Medications that increase lithium levels: nonsteroidal anti-inflammatory drugs, diuretics (thiazides, ethacrynic acid, spironolactone, triamterene), angiotensin-converting enzyme inhibitors, metronidazole, tetracycline. Medications that decrease lithium levels: acetazolamide, theophylline, aminophylline, caffeine, osmotic diuretics.
ABBREVIATION: CYP-450 = cytochrome P-450.

paroxetine in depressed patients with IHD.[250] Both antidepressants were effective in the treatment of depression, but not surprisingly, there were more dropouts because of side effects and more cardiac-related effects with the TCA. Unfortunately, the safety of SSRIs remains to be established in large-scale, randomized treatment trials of post-MI patients with comorbid major depression.[271] The recently completed SADHART study, a randomized, multicenter, double-blind trial of sertraline versus placebo in the treatment of post-MI patients with comorbid major depression, attempted to determine the efficacy and safety of this SSRI in depressed patients with unstable angina and those who are post-MI. Any of the available oral antidepressants usually will produce a clinical therapeutic response (an improvement in depressive symptoms by 50 percent or more) in comparison to pretreatment severity of depressive symptoms in 60 to 70 percent of medically healthy patients provided that the antidepressant is administered in sufficient dosage over a treatment duration of 5 to 6 weeks.

Another somatic treatment modality, electroconvulsive therapy (ECT), is effective in up to 80 percent of patients with either unipolar or bipolar depression[272] over a relatively brief (2- to 3-week) treatment duration. ECT is the initial treatment of choice in depressed patients who are severely ill (e.g., at nutritional risk from severe calorie loss or dehydration) and require a rapid clinical response. ECT also should be considered for patients who have experienced a previous positive response to ECT, do not respond to oral antidepressants, cannot tolerate the associated side effects of antidepressants, or experience depression with psychotic symptoms (hallucinations, delusions, paranoia).

Electroconvulsive therapy produces a seizure by providing a brief pulse (approximately 1 to 2 s in duration) of electrical charge over the scalp in the area of the right parietal lobe (right unilateral ECT) or over both temples (bilateral ECT). This pulse elicits a generalized convulsive seizure that lasts approximately 30 to 60 s. The patient is anesthetized during the procedure with a short-acting barbiturate (e.g., methohexital) and paralyzed with a muscle relaxant such as succinylcholine. Respirations are controlled by masked ventilation, and intubation is not required unless there have been recurrent episodes of aspiration. The morbidity and mortality associated with ECT have decreased dramatically over the past 60 years. The introduction of curare and later succinylcholine decreased the incidence of orthopedic complications from almost 20 percent of cases to being a rare complication. Complications related to cognitive dysfunction, such as delirium and amnesia, also have been decreased through the use of brief pulse (versus sine wave) and unilateral (versus bilateral) ECT. Structural brain studies using magnetic resonance images have shown no evidence of brain damage secondary to ECT.[273] Moreover, most studies of memory problems associated with ECT have reported that patients have transient amnesia and that memory returns to the pre-ECT level of function within 6 months.

Until recently, however, the cardiac complications from ECT resulted in the most serious adverse events. As recently as the 1980s, deaths from ECT were estimated to be approximately 1 per 10,000 treatments (most patients receive 6 to 10 treatments per ECT trial), primarily as a result of cardiac complications. Two major cardiac complications occur in relation to the ECT stimulus: an initial asystole secondary to vagal nerve stimulation followed closely by the release of EPI with tachycardia and hypertension. Although the patient is paralyzed, the ECT electrode that conducts up to 100 J of energy to stimulate the seizure also produces a direct stimulus of the masseter muscles (a bite block is kept in place during the treatments) and the vagus nerve. The stimulation of the vagus can subsequently cause asystole. Within seconds of the vagal stimulation, an adrenergic discharge related to the onset of a generalized seizure causes the release of EPI with tachycardia, hypertension, and the potential for myocardial ischemia or arrhythmias. The tachycardia is relatively brief (1 to 2 min).

Although no absolute contraindications to ECT exist, certain clinical situations increase the risk of complications from a course of ECT, i.e., diseases that affect the CNS and/or the cardiothrombovascular system: a cerebral vascular accident (CVA) during the previous 6 months, any illness that increases intracranial pressure (e.g., brain tumor), medical disorders that disrupt the blood-brain barrier (e.g., meningitis), a cerebral or aortic aneurysm, MI, severe valvular heart disease, a high-grade atrioventricular block, symptomatic ventricular arrhythmias, supraventricular arrhythmias with uncontrolled ventricular rate, and coagulation or bleeding disorders.[274] Implanted cardiac pacemakers and defibrillators are usually not problematic during ECT.[275,276] Some practitioners choose to convert a demand pacemaker to a fixed mode, and an electrophysiologist should be consulted to determine whether the defibrillator's function should be inhibited during each ECT treatment. Electroconvulsive therapy also is tolerated by cardiac transplant patients who have normal cardiac function.[277]

Electroconvulsive therapy can be conceptualized as a cardiac stress test; however, because of the general anesthesia, the patient cannot report symptoms such as chest pain, and the seizure stimulating the tachycardia cannot be terminated abruptly. Therefore, the pre-ECT workup should include a complete review of systems and a screen for exercise intolerance, angina, evidence of congestive heart failure (patients will receive approximately 1 L of fluid per ECT treatment) or diabetes, extent of smoking history, cholesterol level, and other cardiac risk factors. The basic pre-ECT screening includes measurement of serum electrolytes (with particular attention to hydration status and potassium) and hemoglobin and the obtaining of an electrocardiogram (ECG). Chest x-rays are obtained in case of evidence of CHF or pulmonary disease. Patients with a history of back pain are evaluated with spine films; neuroimaging is used to determine whether there has been a recent CVA or increased intracranial pressure in patients with neurologic dysfunction. Although "beta blockers" are used during ECT treatment (see below), cardiovascular screening should determine whether the patient can tolerate transient tachycardia and hypertension. Additional cardiac screening includes a stress test in individuals at significant risk for CAD.

Modern ECT suites are equipped with continuous ECG and blood pressure and heart rate monitors as well as pulse oximetry and an electroencephalograph to record seizure activity. Patients should continue their pulmonary (except theophylline) and cardiac (except lidocaine) medications during a course of ECT treatment. Theophylline and lidocaine are discontinued because of prolongation and reduction of seizure duration, respectively. As a result of the increase in intraocular pressure during an ECT-induced seizure, glaucoma medications generally are continued, except for acetylcholinesterases. Hypoglycemic agents should not be administered the morning of ECT to prevent hypoglycemia in diabetic patients. Patients must not ingest food or fluids before ECT treatments but may receive intravenous fluids as tolerated. In addition to usual ECT medications (methohexital 1 mg/kg and succinylcholine 0.75–1.50 mg/kg), patients with hypertension, CAD, valvular heart disease, and CHF routinely receive prophylactic medication to prevent cardiac complications from the transient hypertension and tachycardia induced by ECT.[278] Such a "cardiac-modified" ECT protocol[279,280] should be utilized for elderly patients and those with cardiac disease. Usually either of two beta blockers, labetalol or esmolol, is utilized to reduce maximal heart rate, mean arterial pressure, and arrhythmia frequency during ECT. Labetalol (selective alpha$_1$- and nonselective beta-adrenergic receptor blockade and elimination half-life of 5 to 8 h) may induce significant hypotension.[281] Esmolol (beta$_1$-selective at the usual doses, rapid onset, and an elimination half-life of 9 min) may replace labetolol if labetolol induces prolonged bradycardia and hypotension. Esmolol, however, has been associated with shortened seizure duration during ECT. If elderly patients pretreated with a beta blocker continue to exhibit transient increases in blood pressure, a calcium channel blocker may be added. Nicardepine has replaced nifedipine as the calcium channel blocker of choice because nicardepine may be administered intravenously and has a shorter duration of action. The ECT protocol also involves adequate hydration before ECT, discontinuation of psychotropic medication whenever possible, and provision of anticholinergic medication (0.4 to 0.8 mg intravenous atropine or 0.2 mg of glycopyrrolate) to decrease oropharyngeal secretions and prevent bradycardias whenever beta blockers are used.[282] Continuous blood pressure monitoring and ECG monitoring should be performed during all treatments, along with monitoring for shortness of breath or chest pain.

The third most common cardiac complication is orthostatic hypotension, which usually occurs in the recovery room, particularly in elderly debilitated patients and patients with medical conditions associated with autonomic dysfunction (e.g., Parkinson's disease). As was noted above, consideration should be given to the utilization of shorter-acting beta blockers that have less alpha-adrenoreceptor blockade (esmolol for labetolol) and/or shorter-acting calcium channel blockers (nicardepine for nifedipine). After each ECT treatment, patients recover for over an hour in a setting similar to an outpatient surgical suite. Patients remain on a cardiac monitor with intravenous fluids and supplemental oxygen provided until they are oriented and exhibit no orthostatic hypotension (approximately 20 to 30 min). They are then dressed and asked to be seated upright in a chair until they are fully alert and able to ingest fluids orally (approximately 20 to 30 min in duration).

In summary, the magnitude of the risks associated with ECT are approximately equivalent to those of general anesthesia. The incidence of delirium during ECT can be reduced to less than 5 percent in elderly patients through the administration of twice-weekly ECT treatments and the use of unilateral electrode placement on the right temporal area in patients at risk (patients with structural brain changes, concomitant medical illness, Alzheimer's disease, Parkinson's disease, advanced age, and concomitant administration of psychotropic medications).[282] Cardiac complications are not uncommon with ECT but are reduced significantly with a cardiac ECT protocol. Although generally a safe and effective treatment, ECT in elderly patients with cardiovascular disease requires a multispecialty coordinated effort among a specially trained ECT-nursing service, psychiatrist, anesthesiologist, and cardiologist.

FUTURE DIRECTIONS FOR RESEARCH

Usually underdiagnosed and undertreated, major depression and anxiety disorders are encountered commonly in patients with CAD and patients referred for evaluation of chest pain. However, a burgeoning literature on the importance of major depression and anxiety disorders in patients with heart disease has accumulated over the past two decades. Several studies have shown depression and its associated symptoms to be a major risk factor in both the development of CVD and death after an index MI. Further evidence is accumulating regarding the increased risk of patients with anxiety disorders or anxiety symptoms for the development of IHD, although currently there is a dearth of information about the prevalence of anxiety disorders in patients with CAD or CHF. An intriguing area of investigation involves the possible effects of anxiety disorders on the thrombovascular system and the "reciprocal" cardiovascular contributions to anxiety symptoms or anxiety syndromes, such as panic disorder. Although treatment of depression in many patients with CVD improves their dysphoria and other signs and symptoms of depression, are these agents safe and effective in the treatment of anxiety disorders as well? One of many important questions to be answered is whether aggressive and consistent treatment of anxiety and depressive syndromes in patients with CVD not only improves their quality of life but diminishes cardiovascular-related morbidity and improves survival. Which treatment modalities (psychotherapeutic versus psychopharmacologic or a combination) will be most effective in patients with recurrent or more severe depression remains to be determined. Treatment studies also may assess the relation between depression and subsequent compliance with medication and modification of risk factors for CVD.[31] Future studies undoubtedly should include women to assess whether there are gender-specific psychiatric and psychobiological differences in the response to treatment[198,283–285] because women are more vulnerable to depression and because CVD is the leading cause of death among adult women in the United States.

The associations between diseases of the CNS (anxiety and depressive disorders) and disorders of peripheral "end organs" such as the heart raise intriguing questions regarding what is "cardiovascular" or "psychiatric." Illumination of the interplay between anxiety disorders, depressive syndromes, and the thrombovascular system, particularly in patients with CVD, undoubtedly will lead to the development of new treatment modalities that not only will improve patients' quality of life but potentially will decrease their morbidity and improve long-term survival rates.

ACKNOWLEDGMENTS

This research was supported by grants MH-01399, NIMH 156617-03, MH-42088, MH-49523, and RR-00039 from the National Institutes of Health, Bethesda, MD, an Established Investigator Award from the National Alliance for Research on Schizophrenia and Depression (Dr. Nemeroff), and a Research Award from the Dana Foundation (Dr. Musselman).

References

1. Hayward C. Psychiatric illness and cardiovascular disease risk. *Epidemiol Rev* 1995; 17:129–138.
2. Dimsdale JE. A perspective on Type A behavior and coronary disease. *N Engl J Med* 1988; 318:110–112.
3. American Psychiatric Association. *Diagnostic and Statistical Manual of Mental Disorders,* 4th ed. Washington, DC: American Psychiatric Association; 1994.
4. Kessler RC, McGonagle KA, Zhao S, et al. Lifetime and 12-month prevalence of DSM-III-R psychiatric disorders in the United States. *Arch Gen Psychiatry* 1994; 51:8–19.
5. Leeper J, Badger L, Milo T. Mental disorders among physical disability determination patients. *Am J Public Health* 1985; 75: 78–79.
6. Blacker CVR, Clare AW. Depressive disorder in primary care. *Br J Psychiatry* 1987; 150:737–751.
7. Barrett JE, Barrett JA, Oxman TE, Gerber PD. The prevalence of psychiatric disorders in a primary care practice. *Arch Gen Psychiatry* 1988; 45:1100–1106.
8. Von Korff M, Shapiro S, Burke JD, et al. Anxiety and depression in a primary care clinic: Comparison of Diagnostic Interview Schedule, General Health Questionnaire, and practitioner assessments. *Arch Gen Psychiatry* 1987; 44:152–156.
9. Cohen-Cole SA, Kaufman KG. Major depression in physical illness: Diagnosis, prevalence, and antidepressant treatment (a ten year review: 1982–1992). *Depression* 1993; 1:181–204.
10. Magni G, Schifano F, DeLeo D. Assessment of depression in an elderly medical population. *J Affect Disord* 1986; 11:121–124.
11. Feldman E, Mayou R, Hawton K, et al. Psychiatric disorder in medical inpatients. *Q J Med* 1987; 63:405–412.
12. Blazer D, Swartz M, Woodbury M, et al. Depressive symptoms and depressive diagnoses in a community population: Use of a new procedure for analysis of psychiatric classification. *Arch Gen Psychiatr* 1988; 45:1078–1084.
13. Bebbington P, Katz R, McGuffin P, et al. The risk of minor depression before age 65: Results from a community survey. *Psychol Med* 1989; 19:393–400.
14. Broadhead WE, Blazer DG, George LK, Tse CK. Depression, disability days, and days lost from work in a prospective epidemiologic survey. *JAMA* 1990; 264:2524–2528.
15. Johnson J, Weissman MM, Klerman GL. Service utilization and social morbidity associated with depressive symptoms in the community. *JAMA* 1992; 267:1478–1483.
16. Kessler LG, Cleary PD, Burke JD Jr. Psychiatric disorders in primary care: Results of a follow-up study. *Arch Gen Psychiatry* 1985; 42:583–587.
17. Ormel J, Koeter MWJ, van den Brink W, van de Willige G. Recognition, management, and course of anxiety and depression in general practice. *Arch Gen Psychiatry* 1991; 48:700–706.
18. Kurosawa H, Shimizu Y, Nishimatsu Y, et al. The relationship between mental disorders and physical severities in patients with acute myocardial infarction. *Jpn Circ J* 1983; 47:723–725.
19. Mayou R, Foster A, Williamson B. Medical care after myocardial infarction. *J Psychos Res* 1979; 23:23–26.
20. Carney RM, Rich MW, teVelde A, et al. Major depressive disorder in coronary artery disease. *Am J Cardiol* 1987; 60:1273–1275.

21. Schlelfer SJ, Macarini-Hinson MM, Coyle DA, et al. The nature and course of depression following myocardial infarction. *Arch Intern Med* 1989; 149:1785–1789.
22. Frasure-Smith N, Lesperance F, Talajic M. Depression following myocardial infarction: Impact on 6-month survival. *JAMA* 1993; 270:1819–1861.
23. Blumenthal JA, Williams RS, Wallace AG, et al. Physiological and psychological variables predict compliance to prescribed exercise therapy in patients recovering from myocardial infarction. *Psychosom Med* 1982; 44:519–527.
24. Stern JJ, Pascale L, Ackerman A. Life adjustment postmyocardial infarction: Determine predictive variables. *Arch Intern Med* 1977; 137:1680–1685.
25. Mayou R, Foster A, Williamson B. Psychosocial adjustment in patients one year after myocardial infarction. *J Psychosom Res* 1978; 22:447–453.
26. Skodol AE, Schwartz S, Dohrenwend BP, et al. Minor depression in a cohort of young adults in Israel. *Arch Gen Psychiatry* 1994; 51:542–551.
27. Wells KB, Stewart A, Hayes RD, et al. The functioning and well-being of depressed patients: Results of the Medical Outcomes Study. *JAMA* 1989; 262:914–919.
28. Carney RM, Rich MW, Freedland KE, Saini J. Major depressive disorder predicts cardiac events in patients with coronary artery disease. *Psychosom Med* 1988; 50:627–633.
29. Aromaa A, Raitasalo R, Reunanen A, et al. Depression and cardiovascular diseases. *Acta Psychiatr Scand* 1994; 377:77–82.
30. Ahern DK, Gorkin L, Anderson JL, et al. Biobehavioral variables and mortality or cardiac arrest in the Cardiac Arrhythmia Pilot Study (CAPS). *Am J Cardiol* 1990; 66:59–62.
31. Frasure-Smith N, Lesperance F, Talajic M. Depression and 18-month prognosis after myocardial infarction. *Circulation* 1995; 91:999–1005.
32. Wynn A. Unwarranted emotional distress in men with ischaemic heart disease. *Med J Aust* 1967; 2:847–851.
33. Hackett TP, Cassem NH, Wishnie HA. The coronary-care unit: An appraisal of its psychologic hazards. *N Engl J Med* 1968; 279:1365–1370.
34. Cay EL, Vetter N, Philip AE, Dugard P. Psychological status during recovery from an acute heart attack. *J Psychosom Res* 1972; 16:425–435.
35. Robins LN, Helzer JE, Croughan JL, et al. The NIMH Diagnostic Interview Schedule, Version III. Washington DC: Public Health Service (HSS), ADM-T-42-3 (5-81, 8-81); 1981.
36. Endicott J, Spitzer RL. A diagnostic interview: The Schedule for Affective Disorders and Schizophrenia. *Arch Gen Psychiatry* 1978; 35:837–844.
37. Freedland KE, Carney RM, Rich MW, et al. Depression in elderly patients with heart failure. *J Geriatr Psychiatry* 1991; 24: 59–71.
38. Gonzalez MB, Snyderman TB, Colket JT, et al. Depression in patients with coronary artery disease. *Depression* 1996; 4:57–62.
39. Koenig HG. Depression in hospitalized older patients with congestive heart failure. *Gen Hosp Psychiatry* 1998; 20:29–43.
40. Ostfeld AM, Lebovits BZ, Shekelle RB, Paul O. A prospective study of the relationship between personality and coronary heart disease. *J Chronic Dis* 1964; 17:265–276.
41. Hathaway SR, McKinley JC. *Minnesota Multiphasic Personality Inventory Manual*, rev. ed. New York: Psychological Corporation; 1951.
42. Cattell RB, Saunders DR, Stice G. *Handbook for the Sixteen Personality Factor Questionnaire.* Champaign, IL: Institute for Personality and Ability Testing; 1957.
43. Brozek J, Keyes A, Blackburn H. Personality differences between potential coronary and noncoronary subjects. *Ann NY Acad Sci* 1966; 134:1057–1064.
44. Goldberg EL, Comstock GW, Hornstra RK. Depressed mood and subsequent physical illness. *Am J Psychiatry* 1979; 136: 530–534.
45. Radloff LS. The CES-D scale: A self-report depression scale for research in the general population. *J Appl Psychol Meas* 1977; 1:385–401.
46. Murphy JM, Monson RR, Olivier DC, et al. Affective disorders and mortality. *Arch Gen Psychiatry* 1987; 44:473–480.
47. Murphy JM, Neff RK, Sobol AM, et al. Computer diagnosis of depression and anxiety: The Stirling County Study. *Psychol Med* 1985; 15:99–112.
48. Anda R, Williamson D, Jones D, et al. Depressed affect, hopelessness, and the risk of ischemic heart disease in a cohort of U.S. adults. *Epidemiology* 1993; 4:285–294.
49. Dupuy HJ. A concurrent validational study of the NCHS General Well-Being Schedule. *Vital Health Stat* 1977; 73.
50. Wing JK, Cooper JE, Sartorius N. *The Measurement and Classification of Psychiatric Symptoms.* London: Cambridge University Press; 1974.
51. Vogt T, Pope C, Mullooly JJH. Mental health status as a predictor of morbidity and mortality: A 15-year follow-up of members of a health maintenance organization. *Am J Public Health* 1994; 84:227–231.
52. McFarland BH, Freeborn DK, Mullooly JP, Pope CR. Utilization patterns among long-term enrollees in a prepaid group practice health maintenance organization. *Med Care* 1985; 23:1221–1233.
53. Simonsick EM, Wallace RB, Blazer DG, Berkman LF: Depressive symptomatology and hypertension-associated morbidity and mortality in older adults. *Psychosom Med* 1995; 57:427–435.
54. Everson SA, Goldberg DE, Kaplan GA, et al. Hopelessness and risk of mortality and incidence of myocardial infarction and cancer. *Psychosom Med* 1996; 58:113–121.
55. Barefoot JC, Schroll M. Symptoms of depression, acute myocardial infarction, and total mortality in a community sample. *Circulation* 1996; 93:1976–1980.
56. Greene RL. *The MMPI-2/MMPI: An Interpretive Manual.* Boston: Allyn and Bacon; 1991.
57. Pratt LA, Ford DE, Crum RM, et al. Depression, psychotropic medication, and risk of myocardial infarction: Prospective data from the Baltimore ECA follow-up. *Circulation* 1996; 94:3123–3129.
58. Wassertheil-Smoller S, Applegate WB, Berge K, et al. Change in depression as a precursor of cardiovascular events. *Arch Intern Med* 1996; 156:553–561.
59. Callahan CM, Wolinsky FD, Stump TE, et al. Mortality, symptoms, and functional impairment in late-life depression. *J Gen Intern Med* 1998; 13:746–752.
60. Mendes de Leon CF, Krumholz HM, Seeman TS, et al. Depression and risk of coronary heart disease in elderly men and women: New Haven EPESE, 1982–1991. *Arch Intern Med* 1998; 158:2341–2348.
61. Ford DE, Mead LA, Chang PP, et al. Depression is a risk factor for coronary artery disease in men: The Precursors Study. *Arch Intern Med* 1998; 158:1422–1426.
62. Vingerhoets A. *Psychosocial Stress: An Experimental Approach.* Groningen, Netherlands: Swets & Zeitlinger; 1985.
63. Selye H. *The Stress of Life.* New York: McGraw Hill; 1956.
64. Nemeroff CB, Widerlov E, Bissette G, et al. Elevated concentrations of CSF corticotropin-releasing factor-like immunoreactivity in depressed patients. *Science* 1984; 226:1342–1344.
65. Arato M, Banki CM, Nemeroff CB, Bissette G. Hypothalamic-pituitary-adrenal axis and suicide. *Ann NY Acad Sci* 1986; 487: 263–270.
66. Banki CM, Bissette G, Arato M, et al. Cerebrospinal fluid corticotropin-releasing factor-like immunoreactivity in depression and schizophrenia. *Am J Psychiatry* 1987; 144:873–877.
67. Banki CM, Karmasci L, Bissette G, Nemeroff CB. CSF corticotropin-releasing and somatostatin in major depression: Response to

antidepressant treatment and relapse. *Eur Neuropsychopharmacol* 1992; 2:107–113.

68. France RD, Urban B, Krishnan KRR, et al. CSF corticotropin-releasing factor-like immunoreactivity in chronic pain patients with and without major depression. *Biol Psychiatry* 1988; 23: 86–88.
69. Risch SC, Lewine RJ, Kalin NH, et al. Limbic-hypothalamic-pituitary-adrenal axis activity and ventricular-to-brain ratio studies in affective illness and schizophrenia. *Neuropsychopharmacology* 1992; 6:95–100.
70. Raadsheer FC, Hoogendijk WJG, Stam FC, et al. Increased numbers of corticotropin-releasing hormone expressing neurons in the hypothalamic paraventricular nucleus of depressed patients. *Neuroendocrinology* 1994; 60:436–444.
71. Raadsheer FC, van Heerikhuize JJ, Lucassen PJ, et al. Corticotropin-releasing hormone mRNA levels in the paraventricular nucleus of patients with Alzheimer's disease and depression. *Am J Psychiatry* 1995; 152:1372–1376.
72. Bjorkerud S. Effect of adrenocortical hormones on the integrity of rat aortic endothelium. In: Schettler G, Weizel A, eds. *Proceedings of the 3rd International Symposium on Atherosclerosis III.* Berlin: Springer-Verlag; 1973:245.
73. Nahas GG, Brunson JG, King WM, Cavert HM. Functional and morphologic changes in heart lung preparations following administration of adrenal hormones. *Am J Clin Pathol* 1958; 34: 717–729.
74. Valigorsky JM. Metaplastic transformation of aortic smooth muscle cells in cortisone-induced dissecting aneurysms in hamsters. *Fed Proc* 1969; 28:802.
75. Kemper JW, Baggenstoss AH, Slocumb CH. The relationship of therapy with cortisone to the incidence of vascular lesions in rheumatoid arthritis. *Ann Intern Med* 1957; 46:831–851.
76. Ross R, Harker L. Hyperlipidemia and atherosclerosis. *Science* 1976; 193:1094–1100.
77. Troxler RG, Sprague EA, Albanese RA, et al. The association of elevated plasma cortisol and early atherosclerosis as demonstrated by coronary angiography. *Atherosclerosis* 1977; 26: 151–162.
78. Swanson LW, Sawchenko PE. Organization of ovine corticotropin-releasing factor immunoreactive cells and fibers in the rat brain: An immunohistochemical study. *Neuroendocrinology* 1983; 36:165–186.
79. Merchenthaler I, Vigh S, Petruscz P, Schally AV. Immunocytochemical localization of corticotropin-releasing factor (CRF) in the rat brain. *Am J Anat* 1982; 165:385–396.
80. Cummings S, Elde R, Ellis J, Lindall A. Corticotropin-releasing factor immunoreactivity is widely distributed with the central nervous system of the rat: An immunohistochemical study. *J Neurosci* 1983; 8:1355–1368.
81. Wyatt RJ, Portnoy B, Kupfer DJ, et al. Resting plasma catecholamine concentrations in patients with depression and anxiety. *Arch Gen Psychiatry* 1971; 24:24:65–70.
82. Louis WJ, Doyle AE, Anavekar SN. Plasma noradrenaline concentration and blood pressure in essential hypertension, phaeochromocytoma and depression. *Clin Soc* 1975; 48:239S–242S.
83. Roy A, Pickar D, DeJong J, et al. Norepinephrine and its metabolites in cerebrospinal fluid, plasma and urine: Relationship to hypothalamic-pituitary-adrenal axis function in depression. *Arch Gen Psychiatry* 1988; 45:849–857.
84. Veith RC, Lewis L, Linares OA, et al. Sympathetic nervous system activity in major depression: Basal and desipramine-induced alterations in plasma NE kinetics. *Arch Gen Psychiatry* 1994; 51:411–422.
85. Roy A, Guthrie S, Pickar D, Linnoila M. Plasma NE responses to cold challenge in depressed patients and normal controls. *Psychiatry Res* 1987; 21:161–168.
86. Charney DS, Menkes DB, Henninger GR. Receptor sensitivity and the mechanism of action of antidepressant treatment. *Arch Gen Psychiatry* 1981; 38:1160–1180.
87. Golden RN, Markey SP, Risby ED, et al. Antidepressants reduce whole-body norepinephrine turnover while enhancing 6-hydroxymelatonin output. *Arch Gen Psychiatry* 1988; 45:150–154.
88. Linnoila M, Karoum F, Calil HM, et al. Alteration of NE metabolism with desipramine and zimelidine in depressed patients. *Arch Gen Psychiatry* 1982; 39:1025–1028.
89. Linnoila M, Guthrie S, Lane EA, et al. Clinical studies on NE metabolism: How to interpret the numbers. *Psychiatry Res* 1986; 17:229–239.
90. Scubee-Moreau JJ, Dresse AE. Effect of various antidepressant drugs on the spontaneous firing rate of locus coeruleus and raphe dorsalis neurons of the rat. *Euro J Pharmacol* 1979; 57:219–225.
91. Sulser F, Vetulani J, Mobley PL. Mode of action on antidepressant drugs. *Biochem Pharmacol* 1978; 27:257–261.
92. Anfossi G, Trovati M. Role of catecholamines in platelet function: Pathophysiological and clinical significance. *Euro J Clin Invest* 1996; 26:353–370.
93. Gerritsen ME. Physiological and pathophysiological roles of eicosanoids in the microcirculation. *Cardiovas Res* 1996; 32:720–732.
94. Goldstein DS. Plasma catecholamines and essential hypertension: An analytical review. *Hypertension* 1983; 5:86–99.
95. Lund-Johansen P. Hemodynamic alterations in early essential hypertension: Recent advances. In: Gross F, Strasser T, eds. *Mild Hypertension: Recent Advances.* New York: Raven Press; 1983:237.
96. Lechin F, van der Dijs B, Orozco B, et al. Plasma neurotransmitters, blood pressure, and heart rate during supine-resting, orthostasis, and moderate exercise conditions in major depressed patients. *Biol Psychiatry* 1995; 38:166–173.
97. Akselrod S, Gordon D, Ubel FA, et al. Power spectrum analysis of heart rate fluctuation: A quantitative probe of beat-to-beat cardiovascular control. *Science* 1981; 213:220–222.
98. Low PA. Autonomic nervous system function. *J Clin Neurophysiol* 1993; 10:14–27.
99. Spyer KM. Central nervous system control of the cardiovascular system. In: Bannister R, ed. *Autonomic Failure: A Textbook of Clinical Disorders of the Autonomic Nervous System.* Oxford, UK: Oxford University Press; 1988:56.
100. Shields RW. Functional anatomy of the autonomic nervous system. *J Clin Neurophysiol* 1993; 10:2–13.
101. Dalack GW, Roose SP. Perspectives on the relationship between cardiovascular disease and affective disorder. *J Clin Psychiatry* 1990; 51(suppl 7):4–9, 10–11.
102. Wolf M, Varigos G, Hunt D, Sloman JG. Sinus arrhythmia in acute myocardial infarction. *Med J Aust* 1978; 2:52–53.
103. Billman GE, Schwartz PJ, Stone HL. Baroreceptor reflex control of heart rate: A predictor of sudden cardiac death. *Circulation* 1982; 66:874–880.
104. Kleiger RE, Miller PJ, Bigger TJ, et al. Decreased heart rate variability and its association with increased mortality after acute myocardial infarction. *Am J Cardiol* 1987; 39:256–262.
105. Bigger JT, Kleiger RE, Fleiss JL, et al. Components of HR variability measured during healing of acute myocardial infarction. *Am J Cardiol* 1988; 61:208–215.
106. LaRovere MT, Specchia G, Mortana A, Schwartz PJ. Baroreflex sensitivity, clinical correlates, and cardiovascular mortality among patients with a first myocardial infarction: A prospective study. *Circ* 1988; 78:816–824.
107. Cripps T, Malik M, Farrell T, Camm AJ. Prognostic value of reduced heart rate variability after myocardial infarction: Clinical evaluation of a new analysis method. *Br Heart J* 1991; 65:14–19.
108. Viskin S, Belhassen B. Noninvasive and invasive strategies for the prevention of sudden death after myocardial infarction: Value, limitations and implications for therapy. *Drugs* 1992; 44:336–355.
109. Araya-Gomez V, Gonzalez-Hermosillo J, Casanova-Garces J, et

al. Identification of patients at risk of malignant arrythmia in the 1st year after myocardial infarction. *Arch Inst Cardiol Mex* 1994; 64:145–159.

110. Campbell RWF. Can analysis of heart rate variability predict arrhythmias and antiarrhythmic effects? In: Oto AM, ed. *Practice and Progress in Cardiac Pacing and Electrophysiology.* Dordrecht, Netherlands: Kluwer; 1996:63.
111. Sayers BM. Analysis of heart rate variability. *Ergonomics.* 1973; 16:17–32.
112. Pomeranz B, Macaulay RJB, Caudill MA, et al. Assessment of autonomic function in humans by heart rate spectral analysis. *Am J Physiol* 1985; 248:H151–H153.
113. Pagani M, Lombardi F, Guzzetti S, et al. Power spectral analysis of heart rate and arterial pressure variabilities as a marker of sympathovagal interaction in man and conscious dog. *Circ Res* 1986; 59:178–193.
114. Koizumi K, Terui N, Kollai M. Effect of cardiac vagal and sympathetic nerve activity on heart rate in rhythmic fluctuations. *J Auton Nerv Sys* 1985; 12:251–259.
115. Katona PG, Jih F. Respiratory sinus arrhythmia: Noninvasive measure of the parasympathetic cardiac control. *J Appl Physiol* 1975; 39:801–805.
116. Fouad FM, Tarazzi RC, Gerrario CM, et al. Assessment of parasympathetic control of heart rate by a noninvasive method. *Am J Physiol* 1984; 246:H838–H842.
117. Bigger TJJ, Fleiss JL, Steinman RC, et al. Frequency domain measures of heart period variability and mortality after myocardial infarction. *Circulation* 1992; 85:164–171.
118. Miyawaki E, Salzman C. Autonomic nervous system tests in psychiatry: Implications and potential uses of heart rate variability. *Integr Psychiatry* 1991; 7:21–28.
119. Yeragani VK, Pohl R, Ramesh C, et al. Effect of imipramine treatment on heart rate variability measures. *Neuropsychobiology* 1992; 26:27–32.
120. Rechlin T, Weis MDC. Heart rate variability in depressed patients and differential effects of paroxetine and amitriptyline on cardiovascular autonomic functions. *Pharmacopsychiatry* 1994; 27:124–128.
121. Carney RM, Saunders RD, Freedland KE, et al. Association of depression with reduced heart rate variability in coronary artery disease. *Am J Cardiol* 1995; 76:562–564.
122. Roose SP, Glassman AH, Dalack GW. Depression, heart disease, and tricyclic antidepressants. *J Clin Psychiatry* 1989; 50(suppl 7):12–16.
123. Severus WE, Ahrens B, Stoll AL. Omega-3 fatty acids—the missing link? (letter). *Arch Gen Psychiatry* 1999; 56:380–381.
124. Edwards R, Peet M, Shay J, Horrobin D. Omega-3 polyunsaturated fatty acid levels in the diet and in red blood cell membranes of depressed patients. *J Affect Dis* 1998; 48:149–155.
125. Adams PB, Lawson S, Sanigorski A, Sinclair AJ. Arachidonic acid to eicosapentaenoic acid ratio in blood correlates positively with clinical symptoms of depression. *Lipids* 1996; 31:S157–S161.
126. Maes M, Smith R, Christophe A, et al. Fatty acid composition in major depression: Decreased omega 3 fractions in cholesteryl esters and increased C20:4 omega-6/C20:5 omega-3 ratio in cholesteryl esters and phospholipids. *J Affect Dis* 1996; 38: 35–46.
127. Albert CM, Hennekens CH, O'Donnell CJ, et al. Fish consumption and risk of sudden cardiac death. *JAMA* 1998; 279:23–28.
128. Siscovick DS, Raghunathan TE, King I, et al. Dietary intake and cell membrane levels of long-chain n-3 polyunsaturated fatty acids and the risk of primary cardiac arrest. *JAMA* 1995; 274:1363–1367.
129. Burr ML, Fehily AM, Gilbert JF, et al. Effects of changes in fat, fish and fibre intake on death and myocardial reinfarction: Diet and reinfarction trial. *Lancet* 1989; 2:757–761.
130. Sellmayer A, Witzgall H, Lorenz RL, Weber PC. Effects of dietary fish oil on ventricular premature complexes. *Am J Cardiol* 1995; 76:974–977.
131. Christensen JH, Gustenhoff P, Korup E, et al. Effect of fish oil on heart rate variability in survivors of myocardial infarction: A double blind randomised controlled trial. *Brit Med J* 1996; 312:677–678.
132. Christensen JH, Korup E, Aaroe J, et al. Fish consumption, n-3 fatty acids in cell membranes, and heart rate variability in survivors of myocardial infarction with left ventricular dysfunction. *Am J Cardiol* 1997; 79:1670–1673.
133. Balogh S, Fitzpatrick DF, Hendricks SE, Paige SR. Increases in heart rate variability with successful treatment in patients with major depressive disorder. *Psychopharmacol Bull* 1993; 29:201–206.
134. Markovitz JH, Matthews KA. Platelets and coronary heart disease: Potential psychophysiologic mechanism. *Psychosom Med* 1991; 53:643–668.
135. Morris PLP, Robsin RG, Andrzejewski P, et al. Association of depression with 10-year poststroke mortality. *Am J Psychiatry* 1993; 150:124–129.
136. Lefkovits J, Plow EF, Topol EJ. Platelet glycoprotein IIb/IIIa receptors in cardiovascular medicine. *N Engl J Med* 1995; 332:1553–1559.
137. Hess H, Mietaschk A, Deichsel G. Drug-induced inhibition of platelet function delays progression of peripheral occlusive arterial disease: A prospective double-blind arteriographically controlled trial. *Lancet* 1985; 1:415–419.
138. Antiplatelet Trialists' Collaboration. Secondary prevention of vascular disease by prolonged antiplatelet treatment. *Brit Med J (Clinical Research Edition)* 1988; 296:320–331.
139. Verstraete M. Risk factors, interventions and therapeutic agents in the prevention of atherosclerosis-related ischaemic diseases. *Drugs* 1991; 42(suppl 5):22–38.
140. Ridker PM, Manson JE, Burning JE, et al. The effect of chronic platelet inhibition with low-dose aspirin on atherosclerotic progression and acute thrombosis: Clinical evidence from the Physicians' Health Study. *Am Heart J* 1991; 122:1588–1592.
141. Second International Trial of Infarct Survival Collaborative Group. Randomized trial of intravenous streptokinase, oral aspirin, both, or neither among 17,187 cases of suspected acute myocardial infarction: ISIS-2. *Lancet* 1988; 2:349–360.
142. Antiplatelet Trialists' Collaboration. Collaborative overview of randomized trials of antiplatelet therapy: I. Prevention of death, myocardial infarction, and stroke by prolonged antiplatelet therapy in various categories of patients. *Brit Med J* 1994; 308: 81–106.
143. Musselman DL, Tomer A, Manatunga AK, et al. Exaggerated platelet reactivity in major depression. *Am J Psychiatry* 1996; 153:1313–1317.
144. Laghrissi-Thode F, Wagner WR, Pollock BG, et al. Elevated platelet factor 4 and β-thromboglobulin plasma levels in depressed patients with ischemic heart disease. *Biol Psychiatry* 1997; 42:290–295.
145. Weyrich AS, Solis GA, Li KS, et al. Platelet amplification of vasospasm. *Am J Physiol* 1992; 263:H349–H358.
146. DeClerck F. Effects of serotonin on platelets and blood vessels. *J Cardiovasc Pharmacol* 1991; 17(suppl 5):S1–S5.
147. Owens MJ, Nemeroff CB. Role of serotonin in the pathophysiology of depression: Focus on the serotonin transporter. *Clin Chem* 1994; 40:288–295.
148. Osim EE, Wyllie JH. Evidence for loss of 5-hydroxytryptamine from circulating platelets. *J Physiol (Lond)* 1982; 326:25P–26P.
149. Ashton JH, Benedict CR, Fitzgerald C, et al. Serotonin as a mediator of cyclic flow variations in stenosed canine coronary arteries. *Circulation* 1986; 73:572–578.
150. Ashton JH, Ogletree ML, Michel IM, et al. Cooperative mediation by serotonin S2 and thromboxane S2/prostaglandin H2 receptor

activation of cyclic flow variation in dogs with severe coronary artery stenosis. *Circulation* 1987; 76:952–959.
151. Biegon A, Weizman A, Karp L, et al. Serotonin 5-HT2 receptor binding on blood platelets—a peripheral marker for depression? *Life Sci* 1987; 41:2485–2492.
152. Biegon A, Grinspoon A, Blumenfelt B, et al. Increased serotonin 5-HT2 receptor binding on blood platelets on suicidal men. *Psychopharmacology* 1990; 100:165–167.
153. Biegon A, Essar N, Israeli M, et al. Serotonin 5-HT2 receptor binding on blood platelets as a state dependent marker in major affective disorder. *Psychopharmacology* 1990; 102:73–75.
154. Arora RC, Meltzer HY. Increased serotonin (5-HT2) receptor binding as measured by 3H-LSD in the blood platelets of depressed patients. *Life Sci* 1989; 44:725–734.
155. Pandey GN, Pandey SC, Janicak PG. Platelet serotonin-2 binding sites in depression and suicide. *Biol Psychiatry* 1990; 28:215–222.
156. Briley MS, Langer SZ, Raisman R, et al. Tritiated imipramine binding sites are decreased in platelets of untreated depressed patients. *Science* 1980; 209:303–305.
157. Langer SZ, Arifian E, Briley MS, et al. High-affinity binding of 3H-imipramine in brain and platelets and its relevance to the biochemistry of affective disorders. *Life Sci* 1981; 29:211–218.
158. Paul SM, Rehavi M, Skolnick P, et al. Depressed patients have decreased binding of tritiated imipramine to platelet serotonin "transporter." *Arch Gen Psychiatry* 1981; 38:1315–1317.
159. Nemeroff CB, Knight DL, Franks J, et al. Further studies on platelet transporter binding in depression. *Am J Psychiatry* 1994; 151:1623–1625.
160. Cerrito F, Lazzaro MP, Gaudio E, et al. 5HT2-receptors and serotonin release: Their role in human platelet aggregation. *Life Sci* 1993; 53:209–215.
161. Kusumi I, Koyama T, Yamashita I. Serotonin-stimulated Ca^{2+} response is increased in the blood platelets of depressed patients. *Biol Psychiatry* 1991; 30:310–312.
162. Mikuni M, Kusumi I, Kagaya A, et al. Increased 5-HT2 receptor function as measured by serotonin-stimulated phosphoinositide hydrolosis in platelets of depressed patients. *Prog Neuropsychopharmacol Biol Psychiatry* 1991; 15:49–61.
163. Eckert A, Gann H, Riemann D, et al. Elevated intracellular calcium levels after 5-HT2 receptor stimulation in platelets of depressed patients. *Biol Psychiatry* 1993; 34:565–568.
164. Plein H, Berk M, Eppel S, Butkow N. Augmented platelet calcium uptake in response to serotonin stimulation in patients with major depression measured using Mn^{2+} influx and $^{45}CA^{2+}$ uptake. *Life Sci* 1999; 66:425–431.
165. Ware JA, Smith M, Salzman EW. Synergism of platelet aggregating agents: Role of elevation of cytoplasmic calcium. *J Clin Invest* 1987; 80:267–271.
166. Verrier RL. Behavioral stress, myocardial ischemia, and arrhythmias. In: Zipes DP, Jalife J, eds. *Cardiac Electrophysiology from Cell to Bedside.* Toronto: Saunders; 1990:343.
167. Jiang W, Babyak M, Krantz DS, et al. Mental stress-induced myocardial ischemia and cardiac events. *JAMA* 1996; 21:1651–1656.
168. Lown B, DeSilva RA, Reich P, Murawski BJ. Psychophysiologic factors in sudden cardiac death. *Am J Psychiatry* 1980; 137:1325–1335.
169. Lown B, Verrier RL. Neural activity and ventricular fibrillation. *N Engl J Med* 1976; 294:1165–1170.
170. Zaza A, Schwartz PJ. Role of the autonomic nervous system in the genesis of early ischemic arrhythmias. *J Cardiovasc Pharmacol* 1985; 7(suppl 5):S8–S12.
171. *Stedman's Medical Dictionary.* Baltimore: Williams & Wilkins; 1982.
172. Heit S, Owens MJ, Plotsky P, Nemeroff CB. Corticotropin-releasing factor, stress, and depression. *Neuroscientist* 1997; 3:186–194.
173. Tavazzi L, Zotti AM, Rondanelli R. The role of psychologic stress in the genesis of lethal arrhythmias in patients with coronary artery disease. *Eur Heart J* 1986; 7(suppl A):99–106.
174. Follick MJ, Gorkin L, Capone RJ, et al. Psychological distress as a predictor of ventricular arrhythmias in a post-myocardial infarct population. *Am Heart J* 1988; 116:32–36.
175. Gold PW, Goodwin FK, Chrousos GP. Clinical and biochemical manifestations of depression: Relation to the neurobiology of stress. *N Engl J Med* 1988; 319:413–420.
176. Valentino RJ, Foote SL, Page ME. The locus coeruleus as a site for integrating corticotropin-releasing factor and noradrenergic mediation of stress responses. *Ann NY Acad Sci* 1993; 697: 173–188.
177. Curtis AL, Pavcovich LA, Grigoriadis DE, Valentino RJ. Previous stress alters corticotropin-releasing factor neurotransmission in the locus coeruleus. *Neuroscience* 1995; 65:541–550.
178. Chrousos GP, Gold PW. The concepts of stress and stress system disorders: Overview of physical and behavioral homeostasis. *JAMA* 1992; 267:1244–1252.
179. Paykel E. Causal relationships between clinical depression and life events. In: Barrett JE, ed. *Stress and Mental Disorder.* New York: Raven Press; 1979.
180. Kendler KS, Kessler RC, Neale MC, et al. The prediction of major depression in women: Toward an integrated etiologic model. *Am J Psychiatry* 1993; 150:1139–1148.
181. Echt DS, Liebson PR, Mitchell LB, et al. Mortality and morbidity in patients receiving encainide, flecainide or placebo: The Cardiac Arrythmia Suppression Trial. *N Engl J Med* 1991; 324: 781–788.
182. Thomas SA, Friedmann E, Wimbush F, Shron E. Psychosocial factors and survival in the Cardiac Arrhythmia Suppression Trial (CAST): A reexamination. *Am J Crit Care* 1997; 6:116–126.
183. Fifer SK, Mathias SD, Patrick DL, et al. Untreated anxiety among adult primary care patients in a health maintenance organization. *Arch Gen Psychiatry* 1994; 51:740–750.
184. Sullivan MD, LaCroix AZ, Baum C, et al. Functional status in coronary artery disease: A one-year prospective study of the role of anxiety and depression. *Am J Med* 1997; 103:348–356.
185. Boyd JH. Use of mental health services for the treatment of panic disorder. *Am J Psychiatry* 1986; 143:1569–1574.
186. Klerman G, Weissman MM, Ouellette R, et al. Panic attacks in the community: Social morbidity and health care utilization. *JAMA* 1991; 265:742–746.
187. Markowitz JS, Weissman MM, Ouellette R, et al. Quality of life in panic disorder. *Arch Gen Psychiatry* 1989; 46:984–992.
188. Noyes R. The comorbidity and mortality of panic disorder. *Psychiatr Med* 1990; 8:41–66.
189. Sherbourne CD, Jackson CA, Meredith LS, et al. Prevalence of comorbid anxiety disorders in primary care outpatients. *Arch Family Med* 1996; 5:27–34.
190. Lum LC. Hyperventilation syndrome in medicine and psychiatry: A review. *J R Soc Med* 1987; 80:229–231.
191. Beck JG, Berisford MA, Taegtmeyer H. The effects of voluntary hyperventilation on patients with chest pain without coronary artery disease. *Behav Res Ther* 1991; 29:611–621.
192. Bass CM. Functional and cardiorespiratory symptoms. In: Bass CM, ed. *Somatization: Physiological and Psychologic Illness.* London: Blackwell; 1990:171.
193. Lynch P, Bakal DA, Whitelaw W, Fung T. Chest muscle activity and panic anxiety: A preliminary investigation. *Psychosom Med* 1991; 53:80–89.
194. Bass C, Wade C. Chest pain in normal coronary arteries: A comparative study of psychiatric and social morbidity. *Psychol Med* 1984; 14:51–61.
195. Goldberg DP, Cooper B, Eastwood MR, et al. A standardised psychiatric interview for use in community surveys. *Br J Prevent Social Med* 1970; 24:18–23.
196. Katon W, Hall ML, Russo J, et al. Chest pain: Relationship of psy-

chiatric illness to coronary arteriographic results. *Am J Med* 1988; 84:1–9.

197. Haines AP, Imeson JD, Meade TW. Phobic anxiety and ischaemic heart disease. *Brit M J (Clinical Research Edition)* 1987; 295: 297–299.
198. Eaker ED, Pinsky J, Castelli WP. Myocardial infarction and coronary death among women: Psychosocial predictors from a 20-year follow-up women in the Framingham Study. *Am J Epidemiol* 1992; 135:854–864.
199. Kawachi I, Colitz GA, Ascherio A. Prospective study of phobic anxiety and risk of coronary heart disease in men. *Circulation* 1994; 89:1992–1997.
200. Kawachi I, Sparrow D, Vokonas PS, et al. Symptoms of anxiety and risk of coronary heart disease: The normative aging study. *Circulation* 1994; 90:2225–2229.
201. Davis M. The role of the amygdala in fear-potentiated startle: Implications for animal models of anxiety. *Trends Pharmacol Sci* 1992; 13:35–41.
202. Ninan PT. The functional anatomy, neurochemistry, and pharmacology of anxiety. *J Clin Psychiatry* 1999; 60(suppl 22):12–17.
203. Stein MB, Uhde TW. Biology of anxiety disorders. In: Schatzberg AF, Nemeroff CB, eds. *The American Psychiatric Association Textbook of Psychopharmacology*, 2d ed. Washington, DC: American Psychiatric Association; 1998:609.
204. Klein DF. False suffocation alarms, spontaneous panics, and related conditions: An integrative hypothesis. *Arch Gen Psychiatry* 1993; 50:306–317.
205. McNally RJ, Eke M. Anxiety sensitivity, suffocation fear, and breath-holding duration as predictors of response to carbon dioxide challenge. *J Abnorm Psychol* 1996; 105:146–149.
206. Torgersen S. Twin studies in panic disorder. In: Ballenger J, ed. *Neurobiology of Panic Disorder.* New York: Liss; 1990:51.
207. Stein MB, Millar TW, Larsen DK, et al. Irregular breathing during sleep in patients with panic disorder. *Am J Psychiatry* 1995; 152:1168–1173.
208. Martinez JM, Papp LA, Coplan JD, et al. Ambulatory monitoring of respiration during anxiety. *Anxiety* 1996; 2:296–302.
209. Bremner JD, Licinio J, Darnell A, et al. Elevated CSF corticotropin-releasing factor concentrations in posttraumatic stress disorder. *Am J Psychiatry* 1997; 154:624–629.
210. Baker DG, West SA, Nicholson WE, et al. Serial CSF corticotropin-releasing hormone levels and adrenocortical activity in combat veterans with posttraumatic stress disorder. *Am J Psychiatry* 1999; 156:585–588.
211. Smith MA, Davidson J, Ritchie JC, et al. The corticotropin-releasing hormone test in patients with posttraumatic stress disorder. *Biol Psychiatry* 1989; 26:349–355.
212. Yehuda R, Southwick SM, Nussbaum G, et al. Low urinary cortisol excretion in PTSD. *J Nerv Ment Dis* 1990; 178:366–369.
213. Yehuda R, Teicher MH, Levengood RA, et al. Low urinary cortisol excretion in Holocaust survivors with posttraumatic stress disorder. *Am J Psychiatry* 1995; 152:982–986.
214. Yehuda R, Boisoneau D, Lowy MT, et al. Dose-response changes in plasma cortisol and lymphocyte glucocorticoid receptors following dexamethasone administration in combat veterans with and without posttraumatic stress disorder. *Arch Gen Psychiatry* 1995; 52:583–593.
215. Boscarino JA. Posttraumatic stress disorder, exposure to combat, and lower plasma cortisol among Vietnam veterans: Findings and clinical implications. *J Consultat Clin Psychol* 1996; 64: 191–201.
216. Stein MB, Yehuda R, Koverola C, et al. Enhanced dexamethasone suppression of plasma cortisol in adult women traumatized by childhood sexual abuse. *Biol Psychiatry* 1997; 42:680–686.
217. Linares OA, Zech LA, Jacquez JA, et al. Effect of sodium-restricted diet and posture on norepinephrine kinetics in humans. *Am J Physiol* 1988; 254:E222–E230.
218. Villacres EC, Hollifield M, Katon WJ, et al. Sympathetic nervous system activity in panic disorder. *Psychiatry Res* 1987; 21:313–321.
219. Wilkinson DJC, Thompson JM, Lambert GW, et al. Sympathetic activity in patients with panic disorder at rest, under laboratory mental stress, and during panic attacks. *Arch Gen Psychiatry* 1998; 55:511–520.
220. Weissman MM, Markowitz JS, Ouellette R, et al. Panic disorder and cardiovascular/cerebrovascular problems: Results from a community survey. *Am J Psychiatry* 1990; 147:1504–1508.
221. Coryell W, Noyes R, Clancy J. Excess mortality in panic disorder: A comparison with primary unipolar depression. *Arch Gen Psychiatry* 1982; 39:701–703.
222. Markovitz JH, Matthews KA, Wing RR, et al. Psychological, biological and health behavior predictors of blood pressure changes in middle-aged women. *J Hypertens* 1991; 9:399–406.
223. Markovitz JH, Matthews KA, Kannel WB, et al. Psychological predictors of hypertension in the Framingham Study: Is there tension in hypertension? [see comments]. *JAMA* 1993; 270:2439–2443.
224. Jonas BS, Franks P, Ingram DD. Are symptoms of anxiety and depression risk factors for hypertension? Longitudinal evidence from the national Health and Nutrition Examination Survey I Epidemiologic Follow-Up Study. *Arch Family Med* 1997; 6:43–49.
225. Kubzansky LD, Kawachi I, Weiss ST, Sparrow D. Anxiety and coronary heart disease: A synthesis of epidemiological, psychological, and experimental evidence. *Ann Behav Med* 1998; 20:47–58.
226. Sheehan DV, Coleman JH, Greenblatt DJ, et al. Some biochemical correlates of panic attacks with agoraphobia and their response to a new treatment. *J Clin Psychopharmacol* 1984; 4:66–75.
227. Girotti LA, Crosatto JR, Messuti H, et al. The hyperventilation test as a method for developing successful therapy in Prinzmetal angina. *Am J Cardiol* 1982; 49:834–841.
228. Freeman IJ, Nixon PGF. Are coronary artery spasm and progressive damage to the heart associated with the hyperventilation syndrome? *Brit Med J* 1985; 291:851–852.
229. Rasmussen K, Ravnsbaek J, Funch-Jensen P, et al. Oesophageal spasm in patients with coronary artery spasm. *Lancet* 1986; 1:174–176.
230. Myerburg RJ, Kessler KM, Mallon SM, et al. Life-threatening ventricular arrhythmias in patients with silent myocardial ischemia due to coronary artery spasm. *N Engl J Med* 1992; 326:1451–1455.
231. Friedman BH, Thayer JF. Heart rate variability and anxiety: Excess lability or flexibility? [Abstract]. *Psychophysiology* 1993; 30:S10.
232. Thayer JF, Friedman BH. Assessment of anxiety using heart rate nonlinear dynamics. In: Ditto W, ed. *Chaos in Biology and Medicine: SPIE Proceedings*. Bellingham, Washington: Society of Photo-optical Instrumentation Engineers; 1993:42–48.
233. Yeragani VK, Balon R, Pohl R, et al. Decreased R-R variance in panic disorder patients. *Acta Psychiatr Scand* 1990; 81:554–559.
234. Yeragani VK, Pohl R, Berger R, et al. Decreased heart rate variability in panic disorder patients: A study of power-spectral analysis of heart rate. *Psychiatry Res* 1993; 46:89–103.
235. Lyonsfield JD. An examination of image and thought processes in generalized anxiety. Association for the Advancement of Behavior Therapy. New York; 1991.
236. Thayer JF, Friedman BH, Borkovec TD. Autonomic characteristics of generalized anxiety disorder and worry. *Biol Psychiatry* 1996; 39:255–266.
237. Shear MK, Kligfield P, Harshfield G, et al. Cardiac rate and rhythm in panic patients. *Am J Psychiatry* 1987; 144:633–637.
238. Chignon J-M, Lepine J-P, Ades J. Panic disorder in cardiac outpatients. *Am J Psychiatry* 1993; 150:780–785.
239. Winkle RA. The relationship between ventricular ectopic beat frequency and heart rate. *Circulation* 1982; 66:633–637.
240. Katz C, Martin RD, Landa B, Chadda KD. Relationship of psychologic factors to frequent symptomatic ventricular arrhythmia. *Am J Med* 1985; 78:589–594.

241. Orth-Gomer K, Edwards ME, Erhardt L, et al. Relation between ventricular arrhythmias and psychological profile. *Acta Med Scand* 1980; 207:31–36.
242. Freeman AM, Cohen-Cole S, Fleece L, et al. Psychiatric symptoms, Type A behavior and arrhythmias following coronary bypass. *Psychosomatics* 1984; 25:586–589.
243. Follick MJ, Ahern DK, Gorkin L, et al. Relation of psychosocial and stress reactivity variables to ventricular arrhythmias in the Cardiac Arrhythmia Pilot Study (CAPS). *Am J Cardiol* 1990; 66:63–67.
244. Frasure-Smith N, Prince R. The ischemic heart disease life stress monitoring program: Impact on mortality. *Psychosom Med* 1984; 47:431–445.
245. Friedman M, Thoresen CE, Gill JJ, et al. Alteration of type A behavior and its effect on cardiac recurrences in postmyocardial infarction patients: Summary results of the recurrent coronary prevention project. *Am Heart J* 1986; 112:653–665.
246. Frasure-Smith N. In-hospital symptoms of psychological stress as predictors of long-term outcome after acute myocardial infarction in men. *Am J Cardiol* 1991; 67:121–127.
247. Frasure-Smith N, Lesperance F, Juneau M. Differential long-term impact of in-hospital symptoms of psychological stress after non-Q-wave and Q-wave myocardial infarction. *Am J Cardiol* 1992; 69:1128–1134.
248. Jones DA, West RR. Psychological rehabilitation after myocardial infarction: Multicentre randomised controlled trial. *Brit Med J* 1996; 313:1517–1521.
249. Frasure-Smith N, Lesperance F, Prince RH, et al. Randomised trial of home-based psychosocial nursing intervention for patients recovering from myocardial infarction. *Lancet* 1997; 350:473–479.
250. Roose SP, Laghriss-Thode F, Kennedy JS, et al. Comparison of paroxetine and nortriptyline in depressed patients with ischemic heart disease. *JAMA* 1998; 279:287–291.
251. Shapiro PA, Lesperance F, Frasure-Smith N, et al. An open-label preliminary trial for the treatment of major depression after acute-myocardial infarction (the SADHAT Trial). *Am Heart J* 1999; 137:1100–1106.
252. Muskin PR, Glassman AH. The use of tricyclic antidepressants in a medical setting. In: Finkel JB, ed. *Consultation-Liaison Psychiatry: Current Trends and Future Perspectives.* New York: Grune & Stratton; 1983:137.
253. Roose SP, Dalack GW. Treating the depressed patient with cardiovascular problems. *J Clin Psychiatry* 1992; 53:25–31.
254. Arana GW, Hyman SE. *Handbook of Psychiatric Drug Therapy.* 2d ed. Boston: Little, Brown; 1995:61.
255. Roose SP, Glassman AH, Siris SG, et al. Comparison of imipramine- and nortriptyline-induced orthostatic hypotension: A meaningful difference. *J Clin Psychopharmacol* 1981; 1:316–319.
256. Thayssen P, Bjerre M, Kragh-Sorensen P, et al. Cardiovascular effects of imipramine and nortriptyline in elderly patients. *Psychopharmacology (Berl)* 1981; 74:360–364.
257. Feder R. Bradycardia and syncope induced by fluoxetine (letter). *J Clin Psychiatry* 1991; 52:139.
258. Hyman SE, Arana GW, Rosenbaum JF. *Handbook of Psychiatric Drug Therapy.* Boston: Little, Brown; 1995.
259. Robinson DS, Roberts DL, Smith JM, et al. The safety profile of nefazodone. *J Clin Psychiatry* 1996; 57(suppl 2):31–38.
260. Franco-Brunson K. The management of treatment-resistant depression in the medically ill. *Psychiatr Clin North Am* 1996; 19:329–350.
261. Feighner JP. Cardiovascular safety in depressed patients: Focus on venlafaxine. *J Clin Psychiatry* 1995; 56:574–579.
262. Ellison JM, Milofsky JE, Ely E. Fluoxetine-induced bradycardia and syncope in two patients. *J Clin Psychiatry* 1990; 51:385–386.
263. Enemark B. The importance of ECG monitoring in antidepressant treatment. *Nordic J Psychiatry* 1993; 47(suppl 30):57–65.
264. Humphries JE, Wheby MS, VandenBerg SR. Fluoxetine and the bleeding time. *Arch Pathol Lab Med* 1990; 114:727–728.
265. Evans TG, Buys SS, Rodgers GM. Letter to the editor. *N Engl J Med* 1991; 324:1671.
266. Yaryura-Tobias JA, Kirschen H, Ninan P, Mosberg HF. Fluoxetine and bleeding in obsessive-compulsive disorder (letter). *Am J Psychiatry* 1991; 148:949.
267. Alderman CP, Moritz CK, Ben-Tovim DI. Abnormal platelet aggregation associated with fluoxetine therapy. *Ann Pharmacother* 1992; 26:1517–1519.
268. Callahan AM, Marangell LB, Ketter TA. Evaluating the clinical significance of drug interactions: A systematic approach. *Harvard Rev Psychiatry* 1996; 4:153–158.
269. Roose SP, Dalack GW, Glassman AH, et al. Cardiovascular effects of buproprion in depressed patients with heart disease. *Am J Psychiatry* 1991; 148:512–516.
270. Roose SP, Glassman AH, Attia E, et al. Cardiovascular effects of fluoxetine in depressed patients with heart disease. *Am J Psychiatry* 1998; 155:660–665.
271. Roose SP, Glassman AH, Attia E, Woodring S. Comparative efficacy of selective serotonin reuptake inhibitors and tricyclics in the treatment of melancholia. *Am J Psychiatry* 1994; 151:1735–1739.
272. American Psychiatric Association Task Force on Electroconvulsive Therapy. *The Practice of Electroconvulsive Therapy.* Washington, DC: American Psychiatric Association Press; 1990.
273. Weiner RD. Does electroconvulsive therapy cause brain damage? *Behav Brain Sci* 1984; 7:1–53.
274. Applegate RJ. Diagnosis and management of ischemic heart disease in the patient scheduled to undergo electroconvulsive therapy. *Convulsive Ther* 1997; 13:128–144.
275. Alexopoulos GS, Shamoian CJ, Lucas J, et al. Medical problems of geriatric psychiatric patients and younger controls during electroconvulsive therapy. *J Am Geriatr Soc* 1994; 32:651–654.
276. Pornnoppadol C, Isenberg K. ECT and the implantable converter defibrillator. *J Electroconvuls Ther* 1998; 14:124–126.
277. Block M, Admon D, Bonne O, Lerer B. Electroconvulsive therapy in depressed cardiac transplant patients. *Convuls Ther* 1992; 8:290–293.
278. Maneksha FR. Hypertension and tachycardia during electroconvulsive therapy: To treat or not to treat. *Convuls Ther* 1991; 70:28–35.
279. Figiel GS, deLeo B, Zorumski CF, et al. Combined use of labetalol and nifedipine in controlling the cardiovascular response from ECT. *J Geriatr Psychiatry Neurol* 1993; 6:20–24.
280. Figiel GD, McDonald L, LaPlante R. Cardiac modified ECT in the elderly (letter). *Am J Psychiatry* 1994; 151:790–791.
281. Stoudemire A, Knos G, Gladson M, et al. Labetalol in the control of cardiovascular responses to electroconvulsive therapy in high-risk depressed medical patients. *J Clin Psychiatry* 1990; 51:508–512.
282. Figiel G, McDonald WM, McCall WV, Zorumpski C. Electroconvulsive therapy. In: Schatzberg AF, Nemeroff CB, eds. *American Psychiatric Association Textbook of Psychopharmacology.* 2d ed. Washington, DC: American Psychiatric Association; 1998:523.
283. Lesperance F, Frasure-Smith N, Talajic M. Major depression before and after myocardial infarction: Its nature and consequences. *Psychosom Med* 1996; 58:99–110.
284. Grodstein F, Stampfer MJ. The epidemiology of coronary heart disease and estrogen replacement in postmenopausal women. *Progr Cardiovasc Dis* 1995; 38:199–210.
285. Kon Koh K, Mincemoyer R, Bui MN, et al. Effects of hormone-replacement therapy on fibrinolysis in postmenopausal women. *N Engl J Med* 1997; 336:683–690.

CHAPTER 81

ADVERSE CARDIOVASCULAR DRUG INTERACTIONS AND COMPLICATIONS

Lionel H. Opie / William H. Frishman

Toxicities from drug interactions have been shown to be a cause of morbidity and death in patients,[1] and these interactions often are associated with the loss of individual drug efficacy.[2] Recent technologies have resulted in an explosion of information concerning the cytochrome P450 isoenzyme system involved in the metabolism of cardiovascular drugs.[3–10] In addition to the isoenzyme inhibition and induction by various drugs, microsomal drug metabolism is affected by genetic polymorphisms,[9] age, nutrition, gender,[6] and hepatic diseases.[3,4,7] P-glycoprotein, which mediates the transcellular transport of many drugs, may also play an important role in clinically significant drug-drug interactions.[5]

Today, a knowledge of cardiovascular drug interactions is regarded as basic to our understanding of the pharmacologic properties of cardiovascular drugs. Such interactions can be either pharmacokinetic, whereby one agent interferes with the metabolism of another, or pharmacodynamic, whereby the hemodynamic properties of one agent are additive or subtractive to those of another (Fig. 81-1). An example of pharmacokinetic interaction is the decreased rate of hepatic metabolism of lidocaine during cimetidine therapy, with a possible risk of lidocaine toxicity. An example of a pharmacodynamic interaction arises when nifedipine is added to beta-adrenergic blockade in the therapy of severe angina, sometimes with excess hypotension as a side effect.

This chapter includes discussions of the drug interactions of the major classes of cardiovascular drugs, following an established sequence of these drugs.[11,12]

BETA-ADRENERGIC–BLOCKING DRUGS

Beta-adrenergic blockers demonstrate relatively few serious drug interactions (Table 81-1). An example of a pharmacokinetic interaction is that with cimetidine,[13] which reduces hepatic metabolism and therefore increases blood levels of carvedilol, propranolol, labetalol, and metoprolol, which are metabolized in the liver by the cytochrome oxidase system (Fig. 81-2). However, there is no interaction of cimetidine with beta blockers

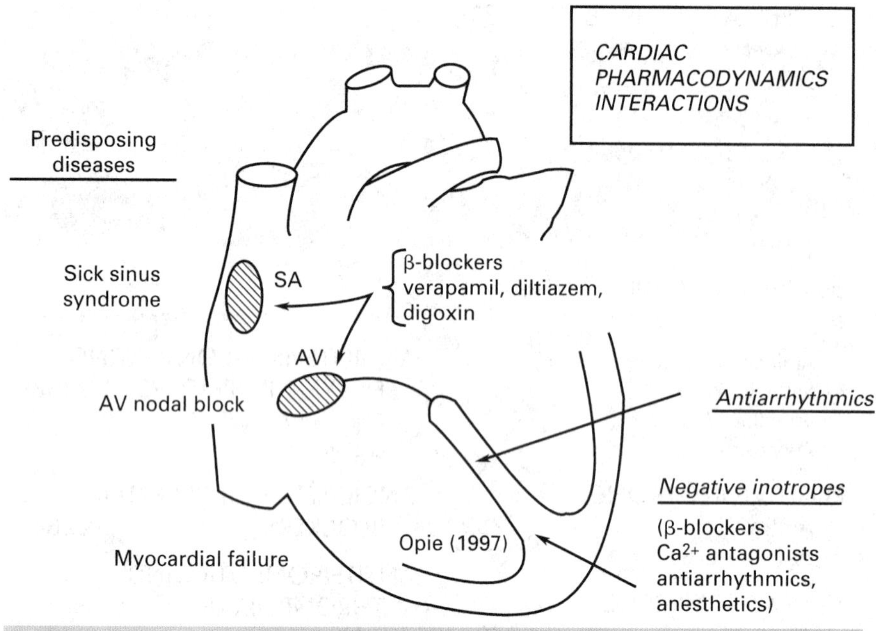

FIGURE 81-1 Cardiac pharmacodynamic interactions at the levels of the SA node, AV node, conduction system, and myocardium. The predisposing disease conditions are shown on the left. (Figure copyrighted by LH Opie.)

such as atenolol, sotalol, and nadolol, which are not metabolized in the liver. Another pharmacokinetic interaction is when verapamil raises blood levels of metoprolol through a hepatic interaction[14]; presumably, other beta blockers metabolized by the liver may be subject to a similar interaction.

Now used with increasing frequency in the acute phase of myocardial infarction, beta blockers may depress hepatic blood flow, thereby decreasing the hepatic inactivation of lidocaine.[15] Thus, beta blockade increases lidocaine blood levels, with an enhanced risk of toxicity. An example of a pharmacodynamic interaction with beta blockers is that seen with nonsteroidal anti-inflammatory drugs (NSAIDs), including indomethacin, which may attenuate the antihypertensive effects of beta blockers, possibly by decreasing the formation of vasodilatory prostaglandins.[16]

NITRATES

The chief drug interactions of nitrates are pharmacodynamic (Table 81-2). For example, during triple therapy of angina pectoris (nitrates, beta blockers, and calcium antagonists), the overall efficacy of the combination may be lessened because each drug can predispose patients to excess hypotension.[17] Even two components of triple therapy, such as diltiazem and nitrates, may interact adversely to cause moderate hypotension.[18] Nonetheless, high doses of diltiazem can improve persistent effort angina when added to maximum doses of propranolol and isosorbide dinitrate without any report of significant hypotension.[19] Therefore, individual patients vary greatly in their susceptibility to the hypotension of triple therapy. A dangerous drug-drug interaction is that of nitrates with sildenafil, an anti-impotence drug that can intensify the hypotensive effects of nitrates.[20] Sildenafil should not be used within 24 h of nitrate use. There is a reported beneficial interaction between nitrates and hydralazine whereby the latter drug appears to lessen nitrate tolerance.[21]

Unexpectedly, high doses of nitroglycerin may induce heparin resistance by altering the activity of antithrombin III.[22] Nitroglycerin can also lessen the therapeutic effects of the tissue plasminogen activator alteplase.

CALCIUM ANTAGONISTS

Many of the interactions of calcium antagonists are pharmacodynamic (Table 81-2),[23,24] such as added effects on the atrioventricular (AV) or sinus nodes (verapamil or diltiazem plus beta blockers, excess digitalis, or amiodarone), or on the systemic vascular resistance (e.g., nifedipine plus beta blockers causing excess hypotension). However, it is now increasingly recognized that verapamil and diltiazem (but probably not nifedipine) inhibit the hepatic oxidation of some drugs, the blood levels of which consequently increase. Such agents include cyclosporine (diltiazem), the antiepileptic carbamazepine (verapamil), prazosin (verapamil), lovastatin, atorvastatin and simvastatin (diltiazem), theophylline (verapamil), some HIV protease inhibitors (diltiazem), and quinidine (verapamil). In addition, nifedipine especially and also verapamil tend to increase hepatic blood flow, potentially leading to enhanced first-pass metabolism of agents such as propranolol, resulting in decreased beta blocker blood levels.[7] The effects of some dihydropyridine calcium channel blockers (e.g., felodipine and nifedipine) are potentiated by concomitant grapefruit juice ingestion.[25] The number of potentially toxic drug–drug interactions with bepridil are so great that it is used only as a last resort.[26,27]

Verapamil and Beta Blockers

Intravenous verapamil added to beta-adrenergic blockade has the additional risk of added hypotension or added nodal inhibition.[28,29] In patients with angina pectoris already receiving beta blockers, verapamil given intravenously[30] or orally[31] can reduce myocardial contractility,[31] increase heart size,[32] and cause sinus bradycardia.[33] By a hepatic pharmacokinetic interaction,[7,34] verapamil may raise blood levels of the beta blockers metabolized by the liver. Despite such hepatic interactions (e.g., verapamil with propranolol) in normal subjects, pharmacodynamic changes are more important.[35] The combination of verapamil and beta blockade in the therapy of angina pectoris must be used with care with preexisting depression of the sinoatrial (SA) or AV nodes and clinically detectable myocardial failure. The combination of verapamil and beta blockers improves myocardial function during exercise more than either agent alone.[36] Verapamil plus a beta blocker may have an additive therapeutic effect in hypertension, but with a small risk of excess inhibition of sinus rate, AV conduction, or left ventricular function.[37]

TABLE 81-1 Drug Interactions of Beta-Adrenergic–Blocking Agents

Cardiac Drug	Interacting Drugs	Mechanism	Consequence	Prophylaxis
		HEMODYNAMIC INTERACTIONS		
All beta blockers	Calcium antagonists, especially nifedipine	Added hypotension	Risk of myocardial ischemia	Blood pressure control, adjust doses
	Verapamil or diltiazem	Added negative inotropic effect	Risk of myocardial failure	Check for CHF, adjust doses
	Flecainide		Hypotension	Check LV function flecainide levels
	Sympathomimetics (S)	Opposing effects	Loss of clinical benefit	Avoid S
		ELECTROPHYSIOLOGICAL INTERACTIONS		
All beta blockers	Verapamil	Added inhibition of SA, AV nodes	Bradycardia, asystole, complete heart block	Exclude "sick-sinus" syndrome, AV nodal disease; adjust dose, exclude predrug LV failure
	Diltiazem	Added negative inotropic effect	Excess hypotension	
		HEPATIC INTERACTIONS		
Propranolol (P)	Cimetidine (C)	C decreases P metabolism	Excess propranolol effects	Reduce both drug doses
	Lidocaine	Low hepatic blood flow	Excess lidocaine effects	Reduce lidocaine dose
Metoprolol (M)	Verapamil (V)	V decreases M metabolism	Excess M effects	Reduce M dose
	Cimetidine (C)	C decreases M metabolism	Excess M effects	Reduce both drug doses
Labetalol (L)	Cimetidine (C)	C decreases L metabolism	Excess L and C effects	Reduce both drug doses
Carvedilol (CV)	Cimetidine (C)	C decreases CV metabolism	Excess CV effects	Reduce both drug doses
		ANTIHYPERTENSIVE INTERACTIONS		
Beta blockers	Indomethacin (I), NSAIDs	I inhibits vasodilatory prostaglandins	Decreased antihypertensive effect	Omit indomethacin; use alternative drugs
		IMMUNE INTERACTING DRUGS		
Acebutolol	Other drugs altering immune status: procainamide, hydralazine, captopril	Theoretical risk of additive immune effects	Theoretical risk of lupus or neutropenia	Check antinuclear factors and neutrophils; low doses during cotherapy

ABBREVIATION: LV = left ventricular.

Verapamil and Digoxin

Verapamil can increase blood digoxin levels by over 50 percent.[38] The dose of digoxin must be cut to about half, and blood levels of digoxin must then be rechecked. In digitalis toxicity, rapid intravenous verapamil is absolutely contraindicated because the sum of the inhibitory effects of these two agents on the AV node can be fatal. Experimentally, verapamil can inhibit the calcium-dependent delayed afterdepolarizations, which cause the ventricular automaticity found in digitalis toxicity. Oral verapamil and digitalis can, however, be combined in the absence of digitalis toxicity or AV block, because their pharmacologic sites of action are different; nevertheless, the digoxin level needs monitoring. The combination is often used for the management of supraventricular tachycardias.

Verapamil and Prazosin

The combination of verapamil with prazosin for hypertension provides added and synergistic activities.[39] A hepatic pharmacokinetic interaction with enhanced bioavailability of prazosin may explain these effects.[40,41]

Verapamil and Quinidine

Verapamil and quinidine may interact to cause excess hypotension,[42] either by combined inhibition of peripheral receptors or

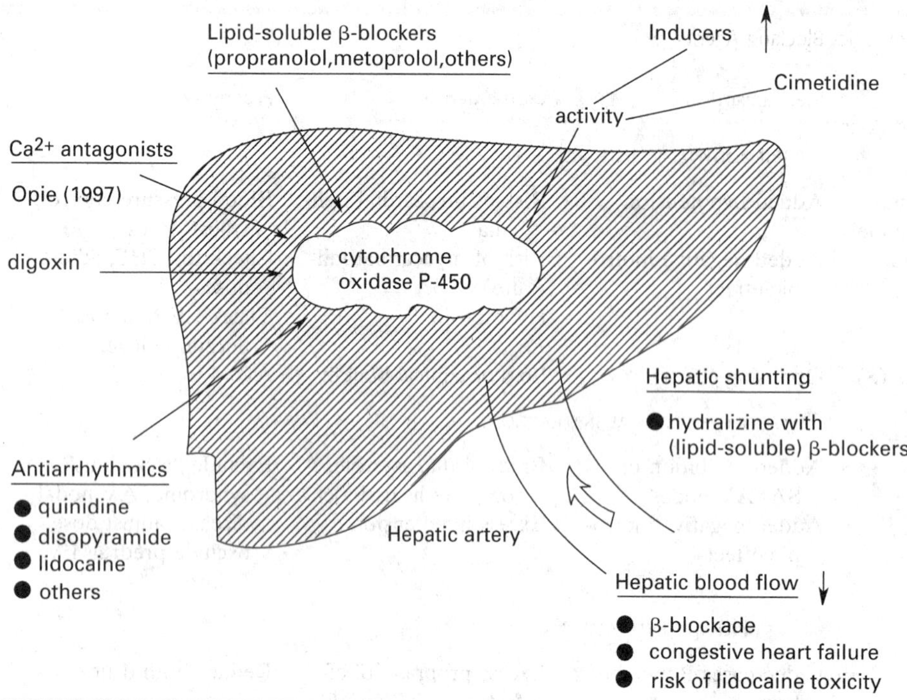

FIGURE 81-2 Potential hepatic pharmacokinetic interactions at the level of cytochrome oxidase P450 and potential pharmacodynamic interactions due to altered hepatic blood flow. (Figure copyrighted by LH Opie.)

by increase of quinidine levels.[43] The latter may be a hepatic interaction.

Verapamil and Disopyramide

Both verapamil and disopyramide are powerful negative inotropes. Thus, the combination can only be given when left ventricular function is good prior to initiation of therapy and can be closely monitored.

Verapamil and Theophylline

Verapamil may inhibit the hepatic metabolism of theophylline and lead to increased blood theophylline levels.[44]

Verapamil and Protease Inhibitors

Verapamil may inhibit the hepatic metabolism of the human immunodeficiency virus (HIV) protease inhibitors, causing decreased drug clearance of these agents and increased exposure to active drug.[24] No known toxicity has been observed at this time.[24]

Nifedipine

The combination of nifedipine with beta blockade is generally well tolerated except for the risk of hypotension.[45] Nifedipine and propranolol may have a pharmacokinetic interaction whereby blood levels of propranolol are increased; it is thought that nifedipine increases the hepatic blood flow so that propranolol breakdown in the liver is increased.[46] Although nifedipine is an afterload reducer, it also has a direct negative inotropic effect. Hence, combination with beta blockers, disopyramide, or any other negative inotropic agent should be undertaken with caution. Nifedipine combined with prazosin hydrochloride may cause excess hypotension[47]; thus, low initial additive doses are recommended (see "Prazosin, Doxazosin, and Terazosin," below).

Diltiazem

Diltiazem, like verapamil, may increase blood digoxin levels; however, the rise is likely to be much less, and some studies report no increase at all. Diltiazem plus long-acting nitrates occasionally causes excess hypotension.[18] Similar effects have been seen when diltiazem is combined with nifedipine.[48] The combination of high-dose diltiazem with beta blockade may cause bradycardia or hypotension.[49] Relatively few life-threatening interactions have been described for intravenous diltiazem. However, it can be expected to produce a spectrum of drug interactions similar to that of intravenous verapamil. As diltiazem is metabolized by the liver, it interacts with both cyclosporine and cilostazol, resulting in increased blood levels of both drugs.[50,51] Blood levels of some statins increase (Table 81-2).

ANTIARRHYTHMIC AGENTS

During antiarrhythmic therapy, numerous drug interactions are possible that are sometimes serious (Table 81-3).[52,53] Patients with serious ventricular arrhythmias frequently have associated angina pectoris (potentially necessitating treatment with calcium antagonists or beta blockers) or heart failure (requiring digitalis and diuretics). Nausea, a common symptom of patients with chronic cardiac conditions, may require cimetidine, with a risk of hepatic interactions (Table 81-3). The most frequent antiarrhythmic drug interactions are with digoxin (the levels of which increase with quinidine and verapamil), with diuretics (there is risk of ECG QT prolongation with antiarrhythmics, such as quinidine, disopyramide, amiodarone, and sotalol, which prolong duration of the action potential), and at the level of hepatic enzyme induction (cimetidine decreases hepatic metabolism of quinidine[54]; phenytoin and barbiturates have an opposite effect). There is also the risk of antiarrhythmic drug–drug interactions. Thus, amiodarone, when added to quinidine, enhances the risk of QT prolongation, while quinidine levels increase, so that quinidine toxicity is also more likely.[53] The combination of arrhythmic drugs, such as amiodarone and beta blockers, can also lead to life-threatening bradycardia. Type I antiarrhythmic drugs should not be used with certain macrolide antibiotics (erythromycin) because both drugs can prolong the QT interval, precipitating torsades de pointes, especially in

TABLE 81-2 Drug Interactions of Nitrates and Calcium Channel Blocking Agents

Cardiac Drug	Interacting Drugs	Mechanism	Consequence	Prophylaxis
		HEMODYNAMIC INTERACTIONS		
All nitrates	Calcium antagonists	Excess vasodilation	Syncope, dizziness	Monitor BP
	Prazosin (PZ)	Excess vasodilation	Syncope, dizziness	Check BP, low initial PZ doses
	Sildenafil (S)	Excess vasodilation	Syncope, dizziness	Avoid S
		CALCIUM ANTAGONIST DRUGS		
Verapamil (V)	Beta blockers	SA and AV nodal inhibition; myocardial failure	Added nodal and negative inotropic effects	Care during cotherapy Check ECG, BP, heart size
	Cimetidine	Hepatic metabolic interaction	Blood V rises	Adjust dose
	Digitalis poisoning	Added SA and AV nodal inhibition	Asystole; complete heart block after IV V	Avoid IV V in digitalis poisoning
	Digoxin (D)	Decreased digoxin clearance	Risk of D toxicity	Halve D dose; blood D level
	Disopyramide	Pharmacodynamic	Hypotension, constipation	Check BP, LV, and gut
	Flecainide (F)	Added negative inotropic effect	Hypotension	Check LV, F levels
	Prazosin	Hepatic interaction	Excess hypotension	Check BP during cotherapy
	Quinidine (Q)	Added alpha-receptor inhibition; V decreases Q clearance	Hypotension; increased Q levels	Check Q levels and BP
	Theophylline (T)	Inhibition of hepatic metabolism	Increased blood T levels	Reduce T, check levels
Nifedipine (N)	Beta blockers	Added negative inotropism	Excess hypotension	Check BP, use test dose of N
	Cimetidine	Hepatic metabolic interaction	Increased blood N levels	Decreased N dosage by 40%
	Digoxin (D)	Minor/modest changes in digoxin	Increased digoxin levels	Check D levels
	Prazosin (PZ)	PZ blocks alpha reflex to N	Postural hypotension	Test dose of N or PZ
	Propranolol (P)	N and P have opposite effects on blood liver flow	N decreases P levels; P increases N levels	Readjust P and N doses if needed
	Quinidine (Q)	N improves poor LV function; Q clearance faster	Decreased Q effect	Check Q levels
	Diltiazem	Hepatic metabolism of N inhibited	Increased hypotension	Decrease N levels
Diltiazem (D)	Beta blockers	Added SA nodal inhibition; negative inotropism	Bradycardia, hypotension	Check ECG and LV function
	Cimetidine	Hepatic metabolic interaction	Increased D levels	Reduce D dose by one-third
	Cyclosporine (C)	Hepatic metabolism of C inhibited	Increased blood C levels	Decrease C dose
	Digoxin (D)	Some fall in D clearance	Only in renal failure	Check D levels
	Flecainide (F)	Added negative inotropic effect	Hypotension	Check LV; F levels
	Cilostazol (Ci)	Hepatic metabolism of Ci inhibited	Increased Ci levels	Decrease Ci dose
	Simvastatin (Si) Lovastatin (L) Atorvastatin (A)	Hepatic metabolism of L inhibited	Increased L levels	Decrease Si, L, and A doses
Nicardipine (see also nifedipine)	Cyclosporine (C)	Hepatic metabolism of C inhibited	Increased blood C levels	Decrease C dose
	Digoxin (D)	Decreased D clearance	Blood D doubles	Decrease D, D levels

ABBREVIATIONS: BP = blood pressure; ECG = electrocardiogram; IV = intravenous; LV = left ventricle.

TABLE 81-3 Drug Interactions of Antiarrhythmic Drugs

Cardiac Drug	Interacting Drugs	Mechanism	Consequence	Prophylaxis
		CLASS 1A		
Quinidine (Q)	Amiodarone	Added QT effects; blood O rises	Torsades de pointes	Check QT, potassium
	Antibiotics (some)	Quinidine inhibits muscarinic receptors	Increased antibiotic-induced muscular weakness	Clinical care, drug levels
	Anticholinesterases	Quinidine inhibits muscarinic receptors	Decreased Ach efficacy in myasthenia gravis	Avoid Q if possible
	Antihypertensive agents Beta blockers	Added hypotensive and added SA nodal effects	Hypotension, excess bradycardia	Regulate BP Check BP ECG
	Cimetidine (C)	C inhibits oxidative metabolism of Q	Increased Q levels, risk of toxicity	Q levels, consider ranitidine
	Coumarin anticoagulants	Hepatic interaction with Q	Bleeding	Check prothrombin time
	Digoxin (Dig)	Decreased Dig clearance	Risk of Dig toxicity	Check Dig dose levels
	Diltiazem	Added inhibition of SA node	Excess bradycardia	Check ECG, heart rate
	Disopyramide	Added QT prolongation	Torsades de pointes	Check QT, potassium
	Diuretic, potassium losing	Hypokalemia and QT prolongation	Torsades de pointes	Check QT, potassium
	Hepatic enzyme inducers (phenytoin, barbiturates, rifampin)	Increased Q hepatic metabolism	Decreased Q levels	Q levels, doses
	Nifedipine	Increased Q clearance	Decreased Q levels	Q levels, doses
	Sotalol	Added QT prolongation	Torsades de pointes	Check QT, potassium
	Verapamil	Decreased Q clearance	Excess bradycardia	Check ECG, Q levels
	Warfarin	Hepatic interaction with Q	Bleeding	Check prothrombin time
Procainamide (P)	Captopril	Combined immune effects	Theoretical risk of neutropenia	Cotherapy with care
	Cimetidine	Decreased renal P clearance	Prolonged P half-life, excess P effect	Reduce P dose; consider ranitidine
Disopyramide (D)	Agents prolonging APD (quinidine, amiodarone, sotalol)	Added QT prolongation, especially if hypokalemic	Torsades de pointes	Check QT, potassium
	Beta blockers	Combined negative inotropism	Hypotension	Low doses
	Cimetidine	Hepatic D metabolism falls	Increased blood D levels	
	Digitalis toxicity	Added SA, AV nodal depression	SA, AV block	Avoid D in digitalis toxicity
	Hepatic enzyme inducers (phenytoin, rifampin, barbiturates)	Enhanced D hepatic metabolism	Blood D levels fall; readjust D dose	Readjust D dose

TABLE 81-3 Drug Interactions of Antiarrhythmic Drugs (*Continued*)

Cardiac Drug	Interacting Drugs	Mechanism	Consequence	Prophylaxis
	Drugs inhibiting SA or AV nodes/conduction system (quinidine, beta blockers, methyldopa, digoxin)	Pharmacodynamic additive effects	SA, AV block; conduction block	Check ECG; decrease doses
	Pyridostigmine (Py)	Inhibition of cholinesterase activity	Beneficial effect of Py on D; harmful effect of D on P	In myasthenia gravis, avoid D
		CLASS 1B		
Lidocaine (L)	Verapamil (V), Diltiazem (Di)	Combined negative inotropism	Hypotension	Avoid IV Di or V cotherapy
	Cimetidine	Decreased hepatic metabolism	Increased L levels	Decrease L infusion rate
	Halothane	Decreased hepatic blood flow	Increased L levels	Decrease L infusion rate
	Propranolol	Decreased hepatic blood flow	Increased L levels	Decrease L infusion rate
	Other beta blockers	Decreased hepatic blood flow	Increased L levels	Decrease L infusion rate
Mexiletine (M)	Hepatic enzyme inducers (phenytoin, barbiturates, rifampin)	Increased hepatic metabolism	Decreased plasma M levels	Increase M dose
		CLASS 1C		
Flecainide (F)	Amiodarone	Unknown	Blood F rises, added effect on nodes, myocardium	Decrease F dose
	Digoxin (Dig)	Decreased Dig clearance	Blood Dig rises slightly	Check Dig level
	Drugs inhibiting SA or AV nodes, IV conduction or myocardial function	Pharmacodynamic additive effects	SA, AV block; conduction block, cardiogenic shock	Avoid combinations Decrease doses
	Cimetidine	Decreased hepatic F loss	Blood F rises	Check F dose
Propafenone	Digoxin (Dig)	Pharmacokinetic	Increased Dig level	Decrease Dig dose
Moricizine (Mo)	Cimetidine	Decreased Mo metabolism	Blood Mo rises	Decrease Mo dose
		CLASS III		
Amiodarone (A)	Drugs prolonging QT interval (quinidine, disopyramide, phenothiazines, tricyclic antidepressants, thiazide diuretics, sotalol)	Pharmacodynamic additive effects	Torsades de pointes	Avoid low K^+; avoid combinations
	Quinidine (Q)	Pharmacokinetic	Blood Q rises	Check Q levels
	Procainamide (P)	Pharmacokinetic	Blood P rises	Check P dose
Sotalol	Procainamide	Hypokalemia plus class III action	Torsades de pointes	Exclude low K^+; use K^+-retaining diuretic

ABBREVIATIONS: Ach = acetylcholine; APD = action potential duration; BP = blood pressure; ECG = electrocardiogram; IV = intravenous.

women.[55-57] Other drugs that prolong the QT interval are shown in Fig. 81-2.

Quinidine

Because quinidine increases blood digoxin levels, the dose of quinidine must be decreased and blood digoxin levels checked.[58] Quinidine may enhance the effects of other hypotensive agents, including verapamil,[42] or of agents inhibiting the sinus node (beta blockers, verapamil, diltiazem, and methyldopa). Quinidine increases the effects of coumarin anticoagulants by a hepatic interaction.[59] When hepatic enzymes are induced by drugs such as phenytoin, phenobarbital, and rifampin (rifampicin), the hepatic metabolism of quinidine may markedly increase, with decreased steady-state concentrations of quinidine.[60,61] Conversely, cimetidine can inhibit hepatic enzymes to decrease the metabolism of quinidine with opposite effects. It appears that ranitidine has no such effects.[62] Verapamil may increase quinidine levels. Conversely, nifedipine may lower plasma quinidine levels, probably by improving left ventricular systolic function.[62-64]

Hypokalemia decreases the antiarrhythmic effect of quinidine and predisposes to QT prolongation by quinidine. When quinidine is combined with other drugs that also prolong the QT interval, such as amiodarone, sotalol, or thiazide diuretics, careful monitoring of the QT interval is required.[65]

Quinidine is a vagolytic drug and reduces the effects of procedures that enhance vagal activity, such as carotid sinus massage. Quinidine also inhibits muscarinic receptors to reduce the effects of anticholinesterases in myasthenia gravis.

Procainamide

Cimetidine inhibits the renal clearance of procainamide. Since the elimination half-life lengthens, the dose of procainamide needs reduction.[66]

Disopyramide

Since disopyramide is negatively inotropic, there is a potential danger of reduction of the cardiac output in patients already receiving other negative inotropes, such as the calcium antagonists—verapamil,[67] beta blockers, or flecainide—and in patients with preexisting myocardial failure. It is also potentially dangerous to combine disopyramide with other drugs likely to depress nodal or conduction tissues, such as quinidine, digoxin, beta blockers, and methyldopa. Disopyramide is ineffective in digitalis toxicity and should be avoided. There is no interaction between disopyramide and lidocaine. The concomitant use of disopyramide with other type I antiarrhythmic agents or beta blockers should be reserved for life-threatening arrhythmias because of a risk of bradycardia and hypotension. The risk of QT prolongation requires that disopyramide not be combined with other drugs prolonging the QT interval, such as the tricyclic antidepressants, and certain other antiarrhythmic agents, such as amiodarone or sotalol. Phenytoin[68] and other inducers of hepatic enzymes (e.g., barbiturates and rifampin) may lower disopyramide plasma levels. Pyridostigmine bromide may interact beneficially with disopyramide by inhibiting cholinesterase activity, reducing the anticholinergic side effects of disopyramide.[69]

Lidocaine

In patients receiving cimetidine,[70] propranolol,[15] or halothane,[71] the hepatic clearance of lidocaine is reduced, and toxicity may occur more readily. Lidocaine may cause SA arrest, especially during coadministration of other agents potentially depressing nodal function,[72] including beta blockers.

Tocainide

There are currently no known adverse drug interactions involving tocainide.

Dofetilide and Ibutilide

There are presently no known adverse drug interactions involving dofetilide or ibutilide. However, drugs known to directly prolong the QT interval and induce torsades de pointes (e.g., tricyclic antidepressants, antiarrhythmics, cisapride, astemizole, erythromycin, haloperidol, and protease inhibitors) should be avoided.[73]

Mexiletine

Narcotics delay the gastrointestinal absorption of mexiletine. Rifampin, barbiturates, and phenytoin all induce hepatic enzymes, reducing the plasma levels of mexiletine. Cimetidine inhibits the CYD 26 hepatic isoform that breaks down mexilitine. It should, but does not, increase plasma levels of mexiletine.[74] Rather, cimetidine has a beneficial side effect of decreasing the gastrointestinal symptoms associated with mexiletine. Disopyramide and mexiletine given together may predispose to a negative inotropic effect.[75] Mexiletine may, however, be combined with quinidine,[76,77] beta-adrenergic blockers,[78] and amiodarone,[79] provided that the appropriate contraindications for each drug are observed and the patient is closely monitored for heart failure.

Flecainide

Since flecainide inhibits the sinus and AV nodal function, its combination with beta blockers, verapamil, diltiazem, and digitalis can cause bradycardia and requires care. Flecainide also has additive negative inotropic effects that may exaggerate those of beta blockers,[80] verapamil, or disopyramide. Combined inhibitory effects on His-Purkinje conduction may arise during cotherapy with quinidine or procainamide and to a lesser extent with disopyramide. Flecainide blood levels are increased by amiodarone; when both of these drugs are used, the flecainide dose should be decreased by about one-third.[81] Studies of healthy volunteers suggest that (1) cimetidine delays the clearance of flecainide[82] and (2) flecainide increases blood digoxin levels.[80]

Propafenone

Propafenone is a class IC antiarrhythmic drug; therefore, it may interact adversely with other drugs, depressing nodal function, intraventricular conduction, or the inotropic state. Nonetheless, propafenone can be combined with quinidine or procainamide at reduced doses of both drugs.[74] Propafenone substantially increases serum digoxin levels.[83]

Amiodarone

The most serious interaction of amiodarone[65] is the potential for an additive proarrhythmic effect with other drugs that prolong the QT interval, such as class IA antiarrhythmic agents, sotalol, phenothiazines, tricyclic antidepressants, and thiazide diuretics. Amiodarone does not normally depress the sinus node, but it may do so when it is combined with beta blockers or calcium antagonists such as verapamil or diltiazem.[23] In patients receiving warfarin, amiodarone further prolongs the prothrombin time and, if not monitored closely, can lead to excessive bleeding.[84] Amiodarone may double digoxin levels (Table 81-3).

Sotalol

Cotherapy with any other agents that may cause hypokalemia (e.g., diuretics) or prolong the action potential duration (e.g., quinidine, disopyramide, amiodarone, tricyclic antidepressants, or probucol) may precipitate torsades de pointes.

Bretylium

Experimentally, bretylium may worsen digitalis-induced ventricular tachycardia.[85] Nonetheless, the drug may be lifesaving for patients with ventricular fibrillation thought to be induced by digitalis.[86]

Adenosine

Adenosine has an indirect effect, similar to that of the calcium antagonist verapamil, by enhancing the flow of the current $I_{k(ACh)}$. Aminophylline or theophylline, by competing with adenosine for the receptor sites, completely inhibits the adenosine-induced effect on AV conduction. Dipyridamole, on the other hand, inhibits the breakdown of adenosine and/or its uptake into the tissues, so that the amount of adenosine available for the antiarrhythmic effect is enhanced.[12] Effective doses of adenosine in patients receiving sustained dipyridamole therapy may only be one-quarter to one-eighth of the normal doses.

POSITIVE INOTROPIC AGENTS

Drug interactions of digitalis and other positive inotropic agents are shown in Table 81-4.

TABLE 81-4 Drug Interactions of Digitalis and Other Positive Inotropic Agents

Cardiac Drug	Interacting Drugs	Mechanism	Consequence	Prophylaxis
		POSITIVE INOTROPIC AGENTS		
Digitoxin	Verapamil	Nonrenal clearance of digitoxin falls	Digitoxin levels up by one-third	Check digitoxin levels
	Other drugs interacting with digoxin	Altered digitoxin clearance (?)	Digitoxin levels increase (?)	Check digitoxin levels
Digoxin (D)	Amiodarone	Reduced renal clearance of D	D level may double	Check D level; halve dose
	Captopril	Reduced D clearance	Blood D increases	Check D dose
	Diltiazem	Variable decrease of D clearance	Variable blood D increases	Check D level
	Diuretics; potassium-sparing amiloride/triamterene, spironolactone (S)	Reduced extrarenal D clearance S reduces renal D clearance	D levels up by 20% D levels increase	Check D level Complex effects; check D levels
	Nifedipine	Variable fall of D clearance	Variable blood D rises	Check D level
	Nitrendipine	Reduced D clearance	Blood D doubles	Check D level; halve dose
	Prazosin (PZ)	PZ displaces D from binding sites	Blood D rises	Needs confirmation in humans
	Propafenone	Not defined	D level increases	Check D level
	Quinidine, quinine	Reduced D clearance	Blood D doubles	Check D level; halve dose
	Verapamil	Reduced D clearance	Blood D doubles or more	Check D level; halve dose
		SYMPATHOMIMETIC INOTROPES		
Dobutamine Amrinone Milrinone	Thiazide diuretics	Additive hypokalemic effects	Arrhythmias	Check blood potassium

Digoxin

The quinidine-digoxin interaction is best known (Fig. 81-3). Quinidine approximately doubles the blood digoxin levels, decreasing both renal and extrarenal clearance.[38,86–88] The previous dose of digoxin should be halved and the plasma digoxin rechecked. Quinine given for muscle cramps acts likewise. Recent evidence indicates that quinidine inhibits digoxin transport across epithelial cell membranes (especially in the kidney) owing to its high affinity for p-glycoprotein on the ATP-dependent efflux pump encoded by the *mdrla* gene.[88–90]

The verapamil-digoxin interaction is equally significant; digoxin levels increase by 60 to 90 percent.[38,91] The other calcium antagonists, nifedipine and diltiazem, increase digoxin levels much less than does verapamil.[87,92,93] Adjustment of the digoxin dose with these agents is usually not necessary except in the presence of renal failure (which decreases digoxin excretion). Nicardipine causes only a modest rise of digoxin levels.[94] Nitrendipine, however, resembles verapamil in approximately doubling the digoxin levels.[94] Thus, there are no simple rules to explain which class of calcium antagonists or which specific agent is likely to increase digoxin levels significantly.

Among other vasodilators, prazosin increases digoxin levels in dogs by reduction of plasma and tissue binding.[95] Among antiarrhythmics other than quinidine or verapamil, amiodarone and propafenone[83] also elevate serum digoxin levels. Other antiarrhythmics, including procainamide and mexiletine, have no interaction with digoxin except for a relatively small rise of digoxin levels with flecainide.[80] When cotherapy elevates digoxin levels, the features of digitalis toxicity may depend on the agent added. With quinidine, tachyarrhythmias become more likely; amiodarone and verapamil seem to repress the ventricular arrhythmias of digitalis toxicity, making bradycardia and AV block more likely.[96]

Diuretics may indirectly precipitate digitalis toxicity by causing hypokalemia, which, when really severe (plasma potassium below 2 to 3 meq/L), may stop the tubular secretion of digoxin. Potassium-sparing diuretics (amiloride, triamterene, and spironolactone)[97] as well as captopril decrease digoxin clearance by about 20 to 30 percent and may also elevate serum K^+ levels. When these combinations with digoxin are used in the therapy of congestive heart failure, the blood digoxin level must be watched. Unexpectedly, spironolactone and its metabolite canrenone may decrease features of digitalis toxicity,[98] probably through increased K^+ levels resulting from aldosterone inhibition. Nonetheless, the combination digoxin-quinidine-spironolactone markedly elevates digoxin levels.[99]

The gastrointestinal absorption of digoxin may be decreased by cholestyramine, probably because of the binding of digoxin to the resin; digoxin should therefore be given several hours before the resin, or else digoxin capsules may be used (Lanoxicaps; 0.2 mg = 0.25 mg of digoxin). Digoxin capsules also decrease interaction with kaolin pectate and acarbose,[100] which reduces digoxin absorption, and with erythromycin and tetracycline, which inhibit gastrointestinal flora that inactivate digoxin and thereby increase digoxin blood levels. Cancer chemotherapeutic agents may damage intestinal mucosa to depress digoxin absorption. NSAIDs decrease the renal clearance of digoxin, thereby increasing plasma digoxin levels. Rifampin and phenobarbital, through hepatic enzyme induction, can reduce plasma digoxin levels.[90]

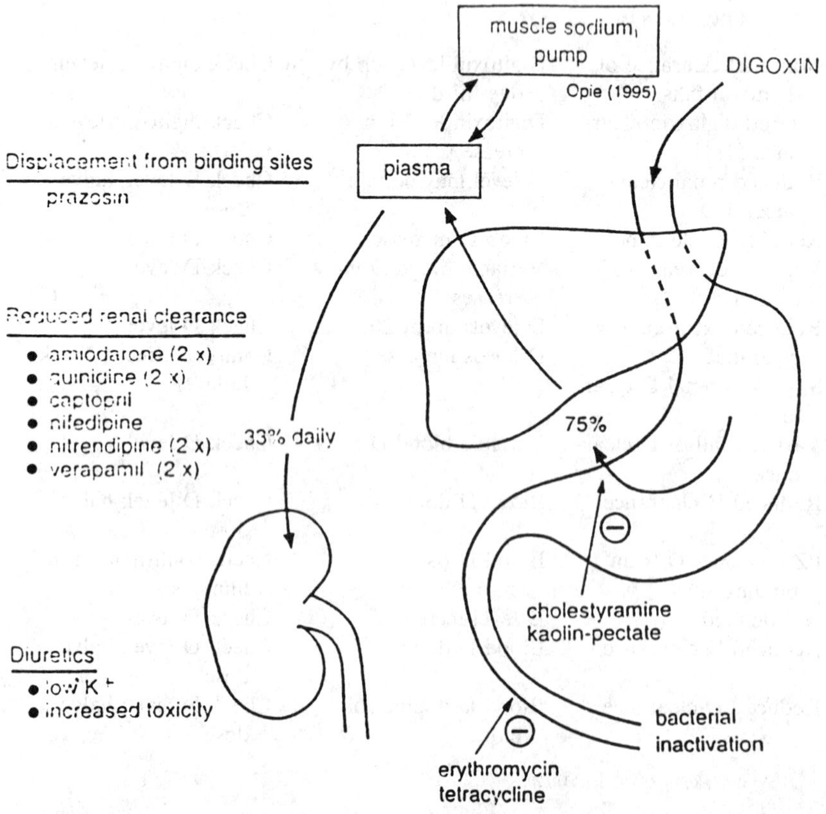

FIGURE 81-3 Potential site of digoxin interactions. Note the importance of reduced renal clearance. 2× means that an approximate doubling of digoxin blood levels has been reported. (Figure copyrighted by LH Opie.)

SYMPATHOMIMETIC AGENTS

Dopamine

Dopamine is contraindicated during the use of cyclopropane or halogenated hydrocarbon anesthetics (enhanced risk of arrhythmias). Monoamine oxidase inhibitors decrease the rate of dopamine metabolism by the tissues; the dose of dopamine should therefore be cut to one-tenth of usual.

Dobutamine

Dobutamine decreases plasma potassium levels and should be given with care together with diuretics, especially intravenous loop diuretics.

PHOSPHODIESTERASE INHIBITORS

Amrinone and Milrinone

Amrinone and milrinone are phosphodiesterase inhibitors that can also provoke arrhythmias. During diuretic therapy, plasma potassium levels need monitoring. When these drugs are combined with digitalis, the digoxin level does not change, but digoxin toxicity should be guarded against because of multiple mechanisms for arrhythmia development.

DIURETICS

Drug interactions with diuretics are summarized in Table 81-5.

Loop Diuretics

Hypokalemia, which may occur when loop diuretics are given acutely and intravenously, may precipitate digitalis toxicity. An interesting and complex set of interactions between furosemide and captopril has emerged. On the one hand, captopril decreases the renal excretion of furosemide, which is required for the diuretic effect of the latter. This may explain why captopril reduces furosemide-induced natriuresis to less than half.[101] This effect of captopril in altering furosemide excretion seems not to be shared by other angiotensin-converting enzyme (ACE) inhibitors.[102] There is an important pharmacodynamic interaction between captopril and furosemide. Both agents are able to dilate the postglomerular efferent arterioles. When captopril is given in a standard dose of 25 mg, furosemide has little or no diuretic effect. On the other hand, only minute doses of captopril, such as 1 mg, enhance the diuretic effect of furosemide.[103] The proposed mechanism is that the very low dose of captopril still allows sufficient circulating angiotensin II to maintain efferent arteriolar tone and thereby to keep the glomerular filtration rate sufficiently high for the furosemide to act. Both of these pharmacokinetic and pharmacodynamic interactions, therefore, argue for a low-dose captopril combination with furosemide. In patients with a low serum sodium level, which is an indirect indicator of a high-renin state, it is the high aldosterone level that retains sodium and stimulates vasopressin secretion, the latter causing the hyponatremia. Therapy of such patients by furosemide alone is ineffective, and the addition of captopril in a standard dose may achieve improvement.[12]

Quite apart from the complex interactions described above, it is generally regarded as a wise precaution to reduce the diuretic dose of patients with congestive heart failure (CHF) before adding an ACE inhibitor. The aim of this procedure is to lessen excessive first-dose hypotension. Overdiuresis tends to result in activation of the renin-angiotensin system and greater sensitivity to ACE inhibition.

Thiazide Diuretics

Steroids, estrogens, and indomethacin and other NSAIDs lessen the antihypertensive effect of thiazide diuretics and may worsen congestive heart failure.[104,105] ACE inhibitors tend to be potassium-retaining and may cause hyperkalemia if combined with other potassium retainers. The angiotensin II receptor blockers may have a weaker potassium-conserving effect. Diuretic-induced hypokalemia may predispose to ventricular arrhythmias, including torsades de pointes; when that happens, usually an antiarrhythmic agent, such as sotalol,[106] quinidine, or amiodarone (all of which may prolong the QT interval), is being used. Probenecid interferes with the urinary excretion of thiazide and loop diuretics, reducing diuretic efficacy. Since diuretics may impair the renal clearance of lithium, the blood level of lithium rises, with a risk of lithium toxicity.[107]

Potassium-Sparing Diuretics

Drugs that conserve potassium (e.g., ACE inhibitors, angiotensin II receptor blockers, and trimethoprim)[108,109] may potentiate hyperkalemia when used with potassium-sparing diuretics.

VASODILATORS

Drug interactions of vasodilators, ACE inhibitors, and angiotensin II receptor blockers are given in Table 81-6.

Nitroprusside and Hydralazine

Nitroprusside and hydralazine may decrease digoxin levels, possibly as a result of increased tubular excretion, by improving CHF, renal plasma flow, and renal excretion of digoxin.[110] Hy-

TABLE 81-5 Drug Interactions of Diuretics

Cardiac Drug	Interacting Drugs	Mechanism	Consequence	Prophylaxis
Loop and thiazide diuretics	Indomethacin and other NSAIDs	Pharmacodynamic	Decreased antihypertensive effect	Adjust diuretic dose or add another agent
	Probenecid	Decreased intratubular secretion of diuretic	Decreased diuretic effect	Increase diuretic dose
	ACE inhibitors	Excess diuretics, high renins	Excess hypotension; prerenal uremia	Lower diuretic dose; test dose ACE inhibitor
Furosemide (F)	Captopril	Possible interference with tubular secretion of F; added efferent arteriolar vasodilator	Loss of diuretic efficacy of F; decreased glomerular flow; diuretic effect of F less	Increase F dose (?); ultra low-dose captopril (?); Avoid Captopril (?)
K^+-retaining diuretics	ACE inhibitors AII receptor blockers	Added K^+ retention	Hyperkalemia	Check K^+ levels

ABBREVIATION: A II = angiotensin II.

TABLE 81-6 Drug Interactions of Vasodilators, Angiotensin Converting Enzyme Inhibitors, and Angiotensin II Receptor Blockers

Cardiac Drug	Interacting Drugs	Mechanism	Consequence	Prophylaxis
		VASODILATORS		
Hydralazine	Beta blockers (BB) (hepatic metabolized)	Hepatic shunting	BB metabolism ↓ Blood levels ↑	Propranolol, metoprolol dose ↓ (beneficial)
Hydralazine	Nitrates (N)	Renal blood flow ↑	Less N tolerance	
Hydralazine/ nitroprusside	Digoxin (D)	Increased renal D excretion	Decreased D levels	Check D levels
Prazosin (P)	Nifedipine (Nif)	Pharmacodynamic	Excess hypotension	Test dose of Nif
	Nitrates	Pharmacodynamic	Syncope, hypotension	Decrease P dose
	Verapamil	Hepatic metabolism	Synergistic antihypertensive effect	Adjust doses
Cilostazol (Ci)	Diltiazem	↓ hepatic metabolism	Increased Ci levels	Lower Ci dose
		ANGIOTENSIN-CONVERTING ENZYME INHIBITORS (ACEI)		
ACEI (class effect)	Diuretics	High renin levels in overdiuresed patients	"First" dose hypotension; risk of renal failure	Low test dose
ACEI (class effect)	Potassium-sparing diuretics	Added potassium retention	Hyperkalemia	Avoid combination
ACEI (class effect)	Indomethacin	Less vasodilation	Less BP ↓; less antifailure effects	Avoid if possible
ACEI (class effect ?)	Aspirin	Less vasodilation	Less antifailure effects	Low-dose aspirin
Captopril	Loop diuretic	Possible interference with tubular secretion	Lessened diuretic effect of furosemide	Consider alternate ACE inhibitor drug
Captopril	Immunosuppressive drugs, procainamide, hydralazine, possibly acebutolol	Added immune effects	Increased risk of neutropenia	Avoid combination; check neutrophils
	Probenecid (P)	P inhibits tubular secretion of C	Small risk in C levels	Decrease dose of C
		ANGIOTENSIN II RECEPTOR BLOCKERS (ARBs)		
ARBs (class effect)	Diuretics	High renin levels in overdiuresed patients	First dose hypotension, risk of renal failure	Low test dose
	Potassium sparing diuretics	Added potassium retention	Hyperkalemia	Avoid combination

ABBREVIATION: BP = blood pressure.

dralazine, by creating hepatic shunts, may substantially increase the blood levels of those beta blockers that undergo hepatic metabolism, such as propranolol and metoprolol.[111] Hydralazine interacts beneficially with nitrates, helping to lessen nitrate tolerance.[21]

Prazosin, Doxazosin, and Terazosin

There is an interaction between prazosin and the calcium antagonists verapamil and nifedipine, resulting in excessive hypotension. In the case of verapamil, part of the effect may be explained by a pharmacokinetic hepatic interaction. Both nitrates and prazosin may cause syncope, and these agents should be combined with care. Experimentally, prazosin may increase the plasma digoxin level. Similar interactions may hold for the other agents in this group.

ANGIOTENSIN-CONVERTING ENZYME INHIBITORS

In general, ACE inhibitors have few drug interactions (Table 81-6). In patients with CHF, excessive first-dose hypotension should be avoided to lessen the risk of renal impairment, which may lead to accumulation and interaction of renal-excreted drugs.

Because of potential hyperkalemia with potassium-sparing

TABLE 81-7 Drug Interactions of Antithrombotic Agents

Cardiac Drug	Interacting Drugs	Mechanism	Consequence	Prophylaxis
Aspirin (A)	ACE inhibitors	Vasodilation ↓	Less antifailure effect	Very low A dose
	Hepatic enzyme inducers (barbiturates, phenyton, rifampin)	Increased A metabolism	Decreased A effect	Adjust A dose; check A side effects
	Sulfinpyrazone (S), probenecid (P)	A decreases urate excretion	Decreased uricosuric effect of S or P	Increase dose of S or P
	Thiazide diuretics	A decreases urate excretion	Hyperuricemia	Check blood urate
	Warfarin	A is antithrombotic	Excess bleeding	Check INR or prothrombin time
Sulfinpyrazone (S)	Warfarin (W)	S displaces W from plasma proteins	Excess bleeding	Check INR or prothrombin time
Warfarin	Potentiating drugs			
	Allopurinol	Mechanism unknown	Excess bleeding	Check INR or prothrombin time
	Amiodarone	Mechanism unknown	Sensitizes to W for months	Avoid combination
	Aspirin	Added bleeding tendency	Excess bleeding	Check INR or prothrombin time
	Cimetidine	Decreased W degradation	Excess bleeding	Check INR or prothrombin time
	Quinidine	Hepatic interaction	Excess bleeding	Check INR or prothrombin time
	Statins	Hepatic interaction (?)	Excess bleeding	Check INR or prothrombin time
	Sulfinpyrazone	Displaces W from plasma proteins	Excess bleeding	Check INR or prothrombin time
	Acetaminophen	Hepatic interaction	Excess bleeding	Check INR or prothrombin time
	Inhibitory drugs			
	Cholestyramine, colestipol	Decrease absorption of W	Decreased W effect	Check INR or prothrombin time
Alteplase, tPA	Nitrates	Decreased tPA effect	Less thrombolytic benefit	Avoid; ? increase tPA dose

ABBREVIATION: INR = international normalized ratio.

diuretics, the ideal combination with an ACE inhibitor is a thiazide diuretic or furosemide, but without a potassium-retaining component.[12] In patients receiving NSAIDs, which tend to decrease renal plasma flow in their own right, addition of an ACE inhibitor can further decrease the glomerular filtration rate, with an added risk of hyperkalemia.[12] Captopril may interact with probenecid, which inhibits its tubular excretion, and, as mentioned earlier, there is a serious interaction with the loop diuretic furosemide.[101]

In patients with severe CHF, the acute combination of aspirin and an ACE inhibitor decreases the peripheral vasodilatation,[112] an effect not seen with ticlopidine.[113–115] Lower aspirin doses seem to have little or no hemodynamic interference,[116,117] but there are no true dose-response or chronic studies. It is best to keep the dose of aspirin as low as possible when combined with ACE inhibitors.

Captopril

Cotherapy of high-dose captopril with other drugs that alter or impair the immune status (e.g., hydralazine and procainamide) may predispose to neutropenia. Probenecid inhibits the renal tubular excretion of captopril, thereby increasing blood captopril levels[118]; doses of captopril may need downward adjustment. Captopril may decrease digoxin clearance by 20 to 30 percent.[97]

Enalapril

Drug interactions of enalapril are similar to those of captopril, except that the risk of neutropenia is less. It must be considered that enalapril has a longer duration of action; adverse hypotensive interactions with diuretics are therefore potentially more serious.

ANGIOTENSIN II RECEPTOR BLOCKERS

No significant drug–drug pharmacokinetic interactions have been found in interaction studies with hydrochlorothiazide, digoxin, warfarin, cimetidine, and phenobarbital (Table 81-6).[119] Moreover, in vitro studies show significant inhibition of the formation of the active metabolites by inhibitors of P450,3A4 or 2C9. Potent inhibitors of cytochrome P450,3A4 and 2C9 have been studied in patients, with no interaction with angiotensin II blockers observed.[120]

As with other drugs that block angiotensin II or its effects, concomitant use of potassium-sparing diuretics, potassium supplements, or salt substitutes containing potassium may lead to increases in serum potassium levels.

ANTITHROMBOTIC AND THROMBOLYTIC AGENTS

Table 81-7 summarizes the drug interactions of antithrombotic agents.

Aspirin

Since blood levels of uric acid may be increased by both aspirin and thiazide diuretics, special care is required in patients with a history of gout.[121] Conversely, aspirin may decrease the uricosuric effects of sulfinpyrazone and probenecid. Aspirin has some effects similar to those of the NSAIDs, inhibiting the effects of vasodilatory prostaglandins (Fig. 81-4). Thus, aspirin can reduce the natriuretic effect of spironolactone and some of the benefits of ACE inhibitors in CHF. Aspirin-induced gastrointestinal bleeding may be a greater hazard in patients receiving other NSAIDs or corticosteroid therapy. Antacids, by altering the pH of the stomach, may decrease the efficacy of enteric-coated preparations.

Inducers of the hepatic cytochrome oxidase system (e.g., barbiturates, phenytoin, and rifampin) increase aspirin breakdown. Aspirin tends to cause hypoglycemia in patients receiving oral hypoglycemics or insulin. Aspirin, especially in high doses, may exaggerate a bleeding tendency and anticoagulant-induced bleeding.[122] The dipyridamole-warfarin combination causes less bleeding than the aspirin-warfarin combination in patients who have undergone bypass surgery.[123] All these drug interactions should be less intense if the aspirin doses are kept low, as is the current trend.

Sulfinpyrazone

Sulfinpyrazone is highly bound to plasma proteins (98 to 99 percent) and may displace warfarin to precipitate bleeding. Like aspirin, sulfinpyrazone may sensitize patients who are given sulfonylureas and insulin to hypoglycemia.

Dipyridamole

Dipyridamole is a potent vasodilator. Thus, care is required when it is used in combination with other vasodilators. Note the interaction with adenosine, as discussed above.

Ticlopidine

Ticlopidine is an antiplatelet drug that interferes with ATP-induced platelet aggregation and does not appear to interfere with the vasodilating activity of ACE inhibitor drugs.[115]

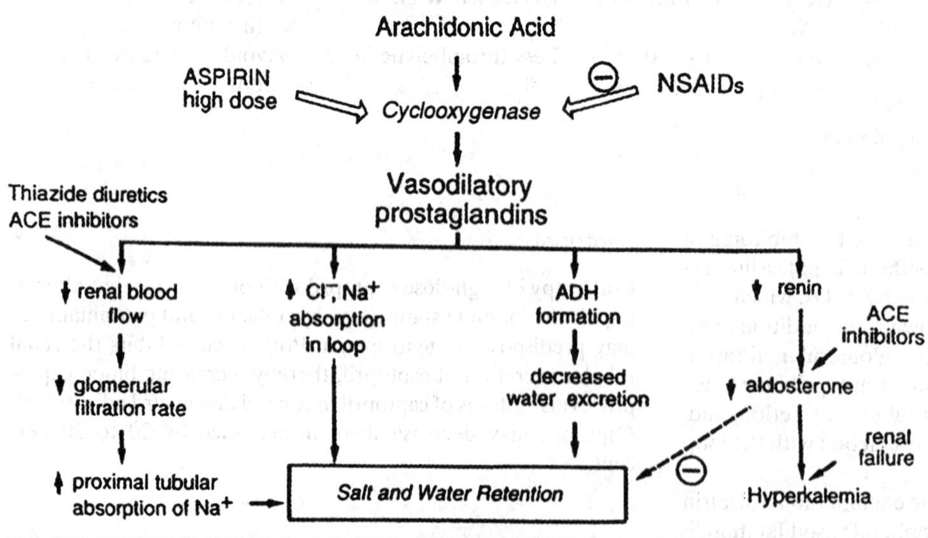

FIGURE 81-4 Possible mechanism whereby NSAIDs and aspirin block the cyclooxygenase pathway and thereby inhibit formation of vasodilatory prostaglandins. The resultant salt and water retention may decrease the effects of almost all antihypertensives, including ACE inhibitors. In addition, NSAIDs decrease renin and aldosterone through an entirely different mechanism, which would tend to lessen salt and water retention. (Adapted from Houston MC: Nonsteroidal anti-inflammatory drugs and antihypertensives. *Am J Med* 1991; 90(suppl 5A):42S–47S. Reproduced with permission from the publisher and authors.)

Warfarin

Warfarin may be subject to many (up to 80) drug interactions.[12] A good rule is to suspect interactions unless one can be sure. The safest rule is to tell patients having oral anticoagulation not to use any new or over-the-counter drugs without consultation and for the physician to carefully check out any added compounds. More frequent measurements of the prothrombin time and dose adjustments are required when potentially interfering drugs are added.

Interfering drugs include those that reduce absorption of vitamin K or warfarin, such as cholestyramine.[12] Sulfinpyrazone increases warfarin levels by displacing it from plasma proteins. Other interfering drugs are inducers of the hepatic cytochrome oxidase system, which increase the rate of warfarin metabolism in the liver.

TABLE 81-8 Drug Interactions of Lipid-Lowering Agents

Cardiac Drug	Interacting Drugs	Mechanism	Consequence	Prophylaxis
Fibric acids (gemfibrozil, clofibrate, bezafibrate, fenofibrate)	Warfarin	Hepatic interference	Risk of bleeding	Check prothrombin time
Bile acid sequestrants (cholestyramine, colestipol)	Warfarin (W)	Decreased absorption	Decreased W effect	Check prothrombin time
HMG-CoA reductase inhibitors (statins) (lovastatin, simvastatin, pravastatin) atorvastatin, cerivastatin, fluvastatin	Fibrates, cyclosporine, erythromycin, niacin, antifungal azoles	Added damage to muscle with myositis	Rhabdomyolysis and risk of renal failure	Check creatine phosphokinase levels
Statins	Warfarin	Hepatic interaction	Increased risk of bleeding	Check INR or prothrombin time (beneficial)
Pravastatin	Cyclosporine	Hepatic interaction (?)	Enhanced immunosuppression	

Yet, other drugs decrease the hepatic degradation of warfarin to increase the anticoagulant effect, including antibiotics, such as metronidazole and cotrimoxazole. Cimetidine likewise inhibits hepatic degradation. Ranitidine does not do likewise. Other potentiating cardiovascular agents are allopurinol, clofibrate, quinidine, and amiodarone.[12,124] Amiodarone is especially dangerous because its very long half-life means a very long potentiation of warfarin. Heparin or aspirin may potentiate bleeding, although there are large interindividual variations.[125] Very high doses of aspirin impair synthesis of clotting factors.

It must be reemphasized that sulfinpyrazone has a powerful effect in displacing warfarin from blood proteins; thus, the dose of warfarin required may be reduced to only 1 mg.[103]

Heparins

Physically, heparin, including the low-molecular-weight heparins, is incompatible in a water solution with certain substances, including antibiotics, antihistamines, phenothiazides, and hydrocortisone.

TABLE 81-9 Herbal Medicines Associated with Drug Interactions

ANTICOAGULANTS		
Angelica	Fenugreek	Lungwort
Black haw	Garlic	Pau d'arco
Bogbean	Ginger	Poplar
Buchu	Gingko	Prickly ash
Cat's claw	Horse chestnut	Red clover
Chamomile	Irish moss	Tonkas bean
Chondroitin	Kelp	Wintergreen
Dong quai	Khella	Yarrow
ANTIHYPERTENSIVES		
Arnica	Dandelion	
Betony	Goldenseal	
Black cohosh	Kelp	
Blue cohosh	Khella	
Capsicum	Queen Ann's lace	
Cat's claw	Yarrow	
SPECIFIC DRUGS		
Broom (and beta blockers)		Fumitory (and digoxin)
Fumitory (and beta blockers)		Goldenseal (and digoxin)
Cowslip (and diuretics)		Aloe (and digoxin)
Cucumber (and diuretics)		St. John's wort (and digoxin)
Horsetail (and diuretics)		Queen Ann's lace (and digoxin)
Licorice (and diuretics)		
Dandelion (and diuretics)		

However, direct pharmacokinetic or pharmacodynamic drug interactions have not been described, except for a controversial interaction with nitrates.[126]

Tissue-Type Plasminogen Activator

Concurrent use of intravenous nitroglycerin diminishes the efficacy of recombinant tissue-type plasminogen activator (tPA or alteplase), possibly because of increased hepatic blood flow and enhanced catabolism of tPA.[127]

LIPID-LOWERING AGENTS

There are not many serious interactions with lipid-lowering agents (Table 81-8). A number of lipid-lowering agents may interact with warfarin, either by decreased absorption (cholestyramine) or by hepatic interference (clofibrate, bezafibrate, fenofibrate, or gemfibrozil). The precise mechanism is not clear. Clofibrate, fenofibrate, gemfibrozil, and many of the statins increase the effects of warfarin.

Simvastatin, lovastatin, and atorvastatin are metabolized by cytochrome P450,3A4. Clinical experience has shown that the risk of myopathy with these statins is increased substantially by concomitant use of the few drugs that substantially inhibit P450,3A4, including cyclosporine and erythromycin.[128] Calcium channel blockers and grapefruit juice are weak inhibitors of P450,3A4.[129]

Probucol, in the presence of additional agents, such as thiazide diuretics or group IA or III antiarrhythmics, may prolong the QT interval and theoretically precipitate torsades de pointes. The hydroxymethylglutaryl coenzyme A (HMG-CoA) reductase inhibitors, such as atorvastatin, cerivastatin, lovastatin, simvastatin, pravastatin, and fluvastatin, should ideally not be combined with the fibrates because of the higher risk of myositis with rhabdomyolysis and possible renal failure. Likewise, concurrent therapy with niacin, cyclosporine, or erythromycin may also carry a small risk of rhabdomyolysis. Adding an antifungal azole (a group that includes ketoconazole, used in transplantation) has precipitated myolysis in a patient already receiving a statin and niacin.[130] Yet, in clinical practice, the advantages of better lipid control with combined therapy seems to outweigh these risks. Furthermore, a positive interaction of pravastatin with cyclosporine is reported, whereby there appears to be increased immunosuppression.[131] Serum creatine kinase levels should be checked periodically, especially after increasing doses or after starting combination therapy.

ANTIHYPERTENSIVE DRUGS

Interactions for diuretics, beta-adrenergic blockers, calcium antagonists, ACE inhibitors, and alpha$_1$-adrenergic blockers have already been considered. In general, NSAIDs interfere severely with the antihypertensive efficacy of all antihypertensives.[132,133] An exception is nifedipine (and, presumably, other dihydropyridines).[134] Unlike other NSAIDs, aspirin[16] and sulindac may give relative protection from the negative interaction.[132] When calcium antagonists are used as antihypertensives, part of their effect is by natriuresis; thus, adding a diuretic is often relatively ineffective.[135]

HERBAL MEDICINE

Herbal supplements are commonly used by patients for various cardiac conditions.[136] Many of the herbs cause cardiac toxicity or can interact unfavorably with known cardiac drugs (Table 81-9).

Chamomile has antispasmodic actions and warfarin-like effects. Feverfew, garlic, and ginger have antiplatelet actions and can pose safety problems in patients taking warfarin. Gingko and ginseng should be avoided in patients receiving warfarin and heparin. Herbal acquertics can inhibit the activity of diuretics or other antihypertensive therapy. Gossypol and licorice are associated with renal loss of potassium and should not be used with thiazide and loop diuretics or digoxin. Plantain and hawthorn berries can mimic or potentiate digitalis toxicity. Kelp can interfere with the antiarrhythmic effects of amiodarone. St. John's wort can lower serum digoxin levels by reducing digoxin absorption, possibly by inducing p-glycoprotein in the gut.[137,138]

References

1. Doucet J, Chassagne P, Trivalle C, et al. Drug-drug interactions related to hospital admissions in older adults: A prospective study of 1000 patients. *J Am Geriatr Soc* 1996; 44:944–948.
2. Lacombe PS, Garcia Vicente JA, Costa Pagès J, Morselli PL: Causes and problems of nonresponse or poor response to drugs. *Drugs* 1996; 51:552–570.
3. Michalets EL. Update: Clinically significant cytochrome P-450 drug interactions. *Pharmacotherapy* 1998; 18:84–112.
4. Cheng JWM. Cytochrome P450 mediated cardiovascular drug interactions. *Heart Dis* 2000; 2:254–258.
5. Yu DK. The contribution of p-glycoprotein to pharmacokinetic drug-drug interactions. *J Clin Pharmacol* 1999; 39:1203–1211.
6. Tran C, Knowles SR, Liu BA, Shear NH. Gender differences in adverse drug reactions. *J Clin Pharmacol* 1998; 38:1003–1009.
7. Sokol SI, Cheng-Lai A, Frishman WH, Kaza CS. Cardiovascular drug therapy in patients with hepatic diseases and patients with congestive heart failure. *J Clin Pharmacol* 2000; 40:11–30.
8. Be alert for interactions between prescription and OTC drugs. *Drugs Ther Perspect* 1996; 7:12–14.
9. Huang J-D, Chuang S-K, Cheng C-L, Lai M-L. Pharmacokinetics of metoprolol enantiomers in Chinese subjects of major CYP2D6 genotypes. *Clin Pharmacol Ther* 1999; 65:402–407.
10. Strayhorn VA, Baciewicz AM, Self TH. Update on rifampin drug interactions: III. *Arch Intern Med* 1997; 157:2453–2458.
11. Opie LH, ed. *Drugs for the Heart,* 4th ed. Philadelphia: Saunders; 1995.
12. Opie LH. Cardiovascular drug interactions. In: Frishman WH, Sonnenblick EH, eds. *Cardiovascular Pharmacotherapeutics.* New York: McGraw Hill; 1997:1383.
13. Kirch W, Spahn H, Kohler H, Mutschler E. Influence of β-receptor antagonists on pharmacokinetics of cimetidine. *Drugs* 1983; 25(suppl 2):127–130.
14. McLean AJ, Knight R, Harrison PM, Harper RW. Clearance-based oral drug interaction between verapamil and metoprolol and comparison with atenolol. *Am J Cardiol* 1985; 55:1628–1629.
15. Ochs HR, Carstens G, Greenblatt DJ. Reduction in lidocaine clearance during continuous infusion and by coadministration of propranolol. *N Engl J Med* 1980; 303:373–377.
16. Webster J. Interactions of NSAIDs with diuretics and β-blockers: Mechanism and clinical implications. *Drugs* 1985; 30:32–41.

17. Tolins M, Weir K, Chesler E, Pierpont GL. "Maximal" drug therapy is not necessarily optimal in chronic angina pectoris. *J Am Coll Cardiol* 1984; 3:1051–1057.
18. Bruce RA, Hossack KF, Kusumi F, et al. Excessive reduction in peripheral resistance during exercise and risk of orthostatic symptoms with sustained-release nitroglycerin and diltiazem treatment of angina. *Am Heart J* 1985; 109:1020–1026.
19. Boden WE, Bough EW, Reichman MJ, et al. Beneficial effects of high-dose diltiazem in patients with persistent effort angina on β-blockers and nitrates: A randomized, double-blind, placebo-controlled, cross-over study. *Circulation* 1985; 71:1197–1205.
20. Cheitlin MD, Hutter AM Jr, Brindis RG, et al. ACC/AHA Expert Consensus Document: Use of sildenafil (Viagra) in patients with cardiovascular disease. *J Am Coll Cardiol* 1999; 33:273–282.
21. Gogia H, Mehra A, Parikh S, et al. Prevention of tolerance to hemodynamic effects of nitrates with concomitant use of hydralazine in patients with chronic heart failure. *J Am Cardiol* 1995; 26:1575–1580.
22. Becker RC, Corrao JM, Bovill EG, et al. Intravenous nitroglycerin-induced heparin resistance: A qualitative antithrombin III abnormality. *Am Heart J* 1990; 119:1254–1261.
23. Reicher-Reiss H, Neufeld HN, Ebner FX. Calcium antagonists: Adverse drug interactions. *Cardiovasc Drug Ther* 1987; 1: 403–409.
24. Abernethy DR, Schwartz JB. Calcium antagonist drugs. *N Engl J Med* 1999; 341:1447–1457.
25. Abernethy DR. Grapefruits and drugs: When is statistically significant clinically significant? *J Clin Invest* 1997; 10:2297–2298.
26. Frishman WH. Comparative efficacy and concomitant use of bepridil and beta blockers in the management of angina pectoris. *Am J Cardiol* 1992; 69(suppl):50D–60D.
27. Mullins ME, Horowitz Z, Linden DHJ, et al. Life-threatening interaction of mibefradil and β blockers with dihydropyridine calcium channel blockers. *JAMA* 1998; 280:157–158.
28. Yeh R, Gulamhusein SS, Klein GJ. Combined verapamil and propranolol for supraventricular tachycardia. *Am J Cardiol* 1984; 53:757–763.
29. Ellrodt AG, Ault MJ, Riedinger MS, Murati GH. Efficacy and safety of sublingual nifedipine in hypertensive emergencies. *Am J Med* 1985; 79(suppl 4A):19–25.
30. Kieval J, Kirsten EB, Kessler KM, et al. The effects of intravenous verapamil on hemodynamic status of patients with coronary artery disease receiving propranolol. *Circulation* 1982; 65:653–659.
31. Packer M, Meller J, Medina N, et al. Hemodynamic consequences of combined beta-adrenergic and slow calcium channel blockade in man. *Circulation* 1982; 65:660–668.
32. Johnston DL, Lesoway R, Humen DP, Kostuk WJ. Clinical and hemodynamic evaluation of propranolol in combination with verapamil, nifedipine and diltiazem in exertional angina pectoris: A placebo-controlled, double-blind, randomized, cross-over study. *Am J Cardiol* 1985; 55:680–687.
33. Winniford MD, Fulton KL, Corbett JR, et al. Propranolol-verapamil versus propranolol-nifedipine in severe angina pectoris of effort: A randomized, double-blind, cross-over study. *Am J Cardiol* 1985; 55:281–285.
34. Hamann SR, Kaltenborn KE, Vore M, et al. Cardiovascular pharmacokinetic consequences of combined administration of verapamil and propranolol in dogs. *Am J Cardiol* 1985; 56:147–156.
35. Murdoch DL, Thomson GD, Thompson GG, et al. Evaluation of potential pharmacodynamic and pharmacokinetic interactions between verapamil and propranolol in normal subjects. *Br J Clin Pharmacol* 1991; 31:323–332.
36. Johnston DL, Gebhardt VA, Donald A, Kostuk WJ. Comparative effects of propranolol and verapamil alone and in combination on left ventricular function in patients with chronic exertional angina: A double-blind, placebo-controlled, randomized, cross-over study with radionuclide ventriculography. *Circulation* 1983; 68:1280–1289.
37. McInnes GT, Findlay IN, Murray G, et al. Cardiovascular responses to verapamil and propranolol in hypertensive patients. *J Hypertens* 1985; 3(suppl 3):S219–S221.
38. Pedersen KE. Digoxin interactions: The influence of quinidine and verapamil on the pharmacokinetics and receptor binding of digitalis glycosides. *Acta Med Scand* 1985; 697(suppl):12–40.
39. Elliott HL, Pasanisi F, Meredith PA, Reid JL. Acute hypotensive response to nifedipine added to prazosin. *Br Med J* 1984; 288:238.
40. Pasanisi F, Elliott HL, Meredith PA, et al. Combined alpha-adrenoceptor antagonism and calcium channel blockade in normal subjects. *Clin Pharmacol Ther* 1984; 36:716–723.
41. Reid JL, Meredith PA, Pasanisi F. Clinical pharmacological aspects of calcium antagonists and their therapeutic role in hypertension. *J Cardiovasc Pharmacol* 1985; 7(suppl 4):S18–S20.
42. Maisel AS, Motulsky HJ, Insel PA. Hypotension after quinidine plus verapamil: Possible additive competition at alpha-adrenergic receptors. *N Engl J Med* 1985; 312:167–171.
43. Trohman RG, Estes DM, Castellanos A, et al. Increased quinidine plasma concentrations during administration of verapamil: A new quinidine-verapamil interaction. *Am J Cardiol* 1986; 57:706–707.
44. Hansten PD, Horn JR. Calcium channel blocker-induced drug interactions: Evidence for metabolic inhibition. *Drug Interact Newsl* 1986; 6:35–40.
45. Opie LH, White DA. Adverse interaction between nifedipine and beta blockade. *Br Med J* 1980; 281:1462–1464.
46. Kleinbloesem CH, van Brummelen P, Sandberg TH, et al. Kinetic and haemodynamic interactions between nifedipine and propranolol in healthy subjects utilizing controlled rates of drug input. In: Kleinbloesem CH, ed. *Nifedipine: Clinical Pharmacokinetics and Haemodynamic Effects.* The Hague: Drukkerij JH Pasmans BV; 1985:151.
47. Kiss I, Farsang C. Nifedipine-prazosin interaction in patients with essential hypertension. *Cardiovasc Drugs Ther* 1989; 3:413–415.
48. Frishman WH, Charlap S, Kimmel B, et al: Diltiazem compared to nifedipine and combination treatment with stable angina: Effects on angina, exercise tolerance and the ambulatory ECG. *Circulation* 1988; 77:774–786.
49. Hung J, Lamb IH, Connolly SJ, et al. The effect of diltiazem and propranolol, alone and in combination, on exercise performance and left ventricular function in patients with stable effort angina: A double-blind, randomized, and placebo-controlled study. *Circulation* 1983; 68:560–567.
50. Grino JM, Sabate I, Castelao AM, Alsina J. Influence of diltiazem on cyclosporin clearance. *Lancet* 1986; 2:1387.
51. Cheng JWM. Cilostazol. *Heart Dis* 1999; 1:182–186.
52. Bigger JT, Giardina EG. Drug interactions in antiarrhythmic therapy. *Ann NY Acad Sci* 1984; 427:140–161.
53. Jaillon P. Antiarrhythmic drug interactions: Are they important? *Eur Heart J* 1987; 8(suppl A):127–132.
54. Hardy BG, Zador IT, Golden L, et al. Effects of cimetidine on the pharmacokinetics of quinidine. *Am J Cardiol* 1983; 52:172–175.
55. Drici M-D, Knollman BC, Wang W-X, Woosley RL. Cardiac actions of erythromycin: Influence of female sex. *JAMA* 1998; 280:1774–1776.
56. Mishra A, Friedman HS, Sinha AK. The effects of erythromycin on the electrocardiogram. *Chest* 1999; 115:983–986.
57. Lee KL, Jim M-H, Tang SC, Tai Y-T. QT prolongation and Torsades de Pointes associated with clarithromycin. *Am J Med* 1998; 104:395–396.
58. Hager WD, Fenster P, Mayersohn M, et al. Digoxin-quinidine interaction: Pharmacokinetic evaluation. *N Engl J Med* 1979; 300:1238–1241.
59. Koch-Weser J. Quinidine-induced hypoprothrombinemic hemor-

rhage in patients on chronic warfarin therapy. *Ann Intern Med* 1968; 68:511–517.
60. Dada JL, Wilkinson GR, Nies AJ. Interaction of quinidine with anticonvulsant drugs. *N Engl J Med* 1976; 294:699–702.
61. Twum-Barima Y, Carruthers SG. Quinidine-rifampicin. *N Engl J Med* 1981; 304:1466–1469.
62. Farringer JA, McWay-Hess K, Clementi WA. Cimetidine-quinidine interaction. *Clin Pharmacol* 1984; 3:81–83.
63. Green JA, Clementi WA, Porter C, Stigelman W. Nifedipine-quinidine interaction. *Clin Pharmacol* 1983; 2:461–465.
64. Van Lith RM, Appleby DH. Quinidine-nifedipine interaction. *Drug Intell Clin Pharm* 1985; 19:829–830.
65. Marcus FI. Drug interactions with amiodarone. *Am Heart J* 1983; 106:924–930.
66. Christian CO, Meredith CG, Speeg KV. Cimetidine inhibits procainamide clearance. *Clin Pharmacol Ther* 1984; 36:221–227.
67. Lee JT, Davy JM, Kates RE. Evaluation of combined administration of verapamil and disopyramide in dogs. *J Cardiovasc Pharmacol* 1985; 7:501–507.
68. Kapil RP, Axelson JE, Mansfield IL, et al. Disopyramide pharmacokinetics and metabolism: Effect of inducers. *Br J Clin Pharmacol* 1987; 24:781–791.
69. Teichman SL, Fisher JD, Matos JA, Kim SG. Disopyramide-pyridostigmine: Report of a beneficial drug interaction. *J Cardiovasc Pharmacol* 1985; 7:108–113.
70. Feely J, Wilkinson GR, McAllister CB, Wood AJ. Increased toxicity and reduced clearance of lidocaine by cimetidine. *Ann Intern Med* 1982; 96:592–594.
71. Boyce JR, Cervenko FW, Wright FJ. Effects of halothane on the pharmacokinetics of lidocaine in digitalis-toxic dogs. *Can Anaesth Soc J* 1978; 25:323–328.
72. Jeresaty RM, Kahn AH, Landry AB. Sinoatrial arrest due to lidocaine in a patient receiving quinidine. *Chest* 1972; 61:683–685.
73. Frishman WH, Cheng-Lai A, Chen J, eds. Antiarrhythmic agents. In: *Current Cardiovascular Drugs,* 3d ed. Philadelphia: Current Medicine; 2000:54.
74. Klein R, Huang SK, Group Southwest Cardiology Research. Combination therapy of propafenone with quinidine or procainamide: Enhanced efficacy and reduced side-effects [abstr]. *J Am Coll Cardiol* 1985; 5:423.
75. Breithardt G, Selpel L, Abendroth RR. Comparative cross-over study of the effects of disopyramide and mexiletine on stimulus-induced ventricular tachycardia [abstr]. *Circulation* 1980; 62(suppl 3):153.
76. Duff HJ, Roden D, Primm RK, et al. Mexiletine in the treatment of resistant ventricular arrhythmias: Enhancement of efficacy and reduction of dose-related side-effects by combination with quinidine. *Circulation* 1983; 67:1124–1128.
77. Greenspan AM, Spielman SR, Webb CR, et al. Efficacy of combination therapy with mexiletine and a type 1A agent for inducible ventricular tachyarrhythmias secondary to coronary artery disease. *Am J Cardiol* 1985; 56:277–284.
78. Leahey EB, Heissenbuttel RH, Giardina EG, Bigger JT. Combined mexiletine and propranolol treatment of refractory ventricular tachycardia. *Br Med J* 1980; 2:357–358.
79. Waleffe A, Mary-Rabine L, Legrand V, et al. Combined mexiletine and amiodarone treatment of refractory recurrent ventricular tachycardia. *Am Heart J* 1980; 100:788–793.
80. Lewis GP, Holtzman JL. Interaction of flecainide with digoxin and propranolol. *Am J Cardiol* 1984; 53:52B–57B.
81. Shea P, Lal R, Kim SS, et al. Flecainide and amiodarone interaction. *J Am Coll Cardiol* 1986; 7:1127–1130.
82. Maga TB, Verbesselt R, Van Hecken A, et al. Oral flecainide elimination kinetics: Effects of cimetidine [abstr]. *Circulation* 1983; 68(suppl 3):416.
83. Hodges M, Salerno D, Granrud G. Double-blind placebo-controlled evaluation of propafenone in suppressing ventricular ectopic activity. *Am J Cardiol* 1984; 54:45D–50D.
84. Martinowitz U, Rabinovich J, Goldfarb D, et al. Interaction between warfarin sodium and amiodarone. *N Engl J Med* 1981; 304:671–672.
85. Gillis RA, Clancy MM, Anderson RJ. Deleterious effects of bretylium in cats with digitalis-induced ventricular tachycardia. *Circulation* 1973; 47:974–983.
86. Vincent JL, Dufaye P, Berre J, Kahn RJ. Bretylium in severe ventricular arrhythmias associated with digitalis intoxication. *Am J Emerg Med* 1984; 2:504–506.
87. Peipho RW, Culbertson VL, Rhodes RS. Drug interactions with the calcium-entry blockers. *Circulation* 1987; 75:181–194.
88. Hauptman PJ, Kelley RA. Digitalis. *Circulation* 1999; 99:1265–1270.
89. Greiner B, Eichelbaum M, Fritz P, et al. The role of intestinal p-glycoprotein in the interaction of digoxin and rifampin. *J Clin Invest* 1999; 104:147–153.
90. Haas GJ. How best to use digoxin in the treatment of CHF: Strategies and practical tips learned from clinical trials. *J Crit Illness* 1999; 14:484–491.
91. Lessem J, Bellinetto A. Interaction between digoxin and the calcium antagonists nicardipine and tiapamil. *Clin Ther* 1983; 5:595–602.
92. Kirch W, Hutt HJ, Dylewicz P, Ohnhaus EE. Dose-dependence of the nifedipine–digoxin interaction. *Clin Pharmacol Ther* 1986; 39:35–39.
93. Lessem JN. Interaction between Ca^{2+} antagonists and digitalis. *Cardiovasc Drugs Ther* 1988; 1:441–446.
94. Kirch W, Hutt HJ, Heidemann H, et al. Drug interactions with nitrendipine. *J Cardiovasc Pharmacol* 1984; 6:S982–S985.
95. Plunkett LM, Gokhale RD, Vallner JJ, Tackett RL. Prazosin alters free and total plasma digoxin levels in dogs. *Am Heart J* 1985; 109:847–851.
96. Marcus FI. Pharmacokinetic interactions between digoxin and other drugs. *J Am Cardiol* 1985; 5:82A–90A.
97. Waldorff S, Andersen JD, Heeboil-Nielsen N, et al. Spironolactone-induced changes in digoxin kinetics. *Clin Pharmacol Ther* 1978; 24:162–167.
98. Waldorff S, Hansen PB, Egeblad H, et al. Interactions between digoxin and potassium-sparing diuretics. *Clin Pharmacol Ther* 1983; 33:418–423.
99. Fenster PE, Hager WD, Goodman MM. Digoxin-quinidine-spironolactone interaction. *Clin Pharmacol Ther* 1984; 36:70–73.
100. Miura T, Ueno K, Tanaka K, et al. Impairment of absorption of digoxin by acarbose. *J Clin Pharmacol* 1998; 38:654–657.
101. McLay JS, McMurray JJ, Bridges AB, et al. Acute effects of captopril on the renal actions of furosemide in patients with chronic heart failure. *Am Heart J* 1993; 126:879–886.
102. Van Hecken AM, Verbresselt R, Buntinx A, et al. Absence of a pharmacokinetic interaction between enalapril and furosemide. *Br J Clin Pharmacol* 1987; 23:84.
103. Motwani JG, Fenwick MK, Morton JJ, Struthers AD: Furosemide-induced natriuresis is augmented by ultra-low-dose captopril but not by standard dose of captopril in chronic heart failure. *Circulation* 1992; 86:439.
104. Dzau VJ, Packer M, Lilly LS, et al. Prostaglandins in severe congestive heart failure: Relation to activation of the renin-angiotensin system and hyponatremia. *N Engl J Med* 1984; 310:347–352.
105. Heerdink ER, Leufkens HG, Herings RMC, et al. NSAIDs associated with increased risk of congestive heart failure in elderly patients taking diuretics. *Arch Intern Med* 1998; 158:1108–1112.
106. McKibbin JK, Pocock WA, Barlow JB, et al. Sotalol, hypokalaemia, syncope, and torsades de pointes. *Br Heart J* 1984; 51:157–162.
107. Jefferson JW, Kalin NH. Serum lithium levels and long-term diuretic use. *JAMA* 1979; 241:1134–1136.

108. Ruddy MC, Kostis JB, Frishman WH. Drugs that affect the renin-angiotensin system. In: Frishman WH, Sonnenblick EH, eds. *Cardiovascular Pharmacotherapeutics.* New York: McGraw-Hill; 1997:131.
109. Perazella MA. Trimethoprim is a potassium-sparing diuretic like amiloride and causes hyperkalemia in high-risk patients. *Am J Ther* 1997; 4:343–348.
110. Cogan JJ, Humphreys MH, Carlson CJ, et al. Acute vasodilator therapy increases renal clearance of digoxin in patients with congestive heart failure. *Circulation* 1981; 64:973–976.
111. Schneck DW, Vary JE. Mechanism by which hydralazine increases propranolol bioavailability. *Clin Pharmacol Ther* 1984; 35:447–453.
112. Hall D, Zeitler H, Rudolph W. Counteraction of the vasodilator effects of enalapril by aspirin in severe heart failure. *J Am Coll Cardiol* 1992; 20:1549–1555.
113. Teerlink JR, Massie BM. The interaction of ACE inhibitors and aspirin in heart failure: Torn between two lovers [editorial]. *Am Heart J* 1999; 138:193–197.
114. Guazzi M, Pontone G, Agostoni P. Aspirin worsens exercise performance and pulmonary gas exchange in patients with heart failure who are taking angiotensin-converting enzyme inhibitors. *Am Heart J* 1999; 138:254–260.
115. Spaulding C, Charbonnier B, Cohen-Solal A, et al. Acute hemodynamic interaction of aspirin and ticlopidine with enalapril: Results of a double-blind, randomized comparative trial. *Circulation* 1998; 98:757–765.
116. Van Wijngaarden J, Smit AJ, deGraeff PA, et al. Effects of acetylsalicylic acid on peripheral hemodynamics in patients with chronic heart failure treated with angiotensin-converting enzyme inhibitors. *J Cardiovasc Pharmacol* 1994; 23:240–245.
117. Baur LHB, Schipperheyn JJ, van der Laarse A, et al. Combining salicylate and enalapril in patients with coronary artery disease and heart failure. *Br Heart J* 1995; 73:227–236.
118. Singhvi SM, Duchin KL, Willard DA, et al. Renal handling of captopril: Effect of probenicid. *Clin Pharmacol Ther* 1982; 32:182–189.
119. Kazierad DJ, Martin DE, Ilson B, et al. Eprosartan does not affect the pharmacodynamics of warfarin. *J Clin Pharmacol* 1998; 38:649–653.
120. Meadowcroft AM, Williamson KM, Patterson H, et al. The effects of fluvastatin, a CYP2C9 inhibitor, on losartan pharmacokinetics in healthy volunteers. *J Clin Pharmacol* 1999; 39:418–424.
121. Grayzel AI, Liddle L, Seegmiller JE. Diagnostic significance of hyperuricemia in arthritis. *N Engl J Med* 1961; 265:763–768.
122. Moroz L. Increased blood fibrinolytic activity after aspirin ingestion. *N Engl J Med* 1977; 296:525–529.
123. Chesebro JH, Fuster V, Elveback LR, et al. Trial of combined warfarin plus dipyridamole or aspirin therapy in prosthetic heart valve replacement: Danger of aspirin compared with dipyridamole. *Am J Cardiol* 1983; 51:1537–1541.
124. Lin JC, Ito MK, Stolley SN, et al. The effect of converting from pravastatin to simvastatin on the pharmacodynamics of warfarin. *J Clin Pharmacol* 1999; 39:86–90.
125. O'Reilly RA, Sahud MA, Aggeler PM. Impact of aspirin and chlorthalidone on the pharmacodynamics of oral anticoagulant drugs in man. *Ann NY Acad Sci* 1971; 179:173–186.
126. Koh KK, Park GS, Song JH, Moon TH. Interaction of intravenous heparin and organic nitrates in acute ischemic syndromes. *Am J Cardiol* 1995; 76:706–709.
127. Romeo F, Rosano GM, Martuscelli E, De Luca F. Concurrent nitroglycerin administration reduces the efficacy of recombinant tissue-type plasminogen activator in patients with acute anterior wall myocardial infarction. *Am Heart J* 1995; 130:692–697.
128. Gruer PJK, Vega JM, Mercuri MF, et al. Concomitant use of cytochrome P450, 3A4 inhibitors and simvastatin. *Am J Cardiol* 1999; 84:811–815.
129. Rogers JD, Zhao J, Liu L, et al. Grapefruit juice has minimal effects on plasma concentrations of lovastatin-derived 3-hydroxy-3-methylglutaryl coenzyme A reductase inhibitors. *Clin Pharmacol Ther* 1999; 66:358–366.
130. Lees RS, Lees AM. Rhabdomyolysis from the coadministration of lovastatin and the antifungal agent itraconazole. *N Engl J Med* 1995; 333:664–665.
131. Keogh A, Spratt P, McCosker C, et al. Ketoconazole to reduce the need for cyclosporine after cardiac transplantation. *N Engl J Med* 1995; 333:628–633.
132. Houston MC. Nonsteroidal anti-inflammatory drugs and antihypertensives. *Am J Med* 1991; 90(suppl 5A):42S–47S.
133. NSAIDs and hypertension: Is it clinically important? *Drugs Ther Perspect* 1998; 11:14–16.
134. Salvetti A, Magagna A, Abdel-Haq B, et al. Nifedipine interactions in hypertensive patients. *Cardiovasc Drugs Ther* 1990; 4:963–968.
135. Weinberger MH. The relationship of sodium balance and concomitant diuretic therapy to blood pressure response with calcium channel entry blockers. *Am J Med* 1991; 90(suppl 5A):15S–20S.
136. Lin GI, Frishman WH. Use of alternative medications in treating cardiovascular disease. In: Frishman WH, Sonnenblick EH, eds. *Cardiovascular Pharmacotherapeutics.* New York: McGraw-Hill; 1997:989.
137. Johne A, Brockmöller Bauer S, Maurer A, et al. Pharmacokinetic interaction of digoxin with an herbal extract from St. John's wort (*Hypericum perforatum*). *Clin Pharmacol Ther* 1999; 66: 338–345.
138. Yu DK. The contribution of p-glycoprotein to pharmacokinetic drug–drug interactions. *J Clin Pharmacol* 1999; 39:1203–1211.

CHAPTER 82

HEART DISEASE AND PREGNANCY

John H. McAnulty / James Metcalfe / Kent Ueland

INTRODUCTION

The remarkable decrease in maternal morbidity and mortality over the last century is a high achievement. At the beginning of the twenty-first, cardiovascular disease still has significant consequences. This chapter describes how pregnancy affects the cardiovascular system and how the heart and heart disease affect pregnancy. Even if there were no heart disease, an understanding of the cardiovascular changes of a normal pregnancy is important for optimal care. But pregnancy in patients with heart disease is becoming more common. This is not because of a failure of health care. Rather, treatment of heart disease during childhood, usually with surgery, has led an increasing number of women with treated heart disease to survive to the age of childbearing and to be able to conceive. Because of this and because failure to treat heart disease may adversely affect both the mother and the child, the person caring for a pregnant woman must recognize heart disease and direct care accordingly.

HEART DISEASE ISSUES UNIQUE TO PREGNANCY

In the case of a woman with heart disease during pregnancy, some issues are always important. These are outlined below.

Health Priorities

Mother and child—the health of one importantly influences that of the other. The well-being of the fetus should be considered, but the safety of the mother is always the highest priority. Ideally, treatment of the mother with drugs, diagnostic studies, or surgery should be avoided. If required for maternal safety, however, they should be used.

Maternal Fragility

Despite advances in the recognition and management of heart disease, pregnancy puts the mother at risk. The normal hemodynamic changes of pregnancy may result in disability or death. The risk[1] is so great with some cardiovascular abnormalities that a recommendation of avoidance or interruption of pregnancy is supportable (Table 82-1).[2] Emotional stability is also threatened by pregnancy in the woman with heart disease. Misconceptions and apprehension are common. The following previously described case provides one example of the need to keep a pregnant woman and her family informed and comfortable:[3]

> A cardiac care unit nurse for 10 years, always logical and calm, and 7 months into her second pregnancy—could she be this frightened? She is, and it's about what the pregnancy will do to her heart and what her heart will

TABLE 82-1 Cardiovascular Abnormalities Placing a Mother and Infant at Extremely High Risk

Advise *avoidance* or *interruption of pregnancy*
Pulmonary hypertension
Dilated cardiomyopathy with congestive failure
Marfan's syndrome with dilated aortic root
Cyanotic congenital heart disease
Pregnancy counseling and close clinical follow-up required
Prosthetic valve
Coarctation of the aorta
Marfan's syndrome
Dilated cardiomyopathy in asymptomatic women
Obstructive lesions

SOURCE: Modified from McAnulty JH, et al.[2] Reproduced with permission from the publisher and authors.

do to her pregnancy. She, of course, knows too much. She has heard of a peripartum cardiomyopathy and is for some reason convinced that her labor will cause it. She is wrong about that (we believe), but she still is an appropriate representative of a prospective parent—easily worried about the effects of pregnancy on her health and worried about the baby. She knows about her ventricular ectopy. It has to be bad for the baby! She's probably wrong, but again, this is an example of how pregnancy raises issues that we ordinarily do not consider when taking care of a patient: an example of the apprehension that surrounds heart disease and pregnancy.

Fetal Vulnerability

The fetus depends on its mother for a continuous supply of oxygen and adequate nutrients. The mother must also remove the products of fetal metabolism, including heat. The maternal commitment to the fetus is exceptional, but if the mother requires a redistribution of volume for her own safety, blood is preferentially diverted away from the uterus. In the woman with a normal cardiovascular system, blood flow to the fetus seems to be adequate, even during periods of physical and emotional stress. In the woman with heart disease, however, where uterine blood flow may already be compromised, the chance of inadequate uterine perfusion increases. Treatment of maternal heart disease may also jeopardize the fetus. Diagnostic studies, drugs, or surgery may increase fetal loss, result in teratogenicity, or alter fetal growth.

Newborn Infant Vulnerability

The health of a newborn infant is a concern when the mother has heart disease. This fragility may be due to a marginal uterine blood flow during pregnancy or to lingering effects of the medications used to treat the mother. Additionally, the live-born infant of a parent with congenital heart disease will have an increased incidence of congenital heart disease (Table 82-2). Early infant nourishment may be jeopardized if maternal heart disease is severe enough to interfere with breast-feeding. Even if the mother is capable of breast-feeding, cardiovascular medications may be transmitted to the infant in breast milk. Finally, the infant is at risk of losing a parent, since life expectancy with many forms of heart disease is significantly less than normal.

Maternal Heart Disease May Not Be "Typical"

Many women with heart disease who become pregnant have a form of heart disease that is relatively new, having existed for less than 50 years. They have mechanically "altered" heart disease. Although much has been learned about hearts that have been altered by surgery (or a catheter), there is still much that is unknown. It is best not to consider a previous lesion mechanically "corrected," because there is always some residual disease. In some cases, the residual disease (a shunt, ventricular dysfunction, an arrhythmia redisposition, or persistent obstruc-

TABLE 82-2 Congenital Heart Disease in the Offspring of a Parent with Congenital Heart Disease

Congenital Heart Defect in a Parent	Risk of Congenital Heart Disease in Offspring If One Parent Is Affected,[a,b] Percentage
Intracardiac shunts	
Atrial septal defect	3–11
Ventricular septal defect	4–22
Patent ductus arteriosus	4–11
Obstruction to flow	
Left-sided obstruction[c]	3–26
Right-sided obstruction	3–22
Complex abnormalities	
Tetralogy of Fallot	4–15
Ebstein's anomaly	Uncertain
Transposition of the great arteries	Uncertain
Hypertrophic cardiomyopathy with asymmetric septal hypertrophy	50
Marfan's syndrome	50

[a]The higher number in each range comes from one large series.[159,162] The incidence of congenital heart disease in the offspring tends to be closer to the lower number for most other reported series.[155,156]
[b]The risk in obstructive lesions is decreased by corrective surgery prior to pregnancy.[160]
[c]Includes coarctation, aortic stenosis, discrete subaortic stenosis, supravalvular stenosis.

SOURCE: Modified from McAnulty JH, Metcalfe J, Ueland K: Cardiovascular disease. In: Burrow GN, Ferris TF, eds. *Medical Complication during Pregnancy.* Philadelphia: Saunders; 1988. Reproduced with permission from the publisher and authors.

tion) may adversely affect the mother and, in turn, may harm the fetus.

CARDIOVASCULAR ADJUSTMENTS DURING A NORMAL PREGNANCY

Maternal adaptation to pregnancy includes remarkable cardiovascular changes. These explain in part why some cardiac abnormalities are not well tolerated during pregnancy (see Table 82-1) and may result in symptoms and signs, even in a normal pregnancy, that are difficult to distinguish from those occurring with heart disease.

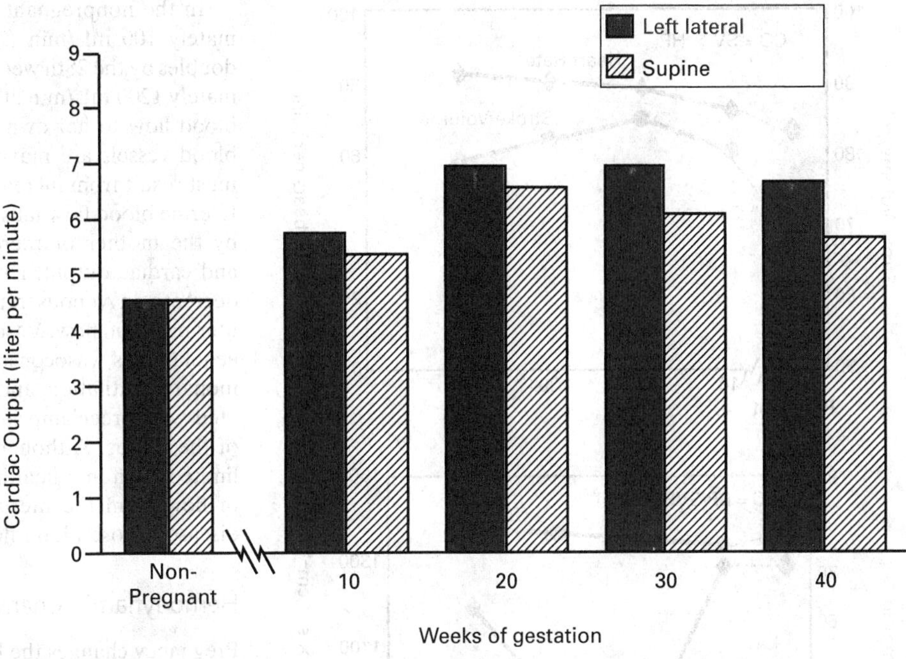

FIGURE 82-1 Cardiac output values during normal pregnancy when measured in the supine and left lateral positions. The values are derived from measurements made in many studies.[5–10] (From Neill and Swanson.[167] Reproduced with permission from the publisher and authors.)

Hemodynamic Changes at Rest

Resting cardiac output increases by over 40 percent during pregnancy. The increase begins early, with the cardiac output reaching its highest levels by the 20th week. In the last half of pregnancy, cardiac output is significantly affected by body position (Fig. 82-1), as the enlarged uterus diminishes venous return from the lower extremities.[4–9] Compared with measurements made near term, when the woman is in the left lateral position, cardiac output is lower by an average of 0.6 L/min when a woman is supine and by 1.2 L/min when she assumes the upright position.[8] In general, this results in few or no symptoms, but in some women, maintenance of the supine position may result in symptomatic hypotension, possibly in those whose collateral vessels are not well developed.[9–11] Symptoms of this "supine hypotensive syndrome of pregnancy" can be corrected by having the woman turn onto her side.

The hemodynamic changes associated with or causing the variation in cardiac output also change dramatically (Fig. 82-2). Cardiac output is the product of heart rate times stroke volume. Its early rise is due mainly to an increase in stroke volume.[4,7] By the 20th week, stroke volume gradually begins to fall because of obstruction of the vena cava by the enlarged uterus and increased dilation of the venous bed. The heart rate increases gradually throughout pregnancy, reaching a level that is approximately 25 percent above the nonpregnant levels by the time of delivery.

Cardiac output is also directly related to the mean blood pressure and inversely related to the systemic vascular resistance. There is a fall in blood pressure early in pregnancy, with a gradual return to nonpregnant levels by term. The fall in systemic vascular resistance is more marked, decreasing to two-thirds of resting nonpregnant values at about the 20th week of pregnancy and then gradually rising through the remainder of pregnancy, although not achieving nonpregnant levels until a few weeks after delivery.[4,7]

Finally, the cardiac output is equal to the oxygen consumption divided by the systemic arterial venous oxygen difference. The mother's oxygen consumption (which includes that of her fetus) increases by 20 percent within the first 20 weeks of pregnancy and increases steadily to a level that is approximately 30 percent above the nonpregnant levels by the time of delivery.[7] This increase is due both to the metabolic needs of the fetus and the increased metabolic needs of the mother. The increase in cardiac output occurs earlier than the rise in oxygen consumption; thus the arteriovenous oxygen difference narrows early in pregnancy with a gradual increase in oxygen extraction throughout pregnancy, so that by term, the systemic arteriovenous oxygen difference exceeds nonpregnant values.

At the beginning of labor, cardiac output measured in the supine position increases to over 7 L/min (Fig. 82-3). With each uterine contraction, this rises by still another 34 percent as a result of increases in heart rate as well as an increment in stroke volume resulting from extrusion of approximately 500 mL of blood into the central venous system with each contraction. Thus, at these times, the cardiac output can be as great as 9 L/min.[12] Administration of epidural anesthesia reduces this cardiac output to about 8 L/min, and the use of general anesthesia reduces it still further. Following delivery, there is a transient, marked elevation in cardiac output that approaches 10 L/min[12] (7 to 8 L/min with cesarean section),[13] with the cardiac output falling rapidly to near-normal, nonpregnant values within a few weeks after delivery, although there is a slight elevation that can persist for as long as a year.[14]

The increase in maternal cardiac output in women with twins or triplets is slightly greater than that in women with single pregnancies.[15]

The distribution of blood flow is not fully understood; it is affected by changes in local vascular resistance[16] (Fig. 82-4). Renal blood flow increases by approximately 30 percent in the first trimester and stays at about that level or declines slightly

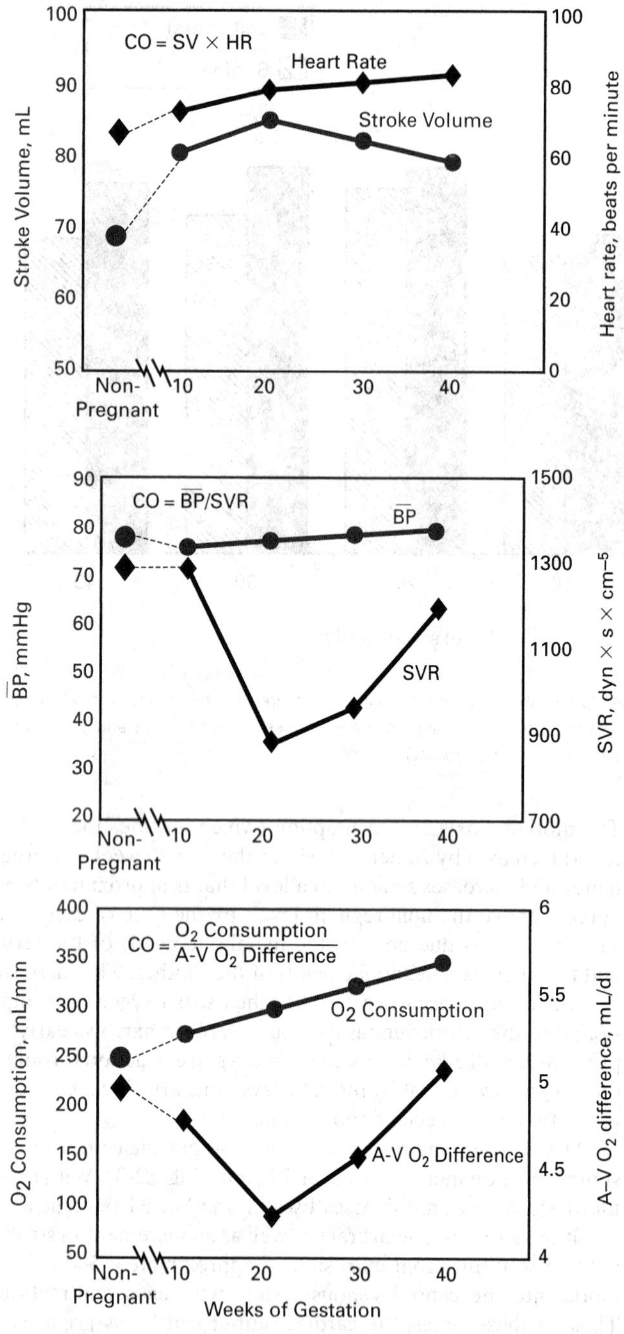

FIGURE 82-2 The cardiac output (CO) can be determined from other parameters in at least 3 ways: CO = heart rate (HR) × stroke volume (SV); CO = mean arterial pressure (BP) minus the RA pressure/systemic vascular resistance (SVR); CO = oxygen (O_2) consumption/arteriovenous (AV) O_2 difference. The expected values for these parameters measured in the supine position during pregnancy are based on information acquired from many studies.[5–8] (From Neill and Swanson.[167] Reproduced with permission from the publisher and authors.)

throughout the pregnancy. Nonpregnant mammary blood flow is usually less than 1 percent of the cardiac output but can be approximately 2 percent of the cardiac output at term. Blood flow to the skin increases by 40 to 50 percent—a mechanism for heat dissipation.

In the nonpregnant woman, uterine blood flow is approximately 100 mL/min (2 percent of the cardiac output). This doubles by the 28th week of pregnancy and increases to approximately 1200 mL/min at term, a value approaching the mother's blood flow to her own kidneys.[17–19] During pregnancy, uterine blood vessels are maximally dilated; flow can increase, but it must result from increased maternal arterial pressure and flow. Uterine blood flow falls if redistribution of total flow is required by the mother or there is a fall in maternal blood pressure and cardiac output. Excitement, heat, anxiety,[20] exercise, and decrease in venous return have all been shown to decrease uterine blood flow. Vasoconstriction caused by endogenous catecholamines, vasoconstrictive drugs, maternal mechanical pulmonary ventilation, and some anesthetics as well as that associated with preeclampsia and eclampsia can decrease perfusion of the uterus. Although uterine blood flow can potentially be limited even in a healthy woman, the concern about diversion of flow from the uterus is greater in the mother with heart disease, whose blood flow may already be compromised.

Hemodynamic Changes with Exercise

Pregnancy changes the hemodynamic response to exercise. For any given level of exercise in the sitting position, the cardiac output is greater than in nonpregnant women, and maximum cardiac output is reached at lower exercise levels. The increase in cardiac output is relatively greater than the increase in oxygen consumption, so the arteriovenous oxygen difference is wider than that produced by the same exercise in the nonpregnant woman. This suggests that oxygen delivery to the periphery is somewhat less efficient during pregnancy.[21] In a nonpregnant woman, training or conditioning results in a greater increase in stroke volume and a smaller increment in heart rate with exercise than would occur in an untrained individual. During pregnancy, this training effect is not seen—possibly because the increase in stroke volume is limited as a result of compression of the inferior vena cava or the increased venous distensibility.[22]

Exercise during pregnancy is not clearly any more dangerous or beneficial to the mother with heart disease than it would be when she was not pregnant. It does affect the fetus. In animal models, maternal exercise has been associated with a fall in uterine blood flow. In humans, it is known that the type of exercise affects maternal hemodynamics and uterine perfusion.[23,24] As an example, maximal exercise by swimming causes less fetal bradycardia (a marker of uterine blood flow) than the same level of cycling.[25] Additionally, regular aerobic endurance exercise during pregnancy has been associated with a reduction in birth weight. Since most of the reduction is due to a decrease in neonatal fat mass, it is not clear if this is detrimental.[26]

Infants born to mothers who work in a standing position may be abnormally small at birth.[27] Although the long-term effects of this are not clear, the implications in relation to exercise and work in the upright position would seem to be greater for women with heart disease.[28,29] This question, relating to exercise and the effect on the fetus, has become more important with an increasing enthusiasm for recreational exercise in the United States. Although there is not enough evidence available to suggest that the healthy pregnant woman should avoid recreational exercise, an argument can be made for advising the woman with heart disease to keep the exercise level below that which causes symptoms.

Mechanisms for Hemodynamic Changes

The mechanisms evoking the hemodynamic adaptation to pregnancy are not fully understood. They may in part be due to volume changes. Total body water increases steadily throughout pregnancy by 6 to 8 L (most is extracellular).[30] Sodium retention results in an excess accumulation of 500 to 900 meq by the time of delivery. As early as 6 weeks after conception, plasma volume increases, approaching its maximum of 1½ times normal by the second trimester, where it stays throughout the pregnancy.[31] The red blood cell mass also increases, but not to the same degree as the increase in plasma volume. As a result, the hematocrit falls, though rarely to less than 30 percent. Peak hemodilution occurs at 24 to 26 weeks; then the hematocrit gradually increases.

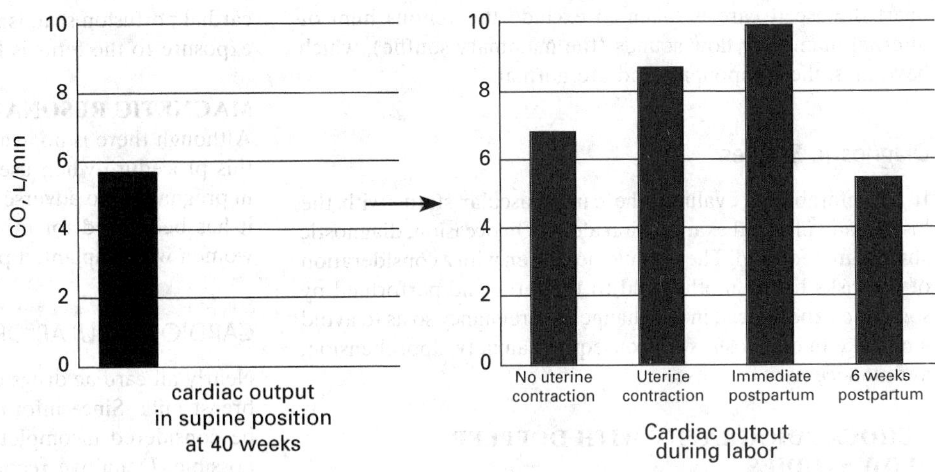

FIGURE 82-3 Cardiac output measured in the supine position is high at 40 weeks (*A*), increased during labor (*B*), particularly with contractions, and even higher in the minutes to hours following a vaginal delivery.[13,15] (From Neill and Swanson.[167] Reproduced with permission from the publisher and authors.)

Vascular alterations also contribute to the hemodynamic changes of pregnancy. Arterial compliance is increased,[32,33] and there is an increase in venous vascular capacitance.[33–35] These changes are advantageous in maintaining the hemodynamics of a normal pregnancy. There may be disadvantages as well. The arterial changes are associated with increased fragility; vascular accidents, when they occur in women, frequently do so during pregnancy.[36–40] The venous changes may explain in part the increase in thromboemboli during pregnancy.[41]

Intrinsic cardiac changes can also explain some of the hemodynamic changes.[42–44] The stroke volume increases by approximately 25 percent. The ejection fraction does not change; thus the heart has to enlarge (since the ejection fraction is the stroke volume divided by the end-diastolic volume). Since the increases in left ventricular end-diastolic and systolic volumes are small and not adequate to explain the constant ejection fraction, the heart must become reconfigured as well. If so, this occurs with only a 10 to 15 percent increase in myocardial mass during pregnancy.[45]

The ultimate cause (or causes) for these recognized changes is uncertain. Complex interactions of the renin-angiotensin-aldosterone system, the reproductive hormones, prostaglandins, and atrial natriuretic factor contribute to the fluid and sodium changes.[46,47] At the present time, the effects of the increased level of circulating steroid hormones seem to explain the vascular and myocardial changes satisfactorily.

DIAGNOSIS OF HEART DISEASE

Clinical Evaluation

The recognition and definition of heart disease are difficult at any time. This is particularly true during pregnancy. Symptoms suggesting heart disease—fatigue, dyspnea, orthopnea, pedal edema, and chest discomfort—occur commonly in pregnant women with normal hearts. Although they should alert a caregiver to the possibility of heart disease, the concern should increase if the dyspnea or orthopnea is progressive and limiting or if a woman develops hemoptysis, syncope with exertion, or chest pain clearly related to effort. Common examination features of a normal pregnancy include pedal edema, basilar pulmonary rales, a third heart sound, a systolic murmur, and visible neck vein pulsations. However, cyanosis or clubbing, a loud systolic murmur (≥3/6), cardiomegaly, a "fixed split" second heart sound, or evidence for pulmonary hypertension (a left parasternal lift and loud P_2) do not occur as part of a normal pregnancy and deserve attention. A diastolic murmur is unusual enough during pregnancy that its presence is an indication of

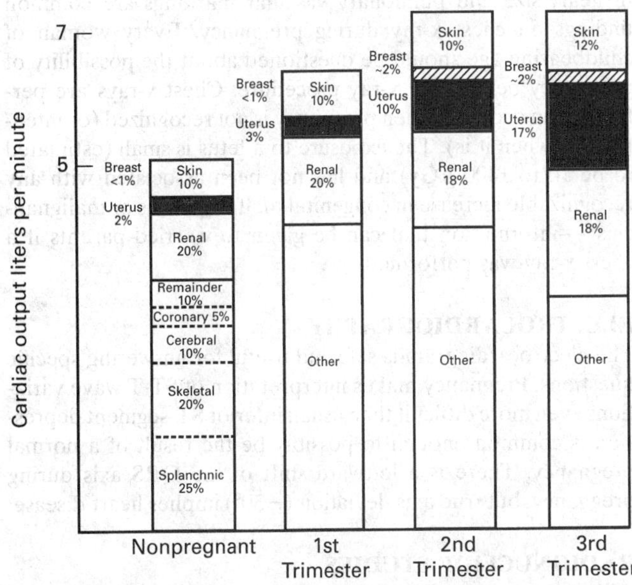

FIGURE 82-4 The changes in cardiac output and its distribution at rest in nonpregnant and pregnant women are depicted. Data used in this graph are fragmentary, especially early in pregnancy. (From Neill and Swanson.[167] Reproduced with permission from the publisher and authors.)

heart disease if care is taken to exclude the venous hum or internal mammary flow sounds (the mammary souffle), which have diastolic components and are normal.

Diagnostic Studies

It is preferable to evaluate the cardiovascular status with the history and physical examination alone. On occasion, diagnostic studies are required. They should be chosen with a consideration of the risks to the mother and to the fetus and performed by someone experienced in the changes of pregnancy so as to avoid a mistake in diagnosis, with consequent anxiety, apprehension, and unnecessary expense.

ECHOCARDIOGRAPHY WITH DOPPLER FLOW STUDIES

Echocardiography with evaluation of flow by Doppler is so safe, with no known risk to the mother or fetus, and is so diagnostically useful that overuse is the only significant concern (Chap. 13). Expense and potential misinterpretation are reasons to consider its use only when required to answer a specific question. The safety of transesophageal echocardiography has not been assessed in pregnancy. The use of anesthetic agents during the procedure would seem to create the greatest risk, and this is minor.

RADIOGRAPHIC PROCEDURES

All x-ray procedures should generally be avoided, particularly early in pregnancy. They increase the risk of abnormal fetal organogenesis or of a subsequent malignancy in the child, particularly leukemia. If a study is required, it should be delayed to as late in pregnancy as possible, the radiation dose should be kept to a minimum, and shielding of the fetus should be optimal. Interpretation should take into consideration the changes expected in a normal pregnancy. As an example, some increase in heart size and pulmonary vascular markings are common findings on chest x-ray during pregnancy. Every woman of childbearing age should be questioned about the possibility of pregnancy before any x-ray procedure. Chest x-rays are performed on occasion when pregnancy is not recognized (or intentionally when it is). The exposure to a fetus is small (estimated to be 10 to 1400 μGy) and has not been associated with any recognizable increase in congenital malformations or malignancies[48]—information that can be given to worried parents if a chest x-ray was performed.

ELECTROCARDIOGRAPHY

The electrocardiogram is safe and useful for answering specific questions. Pregnancy makes interpretation of ST-T wave variations even more difficult than usual; inferior ST-segment depression is common enough to possibly be the result of a normal pregnancy. There is a leftward shift of the QRS axis during pregnancy, but true axis deviation (−30°) implies heart disease.

RADIONUCLIDE STUDIES

Although many radionuclides should attach to albumin and thus not reach the fetus, separation can occur and fetal exposure is possible. It is preferable to avoid these studies. On occasion, a pulmonary ventilation/perfusion scan or even a thallium myocardial perfusion scan is required during pregnancy. Estimated exposure to the fetus is low (400 μGy).[41]

MAGNETIC RESONANCE IMAGING

Although there is no available information about the safety of this procedure when used for the evaluation of heart disease in pregnancy, no adverse fetal effects have been reported when it has been used for other purposes. It should be avoided in women with implanted pacemakers or defibrillators.

CARDIOVASCULAR DRUGS AND PREGNANCY

Nearly all cardiac drugs cross the placenta and are secreted in breast milk. Since information about the use of any drug can be considered incomplete, it is best to avoid their use when possible. Definitive recommendations about the use of drugs in pregnancy is difficult, but if required for maternal safety, they should not be withheld.[49,50]

Diuretics

Diuretics can and should be used for treatment of congestive heart failure that is uncontrolled by sodium restriction, and they remain front-line therapy for the treatment of hypertension. No one agent is clearly contraindicated—experience is greatest with the thiazide diuretics and with furosemide.[50,51] Diuretics should not be used for prophylaxis against toxemia or for treatment of pedal edema.

Inotropic Agents

The indications for the use of digitalis are not changed by pregnancy. Digoxin and digitoxin cross the placenta, and fetal serum levels approximate those in the mother. The same dose of digoxin in general will yield lower maternal serum levels during pregnancy than in the nonpregnant state.[52] If the desired clinical effect is not achieved, it may be helpful to measure levels (if the assay used is not affected by an immunoreactive substance of pregnancy).[53] Digitalis may shorten the duration of gestation and labor due to an effect on the myometrium similar to the inotropic effect on the myocardium.

When intravenous inotropic or vasopressor agents are required, the standard agents (dopamine, dobutamine, and norepinephrine) may be used, but the fetus is jeopardized because all result in decreased uterine blood flow and may stimulate uterine contractions. Ephedrine is an appropriate initial vasopressor drug as, at least in animal models, it does not adversely affect uterine blood flow.

There is no available information about the efficacy or safety of the phosphodiesterase inhibitors (amrinone, milrinone).

Adrenergic Receptor Blocking Agents

Observations that beta blockers may decrease umbilical blood flow, initiate premature labor, and result in a small and infarcted placenta with the potential for low-birth-weight infants have led to concerns about their use.[54] Large studies have not confirmed these concerns, however, and beta-blocking drugs have been used in a large number of pregnant women without adverse effects. Their use for the usual clinical indications is reasonable.[54–56] All the available beta-blocking agents cross the placenta, are present in human breast milk, and can reach significant levels in the fetus or the newborn. Recent concerns about low birth weights from maternal use of atenolol early in pregnancy[57,58] make use of alternative $beta_1$-selective agents preferable. If these agents are used during pregnancy, it is appropriate to monitor fetal heart rate as well as the newborn infant's heart rate, blood sugar, and respiratory status immediately after delivery.

Experience with the alpha-blocking agents phenoxybenzamine and phentolamine is sparse. Clonidine, prazosin, and labetalol, with their mixed alpha- and beta-blocking effects, have been used for treatment of hypertension without clear detrimental effects.[59]

Calcium Channel Blocking Drugs

Nifedipine, verapamil, diltiazem, nicardipine, and isradipine have been used to treat hypertension and arrhythmias without an adverse effect on the fetus or newborn infant.[50,60] The drugs cause relaxation of the uterus; nifedipine has been used for this purpose.

Antiarrhythmic Agents

Atrioventricular (AV) node blockade is occasionally required during pregnancy. This can be achieved with digoxin, beta blockers, and calcium blockers. Early reports suggest that adenosine can also be safely used as a node-blocking agent.[61]

As a general rule, it is preferable to avoid the standard antiarrhythmic drugs in any patient. This is true during pregnancy as well. When essential for recurrent arrhythmias or for maternal safety, they should be used; however, there is insufficient accumulated information to know whether or not these drugs increase the risk to the fetus or child.[50,62,63] If intravenous drug therapy is required, lidocaine is reasonable first-line therapy. There has been demonstration of transient neonatal depression when the neonate's blood level exceeds 2.5 μg/L, a reason to recommend keeping maternal blood levels below 4 μg/L (since fetal levels are 60 percent of maternal levels).[50,64] Intravenous procainamide and quinidine may cause hypotension; there is no available information about intravenous amiodarone. Based on its effects on maternal blood pressure, bretylium would seem likely to decrease uterine perfusion.

If oral antiarrhythmic therapy is necessary, it may still be appropriate to begin with quinidine since, given its long-term availability, it has been most frequently used without clear adverse fetal effects.[50,54,65] There is some information about procainamide,[66] disopyramide,[67] mexiletine,[68] flecainide,[69,70] and sotalol,[71] but it is insufficient to recommend their use unless it would be essential for the mother. The early available information concerning amiodarone would suggest an increased likelihood of fetal loss and deformity.[72–74]

Vasodilator Agents

When needed for a hypertensive crisis or emergency afterload and preload reduction, nitroprusside is the vasodilator drug of choice. Despite a paucity of information about its use during pregnancy, this controversial recommendation is made because the drug is highly effective, works instantly, and is easily tolerated; moreover, its effects dissipate immediately when the drug is stopped. The concern about the use of this drug is that its metabolite, cyanide, can be detected in the fetus, but this has not been demonstrated to be a significant problem in humans.[75,76] This metabolite is a reason to limit the duration of use of this drug whenever possible. Intravenous hydralazine, nitroglycerin, or labetalol are options for parenteral therapy.

Chronic afterload reduction to treat hypertension, aortic or mitral regurgitation, or ventricular dysfunction during pregnancy has been achieved with the calcium blocking drugs, hydralazine, and methyldopa.[59,77] Adverse fetal effects have not been reported. The *angiotension-converting enzyme* (ACE) inhibitors are contraindicated in pregnancy.[59,77,78] They increase the risk of abnormalities in fetal renal development. There are no data available on losartin and valsartin, the new angiotensin II blockers.

Antithrombotic Agents

The chronic use of warfarin is associated with a 1 to 5 percent chance per year of significant bleeding. More importantly, in considering its use during pregnancy, one must keep in mind that warfarin crosses the placenta, and fetal exposure during the first 3 months is associated with a 5 to 25 percent incidence of malformations that comprise the "warfarin embryopathy syndrome" (facial abnormalities, optic atrophy, digital abnormalities, epithelial changes, and mental impairment).[75–81] Women receiving the drug during the 7th to 12th week of gestation are particularly prone to having children with this syndrome.[82,83] The syndrome may be dose-related, with one study suggesting that it occurs only with doses greater than 5 mg per day.[84] Warfarin use at any time during pregnancy increases the risk of fetal bleeding or maternal uterine hemorrhage.

In women who require anticoagulation, heparin is preferable to warfarin. Self-administered subcutaneous high-dose heparin (16,000 to 24,000 units per day) has been proven feasible and efficacious.[85–88] This drug does not cross the placenta. Accumulating data suggest that low-molecular-weight heparin, while currently more expensive, is effective, easier to use (once or twice daily without the need to follow serial blood tests), and as safe as standard heparin therapy. Although evaluated for venous thrombosis prophylaxis,[89,90] its value in preventing thromboemboli in patients with mechanical prostheses has not been proven. (See Chap. Chap. 61.)

When anticoagulation is required, some have advocated using heparin for the first trimester and warfarin for the next 5 months, with a return to heparin prior to labor and delivery. Although successful pregnancy has been achieved with this approach, the authors favor avoidance of warfarin during pregnancy.

Antiplatelet agents increase the chance of maternal bleeding and they cross the placenta. The most commonly used, aspirin, has some observed and theoretical disadvantages.[91] It is associated with an increased incidence of abortion and fetal growth retardation, and its inhibition of prostaglandin synthesis may result in closure of the ductus arteriosis during fetal life.[92] Still, it has been frequently used and even recommended by some for specific indications and as prophylaxis against preeclampsia.[93]

These trade-offs are difficult to evaluate; thus aspirin should be avoided unless necessary. There are no data available on the effects of clopidogrel or ticlopidine during pregnancy.

Obstetric Drugs and Anesthetic Agents Used During Pregnancy

Drugs used specifically for pregnancy can cause hemodynamic alterations. Although there is some question as to their value,[94] beta-sympathetic amines are used to stop premature labor. All cause maternal tachycardia. Ritodrine and terbutaline have been associated with pulmonary edema, usually when glucocorticoids are being administered concurrently to promote fetal lung maturation. This pulmonary edema responds abruptly to cessation of the drugs and initiation of diuretic therapy. On other occasions, prostaglandins E_2 and F_2 are used to induce labor and have no significant hemodynamic effects.

Synthetic oxytocin (pitocin) is given to minimize blood loss after delivery. The synthetic preparation prevents vasoconstriction, but it has been associated, in turn, with transient hypotension.

Anesthesia for surgery during pregnancy and at the time of labor and delivery can adversely affect a woman with heart disease. In most cases, lumbar epidural anesthesia with a pudendal nerve block to minimize pain is effective and least likely to result in hemodynamic compromise.[95]

MANAGEMENT OF CARDIOVASCULAR SYNDROMES

Cardiovascular complications can occur with any form of heart disease. Management of each patient has to be individualized, but some recommendations are applicable in most cases.

Low-Cardiac-Output Syndrome

A low cardiac output is an ominous sign in any patient, and this is particularly true in pregnancy. It results in signs of poor perfusion (mental obtundation, peripheral vascular constriction, low urine output, and often a low blood pressure). Although potentially treatable causes such as tamponade or severe valvular stenosis should be considered, it is most often due to intravascular volume depletion. This should be prevented when possible and corrected when recognized. Although it is a concern in any pregnant woman, volume depletion is particularly dangerous in those with lesions that limit blood flow, such as pulmonary hypertension, aortic or pulmonic valve stenosis, hypertrophic cardiomyopathy, or mitral stenosis. Measures to prevent or treat a fall in central blood volume are outlined in Table 82-3.

TABLE 82-3 Measures to Protect Against a Fall in Central Blood Volume

Position
- 45–60° left lateral
- 10° Trendelenburg

Full-leg stockings

Volume preloading for surgery and delivery 1500 mL of glucose-free normal saline

Drugs
- Avoid vasodilator drugs
- Ephedrine for hypotension unresponsive to fluid replacement
- Anesthetics (if required)
  - Regional: serial small boluses
  - General: emphasis on benzodiazepines and narcotics, low-dose inhalation agents

Congestive Heart Failure

Management of congestive heart failure during pregnancy should not differ greatly from that at other times. Attention to reduction in salt intake and limitation of activity to a level below that which causes symptoms are appropriate. In a woman with significant symptoms or pulmonary edema, standard therapy can be used with the concerns about the drugs as outlined earlier (remembering particularly that ACE inhibitors should be avoided). Congestive heart failure is one situation where maintaining a woman in the supine position may be beneficial by causing preload reduction with obstruction of return of blood from the inferior vena cava to the heart.

Thromboembolic Complications

The risk of venous thromboemboli increases fivefold during and immediately after pregnancy,[41,96,97] and there is arguably an increase in arterial emboli as well.[98,99] Both may be the result of a woman's hypercoagulable status during pregnancy, and the likelihood of venous thrombosis is increased by venous stasis. Prevention is optimal, and prophylactic full-dose heparin or low-molecular-weight heparin[100] is indicated in those at high risk of a thromboembolic complication, including women with thromboemboli during a previous pregnancy (a risk of 4 to 15 percent), antithrombin III deficiency (a risk of 70 percent), protein C deficiency (a risk of 33 percent), protein S deficiency (17 percent), and the anticardiolipin antibody syndrome.[41] Prothrombin gene mutations and factor V mutation resulting in the resistance to activated protein C (found in 3 to 5 percent of the population) may eventually be shown to be a reason for prophylaxis as well.[101,102]

If a thrombus or embolus is identified, 5 to 10 days of intravenous heparin therapy followed by full-dose subcutaneous heparin is recommended.[41] If a thromboembolus is life-threatening (e.g., a massive pulmonary embolus or a thrombosed prosthetic valve), thrombolytic therapy can be used.[103]

Hypertension

Hypertension can be present before pregnancy (in 1 to 5 percent) and persist throughout pregnancy, or it can develop with pregnancy.[59,104] When normotensive women become pregnant, 5 to 7 percent will develop hypertension. Because of the marked early fall in systemic vascular resistance, this often does not occur until the second half of pregnancy. It has been called *pregnancy-induced* or *gestational hypertension* or *toxemia*. When associated with proteinuria, pedal edema, central nervous system (CNS) irritability, elevation of liver enzymes, and coagulation disturbances, the hypertension syndrome is called *preeclampsia*. If convulsions occur, the diagnosis is *eclampsia*. It is not clear that hypertension alone puts the mother or fetus at risk during pregnancy, but preeclampsia increases maternal risk (approximately 1 to 2 percent chance of CNS bleed, convulsions, or other severe systemic illness) and may cause fetal growth retardation (10 to 15 percent). Maternal and fetal morbidity and mortality increase still further with eclampsia.

Guidelines for the level of blood pressure control are not well established. Until more is known, an argument can be made for keeping the systolic pressure below 160 mmHg and the diastolic pressure below 100 mmHg. This may provide a margin of safety against severe hypertensive episodes and possibly will improve fetal survival. Nonpharmacologic therapy is preferable when possible, although it is not clearly defined. While strict bed rest may achieve blood pressure lowering, it is not generally recommended, although limitation of activity and reduction of stress is commonly advised.[77,104] Unless the patient has previously demonstrated salt-sensitive hypertension, sodium restriction is generally inadvisable, since pregnant women with hypertension have lower plasma volumes than normotensive women. If drug treatment is required, experience is greatest with methyldopa.[59,105,106] This otherwise infrequently used antihypertensive agent has been demonstrated to promote fetal survival and to result in children with normal mental and physical development. It may be that other drugs will achieve the same goal, but they have not been studied adequately. Initial therapy could also include a β_1 selective beta blocker or a diuretic. Calcium channel blockers have been proven to be effective.[60] As mentioned earlier, ACE inhibitors should not be used, and the safety of angiotension II blocking agents is undefined.

Pulmonary Hypertension

Whether pulmonary hypertension (Chap. 52) is primary or secondary to prolonged left-to-right shunting (Eisenmenger's syndrome), drug abuse, a primary vascular disease syndrome, or recurrent pulmonary emboli, maternal mortality ranges from 30 to 70 percent.[107,108] Even with maternal survival, fetal loss exceeds 40 percent. Maternal death can occur at any time during pregnancy, but the mother is most vulnerable during the time of labor and delivery and in the first postpartum week. If recognized early in pregnancy, interruption is advised. If this is declined, or if the pulmonary hypertension is recognized late in pregnancy, close follow-up is required. Intravascular volume depletion puts these patients at greatest risk. For this group in particular, the measures outlined in Table 82-3 are important. Systemic vascular resistance and pressure must be maintained in patients with pulmonary hypertension who have a right-to-left shunt (to minimize still further shunting), and meticulous attention to avoidance of air or thrombus emboli from intravenous catheters is essential to avoid systemic emboli in these patients. At the time of labor and delivery, a central venous line allows adequate fluid administration, and a radial artery catheter makes determinations of blood pressure and oxygen saturation easier. These lines should be used for 48 to 72 h postdelivery.

Arrhythmias

In the woman with dizziness, palpitations, and light-headedness, pregnancy offers many other explanations, but arrhythmias should be considered as a possible cause (Chap. 24). The rules for treatment should be the same as in the nonpregnant patient with the possible exception that a rhythm causing hemodynamic instability should be treated somewhat more rapidly and aggressively because of the concern about diversion of blood flow away from the uterus. As always, if a potentially reversible cause can be identified, it should be corrected. If treatment is required, it should never be instituted without electrocardiographic documentation of the rhythm.

Tachyarrhythmias are as frequent during pregnancy as at other times. As always, the presence of *atrial* or *ventricular premature beats* or of *sinus tachycardia* is a reason to look for and to correct the cause but not a reason to institute specific treatment for arrhythmias.

Paroxysmal supraventricular tachycardia may occur somewhat more frequently during pregnancy than in the nonpregnant state, whether because of the mechanism of AV node reentry ("dual AV node mechanism") or owing to atrial ventricular reentry ("accessory pathway mechanism").[109–111] This is the most common sustained abnormal rhythm occurring with pregnancy. Initial treatment with vagal maneuvers is as appropriate as at other times. If medical treatment is required, intravenous adenosine or verapamil is effective. Cardioversion can be used if required, remembering that the rule "never cardiovert an awake patient" is just as applicable during pregnancy as at any other time.[112] If recurrent episodes require a chronic day-to-day drug, verapamil or a beta blocker would seem to be an optimal choice; digoxin may be effective, although it should be avoided if the patient has preexcitation. Management of *atrial fibrillation* and *flutter* should be as in the nonpregnant woman. If these rhythms occur in a woman with mitral stenosis, severe left ventricular dysfunction, or a previous thromboembolic event, antithrombotic therapy with heparin is indicated.

Ventricular tachycardia may occur during pregnancy.[113,114] If it is suggestive of a right ventricular outflow tract tachycardia (a left bundle branch block with vertical axis morphology), beta-blocker therapy may be effective. If a fascicular ventricular tachycardia (often with a right bundle branch block and left axis deviation), verapamil or diltiazem may be effective treatment. Emergency management of rapid ventricular tachycardia or ventricular fibrillation should be as recommended for the nonpregnant woman.[115,116] If possible, the pelvis should be rolled to the left to enhance blood return from the lower extremities. If pregnancy has proceeded beyond 24 weeks and maternal survival is in question, emergency cesarean section could be considered.

A prolonged QT-interval syndrome can be diagnosed first during pregnancy.[117,118] If this is recognized and it is an acquired form (of course, almost always from drugs), the offending cause should be eliminated. If the syndrome is congenital, beta-blocker therapy during pregnancy is warranted. Implantable defibrillators have been used with recurrent ventricular arrhythmias, but their value remains unproven in this syndrome, even when it is unrelated to pregnancy. In patients with a congenital syndrome, transmission with autosomal dominance can affect the child.

Bradyarrhythmias may also occur during pregnancy. Although they are a reason to look for a reversible cause, treatment is generally not required unless the patient has clear hemodynamic compromise. Complete heart block, which in this age group is most likely to be congenital in origin, is consistent with a successful pregnancy.[119] If required, a permanent pacemaker can be inserted.

Loss-of-Consciousness Spells

Pregnancy makes an assessment of a loss-of-consciousness spell even more difficult than usual. If a seizure disorder cannot be excluded as a cause, appropriate evaluation with electroencephalography is indicated. If a seizure is unlikely or excluded, the syndrome of syncope should include a consideration of the usual causes.

Endocarditis

Infective endocarditis can occur during pregnancy in women without a recognized heart abnormality, but structural abnormalities place individuals at much greater risk (Chap. 73). The clinical presentation of endocarditis is the same during pregnancy as at other times.[120,121] *Streptococcus* is the most common cause. Intravenous drug abusers are more likely to have staphylococcal infections, and women with genitourinary tract infections are more likely to have gram-negative infections, most commonly due to *Escherichia coli*. Optimal management includes prevention. Although it is not the recommendation of the American Heart Association committee addressing this issue,[122] most physicians caring for women with heart disease recommend antibiotic prophylaxis at the time of dental or surgical procedures or at labor and delivery. If endocarditis does occur, it should be treated aggressively with medical therapy, and the usual indications for surgery are appropriate during pregnancy. If open-heart surgery is required late in pregnancy, simultaneous cesarean section should be considered.

Surgery

Although not exactly a complication of pregnancy, pregnant women with recent disease have the same 0.5 to 2.0 percent chance of requiring surgery as in those who are not pregnant. A number of rules are appropriate to consider. Venous return must be maintained, and, when possible, surgery should be performed in the left lateral position. Unless there is severe congestive heart failure, volume loading with 1500 mL of normal saline prior to surgery or labor and delivery is important. This fluid should not include glucose at the time of labor and delivery, because it can cause subsequent hypoglycemia in the newborn. In the woman who requires assisted ventilation, hyperventilation should be avoided, as it decreases venous return. Pain relief should be assured to minimize the rise in catecholamine levels that would, in turn, decrease uterine blood flow. Fetal monitoring should be performed. If it is essential to perform heart surgery during pregnancy, the risks are greater than in the nonpregnant woman and fetal risk is high.[123]

SPECIFIC FORMS OF HEART DISEASE

Other sections of this book discuss each of the following cardiovascular abnormalities in detail. The remainder of this chapter relates the specific abnormalities to pregnancy and considers the potential problems during pregnancy, the demonstrated risk to the mother and fetus, and the management of both mother and fetus during pregnancy. As discussed earlier, with each abnormality, antibiotic prophylaxis against endocarditis with dental or surgical procedures is as appropriate during pregnancy as at other times[122] and is recommended at labor and delivery.

Rheumatic Heart Disease

Worldwide, rheumatic fever remains a common and virulent disease (see Chap. 55). The resultant valve and myocardial disease is probably the most common cause of heart disease during pregnancy.[123] In the United States, clinically recognized rheumatic fever is uncommon and, when it does occur, appears to be associated with less severe heart disease.[124] Still, even in this country, there are regions where its incidence is increasing.[125] In a woman presenting with myocarditis, rheumatic fever as a cause should be considered, particularly if it is associated with fever, joint discomfort, subcutaneous nodules, erythema marginatum, or chorea and if there is evidence of a group A streptococcal infection.[126] Rheumatic fever is the cause of almost all mitral stenosis; of some isolated mitral, aortic, or tricuspid regurgitation; and of some double- and triple-valve disease. Definition of valve morphology by echocardiography can help to clarify the etiology. Recognition of rheumatic fever as the cause of heart disease is important because it identifies those who need antibiotic prophylaxis to prevent recurrence of the disease; people at highest risk of developing rheumatic fever are those who have had it in the past. Twice-daily penicillin is the treatment regimen of choice, and this should be continued throughout pregnancy.[127]

Valve Disease

MITRAL STENOSIS

When present, mitral stenosis is caused almost exclusively by rheumatic fever, and the lesion is more common in women than in men (Chap. 57). The increased cardiac output, tachycardia, and fluid retention of pregnancy may double the resting pressure gradient across a stenotic mitral valve.[128] Symptoms attributable to an increase in left atrial pressure, with associated pulmonary vascular congestion and bronchial vein distention, occur in up to 25 percent of patients with mitral stenosis during pregnancy.[129,130] They usually become apparent by the 20th week and may be aggravated still further at the time of labor and delivery, with the associated increases in heart rate and cardiac output. Maternal death is rare when there is careful attention to the management of congestive heart failure. Although potentially at risk from the elevated left atrial pressure, the patient with mitral stenosis also depends on this pressure to fill the left ventricle and maintain cardiac output. Because the pregnant woman is especially liable to sudden shifts in the distribution of blood volume, preservation of an adequate intravascular volume is essential to prevent a dramatic fall in cardiac output.

If a woman contemplating pregnancy has symptomatic mitral valve stenosis, balloon dilation or valve surgery is appropriate before conception. If mitral stenosis is first recognized during pregnancy and symptoms develop, standard medical therapy is appropriate. If this does not control symptoms, balloon valvuloplasty can be performed (with appropriate radiation shielding of the fetus).[131,132] Mitral valve surgical commissurotomy or valve replacement has been performed, but fetal loss exceeds 30 percent.[123,133,134] Atrial fibrillation is of particular concern during pregnancy. The usual rapid ventricular response further compromises diastolic flow time and can result in pulmonary edema. Emergency treatment should include intravenous verapamil or cardioversion.

MITRAL REGURGITATION

Mitral regurgitation may be due to rheumatic fever, but unlike mitral stenosis, the majority of cases are due to other causes. Whatever the cause, in general it is well tolerated during pregnancy. If symptoms do occur, fatigue or dyspnea is most common. Treatment for congestive heart failure should be as described earlier. Afterload reduction is an important component of this therapy, remembering that ACE inhibitors should not be used. One cause of mitral regurgitation is *mitral valve prolapse* (Chap. 58). This deserves discussion not because it carries any particular risk during pregnancy but because it is so common, occurring in 5 to 10 percent of young adults. The volume and pressure changes of pregnancy may alter examination findings in a woman with mitral valve prolapse. Associated arrhythmias, endocarditis, cerebral emboli, and hemodynamically significant regurgitation may be rare complications and are no more likely to occur during pregnancy than at other times.[135–138] The physical examination is sufficient for diagnosis—diagnostic studies, including an echocardiogram, do little to benefit the patient. Antibiotic prophylaxis at the time of labor and delivery is recommended in those with a heart murmur.

AORTIC STENOSIS

More common in males, aortic valve stenosis is an unusual finding in pregnancy, but it does occur. The diagnostic criteria are the same during pregnancy as at other times. Concerns from an early review indicating high maternal and fetal mortality rates[139] should be tempered by more recent information (although still involving only small numbers) demonstrating that pregnancy can be carried through with little or no maternal mortality and with no clear increase in fetal loss.[140–143] The offspring can have as high as a 20 percent incidence of congenital heart disease, a value that interestingly can potentially be halved by correcting the outflow tract obstruction prior to pregnancy.[144]

If severe stenosis is recognized before pregnancy, balloon valvotomy or a surgical commissurotomy is recommended prior to conception (Chap. 56). If pregnancy does occur in the presence of severe aortic stenosis, measures to avoid hypovolemia are particularly important (see Table 82-3). If congestive heart failure develops, it can be treated as previously described, with emphasis, again, on the need to avoid excessive diuresis. If severe symptoms persist, a balloon valvuloplasty or aortic valve surgery can be performed during pregnancy,[123,145,146] the latter being associated with increased fetal loss.

AORTIC REGURGITATION

Unlike aortic stenosis, which is almost always congenital in etiology, aortic regurgitation has other causes and is encountered more frequently during pregnancy. These causes include rheumatic fever, endocarditis, dilation of the aortic root, or, more ominously, aortic dissection. A dilated root or dissection should raise the consideration of Marfan's syndrome as a cause. Aortic regurgitation is generally well tolerated during pregnancy. Congestive heart failure may occur but responds to treatment, with an emphasis on afterload reduction—again with a warning to avoid ACE inhibitors. If endocarditis should occur and the infection is not rapidly controlled, mortality with medical therapy is high and surgical therapy is indicated. If this occurs late in pregnancy, consideration of associated cesarean section is appropriate.

PULMONIC VALVE DISEASE

Many women with pulmonic valve disease will have had previous valve comissurotomy or balloon valvuloplasty for valve stenosis or as part of the correction of tetralogy of Fallot. The residual stenosis and invariable regurgitation are potential concerns but in general do not adversely affect the outcome of pregnancy. The occasional patient with significant pulmonic valve stenosis who has not been treated appears to tolerate pregnancy well. Intravascular volume depletion should be avoided. If severe symptoms (recurrent syncope, uncontrolled dyspnea, and chest pain) occur, balloon valvuloplasty can be performed.

TRICUSPID VALVE DISEASE

Significant tricuspid valve disease is also uncommon during pregnancy (Chap. 54). The incidence of regurgitation has increased because of intravenous drug use, with its resultant right-sided endocarditis. This regurgitation requires no specific therapy during pregnancy. Tricuspid stenosis is rare. If it is encountered, avoidance of intravascular volume depletion would seem to be important.

PROSTHETIC VALVE DISEASE

An artificial valve can perhaps be considered the ultimate form of valve disease. Although many have benefited from these valves, all are left with "prosthetic heart valve disease." One or more of its major associated complications—thromboemboli, bleeding (from anticoagulation), endocarditis, valve dysfunction, reoperation, or death—affects patients at a rate of greater than 5 percent per year throughout their lives.[147,148] Pregnancy increases the risk of each of these complications, and the prosthetic valve and its treatment can adversely affect the fetus.[88,149–153] All these are reasons that a prosthetic valve is a relative contraindication to pregnancy. Still, women with prosthetic valves often become pregnant. Anticoagulation is required in those with a *mechanical* prosthesis. Although some clinicians have suggested that warfarin is acceptable anticoagulation,[151] most would advise avoidance, particularly in the first and third trimesters.[153] Full-dose subcutaneous heparin is the therapy of choice, maintaining anticoagulation at the "high therapeutic level" by following levels of factor Xa; partial thromboplastin levels are unreliable during pregnancy. Low-molecular-weight heparin once a day may be a reasonable alternative but has not been evaluated in patients with prosthetic valves and thus cannot be recommended. A *heterograft* or *homograft* prosthesis is an alternative to a mechanical prosthesis. Because of the inherently lower thromboembolic rates associated with these tissue prostheses, anticoagulation is not needed. This opportunity to avoid anticoagulation therapy is a logical argument for using these prostheses in young women who are contemplating pregnancy. However, these valves do not completely eliminate the concern about thromboemboli, and the rate of heterograft degeneration is high in young women, resulting in the need for early valve replacement[154] (see Chap. 61).

Congenital Heart Disease

Congenital heart disease is now the most common heart disease encountered in women of childbearing age in the United States. In most, it has been altered by surgery (Chap. 64). Each abnormality is unique, but there are some issues that should be considered with all of them. First, some abnormalities significantly increase the risk of maternal morbidity and mortality during pregnancy (see Table 82-1). Second, there is an increased risk of fetal death, which increases with the severity of the maternal lesions. Third, the presence of a congenital cardiac abnormality in either parent or in a sibling increases the risk of cardiac and other congenital abnormalities in the fetus. Congenital heart disease is recognized in 0.8 percent of all live births in the United States.[155,156] Its presence in a parent increases this risk to 2 to 15 percent (see Table 82-2).[156–163] Although some have shown that the risk is two to three times greater if it is the mother rather than the father who has congenital heart disease,[161,163] this finding has not been universal.[162] Actually, the risk that a child will have heart disease can reach 50 percent when the abnormality is transmitted as an autosomal dominant trait, as in the case of Marfan's syndrome, the congenital long-QT syndrome, or hypertrophic cardiomyopathy. When recognized, maternal congenital heart disease should be corrected prior to surgery. In some cases, this will make the pregnancy safer for the mother and may provide a better intrauterine environment for fetal development. Fourth, the implications of residual or inoperable lesions must be clearly understood before pregnancy is undertaken. Finally, as with valve disease, antibiotic prophylaxis against endocarditis is as appropriate during pregnancy as at other times in patients with lesions that render them susceptible to this complication.

LEFT-TO-RIGHT SHUNTS

Some women with left-to-right shunts reach adulthood and become pregnant often without previous recognition of their disease. Although left-to-right shunting increases the chances of pulmonary hypertension, right ventricular failure, arrhythmias, and emboli, it is not clear that these complications are made more likely by a pregnancy. The degree of shunting is affected by the relative resistances of the systemic and pulmonary vascular circuits, both of which fall to a similar degree during pregnancy.[164] In general, there is no significant alteration in the degree of shunting with pregnancy. The right ventricular volume overload associated with the shunts is generally well tolerated during pregnancy.

In the United States, most patients with left-to-right shunts will have undergone surgical correction prior to pregnancy. If anything, this surgery makes pregnancy safer, and there is no clear increase in mortality in these patients with pregnancy as compared with women who have normal hearts.[165] The surgery does not influence the incidence of congenital heart disease in the offspring.

Atrial Septal Defect The symptoms and signs of an atrial septal defect can be subtle and the abnormality may not be recognized before pregnancy. In women with an ostium secundum defect, pregnancy is generally well tolerated by the mother and the fetus. When either parent has an atrial septal defect, 5 to 10 percent of their children will have congenital heart disease. This is not affected by corrective surgery in the mother.[161,162] Ostium primum defects are equally well tolerated during pregnancy unless they are associated with other significant congenital cardiovascular abnormalities.

Ventricular Septal Defect Over half of ventricular septal defects close in childhood, and since the murmur is usually detected in those in whom the lesion persists, an unrecognized defect at the time of pregnancy is uncommon. If such a defect is present, however, pregnancy is generally well tolerated. The occasional congestive heart failure or arrhythmias developing during pregnancy can be managed as described previously. If there is no associated pulmonary hypertension, there is no increase in maternal mortality with pregnancy. Fetal loss in women with uncorrected lesions may approach 20 percent. The child of such a mother has a 5 to 8 percent chance of being born with a cardiac defect; again, this incidence is not altered by previous surgical correction of the defect.[164]

Patent Ductus Arteriosus Like the other left-to-right shunts, a patent ductus is tolerated well during pregnancy. On occasion, congestive heart failure can occur, but standard treatment is effective. Antibiotic prophylaxis against endocarditis is recommended. Fetal loss is not clearly greater than that occurring in women without heart disease.

RIGHT-TO-LEFT SHUNT ("CYANOTIC" HEART DISEASE)

Right-to-left shunting can occur through an atrial or ventricular septal defect or a patent ductus arteriosus when pulmonary vascular resistance exceeds systemic vascular resistance or when there is an obstruction to right ventricular outflow and pulmonary vascular resistance is normal. All are forms of "cyanotic" heart disease. The presence of cyanosis, especially when sufficient to result in elevated hemoglobin levels, is associated with high fetal loss, prematurity, and reduced infant birth weights (see Fig. 82-5).[144,166,167] The situation of elevated pulmonary vascular resistance, or Eisenmenger's syndrome, has been discussed earlier under "Pulmonary Hypertension," but it is worth repeating that with this problem it is advisable to avoid or interrupt pregnancy. When the cyanosis is not due to Eisenmenger's syndrome, maternal mortality is less, but women are at increased risk of heart failure (approximately 15 percent) from thromboemboli, arrhythmias, and endocarditis (4.5 percent).[166]

Tetralogy of Fallot This is the most common form of right-to-left shunting resulting from obstruction to pulmonary flow when pulmonary vascular resistance is normal. If it is uncorrected, successful pregnancy can be achieved, but maternal mortality is high and fetal loss can exceed 50 percent. After surgical correction of the defect, maternal mortality does not clearly exceed that of a woman without heart disease;[165,168] the offspring have a 5 to 10 percent chance of having congenital heart disease.

OBSTRUCTIVE LESIONS

Two recommendations apply in women with obstructive cardiac lesions. First, volume depletion should be avoided, since it can result in a significant fall in cardiac output whether the obstruction is on the left or right side of the heart. Second, surgical or catheter treatment for the obstructive lesion is recommended prior to pregnancy, not only to increase maternal safety but

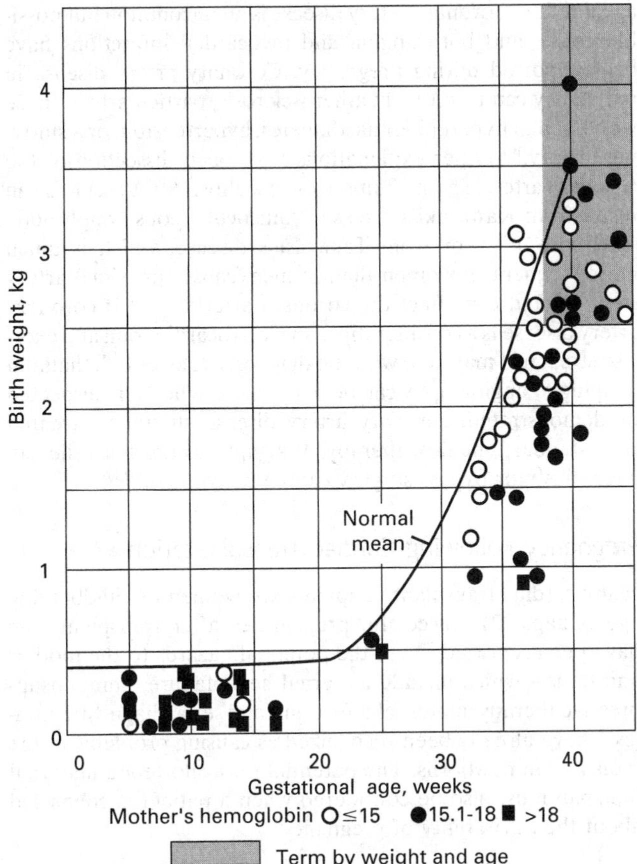

FIGURE 82-5 This figure shows that the severity of maternal cyanosis as manifest by the hemoglobin level relates directly to fetal loss (gestational age <20), prematurity, and infant birth weight. (From Neill and Swanson.[167] Reproduced with permission from the publisher and authors.)

also to decrease the chance of congenital heart disease in the offspring.[160]

Obstruction to flow from the *right ventricle* is preferably corrected prior to pregnancy. This approach will decrease maternal morbidity and may decrease the incidence of congenital heart disease in the offspring.[160] If an obstructive lesion persists into pregnancy, prevention of intravascular volume depletion is important.

Obstructive lesions to the left side of the heart include aortic valve stenosis, described previously. There is very little experience with isolated supravalvular aortic stenosis, bands or with subvalvular bands, but the approach recommended for aortic valve stenosis would seem applicable. Two other left ventricular obstructive disease processes warrant some discussion: coarctation of the aorta and hypertrophic obstructive cardiomyopathy.

Coarctation of the Aorta This condition is more common in men but may occur in women and, as in men, may be associated with a bicuspic aortic valve (Chap. 64). Affected individuals may reach childbearing age and may conceive. Maternal mortality rates range from 3 to 8 percent.[169] Surgical correction prior to pregnancy reduces the risk of aortic dissection or rupture—and thus death—to less than 1 percent.[170,171] If pregnancy occurs in a woman with a coarctation, blood pressure control, as described previously, is appropriate. Antibiotic prophylaxis is needed because of the associated bicuspic aortic valve. The effects of catheter dilation of a coarctation on subsequent pregnancies are uncertain, but it would seem that they are as likely to decrease the risks associated with pregnancy as the surgical procedure. It is not clear whether mechanical treatment decreases the rate of rupture of associated intracranial aneurisms.

Hypertrophic Obstructive Cardiomyopathy *Hypertrophic obstructive cardiomyopathy* (HOCM) (also called idiopathic hypertrophic subaortic stenosis, or IHSS) is inherited as an autosomal dominant trait with variable penetrance; thus offspring have a 50 percent chance of having the same abnormality (see Chaps. 4 and 67). The fall in peripheral vascular resistance and peripheral pooling of blood can cause hypotension, and the intermittent high catecholamine state of pregnancy can increase left ventricular outflow tract obstruction. An increase in the symptoms of dyspnea, chest discomfort, and palpitations has been noted during pregnancy.[172,173] It is not clear that pregnancy increases the approximately 1 to 3 percent chance per year of sudden death, although a death has been reported with this syndrome during pregnancy.[174] This is another obstructive lesion where it is important to avoid hypovolemia. Beta-blocker therapy has been recommended at the time of labor and delivery; the concept makes sense, although it is of unproven value.

COMPLEX CONGENITAL LESIONS

Predicting the outcome of pregnancy becomes more difficult as maternal abnormalities become more complex. In general, maternal and fetal morbidity and mortality are high, particularly when the abnormality results in maternal cyanosis. Still, surgery has made pregnancy a consideration, even in women with the most severe disease, such as a functional single-ventricle or tricuspid atresia.[175]

Transposition of the Great Vessels Women with d-transposition of the great arteries (some with single ventricles) may become pregnant. The little available information available indicates a very poor maternal and fetal outcome.[176] Partial or complete surgical correction of the lesion prior to pregnancy improves the outcome for the mother as well as the fetus.[176,178] If l-transposition ("corrected" transposition) is not complicated by cyanosis, ventricular dysfunction, or heart block, pregnancy should be well tolerated.[179]

Ebstein's Anomaly of the Tricuspid Valve This condition may be mild and unrecognized during pregnancy. Increasing problems of right ventricular dysfunction, obstruction to right-sided heart flow, and right-to-left shunting resulting in cyanosis increase the risk to the woman during pregnancy. Maternal morbidity and mortality are low if the patient does not have severe disease, and fetal loss is approximately 25 percent: significant right-to-left shunting is a reason to avoid pregnancy.[180,181]

Marfan's Syndrome It may be difficult to make the diagnosis of Marfan's syndrome, but it is important to do so because pregnancy is particularly dangerous for affected women. First, the risk of death from aortic rupture or dissection is high during pregnancy, particularly if the aortic root is enlarged (greater than 40 mm by echocardiography).[40,182,183] Second, the expected life span of the woman with Marfan's syndrome is reduced to about half of normal, implying that her years of motherhood will be limited. Third, half of the offspring will be affected with the syndrome. These are reasons that women with Marfan's syndrome should be advised to avoid pregnancy. The risks are sufficient to recommend interruption if pregnancy has occurred. Should the parents elect to continue the pregnancy, activity should be restricted and hypertension prevented. Beta blockade has not yet been clearly proved to be of value when used on a prophylactic basis, but its use in pregnant patients with Marfan's syndrome seems reasonable. This is the one cardiovascular syndrome where cesarean delivery is recommended in order to avoid the hemodynamic stresses of labor.

Myocardial Disease

HYPERTROPHIC CARDIOMYOPATHY

The hypertrophic cardiomyopathies are characterized as "concentric" or "asymmetric (Chap. 67)." The asymmetric form [hypertrophic obstructive cardiomyopathy" (or HOCM)] has been discussed as an obstructive lesion. A concentric hypertrophic cardiomyopathy may be the result of aortic stenosis or hypertension. When *not* due to either of these, the cause, prognosis, and management are often unclear, even unrelated to pregnancy. If congestive heart failure or abnormal rhythms occur, standard therapy is appropriate. Again, hypovolemia should be avoided.

DILATED CARDIOMYOPATHY

The cause of a dilated cardiomyopathy is often unclear, but up to 30 to 50 percent of these cases are familial.[184,185] Its occurence is a reason to suggest that pregnancy should be avoided. This strong recommendation is not supported by data from prospective trials but is given because myocardial dysfunction is the feature associated with increased maternal and fetal mortality in many forms of heart disease. It also comes from the observations of those who develop this problem as a result of pregnancy. This *peripartum cardiomyopathy* may simply be a dilated cardiomyopathy occurring in pregnancy, but the fact that it seems to occur almost exclusively in the third trimester or in the first 6 postpartum weeks suggests that it may be a unique entity.[186–189] Case reports have suggested that myocarditis may be a part of this disease and that, when it is proven by endomyocardial biopsy, treatment with anti-inflammatory drugs may affect outcome favorably.[190] It is not clear, however, that myocarditis is more common in this form of cardiomyopathy,[191] and a large prospective trial in other myocarditis situations has failed to support the value of treatment.[192] Small studies have suggested a possible role for treatment with immune globulin.[193] In the woman with a dilated cardiomyopathy during pregnancy, standard treatment for heart failure, thromboemboli, and arrhythmias is appropriate.

If ventricular function does not return to normal after pregnancy, subsequent pregnancies have been associated with maternal mortality rates approaching 50 percent (Chap. 66). When ventricular function returns to normal, a subsequent pregnancy is possible, but maternal mortality still approaches 10 percent.[188–190,193]

Coronary Artery Disease

Chest discomfort is common during a normal pregnancy and for the most part is due to abdominal distension or gastroesophageal reflux. Coronary artery disease is an uncommon but possible cause, and both angina and myocardial infarctions have been reported during pregnancy. Coronary artery disease in pregnancy can result from atherosclerosis, particularly in those with familial hyperlipidemia, diabetes, hypertension, or a smoking history.[194] Other explanations have been dissection of the coronary artery, spasm, emboli, or vasculitis.[194–197] Vasculitis can result from Kawasaki's disease ("mucocutaneous lymph node syndrome")[198,199] or from Takayasu's disease, which is much more frequent in women than in men, causes proximal artery stenosis, and can affect the coronary arteries.[200,201] If coronary artery disease is a consideration, an electrocardiogram and exercise stress test may help with the diagnosis. If essential, thallium imaging or angiography can be performed. When it is suspected or demonstrated, coronary artery disease should be treated with standard medical therapy. If symptoms are not relieved, angioplasty or bypass surgery can be performed.[202,203]

Pregnancy Following Cardiac Transplantation

Many cardiac transplant recipients are women of childbearing age (Chap. 22). Successful pregnancies after transplantation have been reported,[204] but the potential hazards to the mother and fetus—which include maternal heart failure, immunosuppressive therapy, maternal infections, and serial diagnostic studies—have already been recognized as causing problems in the fetus and in newborns. The potential for a shortened maternal life span must also be considered when a patient is counseled about the advisability of pregnancy.

References

1. Siu SC, Sermer M, Harrison DA, et al. Risk and predictors for pregnancy-related complications in women with heart disease. *Circulation* 1997; 96:2789–2794.
2. McAnulty JH, Morton MJ, Ueland K. The heart and pregnancy. *Curr Probl Cardiol* 1988; 13:589–665.
3. McAnulty JH. Heart diseases in pregnancy. In: Kloner RA, ed. *Guide to Cardiology*. New York: LeJacq Communications; 1995.
4. Ueland K, Novy MJ, Peterson EN, Metcalfe J. Maternal cardiovascular dynamics: IV. The influence of gestational age on the maternal cardiovascular response to posture and exercise. *Am J Obstet Gynecol* 1969; 104:856–864.
5. Capeless EL, Clapp JF. Cardiovascular changes in early phase of pregnancy. *Am J Obstet Gynecol* 1989; 161:1449–1453.
6. Easterling TR, Benedetti TJ, Schmucher BC, Millard SP. Maternal hemodynamics in normal and preeclamptic pregnancies: A longitudinal study. *Obstet Gynecol* 1990; 76:1061–1069.
7. Robson SC, Hunter S, Boys RJ, Dunlop W. Serial study of factors influencing changes in cardiac output during human pregnancy. *Am J Physiol* 1989; 256:H1060–H1065.
8. Clark SL, Cotton DB, Pivarnik JM, et al. Position change and central hemodynamic profile during normal third-trimester pregnancy and postpartum. *Am J Obstet Gynecol* 1991; 164:883–887.
9. Sady MA, Haydon BB, Sady SP, et al. Cardiovascular response to maximal cycle exercise during pregnancy and at two and seven months postpartum. *Am J Obstet Gynecol* 1990; 162:1181–1185.
10. Kerr MG. The mechanical effects of the gravid uterus in late pregnancy. *J Obstet Gynaecol Br Commonw* 1965; 72:513–529.
11. Kinsella SM, Lohmann G. Supine hypotensive syndrome (review). *Obstet Gynecol* 1994; 83:774–788.
12. Robson S, Dunop W, Boys R, Hunter S. Cardiac output during labor. *BMJ* 1987; 295:1169–1172.
13. James C, Banner T, Caton D. Cardiac output in women undergo-

ing cesarean section with epidural or general anesthesia. *Am J Obstet Gynecol* 1989; 160:1178–1183.

14. Clapp JF III, Capeless E. Cardiovascular function before, during, and after the first and subsequent pregnancies. *Am J Cardiol* 1997; 80:1469–1473.
15. Rovinsky JJ, Jaffin H. Cardiovascular hemodynamics in pregnancy: II. Cardiac output and left ventricular work in multiple pregnancy. *Am J Obstet Gynecol* 1966; 95:781–784.
16. Metcalfe J, McAnulty JH, Ueland K. *Heart Disease in Pregnancy: Physiology and Management.* Boston: Little, Brown; 1986:1–54.
17. Thoresen M, Wesche J. Doppler measurements of changes in human mammary and uterine blood flow during pregnancy and lactation. *Acta Obstet Gynecol Scand* 1988; 67:741–745.
18. Lunell NO, Nylund LE, Lewlander R, Sarby B. Uteroplacental blood flow in preeclampsia, measurement with indium-113m and a computer-linked gamma camera. *Clin Exp Hypertens (B)* 1982; 1:105–117.
19. Thaler I, Manor D, Itskovitz J, et al. Changes in uterine blood flow during human pregnancy. *Am J Obstet Gynecol* 1990; 162:121–125.
20. Teixerira JM, Fisk NM, Glover V. Association between maternal anxiety in pregnancy and increased uterine artery resistance index: Cohort based study. *BMJ* 1999; 318:1288–1289.
21. Guzman CA, Caplan R. Cardiorespiratory response to exercise during pregnancy. *Am J Obstet Gynecol* 1970; 108:600–607.
22. Morton MJ, Paul MS, Campos GR, et al. Exercise dynamics in late gestation: Effects of physical training. *Am J Obstet Gynecol* 1985; 152:91–97.
23. Veille JC, Hellerstein HK, Bacevice AE. Maternal left ventricular performance during bicycle exercise. *Am J Cardiol* 1992; 69:1506–1508.
24. Rauramo I, Forss M. Effect of exercise on maternal hemodynamics and placental blood flow in healthy women. *Acta Obstet Gynecol Scand* 1988; 67:21–25.
25. Watson WJ, Katz VL, Hackney AC, et al. Fetal responses to maximal swimming and cycling exercise during pregnancy. *Obstet Gynecol* 1991; 77:382–386.
26. Clapp JF III, Capeless EL. Neonatal morphometrics after endurance exercise during pregnancy. *Am J Obstet Gynecol* 1990; 163:1805–1811.
27. Naeye RL, Peters EC. Working during pregnancy: Effects on the fetus. *Pediatrics* 1982; 69:724–727.
28. Clapp JF III. Pregnancy outcome: Physical activities inside versus outside the workplace. *Semin Perinatol* 1996; 20(1):70–76.
29. Sternfeld B. Physical activity and pregnancy outcome: Review and recommendations. *Sports Med* 1997; 23(1):33–47.
30. Lindheimer MC, Katz AL. Sodium and diuretics in pregnancy. *N Engl J Med* 1973; 299:891–894.
31. Chesley LC. Plasma and red cell volumes during pregnancy. *Am J Obstet Gynecol* 1972; 112:440–450.
32. Hart MV, Morton MJ, Hosenpud JD, Metcalfe J. Aortic function during normal human pregnancy. *Am J Obstet Gynecol* 1986; 154:887–891.
33. Poppas A, Shroff SG, Korcarz CE, et al. Serial assessment of the cardiovascular system in normal pregnancy: Role of arterial compliance and pulsatile arterial load. *Circulation* 1997; 95:2407–2415.
34. Rovinsky JJ, Jaffin H. Cardiovascular hemodynamics in pregnancy: III. Cardiac rate, stroke volume, total peripheral resistance, and central blood volume in multiple pregnancy. Synthesis of results. *Am J Obstet Gynecol* 1966; 95:784–787.
35. Clark-Pearson DL, Jelovsek RD. Alterations of occlusive cuff impedance plethysmography results in the obstetric patient. *Surgery* 1981; 89:594–598.
36. Barrett JM, Vanhooydonk JD, Bochm FH. Pregnancy related rupture of arterial aneurysms. *Obstet Gynecol Surv* 1982; 37:557–566.
37. Anderson RA, Fineron PW. Aortic dissection in pregnancy: Importance of pregnancy-induced changes in the vessel wall and bicuspid aortic valve in pathogenesis. *Br J Obstet Gynaecol* 1994; 101:1085–1088.
38. Nolte JE, Rutherford RB, Nawaz S, et al. Arterial dissections associated with pregnancy (review). *J Vasc Surg* 1995; 21:515–520.
39. Elkayam U, Ostrzega E, Shotan A, Mehra A. Cardiovascular problems in pregnant women with the Marfan syndrome (review). *Ann Intern Med* 1995; 123:117–122.
40. Lipscomb KJ, Smith JC, Clarke B, et al. Outcome of pregnancy in women with Marfan's syndrome. *Br J Obstet Gynecol* 1997; 104(2):201–206.
41. Toglia MR, Weg JH. Venous thromboembolism during pregnancy. *N Engl J Med* 1996; 335:108–113.
42. Rubler S, Damani PM, Pinto ER. Cardiac size and performance during pregnancy estimated with echocardiography. *Am J Cardiol* 1977; 50:534–540.
43. Katz R, Karliner JS, Resnik R. Effects of a natural volume overload state (pregnancy) on left ventricular performance in normal human subjects. *Circulation* 1978; 58:434–441.
44. Sadaniantz A, Kocheril AG, Emans SP, et al. Cardiovascular changes in pregnancy evaluated by two-dimensional and Doppler echocardiography. *J Am Soc Echo* 1992; 5:253–258.
45. Morton MJ, Tsang H, Hohimer AR, et al. Left ventricular size, output and structure during guinea pig pregnancy. *Am J Physiol* 1984; 246:R40–R48.
46. Milsom I, Hedner J, Hedner T. Plasma atrial natriuretic peptide (ANP) and maternal hemodynamic changes during normal pregnancy. *Acta Obstet Gynecol Scand* 1988; 67:717–722.
47. Schrier RW. Pathogenesis of sodium and water retention in high-output and low-output cardiac failure, nephrotic syndrome, cirrhosis and pregnancy. *N Engl J Med* 1988; 319:1065–1072.
48. Ginsberg JS, Hirsh J, Rainbow AG, Coastes G. Risks to the fetus of radiographic procedures used in the diagnosis of maternal venous thromboembolic disease. *Thromb Haemost* 1989; 61: 189–196.
49. Committee on Drugs, American Academy of Pediatrics. The transfer of drugs and other chemicals into human breast milk. *Pediatrics* 1994; 93:137.
50. Cox JL, Gardner MJ. Cardiovascular drugs in pregnancy and lactation. In: Gleicher N, Gall SA, Sibai BM, et al, eds. *Principles and Practice of Medical Therapy in Pregnancy*, 3rd ed. Norwalk, CT: Appleton & Lange; 1998:911–926.
51. Collins R, Yusuf S, Peto R. Overview of randomized trials of diuretics in pregnancy. *BMJ* 1985; 290:17–23.
52. Rogers MC, Willerson JT, Goldblatt A, Smith TW. Serum digoxin concentrations in the human fetus, neonate and infant. *N Engl J Med* 1972; 287:1010–1013.
53. Gonzalez AR, Phelps EJ, Cochran EB, Sibai BM. Digoxin-like immunoreactive substance in pregnancy. *Am J Obstet Gynecol* 1987; 157:660–664.
54. Ueland K, McAnulty JH, Ueland FR. Special considerations in the use of cardiovascular drugs. *Clin Obstet Gynecol* 1981; 24:809–823.
55. Rubin PC. Beta blockers in pregnancy. *N Engl J Med* 1982; 305:1323–1326.
56. Frishman WH, Chesner M. Beta-andrenergic blockers in pregnancy. *Am Heart J* 1988; 115:147–152.
57. Lip GY, Beevers M, Churchill D, Shaffer LM, Beevers DG. Effect of atenolol on birth weight. *Am J Cardiol* 1997; 79:1436–1438.
58. Lydakis C, Lip GY, Beevers M, Beevers DG. Atenolol and fetal growth in pregnancies complicated by hypertension. *Am J Hypertension* 1999; 12:541–547.
59. Sibai BM. Treatment of hypertension in pregnant women (review). *N Engl J Med* 1996; 335:257–265.
60. Wide-Swensson DH, Ingemarsson I, Lunell NO, et al. Calcium channel blockade (isradipine) in treatment of hypertension in

pregnancy: A randomized placebo-controlled study. *Am J Obstet Gynecol* 1995; 173:872–878.
61. Elkayam U, Goodwin TM. Adenosine therapy for supraventricular tachycardia during pregnancy. *Am J Cardiol* 1995; 75:521–523.
62. Cox JL, Gardner JM. Treatment of cardiac arrhythmias during pregnancy. *Prog Cardiovasc Dis* 1993; 36:137–178.
63. Page RL. Treatment of arrhythmias during pregnancy (review). *Am Heart J* 1995; 130:871–876.
64. Juneja MM, Ackerman WE, Kaczorowski DM, et al. Continuous epidural lidocaine infusion in the parturient with paroxysmal ventricular tachycardia. *Anesthesiology* 1989; 71:305–308.
65. Hill LM, Malkasian GD Jr. The use of quinidine sulfate throughout pregnancy. *Obstet Gynecol* 1979; 54:366.
66. Allen NM, Page RL. Procainamide administration during pregnancy. *Clin Pharm* 1993; 12:58–60.
67. Leonard RF, Braun TE, Levy AM. Initiation of uterine contractions by disopyramide during pregnancy. *N Engl J Med* 1978; 299:84.
68. Lownes HE, Ives TJ. Mexiletine use in pregnancy and lactation. *Am J Obstet Gynecol* 1987; 157:446–447.
69. Perry JC, Ayres NA, Carpenter RJ Jr. Fetal supraventricular tachycardia treated by flecainide acetate. *J Pediatr* 1991; 118: 303–305.
70. Connaughton M, Jenkins BS. Successful use of flecainide to treat new onset maternal ventricular tachycardia in pregnancy. *Br Heart J* 1994; 72:297.
71. Wagner X, Jouglard J, Moulin M, et al. Coadministration of flecainide acetate and sotalol during pregnancy. *Am Heart J* 1990; 119:700–702.
72. Foster CJ, Love HG. Amiodarone in pregnancy: Case report and review of the literature. *Int J Cardiol* 1988; 20:307–316.
73. Ovadin M, Brito M, Hoyer GL, Marcus FI. Human experience with amiodarone in the embryonic period. *Am J Cardiol* 1994; 73:316–317.
74. Magee LA, Downar E, Sermer M, et al. Pregnancy outcome after gestational exposure to amiodarone in Canada. *Am J Obstet Gynecol* 1995; 172:1307–1311.
75. Stempel JE, O'Grady JP, Morton MJ, Johnson KA. Use of sodium nitroprusside in complications of gestational hypertension. *Obstet Gynecol* 1982; 60:533–538.
76. Shoemaker CT, Meyers M. Sodium nitroprusside for control of severe hypertensive disease of pregnancy: A case report and discussion of potential toxicity. *Am J Obstet Gynecol* 1984; 149:171–173.
77. Cunningham FG, Lindheimer MD. Hypertension in pregnancy. *N Engl J Med* 1992; 326:927–932.
78. Hanssens M, Keirse MJ, Vankelecom F, et al. Fetal and neonatal effects of treatment with angiotensin converting enzyme inhibitors in pregnancy. *Obstet Gynecol* 1991; 78:128–135.
79. Fillmore SJ, McDevitt E. Effects of coumarin compounds on the fetus. *Ann Intern Med* 1970; 73:731–735.
80. Hall JT, Pauli RM, Wilson KM. Maternal and fetal sequelae of anticoagulation during pregnancy. *Am J Med* 1980; 68:122.
81. Stevenson RE, Burton M, Frelauto GH, Taylor HA. Hazards of oral anticoagulants during pregnancy. *JAMA* 1985; 243:1549–1551.
82. Iturbe-Alessio I, Fonseca MC, Mutchinik O, et al. Risks of anticoagulant therapy in pregnant women with artificial heart valves. *N Engl J Med* 1986; 315:1390–1393.
83. Brabeck MC. Ambulatory management of thromboembolic diseases during pregnancy with continuous infusion of heparin. *JAMA* 1987; 257:1790–1791.
84. Vitale N, De Feo M, De Santo LS, et al. Dose-dependent fetal complications of warfarin in pregnant women with mechanical heart valves. *J Am Coll Cardiol* 1999; 33:1637–1641.
85. Ginsberg JS, Hirsh J. Use of antithrombotic agents during pregnancy: A series of eight cases. *Can J Anaesth* 1994; 41:502–512.
86. Ginsbert JS, Kowalchuk G, Hirsh J, et al. Heparin therapy during pregnancy. *Arch Intern Med* 1989; 149:2233–2236.
87. Anderson DR, Ginsburg JS, Brill-Edwards P, et al. The use of an indwelling Teflon catheter for subcutaneous heparin administration during pregnancy. *Arch Intern Med* 1993; 153:841–844.
88. Elkayam U. Anticoagulation in pregnant women with prosthetic heart valves: A double jeopardy (editorial). *J Am Coll Cardiol* 1996; 27:1704–1706.
89. Nelson-Piercy C, Letsky EA, De Sweit M. Low-molecular weight heparin for obstetric thromboprophylaxis: Experience of sixty-nine pregnancies in sixty-one women at high risk. *Am J Obstet Gynecol* 1997; 176:1062–1068.
90. Sanson BJ, Lensing AW, Prins MH, et al. Safety of low-molecular weight heparin in pregnancy: A systematic review. *Thromb Hemost* 1999; 81:668–672.
91. Corby DG. Aspirin in pregnancy and fetal effects. *Pediatrics* 1978; 62:930–937.
92. Werler MM, Mitchell AA, Shapiro S. The relation of aspirin use during the first trimester of pregnancy to congenital cardiac defects. *N Engl J Med* 1989; 321:1639–1642.
93. DuBard MB, Cutter GR. Low-dose aspirin therapy to prevent preeclampsia. *Am J Obstet Gynecol* 1993; 168:1083–1091.
94. The Canadian Preterm Labor Investigators Group. Treatment of preterm labor with the beta-adrenergic agonist ritodrine. *N Engl J Med* 1992; 327:308–312.
95. McAnulty JH. Anesthesia during pregnancy in the patient with heart disease. In: Bonica JJ, McDonald JS, eds. *Principles and Practice of Obstetric Analgesia and Anesthesia*. Philadelphia: Lea & Febiger; 1994:1013–1039.
96. Haemostatis and Thrombosis Task Force. Guidelines on the prevention, investigation and management of thrombosis associated with pregnancy: Maternal and neonatal haemostasis working papers of the Haemostasis and Thrombosis Task Force. *J Clin Pathol* 1993; 46:489–496.
97. Greer IA. Thrombosis in pregnancy: Maternal and fetal issues. *Lancet* 1999; 353:1258–1265.
98. Kittner SJ, Stern BJ, Feeser BR, et al. Pregnancy and the risk of stroke. *N Engl J Med* 1996; 335:768–774.
99. Donaldson JO, Lee NS. Arterial and venous stroke associated with pregnancy. *Neurol Clin* 1994; 12:583–599.
100. Sturridge F, de Swiet M, Letsky E. The use of low molecular weight heparin for thrombophylaxis in pregnancy. *Br J Obstet Gynaecol* 1994; 101:69–71.
101. Hellgren M, Svensson PJ, Dahlback B. Resistance to activated protein C as a basis for venous thromboembolism associated with pregnancy and oral contraceptives. *Am J Obstet Gynecol* 1995; 173:210–213.
102. Gerhart A, Scharf RE, Beckmann MW, et al. Prothrombin and factor V mutations in women with a history of thrombosis during pregnancy and the puerperium. *N Engl J Med* 2000; 342:374–380.
103. Turrentine MA, Braems G, Ramirez MM. Use of thrombolytics for the treatment of thromboembolic disease during pregnancy (review). *Obstet Gynecol Surv* 1995; 50:534–541.
104. National High Blood Pressure Education Program. Working Group report on high blood pressure in pregnancy. *Am J Obstet Gynecol* 1990; 163:1691–1712.
105. Rey E, LeLorier J, Burgess E, et al. Report of the Canadian Hypertension Society Consensus Conference: 3. Pharmacologic treatment of hypertensive disorders in pregnancy. *Can Med Assoc J* 1997; 157:1245–1254.
106. Witlin AG, Sibai BM. Hypertension. *Clin Obstet Gynecol* 1998; 41:533–544.
107. Avila S, Grinberg M, Snitcowsky R, et al. Maternal and fetal outcome in pregnant women with Eisenmenger's syndrome. *Eur Heart J* 1995; 16:460–464.
108. Weiss BM, Hess OM. Pulmonary vascular disease and pregnancy:

Current controversies, management strategies, and perspectives. *Eur Heart J* 2000; 21:104–115.

109. Widerhorn J, Woderhorn AL, Rahimtoola SH, Elkayam U. WPW syndrome during pregnancy: Increased incidence of supraventricular arrhythmias. *Am Heart J* 1992; 123:796–798.
110. Tawam M, Levine J, Mendelson M, et al. Effect of pregnancy on paroxysmal supraventricular tachycardia. *Am J Cardiol* 1993; 72:838–840.
111. Lee SH, Chan SA, Wu TJ, et al. Effects of pregnancy on first onset and symptoms of paroxysmal supraventricular tachycardia. *Am J Cardiol* 1995; 76:675–678.
112. Rosemond RL. Cardioversion during pregnancy. *JAMA* 1993; 269:3167.
113. Brodsky M, Doria R, Allen V, Sato D. New onset ventricular tachycardia during pregnancy. *Am Heart J* 1992; 123:933–941.
114. Varon ME, Sherer DM, Abramowicz JS, Akiyama T. Maternal ventricular tachycardia associated with hypomagnesemia. *Am J Obstet Gynecol* 1992; 167:1352–1355.
115. Lee RV, Rodgers BD, Shite LM, Harvey RC. Cardiopulmonary resuscitation of pregnant women. *Am J Med* 1986; 81:311–318.
116. Dildy GA, Clark SL. Cardiac arrest during pregnancy. *Obstet Gynecol Clin North Am* 1995; 22:303–314.
117. Nakazato Y, Nakata Y, Tokano T, et al. Long-term follow-up study of three patients with the long QT syndrome. *Jpn Circ J* 1992; 56:1025–1031.
118. McCurdy CM, Rutherford SE, Coddington CC. Syncope and sudden arrhythmic death complicating pregnancy: A case report of Ramano-Ward syndrome. *J Reprod Med* 1993; 38:233–234.
119. Dalvi BV, Chaudhuri A, Kulkarni HL, Kale PA. Therapeutic guidelines for congenital complete heart block presenting in pregnancy. *Obstet Gynecol* 1994; 79:802–804.
120. Seaworth BJ, Durack DT. Infective endocarditis in obstetric and gynecologic practice. *Am J Obstet Gynecol* 1986; 154:180–188.
121. Ebrahimi R, Leung CY, Elkayam U, Reid CL. Infective endocarditis. In: Gleicher N, ed. *Principles and Practice of Medical Therapy in Pregnancy*, 2d ed. Norwalk, CT: Appleton & Lange; 1992:795–801.
122. Dajani AS, Taubert KA, Wilson W, et al. Prevention of bacterial endocarditis—Recommendations by the American Heart Association. *JAMA* 1997; 277:1794–1801.
123. McAnulty JH. Rheumatic heart disease. In: Gleicher N, Gall SA, Sibai BM, et al, eds. *Principles and Practice of Medical Therapy in Pregnancy*, 2d ed. Norwalk, CT: Appleton & Lange; 1992:783–788.
124. Massell BF, Chute CG, Walker AM, Kurland GS. Penicillin and the marked decrease in morbidity and mortality from rheumatic fever in the United States. *N Engl J Med* 1988; 318:280–286.
125. Veasy LG, Widemeier SE, Orsmond GS, et al. Resurgence of acute rheumatic fever in the intermountain area of the United States. *N Engl J Med* 1987; 316:421–427.
126. Special Writing Group of the Committee on Rheumatic Fever, Endocarditis, and Kawasaki Disease of the Council on Cardiovascular Disease in the Young of the American Heart Association. Guidelines for the diagnosis of rheumatic fever: Jones criteria, 1992 update. *JAMA* 1992; 268:2069–2073.
127. Dajani AS, Bisno AL, Chung KJ, et al. Prevention of rheumatic fever. *Circulation* 1988; 78:1082–1086.
128. Bryg RJ, Gordon PR, Kudesia VS, Bhatia RK. Effect of pregnancy on pressure gradient in mitral stenosis. *Am J Cardiol* 1989; 63:384–386.
129. Ueland K, Metcalfe J. Acute rheumatic fever in pregnancy. *Am J Obstet Gynecol* 1966; 95:586–587.
130. Stephen SJ. Changing patterns of mitral stenosis in childhood and pregnancy in Sri Lanka. *J Am Coll Cardiol* 1992; 19:1276–1284.
131. Gupta A, Lokhandwala YY, Satoskar PR, Salvi VS. Balloon mitral valvotomy in pregnancy: Maternal and fetal outcomes. *J Am Coll Surg* 1998; 187:409–415.
132. Martinez-Reding J, Cordero A, Kuri J, et al. Treatment of severe mitral stenosis with percutaneous balloon valvotomy in pregnant patients. *Clin Cardiol* 1998; 21:659–663.
133. Commerford PJ, Hastie T, Beck W. Closed mitral valvotomy: Actuarial analysis of results in 654 patients over 12 years and analysis of preoperative predictors of long-term survival. *Ann Thorac Surg* 1982; 33:473–479.
134. Chambers CE, Clark SL. Cardiac surgery during pregnancy (review). *Clin Obstet Gynecol* 1994; 37:316–323.
135. Shapiro EP, Trible EL, Robinson JC, et al. Safety of labor and delivery in women with mitral valve prolapse. *Am J Cardiol* 1985; 56:806–807.
136. Degani S, Abinader EG, Scharf M. Mitral valve prolapse and pregnancy: A review. *Obstet Gynecol Surv* 1989; 72:113–118.
137. Cowles T, Gonik B. Mitral valve prolapse in pregnancy. *Semin Perinatol* 1990; 14:34–41.
138. Nishimura RA, McGoon MD. Perspectives on mitral-valve prolapse. *N Engl J Med* 1999; 341(1):48–59.
139. Arias F, Pineda J. Aortic stenosis and pregnancy. *J Reprod Med* 1978; 20:229–232.
140. Easterling TR, Chadwick HS, Otto CM, Benedetti TJ. Aortic stenosis in pregnancy. *Obstet Gynecol* 1988; 72:113–118.
141. Lao TT, Sermer M, McGee L, et al. Congenital aortic stenosis and pregnancy—A reappraisal (review). *Am J Obstet Gynecol* 1993; 169:540–545.
142. Banning AP, Pearson JF, Hall RJ. Role of balloon dilatation of the aortic valve in pregnant patients with severe aortic stenosis. *Br Heart J* 1993; 70:544–545.
143. American College of Cardiology/American Heart Association Task Force on Practice Guidelines (Committee on Management of Patients with Valvular Heart Disease). ACC/AHA Guidelines for the management of patients with valvular heart disease. *J Am Coll Cardiol* 1998; 32:1486–1588.
144. Whittemore R, Hobbins JC, Engle MA. Pregnancy and its outcome in women with and without surgical treatment of congenital heart disease. *Am J Cardiol* 1982; 50:641–651.
145. Lao TT, Adelman AG, Sermer M, Colman JM. Balloon valvuloplasty for congenital aortic stenosis in pregnancy. *Br J Obstet Gynaecol* 1993; 100:1141–1142.
146. Sullivan HJ. Valvular heart surgery during pregnancy (review). *Surg Clin North Am* 1995; 75:59–75.
147. Bloomfield P, Wheatley DJ, Prescott RJ, Miller HC. Twelve-year comparison of a Bjork-Shirley mechanical heart valve with porcine bioprostheses. *N Engl J Med* 1991; 324:573–579.
148. Hammermeister KE, Sethi GK, Henderson WG, et al. A comparison of outcomes in men 11 years after heart-valve replacement with a mechanical valve or bioprosthesis. *N Engl J Med* 1993; 328:1289–1296.
149. Sareli P, England MJ, Berk MR, et al. Maternal and fetal sequelae of anticoagulation during pregnancy in patients with mechanical heart valve prostheses. *Am J Cardiol* 1989; 63:1462–1465.
150. Born D, Martinez EE, Almeida PA, et al. Pregnancy in patients with prosthetic heart valves: The effects of anticoagulation on mother, fetus, and neonate. *Am Heart J* 1992; 124:413–417.
151. Salazar E, Izaguirre R, Verdejo J, Mutchinick O. Failure of adjusted doses of subcutaneous heparin to prevent thromboembolic phenomena in pregnant patients with mechanical cardiac valve prostheses. *J Am Coll Cardiol* 1996; 27:1698–1703.
152. North RA, Sadler L, Stewart AW, et al. Long-term survival and valve-related complications in young women with cardiac valve replacements. *Circulation* 1999; 99:2669–2676.
153. Elkayam U. Pregnancy through a prosthetic valve. *J Am Coll Cardiol* 1999; 33:1643–1645.
154. Jamieson WR, Miller DC, Akins CW, et al. Pregnancy and bioprostheses: Influence on structural valve deterioration. *Ann Thorac Surg* 1995; 60:S282–S286.
155. Mitchell SC, Korones SB, Berendes HW. Congenital heart dis-

ease in 56,109 births: Incidence and natural history. *Circulation* 1971; 43:323–332.
156. Nora JJ, Nora AH. The evolution of specific genetic and environmental counseling in congenital heart disease. *Circulation* 1978; 57:205–213.
157. Roberts N. A predictive study of congenital heart disease and need for care. *West J Med* 1978; 120:19–25.
158. McFaul PB, Dornan JC, Lamki H, Boyle D. Pregnancy complicated by maternal heart disease: A review of 519 women. *Br J Obset Gynaecol* 1988; 95:861–867.
159. Nora JJ, Nora AH. Maternal transmission of congenital heart diseases: New recurrence risk figures and the questions of cytoplasmic inheritance and vulnerability to teratogens. *Am J Cardiol* 1987; 59:459–463.
160. Whittemore R, Hobbins JC, Engle MA. Pregnancy and its outcome in women with and without surgical treatment of congenital heart disease. *Am J Cardiol* 1982; 50:641–651.
161. Morris CD, Menashe VD. Evidence for maternal transmission of congenital heart defects. *Circulation* 1993; 88(suppl):1–98.
162. Whittemore R, Wells JA, Castellsagne X. A second-generation study of 427 probands with congenital heart defects and their 837 children. *J Am Coll Cardiol* 1994; 23:1459–1467.
163. Nora J. From generational studies to a multilevel genetic-environmental interaction (editorial). *J Am Coll Cardiol* 1994; 23:1468–1471.
164. Metcalfe J, Ueland K. Maternal cardiovascular adjustments to pregnancy. *Prog Cardiovasc Dis* 1974; 16:363–374.
165. Morris CD, Manashe VD. 25-year mortality after surgical repair of congenital heart defect in childhood: A population-based cohort study. *JAMA* 1991; 266:3447–3452.
166. Presbytero P, Sommerville J, Stone S, et al. Pregnancy and cyanotic congenital heart disease, outcome of mother and fetus. *Circulation* 1994; 89:2673–2676.
167. Neill CA, Swanson S. Outcome of pregnancy in congenital heart disease. *Circulation* 1961; 24:1003–1011.
168. Zellers TM, Driscoll DJ, Michaels VV. Prevalence of significant congenital heart defects in children of parents with Fallot's tetralogy. *Am J Cardiol* 1990; 65:523–526.
169. Deal D, Wooley CF. Coarctation of the aorta and pregnancy. *Ann Intern Med* 1973; 78:706–710.
170. Connolly HM, Ammash NM, Warnes CA. Pregnancy in women with coarctation of the aorta (abstr). *J Am Coll Cardiol* 1996; 27(suppl A):43A.
171. Pitkin RM, Perloff JK, Koos BJ, Beall MH. Pregnancy and congenital heart disease. *Ann Intern Med* 1990; 112:445–454.
172. Oakley GD, McGarry K, Limb DG, Oakley CM. Management of pregnancy in patients with hypertrophic cardiomyopathy. *BMJ* 1979; 1:1749–1750.
173. Piacenza JM, Kirkorian G, Audra PH, Mellier G. Hypertrophic cardiomyopathy and pregnancy. *Eur J Obstet Gynecol Reprod Biol* 1998; 80(1):17–23.
174. Shah DM, Sunderji SG. Hypertrophic cardiomyopathy and pregnancy: Report of a maternal mortality and review of literature. *Obstet Gynecol Surv* 1985; 40:444–448.
175. Conobbio MM, Mair DD, Velde M, Koos BJ. Pregnancy outcomes after the Fontan repair. *J Am Coll Cardiol* 1996; 28: 763–767.
176. Patton DE, Lee W, Cotton DB, et al. Cyanotic maternal heart disease in pregnancy. *Obstet Gynecol Surv* 1990; 45:594–600.
177. Clarkson PM, Wilson NJ, Neutze JM, et al. Outcome of pregnancy after the Mustard operation for transposition of the great arteries with intact ventricular septum. *J Am Coll Cardiol* 1994; 24: 190–193.
178. Perloff JK. Pregnancy and congenital heart disease. *J Am Coll Cardiol* 1991; 18:340–342.
179. Connolly H, Grogan M, Warnes CA. Pregnancy among women with congenitally corrected transposition of great arteries. *J Am Coll Cardiol* 1999; 33:1692–1695.
180. Wooley CF, Sparks EH. Congenital heart disease, heritable cardiovascular disease, and pregnancy. *Prog Cardiovasc Dis* 1992; 35:41–60.
181. Connolly HM, Warnes CA. Ebstein's anomaly: Outcome of pregnancy. *J Am Coll Cardiol* 1994; 23:1194–1198.
182. Mor-Yosef S, Younis J, Granat M, et al. Marfan's syndrome in pregnancy. *Obstet Gynecol Surv* 1988; 43:382–385.
183. Pyeritz RE. Maternal and fetal complications of pregnancy in the Marfan syndrome. *Am J Med* 1981; 71:784–790.
184. Grunig E, Tasman JA, Kucherer H, et al. Frequency and phenotypes of familial dilated cardiomyopathy. *J Am Coll Cardiol* 1998; 31:86–94.
185. Olson TM, Michels VV, Thibodeau SN, et al. Actin mutations in dilated cardiomyopathy, a heritable form of heart failure. *Science* 1998; 280:750–752.
186. Damakil JG, Rahimtoola SH, Sutton GC, et al. Natural course of peripartum cardiomyopathy. *Circulation* 1971; 44:1053–1061.
187. O'Connell JB, Costanzo-Mordin MR, Surbranian R, et al. Peripartum cardiomyopathy: Clinical, hemodynamic, histologic and prognostic characteristics. *J Am Coll Cardiol* 1986; 8:52–56.
188. Lampert MB, Lang RM. Peripartum cardiomyopathy. *Am Heart J* 1995; 130:860–870.
189. Heider AL, Kuller JA, Strauss RA, Wells SR. Peripartum cardiomyopathy: A review of the literature. *Obstet Gynecol Surv* 1999; 54: 526–531.
190. Melvin KR, Richardson PJ, Olsen EG, et al. Peripartum cardiomyopathy due to myocarditis. *N Engl J Med* 1982; 308:731–734.
191. Rizeq MN, Rickenbacher PR, Fowler MB, Billingham ME. Incidence of myocarditis in peripartum cardiomyopathy. *Am J Cardiol* 1994; 74:474–477.
192. Parrilo JE, Cunnion RE, Epstein SE, et al. A prospective, randomized, controlled trial of prednisone for dilated cardiomyopathy. *N Engl J Med* 1989; 321:1061–1068.
193. Sutton MS, Cole P, Plappert M, et al. Effects of subsequent pregnancy on left ventricular function in peripartum cardiomyopathy. *Am Heart J* 1991; 121:1776–1778.
194. Roth A, Elkayam U. Acute myocardial infarction associated with pregnancy. *Ann Intern Med* 1996; 125:751–762.
195. Ciraulo DA, Markovitz A. Myocardial infarction in pregnancy associated with a coronary artery thrombus. *Arch Intern Med* 1979; 139:1046–1047.
196. Ahronheim JH. Isolated coronary periarteritis: Report of a case of unexpected death in a young pregnant woman. *Am J Cardiol* 1977; 40:287–290.
197. Jewett J. Two dissecting coronary-artery aneurysms post partum. *N Engl J Med* 1978; 298:1255–1256.
198. Nolan TE, Savage RW. Peripartum myocardial infarction from presumed Kawasaki's disease. *South Med J* 1990; 83:360–361.
199. Taubert KA, Rowley AH, Shulman ST. Nationwide survey of Kawasaki disease and acute rheumatic fever. *J Pediatr* 1991; 119:279–282.
200. Ishikawa A, Matsura S. Occlusive thromboaortopathy (Takayasu's disease) and pregnancy. *Am J Cardiol* 1982; 50:1293–1300.
201. Railton A, Allen DG. Takayasu's arteritis in pregnancy: A report of 4 cases. *S Afr Med J* 1988; 73:123–127.
202. Cowan NC, de Belder MA, Rothman MT. Coronary angioplasty in pregnancy. *Br Heart J* 1988; 59:588–592.
203. Garry D, Leikin E, Fleisher AG, Tejani N. Acute myocardial infarction in pregnancy with subsequent medical and surgical management. *Obstet Gynecol* 1996; 87(5 pt 2):802–804.
204. Morini A, Spina V, Aleandri V, et al. Pregnancy after heart transplant: Update and case report. *Hum Reprod* 1998; 13: 749–757.

CHAPTER 83

THE HEART AND OBESITY

Paul Poirier / Robert H. Eckel

INTRODUCTION

Very fat people were apt to die earlier than those who were slender.

Hippocrates (Aphorism 44)

Populations in industrialized countries are becoming more overweight as a result of changes in lifestyle. Both overweight and obesity must be regarded as serious current medical problems. Increased body fat is associated with an increased risk of heart disease, stroke, hypertension, dyslipidemia, type 2 diabetes mellitus, gallbladder disease, osteoarthritis, sleep apnea and respiratory problems, and endometrial, breast, prostate, and colon cancers.[1,2] Moreover, obesity is associated with reduced life expectancy.[3] The incidence of obesity in the United States has increased progressively since 1960, and the prevalence of obesity is three times higher in the United States than it is in France and one and a half times higher than in Great Britain.[4]

After a follow-up of 26 years, the Framingham Heart Study and the Manitoba Study have documented that obesity represents an independent predictor of cardiovascular disease, particularly among women.[5,6] Cardiovascular disease was defined as an incidence of coronary disease, coronary death, and congestive heart failure. This relation was independent of age, cholesterol, systolic blood pressure, cigarette smoking, left ventricular hypertrophy (LVH), and glucose intolerance. It is noteworthy that this association was more pronounced in individuals younger than age 50 years. These data have led the American Heart Association to state that obesity is a major modifiable risk factor for heart disease.[7,8] A regulatory system that maintains constant energy storage is likely to involve complex interactions among humoral, neural, metabolic, and psychological factors, among others. Thus, overweight/obesity is a complex multifactorial chronic disorder that develops from an interaction between genotype and the environment.[2,9] Because weight reduction is difficult to achieve and maintain, obesity is a self-perpetuating condition in which homeostatic mechanisms restrain further weight loss.

There are several definitions of overweight and obesity.[10] Although body weight that exceeds ideal standards as determined by age, sex, and height may be accounted for by greater muscle mass or bone mass, most individuals who weigh over their calculated ideal body weights have excessive adipose tissue mass. Because body mass index (BMI) is an assessment of total fat content that does not derive from frame size and gender, it has replaced relative weight as an index of body composition.[2] From a clinical viewpoint, overweight is defined as a body mass index (weight in kilograms divided by the square of height in meters) of 25 to 29.9 kg/m^2 and obesity as a BMI $\geq$30 kg/m^2 [2] (Table 83-1). Importantly, the number of overweight and obese individuals has risen since 1960; in the last decade, the percentage of people in these categories has increased to over 50 percent of adults age 20 years and older. Currently, all overweight and obese adults (age >18 years with a BMI $\geq$25 kg/m^2) are considered at risk for developing comorbidities such as hypertension, dyslipidemia, type 2 diabetes mellitus, and coronary heart disease.

Adipose tissue should not be regarded as merely a passive storehouse for fat but instead as a diffuse vascular organ in which the synthesis of a variety of molecules important to cardiovascular medicine is carried out. Although activated leukocytes, fibroblasts, and endothelial cells are assumed widely to be the major source of circulating interleukin-6 (IL-6), it has been estimated that in vivo, ~30 percent of total circulating

TABLE 83-1 Classification of Overweight and Obesity by Percentage of Body Fat, Body Mass Index (BMI), Waist Circumference, and Associated Disease Risk

	BMI, kg/m^2	Disease Risk[a] Relative to Normal Weight and Waist Circumference: Men, ≤102 cm Women, ≤88 cm	Men, >102 cm Women, >88 cm
Underweight	<18.5		
Normal	18.5–24.9		
Overweight	25.0–29.9	Increased	High
Obesity, class			
I	30.0–34.9	High	Very high
II	35.0–39.9	Very high	Very high
III (extreme obesity)	≥40	Extremely high	Extremely high

[a]Disease risk for type 2 diabetes, hypertension, and cardiovascular disease.
SOURCE: From Clinical Guidelines on the Identification, Evaluation, and Treatment of Overweight and Obesity in Adults.[2]

concentrations of IL-6 originate from adipose tissue.[11,12] This is important since IL-6 modulates the production of C-reactive protein in the liver and that protein may be an independent predictor of cardiovascular disease events.[13] Also, adipose tissue is a major source of tumor necrosis factor-alpha (TNF-alpha)[14,15] and plasminogen activator inhibitor-1 (PAI-1),[16] and circulating concentrations of PAI-1, angiotensin II, C-reactive protein, fibrinogen, and TNF-alpha are all related to BMI.[11,17] This is important because PAI-1 levels parallel the concentration of triglycerides, cytokines are implicated in endothelial cell dysfunction, and increases in angiotensin II may contribute to hypertension and heart failure, which are seen more often in obese persons.

ADAPTATION OF THE CARDIOVASCULAR SYSTEM IN OBESITY

Adipose Tissue Circulation

From morphologic studies, it has been shown that an extensive capillary network surrounds adipose tissue. The adipocytes are located close to vessels with the highest permeability, the lowest hydrostatic pressure, and the shortest distance for transport of molecules from adipocytes.[18] Resting blood flow is usually between 2 and 3 mL/min per 100 grams of adipose tissue,[19,20] whereas maximal blood flow amounts to only 25 to 30 mL/min per 100 grams of adipose tissue compared with 50 to 75 mL/min in skeletal muscle.[21] The interstitial space of adipose tissue accounts for approximately 10 percent of tissue wet weight.[22] Since a large part of body weight consists of adipose tissue, significant quantities of fluid are present in the interstitial space of adipose tissue and could be important in the regulation of blood volume if mobilized into the blood. For example, in a 100-kg person with 25 to 30 percent of body fat, 2 to 3 L of fluid may be present in this compartment. Clinically, this can have important repercussions in cardiologically compromised individuals if the extra volume is repartitioned in the circulation.

The function of adipose tissue is more severely impaired by hypovolemia, i.e., hemorrhagic shock, than is that of most other tissues. Interestingly, the beta-adrenoceptors that mediate vasodilatation in adipose tissue are mainly the beta$_1$ type, in contrast to those of skeletal muscle, which are mainly beta$_2$. This explains why during hemorrhagic shock increased epinephrine levels decrease blood flow much more in adipose tissue than they do in skeletal muscle.[18] More specifically, blood flow in subcutaneous adipose tissue is reduced to about 10 percent of resting blood flow, whereas in skeletal muscle, liver, myocardium, and hypothalamus, blood flow falls to about 60 percent of resting flow and renal cortical flow falls to about 40 percent.[18] As a consequence of this dramatic decrease in blood flow in adipose tissue, the fluid present in the interstitial compartment is not readily accessible to restore volemia.

While there are differences between blood flow in adipose tissue and that in other organs, the increment in blood flow with increasing adiposity is not proportional to the increment in adipose tissue mass; therefore, perfusion per unit of adipose tissue decreases significantly with increasing obesity, i.e., from 2.36 mL/min per 100 grams to 1.53 mL/min of adipose tissue in patients who have 15 to 26 percent body fat to >36 percent body fat, respectively.[20] Thus, increases in total body fat result in higher total blood flow secondary to the enlarged vascular bed, but the adipose tissue is less vascularized than lean tissue with increasing obesity. Thus, the increase in systemic blood flow seen in obesity[23] cannot be explained solely by increased requirements resulting from adipose tissue perfusion but most probably is caused by the concomitant increase in lean body mass in these individuals.

Cardiac Output

Any increase in body mass from adipose tissue or muscular tissue requires a higher cardiac output and expanded intravascular volume to meet the higher metabolic demand. Because of the need to move excess body weight, at any given level of activity, the cardiac workload is greater for obese subjects than it is for nonobese individuals. Thus, obese subjects are known to have higher cardiac output and a lower total peripheral resistance.[23] The high cardiac output is attributable to increased stroke volume, while heart rate is usually unchanged.[24] The increase in blood volume and cardiac output in obesity is in proportion to the amount of excess body weight and the duration of obesity. In the setting of this increase in cardiac output, cerebral blood flow, oxygen uptake, and cerebral arteriovenous O_2 difference did not differ from those in nonobese individuals.[25] This implies that the fraction of the cardiac output distributed to the brain is lower than normal in obesity.[25] In the same study, renal blood flow was normal or slightly reduced in obesity.

Thus, the percentage of total cardiac output to the kidney was about 20 percent lower than that in the splanchnic vascular flow bed, which approximated normal.[25] The increase in splanchnic flow was not sufficient to account for the observed increases in cardiac output. Also, in obesity, left ventricular filling pressure and volume increase, shifting left ventricular function to the left on the Frank-Starling curve and inducing chamber dilatation. The volume of the dilated chamber increases inappropriately to the stress on the left ventricular wall. Thus, the myocardium adapts by increasing contractile elements and subsequently myocardial mass. The end product is left ventricular hypertrophy, often of the eccentric type.[26,27] If this hemodynamic burden is sustained, premature impairment of left ventricular contractile function may result. Left atrial enlargement is also common in normotensive obese individuals and is associated with increased left ventricular mass. Importantly, left atrial enlargement is not necessarily mediated through impairment of left ventricular diastolic function and may simply reflect a physiologic adaptation to the expanded blood volume.[28]

If arterial pressure does not change, the increase in cardiac output is associated with a decrease in vascular resistance. Therefore, for any given level of arterial pressure, cardiac output is higher and vascular resistance is lower in an obese person than it is in a nonobese individual. However, obesity and hypertension often are associated. When both are present, obesity increases preload and hypertension increases postload. The heart of an obese hypertensive individual is now confronted with a double burden, and this may result in early left ventricular dysfunction and premature heart failure.

To examine the impact of obesity on the circulation, data have been obtained before and after surgically induced weight reduction at rest and during exercise by using right heart catheterization.[29] Resting oxygen consumption and cardiac output fell in proportion to weight loss.[29,30] Stroke volume fell in parallel to the decrease in blood volume and heart volume. Systemic arterial pressure declined, while systemic arterial resistance did not change. Left ventricular stroke work diminished. Filling pressures of the right and left sides of the heart decreased but were still higher in relation to cardiac output than they were in normal-weight subjects. Left ventricular dysfunction persisted, as evidenced by reduced myocardial wall compliance.[29] Right ventricular systolic pressure was lowered by 5 mmHg, and pulmonary arterial pressures by about 6 mmHg, but wedge pressure did not change.[29] At any given cardiac output, all pressures in the right ventricle, pulmonary artery, and pulmonary capillary venous position were higher than they were in normal-weight subjects,[29] with relative increases in left ventricular end-diastolic pressure.[24]

Obesity also is associated with persistence of elevated cardiac filling pressures during exercise.[29,31] Moreover, the average left ventricular filling pressure rose with exercise similarly (~20 mmHg) after weight loss. The average resting left ventricular filling pressure is within the upper limits of normal but is increased abnormally with increased venous return of passive leg raising and is increased further with exercise.[24] This is consistent with centralization of the circulating volume. With the increased venous return of passive leg raising, small increments of central blood volume were associated with a significant increase in left ventricular end-diastolic pressure. Normally, this intervention in healthy individuals would not cause any increase in diastolic filling pressures or would cause only a minimal change of 1 to 2 mmHg. This is consistent with a reduced distensibility of the central circulation in these patients. A decrease in central blood volume accompanies weight reduction, and when present, relief of edema and dyspnea accompanies this improvement.[24] However, myocardial hypertrophy and reduced ventricular compliance characterized by left ventricular diastolic dysfunction during exercise did not always regress with weight loss.[29,31]

FREQUENTLY PERFORMED PROCEDURES IN CARDIOLOGY AND OBESITY

Physical Examination

Fat mass is distributed differently in men and in women. The android, or male, pattern is characterized by fat distributed predominantly in the upper body above the waist, whereas the gynecoid, or female, pattern is characterized by fat predominantly in the lower body, that is, the lower abdomen, buttocks, hips, and thighs.

Although obesity often is described as an endocrine disease, fewer than 1 percent of obese patients have any significant endocrine dysfunction; hypothalamic (inflammation, trauma, tumor), pituitary (Cushing's disease), thyroid (hypothyroidism), adrenal (Cushing's syndrome), and ovarian (polycystic ovarian syndrome) dysfunctions have all been related to obesity. Obesity is the most common manifestation of Cushing's disease/syndrome, and weight gain is usually the initial symptom. Obesity is classically central, affecting mainly the face (moon facies), neck (buffalo hump), trunk, and abdomen, with relative sparing of the extremities. Hypogonadism also is associated with redistribution of body fat characterized by a lower abdominal–pelvic girdle fat distribution in patients who develop androgen deficiency.

In some ways, the presence of obesity may limit the accuracy of the physical examination. Jugular venous pulse often is not seen, and heart sounds are usually distant. A common finding in massive obesity is pedal edema, which can occur in part as a consequence of elevated ventricular filling pressure despite an elevation in cardiac output.[32,33] Obese individuals also can have increases in the demand for ventilation and breathing workload, especially in the supine position. At one time it was thought that Cheyne-Stokes breathing was pathognomonic of the cardiomyopathy of obesity.[34] Accurate blood pressure measurement is crucial, since many obese patients are hypertensive. A small cuff size can cause considerable increases in blood pressure.[35] This could result in incorrect classification of up to 35 percent of normotensive individuals as hypertensive in the presence of obesity.[35] When the bladder within the cuff is not long enough to encircle at least 80 percent of the arm, a wider cuff should be used. However, if the cuff is too wide, the pressure may be underestimated. One should always evaluate the presence of cor pulmonale when examining an obese individual. In the majority of individuals, splitting of the S_2 sound is most often heard at the second or third left interspace parasternally. However, in obese patients, the split S_2, when either inaudible or very poorly defined in the second interspace, often is best heard at the first left interspace.[36] Therefore, an increase in the intensity of P_2 suggestive of pulmonary hypertension may be missed at the bedside.

Surface Electrocardiogram

Obesity has the potential to affect the electrocardiogram (ECG) in several ways: (1) displacing the heart by elevating the diaphragm in the supine position, (2) increasing the cardiac workload, and (3) increasing the distance between the heart and the recording electrodes.

The voltage of the QRS complexes is attenuated by its passage through a fat-laden chest wall and is related to several factors, including the anatomy of the thorax, the degree of fatty infiltration of the heart, the degree of associated chronic lung disease, the increase in left ventricular muscle mass, and, most important, the selection of the ECG leads for measuring voltage. Overall, the effect of weight loss in obese patients on the QRS voltage is a source of controversy in the literature; studies have reported a decrease,[37–39] no change,[40] or an increase in the QRS amplitude after weight reduction.[41,42] Several factors, probably acting in different directions, are responsible for the ECG changes associated with weight reduction. In some instances, low QRS voltage after drastic weight loss could be secondary to lean mass loss and myocardial atrophy.[39,43,44] One must bear in mind that weight loss with modifications in the anatomy of the thorax (decrease in the amount of fat mass) may counterbalance a real decrease in left ventricular mass. These factors acting in opposite directions may affect the resultant QRS amplitudes differently.

In a study of over 1000 obese individuals, the heart rate, PR interval, QRS interval, QRS voltage, and QTc interval all showed an increase with increasing obesity.[45] Although the prolongation of the PR interval and the QRS interval probably was not clinically important, it is noteworthy that 8 percent of these patients presented with a QTc >0.44 s. Although the QRS axis also tended to shift leftward, fewer than 1 percent of the patients displayed an abnormal axis deviation. Interestingly, only 4 percent of this population had low QRS voltage and 19 percent presented with bradycardia.[45] Weight loss induced a rightward shift of the QRS axis.[41]

One study reported an increased incidence of false-positive criteria for inferior myocardial infarction in both obese individuals and women in the final trimester of pregnancy, presumably because of diaphragmatic elevation.[46] Several studies have documented nonspecific flattening of the T wave in the inferolateral leads in obese subjects.[42,47] In contrast, most conduction intervals, i.e., duration of the P wave, QRS complex, and the PQ interval in lead II, are not affected by weight loss.[41]

Since LVH is strongly associated with cardiac morbidity and mortality,[48] better ECG detection of LVH is mandatory in obese individuals. As left ventricular mass increases, electrical forces usually become more posteriorly oriented, and the S wave in lead V_3 may be the most representative voltage for evaluating posterior forces. In addition, it has been shown that with increasing LVH, the heart is oriented more horizontally, and this may explain the usefulness of the R wave in aV_L as an important determinant of LVH. Thus, it was proposed that for men at all ages, LVH is present by QRS voltage alone when the amplitude of the R wave in lead aV_L and the S wave in lead V_3 are >35 mm. For women of all ages, the same criteria were set at >25 mm.[49] When slightly different ECG voltage criteria in the same leads were compared with left ventricular mass estimated by echocardiography, a sensitivity of 49 percent, a specificity of 93 percent, and an overall accuracy of 76 percent were revealed. These percentages are higher than most widely used criteria, such as the Romhilt-Estes point score and the Sokolow-Lyon voltage (Table 83-2). Additionally, another study suggested that for simple LVH detection criteria, Sokolow-Lyon voltage should be avoided in obese hypertensive patients and replaced by the Cornell voltage criteria, which seems to be influenced less by the presence of obesity.[50]

Radiology

In obesity, the chest x-ray generally shows an elevated diaphragm with a widened heart in a horizontal direction, with the apex displaced outward to the left.[47] The heart appears enlarged and the left ventricle hypertrophied, based on the criteria of a total transverse diameter of the heart more than half the maximum internal thoracic diameter (Fig. 83-1). This is often discordant with the findings on the surface ECG (see above). The apex or the lower portion of the left border of the heart may be hazy in outline owing to the presence of apical pericardial fat.[47] Moreover, portable bedside radiographs are usually of very poor quality in obese patients, limiting the value of this important diagnostic tool in an emergency situation. Also, many computed tomography (CT) scan tables have weight restrictions (about 160 kg) that prohibit imaging of severely obese patients.

Echocardiography

Transthoracic echocardiography can be technically difficult in obese patients, and obtaining a good echocardiographic window is often difficult. This is important in evaluating the presence of left ventricular diastolic dysfunction. Although the evaluation of the presence of left ventricular diastolic dysfunction is important in obese subjects, complete echocardiogram studies are feasible in only 10 to 50 percent of patients.[51–53] Pulmonary venous Doppler evaluation may be used, but if it is not technically accessible, transmitral Doppler imaging with the use of the Valsalva maneuver may properly evaluate the presence of left ventricular diastolic dysfunction.[54,55]

Another feature of the echocardiographic assessment in obese

TABLE 83-2 Detection of Left Ventricular Hypertrophy by QRS Voltage in Obesity

	Sensitivity in Obesity, %	Specificity in Obesity, %	Accuracy in Obesity, %
Sokolow-Lyon	20	93	65
Romhilt-Estes point score ≥4	31	83	63
Cornell	49	93	76

Sokolow-Lyon voltage criteria: R in V_5 or V_6 plus S in V_1 >35 mm.
Romhilt-Estes point score; *Am Heart J* 1968; 75:752–758.
Cornell voltage criteria: R in aV_L plus S in V_3 >28 mm in men, >20 mm in women.
SOURCE: Adapted from Casale et al.[49]

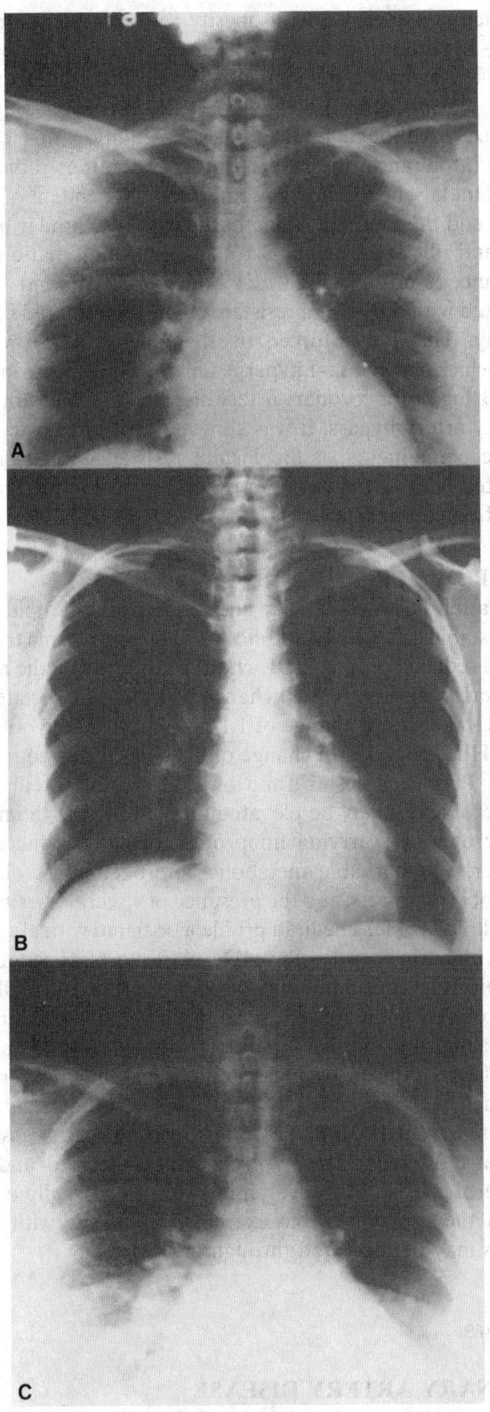

FIGURE 83-1 Chest films of a woman first presenting with severe pulmonary and systemic congestion. *A*. At age 20, weight is 184 kg. *B*. At age 31, weight reduction to 157 kg was associated with decrements in heart size as well as pulmonary congestion. *C*. Recurrence of cardiomegaly and pulmonary congestion attended regained weight at age 37. At age 43, weight 195 kg, echocardiogram demonstrated normal left ventricular systolic performance, with ejection fraction 64 percent, mean velocity of circumferential fiber shortening 1.36 cir/s. Left ventricular septal and posterior wall thickness were increased to 1.7 and 2.0 cm, respectively, and E-F slope was reduced to 30 mm/s, suggesting reduced left ventricular compliance. Left atrial dimension was enlarged to 5.2 cm. By age 48, atrial fibrillation had developed. (From Alexander JK. The cardiomyopathy of obesity. *Prog Cardiovasc Dis* 1985; 27:325–334. Reproduced with permission from Grune & Stratton, Inc., and the author.)

patients is the differentiation between subepicardial adipose tissue and pericardial effusion, which at times can be difficult. Epicardial adipose tissue is known to be a common cause of pseudopericardial effusion, and this adipose tissue depot may cause an underestimation of the amount of pericardial fluid.[56] Another issue is the presence of fat within the heart. Fat can accumulate in a variety of places, but the predominant site tends to be the interatrial septum. Lipomatous hypertrophy of the interatrial septum should be suspected in the presence of a dumb-bell-shaped appearance of the septum with thick echogenic tissue surrounding a thin echo at the level of the fossa ovalis.[57] In addition, an accumulation of fat may simulate a mass.

In the evaluation of the presence of LVH, it is customary to correct left ventricular mass by body surface area, and this is widely done clinically. However, even if indexation of left ventricular mass by body surface area is well adapted in nonobese subjects, evaluation of LVH prevalence in obesity, using a threshold equivalent to the one applied to the nonobese, would underestimate obesity as a predictor of increased left ventricular mass. To avoid this problem, some investigators have proposed that it is preferable to adjust left ventricular mass for height, height$^{2.13}$ or height$^{2.7}$.[58,59] This may reduce the variability in left ventricular mass associated with body size and sex. Of clinical importance, the application of different echocardiographic indexation methods to assess left ventricular mass did not modify the performance of the ECG criteria of Cornell.[50]

It is possible that these indexations may be more adapted for evaluating left ventricular mass in obese persons than is normalization for body surface area or even height.[60,61] Another potential way to normalize the left ventricular mass is with lean body mass.[62] Interestingly, after this indexation, there were no gender differences in left ventricular mass and the relative effects of adiposity and blood pressure on left ventricular mass were of similar amplitude.[62] Undoubtedly, the adiposity status has an impact on heart size, but the best indexation criteria to define LVH after an echocardiographic study in obese individual need to be refined and confirmed.

Nuclear Medicine

Cardiac function can be assessed adequately in severely obese subjects by using nuclear cardiology imaging techniques.[63–65] Because of the obvious limitations, a dipyridamole thallium-201 or technetium-99m perfusion scan may be used instead of exercise testing in very obese patients to evaluate the presence of ischemic heart disease. In spite of the attenuation factor caused by obesity, prolonged transmission scanning with thallium-201 is not required in obese compared with normal-size patients,[66] and triple-head simultaneous emission transmission tomography using technetium-99m is also accurate in obesity.[67]

Cardiac Catheterization

Obese individuals may have several limitations in the catheterization laboratory. The catheterization laboratory table usually does not accommodate subjects weighing more than 160 kg. Moreover, vascular access to the femoral vein and artery may be difficult. The percutaneous radial approach has advantages in very obese patients, in whom the percutaneous femoral technique may be technically difficult and bleeding may be hard to control after catheter removal. Indeed, the frequency of complications with the use of the percutaneous radial technique is very low and should be contemplated when the evaluation of extremely obese individuals is necessary in the catherization laboratory.[68]

OBESITY AND CARDIOVASCULAR DISEASE

Metabolic

VISCERAL OBESITY

Accumulation of intraabdominal (visceral) fat, located in the mesenterium and omentum, is associated with type 2 diabetes mellitus, hypertension, and coronary artery disease (Table 83-1). There is ample evidence to suggest that increased cardiovascular risk is at least partly accounted for by the metabolic and hemodynamic abnormalities associated with excessive abdominal fat distribution.[69] Indeed, disturbances in lipoprotein metabolism and plasma insulin-glucose homeostasis and elevations of blood pressure, which are risk factors for cardiac disease, have been reported in subjects with an excessive deposition of adipose tissue in the abdomen.[17,70] In addition, abdominal distribution of body fat is associated with increased plasma levels of fibrinogen, factor VII, and factor VIIIc coagulant activities and tissue plasminogen activator (TPA) antigen and PAI-1 antigen and activity.[17,70–72] This hypercoagulable state that accompanies excessive central fat deposition also may be associated with left ventricular dysfunction.[72] There is a beneficial impact of weight loss on plasma PAI-1 activity and other hemostatic factors in overweight individuals;[70,71] however, exercise seems to confer no additional benefit of the weight loss regimen on hemostatic factors.[70]

The presence of excess fat in the abdomen in proportion to total body fat is an independent predictor of coronary heart disease (CHD). Waist circumference is positively correlated with abdominal fat content and is the most practical anthropometric measurement for assessing a patient's abdominal fat content.[73] The waist circumference cutoffs lose their incremental predictive power in patients with a BMI $\geq$35 kg/m^2.[2] When obese subjects are matched for their levels of total body fat, subjects with high levels of visceral fat have dyslipidemia.[74] This further implicates visceral fat as a deleterious atherogenic factor.

BLOOD GLUCOSE AND HYPERINSULINEMIA

The increased risk of diabetes mellitus as weight increases has been shown in prospective studies in numerous countries.[75–77] The development of type 2 diabetes has been found to be associated with weight gain after age 18 in both men and women. The relative risk of diabetes increases approximately 25 percent for each additional unit of BMI over 22 kg/m^2.[78] Moreover cross-sectional and longitudinal studies have shown that abdominal obesity is a major risk factor for type 2 diabetes.[69,79,80] There is strong evidence that weight loss reduces blood glucose levels and hemoglobin A_{1c} levels in patients with type 2 diabetes, and it has been reported in three European cohorts (>17,000 men) followed for over 20 years that nondiabetic men with higher blood glucose had a significantly higher risk of death from cardiovascular and coronary heart disease.[81] In addition, it was demonstrated in the Framingham offspring cohort that metabolic factors associated with obesity (overall and central), including hypertension, low levels of high-density lipoprotein (HDL)-cholesterol, and increased levels of triglycerides and insulin, worsen continuously across the spectrum of glucose tolerance.[82] Although BMI increased steadily with increasing glucose intolerance, the association between most other measures of metabolic risk and glycemia was independent of overall obesity and the gradient of increasing risk was similar for nonobese and obese participants.[82,83] Thus, asymptomatic glucose intolerance is not a benign metabolic condition, and features associated with the insulin resistance syndrome should be taken seriously. This is reinforced by the Quebec Cardiovascular Study, which showed that hyperinsulinemia may be an independent risk factor for coronary artery disease.[84] Furthermore, after coronary artery bypass, it was shown after a 5-year follow-up that the components of the insulin resistance syndrome are associated with angiographic progression of atherosclerosis in nongrafted coronary arteries.[85]

DYSLIPIDEMIA

The relation between obesity and altered plasma lipid profile is well established. Generally, increased fasting plasma triglycerides and reduced plasma HDL-cholesterol levels on the average characterize obesity. A BMI change of 1 unit is associated with an HDL-cholesterol change of 1.1 mg/dL for young adult men and an HDL-cholesterol change of 0.69 mg/dL for young adult women.[2] Plasma cholesterol and low-density lipoprotein (LDL)-cholesterol levels may be elevated marginally, but the number of apoprotein B–carrying lipoproteins usually is increased.[74] However, a remarkable metabolic heterogeneity is observed among obese subjects, and the presence of visceral obesity worsens the lipid profile. The lipid profile associated with abdominal obesity, high triglycerides, low HDL-cholesterol, elevated apolipoprotein B levels, and an increased proportion of small dense LDL probably is the main contributor to the increase in CHD in this subgroup of obese patients.[74] There is evidence that weight loss produced by lifestyle modifications in overweight individuals is accompanied by reductions in serum triglycerides and increases in HDL-cholesterol.[86] Weight loss occasionally produces some reductions in serum total cholesterol and LDL-cholesterol levels.[87] Moreover, improvement in the lipid profile through the use of aerobic exercise in subjects with type 2 diabetes may be mediated through fat loss.[88]

Structural

CORONARY ARTERY DISEASE

Obesity may be an independent risk factor for ischemic heart disease. However, numerous studies have not been able to confirm this because of the short time period of observation. Indeed, the association between obesity and ischemic heart disease seems evident only after two decades of follow-up.[6] This relation was also stronger in younger individuals.[5,6] A high BMI was significantly associated with the development of myocardial infarction, coronary insufficiency, and sudden death, and among those adverse events, the association was strongest with sudden death.[6] In the Nurses Health Study, weight gains of 5 to 8 kg increased CHD risk (nonfatal myocardial infarction and CHD death) 25 percent and weight gains of $\geq$20 kg increased that risk more than 2.5 times in comparison with women whose weight was stable within a range of 5 kg.[89] In British men, an increase of 1 BMI unit was associated with a 10 percent increase in the rate of coronary events.[90] Although, obesity per se is considered a major modifiable risk factor for ischemic heart disease,[8] it is important to remember that overweight individuals present a cluster of other traditional and nontraditional risk factors, i.e., dyslipidemia, hypertension, type 2 diabetes mellitus, the prothrombotic state, hyperinsulinemia, hypertriglyceridemia, and elevated apolipoprotein B, that are all potentially deleterious. In the ECAT angina pectoris study, there was a strong relation between obesity and the fibrinolytic system even after adjusting for total triglycerides, cholesterol, age, and sex.[91] Thus, the detrimental impact of overweight/obesity as a risk factor for ischemic heart disease involves multiple mechanisms that accompany the obese state.

HYPERTENSION

The majority of patients with high blood pressure are overweight, and hypertension is about six times more common in obese than it is in lean subjects.[92] Not only is hypertension more common in obese subjects, weight gain in young people is an important risk factor for the subsequent development of hypertension. A 10-kg higher body weight is associated with a 3.0 mmHg higher systolic and a 2.3 mmHg higher diastolic blood pressure. These increases translate into an estimated 12 percent increase in risk for CHD and a 24 percent increase in risk for stroke.[2]

In the Framingham Heart Study, obesity was significantly correlated with increased left ventricular mass,[93] and it has been shown that a 10 percent reduction in weight in obese hypertensive patients not only reduced blood pressure but also decreased left ventricular wall thickness and left ventricular mass.[94] The effect on left ventricular mass was seen in both hypertensive[94] and nonhypertensive patients.[51] Moreover, it has been shown that weight reduction using modest amounts of exercise and a hypocaloric intake decreases left ventricular mass regardless of blood pressure level in obese subjects.[95] There is strong and consistent evidence from lifestyle trials in overweight hypertensive and nonhypertensive patients that weight loss produced by lifestyle modifications reduces blood pressure levels. Weight reduction is one of the rare antihypertensive strategies that decrease blood pressure in normotensive as well as hypertensive persons.[2,96]

Some investigators have suggested that reductions in blood pressure are attributable to reductions in salt intake concomitant with caloric restriction, but it has been established that reductions in blood pressure do not necessarily result from the reduction in salt intake.[95,97] Although the pathophysiologic mechanisms in the lowering of blood pressure with weight loss are not clear, numerous factors probably are involved. The reduction in blood pressure also could be attributable to reductions in total circulating and cardiopulmonary blood volume as well as reductions in sympathetic nervous system activity.[97] The reduction in plasma catecholamines and plasma renin activity that is associated with decreased sympathetic activity, also probably plays a role.[98,99]

Although both normotensive and hypertensive individuals have elevated cardiac output and blood volume compared with nonobese subjects,[100] normotensive obese patients have diminished vascular resistance whereas hypertensive obese patients have normal vascular resistance. However, estimates of cardiac output could be misleading in obesity. Cardiac output probably is better expressed in actual values rather than being related to body surface area (cardiac index) because when cardiac output (rather than cardiac index) is used to calculate total peripheral resistance, it is often normal or reduced in hypertensive obese patients.[101,102] Therefore, peripheral resistance and intravascular volume may be normal in mildly hypertensive obese patients because of the mutually opposing effects of the increase in arterial pressure and the increase in body weight.

LEFT VENTRICULAR DIASTOLIC DYSFUNCTION

A longer duration of obesity is associated with higher left ventricular mass, poorer left ventricular systolic function, and greater impairment of left ventricular diastolic function.[103] Obese subjects often present with abnormal left ventricular diastolic filling with a greater peak atrial velocity and a longer late diastolic flow time compared with nonobese subjects.[27] It has been shown by echocardiography that the eccentric left ventricular hypertrophy in obese subjects causes an abnormal left ventricular diastolic filling pattern similar to concentric left ventricular hypertrophy of hypertension. However, the increased intravascular volume in obesity may mask the Doppler-derived abnormalities of diastolic filling. It is interesting to note that the abnormal filling patterns seen in obese subjects are present despite hemodynamics that are unfavorable for detection.

Left ventricular diastolic dysfunction and increased left ventricular mass may be attributable to a disproportionate accumulation of collagen in the interstitial space of the hypertrophied left ventricle, a consequence that is secondary to pressure overload. However, in normotensive obese persons, the increase in left ventricular mass is not always accompanied by myocardial fibrosis,[104] and normal diastolic function is commonly found.[53] In addition, it was reported that only obese subjects with increased left ventricular mass appeared to have impaired left ventricular diastolic dysfunction, and that group of subjects had improvements in left ventricular function after weight lost.[53,105] Substantial weight loss may improve the abnormal pattern of ventricular filling and increased left ventricular dimension in diastole.[53] In another study involving hypertensive obese subjects, weight loss was associated with a greater decrease in ventricular and posterior wall thickness and left ventricular mass than was seen in subjects treated with metoprolol, suggesting that changes in weight, independent of changes in blood pressure, were directly associated with changes in left ventricular mass.[94]

LEFT VENTRICULAR HYPERTROPHY AND CONGESTIVE HEART FAILURE

As was stated previously, cardiac adaptation to obesity results in cardiac hypertrophy of the concentric [106,107] or eccentric type.[108] Pathologically, there is a proportionality between heart weight and body weight[106,109] (Fig. 83-2), and echocardiographic studies have shown that left ventricular end-diastolic dimension and septal and posterior wall dimensions are greater in obese subjects.[27] Possible explanations are that the reduction in left ventricular mass may be secondary to the reduction in blood pressure associated with weight loss or simply to the reduction in body weight. Indeed, 14 to 25 percent of the reduction in left ventricular mass could be explained by the change in body weight.[94,95] Work by Messerli and associates[108] suggests that the

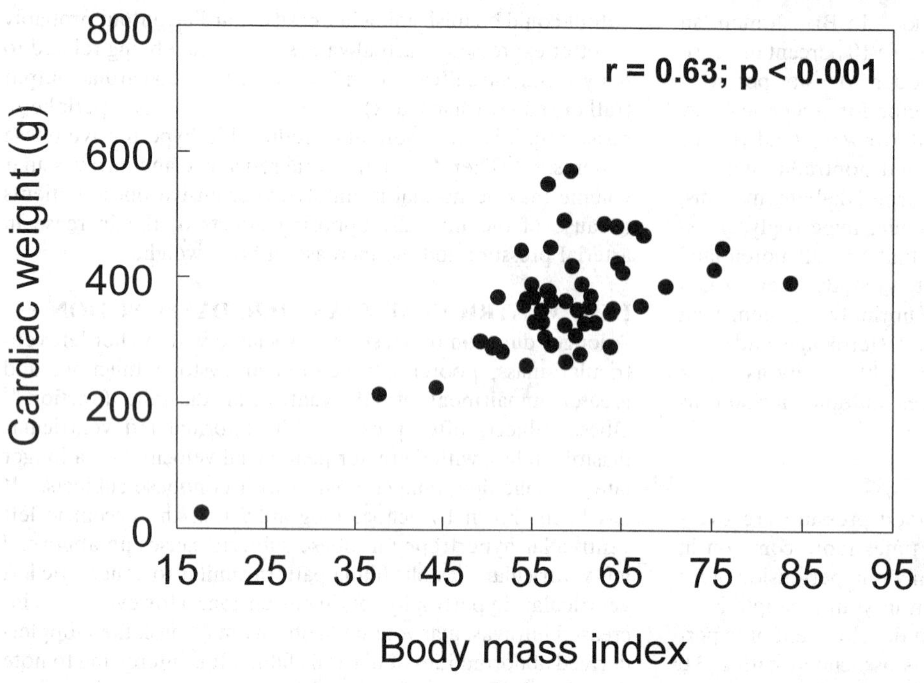

FIGURE 83-2 Relation between cardiac weight (g) and body mass index (BMI) from autopsies of 52 cases of obesity without demonstrable evidence of heart disease. (Adapted from Smith and Willius.[109])

combination of obesity and hypertension results in myocardial hypertrophy with left ventricular dilatation. Premature ventricular complex increases with body weight and is 30 times higher in obese patients with eccentric left ventricular hypertrophy than it is in lean subjects.[23] This could be one of the mechanisms that explain the importance of left ventricular hypertrophy as a parameter associated with cardiac morbidity and mortality in this population. Of note, the combination of obesity and hypertension burdens the heart with high preload and high afterload, greatly enhancing the risk of congestive heart failure. Sympathetic mechanisms have been implicated in the development of LVH,[48] and weight reduction in obese subjects reduces indexes of sympathetic activity such as plasma norepinephrine, urinary norepinephrine excretion, and resting heart rate. The renin-angiotensin system also may be involved in the pathogenesis of LVH, and weight reduction may decrease plasma renin activity and aldosterone levels.[98] The improvement in hyperinsulinemia also may contribute to the reduction in left ventricular mass in hypertensive obese subjects, since insulin resistance is an important independent contributing factor to left ventricular mass in normotensive nondiabetic obese subjects.[110] Nevertheless, the role of all these neurohumoral factors in the regression of cardiac hypertrophy associated with weight reduction merits further investigation.

OBSTRUCTIVE SLEEP APNEA, HYPOVENTILATION, PULMONARY HYPERTENSION, RIGHT VENTRICULAR FAILURE

There are numerous respiratory complications of obesity, including an increased breathing workload, respiratory muscle inefficiency, decreased functional reserve capacity and expiratory reserve volume, and closure of peripheral lung units. These complications often result in a ventilation-perfusion mismatch, especially in the supine position. Obesity is a classic cause of alveolar hypoventilation. Historically, the obesity-hypoventilation syndrome has been described as the "pickwickian" syndrome, and obstructive apnea was first observed in patients with severe obesity. Sleep apnea is defined as repeated episodes of obstructive apnea and hypopnea during sleep, together with daytime somnolence and/or altered cardiopulmonary function.[111] The prevalence of sleep-disordered breathing and sleep disturbances rises dramatically in obese subjects,[112] and obesity is by far the most important modifiable risk factor in sleep-disordered breathing.[113,114] It has been estimated that 40 million Americans suffer from sleep disorders and that the vast majority of these patients remain undiagnosed.[113,114]

Despite careful screening by history and physical examination, sleep apnea is revealed only by polysomnography in most patients.[115] Although, some clinical features could be useful in screening for sleep apnea, the diagnostic accuracy is inadequate.[116]

Patients with sleep apnea have an increased risk of diurnal hypertension, nocturnal dysrhythmias, pulmonary hypertension, right and left ventricular failure, myocardial infarction, stroke, and mortality.[117] The prevalence of pulmonary hypertension in subjects with obstructive sleep apnea is 15 to 20 percent; however, pulmonary hypertension rarely is observed in the absence of daytime hypoxemia.[118,119] According to Kessler and colleagues,[118] the extent of pulmonary hypertension in patients with obstructive sleep apnea is generally mild to moderate (pulmonary artery pressures ranging between 20 and 35 mmHg) and does not necessitate specific treatment.

Although there is a link between sleep apnea and systemic hypertension, the association of obesity with both disorders confounds the relationship. A physician who evaluates an obese patient who has been referred for hypertension should address related symptoms such as habitual snoring, nocturnal gasping or choking, witnessed episodes of apnea, and daytime sleepiness.[113,114,120] It is important to remember, however, that the clinical and ECG signs of cor pulmonale appear later than do those of pulmonary hypertension (assessed by right heart catheterization). Numerous treatments are available for sleep apnea, but weight loss in obese patients should always be advocated.[111]

AUTONOMIC NERVOUS SYSTEM ACTIVITY

The autonomic nervous system, an important contributor to the regulation of both the cardiovascular system and energy expenditure, is assumed to play a role in the pathophysiology of obesity and related complications.[121] Numerous techniques, e.g., heart rate variability, microneurography, and catecholamine turnover, have been used to examine the variation in the autonomic nervous system induced by diet and weight change in humans. However, the exact role of the sympathetic and parasympathetic nervous systems in obesity and weight loss is unclear. According to Peterson and coworkers,[121] both parasympathetic activity and sympathetic activity decrease as the percentage of body fat increases. This is in contrast to the findings of others who have used more invasive techniques to demonstrate that obesity is associated with predominantly sympathetic activation.[122] A 10 percent increase in body weight is associated with a decline in parasympathetic tone accompanied by a rise in mean heart rate, but heart rate declines during weight reduction.[123] Such reductions in vagal activity with increments in weight may be one mechanism for the arrhythmia and other cardiac abnormalities that accompany obesity. Discrepancies between studies of the impact of the autonomic nervous system in obesity can be explained in part by the techniques used to evaluate that system.[124] In addition, confounding conditions such as obstructive sleep apnea may be important.[114] In sleep apnea patients, sympathetic activity is increased,[115,125] and using microneurography, obesity per se (in the absence of obstructive sleep apnea) was not accompanied by increased sympathetic activity.[115]

ARRHYTHMIA, SUDDEN DEATH, AND QT INTERVAL

Hippocrates presumably stated, "Sudden death is more common in those who are naturally fat than in the lean." Obese subjects, even without dieting, have an increased risk of arrhythmias and sudden death in the absence of cardiac dysfunction.[23,126] In the Framingham study, the risk of sudden cardiac death with increasing weight was seen in both sexes.[6] Hence, the annual sudden cardiac mortality rate in obese men and women has been estimated to be 65 per 100,000 patients, about 40 times higher than the rate of unexplained cardiac arrest in a matched nonobese population.[127] In severely obese men age 25 to 34 years, a 12-fold excess mortality rate was seen, whereas in men age 35 to 44 years, a substantial risk with a sixfold excess mortality rate was demonstrated.[3]

Prolongation of the QTc interval is a risk factor for ventricular arrhythmias and sudden death. Importantly, there is a correlation between BMI and QTc, with longer intervals observed in obese subjects.[128] The relation between fatness and the QTc interval persisted even after absolute QT intervals were adjusted for heart rate using different formulas (Bazett, Framingham, Fridericia) and by multiple regression analysis.[128] Therefore, a prolonged QT interval is observed in a relatively high percentage of obese subjects, and the association between abnormal QTc and BMI is most evident in the severely obese.[40,128] Weight loss through starvation,[37,39] liquid protein diets,[43,44] very low calorie diets, or even obesity surgery[107] can be associated with prolongation of the QTc interval. To some extent, this occurs irrespective of the biological value of the constituent protein or the addition of mineral and trace supplements.[43] In addition, it has been shown that liquid protein diets frequently are associated with potentially life-threatening arrhythmias, a relationship documented by 24-h Holter recording but not in a study using routine ECG.[129] Ventricular tachycardia (torsades de pointes) and fibrillation often have been documented in subjects who died under observation.[43,130] Drug treatment with lidocaine, propranolol, phenytoin, mexiletine, disopyramide, and procainamide is usually ineffective.[37,43] Infusion of potassium, calcium, magnesium, bicarbonate, or glucagon and even ventricular overdrive pacing or open chest cardiac massage are ineffective in controlling the refractory arrhythmia.[43,107,130]

ECG changes in the course of weight loss in obese patients appear to be common. However, histologic findings in the hearts of those dying while ingesting liquid modified protein diets and a group of cachectic patients dying from malignant disease were similar[44] despite a lack of ECG abnormalities in the latter and QT prolongation in the former. Thus, the underlying mechanism and, in particular, the clinical significance of obesity-associated QT prolongation remain speculative. Also, a variety of arrhythmogenic factors have been implicated; acute heart failure with stretching of the myocardium that decreases the electric threshold in myocytes and facilitates spontaneous depolarization, myocyte hypertrophy, and multiple intercalated disks may facilitate the current flow and cause reentrant arrhythmias, and increased myocardial oxygen demand and impaired vasodilatory reserve may cause acute myocardial ischemia in the absence of coronary artery disease. Fatty infiltration of the myocardium is unlikely to be involved in the majority of cases. Because extremely obese patients often have a dilated cardiomyopathy, fatal arrhythmias may be the most common cause of death in those patients.[23,108]

CARDIAC SURGERY

Health care professionals often cite obesity as a risk factor for perioperative morbidity and mortality. The presence of hypertension, coronary artery disease, dyslipidemia, and type 2 diabetes mellitus and the technical difficulties inherent in the surgical and postsurgical care of the obese patients probably contribute to this perception. In contrast, obesity is not associated with increased mortality or postoperative cerebrovascular accidents after coronary artery bypass surgery.[131] However, sternal wound infection is increased in obese patients.[131] The large and poorly vascularized panniculus, the higher incidence of hyperglycemia in the obese, and the difficulty in wound surveillance may predispose to wound infections.[131]

Obesity also has been identified as a risk factor for superficial wound infection, saphenous vein harvest site infection, and atrial dysrhythmias.[132] These complications increase with increasing BMI. In accordance, obesity (defined by a BMI >30 kg/m^2) was not associated with an increase risk of operative mortality, stroke, renal failure, acquired respiratory distress syndrome, prolonged mechanical ventilation, pneumonia, sepsis, pulmonary embolism, or ventricular arrhythmias.[132] In contrast to other findings, the risk of mediastinitis was not increased.[131] Strangely, despite well-documented alterations in respiratory physiology in obese patients, pulmonary complications were comparable to those seen in nonobese patients.[131,132] Obese patients have been shown to have a higher incidence of postoperative thromboembolic disease in noncardiac surgery.[133] The discrepancy between these results may reflect different treatment attitudes in the postoperative period, with more vigorous pulmonary cleansing being performed by the nursing staff or more vigilance being taken in enforcing postoperative use of incentive spirometry and early ambulation in patients undergoing cardiac surgery. Nevertheless, the high risk of thromboembolic disease in obese patients may warrant an aggressive approach to deep venous thrombosis prophylaxis.[133] Although major unanticipated problems with ventilation are relatively rare in the postanesthesia period, obesity is a risk factor for this complication.[134]

VASCULAR ACCESS

Poor peripheral venous access in obese patients may necessitate more frequent use of central venous lines. A short stubby neck, loss of physical landmarks, and a greater skin–blood vessel distance make internal jugular and subclavian vein cannulation in the coronary care unit technically more difficult.[133] This could result in multiple skin punctures and a higher incidence of catheter malpositioning. Femoral access may not be possible not only because of the volume of adipose tissue but also because of the presence of intertrigo.

CARDIOMYOPATHY OF OBESITY (ADIPOSITAS CORDIS)

Cardiomyopathy associated with obesity without evidence of other heart disease was recognized as early as 1818.[34] This case is of historical interest not only because it is a carefully recorded documentation of a fatty heart but also because it was the first reported case in which a specific type of respiration, now recognized as Cheyne-Stokes respiration, was described.[34] Subsequently, Smith and Willius[109] described excess epicardial fat and fatty infiltration of the myocardium in the hearts of obese subjects that might have interfered with cardiac function. Other groups have demonstrated the same findings showing increased fat in the atrioventricular sulci and the atrial septum.[135] Characteristically, the thickness of the atrial septum is increased (lipomatous hypertrophy). Of interest, myocardial fatty infiltration also has been described without a relationship to obesity.[136]

Myocardial fat infiltration is an uncommon autopsy finding, with an incidence of approximately 3 percent.[137] This condition is more prevalent in women.[137,138] The presence of excess adipose tissue on the surface of the right ventricle represents an exaggeration of the normal architecture. Thus, at least at first, the fatty heart is probably not an infiltrative process but most likely a metaplastic phenomenon.

With time, fat can infiltrate between muscle fibers and/or result in myocyte degeneration. With progressive disease, fatty heart can result in cardiac conduction defects.[139,140] Associated with fat infiltration of the right ventricle, there can be extensive fatty replacement of the sinus node musculature and, to a lesser degree, infiltration of the atrioventricular node and the right bundle branch[139] while the entire myocardium of the atrioventricular region is replaced by fat.[140] Fatty heart also can result in a restrictive cardiomyopathy.[136,141] Here, small irregular aggregates and bands of adipose tissue separate myocardial cells. The fibers often are reduced in diameter, presumably as a result of pressure-induced atrophy from the intervening fat.[141] In general, the right ventricle is more likely to be involved than is the left ventricle and the anterior wall is involved to a greater extent than is the posterior wall. Most of the time, cardiac hypertrophy is a direct reflection of BMI and the hypertrophy results from myocyte change, not from excessive fat infiltration or fibrosis.[104]

TREATMENT

The general goals of weight loss and management are at a minimum to prevent further weight gain, reduce body weight, and maintain a lower body weight indefinitely. Patients should have their BMI and levels of abdominal fat measured with the goal of weight reduction established to favorably affect outcomes, including cardiovascular health. Obesity management and treatment include counseling,[96] diet,[142] exercise,[142,143] drugs,[144] and surgery.[145]

Lifestyle Modifications

BEHAVIORAL

Behavioral strategies to reinforce changes in diet and physical activity in obese adults can produce weight loss in the range of 10 percent over a period of 6 months.[96] Although no single behaviorial therapy appears superior to any other in general, a combination of strategies appears to work best and interventions with the greatest intensity appear to be associated with the greatest benefit. Weight loss programs that result in slow but steady weight reduction, e.g., 1 to 2 lb/week, may be more effective than are those which result in rapid weight loss.[146] Long-term follow-up results in patients undergoing behavior therapy show a return to baseline weight for the majority of subjects in the absence of continued behavior intervention.[147–149] In obese patients who smoke, smoking cessation is mandatory. However, a major obstacle to cessation has been the attendant weight gain observed in about 80 percent of quitters.[150–152] Weight gain that accompanies smoking cessation has been quite resistant to most dietary, behavioral, and physical activity interventions. Importantly, the weight gain with smoking cessation is less likely to produce negative health consequences than is continued smoking.[96]

DIET

Weight reduction depends on an energy intake less than it does on energy expenditure. Here, energy density of the diet is important. In general, foods high in fat (9 kcal/g) and sugar are energy-dense. Thus, diets for weight reduction should be restricted not only in total calories but also in fat and sugar. Approximately 1 lb per week can be lost with no change in physical activity if 500 kcal/day is eliminated. Such diets would continue to include foods that are low in saturated fat and cholesterol but enriched in nutrients that are associated with a reduced risk for cardiovascular disease, e.g., fruits, vegetables, legumes, and whole-grain products.[153] Although diets high in fat and protein have become popular, there is concern about the long-term efficacy and safety of these diets. Unquestionably, weight reduction occurs and can be rapid on such carbohydrate-restricted diets.[154] Nevertheless, no evidence suggests that these diets are any more effective than are fat-restricted diets months to years after intervention, and some of these diets raise questions about enhanced atherogenesis and renal and skeletal complications if they are sustained.

EXERCISE

Aerobic exercise alone produces a modest weight reduction, generally 2 to 3 percent; however, it is extremely important to sustain the weight-reduced state.[155–157] Fat loss through dieting and/or exercise produces comparable and favorable changes in HDL-cholesterol and its subfractions HDL_2 and HDL_3 and triglycerides.[86,142] Furthermore, long-term aerobic exercise training can normalize the metabolic profile of obese subjects even if those subjects remain very obese at the end of the program (41 percent of body fat).[143] Even if weight loss is minimal, physically fit obese individuals are less prone to mortality from cardiovascular disease than are lean subjects who are not physically fit.[158] Initially, moderate levels of physical activity for 30 to 45 min, 3 to 5 days a week, should be encouraged. Thereafter, all adults should set a long-term goal of doing 30 min or more of moderate-intensity physical activity on most, and preferably all, days of the week.[159]

A combined intervention of behavior therapy, a low-calorie diet, and increased physical activity provides the most successful therapy for weight loss and weight maintenance. In overweight/obese patients who are psychologically ready for weight loss, this approach should be emphasized and sustained for at least 6 months before pharmacotherapy is considered.

Drugs

Weight loss drugs can be useful adjuncts to dietary therapy and physical activity for some patients, i.e., those with a BMI ≥30 kg/m^2 with or without concomitant comorbidities, and for patients with a BMI ≥27 kg/m^2 with concomitant risk factors or diseases.[2,96] The comorbidities considered sufficiently important to warrant pharmacotherapy at a BMI of 27 to 29.9 kg/m^2 are hypertension (≥140/90 mmHg), dyslipidemia (LDL ≥160 mg/dl, HDL <35 mg/dL), coronary artery disease, type 2 diabetes, and obstructive sleep apnea.[2,96] The two main categories of obesity drugs are anorectics that act centrally in the brain on adrenergic or serotonergic pathways and nutrient absorption inhibitors that decrease macronutrient absorption from the gastrointestinal tract.

Fenfluramine and dexfenfluramine, which reduce appetite by enhancing serotonin at nerve terminals in the hypothalamus, were removed from the marketplace in the United States after reports of cardiac valve disorders,[160] particularly aortic and mitral insufficiency. An increased risk of primary pulmonary hypertension also was associated with these agents.[161–164] The valvular abnormalities produced by fenfluramine and dexfenfluramine were histopathologically similar to those noted in patients with the carcinoid syndrome.[165,166] Of importance, the development of valvulopathy was correlated with the duration of exposure.[167] There were no cases reported of cardiac valve abnormalities associated with the use of phentermine alone,[168] and regression of valvular disease after the cessation of fenfluramine or dexfenfluramine is possible.[169] Unlike fenfluramine or dexfenfluramine, phentermine is a sympathomimetic drug that reduces food intake through its effects on adrenergic receptors in the hypothalamus.

Sibutramine hydrochloride promotes a sense of satiety by blocking the reuptake of both norepinephrine and serotonin in nerve terminals. Sibutramine also has a moderate effect on energy expenditure by attenuating the decrease in energy output during rest.[170] This drug has been approved for long-term use. It has limited but definite effects on weight loss and can facilitate weight loss maintenance.[170] In one study, the prevalence of cardiac valve dysfunction was not increased in 133 obese patients who were treated with sibutramine for an average of 7.6 months.[171] Increases in blood pressure and heart rate may occur with the use of this drug.[144] Like phentermine, sibutramine should not be used in patients with untreated hypertension, coronary heart disease, congestive heart failure, arrhythmias, or stroke.[170]

Orlistat reduces the absorption of dietary fat (approximately 30 percent reduction) by binding to pancreatic lipase in the intestinal lumen and inhibiting its action. Orlistat has an advantage over drugs that act on the central nervous system because it is not absorbed.[144,172] The major side effect is symptoms associated with steatorrhea. With long-term use, fat-soluble vitamins may need to be replaced.[173]

Surgery

Weight loss surgery that includes gastric plication and gastric bypass with a Roux-en-Y anastomosis is an option in a limited number of patients with extreme obesity, i.e., BMI ≥40 kg/m^2 or BMI ≥35 kg/m^2, with comorbid conditions.[2] Weight loss surgery should be reserved for patients who have extreme obesity in whom efforts at medical therapy have failed. An acceptable operative risk also must be present. Furthermore, lifelong medical surveillance after surgery is necessary.

CONCLUSIONS

Obesity is a chronic metabolic disorder that is associated with cardiovascular disease and increased morbidity and mortality. When the BMI is ≥30 kg/m^2, mortality rates from all causes, especially cardiovascular disease, are increased 50 to 100 percent. There is strong evidence that weight loss in overweight and obese individuals reduces risk factors for diabetes and cardiovascular disease. Additional evidence indicates that weight loss and the associated diuresis reduce blood pressure in overweight hypertensive and nonhypertensive individuals, reduce serum triglyceride levels, and increase high-density lipoprotein cholesterol (HDL-C) levels, and may produce some reduction in low-density lipoprotein cholesterol (LDL-C) levels. Weight loss also reduces blood glucose levels and hemoglobin A_{1c} levels in patients with type 2 diabetes, signs and symptoms of left ventricular failure, and obstructive sleep apnea. Although no prospective trials have convincingly shown changes in mortality with weight loss in obese patients, reductions in risk factors at least would predict a reduced incidence of cardiovascular disease and perhaps cardiovascular disease–related mortality.

References

1. Calle EE, Thun MJ, Petrelli JM, et al. Body-mass index and mortality in a prospective cohort of U.S. adults. *N Engl J Med* 1999; 341:1097–1105.
2. Clinical Guidelines on the Identification, Evaluation, and Treatment of Overweight and Obesity in Adults—The Evidence Report: National Institutes of Health. *Obes Res* 1998; (suppl 2):51S–209S.
3. Drenick EJ, Bale GS, Seltzer F, Johnson DG. Excessive mortality and causes of death in morbidly obese men. *JAMA* 1980; 243:443–445.
4. VanItallie TB. Prevalence of obesity. *Endocrinol Metab Clin North Am* 1996; 25:887–905.
5. Hubert HB, Feinleib M, McNamara PM, Castelli WP. Obesity as an independent risk factor for cardiovascular disease: A 26-year follow-up of participants in the Framingham Heart Study. *Circulation* 1983; 67:968–977.
6. Rabkin SW, Mathewson FA, Hsu PH. Relation of body weight to development of ischemic heart disease in a cohort of young North American men after a 26 year observation period: The Manitoba Study. *Am J Cardiol* 1977; 39:452–458.
7. Eckel RH. Obesity and heart disease: A statement for healthcare

professionals from the Nutrition Committee, American Heart Association. *Circulation* 1997; 96:3248–3250.
8. Eckel RH, Krauss RM. American Heart Association call to action: Obesity as a major risk factor for coronary heart disease: AHA Nutrition Committee. *Circulation* 1998; 97:2099–2100.
9. Bouchard C, Després JP, Mauriège P. Genetic and nongenetic determinants of regional fat distribution. *Endocr Rev* 1993; 14:72–93.
10. Bray GA, Bouchard C, James WPT. *Handbook of Obesity*. New York: Marcel Dekker; 1998:31.
11. Yudkin JS, Stehouwer CD, Emeis JJ, Coppack SW. C-reactive protein in healthy subjects: Associations with obesity, insulin resistance, and endothelial dysfunction: A potential role for cytokines originating from adipose tissue? *Arterioscler Thromb Vasc Biol* 1999; 19:972–978.
12. Mohamed-Ali V, Goodrick S, Rawesh A, et al. Subcutaneous adipose tissue releases interleukin-6, but not tumor necrosis factor-alpha, in vivo. *J Clin Endocrinol Metab* 1997; 82:4196–4200.
13. Ridker PM. Novel risk factors and markers for coronary disease. *Adv Intern Med* 2000; 45:391–418
14. Kern PA, Saghizadeh M, Ong JM, et al. The expression of tumor necrosis factor in human adipose tissue: Regulation by obesity, weight loss, and relationship to lipoprotein lipase. *J Clin Invest* 1995; 95:2111–2119.
15. Hotamisligil GS, Arner P, Caro JF, et al. Increased adipose tissue expression of tumor necrosis factor-alpha in human obesity and insulin resistance. *J Clin Invest* 1995; 95:2409–2415.
16. Lundgren CH, Brown SL, Nordt TK, et al. Elaboration of type-1 plasminogen activator inhibitor from adipocytes: A potential pathogenetic link between obesity and cardiovascular disease. *Circulation* 1996; 93:106–110.
17. Cigolini M, Targher G, Bergamo AI, et al. Visceral fat accumulation and its relation to plasma hemostatic factors in healthy men. *Arterioscler Thromb Vasc Biol* 1996; 16:368–374.
18. Rosell S, Belfrage E. Blood circulation in adipose tissue. *Physiol Rev* 1979; 59:1078–1104.
19. Larsen OA, Lassen NA, Quaade F. Blood flow through human adipose tissue determined with radioactive xenon. *Acta Physiol Scand* 1966; 66:337–345.
20. Lesser GT, Deutsch S. Measurement of adipose tissue blood flow and perfusion in man by uptake of 85Kr. *J Appl Physiol* 1967; 23:621–630.
21. Oberg B, Rosell S. Sympathetic control of consecutive vascular sections in canine subcutaneous adipose tissue. *Acta Physiol Scand* 1967; 71:47–56.
22. Linde B, Chisolm G. The interstitial space of adipose tissue as determined by single injection and equilibration techniques. *Acta Physiol Scand* 1975; 95:383–390.
23. Messerli FH, Nunez BD, Ventura HO, Snyder DW. Overweight and sudden death: Increased ventricular ectopy in cardiopathy of obesity. *Arch Intern Med* 1987; 147:1725–1728.
24. Kaltman AJ, Goldring RM. Role of circulatory congestion in the cardiorespiratory failure of obesity. *Am J Med* 1976; 60:645–653.
25. Alexander JK, Dennis EW, Smith WG, et al. Blood volume, cardiac output, and distribution of systemic blood flow in extreme obesity. *Cardiovasc Res Cent Bull* 1963; 1:39–44.
26. Messerli FH. Cardiopathy of obesity—A not-so-Victorian disease. *N Engl J Med* 1986; 314:378–380.
27. Ku CS, Lin SL, Wang DJ, et al. Left ventricular filling in young normotensive obese adults. *Am J Cardiol* 1994; 73:613–615.
28. Sasson Z, Rasooly Y, Gupta R, Rasooly I. Left atrial enlargement in healthy obese: Prevalence and relation to left ventricular mass and diastolic function. *Can J Cardiol* 1996; 12:257–263.
29. Backman L, Freyschuss U, Hallberg D, Melcher A. Reversibility of cardiovascular changes in extreme obesity: Effects of weight reduction through jejunoileostomy. *Acta Med Scand* 1979; 205:367–373.
30. Backman L, Freyschuss U, Hallberg D, Melcher A. Cardiovascular function in extreme obesity. *Acta Med Scand* 1973; 193: 437–446.
31. Alexander JK, Peterson KL. Cardiovascular effects of weight reduction. *Circulation* 1972; 45:310–318.
32. De Divitiis O, Fazio S, Petitto M, et al. Obesity and cardiac function. *Circulation* 1981; 64:477–482.
33. Nakajima T, Fujioka S, Tokunaga K, et al. Correlation of intraabdominal fat accumulation and left ventricular performance in obesity. *Am J Cardiol* 1989; 64:369–373.
34. Cheyne J. A case of apoplexy in which the fleshy part of the heart was converted into fat. *Dublin Hosp Rep* 1818; 2:216–223.
35. Maxwell MH, Waks AU, Schroth PC, et al. Error in blood-pressure measurement due to incorrect cuff size in obese patients. *Lancet* 1982; 2:33–36.
36. Nelson WP, North RL. Splitting of the second heart sound in adults forty years and older. *Am J Med Sci* 1967; 254:805–807.
37. Pringle TH, Scobie IN, Murray RG, et al. Prolongation of the QT interval during therapeutic starvation: A substrate for malignant arrhythmias. *Int J Obes* 1983; 7:253–261.
38. Sandhofer F, Dienstl F, Bolzano K, Schwingshackl H. Severe cardiovascular complication associated with prolonged starvation. *Br Med J* 1973; 1:462–463.
39. Garnett ES, Barnard DL, Ford J, et al. Gross fragmentation of cardiac myofibrils after therapeutic starvation for obesity. *Lancet* 1969; 1:914–916.
40. Rasmussen LH, Andersen T. The relationship between QTc changes and nutrition during weight loss after gastroplasty. *Acta Med Scand* 1985; 217:271–275.
41. Pidlich J, Pfeffel F, Zwiauer K, et al. The effect of weight reduction on the surface electrocardiogram: A prospective trial in obese children and adolescents. *Int J Obes Relat Metab Disord* 1997; 21:1018–1023.
42. Eisenstein I, Edelstein J, Sarma R, et al. The electrocardiogram in obesity. *J Electrocardiol* 1982; 15:115–118.
43. Sours HE, Frattali VP, Brand CD, et al. Sudden death associated with very low calorie weight reduction regimens. *Am J Clin Nutr* 1981; 34:453–461.
44. Isner JM, Sours HE, Paris AL, et al. Sudden, unexpected death in avid dieters using the liquid-protein-modified-fast diet: Observations in 17 patients and the role of the prolonged QT interval. *Circulation* 1979; 60:1401–1412.
45. Frank S, Colliver JA, Frank A. The electrocardiogram in obesity: Statistical analysis of 1,029 patients. *J Am Coll Cardiol* 1986; 7:295–299.
46. Starr JW, Wagner GS, Behar VS, et al. Vectorcardiographic criteria for the diagnosis of inferior myocardial infarction. *Circulation* 1974; 49:829–836.
47. Master AM, Oppenheimer ET. A study of obesity: Circulatory, roentgen-ray and electrocardiographic investigations. *JAMA* 1929; 92:1652–1656.
48. Benjamin EJ, Levy D. Why is left ventricular hypertrophy so predictive of morbidity and mortality? *Am J Med Sci* 1999; 317:168–175.
49. Casale PN, Devereux RB, Kligfield P, et al. Electrocardiographic detection of left ventricular hypertrophy: Development and prospective validation of improved criteria. *J Am Coll Cardiol* 1985; 6:572–580.
50. Abergel E, Tase M, Menard J, Chatellier G. Influence of obesity on the diagnostic value of electrocardiographic criteria for detecting left ventricular hypertrophy. *Am J Cardiol* 1996; 77: 739–744.
51. Alpert MA, Lambert CR, Terry BE, et al. Effect of weight loss on left ventricular mass in nonhypertensive morbidly obese patients. *Am J Cardiol* 1994; 73:918–921.
52. Chakko S, Mayor M, Allison MD, et al. Abnormal left ventricular

diastolic filling in eccentric left ventricular hypertrophy of obesity. *Am J Cardiol* 1991; 68:95–98.

53. Alpert MA, Lambert CR, Terry BE, et al. Effect of weight loss on left ventricular diastolic filling in morbid obesity. *Am J Cardiol* 1995; 76:1198–1201.
54. Rakowski H, Appleton C, Chan KL, et al. Canadian consensus recommendations for the measurement and reporting of diastolic dysfunction by echocardiography: From the Investigators of Consensus on Diastolic Dysfunction by Echocardiography. *J Am Soc Echocardiogr* 1996; 9:736–760.
55. Dumesnil JG, Gaudreault G, Honos GN, Kingma JG Jr. Use of Valsalva maneuver to unmask left ventricular diastolic function abnormalities by Doppler echocardiography in patients with coronary artery disease or systemic hypertension. *Am J Cardiol* 1991; 68:515–519.
56. House AA, Walley VM. Right heart failure due to ventricular adiposity: "Adipositas cordis"—An old diagnosis revisited. *Can J Cardiol* 1996; 12:485–489.
57. Jornet A, Batalla J, Uson M, et al. Lipomatous hypertrophy of the interatrial septum. *Echocardiography* 1992; 9:501–503.
58. Levy D, Savage DD, Garrison RJ, et al. Echocardiographic criteria for left ventricular hypertrophy: The Framingham Heart Study. *Am J Cardiol* 1987; 59:956–960.
59. Levy D, Anderson KM, Savage DD, et al. Echocardiographically detected left ventricular hypertrophy: Prevalence and risk factors: The Framingham Heart Study. *Ann Intern Med* 1988; 108:7–13.
60. De Simone G, Daniels SR, Devereux RB, et al. Left ventricular mass and body size in normotensive children and adults: Assessment of allometric relations and impact of overweight. *J Am Coll Cardiol* 1992; 20:1251–1260.
61. Lauer MS, Anderson KM, Larson MG, Levy D. A new method for indexing left ventricular mass for differences in body size. *Am J Cardiol* 1994; 74:487–491.
62. Hense HW, Gneiting B, Muscholl M, et al. The associations of body size and body composition with left ventricular mass: Impacts for indexation in adults. *J Am Coll Cardiol* 1998; 32:451–457.
63. Alaud-din A, Meterissian S, Lisbona R, et al. Assessment of cardiac function in patients who were morbidly obese. *Surgery* 1990; 108:809–818.
64. Gal RA, Gunasekera J, Massardo T, et al. Long-term prognostic value of a normal dipyridamole thallium-201 perfusion scan. *Clin Cardiol* 1991; 14:971–974.
65. Ferraro S, Perrone-Filardi P, Desiderio A, et al. Left ventricular systolic and diastolic function in severe obesity: A radionuclide study. *Cardiology* 1996; 87:347–353.
66. Prvulovich EM, Lonn AH, Bomanji JB, et al. Transmission scanning for attenuation correction of myocardial 201TI images in obese patients. *Nucl Med Commun* 1997; 18:207–218.
67. Barnden LR, Ong PL, Rowe CC. Simultaneous emission transmission tomography using technetium-99m for both emission and transmission. *Eur J Nucl Med* 1997; 24:1390–1397.
68. Barbeau GR, Gleeton O, Juneau C, et al. Transradial approach for coronary angiography and interventions: Procedural results and vascular complications from a series of 7049 procedures. *Circulation* 1999; 100:I-306.
69. Lemieux S, Després JP. Metabolic complications of visceral obesity: Contribution to the aetiology of type 2 diabetes and implications for prevention and treatment. *Diabetes Metab* 1994; 20:375–393.
70. Svendsen OL, Hassager C, Christiansen C, et al. Plasminogen activator inhibitor-1, tissue-type plasminogen activator, and fibrinogen: Effect of dieting with or without exercise in overweight postmenopausal women. *Arterioscler Thromb Vasc Biol* 1996; 16:381–385.
71. Folsom AR, Qamhieh HT, Wing RR, et al. Impact of weight loss on plasminogen activator inhibitor (PAI-1), factor VII, and other hemostatic factors in moderately overweight adults. *Arterioscler Thromb* 1993; 13:162–169.
72. Licata G, Scaglione R, Avellone G, et al. Hemostatic function in young subjects with central obesity: Relationship with left ventricular function. *Metabolism* 1995; 44:1417–1421.
73. Pouliot MC, Després JP, Lemieux S, et al. Waist circumference and abdominal sagittal diameter: Best simple anthropometric indexes of abdominal visceral adipose tissue accumulation and related cardiovascular risk in men and women. *Am J Cardiol* 1994; 73:460–468.
74. Després JP. Dyslipidaemia and obesity. *Baillieres Clin Endocrinol Metab* 1994; 8:629–660.
75. Westlund K, Nicolaysen R. Ten-year mortality and morbidity related to serum cholesterol: A follow-up of 3751 men aged 40–49. *Scand J Clin Lab Invest* 1972; 127:1–24.
76. Lew EA, Garfinkel L. Variations in mortality by weight among 750,000 men and women. *J Chronic Dis* 1979; 32:563–576.
77. Larsson B, Bjorntorp P, Tibblin G. The health consequences of moderate obesity. *Int J Obes* 1981; 5:97–116.
78. Colditz GA, Willett WC, Rotnitzky A, Manson JE. Weight gain as a risk factor for clinical diabetes mellitus in women. *Ann Intern Med* 1995; 122:481–486.
79. Chan JM, Rimm EB, Colditz GA, et al. Obesity, fat distribution, and weight gain as risk factors for clinical diabetes in men. *Diabetes Care* 1994; 17:961–969.
80. Sparrow D, Borkan GA, Gerzof SG, et al. Relationship of fat distribution to glucose tolerance: Results of computed tomography in male participants of the Normative Aging Study. *Diabetes* 1986; 35:411–415.
81. Balkau B, Shipley M, Jarrett RJ, et al. High blood glucose concentration is a risk factor for mortality in middle-aged nondiabetic men: 20-year follow-up in the Whitehall Study, the Paris Prospective Study, and the Helsinki Policemen Study. *Diabetes Care* 1998; 21:360–367.
82. Meigs JB, Nathan DM, Wilson PW, et al. Metabolic risk factors worsen continuously across the spectrum of nondiabetic glucose tolerance: The Framingham Offspring Study. *Ann Intern Med* 1998; 128:524–533.
83. Fuller JH, Shipley MJ, Rose G, et al. Mortality from coronary heart disease and stroke in relation to degree of glycaemia: The Whitehall study. *Br Med J* 1983; 287:867–870.
84. Després JP, Lamarche B, Mauriège P, et al. Hyperinsulinemia as an independent risk factor for ischemic heart disease. *N Engl J Med* 1996; 334:952–957.
85. Korpilahti K, Syvanne M, Engblom E, et al. Components of the insulin resistance syndrome are associated with progression of atherosclerosis in non-grafted arteries 5 years after coronary artery bypass surgery. *Eur Heart J* 1998; 19:711–719.
86. Eckel RH, Yost TJ. HDL subfractions and adipose tissue metabolism in the reduced-obese state. *Am J Physiol* 1989; 256:E740–E746.
87. Eckel RH. The importance of timing and accurate interpretation of the benefits of weight reduction on plasma lipids. *Obes Res* 1999; 7:170–178.
88. Poirier P, Catellier C, Tremblay A, Nadeau A. Role of body fat loss in the exercise-induced improvement of the plasma lipid profile in non-insulin-dependent diabetes mellitus. *Metabolism* 1996; 45:1383–1387.
89. Willett WC, Manson JE, Stampfer MJ, et al. Weight, weight change, and coronary heart disease in women: Risk within the "normal" weight range. *JAMA* 1995; 273:461–465.
90. Shaper AG, Wannamethee SG, Walker M. Body weight: Implications for the prevention of coronary heart disease, stroke and diabetes mellitus in a cohort study of middle aged men. *Br Med J* 1997; 314:1311–1317.
91. ECAT angina pectoris study: Baseline associations of haemostatic factors with extent of coronary arteriosclerosis and other

coronary risk factors in 3000 patients with angina pectoris undergoing coronary angiography. *Eur Heart J* 1993; 14:8–17.
92. Stamler R, Stamler J, Riedlinger WF, et al. Weight and blood pressure: Findings in hypertension screening of 1 million Americans. *JAMA* 1978; 240:1607–1610.
93. Lauer MS, Anderson KM, Kannel WB, Levy D. The impact of obesity on left ventricular mass and geometry: The Framingham Heart Study. *JAMA* 1991; 266:231–236.
94. MacMahon SW, Wilcken DE, Macdonald GJ. The effect of weight reduction on left ventricular mass: A randomized controlled trial in young, overweight hypertensive patients. *N Engl J Med* 1986; 314:334–339.
95. Himeno E, Nishino K, Nakashima Y, et al. Weight reduction regresses left ventricular mass regardless of blood pressure level in obese subjects. *Am Heart J* 1996; 131:313–319.
96. Executive summary of the clinical guidelines on the identification, evaluation, and treatment of overweight and obesity in adults. *Arch Intern Med* 1998; 158:1855–1867.
97. Reisin E, Frohlich ED, Messerli FH, et al. Cardiovascular changes after weight reduction in obesity hypertension. *Ann Intern Med* 1983; 98:315–319.
98. Tuck ML, Sowers J, Dornfeld L, et al. The effect of weight reduction on blood pressure, plasma renin activity, and plasma aldosterone levels in obese patients. *N Engl J Med* 1981; 304:930–933.
99. Tuck ML, Sowers JR, Dornfeld L, et al. Reductions in plasma catecholamines and blood pressure during weight loss in obese subjects. *Acta Endocrinol (Copenh)* 1983; 102:252–257.
100. Alexander JK. Obesity and the circulation. *Mod Concepts Cardiovasc Dis* 1963; 32:799–803.
101. Frohlich ED, Messerli FH, Reisin E, Dunn FG. The problem of obesity and hypertension. *Hypertension* 1983; 5:III71–III78.
102. Messerli FH. Cardiovascular effects of obesity and hypertension. *Lancet* 1982; 1:1165–1168.
103. Alpert MA, Lambert CR, Panayiotou H, et al. Relation of duration of morbid obesity to left ventricular mass, systolic function, and diastolic filling, and effect of weight loss. *Am J Cardiol* 1995; 76:1194–1197.
104. Duflou J, Virmani R, Rabin I, et al. Sudden death as a result of heart disease in morbid obesity. *Am Heart J* 1995; 130:306–313.
105. Caviezel F, Margonato A, Slaviero G, et al. Early improvement of left ventricular function during caloric restriction in obesity. *Int J Obes* 1986; 10:421–426.
106. Amad KH, Brennan JC, Alexander JK. The cardiac pathology of chronic exogenous obesity. *Circulation* 1965; 32:740–745.
107. Drenick EJ, Fisler JS. Sudden cardiac arrest in morbidly obese surgical patients unexplained after autopsy. *Am J Surg* 1988; 155:720–726.
108. Messerli FH, Sundgaard-Riise K, Reisin ED, et al. Dimorphic cardiac adaptation to obesity and arterial hypertension. *Ann Intern Med* 1983; 99:757–761.
109. Smith HL, Willius FA. Adiposity of the heart: A clinical and pathologic study of one hundred and thirty-six obese patients. *Arch Intern Med* 1933; 52:911–931.
110. Sasson Z, Rasooly Y, Bhesania T, Rasooly I. Insulin resistance is an important determinant of left ventricular mass in the obese. *Circulation* 1993; 88:1431–1436.
111. Strollo PJJ, Rogers RM. Obstructive sleep apnea. *N Engl J Med* 1996; 334:99–104.
112. Vgontzas AN, Tan TL, Bixler EO, et al. Sleep apnea and sleep disruption in obese patients. *Arch Intern Med* 1994; 154:1705–1711.
113. Bearpark H, Elliott L, Grunstein R, et al. Snoring and sleep apnea: A population study in Australian men. *Am J Respir Crit Care Med* 1995; 151:1459–1465.
114. Young T, Palta M, Dempsey J, et al. The occurrence of sleep-disordered breathing among middle-aged adults. *N Engl J Med* 1993; 328:1230–1235.
115. Narkiewicz K, van de Borne PJ, Cooley RL, et al. Sympathetic activity in obese subjects with and without obstructive sleep apnea. *Circulation* 1998; 98:772–776.
116. Viner S, Szalai JP, Hoffstein V. Are history and physical examination a good screening test for sleep apnea? *Ann Intern Med* 1991; 115:356–359.
117. Partinen M, Jamieson A, Guilleminault C. Long-term outcome for obstructive sleep apnea syndrome patients: Mortality. *Chest* 1988; 94:1200–1204.
118. Kessler R, Chaouat A, Weitzenblum E, et al. Pulmonary hypertension in the obstructive sleep apnoea syndrome: Prevalence, causes and therapeutic consequences. *Eur Respir J* 1996; 9:787–794.
119. Laaban JP, Cassuto D, Orvoen-Frija E, et al. Cardiorespiratory consequences of sleep apnoea syndrome in patients with massive obesity. *Eur Respir J* 1998; 11:20–27.
120. Phillipson EA. Sleep apnea—A major public health problem. *N Engl J Med* 1993; 328:1271–1273.
121. Peterson HR, Rothschild M, Weinberg CR, et al. Body fat and the activity of the autonomic nervous system. *N Engl J Med* 1988; 318:1077–1083.
122. Scherrer U, Randin D, Tappy L, et al. Body fat and sympathetic nerve activity in healthy subjects. *Circulation* 1994; 89:2634–2640.
123. Hirsch J, Leibel RL, Mackintosh R, Aguirre A. Heart rate variability as a measure of autonomic function during weight change in humans. *Am J Physiol* 1991; 261:R1418–R1423.
124. Vaz M, Jennings G, Turner A, et al. Regional sympathetic nervous activity and oxygen consumption in obese normotensive human subjects. *Circulation* 1997; 96:3423–3429.
125. Carlson JT, Hedner J, Elam M, et al. Augmented resting sympathetic activity in awake patients with obstructive sleep apnea. *Chest* 1993; 103:1763–1768.
126. Kannel WB, Plehn JF, Cupples LA. Cardiac failure and sudden death in the Framingham Study. *Am Heart J* 1988; 115:869–875.
127. Alexander JK. The cardiomyopathy of obesity. *Prog Cardiovasc Dis* 1985; 27:325–334.
128. El-Gamal A, Gallagher D, Nawras A, et al. Effects of obesity on QT, RR, and QTc intervals. *Am J Cardiol* 1995; 75:956–959.
129. Lantigua RA, Amatruda JM, Biddle TL, et al. Cardiac arrhythmias associated with a liquid protein diet for the treatment of obesity. *N Engl J Med* 1980; 303:735–738.
130. Singh BN, Gaarder TD, Kanegae T, et al. Liquid protein diets and torsade de pointes. *JAMA* 1978; 240:115–119.
131. Birkmeyer NJ, Charlesworth DC, Hernandez F, et al. Obesity and risk of adverse outcomes associated with coronary artery bypass surgery: Northern New England Cardiovascular Disease Study Group. *Circulation* 1998; 97:1689–1694.
132. Moulton MJ, Creswell LL, Mackey ME, et al. Obesity is not a risk factor for significant adverse outcomes after cardiac surgery. *Circulation* 1996; 94:II87–II92.
133. Marik P, Varon J. The obese patient in the ICU. *Chest* 1998; 113:492–498.
134. Rose DK, Cohen MM, Wigglesworth DF, DeBoer DP. Critical respiratory events in the postanesthesia care unit: Patient, surgical, and anesthetic factors. *Anesthesiology* 1994; 81:410–418.
135. Roberts WC, Roberts JD. The floating heart or the heart too fat to sink: Analysis of 55 necropsy patients. *Am J Cardiol* 1983; 52:1286–1289.
136. De Scheerder I, Cuvelier C, Verhaaren R, et al. Restrictive cardiomyopathy caused by adipositas cordis. *Eur Heart J* 1987; 8:661–663.
137. Carpenter CL. Myocardial fat infiltration. *Am Heart J* 1962; 63:491–496.
138. Saphir O, Corrigan M. Fatty infiltration of the myocardium. *Arch Intern Med* 1933; 52:410–428.

139. Balsaver AM, Morales AR, Whitehouse FW. Fat infiltration of myocardium as a cause of cardiac conduction defect. *Am J Cardiol* 1967; 19:261–265.
140. Spain DM, Cathcart RT. Heart block caused by fat infiltration of the interventricular septum (cor adiposum). *Am Heart J* 1946; 32:659–664.
141. Dervan JP, Ilercil A, Kane PB, Anagnostopoulos C. Fatty infiltration: Another restrictive cardiomyopathic pattern. *Cathet Cardiovasc Diagn* 1991; 22:184–189.
142. Wood PD, Stefanick ML, Dreon DM, et al. Changes in plasma lipids and lipoproteins in overweight men during weight loss through dieting as compared with exercise. *N Engl J Med* 1988; 319:1173–1179.
143. Tremblay A, Després JP, Maheux J, et al. Normalization of the metabolic profile in obese women by exercise and a low fat diet. *Med Sci Sports Exerc* 1991; 23:1326–1331.
144. Atkinson RL. Use of drugs in the treatment of obesity. *Annu Rev Nutr* 1997; 17:383–403.
145. Marceau P, Hould FS, Potvin M, et al. Biliopancreatic diversion (doudenal switch procedure). *Eur J Gastroenterol Hepatol* 1999; 11:99–103.
146. Wadden TA, Foster GD, Letizia KA. One-year behavioral treatment of obesity: Comparison of moderate and severe caloric restriction and the effects of weight maintenance therapy. *J Consult Clin Psychol* 1994; 62:165–171.
147. Wadden TA, Sternberg JA, Letizia KA, et al. Treatment of obesity by very low calorie diet, behavior therapy, and their combination: A five-year perspective. *Int J Obes* 1989; 13:39–46.
148. Wadden TA, Stunkard AJ. Controlled trial of very low calorie diet, behavior therapy, and their combination in the treatment of obesity. *J Consult Clin Psychol* 1986; 54:482–488.
149. Perri MG, Nezu AM, Patti ET, McCann KL. Effect of length of treatment on weight loss. *J Consult Clin Psychol* 1989; 57:450–452.
150. Gerace TA, Hollis J, Ockene JK, Svendsen K. Smoking cessation and change in diastolic blood pressure, body weight, and plasma lipids: MRFIT Research Group. *Prev Med* 1991; 20:602–620.
151. Klesges RC, Meyers AW, Klesges LM, La Vasque ME. Smoking, body weight, and their effects on smoking behavior: A comprehensive review of the literature. *Psychol Bull* 1989; 106:204–230.
152. Williamson DF, Madans J, Anda RF, et al. Smoking cessation and severity of weight gain in a national cohort. *N Engl J Med* 1991; 324:739–745.
153. Krauss RM, Deckelbaum RJ, Ernst N, et al. AHA Dietary guidelines for healthy American adults. *Circulation* 1996; 94:1795–1800.
154. Cahill GFJ. Starvation in man. *Clin Endocrinol Metab* 1976; 2:397–415.
155. McGuire MT, Wing RR, Klem ML, Hill JO. Behavioral strategies of individuals who have maintained long-term weight losses. *Obes Res* 1999; 4:334–341.
156. Doucet E, Imbeault P, Almeras N, Tremblay A. Physical activity and low-fat diet: Is it enough to maintain weight stability in the reduced-obese individual following weight loss by drug therapy and energy restriction? *Obes Res* 1999; 4:323–333.
157. Tremblay A, Doucet E, Imbeault P, et al. Metabolic fitness in active reduced-obese individuals. *Obes Res* 1999; 6:556–563.
158. Lee CD, Blair SN, Jackson AS. Cardiorespiratory fitness, body composition, and all-cause and cardiovascular disease mortality in men. *Am J Clin Nutr* 1999; 69:373–380.
159. Pate RR, Pratt M, Blair SN, et al. Physical activity and public health: A recommendation from the Centers for Disease Control and Prevention and the American College of Sports Medicine. *JAMA* 1995; 273:402–407.
160. From the Centers for Disease Control and Prevention. Cardiac valvulopathy associated with exposure to fenfluramine or dexfenfluramine: US Department of Health and Human Services interim public health recommendations. *JAMA* 1997; 278:1729–1731.
161. Connolly HM, Crary JL, McGoon MD, et al. Valvular heart disease associated with fenfluramine-phentermine. *N Engl J Med* 1997; 337:581–588.
162. Weissman NJ, Tighe JFJ, Gottdiener JS, Gwynne JT. An assessment of heart-valve abnormalities in obese patients taking dexfenfluramine, sustained-release dexfenfluramine, or placebo: Sustained-Release Dexfenfluramine Study Group. *N Engl J Med* 1998; 339:725–732.
163. Khan MA, Herzog CA, St Peter JV, et al. The prevalence of cardiac valvular insufficiency assessed by transthoracic echocardiography in obese patients treated with appetite-suppressant drugs. *N Engl J Med* 1998; 339:713–718.
164. Abenhaim L, Moride Y, Brenot F, et al. Appetite-suppressant drugs and the risk of primary pulmonary hypertension: International Primary Pulmonary Hypertension Study Group. *N Engl J Med* 1996; 335:609–616.
165. Robiolio PA, Rigolin VH, Wilson JS, et al. Carcinoid heart disease: Correlation of high serotonin levels with valvular abnormalities detected by cardiac catheterization and echocardiography. *Circulation* 1995; 92:790–795.
166. Redfield MM, Nicholson WJ, Edwards WD, Tajik AJ. Valve disease associated with ergot alkaloid use: Echocardiographic and pathologic correlations. *Ann Intern Med* 1992; 117:50–52.
167. Ryan DH, Bray GA, Helmcke F, et al. Serial echocardiographic and clinical evaluation of valvular regurgitation before, during, and after treatment with fenfluramine or dexfenfluramine and mazindol or phentermine. *Obes Res* 1999; 7:313–322.
168. Jick H, Vasilakis C, Weinrauch LA, et al. A population-based study of appetite-suppressant drugs and the risk of cardiac-valve regurgitation. *N Engl J Med* 1998; 339:719–724.
169. Cannistra LB, Cannistra AJ. Regression of multivalvular regurgitation after the cessation of fenfluramine and phentermine treatment. *N Engl J Med* 1998; 339:771.
170. McNeely W, Goa KL. Sibutramine: A review of its contribution to the management of obesity. *Drugs* 1998; 5:1093–1244.
171. Bach DS, Rissanen AM, Mendel CM, et al. Absence of cardiac valve dysfunction in obese patients treated with sibutramine. *Obes Res* 1999; 7:363–369.
172. Zhi J, Mulligan TE, Hauptman JB. Long-term systemic exposure of orlistat, a lipase inhibitor, and its metabolites in obese patients. *J Clin Pharmacol* 1999; 39:41–46.
173. Melia AT, Koss-Twardy SG, Zhi J. The effect of orlistat, an inhibitor of dietary fat absorption, on the absorption of vitamins A and E in healthy volunteers. *J Clin Pharmacol* 1996; 36: 647–653.

CHAPTER 84

THE HEART AND KIDNEY DISEASE

Stephen O. Pastan / William E. Mitch

Almost half of deaths in end-stage renal disease (ESRD) patients treated with chronic dialysis in the United States are caused by cardiovascular disease; acute myocardial infarctions cause 20.8 deaths per 1000 patient-years.[1,2] The cardiovascular mortality rate in ESRD patients on dialysis is approximately 10 to 20 times higher than it is in the general population (see Fig. 84-1).[3]

Specific risk factors for coronary artery disease and cardiovascular morbidity in dialysis patients include the high prevalence of hypertension and diabetes mellitus, hyperlipidemia, hypotension during hemodialysis, and abnormalities in calcium and phosphate metabolism causing hyperparathyroidism with vascular calcification. Pericardial disease, infective endocarditis, and fluid and electrolyte disturbances can also contribute significantly to cardiac dysfunction in ESRD.

CARDIOVASCULAR RISK FACTORS IN CHRONICALLY UREMIC PATIENTS

Systemic Arterial Hypertension

Some 60 to 90 percent of patients with progressive chronic renal failure develop systemic hypertension before beginning dialysis therapy.[4] Both an expanded extracellular fluid volume (ECV)[5,6] and vasoconstriction, mediated by sympathetic overactivity and by the renin-angiotensin axis,[6–9] play roles in the pathogenesis of hypertension in patients with kidney disease, including those with ESRD.

Hypertension due to sodium retention with ECV expansion in kidney disease (and especially, ESRD) is associated with an increased cardiac output and generally an increased total peripheral vascular resistance.[10] This differs from the situation in hypertensive subjects with normal renal function, who usually have a normal cardiac output and a high peripheral resistance (see Chap. 51). The difference may be related to anemia, which causes a secondary increase in cardiac output. Echocardiographic evidence of left ventricular hypertrophy, which results from hypertension and a contribution from anemia, is found in over 50 percent of dialysis patients.

Direct evidence that ECV expansion plays a critical role in the hypertension of chronic renal failure is found in studies demonstrating rapid resolution of hypertension in most patients when the ECV is reduced by diuretics or vigorous dialysis.[6,7,11] This is not the sole cause, because a small group (10 to 20 percent) of ESRD patients exhibit dialysis-resistant hypertension with high levels of plasma renin activity. Control of their hypertension requires drugs inhibiting the renin-angiotensin axis, but some patients may require bilateral nephrectomy.[6,12]

The mechanisms for arterial vasoconstriction may be more complicated than activation of the renin system alone. It has been proposed that circulating inhibitors of Na^+-K^+-ATPase increase peripheral vascular resistance by causing an increase in intracellular sodium, resulting in an increase in intracellular calcium and, hence, contraction of vascular smooth muscle cells.[13,14] Overactivity of the sympathetic nervous system has also been observed in chronic renal failure. This increase in activity is reversed by nephrectomy,[15] suggesting it is mediated by an afferent signal from the kidneys. Enalapril was shown to reduce sympathetic hyperactivity in patients with chronic renal failure,[8] implying this afferent signal is mediated by the renin-angiotensin system, possibly through activation of cerebral circumventricular receptors by angiotensin II.[16] Other proposed mechanisms causing hypertension in patients with chronic renal failure include a decrease in the production of vasodilator prostaglandins[17] or nitric oxide, an increase in the levels of plasma endothelin, a vasoconstrictor,[18] and hyperparathyroidism.[19]

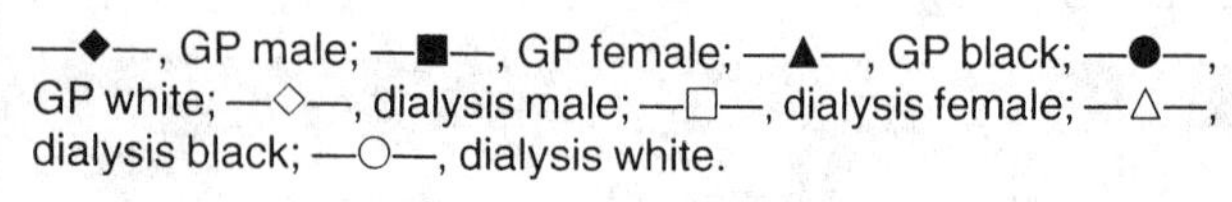

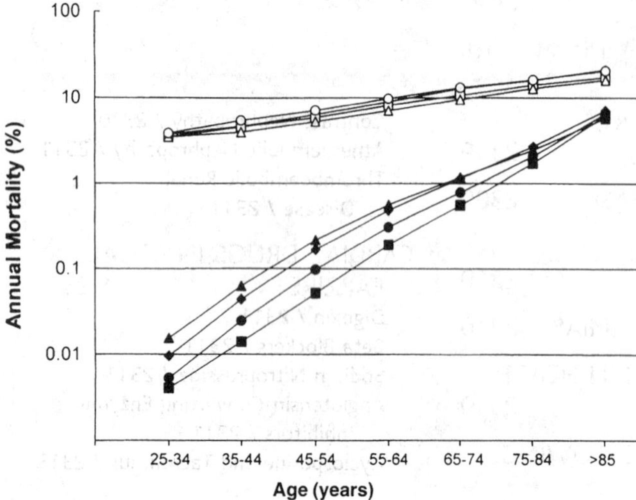

FIGURE 84-1 Cardiovascular mortality defined by death due to arrhythmias, cardiomyopathy, cardiac arrest, myocardial infarction, atherosclerotic heart disease, and pulmonary edema in the general population (GP) compared to ESRD treated by dialysis. Data is stratified by age, race, and gender. [Reproduced with permission from the *American Journal of Kidney Diseases* 1998; 32(5):(Suppl 3):S115, Fig. 1; Copyright © 1998 by the National Kidney Foundation.]

The use of recombinant human erythropoietin (EPO) to correct the anemia associated with ESRD worsens hypertension in approximately 20 to 30 percent of dialysis patients.[20] The proposed mechanism is that increasing hemoglobin is associated with a decline in cardiac output and an increase in peripheral vascular resistance; there may also be an increase in blood viscosity.[21]

The most common reason for *dialysis-resistant* hypertension is ECV expansion because of inadequate fluid removal by dialysis and ultrafiltration. Consequently, the cornerstone of managing hypertension in dialysis patients must be a reduction in the ECV to obtain a true "dry weight." The dry weight of a dialysis patient is defined as that weight at which there is no ECV expansion (e.g., edema or effusions), but there is a normal blood pressure. Unfortunately, this goal is difficult to achieve because patients become symptomatically hypotensive or develop leg cramps before the dry weight is achieved. Consequently, antihypertensive drugs are often required.

In patients who have persistent hypertension despite ECV depletion, antihypertensive medications that inhibit the renin-angiotensin axis [beta blockers or angiotensin converting enzyme (ACE) inhibitors] are the logical choice because of their "cardioprotective" properties. If these are ineffective, calcium channel blockers, clonidine or minoxidil, can be used but only after the ECV has been reduced. The dosage of antihypertensive drugs should be adjusted for the degree of renal failure: generally, antihypertensive drugs are withheld on the day of hemodialysis to prevent hypotension from occurring. Bilateral nephrectomy is occassionally used to treat dialysis-resistant hypertension.[22]

Diabetes Mellitus

Approximately 30 percent of all patients who begin maintenance dialysis therapy have diabetes. They have a significantly higher mortality rate than age-matched patients who do not have diabetes. The most significant factor contributing to their high death rate is coronary artery disease[2] (see also Chap. 78).

Hyperlipidemia

Hyperlipidemia is more common in patients with chronic renal failure than it is in the general population, but the types of abnormalities vary.[23] An elevated low density lipoprotein is common in nephrotic patients, as well as in those treated with chronic ambulatory peritoneal dialysis (CAPD) or patients with a renal transplant and the degree of LDL elevation is correlated with the tendency for cardiovascular disease. Hypertriglyceridemia is the most common lipid abnormality in patients with chronic renal failure or ESRD patients and is often found in association with a low HDL (but may occur in the absence of an elevated LDL).[23] Impaired degradation of very low density lipoprotein by lipoprotein lipase appears to be the major mechanism causing hypertriglyceridemia.[24] In patients treated with chronic ambulatory peritoneal dialysis, the high concentration of glucose in the dialysate worsens the serum triglyceride level because glucose increases the production of triglycerides.[25] About 50 to 80 percent of patients undergoing renal transplantation develop hypercholesterolemia.[23]

Other factors that may contribute to hyperlipidemia in patients with chronic renal failure or ESRD patients include the use of diuretics and beta blockers,[26,27] and possibly carnitine deficiency.[28] Heparin, given to prevent clotting within the dialyzer cartridge, will cause a transient fall in serum triglycerides by increasing the activity of lipoprotein lipase.[29] In order to standardize the measurement of plasma lipids, the blood sample should be obtained after a 12-h fast and before the patient is given heparin for dialysis.

At present, there is no definite evidence that lowering plasma triglycerides improves survival.[30] Strategies for lowering triglycerides and LDL cholesterol include restricting dietary fat, exercise, giving fish-oil supplements, and avoiding alcohol or treatment with beta blockers or diuretics[26,27,31–33] (see Chap. 38). The 3-hydroxy-3-methylglutaryl coenzyme A (HMG-CoA) reductase inhibitors are the preferred agents for drug therapy of triglycerides and LDL-cholesterol. They appear to be safe in ESRD patients but the dose must be reduced for patients taking cyclosporine or tacrolimus after renal transplantation. Clofibrate or gemfibrozil may be effective, but their use has been associated with an increased incidence of myositis and hepatotoxicity in dialysis patients (see Chap 38). Again, it is particularly important to adjust the dosage for the degree of renal failure; for instance, clofibrate should be reduced to 25 to 50 percent of the usual dose. Although definitive evidence that drug treatment prevents atherosclerosis in dialysis patients is lacking, attempts at treatment seem prudent.[31] The National Cholesterol Education Program Adult Treatment Panel guidelines are recommended for classifying and treating lipid abnormalities in patients with chronic renal disease.[34]

Homocysteine

Plasma levels of homocysteine are often elevated in patients with chronic renal failure (see Fig. 84-2). The exact mechanism

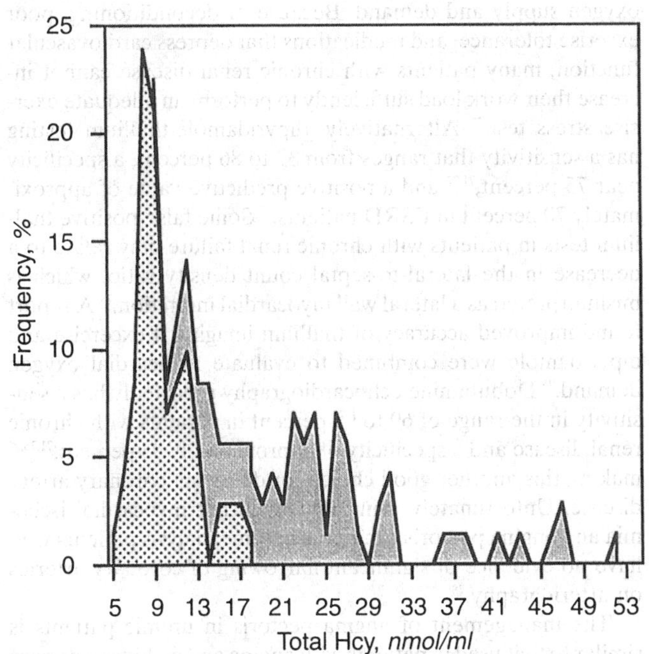

FIGURE 84-2 Distributions of fasting total homocysteine levels in ($N = 71$) dialysis-dependent ESRD patients; and ($N = 71$) age, sex, and race matched Framingham Offspring/Omni Study controls free of renal disease with serum creatinine levels <1.5 mg/dL. Symbols are: (▩) control; (■) ESRD. [Reproduced with permission from *Kidney International* 1997; 52(1):13, Fig. 2; Copyright © 1997 by the International Society of Nephrology.]

of homocysteine elevation is unknown, although reduced renal clearance appears to play a role.[35-37] Preliminary studies indicate that homocysteine is a risk factor for cardiovascular morbidity and mortality in patients with ESRD,[38] but larger studies that take into account the influence of other comorbid conditions are needed for confirmation.[36] Supplementation of patients with kidney diseases using folic acid (5 mg per day), vitamin B_{12} (0.4 mg per day) and vitamin B_6 (50 mg per day) can lower homocysteine levels by about 25 percent.[35,36] Such treatments may normalize levels in patients with chronic renal failure, but not in most ESRD patients on dialysis. The benefit of this type of vitamin supplementation on cardiovascular outcomes is not known.

Hemodialysis-Associated Hypotension

Clinically significant hypotension occurs in approximately 25 percent of hemodialysis sessions.[39] Usually, the consequences are minor, but acute myocardial and cerebral ischemia can occur. Excessive ultrafiltration and ECV depletion is the most common cause of hypotension during dialysis due to reduced cardiac output.[40] Rapid lowering of plasma osmolality during the removal of urea and other molecules also causes a shift of fluid from the ECV to the intracellular compartment, as these molecules do not move out of cells as rapidly as dialysis removes them from blood.[41,42] Finally, diffusion of acetate from an acetate-based dialysate into the patient can cause vasodilatation that interferes with the hemodynamic vasoconstriction that should occur when ECV is reduced.

The concentration of sodium in the dialysate is an important factor governing changes in plasma osmolality. Dialyzers currently in use can achieve high rates of fluid removal (i.e., ultrafiltration) but even so, a higher concentration of sodium in the dialysate can reduce the number of hypotensive episodes by removing more fluid from the intracellular compartment.[43]

Hypotension can occur when complement is activated by the dialyzer membranes leading to intrapulmonary shunting of blood and hypoxemia. This response is most often observed with cuprophane dialyzer membranes[44]; newer dialysis membranes cause less activation of the complement cascade.[45] Hypersensitivity to ethylene oxide, which is used to sterilize dialyzers, can also cause hypotension and, rarely, anaphylaxis.[46] Finally, ACE inhibitors may be associated with profound hypotension when polyacrylonitrile dialysis membranes are used because this membrane has a high negative surface charge that stabilizes enzymes that generate bradykinin.[47] Since ACE inhibitors block kininases, the high levels of bradykinin cause anaphylactoid reactions.

Other factors favoring hypotension during hemodialysis include (1) cardiac dysfunction from long-standing hypertension, ischemic or valvular heart disease, cardiomyopathy, or pericardial tamponade; (2) a rapid reduction in serum potassium and calcium depressing cardiac contractility; (3) autonomic neuropathy (particularly in diabetic patients); (4) sepsis; (5) occult hemorrhage (e.g., retroperitoneal hemorrhage after femoral vein catheterization to place a dialysis access catheter); (6) eating prior to or during dialysis resulting in splanchnic vasodilation; and (7) use of antihypertensive medications on the day of dialysis. Rarely a patient may develop a paradoxical withdrawal of sympathetic nervous system activity during hemodialysis resulting in a slowing of heart rate and a reduction in systemic vascular resistance and profound hypotension.[48]

To reduce the incidence of hypotension, a high-sodium and bicarbonate-buffered (rather than acetate-buffered) dialysate should be used and the rate and extent of ultrafiltration monitored carefully; antihypertensive medications should be avoided on hemodialysis days. "Sodium Modeling," the practice of lowering an initially hypertonic dialysis solution to isotonic levels during the dialysis session, may reduce the frequency of hypotensive events by offsetting fluid shifts from the ECV (see above).[49] Management of hypotension includes reducing the ultrafiltration rate, placing the patient in the Trendelenburg position, and administering saline through the arteriovenous access. Oxygen administration may be useful in patients with ischemic heart disease. Lowering the dialysate temperature can also reduce the incidence of hypotension in patients who have this reaction repeatedly.[50]

Hyperparathyroidism

Secondary hyperparathyroidism is virtually universal in dialysis patients.[51] Hyperphosphatemia due to the failure to excrete phosphate plays a major role in the pathogenesis of secondary hyperparathyroidism. Hyperphosphatemia reduces the plasma-ionized calcium concentration by direct complexing of calcium with phosphates which stimulates parathyroid hormone secretion. Hyperphosphatemia and the loss of kidney tissue also decrease the activity of 1 -hydroxylase in proximal tubule cells, leading to limited production of 1,25-dihydroxyvitamin D_3, the most active vitamin D analogue.[51,52] Finally, reduced levels of both the vitamin D and calcium receptors have been found in patients with uremic hyperparathyroidism, particularly in areas of nodular hyperplasia.[53,54] Receptor downregulation is likely to play an important role in the abnormal patterns of parathyroid hormone secretion and cellular growth.

All of these factors reduce the level of ionized calcium, which stimulates parathyroid hormone secretion. A deficiency of 1,25-dihydroxyvitamin D_3 also limits the ability of ionized calcium to suppress parathyroid hormone secretion.[55,56]

It is often taught that a high calcium × phosphate product (>60 mg^2/dL^2) is an independent risk factor for mortality and morbidity,[62] but it is almost certain that the pathophysiologic mechanism is due solely to a high serum phosphorus level. When the serum phosphorous level is high, the risk of vascular and soft tissue calcification rises sharply.[57,58] Calcification can occur in coronary and peripheral arteries[59] and in the myocardium.[60] Extensive valvular calcification can also impair native or prosthetic valve function.[61] Finally, it has been proposed that parathyroid hormone itself can directly impair myocardial function,[62] but not all investigators agree.[63]

Prevention or treatment of secondary hyperparathyroidism must be based on correcting hyperphosphatemia. This can be accomplished only if patients adhere to a diet containing less than 1 g of phosphorus per day. But even with compliance, many patients will need to take phosphate binders after meals. Calcium carbonate or calcium acetate are the preferred agents, because they also increase calcium intake and avoid the risk of aluminum toxicity (including aluminum-induced osteomalacia, anemia, and encephalopathy). Another agent, RenaGel, a non-calcium non-aluminum containing phosphorus binder, shows promise for the management of hyperphosphatemia.[64] If hypocalcemia persists and serum phosphorus is normal (especially if there is evidence of secondary hyperparathyroidism) intravenous administration of 1,25-dihydroxyvitamin D_3 (calcitriol) can be useful therapeutically. Vitamin D can also be given orally, but with somewhat greater risk of hypercalcemia. Vitamin D analogues, such as 19-Nor-1,25-dihydroxyvitamin D_2 (paricalcitol) have more specificity for parathyroid tissue and should result in fewer complications of hypercalcemia or worsening hyperphosphatemia.[65] Just as it is rarely necessary to perform bilateral nephrectomy to manage hypertension, subtotal parathyroidectomy should also be rare since severe hyperparathyroidism can be avoided. Prevention of hyperphosphatemia, hypocalcemia, and hyperparathyroidism is critical because hypocalcemia after parathyroidectomy is serious and requires that a patient take many calcium and vitamin D tablets.

ISCHEMIC HEART DISEASE

The prevalence of coronary artery disease approaches 40 percent in ESRD patients.[66] At autopsy, acute myocardial infarctions were noted in about 25 percent of dialysis patients.[67,68] Risk factors for coronary artery disease include smoking, hypertension, left ventricular hypertrophy, insulin-dependent or non-insulin-dependent diabetes mellitus, hyperlipidemia, and hyperparathyroidism[6,23,69] (see also Chap. 38). Factors increasing the risk of myocardial infarction include hypertension, ECV overload, anemia, hypotension and hypoxia during hemodialysis, and increased blood flow through the arteriovenous fistula.[70] These factors adversely affect the balance between myocardial oxygen supply and demand. Because of deconditioning, poor excerise tolerance, and medications that depress cardiovascular function, many patients with chronic renal disease cannot increase their work load sufficiently to perform an adequate exercise stress test.[71] Alternatively, dipyridamole-thallium testing has a sensitivity that ranges from 37 to 86 percent, a specificity near 75 percent,[71,72] and a positive predictive value of approximately 70 percent in ESRD patients.[73] Some false-positive thallium tests in patients with chronic renal failure may relate to a decrease in the lateral-to-septal count density ratio, which is misinterpreted as a lateral wall myocardial infarction.[74] A report found improved accuracy of thallium imaging if excercise and dipyridamole were combined to evaluate myocardial oxygen demand.[75] Dobutamine echocardiography reportedly has a sensitivity in the range of 69 to 95 percent in patients with chronic renal disease and a specificity of approximately 95 percent,[71,76,77] making this another good choice for detecting coronary artery disease. Unfortunately, clinically significant myocardial ischemia and angina pectoris can occur in some dialysis patients who have no evidence of significant narrowing of coronary arteries on arteriography.[78]

The management of angina pectoris in uremic patients is similar to that used in patients with angina and no kidney disease except that drug dosages often have to be reduced (see Chap. 40). Nitrates, beta blockers, and calcium channel blockers are well tolerated but usually are withheld before dialysis to avoid hypotension during the procedure. Exercise tolerance has been shown to improve in hemodialysis patients with coronary artery disease if anemia is corrected with erythropoietin: for this reason, the hematocrit should be maintained above 30 percent.[79] When using erythropoetin, attention must be paid to repleting iron stores and to hypertension as well as ECV overload. Hyperparathyroidism should be prevented for optimal control of coronary artery disease.

Treatment of angina pectoris that develops during hemodialysis includes (1) stopping ultrafiltration to avoid ECV depletion; (2) reducing blood flow through the dialyzer; and (3) administering oxygen. If there is hypotension, the patient should be placed in the Trendelenburg position and saline infused through the venous line before administering sublingual nitroglycerin (which could cause further hypotension). If there is no hypotension, nitroglycerin can be administered immediately but the blood pressure must be monitored repeatedly. Finally, it should be emphasized that changes in serum potassium and ionized calcium during dialysis and between dialysis treatments may complicate interpretation of the ECG. Electrocardiograms obtained during angina while on dialysis can differ from prior tracings taken between dialysis sessions.

In ESRD patients, acute and long-term management of myocardial infarction is similar to that in nonuremic patients except that controlling the degree of changes in ECV is more critical and requires restriction of salt and fluid intake plus judicious ultrafiltration to prevent hemodynamic instability. Hypertension and anemia should be managed as discussed. The concentration of potassium in the dialysate is generally 2 meq/L, but can be raised to 3 to 3.5 meq/L to stabilize serum potassium or prevent arrhythmias in patients receiving digoxin. Dietary potassium must be restricted in all dialysis patients, and potassium infusions must be avoided to prevent hyperkalemia. Patients with kidney disease are particularly prone to developing hyperkalemia and unnecessary dialysis treatments with the cardiovascular stress required should be avoided. The use of antiarrhythmic drugs should be carefully monitored by measuring serum levels.

The decision to perform coronary arteriography is based upon the same criteria as for patients without kidney disease (see Chaps. 40 to 42). However, the dose of contrast dye for kidney patients should be minimized and means taken to prevent loss of residual renal function. This is especially true for diabetic patients or patients with proteinuria. It is not necessary to dialyze patients immediately after arteriography unless there is concern about the consequences of excess fluid or heart failure.

Coronary artery bypass grafting has a mortality rate of approximately 10 percent in dialysis patients,[71,80] as well as an increased perioperative morbidity.[81] These data emphasize the importance of ensuring that there will be improved quality of life after coronary artery bypass grafting before recommending this operation for a dialysis patient. Dialysis should be performed just before cardiac surgery to optimize ECV status and avoid hyperkalemia. Interestingly, percutaneous transluminal coronary angioplasty has an unacceptably high rate of restenosis despite good initial angiographic success.[71,82,83] Therefore it should be reserved for dialysis patients who are not candidates for coronary artery bypass grafting. Preliminary data suggest that coronary stenting may improve coronary patency and survival compared with angioplasty alone.[83]

CONGESTIVE HEART FAILURE

Congestive heart failure accounts for 20 to 30 percent of the mortality occurring in ESRD patients.[3,84] Echocardiograms reveal a high prevalence of "hypertrophic cardiomyopathy" characterized by left ventricular hypertrophy, asymmetric septal hypertrophy, and/or impaired contractility,[85–87] as well as dilated cardiomyopathy.[88] Concentric left ventricular hypertrophy occurs in patients with current or previous systemic hypertension.[89] Risk factors for myocardial failure in dialysis patients include hypertension, persistent ECV expansion, anemia, arteriovenous fistula,[70] ischemic heart disease, metabolic acidosis, electrolyte disturbances (hyperkalemia, hypocalcemia), hyperparathyroidism,[90] and possibly the uremic state itself. Hemodialysis can improve cardiac function dramatically,[91–93] presumably by controlling hypertension, correcting volume overload, removing uremic toxins, and normalizing blood pH and electrolyte levels (particularly, ionized calcium[94] and potassium[95]).

In uremic patients who develop pulmonary edema, the pulmonary capillary pressure is lower than it is in nonuremic patients and is less than the plasma oncotic pressure. Thus, pulmonary capillary permeability must be increased, further complicating management.[96]

The prevention of heart failure in dialysis patients requires strict control of ECV and hypertension. Salt and fluid restriction must be combined with adequate fluid removal by diuretics or dialysis to maintain the patient's weight as close as possible to the estimated "dry weight." Reasons for an erroneous assessment of dry weight include an unsuspected loss of muscle mass (e.g., catabolic weight loss) that is unrecognized because the measured body weight does not change if fluid is retained. Finally, the adverse influence of the arteriovenous fistula can be tested by occluding it and determining whether or not the heart rate slows (Branham's sign). When this occurs, revision of the fistula may be required to decrease excessive blood flow and oxygen demands of the heart.[97]

Management of heart failure includes bed rest and oxygen therapy plus removal of excess fluid by ultrafiltration while excluding other causes of heart failure such as myocardial infarction, arrhythmias, or infective endocarditis. If digitalis is used, appropriate adjustment of dosage and frequent monitoring of plasma levels are necessary.

Left ventricular hypertrophy has been found to improve after using recombinant human erythropoietin to correct anemia in dialysis patients. Left ventricular muscle mass can decrease by an average of 18 percent over 45 weeks as the hematocrit increases to 32 percent.[20] Complete normalization of left ventricular hypertrophy is, however, uncommon, and it is unknown whether a decrease in left ventricular wall thickness will result in improved patient survival.[21,98]

PERICARDIAL DISEASE

Before dialysis was widely available, pericarditis was regarded as a preterminal event in uremic patients. The current incidence of clinically apparent pericarditis has decreased from 50 percent to 5 to 20 percent since the predialysis era.[99,100] The cause of pericarditis in dialysis patients is unknown but may be related to inadequate removal of uremic toxins; coincident diseases such as viral infections,[101] tuberculosis, systemic lupus erythematosus; or to drugs such as minoxidil.[102] Pericarditis appears to occur less frequently in peritoneal dialysis patients than it does in hemodialysis patients. This difference has been attributed to a higher clearance of "middle molecules" by peritoneal dialysis.[103]

The primary treatment for dialysis-associated pericarditis is intensive dialysis (e.g., daily hemodialysis for 1 to 2 weeks) and elimination of heparin in order to avoid pericardial hemorrhage and tamponade. Unfortunately, intensive dialysis for pericarditis can cause hypokalemia, hypophosphatemia, and volume depletion. Besides intensive dialysis, oral or intrapericardial administration of corticosteroids[104,105,112] and indomethacin[106] have been tried. The efficacy of indomethacin is questionable; results from a prospective, double-blind study led to the conclusion that the predominant effect of indomethacin is to reduce fever.[107]

Pericardial effusion frequently complicates pericarditis, but cardiac tamponade is rare; the exact frequency is unknown. An important clue to the development of cardiac tamponade is severe hypotension during dialysis, especially in the absence of volume depletion. Small pericardial effusions are found in 15 to 20 percent of stable, asymptomatic dialysis patients.[108] It is unclear whether or not daily dialysis is beneficial in these patients, but frequent evaluation of the size and hemodynamic importance of the effusion is prudent. Treatment of a large pericardial effusion by intensification of dialysis may result in improvement,[100,101] but if there is no improvement, or if hemodynamic compromise occurs, surgical drainage[100,109–111] of the pericardial effusion by subxiphoid pericardiotomy and creation of a pericardial "window" is the preferred procedure. This can be performed under local anesthesia,[112] and it is usually well tolerated (see Chap. 72). Although pericardiectomy is the definitive treatment for patients with pericarditis and clinically significant effusion, this more invasive procedure is not usually necessary.[100]

Constrictive pericarditis is rare in dialysis patients, even those with pericarditis.[113] It should be suspected when there is intractable right-sided heart failure in patients with a normal-sized or small heart. Cardiac catheterization will verify the diagnosis, and pericardiectomy is the definitive treatment (see Chap. 72).

INFECTIVE ENDOCARDITIS

Bacteremia occurs in approximately 10 to 20 percent of hemodialysis patients;[114–116] the incidence of *Staphylococcus aureus* bacteremia is about 1.2 episodes per 100 patient months.[115] *Staph. aureus* is the most frequent organism causing endocarditis,[114,117,118,125,126] although other microbes, including *Staph. epidermidis, Streptococcus viridans,* enterococci, and gram-negative organisms are also reported. Several factors predispose dialysis patients to infective endocarditis, which can have an incidence of 3 to 5 percent.[114,117,118] These include uremia-associated immunocompromise,[119,120] repeated puncture of the arteriovenous fistula, or an indwelling dialysis catheter. Other factors are aortic valve calcifications, found in 28 to 55 percent, and mitral valve calcifications in 10 to 40 percent of dialysis patients.[59,61,121,122] Calcified valves may serve as a nidus for infection; in this case, the aortic valve is involved in over 80 percent of cases.[114]

The diagnosis of infective endocarditis may be difficult in uremic patients because of the frequency of bacteremia and because systolic and diastolic murmurs are common (see also Chap. 73). Repeated blood cultures, physical examination, and an echocardiographic assessment are mandatory when infective endocarditis is suspected. Treatment of infective endocarditis consists of 4 to 6 weeks of parenteral antibiotics (see Chap. 73). Survival of hemodialysis patients undergoing valve replacement for endocarditis is poor.[123]

CARDIAC ARRHYTHMIAS

Risk factors for cardiac arrhythmias in dialysis patients include ischemic heart disease, calcification of the conduction system from secondary hyperparathyroidism and/or pericarditis, hemodialysis-associated hypotension, dialysis-induced acid-base and electrolyte disturbances (hyper- and hypokalemia, hyper- and hypocalcemia, and hypermagnesemia), and hypoxemia. Fortunately, serious arrhythmias are uncommon except in patients with underlying heart disease, those receiving digitalis, or those with severe hypokalemia.[124–126] Dialysis patients receiving digitalis have an excessive risk for atrial and ventricular arrhythmias during dialysis because of rapid shifts of potassium. Therefore, digitalis should be used only when necessary and in the lowest dosage. While the potassium concentration in the dialysate can be raised to decrease the risk of digitalis-toxic arrhythmias, there also must be strict restriction of dietary potassium to prevent hyperkalemia between dialyses. Hyperkalemia is believed to be responsible for a significant fraction of the 10 percent death rate from cardiac arrest in dialysis patients.

RENAL FUNCTION IN HEART FAILURE

In heart failure, enhanced sympathetic activity and activation of the renin-angiotensin-aldosterone axis enhance salt reabsorption by the kidney. Excess vasopressin release and increases in aquaporin-2 water channels augment water retention.[127,128] These responses expand the ECV and plasma volume leading to increased end-diastolic volume plus edema.[129] Circulating atrial natriuretic peptide levels are increased in heart failure[127,130]; possibly, atrial natriuretic peptide modulates the antinatriuretic effects caused by sympathetic and renin system activation. Excessive vasopressin-induced water reabsorption, coupled with increased water intake (possibly related to angiotensin-II-stimulated central thirst receptors) can cause hyponatremia. Hyponatremia is an important indicator of a poor prognosis.[131]

Renal vasoconstriction in heart failure patients can be sufficiently severe to cause prerenal azotemia, characterized by a blood urea nitrogen-creatinine ratio that is greater than the expected, normal of 10:1. Renal vasoconstriction causes a selective decrease in urea clearance resulting from enhanced sodium reabsorption and a secondary increase in urea reabsorption in the proximal tubule. The increase in salt and water reabsorption both reduces urine flow and causes a low urinary sodium excretion, as well as a high urine specific gravity and osmolality. In terms of diagnosis, the urinalysis is normal and there are no cellular or granular casts indicating kidney damage. Diuretic therapy can mask these characteristics by increasing urine flow and sodium excretion, thereby reducing the urine specific gravity and osmolality and diluting the presence of cellular or granular casts. Factors that can precipitate or exacerbate renal failure include excessive diuresis, use of ACE inhibitors or nonsteroidal anti-inflammatory drugs, and worsening cardiac function. The basis for renal insufficiency in these cases is that renal perfusion is reduced by heart failure. Consequently, the glomerular filtration rate becomes dependent on angiotensin-II-induced efferent glomerular arteriolar constriction. By blocking this response, ACE inhibitors can markedly decrease the glomerular filtration rate.[132] Non-steroidal anti-inflammatory drugs reduce the glomerular filtration rate by blocking the release of prostaglandins, which in turn, reduce activation of the renin-angiotensin system.[133] The ACE inhibitors and other antihypertensive agents (e.g., hydralazine) can also reduce glomerular filtration by causing systemic hypotension and reducing renal perfusion pressure.

The management of renal insufficiency in heart failure patients is aimed primarily at improving cardiac function (see Chap. 21). Non-steroidal anti-inflammatory drugs should be avoided, and diuretics should be used judiciously because excessive diuresis can predispose the patient to any factor that lowers blood pressure or that interrupts the glomerular efferent arteriolar vasoconstriction (e.g., an ACE inhibitor). Careful attention to changes in the blood urea nitrogen relative to serum creatinine and potassium is mandatory to avoid these problems. It should be emphasized that ACE inhibitor therapy may sharply reduce renal clearance (i.e., cause a sharp rise in serum creatinine) in heart failure patients that have an activation of the renin system. Often, this is a transient physiologic response and the serum creatinine will return to pretreatment values. If it does not, the drug should be withdrawn and a diagnosis of renal artery stenosis considered.

RENAL FAILURE FOLLOWING CARDIAC CATHETERIZATION

Contrast Nephropathy

The risk of renal damage following radiocontrast dye is high in patients with diabetes mellitus, multiple myeloma, preexisting renal failure, and, especially, proteinuria, volume depletion, heart failure, and with large amounts of contrast dye.[134–136] Renal failure after contrast dye is typically brief (approximately 5 to 7 days) unless there is preexisting renal damage. Interestingly, renal insufficiency in contrast-dye nephropathy can be associated with excessive edema (from reduced urinary sodium excretion) and hyperkalemia.[137] In high-risk patients, contrast dye studies should be avoided and noninvasive studies used to assess ventricular function and anatomy; at the very least, the amount of contrast dye should be minimized. Extracellular fluid volume expansion with saline prior to the studies reduces the incidence of contrast nephropathy to approximately 10 percent.[138]

Atheroembolic Nephropathy

This complication usually occurs in elderly patients with erosive aortic atherosclerosis. They develop cholesterol emboli to the kidneys, and this is most commonly detected after arterial catheterization.[134,139] Serum creatinine rises progressively and usually does not return to basal levels, and often renal insufficiency progresses to ESRD. Hypertension due to activation of the renin-angiotensin system may be present.[140] The urinalysis typically does not contain cellular or granular casts (the signs of acute tubular damage). Atheroembolization to other organs such as the eyes (cholesterol plaques seen by fundoscopy), pancreas (pancreatitis), and skin (livedo reticularis or gangrene) may be present, suggesting the diagnosis.[141] Occasionally, immunologic activation may occur yielding an "active" urinary sediment with hematuria and cellular casts, hypocomplementemia, eosinophilia, and a high sedimentation rate.[142–144] Biopsy of an affected organ (e.g., skin or kidney) can help establish the diagnosis, but the absence of atheroemboli in a kidney biopsy does not exclude the diagnosis since the affected vessels may be missed. There is no specific treatment.

Thromboembolic Renal Disease

In contrast to atheroembolic renal disease, thromboembolic renal arterial disease (e.g., in patients with atrial fibrillation or after myocardial infarction) can cause renal infarction. Such patients may present with flank pain, proteinuria, and hematuria; the serum lactate dehydrogenase level is increased and renal failure leads to an increased serum creatinine, particularly if both kidneys are affected.[145–147] A radioisotope scan or renal arteriography may confirm the diagnosis. Therapy includes anticoagulation, thrombolysis, and possibly surgical intervention.

CARDIAC DRUGS IN RENAL FAILURE

Many drugs used in the treatment of cardiovascular diseases are eliminated (i.e., cleared) by the kidneys. In order to avoid toxic side effects, the doses of these drugs must be modified depending on the level of the patient's glomerular filtration rate (see also Chap. 81). Dosing guidelines for commonly prescribed cardiovascular drugs in patients with diminished renal function are listed in Table 84-1. Specific drugs are discussed in more detail later.

Digoxin

The volume of distribution of digoxin is reduced 30 to 50 percent in ESRD patients; therefore the loading dose of digoxin should be reduced. The maintenance dosage should also be decreased because the primary route of elimination is by glomerular filtration of unmetabolized digoxin. Because of individual variation in digoxin pharmacokinetics, only general guidelines for maintenance dosages are available: 0.0625 to 0.125 mg every other day can result in a therapeutic plasma level but regular monitoring of the plasma digoxin level is still required. If a loading dose is not administered or if adjustments are made in the maintenance dose, the time required to attain a new steady state can be prolonged to approximately 3 weeks because of the longer half-life of digoxin in renal failure (4.4 days versus 1.6 days in normal subjects[148]). Concomitant administration of quinidine or verapamil can increase plasma digoxin levels and produce clinical toxicity.

Beta Blockers

Since atenolol (Tenormin) and nadolol (Corgard) are eliminated primarily by the kidneys, a dose reduction of 50 to 70 percent is necessary for patients with chronic renal failure.[149] These drugs should be withheld on the morning of a hemodialysis treatment because a significant fraction is removed by the dialysis procedure. The usual dose is then given after dialysis (Table 84-1).

Sodium Nitroprusside

In dialysis or predialysis patients, thiocyanate will accumulate when sodium nitroprusside is infused.[150] Thiocyanate can cause neurologic toxicity such as confusion, hyperreflexia, and seizures. Therefore the dose of nitroprusside for patients with chronic renal failure should be minimized and the drug given for as short a period as possible. Both the cyanide and thiocyanate levels in plasma should be monitored to avoid toxicity. Fenoldopam, a dopamine$_1$ recepter agonist, increases renal blood flow and glomerular filtration rate; this agent may be a good alternative to nitroprusside for the treatment of severe hypertension in patients with renal disease.[151]

Angiotensin-Converting Enzyme Inhibitors

The doses of ACE inhibitors should be reduced by approximately 50 percent in dialysis patients because they and their metabolites are excreted by the kidney. Accumulation of converting enzyme inhibitors can cause hematologic toxicity. These drugs have two other types of toxic effects in predialysis patients. First, in patients who are not treated by dialysis, they can cause hyperkalemia by blocking angiotensin-stimulated aldosterone release, resulting in decreased potassium excretion and hyperkalemia. Second, they can cause rapid loss of renal function in patients with renal artery stenosis or other conditions associated with activation of the renin-angiotensin system, including congestive heart failure.[132] The mechanism for the decrease in glomerular filtration rate is inhibition of angiotensin-induced constriction of the efferent glomerular arterioles. The resulting dilation leads to a decrease in the hydrostatic pressure across the glomerular capillary wall. These drugs, like other antihypertensive agents, should be withheld on the morning of a hemodialysis treatment to avoid hypotension.

TABLE 84-1 Dosing of Selected Cardiovascular Drugs in Renal Failure

Drug	Method of Modification	GFR >50	GFR 10–50	GFR <10	Supplemental Dose after Hemodialysis
			ADRENERGIC AGENTS		
Clonidine	D	100%	100%	100%	No
Doxazosin	D	100%	100%	100%	No
Methyldopa	I	q8h	q8–q12h	q12–q24h	250 mg
Prazosin	D	100%	100%	100%	No
Terazosin	D	100%	100%	100%	?
			ANGIOTENSIN-CONVERTING ENZYME INHIBITORS		
Benazepril	D	100%	75–100%	50%	No
Captopril	D	100%	75%	50%	25–30%
Cilazapril	D	75%	50%	10–25%	No
	I	q24h	q24–48h	q72h	
Enalapril	D	100%	75–100%	50%	20–25%
Fosinopril	D	100%	100%	75%	No
Lisinopril	D	100%	50–75%	25–50%	20%
Pentopril	D	100%	50–75%	50%	?
Perindopril	D	100%	75%	50%	25–50%
Quinapril	D	100%	75–100%	50%	25%
Ramapril	D	100%	50–75%	25–50%	20%
			ANGIOTENSIN-II-RECEPTOR ANTAGONISTS		
Losartan	D	100%	100%	100%	?
Valsartan	D	100%	100%	50%	?
			ANTIARRHYTHMICS		
Amiodarone	D	100%	100%	100%	No
Bretylium	D	100%	25–50%	25%	No
Disopyramide	I	q8h	q12–24h	q24–48h	No
Flecainide	D	100%	100%	50–75%	No
Lidocaine	D	100%	100%	100%	No
Mexiletine	D	100%	100%	50–75%	No
N-Acetyl-procainamide	D	100%	50%	25%	No
	I	q6–8h	q8–q12h	q12–q18h	
Procainamide	I	q4h	q6–12h	q8–24h	200 mg
Propafenone	D	100%	100%	100%	No
Quinidine	D	100%	100%	75%	100–200 mg
Tocainide	D	100%	100%	50%	200 mg
			BETA BLOCKERS		
Acebutolol	D	100%	50%	30–50%	No
Atenolol	D	100%	50%	30–50%	25–50 mg
	I	q24h	q48h	q96h	
Betaxolol	D	100%	100%	50%	No
Bisoprolol	D	100%	75%	50%	?
Carvedilol	D	100%	100%	100%	No
Labetalol	D	100%	100%	100%	No
Metoprolol	D	100%	100%	100%	50 mg
Nadolol	D	100%	50%	25%	40 mg
Pindolol	D	100%	100%	100%	No
Propranolol	D	100%	100%	100%	No
Sotalol	D	100%	30%	15–30%	80 mg
Timolol	D	100%	100%	100%	No

TABLE 84-1 Dosing of Selected Cardiovascular Drugs in Renal Failure (*Continued*)

Drug	Method of Modification	GFR >50	GFR 10–50	GFR <10	Supplemental Dose after Hemodialysis
CALCIUM CHANNEL BLOCKERS—NO ADJUSTMENT NECESSARY					
CARDIAC GLYCOSIDES					
Digitoxin	D	100%	100%	50–75%	No
Digoxin	D	100%	25–75%	10–25%	No
	I	q24h	q36h	q48h	
IONOTROPIC AGENTS					
Amrinone	D	100%	100%	50–75%	?
Dobutamine	D	100%	100%	100%	?
Milrinone	D	100%	100%	50–75%	?
VASODILATORS					
Hydralazine	I	q8h	q8h	q16h	No
Fenoldopam	D	100%	100%	100%	No
Minoxidil	D	100%	100%	50–75%	No
Nitroprusside	D	100%	100%	50–75%	No

ABBREVIATIONS: GFR = glomerular filtration rate; D = Dose; I = interval; ? = unknown.
SOURCE: Adapted from Aronoff GR, Berns JS, Brier ME, et al. *Drug Prescribing in Renal Failure: Dosing Guidelines for Adults*, 4th ed. Philadelphia: American College of Physicians: 1999.

Cyclosporine and Tacrolimus

The use of cyclosporine A and tacrolimus in heart transplant recipients is often associated with acute reduction in renal function, which progresses to chronic renal failure in some patients[152] (see also Chap. 22). These agents constrict both afferent and efferent glomerular arterioles, resulting in a reduced blood flow and, ultimately, the glomerular filtration rate. Proximal tubular injury—with vacuolar changes, inclusion bodies, and giant mitochondria—has also been noted. Hyperkalemia and renal tubular acidosis can occur, but these acute effects are usually reversible if the dose is reduced or the drug is discontinued. Chronic irreversible nephrotoxicity associated with tubulointerstitial fibrosis, tubular atrophy, hyaline arteriolar degeneration, and glomerular sclerosis results in long-term renal damage with chronic renal failure. Although chronic renal failure remains stable in many patients, approximately 7 percent of heart transplant patients treated with cyclosporine A progress to ESRD.[153] Hemolytic uremic syndrome, presumably due to endothelial cell damage, has also been described with these agents but this is uncommon.[154]

References

1. Levey AS. Controlling the epidemic of cardiovascular disease in chronic renal disease: Where do we start? *Am J Kidney Dis* 1998; 32(Suppl 3):S5.
2. Causes of Death. United States Renal Data System 1999 Annual Report. *Am J Kidney Dis* 1999; 34(Suppl 1):S87.
3. Foley RN, Parfrey PS, Sarnak MJ. Clinical epidemiology of cardiovascular disease in chronic renal disease. *Am J Kidney Dis* 1998; 32(Suppl 3):S112.
4. Mailloux LU, Levey AS. Hypertension in patients with chronic renal disease. *Am J Kidney Dis* 1998; 32(Suppl 3):S120.
5. Ritz E, Charra B, Leunissen KML, et al. How important is volume excess in the etiology of hypertension in dialysis patients? *Sem Dialysis* 1999; 12:296.
6. Vertes V, Cangiano JL, Berman LB, et al. Hypertension in end-stage renal disease. *N Engl J Med* 1991; 280:978.
7. Weidmann P, Maxwell MH, Lupu AN, et al. Plasma renin activity and blood pressure in terminal renal failure. *N Engl J Med* 1991; 285:757.
8. Ligtenberg G, Blankestijn PJ, Oey PL, et al. Reduction of sympathetic hyperactivity by enalapril in patients with chronic renal failure. *N Engl J Med* 1999; 340:1321.
9. Kim KE, Onesti G, Schwartz AB, et al. Hemodynamics of hypertension in chronic end-stage renal disease. *Circulation* 1972; 46:452.
10. Kim KE, Onesti G, DelGuercio ET, et al. Sequential hemodynamic changes in end-stage renal disease and the anephric state during volume expansion. *Hypertension* 1991; 2:102.
11. Charra B, Calemarad E, Ruffet M, et al. Survival as an index of adequacy of dialysis. *Kidney Int* 1992; 41:1286.
12. Vaughan ED, Carey RM, Ayers CR, et al. Hemodialysis-resistant hypertension: Control with an orally active inhibitor of angiotensin-converting enzyme. *J Clin Endocrinol Metab* 1991; 48:869.
13. Kelly RA, O'Hara DS, Mitch WE, et al. Endogenous digitalis-like factors in hypertension and chronic renal insufficiency. *Kidney Int* 1986; 30:723.
14. Glatter KA, Graves SW, Hollenberg NK, et al. Sustained volume expansion and (Na-K) ATPase inhibition in chronic renal failure. *Am J Hypertension* 1994; 7:1016.
15. Converse RL Jr, Jacobsen TN, Toto RD, et al. Sympathetic overactivity in patients with chronic renal failure. *N Engl J Med* 1992; 327:1912.
16. Remuzzi, G. Sympathetic overactivity in hypertension patients with chronic renal disease. *N Engl J Med* 1999; 340:1360.
17. Cinotti GA, Pugliese F. Prostaglandins in blood pressure regulation. *Kidney Int* 1988; 35(suppl 25):57.
18. Shichiri M, Hirata Y, Ando K, et al. Plasma endothelin levels in patients with uremia. *Hypertension* 1990; 15:493.

19. Goldsmith DJA, Covic AA, Venning MC, et al. Blood pressure reduction after parathyroidectomy for secondary hyperparathyroidism: Further evidence implicating calcium homeostasis in blood pressure regulation. *Am J Kidney Dis* 1996; 27:819.
20. Radermacher J, Koch KM. Treatment of renal anemia by erythropoietin substitution: The effects on the cardiovascular system. *Clin Nephrol* 1995; 44(suppl 1):S56.
21. Mann JFE. Hypertension and cardiovascular effects–Long-term safety and potential long-term benefits of r-HuEPO. *Nephrol Dial Transplant* 1995; 10(suppl 2):80.
22. Zazgornik J, Biesenbach G, Janko O, et al. Bilateral nephrectomy: The best, but often overlooked, treatment for refractory hypertension in hemodialysis patients. *Am J Hypertension* 1998; 11:1364.
23. Kaski BL. Hyperlipidemia in patients with chronic renal disease. *Am J Kidney Dis* 1998; 32(Suppl 3):S142.
24. Chan MK, Persaud J, Varghese Z, et al. Pathogenic roles of post-heparin lipases in lipid abnormalities in hemodialysis patients. *Kidney Int* 1991; 25:812.
25. Lindholm B, Norbeck HE. Serum lipids and lipoproteins during continuous ambulatory peritoneal dialysis. *Acta Med Scand* 1986; 220:143.
26. Ames RP, Hill P. Elevation of serum lipid levels during diuretic therapy of hypertension. *Am J Med* 1976; 61:748.
27. Tanaka N, Sakaguchi S, Oshige K, et al. Effect of chronic administration of propranolol on lipoprotein composition. *Metabolism* 1976; 25:1071.
28. Lacour B, Chanard J, Haguet M, et al. Carnitine improves lipid anomalies in haemodialysis patients. *Lancet* 1980; 2:763.
29. Wessel-Aas T, Blomhoff JP, Wideroe T-E, et al. The effect of systemic heparinization on plasma lipoproteins and toxicity in patients on hemodialysis and continuous ambulatory peritoneal dialysis. *Acta Med Scand* 1984; 216:85.
30. Ritz E, Augustin J, Bommer J, et al. Should hyperlipemia of renal failure be treated? *Kidney Int* 1985; 28:S-84.
31. Golper TA. Therapy for uremic hyperlipidemia. *Nephron* 1991; 38:217.
32. Goldberg AP, Hagberg JM, Delez JA, et al. Metabolic effects of exercise training in hemodialysis patients. *Kidney Int* 1980; 18:754.
33. Hamazaki T, Nakazawa R, Tateno S, et al. Effects of fish oil rich in eicosapentaenoic acid on serum lipid in hyperlipidemic hemodialysis patients. *Kidney Int* 1984; 26:81.
34. Expert panel on detection evaluation and treatment of high blood cholesterol in adults: Summary of the second report of the National Cholesterol Education Program (NCEP) (Adult treatment panel II). JAMA 1993; 269:3015.
35. Bostom AG, Lathrop L. Hyperhomocysteinemia in end-stage renal disease: Prevalence, etiology, and potential relationship to arteriosclerotic outcomes. *Kidney Int* 1997; 52:10.
36. Beto JA, Bansal VK. Interventions for other risk factors: tobacco use, physical inactivity, menopause, and homocysteine. *Am J Kidney Dis* 1998; 32(Suppl 3):S172.
37. Guttormsen AB, Ueland PM, Svarstad E, et al. Kinetic basis of hyperhomocysteinemia in patients with chronic renal failure. *Kidney Int* 1997; 52:495.
38. Moustapha A, Naso A, Nahlawi M, et al. Prospective study of hyperhomocysteinemia as an adverse cardiovascular risk factor in end-stage renal disease [published erratum appears in *Circulation* 1998; 97:711]. *Circulation* 1998; 97:138.
39. Passaver J, Bussemaker E, Gross P. Dialysis hypotension: Do we see light at the end of the tunnel? *Nephrol Dial Transp* 1999; 13:3024.
40. Daugirdas JT. Dialysis-induced hypotension: A fresh look at pathophysiology. *Kidney Int* 1991; 39:233.
41. Rosa AA, Shideman J, McHugh R, et al. The importance of osmolality fall and ultrafiltration rate on hemodialysis side effects. *Nephron* 1981; 27:134.
42. Keshaviah P, Shapiro F. A critical examination of dialysis-induced hypotension. *Am J Kidney Dis* 1982; 2:290.
43. Henrich WL, Woodard TD, McPhaul JJ Jr. The chronic efficacy and safety of high sodium dialysate: Double-blind, crossover study. *Am J Kidney Dis* 1982; 2:349.
44. Hakim RM, Breillatt J, Lazarus JM, et al. Complement activation and hypersensitivity reactions to dialysis membranes. *N Engl J Med* 1984; 311:878.
45. Pastan S, Bailey J. Dialysis therapy. *N Eng J Med* 1998; 338:1428.
46. Dolovich J, Marshall CP, Smith EKM, et al. Allergy to ethylene oxide in chronic hemodialysis patients. *Artif Organs* 1984; 8:334.
47. Verresen L, Fiink E, Lemke HD, et al. Bradykinin is a moderator of anaphylactoid reactions during hemodialysis with AN69 membranes. *Kidney Int* 1994; 45:1497.
48. Converse RL Jr, Jacobsen TN, Jost CMT, et al. Paradoxical withdrawal of reflex vasoconstriction as a cause of hemodialysis-induced hypotension. *J Clin Invest* 1992; 90:1657.
49. Sang GL, Kovithavongs C, Ulan R, et al. Sodium ramping in hemodialysis: A study of beneficial and adverse effects. *Am J Kidney Dis* 1997; 29:669.
50. Cruz DN, Mahnesmith RL, Brickle HM, et al. Midrodrine and cool dialysate are effective therapies for symptomatic intradialytic hypotension. *Am J Kidney Dis* 1997; 33:920.
51. Felsenfeld AJ. Considerations for the treatment of secondary hyperparathyroidism in renal failure. *J Am Soc Nephrol* 1997; 8:993.
52. Portale AA, Halloran BP, Murphy MM, et al. Oral intake of phosphorus can determine the serum concentration of 1,25-dihydroxyvitamin D by determining its production rate in humans. *J Clin Invest* 1986; 77:7.
53. Fukuda N, Tanaka H, Tominaga Y, et al. Decreased 1,25-dihydroxyvitamin D3 receptor density is associated with a more severe form of parathyroid hyperplasia in chronic uremic patients. *J Clin Invest* 1993; 92:1436.
54. Gogusev J, Duchambon P, Hory B, et al. Depressed expression of calcium receptor in parathyroid gland tissue of patients with hyperparathyroidism. *Kidney Int* 1997; 51:328.
55. Delmez JA, Tindira C, Grooms P, et al. Parathyroid hormone suppression by intravenous 1,25-dihydroxyvitamin D. *J Clin Invest* 1991; 83:1349.
56. Silver J, Russell J, Sherwood LM. Regulation by vitamin D metabolites of messenger ribonucleic acid for preproparathyroid hormone in isolated bovine parathyroid cells. *Proc Natl Acad Sci USA* 1985; 82:4270.
57. Kuzda DC, Huffer WE, Conger JD, et al. Soft tissue calcification in chronic dialysis patients. *Am J Pathol* 1977; 86:403.
58. Goldsmith DG, Covic A, Sambrook PA, et al. Vascular calcification in long-term hemodialysis patients in a single unit: A retrospective analysis. *Nephron* 1977; 77:37.
59. Braun J, Oldendorf N, Moshage W, et al. Electron beam computed tomography in the evaluation of cardiac calcification in chronic dialysis patients. *Am Journal Kidney Dis* 1996; 27:394.
60. Llach F. Cardiac calcification: dealing with another risk factor in patients with kidney failure. *Sem Dial* 1999; 12:293.
61. Ribeiro S, Ramos A, Brandao A, et al. Cardiac valve calcification in haemodialysis patients: Role of calcium-phosphate metabolism. *Nephrol Dial Transplant* 1998; 13:2037.
62. McGonigle RJS, Fowler MB, Timmis AB, et al. Uremic cardiomyopathy: Potential role of vitamin D and parathyroid hormone. *Nephron* 1984; 36:94.
63. Gafter U, Battler A, Eldar M, et al. Effect of hyperparathyroidism on cardiac function in patients with end-stage renal disease. *Nephron* 1985; 41:30.
64. Slatopolsky EA, Burke SK, Dillon MA. RenaGel, a nonabsorbed calcium- and aluminum-free phosphate binder, lowers serum phosphorus and parathyroid hormone. The RenaGel Study Group. *Kidney Int* 1999; 55:299.

65. Llach F, Slatopolsky E, eds. New vitamin D analogues in the treatment of secondary hyperparathyroidism. *Am J Kid Dis* 1998; 32(Suppl 2):S1.
66. U.S. Renal Data System 1992, Annual Report. IV. Comorbid conditions and correlations with mortality risk among 3,399 incident hemodialysis patients. *Am J Kidney Dis* 1992; 20(Suppl 2):S32.
67. Ansari A, Kaupke CJ, Vaziri ND, et al. Cardiac pathology in patients with end-stage renal disease maintained on hemodialysis. *Int J Artif Organs* 1993; 64:560.
68. Wing AJ, Brunner FP, Brynger H, et al. Cardiovascular-related causes of death and the fate of patients with renovascular disease. *Contrib Nephrol* 1984; 41:306.
69. Manske CL. Hyperglycemia and intensive glycemic control in diabetic patients with chronic renal disease. *Am J Kidney Dis* 1998; 32(Suppl 3):S159.
70. Ori Y, Korets A, Katz M, et al. Hemodialysis arteriovenous access—A prospective hemodynamic evaluation. *Nephrol Dial Transplant* 1996; 14(Suppl 1):94.
71. Murphy SW, Foley RN, Parfrey PS. Screening and treatment for cardiovascular disease in patients with chronic renal disease. *Am J Kidney Dis* 1998; 32(Suppl 3):S184.
72. Dahan M, Lagallicier B, Himbert D, et al. Diagnostic value of myocardial thallium stress scintigraphy in the selection of CAD in patients undergoing chronic hemodialysis. *Arch Mal Coeur* 1995; 88:1121.
73. Brown JH, Vites NP, Testa HJ, et al. Value of thallium myocardial imaging in the prediction of future cardiovascular events in patients with end-stage renal failure. *Nephrol Dial Transplant* 1993; 8:433.
74. DePuey EG, Guertler-Krawczynska E, Perkins JV, et al. Alterations in myocardial thallium-201 distribution in patients with chronic systemic hypertension undergoing single-photon emission computed tomography. *Am J Cardiol* 1988; 62:234.
75. Dahan M, Viron BM, Faraggi M, et al. Diagnostic accuracy and prognostic value of combined dipyridamole-exercise thallium imaging in hemodialysis patients. *Kidney Int* 1998; 54:255.
76. Resis G, Marcovitz PA, Leichtman AB, et al. Usefulness of dobutamine stress echocardiography in detecting CAD in end-stage renal disease. *Am J Cardiol* 1995; 75:707.
77. Bates JR, Sawada SG, Segar DS, et al. Evaluation using dobutamine stress echocardiography in patients with insulin dependent diabetes mellitus before kidney and/or pancreas transplant. *Am J Cardiol* 1996; 77:175.
78. Roig E, Betriu A, Castaner A, et al. Disabling angina pectoris with normal coronary arteries in patients undergoing long-term hemodialysis. *Am J Med* 1981; 71:431.
79. Wizemann V, Kaufmann J, Kramer W. Effect of erythropoietin on ischemia tolerance in anemic hemodialysis patients with confirmed coronary artery disease. *Nephron* 1992; 62:161.
80. Francis GS, Sharma B, Collins AJ, et al. Coronary-artery surgery in patients with end-stage renal disease. *Ann Intern Med* 1980; 92:499.
81. Batiuk TD, Kurtz SB, Oh JK, et al. Coronary artery bypass operation in dialysis patients. *Mayo Clin Proc* 1991; 66:45.
82. Schoebel FC, Gradaus F, Ivens K, et al. Restenosis after elective coronary balloon angioplasty in patients with end-stage renal disease: A case-control study using quantitative coronary angiography. *Heart* 1997; 78:337.
83. Herzog CA, Ma JZ, Collins AJ. Long-term survival of dialysis patients in the United States after coronary artery bypass surgery, coronary angioplasty, and coronary stenting. *J Am Soc Nephrol* 1999; 10:166A.
84. Harnett JD, Foley RN, Kent GM, et al. Congestive heart failure in dialysis patients: Prevalence, incidence, prognosis and risk factors. *Kidney Int* 1995; 47:884.
85. Bernardi D, Bernini L, Cini G, et al. Asymmetric septal hypertrophy and sympathetic overactivity in normotensive hemodialyzed patients. *Am Heart J* 1985; 109:539.
86. Levin A, Singer J, Thompson CR, et al. Prevelant left ventricular hypertrophy in the predialysis population: Identifying opportunities for intervention. *Am J Kid Dis* 1996; 27:347.
87. Wizemann V, Blank S, Kramer W. Diastolic dysfunction of the left ventricle in dialysis patients. *Contrib Nephrol* 1994; 106:106.
88. Foley RN, Parfrey PS, Kent GM, et al. Long-term evolution of cardiomyopathy in dialysis patients. *Kidney Int* 1998; 54:1720.
89. Tucker B, Fabbian F, Giles M, et al. Left ventricular hypertrophy and ambulatory blood pressure monitoring in chronic renal failure. *Nephrol Dial Transplant* 1997; 12:724.
90. London GM, De Vernejoul M-C, Fabiani F, et al. Secondary hyperparathyroidism and cardiac hypertrophy in hemodialysis patients. *Kidney Int* 1987; 32:900.
91. Nixon JV, Mitchell JH, McPhaul JJ Jr, et al. Effect of hemodialysis on left ventricular function. *J Clin Invest* 1983; 71:377.
92. Hung J, Harris PJ, Uren RF, et al. Uremic cardiomyopathy—Effect of hemodialysis on left ventricular function in end-stage renal failure. *N Engl J Med* 1980; 230:547.
93. Madsen BR, Alpert MA, Whiting RB, et al. Effect of hemodialysis on left ventricular performance. *Am J Nephrol* 1984; 4:86.
94. Van der Sande FM, Cheriex EC, van Kuijk WH, et al. Effect of dialysate calcium concentration on intradialytic blood pressure course in cardiac-compromised patients. *Am J Kid Dis* 1998; 32:125.
95. Chaignon M, Chen W-T, Tarazi RC, et al. Acute effects of hemodialysis on echographic-determined cardiac performance: Improved contractility resulting from serum increased calcium with reduced potassium despite hypovolemic-reduced cardiac output. *Am Heart J* 1982; 103:374.
96. Rackow EC, Fein IA, Sprung C, et al. Uremic pulmonary edema. *Am J Med* 1978; 64:1084.
97. Young PR Jr, Rohr MS, Marterre WF Jr. High output cardiac failure secondary to brachiocephalic arteriovenous hemodialysis fistula: Two cases. *Am Surg* 1998; 64:239.
98. Eckardt K. Cardiovascular consequences of renal anemia and erythropoietin therapy. *Nephrol Dial Transplant* 1999; 14:1317.
99. Wacker J, Merrill JP. Uremic pericarditis in acute and chronic renal failure. *JAMA* 1954; 156:764.
100. Rostand SG, Rutsky EA. Pericarditis in end-stage renal disease. *Cardiol Clin* 1990; 8:701.
101. Osanloo E, Shalhoub RJ, Cioffi RF, et al. Viral pericarditis in patients receiving hemodialysis. *Arch Intern Med* 1979; 139:301.
102. Houston MC, McChesney JA, Chatterjee K. Pericardial effusion associated with minoxidil therapy. *Arch Intern Med* 1981; 141:69.
103. Silverberg S, Oreopoulos DG, Wise DJ, et al. Pericarditis in patients undergoing long-term hemodialysis and peritoneal dialysis. *Am J Med* 1977; 63:874.
104. Eliasson G, Murphy JF. Steroid therapy in uremic pericarditis. *JAMA* 1974; 229:1634.
105. Buselmeier TJ, Simmons RL, Najarian JS, et al. Uremic pericardial effusion. *Nephron* 1976; 16:371.
106. Minuth NW, Nottebohm GA, Eknoyan G, et al. Indomethacin treatment of pericarditis in chronic hemodialysis patients. *Arch Intern Med* 1975; 135:807.
107. Spector D, Alfred H, Siedlecki M, et al. A controlled study of the effect of indomethacin in uremic pericarditis. *Kidney Int* 1983; 24:663.
108. Goldberg M, Lazarus JM, Gottlieb MN, et al. Treatment of uremic pericardial effusion. *Proc Clin Dial Transplant Forum* 1975; 5:20.
109. Luft FC, Kleit SA, Smith RN, et al. Management of uremic pericarditis with tamponade. *Arch Intern Med* 1974; 134:488.
110. Daugirdas JT, Leehey DJ, Popli S, et al. Subxiphoid pericardiostomy for hemodialysis-associated pericardial effusion. *Arch Intern Med* 1986; 146:1113.

111. Peraino RA. Pericardial effusion in patients treated with maintenance dialysis. *Am J Nephrol* 1983; 3:319.
112. Figueroa W, Alankar S, Pai N, et al. Subxiphoid pericardial window for pericardial effusion in end-stage renal disease. *Am J Kidney Dis* 1996; 27:664.
113. Moraski RE, Bousvaros G. Constrictive pericarditis due to chronic uremia. *N Engl J Med* 1969; 281:542.
114. Robinson DL, Fowler VG, Sexton DJ, et al. Bacterial endocarditis in hemodialysis patients. *Am J Kidney Dis* 1997; 30:521.
115. Marr KA, Kong L, Fowler VG, et al. Incidence and outcome of *Staphylococcus aureus* bacteremia in hemodialysis patients. *Kidney Int* 1998; 54:1684.
116. Nsouli KA, Lazarus JM, Schoenbaum SC, et al. Bacteremic infection in hemodialysis. *Arch Intern Med* 1979; 139:1255.
117. Leonard A, Raij L, Shapiro FL. Bacterial endocarditis in regularly dialyzed patients. *Kidney Int* 1973; 4:407.
118. Cross AS, Steigbigel RT. Infective endocarditis and access site infections in patients on hemodialysis. *Medicine* 1976; 55:453.
119. Haag-Weber M, Horl WH. Uremia and infection: Mechanisms of impaired cellular host defense. *Nephron* 1993; 63:125.
120. Ruiz P, Gomez F, Schrieber AD. Impaired function of macrophage Fc gamma receptors in end-stage renal disease. *N Engl J Med* 1990; 322:717.
121. Forman MB, Virmani R, Robertson RM, et al. Mitral annular calcification in chronic renal failure. *Chest* 1984; 85:367.
122. Straumann E, Meyer B, Mastroli M, et al. Aortic and mitral valve disease in patients with end-stage renal failure on hemodialysis. *Br Heart J* 1992; 67:236.
123. Baglin A, Hanslik T, Vaillant JN, et al. Severe valvular heart disease in patients on chronic dialysis: A five-year multicenter French survey. *Ann Med Int* 1997; 148:521.
124. Kyriakidis M, Voudiclaris S, Kremastinos D, et al. Cardiac arrhythmias in chronic renal failure. *Nephron* 1984; 38:26.
125. Weber H, Schwarzer C, Stummvoll HK, et al. Chronic hemodialysis: High risk patients for arrhythmias? *Nephron* 1984; 37:180.
126. Wizeman V, Kramer W, Funke T, et al. Dialysis-induced cardiac arrhythmias: Fact or fiction? *Nephron* 1985; 39:356.
127. Dzau VJ. Renal and circulatory mechanisms in congestive heart failure. *Kidney Int* 1987; 31:1402.
128. Xu DL, Martin PY, Ohara M, et al. Upregulation of aquaporin-2 water channel expression in chronic heart failure rat. *J Clin Invest* 1997; 99:1500.
129. Schrier RW, Abraham WT. Hormones and hemodynamics in heart failure. *N Engl J Med* 1999; 341:577.
130. Abraham WT. Natriuretic peptides in heart failure. *Congestive Heart Fail* 1998; 4:23.
131. Lee WH, Packer M. Prognostic importance of serum sodium concentration and its modification by converting-enzyme inhibition in patients with severe chronic heart failure. *Circulation* 1986; 73:257.
132. Suki WN. Renal hemodynamic consequences of angiotensin-converting enzyme inhibition in congestive heart failure. *Arch Intern Med* 1989; 149:669.
133. Dzau VJ, Packer M, Lilly LS, et al. Prostaglandins in severe congestive heart failure. *N Engl J Med* 1984; 310:347.
134. Rudnick MR. Nephrotoxic risks of renal angiography: Contrast media-associated nephrotoxicity and atheroembolism—A critical review. *Am J Kidney Dis* 1994; 24:713.
135. Taliercio CP, Vlietstra RE, Fisher LD, et al. Risks for renal dysfunction with cardiac angiography. *Ann Intern Med* 1986; 104:501.
136. Solomon R. Contrast-medium-induced acute renal failure. *Kidney Int* 1998; 53:230.
137. Fang LST, Sirota RA, Ebert TH, et al. Low fractional excretion of sodium with contrast media-induced acute renal failure. *Arch Intern Med* 1980; 140:531.
138. Solomon R, Werner C, Mann D, et al. Effects of saline, mannitol, and furosemide on acute decreases in renal function induced by radiocontrast agents. *N Engl J Med* 1994; 331:1416.
139. Thadhani RI, Camargo CA Jr. Atheroembolic renal failure after invasive procedures: Natural history based on 52 histologically proven cases. *Medicine* 1995; 74:350.
140. Dalakos TG, Streeten DHP, Jones D, et al. "Malignant" hypertension resulting from atheromatous embolization predominantly of one kidney. *Am J Med* 1974; 57:135.
141. McGowan JA, Greenberg A. Cholesterol atheroembolic renal disease. *Am J Nephrol* 1986; 6:135.
142. Richards AM, Eliot RS, Kanjuh VI, et al. Cholesterol embolism: A multiple-system disease masquerading as polyarteritis nodosa. *Am J Cardiol* 1965; 15:696.
143. Scully RE, Mark EJ, McNeely BU. Case records of the Massachusetts General Hospital. *N Engl J Med* 1986; 315:308.
144. Cosio FG, Zager RA, Sharma HM. Atheroembolic renal disease causes hypocomplementaemia. *Lancet* 1985; 2:118.
145. Lessman RK, Johnson SF, Coburn JW. Renal artery embolism. *Ann Intern Med* 1978; 89:477.
146. Winzelberg GG, Hull JD, Agar JWM, et al. Elevation of serum lactate dehydrogenase levels in renal infarction. *JAMA* 1979; 242:268.
147. London IL, Hoffstein P, Perkoff GT, et al. Renal infarction. *Arch Intern Med* 1968; 121:87.
148. Jelliffe RW. An improved method of digoxin therapy. *Ann Intern Med* 1968; 69:703.
149. Kirch W, Gorg ER. Clinical pharmacokinetics of atenolol–A review. *Eur J Drug Metab Pharmacokinet* 1982; 7:81.
150. Cohn JN, Burke LP. Nitroprusside. *Ann Intern Med* 1979; 91: 752.
151. Oparil S, Aronson S, Deeb GM, et al. Fenoldopam: A new parenteral antihypertensive: consensus roundtable on the management of perioperative hypertension and hypertensive crises. *Am J Hypertension* 1999; 12:653.
152. Ader JL, Rostaing L. Cyclosporin nephrotoxicity: Pathophysiology and comparison with FK-506. *Curr Opin Nephrol Hypertension* 1998; 7:539.
153. Goldstein DJ, Zuech N, Sehgal V, et al. Cyclosporin-associated end-stage nephropathy after cardiac transplantation. *Transplantation* 1997; 63:664.
154. De Mattos AM, Olyaei AJ, Bennett WM. Pharmacology of immunosuppressive medications used in renal diseases and transplantation. *Am J Kid Dis* 1996; 28:631.

CHAPTER 85

EXERCISE AND THE CARDIOVASCULAR SYSTEM: ACUTE HEMODYNAMICS, CONDITIONING TRAINING, THE ATHLETE'S HEART, AND SUDDEN DEATH

Gerald F. Fletcher / Thomas R. Flipse

Exercise for the cardiovascular system has evolved in recent years as an important component of preventive and maintenance health care. Exercise, defined as properly prescribed physical activity, can provide health benefits for asymptomatic, healthy individuals as well as for those who are at high risk for or have established cardiovascular disease. This chapter addresses the topics of acute hemodynamics, conditioning training and implementation, the athlete's heart, and sudden death with exercise.

ACUTE HEMODYNAMICS

During physical activity, body energy expenditure increases, requiring appropriate adjustments in blood flow that affect the entire cardiovascular system. These changes are the result of a combination and integration of neural, chemical, and other physiologic factors.

The cardiovascular "control center" is believed to be in the ventrolateral medulla of the brain and receives input that modulates its activity. Central impulses are provided by the somatomotor centers of the brain. Peripheral impulses are generated by the mechanoreceptors found in muscles, joints, and the vascular system; the chemoreceptors from the muscles and vascular system; and the vascular baroreceptors. These impulses arrive at the control center through autonomic afferent fibers. The control center regulates the output of blood from the heart and its preferential distribution to other organs and tissues in need.

The "feed-forward" command system, located in the higher areas of the brain, provides a coordinated and rapid response of the cardiovascular system to optimize tissue perfusion and maintain central blood pressure in relation to motor cortex activity. The central command provides the greatest control over heart rate during exercise[1] and is also involved in the preexercise anticipatory period.[2] The effect of the stimulating input from the higher command centers is an alteration of the autonomic tone. The involvement of the central command in cardiovascular regulation may explain in part the influence of one's emotional state on the cardiovascular response.

The cardiovascular control center also receives input from peripheral receptors in muscles, joints, and blood vessels. Stretch and tension of muscular and articular mechanoreceptors trigger afferent impulses. Impulses triggered by the stimulation of muscle chemoreceptors resulting from products of metabolism influence the control center as well. This reflex neural input, termed the exercise pressor reflex, provides rapid feedback that modifies the parasympathetic or sympathetic outflow to adjust the cardiovascular response to physical activity.[3] Input from mechanoreceptors in the muscles and joints is important in the regulation of the circulatory response during dynamic exercise.[4]

Baroreceptors are located in the aortic arch and carotid sinuses and respond to changes in arterial blood pressure, and regulate heart rate by reciprocal changes in activity of the two divisions of the autonomic nervous system. The arterial baroreceptors protect the cardiovascular system against relatively short-term changes in blood pressure, as seen during physical exercise. The cardiopulmonary mechanoreceptors in the atria, ventricles, and pulmonary vessels are tonically active and participate in the regulation of the circulatory responses through the autonomic nervous system. An increase in blood pressure results in a reflex slowing of the heart, and the converse applies during hypotension. During physical activity, this feedback mechanism is "reset" so that blood pressure is permitted to rise to the higher levels observed during exercise. The aortic and carotid bodies contain chemoreceptors sensitive to arterial oxygen, carbon dioxide, and hydrogen ion concentrations—indices that may be altered during physical activity. Decreased arterial oxygen levels cause an increase in the arterial pressure, while changes in carbon dioxide and hydrogen ion concentration have a relatively small effect by this pathway.

Circulatory Adjustments with Exercise

The circulatory response to exercise involves a complex series of adjustments resulting in an increase in cardiac output (CO) that is proportional to the increased metabolic demands placed on the body. These changes ensure that the metabolic needs of exercising muscles are met, that hyperthermia does not occur, and that blood flow to essential organs is protected. Certain major changes occur during exercise that provide blood flow required by the muscles. These are the increase in CO and the redistribution of blood flow, with a relative increase in flow to the exercising muscles. (CO is defined as the product of stroke volume and heart rate. The average CO at rest is about 5 L/min for both trained and untrained men. In women the value is usually 25 percent lower.)

Resting CO increases immediately before the onset of physical exercise as a result of anticipatory changes in the autonomic nervous system resulting in tachycardia and increased venous return. After the onset of exercise, CO may increase rapidly until steady-rate exercise is reached; this is followed by a gradual rise until a plateau is achieved. The magnitude of the hemodynamic response during physical activity depends on the intensity of exercise and the muscle mass involved. In sedentary individuals, the CO during maximal exercise increases approximately four times, to an average of 20 to 22 L/min. In elite-class athletes, however, the CO may rise eightfold, to values of 35 to 40 L/min.

HEART RATE RESPONSE TO EXERCISE

At the transition from rest to strenuous exercise, the heart rate increases rapidly to levels of 160 to 180 beats per minute. During short periods of maximal exercise, rates of 240 beats per minute have been recorded. The initial rapid increase is believed to be the result of central command influences or a rapid reflex from muscle mechanoreceptors. The almost instant acceleration in heart rate is due more to vagal withdrawal than to an increase in sympathetic tone. Later increases result from reflex activation of the pulmonary stretch receptors, which trigger increased sympathetic tone and more parasympathetic withdrawal. Increased circulating catecholamines play a role as well. It has been shown that during exercise the heart rate increase accounts for a greater percentage of the increase in CO than does the increase in stroke volume. For instance, the stroke volume normally reaches its maximum when the CO has increased to only one-half of its maximum. Any further increase in CO occurs by an increase in the heart rate.

STROKE VOLUME CHANGES WITH EXERCISE

Two physiologic mechanisms influence the stroke volume of the heart. The first is intrinsic to the myocardium and involves enhanced cardiac filling in diastole secondary to increased venous return followed by a more forceful systolic contraction. The second mechanism involves normal ventricular filling with a forceful contraction secondary to neurohormonal influences, which leads to more complete emptying.

ENHANCED DIASTOLIC FILLING

Greater ventricular filling during diastole, or preload, is caused by factors that slow heart rate and increase venous return. Increased end-diastolic volume stretches myocardial fibers and causes a greater contraction with a larger stroke volume. As myocardial fibers stretch, there is a more optimal arrangement of the myofilaments of the sarcomere, which results in enhanced contractility. It is believed that this mechanism is responsible for the increased stroke volume during transition from rest to exercise or from the upright to the supine position. CO and stroke volume are the highest in the supine position. In this position, the stroke volume is nearly maximal at rest and increases only slightly during exercise. In the upright position, at rest, the venous return to the heart is diminished, resulting in a smaller stroke volume and CO. During upright exercise, however, stroke volume can increase to the point where it approaches the maximum stroke volume observed in the recumbent position, usually without an increase in ventricular diastolic dimensions.[5]

IMPROVED SYSTOLIC EMPTYING

Although experimental findings are not always consistent, it seems that increases in stroke volume during upright exercise occur through the combined effect of enhanced diastolic filling and a more complete emptying during systole. The improved myocardial inotropy during exercise is the result of the increased levels of catecholamines. In the normal supine individual, increased CO with exercise results predominantly from an increase in heart rate, with little improvement of stroke volume. In the upright position, in the early phase of exercise CO rises due to a simultaneous increase in stroke volume and heart rate. In the later phases of exercise, the increase in heart rate is primarily responsible for the further increase in CO.

DISTRIBUTION OF CARDIAC OUTPUT DURING EXERCISE

Blood flow to various tissues is generally proportional to metabolic activity, but certain organs have blood flow variations with the metabolic demands of exercising muscle. At rest, about 20 percent of the 5 L/min CO is distributed to the skeletal muscle. This accounts for approximately 4 to 7 mL of blood delivered each minute to every 100 g of muscle. During physical activity, regional blood flow depends on the type of exercise, environmental conditions, and level of fatigue. Still, the majority (up to 85 percent) of the increased CO is diverted to the working muscles. This represents about 50 to 75 mL blood every minute per 100 g of muscle. Even within active muscle, the increased blood flow is highly regulated, so that the greatest amount is delivered to the oxidative portions of the muscle at the expense of the tissue with high glycolytic capacity.

Two factors are responsible for the increased muscle flow during exercise: increased CO and redistribution of blood flow. Local metabolic conditions and neural and hormonal vascular regulation control the shunting of blood from various tissues to active muscles. The local response is due primarily to the buildup of vasodilatory metabolites in the exercising muscle, the increase in skeletal muscle flow being directly proportional to the increase in body oxygen consumption ($\dot{V}O_2$).

During exertion, parasympathetic activity is withdrawn and sympathetic discharge is maximal. These changes result in increased release of norepinephrine from the sympathetic postganglionic nerve endings. Plasma epinephrine levels are also increased. As a result, the majority of the vascular beds of the body are constricted, except those in exercising muscles and in the coronary and cerebral circulation. Blood flow to the skin increases during light and moderate exercise, favoring body cooling. Further increases in workload cause a progressive decrease in skin flow as the rising cutaneous sympathetic vascular tone overcomes the thermoregulatory vasodilatory response.[2] The kidneys and splanchnic tissues use only 10 to 25 percent of the oxygen available in the blood supply. Consequently, considerable reductions in blood flow to these tissues can be tolerated because of increased extraction of oxygen from the available blood supply.[6] Some tissues cannot, however, compromise their blood supply. At rest, the heart extracts about 75 percent of the oxygen in the coronary blood flow. Because of a limited margin of reserve, increased myocardial demands during exercise are met mainly by a fourfold increase in coronary blood flow. Cerebral blood flow also increases during exercise by approximately 25 to 30 percent compared to the resting flow.[7] During maximal exercise, however, cerebral flow may also decrease in association with hyperventilaton and respiratory alkalosis.

TABLE 85-1 Types of Exercise

	Isotonic	Isometric	Resistance
Alternative terminology	Dynamic	Static	Resistive
Example	Running	Static hand grip	Weight lifting
Oxygen uptake	Greatest	Least	Intermediate
CO	Greatest	Least	Intermediate
Peripheral resistance	Greatest decrease	Least decrease	Intermediate
Blood pressure	Decreases	Increases	Increases

ABBREVIATION: CO = cardiac output.

On cessation of exercise, there is an abrupt decrease in heart rate and CO secondary to removal of the sympathetic drive and reactivation of vagal activity. In contrast, systemic vascular resistance remains lower for some time due to persistent vasodilatation in the muscles. As a result, arterial pressure falls, often below preexercise levels, for periods up to 12 h into recovery.[8] Blood pressure is then stabilized at normal levels by the baroreceptor reflexes.

Exercise Type and Cardiovascular Response

Different types of exercise impose various loads on the cardiovascular system. Isotonic (dynamic) exercise is defined as muscular contraction of large muscle groups resulting in movement. It primarily induces a volume load to the heart. Isometric (static) exercise is defined as a constant muscular contraction of smaller muscle group without movement. It provokes more pressure than volume load to the heart. Significant increases in both CO and oxygen consumption and a fall in systemic vascular resistance characterize the acute load posed by isotonic exercise. In contrast, isometric exercise increases systemic vascular resistance while producing only minimal changes in CO and oxygen consumption.[9] A third type of exercise is resistance exercise. This is a combination of isometric and isotonic exercise evoked by using muscular contraction with movement, as in free-weight lifting. Most activities, such as sports or employment-related activities, usually combine all three types of exercise (see Table 85-1).

ISOTONIC (DYNAMIC) EXERCISE

The acute cardiovascular response to isotonic exercise is accomplished through both central and peripheral adaptations that result in increased oxygen delivery to and extraction by the exercising muscles. In normal sedentary individuals, $\dot{V}O_2$ typically increases tenfold from rest to maximal exertion,[10] while in world-class athletes the increase can be even greater. Maximal $\dot{V}O_2$ is considered an indicator of the level or degree of exercise training.[11]

During acute isotonic exercise, such as running, total peripheral vascular resistance falls as a result of marked vasodilatation of vessels in the exercising muscles, which overcomes the vasoconstriction of the splanchnic and renal vessels. This effect is pronounced at minimal levels of exercise, with little further change as exercise increases. As a result, afterload decreases and CO is redistributed mainly to the active muscles. These changes result from local autoregulation and are mediated by local factors related to the level of tissue metabolism (hypoxia, acidic pH, and increased local temperature), stimulation of sympathetic vasodilatory nerve endings, and the effects of circulating catecholamines.

During prolonged dynamic exercise, skeletal muscle metabolism is primarily aerobic and requires a significant increase in oxygen supply to meet the increased demand for adenosine triphosphate generation. The increased oxygen requirements are met by an augmentation of the local blood flow and improved oxygen extraction.

ISOMETRIC (STATIC) EXERCISE

The acute cardiovascular responses to isometric exercise are different from the responses to isotonic exercise. The oxygen requirements needed to sustain the contraction of a smaller muscle group without performing external work are lower.

With isometric exercise, the necessary $\dot{V}O_2$ is maintained with a smaller increase in CO. An increase in regional blood flow is limited because local vasodilatation is impeded by the mechanical compression of the blood vessels during the sustained muscular contraction.[12] Actually, regional blood flow may decrease. In order to maintain regional perfusion, a pressor response is evoked, which is thought to be, at least in part, mediated locally by reflexes originating in the muscles.[13] The amplitude of the increase in blood pressure is proportional both to the relative muscle tension and the mass of the muscle groups involved.

As a result of the increase in blood pressure and in the absence of an increase in venous return, stroke volume usually declines. In its "pure state," static exercise represents a pressure, or systolic, load. In order to maintain the higher CO, the heart rate must increase, often out of proportion to the metabolic needs of the active muscle groups.

RESISTANCE (RESISTIVE) EXERCISE

Resistance exercises are activities that use low or moderate repetition movements against a resistance, generating a rise in muscle tension. The acute cardiovascular response to resistance exercise is determined by the extent of both the isotonic and isometric components.

Weight lifting is considered the prototype resistance exercise and is thought to have a high isometric component. Blood pressure and heart rate responses during weight lifting are proportional to the relative intensity of muscle contraction, the mass of the muscle groups involved, and the duration of the contraction.[14] Weight-training exercises have been shown to cause an acute increase in blood pressure.[15] This is thought to be the result of the restricted muscle blood flow and a centrally mediated pressor response caused by increased muscle tension. The heart rate response during maximal upper body resistance exercise is lower than that seen during maximal isotonic exercise.[16] This is believed to be one of the factors to explain why the heart rate–blood pressure product during maximal resistance exercise is lower than that observed during maximal dynamic exercise.

Previous concerns regarding the safety of resistance training have been rebutted by several reports that reveal that moderate resistance training programs are safe even in subjects with cardiac disease.[17,18] At this time, it is believed that resistance training is useful for promoting muscle strength and flexibility but probably contributes less significantly than isotonic exercise to overall cardiovascular health.

CONDITIONING TRAINING

Physical conditioning or exercise training affects the cardiovascular and skeletal muscle systems in a variety of ways that improve work performance or exercise capacity. The response of the cardiovascular system to regular exercise is an increase in its capacity to deliver oxygen to active muscle. Physical training also improves the ability of the muscles to utilize oxygen. It is believed that, through conditioning induced by repetitive periods of dynamic exercise, the maximal $\dot{V}O_2$ may increase to two- to threefold. About half of this increase is due to increased CO and half to peripheral adaptations that improve oxygen extraction.[19] Through physical training, an individual can increase maximal exercise intensity and duration and achieve submaximal work loads with less cardiovascular effort. This aspect of exercise conditioning has the broadest therapeutic impact.

With conditioning, cardiac stroke volume increases, with exercise secondary to alterations in cardiac structure and function. At rest, CO, however, is similar for both trained and untrained individuals. Endurance training induces an increase in the resting parasympathetic tone, associated with a concomitant reduction in resting sympathetic activity. The effect is a bradycardia, with recorded heart rates averaging about 50 beats per minute, although values below 30 beats per minute have been recorded for healthy athletes. The CO is maintained by an increase in stroke volume. The underlying physiologic mechanisms are not fully understood, but it is believed that increased blood volume associated with training and intrinsic myocardial factors are responsible (Table 85-2). During exercise, trained individuals achieve a larger maximal CO than do sedentary persons. In the untrained person, there is only a small increase in stroke volume during the transition from rest to exercise, while the major augmentation in CO is induced by tachycardia. The improved cardiac performance after conditioning is secondary to both the Frank-Starling mechanism and augmented myocardial contraction and relaxation.

TABLE 85-2 Clinical Effects of Exercise Training

Increase in oxygen consumption
Increase in cardiac stroke volume
Increase in maximal exercise CO
Increase in resting parasympathetic tone
Decrease in resting sympathetic tone
Decrease in resting heart rate

ABBREVIATION: CO = cardiac output.

It has been shown that, in previously sedentary individuals, 8 weeks of aerobic training will increase stroke volume. This change results from increased end-diastolic dimensions of the ventricular cavity with preservation or even reduction of the end-systolic size.[20] The values are, however, much lower than those of well-trained athletes.[21] It is not known whether this is the result of prolonged training, genetic factors, or a combination of both. After cessation of training, these changes largely regress within 3 weeks.

Several factors contribute to the chronic adaptations seen with training. An increased parasympathetic tone induces bradycardia, which prolongs diastolic filling time, resulting in ventricular dilatation. In trained individuals, there is an increased preload, attributed to an expanded plasma volume in response to aerobic training.[22] Some studies have shown that endurance training results in increased compliance of the left ventricle.[23] This is probably due to enhanced early diastolic filling and increased peak myocardial lengthening during exercise.[24,25] These findings are in contrast to those in pressure overload conditions, when peak shortening and relaxation rates are diminished (Table 85-2).

These physiologic changes are accompanied by biochemical and ultrastructural alterations of the myocardial fibers, which have been demonstrated in the hearts of physically conditioned animals. There is an increase in lactic dehydrogenase and pyruvate kinase activity, which enhances the respiratory capacity of the cardiac myocytes. The size of the myocardial cells increases, as well as the number of mitochondria and myofibrils. In addition, changes in the sarcolemma and sarcoplasmic reticulum have been noted. These cellular organelles are implicated in the utilization of intracellular calcium, and the associated changes may explain the improved diastolic function of the conditioned heart.

It has been demonstrated that the cross-sectional area of the epicardial coronary arteries increases in response to exercise. Alterations in the microcirculation have been identified in animal studies, revealing an increased capillary density with an increased capillary-to-fiber ratio and a decrease in the diffusion distance between the capillaries and the mitochondria of myocytes.[26] Some data suggest that conditioning can promote coronary collateral formation to a potentially ischemic vascular bed.[27] These adaptations may enable the heart to better tolerate and recover from transient episodes of ischemia and to function at a lower percentage of its total oxidative capacity during exercise.[28] It is therefore likely that training-induced myocardial adaptations can provide protection from myocardial ischemia of coronary artery disease.

Skeletal muscle also undergoes adaptations with training that favor enhanced oxygen extraction. With long-term training, capillary density and capillary-to-fiber ratio in skeletal muscles increase.[29] The number of mitochondria increases, as do the oxidative enzyme levels in the mitochondria. It appears that other cellular adaptations occur with physical conditioning, including increases in myoglobin levels, in the levels of enzymes involved in lipid metabolism, and in ATPase activity with physical conditioning.[30] It is estimated that improved peripheral oxygen extraction accounts for approximately 50 percent of the increased maximal $\dot{V}O_2$ observed during exercise. The proportion may be even higher when CO has a limited capability to increase, which is of practical benefit for individuals with a limited cardiac reserve.

Gender Differences

Few studies have assessed the physiologic responses of women to exercise, but the qualitative aspects of these responses are similar to those seen in men, and basically the same physiologic changes occur in response to acute dynamic or static exercise. There have been some basic quantitative differences, in that teenage girls have a 5 to 10 percent greater CO at any level of submaximal oxygen uptake than do boys.[31] This is likely explained by the 10 percent lower hemoglobin concentration in women than in men. In order to deliver the same amount of oxygen, there is a compensatory proportionate increase in CO. The maximal aerobic capacity in women is approximately 50 percent lower than in men.[32] If adjusted to lean body mass, the difference is reduced to about 10 to 15 percent, which probably represents a true gender-specific difference.

The absolute number of muscle fibers and the fiber-type distribution are similar in women and men.[33] For reasons that are unclear, muscle fibers in men are hypertrophied, resulting in a cross-sectional muscle mass that is higher than in women. The increased muscle mass in men explains the greater isometric strength, while strength adjusted to cross-sectional muscle area is similar.[34]

Another gender difference with potentially significant clinical implications is the mechanism through which stroke volume is increased during acute dynamic exercise. In men there is a progressive increase in ejection fraction with little or no increase in end-diastolic volume. In contrast, women tend to increase end-diastolic volume without a significant increase in ejection fraction,[35] which results in a plateau of ejection fraction during stress testing compared to the continued increase in men.

Aging Differences

Aging results in changes in cardiovascular structure and function and varies significantly among individuals. An increased frequency of acquired heart disease occurs during aging, and there needs to be a differentiation between normal aging and the interplay of aging and disease.

Left ventricular hypertrophy and prolongation of the isovolumic relaxation period in aging can cause a decrease in early left ventricular diastolic compliance similar to the changes seen in the hypertensive heart.[36] An augmented atrial contraction ensures enhanced ventricular filling later in diastole.[37] As a result, left ventricular end-diastolic volume does not decrease with age; the end-diastolic pressure is often higher in older subjects.[38] The resting ejection fraction remains stable in healthy subjects with aging,[39] while the resting CO decreases or remains unchanged.[40] Exercise-induced alterations in cardiovascular function of the elderly may be attributed in part to the effect of age on intrinsic cellular mechanisms or to the autonomic modulation of these mechanisms.[41]

It has been noted that exercise capacity and maximal $\dot{V}O_2$ decrease with aging.[42] When adjusted for lean body mass, however, the age difference in maximal $\dot{V}O_2$ is minimized.[43] Measurements of CO during exercise have failed to substantiate that a failure of CO to increase limits peak $\dot{V}O_2$ or work capacity in older subjects. There is no clear explanation for the decline in maximal work performance and reduced maximal $\dot{V}O_2$, with aging; however, there are several mechanisms that have been proposed to influence this process. These proposed mechanisms include skeletal muscle fatigue, increased work of breathing or overall decrease in pulmonary function, differences in muscle mass, reduced blood flow to skeletal muscle, decreased oxygen extraction, or psychological factors. These age-related changes can be overcome to some extent through physical conditioning. Healthy elderly individuals undergoing 1 year of conditioning have shown a significant rise in maximum $\dot{V}O_2$.[44] Potential mechanisms for this improvement include an improved beta-adrenergic sensitivity and/or a decrease in afterload.

With regard to the effect of exercise on the cardiovascular system in the elderly, there are certain significant changes. In the elderly there is a decrease in the maximal heart rate response during exercise at any work load, and this observation is likely explained by a decreased sympathetic response. The end-systolic volume, also fails to decrease with exercise, as it does in youth. This is thought to represent a diminished cardiac inotropy and increased impedance to ejection. These alterations are not attributable to decreased circulating catecholamine production, since the plasma levels of catecholamines in the elderly are actually higher during exercise.[45] Another difference from younger individuals is a greater increase in end-diastolic volume. The stroke volume is augmented secondary to utilization of the Frank-Starling mechanism. These changes result in a similar CO in elderly and younger individuals at any specific exercise load. However, the mechanisms for achieving the augmented CO differ markedly. While in young individuals CO is augmented by utilizing adrenergically mediated responses (increased heart rate, decreased end-systolic volume, and decreased impedance to left ventricle ejection), the elderly rely mainly on the effective utilization of the Frank-Starling mechanism, which compensates for the age-related decrease in beta-adrenergic responsiveness.

The ejection fraction at rest and during exercise is used clinically in the identification of heart disease and in assessing its severity and prognosis. Ejection fraction at rest is unchanged with age and increases during exercise in both young and old healthy subjects. This increase is less in older individuals due to a smaller decrease in end-systolic volume. In all individuals, however, a decrease in ejection fraction during exercise is abnormal and suggestive of a pathologic condition.

Implementation of Exercise Training

The type of activity, frequency, duration, intensity, and progression are important variables that influence the benefit obtained from different types of physical activity. The epidemiologic literature suggests that moderate-intensity activities, such as brisk walking, performed on a regular basis confer cardioprotection.[46–48] More vigorous activity and higher levels of conditioning may confer greater cardioprotection,[49] but this issue has not been clearly resolved. High-intensity exercise programs are often associated with poor compliance rates and more musculoskeletal injuries. For these reasons, a highly structured program of vigorous exercise, especially in the elderly, is not generally recommended. Health benefits can be gained by performing moderate-intensity activity in less formal settings.

Current guidelines recommend that persons of all ages perform exercise of moderate intensity for 30 to 60 min, four to six times weekly or at least 30 min of moderate-intensity physical activity on a near-daily basis.[50–53] At the present, only 10 to 20 percent of the population meets this recommendation.[51,54] Since only a small percentage of the population is employed in a physically demanding occupation, most need to perform this activity in their leisure time. Examples of recommended activities include brisk walking, cycling, swimming, and yard work. Daily activity does not need to be continuous. The duration of any period of activity should be at least 10 min, and the accumulated daily duration should be at least 30 min. Those who are sedentary should be encouraged to initially perform a duration of activity that is comfortable and to gradually increase to 30 to 60 min of daily activity. People who meet these daily standards and who wish to increase their activity further should be encouraged to do so. Figure 85-1 displays an exercise training model protocol for beginning and maintaining an effective training program. Resistance exercises can be added to the activity program to increase muscle strength. Resistance training using 8 to 10 different exercise sets with 10 to 15 repetitions each (arms, shoulders, chest, trunk, back, hips, and legs) performed at a moderate to high intensity (e.g., 10 to 15 pounds of free weight) for a minimum of 2 days per week is recommended.

Physicians and other health professionals should encourage the general public and their patients to follow these guidelines. Many physicians believe they lack adequate training in physical activity counseling, and implementation of preventive services into medical practice can be difficult due to time and financial constraints. To address these issues, the Centers for Disease Control and Prevention developed the Physician-Based Assessment and Counseling for Exercise (PACE) project.[55] This system includes a simple discussion of physical activity counseling and illustrates how a clinician can efficiently incorporate physical activity counseling into a busy clinical practice through the use of paramedical personnel, such as nurses.

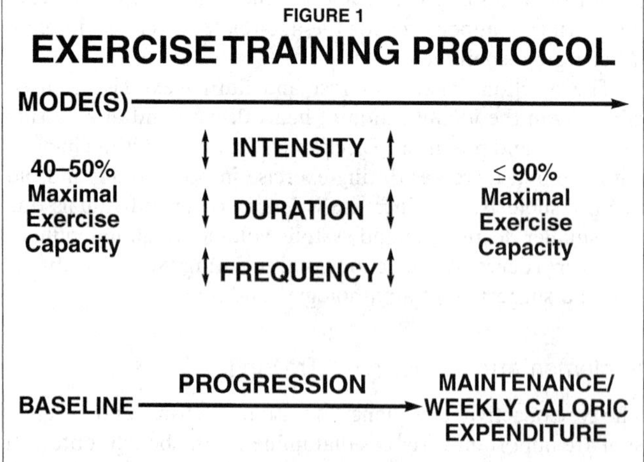

FIGURE 85-1 Exercise training model protocol. *Mode* refers to the type of exercise, such as walking, jogging, swimming, or biking. *Maximal exercise capacity* refers to that achieved at peak exercise testing and can be expressed in terms of oxygen consumption, metabolic units, heart rate, caloric expenditure, or perceived exertion. Intensity, duration, and frequency are each increased or decreased appropriately to ultimately achieve a maintenance level of total weekly caloric expenditure.

THE ATHLETE'S HEART

The structural characteristics of the hearts of apparently healthy, highly trained athletes differ considerably from those of normal individuals. Regardless of age, exercise training is followed by an increase in heart size, and this cardiac hypertrophy is viewed as a normal biologic response to an increased workload.

The duration of training affects cardiac size and structure. Short-term training is not associated with changes in cardiac dimensions, even though there is an improvement in maximal $\dot{V}O_2$ and submaximal heart response.[56,57] Prolonged endurance training is followed by left ventricular enlargement, which regresses to a pretraining level after cessation of the exercise training program. This involution is not apparently associated with any deleterious effects.[58] There is considerable variability among individuals in terms of the structural response of the heart to various forms of training. It is apparent that the structural and dimensional differences among the hearts of athletes reflect specific training demands.[59]

Isotonically trained athletes undergo an eccentric hypertrophy characterized by a slight increase in wall thickness and an increased end-diastolic volume with a normal ratio of volume to thickness. Endurance athletes have a higher prevalence of multivalvular regurgitation. The cause is not entirely clear but may reflect higher end-systolic annuli sizes of the tricuspid and mitral valves in these athlete's hearts.[60] In contrast, athletes involved in isometric training show a concentric hypertrophy defined by symmetrically thickened intraventricular septum and ventricular wall and little difference in end-diastolic volume compared to sedentary persons. The concentric hypertrophy with isometric training is not associated with changes in ventricular compliance.[61] It is interesting to note that measurements of diastolic filling in isometrically trained athletes who used anabolic steroids are significantly abnormal.[61,62] These studies suggest that anabolic steroids alter the normal physiologic hypertrophy, leading to increased myocardial stiffness.

The implications of these changes for myocardial blood flow and long-term cardiovascular health are unknown. The functional hypertrophy that occurs in response to exercise training is different from the pathologic hypertrophy secondary to chronic disease states. During exercise training, the myocardial overload is only temporary, allowing for a "recuperative period" between exercise sessions. The cardiac hypertrophy associated with training is not accompanied by "weakening" of the left ventricle, which is usually seen with chronic pathologic pressure loads. Even though the hearts of elite athletes are larger than the hearts of sedentary control subjects, the size is usually within the upper range of normal limits in relation to body size or to the increased end-diastolic volume. One study of highly trained athletes[63] revealed that left ventricular cavity dimension varied widely but was increased to a degree compatible with dilated cardiomyopathy in almost 15 percent of subjects. Because of the absence of systolic dysfunction, this cavitary enlargement is most likely the result of an extreme physiologic adaptation, of which the long-term consequences and significance are not known. At this time, there is no compelling scientific evidence to indicate that specific forms of exercise training can "harm" a normal heart. To the contrary, the cardiac functional capacity of the athlete is much greater, in terms of stroke volume and maximal CO, than that of healthy sedentary individuals.

The cardiovascular examination results for an athlete have distinctive features. There is resting bradycardia, with pulse rates as low as 30 to 40 beats per minute, and an exaggerated normal respiratory variation in heart rate. The bradycardia is due to increased vagal tone associated with conditioning and represents a physiologic adaptation requiring no specific intervention if the athlete is otherwise asymptomatic. The apical impulse may be slightly displaced due to left ventricular enlargement, but wide displacements suggest concurrent cardiac pathology. Both ventricular and atrial "gallop sounds" are not uncommonly encountered in athletes, especially in the supine position, but are considered normal. Short systolic murmurs are also relatively common, reflecting a larger stroke volume or functional regurgitation due to enlarged annuli of the atrioventricular valves.

Electrocardiographic abnormalities are often seen in the highly trained athlete (Table 85-3). These include sinus bradycardia with sinus arrhythmia, sinus pauses with occasional junctional escape beats, first-degree atrioventricular block, and even periods of Möbitz type I second-degree atrioventricular block.[64] These are likely vagally mediated and disappear with exercise or atropine administration. Morphologic P-wave changes are frequently noticed as a result of atrial enlargement. QRS voltage changes suggesting ventricular hypertrophy are often seen associated with T-wave inversion in the inferior leads. Juvenile T-wave pattern (T-wave inversions in the anterior leads) and elevated early "takeoff" of the T-wave are seen frequently. "Strain" patterns, with downsloping ST-T changes indicating abnormal repolarization, are not common but can be seen in athletes who perform isometric exercise.[65]

Chest roentgenograms may reveal symmetric globular cardiomegaly with a cardiothoracic ratio between 0.5 and 0.6. Such findings are not considered pathologic.

Echocardiography is the best tool for assessing cardiac hypertrophy associated with physical conditioning and is useful in differentiating functional hypertrophy from hypertrophic cardiomyopathy. At times, left ventricular wall thickness of greater than 13 mm or asymmetric septal hypertrophy (both rare occurrences in physiologic hypertrophy) pose diagnostic challenges. The distinction is important because hypertrophic cardiomyopathy may confer a risk of sudden death during exercise. In these cases, screening of relatives and/or a period of deconditioning, which would induce a regression of hypertrophy in cases of physiologic hypertrophy, may be indicated. The clinician's role is to recognize the physiologic adaptation to the conditioned state and distinguish such adaptation from pathologic conditions, which occur in athletes in the same frequency as in the general population.

TABLE 85-3 Electrocardiographic Changes Seen in Highly Trained Athletes

Sinus bradycardia and sinus pauses
Atrioventricular block
  First degree
  Type I second degree
Morphologic P-wave changes
QRS voltage of left ventricular hypertrophy
T-wave changes

SUDDEN DEATH

Sudden death in the athlete occurs rarely but invariably captures public attention, especially when the victim is young, vigorous, and apparently healthy. Through the efforts of the American Heart Association and similar organizations, regular exercise has been encouraged as part of a healthy lifestyle. Consequently, physicians and other health care workers may be asked to defend their recommendations in the face of media attention, and may find themselves addressing the anxieties of athletes, parents, and coaches when sudden death occurs. Fortunately, sudden death with exercise is a rare phenomenon; accidents, homicides, and illicit drug use among adolescents and young adults puts them at much greater risk.[66]

One of the earliest reports of sudden death during exercise dates back to 490 B.C. when Phidippides died after running the 26 miles from Marathon to Athens to report the defeat of the Persian army. The number of modern-day reports of sudden death in exercise is small. Each year there are approximately 4 million competitive high school athletes, 500,000 collegiate athletes, and 5000 professional athletes participating in sports.[67] In one review,[68] Maron reported 134 deaths in young competitive athletes over a 10-year period. While the number of reported cases of sudden death in young athletes is probably less than the actual figure, it remains a rare event. It is estimated that sudden death from cardiovascular disease in the high school and college athlete occurs in 1:200,000 to 1:300,000 individual athletes per academic year, and 1:70,000 over a 3-year high school career.[66]

The incidence of sudden death during exercise in older athletes (over 35 years of age) is higher. In one review in Seattle, 11 percent of 316 consecutive victims of sudden death died during or immediately after exercise, and, in Miami, 17 percent of 150 patients had exertion-related sudden death.[69] The majority of these victims had coronary artery disease. In Rhode Island, the incidence of sudden death while jogging for middle-aged men was 13 deaths per 100,000 joggers per year.[70] Nationally, the frequency of sudden death in apparently healthy men is 1:15,000 joggers, and 1:50,000 marathoners.[67] There appears to be a causal relationship between exertion and sudden death. When reexamined, the same data from Rhode Island revealed 1 death per 396,000 h of jogging, while the death rate for nonvigorous activity was 1 death per 3 million person-hours.[69]

There may be an association between sudden death and the intensity of exercise. In Seattle, the incidence of exercise-related sudden death is estimated at 5.4 per 100,000, but during vigorous activity the incidence is 5 times higher for men who exercise frequently and 56 times higher for men who exercise infrequently.[71] Among men who participate regularly in high-intensity exercise, the increase in risk during athletic training and competition is outweighed by a decrease in risk of sudden cardiac death at other times; therefore, their overall risk of sudden death was lower.[72]

Gender differences are present when evaluating the incidence of sudden death. Approximately 10 percent of events occur in women athletes, and several potential explanations exist. In the past, women have been less likely to participate in high school and college sports and have been subjected to less intensive training demands than men, although these trends are changing. At present, women do not participate as frequently as men in sports associated with the greatest risk for sudden cardiac death, and they less commonly have hypertrophic cardiomyopathy.[66] Racial differences also exist, which may be due to differences in access to health care. Hypertrophic cardiomyopathy is a significant cause of sudden death in African-American men, yet this finding is comparatively underreported in this subset of the population.[66]

In Maron's series of 134 athletes with sudden death, 52 percent were white, 44 percent were African-American, and the majority of events occurred during high school years, with a median age of 17 years. Basketball, football, and track were the most common sports associated with sudden death, and 63 percent of all cases of sudden death occurred between 3 P.M. and 9 P.M., coinciding with the peak participation time for these sports.[68] Ninety percent of victims collapse during or immediately after a training session. A prodromal complaint, such as chest pain, shortness of breath, or lightheadedness, was present in 90 percent of victims immediately prior to the event, and 18 percent had symptoms in the 3 years before their death.[68]

Sudden cardiac death may be due to mechanical abnormalities, but the majority of cases are due to dysrhythmias, namely, ventricular fibrillation. The healthy heart does not appear to be vulnerable to exercise-induced ventricular arrhythmias, except in cases of significant electrolyte abnormalities, drug use, heat stroke, or blunt trauma to the chest wall.[73] The proper substrate is needed, and this is usually a heart with a structural abnormality. An ill-timed ventricular ectopic beat is usually the trigger for a ventricular fibrillation, but exercise is believed to have significant influence on the development of ventricular fibrillation, and this may be due to transient myocardial ischemia. Other factors that may exert an influence include hypoxia due to an increase in myocardial oxygen demand in the setting of a shortened diastolic period and reduced coronary perfusion time. Alterations in autonomic tone, enhanced coagulability, and release of coronary vasoconstrictor substances, including thromboxane A_2, may play a role. Acidosis, electrolyte derangements, a rise in body temperature, and elevated circulating free fatty acid levels may also be responsible.[73] Finally, medications may play a role in some instances.

The most frequent cause of sudden death in athletes over 35 is coronary artery disease. The majority of these victims at necropsy do not have any evidence of acute thrombi, suggesting that transient myocardial ischemia may result from myocardial oxygen demands not being met during exercise during a fixed obstruction or perhaps due to coronary vasospasm.[73] Coronary artery thrombi are seen in only 25 percent of victims with coronary artery disease.[74] The true incidence may be greater. Plaque rupture may occur due to twisting of epicardial arteries as a result of exaggerated changes in systolic and diastolic dimensions during exercise, or the rise in systolic blood pressure may cause an increase in shear forces. Catecholamine-induced platelet aggregation may also play a role.[71] The majority of exercise-related sudden death due to coronary artery disease occurs in victims who had risk factors for this condition or prodromal symptoms, including chest pain.[70,74,75] This suggests that efforts directed at screening and counseling patients on symptoms may be effective at preventing sudden death in this patient population of patients.

For younger athletes (under 35 years of age), coronary artery disease is a very rare cause of exercise-induced sudden death. The majority of these deaths are due to congenital cardiac anomalies, and hypertrophic cardiomyopathy is the most common cause in this age group. It is present in 0.2 percent of the general population but accounts for 36 percent of the cases of sudden death in this subgroup.[66,68] Patients with this condition have a propensity for malignant ventricular arrhythmias, and exercise-induced alterations in circulating catecholamines, blood volume, and electrolytes contribute to the risk of sudden death with exertion.[66] Sudden cardiac death with exercise may be more likely if there is a family history of sudden death, a systolic pressure gradient greater than 50 mmHg, marked left ventricular hypertrophy, ventricular or atrial arrhythmias, or a history of syncope.[73] However, the heterogeneity of this disorder makes accurate stratification of the risk of sudden death difficult.[66] Therefore, the Twenty-Sixth Bethesda Conference report recommended that athletes with a diagnosis of hypertrophic cardiomyopathy avoid intense athletic training and competition.[76] (For a list of conditions associated with sudden cardiac death, see Table 85-4.)

Screening young athletes for sudden death is difficult because it is an infrequent event, with only a very few participants in sports at risk. Cardiac abnormalities known to cause sudden death in this age range occur infrequently in the general population,[67] and large-scale screening strategies must be designed with this in mind. In Italy, government legislation mandates that all persons between 12 to 35 years of age participating in sports must have annual medical clearance. In addition to a history and physical examination, an electrocardiogram, exercise test, and pulmonary function test are required. Echocardiograms are required in selected professional sports.[66] In the United States, there are no accepted standards for screening high school and college athletes. Five states do not require an examination, and 11 states do not have a standard medical form.[67] In addition to nurses and physician assistants, some states allow chiropractors and "naturopathic" clinicians to per-

TABLE 85-4 Cardiovascular Abnormalities Associated with Sudden Death

Coronary artery disease
Congenital malformations of the coronary arteries
Myocardial bridging of coronary arteries
Idiopathic left ventricular hypertrophy
Idiopathic dilated cardiomyopathy
Hypertrophic cardiomyopathy
Mitral valve prolapse
Aortic stenosis
Marfan syndrome
Coarctation of the aorta
Long-QT syndrome
Wolff-Parkinson-White syndrome
Idiopathic ventricular tachycardia
Arrhythmogenic right ventricular dysplasia
Sarcoidosis
Kawasaki's disease
Commotio cordis
Drug-related morphologic changes
Myocarditis

form preparticipation examinations.[66] The American Heart Association has recommended a national standard for preparticipation evaluations and that they be performed by a physician or, in select instances, a registered nurse or physician assistant. In any cases, the individual performing the evaluation should have the training and skills to perform the history and physical examination and to recognize potential heart disease.[67]

The American Heart Association has also recommended that a screening history and physical examination be performed on everyone before participating in high school and collegiate sports. In high school, the screening should be repeated every 2 years, with an interim history obtained in the intervening years. For collegiate athletes, an interim history and blood pressure measurement should be obtained in the third or fourth year, but repeated screening is not necessary.[67,77] The cardiovascular history should inquire about chest pain, syncope, unexplained shortness of breath, or diminished exercise tolerance. The athlete should be asked about a history of heart murmur or hypertension and any family history of premature death or significant cardiovascular conditions. At a minimum, the cardiovascular examination should include brachial blood pressure in the sitting position, assessment of femoral pulses to exclude coarctation of the aorta, recognition of the physical stigmata of Marfan syndrome, and precordial auscultation in supine and standing positions to identify a murmur associated with dynamic left ventricular outflow obstruction.[67] If a cardiovascular abnormality is suspected, the athlete should be referred to a cardiologist for evaluation.

The routine use of diagnostic tests as part of preparticipation screening evaluations is limited by low specificity and cost considerations. The electrocardiogram is abnormal in hypertrophic cardiomyopathy in approximately 95 percent of cases, and it proved useful in helping to identify this condition in a large series from Italy.[78] It is often abnormal in athletes with coronary anomalies and may identify the long-QT syndrome. However, it has a low specificity in the athletic population because of an increased frequency of ECG changes due to the physiologic adaptations of training (see Table 85-3).[67] The routine use of exercise testing to detect coronary artery disease in older athletes is not justified because of its low specificity as well. However, for an athlete with an intermediate pretest probability of coronary artery disease, exercise testing is useful. Echocardiograms are very accurate in the detection of hypertrophic cardiomyopathy, valvular heart disease, aortic root dilation, and left ventricular dysfunction. Although the routine use of the electrocardiogram, the echocardiogram, and other diagnostic testing would improve the diagnosis of hypertrophic cardiomyopathy and other cardiovascular abnormalities, the practical application on a national scale is limited by the cost of screening such a large number of athletes and by the infrequent occurrence of these cardiovascular abnormalities in the general population. The potential for false-positive test results, unnecessary disqualification from athletic participation, and heightened anxiety should be considered as well.

There are inherent limits to large-scale screening efforts, due to the nature of the cardiovascular abnormalities involved and the size of the athletic population in the United States. In retrospective studies, cardiovascular abnormalities were suspected by screening history and physical examinations in only 3 percent of athletes who died suddenly of cardiovascular abnormalities.[66] Even with the addition of noninvasive testing, it would not be possible to identify all athletes at risk. However, a uniform screening process such as the one outlined by the American Heart Association would be expected to identify more cardiovascular abnormalities in athletes and, by disqualifying such individuals from intense athletic activity, may decrease the incidence of sudden death.[66]

References

1. Williamson JW, Nobrega AC, Garcia JA, et al. Cardiovascular responses at the onset of static exercise in patients with dual-chamber pacemakers. *J Appl Physiol* 1995; 79:1668–1672.
2. Rowell LB. *Human Cardiovascular Control*. New York: Oxford University Press; 1993:xv, 500.
3. Rowell LB, O'Leary DS. Reflex control of the circulation during exercise: Chemoreflexes and mechanoreflexes. *J Appl Physiol* 1990; 69:407–418.
4. Strange S, Secher NH, Pawelczyk JA, et al. Neural control of cardiovascular responses and of ventilation during dynamic exercise in man. *J Physiol* (*Lond*) 1993; 470:693–704.
5. Bevegard S, Holmgren A, Jonsson B. Circulatory studies in well-trained athletes at rest and during heavy exercise, with special reference to stroke volume and the influence of body position. *Acta Physiol Scand* 1963; 57:26–50.
6. Musch TI, Haidet GC, Ordway GA, et al. Training effects on regional blood flow response to maximal exercise in foxhounds. *J Appl Physiol* 1987; 62:1724–1732.
7. Thomas SN, Schroeder T, Secher NH, Mitchell JH. Cerebral blood flow during submaximal and maximal dynamic exercise in humans. *J Appl Physiol* 1989; 67:744–748.
8. Pescatello LS, Fargo AE, Leach CN Jr, Scherzer HH. Short-term effect of dynamic exercise on arterial blood pressure. *Circulation* 1991; 83:1557–1561.
9. Bechuza GR, Lenser MC, Hanson PG, Nagle FJ. Comparison of hemodynamic responses to static and dynamic exercise. *J Appl Physiol* 1982; 53:1589–1593.
10. Bruce RA, Kusumi F, Hosmer D. Maximal oxygen intake and normographic assessment of functional aerobic impairment in cardiovascular disease. *Am Heart J* 1973; 85:546–562.
11. Saltin B, Astrand PO. Maximal oxygen uptake in athletes. *J Appl Physiol* 1967; 23:353–358.
12. Asmussen E. Similarities and dissimilarities between static and dynamic exercise. *Circ Res* 1981; 48:I3–I10.
13. Hanson P, Nagle F. Isometric exercise: Cardiovascular responses in normal and cardiac populations. In: Hanson P, ed. *Exercise and the Heart: Cardiology Clinics*. Philadelphia: Saunders; 1987:157.
14. Seals DR, Washburn RA, Hanson PG, et al. Increased cardiovascular response to static contraction of large muscle groups. *J Appl Physiol* 1983; 54:434–437.
15. Wescott W, Howeff B. Blood pressure response during weight training exercises. *NSCA J* 1983; 5:67–71.
16. DeBusk RF, Valdez R, Houston N, Haskell W. Cardiovascular responses to dynamic and static effort soon after myocardial infarction: Application to occupational work assessment. *Circulation* 1978; 58:368–375.
17. Ghilarducci LE, Holly RG, Amsterdam EA. Effects of high resistance training in coronary artery disease. *Am J Cardiol* 1989; 64:866–870.
18. Sparling PB, Cantwell JD, Dolan CM, Niederman RK. Strength training in a cardiac rehabilitation program: A six-month follow-up. *Arch Phys Med Rehabil* 1990; 171:148–152.
19. Rowell LB. Human cardiovascular adjustments to exercise and thermal stress. *Physiol Rev* 1974; 54:75–159.
20. Ehsani AA, Hagberg JM, Hickson RC. Rapid changes in ventricular dimensions and mass in response to physical conditioning and deconditioning. *Am J Cardiol* 1972; 42:52–56.

21. Saltin B. Physiologic effects on physical conditioning. *Med Sci Sports* 1969; 1:50–56.
22. Convertino VA. Blood volume: Its adaptation to endurance training. *Med Sci Sports Exerc* 1991; 23:1338–1348.
23. Levy WC, Cerqueira MD, Abrass IB, et al. Endurance exercise training augments diastolic filling at rest and during exercise in healthy young and older men. *Circulation* 1993; 88:116–126.
24. Matsuda M, Sugishita Y, Koseki S, et al. Effect of exercise on left ventricular diastolic filling in athletes and nonathletes. *J Appl Physiol* 1983; 55:323–328.
25. Granger CB, Karimeddini MK, Smith VE, et al. Rapid ventricular filling in left ventricular hypertrophy: I. Physiologic hypertrophy. *J Am Coll Cardiol* 1985; 5:862–868.
26. Anversa P, Levicky V, Beghi C, et al. Morphometry of exercise-induced right ventricular hypertrophy in the rat. *Circ Res* 1983; 52:57–64.
27. Froelicher V, Jensen D, Atwood JE, et al. Cardiac rehabilitation: Evidence for improvement in myocardial perfusion and function. *Arch Phys Med Rehabil* 1980; 61:517–522.
28. Starnes JW, Bowles DK. Role of exercise in the cause and prevention of cardiac dysfunction. *Exerc Sport Sci Rev* 1995; 23:349–373.
29. Hermansen L, Wachtlova M. Capillary density of skeletal muscle in well-trained and untrained men. *J Appl Physiol* 1971; 30: 860–863.
30. Holloszy JO, Booth FW. Biochemical adaptations to endurance exercise in muscle. *Annu Rev Physiol* 1976; 38:273–291.
31. Bar-Or O, Shephard RJ, Allen CL. Cardiac output of 10- to 13-year-old boys and girls during submaximal exercise. *J Appl Physiol* 1971; 30:219–223.
32. Drinkwater BL. Women and exercise: Physiological aspects. *Exerc Sport Sci Rev* 1984; 12:21–51.
33. Costill DL, Daniels J, Evans W, et al. Skeletal muscle enzymes and fiber composition in male and female track athletes. *J Appl Physiol* 1976; 40:149–154.
34. Astrand PO, Rodahl K. *Textbook of work physiology: Physiological basis of exercise.* New York: McGraw-Hill; 1986:756.
35. Higginbotham MB, Morris KG, Coleman RE, Cobb FR. Sex-related differences in the normal cardiac response to upright exercise. *Circulation* 1984; 70:357–366.
36. Lakatta EG. Do hypertension and aging have a similar effect on the myocardium? *Circulation* 1987; 75:I69–I77.
37. Miyatake K, Okamoto M, Kinoshita N, et al. Augmentation of atrial contribution to left ventricular inflow with aging as assessed by intracardiac Doppler flowmetry. *Am J Cardiol* 1984; 53:586–589.
38. Nixon JV, Hallmark H, Page K, et al. Ventricular performance in human hearts aged 61 to 73 years. *Am J Cardiol* 1985; 56:932–937.
39. Gerstenblith G, Frederiksen J, Yin FC, et al. Echocardiographic assessment of a normal adult aging population. *Circulation* 1977; 56:273–278.
40. Raven PB, Mitchell J. The effect of aging on the cardiovascular response to dynamic and static exercise. *Aging* 1980; 12:269–296.
41. Lakatta EG. Health, disease and cardiovascular aging. In: Committee on an Aging Society, Institute of Medicine and National Research Council, ed. *Health in an Older Society.* Washington: National Academy Press; 1985:73–104
42. Bruce RA, Hornsten TR. Exercise stress testing in evaluation of patients with ischemic heart disease. *Prog Cardiovasc Dis* 1969; 11:371–390.
43. Fleg JL, Lakatta EG. Role of muscle loss in the age-associated reduction in $\dot{V}O_2$ max. *J Appl Physiol* 1988; 65:1147–1151.
44. Ehsani AA, Ogawa T, Miller TR, et al. Exercise training improves left ventricular systolic function in older men. *Circulation* 1991; 83:96–103.
45. Fleg JL, Tzankoff SP, Lakatta EG. Age-related augmentation of plasma catecholamines during dynamic exercise in healthy males. *J Appl Physiol* 1985; 59:1033–1039.
46. Powell KE, Thompson PD, Caspersen CJ, Kendrick JS. Physical activity and the incidence of coronary heart disease. *Annu Rev Public Health* 1987; 8:253–287.
47. Berlin JA, Colditz GA. A meta-analysis of physical activity in the prevention of coronary heart disease. *Am J Epidemiol* 1990; 132:612–628.
48. O'Connor GT, Buring JE, Yusuf S, et al. An overview of randomized trials of rehabilitation with exercise after myocardial infarction. *Circulation* 1989; 80:234–244.
49. Lee IM, Hsieh CC, Paffenbarger RS Jr. Exercise intensity and longevity in men: The Harvard Alumni Health Study. *JAMA* 1995; 273:1179–1184.
50. Fletcher GF, Balady G, Blair SN, et al. Statement on exercise: Benefits and recommendations for physical activity programs for all Americans, a statement for health professionals by the Committee on Exercise and Cardiac Rehabilitation of the Council on Clinical Cardiology, American Heart Association. *Circulation* 1996; 94:857–862.
51. U.S. Department of Health and Human Services, National Center for Chronic Disease Prevention and Health Promotion. *Physical Activity and Health: A Report of the Surgeon General.* Pittsburgh: President's Council on Physical Fitness and Sports; 1996:278.
52. Pate RR, Pratt M, Blair SN, et al. Physical activity and public health: A recommendation from the Centers for Disease Control and Prevention and the American College of Sports Medicine. *JAMA* 1995; 273:402–407.
53. NIH Consensus Development Panel: Physical activity and cardiovascular health. *JAMA* 1996; 276:241–246.
54. Caspersen CJ, Christenson GM, Pollard RA. Status of the 1990 physical fitness and exercise objectives: Evidence from NHIS 1985. Public Health Report 1986; 101:587–592.
55. Patrick K, Calfas KJ, Sallis JF, Long B. Basic principles of physical activity counseling: Project PACE. In: Thomas R, ed. *The Heart and Exercise.* New York: Igaku-Shoin; 1996:33.
56. Ricci G, Lajoie D, Petitclerc R, et al. Left ventricular size following endurance, sprint, and strength training. *Med Sci Sports Exerc* 1982; 14:344–347.
57. Thompson PD, Lewis S, Varady A, et al. Cardiac dimensions and performance after either arm or leg endurance training. *Med Sci Sports Exerc* 1981; 13:303–309.
58. Dickhuth HH, Horstmann T, Staiger J, et al. The long-term involution of physiological cardiomegaly and cardiac hypertrophy. *Med Sci Sports Exerc* 1989; 21:244–249.
59. Maron BJ. Structural features of the athlete heart as defined by echocardiography. *J Am Coll Cardiol* 1986; 7:190–203.
60. Douglas PS, Berman GO, O'Toole ML, et al. Prevalence of multivalvular regurgitation in athletes. *Am J Cardiol* 1989; 64:209–212.
61. Pearson AC, Schiff M, Mrosek D, et al. Left ventricular diastolic function in weight lifters. *Am J Cardiol* 1986; 58:1254–1259.
62. Urhausen A, Holpes R, Kindermann W. One- and two-dimensional echocardiography in bodybuilders using anabolic steroids. *Eur J Appl Physiol* 1989; 58:633–640.
63. Pelliccia A, Culasso F, Di Paolo FM, Maron BJ. Physiologic left ventricular cavity dilatation in elite athletes. *Ann Intern Med* 1999; 130:23–31.
64. Zehender M, Meinertz T, Keul J, Just H. ECG variants and cardiac arrhythmias in athletes: Clinical relevance and prognostic importance. *Am Heart J* 1990; 119:1378–1391.
65. Buttrick PM, Scheuer J. Exercise and the heart: Acute hemodynamics, conditioning training, the athlete's heart, and sudden death. In: Schlant RC, Alexander RW, eds. *Hurst's the Heart*, 8th ed. New York: McGraw-Hill; 1994:2057.
66. Maron BJ. Cardiovascular risks to young persons on the athletic field. *Ann Intern Med* 1998; 129:379–386.
67. Maron BJ, Thompson PD, Puffer JC, et al. Cardiovascular preparticipation screening of competitive athletes: A statement for health professionals from the Sudden Death Committee (clinical cardiology) and Congenital Cardiac Defects Committee (cardiovascular

disease in the young), American Heart Association. *Circulation* 1996; 94:850–856.
68. Maron BJ, Shirani J, Poliac LC, et al. Sudden death in young competitive athletes: Clinical, demographic, and pathological profiles. *JAMA* 1996; 276:199–204.
69. Cobb LA, Weaver WD. Exercise: A risk for sudden death in patients with coronary heart disease. *J Am Coll Cardiol* 1986; 7:215–219.
70. Thompson PD, Funk EJ, Carleton RA, Sturner WQ. Incidence of death during jogging in Rhode Island from 1975 through 1980. *JAMA* 1982; 247:2535–2538.
71. Thompson PD. The cardiovascular complications of vigorous physical activity. *Arch Intern Med* 1996; 156:2297–2302.
72. Siscovick DS, Weiss NS, Fletcher RH, Lasky T. The incidence of primary cardiac arrest during vigorous exercise. *N Engl J Med* 1984; 311:874–877.
73. Franklin BA, Fletcher GF, Gordon NF, et al. Cardiovascular evaluation of the athlete: Issues regarding performance, screening and sudden cardiac death. *Sports Med* 1997; 24:97–119.
74. Virmani R, Burke AP, Farb A, Kark JA. Causes of sudden death in young and middle-aged competitive athletes. *Cardiol Clin* 1997; 15:439–466.
75. Northcote RJ, Ballantyne D. Sudden cardiac death in sport. *Br Med J (Clin Res Ed)* 1983; 287:1357–1359.
76. Maron BJ, Mitchell JH. 26th Bethesda Conference: Recommendations for determining eligibility for competition in athletes with cardiovascular abnormalities. *J Am Coll Cardiol* 1994; 24:845–899.
77. Maron BJ, Thompson PD, Puffer JC, et al. Cardiovascular preparticipation screening of competitive athletes: An addendum to a statement for health professionals from the Sudden Death Committee (Council on Clinical Cardiology) and the Congenital Cardiac Defects Committee (Council on Cardiovascular Disease in the Young), American Heart Association. *Circulation* 1998; 97: 2294.
78. Corrado D, Basso C, Schiavon M, Thiene G. Screening for hypertrophic cardiomyopathy in young athletes. *N Engl J Med* 1998; 339:364–369.

CHAPTER 86

CARDIOVASCULAR AGING IN HEALTH AND THERAPEUTIC CONSIDERATIONS IN OLDER PATIENTS WITH CARDIOVASCULAR DISEASES

Edward G. Lakatta / Steven P. Schulman / Gary Gerstenblith

CARDIOVASCULAR AGING IN HEALTH

Introduction

The proportion of older persons that constitute populations worldwide is increasing. It is estimated that, by the year 2035, nearly one in four individuals will be 65 years of age or older. Cardiovascular diseases, such as coronary arterial atherosclerosis and hypertension, and resultant chronic heart failure reach epidemic proportions among older persons. The clinical manifestations and prognosis of these diseases as well as heart failure also worsen with increasing age. It is hypothesized that one reason for this is that specific pathophysiologic mechanisms causing clinical disorders in older persons become superimposed on heart and vascular substrates that are modified by the aging process per se. In this regard, quantitative information on age-associated alterations in cardiovascular structure and function in health is essential to define and target the specific characteristics of cardiovascular aging that render it such a major risk factor for cardiovascular diseases. Such information is also required to differentiate between the limitations of an elderly person that relate to disease and those that are within expected normal limits.

During the past two decades, a sustained effort has been applied to characterize the effects of aging in health on multiple aspects of cardiovascular structure and function in a single study population. In the Baltimore Longitudinal Study on Aging (BLSA), community-dwelling volunteers are rigorously screened to detect both clinical and occult cardiovascular disease and are characterized with respect to lifestyle (e.g., exercise habits) in an attempt to clarify the interactions of these factors and those changes that result from aging, per se. Perspectives gleaned from these studies will be emphasized throughout this section of the chapter, as will relevant information from studies in animal models.

Cardiovascular Structure

CARDIAC STRUCTURE

Cross-sectional studies of sedentary BLSA volunteer subjects without cardiovascular disease indicate that the left ventricular (LV) wall thickness, measured via M-mode (one-dimensional) echocardiography, increases progressively with age in both sexes (Fig. 86-1*A*).[1] This is mostly due to an increase in average myocyte size. In older, hospitalized patients without apparent cardiovascular disease, autopsy overall LV mass decreased with age, and cardiac myocyte enlargement was observed concurrently with an estimated decrease in myocyte number.[2] The observed frequency of apoptotic myocytes is higher in older male than female hearts.[3] An increase in the amount and a change in the physical properties of collagen (purportedly due to nonenzymatic cross-linking) also occur within the myocardium with aging. However, the cardiac myocyte-to-collagen ratio in the older heart either remains constant or increases.

There is an increase in elastic and collagenous tissue in all parts of the conduction system with advancing age. Fat accumulates around the sinoatrial node, sometimes producing a partial or complete separation of the node from the atrial musculature. There may be a pronounced decrease in the number of pace-

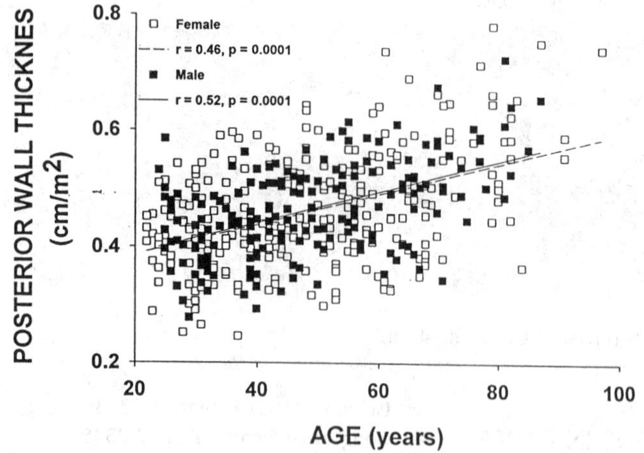

A

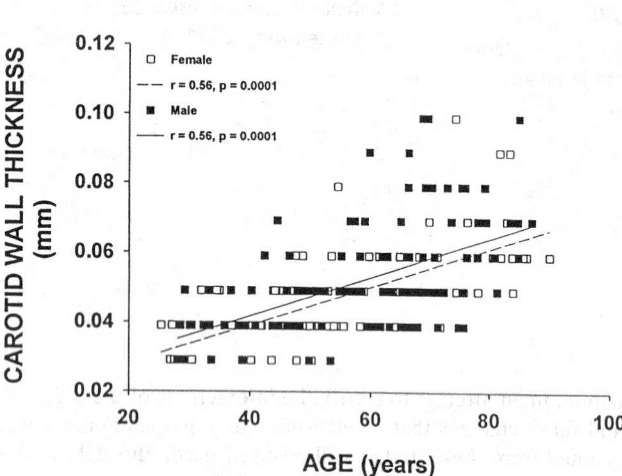

B

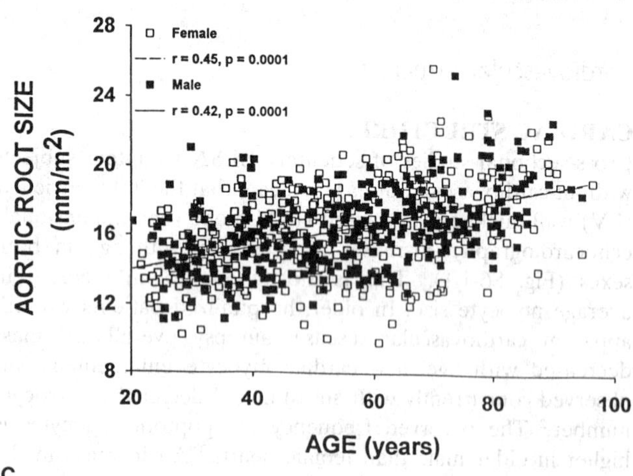

C

FIGURE 86-1 *A.* Aortic root diameter, measured via M-mode echocardiography. (From *Circulation* 1997; 56:273. Reproduced with permission from the publisher and authors.) *B.* Carotid intimal-medial wall thickness measured via echo Doppler techniques. (From *Circulation* 1998; 98: 1504. Reproduced with permission from the publisher and authors.) *C.* Left ventricular posterior wall thickness, measured by M-mode echocardiography, increases with age in healthy men and women from the Baltimore Longitudinal Study on Aging. (From *Circulation* 1997; 56:273, 1997. Reproduced with permission from the publisher and authors.)

maker cells in the sinoatrial node beginning at age 60, and by age 75 less than 10 percent of the cell number found in the young adult remains. A variable degree of calcification of the left side of the cardiac skeleton, which includes the aortic and mitral annuli, the central fibrous body, and the summit of the interventricular septum, also occurs with aging. Because of their proximity to these structures, the atrioventricular (AV) node, AV bundle, bifurcation, and proximal left and right bundle branches may be affected by this process.

The altered cardiac structural phenotype with aging in rodents in addition to an increase in LV mass, due to enlargement of myocyte size,[4] includes proliferation of the matrix in which the myocytes reside, which is focal in nature and may be linked to an altered cardiac fibroblast number or function.

With advancing age in rodents, the number of cardiac myocytes, which are postmitotic, terminally differentiated cells, also becomes reduced.[5] Putative stimuli for cardiac cell growth enlargement with aging in rodents are an age-associated increased vascular load, due to arterial stiffening (see below), and an additional load due to stretching of cells caused by dropout of neighboring myocytes. The reduction in myocyte number may be attributable to apoptosis as well as necrosis.[6] In fact, stretch, per se, is linked to cardiac myocyte apoptosis.[7] Stretch of cardiac myocytes and fibroblasts releases growth factors, one of which is angiotensin II, which in addition to modulating cell growth and matrix collagen production and, therefore, cell size, also leads to apoptosis.[8] Enhanced secretion of molecules like atrial natriuretic[9] and opioid[10] peptides, molecules that are usually produced in response to stress, is also observed in the senescent rodent heart.

VASCULAR STRUCTURE

With advancing age in healthy humans, the large arteries dilate (Fig. 86-1*A*), their walls, particularly the intima, become thickened (Fig. 86-1*B*), and changes occur within the vascular intima that appear to resemble those that occur during early atherosclerosis. Collagen content increases, and elastin becomes frayed. An increased elastase activity with aging may contribute to both elastin fragmentation and a reduction in its content with aging.[11]

Whereas the macroscopic changes in vascular cells and the matrix of large vessels in humans are well described, the specific molecular mechanisms that lead to vascular stiffening and a thickened intima remain to be elucidated. In general, changes in resistance vessels with aging in healthy individuals are less well studied but are apparently less marked than those in conduit arteries.

Age-associated macroscopic changes within large blood vessels in rodents are similar in many ways to those that occur in humans. Arterial remodeling with adult aging in rodents consists of dilation, medial thickening, and formation of an intima.[12–15] Chronic morphologic and biochemical modifications in the aortic intima of aging rats, i.e., fragmentation of the internal elastic membrane and intimal thickening, and localized increases in growth factors and collagenase activity appear as a muted version of alterations associated with chronic hypertension. Vascular smooth muscle (VSM) and endothelial cells are not terminally differentiated. VSM cells are subject to phenotypic modulation during which they revert to a proliferative, secretory and migratory mode. This *modulated* VSM phenotype repairs vascular damage and participates in vascular pathologies such as hypertension and atherosclerosis.

The thickened intima in older rats is composed of matrix molecules, including collagen and proteoglycan, and VSM cells and contains markedly higher levels of the matrix metalloproteinase, MMP-2, than do younger vessels.[16] The metalloproteinases can mediate tissue breakdown and remodeling. The intimal growth occurring during aging resembles, in some ways, neointimal formation in response to arterial balloon catheter-induced injury. In fact, neointimal growth in response to endothelial injury is markedly enhanced in old versus young rats, and this response is due to factors intrinsic to the vessel wall.[17] Ample evidence indicates the occurrence of discontinuities of the internal elastic lamina in the aorta with advancing age, in the absence of externally imposed experimental injury. Degradation of elastin by elastases and gelatinases (e.g., MMP-2 and MMP-9) may be implicated in elastic membrane breaks.[18]

The cytokine, transforming growth factor β (TGF-β), accumulates in the same regions of intima of old rats, as does MMP-2. TGF-β, which suppresses protease activity and activates tissue inhibitors of MMP,[19] is a potent factor for the synthesis of extracellular matrix proteins[13,20,21] and its expression can lead to excessive fibrosis.[19] Accumulation of TGF-β in the aortic wall of aged rats occurs with adult aging and may account for the concomitant increase in fibronectin.[16,22] There is some evidence to indicate that the collagenolytic[23] and antiproliferative actions of TGF-β decrease with aging.[24] Both fibronectin and TGF-β expression are regulated by angiotensin II,[25] and chronic administration of an angiotensin-converting enzyme inhibitor substantially reduces and delays the matrix and intimal changes associated with aging or hypertension.[12] This suggests that *age-associated changes in local vascular angiotensin regulation may have a role in the age-associated changes observed in TGF-β, fibronectin, and collagen deposition.*

Cardiovascular Function

CARDIAC VOLUMES AND EJECTION

Left Ventricular Filling and Preload Factors that determine ventricular volume (i.e., fiber stretch, end-diastolic blood volume, and filling pressure) are sometimes referred to as *preload*, which is a preexcitation determinant of myocardial function and pump performance, determined, in part, by ventricular filling characteristics. The latter are determined by the diastolic AV pressure gradient, one determinant of which is LV compliance (inverse of stiffness). Contrary to much that has been written on the subject, a reduction in ventricular compliance with age remains unproven because its measurement requires the simultaneous determination of pressure and volume, which have not been characterized in healthy younger and older persons. The early diastolic filling rate progressively slows after the age of 20 years, however, so that, by 80 years, the rate is reduced up to 50 percent (Fig. 86-2). This reduction in filling rate (demonstrated by echocardiography,[26] radionuclide angiography,[27] and Doppler ultrasonography[28] is likely attributable either to structural (fibrous) changes within the LV myocardium or to residual myofilament Ca^{2+} activation from the preceding systole (see below).

Despite the slowing of LV filling early in diastole, more filling occurs in late diastole, due, in part, to a more vigorous atrial contraction.[27] The augmented atrial contraction is accompanied by atrial enlargement and is manifested on auscultation as a fourth heart sound (atrial gallop).

Despite the age-associated changes in the diastolic filling pattern in older men, their LV end-diastolic volume index—i.e., normalized for body surface area (EDVI)—in the supine position, does not substantially differ from those in their younger counterparts (Fig. 86-3*A*). The acute reserve capacity of specific functions (e.g., EDV) that determine cardiac performance can be conveniently illustrated by depicting these over a wide range of demand for blood flow and pressure regulation, e.g., assumption of the sitting posture and during submaximal and exhaustive (max) upright exercise (Figs. 86-2*A* and 86-3). The lines depicted in these figures are the least-square linear regression on age of a given function in the steady state at different levels of effort in healthy, sedentary BLSA males. The overall magnitude of the acute, dynamic range of reserve of a given function in younger versus older subjects can quickly be gleaned from the length of the brackets depicted at the extremes of the regression lines.

Assumption of the sitting position reduces EDVI in younger but not in older individuals (Fig. 86-3*A*); during submaximal cycle-seated exercise EDVI increases equivalently at all ages, but during exhaustive exercise EDVI drops to the seated rest level in young men but remains elevated in older men (Fig. 86-3*A*). Thus, for EDVI, the average, acute, dynamic EDV reserve range during the postural change and during graded upright exercise is moderately *greater* at 85 than at 20 years. This does not support the widely held concept that the dynamic range of filling volumes is compromised in older hearts despite a reduction in LV early diastolic filling rate (Fig. 86-2*A*). In fact, during vigorous exercise (max), the LV at end diastole becomes acutely dilated in healthy, older but not younger persons. The interindividual variation of EDVI within the age-associated patterns depicted during exhaustive exercise (max) by the regression line for men in Fig. 86-3*A* is illustrated for both men and women in Fig. 86-4*A*.

Whether the capacity for *further* acute dilation of the LV of older persons beyond that observed in Figs. 86-1 to 86-3*A* and 86-4*A* is compromised cannot be readily determined either. In older BLSA persons with occult silent coronary disease, however, as evident by both ECG evidence and thallium scan perfusion deficits during exhaustive exercise, but not at rest, the LV EDVI at maximum exercise is greater than that in healthy age-matched subjects [as is the increase in LV end-systolic volume index (ESVI) and reduction in ejection fraction[28]]. Thus, at least in older patients with silent ischemia, the capacity exists for further acute EDVI dilation during exercise than that observed in healthy individuals.

Left Ventricular Ejection Figure 86-3*B* illustrates a remarkable age-associated reduction in the range of reserve in the ESVI: in younger men, the ESVI becomes progressively reduced with increasing demands for cardiovascular perfusion from supine rest to maximum upright exercise, but the range of acute ESV reserve at age 85 is only about a fifth of that at age 20. The age-associated failure in ESV regulation across the various levels of demand depicted in Fig. 86-3*B* causes a similar age-associated loss of ejection fraction regulation (Fig. 86-3*C*). See Fig. 86-4*B* and *C* for interindividual variations in ESVI and ejection fraction at max exercise in both males and females.

As a result of the age-associated changes in EDVI and ESVI

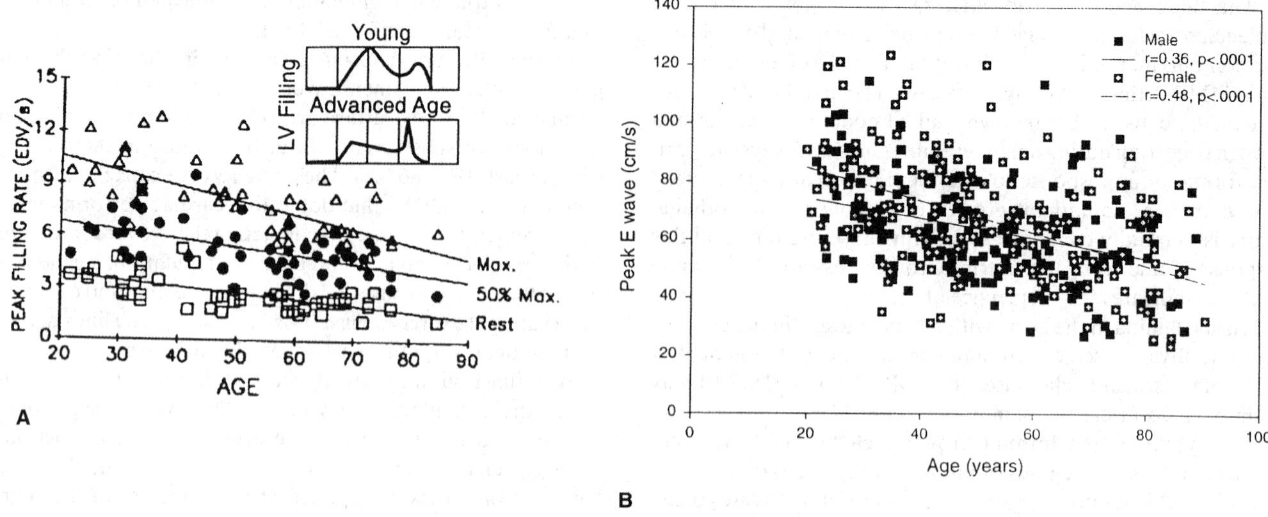

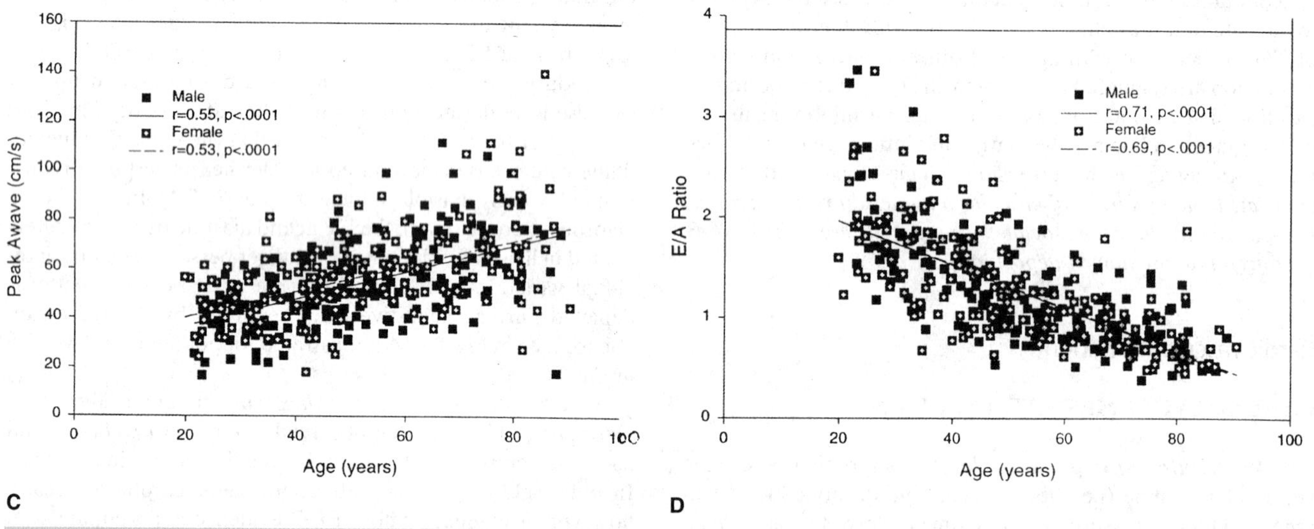

FIGURE 86-2 *A*. Maximum left ventricular filling rate assessed via equilibrium gated blood-pool scans in healthy volunteers from the Baltimore Longitudinal Study on Aging. (From *Am J Physiol* 1992; 263:H1932. Reproduced with permission from the publisher and authors.) Age-associated changes in the early diastolic left ventricular filling rate, E (*B*), the atrial contribution to filling, A (*C*), and the ratio of early to atrial filling rates (*D*). EDV = end-diastolic volume. (From *Am J Cardiol* 1992; 69: 823. Reproduced with permission from the publisher and authors.)

FIGURE 86-3 Least-squares linear regression on age of left ventricular values, ejection fraction (EF), heart rate (HR), and cardiac index (CI), at rest and during graded cycle exercise in 149 healthy males from the Baltimore Longitudinal Study on Aging (BLSA), who exercised to at least a 100-W workload. The *asterisk* indicates that regression on age is statistically significant. The overall magnitude of the acute, dynamic range of reserve of a given function in younger compared with older subjects can quickly be gleaned from the length of the *brackets* depicted at the extremes of the regression lines. For end-diastolic volume index (EDVI), the average, acute, dynamic EDV reserve range during the postural change and during graded upright exercise is moderately *greater* at 85 than at 20 years. (*A*) There is a remarkable age-associated reduction in the range of reserve in the end-systolic volume index (ESVI) (*B*) which causes a similar age-associated loss of EF regulation (*C*). The stroke volume index (SVI) is preserved in older persons over a wide range of performance (*D*). During progressive exhaustive exercise, however, when in older men the failure to reduce ESVI (*B*) impairs the EF (*C*), SVI is not augmented in older compared with younger men, as would be anticipated on the basis of their augmented EDVI. The maximum acute dynamic reserve range of HR is reduced by about one-third between 20 and 85 years of age (*E*). The loss of acute cardiac output reserve from seated rest to exhaustive, seated cycle exercise averages about 30 percent in healthy, community-dwelling BLSA volunteer men (*F*). This reduction is entirely due to a reduction in HR reserve, as SVI at max exercise is preserved. At max exercise, the age-associated increase in EDVI is of borderline statistical significance in women, but the change in EDVI from rest to max exercise in a given individual (not shown) significantly increases with age and is nearly identical in both men and women. (From *J Appl Physiol* 1995; 78:890. Reproduced with permission from the publisher and authors.)

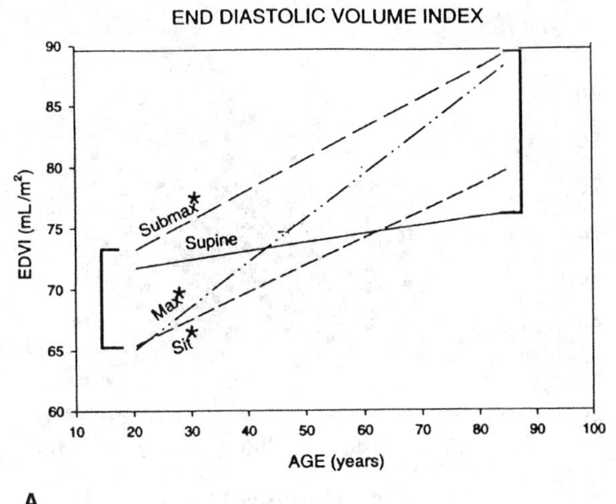
END DIASTOLIC VOLUME INDEX
EDVI (mL/m²)
Submax*
Supine
Max*
Sit*
AGE (years)
A

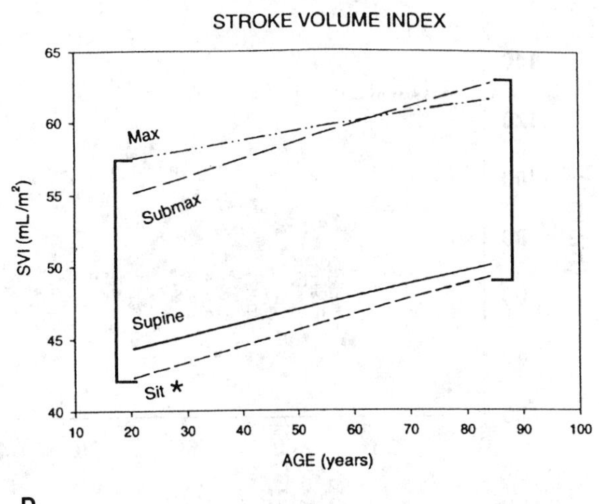
STROKE VOLUME INDEX
SVI (mL/m²)
Max
Submax
Supine
Sit *
AGE (years)
D

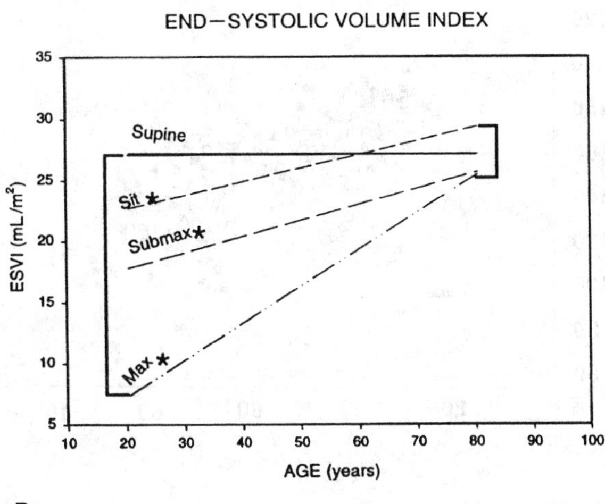
END–SYSTOLIC VOLUME INDEX
ESVI (mL/m²)
Supine
Sit *
Submax*
Max *
AGE (years)
B

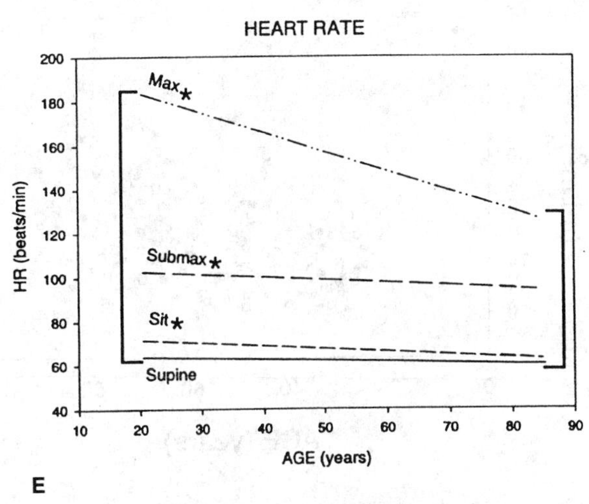
HEART RATE
HR (beats/min)
Max*
Submax*
Sit*
Supine
AGE (years)
E

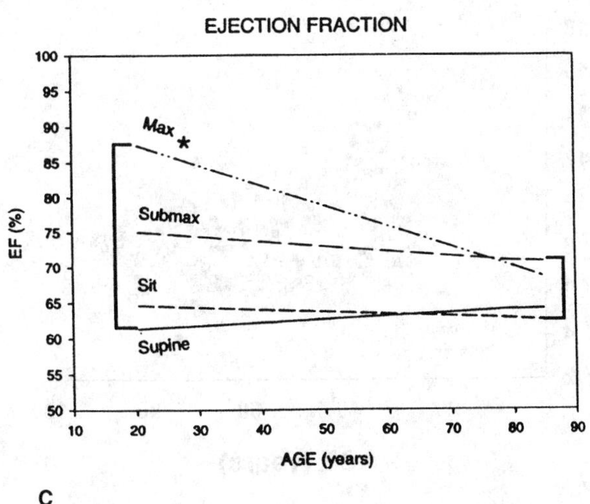
EJECTION FRACTION
EF (%)
Max *
Submax
Sit
Supine
AGE (years)
C

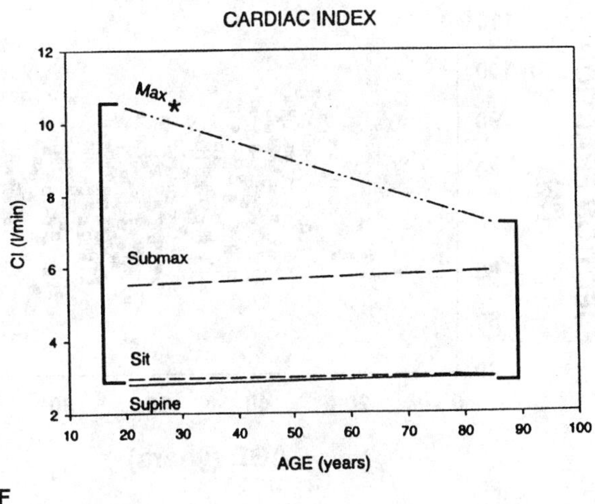
CARDIAC INDEX
CI (l/min)
Max*
Submax
Sit
Supine
AGE (years)
F

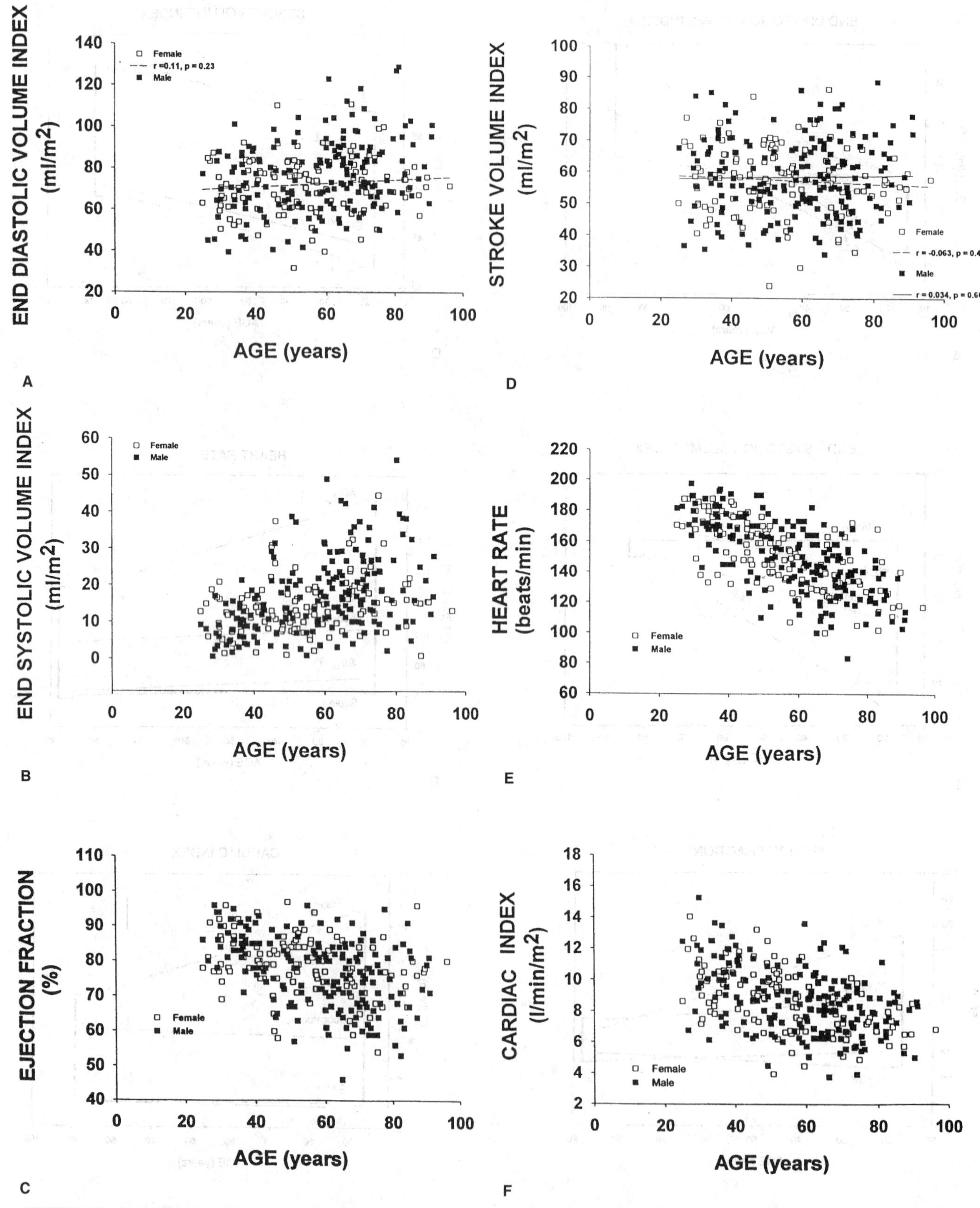

FIGURE 86-4 Scatter plots of heart rate and cardiac volumes, ejection fraction, and cardiac index in healthy sedentary men from the Baltimore Longitudinal Study on Aging (BLSA) depicted in Fig. 86-3 and for 113 BLSA women who exercised to a 75-W workload. Illustrated is the heterogeneity among individuals at a given age. In some instances (e.g., end-systolic volume index and ejection fraction), the heterogeneity increases with age. (From *J Appl Physiol* 1995; 78:80. Reproduced with permission from the publisher and authors.)

regulation depicted in Fig. 86-3*A* and *B,* the stroke volume index (SVI) is preserved in older persons over a wide range of performance (Fig. 86-3*D*). Specifically, the Frank-Starling mechanism is utilized in older men with the assumption of an upright, seated posture at rest (Fig. 86-3*A*) to produce a modest age-associated increase in SVI (Fig. 86-3*D*). During progressive exhaustive exercise, however, when in older men the failure to reduce ESVI (Fig. 86-3*B*) impairs the ejection fraction (Fig. 86-3*C*), SVI is not augmented in older compared with younger men, as would be anticipated on the basis of their augmented EDVI. In other words, *while healthy older persons utilize the Frank-Starling mechanism during vigorous exercise, this mechanism is impaired due to impaired LV ejection.* See Fig. 86-4*D* for interindividual variation of SVI in both men and women at maximum effort.

HEART RATE

In the supine position at rest, the heart rate in healthy BLSA men is not age related (Fig. 86-3*E*). In other populations, a reduction in the spontaneous and respiratory variations in resting heart rate is observed and reflects altered autonomic modulation with aging (see below). With assumption of the seated resting position, heart rate increases slightly less in older than in younger men (Fig. 86-3*E*). The magnitude of this age-associated reduction increases progressively during exercise. The net result is that maximum acute dynamic reserve range of heart rate is reduced by about one-third between 20 and 85 years of age. See Fig. 86-4*E* for individual variation in heart rate in both men and women at maximum effort.

CARDIAC OUTPUT

The *cardiac index,* as expected from the behavior of the SVI and heart rate functions in Fig. 86-3*D* and *E,* does not vary with age in either posture at rest (Fig. 86-3*E*), but *is reduced at max exercise in older men due to the age-associated decline in max heart rate.* The loss of acute cardiac output reserve from seated rest to exhaustive, seated cycle exercise averages about 30 percent in healthy, community-dwelling BLSA volunteer men. This reduction is entirely due to a reduction in heart rate reserve, as SVI at max exercise is preserved in healthy men rigorously screened to exclude occult coronary disease at older age. Alternatively stated, *subjects at the older end of the age range can augment their cardiac index 2.5-fold over seated rest, whereas those at the younger end of the spectrum can increase their cardiac index 3.5-fold.*

The hemodynamic patterns measured across the range of demands as illustrated in Fig. 86-3 for males are nearly identical in females. Exceptions are that, at seated rest, females do not exhibit a modest age-associated increase in EDVI because, unlike males, assumption of the upright posture does not produce a greater reduction in EDVI in younger than in older women. Due to the absence in women of an age-associated increase in EDVI in the seated position, the SVI does not increase with age at seated rest, and, in contrast to males, the calculated cardiac index at seated rest decreases modestly with age in women. At max exercise, the age-associated increase of EDVI is of borderline statistical significance in women. However, the change in EDVI from rest to max exercise in a given individual (not shown) significantly increases with age and is nearly identical, in both men and women.[29]

In summary, Figs. 86-3 and 86-4 illustrate that when cardiovascular function in adult volunteer community-dwelling subjects ranging in age from 20 to 85 years is compared, *impaired LV ejection reserve capacity is the most dramatic change in cardiac pump function with aging in health,* as indicated by the failure of older persons to regulate ESV (Figs. 86-3*B* and 86-4*B*) as effectively as younger ones do. *This impaired ESV regulation is accompanied by diminished cardioacceleration, LV dilation at end diastole* (Figs. 86-3 and 86-4*A* and *D*) *and an altered diastolic filling pattern* (Fig. 86-2). See Fig. 86-4 for interindividual variation in the maximum cardiac output in both BLSA men and women.

AEROBIC CAPACITY

The peak (max) upright, seated cycle aerobic capacity estimated by either peak oxygen consumption or work capacity (accompanying the hemodynamic pattern in Figs. 86-3 and 86-4) declines approximately 50 percent. Thus, in this study population, *the age-associated reduction in the cardiac component accounts for roughly half of the age-associated decline in aerobic capacity, the remainder being attributable to age-associated differences in oxygen utilization.* Such reductions in O_2 utilization during vigorous exercise result from age-associated reduction in muscle mass[30] and from a reduction in the shunting of blood from viscera to working muscles during exercise,[31] and the amount of O_2 consumed per unit of working muscle mass per amount of O_2 delivered to the muscle. The extent to which the maximum aerobic capacity declines with aging, and its suspected underlying mechanisms, vary among studies (see Lakatta[32] for a review).

Mechanisms of Deficient Cardiovascular Regulation with Aging in Otherwise Healthy Persons

The ESV is regulated across the range of demands for blood flow encountered in Fig. 86-3 by changes in intrinsic myocardial contractility, afterload, and autonomic modulation of both, with parasympathetic influences diminishing and sympathetic influences becoming more predominant with increasing demands for cardiovascular performance. The max heart rate is regulated, in large part, by the effectiveness of sympathetic modulation. The EDV is regulated by the venous return, by determinants of the AV pressure gradient, including distensibly characteristics of the LV, during exercise, by the filling time, and by the strength of the atrial contraction. Neither the AV pressure gradient nor the end-diastolic pressure either at rest or during the other demand levels depicted in Fig. 86-3 have been measured in a sufficient number of individuals of any study population due to experimental constraints in healthy volunteers.

MYOCARDIAL CONTRACTILITY

In humans, information as to how aging affects factors that regulate intrinsic myocardial contractility is incomplete because the effectiveness of intrinsic myocardial contractility in the intact circulation is difficult to separate from loading and autonomic modulatory influences on contractility. A deficit in maximal intrinsic contractility of older persons might be expected on the basis of the reduced maximum heart rate, as the heart rate, per se, is a determinant of the myocardial contractile state. Additional supporting evidence for reduced LV contractility with aging comes from studies in which the LV of older but not younger healthy BLSA men in the presence of β-adrenergic blockade dilates at end diastole in response to a given increase in afterload.[33]

The most reliable estimate of myocardial contractility, the slope of the ESP/ESV coordinates measured across a range of EDVs at rest, has not been estimated in a homogeneous, healthy study population across a broad age range, and by convention cannot be accessed during exercise. A single point, depicting ESP/ESV as a *contractility* index at each overall cardiovascular level of performance in Fig. 86-3, provides an age-associated pattern of myocardial contractile reserve that is nearly indentical to the ejection fraction in Fig. 86-3*C*.[29]

Most of our current information regarding age-associated changes in factors that regulate cardiac muscle or myocyte function is derived from studies in rodents. Coordinated changes in gene expression or in protein function that modify several key steps of cardiac muscle excitation-Ca^{2+} release-contraction relaxation coupling occur in rodent hearts with aging and result in a prolonged action potential, a prolonged Ca_i transient, and a prolonged contraction. A twofold prolongation of the action potential in cardiac muscle isolated from senescent 24-month rats, compared with that in myocardium of younger adult 6- to 8-month rats, is not due to an age-associated increase in the L-type sarcolemmal Ca^{2+} current density; however, the L-type current inactivates more slowly, and this could account, in part, for the prolonged action potential.[34] It is likely that reductions in outwardly directed K^+ currents with aging also substantially contribute to prolongation of the action potential.[34] The rate of Ca^{2+} sequestration by the sarcoplasmic reticulum decreases in senescent myocardium and may, in part, explain the prolonged Ca_i transient.[35] An age associated reduction in the transcription of the gene coding for the sarcoplasmic reticulum Ca^{2+} pump, Serca2,[36] could account for a decrease in the sarcoplasmic reticulum pump site density.[37] The cardiac Na^+-Ca^{2+} exchanger (NCX1) serves as the main transsarcolemmal Ca^{2+} extrustion mechanism. It has been suggested that the Na^+-Ca^{2+} exchanger is more active in ejecting Ca^{2+} from cells of older than younger hearts during diastole, and an increased NCX1 expression may compensate partly for a reduced sarcoplasmic reticulum pump function. The supporting evidence is that the abundance of cardiac Na^+-Ca^{2+} exchanger transcripts increases about 50 percent in senescent (24 month) compared with the young adult (6 month) rat heart.[38]

The contractile force of isolated cardiac muscle generated by a given increase in cell Ca^{2+} at low rates of electrical stimulation is not altered by age. In rodents, however, marked shifts occur in the myosin heavy-chain isoforms, i.e., the β isoform becomes predominant in senescence rats.[37,39] The myosin Ca^{2+}-ATPase activity declines with the decline in α myosin heavy chain (αMHC) content.[39,40] The altered cellular profile, which results in a contraction that exhibits reduced velocity and a prolonged time course, can be considered to be adaptive rather than degenerative, because the reduced velocity is energy efficient and a prolonged contraction permits continued ejection for a longer period into the stiffened vasculature that accompanies advancing age (vide infra).

Aggregate, age-associated alterations in the kinetics of the cytosolic Ca^{2+} transient, the Na-Ca exchanger,[41] Na-K pump, and the sarcoplasmic reticulum Ca^{2+} pump function, possibly in conjunction with nonspecific changes in sarcolemmal membrane composition ionic permeability,[42] may predispose senescent myocardium to altered cell Ca^{2+} homeostasis. Intriguingly, aged myocardium (and also that of young rodents chronically exposed to pressure overload) is more susceptible to Ca^{2+} overload and spontaneous sarcoplasmic reticulum Ca^{2+} release than is young adult myocardium.[43] Specifically, aged myocardium demonstrates a reduced threshold for Ca^{2+}-dependent diastolic aftercontractions and afterdepolarizations and for ventricular fibrillation during situations that increase cell Ca^{2+} loading[43] as well as the likelihood for the occurrence of spontaneous oscillatory sarcoplasmic reticulum Ca^{2+} release.[44] During higher pacing rates in older but not in younger hearts or cardiac myocytes[45] temporally summated, asynchronous spontaneous Ca^{2+} release occurring within and among cells, or a steady increase in diastolic Ca^{2+} within the cytosol, leads to incomplete diastolic myofilament relaxation and contributes to an increase in diastolic tone.

Many of the multiple changes in cardiac excitation, myofilament activation, contraction mechanisms, and gene expression that occur with aging can be interpreted as adaptive in nature, because they also occur in the hypertrophied myocardium of younger animals adapted to experimentally induced chronic hypertension.[32] Evidence suggests that the adaptive response to chronic pressure loading is reduced in older animals, possibly because some of the adaptive capacity of the heart is used as a response to the aging process.[32]

AFTERLOAD

Cardiac afterload has two components, one generated by the heart itself and the other by the vasculature. The cardiac component of afterload can be expected to increase as a function of ventricular volume, e.g., it increases acutely as the heart size increases during the various maneuvers listed in Figs. 86-3 and 86-4. Considerable evidence indicates that at rest the vascular load on the LV increases with age. The vascular load on the heart has four components: conduit artery compliance characteristics, reflected pulse waves, inertance, and resistance.

FIGURE 86-5 Considerable evidence indicates that at rest the vascular load on the left ventricle increases with age. The age-associated structural changes in compliance arteries (Fig. 86-1*A* and *B*) lead to a reduction in arterial compliance with aging. One manifestation of this is increased pulse-wave velocity (*A*), which causes reflected pulse waves to reach the base of aorta earlier (i.e., prior to closure of the aortic value), producing a late-systolic augmentation of the central pressure pulse contour (*B*). Early reflected pulse waves in conjunction with a resetting of the baroflex lead to an increase in the resting systolic pressure with aging, which by definition, in normotensives, occurs within the clinically normal range (*E*). On average, the diastolic pressure does not increase after middle age (*F*) and, in many older persons, becomes reduced, due to the reduced conduit artery compliance and early reflected pulse waves occurring centrally in late systole rather than in diastole. *The net result is a dramatic increase in pulse pressure with increasing older age.* Thus, the pulse pressure/stroke volume index (PP/SVI), an index of large-vessel stiffness, increases with aging (*D*). The total systemic vascular resistance calculated from the resting mean arterial pressure and cardiac output increases modestly or does not appreciably change at rest with aging in otherwise healthy persons (*C*). (*A* and *B* from *Circulation* 1993; 88:1456; *C* and *D* from *J Appl Physiol* 1995; 78:890; *E* and *F* from *J Gerontol* 1997; 52:M177. Each is reproduced with permission from the publisher and authors.)

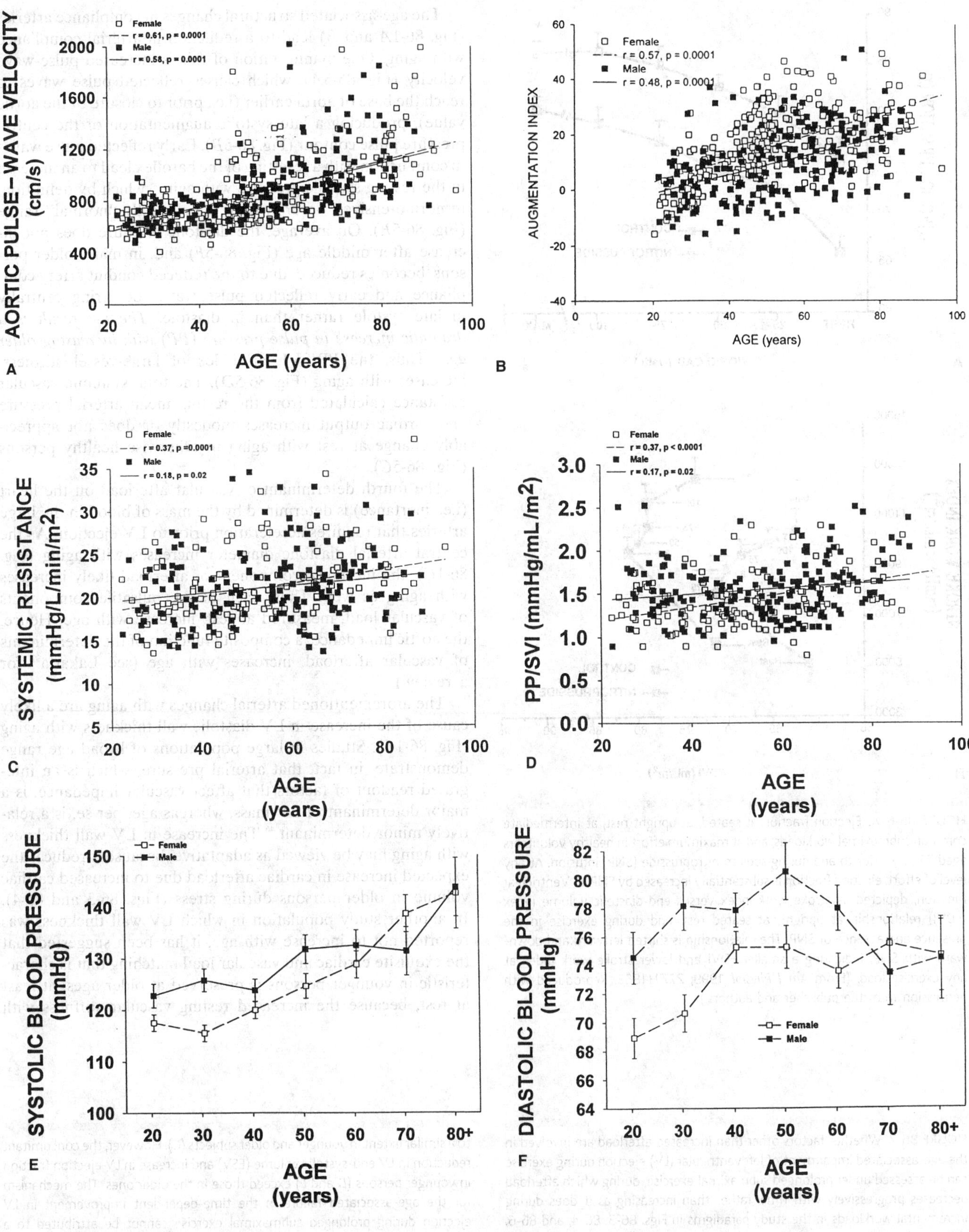
A
AORTIC PULSE–WAVE VELOCITY (cm/s)
AGE (years)
Female
r = 0.61, p = 0.0001
Male
r = 0.58, p = 0.0001
B
AUGMENTATION INDEX
AGE (years)
Female
r = 0.57, p = 0.0001
Male
r = 0.48, p = 0.0001
C
SYSTEMIC RESISTANCE (mmHg/L/min/m2)
AGE (years)
Female
r = 0.37, p =0.0001
Male
r = 0.18, p = 0.02
D
PP/SVI (mmHg/mL/m2)
AGE (years)
Female
r = 0.37, p < 0.0001
Male
r = 0.17, p = 0.02
E
SYSTOLIC BLOOD PRESSURE (mmHg)
AGE (years)
Female
Male
F
DIASTOLIC BLOOD PRESSURE (mmHg)
AGE (years)
Female
Male

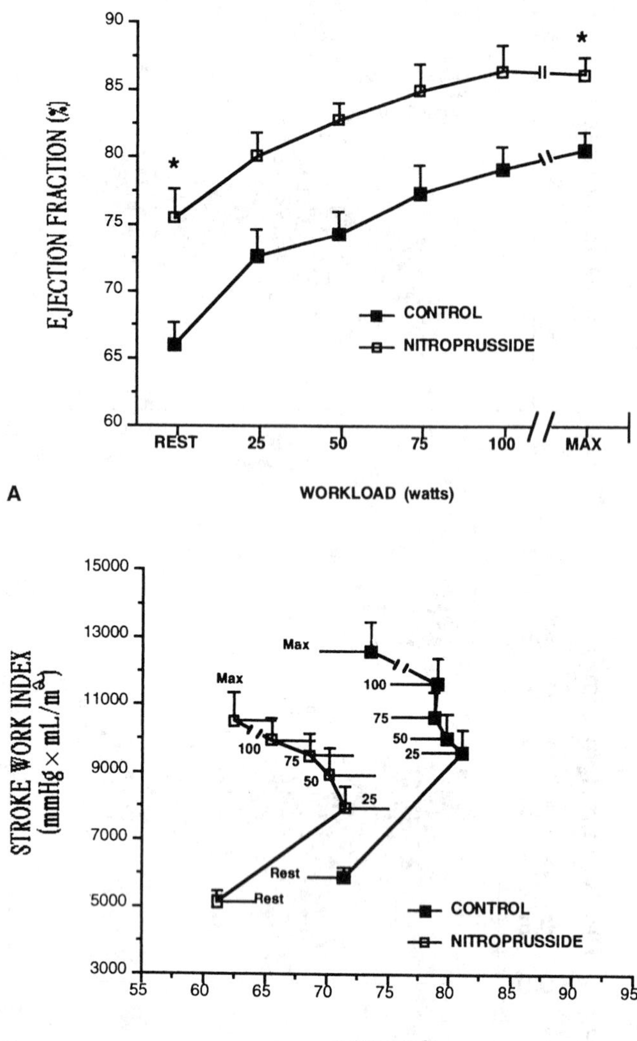

FIGURE 86-6 *A*. Ejection fraction at seated, at upright rest, at intermediate common submaximal workloads, and at maximum effort in healthy volunteers aged 71 ± 7 prior to and during sodium nitroprusside (SNP) infusion. At any level of effort, ejection fraction is substantially increased by SNP. *B*. Ventricular function, depicted as stroke work index versus end-diastolic volume index (EDVI) relationship at upright, at seated rest, and during exercise in the presence and absence of SNP. The relationship is shifted leftward and downward with SNP, indicating a smaller EDVI and lower stroke work index at any exercise load. (From *Am J Physiol* 1999; 277:H1863. Reproduced with permission from the publisher and authors.)

The age-associated structural changes in compliance arteries (Fig. 86-1*A* and *B*) lead to a reduction in arterial compliance with aging. One manifestation of this is increased pulse-wave velocity (Fig. 86-5*A*), which causes reflected pulse waves to reach the base of aorta earlier (i.e., prior to closure of the aortic value), producing a late systolic augmentation of the central pressure pulse contour (Fig. 86-5*B*). Early reflected pulse waves in conjunction with a resetting of the baroflex lead to an increase in the resting systolic pressure with aging, which by definition, in normotensives, occurs within the clinically "normal" range (Fig. 86-5*E*). On average, the diastolic pressure does not increase after middle age (Fig. 86-5*F*) and, in many older persons, becomes reduced, due to the reduced conduit artery compliance and early reflected pulse waves occurring centrally in late systole rather than in diastole. *The net result is a dramatic increase in pulse pressure (PP) with increasing older age.* Thus, the PP/SVI, an index of large-vessel stiffness, increases with aging (Fig. 86-5*D*). The total systemic vascular resistance calculated from the resting mean arterial pressure and cardiac output increases modestly or does not appreciably change at rest with aging in otherwise healthy persons (Fig. 86-5*C*).

The fourth determinant of vascular afterload on the heart (i.e., inertance) is determined by the mass of blood in the large arteries that requires acceleration prior to LV ejection. As the central arterial diastolic diameter increases with aging (Fig. 86-1*C*), the inertance component of afterload likely increases with aging as well. Thus, each of the pulsatile components of vascular load, measured at rest, increase with age. Hence, the aortic impedance, a composite function of the determinants of vascular afterload, increases with age (see Lakatta[32] for a review).

The aforementioned arterial changes with aging are a likely cause of the increase in LV diastolic wall thickness with aging (Fig. 86-1*C*). Studies in large populations of broad age range demonstrate, in fact, that arterial pressure, which is an integrated readout of factors that affect vascular impedance, is a major determinant of LV mass, whereas age, per se, is a relatively minor determinant.[46] The increase in LV wall thickness with aging may be viewed as adaptative, because it reduces the expected increase in cardiac afterload due to increased cardiac volume in older persons during stress (Figs. 86-3 and 86-4). In another study population in which LV wall thickness was reported not to increase with age, it has been suggested that the exquisite cardiac and vascular load matching that is characteristic in younger persons is preserved at older ages, at least at rest, because the increased resting vascular stiffness with

FIGURE 86-7 Whether factors other than increased afterload are involved in the age-associated impairment of left ventricular (LV) ejection during exercise can be assessed under prolonged submaximal exercise, during which afterload decreases progressively with time, rather than increasing as it does during incremental workloads in the study paradigms in Figs. 86-3, 86-4, and 86-6. When individuals exercise at a constant submaximal work rate (50 percent of age-matched VO_2 max) for prolonged times (i.e., 60 min or longer), arterial pressure drops with time (*A* and *B*), and the estimate of arterial stiffness—pulse pressure/stroke volume index (PP/SVI)—decreases with time, both changing to a similar extent in younger and older subjects (*C*). However, the concomitant reduction in LV end-systolic volume (ESV) and increase in LV ejection fraction in younger persons (*D* and *E*) exceed those in the older ones. The mechanism for the age-associated failure in the time-dependent improvement in LV ejection during prolonged submaximal exercise cannot be attributed to a failure of afterload reduction to occur with time, and thus other mechanisms limit the acute LVESV reserve in these healthy, older persons (From *Circ Suppl* 1999; 100:I-141. Reproduced with permission from the publisher and authors.)

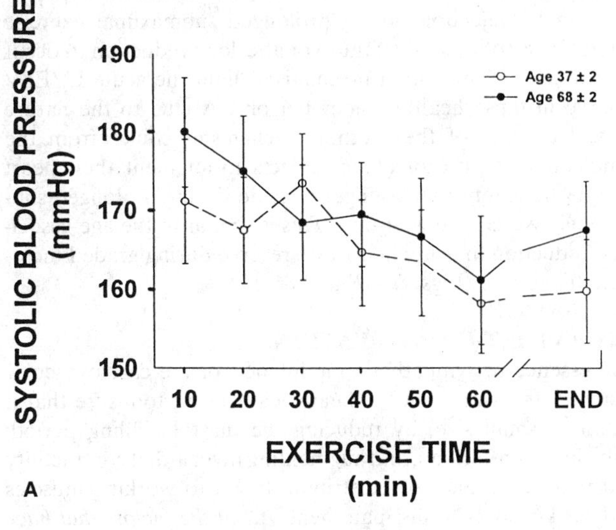
SYSTOLIC BLOOD PRESSURE
(mmHg)
190
180
170
160
150
Age 37 ± 2
Age 68 ± 2
10 20 30 40 50 60 END
EXERCISE TIME
(min)
A

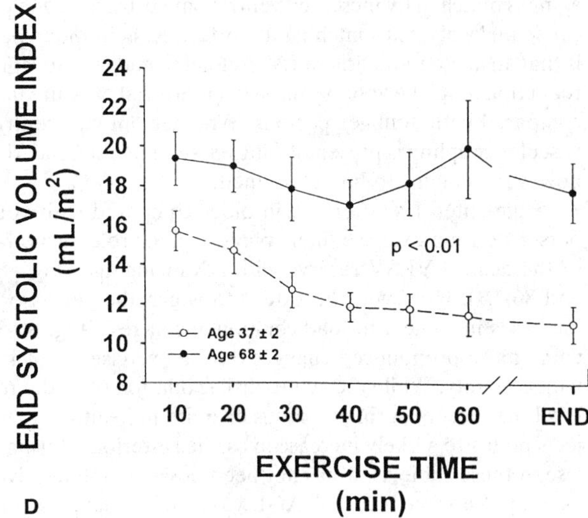
END SYSTOLIC VOLUME INDEX
(mL/m^2)
24
22
20
18
16
14
12
10
8
$p < 0.01$
Age 37 ± 2
Age 68 ± 2
10 20 30 40 50 60 END
EXERCISE TIME
(min)
D

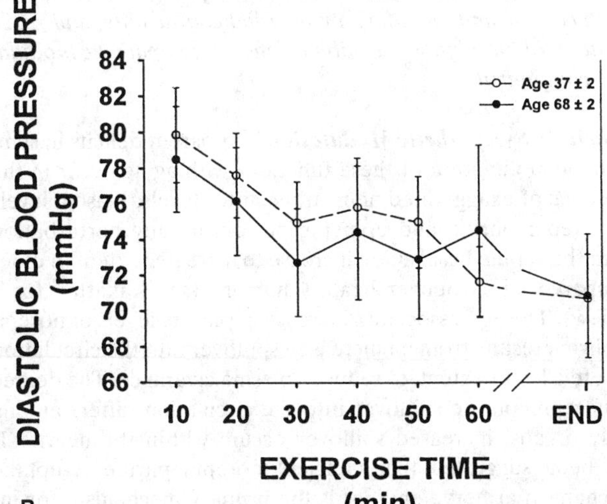
DIASTOLIC BLOOD PRESSURE
(mmHg)
84
82
80
78
76
74
72
70
68
66
Age 37 ± 2
Age 68 ± 2
10 20 30 40 50 60 END
EXERCISE TIME
(min)
B

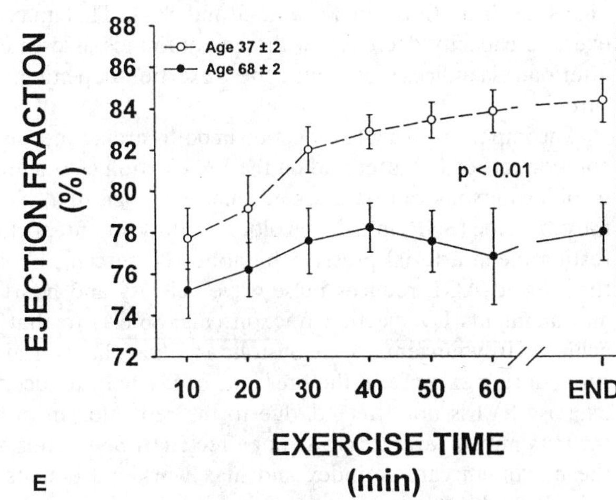
EJECTION FRACTION
(%)
88
86
84
82
80
78
76
74
72
Age 37 ± 2
Age 68 ± 2
$p < 0.01$
10 20 30 40 50 60 END
EXERCISE TIME
(min)
E

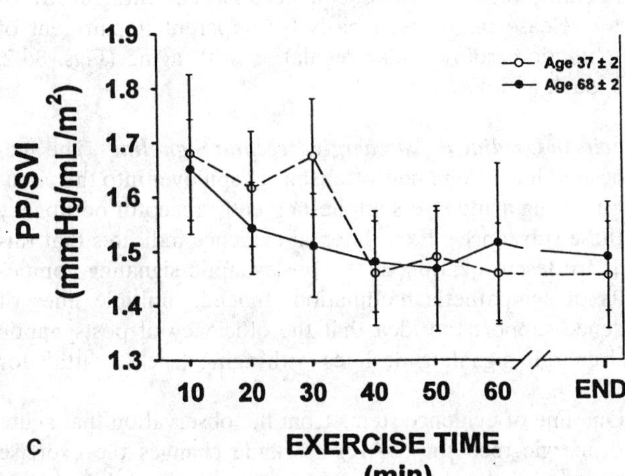
PP/SVI
($mmHg/mL/m^2$)
1.9
1.8
1.7
1.6
1.5
1.4
1.3
Age 37 ± 2
Age 68 ± 2
10 20 30 40 50 60 END
EXERCISE TIME
(min)
C

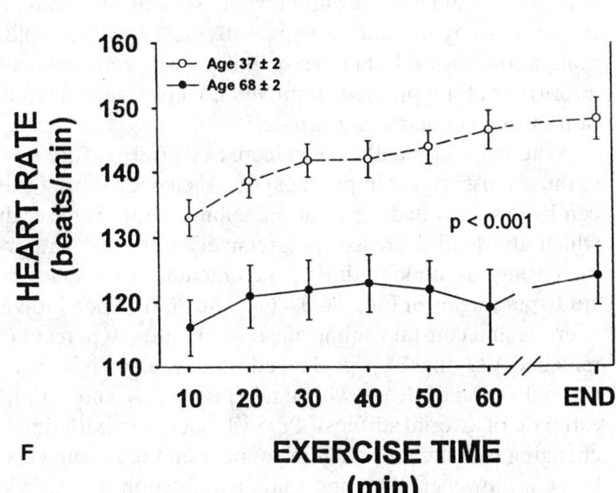
HEART RATE
(beats/min)
160
150
140
130
120
110
Age 37 ± 2
Age 68 ± 2
$p < 0.001$
10 20 30 40 50 60 END
EXERCISE TIME
(min)
F

aging is matched by increased ventricular stiffness.[45] One practical sequela of such matching at stiffer levels in older persons is that an acute reduction in LV preload would lead to a greater reduction in stroke volume and systolic arterial pressure in older compared with younger persons. Whether optimal ventricular vascular coupling is present during exercise in older individuals, however, remains to be determined.

Augmented LV afterload in older compared with younger persons during exercise likely plays a major role in the failure of the acute LVESV reserve with advancing age (Figs. 86-3*B* and 86-4*B*). However, the extent to which the age-associated increases in some afterload components at rest (Fig. 86-5) become more pronounced changes during exercise is not known with certainty. While the acute cardiac dilation from the resting level that occurs during vigorous exercise in healthy older subjects points to a likely increase in cardiac afterload during exercise in these subjects, it has not been possible noninvasively to assess pulse-wave velocity, AGI, vascular diameter, or impedance during exercise. While some manifestations of afterload [e.g., arterial pressure and total systemic vascular resistance (TSVR)] have been measured during exercise, the range of these varies with the degree of effort achieved in exercise paradigms, such as those in Figs. 86-3 and 86-4. That maximum exercise capacity decreases with age confounds assessment of afterload via indices that require these exertion-dependent measures.

The impact of an acute reduction in both cardiac and vascular components of LV afterload on the LV ejection characteristics of older persons can be assessed pharmacologically.[47] Sodium nitroprusside (SNP) infusion in older, healthy volunteers lowers resting mean arterial pressure by about 12 percent, abolishes the carotid AGI, reduces pulse-wave velocity and heart size, and augments LV ejection fraction (Fig. 86-6*A*) to that level achieved by younger persons. Systolic and diastolic arterial pressures during exercise in the presence of SNP are reduced, but exercise SVI is not affected, due to the reduction in preload; the maximum heart rate is also not affected by SNP. Thus, while the maximum cardiac index and max workload deficits with aging in healthy persons are not reduced because of concomitant reductions in preload and afterload by SNP, the LV of older persons could, nevertheless, deliver the same SV stroke work (Fig. 86-6*B*) and cardiac output while working at a smaller size. A recent study in another apparently healthy older volunteer population showed that verapamil, which reduced exercise afterload but not preload, improved LV ejection and O_2 utilization during submaximal exercise.[48]

Whether factors other than increased afterload are involved in the age-associated impairment of LV ejection during exercise can be assessed under prolonged submaximal exercise, during which afterload decreases progressively with time, rather than increasing, as it does during incremental work loads in the study paradigms in Figs. 86-3, 86-4, and 86-6. When individuals exercise at a constant submaximal work rate (50 percent of age matched VO_2 max) for prolonged times (i.e., 60 min or more), arterial pressure drops with time (Fig. 86-7*A* and *B*) and the estimate of arterial stiffness, PP/SVI, decreases with time, both changing to a similar extent in younger and older subjects (Fig. 86-7*C*). However, the concomittant reduction in LVESV and increase in LV ejection fraction in younger persons (Fig. 86-7*D* and *E*) exceed those in the older ones. The mechanism for the age-associated failure in the time-dependent improvement in LV ejection during prolonged submaximal exercise cannot be attributed to a failure of afterload reduction to occur with time, and thus other mechanisms limit the acute LVESV reserve in these healthy, older persons. A clue to the nature of at least one of these other mechanisms comes from the concomitant failure of older subjects to augment their heart rate to the extent that younger ones do during prolonged submaximal exercise (Fig. 86-7*F*). This is similar to the age-associated reduction in acute heart rate reserve during graded incremental exercise (Figs. 86-3*E* and 86-4*E*).

SYMPATHETIC MODULATION

The essence of sympathetic modulation of the cardiovascular system is to insure that the heart beats faster; to insure that it retains a small size, by reducing the diastolic filling period, reducing LV afterload, and augmenting myocardial contractility and relaxation; and to redistribute blood to working muscles and to skin so as to dissipate heat. *All of the factors that have been identified to play a role in the deficient cardiovascular regulation with aging—i.e., heart rate (and thus filling time), afterload (both cardiac and vascular), myocardial contractility, and redistribution of blood flow—exhibit a deficient sympathetic modulatory component.*

Deficits in Sympathetic Modulation Apparent deficits in sympathetic modulation of these functions with aging occur in the presence of exaggerated neurotransmitter levels. Plasma levels of norepinephrine and epinephrine, during any perturbation from the supine basal state, increase to a greater extent in older compared with younger healthy humans (see Lakatta[49] for a review). The age-associated increase in plasma levels of norepinephrine results from an increased spillover into the circulation and, to a lesser extent, to reduced plasma clearance. The degree of norepinephrine spillover into the circulation differs among body organs; increased spillover occurs within the heart.[50] It has been suggested that deficient norepinephrine re-uptake mechanism at nerve endings is the primary mechanism for increased spillover. During prolonged exercise, however, diminished neurotransmitter re-uptake might also be associated with depletion and reduced release and spillover.[51] Thus, depending on the duration of the stress, enhanced or deficient neurotransmitter release might be a basis for apparent impairment of sympathetic cardiovascular regulation with aging (Figs. 86-2, 86-3, 86-4, and 86-7).

Deficits in Cardiac β-Adrenergic Receptor Signaling The age-associated increase in neurotransmitter spillover into the circulation during acute stress implies a greater receptor occupancy by these substances. Experimental evidence indicates that this leads to desensitization of the postsynaptic signaling components of sympathetic modulation. Indeed, multiple lines of evidence support the idea that the efficiency of postsynaptic β-adrenergic signaling declines with aging (see Lakatta[49] for a review).

One line of evidence stems from the observation that acute β-adrenergic receptor (βAR) blockade changes the exercise hemodynamic profile of younger persons to resemble that of older ones. The age-associated deficits in LV early diastolic filling rate both at rest and during exercise (Fig. 86-8*C*) also

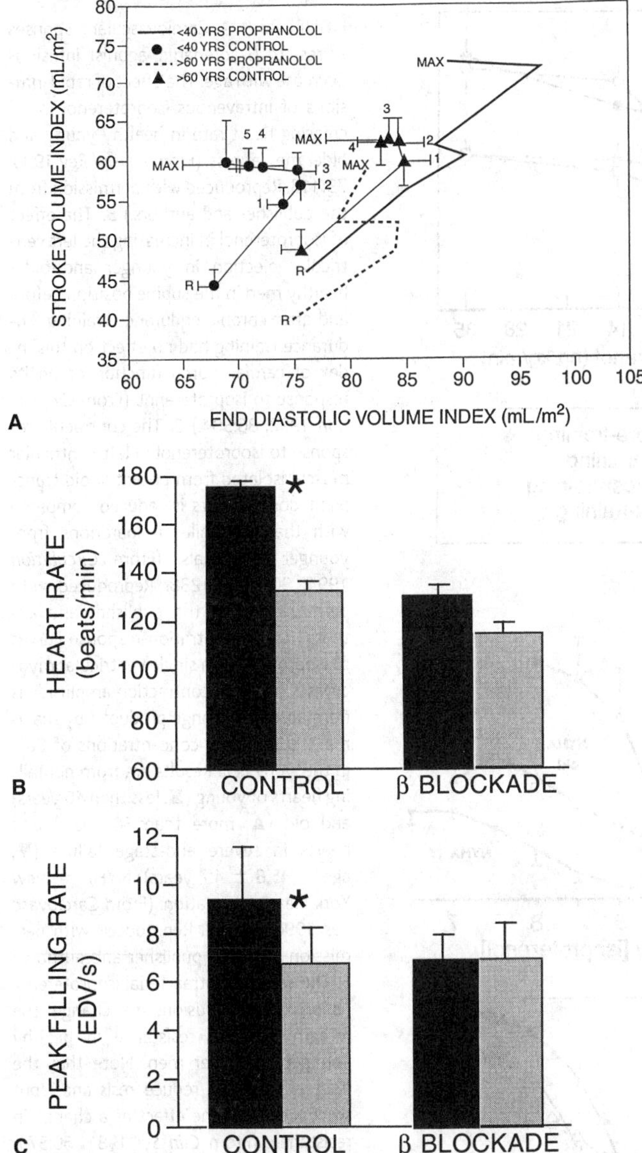

FIGURE 86-8 *A*. Stroke volume index as a function of end-diastolic volume (EDV) index at rest (R) and during graded cycle workloads in the upright seated position in healthy men from the Baltimore Longitudinal Study on Aging (BLSA), in the presence and absence (dashed line) of β-adrenergic blockade. R = seated rest; 1–4 or 5 = graded submaximal workloads on cycle ergometer; max = maximum effort. Stroke volume/end-diastolic functions with symbols are those measured in the absence of propranolol; *dashed and solid line* functions without symbols are the stroke volume compared with end-diastolic function measured in the presence of propranolol. Note that, in the absence of propranolol, the stroke volume versus EDV relation in older persons (▲) is shifted rightward from that in younger ones (●). This indicates that the left ventricle of older persons in the sitting position compared with that of younger ones operates from a greater preload both at rest and during submaximal and max exercise. Propranolol markedly shifts the stroke volume/EDV relationship in younger persons (*solid line without points*) rightward but does not markedly offset the curve in older persons (*dashed line without points*). Thus, with respect to this assessment of ventricular function curve, β-adrenergic blockade with propranolol makes younger men appear like older ones. The abolition of the age-associated differences in the left ventricular (LV) function curve after propranolol are accompanied by a reduction or abolition of the age-associated reduction in heart rate, which, at max, is shown in *B*. Note, however, that β-adrenergic blockade in younger individuals in this figure causes stroke volume index to increase to a greater extent than during β blockade in older ones, suggesting that mechanisms other than deficient β-adrenergic regulation compromise LV ejection. One potential mechanism is an age-associated decrease in *maximum intrinsic* myocardial contractility. Another likely mechanism is enhanced vascular afterload, due to the structural changes in compliance arteries noted above and possibly also to impaired vasorelaxation during exercise. (From *Circulation* 1994; 90:2333. Reproduced with permission from the publisher and authors.) *B*. Peak exercise heart rate in the same subjects as in *A* in the presence and absence of acute β-adrenergic blockade by propranolol. *C*. The age-associated reduction in peak LV diastolic filling rate at max exercise in healthy BLSA subjects is abolished during exercise in the presence of β-adrenergic blockade with propranolol. Solid = less than 40 years; light = more than 60 years. (From *Am J Physiol* 1992; 73:H1932. Reproduced with permission from the publisher and authors.)

are abolished by acute β-adrenergic blockade.[52] The heart rate reduction during exercise in the presence of acute β-adrenergic blockade is greater in younger than in older subjects (Fig. 86-8*B*), and significant β blockade-induced LV dilatation occurs only in younger subjects (Fig. 86-8*A*). Note, however, that β-adrenergic blockade in younger individuals in Fig. 86-8 causes SVI to increase to a greater extent than in β blockade in older ones, suggesting that mechanisms other than deficient β-adrenergic regulation compromise LV ejection. One potential mechanism is an age-associated decrease in *maximum intrinsic* myocardial contractility. Another likely mechanism is enhanced vascular afterload due to the structural changes in compliance arteries noted above and possibly also to impaired vasorelaxation during exercise. In this regard, it has been observed that the increase in impedance during exercise in old dogs is abolished by β-adrenergic blockade.[53]

The second type of evidence for a diminished efficacy of synaptic βAR signaling is that cardiovascular responses at rest to β-adrenergic agonist infusions decrease with age (Fig. 86-9). Cellular mechanisms for the deficiency in βAR signaling in humans include a reduction in receptor number, and affinity and coupling to adenyl cyclase via G_s proteins. There is evidence that other G protein-coupled receptor signaling may also deteriorate in humans with aging (see Lakatta[49] for a review). The efficacy of βAR (i.e., β_1 vs. β_2 vs. β_3) signaling has not yet been studied in humans. Studies in rodent models have delineated additional age-associated deficits in the β-adrenergic signaling cascade. A reduced contractile response to both β_1AR and β_2AR stimulation occurs with aging in rodent isolated LV muscle and in individual rat ventricular cardiocytes.[54,55] This is due to failure of βAR stimulation to augment the intracellular Ca^{2+} transient to the same extent in cells of senescent hearts to which it does in cells from younger adult hearts.[54] The blunted increase in the Ca^{2+} transient following βAR stimulation in cells from older compared with younger adult hearts is attributable to a decrease in the ability of either β_1AR and β_2AR stimulation to increase L-type sarcolemmal Ca^{2+} channel availability and thus to a lesser increase in Ca^{2+} influx via these channels during the action potential. The richly documented age-associated reduction in the postsynaptic response of myocardial cells to β_1AR stimulation appears to be due to multiple changes in molecular and biochemical receptor coupling and postreceptor mechanisms. However, the major limiting modification of this signaling

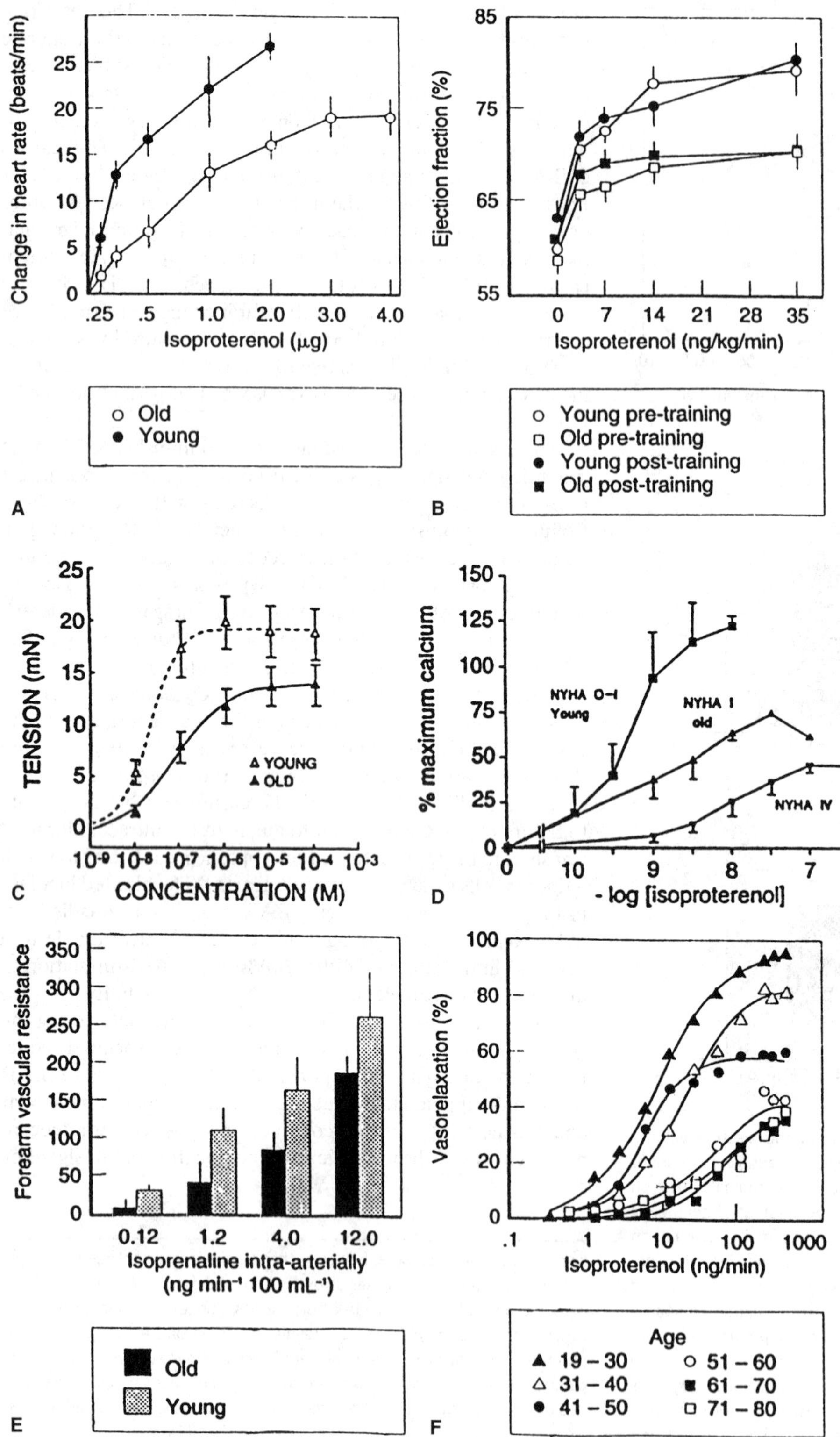

FIGURE 86-9 *A.* Cardiovascular responses at rest to β-adrenergic agonist infusions decrease with age. The effect of rapid infusions of intravenous isoproterenol in increasing heart rate in healthy young and older men at rest. (From *Physiol Rev* 1993; 73:413. Reproduced with permission from the publisher and authors.) *B.* The effect of isoproterenol in increasing the left ventricular ejection in younger and older healthy men in the supine position before and after chronic endurance training. Endurance training had no effect on this index of cardiac pump function or on its response to isoproterenol. (From *Circulation* 1992; 86:504.) *C.* The contractile response to isoproterenol in left ventricular muscle isolated from potential old transplant donor hearts is reduced compared with that in similar preparations from younger individuals. (From *Circulation* 1994; 90:1225–1238. Reproduced with permission from the publisher and authors.) *D.* Concentration-response curves to isoproterenol in single ventricular myocytes. Change in contraction amplitude is normalized to change produced by maximally stimulating concentrations of Ca^{2+} in the same cell. Results are from nonfailing hearts of young (■, less than 40 years) and old (▲, more than 50 years) and hearts in severe end-stage failure (▼, age = 45.8 ± 4.7 years). NYHA = New York Heart Association. (From *Cardiovasc Res* 1996; 31:152. Reproduced with permission from the publisher and authors.) *E.* The effect of intraarterial isoproterenol (isoprenaline) infusions to change the forearm vascular resistance in healthy younger and older men. Note that the drug effect is to reduce resistance, but the figure plots the effect as a change in resistance. (From *Clin Sci* 1981; 60:571. Reproduced with permission from the publisher and authors.) *F.* The effect of intravenous arterial infusion of isoproterenol in relaxing dorsal hand veins, previously constricted by phenylephrine, in men of varying ages. (From *J Pharmacol Exp Ther* 1986; 239:802. Reproduced with permission from the publisher and authors.)

pathway with advancing age appears to be at the coupling of the β-adrenergic receptor to adenyl cyclase via the G_s protein[55] and to changes in adenyl cyclase protein, per se, leading to a reduction in the ability to augment cell cAMP sufficiently to drive the phosphorylation of key proteins[56] that is required to alter protein function and augment cardiac contractility. The apparent desensitization of β_1AR and β_2AR signaling with aging is not mediated via increased β-adrenergic receptor kinase or increased G_i activity.[55]

PHYSICAL DECONDITIONING

A marked reduction in physical activity accompanies advancing age in a majority of adults. Thus, it may be hypothesized that a reduction in physical *conditioning* might be implicated as a factor in the reduced cardiovascular reserve of older, healthy sedentary individuals, as discussed. Alternatively, the issue arises as to whether physical conditioning via aerobic training of sedentary older persons can affect deficits in cardiovascular reserve capacity due to an *aging process,* per se.

It has been amply documented that physical conditioning of older persons can substantially increase their maximum aerobic work capacity and peak oxygen consumption. The extent to which this conditioning effect results from enhanced central cardiac performance or from augmented peripheral circulatory and O_2 utilization mechanisms, including changes in skeletal muscle mass, varies with the type and degree of conditioning achieved, gender, body position during study (see Lakatta[32] for a review), and likely genetic factors. A longitudinal study of older males in the upright position indicates that an enhanced physical conditioning status increases O_2 consumption and work capacity, in part by increases in the maximum CO by increasing the maximum SV, and in part by increasing the estimated total body (AV) O_2 utilization.[57] The augmentation of maximum SVI is due to an augmented reduction of LVESV (Fig. 86-10*A*) and, thus, a concomitant increase in LV ejection fraction, as the effect of conditioning status to increase LVEDI exercise is minimal (recall that LVEDI during acute vigorous exercise is already appreciably increased in older, sedentary, preconditioned men). This minor effect of physical conditioning on LVEDVI in older persons is in contrast to the effect of physical conditioning in younger persons, which substantially increases EDVI and SVI on the basis of the Frank-Starling mechanism, as well as via an enhanced LV ejection fraction. In contrast to the improved LV ejection, the max heart rate of older persons did not vary with physical conditioning status (Fig. 86-10*A*). *There is no strong evidence at hand that physical conditioning of older persons can offset the deficiency in sympathetic modulation.* Rather, conditioning effects to increase LV ejection appear to relate to the reduction in vascular afterload, as reflected in a reduced carotid AGI in older athletes compared with sedentary controls (Fig. 86-10*B*), and possibly to an augmentation of the maximum *intrinsic* myocardial contractility. In animal models, some, but not all, studied determinants of the latter are affected by physical conditioning status (see Lakatta[32] for a review).

Summary

In summary, an age-associated increase in vascular afterload on the heart is due to arterial stiffening and is reflected in the age-associated modest increase in systolic blood pressure at rest. In healthy individuals, these vascular changes are compen-

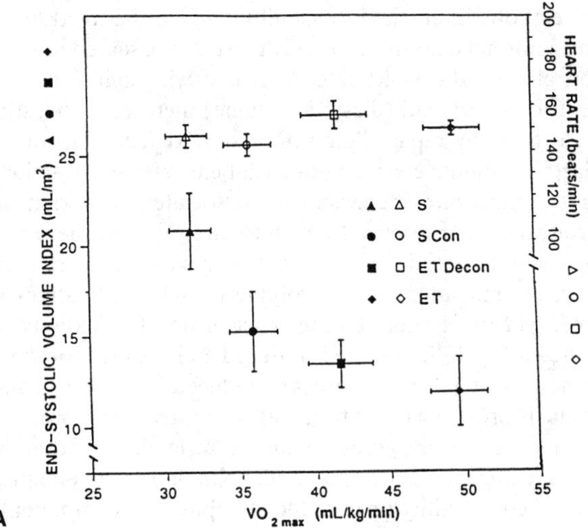

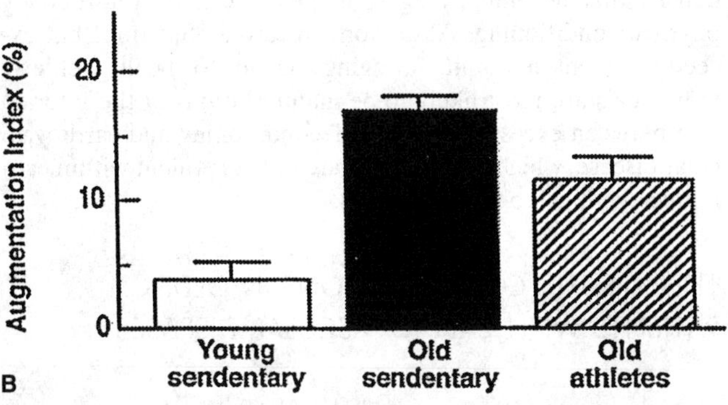

FIGURE 86-10 *A.* Heart rate and end-systolic volume during peak seated, upright exercise on a cycle ergometer across a broad range of aerobic capacity in healthy males who have been exercise conditioned or deconditioned. S = sedentary; ET = exercise trained; SCon = sedentary men after conditioning; ET Decon = men who had been exercise trained but stopped their training for the study to become detrained or deconditioned (DeCon). The figure shows that the extent to which the left ventricle empties, as manifest by the end-systolic volume, varies with the level of aerobic capacity (VO_2 max), which was varied among the four groups by either conditioning or deconditioning protocols. In contrast, the peak heart rate achieved does not vary with aerobic capacity. (From *Circulation* 1996; 94:359. Reproduced with permission from the publisher and authors.) *B.* With increasing age, the carotid pressure pulse exhibits a late peak, often observed as a second component. This is due to early reflected waves from peripheral sites, which, in part, are attributable to a reduced aortic compliance that causes the pulse-wave velocity to increase. The ratio of amplitude of the late component of the pressure pulse to the amplitude of the total pressure pulse is defined as an *augmentation index.* The increase in carotid augmentation index in highly trained older men (aged 60 to 85 years) is only about half of that expected on the basis of age. Thus, physical conditioning has an effect to alter the reflected waves in these older men. The effect may occur via a reduction in aortic stiffness, as the pulse-wave velocity is also reduced by conditioning (not shown). (From *Circulation* 1993; 881456. Reproduced with permission from the publisher and authors.)

sated for, in large part, by the age-associated changes in the architecture and contractile properties of the heart, which, despite reductions in aortic distensibility, enable the aged heart to pump a normal quantity of blood at rest. In the seated upright position at rest, the heart rate decreases with aging in men and ventricular preload (diastolic volume) increases modestly, although the early rapid filling rate is slowed. The fraction of end-diastolic volume ejected with each beat (ejection fraction) does not decline with age. Major age-associated alterations in the cardiovascular response to exercise are evident: there is a striking age-associated decrease in the maximum heart rate; however, the maximum stroke volume in older individuals is preserved via the Frank-Starling mechanism. The extents to which the end-systolic volume is reduced and the ejection fraction increases at peak exercise are reduced with aging, and these deficits probably result from deficient intrinsic myocardial performance and from an augmented afterload, both due, in part, to a deficiency in β-adrenergic stimulation to enhance myocardial contractility or to reduce the pulsatile components of vascular afterload. A decrease in the maximum capacity for physical work with aging is due to both diminished cardiac (heart rate) and peripheral factors. Some of the cardiovascular deficits that accompany aging in health can be retarded by physical conditioning. Alterations in cardiac function that exceed the identified limits for aging changes for healthy elderly individuals are most likely to be manifestations of the interaction between excessive physical deconditioning and cardiovascular disease, which are, unfortunately, so prevalent within economically developed populations.

THERAPEUTIC CONSIDERATIONS IN OLDER PATIENTS WITH CARDIOVASCULAR DISEASES

Cardiovascular Disease in Elderly Individuals

More successful recognition and treatment of cardiovascular risk factors and diseases continue to decrease age-adjusted cardiovascular mortality[58] and to increase the number and proportion of the cardiac patient population who are considered elderly. In the United States, cardiovascular disease is the leading cause of mortality, accounting for over 40 percent of deaths in those aged 65 years and older. Over 80 percent of all cardiovascular deaths occur in the same age group.[59] These data indicate that *age is the major risk factor for cardiovascular disease.*

One way to conceptualize why the clinical manifestations and the prognosis of these diseases worsen with age is that in older individuals the specific pathophysiologic mechanisms that cause clinical disorders are superimposed on heart and vascular substrates that are modified by aging per se (Fig. 86-11). The horizontal line separating the lower and upper parts of Fig. 86-11 represents the clinical practice *threshold* for disease recognition. Thus, entities above the line are presently classified as *diseases* that lead to heart and brain failure. The vascular and cardiac changes presently thought to occur as a result of the *normal* or *physiologic* aging process (i.e., those addressed in the previous sections) are depicted below the line. These age-associated changes in cardiac and vascular properties alter the substrate upon which cardiovascular disease is superimposed in several ways (Table 86-1). First, they lower the extent of disease severity required to cross the threshold that results in clinically significant signs and symptoms. For example, a mild degree of ischemia-induced relaxation abnormalities that may be asymptomatic in a younger individual may cause dyspnea in an older individual, who, by virtue of age alone, has preexisting slowed and delayed early diastolic relaxation.

Age-associated changes may also alter the manifestations and presentation of common cardiac diseases. This usually occurs in patients with acute infarction in whom the diagnosis is delayed because of atypical symptoms resulting in increased time to onset of therapy. Age-associated changes, including those in β-adrenergic responsiveness and in vascular stiffness also influence the response to and therefore the selection of different therapeutic inventions in older individuals with cardiovascular disease. Thus, in one sense, those processes below the line in Fig. 86-11 ought not to be considered to reflect normal or physiologic aging. Rather, they might be construed as specific risk factors for the diseases that they relate to, and thus might be targets of interventions designed to decrease the occurrence and/or manifestations of cardiovascular disease at later ages. Such a strategy would thus advocate treating "normal" aging. However, additional studies of the specific risks of each "normal" age-associated change and the effectiveness of treatment regimens to delay or prevent each change are required for this strategy to be put into practice. In the following section, the question of how aging influences the presentation and approach to the treatment of common cardiovascular diseases is considered, focusing on the influence and impact of the age-associated changes described previously.

Ischemic Heart Disease

In general, advancing age is associated with increasingly severe, diffuse atherosclerosis and with damage to the left ventricle. Therefore, almost all clinical manifestations of ischemic heart disease have a higher mortality rate and a worse outcome in the older population. The clinical assessment of elderly patients with coronary artery disease is often limited by the coexistence of diseases that make interpretation of symptoms difficult.[60] Thus, in the elderly, a high clinical index of suspicion plus the use of objective parameters such as stress test results are important in assessing and diagnosing ischemic heart disease. Treadmill testing is also useful to detect silent ischemia, which occurs with increasing frequency in the elderly and is a strong risk factor for the development of future symptomatic cardiac disease.[61]

ACUTE CORONARY SYNDROMES

Older patients with acute myocardial infarction are more likely to be female, have a preexisting history of angina and experience a non-Q-wave myocardial infarction[62,63] (see Chap. 42). Older patients are also more likely to present with atypical symptoms of acute myocardial ischemia and infarction, such as shortness of breath, confusion, and failure to thrive.[64] Furthermore, nearly one-half of myocardial infarctions in the elderly are unrecognized clinically.[64] Age is a powerful independent predictor of short-term and long-term mortality in patients with an acute myocardial infarction.[63-66] In patients admitted with a first ST-segment elevation myocardial infarction and treated with thrombolytic therapy, in-hospital mortality increases exponentially as a function of age from 1.9 percent among patients 40

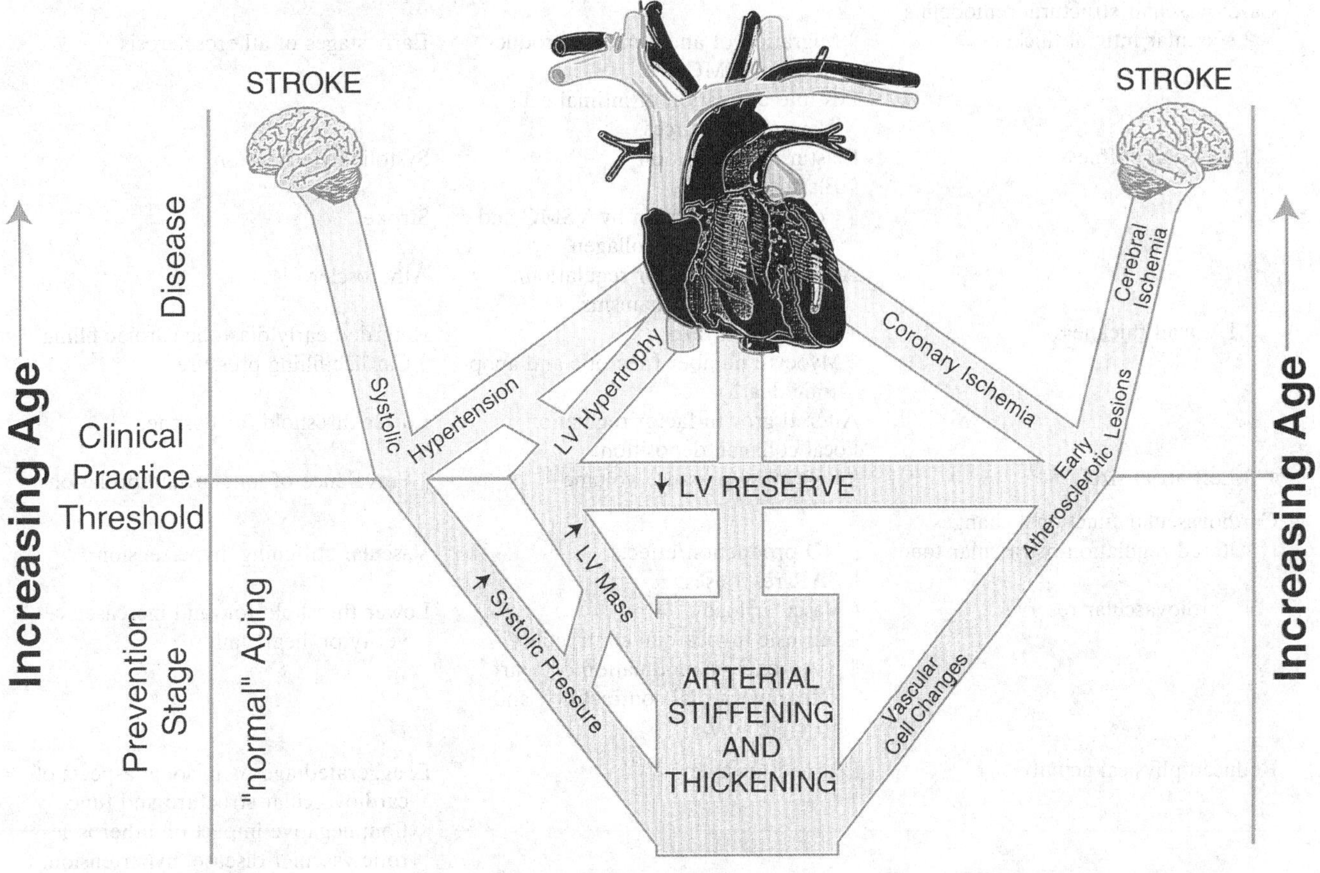

FIGURE 86-11 Changes in the vasculature and heart with aging in health may also be construed as risk factors for cardiovascular disease leading to heart and brain disorders in older age (see the text for details). LV = left ventricular. (From E. Braunwald, ed. *Heart Disease: A Textbook of Cardiovascular Medicine*, 5th ed. New York: WB Saunders; 1996:1687. Reproduced with permission from the publisher and authors.)

years or younger to 31.9 percent among patients older than 80 years.[65] Similarly, in the Global Utilization of Streptokinase and Tissue Plasminogen Activator for Occluded Arteries (GUSTO-1) Trial, 30-day mortality following a ST-segment elevation myocardial infarction increased from 3 percent in patients under 65 years of age to 19.6 percent in patient 75 to 85 years of age and to 30.3 percent in patients over 85 years of age.[67] *Age was the most powerful predictor of in-hospital and 30-day mortality in this trial.* Age is also a powerful predictor of recurrent ischemia and 30-day mortality in patients with non-ST-segment elevation acute coronary syndromes.[68] Hospital volume for acute coronary syndromes also influences outcome in the elderly.[69] Older patients admitted to hospitals with larger patient volumes for acute myocardial infarction have improved survival compared with lower-volume hospitals.

Elderly acute infarct patients experience a much greater incidence of heart failure and cardiogenic shock even though indices of infarct size, such as creatinine phosphokinase levels and QRS scores, do not change with age.[63,65] The risks of heart failure and shock increase three- to fourfold in patients older than 85 compared with those younger than 65.[67] The higher incidences of heart failure and shock may result from age-related changes in diastolic filling, aortic compliance, and decreased sensitivity to catecholamine stimulation, resulting in diminished cardiac reserve and afterload mismatch following ischemic damage. Mortality in older patients with myocardial infarction is less likely to result from ventricular fibrillation compared with younger patients but is much more likely to result from electromechanical dissociation and a finding of cardiac rupture on autopsy. The risk of death following hospital discharge also increases exponentially with increasing age, by almost 6 percent per year.[65]

The high morbidity and mortality associated with acute ischemic syndromes in the elderly dictate an aggressive management approach. Thrombolytic therapy in acute myocardial infarction reduces mortality, and data suggest a possible benefit in the elderly. In a meta-analysis of large randomized trials of thrombolytic therapy, subset analyses of the nearly 5800 patients older than 74 years showed a nonsignificant trend toward thrombolytic benefit, with a net saving of 1.0 life per 100 patients treated at 35 days after infarction. Although the percent decrease in mortality is less in older compared with younger pa-

TABLE 86-1 Relationship of Cardiovascular Human Aging in Health to Cardiovascular Disease

Age-Associated Changes	Plausible Mechanisms	Possible Relation to Human Disease
Cardiovascular structural remodeling		
⇑ Vascular intimal thickness	⇑ Migration of and ⇑ matrix production by VSMC	Early stages of atherosclerosis
	Possible derivation of intimal cells from other sources	
⇑ Vascular stiffness	Elastin fragmentation	Systolic hypertension
	⇑ Elastase activity	
	⇑ Collagen production by VSMC and ⇑ cross-linking of collagen	Stroke
	Altered growth factor regulation/ tissue repair mechanisms	Atherosclerosis
⇑ LV wall thickness	⇑ LV myocyte size	Retarded early diastolic cardiac filling
	⇓ Myocyte number (necrotic and apoptotic death)	⇑ Cardiac filling pressure
	Altered growth factor regulation	Lower threshold for dyspnea
	Focal collagen deposition	
⇑ Left atrial size	⇑ Left atrial pressure/volume	⇑ Prevalence of lone atrial fibrillation
Cardiovascular functional changes		
Altered regulation of vascular tone	⇓ NO production/effects	Vascular stiffening; hypertension
	⇓ βAR responses	
⇓ Cardiovascular reserve	⇑ Vascular load	Lower threshold for, and increased severity of, heart failure
	⇓ Intrinsic myocardial contractility	
	⇓ β-Adrenergic modulation of heart rate, myocardial contractility, and vascular tone	
Reduced physical activity	Learned lifestyle	Exaggerated age Δs in some aspects of cardiovascular structure and function; negative impact on atherosclerotic vascular disease, hypertension, and heart failure

ABBREVIATIONS: VSMC = vascular smooth muscle cell; LV = left ventricular; NO = nitric oxide; βAR = β-adrenergic receptor.

tients treated with thrombolytics, the absolute benefit in terms of number of lives saved with treatment is similar.[70] In the GUSTO-1 trial,[67,71] subgroup analysis of 3655 patients over 75 years of age showed a similar absolute benefit compared with younger patients for accelerated dosed tissue plasminogen activator compared with steptokinase for the end point of death and nonfatal disabling stroke, although this subgroup comparison was not statistically significant. The use of accelerated tissue plasminogen activator appears relatively cost effective in the elderly.[72] In spite of these data, large registry data in the United States indicate that thrombolytic-eligible patients older than 75 are significantly less likely to receive reperfusion therapy than are patients younger than 65, with an odds ratio of 0.4.[73] Part of the reluctance of physicians to use thrombolytic agents in this age group arises from the concerns about intracranial hemorrhage. Age is an important predictor of hemorrhagic stroke with thrombolytic therapy and occurs more frequently with tissue plasminogen activator than with streptokinase.[67,74] Other comorbid conditions, such as cerebral vascular disease, hypertension, and body weight, must be considered, and age alone is not a criterion to exclude a patient from receiving thrombolytic therapy.[74]

Primary angioplasty is compared with thrombolytic therapy in several trials and may have beneficial effects on mortality, recurrent myocardial infarction, and recurrent ischemia.[75,76] Data from meta-analyses suggest a decrease in short-term death and nonfatal reinfarction in patients with ST-segment elevation myocardial infarction treated with primary angioplasty compared with thrombolytic therapy, with a particular benefit in the elderly.[77] Patients treated with direct angioplasty have a lower overall stroke and hemorrhagic stroke risk compared with thrombolytic-treated patients. Caveats from these studies include the short follow-up, operator expertise, and the importance of time delay prior to treatment; the delay is usually significantly longer with angioplasty than with thrombolytic therapy. Although elderly subjects treated with thrombolytic therapy will more often have multivessel coronary disease than will younger subjects, routine angioplasty following thrombolytic therapy does not decrease rates of death or recurrent myocardial infarction.[78] Angioplasty can be very effective, however, in relieving ischemia in elderly patients with postinfarction angina and unstable angina.[79,80]

In the Cooperative Cardiovascular Project, investigators reviewed records of approximately 200,000 Medicare beneficiaries who suffered a myocardial infarction. Only 34 percent of this elderly cohort were discharged home on a β-blockade.[81] Paradoxically, patients leaving hospital without β-blockade therapy have comorbidities that place them at the highest mortality risk. All subgroups of patients in this data base had a large survival advantage (approximately 40 percent reduction in 2-year mortality rate) with β-blockade therapy. Similarly, aspirin therapy decreases mortality rates in elderly infarct subjects and reduces recurrent ischemic pain in older unstable angina patients.[82] Nevertheless, among 10,000 Medicare beneficiaries with an acute myocardial infarction with no contraindication to aspirin therapy, only 61 percent of those received it within the first 2 hospital days.[83] Aspirin therapy in this large group of elderly infarct patients was independently associated with a lower 30-day mortality rate. Furthermore, only 76 percent of elderly subjects without any contraindications were discharged home on aspirin therapy after a myocardial infarction.[84] Aspirin use is independently associated with improved 6-month outcomes in this group. Angiotensin-converting enzyme (ACE) inhibitor therapy following acute myocardial infarction was evaluated in two groups of patients. First, patients with myocardial infarction started within 24 h of symptom onset and, second, in high-risk patients (LV dysfunction or congestive heart failure) with initiation of ACE inhibitor therapy 3 to 16 days after the infarction. A recent meta-analysis of the four large randomized placebo and open controlled trials evaluating the effects of ACE inhibitor therapy on early postinfarction mortality in approximately 100,000 patients[85] recently reported that 30-day mortality rate was significantly lower among the ACE inhibitor-treated patients (7.11 versus 7.59 percent). Thirty percent of the population was aged 65 to 74 years and 15 percent aged 75 years and older. Thirty-day mortality was 10.8 percent lower in the former group of patients treated with an ACE inhibitor as compared with the cohort not treated with ACE inhibitor. In patients 75 years of age and older, 30-day mortality was not reduced compared with the control group. In the trials that involved high-risk patients with LV dysfunction or clinical congestive heart failure, there is a large survival benefit among patients randomized to ACE inhibitor therapy.[86,87] In the Acute Infarction Ramipril Efficacy Study, in which ramipril was compared with placebo in 2006 postinfarction patients with clinical congestive heart failure, the mean age of the population was 65 years.[86] Treatment was initiated between days 3 and 10 after myocardial infarction. After an average of 15 months' follow-up, mortality was reduced from 23 percent in the placebo group to 17 percent in the ramipril group. Patients over 65 years of age had a larger survival advantage with the ACE inhibitor than did those under 65 years of age. In the 1749 postinfarct patients (mean age, 67.7 years) with echocardiographic evidence of LV dysfunction and randomized to the ACE inhibitor trandolapril versus placebo, long-term survival was significantly improved with ACE inhibitor therapy.[87] The 1121 patients at least 65 years of age had a relative risk of death of 0.83 with trandolapril compared with placebo. Therefore, *older patients with large infarctions, LV dysfunction, or clinical heart failure have a large survival advantage with long-term ACE inhibitor therapy.* For lower-risk elderly patients, the benefits are clearly less, and individualized treatment because of risk of hypotension and renal insufficiency, should be considered in this lower-risk, less benefiting group. Finally, lipid-lowering therapy also reduces morbidity and mortality among older patients after acute myocardial infarction. In the Cholesterol and Recurrent Events Trial evaluating either 40 mg of pravastatin or placebo over 5 years in 4159 patients with a myocardial infarction who had total cholesterol levels below 240 mg/dL and low-density lipoprotein levels between 115 and 174 mg/dL, 1283 patients were aged 65 to 75 years of age.[88] In this group, lipid-lowering therapy reduced the primary end point of cardiac death or nonfatal myocardial infarction by 39 percent. The individual secondary end points of cardiac death, nonfatal reinfarction, stroke, and need for coronary artery bypass surgery, were also reduced.

In patients with unstable angina or non-Q-wave myocardial infarction, recent studies show that the addition of a parenteral glycoprotein (GP) IIb/IIIa inhibitor to standard anti-ischemic therapy including aspirin and heparin reduces short-term risks of death, myocardial infarction, and refractory angina[89–125] (see Chap. 41). In a large randomized trial evaluating the GPIIb/IIIa inhibitor eptifibatide,[90] the mean age of the patient population was 64 years. In this nearly 11,000-patient trial, 30-day risk of death or nonfatal myocardial infarction was reduced from 15.7 percent in the placebo group to 14.2 percent in the eptifibatide-treated patients. In the subgroup of patients at least 65 years of age, there was no benefit for this GPIIb/IIIa inhibitor compared with placebo. In the randomized trial evaluating the GPIIb/IIIa inhibitor tirofiban compared with placebo,[91] patients treated with this GPIIb/IIIa inhibitor also benefited compared with aspirin and heparin alone, with the main end point of death, myocardial infarction, or refractory ischemia reduced from 17.9 percent to 12.9 percent at 7 days. In this 1915-patient trial, the mean age of the patients was 63 years. Both patients younger and older than 65 years of age benefited from GPIIb/IIIa inhibitor therapy: The composite event rate in the older group was reduced from 23.5 percent in the placebo group to 17.8 percent in the tirofiban group. Although bleeding is more common with GPIIb/IIIa inhibitor therapy than with placebo, bleeding is generally mild, with no increase in stroke rate or risk of intracranial hemorrhage. Therefore, *age should not exclude the addition of a GPIIb/IIIa inhibitor to standard anti-ischemic therapy in patients with unstable angina or non-Q-wave myocardial infarction.*

CHRONIC CORONARY DISEASE

The use of percutaneous transluminal angioplasty or coronary artery bypass surgery as therapy for chronic ischemic heart disease in the elderly has increased significantly over the last decade.[92] Revascularized Medicare patients are increasingly older, with a greater number of comorbid conditions. Nevertheless, 30-day and 1-year mortality rates have decreased significantly from 1987 to 1990 for both revascularization procedures in the elderly. The improved mortality rate likely represents improved technical approaches with angioplasty and bypass surgery, including increased use of internal mammary grafts.

Use of bypass surgery has also increased in the very elderly, increasing 67 percent in octogenarians from 1987 to 1990.[93] Thirty-day and 1-year mortality rates averaged 11.5 and 19.2 percent, respectively, both 2.5-fold greater than the corresponding operative mortality rate in the 65 to 70 year olds. Independent predictors of short-term and long-term mortality rates included increasing age, female gender, admission with acute myocardial infarction, congestive heart failure, cerebral or peripheral vascular disease, and chronic renal disease. Increasing age is also a significant independent predictor of stroke, which occurs in about 8 percent of the very elderly who undergo bypass surgery.[94] In spite of the high short-term morbidity and mortality rates, the 3-year mortality rate of this group was similar to that of the general octogenarian population. No randomized trial of medicine compared with bypass surgery has included the elderly, although significant improvement in quality of life with relief of medically refractory angina is achieved in many elderly bypass patients.[95,96] Therefore, the risk and benefits of bypass surgery should be assessed carefully, including consideration of comorbid conditions.

Angioplasty techniques and results have improved as well over the last several years.[97] Compared with prior data bases, elderly patients receiving the procedure more recently are older, with a more frequent history of a myocardial infarction, prior bypass surgery, and diabetes mellitus. In spite of the greater age and comorbidities, the procedural success rate has improved significantly in the elderly, to 93.5 percent, with a significant reduction in procedural complications, including death and myocardial infarction. The most dramatic decrease in complications was in the need for emergent bypass surgery, dropping to 0.65 percent, likely because of the introduction of coronary stents.[97] Although no trial randomized elderly subjects with multivessel disease to angioplasty compared with bypass surgery, the number of vessels with critical coronary artery disease and completeness of revascularization are powerful predictors of both short-term and long-term event-free survival in elderly patients after angioplasty and should be an important factor in deciding between angioplasty and bypass surgery.[98,99]

Cholesterol lowering is beneficial for elderly patients with chronic coronary artery disease. The Scandinavian Simvastatin Survival Study (4S) included 1848 patients 65 to 70 years of age with chronic coronary artery disease and an elevated baseline total cholesterol.[100] After 5.4 years of follow-up, cholesterol lowering with simvastatin resulted in significant decreases in total mortality, coronary heart disease mortality, major coronary events, and revascularization procedures. Therefore, *lipid-lowering therapy should be a goal in elderly patients with established coronary disease and elevated total cholesterol and low-density lipoprotein cholesterol.* Finally, observational data suggest that postmenopausal women benefit from the addition of hormone replacement therapy, with large reductions in future cardiovascular morbidity and mortality rates. This benefit was hypothesized to be due to not only the lipid-lowering effects of hormone replacement therapy, but also to the direct effects of estrogen on the coronary endothelium, likely via an increase in nitric oxide.[101] In a randomized, placebo-controlled trial evaluating premarin plus progesterone, however, there was no decrease in coronary death or nonfatal myocardial infarction among women with established coronary artery disease randomized to hormone therapy.[102] There are several potential explanations of why this was a negative trial, including data suggesting that, with increasing age and with atherosclerosis, there is less vascular expression of the estrogen receptor, likely due to methylation of the estrogen gene.[103,104] Further studies are in progress to determine whether there is a role for hormone replacement therapy in older women with coronary artery disease. Currently, *initiation of estrogen therapy is not recommended for the treatment of coronary artery disease in postmenopausal women.*

Congestive Heart Failure

In contrast to other cardiovascular disorders, the prevalence of chronic heart failure (CHF) is dramatically increasing. Approximately 4.7 million Americans have CHF, and each year 400,000 new cases are diagnosed.[105] The incidence of heart failure doubles with each decade of life, and the prevalence rises from 2 to 5 percent of those 70 to 79 years of age, and to almost 10 percent of those older than 80 years.[106] This is, in part, because heart failure represents a final common pathway for most other cardiac disorders and, in part, because of the more successful treatments of acute ischemic disease. These successes increase the numbers surviving, albeit with, or at increased risk for, heart failure. Although the etiology of CHF is ischemic in most patients, hypertension is also a common etiology, especially among African-Americans.[107]

CHF is also a highly lethal condition, with significant mortality, morbidity, and associated costs. Framingham investigators report a median survival of 1.66 years among men and 3.17 years among women in the community setting.[106] More than 90 percent of CHF deaths occur among adults older than 65 years.[108] CHF is also the leading cause of hospitalization in Medicare beneficiaries,[109] and hospitalization of these patients is itself a major risk factor for subsequent rehospitalization, mortality, and functional decline[110] (see also Chaps. 20 and 21).

The importance of the individual patient's role as a partner in his or her care and of individualizing treatment and monitoring plans cannot be overemphasized. Although patients may carry the same heart failure diagnosis, they differ markedly in terms of disease severity and complexity, associated comorbidities, social support, education, ingrained habits, access to medical personnel and knowledge, and understanding of health care information and directions. Noncompliance with medications or diet is often cited as a major factor contributing to hospitalization in heart failure patients. In a study of 7,247 elderly outpatients with CHF who were newly prescribed digoxin, only 10 percent filled enough prescriptions to have daily digoxin available for an entire year.[111] In 161 prospectively studied patients 70 years or older admitted with heart failure, 47 percent were readmitted within 90 days, and 38 percent of these readmissions were felt to have been possibly preventable.[112] The most common factors contributing to possibly preventable readmissions were noncompliance, failure to seek help promptly, and poor social support.

Age-associated biologic factors themselves are unlikely to result in heart failure but increase the likelihood for the development of symptoms in the presence of ischemic or hypertensive disease. Increased vascular load due to increased central vascular stiffness[113] and decreased endothelium-dependent vasodilatation[114] increase the likelihood of progressive LV dysfunction, adverse clinical outcomes, and a more variable and complicated response to conventional therapeutic interventions in older individuals with ischemic or hypertensive-induced LV damage.[115–117] In addition, the age-associated decrease in sympathetic responsiveness limits the ability of older people to augment heart rate and cardiac function in the presence of superimposed heart disease, particularly in the setting of acute depression of LV function. Finally, the decrease in early LV filling and the presumptive increase in LV filling pressures during exercise may worsen heart failure symptoms, especially in association with diseases that also impair LV filling, such as coronary artery disease and systemic arterial hypertension.

Evaluation of older patients with heart failure symptoms should include a noninvasive study to determine whether the primary problem is systolic dysfunction. *Up to 40 percent of older individuals with heart failure have normal systolic function.*[118] If ischemic, hypertensive, or valvular disease is responsible for failure, they should be specifically treated. Otherwise, *diuretics are particularly useful in patients with increased vascular stiffness presenting with acute congestive symptoms, since significant reductions in pressure occur with relatively small changes in intravascular volume.* Digitalis may improve signs and symptoms of heart failure without affecting overall survival in patients with systolic dysfunction and sinus rhythm.[119] However, the maintenance dose should be reduced to 0.125 mg/day because of the age-associated decreased volume of distribution and creatinine clearance. ACE inhibitors are a cornerstone of therapy in patients with systolic dysfunction, and their benefit extends to the elderly, as well.[120] Recent studies indicating the value of the β-blockades carvedilol[121] and metoprolol,[122] as well as aldosterone inhibition[123] in patients with continued symptoms despite ACE-I therapy, probably extend to the older population. It is possible to predict which older heart failure patients are at increased risk for early readmission. In this group, Rich et al.[124] and Stewart et al.[125] demonstrated that a multidisciplinary team approach including simplification of the medical regimen, close monitoring, and intensive patient education can decrease hospital admission and improve quality of life.

Arrhythmias

Supraventricular and ventricular arrhythmias increase in frequency with aging,[126] probably due to age-associated changes in the impulse formation and conduction system, including loss of pacemaker and conducting cell and fibrosis,[127] as well as increased incidence of mitral annular and aortic calcification, hypertension, and ischemic disease. Other illnesses may frequently present with arrhythmias in the elderly as well, including hyperthyroidism, anemia, hypoxia, electrolyte imbalance, infections, and hypotension or hypertension. Evaluation of older patients with symptomatic or asymptomatic arrhythmias, therefore, should include a search for these illnesses as well as other presenting triggers such as chest pain, exercise, smoking, caffeine, and medicine and alcohol ingestion (see Chap. 24). Long-term ambulatory electrocardiographic monitoring during the patient's normal activities is most likely to determine the nature and severity of the arrhythmia. Loop recorders, which enable continuous monitoring and recording when activated, may be particularly useful. These devices may be activated by the patient, which depends on the arrhythmia not being severe enough to preclude patient activation, or activated by the presence of the arrhythmia itself, which depends on the ability and reliability of the detection device. Invasive electrophysiology studies can be used to not only diagnose the arrhythmia but also to determine its mechanism, obtain prognostic information, and determine the suitability of different therapeutic approaches. The prognostic significance of an arrhythmia depends on the ventricular rate, the presence of atrial/ventricular synchrony, the duration of the arrhythmia, and the underlying cardiovascular substrate. Age-associated changes in both passive-state and active-state diastolic properties, as well as decreased systolic reserve (see above), may increase the likelihood that an older individual will develop hemodynamic compromise and/or ischemia during an arrhythmic episode.

Atrial fibrillation is common among the elderly. In the population-based Cardiovascular Health Study of 5201 men and women aged older than 65 years, 4.8 percent of women and 6.2 percent of men had atrial fibrillation.[128] In five randomized trials of anticoagulation for the prevention of stroke in atrial fibrillation, the mean age of enrolled patients was 69 years, with 25 percent over age 75.[129] Atrial fibrillation in this elderly cohort was associated with increasing age, heart failure, valvular heart disease, stroke, diabetes, and hypertension. Older individuals are more likely to experience hemodynamic compromise resulting from the increased ventricular rate and loss of atrial/ventricular synchrony accompanying the arrhythmia, because of the age-associated changes in relaxation properties and increased dependence on atrial contribution. Because of the increased likelihood of coronary disease, the higher rate is also more likely to be associated with myocardial ischemia. Atrial fibrillation may also result in atrial remodeling, which increases the likelihood of maintenance of the arrhythmia,[130] and lower output related to the irregularity of the rhythm.[131] The risk of embolic stroke in atrial fibrillation also increases with age. The Framingham Study reported that the risk of stroke attributed to atrial fibrillation rose from 7.3 percent in those 60 to 69 years of age to 30.8 percent in those aged 80 to 89 years.[132]

Therapeutic goals in patients with atrial fibrillation include stroke prevention, rate control, and possibly rhythm control. In randomized trials of anticoagulation versus placebo for the prevention of embolic strokes in atrial fibrillation, a significant reduction is seen generally with anticoagulation therapy, as well as in patients over 75 years of age.[133] This benefit of anticoagulation is greater than treatment with aspirin in the elderly, although there is a higher rate of intracranial hemorrhage.[134] Careful monitoring of the international normalized ratio (INR) is important, as most embolic strokes in the elderly occur when the ratio is under 2.0 and most cerebral hemorrhages occur when the ratio is above 3.0. Although the benefits of aspirin are less significant, it can be used in older patients who have a contraindication to warfarin therapy, including an inability to monitor the INR carefully. Rate control in patients without systolic dysfunction may be attempted with diltiazem, verapamil, and β-blockades; in patients with systolic dysfunction, β-blockades and digitalis may be used. In a recent randomized trial, the combination of atenolol and digitalis was found to be most effective in controlling both rest and exercise heart rates in atrial fibrillation patients.[135] If patients are intolerant of medical therapy, or if medical therapy is ineffective, AV node ablation and pacemaker insertion is highly safe and effective.[136] Cardioversion should be attempted in patients who are hemodynamically compromised, in acute atrial fibrillation, and for those who are at low likelihood of reversion to atrial fibrillation if conversion does occur. This can be attempted with electrical or pharmacologic[137] approaches (see also Chap. 24). Otherwise, the value of attempted conversion to sinus rhythm is not clear. If attempted, flecanide and propafenone are generally well tolerated by patients without ischemic or structural heart disease. Those with suspected tachycardia/bradycardiac syndrome, however, should be monitored for bradycardiac side effects. In patients with ischemic disease and preserved ventricular function, sotalol may be used. In patients with structural heart disease, the probability of pro-arrythmic effects is increased with all drugs. Potential side effects require close monitoring, therefore, when instituting agents other than amiodarone in these patients. In patients with heart failure, dofetilide, under careful monitoring conditions, was recently demonstrated to increase the likelihood of conversion to, and maintenance of, sinus rhythm[138] without the increase in mortality associated with some other antiarrhythmic agents in patients with heart failure. Experimental approaches include the Maze surgical procedure,[139] catheter ablation of atrial foci,[140] and the use of implantable defibrillators[141] to terminate atrial fibrillation. A more detailed discussion of the management of atrial fibrillation is presented in Chap. 24.

The use of programmable pacemakers to time atrial and ventricular systole appropriately may be particularly useful in older patients because diastolic filling and cardiac output are more dependent on atrial contribution. In the Medicare population, dual-chamber pacing was associated with improved 1- and 2-year survival, when compared with single-chamber pacing, after adjustment for confounding patient characteristics.[142]

Ventricular arrhythmias in the elderly are to be approached in the same fashion as in younger individuals, i.e., those that are asymptomatic and those unassociated with evidence of cardiac disease can be viewed as less serious than ventricular arrhythmias associated with evidence of LV dysfunction and/or ischemia. Both older and younger postmyocardial infarction patients benefit from β-blockade therapy, with a reduction in the rate of sudden death.[81] Life-threatening ventricular arrhythmias are common among elderly patients with severe coronary disease and LV dysfunction. As in younger subjects, aggressive management of elderly survivors of cardiac arrest or of those with hypotensive ventricular tachycardia is justified.[143] Antiarrhythmic therapy selected with electrophysiologic testing and/or placement of the implantable cardioverter defibrillator are well tolerated by the elderly and lead to improved survival.[144] Ventricular arrhythmias are discussed in detail in Chap. 24.

Valvular Heart Disease

The most frequent clinically significant valvular heart disease in the elderly is calcific aortic stenosis.[145] The development of clinically significant aortic stenosis may be very rapid in this age group (6 to 18 months), as calcification and severe scarring occur rather abruptly. Also, animal studies show that there is less compensatory hypertrophy in response to increased impedance to LV ejection in the elderly, which could also contribute to the development of heart failure.[146]

Clinical recognition of valvular aortic stenosis may be difficult in the elderly, and the features differ from those of isolated aortic stenosis in younger subjects (Table 86-2).[147] Aortic stenosis should be suspected in elderly patients presenting with congestive heart failure. By far, the most helpful study one can perform in screening an elderly subject for significant aortic stenosis is a Doppler echocardiogram looking for severe aortic valve calcification with decreased mobility, a small aortic valve area, and a significant transvalvular gradient. The presence of LV hypertrophy can be assessed as well as LV function. It appears that the condition of asymptomatic elderly patients with significant aortic stenosis by echocardiography can be followed carefully without surgical intervention until the first symptoms appear.[148] It should be noted, however, that if other disease (e.g., arthritis) limits an older patient, he or she might not be able to exercise to the point where symptoms occur, despite the presence of significant disease requiring surgery. These issues are complex and are discussed in greater detail in Chap. 56. To assess the need for bypass grafting at the time of the operation, coronary angiography should be performed in older individuals prior to aortic valve surgery. Aortic valve replacement often results in marked improvement in symptoms and LV function, as well as expected survival in older and even in very old patients.[149,150] Predictors of surgical mortality with aortic valve replacement include low ejection fraction and congestive heart failure, atrial fibrillation, associated surgical procedures, and an emergency procedure, suggesting that aortic valve replacement for symptomatic aortic stenosis should not be delayed merely because a patient is elderly.[151] Percutaneous aortic valvuloplasty in the elderly is associated with poor outcomes, including early restenosis, aortic regurgitation, stroke, high mortality rate, and heart failure.[152] It is useful only for palliation and as a "bridge" to valve replacement in very ill patients.[153]

Chronic aortic regurgitation may occur in elderly individuals secondary to aortic root dilatation. Symptoms include angina, even in patients without significant coronary disease, and congestive heart failure. It is important to recognize, however, that symptoms may not occur until significant LV dysfunction is present; therefore, the onset of dysfunction is enough to prompt surgery, rather than await the occurrence of symptoms. Vasodilator therapy in asymptomatic individuals with normal LV function may be helpful. In a randomized trial, nifedipine was shown to reduce LV volume and mass, increase ejection fraction, and delay the occurrence of systolic dysfunction.[154] Best operative results occur in individuals with no or minimal symptoms, mild to moderate ventricular dysfunction and a brief duration of left ventricular dysfunction[155] (see Chap. 56).

The most common cause of mi-

TABLE 86-2 Frequent Characteristics of Aortic Stenosis

	Older than 65 years	Younger than 65 years
Structure	Tricuspid	Bicuspid
Origin	Degeneration—calcium deposits in sinuses inhibit opening	Congenital bicuspid or deformed cusps—fusion of commissures
Exam	Murmur has a musical component at apex—may mimic mitral regurgitation	Murmur harsh at base
	Carotids may be normal	Carotid upstroke delayed
Gender	Women equal in frequency to men	Men predominate
Presentation	Congestive heart failure	Angina, syncope, and/or congestive heart failure
Rhythm	Atrial fibrillation common	Atrial fibrillation uncommon

tral stenosis in the elderly is rheumatic disease, which at times may not result in symptoms until the patient reaches old age. The diagnosis may be more difficult in the elderly because calcification of the valve may decrease the intensity of the first heart sound and the opening sound, and diminished cardiac output may decrease the intensity of the diastolic rumble. Doppler echocardiography is very useful in diagnosing the presence of significant disease. If symptoms are more than mild, or if pulmonary hypertension develops, surgery or balloon mitral valvuloplasty should be considered. Atrial fibrillation often triggers functional deterioration in older individuals because the dependence of filling on atrial contribution is exaggerated in the presence of mitral stenosis. Balloon mitral valvuloplasty compares favorably with open surgical commissurotomy in appropriate candidates—i.e., those with minimal calcification, good mobility, little subvalvular disease, and only mild mitral regurgitation[156]—and should be considered for elderly patients with symptomatic mitral stenosis.[156,157]

Mitral regurgitation in the elderly is most often related to ischemic heart disease and myxomatous degeneration of the mitral valve. As is true for aortic insufficiency, symptoms may be recognized only after significant LV dysfunction has occurred, and intervention should be considered on the basis of dysfunction, rather than await symptom onset. It should also be remembered that favorable unloading conditions will raise the ejection fraction in the presence of significant mitral regurgitation. Therefore, an ejection fraction of under 0.60 should be considered abnormal and is associated with a poorer postsurgical prognosis.[158] For elderly patients with mitral regurgitation, mitral valve repair is associated with a lower operative mortality and improved late outcomes, eliminates the need for anticoagulation in patients without atrial fibrillation, and results in excellent long-term results.[159,160] Thus, repair, rather than replacement, should be performed, if possible.

For elderly patients requiring valve replacement, the choice of a mechanical valve with the bleeding risk of lifelong anticoagulation must be balanced against a bioprosthetic valve and risk of structural deterioration. Additional factors in the choice include candidacy for anticoagulation and other requirements for anticoagulation, such as atrial fibrillation, age, and valve position. In a series of elderly subjects receiving aortic or mitral mechanical valve replacements, freedom from major anticoagulant-related hemorrhage was 76 percent at 10 years.[161] A bioprosthetic valve in the mitral position deteriorates more rapidly than in the aortic position. In a large series of elderly patients receiving porcine bioprostheses, freedom from structural deterioration at 10 years for the aortic valve bioprostheses was 98 percent and for the mitral valve bioprosthesis was 79 percent, with excellent long-term survival free of major morbidity[162] (see also Chap. 60).

Hypertension

Systolic pressure rises progressively with age, whereas diastolic pressure tends to plateau and even decline after 60 years, as noted. The consequent rise in pulse pressure, due primarily to an increase in central vascular stiffness, is a strong and independent risk factor for cardiovascular events,[163] for adverse consequences following an infarction,[164] and for the development of heart failure.[116] Numerous trials demonstrate the value of antihypertensive therapy in even mild diastolic hypertension in the elderly population.[165] Isolated systolic hypertension is more common in the elderly, and prospective randomized trials demonstrate that diuretic[166] and long-acting dihydropyridine calcium antagonist[167] therapy decrease the risk of stroke, congestive heart failure, and myocardial infarction or death among older patients with this entity. Although the general blood pressure goal is 140/90, lower goals are indicated in the presence of diabetes, target organ damage, or clinical cardiovascular disease.[168] Nonpharmacologic therapy, consisting of restricted salt intake and weight reduction, decreases blood pressure in many elderly hypertensives.[169] The selection of pharmacologic therapy should be based on prospective randomized trials; the presence of associated comorbidities (e.g., ischemia, renal insufficiency, systolic or nonsystolic dysfunction), and the duration of action and side-effect profile of the agent. Despite the widespread choice and effectiveness of proven therapies, the vast majority of hypertensive patients are not at the appropriate blood pressure goal.[168] Many patients require combination therapy to achieve satisfactory blood pressure control, particularly in the presence of diabetes and/or renal insufficiency (see also Chap. 51).

ACKNOWLEDGMENTS

The secretarial assistance of Christina R. Link and Spring Metcalf is greatly appreciated in preparing this chapter.

References

1. Lakatta EG. Cardiovascular aging research: The next horizons [Review]. *J Am Geriatr Soc* 1999; 47:613.
2. Olivetti G, Melissari M, Capasso JM, et al. Cardiomyopathy of the aging human heart: Myocyte loss and reactive cellular hypertrophy. *Circ Res* 1991; 68:1560.
3. Olivetti G, Giordano G, Corradi D, et al. Gender differences and aging: Effects in the human heart. *J Am Coll Cardiol* 1995; 26:1068.
4. Fraticelli A, Josephson R, Danziger R, et al. Morphological and contractile characteristics of rat cardiac myocytes from maturation to senescence. *Am J Physiol* 1989; 257:H259.
5. Anversa P, Palackal T, Sonnenblick EH, et al. Myocyte cell loss and myocyte cellular hyperplasia in the hypertrophied aging rat heart. *Circ Res* 1990; 67:671.
6. Kajstura J, Cheng W, Sarangarajan R, et al. Necrotic and apoptotic myocyte cell death in the aging heart of Fischer 344 rats. *Am J Physiol* 1996; 271:H1215.
7. Cheng W, Li B, Kajstura J, et al. Stretch-induced programmed myocyte cell death. *J Clin Invest* 1995; 96:2247.
8. Cigola E, Kastura J, Li B, et al. Angiotensin II activates programmed myocyte cell death in vitro. *Exp Cell Res* 1997; 231:363.
9. Esler MD, Turner AG, Kaye DM, et al. Ageing effects on human sympathetic neuronal function. *Am J Physiol* 1995; 268:R278.
10. Lakatta EG. Deficient neuroendocrine regulation of the cardiovascular system with advancing age in healthy humans [Point of view] *Circulation* 1993; 87:631.
11. Robert L. Aging of the vascular wall and atherogenesis: Role of the elastin-laminin receptor. *Atherosclerosis* 1996; 123:169.
12. Michel JB, Heudes D, Michel O, et al. Effect of chronic ANGI-converting enzyme inhibition on aging processes: II. Large arteries. *Am J Physiol* 1994; 267(1 pt 2):R124.
13. Fornieri C, Quaglino D, Mori G. Role of the extracellular matrix in age-related modifications of the rat aorta. *Arterioscler Thromb* 1992; 12:1008.
14. Haudenschild CC, Prescott MF, Chobanian AV. Aortic endothe-

lial and subendothelial cells in experimental hypertension and aging. *Hypertension* 1981; 3(suppl I):I-148.
15. Guyton JR, Lindsay KL, Dao DT. Comparison of aortic intima and inner media in young adult versus aging rats. *Am J Pathol* 1983; 111:234.
16. Li Z, Froehlich J, Galis ZS, et al. Increased expression of matrix metalloproteinase-2 in the thickened intima of aged rats. *Hypertension* 1999; 33:116.
17. Hariri RJ, Alonso DR, Hajjar DP, et al. Aging and atherosclerosis: I Development of myointimal hyperplasia after endothelial cell injury. *J Exp Med* 1986; 164:1171.
18. Senior RM, Griffin GL, Fliszar CJ, et al. Human 92- and 72-kilodalton type IV collagenase are elastases. *J Biol Chem* 1991; 266:7870.
19. Border WA, Ruoslahti E. Transforming growth factor-β in disease: The dark side of tissue repair. *J Clin Invest* 1992; 90:1.
20. Majesky MW, Lindner V, Twardzik DR, et al. Production of transforming growth factor β_1 during repair of arterial injury. *J Clin Invest* 1991; 88:904.
21. Battegay EJ, Raines EW, Seifert RA, et al. TGF-β induces bimodal proliferation of connective tissue cells via complex control of an autocrine PDGF loop. *Cell* 1990; 63:515.
22. Takasaki I, Chobanian AV, Sarzani R, et al. Effect of hypertension on fibronectin expression in the rat aorta. *J Biol Chem* 1990; 265:21,935.
23. Millis AJT, Hoyle M, McCue HM, et al. Differential expression of metalloproteinase and tissue inhibitor of metaproteinase genes in aged human fibroblasts. *Exp Cell Res* 1992; 201:373.
24. McCaffrey TA, Falcon DJ. Evidence for an age-associated dysfunction in the antiproliferative response to transforming growth factor-β in vascular smooth muscle cells. *Mol Biol Cell* 1993; 4:315.
25. Crawford DC, Chobanian AV, Brecher P. Angiotensin II induces fibronectin expression associated with cardiac fibrosis in the rat. *Circ Res* 1994; 74:727.
26. Gerstenblith G, Fredricksen J, Yin FCP, et al. Echocardiographic assessment of a normal adult aging population. *Circulation* 1977; 56:273.
27. Swinne CJ, Shapiro EP, Lima SD, et al. Age-associated changes in left ventricular diastolic performance during isometric exercise in normal subjects. *Am J Cardiol* 1992; 69:823.
28. Fleg JL, Schulman SP, Gerstenblith G, et al. Additive effects of age and silent myocardial ischemia on the left ventricular response to upright cycle exercise. *J Appl Physiol* 1993; 75:499.
29. Fleg JL, O'Connor FC, Gerstenblith G, et al. Impact of age on the cardiovascular response to dynamic upright exercise in healthy men and women. *J Appl Physiol* 1995; 78:890.
30. Fleg JL, Lakatta EG. Role of muscle loss in the age-associated reduction in VO_2 max. *J Appl Physiol* 1988; 65:1147.
31. Kenney WL, Ho CW. Age alters regional distribution of blood flow during moderate-intensity exercise. *J Appl Physiol* 1995; 79:1112.
32. Lakatta EG. Cardiovascular regulatory mechanisms in advanced age. *Physiol Rev* 1993; 73:413.
33. Yin FCP, Raizes GS, Guarnieri T, et al. Age-associated decrease in ventricular response to haemodynamic stress during beta-adrenergic blockade. *Br Heart J* 1978; 40:1349.
34. Walker KE, Lakatta EG, Houser SR. Age associated changes in membrane currents in rat ventricular myocytes. *Cardiovasc Res* 1993; 27:1968.
35. Orchard CH, Lakatta EG. Intracellular calcium transients and developed tensions in rat heart muscle: A mechanism for the negative interval-strength relationship. *J Gen Physiol* 1985; 86:637.
36. Lompre AM, Lambert F, Lakatta EG, et al. Expression of sarcoplasmic reticulum Ca^{2+}-ATPase and calsequestrin genes in rat heart during ontogenic development and aging. *Circ Res* 1991; 69:1380.
37. Tate CA, Taffet GE, Hudson EK, et al. Enhanced calcium uptake of cardiac sarcoplasmic reticulum in exercise-trained old rats. *Am J Physiol* 1990; 258:H431.
38. Koban MU, Moorman AFM, Holtz J, et al. Expressional analysis of the cardiac Na/Ca exchanger in rat development and senescence. *Cardiovasc Res* 1998; 37:405.
39. Effron MB, Bhatnagar GM, Spurgeon HA, et al. Changes in myosin isoenzymes, ATPase activity and contraction duration in rat cardiac muscle with aging can be modulated by thyroxine. *Circ Res* 1987; 60:238.
40. Bhatnagar GM, Walford GD, Beard ES, et al. ATPase activity and force production in myofibrils and twitch characteristics in intact muscle from neonatal, adult, and senescent rat myocardium. *J Mol Cell Cardiol* 1984; 16:203.
41. Koban MU, Moorman AFM, Holtz J, et al. Expressional analysis of the cardiac Na-Ca exchanger in rat development and senescence. *Cardiovasc Res* 1998; 37:405.
42. Pepe S, Tsuchiya N, Lakatta EG, et al. PUFA and aging modulate cardiac mitochondrial membrane lipid composition and Ca^{2+} activation of PDH. *Am J Physiol* 1999; 276 (*Heart Circ Physiol.* 45):H149.
43. Hano O, Bogdanov KY, Sakai M, et al. Reduced threshold for myocardial cell calcium intolerance in the rat heart with aging. *Am J Physiol* 1995; 269:H1607.
44. Lakatta EG. Chaotic behavior of myocardial cells: Possible implications regarding the pathophysiology of heart failure. *Perspect Biol Med* 1989; 32:421.
45. Chen C-H, Nakayama M, Nevo E, et al. Coupled systolic-ventricular and vascular stiffening with age implications for pressure regulation and cardiac reserve in the elderly. *J Am Coll Cardiol* 1998; 32:1221.
46. Chen C-H, Ting C-T, Lin S-J, et al. Which arterial and cardiac parameters best predict left ventricular mass? *Circulation* 1998; 98:422.
47. Nussbacher A, Gerstenblith G, O'Connor F, et al. Hemodynamic effects of unloading the old heart. *Am J Physiol* 1999; 277: H1863.
48. Chen C-H, Nakayama M, Talbot M, et al. Verapamil acutely reduces ventricular-vascular stiffening and improves aerobic exercise performance in elderly individuals. *J Am Coll Cardiol* 1999; 33:1602.
49. Lakatta EG. Deficient neuroendocrine regulation of the cardiovascular system with advancing age in healthy humans [Point of view]. *Circulation* 1993; 87:631.
50. Esler MD, Turner AG, Kaye DM, et al. Aging effects on human sympathetic neuronal function. *Am J Physiol* 1995; 268:R278.
51. Seals DR, Dempsey JA. Aging, exercise and cardiopulmonary function. In: Lamb DR, Gisolfi CV, Nadel E, eds. *Perspectives in Exercise Science and Sports Medicine,* vol 8. 1995:237.
52. Fleg JL, Schulman S, O'Connor F, et al. Effects of acute β-adrenergic receptor blockade on age-associated changes in cardiovascular performance during dynamic exercise. *Circulation* 1994; 90:2333.
53. Yin FCP, Weisfeldt ML, Milnor WR. Role of aortic input impedance in the decreased cardiovascular response to exercise with aging in dogs. *J Clin Invest* 1981; 68:28.
54. Xiao R-P, Spurgeon HA, O'Connor F, et al. Age-associated changes in β-adrenergic modulation on rat cardiac excitation-contraction coupling. *J Clin Invest* 1994; 94:2051.
55. Xiao R-P, Tomhave ED, Xiangwu J, et al. Age-associated reductions in cardiac β_1- and β_2-adrenoceptor responses without changes in inhibitory G proteins or receptor kinases. *J Clin Invest* 1998; 101:1273.
56. Jiang MT, Moffat MP, Narayanan N. Age-related alterations in the phosphorylation of sarcoplasmic reticulum and myofibrillar proteins and diminished contractile response to isoproterenol in intact rat ventricle. *Circ Res* 1993; 72:102.
57. Schulman SP, Fleg JL, Goldberg AP, et al. Continuum of cardio-

vascular performance across a broad range of fitness levels in healthy older men. *Circulation* 1996; 94:359.

58. Gillum RF. Trends in acute myocardial infarction and coronary heart disease death in the United States. *J Am Coll Cardiol* 1993; 23:1271.
59. National Center for Health Statistics. *Vital Statistics of the United States, 1988,* vol 2: *Mortality,* part A, tables 1-27, 1-129. Rockville, MD: National Center for Health Statistics; 1991.
60. Frishman WH, DeMaria AN, Ewy GA. Clinical assessment. *J Am Coll Cardiol* 1987; 10(abstr):48A.
61. Fleg JL, Gerstenblith G, Zonderman AB, et al. Prevalence and prognostic significance of exercise-induced silent myocardial ischemia detected by thallium scintigraphy and electrocardiography in asymptomatic volunteers. *Circulation* 1990; 81:428.
62. Nicod P, Gilpin E, Dittrich H, et al. Short- and long-term clinical outcome after Q wave and non-Q wave myocardial infarction in a large population. *Circulation* 1989; 79:528.
63. Goldberg RJ, Gore JM, Gurwitz JH, et al. The impact of age on the incidence and prognosis of initial acute myocardial infarction: The Worcester Heart Attack Study. *Am Heart J* 1989; 117:543.
64. Nadelmann J, Frishman WH, Ooi WL, et al. Prevalence, incidence and prognosis of recognized and unrecognized myocardial infarction in persons aged 75 years or older: The Bronx aging study. *Am J Cardiol* 1990; 66:533.
65. Maggioni AP, Maseri A, Fresco C, et al. Age-related increase in mortality among patients with first myocardial infarctions treated with thrombolysis. *N Engl J Med* 1993; 329:1442.
66. Keller NM, Feit F. Atherosclerotic heart disease in the elderly. *Curr Opin Cardiol* 1995; 10:427.
67. GUSTO Investigators. An international randomized trial comparing four thrombolytic strategies for acute myocardial infarction. *N Engl J Med* 1993; 329:673.
68. Armstrong PW, Fu Yuling, Chang W-C, et al. Acute coronary syndromes in the GUSTO-IIb trial. *Circulation* 1998; 98:1860.
69. Thiemann DR, Coresh J, Oetgen WJ, et al. Association between hospital volume and survival after acute myocardial infarction in the elderly. *N Engl J Med* 1999; 340:1640.
70. Fibrinolytic Therapy Trialists' Collaborative Group. Indications for fibrinolytic therapy in suspected acute myocardial infarction: Collaborative overview of early mortality and major morbidity results from all randomized trials of more than 1000 patients. *Lancet* 1994; 343:311.
71. White HD. Selecting a thrombolytic agent. *Cardiol Clin* 1995; 13:347.
72. Mark DB, Hlatky MA, Califf RM, et al. Cost effectiveness of thrombolytic therapy with tissue plasminogen activator as compared with streptokinase for acute myocardial infarction. *N Engl J Med* 1995; 332:1418.
73. Barron HV, Bowlby LJ, Breen T, et al. Use of reperfusion therapy for acute myocardial infarction in the United States: Data from the National Registry of Myocardial Infarction 2. *Circulation* 1998; 97:1150.
74. Gore JM, Granger CB, Simoons ML, et al. Stroke after thrombolysis: Mortality and functional outcomes in the GUSTO-I Trial. *Circulation* 1995; 92:2811.
75. Grines CL, Browne KF, Marco J, et al. A comparison of immediate angioplasty with thrombolytic therapy for acute myocardial infarction. *N Engl J Med* 1993; 328:672.
76. Zijlstra F, Hoorntje JCA, De Boer M-J, et al. Long-term benefit of primary angioplasty as compared with thrombolytic therapy for acute myocardial infarction. *N Engl J Med* 1999; 341:1413.
77. Weaver WD, Simes RJ, Betriu A, et al. Comparison of primary coronary angioplasty and intravenous thrombolytic therapy for acute myocardial infarction. *JAMA* 1997; 278:2093.
78. Aguirre FV, McMahon RP, Mueller H, et al. Impact of age on clinical outcome and postlytic management strategies in patients treated with thrombolytic therapy: Results from the TIMI II Study. *Circulation* 1994; 90:78.
79. Iniguez A, Macaya C, Hernandez R, et al. Long-term outcome of coronary angioplasty in elderly patients with post-infarction angina. *Eur Heart J* 1994; 15:489.
80. TIMI IIIB Investigators. Effects of tissue plasminogen activator and a comparison of early invasive and conservative strategies in unstable angina and non-Q-wave myocardial infarction: Results of the TIMI IIIB Trial. *Circulation* 1994; 89:1545.
81. Gottlieb SS, McCarter RJ, Vogel RA. Effect of beta-blockade on mortality among high-risk and low-risk patients after myocardial infarction. *N Engl J Med* 1993; 339:489.
82. Forman DE, Bernal JLG, Wei JY. Management of acute myocardial infarction in the very elderly. *Am J Med* 1992; 93:315.
83. Krumholz HM, Radford MJ, Ellerbeck EF, et al. Aspirin in the treatment of acute myocardial infarction in elderly Medicare beneficiaries: Patterns of use and outcomes. *Circulation* 1995; 92:2841.
84. Krumholz HM, Radford MJ, Ellerbeck EF, et al. Aspirin for secondary prevention after acute myocardial infarction in the elderly: Prescribed use and outcomes. *Ann Intern Med* 1996; 124:292.
85. ACE Inhibitor Myocardial Infarction Collaborative Group. Indications for ACE inhibitors in the early treatment of acute myocardial infarction. *Circulation* 1998; 97:2202.
86. Acute Infarction Ramipril Efficacy (AIRE) Study Investigators. Effect of ramipril on mortality and morbidity of survivors of acute myocardial infarction with clinical evidence of heart failure. *Lancet* 1993; 342:821.
87. Kober L, Torp-Pedersen C, Carlsen JE, et al., for the Trandolapril Cardiac Evaluation (TRACE) Study Group. A clinical trial of the angiotensin-converting-enzyme inhibitor trandolapril in patients with left ventricular dysfunction after myocardial infarction. *N Engl J Med* 1995; 333:1670.
88. Lewis SJ, Moye LA, Sacks FM, et al., for the CARE Investigators. Effect of pravastatin on cardiovascular events in older patients with myocardial infarction and cholesterol levels in the average range. *Ann Intern Med* 1998; 129:681.
89. Kong DF, Califf RM, Miller DP, et al. Clinical outcomes of therapeutic agents that block the platelet glycoprotein IIb/IIIa integrin in ischemic heart disease. *Circulation* 1998; 98:2829.
90. Platelet Receptor Inhibition in Ischemic Syndrome Management in Patients Limited by Unstable Signs and Symptoms (PRISM-PLUS) Study Investigators. Inhibition of the platelet glycoprotein IIb/IIIa receptor with tirofiban in unstable angina and non-Q wave myocardial infarction. *N Engl J Med* 1998; 338:1488.
91. PURSUIT Trial Investigators. Inhibition of platelet glycoprotein IIb/IIIa with eptifibatide in patients with acute coronary syndromes. *N Engl J Med* 1998; 339:436.
92. Peterson ED, Jollis JG, Bebchuk MS, et al. Changes in mortality after myocardial revascularization in the elderly: The National Medicare experience. *Ann Intern Med* 1994; 121:919.
93. Peterson ED, Cowper PA, Jollis JG, et al. Outcomes of coronary artery bypass graft surgery in 24461 patients aged 80 years or older. *Circulation* 1995; 92(suppl II):II-85.
94. Freeman WK, Schaff HV, O'Brien PC, et al. Cardiac surgery in the octogenarian: Perioperative outcome and clinical follow-up. *J Am Coll Cardiol* 1991; 18:29.
95. Ko W, Gold JP, Lazzaro R, et al. Survival analysis of octogenarian patients with coronary artery disease managed by elective coronary artery bypass surgery versus conventional medical treatment. *Circulation* 1992; 86(suppl II):II-191.
96. Glower DD, Christopher TD, Milano CA, et al. Performance status and outcome after coronary artery bypass grafting in persons aged 80 to 93 years. *Am J Cardiol* 1992; 70:567.
97. Thompson RC, Holmes DR, Grill DE, et al. Changing outcome of angioplasty in the elderly. *J Am Coll Cardiol* 1996; 27:8.

98. O'Keefe JH, Sutton MB, McCallister BD, et al. Coronary angioplasty versus bypass surgery in patients >70 years old matched for ventricular function. *J Am Coll Cardiol* 1994; 24:425.
99. Thompson RC, Holmes DR, Gersh BJ, et al. Predicting early and intermediate-term outcome of coronary angioplasty in the elderly. *Circulation* 1993; 88:1579.
100. Miettinen TA, Pyorala K, Olsson AG, et al., for the Scandinavian Simvastatin Study Group. Cholesterol-lowering therapy in women and elderly patients with myocardial infarction or angina pectoris. *Circulation* 1997; 96:4211.
101. Mendelsohn ME, Karas RH. The protective effects of estrogen on the cardiovascular system. *N Engl J Med* 1999; 340:1801.
102. Hulley S, Grady D, Bush T, et al., for the Heart and Estrogen/Progestin Replacement (HERS) Study Research Group. Randomized trial of estrogen plus progestin for secondary prevention of coronary heart disease in postmenopausal women. *JAMA* 1998; 280:605.
103. Losordo DW, Kearney M, Kim EA, et al. Variable expression of the estrogen receptor in normal and atherosclerotic coronary arteries of premenopausal women. *Circulation* 1994; 89:1501.
104. Post WS, Goldschmidt-Clermont PJ, Wilhide CC, et al. Methylation of the estrogen receptor gene is associated with aging and atherosclerosis in the cardiovascular system. *Cardiovasc Res* 1999; 43:985.
105. Massie BM, Shah NH. Evolving trends in the epidemiologic factors of heart failure: Rationale for preventive strategies and comprehensive disease management. *Am Heart J* 1997; 133:703.
106. Ho KK, Pinsky JL, Kannel WB, et al. The epidemiology of heart failure: The Framingham Study. *J Am Coll Cardiol* 1993; 22(suppl):6A.
107. Bourassa MG, Gurne O, Bangiwala SI, et al. Natural history and patterns of current practice in heart failure. *J Am Coll Cardiol* 1993; 22(suppl):14A.
108. Centers for Disease Control and Prevention. Changes in mortality from heart failure: United States, 1980–1995. *JAMA* 1998; 280:874.
109. Graves EJ. National hospital discharge survey: Annual summary, 1988. *Vital Health Stat* 1991; 13:1.
110. Wolinsky FD, Smith DM, Stump TE, et al. The sequelae of hospitalization for congestive heart failure among older adults. *J Am Geriatr Soc* 1997; 45:558.
111. Monane M, Bohn RZ, Gurwitz JH, et al. Noncompliance with congestive heart failure therapy in the elderly. *Arch Intern Med* 1994; 154:433.
112. Krumholz HM, Wang Y, Purent EM, et al. Quality of care for elderly patients hospitalized with heart failure. *Arch Intern Med* 1997; 157:2242.
113. Yin FCP. The aging vasculature and its effect on the heart. In: Weisfeldt ML, ed. *The Aging Heart.* New York: Raven; 1980:137.
114. Taddei S, Virdis A, Mattei P, et al. Aging and endothelial function in normotensive subjects and patients with essential hypertension. *Circulation* 1995; 91:1981.
115. Domanski MJ, Nitchell GF, Norman JE, et al. Independent prognostic information provided by sphygmomanometrically determined pulse pressure and mean arterial pressure in patients with left ventricular dysfunction. *J Am Coll Cardiol* 1999; 33:951.
116. Chae CU, Pfeffer MA, Glynn RJ, et al. Increased pulse pressure and risk of heart failure in the elderly. *JAMA* 1999; 281:634.
117. Chen CH, Nakayama M, Nevo E, et al. Coupled systolic-ventricular and vascular stiffening with age: Implications for pressure regulation and cardiac reserve in the elderly. *J Am Coll Cardiol* 1998; 32:1221.
118. Wong WF, Gold S, Fukuyama O, et al. Diastolic dysfunction in elderly patients with congestive heart failure. *Am J Cardiol* 1989; 63:1526.
119. Digitalis Investigation Group. The effect of digoxin on mortality and morbidity in patients with heart failure. *N Engl J Med* 1997; 336:525.
120. CONSENSUS Trial Study Group. Effects of enalapril on mortality in severe congestive heart failure. *N Engl J Med* 1987; 316:1429.
121. Packer M, Bristow MR, Cohn JN, et al. The effect of carvedilol on morbidity and mortality in patients with congestive heart failure. *N Engl J Med* 1996; 334:1349.
122. MERIT-HF Study Group. Effect of metoprolol CR/XL in chronic heart failure: Metoprolol CR/XL randomized intervention trial in congestive heart failure (MERIT-HF). *Lancet* 1999; 353:2001.
123. Pitt B, Zannad F, Remme WJ, et al., for the Randomized Aldactone Study Investigators. The effect of spironolactone on morbidity and mortality in patients with severe heart failure. *N Engl J Med* 1999; 341:709.
124. Rich MW, Beckham V, Wittenberg C, et al. A multidisciplinary intervention to prevent the readmission of elderly patients with congestive heart failure. *N Engl J Med* 1995; 333:1190.
125. Stewart S, Pearson S, Horowitz JD. Effects of a home-based intervention among patients with congestive heart failure discharged from acute hospital care. *Arch Intern Med* 1998; 158:1067.
126. Fleg JL, Kennedy HL. Cardiac arrhythmias in a healthy elderly population: Detection by 24-hour ambulatory electrocardiography. *Chest* 1982; 81:301.
127. Lev M. The pathology of complete atrioventricular block. *Prog Cardiovasc Dis* 1964; 6:31.
128. Furberg CD, Psaty BM, Manolio TA, et al. Prevalence of atrial fibrillation in elderly subjects (the Cardiovascular Health Study). *Am J Cardiol* 1994; 74:236.
129. Alberts GW. Atrial fibrillation and stroke. *Arch Intern Med* 1994; 154:1443.
130. Goette A, Honeycutt C, Langberg JJ. Electrical remodeling in atrial fibrillation: Time course and mechanisms. *Circulation* 1996; 94:2968.
131. Daoud EG, Weiss R, Bahu M, et al. Effect of an irregular ventricular rhythm on cardiac output. *Am J Cardiol* 1996; 78:1433.
132. Wolf PA, Abbott RD, Kannel WB. Atrial fibrillation: A major contributor to stroke in the elderly. *Arch Intern Med* 1987; 147:1561.
133. Atrial Fibrillation Investigators. Risk factors for stroke and efficacy of anti-thrombotic therapy in atrial fibrillation: Analysis of pooled data from five randomized trials. *Arch Intern Med* 1994; 154:1449.
134. Stroke Prevention in Atrial Fibrillation Investigators. Warfarin versus aspirin for prevention of thromboembolism in atrial fibrillation. Stroke Prevention in Atrial Fibrillation II Study. *Lancet* 1994; 343:687.
135. Rosenquist M, Lee MA, Mouliner L, et al. Long-term follow-up of patients after transcatheter direct current ablation of the atrioventricular junction. *J Am Coll Cardiol* 1990; 6:1467.
136. Morady F, Hasse C, Strickberger SA, et al. Long-term follow-up after radiofrequency modification of the atrioventricular node in patients with atrial fibrillation. *J Am Coll Cardiol* 1997; 27:113.
137. Ellenbogen KA, Stambler BS, Wood MA, et al. Efficacy of intravenous ibutilide for rapid termination of atrial fibrillation and atrial flutter: A dose-response study. *J Am Coll Cardiol* 1996; 28:120.
138. Torp-Pedersen C, Moller M, Bloch-Thomsen PE, et al., for the Danish Investigations of Arrhythmia and Mortality on Dofetilide Study Group. Dofetilide in patients with congestive heart failure and left ventricular dysfunction. *N Engl J Med* 1999; 341:857.
139. Cox JL, Schuessler RB, Lappas DG, et al. An 8 1/2 year experience with surgery for atrial fibrillation. *Ann Surg* 1996; 224:267.
140. Jais P, Haissaguerre M, Shah DC, et al. A focal source of atrial fibrillation treated by discrete radiofrequency ablation. *Circulation* 1997; 95:572.
141. Lau C-P, Tse H-F, Lok N-S, et al. Initial clinical experience with an implantable human atrial defibrillator. *PACE* 1997; 20:221.

142. Lamas GA, Pashos CL, Norman SLT, et al. Permanent pacemaker selection and subsequent survival in elderly Medicare pacemaker recipients. *Circulation* 1995; 91:1063.
143. Tresh DD, Platia EV, Guarnier T, et al. Refractory symptomatic ventricular tachycardia and ventricular fibrillation in elderly patients. *Am J Med* 1987; 83:399.
144. Tresh DD, Trouop PH, Thakur RK, et al. Comparison of efficacy of automatic implantable cardioverter defibrillator in patients older and younger than 65 years of age. *Am J Med* 1991; 90:717.
145. Seltzer A. Changing aspects of the natural history of valvular aortic stenosis. *N Engl J Med* 1987; 317:91.
146. Isoyama S, Wei JY, Izumo S, et al. The effect of age on the development of cardiac hypertrophy produced by aortic constriction in the rat. *Circ Res* 1987; 61:337.
147. Roberts WC, Perloff JK, Costantino T. Severe valvular aortic stenosis in patients over 65 years of age. *Am J Cardiol* 1971; 27:497.
148. Pellikka PA, Nushimura RA, Bailey KR, et al. The natural history of adults with asymptomatic hemodynamically significant aortic stenosis. *J Am Coll Cardiol* 1990; 15:1012.
149. Wong JB, Salem DN, Pauker SG. You're never too old. *N Engl J Med* 1993; 328:971.
150. Lindblom D, Lindblom U, Qvist J, Lundstrom H. Long-term relative survival rates after heart valve replacement. *J Am Coll Cardiol* 1990; 15:566.
151. Logeais Y, Langanay T, Roussin R, et al. Surgery for aortic stenosis in elderly patients: A study of surgical risk and predictive factors. *Circulation* 1994; 90:2891.
152. Bernard Y, Etievent J, Mourand JL, et al. Long-term results of percutaneous aortic valvuloplasty compared with aortic valve replacement in patients more than 75 years old. *J Am Coll Cardiol* 1992; 20:792.
153. Carabello BA, Crawford FA. Medical progress: Valvular heart disease. *N Engl J Med* 1997; 337:32.
154. Scognamiglio R, Rahimtoola SH, Fasoli G, et al. Nifedipine in asymptomatic patients with severe aortic regurgitation and normal left ventricular function. *N Engl J Med* 1994; 331:689.
155. Bonow RO. Management of chronic aortic regurgitation. *N Engl J Med* 1994; 331:736.
156. Reyes VP, Raju S, Wynne J, et al. Percutaneous balloon valvuloplasty compared with open surgical commissurotomy for mitral stenosis. *N Engl J Med* 1994; 331:961.
157. Tuzcu EM, Block PC, Griffin BP, et al. Immediate and long-term outcome of percutaneous mitral valvotomy in patients 65 years and older. *Circulation* 1992; 85:963.
158. Enriquez-Sarano M, Tajik AJ, Schaff HV, et al. Echocardiographic prediction of survival after surgical correction of organic mitral regurgitation. *Circulation* 1994; 90:830.
159. Jebara VA, Dervanian P, Acar C, et al. Mitral valve repair using Carpentier techniques in patients more than 70 years old: Early and late results. *Circulation* 1992; 86(suppl II):II-53.
160. Enriquez-Sarano M, Schaff HV, Orsazulak TA, et al. Valve repair improves the outcome of surgery for mitral regurgitation: A multivariate analysis. *Circulation* 1995; 91:1022.
161. Holper K, Ottke M, Lewe T, et al. Bioprosthetic and mechanical valves in the elderly: Benefits and risks. *Ann Thorac Surg* 1995; 60(suppl):S443.
162. Burr LH, Jamieson RE, Munro AI, et al. Porcine bioprostheses in the elderly: Clinical performance by age groups and valve positions. *Ann Thorac Surg* 1995; 60:S264.
163. Franklin SS, Khan SA, Wong ND, et al. Is pulse pressure useful in predicting risk for coronary heart disease? The Framingham Heart Study. *Circulation* 1999; 100:354.
164. Mitchell GF, Moyce LA, Braunwald E, et al. Sphygmomanometrically determined pulse pressure is a powerful independent predictor of recurrent events after myocardial infarction in patients with impaired left ventricular function. *Circulation* 1997; 96:4254.
165. Management Committee of the Australian Therapeutic Trial in Mild Hypertension. Treatment of mild hypertension in the elderly. *Med J Aust* 1981; 2:398.
166. SHEP Cooperative Research Group. Prevention of stroke by antihypertensive drug treatment in older persons with isolated systolic hypertension. *JAMA* 1991; 265:3255.
167. Staessen JA, Fagard R, Thijs L, et al. Randomized double-blind comparison of placebo and active treatment for older patients with isolated systolic hypertension. *Lancet* 1997; 350:757.
168. Sixth Report of the Joint National Committee on Prevention, Detection, Evaluation, and Treatment of High Blood Pressure. Bethesda, MD: National Institutes of Health, National Heart, Lung, and Blood Institute, National High Blood Pressure Education Program. NIH Publ 98-4080; November 1997.
169. Whelton PK, Appel LJ, Espeland MA, et al. Sodium reduction and weight loss in the treatment of hypertension in older persons: A randomized controlled trial of nonpharmacologic interventions in the elderly. *JAMA* 1998; 279:839.

CHAPTER 87

WOMEN AND CORONARY ARTERY DISEASE

Pamela Charney

INTRODUCTION

Only recently has coronary artery disease (CAD) been perceived as a major contributor of morbidity and mortality in women.[1] National acceptance by the public and physicians of the importance of CAD in women has yet to adequately evolve. In a national telephone survey of American women, 58 percent ". . . believed they were as likely or more likely to die of breast cancer than CAD."[2] In this telephone survey, although 86 percent of the women surveyed saw a doctor regularly, almost half of the women reported their physicians had "never talked to them about heart disease."

The increasing focus on women and CAD reflects both greater attention to older populations and enthusiasm for improving women's health. The initial CAD research focus was on middle-aged populations, where middle-aged men have a dramatically higher rate of CAD than middle-aged women. In middle-aged populations around the world, there is a consistent ratio of male-to-female CAD deaths varying from 2.5 to 4.5.[3] The etiology of this excess CAD mortality in men has not been determined, although the variable differences between countries suggest that "sex is not destiny with regard to CHD [coronary heart disease]."[3] Research has only recently included elderly subjects, where differences in mortality rates between women and men are smaller (Fig. 87-1).

In this chapter, prevention, diagnosis and management of women with coronary artery disease are addressed. More detailed discussions can be found in *Coronary Artery Disease in Women: Prevention, Diagnosis and Management*.[1] The section on prevention reviews clinically important gender differences in specific CAD risk factors. The section on diagnosis begins with discussion of the ways that CAD presents in asymptomatic women and then reviews models to assess CAD risk with attention to gender. Finally, symptomatic CAD in women is discussed, including the management of the women with angina and myocardial infarction. The chapter closes with an update on gender differences in sudden death.

PREVENTION: GENDER-SPECIFIC ISSUES

It is especially important to identify women at high risk for CAD for possible primary prevention. Young women with coronary artery mortality[4] are more likely to have a history of tobacco exposure, obesity, hypertension, diabetes, early menopause, or, less often, cocaine abuse.[5] These risk factors are also important in predicting nonfatal myocardial infarction.[1] Gender differences are reviewed in terms of tobacco use and cessation, diabetes, hypertension, lipids, obesity, physical activity and exercise, menopause and hormonal replacement therapy, psychosocial risk factors, and race.

Tobacco

Tobacco is the single most important coronary artery risk factor for women and men, as noted elsewhere.[1,6,7] Cigarette smoking has been associated with an earlier age of first myocardial infarction (see also Chap. 38).[8] The risk of myocardial infarction (fatal and nonfatal) increases 2.5-fold for women who smoke one to four cigarettes daily.[9] Since middle-aged women experience less symptomatic CAD than middle-aged men, the increased risk related to tobacco use on the incidence rates of myocardial infarction and sudden death is greater for women than men. Tobacco use also lowers the age of reported menopause.[10]

Tobacco exposure can occur not only through personal use

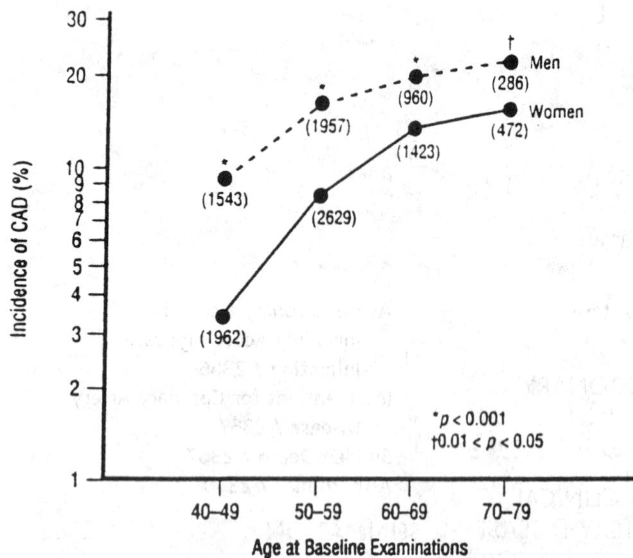

FIGURE 87-1 Framingham data: 10-year incidence of coronary artery disease (angina, myocardial infarction, coronary insufficiency, or death) among women and men by age. (From Eaker ED, Castelli WP. Coronary heart disease and its risk factors among women in the Framingham study. In: Eaker ED, Packard B, Wenger NK, et al., eds. *Coronary Heart Disease in Women: Proceedings of an NIH Workshop*. New York: Haymark Doyma; 1987:122–130. Future directions. In: Charney P, ed. *Coronary Artery Disease in Women*. Philadelphia: American College of Physicians; 576, with permission.)

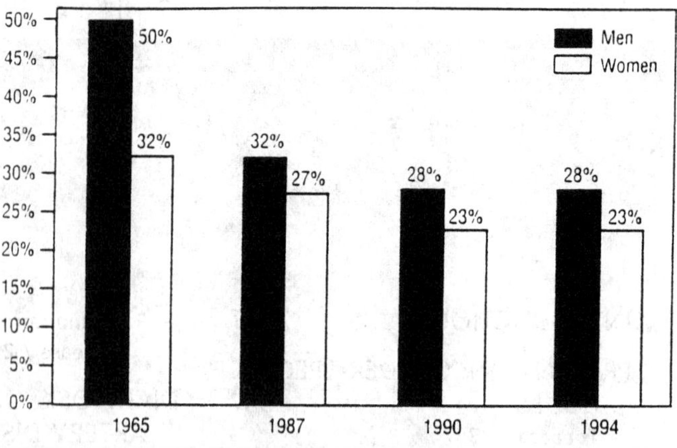

FIGURE 87-2 Prevalence of smoking among men and women in the United States. (Data from the U.S. Department of Health and Human Services. Centers for Disease Control and Prevention, Office of Smoking and Health. *MMWR Morb Mort Wkly Rep* 1995; 45:588–590. In: Ockene JK, Bonollo DP, Adams A. Smoking. In: Charney P, ed. *Coronary Artery Disease in Women*. Philadelphia: American College of Physicians; 1999:42).

of tobacco products but also by inhaling secondhand smoke. In epidemiologic studies, secondhand exposure is also related to an increased risk of CAD events.[7] For both women and men, the relative risks were similar (1.25; 95 percent CI 1.17–1.32). There was a dose-response curve when exposure to more than one package of cigarettes daily was compared with less than one pack cigarettes per day and when number of years of exposure was considered.

Over the last several decades, American women's personal use of cigarettes has not decreased dramatically as has occurred among men (Fig. 87-2). The prevalence of cigarette use among women reflects both higher initiation rates and greater difficulty stopping cigarette use.[6] By the year 2000, it is predicted that 23 percent of women will smoke, compared with 20 percent of men. Of all age and race groups, young white women currently have the highest tobacco initiation rates and are consuming more cigarettes, on average, than men of the same age.[11] Women smokers are more likely than men to report that smoking cigarettes aids in dealing with emotional stress.

Women have more difficulty quitting cigarette use, both initially and in the long term, although successful tobacco cessation for women as for men dramatically decreases the risk of further coronary events.[6] Only recently has exploration of gender and racial differences in tobacco cessation efforts focused on different responses to potential weight gain, social pressures, and physiologic withdrawal symptoms. For women, the frequent weight gain with tobacco cessation is often a substantial barrier to trying to stop smoking cigarettes. An increase in weight is a common consequence of efforts to stop smoking.[6] Smokers who stop cigarettes gain, on average, 7 to 10 lb. Fewer than 10 percent of those who stop smoking gain more than 20 lb. Weight gain tends to be higher among women, blacks, and smokers who inhale more than 25 cigarettes per day. Yet women smokers report that they are unwilling to experience any or minimal weight increase as a result of stopping smoking.[6]

To avoid weight gain with tobacco cessation, several types of interventions have been recommended.[6] It is often helpful for the physician to aid in the development of realistic expectations, encourage exercise, careful choice of snacks, and appropriate pharmacotherapy. Increasing physical activity or participating in exercise programs can increase calories expended and also aid in dealing with emotional stress. Minimizing excess calories is easier to achieve when low-sugar snacks are available to deal with cravings for sweets. Asking patients to begin a weight-reduction program while simultaneously stopping cigarettes is usually not realistic.

Multiple pharmacologic therapies have been explored, including the use of bupropion and nicotine gum, which has been reported to minimize weight gain.[6,12] Bupropion hydrocholorothiazide has been effective in smokers who are not depressed. It is contraindicated in patients with a history of seizures (since it lowers the seizure threshold with a 0.1 percent risk) and similarly in those who have experienced head trauma or are heavy consumers of alcohol. Bupropion can exacerbate symptoms related to anorexia and bulimia and should be avoided with recent use of an monoamine oxidase (MAO) inhibitor.

While social pressures to be thin hinder women's tobacco cessation efforts, social pressures from others are also noted to be an important stimulus for women to stop smoking. Social pressure to stop smoking cigarettes is reported twice as often by women as by men. The source of social pressure also is different, with women reporting pressure from children, while men report pressure from coworkers and friends.[13] Women have been observed in some studies to experience greater withdrawal symptoms than men.[14] In addition, it has been observed that black smokers may have more trouble stopping than white smokers.[15]

Physiologic issues affecting tobacco use and cessation are under exploration. Comparing black and white smokers with similar amounts of tobacco consumption, black smokers had higher cotinine levels than white smokers.[15] Physiologic addiction may have been underestimated previously in black smokers, resulting in undertreatment of nicotine addiction. Descriptions of physiologic symptoms must be considered, not just the number of cigarettes consumed. With improved pharmacologic agents to aid in tobacco cessation, aggressive management of tobacco cessation symptoms is possible.

Physicians are still identifying smoking status at only 67 percent of visits and counseling 50 percent of smokers about cessation, with specialists providing counseling substantially less often than primary care physicians (30 versus 12 percent of visits sampled in 1995).[16] These low physician identification and intervention rates are concerning, especially since surveys reveal that physicians can have a powerful effect on smoking cessation, even with minimal efforts.[6,17] Unfortunately, most programs to aid smokers with CAD have not focused on women's special issues. Programs that promote activities to minimize weight gain, including encouraging exercise and stressing social support may be more effective for women. Additional research is needed. In the meantime "Simple advice by one's physician to stop smoking is more effective than no advice at all, and as the physician-delivered smoking intervention becomes more intensive, the effects are greater."[17]

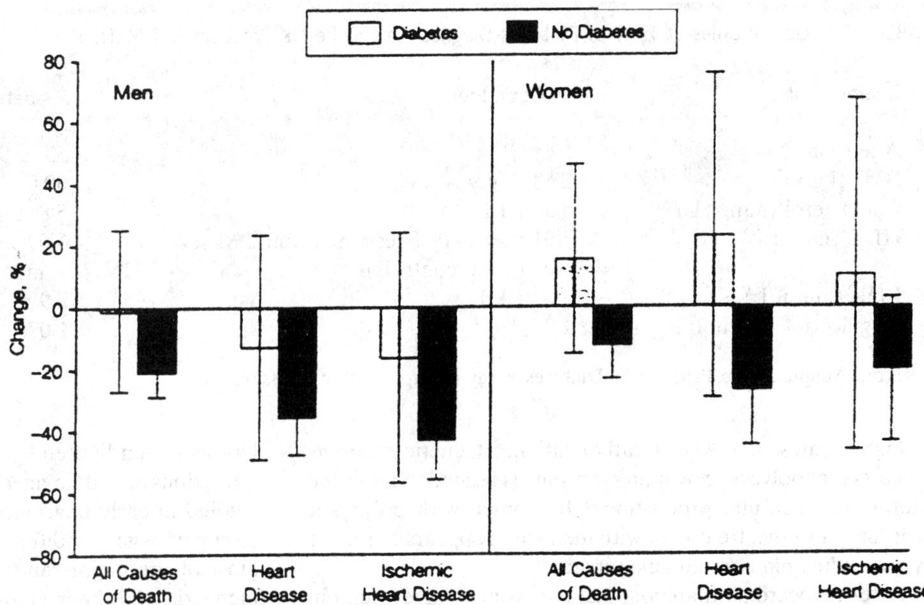

FIGURE 87-3 Change in mortality rates in women and men diabetics compared with nondiabetics. Cohort 1 was defined in 1971–1975 and followed up through 1982–1984, while Cohort 2 was defined in 1982–1984 and followed through 1992–1993. (From Gu K et al.,[20] with permission.)

Diabetes

Diabetic individuals have higher mortality rates from coronary artery disease than nondiabetics[18,19] (see also Chap. 78). Data from two of the National Health and Nutrition Examination Surveys elucidate some important gender differences.[20] The mortality rates from CAD have increased among diabetic women while decreasing among diabetic men (Fig. 87-3). Further research is required to determine whether these observations reflect gender differences in risk factors or natural history or less aggressive CAD prevention in diabetic women.

Diabetic women and men with hypertension have especially high rates of CAD.[18] This is common, since the prevalence of both diseases increases with advancing age. There is substantial variation in prevalence among different populations. Native Americans, Mexican Americans, and black populations have a higher prevalence of both of these disorders than American white populations.[11] Women and men generally have similar incidence rates of diabetes, although with increasing age, more women become hypertensive.

Women at risk for developing diabetes include obese women and those who have experienced gestational diabetes (compared with women who have had a pregnancy without glucose intolerance).[21] Obesity is increasingly common, and with increasing weight there is greater insulin resistance as well as a higher rate of glucose intolerance. For women at risk, regular physical activity[22] and avoiding gaining weight may decrease the chances of developing diabetes. Regular exercise not only decreases the risk of developing

Once a woman is diagnosed with diabetes, her "female advantage" in relation to the risk of CAD is lost.[20,23] Unlike the nondiabetic population, diabetic women have CAD rates similar to those of diabetic men. Diabetic women compared with nondiabetic women are at substantially greater risk of CAD.[18] For example, the 1-year mortality after a first hospitalization with myocardial infarction in a subgroup analysis of the WHO MONICA Project (World Health Organization Multinational Monitoring of Trends and Determinants of Cardiovascular Disease), from Finland, was 44.2 percent in diabetic men, 32.6 percent in nondiabetic men, 36.9 percent in diabetic women, and 20.2 percent in nondiabetic women.[24] The mechanisms for these observations are not fully elucidated and are suspected to be a least partially related to lipid abnormalities as well as insulin resistance.

Lipid abnormalities are common in diabetic patients. At the time of diagnosis of type II diabetes, women have substantially lower high-density lipoprotein (HDL) cholesterol than age-matched diabetic men or nondiabetic women[25] (Table 87-1). Other lipid abnormalities are also present, including elevated triglycerides. Subgroup analysis of diabetic patients treated with HMG-CoA reductase inhibitors within the larger Scandinavian Simvastatin Survival Study (4S) revealed improved lipoprotein patterns with treatment and less CAD events.[26] Larger studies including more women diabetics are in progress.

Insulin resistance is characterized by elevated levels of circulating insulin and is associated with glucose intolerance, higher levels of free fatty acid, central obesity, and hypertension. The relationship between elevated insulin levels and cardiovascular events has been under active investigation.[23] One clinical example is polycystic ovarian syndrome, where increased androgens, lower HDL, and higher triglycerides have been noted as well

TABLE 87-1 Lipid Profiles at Time of Diabetes Diagnosis from the UK Prospective DM Trial

Characteristic	Diabetic Men	Diabetic Women
Age (years)	52 ± 9	53 ± 9
BMI (kg/m²)	28.3 ± 4.9	30.8 ± 6.7
Cholesterol (mmol/L)	5.5 ± 1.1	5.8 ± 1.2
HDL (mmol/L)	1.01 ± 0.24 (9% less than non-DM sex-matched controls)	1.09 ± 0.25 (23% less than non-DM sex-matched controls)
LDL (mmol/L)	3.6 ± 1.0	3.9 ± 1.1
Trigylcerides (mmol/L)	1.8	1.07

SOURCE: Adapted from Prospective Diabetes Study Group,[25] with permission.

as higher rates of CAD at catherization.[27] Genetic mapping suggests that polycystic ovarian syndrome is related to inherited alterations in insulin production.[28] In women with polycystic ovarian syndrome, treatment with metformin appears to reduce hyperinsulinemia and aid amenorrhea.[29]

After myocardial infarction, diabetic women have been observed to have a higher risk of death and congestive heart failure than diabetic men.[19,23] Treatment trials to prevent CAD and its complications in diabetic patients are in progress. The recently completed United Kingdom prospective diabetes study revealed that control of hypertension to below a blood pressure (BP) of 150 systolic as well as maximizing glucose control decreased coronary artery disease events.[29]

Therefore, diabetic women should be considered at high risk for coronary artery disease. Aggressive management of lipoprotein abnormalities[23,26] and hypertension,[29] if present, is beneficial. There is some evidence that glucose control decreases vascular disease. Regular exercise can also improve glucose control[22] and insulin resistance.[30]

Hypertension

The prevalence of hypertension also increases with advancing age, and—since life expectancy is greater for women than men—there are more elderly women with hypertension.[31] At all ages, black women and men have about double the incidence of hypertension as their white counterparts. Generally, women are more likely to have controlled (BP) than men. Both in epidemiologic studies of blood pressure and in treatment trials, lower blood pressure is associated with lower rates of CAD events.

Both systolic and diastolic blood pressures have been found in population and cohort studies to predict coronary events. Framingham data revealed that with a systolic BP greater than 180, the annual incidence of coronary heart disease (angina, coronary insufficiency, myocardial infarction, or death from these diagnoses) in women over 65 years of age is greater than 30 percent, while for older men above age 65, it is about 50 percent.[32] In other epidemiologic studies, higher diastolic blood pressure also predicts greater rates of clinical coronary artery disease.[33]

While treatment trials have also documented that lower blood pressure decreases the incidence of a first myocardial infarction and sudden death, this effect has been less dramatic than the decrease in stroke occurrence with blood pressure control. Analysis of myocardial infarction prevention in women has also been limited by the lower number of first myocardial infarctions in middle-aged women, the age group predominantly studied in early pharmacologic treatment trials.[34] Post hoc assessment of gender differences with individual patient data from most of the major randomized controlled hypertensive treatment trials has been completed.[34] These major treatment trials initiated pharmacologic therapy with thiazides and/or beta blockers versus placebo. Because most participants were middle-aged, the number of coronary events observed among women was smaller than the number of events among men. Since blood pressure control has only a limited impact on the prevention of myocardial infarction, the power to detect a treatment effect on coronary events for women was compromised. In contrast, with a greater reduction in stroke occurrence with treatment, the number of strokes for women and men was equal and adequate in number to reveal a treatment effect, which was similar for women and men. After reviewing the early studies, several authors have stressed the particular importance of identifying and treating hypertension in black women to prevent coronary artery disease events and stroke.[31,35]

Once older subjects were studied in clinical trials, the benefit of treating hypertension to prevent coronary events received greater recognition.[36,37] The number needed to treat (NNT) to prevent one myocardial infarction in representative trials in older and middle-aged women and men are compared in Table 87-2.[38] As Kannel states, ". . . coronary disease is the most common and lethal sequela of hypertension, equaling in incidence all the other cardiovascular outcomes combined."[39]

Gender-specific information about thiazide diuretics and angiotensin-converting enzyme (ACE) inhibitors for the pharmacologic therapy of hypertension is available. Thiazide diuretics are a reasonable first choice in the treatment of hypertension in women as well as men.[40] In epidemiologic studies, thiazide diuretics use has been associated with a lower incidence of hip fracture. In a meta-analysis of several cohort studies, current thiazide use, especially if long-term, was associated with as much as a 20 percent reduction of risk of hip fracture.[41] Evaluation of biochemical variables has suggested potential mechanisms.[42] No prospective treatment trials have explored this relationship. Although ACE drugs are effective in treating hypertension and congestive heart failure as well as preventing the progression of renal disease, these agents should be cautiously utilized in women of reproductive age because they are potentially teratogenic.[43] Cough, a common side effect of first-generation ACE inhibitors, occurs substantially more frequently in women than in men.[44]

Lipids

There are important gender differences in lipoprotein profiles.[45] Total cholesterol peaks in women from age 55 to 64 and in men at around age 50. HDL is usually greater in women than in men, with HDL levels remaining similar with increasing age. Many experts consider HDL more predictive for women than any other lipoprotein component, with the strongest correlation between low HDL levels and CAD events. Low-density lipoprotein (LDL) levels increase with increasing age for both women and men and are especially predictive of events in men. Triglyceride levels may be important in women but have not been shown to be independently important in men.

TABLE 87-2 Numbers Needed to Treat (NNT) to Prevent One Coronary Artery Event in Women and Men from Three Clinical Treatment Trials

		NNT to Prevent One CAD Event	
Treatment Study	Age of Subjects	Women	Men
STOP (25 month)	70–84 years	83	77
SHEP (5 years)	>age 59	50	111
HDFP (5 years)	30–51 years	143	59

ABBREVIATIONS: STOP = Swedish Trial in Older Patients with Hypertension; SHEP = Systolic Hypertension in the Elderly Program; HDFP = Hypertension Detection and Follow-up Program.
SOURCE: From Cohen E, Swiderski D, Wheat ME, Charney P. Hypertension. In: Charney P, ed. *Coronary Artery Disease in Women*. Philadelphia: American College of Physicians; 1999:169.

Many of the initial pharmacologic therapies for hyperlipidemia decreased LDL most effectively and were tested in middle-aged populations. Because women, on average, develop clinical CAD 10 years later than men, there was often inadequate power in primary prevention trials to determine the efficacy of treatment for women. Further data have become available, with older populations being studied and newer agents—such as the HMG-CoA reductase inhibitors, which simultaneously decrease LDL and increase HDL—being used. Secondary prevention studies in a variety of populations, including women, reveal benefit with treatment. Yet these agents are underprescribed after myocardial infarction and target treatment levels are not reached.[46] Most studies have found older age a barrier to prescribing and some researchers have found women less likely to receive treatment than men.[5,19,46]

There has only been adequate power to determine that secondary prevention with pharmacologic treatment of hyperlipidemia decreases CAD events in women. Primary prevention studies have had inadequate power for women because of the small number of observed CAD events. A recent meta-analysis combined primary and secondary treatment trials to reach adequate power for a secondary analysis by gender.[47] Results were dominated by secondary prevention trials. Women at high risk, such as women with diabetes, should be considered candidates for primary prevention with aggressive treatment of lipid abnormalities. There is controversy about aggressive treatment in the woman at low risk for vascular disease while results of further primary prevention clinical trials are pending.

Treatment of hyperlipidemia is discussed in detail in Chap. 38. The choice of agents for the treatment of hyperlipidemia in women includes hormonal therapy. In short-term studies of hyperlipidemia treatment, the HMG-CoA reductase inhibitors have been compared with hormonal replacement therapy regimens.[48,49] Although, both types of agents improve HDL, the HMG-CoA reductase inhibitors are more effective in improving LDL than hormonal therapy. In addition, triglyceride levels often increase with hormonal therapy and decrease with the HMG-CoA reductase inhibitors.[48,49] In a subsequent section, "Menopause and Hormonal Replacement Therapy," the risks and potential benefits of hormonal therapy are further discussed.

Obesity

The prevalence of obesity has been increasing. Over 30 percent of white women and 50 percent of black or Mexican-American women are obese. In a recent third National Health and Nutrition Examination Survey, significantly more of the black and Mexican-American women were obese, with an elevated body mass index (BMI), than the white women (mean BMI for black women was 29.2 kg/m^2, 28.6 for Mexican-American women, and 26.3 kg/m^2 for white women).[50] Racial differences in BMI as well as glycosylated hemoglobin start in childhood, with black and Mexican-American girls having less favorable profiles than white girls.[11]

Obesity is linked to multiple cardiac risk factors (including insulin resistance, diabetes, hypertension, and hyperlipidemia), although it is has not clearly been documented to be independently associated with coronary artery event rates.[51] However, the pattern of weight distribution is predictive of coronary events.[51,52] The "apple" shape, with a greater central or abdominal girth, has been compared with the "pear" shape, with more weight on hips and buttocks. In the Nurses Health Study, both larger waist circumference and waist-hip ratio were independently associated with higher rates of CAD events.[52]

Increasingly, the relationship between greater weight and less physical activity has been elucidated. A study of obese twins revealed that lack of physical activity correlated with which twin was more obese.[53] This is particularly important, since even limited weight loss is associated with a lower risk of CAD events,[54,55] as is increased physical activity (see next section).

Behavioral interventions to decrease weight have been most successful when there is an exercise component.[51,56] One innovative trial for 40 obese women (mean weight 89.2 kg and BMI 32.9 kg) compared a 16-week program with instruction on a low-fat 1200-calorie diet and either training to increase daily physical exertion or addition of an aerobics class.[56] Compared with enrollment, all participants lost weight during the intensive program at the 1-year follow up. Women who had increased their activities of daily living most successfully sustained weight reduction. While new pharmacologic treatments for obesity have been developed, many have been documented to be hazardous.[57]

Physical Activity and Exercise

Gender differences in physiologic response to exercise have been studied.[58] Generally, women have smaller hearts, so cardiac output is increased by raising heart rate. Men, in comparison, accomplish an increase in cardiac output by increasing stroke volume. Women have a smaller work capacity and lower oxygen uptake. There are substantial limitations about what is known about women and physical activity, since—historically—studies have not collected data on housework and child care. Therefore, data about physical exertion in women may underestimate the actual amount of energy expended daily.

Yet in national surveys, sedentary lifestyles are reported by as many as 70 percent of adult women, with higher rates among black and hispanic women and those with less education or lower income.[50] Most studies on physical activity have focused on leisure activities and not included estimates of the energy required for housework or walking.[59] One community survey assessing change in physical activity from 1987 to 1991 found women more likely to exercise regularly if they had prior success with weight loss and exercise and received encouragement from their school-age children.[60] The women were less likely to begin or continue exercising if they worked outside the home. Especially for women, encouraging increased activity during daily activities of living is probably more important than counseling on initiating an exercise program. Recent programs to increase physical activity are cited in the section on obesity, above.

It is well known that overall mortality, CAD, and cancer mortality are inversely related to increasing levels of exercise. Physical activity is also important as secondary prevention. Both women and men are found to benefit from referral to cardiac rehabilitation programs after myocardial infarction.[61] However, fewer women than men are referred (6.9 percent women versus 13.3 percent men).[62]

Menopause and Hormonal Replacement Therapy

The importance of menopause as a risk factor for CAD in women is not fully defined. Women who have experienced early menopause after gynecologic surgery have been considered at higher risk for CAD and osteoporosis on the basis of less years of hormonal exposure.[63] However, a 1999 analysis from the Nurse's Health Study found only women smokers with a younger age of menopause to have a greater risk of CAD.[64]

Medical opinion on the potential benefits and risks of hormonal replacement therapy (HRT) after menopause has been evolving, as discussed elsewhere in this volume (Chaps. 38 and 86). Although population surveys have suggested that hormonal replacement therapy may decrease the risk of coronary artery disease, there are substantial differences between women who chose to take hormones and those who do not. Hormone users have tended to be healthier and wealthier, with less reported tobacco exposure and greater levels of exercise and access to medical care.[65] All these factors decrease the risk of CAD.

Although both retrospective and prospective epidemiologic evidence has suggested that users of hormonal therapy have substantially lower rates of CAD, results from clinical trials have not been confirmatory. The Heart & Estrogen/Progestin Replacement Study (HERS) is the only completed secondary prevention clinical trial of hormonal therapy.[66] Subjects were postmenopausal women with evidence of CAD [myocardial infarction (MI), coronary artery bypass graft (CABG), percutaneous transluminal coronary angioplasty (PTCA) for occlusion greater than 50 percent, or angiography with more than one major coronary artery] who were randomized to conjugated estrogen 0.625 mg plus medroxyprogesterone 2.5 mg or placebo and followed for 4 years. However, recruitment proceeded slowly and there were fewer coronary events than predicted as well as a higher crossover between treatment arms than expected. Results included no overall reduction in CAD events but substantially more venous thrombotic events and gallbladder disease in the group receiving hormonal therapy. Because of these risks, hormonal replacement therapy should be avoided in the setting of acute coronary ischemia. Assessment of hormonal replacement therapy for primary CAD prevention is currently in progress in the Women's Health Initiative.[65]

Multiple potential risks related to HRT have been described; they include increased thrombotic events, as noted in both epidemiologic trials and the HERS Study.[65,66] An increased risk of breast cancer with long-term use (greater than 5 years) is based on a worldwide review of the epidemiologic literature.[67] Other risks of HRT include higher rates of gallbladder disease[66] and elevated triglyceride levels. Vaginal bleeding frequently occurs with HRT and is a common reason why women chose to discontinue treatment.

Although there is controversy about the use of HRT to prevent CAD, there is clearer evidence for control of menopausal symptoms and a decreased rate of hip fracture with long-term use. Data from the Women's Health Initiative will provide evidence from a prospective double-blinded clinical trial. With the current limitations of medical knowledge, it is not surprising that utilization of HRT varies substantially among women potentially eligible for the treatment. In a 1995 national telephone survey of U.S. women, rates of hormonal treatment were shown to vary by geographic region and educational level rather than by medical condition.[68]

Psychosocial Risk Factors

Both socioeconomic and psychological factors affect the prevalence and outcome of CAD.[69] The effect of socioeconomic status on the incidence of CAD has been explored with increasing sophistication in the past decade. Coronary disease morbidity and mortality are greater among those of lower socioeconomic status (SES). Markers for SES have included years of formal education,[70] owning a car,[71] income defined by absolute[72] or relative amount,[73] and parental status.[71] More recently SES has also been defined independently of race.[11,50]

The importance of SES has been considered in a study from the Duke catherization population (consecutive patients with ≥75 percent stenosis of at least one coronary artery at catherization). The most important prognostic factor for CAD was the extent of coronary disease and ejection fraction at catherization, regardless of gender, with a 9-year median follow-up. However, SES and social support were independent risk factors and explained about 12 percent of the prognosis for individual women and men. Those with incomes below $10,000 per year were almost twice as likely to die as those with annual incomes ≥$40,000 within 5 years of follow-up.[72]

Women and men of lower SES from several United Kingdom studies were at increased risk for symptomatic CAD compared to those of a higher SES from the same area.[74-76] Lower SES has also been related to higher rates of tobacco use and higher inpatient mortality after MI.[74] Differences in event rates were greater for women than for men between different socioeconomic classes.

Among the many psychological issues with gender differences that affect outcomes in CAD, there is depression, which is diagnosed twice as often in women as in men.[77] Prospective data from the Baltimore Epidemiologic Catchment Area Study correlated a history of dysphoria or a major depressive episode with an increased risk of myocardial infarction for both women and men.[78] A positive response to a single question was central: "In your lifetime, have you ever had 2 weeks or more during which you felt sad, blue, depressed, or when you lost all interest and pleasure in things that you usually cared about or enjoyed?" The positive answer was associated with a 2.07 odds ratio of self-reporting an MI infarction at 13 years follow-up, compared with those giving a negative response. This odds ratio was independent of other coronary risk factors. Depression diagnosed with a patient interview 5 to 15 days after MI was a significant predictor of mortality at 6 months.[79] Although less women than men agreed to participate in this observation study, depression was more common in women than in men. Subsequent studies have revealed that depression after MI also predicts greater morbidity as well as higher subsequent mortality in women than in men.[80] As early as 1991, the question of whether higher rates of depression in women after MI correlate with sex differences in prognosis was raised;[81] the answer is still unavailable. Although a pharmacologic interventional trial of depression diagnosed after MI has not yet been reported, the selective serotonin reuptake inhibitors are probably safe in the presence of cardiac disease.[80]

Race and Coronary Artery Disease

Race and socioeconomic issues, in addition to traditional CAD risk factors, are important in understanding variations in black and white CAD mortality rates from the limited literature on these issues.[82-84] Social factors particularly important for black women are income, education, occupational status, and place of birth. Combined analysis of data from the 1986 National Mortality Feedback Survey, the 1985 National Health Interview Survey, and the U.S. Bureau of the Census revealed that young black women (age <55) had more than twice the rate of CAD mortality (sudden and nonsudden) than young white Americans.[83] CAD death rates for young black women in this study exceeded rates for young men and white women (Fig. 87-4). Importantly, family income, educational level, and occupational status accounted for more of this observed difference than traditional coronary risk factors.[83] In the Multicenter Investigation of the Limitation of Infarct Size study, black women (n = 63 of 985 randomized subjects) had a higher cumulative 4-year mortality after myocardial infarction than other sex and race groups.[82] The importance of birthplace for black New Yorkers rather than current geographic location has been described.[85,86]

Racial differences in physiology have also begun to be considered. Differences among electrocardiographic findings among black and white healthy subjects was detailed in 1998.[87] Differences in tobacco metabolism—such as slower cotinine

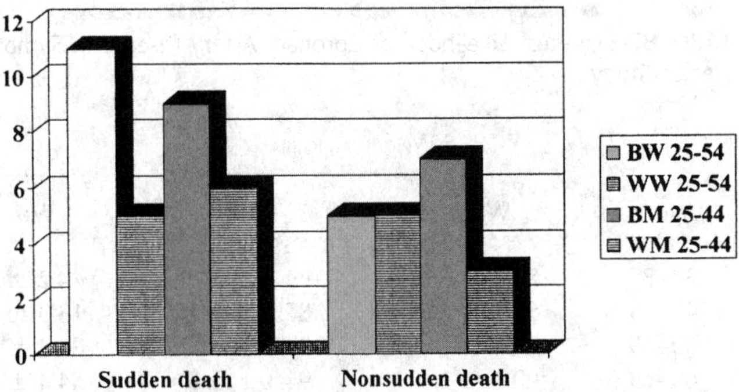

FIGURE 87-4 Coronary artery disease death rates for young adults (women age 25–54 years, men age 25–44 years) by race and gender. BW = black women; WW = white women; BM = black men; WM = white men. (Adapted from Escobedo LG, Giles WH, Anda RF. Socioeconomic status, race and death from coronary heart disease. *Am J Prev Med* 1997; 13:12–130, with permission.)

clearance and higher serum cotinine levels—are seen in black smokers compared with white[88] and Hispanic smokers.[15]

In summary, many important gender differences in specific cardiovascular risk factors have been briefly reviewed. More extensive discussions are available in other individual chapters and in *Coronary Artery Disease in Women.*[1] Models incorporating individual risk factors have been developed to aid in identifying women at higher risk for future CAD events. These models for risk stratification of individual women are discussed in the subsequent section on the management of CAD.

DIAGNOSIS OF CORONARY ARTERY DISEASE IN WOMEN

The biases that affect the diagnosis of CAD in women are explored below. Then, gender differences in noninvasive testing for CAD is discussed. Patterns of referral for coronary catherization are considered, followed by gender differences in cardiac catheterization results.

CAD is often diagnosed clinically by a careful history. The listener's preconceived biases can affect his or her perceptions of risk for CAD. In one study, where an actress portrayed a woman twice with the same script but different clothes and affect, physicians who reviewed the video where the actress described chest pain with "exaggerated emotional presentation style" predicted less CAD than when the same script was presented with a "businesslike affect."[89] More recently, physicians were recruited to view a video of different actors (black and white women and men) accompanied by the same written information. The black woman was least likely to be referred for cardiac catherization.[90] Since the clinical history is essential for the diagnosis of angina and acute coronary syndromes, provider assumptions affect the diagnosis of CAD. If the diagnosis is not considered, then evaluation and management will not occur. The clinical history typical for angina and acute coronary syndromes is reviewed at the beginning of the appropriate sections below as well as elsewhere in this textbook (Chaps. 40–42).

Once CAD is considered as a diagnosis, further evaluation is possible to assess disease presence and severity. Noninvasive stress testing can help to determine which patients with an intermediate risk for CAD will benefit from further interven-

TABLE 87-3 Pretest Likelihood of Coronary Artery Disease in Symptomatic Patients According to Age and Sex from the Cardiovascular Health Study

	Typical Angina		Atypical Angina		Nonanginal Chest Pain	
Age	Women	Men	Women	Men	Women	Men
30–39	25.8 ± 6.6%	69.7 ± 3.2%	4.2 ± 1.3%	21.8 ± 2.4%	0.8 ± 0.3%	5.2 ± 0.8%
40–49	55.2 ± 6.5	87.3 ± 1.0	13.3 ± 2.9	46.1 ± 1.8	2.8 ± 0.7	14.1 ± 1.3
50–59	79.4 ± 2.4	92.0 ± 0.6	32.4 ± 3.0	58.9 ± 1.5	8.4 ± 1.2	21.5 ± 1.7
60–69	90.1 ± 1.0	94.3 ± 0.4	54.4 ± 2.4	67.1 ± 1.3	18.6 ± 1.9	28.1 ± 1.9

SOURCE: From Recommendations of the Task Force of the European Society of Cardiology: Management of stable angina pectoris. *Eur Heart J* 1997:398, with permission.

tions and to assess disease control.[91] Although a more extensive discussion can be found in Chap. 14, potential gender differences in noninvasive testing are discussed briefly here. Unfortunately, each of the noninvasive techniques has limitations in women.[92,93]

Exercise stress testing is the oldest way of assessing CAD risk noninvasively. However, if a completed exercise stress test reveals ST changes and depression greater than 1 mm, especially in younger women (where the prevalence of ST depression is less), this may indicate significant CAD.[94] In comparison, a negative exercise stress test with adequate exertion is often helpful because it decreases the need to consider cardiac catherization.[94] Gender-specific criteria have been proposed to compensate for the generally smaller ST changes seen in women.[95]

As a rule, stress imaging techniques are favored in assessing a woman for possible CAD or staging the severity of disease. Local expertise is an important consideration in deciding whether to use nuclear medicine or echocardiography techniques. Nuclear stress perfusion testing in women can be potentially hindered by soft tissue attenuation from breast tissue with the use of thallium, so technetium may be preferred. Stress echocardiography is highly dependent on operator expertise and may be technically difficult in obese patients. Many authors prefer stress imaging tests with lower false-positive rates than an exercise stress test for women.[94]

Patterns of referral to cardiac catherization may vary by gender, with some appropriate differences.[96,97] Because cardiac catherization is less likely to reveal CAD in women, many clinicians initially evaluate women at intermediate risk with stress imaging techniques. For example, anginal symptoms in women are less predictive of abnormal coronary anatomy than in men (Table 87-3). In the Coronary Artery Surgery Study (CASS), coronary artery disease was diagnosed by cardiac catherization in 63 percent of women with definitive angina, 40 percent in women with probable angina, and 4 percent in women with nonischemic pain.[98] Direct referral to cardiac catheterization should occur with a high suspicion of significant CAD that might benefit from intervention or after an abnormal noninvasive stress test.

MANAGEMENT OF CLINICAL CORONARY ARTERY DISEASE IN WOMEN

Physicians have generally not appreciated some of the gender differences in CAD presentation and management. In a Gallup Survey completed in 1996 in Washington, D.C., "nearly two-thirds of the primary care physicians surveyed (256 internists and family practitioners) said that there is no difference between men and women in the symptoms, signs, or diagnosis of heart disease."[2] Meanwhile, research on CAD is extending our understanding of significant gender differences.[1]

The spectrum of presentations of CAD ranges from an asymptomatic disease phase to chronic angina and acute coronary syndromes including unstable angina, MI, and finally arrhythmia and sudden death. Both women and men may have silent or asymptomatic CAD for many years. Then, as described from Framingham data, the first presentation of symptomatic CAD is typically angina in women and MI in men.[99]

In this section, the entire spectrum of clinical CAD is reviewed, with attention to what is known in relation to caring for women patients. First, the asymptomatic women are considered, for whom coronary artery risk-assessment models have been developed. Then, angina and acute coronary syndromes are discussed. In addition, issues for women related to coronary artery bypass surgery and angioplasty are highlighted. Finally, considerations related to arrhythmias and sudden death are explored. Since women more frequently have atypical symptoms than men, women are more likely to present with occult CAD.

Asymptomatic Women

Some individuals are truly asymptomatic with respect to CAD. Others may have had atypical symptoms that have not yet been diagnosed as possible CAD. When Framingham researchers interviewed patients who had developed evidence of an interim myocardial infarction by electrocardiography (ECG) (25% of all myocardial infarctions), almost 50 percent, in retrospect, reported some symptoms.[100]

For truly asymptomatic women, national guidelines for prevention have been increasingly developed.[101] Important risk factors for both women and men include tobacco use, hypertension, physical inactivity, diabetes, obesity, and hyperlipidemia.[102] Counseling of asymptomatic women about CAD should include a review of the common risk factors, encouragement for implementing a healthy lifestyle, and an outline of the symptoms of CAD. The single most important intervention is avoiding exposure to tobacco.[1,6,7]

Tools to assess CAD risk are receiving increasing attention. Prospective cohort studies have been used to develop models predicting the impact of one or more risk factors on the likelihood of future coronary artery events.[50,103,104] When multiple individual risk factors are present, the cumulative risk of CAD is greater than the sum of its parts.[50,103,105] The prevalence and impact of risk factors are reviewed below—with data on women from the Third National Health and Nutrition Examination Survey,[50] the Chicago Heart Association Detection Project in Industry,[103,105] and the Framingham Heart Study.[104,106]

The Third National Health and Nutrition Examination Survey (NHANES III) explored the intersection between race, SES, and the prevalence of cardiovascular risk factors.[50] Among women, systolic blood pressure, tobacco use, BMI, leisure-time activity, non–high density lipoprotein cholesterol, and the presence of non-insulin-dependent diabetes were assessed in black ($n = 1762$), Mexican-American ($n = 1481$), and white women ($n = 2023$) age 25 to 64 years old. Participants completed both a home questionnaire and a physical examination in a mobile examination center. SES status was defined by the highest educational level attained, and a poverty income ratio was derived from family income and size. Compared with prior studies in which comparisons were attempted, more low-SES white women were included.

Results from NHANES III stressed the importance of race even when SES was included in a CAD risk model. As expected, increasing age was associated with a greater prevalence of all risk factors. However, there were substantial racial variations. Black and Mexican-American women had a higher BMI and systolic blood pressure, more diabetes, and reported more leisure-time activity (as well as lower tobacco use) than white women of a similar SES. With increasing age, black and Mexican-American women had greater prevalence rates of hypertension than white women. In contrast, smoking rates were more stable with increasing age for black and Mexican-American women, while they decreased for white women. Other large cohort studies, including the Chicago Heart Association Detection Project in Industry and cohorts from Framingham and the Lipid Research Clinics, have focused on white populations.

The prevalence and impact of individual and multiple risk factors in the Chicago Heart Association Detection Project in Industry were explored.[103] Employed participants age 40 to 64 years in the Chicago area were surveyed. Smoking status, hypertension, hyperlipidemia, and their relative importance in predicting CAD was assessed among 8686 women and 10,503 men, almost all white, who were followed for 22 years. At the time of enrollment, history of current tobacco use was obtained, a single BP was recorded, and a serum cholesterol was determined. Current tobacco use was reported by 35 percent of women (40 percent of men). Hypertension, defined as BP systolic ≥140, was noted in 53 percent of women (64 percent of men). Hypercholesteremia, defined as cholesterol ≥240 mg/dL, was present in 30 percent of women (22 percent of men). About 80 percent of participants in the Chicago Heart Association Detection Project in Industry had at least one of these risk factors initially. Two risk factors were found in about 34 percent of women and 38 percent of men. Less than 7 percent had all three risk factors. When coronary mortality was considered, those with the most risk factors were at the greatest risk of death. Tobacco use was a significantly more important predictor of mortality in women than in men (RR 2.85 versus 1.68, $p < 0.001$, comparing current smokers with nonsmokers). In a subsequent analysis, the number of risk factors present at screening also directly correlated with the eventual size of Medicare reimbursements.[105] Those without risk factors had the lowest number of Medicare claims.

Similarly, the cardiac risk profile for asymptomatic 50-years-olds in the Framingham cohort was used to predict who would be alive at age 75. For women, survival was associated with lower daily cigarette use and lower systolic blood pressure. In addition, a higher forced vital capacity and parental survival to age 75 were predictive of survival.[104]

Clustering of risk factors was also important on examination in the Framingham Offspring Study (age 30 to 74 years at enrollment) with 16 years of follow-up for coronary artery events (MI or sudden death).[54] On evaluation, 17 percent of all participants had three of the six risk factors (lowest quintile HDL cholesterol, highest quintile cholesterol, BMI, systolic blood pressure, triglycerides, and glucose). There were 79 first coronary artery events among the 1818 women who were initially free of symptomatic CAD, compared with 229 events among the 1759 men. However, CAD events were associated with three or more risk factors for 48 percent of the CAD events in women and 20 percent of the CAD events in men. When Framingham offspring where assessed 8 years apart, weight gain correlated most significantly with changes in blood pressure and lipoproteins for women and men.[106]

A more recent review has considered long-term cardiovascular outcomes among those with a low risk-factor profile, including data on women from the Chicago Heart Association Detection Project in Industry.[107] A low risk-factor profile was defined as follows: not a current smoker, BP ≤120/80, total cholesterol <200, no history of diabetes or MI, and no ECG abnormalities. Only 6.8 percent of the cohort age 40 to 59 years at entry met these criteria. These women had substantially lower CAD mortality with a mean follow up of 22 years (3.5 compared with 14.5 age-adjusted mortality rate per 10,000 person-years, RR 0.21, 95%; CI 0.05 to 0.84).

In summary, these studies indicate that risk factors are additive and that women without traditional cardiovascular risk factors (tobacco, hypertension, high cholesterol, diabetes, physical inactivity, family history, and old age) are at relatively low risk for coronary events. The largest benefit is derived from aggressive preventive measures in women with multiple risk factors or prior coronary events[108–110] (see also Chap. 40).

Angina

The clinical diagnosis of angina can be challenging. Women generally visit physicians more often than men and report more symptoms, including chest pain. In assessing chest symptoms to determine whether angina is the most probable diagnosis, attention to the type and duration of symptoms and their impact on activities of daily living often provide important clues. The chest pain associated with angina classically may be a heavy pressure or squeezing but may also be described as a burning, aching, or stabbing. Typically duration varies between 10 and 20 min, with MI more likely after 30 min of sustained pressure or pain. Often angina is precipitated by exertion. Women compared with men with angina more frequently report angina with emotional or mental stress.[111] Too often older women ascribe their decreased ability to complete housework or walk to "getting old." Therefore regular exploration of a patient's exercise tolerance and consideration of coronary artery disease in the differential when there is a decrease in exercise tolerance are essential.

As discussed under "Diagnosis of Coronary Heart Disease in Women," managing angina in women is complicated by the observation that anginal symptoms in women are less predictive of abnormal coronary anatomy than in men. In CASS, CAD was diagnosed by cardiac catherization in 63 percent of women with definitive angina, 40 percent in women with probable angina, and 4 percent in women with nonischemic pain[98] (Table 87-3). Data on women with unstable angina are discussed below and also reveal lower rates of CAD at cardiac catheterization.

Chronic angina has a generally favorable prognosis in women, with mortality rates of about 2 or 3 percent annually.[112] The management of women with chronic angina requires therapies effective for the prevention of MI in addition to symptom management. Most clinicians begin secondary prevention with the diagnosis of angina, although secondary prevention trials have begun after an MI, not usually after the diagnosis of angina. Secondary prevention treatment goals include tobacco avoidance (both smoking cessation and avoiding secondhand smoke); control of blood pressure, glucose, weight, and emotional stress; and the initiation or continuation of regular physical exercise or exertion.[112] Pharmacologic therapies include the use of aspirin, anti-ischemic agents, and lipid-lowering agents. Most clinicians would hesitate to begin HRT since the recent HERS study, discussed previously.

Potential gender differences in vasospastic responses have been a focus of research. When patients with both a history of chest pain and angiography indicating no more than slight coronary artery abnormalities received acetylcholine by intracoronary infusion, substantial gender differences were noted.[113] Of the 117 patients studied, large-artery spasm (n = 63) occurred predominantly in men (40 men versus 23 women), while microvascular spasm (n = 29) occurred more often in women (20 women versus 9 men). Patients with microvascular spasm had less coronary artery constriction after acetylcholine infusion, although angina (93 percent) and ischemic changes on ECG (83 percent) were often noted. Lactate levels in the coronary sinus were higher after acetylcholine infusion in patients with microvascular spasm (82 percent) than in those with large-artery spasm (53 percent). These types of studies have suggested that patterns of ischemia may vary by gender. More recent reviews of acute coronary syndromes have also suggested clinically important gender differences.

Acute Coronary Ischemia Including Acute Myocardial Infarction

Acute coronary ischemia includes unstable angina and MI; there are substantial gender differences in the presentation and natural history of each. Some differences may be physiologic and others are related to differences in management. Extensive general discussions of acute coronary ischemia syndromes can be found in other chapters within this volume. This section focuses on gender differences in presentation, prognosis, and management.

Gender differences in acute ischemia at the time of presentation and during short-term follow-up have been explored.[114–117] In a recent review of data from the National Registry of Myocardial Infarction–I, women had a higher mortality during the index hospitalization.[114] As in earlier studies, women arrived longer for evaluation after symptoms began; they also received less thrombolytic treatment (e.g., aspirin, beta blockers) as well as less invasive interventions (catherization, PTCA, and CABG). Women had higher mortality rates than men, even at similar ages or after similar interventions, from cardiogenic shock, sudden death, arrhythmias, myocardial rupture, and electromechanical dissociation (in descending order). Complementary results were noted in a Spanish registry of patients less than 80 years of age experiencing a first MI.[115] As well as a later presentation for care, women had higher mortality during hospitalization and within 6 months. Women more often developed acute pulmonary edema or cardiogenic shock (25 percent of women versus 11 percent of men) and less often developed at least one episode of ventricular fibrillation or sustained ventricular tachycardia requiring immediate medical care (15 percent of women versus 24 percent of men).

Prospective subgroup gender analysis of patients enrolled in Global Use of Strategies to Open Occluded Coronary Arteries in Acute Coronary Syndromes (GUSTO IIb) compared initial presentations, evaluation, and 30-day mortality.[116] Although most subjects enrolled had had an acute MI (53.8 percent of women and 67 percent of men), substantial numbers of participants had unstable angina (Table 87-4). At presentation, women were more often diagnosed with unstable angina than men (45.9 versus 35.6 percent, $p < 0.001$; odds ratio 1.51, 95 percent CI 1.34 to 1.69). Women subjects with acute coronary ischemia were older and had more comorbid conditions (diabetes, hypertension, angina, congestive heart failure) than the men, who were more likely to be smokers or have a prior MI, angioplasty, or CABG surgery. With MI, the initial entry ECG in women compared with men was less likely to have ST elevation (27.2 versus 37.0 percent, $p < 0.001$).

In GUSTO IIb, after cardiac catherization (completed in 53 percent of women and 59 percent of men), women were about twice as likely to demonstrate no vessels with CAD compared with men with unstable angina (30.5 versus 13.9 percent, $p < 0.001$), after MI with ST-segment elevation (10.2 versus 6.8 percent, $p < 0.02$) or

TABLE 87-4 Clinical Presentation of Consecutive Enrollees in GUSTO IIb

	Number of Women (Percentage of Women)	Number of Men (Percentage of Men)
MI with ST elevation	997 (27.2)	3134 (37.0)
MI without ST elevation	974 (26.6)	2544 (30.0)
Unstable angina	1690 (46.2)	2801 (33.0)
TOTAL	3661	8479

SOURCE: Adapted from Hochman JS, Tamis JE, Thompson TD. Sex, clinical presentation, and outcome in patients with acute coronary syndromes. *N Engl J Med* 1999; 341:226–232, with permission.

MI without ST-segment elevation (9.1 versus 4.2 percent, $p < 0.001$). These results are similar to those from the National Registry of Myocardial Infarction–II (MITI-II).[117]

Mortality by gender within 30 days after MI has been further elucidated by the GUSTO IIb and MITI-II reports.[116,117] Overall in GUSTO IIb, within 30 days, mortality for women was higher than for men (6.0 versus 4.0 percent, $p < 0.001$) despite similar reinfarction rates (6.2 percent for women, 5.6 percent for men, $p = 0.19$), with the difference explained by baseline variables such as older age and more comorbid conditions.[116] Among those with unstable angina, women had less mortality and reinfarction within 30 days than did men (odds ratio 0.65, 95 percent CI 0.49 to 0.87, $p = 0.003$). Bleeding complications were more common in women, but data analysis could not assess the role of revascularization procedures.

The interaction of gender and age was considered with data available from the National Registry of Myocardial Infarction–II.[117] Women with MI are often older and have more comorbid conditions than do men. Although overall there was a 14 percent early mortality in women after hospitalization for MI compared with 10 percent in men, when age was further considered, the picture became more complex. Upon analysis of the interaction of gender and age, the 30-day mortality after MI was about twice as great for women age 30 to 50 compared with men of the same age and progressively decreased with increasing age until reaching unity at age 75 (Fig. 87-5).

MI can also present as sudden death or without painful symptoms (silent MI). Sudden death is discussed further on, but a high percentage of first MIs are lethal in women. In the Framingham Heart Study, at 30 years of follow-up, the first presentation of MI resulted in death among 39 percent women and 31 percent of men.[100] Silent MI in the Framingham data was common, representing 25 percent of MI when diagnosed on the basis of new Q waves on screening ECG. Despite obtaining further history, almost half of the subjects had no symptoms. Silent MI is more common in women than in men (35 versus 28 percent).[100] The prognosis of silent MI has not been adequately studied. However, sudden death is one possible sequela.[118,119]

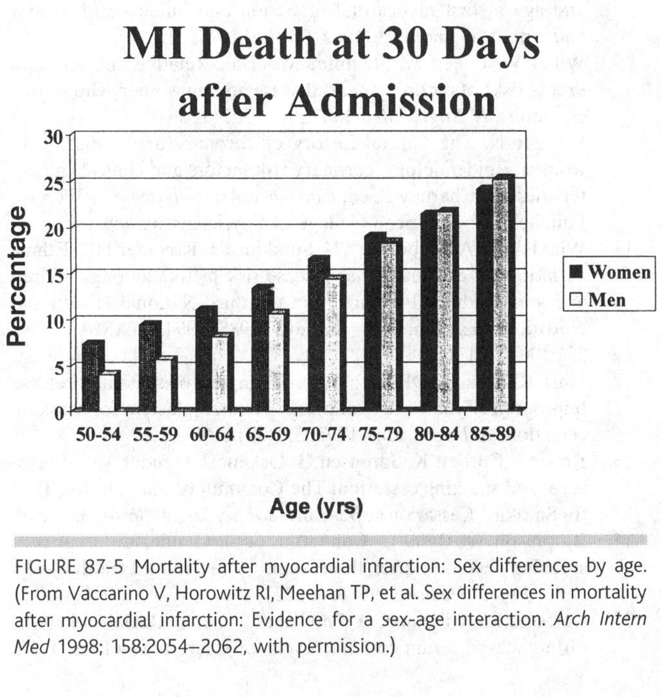

In long-term follow-up after MI, women have more symptoms than men, although long-term mortality is better or similar.[120] Women tend to have more angina and congestive heart failure despite better systolic left ventricular function.[120] Women as well as men most often develop congestive heart failure from ischemic heart disease.[58]

Finally, there has been a substantial lag in translating results of secondary treatment trials for MI into clinical practice. Therapies that are efficacious in women as well as men are often not prescribed—i.e., aspirin and agents to lower cholesterol.[46,104,114,121] Furthermore, treatment goals have often not been met (like achieving an elevated HDL and lower LDL and total cholesterol).[46] Rehabilitation is less often recommended for women, although it is equally effective.[61] To improve the prognosis of women after MI, it is essential to encourage less tobacco exposure (secondary as well as primary exposure) and the use of medications documented to decrease mortality and morbidity (beta blockers, angiotensin-converting enzyme inhibitors, aspirin, etc.) and to address other risk factors.

FIGURE 87-5 Mortality after myocardial infarction: Sex differences by age. (From Vaccarino V, Horowitz RI, Meehan TP, et al. Sex differences in mortality after myocardial infarction: Evidence for a sex-age interaction. *Arch Intern Med* 1998; 158:2054–2062, with permission.)

Interventions for Coronary Artery Disease

Gender differences in the prevalence and complications of angioplasty and CABG surgery are evolving. Both procedures are utilized less in women than in men, and there has been controversy as to whether women are undertreated or men overtreated.[122] Angioplasty initially was associated with a higher complication rate in women. However, with the development of smaller coronary artery catheters, outcomes and complications are similar for women and men.[123]

CABG surgery is more commonly performed in men than women. In the Thoracic Surgeon's National Cardiac Database as in other observational data, about one-quarter of the CABG procedures are completed on women patients.[124] The conduit selected is less often the internal mammary artery in women than in men, although this graft is associated with the best short- and long-term results. Reasons for this might include higher rates of diabetes in women undergoing CABG and the decreased use of internal mammary artery grafting in the setting of osteoporosis.[125] Since women compared to men undergoing CABG tend to be older and have more comorbid conditions, a higher postoperative complication rate, including slower postoperative recovery[126] and higher rates of depression,[127] is not unexpected. Gender differences are less apparent with follow-up after several years.[124]

Sudden Death

In the Framingham study, sudden death was common in both women and men.[100] Within 10 years of an MI, men more often experienced sudden death than did women (12 versus 5 percent).[100] The proportion of sudden death occurring in those without previously documented CAD was greater among women than among men (67 versus 55 percent).[100] Cardiac risk factors for sudden death in one epidemiologic case-controlled study revealed risk factors in white and black women similar to those for MI.[128]

Insights into the pathophysiology of sudden death are revealed in an autopsy study of women's hearts[119] comparing autopsies after sudden death (n = 51) and after trauma (n = 15). Death was witnessed for many of the women with sudden death and significant coronary artery pathology (n = 36, 71 percent). Reported symptoms included chest pain (n = 8), dizziness (n = 3), back pain (n = 2), shortness of breath (n = 1), left shoulder tingling (n = 1), fatigue (n = 1), malaise (n = 1), stomach distention (n = 1), nausea and vomiting (n = 1), and fever and chills (n = 1). Tobacco use was noted in 58 percent of those experiencing sudden death, compared with 50 percent of the controls. Chronic medical problems of the women who experienced sudden death included hypertension (n = 11), history of heart disease (n = 9), and medication for diabetes (n = 5).

On autopsy, healed prior MI was found in 35 percent. Pathologic examination revealed eroded plaque with acute thrombus (n = 18), stable plaque with healed infarct (n = 18), ruptured plaque with acute thrombus (n = 8), and stable plaque without infarction (n = 7). The acute thrombus associated with plaque erosion (often noted in early atherosclerosis) occurred more often in younger women smokers without obesity, high cholesterol, or elevated glycohemoglobin.[119] In comparison, plaque rupture was more often found in older women with elevated cholesterol. Further assessment of women dying with stable plaque without infarction revealed no association with known cardiac risk factors. Although sudden death is rare, tobacco use in young women is an important risk factor. Although only 2 of 51 women had a documented prior MI, on autopsy 35 percent of the sample had evidence of a prior MI. The relationship between sudden death and prior silent MI requires further elucidation.

Arrhythmias

Gender differences in arrhythmia identification, natural history, and management are just beginning to be explored. It is generally known that torsades de pointes occurs more commonly in women.[129,130] Preliminary small studies have considered heart rate variability[131] and QT duration[132] as potential contributors to the development of torsades de pointes. Heart rate variability is different in younger (33 ± 4 years) women and men but similar in more mature (67 ± 3 years) women and men.[131]

Palpitations were reported more commonly by women (17 percent) than men (12 percent) in a Norway population survey.[133] Gender differences were noted among American patients presenting to an emergency department with palpitations.[134] Men were more likely to have irregular beats (57 versus 40 percent) and to have symptoms that lasted more than 5 min (77 versus 61 percent). Although cardiac etiologies for palpitations were most common, psychiatric diagnoses (predominantly panic attacks) were a close second (43 versus 31 percent). After MI, women are more likely to have atrial fibrillation,[116] yet they die less often of arrhythmia than do men.[20] Finally, a German pacemaker registry retrospective review (with 31,913 entries) found that when pacemakers are implanted, women are more likely to receive a single-chamber pacer while men are more likely to receive a dual-chamber pacer.[135]

SUMMATION

Over the past few decades significant differences in individual patient factors that affect diagnosis and management have begun to be futher defined. How differences in sex, race, and SES might affect the care of individual patients is beginning to be explored. With increasing attention to physiologic and social issues, both women and men can receive more appropriate care.

At this juncture it is important to focus on primary and secondary prevention for both women and men, to consider the diagnosis of CAD in women with typical or atypical symptoms, and to manage CAD aggressively in both women and men with an otherwise good prognosis.

References

1. Charney P, ed. *Coronary Artery Disease in Women: Prevention, Diagnosis and Management.* Philadelphia: American College of Physicians; 1999.
2. Legato MJ, Padus E, Slaughter E. Women's perceptions of their general health, with special reference of their risk of coronary artery disease: Results of a national telephone survey. *J Women's Health* 1997; 6(2):189–198.
3. Barrett-Connor E. Sex differences in coronary heart disease: Why are women so superior? The 1995 Ancel Keys Lecture. *Circulation* 1997; 95:252–264.
4. Kreuger DE, Ellenberg SS, Bloom S, et al. Risk factors for fatal heart attack in young women. *Am J Epidemiol* 1981; 113(4):357–370.
5. Collins LJ, Douglas PS. Acute coronary syndromes. In: Charney P, ed. *Coronary Artery Disease in Women.* Philadelphia: American College of Physicians; 1999:403–406.
6. Ockene JK, Bonollo DP, Adams A. Smoking. In: Charney P, ed. *Coronary Artery Disease in Women.* 1999. Philadelphia: American College of Physicians; 1999.
7. He J, Vupputuri S, Allen K, et al. Passive smoking and the risk of coronary heart disease—A meta-analysis of epidemiologic studies. *N Engl J Med* 1999; 340:920–926.
8. Hansen EF, Andersen LT, Von Eyben FE. Cigarette smoking and age at first myocardial infarction and influence of gender and extent of smoking. *Am J Cardiol* 1993; 71:1439.
9. Willet W, Green A, Stampfer M, et al. Relative and absolute excess risks of coronary heart disease among women who smoke cigarettes. *N Engl J Med* 1987; 317:1303–1309.
10. Wenger N. The natural history of coronary artery disease in women: Epidemiology; coronary risk factors and clinical characteristics. In: Charney P, ed, *Coronary Artery Disease in Women.* Philadelphia: American College of Physicians; 1999:8.
11. Winkleby MA, Robinson TN, Sundquist J, Kraemer HC. Ethnic variations in cardiovascular disease risk factors among children and young adults: Findings from the third National Health and Nutrition Examination Survey, 1988–1994. JAMA 1999; 281:1006–1013.
12. Hurt RD, Sachs DP, et al. A comparison of sustained-release bupropion (Zyban and Wellbutrin SR) and placebo for smoking cessation. *N Engl J Med* 1997; 337(17):1195–1202.
13. Royce J, Corbett K, Sorensen G, Ockene J. Gender, social pressure, and smoking cessation: The Community Intervention Trial for Smoking Cessation at Baseline. *Soc Sci Med* 1996; 44: 359–370.
14. Bjoranson W, Rand C, Connett J, et al. Gender differences in smoking cessation after three years in the Lung Health Study. *Am J Public Health* 1995; 85(2):223–230.
15. Carballo RS, Giovino GA, Perchaeck TF, et al. Racial and ethnic differences in serum cotinine levels for cigarette smokers: Third

National Health and Nutrition Examination Survey, 1988–1991. *JAMA* 1998; 280:135–139.

16. Thorndike AN, Rigotti NA, Stafford RS, Singer DE. National patterns in the treatment of smokers by physicians. *JAMA* 1998; 279(8):604–608.
17. Fiore M, Bailey W, Cohen S, et al. *Smoking Cessation: Clinical Practice Guidelines No. 18.* Publication 96-0692. Rockville, MD: USDHHS, PHS, AHCPR; 1996.
18. Sowers JR. Diabetes mellitus and cardiovascular disease in women. *Arch Intern Med* 1998; 158:617–621.
19. Miettinen H, Lehto S, Salomaa V, Mahonen M, et al. Impact of diabetes on mortality after the first myocardial infarction. *Diabetes Care* 1998; 21(1):69–75.
20. Gu K, Cowie CC, Harris MI. Diabetes and decline in heart disease mortality in US adults. *JAMA* 1999; 281:1291–1297.
21. Sullivan M. Criteria for the oral glucose tolerance test in pregnancy. *Diabetes* 1964; 13(13):278–285.
22. Manson JE, Rimm EB, Stampfer MJ, et al. Physical activity and the incidence of non-insulin-dependent diabetes in women. *Lancet* 1991; 338:774–778.
23. Laws A. Diabetes and insulin resistance. In: Charney P, ed. *Coronary Artery Disease in Women*. Philadelphia: American College of Physicians; 1999:70–100.
24. Baldeweg S, Yudkin JS. Implications of the United Kingdom Prospective Diabetes Study. *Primary Care* 1999; 26(4): 809–827.
25. Prospective Diabetes Study Group. United Kingdom Prospective diabetes study 27: Plasma lipids and lipoproteins at diagnosis of NIDDM by age and sex, UK. *Diabetes Care* 1997; 20(11):1683–1687.
26. Pyorala K, Pedersen TR, Kjekshus J, et al. for the Scandinavian Simvastatin Survival Study (4S) Group. Cholesterol lowering with simvastatin improves prognosis of diabetic patients with coronary heart diease: A subgroup analysis of the Scandinavian Simvastatin Survival Study (4S). *Diabetes Care* 1997; 20(4):614–620.
27. Birdall MA, Farquhar CM, White HD. Association between polycystic ovaries and extent of coronary artery disease in women having cardiac catherization. *Ann Intern Med* 1997; 126:32–35.
28. Waterworth DM, Bennett ST, et al. Linkage and association of insulin gene VNTR reglatory polymorphism with polycystic ovarian syndrome. *Lancet* 1997; 349:968–990.
29. Velasquez EM, Mendoza S, Hamer T, et al. Metformin therapy in polycystic ovarian syndrome reduces hyperinsulinemia, insulin resistance, hyperandrogenemia, and systolic blood pressure, while facilitating normal menses and pregnancy. *Metabolism* 1994; 43:647–654.
30. Mayer-Davis EJ, D'Agostino R, Karter AJ, Haffner SM, et al. Intensity and amount of physical activity in relation to insulin sensitivity: The Insulin Resistance Atherosclerosis Study. *JAMA* 1998; 279:669–674.
31. The Women's Caucus, Working Group on Women's Health of the Society of General Internal Medicine. Hypertension in women: What is really known? *Ann Intern Med* 1991; 115:287–293.
32. Sagie A. The natural history of borderline isolated systolic hypertension. *N Engl J Med* 1993; 329:1912–1917.
33. Stamler J, Stamler R, Neaton JD, et al. Blood pressure, systolic and diastolic, and cardiovascular risks: US population data. *Arch Intern Med* 1993; 153:598–615.
34. Gueyffier F, Boutitie F, Boissel Jean-Pierre, et al. Effect of antihypertensive drug treatment on cardiovascular outcomes in women and men: A meta-analysis of individual patient data from randomized, controlled trials. *Am Coll Phys* 1997; 126:761–767.
35. Quan A, Kerlikowske K, Gueyffier F, et al. Efficacy of treating hypertension in women. *J Gen Intern Med* 1999; 14:718–729.
36. SHEP Cooperative Research Group. Prevention of stroke by antihypertensive drug treatment in older persons with isolated systolic hypertension: Final results of the Systolic Hypertension in the Elderly Program (SHEP). *JAMA* 1991; 265(24):3255–3264.
37. Dahlof B, Lindholm LH, Hansson L, et al. Morbidity and mortality in the Swedish Trial in Old Patients with Hypertension (STOP-Hypertension). *Lancet* 1991; 338:1281–1285.
38. Cohen E, Swiderski DM, Wheat ME, Charney P. Hypertension. In: Charney P, ed. *Coronary Artery Disease in Women*. Philadelphia: American College of Physicians; 1999:169.
39. Kannel WB. Blood pressure as a cardiovascular risk factor: Prevention and treatment. *JAMA* 1996; 275:1571–1576.
40. Joint National Committee on Prevention, Detection, Evaluation and Treatment of High Blood Pressure. The Sixth Report of the Joint National Committee on Prevention, Detection, Evaluation and Treatment of High Blood Pressure. *Arch Intern Med* 1997; 157:2413–2446.
41. Jones G, Nguyen T, Sambrook PN, Eismann JA. Thiazide diuretics and fractures: Can meta-analysis help? *J Bone Min Res* 1995; 10:106–111.
42. Peh CA, Horowitz M, Wishart JM, et al. The effect of chorothiazide on bone-related biochemical variables in normal post-menopausal women. *J Am Geriatr Soc* 1995; 41:513–516.
43. Feldkamp M, Jones KL, Ornoy A, et al. Postmarketing surveillance for angiotensin-converting enzyme inhibitor use during the first trimester of pregnancy—United States, Canada and Israel, 1987–1995. *MMWR* 1997; 46:240–242.
44. Os I, Bratland B, Dahlof B, et al. Female sex as an important determinant of lisinopril-induced cough (letter). *Lancet* 1992; 339:372.
45. Walsh ME. Lipids: Natural history and pharmacologic management. In: Charney P, ed. *Coronary Artery Disease in Women.* Philadelphia: American College of Physicians; 1999:101–128.
46. Majumdar SR, Gurwitz JH, Soumerai SB. Undertreatment of hyperlipidemia in the secondary prevention of coronary artery disease. *J Gen Intern Med* 1999; 14:711–717.
47. LaRosa JC, He J, Vupputuri S. Effect of statins on risk of coronary disease: A meta-analysis of randomized controlled trials. *JAMA* 1999; 282:2340–2346.
48. Davidson MH, Testolin LM, Maki KC, et al. A comparison of estrogen replacement, pravastatin, and combined treatment for the management of hypercholesterolemia in postmenopausal women. *Arch Intern Med* 1997; 157:1186–1192.
49. Darling GM, Johns JA, McCloud PI, Davis SR. Estrogen and progestin compared with simvastatin for hypercholesterolemia in postmenopausal women. *N Engl J Med* 1997; 337:595–601.
50. Winkleby M, Kraemer HC, Ahn DK, Varady AN. Ethnic and socioeconomic differences in cardiovascular disease risk factors: Findings for women from the Third National Health and Nutrition Examination Survey, 1988–1994. *JAMA* 1998; 280:356–362.
51. Berenson GS, Charney P, Ramachandaran S, et al. Obesity and other cardiovascular risk factors in young women. In: Charney P, ed. *Coronary Artery Disease in Women: Prevention, Diagnosis and Management.* Philadelphia: American College of Physicians; 1999:188–189.
52. Hennekens CH, Walters EE, Colditz GA, et al. Abdominal adiposity and coronary heart disease in women. *JAMA* 1998; 280 (21):1843–1848.
53. Samaras K, Kelly PJ, Chiano MN, et al. Genetic and environmental influences on total-body and central abdominal fat: The effect of physical activity in female twins. *Ann Intern Med* 1999; 130:873–882.
54. Wilson PWF, Kannel WB, Silbershatz H, D'Agostino RB. Clustering of metabolic factors and coronary heart disease. *Arch Intern Med* 1999; 159:1104–1109.
55. Rexrode KM, Carey VJ, Hennekens CH, Walters EE, et al. Abdominal adiposity and coronary heart disease in women. *JAMA* 1998; 280(21):1843–1848.

56. Andersen RD, Wadden TA, Bartlett SJ, et al. Effects of lifestyle activity vs. structured aerobic exercise in obese women. *JAMA* 1999; 381(4):335–340.
57. Jick H, Vasilakis C, Weinrauch LA, et al. A population-based study of appetite-suppressant drugs and the risk of cardiac-valve regurgitation. *N Engl J Med* 1998; 339(11):719–724.
58. Beniaminovitz A, Mancini D. Congestive heart failure. In: Charney P, ed. *Coronary Artery Disease in Women: Prevention, Diagnosis and Management*. Philadelphia: American College of Physicians; 1999:476–495.
59. Masse LC, Ainsworth BE, Tortolero S, et al. Measuring physical activity in midlife and older and minority women: Issues from an expert panel. *J Women's Health* 1998; 7:57–67.
60. Eaton CB, Reynes J, Assaf AR, et al. Predicting physical activity change in men and women in two New England communities. *Am J Prev Med* 1993; 9:209–219.
61. Fair JM, Berra K, King AC. Excercise as primary and secondary prevention in Charney P, ed. *Coronary Artery Disease in Women: Prevention, Diagnosis and Management*. Philadelphia: American College of Physicians; 1999:209–235.
62. Thomas RJ, Houston Miller N, Lamendola C, et al. National survey on gender differences in cardiac rehabilitation programs. *J Cardiopulm Rehabil* 1996; 16:402–412.
63. Oliver MF, Boyd GS. Effect of bilateral ovariectomy on coronary artery disease and serum lipid levels. *Lancet* 1959; 2:690.
64. Hu FB, Grodstein F, Hennekens CH, et al. Age at natural menopause and risk of cardiovascular disease. *Arch Intern Med* 1999; 159:1061–1066.
65. Blumenthal RS, Bush TL. Hormone replacement therapy and the prevention of coronary artery disease. In: Charney P, ed. *Coronary Artery Disease in Women: Prevention, Diagnosis and Management*. Philadelphia: American College of Physicians; 1999:264–288.
66. Hulley S, Grady D, Bush T, et al. Randomized trial of estrogen plus progestin for secondary prevention of coronary heart disease in postmenopausal women. *JAMA* 1998; 280(7):605–613.
67. Collaborative Group on Hormonal Factors in Breast Cancer. Breast cancer and hormone replacement therapy: Collaborative re-analysis of data from 51 epidemiological studies of 52,705 women with breast cancer and 108,411 women without breast cancer. *Lancet* 1997; 350:1047–1059.
68. Keating NL, Cleary PD, Rossi AS, et al. Use of hormonal replacement therapy by postmenopausal women in the United States. *Ann Intern Med* 1999; 130:545–553.
69. Jacobs SC, Stone PH. Psychosocial isses. In: Charney P, ed. *Coronary Artery Disease in Women*. Philadelphia: American College of Physicians; 1999:496–534.
70. Case RB, Moss AJ, Case N, et al. Living alone after myocardial infarction: Impact on prognosis. *JAMA* 1992; 267(4):515–519.
71. Smith GD, Hart C, Blane D, et al. Lifetime socioeconomic position and mortality: Prospective observational study. *BMJ* 1997; 314:547–552.
72. Williams RB, Barefoot JC, Califf RM, et al. Prognostic importance of social and economic resources among medically treated patients with angiographically documented coronary artery disease. *JAMA* 1992; 267:520–524.
73. Wilkinson RG. *Socioeconomic determinants of health*—Health inequalities: relative or absolute material standards? *BMJ* 1997; 314:591–595.
74. Morrison C, Woodward M, Leslie W, Turnstall-Pedoe H. Effect of socioeconomic group on incidence of, management of, and survival after myocardial infarction and coronary death: Analysis of community coronary event register. *BMJ* 1997; 314:541–546.
75. Bosma H, Marmot MG, Hemingway H, et al. Low job control and risk of coronary heart disease in Whitehall II (prospective cohort) study. *BMJ* 1997; 314:558–565.
76. Marmot MG, Bosma H, Hemingway H, et al. Contribution of job control and other risk factors to social variations in coronary heart disease incidence. *Lancet* 1997; 350:235–239.
77. Jacobs SC, Stone PH. Psychosocial issues. In: Charney P, ed. *Coronary Artery Disease in Women*. Philadelphia: American College of Physicians; 1999:508.
78. Pratt LA, Ford DE, Crum RM, et al. Depression, psychotropic medication, and risk of myocardial infarction: Prospective data from the Baltimore ECA follow-up. *Circulation* 1996; 94:3123–3129.
79. Frasure-Smith N, Lesperance F. Depression following myocardial infarction: Impact on 6-month survival. *JAMA* 1993; 270:1819–1825.
80. Creed F. The importance of depression following myocardial infarction. *Heart* 1999; 82:406–408.
81. Carney RM, Freedland KE, Smith L, et al. Relation of depression and mortality after myocardial infarction in women (letter). *Circulation* 1991; 84(4):1876–1877.
82. Toiler GO, Stone PH, Muller JE, et al. Effects of gender and race on prognosis after myocardial infarction: Adverse prognosis for women, particularly black women. *J Am Coll Cardiol* 1987; 9:473–482.
83. Escobedo LG, Giles WH, Anda RF. Socioeconomic status, race, and death from coronary heart disease. *Am J Prev Med* 1997; 13:123–130.
84. Charney P. Future directions. In: Charney P, ed. *Coronary Artery Disease in Women: Prevention, Diagnosis and Management*. Philadelphia: American College of Physicians; 1999:575–593.
85. Fang J, Madhavan S, Alderman MH. The association between birthplace and mortality from cardiovascular causes among black and white residents of New York City. *N Engl J Med* 1996; 335(21):1545–1551.
86. Shaukat N, Lear J, Lowy A, et al. First myocardial infarction in patients of Indian subcontinent and European origin: Comparison of risk factors, management, and long term outcome. *BMJ* 1997; 314:639–642.
87. Vitelli LL, Crow RS, Shahar E, et al. Electrocardiographic findings in a healthy biracial population. *Am J Cardiol* 1998; 81:453–459.
88. Perez-Stable EJ, Herrera B, Jacob P, Benowitz NL. Nicotene metabolism and intake in black and white smokers. *JAMA* 1998; 280:152–156.
89. Birdwell BG, Herbers JE, Kroenke K. Evaluating chest pain: The patient's presentation style alters the physician's diagnostic approach. *Arch Intern Med* 1993; 153:1991–1995.
90. Schulman KA, Berlin JA, Harless W, et al. The effect of race and sex on physician's recommendations for cardiac catherization. *N Engl J Med* 1999; 340:618–626.
91. Douglas PS, Ginsburg GS. The evaluation of chest pain in women. *N Engl J Med* 1996; 334:1311–1315.
92. Shaw LJ, Peterson ED, Johnson LL. Noninvasive testing techniques for diagnosis and prognosis. In: Charney P, ed. *Coronary Artery Disease in Women*. Philadelphia: American College of Physicians; 1999: 327–350.
93. Kwok Y, Kim C, Grady D, et al. Meta-analysis of excercise testing to detect coronary artery disease in women. *Am J Cardiol* 1999; 83:660–663.
94. Shaw LJ, Peterson ED, Johnson LL. Noninvasive testing techniques for diagnosis and prognosis. In: Charney P, ed. *Coronary Artery Disease in Women*. Philadelphia: American College of Physicians; 1999:327–350.
95. Okin PM, Kligfield P. Gender-specific criteria and performance of the exercise electrocardiogram. *Circulation* 1995; 92(5):1209–1216.
96. Shaw LJ, Peterson ED, Johnson LL. Noninvasive testing techniques for diagnosis and prognosis. In: Charney P, ed. *Coronary Artery Disease in Women*. Philadelphia: American College of Physicians; 1999:341–345.

97. Marwick TH, Miller DD. Influence of gender on the referral of patients to and from coronary angiography. In: Charney P, ed. *Coronary Artery Disease in Women*. Philadelphia: American College of Physicians; 1999:354–356.
98. Weiner DA, Ryan TJ, McCabe CH, et al. Exercise stress testing: Correlations among history of angina, ST segment response and prevalence of coronary artery disease in the Coronary Artery Surgery Study (CASS). *N Engl J Med* 1979; 301:230–235.
99. Lerner DS, Kannel W. Patterns of heart disease morbidity and mortality in the sexes: A 26-year follow-up of the Framingham population. *Am Heart J* 1986; 111:383–390.
100. Kannel WB, Abbott RD. Incidence and prognosis of myocardial infarction in women: The Framingham study. In: Eaker ED, Packard B, Wenger NK, et al., eds. *Coronary Heart Disease in Women: Proceedings of an NIH Workshop*. New York: Haymark Doyma; 1987:208–214.
101. Mosca L, Grundy SM, Judelson D, et al. Guide to preventive cardiology for women. *Circulation* 1999; 99:2480–2484.
102. Turnstall-Pedoe H, Woodward M, Tavendale R, et al. Comparison of the prediction by 27 different factors of coronary heart disease and death in men and women of the Scottish heart health study: A cohort study. *BMJ* 1997; 315:722–729.
103. Lowe LP, Greenland P, Ruth RJ, et al. Impact of major cardiovascular disease risk factors, particularly in combination, on 22-year mortality in women and men. *Arch Intern Med* 1988; 158:2007–2014.
104. Goldberg RJ, Larson M, Levy D. Factors associated with survival to 75 years of age in middle-aged men and women. *Arch Intern Med* 1996; 156:505–509.
105. Daviglus ML, Kiang L, Greenland P, et al. Benefit of a favorable cardiovascular risk-factor profile in middle age with respect to medicare costs. *N Engl J Med* 1998; 339:1122–1129.
106. Hubert HB, Eaker ED, Garrison R, Castelli WP. Life-style correlates of risk factor change in young adults: An eight-year study of coronary heart disease risk factors in the Framingham offspring. *Am J Epdemiol* 1987; 125(5):812–831.
107. Stamler J, Stamler R, Neaton JD, et al. Low risk-factor profile and long-term cardiovascular and noncardiovascular mortality and life expectancy: Findings for 5 large cohorts of young adults and middle-aged men and women. *JAMA* 1999; 282:2012–2018.
108. Grover SA, Paquet S, Levinton C, et al. Estimating the benefits of modifying risk factors of cardiovascular disease: A comparison of primary and secondary prevention. *Arch Intern Med* 1998; 158:655–662.
109. Perlman JA, Wolf PH, Ray R, Lieberknecht G. Cardiovascular risk factors, premature heart disease, and all-cause mortality in a cohort of Northern California women. *Am J Obstet Gynecol* 1988; 158:1568–1574.
110. Newnham HH, Silberberg J. Women's hearts are hard to break. *Lancet* 1997; 349:sl3–sl16.
111. Pepine CJ, Abrams J, Marks RG, et al. Characteristics of a contemporary population with angina pectoris: TIDES investigators. *Am J Cardiol* 1994; 74:226–231.
112. Del Valle N, Frishman WH, Charney P. Angina pectoris. In: Charney P, ed. *Coronary Artery Disease in Women*. Philadelphia: American College of Physicians; 1999:373–400.
113. Mohri M, Koyanagi M, Egashira K, et al. Angina pectoris caused by coronary microvascular spasm. *Lancet* 1998; 351:1165–1169.
114. Chandra NC, Ziegelstein RC, Rogers WJ, et al. Observations of the treatment of women in the United States with myocardial infarction: A report from the National Registry of Myocardial Infarction–I. *Arch Intern Med* 1998; 158:981–988.
115. Marrugat JM, Sala J, Masia R, et al. Mortality differences between men and women following first myocardial infarction. *JAMA* 1998; 280:1405–1409.
116. Hochman JS, Tamis J, Thompson TD, et al. Sex, clinical presentation, and outcome in patients with acute coronary syndromes. *N Engl J Med* 1999; 341:226–232.
117. Vaccarino V, Parsons L, Every NR, et al. Sex-based differences in early mortality after myocardial infarction. *N Engl J Med* 1999; 341:217–225.
118. Burke AP, Farb A, Malcolm GT, et al. Effect of risk factors on the mechanism of acute thrombosis and sudden death in women. *Circulation* 1998; 97:2110–2116.
119. Oparil S. Pathophysiology of sudden coronary death in women: Implications for prevention. *Circulation* 1998: 97:2103–2104.
120. Collins LJ, Douglas PS. Acute coronary syndromes. In: Charney P, ed. *Coronary Artery Disease in Women*. Philadelphia: American College of Physicians; 1999:407–413.
121. Collins LJ, Douglas PS. Acute coronary syndromes. In: Charney P, ed. *Coronary Artery Disease in Women*. Philadelphia: American College of Physicians; 1999:420–422.
122. Bickell NA, Pieper KS, Lee KL, et al. Referral patterns for coronary artery disease treatment: Gender bias or good clinical judgement. *Ann Intern Med* 1992; 116:791–797.
123. Ommen SR, Holmes DR Jr, Bell MR. Percutaneous transluminal coronary angioplasty. In: Charney P, ed. *Coronary Artery Disease in Women*. Philadelphia: American College of Physicians; 1999:463–475.
124. Hartz RS, Charney P. Coronary artery bypass grafting: Is it worth the risk? In: Charney P, ed. *Coronary Artery Disease in Women*. Philadelphia: American College of Physicians; 1999:438–462.
125. Mickleborough L, Takagi Y, Murayama H, et al. Is sex a factor in determining operative risk for aortocoronary bypass? *Circulation* 1995; 90(suppl II):80–84.
126. Moore S. A comparison of women's and men's symptoms during home recovery after coronary artery bypass surgery. *Heart Lung* 1995; 24:495–501.
127. Ai AL, Peterson C, Dunkle RE, et al. How gender affects psychological adjustment one year after coronary artery bypass surgery. *Womens Health* 1997; 26:45–65.
128. Krueger DE, Ellenberg SS, Bloom S, et al. Risk factors for fatal heart attack in young women. *Am J Epidemiol* 1981; 113(4): 357–370.
129. Makkar RR, Fromm BS, Steinman RT, et al. Female gender as a risk factor for torsades de pointes associated with cardiovascular drugs. *JAMA* 1993; 270:2590–2597.
130. Drici D, Knollmann BC, Wang W-X, Woosley RL. Cardiac actions of erythromycin: Influence of female sex. *JAMA* 1998; 280:1774–1776.
131. Stein PK, Kleiger RE, Rottman JN. Differing effects of age on heart rate variability in men and women. *Am J Cardiol* 1997; 80:302–305.
132. Burke JH, Ehlert FA, Kruse JT, et al. Gender-specific differences in the QT interval and the effect of autonomic tone and menstrual cycle in healthy adults. *Am J Cardiol* 1997; 79:178–181.
133. Lochen ML, Snaprud T, Zhang W, Rasmussen K. Arrhythmias in subjects with and without a history of palpitations: The Tromso study. *Eur Heart J* 1994; 15:345–349.
134. Weber BE, Kapoor WN. Evaluation and outcomes of patients with palpitations. *Am J Med* 1996; 100(2):138–148.
135. Schuppel R, Buchele G, Batz L, Koenig W. Sex differences in selection of pacemakers: Retrospective observation study. *BMJ* 1988; 316:492–495.

PART FIFTEEN

DISEASES OF THE GREAT VESSELS AND PERIPHERAL VESSELS

C H A P T E R 88

DIAGNOSIS AND TREATMENT OF DISEASES OF THE AORTA

Joseph Lindsay, Jr.

Structurally a simple conduit, the aorta can manifest disease in only a limited number of ways. When weakened by disease, its wall may dilate, producing an aneurysm, or it may split in its long axis, producing dissection. In either case, fatal rupture may result. Moreover, like all pipes, it may become obstructed. More often than narrowing of the main trunk, however, obstruction at the origin of a main branch is encountered. In contrast to these relatively few clinical manifestations, an array of disease processes can involve the aorta. Not surprisingly, there is considerable overlap in the clinical presentation of these disorders.

This chapter will first discuss the various diseases that involve the aorta together with their pathogenetic mechanisms, characteristic pathologic features, and typical clinical findings. A description of the common clinical manifestations of aortic disease for which there may be several etiologies or for which the etiology is unknown will follow.

ETIOLOGIC AND PATHOGENETIC CONSIDERATIONS IN AORTIC DISEASE

Medial Changes of Aging

Circumferential plates or lamellae of elastin fibers constitute the most conspicuous feature of the aortic media when it is examined histologically. Dispersed between the circular elastic fibers are longitudinally oriented smooth muscle cells, collagen fibers, microfibrils, and ground substance.[1]

Clinicians have long recognized dilatation and elongation of the aorta in the elderly. Characteristic alterations in the structure of the aortic wall accompany these changes. Schlatmann and Becker[2] identified these as fragmentation of elastic fibers and loss of smooth muscle cell nuclei, so-called medionecrosis. Moreover, collagenous tissue and basophilic ground substance deposits are a feature of the aging aorta.[3]

Aortic Atherosclerosis

PATHOLOGIC ANATOMY

By middle life, aortic atherosclerosis is nearly universal in the Western world. Its severity varies from individual to individual. Diabetes, hypercholesterolemia, smoking, and hypertension are among the factors promoting it. The pathology of atherosclerosis is discussed in Chap. 35.

Advanced atherosclerotic changes display a characteristic distribution, and involvement is most severe below the renal arteries in the abdominal aorta, is common but less severe in the descending thoracic segment, and is least severe in the ascending segment.[4] With diabetes mellitus, however, disease is frequently severe throughout. Individuals with familial hypercholesterolemia are a second exception to the rule that the ascending aorta is spared.[5] Also, the aortic root and aortic valve may be severely involved in familial cholesterolemia. Both supravalvular and valvular aortic stenosis may develop.[6] Finally, syphilitic ascending aortitis promotes severe atherosclerosis.

CLINICAL MANIFESTATIONS

Aortic atherosclerosis is manifest as aneurysm, obstruction of the infrarenal aorta, embolization from atheromatous plaques to distal arterial beds, and medial dissection initiated by penetration of a plaque into the media.

Aneurysm Aneurysm of the abdominal aorta has long been presumed to result from penetration into and weakening of the media by atherosclerosis. Thus abdominal aortic aneurysms characteristically appear in individuals with the most severe aortic atherosclerosis in nonaneurysmal segments.[7]

Recent recognition of familial clustering of patients with abdominal aortic aneurysm,[8] the identification of genetic defects in collagen in a family with multiple aneurysms,[9] and the detection of abnormal collagenase and elastase in tissue from aortic aneurysms resected at operation have led some to the assumption that atherosclerosis is invariably the underlying pathophysiologic mechanism. These findings suggest that atherosclerosis represents a secondary response to dilatation of the aorta resulting from medial weakness.[10] This debate will be discussed in greater detail below. Aneurysm of the descending thoracic aorta also traditionally has been attributed to atherosclerosis, since such lesions are commonly accompanied by an infrarenal aneurysm.

Obstruction of the Terminal Aorta. Obstruction of the main aortic channel most often develops in the infrarenal aorta and may extend into the proximal iliac arteries. Obstruction of branch arteries is more common than aortic obstruction.

Atheroembolism The luminal surface of a severely diseased aortic segment is often rough and covered with thrombus. Embolization of plaque material and thrombus from these surfaces now appears to be far more common than was once appreciated.[11–14] Emboli to the brain, the lower extremities, and the coronary, renal, or visceral circulations have been reported.

Transesophageal echocardiography now provides rather startling views of pedunculated thrombus or other atherosclerotic material waving in the aortic blood flow[12] (Fig. 88-1). Aortas with ulcerated plaques, pedunculated or mobile thrombi, or spontaneous echo contrast are more apt to embolize than are those with flat, layered atherosclerosis.[13] Anticoagulant therapy may be protective against future events.[14]

A variation on the theme, the clinical syndrome labeled *cholesterol embolization,* with small atherosclerotic particles obstructing small arteries, is a rare complication of severe aortic atherosclerosis. Clinical signs include mottled skin and "purple toes" in the lower extremities together with renal insufficiency and visceral ischemia in more severe cases.[15] This rarely recognized condition may be spontaneous but is more commonly encountered as a complication of intraaortic catheter manipulation. Because eosinophilia is frequent in the initial phases of this event, an immune reaction to the free particles has been suggested.

Penetrating Atherosclerotic Ulcers Atherosclerotic plaque penetration into the media predisposes to formation of an intramural hematoma.[16] Extension circumferentially and in the long axis of the media may produce a limited medial dissection (Fig. 88-2). Radial extension results in pseudoaneurysm or rupture. Penetrating ulcers are most commonly recognized in the descending thoracic aorta.

The clinical picture resembles that of aortic dissection or of expansion/rupture of a preexisting aneurysm. Sudden onset of severe back pain in a hypertensive patient or one known to have atherosclerosis is typical. Many are identified in the course of imaging for suspected aortic dissection. Since they are more limited in axial length than typical dissection, and since they are located in the descending thoracic aorta, aortic regurgitation and altered pulses are not characteristic features. Surgical treatment is often indicated, although some patients survive without operation.[16]

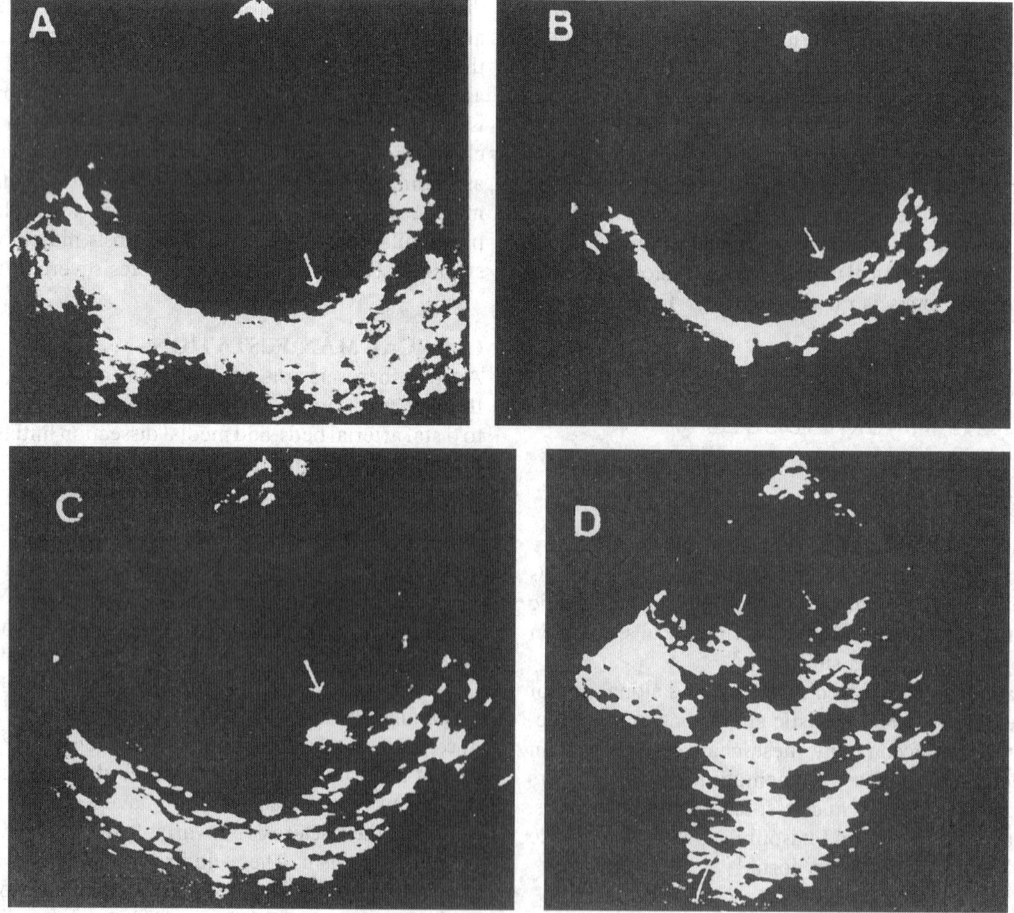

FIGURE 88-1 Panels from transesophageal echocardiographic examinations of the descending thoracic aorta in four patients. Varying degrees of atherosclerotic plaquing are illustrated. A minimal degree is shown in *A* (*upper left*) and a more severe but still moderate degree in *B* (*upper right*). *C* and *D* demonstrate protruding plaques, the configuration with the most serious threat of embolization. (From Lindsay J Jr et al. Diseases of the aorta. In: Schlant RC, Alexander AW, Lipton MJ, eds. *Diagnostic Atlas of the Heart*. New York: McGraw-Hill, 1996:319. Reproduced with permission from the publisher and authors.)

Abnormalities of the Aortic Media

The occurrence of aneurysm and medial dissection reflects a defective aortic media. Although often a component of an acquired process such as atherosclerosis or panaortitis, medial weakness may be genetically determined. Such is the case in aortic disease in a variety of congenital syndromes (e.g., bicuspid aortic valve, coarctation of the aorta) and in heritable disorders of connective tissue (e.g., Marfan's syndrome, polycystic kidney disease, Turner's syndrome, and Ehlers-Danlos syndrome).[17]

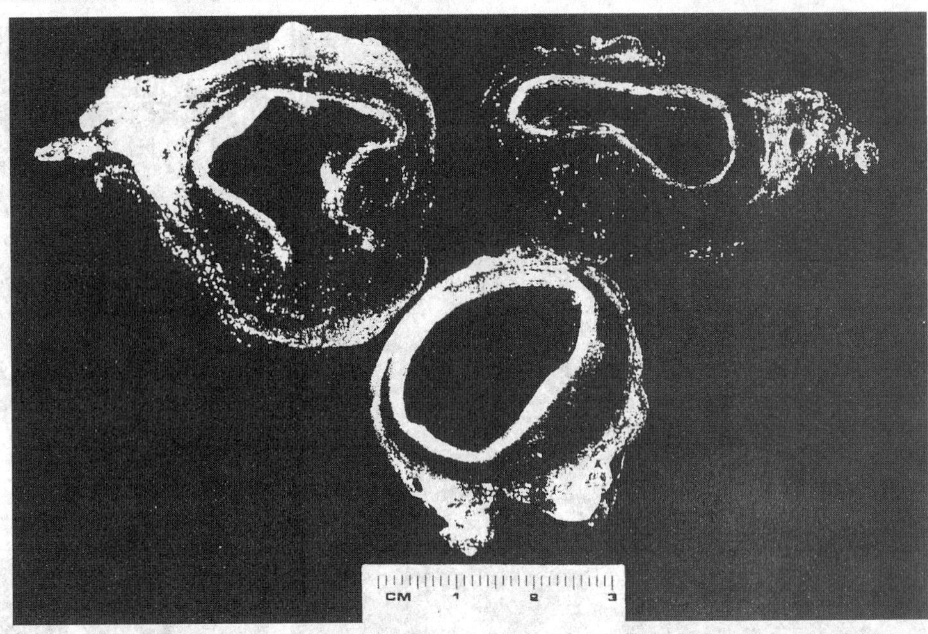

FIGURE 88-2 A necropsy specimen from an elderly woman who died suddenly after having severe back pain suspicious of aortic dissection. It demonstrates a penetrating atherosclerotic plaque (*upper left*) providing communication from the aortic lumen to an adjacent medial hematoma (*bottom*). An aortogram had been negative for dissection, but transesophageal echocardiography revealed the medial hematoma. (From Lindsay J Jr et al. Diseases of the aorta. In: Schlant RC, Alexander AW, Lipton MJ, eds. *Diagnostic Atlas of the Heart*. New York: McGraw-Hill, 1996:321. Reproduced with permission from the publisher and authors.)

CYSTIC MEDIAL DEGENERATION

Microscopic changes in the aortic media, termed *cystic medial necrosis* by Erdheim, were long thought to be diagnostic of medial degeneration. They were identified in Marfan's syndrome, in other instances of aortic aneurysm or dissection,[18,19] and in a variety of familial or congenital syndromes.[17] The features include fragmentation of elastic fibers, disappearance of the nuclei of smooth muscle cells, increase in collagenous fibers, and most characteristically, replacement of the degenerated tissue with interstitial collections ("cysts") of basophilic-staining ground substance.

The fundamental nature of this lesion has been questioned. Hirst and Gore[20] pointed out that the lesion was neither cystic nor necrotic. Recent detailed histologic studies of the media in aortic dissection have failed to demonstrate a close association with this marker of medial degeneration.[21] Schlatmann and Becker[2,19] suggest that qualitatively similar lesions are common with aging, albeit more common and more severe in patients with Marfan's syndrome, with dilatation of the aorta from any cause, or with aortic dissection. They proposed that the observed changes reflect hemodynamic stress. It is noteworthy that the presence of this lesion has been reported in aortas with coarctation of the aorta.[22] Thus, although clearly defective in many cases of aortic aneurysm or dissection, the aortic media often reveals no specific histologic lesion, and the focus now is on subcellular and molecular abnormalities.[17,23] A defect in a microfibrillar constituent of the matrix protein, fibrillin, has been identified in the Marfan's syndrome, and the responsible gene has been identified.[24]

CLINICAL MANIFESTATIONS

Marfan's Syndrome A characteristic aneurysm of the proximal aorta is the cardiovascular hallmark of Marfan's syndrome.[17,18] Aneurysmal dilatation of the ascending aorta extends proximally into the aortic sinuses and ends distally just short of the innominate artery. The result is a "Florence flask" or "onion bulb" deformity. The descriptive term *anuloaortic ectasia* has been applied.[18] Rupture of such aneurysms or the hemodynamic effects of aortic regurgitation, from aortic root dilatation, are responsible for most of the premature deaths from this disorder. Localized or extensive medial dissection is another calamitous complication.

In the most complete presentation of Marfan's syndrome, skeletal, ocular, and cardiovascular anomalies are present, and a family history of similar abnormalities exists[17,18] (see Chaps. 10 and 76). Long extremities, particularly long, thin, hands and feet (arachnodactyly), and sparse muscle mass are typical. Subluxed or frankly dislocated lenses attributable to lax supporting ligaments are characteristic. In addition, myxomatous transformation of the aortic and mitral valves may produce valvular incompetence. Exceptionally, medial degeneration severe enough to result in aneurysm, rupture, or dissection is found in the main pulmonary arteries or in the aorta distal to the ascending segment.

Medial Degeneration Associated with Congenital Aortic or Aortic Valvular Deformity Ascending aortic aneurysm, often in the form of anuloaortic ectasia, and aortic dissection are reported frequently in patients with congenitally deformed aortic valves. The risk of aortic dissection has been estimated to be increased ninefold in subjects with bicuspid or unicuspid valves.[25] There is echocardiographic evidence for increased prevalence of dilatation of the aortic root and ascending aorta in subjects with a biscupid aortic valve[26] (Fig. 88-3). Patients with coarctation are at risk for aortic aneurysm, dissection, and rupture.[17] The strong association of bicuspid aortic valve with

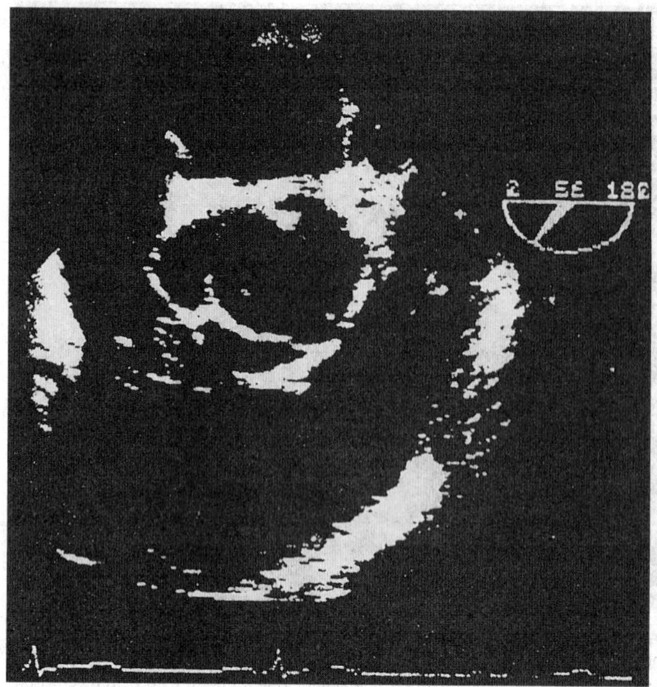

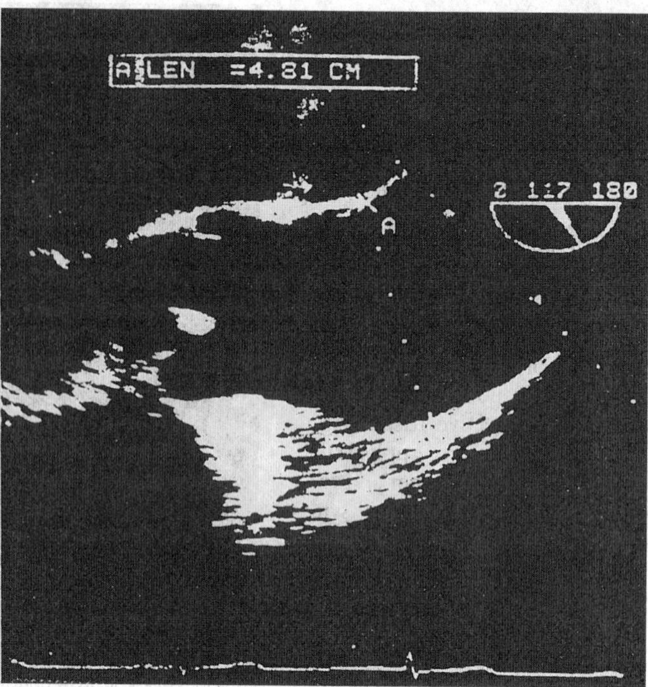

FIGURE 88-3 Transesophageal echocardiographic examination from a patient with bicuspid aortic valve (*left panel*) demonstrating the commonly associated dilatation of the aortic root. (From Lindsay J Jr. Diseases of the aortic root. *Heart Dis Stroke* 1994; 3:377. Reproduced with permission from the publisher and author.)

coarctation, together with clinical observations, is a foundation for the hypothesis that there may be a specific, perhaps genetic medial defect in this spectrum of disease.[27] The fact that Turner's syndrome, with which bicuspid aortic valve, coarctation of the aorta, and aortic dissection are strongly associated bolsters this possibility.[28]

Medial Degeneration in Heritable Disorders of Connective Tissue Reports linking polycystic kidney disease,[29,30] Ehlers-Danlos syndrome,[31] and osteogenesis imperfecta[32] with aortic aneurysm and dissection further support the idea that medial degeneration may have a genetic basis.

Isolated Anuloaortic Ectasia While dilatation of the aortic root and ascending aorta occurs in association with a variety of heritable disorders, it is far more often encountered in individuals with no other manifest disease.[18,33] Isolated anuloaortic ectasia is the most frequent cause of aortic regurgitation requiring valve replacement[34] and is responsible for significant numbers of fatal ruptures or dissections. The finding of fibrillin gene mutations in three patients with anuloaortic ectasia without complete Marfan phenotype suggests that genetic defects of the media may underlie many of these cases.[35]

Infectious Aortitis

A variety of bacterial, mycobacterial, and fungal organisms may infect the walls of the aorta. Microorganisms may gain a foothold through several mechanisms: (1) seeding of the vasa vasorum during hematogenous spread, (2) direct invasion of the wall from the aortic lumen (usually in previously diseased segments or at prosthetic grafts), (3) septic emboli (usually from infective endocarditis) that lodge at a branch point, (4) spread of infection from contiguous structures (e.g., infected cardiac valves or tuberculous periaortic nodes), and (5) traumatic aortic injury with subsequent infection.[36]

SYPHILITIC AORTITIS

Epidemiology Alone among the infectious aortic diseases, treponemal infection produces a chronic aortitis. Clinically evident involvement of the cardiovascular system occurs in about 10 percent of patients with untreated tertiary syphilis of long duration and is the primary cause of death in about the same percentage.[37] Autopsy evidence of the process is more frequent. About half of patients with untreated syphilis for more than 10 years have autopsy evidence of cardiovascular involvement.[37]

Pathology During the spirochetemic phase of primary syphilis, *Treponema pallidum* organisms lodge in the adventitia of the vasa vasorum and initiate an inflammatory response, characteristically a perivascular lymphocytic and plasma cell infiltrate. Later, an obliterative endarteritis develops, resulting in patchy medial necrosis and elastic fiber fragmentation and leading to weakening of the aortic wall and predisposition to aneurysm formation. The intima of the aorta has a characteristic wrinkled appearance, with atherosclerotic plaques frequently superimposed, obscuring the wrinkling and giving the so-called tree bark appearance. Because the infection is seeded through the vasa vasorum, the process is most severe in the ascending aorta and the arch, where vasa density is highest.

Clinical Manifestations *Syphilitic aortitis may present in four ways:*[37] *asymptomatic aortitis, aortic regurgitation, coronary ostial stenosis, and aortic aneurysm.* Asymptomatic aortitis may be unrecognized until necropsy but sometimes can be identified from chest x-ray by linear calcium deposits in the ascending aorta. Aortic regurgitation, present in about 20 to 30 percent of patients with syphilitic aortitis,[37] results primarily from dilatation of the aortic root. Coronary arterial ostial stenosis occurs in 25 to 30 percent of syphilitic aortitis patients, and as many as 85 percent have associated aortic regurgitation.[37] Interestingly, while angina is common in patients with syphilitic ostial stenosis, myocardial infarction is rare.

Aneurysm, the least common manifestation of syphilitic aortitis, is present in 5 to 10 percent of affected patients.[37] About 75 percent are saccular and 25 percent are fusiform. Half are located in the ascending aorta, 30 to 40 percent in the transverse arch, 10 to 15 percent in the proximal descending thoracic aorta, and fewer than 5 percent in the abdominal aorta. Rarely, syphilis causes aneurysm of a sinus of Valsalva. When not treated surgically, syphilitic aortic aneurysms are associated with a 2-year mortality of 80 percent.[37] Thus operation is warranted in patients with large syphilitic aortic aneurysms.

Although antibiotics are indicated for all patients with cardiovascular syphilis, it is unclear if treatment slows progression of syphilitic aortic disease.

Diagnosis The diagnosis of cardiovascular syphilis may be difficult, especially in patients over age 50, when many of the effects of syphilis are mimicked by hypertensive and atherosclerotic disease. Serology can be helpful. Between 40 and 95 percent of patients with cardiovascular syphilis have an elevated venereal disease research laboratory (VDRL) titer, and nearly all have a positive fluorescent treponemal antibody absorption (FTA-ABS) test.[37] Rare, untreated patients have no serologic evidence of the disease. *Thus cardiovascular syphilis must be considered in patients with aortic regurgitation and dilatation of the aortic root, aneurysms of the thoracic aorta, and ostial coronary arterial narrowing (especially when accompanied by aortic regurgitation).* Fortunately, the frequency of cardiovascular syphilis has fallen dramatically over recent decades due to early identification and treatment of the disease.

BACTERIAL AORTITIS COMPLICATING BLOOD-BORNE INFECTIONS

Bacterial aortitis most often presents as an infection of a preexisting aneurysm. Less frequently, the infection may be responsible for initiating an aneurysm or a false aneurysm.

Salmonella species and *Staphylococcus aureus* are the most frequent of a wide spectrum of invading organisms.[38,39] Infections of prosthetic graft material result from agents similar to those causing infective endocarditis (see Chap. 73).

Salmonella organisms have a strong proclivity for invading vascular endothelium. Cohen et al.[40] found a 25 percent prevalence of endothelial infection (arteritis or endocarditis) in patients over age 50 with nontyphoidal *Salmonella* bacteremia. Endothelial invasion was uncommon in patients under age 50 probably because of a lower prevalence of atherosclerosis to serve as a nidus. Thus antibiotic treatment has been recommended for acute *Salmonella* gastroenteritis in patients over age 50.[40]

Clinical Manifestations and Diagnosis Diagnosis of infectious aortitis or aneurysm can be elusive and relies heavily on clinical suspicion prompting further evaluation.[41,42] Symptoms are nonspecific. In abdominal aortic infections, abdominal, back, or flank pain is prominent, whereas chest or shoulder pain is more characteristic of thoracic aortic infections.[43] Physical findings include fever in nearly all patients[44] and a pulsatile abdominal mass in nearly half. Leukocytosis is very common,[44] as are positive blood cultures. In patients with *Salmonella* aortic infection, 83 percent had positive blood cultures and 74 percent had positive stool cultures, even though only a third had gastroenteritis.[43]

There are no specific diagnostic studies for aortic infection. Abdominal ultrasound and computed tomography (CT) are useful to identify an aneurysm and occasionally to show periaortic inflammation or mass. Noncalcified aneurysms and aneurysms with smooth walls seen on aortography or CT scanning are characteristic of an infectious process.[36] Often the diagnosis requires surgery and even at operation may be questionable.

Thus the diagnosis of aortic infection is made most often on the basis of a compatible clinical picture and supporting, if not conclusive, diagnostic tests. Unexplained fever, leukocytosis, and bacteremia (especially Salmonella species) in a patient with a high likelihood of having atherosclerosis should prompt a thorough search for evidence of aortic infection and may be sufficient reason for operative exploration.

Treatment *Infections of the aorta almost always lead to fatal aortic rupture unless treated surgically.* Antibiotics alone are not sufficient. The specific surgical approach is dictated primarily by the extent of involvement of periaortic tissue. If the aortic bed is relatively clean, excision and simple interposition grafting is acceptable. If periaortic infection is widespread, then extraanatomic grafting (e.g., axillobifemoral, thoracic aortobifemoral) is necessary.[41] Some have recommended that essentially all patients with aortic infection be treated, at least initially, with extraanatomic grafting.[36]

INFECTIOUS AORTITIS RESULTING FROM CONTIGUOUS SPREAD

Tuberculous aortitis most often results from spread from infected periaortic nodes. False aneurysm, perforation, or aortoenteric fistula[45,46] may result.

An infection of the aortic valve may invade the valve ring and adjacent structures, producing a perivalvular abscess (sometimes called a *valve ring abscess*). This complication of aortic valvular endocarditis is frequent, especially when infecting organisms are virulent or when patients with prosthetic valves are affected.[47,48] Perivalvular abscesses may compress adjacent structures or rupture into the pericardial space. If the abscess drains into the aortic lumen, a false aneurysm of a sinus of Valsalva may result.[49] Moreover, abscesses may disrupt attachment of the aortic media to the fibrous skeleton of the heart, producing fistulous communications.[48,49]

Nonspecific Aortitis

Narrowing of an aortic segment or of one of its branches, aneurysm formation, or aortic regurgitation may be produced by an arteritis for which no specific etiology can been found. It may occur as an isolated abnormality or be associated with noninfectious inflammatory involvement of other organs as in, for example, lupus erythematosus or rheumatoid arthritis.

TAKAYASU'S DISEASE

The prototypical nonspecific aortitis, Takayasu's arteritis, was named for the Japanese ophthalmologist who first called attention to the funduscopic findings of the disease.[50] Because of its predilection for the brachiocephalic vessels, this arteritis has been labeled *pulseless disease* and *aortic arch syndrome.* The classic form occurs with the greatest frequency in the Orient; however, patients with a similar nonspecific aortitis are encountered worldwide.[51] Whether they represent similar or identical diseases is uncertain.

The description to follow will focus on the prototypical illness described in the Orient. The reader may infer that variations on the theme will be encountered elsewhere.[52]

Etiology The etiology of Takayasu's arteritis is unknown. No infectious agent has been identified, but data support the presence of an "autoimmune" process.[53] Antiendothelial antibodies were identified recently in 18 of 19 patients.[54] A genetic predisposition has been postulated because of clustering of the disorder and of similar histocompatability antigens.[55]

Pathology Histologic examination discloses a granulomatous arteritis during active stages of the disease that is similar to giant cell arteritis and to the aortitis associated with seronegative spondylitis. In later stages, medial degeneration, fibrous scarring, intimal proliferation, and thrombosis result in narrowing of the vessel. Aneurysm formation is observed less commonly than are stenosis and aortic rupture or dissection.

Distribution of stenoses has been defined angiographically.[52] The left subclavian artery, particularly in its midportion, is narrowed in about 90 percent of patients. The right subclavian, the left carotid, and the brachiocephalic trunk follow closely in frequency of stenosis. Thoracic aortic lesions are seen in two-thirds of patients,[52] whereas the abdominal aorta is involved in half, and aortoiliac involvement is present in only 12 percent. Pulmonary arteritis is present in about half of patients. Pulmonary hypertension may be found at catheterization.

Clinical Features Manifestations of the illness appear during the second or third decade in 70 to 80 percent of instances, but it has been reported in childhood and in middle life. Women are eight or nine times more often affected than men.[50–52]

During the early or "prepulseless" period of the illness, constitutional manifestations (e.g., fever, night sweats, malaise, nausea and vomiting, weight loss, arthralgia, and skin rash) are encountered frequently. The patient may experience Raynaud's phenomenon, and splenomegaly may be found on examination. Laboratory study may disclose an elevated erythrocyte sedimentation rate, anemia, and serum protein abnormalities.[50–52]

Claudication or numbness of an upper extremity due to subclavian artery narrowing and evidence of ischemia of the central nervous system occur frequently. Postural dizziness or frank syncope usually reflects cerebral ischemia due to narrowing of the brachiocephalic arteries.[50–52,56]

Hypertension, observed in more than half of aortitis patients, is usually associated with narrowing of the renal arteries or of the aorta proximal to those branches. Difficulty may be encountered in accurately measuring arterial pressure because of arch vessel stenosis.

Cardiac manifestations may result from aortic regurgitation, coronary artery narrowing, or severe hypertension. Dilatation of the aortic root commonly accompanies the aortic valve incompetence. Angina pectoris, heart failure, and myocardial infarction are reported. Pericarditis has been observed clinically, but more commonly healed pericarditis is noted at necropsy.

The retinopathy to which Takayasu first directed attention is believed to result from ischemia of the retina. Ocular ischemia also may be manifested by transient loss of vision, cataracts, corneal opacity, and iridial atrophy. Blindness is a common complication.

Involvement of the visceral arteries occasionally results in splanchnic ischemia, and intermittent claudication due to aortoiliac obstruction may occur.

Recently, attention has been directed toward the special problems that may arise during pregnancy in patients with this disorder.[57] Hypertension is frequent. Good outcomes can result with meticulous obstetrical care.

Diagnosis The American College of Rheumatology has identified *six major criteria for the diagnosis of Takayasu's arteritis.*[58] *Onset of illness by the age of 40 years* was recommended as an obligatory criterion to avoid overlap with patients having giant cell arteritis. Others include *upper extremity claudication, diminished brachial pulses, a 10-mmHg or more difference between the systolic blood pressure in the two arms, a subclavian or aortic bruit, and identification of narrowing of the aorta or a major branch. Identification in a patient of three of these six criteria is associated with high diagnostic sensitivity and specificity.*

Prognosis One-third to one-quarter of patients with severe aortitis at diagnosis will have a significant event or will die within 5 years. Those with few or no ischemic complications at the time of diagnosis fare better and have a good 5- and 10-year outlook. Severe hypertension or cardiac involvement predicts a shortened life expectancy.[56]

Cerebrovascular accidents and blindness are the most common major events. Congestive heart failure and aortic rupture or dissection are less frequent.

Management Adrenocorticoids appear to be effective in suppressing the inflammation of the active phase.[59,60] Immunosuppressive therapy also has been used. Operative treatment may relieve symptoms from arterial obstruction, and percutaneous angioplasty has been used with favorable initial results.[61]

GIANT CELL ARTERITIS

Giant cell arteritis (temporal arteritis, polymyalgia rheumatica) involves extracranial arteries, including the aorta in 10 to 13 percent of cases. Its peak incidence in late life seems to set it apart from other varieties of nonspecific arteritis. Like them, it may produce narrowing of the brachiocephalic arteries, aneurysm of the ascending aorta, aortic regurgitation, and aortic dissection.[62] Unlike Takayasu's arteritis, giant cell arteritis rarely involves the descending thoracic or abdominal aorta.

AORTITIS IN HLA-B27–ASSOCIATED SPONDYLOARTHROPATHIES

Although the etiology of neither ankylosing spondylitis nor Reiter's syndrome is known, more than 90 percent of afflicted individuals have the histocompatibility antigen HLA-B27, which is infrequent in the general population. This observation may provide a clue to a common pathogenetic mechanism.[63]

Aortitis has been demonstrated to accompany a sizable minority of patients with these disorders,[64] especially in those with spondylitis of long duration, in those with peripheral joint complaints in addition to spondylitis, and in patients with associated iritis. Aortitis may be present in some patients with HLA-B27 who are not afflicted with spondyloarthropathy and manifests as lone aortic regurgitation or conduction abnormalities,[63] findings reasonably attributable to inflammation of the aortic root and surrounding regions.

Histologically, the inflammatory aortic lesion in this setting resembles that of syphilis. Focal destruction of the medial elastic tissue is seen. The intima and adventitia, but not the media, are thickened. An obliterative arteritis of the vasa vasorum may be detected.[64]

Unlike syphilis, the process is largely limited to the aortic wall behind and immediately above the sinuses of Valsalva and may extend below the aortic valve to involve the membranous ventricular septum and the base of the anterior leaflet of the mitral valve.[64] The aortic valve cusps are thickened and retracted and their edges rolled. Transesophageal echocardiography shows more thickening of the aortic wall than dilatation.[65]

As in syphilis, aortic regurgitation is the most frequent clinical manifestation of these forms of aortitis. Extension into the interventricular ventricular septum occasionally results in atrioventricular conduction abnormalities. Either condition may be severe and life-threatening.

Congenital Anomalies of the Aorta

Aortic arch anomalies and the complex congenital conditions manifest in infancy or early childhood are discussed in Chap. 63. Coarctation of the aorta and sinus of Valsalva aneurysms are discussed below.

CLINICAL MANIFESTATIONS OF AORTIC DISEASE

Aortic Aneurysm

Aneurysms, areas of focal or diffuse dilatation of the aorta, develop at sites of congenital or acquired medial weakness. Hypertension may expose weakness that might otherwise not be manifest. Once begun, aneurysm formation is progressive because, for any level of intraluminal pressure, tangential wall tension increases with the square of the radius. Thus expansion and rupture are nearly inevitable unless the patient succumbs to intercurrent disease before this can occur.[66]

Fusiform and *saccular* aneurysms are described. In the former, circumferential dilatation, the result of a diffuse area of weakness, produces a spindle-shaped deformity. In the latter, balloon-like dilatation occurs, beginning at a relatively narrow neck. Many aneurysms are not pure examples of either. In both varieties, by the time the aortic wall has been stretched to aneurysmal size, little or no recognizable medial tissue remains; the wall of the aneurysmal sack is composed almost entirely of fibrous tissue.[67]

The lumen of an aneurysm virtually always contains laminated thrombus, which may fill a saccular aneurysm or cover the circumference of a fusiform one. Thus angiographic opacification of the aortic lumen often does not clearly delineate the size or extent of an aneurysm.

Aneurysms may result from a variety of causes. Heritable medial weakness as a basis for aortic dilatation has been discussed. With the declining incidence of syphilis, aneurysms resulting from aortitis, either infectious or nonspecific, are uncommon. Saccular aneurysms are often encountered in regions of the aorta weakened by aortic dissection.[68] Despite alternative etiologic possibilities, the great majority of aortic aneurysms, particularly those of the descending thoracic or abdominal aorta, are generally assumed to be "atherosclerotic"[66] because of the frequent presence of atherosclerosis elsewhere and of its risk factors.

The assumption that atherosclerosis alone is sufficient to produce aneurysm has been challenged.[67] Among other reasons, strong family clustering of abdominal aneurysms, as well as their association with aneurysmal dilatation of other arteries, provides reason to suspect that an underlying genetically determined defect may play an important role in this process, as alluded to earlier.[69–71] It appears likely that both genetically influenced factors and atherosclerosis are involved, perhaps with varying contributions in a given individual.

SINUS OF VALSALVA ANEURYSM

Congenital failure of fusion of the aortic media with the fibrous skeleton of the heart at the aortic valve ring provides a point of weakness through which a sinus of Valsalva aneurysm may develop.[72] Aneurysm of the right coronary sinus is most frequent. Most of the rest protrude from the noncoronary sinus. Congenital aneurysms of the left coronary sinus are rare. In that location, infectious endocarditis is a more frequent cause.

Because the root of the aorta is nearly surrounded by cardiac chambers, sinus of Valsalva aneurysms may intrude on and may rupture into one of them. Those of the right coronary sinus protrude into the right ventricular outflow tract. When they rupture, a fistulous connection between the aorta and right ventricle results. Similarly, an aneurysm of the noncoronary sinus, located posteriorly and to the right of the anterior sinus, typically protrudes into the right atrium and usually ruptures into that structure. The rare aneurysms of the left coronary sinus protrude into the pericardial space from beneath the left main coronary artery.

Some defects in the right coronary sinus are extensive enough to produce undermining of the aortic valve and incompetence of that valve, and some are associated with incomplete closure of the membranous ventricular septum and an interventricular shunt.

Rarely recognized prior to rupture, sinus of Valsalva aneurysm may be detected on imaging of a patient for some other purpose. Rarely, the mass of the unruptured aneurysm may obstruct the right ventricular outflow tract or the left coronary artery.[73] Heart block or other conduction abnormalities may be produced from protrusion into the interventricular septum.

Rupture of a sinus of Valsalva aneurysm usually results in a large shunt from the aorta to the right heart chambers.[73] The patient presents with a continuous murmur and bounding arterial pulses. Often severe heart failure is present. The diagnosis is readily made from the clinical picture and echocardiography. Surgical correction is indicated.

THORACIC AORTIC ANEURYSM

Etiology and Pathologic Anatomy Anuloaortic ectasia, the typical aneurysm resulting from medial degeneration, has its greatest diameter in the proximal ascending aorta, including the aortic sinuses. The diameter quickly tapers, approaching a normal dimension before the takeoff of the innominate artery. Limited or extensive medial dissection may complicate this aneurysm.[17,18,74] The hallmark aortic manifestation of Marfan's syndrome, such lesions are often encountered in individuals with no musculoskeletal or ocular manifestations of that disorder.

Syphilitic aneurysms are still encountered occasionally. They are typically saccular. The ascending aorta and arch are most often affected, but the aortic dilatation often extends into the aortic sinuses and into the descending aortic segment. The abdominal aorta is rarely affected.

Saccular aneurysms of the thoracic aorta frequently follow aortic dissection when operative repair is not carried out. Moreover, they may develop in the descending thoracic aorta even after successful operative repair of a dissection involving the ascending aorta.[68] Such aneurysms may expand gradually over time and require operative treatment months or years after the acute dissection.

About equal in frequency to thoracic aneurysms following dissection are those which have in the past been assumed to be atherosclerotic in origin. They are, however, far less common than infrarenal abdominal aneurysms. Unlike anuloaortic ectasia, these are typically located in the descending thoracic segment and are usually, but not invariably, fusiform. When they extend proximally into the arch or distally into the abdomen, they present a particularly challenging surgical problem. An aneurysm of the abdominal aorta is quite frequently associated and should be sought whenever a thoracic aneurysm is encountered.[75,76]

Clinical Features Aneurysms limited to the ascending aorta rarely produce symptoms directly unless they are undergoing active expansion or rupture. They are commonly recognized in the course of evaluation of a patient with the murmur of aortic regurgitation. Since the aortic root is located within the cardiac silhouette and the entire ascending aorta within the pericardial space, dilatation may not be readily appreciated on a chest radiograph.

Like aneurysms of the ascending aorta, those of the arch and descending segments are often asymptomatic and are detected fortuitously in the course of an incidental imaging study. Those of the arch, however, are more likely than those in other locations to produce symptoms. The arch is fixed by the brachiocephalic arteries, and aneurysms of that segment may compress a variety of mediastinal structures as well as the thoracic spine. Compression of the tracheobronchial tree may be attended by cough or dyspnea. Tracheal deviation or "tug" may be detected on physical examination. Pressure on the esophagus may result in dysphagia, rarely severe. Hoarseness may result from compression of the recurrent laryngeal nerve. Adjacent vascular structures may be compressed, resulting in pulmonary arterial stenosis or superior vena caval obstruction.

Chest pain, described as deep and aching or throbbing, has been the most frequent symptom reported in patients with thoracic aneurysm. Pain may be associated with erosion of the rib cage or vertebrae. The appearance of pain clearly related to an aneurysm must be regarded as a signal of expansion and threatened rupture.[76] It is not unusual for expansion or rupture to be the initial manifestation of a thoracic aneurysm. Massive, usually fatal hemorrhage into the mediastinum, pleural space, esophagus, or tracheobronchial tree ensues. Rupture of an aneurysm of the ascending aorta, because of the intrapericardial location of that structure, results in acute hemopericardium and cardiac tamponade. Hemoptysis may precede by days or weeks fatal hemorrhage in descending thoracic aneurysms that have become adherent to adjacent lung. Rarely, aneurysms may rupture into adjacent vascular structures, producing aortovenous or aortopulmonary fistulas.

Diagnosis The aorta may be imaged by a variety of modalities. Of these, chest x-ray and transthoracic echocardiography are the most readily available and thus most useful for screening purposes. Aortography, computed tomography, magnetic resonance imaging/angiography, and transesophageal echocardiography all provide detailed information regarding the aorta's anatomy.[77]

Natural History and Prognosis Most of the data concerning the natural history of thoracic aortic aneurysms come from retrospective, somewhat dated reports of hospital experience.[75,76] If anuloaortic ectasia and aortic dissection are excluded, the vast majority of cases studied have involved the descending aortic segment. Joyce's classic review[75] suggests a 50 percent 5-year and a 70 percent 10-year mortality. A 5-year mortality of 44 percent was reported more recently.[78]

One-third to one-half of deaths result from rupture of the aneurysm; most of the remainder result from other vascular diseases. The location of the aneurysm does not influence the mortality rate, but advanced age, size more than 6 cm, hypertension, and presence of other cardiovascular disease all increase risk. Symptoms related to the aneurysm itself portend an unfavorable outcome.

To the extent that mortality data in patients with Marfan's syndrome apply to all patients with anuloaortic ectasia, their outlook appears to be worse than for those with aneurysm of the descending aorta. In one early series, 52 of 56 patients with Marfan's syndrome died as a consequence of aortic disease at an average age of 32 years.[79] More recently, the mean age of death in Marfan's patients was found to be 41 years.[80] This improvement may be attributable to advances in surgery or to improved medical therapy (including the use of β-receptor blocking drugs), but different methods of data handling make comparison difficult

Management Until very recently, surgical repair was the only known effective treatment for thoracic aneurysms. The introduction of stent-graft stents offers promise of a less morbid intervention, but experience with this technique is still limited.[81]

Operative intervention is urgently indicated in patients if symptoms suggest expansion or compression of an adjacent structure. Cardiac failure from aortic regurgitation or aortocameral fistula also may necessitate early operative treatment. Available data suggest that in asymptomatic patients, the larger the aneurysm and the more rapid its increase in size, the more likely rupture will occur.[82–84] It is generally agreed that a diameter of 6 cm represents a point at which an operation should be considered.[82–84] For aneurysms in Marfan's patients, a somewhat lower threshold (5 cm) is recommended by some experts. As is true of other aortic aneurysms, the presence of chronic obstructive lung disease is associated with an increased risk of rupture.[85] Compared with the patient who has no other disease, the individual with associated coronary or cerebrovascular disease has a greater operative risk and a smaller risk of dying from rupture of the aneurysm before succumbing to the associated vascular disease.

Traditional surgical treatment consists of replacing the resected aneurysmal segment with a graft attached to relatively normal aorta proximally and distally. Specific surgical procedures vary with the site of the aneurysm and the need for maintaining circulation to distal body parts during aortic occlusion. Accordingly, the surgeon divides thoracic aneurysms into those affecting (1) the ascending aorta, (2) the arch of the aorta containing origins of the brachiocephalic vessels, (3) the descending thoracic aorta arising just distal to the origin of the left subclavian artery, and (4) thoracoabdominal aneurysms, i.e., those arising in the descending thoracic aorta and extending into the abdominal aorta.

For aneurysms of the ascending aorta, total cardiopulmonary bypass is required. The myocardium is protected by cold cardioplegia while the coronary ostia are exposed. The aneurysm is opened, and a graft is sutured in place from within. Finally, the aneurysm is trimmed and sutured around the graft. If the aneurysm is associated with aortic valve incompetence, the leaflets are excised, and a composite graft including a prosthetic valve is sutured in place. The coronary ostia are sutured to an appropriate opening made in the composite graft or to a smaller Dacron graft that is sutured side-to-side to the composite graft.

For aneurysms of the transverse arch of the aorta, total cardiopulmonary bypass is also required, and profound hypothermia is used to protect the brain. A graft is sutured to relatively normal aorta proximally and distally from within the aneurysm, and the brachiocephalic, left common carotid, and left subclavian arteries are attached individually to appropriate openings in the graft. It is often possible to preserve the relatively normal aortic wall segment from which these vessels arise. This segment can be attached to an appropriate opening made in the graft.

For aneurysms arising distal to the left common carotid artery, it is usually desirable to employ atrial-femoral bypass, femoral-femoral partial cardiopulmonary bypass, or various types of shunts during the period of aortic occlusion. Although many techniques to prevent spinal cord ischemia are being studied, there is not as yet convincing evidence that any predictably reduce the incidence of paraparesis associated with these procedures.

The surgical mortality rate for aneurysms of the ascending aorta is about 3 percent.[84] For descending thoracic aortic aneurysms, the rate is approximately 6 percent.[84] It is somewhat higher for those affecting the transverse arch and origins of the brachiocephalic vessels. Late deaths are usually due to associated diseases or other causes, although aneurysms occasionally may develop in other parts of the aorta and require surgical treatment.

Thoracoabdominal aneurysms arise in the descending thoracic aorta and extend distally for varying distances into the abdominal aorta as far as the bifurcation and occasionally into the common iliac arteries. They present a particular challenge to the surgeon because the arteries supplying blood to the abdominal organs arise from this portion of the aorta.

The surgeon must expose the aorta in both the thorax and the abdomen. A left intercostal incision is made and extended down the midline of the abdomen, after which the diaphragm is incised, and the abdominal structures are mobilized retroperitoneally to expose the entire aneurysm. A graft is interposed. In most cases, it is possible to attach the segment of the aorta from which arise the celiac, superior mesenteric, and renal arteries to an opening in the graft and thus avoid the need to use individual grafts to each artery. Occasionally, however, it may be necessary to use a separate graft for one or more of these arteries.

An operative mortality rate of 7 to 11 percent is reported from experienced centers.[84] As in aneurysms of the descending thoracic aorta, paresis or paraplegia is a potential complication.

ABDOMINAL AORTIC ANEURYSM

Rupture of an abdominal aortic aneurysm is the tenth leading cause of death (15,000 annually) for men 55 years of age and older in the United States. Moreover, 40,000 aneurysmectomies are performed each year. In contrast to the well-known decline in age-adjusted deaths from coronary atherosclerosis, the incidence of abdominal aneurysms is increasing.[86] This lesion is particularly treacherous because it is often clinically silent until rupture occurs.

Etiology Until recently, virtually all abdominal aneurysms have been attributed to atherosclerosis,[86] an assumption that is being challenged, as noted earlier. In addition, an occasional traumatic, congenital, or mycotic abdominal aneurysm is encountered, and one is occasionally found as a residual of aortic dissection or in patients with Marfan's syndrome.

Pathologic Anatomy Abdominal aneurysms are, as a rule, fusiform but may be saccular and usually are located distal to the renal arteries but may extend to the aortic bifurcation and involve the iliac arteries. Exceptionally, they extend above the renal arteries. In this case, the origins of not only the renal arteries but also the major visceral arteries may be involved, complicating operative management.[66,86]

Between 5 and 10 percent of abdominal aneurysms are accompanied by an intense inflammatory and fibrotic reaction in the anterior and lateral periaortic tissue,[87,88] a process histologically similar to retroperitoneal fibrosis. These *inflammatory aneurysms* may result from a hypersensitivity reaction to an antigen or antigens in the atherosclerotic plaque. Systemic manifestations, such as weight loss, abdominal pain, and an elevated erythrocyte sedimentation rate, may reflect the inflammatory response. The difficulty of operative repair is increased.

Clinical Features Men are three or four times more likely to have an abdominal aortic aneurysm than women. The typical patient is in the seventh or eighth decade. Most are asymptomatic and are detected in the course of an examination directed at unrelated symptoms.[66,86]

Pain attributable to the aneurysm, especially if it is of recent onset, should be viewed as threatened rupture. Characteristically constant and located in the midabdomen, lumbar region, or pelvis, the pain may be severe and have a boring quality. Detection of an aneurysm that is tender to palpation carries much the same threat of rupture.[87] Because they present with abdominal pain and often a tender abdominal mass, inflammatory aneurysms may mimic threatened rupture.[87,88]

Unless the patient is obese, physical examination almost always discloses an abdominal mass in the epigastrium, slightly to the left of the midline. If definite expansile movement can be detected, the diagnosis of abdominal aneurysm is reasonably secure. Bruits may be audible, and femoral pulses are reduced in some patients.

Rupture may be the initial manifestation. Rapid exsanguination may result from free rupture into the peritoneal cavity. Fortunately, more often the rupture is directed into the retroperitoneal space, where hemorrhage may be retarded. Abdominal pain and evidence of occult blood loss may persist for hours or days, allowing time for diagnosis and operative treatment. Rarely, the rupture is confined for several days to a few weeks. In such instances, the patient may present a puzzling diagnostic picture consisting of abdominal pain, fever, and slight to moderate blood loss.[87,88] Recognition of the nature of the illness can be lifesaving because secondary rupture always ensues.

Rarely, rupture occurs into an adjacent retroperitoneal structure. When a communication develops with the vena cavae or other large vein, a loud continuous murmur in the abdomen and high-output congestive heart failure may ensue.[88] Rupture into the duodenum results in gastrointestinal bleeding,[88] but aortoduodenal fistulas are more common after graft replacement of the infrarenal aorta.

An unruptured aneurysm also may produce serious complications. Acute thrombosis may mimic saddle embolism. Furthermore, embolization of thrombus or atherosclerotic debris from aneurysms (and indeed from severely atherosclerotic, nonaneurysmal segments) to the lower extremities is far more frequent than is generally appreciated.[88,89] Secondary bacterial infection of an aortic aneurysm gives rise to fever, leukocytosis, and abdominal pain and may lead to rupture.

Diagnostic Studies Anteroposterior or cross-table lateral radiographs of the abdomen often confirm the presence of aneurysm by demonstrating the characteristic "egg-shell" calcification of its wall. Imaging with ultrasound provides reproducible measurements of the dimensions of the aneurysm, and computed tomography or magnetic resonance imaging provides more definitive confirmation of the diagnosis. Aortography can be reserved for instances in which additional information regarding the extent of the aneurysm or the degree of involvement of branch arteries is required. The aortogram, a depiction of the luminal contour, may be misleading as to the size of the aneurysm because its lumen is characteristically filled or lined with thrombus.[90]

Management Because of the threat of fatal rupture, frequently in a previously asymptomatic patient, screening of at-risk populations by means of abdominal ultrasound has been proposed. Fewer than 5 percent of those older than age 65 were found to have abdominal aneurysm, and in fewer than 1 percent did it exceed 4 cm in diameter,[91] leading to questioning of the cost-effectiveness of such an approach. The cost-effectiveness of screening could be enhanced by limiting the screening to patients with a family history of aneurysmal disease or patients with atherosclerotic disease in other arteries.[92]

Abdominal aneurysms detected in asymptomatic patients during screening present a sometimes difficult management choice.[93] The risk of fatal rupture must be balanced against the risk of aneurysmectomy, a situation that has spurred efforts to define features predicting high risk for rupture.[66,86,94–96] The larger the aneurysm is, the greater is the risk of rupture. Therefore, when discovered in a patient who is a reasonable operative risk, *aneurysms 5 cm or more in size should be resected, whereas those smaller than 4 cm may be followed safely pending an increase in size.* Aneurysms more than 4 cm but less than 5 cm in size fall into a gray zone in which there is lack of agreement. *The recently reported randomized UK Small Aneurysm Trial, however, suggests that aneurysms smaller than 5.5 cm may be followed safely with serial ultrasound examinations.*[97] In addition to aneurysm size, systemic hypertension and chronic obstructive lung disease are independent predictors of increased risk.

Patients with abdominal aneurysms commonly have coronary and cerebrovascular disease and are more likely to die from these diseases than of rupture and have an increased operative risk for aneurysmectomy.[98] With appropriate preoperative screening for and treatment of coronary disease, the risk of aneurysmectomy is acceptable in experienced centers.[66,99,100]

Symptomatic aneurysms require urgent surgical treatment because early rupture can be confidently predicted.[101] A ruptured abdominal aneurysm is a surgical emergency. Surgery for an abdominal aortic aneurysm does not require maintenance of the distal circulation. The aorta is clamped proximally between the aneurysm and the renal arteries, the iliac arteries are clamped distally, and the aneurysm is opened. From within, the graft is sutured proximally to normal aorta and distally to the aortic bifurcation or individually to the iliac arteries. Finally, the aneurysmal walls are trimmed and sutured over the graft. Operative mortality is less than 5 percent.[66]

Active investigation of the use of endovascular stent-grafts to isolate the aneurysm from the aortic lumen is underway in several centers. Early results suggest that this is both feasible and less morbid than the standard operative approach. Long-term results are not yet available.[102,103]

Aortic Dissection

Aortic dissection is an even more common potentially fatal aortic disease than even rupture of an abdominal aneurysm.[104–106] Every busy general hospital will encounter several each year. *Because fundamental differences exist between the pathogenesis, clinical presentation, and treatment of dissections and those of aneurysms, the confusing term* dissecting aneurysm *should be discarded.*

PATHOLOGIC ANATOMY

Cleavage of the aortic media in its long axis by a column of blood characterizes aortic dissection. The split in the media typically occupies about half the circumference of the aorta and may extend through its entire length. The plane of dissection often follows the greater curvature of the ascending aorta and the arch. In the descending aorta, the path of the dissection is most often located lateral to the true lumen, but it may be medial and may spiral "barber pole" fashion about the long axis.[107]

In classic aortic dissection, the "false channel" created by this medial hematoma communicates with the "true lumen" through an intimal tear located near its proximal end. Such tears typically are single and transverse in orientation, but exceptions are frequent. Multiple secondary ("reentry") tears, located more distally along the false channel, are common.

Two patterns predominate. In about two-thirds of instances the false channel originates in the ascending aorta and the proximal ("entry") tear is located a few centimeters above the aortic valve. The false channel frequently extends to the aortoiliac bifurcation (Fig. 88-4). Dissections that do not involve the ascending aorta account for about a quarter of all cases. In them, the proximal tear most often lies just distal to the left subclavian artery. The medial hematoma begins in proximity to the origin of the left subclavian artery and extends distally for varying distances[104–107] (Fig. 88-5).

The most widely applied nomenclature is that of DeBakey.[104–106] In this classification, dissections involving the ascending aorta are type I, whereas those originating beyond the arch are type III. Type II is limited to the ascending aorta. Apart from length, many type II dissections are indistinguishable from type I, but others originate within chronic fusiform dilatation of the ascending aorta. The Stanford classification applies type A to any dissection involving the ascending aorta and type B to those which do not[106] (Fig. 88-6).

Many medial dissections do not follow these classic patterns. In some, the hematoma is short and limited to the arch or to the descending thoracic or abdominal segments. In another rather frequently encountered variation, an entry tear is located just beyond the left subclavian artery, but the dissection extends proximally into the ascending aorta.

There is a subset of patients with the clinical syndrome of aortic dissection resulting from a medial hematoma but no intimal tear,[108] as demonstrated by computed tomography, transesophageal echocardiography, or magnetic resonance imaging.[109–111] They are now included under the rubric *intramural hematoma.* In one series of patients with medial

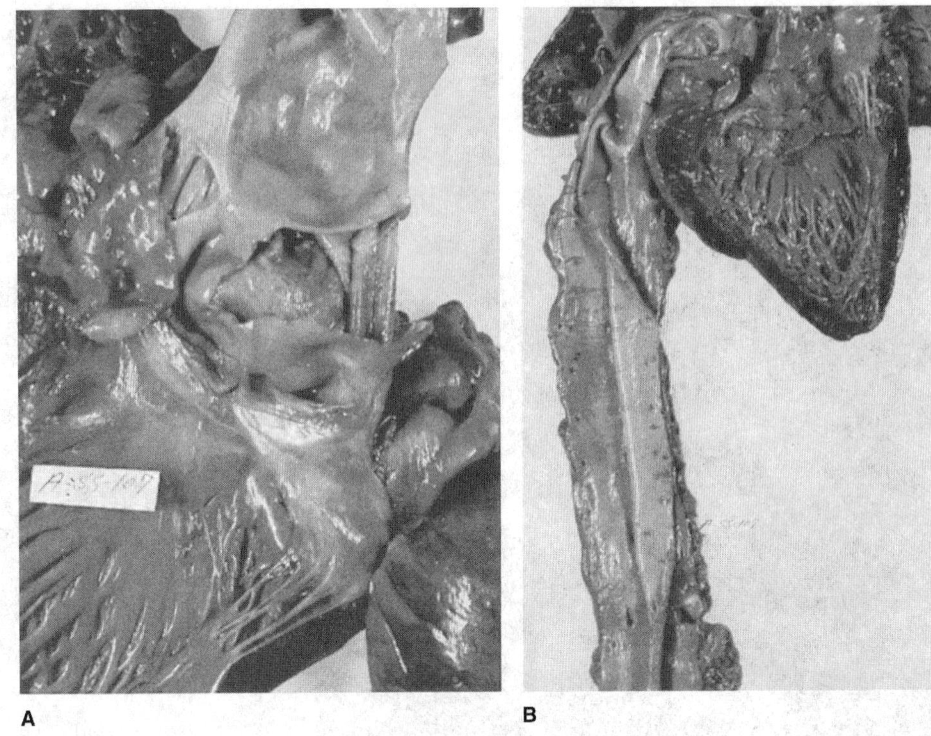

FIGURE 88-4 Necropsy specimen demonstrating the features of a typical proximal aortic dissection. *A*. The large intimal rent may be seen a few centimeters above the aortic cusps. *B*. The false channel created by the dissecting hematoma is shown. Notice the cleanly sheared layers of media.

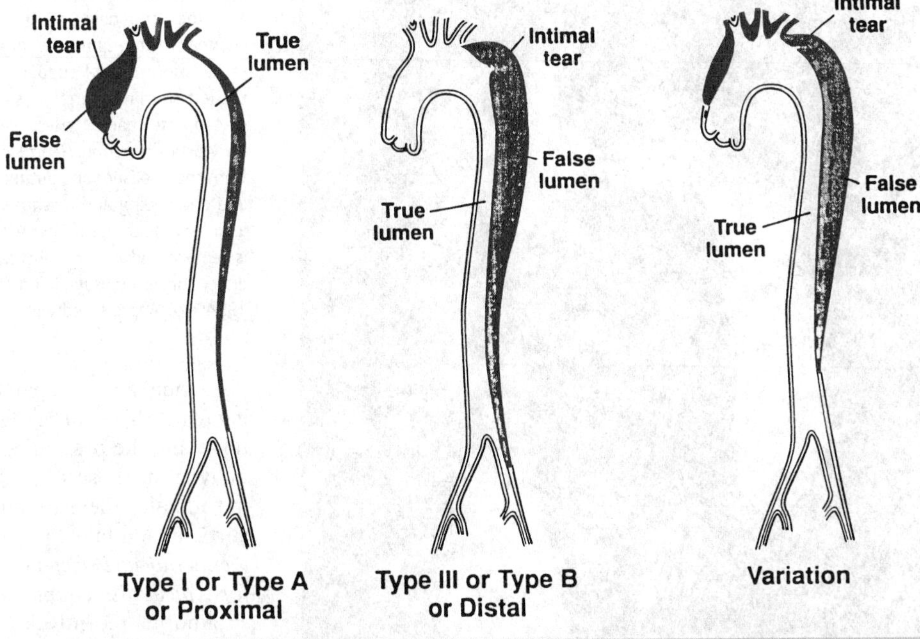

FIGURE 88-5 Artist's depiction of the three major anatomic patterns of aortic dissection. The left panel illustrates the most common variety, in which an intimal tear is located just above the aortic valve, and the medial cleavage plane extends in the long axis for a varying distance, often to the bifurcation. The center panel depicts the second most common variety. An intimal tear is found just beyond the left subclavian artery, and the medial dissection extends distally. The right panel depicts an important, but uncommon, variation. From an intimal tear just distal to the left subclavian artery, the medial dissection extends both antegrade down the thoracic aorta and retrograde into the descending segment. (From Lindsay J Jr. Aortic dissection. *Heart Dis Stroke* 1992; 1:69. Reproduced with permission from the publisher and author.)

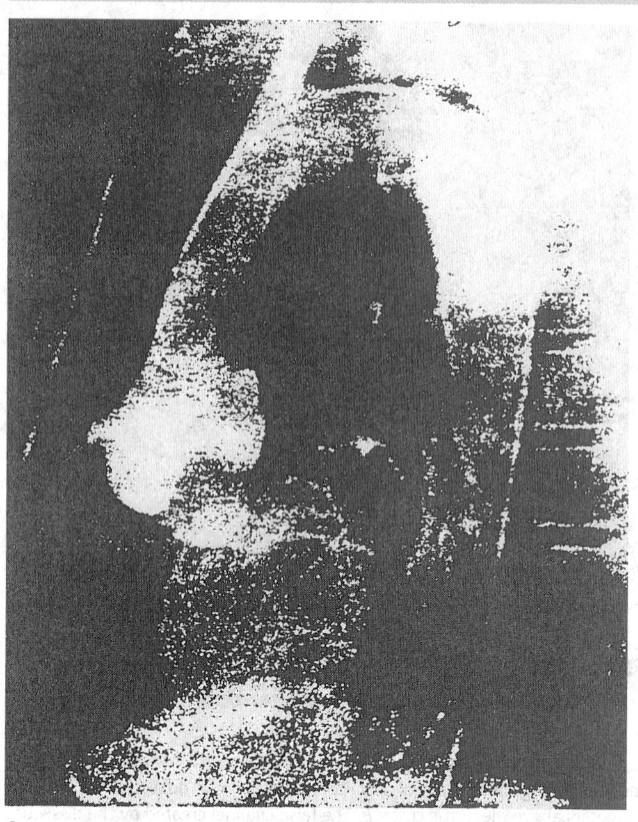

A

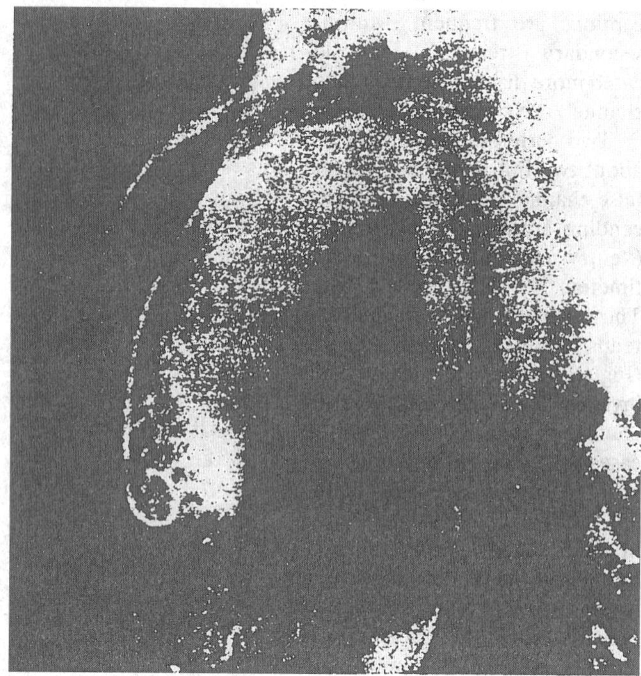

B

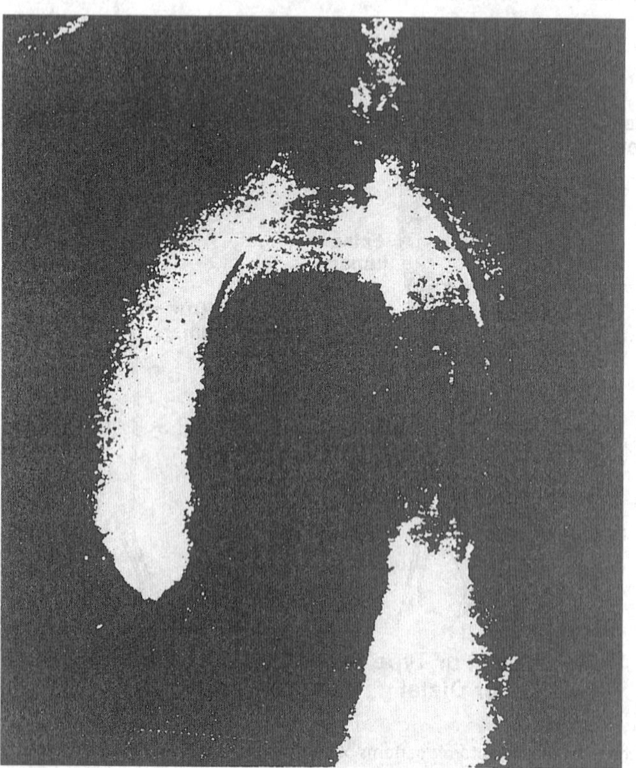

C

FIGURE 88-6 The major anatomic variations of aortic dissection as they appear on aortography. *A.* The dissection originates in the ascending aorta, as in the left panel in the diagram (Fig. 88-5). Note the proximity of the false channel to the right coronary artery as well as the aortic regurgitation that results from loss of support of the valve. *B.* The dissection begins distal to the left subclavian artery, as in the center panel of the diagram. The laterally placed false channel is less well opacified than the true lumen. (From Lindsay J Jr. Aortic dissection. *Heart Dis Stroke* 1992; 1:69. Reproduced with permission from the publisher and author.) *C.* This dissection involves both the ascending and descending aortic segments as well as the intervening arch. At surgery, an intimal tear was found just distal to the left subclavian artery. This variety is represented in the right panel in the diagram. (From Lindsay J Jr. Aortic dissection. In: Lindsay J Jr, ed. *Diseases of the Aorta*. Philadelphia: Lea & Febiger; 1994:137. Reproduced with permission from the publisher and author.)

dissection, about 13 percent had no demonstrable communicating tear.[110] The aortic segments involved with intramural hematoma and the presenting clinical picture do not differ substantially from those of typical dissection.[109–111] Aortography may not identify them because contrast material injected into the aortic lumen fails to enter the medial hematoma.[112] *At present, the therapeutic strategy for intramural hematoma is the same as for typical dissection.*

Another recently described variation involves an intimal tear that exposes the underlying media or adventitia but does not result in a medial hematoma.[113] These lesions are difficult to detect with available imaging techniques.

One additional variety of medial hematoma was described in the section on aortic atherosclerosis. Penetrating atherosclerotic ulcers that have disrupted the aortic media have been demonstrated by imaging techniques and may create a potential for rupture, false aneurysm formation, or dissection by hematoma.[16]

These lesions appear almost exclusively in the middle and distal descending thoracic aorta. Exceptionally, major branch vessels are threatened. The initial presentation of a complication of a penetrating plaque (whether partial rupture or medial dissection) may mimic typical aortic dissection. Surgery may be indicated in selected patients because external rupture is a hazard.[16]

Death from aortic dissection most often occurs from disruption of the outer wall of the false channel opposite the entrance tear.[104–108] Rupture of proximal dissection therefore produces abrupt hemopericardium and cardiac tamponade. Hemorrhage into the mediastinum or either pleural space may occur, whereas external rupture of distal dissection often results in a left hemothorax. Death from external rupture, often abrupt, may be delayed by temporary cessation of hemorrhage attributable to falling arterial pressure and increasing tension in the periaortic tissue. Dramatic clinical syndromes result in those rare instances in which the false channel ruptures into the right heart chambers producing a large left-to-right shunt.[114]

In approximately half of patients with proximal dissection, medial hematoma undermines the support of the aortic valve leaflets, rendering the valve incompetent. Fortunately, very serious hemodynamic consequences of aortic regurgitation appear infrequently during the acute phase.[104–106]

One or more branch vessels of the aorta become obstructed by dissection in about half of patients with type I and in fewer with type III dissection.[104–106] The results may be catastrophic, particularly in patients with type I, in whom the coronary and cerebral circulations are jeopardized. Obstruction by the dissection of the orifice of one of the coronary arteries rarely may produce an acute myocardial infarction. Failure to recognize the underlying process may result in thrombolytic therapy with disastrous results.[115] Obstruction of renal or splanchnic arteries may produce life-threatening complications such as severe hypertension and acute renal failure. The iliac arteries are the branch arteries most frequently compromised. Although not immediately life-threatening, narrowing of these arteries may produce dramatic, painful ischemia of the lower extremities.[116]

The aortic wall containing the medial hematoma is weakened. If it does not rupture during the acute dissection, it is often the site of subsequent aneurysm formation. Rupture of these constitutes a major threat to the survivor of the initial illness.[68,117]

PATHOGENESIS

Arterial hypertension is a major factor in causing aortic dissection in 80 percent of patients.[104–108] In most patients, no conclusive evidence of an underlying medial defect can be identified. Increased arterial pressure must certainly expose any existing weakness of the aortic wall and may, in addition, accentuate medial degeneration.

The frequency with which dissecting hematoma is noted in Marfan's syndrome,[17,18] in certain other congenital and heritable conditions,[17,18] and in experimental lathyrism provides a strong argument for the importance of an underlying medial defect in at least some individuals with this disorder. Indeed, histologic evidence of degeneration of elastin or of smooth muscle cells in the aortic media of such patients has long been noted. As noted previously, considerable doubt on the specificity of the classic histologic findings has been raised. Such findings are frequently absent in patients with dissection and are remarkably similar to changes encountered in older patients without dissection.[21] It seems likely that any fundamental medial defect or defects may be unrecognizable by light microscopy.

The role of the intimal ("entry") tear in the genesis of medial dissection is debated. Many investigators feel that it exposes the media to blood under luminal pressure and that the resulting shear forces initiate and propagate the medial cleavage. Others propose that medial weakness leads to hemorrhage from the vasa vasorum. The resulting intramural hematoma splits the medial layers.[104–108] In this hypothesis the intimal tears are secondary. Instances of medial hematoma in which no intimal tear can be identified support the existence of this mechanism.

CLINICAL FEATURES

Most common in the fifth through the seventh decades of life, aortic dissection has been reported in children as well as the very old. Men are affected at least twice as commonly as women.[104–108]

Predisposing Conditions Certain congenital lesions (e.g., coarctation and bicuspid aortic valve) are associated with increased frequency of dissection.[26] A greater-than-expected incidence is encountered in patients with aortic stenosis even after aortic valve replacement. The same is true with certain heritable disorders such as Marfan's and Turner's syndromes.[17]

Iatrogenic vascular trauma, a complication of cardiac catheterization, coronary bypass surgery, cardiopulmonary bypass, or intraaortic balloon counterpulsation, may produce extensive aortic dissection.

Pregnancy, either because of its effects on the aortic wall or because of attendant hemodynamic stress, has been reported to predispose to medial dissection.[118] This conclusion has been based on the fact that half or more of the reports of aortic dissection in women younger than 40 years have occurred during pregnancy. Since the total number reported is relatively small (certainly in relation to the frequency of pregnancy), and since most reports concern one or a few cases, it is possible that selective reporting accounts for this association.[119]

History Sudden, excruciating pain, presumably attributable to the progress of the medial cleavage, announces the onset of dissection in 90 percent of instances. Patients may describe the pain as "cutting," "ripping," or "tearing," but such vivid descriptors cannot always be elicited.[104–106] Patients will most commonly locate the discomfort in the anterior chest, somewhat less frequently in the interscapular area, in the epigastrium, or in the lumbar region. Since these locations often are the site of pain related to more common processes (e.g., myocardial infarction or cholecystitis), the examiner must be alert to the possibility of aortic dissection in any patient with pain in these sites in whom the more common diagnoses are not immediately obvious.

Two features of the pain of dissection help to separate it from that of other conditions. *The discomfort of dissection typically is at its most intense from its inception and does not build in intensity, as is the case with other disorders producing severe pain in the trunk. Moreover, it often is located either simultaneously or sequentially in more than one of the four sites mentioned earlier.* Suspicion should be aroused particularly by pain occurring both above and below the diaphragm.[104–106]

When pain is not a prominent feature, it is usually because

a sudden neurologic episode has diminished the patient's ability to perceive or report pain. Syncope is the most frequent neurologic event and a particularly ominous sign. It seems always to reflect external rupture, almost always of the ascending aorta into the pericardial space. Less frequently, focal neurologic signs reflect arterial occlusion of the cerebral or spinal circulation.

Unusually, aortic dissection is nearly painless even in the absence of a neurologic event. For example, occlusion of the femoral or the subclavian artery may be the predominant clinical feature, and arterial embolism may be simulated.[104–106] Rarely, the acute episode goes entirely unrecognized by the patient. In such instances, diagnostic study of patients who have an abnormal chest x-ray, aortic regurgitation or obstruction of an arterial branch of the aorta uncovers chronic dissection.

Physical Examination Although none are diagnostic of dissection, physical findings that greatly increase the probability of its presence often can be detected. *The murmur of aortic regurgitation can be heard in about half of all patients with acute type I dissection. Loss or diminution of an arterial pulse also may be detected in half. One or both of these cardinal findings is present in all but a small minority of that subgroup.* In contrast, patients with dissection limited to the descending aorta less frequently have pulse deficits and uncommonly have a murmur of aortic regurgitation.

The frequency with which hypertension underlies aortic dissection has been mentioned. Even those with neither a definitive history of hypertension nor a measurable blood pressure elevation will on examination have left ventricular hypertrophy or vascular changes in the optic fundi indicating a hypotensive history. Extraordinarily high readings can be encountered, particularly in those with type III dissection. Renal ischemia, a consequence of renal artery involvement, has been invoked to explain diastolic blood pressures that may reach 140 to 160 mmHg or more.[104–106]

Twenty percent of patients with dissection involving the ascending aorta present with hypotension. Such a presentation requires immediate consideration of operative treatment because external rupture almost always is responsible.

Diagnostic Studies Of the routine studies, only the chest x-ray provides diagnostic information of much value. The aortic shadow is abnormal in 80 to 90 percent of patients but also may be abnormal in many instances in patients who do not have dissection. Dilatation of the ascending aorta, reflected by protrusion of its shadow from the right side of the mediastinum, is a characteristic finding in proximal dissection. Dilatation of the aortic knob and descending thoracic aorta is typical of distal disease. Certain other findings, e.g., progressive widening of the aortic silhouette on serial films, a lobulated or serrated margin of the aortic shadow, or a "double lumen" effect created by a less radiopaque false channel, are uncommon but more specific. The same may be said for detection of intimal calcification more than 6 mm inside the margin of the aorta.[90]

For confirmation of the diagnosis, either computed tomography after intravenous contrast material or transesophageal echocardiography may be employed. Both have high sensitivity and specificity. Some believe that magnetic resonance imaging is even more accurate; however, its value is limited in acutely ill patients because of the longer imaging time and the relative inaccessibility of patients during the imaging process.[90,120–122]

An aortogram is occasionally required to provide details of branch vessel involvement. Two aortic channels usually can be identified because of the variation in intensity and timing of their opacification (see Fig. 88-6). Moreover, the aortogram may identify a linear lucency representing the aortic intima and media separating the two channels. At times the false channel is not opacified because of thrombosis or because it does not communicate with the true lumen. In such cases, the true lumen may appear to be compressed and to lie at a distance from the margins of the aortic shadow. The resulting appearance of a thickened aortic wall also can be produced by thrombosis within an aneurysm, aortitis, or mediastinal hematoma or tumor. These usually, but not invariably, can be distinguished from dissection because in these the aortic lumen is not significantly compressed.

NATURAL HISTORY AND PROGNOSIS

Older reports of aortic dissection must be used to provide information about its natural history because virtually all patients in the past 30 years have been operated on and/or had aggressive antihypertensive treatment. Thirty-five percent of untreated patients succumb within the initial 24 hours, and 50 percent die within 48 hours, 70 percent by 1 week, and 80 percent by 2 weeks.[108,123]

Certain subgroups with widely differing natural histories can be identified. Hypotension (systolic blood pressure <100 mmHg) usually indicates aortic rupture and nearly certain early death. Almost all such patients have involvement of the ascending aorta; one-quarter of those with such involvement present in this way. Those with distal (type III or type B) dissection are at the other end of the spectrum with regard to their natural history. Older reports indicate that about half survive the acute phase without aggressive treatment. Absent modern therapeutic intervention, the mortality rate of patients with proximal dissection who are hypertensive or normotensive is intermediate between these extremes.

Patients who survive the first 2 weeks continue to experience a high mortality rate in the first year. About half the survivors die within 3 months, and an additional 10 percent die within 1 year of the onset of their illness. The few who pass the first anniversary may expect reasonable longevity. Late deaths may be due to cerebrovascular complications of hypertension, heart failure from severe aortic regurgitation, or rupture of a saccular aneurysm of the residual false channel.[124]

MANAGEMENT

The life-threatening complications of acute aortic dissection include very severe hypertension, cardiac tamponade, massive hemorrhage, severe aortic regurgitation, or ischemic injury to the myocardium, the central nervous system, and kidneys. Optimal management requires close surveillance of vascular pressures, urine flow, mental status, and neurologic signs in an intensive care unit. Pain relief can be difficult even with potent narcotics but usually can be obtained with drug therapy to reduce arterial pressure.[104–106]

A successful outcome requires that progression of the medial cleavage be halted and that external rupture of the weakened aortic wall be prevented. In as much as the aortic defect is structural, operative treatment represents the most effective long-term remedy. Aggressive antihypertensive treatment lessens the stress on the aortic wall and thus the likelihood of progression of the dissection and of rupture. Such therapy is widely employed prior to and, in selected instances, as an alternative to surgical management.[104–106]

In the acute phase, one of several drug regimens may be employed to reduce arterial pressure and its rate of rise. *Aggressive use of a β-blocking agent may be adequate in patients who present with relatively modest levels of hypertension. With more severe hypertension, intravenous nitroprusside combined with a β-blocking agent may be required. Drug therapy should aim to lower systolic arterial pressure to 100 to 120 mmHg. Optimal blood pressure reduction may not be possible if oliguria (<25 mL/h) or mental confusion appears.*

Our intensivists currently prefer *intravenous esmolol as the β-blocking regimen for acute dissection.* Because of its short half-life (9 min), it can be readily titrated in these often unstable patients. *An initial loading dose of 0.5 mg/kg administered over 1 min is followed by an infusion of 0.05 mg/kg per minute. The infusion rate can be increased at 4-min intervals by 0.05 mg/kg per minute. Rates beyond 0.2 mg/kg per minute have not been shown to provide added therapeutic benefit. The substantial amounts of fluid required to maintain this infusion limit the usefulness of this agent in some patients. If there is concern for volume excess, labetalol may be employed. This adrenergic-receptor blocking agent affects both nonselective β and α_1 receptors. A bolus infusion of 0.25 mg/kg over 2 min is recommended. Additional boluses of 0.25 to 0.5 mg/kg may be given every 15 min to effect. A cumulative dose of 300 mg should not be exceeded. A continuous infusion may result in drug accumulation because the half-life of this agent is 5.5 h.* Appropriate oral doses of β-blocking agents can be given for long-term maintenance after the need for acute β blockade has passed.

The ability of *intravenous nitroprusside* to reduce arterial pressure promptly and consistently and the ease with which its hypotensive effects can be titrated recommend it as the *current drug of choice for the patient whose blood pressure does not respond to β blockade. As little as 0.5 μg kg per minute may produce the desired result. Occasionally, as much as 5 μg/kg per minute is necessary. A dose of 10 μg/kg per minute should not be exceeded. A β-blocking agent nearly always should be used in conjunction with nitroprusside* because animal data suggest that when used alone, it does not reduce and may, through reflex mechanisms, enhance the rate of rise of arterial pressure.

Many potent antihypertensive agents (e.g., hydralazine, minoxidil, and diazoxide) cannot be recommended because they produce reflex stimulation of the left ventricle and consequently an increase in the rate of rise of aortic pressure.

Not all patients with acute aortic dissection have elevated blood pressure. Hypotension, it has been noted, may reflect aortic rupture and dictates emergency operation. Some individuals have pressures only slightly higher than the 100- to 120-mmHg target level, and pharmacologic treatment is of dubious value, although β-adrenergic blockade may be tried to reduce the rate of rise of aortic pressure.

As noted earlier, operative treatment must be considered in all patients, but certain subgroups can be recognized whose clinical presentation dictates the timing of the surgery. At one extreme are those who are hypotensive on admission and require emergency operation, as noted. On the other hand, operative treatment may never be an option in those with severe comorbid illness. Further, it may not be justified in those with severe neurologic injury from the dissection. In these inoperable individuals, antihypertensive therapy is continued indefinitely by converting the drug regimen to an oral one that avoids vasodilators.

The appropriateness and urgency of surgery for aortic dissection depend on its location and the clinical picture. *In cases involving the ascending aorta, operative repair should be undertaken as soon as the patient can be stabilized and appropriate diagnostic information compiled.* By contrast, for those with *uncomplicated type III (type B) dissection, it is now believed that operation during the acute phase does not appear to improve survival beyond that achieved with drug treatment unless there is intractable pain, uncontrollable hypertension, or serious organ malperfusion.*[104,106] Those who are relatively good operative risks may benefit from operation in the subacute or chronic phase to protect them from rupture of a residual saccular aneurysm. Risk factors (e.g., age, the presence of chronic obstructive lung disease, size of aneurysms, and its rate of expansion) for such late rupture are similar to those of degenerative thoracic aneurysms.[125]

The surgical technique for aortic dissection varies with the origin and extent of the dissection. The surgeons's *primary goal is always to remove the proximal (i.e., "entry") tear and to close the false channel at that site.* External rupture is most frequent just across from the entrance tear, as noted. For ascending aortic dissection, the procedure consists in transection of the ascending aorta with use of cardiopulmonary bypass, obliteration of the false lumen by approximation of the inner and outer walls of the false channel, and end-to-end anastomosis of the transected aorta. It is usually necessary to restore vascular continuity by means of a patch or tube graft. Aortic valve incompetence secondary to loss of commissural support of the valve leaflets may be corrected when this repair effectively resuspends the valve. Other patients may require prosthetic valve replacement or the use of a composite graft. Surgical mortality approaches 15 to 20 percent but varies with the location and extent of the disease as well as age and comorbid conditions.

Surgical treatment for dissection beginning in the arch or beyond requires much the same operative approach as has been described for aneurysms in these locations. The segment containing the entrance tear is resected, the false channel obliterated by suture closure of the inner and outer layers, and excised segment replaced with a graft. The morbidity and mortality of operative repair of the arch and descending aorta are somewhat greater than when the ascending aorta is treated.

Placement of a stent-graft through an endoluminal approach is being investigated in several centers as a less morbid approach to the treatment of distal dissection.[126]

Aortic Obstruction

COARCTATION OF THE AORTA

In its most common form, aortic coarctation consists of hemodynamically significant narrowing of the aortic isthmus, that segment lying between the left subclavian artery and the insertion of the ductus arteriosus. A common congenital abnormality, it accounts for about 9 percent of all congenital heart disease in children and is the fourth leading cause of symptomatic congenital heart disease in infancy.[127,128] Heart failure in an infant typically announces its presence. Associated, complex cardiac anomalies are frequent contributing factors (see Chaps. 63 and 64). A less complex and often asymptomatic abnormality, bicus-

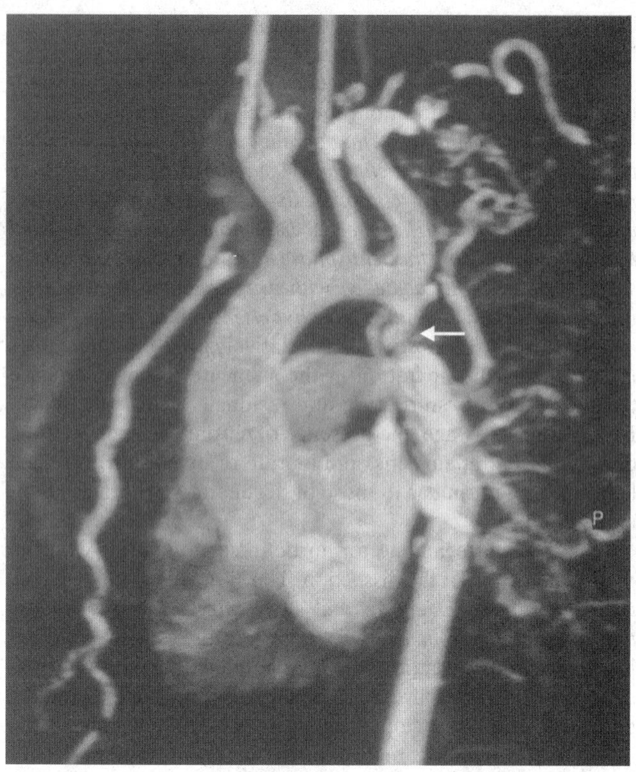

FIGURE 88-7 Magnetic resonance angiographic study from an adult with coarctation of the aorta. The tightly coarcted segment is indicated with an arrow. The collateral circulation is dramatically demonstrated. The left subclavian and innominate arteries, the source of these collaterals, are markedly dilated. (Courtesy of Dr. Karen Kuehl.)

pid aortic valve, is the most frequent associated anomaly. It is present in half or more of patients. Absent the appearance of heart failure in infancy, coarctation may be detected as upper extremity hypertension in an older child or young adult.

Large, tortuous collateral arteries develop in response to the aortic obstruction. These connections between branches of the subclavian and the intercostal arteries deliver blood to the distal aorta (Fig. 88-7). They enlarge, often to near aneurysmal proportions, gradually eroding the undersides of the ribs, producing the characteristic rib notching found on chest x-ray. Flow through these collaterals often produces recognizable bruits over the rib cage.

The natural history of this lesion is grim. Untreated, many patients die in childhood, and 80 percent die by age 50.[127,128] In the older patients, death is precipitated by cerebral hemorrhage (at least in part due to an association with berry aneurysm), aortic dissection or rupture, and infectious endocarditis.

Management Relief of the obstruction is the treatment of choice. Operative repair was first performed in 1945.[129] Currently, resection and end-to-end anastomosis, patch angioplasty, or subclavian flap angioplasty are employed. Catheter-based balloon dilatation or stenting is gaining acceptance as a less morbid option.[130–132]

Resection of the coarcted segment has not been as curative as expected. Persistent hypertension has been a significant problem, and the formation of aneurysms accompanied by dissection or rupture is well known.[129]

PSEUDOCOARCTATION OF THE AORTA

Congenital kinking, so-called pseudocoarctation of the aorta, may be detected during the investigation of a mediastinal mass or of a systolic murmur. An abnormally elongated thoracic aorta tethered to the ligamentum arteriosum produces a silhouette shaped like an S or a 3 on the chest x-ray, resembling true coarctation; however, rib notching is not present. Exclusion of hemodynamically significant coarctation may require sophisticated imaging or the demonstration that no pressure difference exists between the upper and the lower aortic segments. True coarctation may coexist, and congenital cardiovascular anomalies similar to those found in true coarctation may be associated.

Some authorities believe the abnormality to be a sharp downward angulation of the aorta at the attachment of the ligamentum arteriosum as a result of elongation of the fourth aortic arch. Others consider the embryologic defect to be the same as for typical isthmic coarctation, but in these cases the narrowing is not severe enough to result in significant obstruction.[133]

ABDOMINAL AORTIC COARCTATION (MIDDLE AORTIC SYNDROME)

Although rare, hemodynamically significant narrowing of the descending thoracic or abdominal aorta often produces life-threatening hypertension that is surgically correctable.[134–136] Although it often appears to be a congenital lesion, it may result from healed aortitis.[137] For this reason, some writers prefer to avoid the term *coarctation* and label it *middle aortic syndrome.*

Although the narrowed aortic segment typically is focal, diffuse hypoplasia of the abdominal aorta involving the branch arteries may occur. The renal arteries may be stenosed, hypoplastic, or thrombosed, resulting in severe hypertension. Visceral artery narrowing may result in bowel ischemia. Intermittent claudication from involvement of the iliac arteries is more frequent than in patients with typical coarctation.

On examination, upper extremity hypertension will be present together with feeble pulses and hypotension in the legs, findings similar to those of the more common postductal coarctation. Attention may be directed to the unusual location of the stenosis by a bruit in the lumbar or umbilical area.

Operative treatment usually is required because severe hypertension significantly shortens the life expectancy of patients.

CHRONIC OBSTRUCTION OF THE TERMINAL AORTA

Etiology and Pathogenesis Atherosclerosis of the aortoiliac bifurcation is the most common cause of chronic obstruction of the infrarenal aorta.[135,138] Many patients with symptomatic femoropopliteal atherosclerosis also have aortoiliac narrowing. Rarely, infrarenal coarctation, aortitis, clinically silent embolism, or in situ thrombosis produce this situation.

Rupture of atherosclerotic plaques sets the stage for mural thrombus and gradual progression of luminal narrowing and, in many instances, complete occlusion of the terminal aorta. Collateral vessels develop concomitantly, connecting the lumbar and inferior mesenteric arteries to branches of the internal iliac and common femoral arteries. Thus the symptoms of lower extremity ischemia typically progress over months or years, and progression to complete occlusion may not be marked by a clinical event. This indolent course, however, may be punctuated by an abrupt acceleration of symptoms, the result of a sudden increase in the size of the obstructing thrombus or its extension to a significant collateral.[135,138]

Aortoiliac atherosclerosis frequently has unusual features in that patients with aortoiliac narrowing may be younger and have a shorter duration of symptoms than do patients with femoropopliteal obstruction.[135,139] The predilection of atherosclerosis for the terminal aorta may be enhanced in some individuals because they have anatomic variations of the aortoiliac bifurcation that produce an "impedance mismatch." For example, an iliac bifurcation angle more acute than normal has been observed in some patients,[140] and in others, the aorta and iliac arteries are smaller than average.[141]

Clinical Features Men are affected far more often than women. The mean age of patients in most series falls in the sixth decade, but some are much younger. The usual risk factors for atherosclerosis are found frequently.

The original description of the clinical features of distal aortoiliac narrowing by René Leriche[142] (hence the Leriche syndrome) still applies, but variations on the theme are more frequent than the full-blown syndrome. Pain and tiredness in the lower back, buttocks, or thighs produced by exertion and relieved by brief periods of rest are hallmarks. Claudication may occur in the calf or foot in association with the more proximal distress and can be the sole complaint. Men often complain of inability to maintain a penile erection.

Absence of, or reduction in, the femoral pulse is typical. More distal pulses in the legs are reduced or absent, and bruits are commonly audible over femoral arteries and in the midline of the abdomen near the umbilicus. Low skin temperature, diminished hair growth, atrophy of the skin and subcutaneous tissue, and diminished muscle bulk in the lower limbs are common but not universal signs. Frank gangrene is infrequent, and amputation for ischemia is therefore seldom required.[136,139]

The findings in patients with aortoiliac obstruction overlap those in patients with femoropopliteal narrowing. A firm identification of involvement of the aortoiliac segment may be difficult on clinical grounds, and in many patients, obstructing lesions are present at both levels. Modern imaging techniques have made diagnosticians less dependent on clinical findings for the localization of the level of arterial obstruction.[135,138]

Natural History and Prognosis The survival rate for patients with the Leriche syndrome appears to be lower than for those in a control population matched for age and sex, but death rarely results from aortoiliac disease. Coronary and cerebrovascular atherosclerosis are largely responsible for the higher death rate. Significant morbidity or death occasionally follows occlusion of the renal arteries by proximal extension of the thrombotic process.[135,138]

Management End-to-side bypass with a flexible, knitted bifurcation graft is the preferable method of treatment. In the absence of femoropopliteal occlusive disease, this approach is usually successful in restoring normal distal circulation. Even when there is combined aortoiliac and femoropopliteal disease, bypass of the aortoiliac occlusion alone may increase lower extremity flow sufficiently to relieve symptoms.

Percutaneous transluminal angioplasty is being used with increasing frequency in the treatment of iliac and femoropopliteal obstructive atherosclerotic disease. The early success rate appears to be satisfactory, but the long-term patency rate remains to be determined.

ACUTE OBSTRUCTION OF THE TERMINAL AORTA

Etiology Sudden occlusion of the terminal aorta may result from a large ("saddle") embolus, trauma, medial dissection, or in situ thrombosis superimposed on an aneurysm or severe atherosclerosis. With either dissection or trauma, the etiology is usually obvious.[143,144]

Most emboli large enough to occlude the terminal aorta come from the heart, and embolus must be considered in acute aortoiliac occlusion in patients with mitral stenosis, atrial fibrillation, or recent myocardial infarction. Rarely, embolization of a vegetation from fungal endocarditis may be large enough to occlude the aortic bifurcation.[143,144]

In situ thrombosis of an aneurysm or of a severely atherosclerotic aorta may develop when blood flow through these vessels is considerably reduced, as may be the case in shock or congestive heart failure.

Clinical Features Unlike gradually progressive obstruction, abrupt total or near-total interruption of flow through the terminal aorta or common iliac arteries poses an immediate threat to life and limb. Although the clinical picture varies depending on the presence of preexisting collaterals, the full-blown syndrome is characterized by the abrupt onset of pain, typically severe and located in the lumbar area, the buttocks, the perineum, the abdomen, and the legs. Numbness, paresthesia, dysesthesia, and finally paralysis of the affected limb dominate the picture. Pulses are absent in the legs, although at times faint femoral pulsations may be detected. The legs are cold and pale. Unless circulation is restored promptly, massive muscle necrosis may produce myoglobinuria, renal failure, acidosis, and hyperkalemia.

Management In contrast to chronic aortoiliac occlusion, acute obstruction to blood flow does not allow for the formation of collateral circulation. Immediate revascularization is necessary for survival. The procedure used depends on the cause of the occlusion. Moreover, consideration must be given to treatment of the source of the embolus (e.g., mitral stenosis or left ventricular mural thrombus), in order to prevent recurrent embolization to such vital organs as the brain.

Aortoiliac embolectomy may be performed directly through an incision in the distal aorta or proximal iliac arteries but requires laparotomy in a severely ill patient and does not provide the means for removing more distally lodged embolic material. The preferable approach is to expose both common femoral arteries in the groins and, through transverse arteriotomies, to remove, with balloon-tipped Fogarty catheters, the embolic material lodged proximally and distally. Even large amounts of embolic material in the distal aorta itself can be removed safely in this manner. Good circulation usually is restored. Subsequent mortality rates, however, remain high because of the underlying disease.

References

1. Wolinsky H, Glagov S. A lamellar unit of aortic medial structure and function in mammals. *Circulation* 1976; 20:99–111.
2. Schlatmann TJ, Becker AE. Histologic changes in the normal aging aorta: Implications for dissecting aortic aneurysm. *Am J Cardiol* 1977; 39:13–20.
3. Cornwell GG III, Westermark P, Murdoch W, et al. Senile aortic amyloid: A third distinctive type of age-related cardiovascular amyloid. *Am J Pathol* 1982; 108:135–140.
4. Khoury Z, Gottlieb S, Stern S, et al. Frequency and distribution of atherosclerotic plaques in the thoracic aorta as determined by transesophageal echocardiography in patients with coronary artery disease. *Am J Cardiol* 1997; 79:23–27.
5. Kawaguchi A, Miyatake K, Yutani C, et al. Characteristic cardiovascular manifestation in homozygous and heterozygous familial hypercholesterolemia. *Am Heart J* 1999; 137:410–418.
6. Summers RM, Andrasko-Bourgeois J, Feuerstein IM, et al. Evaluation of the aortic root by MRI: Insights from patients with homozygous familial hypercholesterolemia. *Circulation* 1998; 98:509–518.
7. Reed D, Reed C, Stemmermann G, et al. Are aortic aneurysms caused by atherosclerosis? *Circulation* 1992; 85:205–211.
8. Bengtsson H, Norrgard O, Angquist KA, et al. Ultrasonographic screening of the abdominal aorta among siblings of patients with abdominal aortic aneurysms. *Br J Surg* 1989; 76:589–591.
9. Kontusaari S, Tromp G, Kuivaniemi H, et al. A mutation in the gene for type iii procollagen (*COL3A1*) in a family with aortic aneurysms. *J Clin Invest* 1990; 80:1465–1473.
10. Tilson MD. Aortic aneurysms and atherosclerosis. *Circulation* 1992; 85:378–379.
11. Khatibzadeh M, Mitusch R, Stierle U, et al. Aortic atherosclerotic plaques as a source of systemic embolism. *J Am Coll Cardiol* 1996; 27:664–669.
12. Davila-Roman VG, Murphy SF, Nickerson NJ, et al. Atherosclerosis of the ascending aorta is an independent predictor of long-term neurologic events and mortality. *J Am Coll Cardiol* 1999; 33:1308–1316.
13. Finkelhor RS, Youssefi ME, Lamont WE, et al. Embolic risk based on aortic atherosclerotic morphologic features and aortic spontaneous echocardiographic contrast. *Am Heart J* 1999; 137:1088–1093.
14. Ferrari E, Vidal R, Chevallier T, et al. Atherosclerosis of the thoracic aorta and aortic debris as a marker of poor prognosis: Benefit of oral anticoagulants. *J Am Coll Cardiol* 1999; 33:1317–1322.
15. Om A, Ellahham S, DiSciascio G. Cholesterol embolism: An underdiagnosed clinical entity. *Am Heart J* 1992; 124:1321–1326.
16. Vilacosta I, San Roman JA, Aragoncillo P, et al. Penetrating atherosclerotic ulcer: Documentation by transesophageal echocardiography. *J Am Coll Cardiol* 1998; 32:83–89.
17. Roman MJ, Devereux RB. Heritable aortic disease. In: Lindsay J Jr, ed. *Diseases of the Aorta*. Philadelphia: Lea and Febiger; 1994:55–74.
18. Savunen T. Annulo-aortic ectasia: A clinical, structural and biochemical study. *Scand J Thorac Cardiovasc Surg Suppl* 1986; 37:1–45.
19. Schlatmann TJ, Becker AE. Pathogenesis of dissecting aneurysm of the aorta: Comparative histopathologic study of significance of medial changes. *Am J Cardiol* 1977; 39:21–26.
20. Hirst AE, Gore I. Is cystic medionecrosis the cause of dissecting aortic aneurysm? *Circulation* 1976; 53:915–916.
21. Nakashima Y, Kurozumi T, Sueishi K, et al. Dissecting aneurysm: A clinicopathologic and histopathologic study of 111 autopsied cases. *Hum Pathol* 1990; 21:291–296.
22. Isner JM, Donaldson RF, Fulton D, et al. Cystic medial necrosis in coarctation of the aorta. *Circulation* 1987; 75:689–695.
23. Bonderman D, Gharehbaghi-Schnell E, Wollenek G, et al. Mechanisms underlying aortic dilatation in congenital aortic valve malformation. *Circulation* 1999; 99:2138–2143.
24. Tsipouras P, Del Mastro R, Sarfarazi M, et al. Genetic linkage of the Marfan syndrome, ectopia lentis, and congenital contractural arachnodactyly to the fibrillin genes on chromosomes 15 and 5. *N Engl J Med* 1992; 326:905–909.
25. Roberts CS, Roberts WC. Dissection of the aorta associated with congenital malformation of the aortic valve. *J Am Coll Cardiol* 1991; 17:712–716.
26. Nistri S, Sorbo MD, Marin M, et al. Aortic root dilatation in young men with normally functioning bicuspid valves. *Heart* 1999; 82:19–22.
27. Lindsay J Jr. Coarctation of the aorta, bicuspid aortic valve and abnormal ascending aortic wall. *Am J Cardiol* 1988; 61:182–184.
28. Subramaniam PN. Turner's syndrome and cardiovascular abnormalities: A case report and review of the literature. *Am J Med Sci* 1989; 297:260–262.
29. Nunez L, O'Connor LF, Pinto AG, et al. Annuloaortic ectasia and adult polycystic kidney: A frequent association. *Chest* 1986; 90:299–300.
30. Biagini A, Maffei S, Baroni M, et al. Familial clustering of aortic dissection in polycystic kidney disease. *Am J Cardiol* 1993; 72:741–742.
31. Leier CV, Call TD, Fulkerson PK, et al. The spectrum of defects in the Ehlers-Danlos syndrome, types I and III. *Ann Intern Med* 1980; 92:171–178.
32. Hortop J, Tsipouras P, Hanley JA, et al. Cardiovascular involvement in osteogenesis imperfecta. *Circulation* 1986; 73:54–61.
33. Marsalese DL, Moodie DS, Lytle BW, et al. Cystic medial necrosis of the aorta in patients without Marfan's syndrome: Surgical outcome and long-term follow-up. *J Am Coll Cardiol* 1990; 16:68–73.
34. Roman MJ, Devereux RB, Niles NW, et al. Aortic root dilatation as a cause of isolated, severe aortic regurgitation. *Ann Intern Med* 1987; 106:800–807.
35. Milewicz DM, Michael K, Fisher N, et al. Fibrillin-1 (*FBN1*) mutations in patients with thoracic aortic aneurysms. *Circulation* 1996; 94:2708–2711.
36. Ewart JM, Burke ML, Bunt TJ. Spontaneous abdominal aortic infections: Essentials of diagnosis and management. *Am Surg* 1983; 49:37–50.
37. Jackman JD, Radolf JD. Cardiovascular syphilis. *Am J Med* 1989; 87:425–433.
38. Atnip RG. Mycotic aneurysms of the suprarenal abdominal aorta: Prolonged survival after in situ aortic and visceral reconstruction. *J Vasc Surg* 1989; 10:635–641.
39. Oz MC, McNicholas KW, Serra AJS, et al. Review of *Salmonella* mycotic aneurysms of the thoracic aorta. *J Cardiovasc Surg* 1989; 30:99–103.
40. Cohen PS, O'Brien TF, Schoenbaum SC, Medeiros AA. The risk of endothelial infection in adults with salmonella bacteremia. *Ann Intern Med* 1978; 89:931–932.
41. Johansen K, Devin J. Mycotic aortic aneurysms: A reappraisal. *Arch Surg* 1983; 118:583–641.
42. Sessa C, Farah I, Voirin L, et al. Infected aneurysms of the infrarenal abdominal aorta: Diagnostic criteria and therapeutic strategy. *Ann Vasc Surg* 1997; 11:453–463.
43. Oskoui R, Davis WA, Gomes MN. *Salmonella* aortitis: A report of a successfully treated case with a comprehensive review of the literature. *Arch Intern Med* 1993; 153:517–525.
44. Bennett DE. Primary mycotic aneurysms of the aorta. *Arch Surg* 1967; 94:758–765.
45. Allins AD, Wagner WH, Cossman DV, et al. Tuberculous infection of the descending thoracic and abdominal aorta: Case report and literature review. *Ann Vasc Surg* 1999; 13:439–444.
46. Golzarian J, Cheng J, Giron F, et al. Tuberculous pseudoaneu-

rysm of the descending thoracic aorta. *Tex Heart Inst J* 1999; 26:232–235.

47. Arnett EN, Roberts WC. Valve ring abscess in active infective endocarditis: Frequency, location, and clues to clinical diagnosis from the study of 95 necropsy patients. *Circulation* 1976; 54:140–145.
48. Daniel WG, Mugge A, Martin RP, et al. Improvement in the diagnosis of abscesses associated with endocarditis by transesophageal echocardiography. *N Engl J Med* 1991; 324:795–800.
49. Feigl D, Feigl A, Edwards JE. Mycotic aneuryms of the aortic root: A pathologic study of 20 cases. *Chest* 1986; 90:553–557.
50. Ito I. Aortitis syndrome (Takayasu's arteritis): A historical perspective. *Jpn Heart J* 1995; 36:273–281.
51. Kerr GS, Hallahan CW, Giordano J, et al. Takayasu Arteritis. *Ann Intern Med* 1994; 120:919–929.
52. Ishikawa K. Diagnostic approach and proposed criteria for the clinical diagnosis of Takayasu's arteriopathy. *J Am Coll Cardiol* 1988; 12:964–972.
53. Noris M, Daina E, Gamba S, et al. Interleukin-6 and RANTES in Takayasu's arteritis: A guide for therapeutic decisions. *Circulation* 1999; 100:55–60.
54. Eichorn J, Sima D, Thiele B, et al. Anti-endothelial cell antibodies in Takayasu's arteritis. *Circulation* 1996; 94:2396–2401.
55. Takeuchi Y, Matsuki K, Saito Y, et al. HLA-D region genomic polymorphism associated with Takayasu's arteritis. *Angiology* 1990; 41:421–426.
56. Ishikawa K, Maetani S. Long-term outcome for 120 Japanese patients with Takayasu's disease. *Circulation* 1994; 90:1855–1860.
57. Wong VCW, Wang RYC, Tse TF. Pregnancy and Takayasu's arteritis. *Am J Med* 1983; 75:597–601.
58. Arend WP, Michel BA, Bloch DA, et al. The American College of Rheumatology 1990 criteria for the classification of Takayasu arteritis. *Arthritis Rheum* 1990; 33:1129–1134.
59. Ishikawa K. Effects of prednisolone therapy on arterial angiographic features in Takayasu's disease. *Am J Cardiol* 1991; 68:410–413.
60. Fraga A, Mintz G, Valle L, et al. Takayasu's arteritis: Frequency of systemic manifestations (study of 22 patients) and favorable response to maintenance corticosteroid therapy with adrenocorticosteroids (12 patients). *Arthritis Rheum* 1972; 15:617–624.
61. Tyagi S, Singh B, Kaul UA, et al. Balloon angioplasty for renovascular hypertension in Takayasu's arteritis. *Am Heart J* 1993; 125:1386–1393.
62. Evans JM, O'Fallon WM, Hunder GG. Increased incidence of aortic aneurysm and dissection in giant cell (temporal) arteritis. *Ann Intern Med* 1995; 122:502–507.
63. Bergfeldt L, Insulander P, Lindblom D, et al. HLA-B27: An important genetic risk factor for lone aortic regurgitation and severe conduction system abnormalities. *Am J Med* 1988; 85:12–18.
64. Bulkley BH, Roberts WC. Ankylosing spondylitis and aortic regurgitation: Description of the characteristic cardiovascular lesion from study of eight necropsy patients. *Circulation* 1973; 48:1014–1027.
65. Roldan CA, Chavez J, Wiest PW, et al. Aortic root disease and valve disease associated with ankylosing spondylitis. *J Am Coll Cardiol* 1998; 32:1397–1404.
66. Kent KC, Boyce SW. Aneurysms of the aorta. In: Lindsay J Jr, ed. *Diseases of the Aorta*. Philadelphia: Lea and Febiger; 1994:109–125.
67. Patel MI, Hardman DTA, Fisher CM. Current views on the pathogenesis of abdominal aortic aneurysms. *J Am Coll Surg* 1995; 181:371–382.
68. Heinemann M, Laas J, Karck M, et al. Thoracic aortic aneurysm after acute type A aortic dissection: Necessity for follow-up. *Ann Thorac Surg* 1990; 49:580–584.
69. Verloes A, Sakalihasan N, Koulischer L, et al. Aneurysms of the abdominal aorta: Familial and genetic aspects in three hundred thirteen pedigrees. *J Vasc Surg* 1995; 21:646–655.
70. Salo JA, Soisalon-Soininen S, Bondestam S, et al. Familial occurrence of abdominal aneurysm. *Ann Intern Med* 1999; 130: 637–642.
71. Davies MJ. Aortic aneurysm formation. *Circulation* 1998; 98:193–195.
72. Sakakibara S, Konno S. Congenital aneurysm of the sinus of Valsalva: Anatomy and classification. *Am Heart J* 1962; 63:405–424.
73. Lindsay J Jr. Anatomic and pathogenetic bases for some uncommon clinical syndromes from aortic disease. In: Lindsay J Jr, ed. *Diseases of the Aorta*. Philadelphia: Lea and Febiger; 1994:165–177.
74. Smith JA, Fann JI, Miller DC, et al. Surgical management of aortic dissection in patients with the Marfan syndrome. *Circulation* 1994; 90(2):II235–II242.
75. Joyce JW, Fairbairn JF II, Kincaid OW, et al. Aneurysms of the thoracic aorta: A clinical study with special reference to prognosis. *Circulation* 1964; 29:176–181.
76. Pressler V, McNamara JJ. Thoracic aortic aneurysm: Natural history and treatment. *J Thorac Cardiovasc Surg* 1980; 79:489–498.
77. Goldstein SA, Lindsay J Jr. Thoracic aortic aneurysms: Role of echocardiography. *Echocardiography* 1996; 13:213–232.
78. Clouse WD, Hallett JW Jr, Schaff HV, et al. Improved prognosis of thoracic aortic aneurysms. *JAMA* 1998; 280:1926–1929.
79. Murdoch JL, Walker BA, Halpern BL, et al. Life expectancy and causes of death in the Marfan syndrome. *N Engl J Med* 1972; 286:804–808.
80. Silverman DI, Burton KJ, Gray J, et al. Life expectancy in the Marfan Syndrome. *Am J Cardiol* 1995; 75:157–160.
81. Dake MD, Miller DC, Mitchell RS, et al. The "first generation" of endovascular stent-grafts for patients with aneurysms of the descending thoracic aorta. *J Thorac Cardiovasc Surg* 1998; 116:689–704.
82. Dapunt OE, Galla JD, Sadeghi AM, et al. The natural history of thoracic aortic aneurysms. *J Thorac Cardiovasc Surg* 1994; 107:1323–1333.
83. Kouchoukos NT, Dougenis D. Surgery of the thoracic aorta. *N Engl J Med* 1997; 336:1876–1888.
84. Coady MA, Rizzo JA, Hammond GL, et al. What is the appropriate size criterion for resection of thoracic aortic aneurysms? *J Thorac Cardiovasc Surg* 1997; 113:476–491.
85. Juvonen T, Ergin MA, Galla JD, et al. Prospective study of the natural history of thoracic aortic aneuryms. *Ann Thorac Surg* 1997; 63:1533–1545.
86. Ernst CB. Abdominal aortic aneurysm. *N Engl J Med* 1993; 328:1167–1172.
87. Sterpetti AV, Hunter WJ, Feldhaus RJ, et al. Inflammatory aneurysms of the abdominal aorta: Incidence, pathologic, and etiologic considerations. *J Vasc Surg* 1989; 9:643–650.
88. Leseche G, Schaetz A, Arrive L, et al. Diagnosis and management of 17 consecutive patients with inflammatory abdominal aortic aneurysms. *Am J Surg* 1992; 164:39–44.

88a. Sullivan CA, Rohrer MJ, Cutler BS. Clinical management of the symptomatic but unruptured abdominal aortic aneurysm. *J Vasc Surg* 1990; 11:799–803.

88b. Bower TC, Cherry KJ Jr, Pairolero PC. Unusual manifestations of abdominal aortic aneurysms. *Surg Clin North Am* 1989; 69:745–754.

89. Keen RR, McCarthy WJ, Shireman PK, et al. Surgical management of atheroembolization. *J Vasc Surg* 1995; 21:773–781.
90. Dolmatch BL, Gray RJ, Horton KM, et al. Diagnostic imaging in the evaluation of aortic disease. In: Lindsay J Jr, ed. *Diseases of the Aorta*. Philadelphia: Lea and Febiger; 1994:197–250.
91. Scott RAP, Wilson NM, Ashton HA, et al. Is surgery necessary

for abdominal aneurysm less than 6 cm in diameter? *Lancet* 1993; 342:1395–1396.

92. Vazquez C, Sakalihasan N, D'Harcour J-B, et al. Routine ultrasound screening for abdominal aortic aneurysm among 65- and 75-year-old men in a city of 200,000 inhabitants. *Ann Vasc Surg* 1998; 12:544–549.
93. Lederle FA. Management of small abdominal aortic aneurysms. *Ann Intern Med* 1990; 113:731–732.
94. Nevitt MP, Ballard DJ, Hallett JW Jr. Prognosis of abdominal aortic aneurysm: A population-based study. *N Engl J Med* 1989; 321:1009–1014.
95. Guiruis EM, Barber GG. The natural history of abdominal aortic aneurysms. *Am J Surg* 1991; 162:481–483.
96. Nehler MR, Taylor LM Jr, Moneta GL, et al. Indications for operation for infrarenal abdominal aneurysms: Current guidelines. *Semin Vasc Surg* 1995; 8:108–114.
97. UK Small Aneurysm Trial Participants. Mortality results for randomised controlled trial of early elective surgery or ultrasonographic surveillance for small abdominal aortic aneurysms. *Lancet* 1998; 352:1649–1655.
98. Roger VL, Ballard DJ, Hallett JW Jr, et al. Influence of coronary artery disease on morbidity and mortality after abdominal aortic aneurysmectomy: A population-based study, 1971–1987. *J Am Coll Cardiol* 1989; 14:1245–1252.
99. Graor RA. Preoperative evaluation and management of coronary and carotid artery occlusive disease in patients with abdominal aortic aneurysms. *Surg Clin North Am* 1989; 69:737–743.
100. Cambria RP, Eagle K. Cardiac screening before abdominal aortic aneurysm surgery: A reassessment. *Semin Vasc Surg* 1995; 8:93–102.
101. Koskas F, Kieffer E, for the AURC. Surgery for ruptured abdominal aortic aneurysm: Early and late results of a prospective study by the AURC in 1989. *Ann Vasc Surg* 1997; 11:473–481.
102. Zarins CK, White RA, Schwarten D, et al. Aneux stent graft versus open surgical repair of abdominal aortic aneurysms: Multicenter prospective trials. *J Vasc Surg* 1999; 29:292–308.
103. Seelig MH, Oldenburg WA, Hakaim AG, et al. Endovascular repair of abdominal aortic aneurysms: Where do we stand? *Mayo Clin Proc* 1999; 74:999–1010.
104. Spittell PC, Spittell JA Jr, Joyce JW, et al. Clinical features and differential diagnosis of aortic dissection: Experience with 236 cases (1980–1990). *Mayo Clin Proc* 1993; 68:642–651.
105. Crawford ES. The diagnosis and management of aortic dissection. *JAMA* 1990; 264:2537–2541.
106. Lindsay J Jr. Aortic dissection. In: Lindsay J Jr, ed. *Diseases of the Aorta*. Philadelphia: Lea and Febiger; 1999:127–142.
107. Roberts WC. Aortic dissection: Anatomy, consequences, and causes. *Am Heart J* 1981; 101:195–214.
108. Hirst AE Jr, Johns VJ Jr, Kime SW Jr. Dissecting aneurysms of the aorta: A review of 505 cases. *Medicine* 1958; 37:217–279.
109. Mohr-Kahaly S, Erbel R, Kearney P, et al. Aortic intramural hemorrhage visualized by transesophageal echocardiography: Findings and prognostic implications. *J Am Coll Cardiol* 1994; 23:658–664.
110. Nienaber CA, von Kodolitsch Y, Peterson B, et al. Intramural hemorrhage of the thoracic aorta: Diagnostic and therapeutic implications. *Circulation* 1995; 92:1465–1472.
111. Harris KM, Braverman AC, Gutierrez FR, et al. Transesophageal echocardiographic and clinical features of aortic intramural hematoma. *J Thorac Cardiovasc Surg* 1997; 114:619–626.
112. Bansal RC, Chandrasekaran K, Ayala K, et al. Frequency and explanation of false negative diagnosis of aortic dissection by aortography and transesophageal echocardiography. *J Am Coll Cardiol* 1995; 25:1393–1401.
113. Svensson LG, Labib SB, Eisenhauer AC, et al. Intimal tear without hematoma: An important variant of aortic dissection that can elude current imaging techniques. *Circulation* 1999; 99:1331–1336.
114. Lindsay J Jr. Aortocameral fistula: A rare complication of aortic dissection. *Am Heart J* 1993; 126:441–443.
115. Kamp TJ, Goldschmidt-Clermont PJ, Brinker JA, et al. Myocardial infarction, aortic dissection, and thrombolytic therapy. *Am Heart J* 1994; 128:1234–1237.
116. Hughes JD, Bacha EA, Dodson TF, et al. Peripheral vascular complications of aortic dissection. *Am J Surg* 1995; 170:209–212.
117. Moore NR, Parry AJ, Trottman-Dickenson B, et al. Fate of the native aorta after repair of acute type A dissection: A magnetic resonance imaging study. *Heart* 1996; 75:62–66.
118. Williams GM, Gott VL, Brawley RK, et al. Aortic disease associated with pregnancy. *J Vasc Surg* 1988; 8:470–475.
119. Oskoui R, Lindsay J Jr. Aortic dissection in women less than 40 years of age and the unimportance of pregnancy. *Am J Cardiol* 1994; 73:821–822.
120. Keren A, Kim CB, Hu BS, et al. Accuracy of biplane and multiplane transesophageal echocardiography in diagnosis of typical acute aortic dissection and intramural hematoma. *J Am Coll Cardiol* 1996; 28:627–636.
121. Cigarroa JE, Isselbacher EM, DeSanctis RW, et al. Diagnostic imaging in the evaluation of suspected aortic dissection. *N Engl J Med* 1993; 328:35–43.
122. Armstrong WF, Bach DS, Carey LM, et al. Clinical and echocardiographic findings in patients with suspected acute aortic dissection. *Am Heart J* 1998; 136:1051–1060.
123. Lindsay J Jr, Hurst JW. Clinical features and prognosis in dissecting aneurysm of the aorta: A reappraisal. *Circulation* 1967; 35:880–888.
124. Doroghazi RM, Slater EE, DeSanctis RW, et al. Long-term survival of patients with treated aortic dissection. *J Am Coll Cardiol* 1984; 3:1026–1034.
125. Juvonen T, Ergin MA, Galla JD, et al. Risk factors for rupture of chronic type-B dissections. *J Thorac Cardiovasc Surg* 1999; 117:776–786.
126. Nienaber CA, Fattori R, Lund G, et al. Nonsurgical reconstruction of thoracic aortic dissection by stent-graft placement. *N Engl J Med* 1999; 340:1539–1545.
127. Reifenstein GH, Levine SA, Gross RE. Coarctation of the aorta. *Am Heart J* 1947; 33:146–168.
128. Liberthson RR, Pennington DG, Jacobs ML, et al. Coarctation of the aorta: Review of 234 patients and clarification of management problems. *Am J Cardiol* 1979; 43:835–840.
129. Maron BJ, Humphries JO, Rowe RD, et al. Prognosis of surgically corrected coarctation of the aorta: A 20-year postoperative appraisal. *Circulation* 1973; 47:119–126.
130. McCrindle BW, Jones TK, Morrow WR, et al. Acute results of balloon angioplasty of native coarctation versus recurrent aortic obstruction are equivalent. *J Am Coll Cardiol* 1996; 28:1810–1817.
131. Eid Fawzy M, SivanandamV, Galal O, et al. One- to ten-year follow-up results of balloon angioplasty of native coarctation of the aorta in adolescents and adults. *J Am Coll Cardiol* 1997; 30:1542–1546.
132. Ebeid MR, Prieto LR, Latson LA. Use of balloon-expandable stents for coarctation of the aorta: Initial results and intermediate-term follow-up. *J Am Coll Cardiol* 1997; 30:1847–1852.
133. Hoeffel JC, Henry M, Mentre B, et al. Pseudocoarctation or congenital kinking of the aorta: Radiologic considerations. *Am Heart J* 1975; 89:428–436.
134. Bergamini TM, Bernard JD, Mavroudis C, et al. Coarctation of the abdominal aorta. *Ann Vasc Surg* 1995; 9:352–356.
135. Lindsay J Jr. Acquired obstructive disease of the aorta. In: Lindsay J Jr, ed. *Diseases of the Aorta*. Philadelphia: Lea and Febiger; 1994:145–156.
136. Mickley V, Fleiter T. Coarctations of the descending and abdomi-

nal aorta: Long-term results of surgical therapy. *J Vasc Surg* 1998; 28:206–214.

137. Lande A. Takayasu's arteritis and congenital coarctation of the descending thoracic and abdominal aorta: A critical review. *AJR* 1976; 127:227–233.
138. Brewster DC. Clinical and anatomical considerations for surgery in aortoiliac disease and results of surgical treatment. *Circulation* 1991; 83(suppl I):I-42–52.
139. Stubbs DH, Kasulke RJ, Kapsch DN, et al. Populations with the Leriche syndrome. *Surgery* 1981; 89:612–616.
140. Sharp WV, Donovan DL, Teague PC, et al. Arterial occlusive disease: A function of vessel bifurcation angle. *Surgery* 1982; 91:680–685.
141. Palmaz JC, Carson SN, Hunter G, et al. Male hypoplastic infrarenal aorta and premature atherosclerosis. *Surgery* 1983; 94: 91–94.
142. Leriche R, Morel A. The syndrome of thrombotic obliteration of the aortic bifurcation. *Ann Surg* 1948; 127:193–204.
143. Busuttil RW, Keehn G, Milliken J, et al. Aortic saddle embolus: A twenty-year experience. *Ann Surg* 1983; 197:698–706.
144. Webb KH, Jacocks MA. Acute aortic occlusion. *Am J Surg* 1988; 155:405–407.

CHAPTER 89

CEREBROVASCULAR DISEASE AND NEUROLOGIC MANIFESTATIONS OF HEART DISEASE

Louis R. Caplan

Most vascular diseases affect both the heart and the brain. Heart diseases often lead to lesions and dysfunction within the brain, and central nervous system (CNS) diseases influence the heart and its function.

BRAIN AND CEREBROVASCULAR COMPLICATIONS OF HEART DISEASE

Cerebral complications occur when (1) the heart pumps unwanted materials into the circulation that reach the brain (embolism), (2) pump function fails and the brain is hypoperfused, and (3) drugs given to treat cardiac disease have neurologic side effects.

Cardiogenic Brain Embolism

ETIOLOGY

The diagnostic criteria for cardiogenic embolism were formerly very restrictive. Embolism was diagnosed when sudden focal neurologic signs, maximal at onset, developed in patients with peripheral systemic embolism and recent myocardial infarction or rheumatic mitral stenosis.[1] With the use of these criteria, cardiogenic embolism was diagnosed in only 3 to 8 percent of stroke patients.[2–5] None of these criteria are secure. In various stroke registries, about 10 to 20 percent of patients did not have maximal symptoms at onset.[5–7] Many other cardiac lesions are now well-accepted sources of emboli, e.g., atrial fibrillation. Only about 2 percent of patients with a cardiogenic brain embolism have clinically recognized peripheral emboli. In necropsy studies of patients with brain embolism, however, infarcts are found commonly in the spleen and kidneys and in other organs. The symptoms of peripheral embolism are often so minor and nonspecific (transient abdominal discomfort, leg cramp, etc.) that they seldom are diagnosed correctly.

Before the advent of echocardiography, 30 percent of stroke patients were considered likely to have a cardiogenic embolism.[5,6] Later studies using stricter criteria attributed up to 22 percent[8] of strokes to a cardiogenic embolism. With more advanced diagnostic techniques, more cardiac abnormalities are recognized; in the Lausanne Stroke Registry, 23 percent of patients with a first stroke had a potential cardiac source of embolism.[9] Because many patients have coexisting cardiac and extracranial vascular disease,[9] criteria for the diagnosis of cardiac embolism remain controversial.

Cardiac sources can be divided into three groups:[1] (1) *cardiac wall and chamber abnormalities*, e.g., cardiomyopathies, hypokinetic and akinetic ventricular regions after myocardial infarction, atrial septal aneurysms, ventricular aneurysms, atrial myxomas, papillary fibroelastomas and other tumors, septal defects, and patent foramen ovale, (2) *valve disorders*, e.g., rheumatic mitral and aortic disease, prosthetic valves, bacterial endocarditis, fibrous and fibrinous endocardial lesions, mitral valve prolapse, and mitral annulus calcification, and (3) *arrhythmias*, especially atrial fibrillation and "sick-sinus" syndrome.

Some cardiac sources have much higher rates of initial and

recurrent embolism. The Stroke Data Bank[10] divided potential sources into *strong sources* (prosthetic valves, atrial fibrillation, sick-sinus syndrome, ventricular aneurysm, akinetic segments, mural thrombi, cardiomyopathy, diffuse ventricular hypokinesia) and *weak sources* (myocardial infarct over 6 months old, aortic and mitral stenosis and regurgitation, congestive failure, mitral valve prolapse, mitral annulus calcification, hypokinetic ventricular segments).

The risk of embolism varies within individual cardiac abnormalities, depending on many factors. For example, in patients with atrial fibrillation, associated heart disease, patient age, duration, chronic versus intermittent fibrillation, and atrial size all influence embolic risk. The presence of a potential cardiac source of embolism does not mean that a stroke was caused by an embolus from the heart. Coexistent occlusive cerebrovascular disease is common. In the Lausanne registry, among patients with potential cardiac embolic sources, 11 percent had severe cervicocranial vascular occlusive disease (>75 percent stenosis) and 40 percent had mild to moderate stenosis proximal to brain infarcts.[9]

Mitral valve prolapse (MVP) as a source of embolism continues to be controversial[1] (see Chap. 58). Clinical studies indicate that MVP is associated with stroke.[11,12] Morphologic lesions such as thrombi and fibrous lesions clearly suggest embolism;[13] fibrin-platelet depositions on the surfaces of the mitral leaflets have been noted,[13] as well as thrombi in the angle between the posterior mitral valve leaflet and the left atrial wall.[12,14] Patients with MVP also have other disorders, such as atrial fibrillation, syncope, and migraine. The rate of recurrence of stroke in patients with MVP as the only known cause is very low.[11,12] In light of the very high incidence of MVP, the frequency of MVP-related stroke is extremely low.[12,14,15] Most neurologists feel that warfarin anticoagulants ordinarily are not indicated in prophylaxis of patients with MVP even after an initial stroke. Aspirin prophylaxis (80 to 325 mg/day) is, however, advisable. Demonstration of an intracardiac thrombus by echocardiography would change that recommendation to warfarin.

Mitral annulus calcification (MAC) is an important and often unrecognized cause of embolism. Ulceration and extrusion of calcium through overlapping cusps have been seen at necropsy,[16] thrombi have been found on valves attached to the ulcerative process,[17] and calcific emboli have been seen in surgical embolectomies.[12,16] Several series have shown a convincing relationship between MAC and brain emboli and stroke.[1,18,19] Bacterial endocarditis also can develop on a MAC.

More patients have cardiogenic embolism than are diagnosed. Clinical features and brain investigations such as computed tomography (CT), magnetic resonance imaging (MRI), and angiography (CT, MRI, and digital subtraction) may suggest emboli, but often a source is not identified. These cases, which are termed *infarcts of unknown causes* (IUC) in the Stroke Data Bank,[6,20] include as many as 40 percent of patients.

Some disorders are associated with *fibrous and fibrinous lesions of the heart valves and endocardium.*[1] Similar valve lesions occur in patients with systemic lupus erythematosus (Libman-Sachs endocarditis[21]), the antiphospholipid antibody syndrome,[22] and cancer and other debilitating diseases (nonbacterial thrombotic endocarditis). Mobile fibrous strands also are found frequently during echocardiography.[1,23,24] Fibrin-platelet aggregates may attach to these fibrous and fibrinous lesions. Warfarin anticoagulants are ineffective in preventing embolism in these conditions.

Embolic complications are common in patients who have *infective endocarditis.*[1,25] Mycotic aneurysms can cause fatal subarachnoid bleeding. Bleeding also can result from vascular necrosis caused by an infected embolus.[25] Embolization usually stops when infection is controlled.[25] Warfarin does not prevent embolization and probably is contraindicated unless there are other important lesions, such as prosthetic valves and life-threatening pulmonary embolism (see Chap. 73). In children and young adults with congenital heart defects, especially those with right-to-left shunts and polycythemia, brain abscess is an important complication (see Chap. 63).

Emboli often arise from sources other than the heart, such as the aorta, proximal arteries (intraarterial or so-called local embolism), leg veins (paradoxical emboli), fat in the liver or bones (fat embolism), and materials introduced by the patient or physician (drug particles or air).[1] The type of embolic material also varies (Table 89-1).[1,26] *Atheromatous plaques in the aortic arch and ascending aorta are a very important and previously neglected source of embolism to the brain* (Figs. 89-1 and 89-2). Ulcerated atheromatous plaques often are found at necropsy in patients with ischemic strokes, especially patients in whom the stroke etiology was not determined during life.[27] Transesophageal echocardiography (TEE) often shows these atheromas, but technical factors limit visualization of the entire arch (see Chap. 13). The aorta also can be insonated by B-mode ultrasound probes placed in the supraclavicular fossa on each side.[28] *Large (>4 mm), protruding mobile aortic atheromas are especially likely to cause embolic strokes and are associated with a high rate of recurrent strokes.*[29]

CLINICAL FINDINGS

Anterior Circulation Recipient Sites Balloons placed into the circulation tend to follow the same flow patterns;[30] anterior circulation material reaches the middle cerebral arteries (MCA) and their branches.[30] The most common sites are the mainstem MCA, the upper or lower divisions of the MCA, and their branches. The upper division of the MCA supplies the frontal and parietal lobes above the sylvian fissure, and the lower division supplies the convexal temporal and inferior parietal lobes. Resultant neurologic deficits include the following.

MCA UPPER DIVISION Contralateral hemiparesis, hemisensory loss; aphasia (left hemisphere); lack of awareness of deficit, neglect of the left visual space, and motor impersistence[31] (right hemisphere).

MCA INFERIOR DIVISION Wernicke-type fluent aphasia, agitation, right-upper-quadrantanopia (left hemisphere); agitation and hyperactivity, left neglect, poor drawing and copying (right hemisphere).[32]

MCA MAINSTEM Findings include features of both upper and lower division infarcts.

Posterior Circulation Recipient Sites Vertebrobasilar territory symptoms usually are attributed to local disease within that circulation without consideration of a possible cardiogenic

TABLE 89-1 Embolic Materials

Cardiac	Intraarterial
1. Red fibrin-dependent thrombi	1. Red fibrin-dependent thrombi
2. White platelet-fibrin nidi	2. White platelet-fibrin nidi
3. Material from marantic endocarditis	3. Combined fibrin-platelet and fibrin-dependent clots
4. Bacteria from vegetations	4. Cholesterol crystals
5. Calcium from valves and mitral annulus calcification	5. Atheromatous plaque debris
6. Myxoma cells and debris	6. Calcium from vascular calcifications
	7. Air
	8. Mucin from tumors
	9. Talc or microcrystalline cellulose from injected drugs

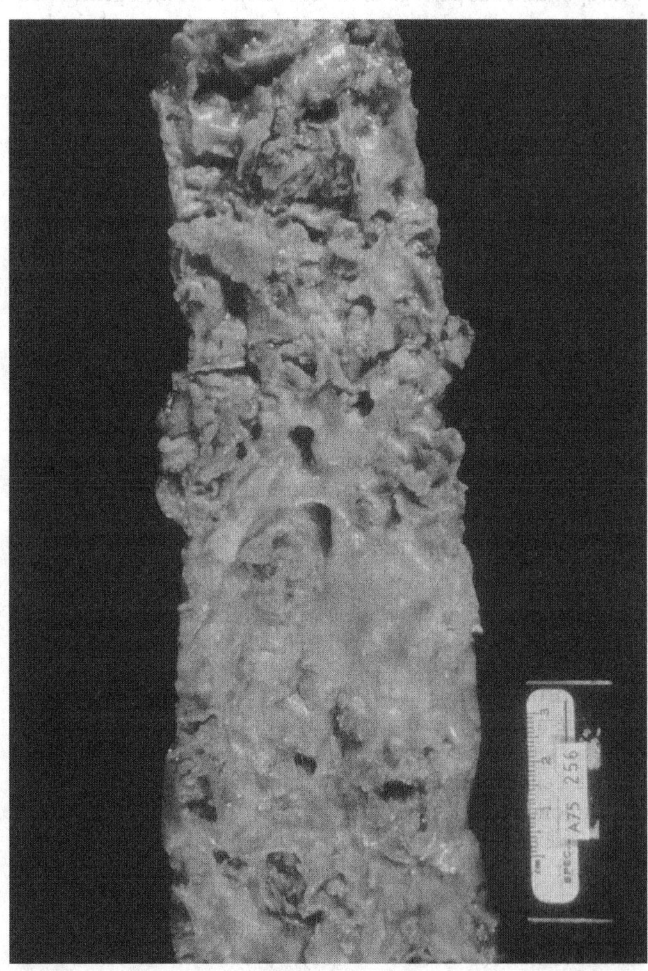

FIGURE 89-1 Descending aorta at necropsy from a patient in whom TEE before surgery showed severe disease of the ascending aorta and aortic arch with mobile protruding plaques. This patient died after CAB surgery, having never awakened after the procedure. Submitted by Dr. Denise Barbut. (From Caplan LR. *Stroke: A Clinical Approach*, 3d ed. Boston: Butterworth-Heinemann; 2000, with permission.)

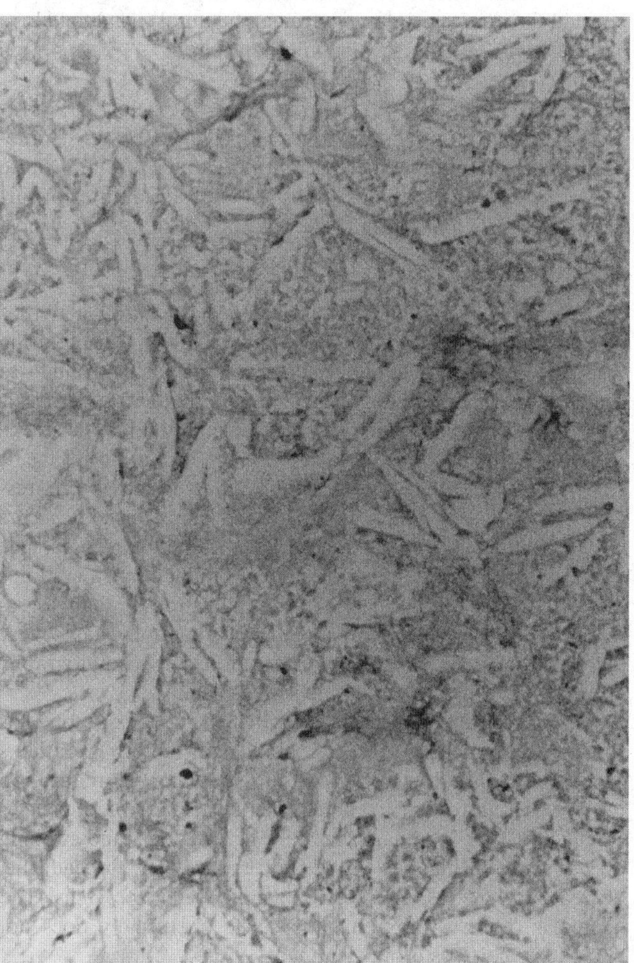

FIGURE 89-2 Cholesterol crystals and other particulate debris are caught in a filter placed in the aorta at the time when aortic clamps are removed. Submitted by Dr. Denise Barbut. (From Caplan LR. *Stroke: A Clinical Approach*, 3d ed. Boston: Butterworth-Heinemann; 2000, with permission.)

embolism. In the major stroke registries,[1,5,9] however, about 20 percent of emboli of cardiac origin go to the posterior circulation. Twenty percent is expected, as about one-fifth of cerebral blood flow goes to this circulation. In the posterior circulation, certain recipient sites are favored.

POSTERIOR CEREBRAL ARTERY (PCA)[33,34] Particles and clots go to the most distal part of the system; the PCA is the terminal vessel in the vertebrobasilar circuit. The hallmark of PCA lesions is hemianopia and/or hemisensory loss contralateral to the infarct. Patients with left-PCA territory infarcts also often cannot read or name colors but retain the ability to write and spell. Amnesia is sometimes prominent and may last up to 6 months. Right-PCA territory infarction often is associated with left visual neglect.

TOP OF THE BASILAR ARTERY[35] The major clinical features are apathy and sleepiness; abnormal vertical gaze; and hallucinations, unusual reports, and other behavioral abnormalities. Bilateral PCA territory infarction causes bilateral visual field loss, amnesia, and severe agitation and delirium.

VERTEBRAL ARTERY (VA) INTRACRANIALLY AND ITS POSTERIOR INFERIOR CEREBELLAR ARTERY (PICA) BRANCH Somewhat larger emboli may occlude an intracranial VA and cause cerebellar infarction involving mostly the posterior inferior surface.[36] Ataxia, vomiting, and occipital headache are the most common signs.

Onset and Course Most embolic events occur during activities of daily living, but some embolic strokes have their onset during rest or sleep. Sudden coughing, sneezing, or arising at night to urinate can precipitate an embolism.[1,5] Although the deficit is most often maximal at the outset, 11 percent of embolic stroke patients in the Harvard Stroke Registry had a stuttering or stepwise course, whereas 10 percent had fluctuations or progressive deficits. Later progression, if it develops, usually occurs within the first 48 h. Progression usually is due to distal passage of emboli. "Nonsudden embolism" is explained by an embolus moving from its initial location, as demonstrated by angiography, to a more distal branch.[1] Early angiography has a very high rate of showing intracranial emboli,[6,37] but angiography after 48 h shows a much lower rate of blockage.

More recently, transcranial Doppler (TCD) sonography has shown a high incidence of MCA blockage acutely in patients with sudden-onset hemispheric strokes, but later, recanalization of the MCA and normalization of the intracranial blood velocities occur.[1,38] As in all large infarcts, brain edema and swelling may develop during the 24 to 72 h after a stroke, with headache, decreased alertness, and worsening of neurologic signs. The edema is often cytotoxic (inside cells) and usually does not respond to corticosteroid treatment.

DIAGNOSTIC TESTING

Emboli usually cause occlusion of distal branches and produce surface infarcts that are roughly triangular, with the apex of the triangle pointing inward. CT and MRI findings can suggest the presence of embolism by the location and shape of the lesion,[39] the presence of superficial wedge-shaped infarcts in multiple different vascular territories, hemorrhagic infarction, and visualization of thrombi within arteries. Among 60 patients with cardiogenic sources of embolism studied by CT in whom occlusive atherosclerotic cerebrovascular disease had been excluded, 56 had superficial large or small cortical or subcortical infarcts and only 4 had deep infarcts.[39] Emboli can block the MCA and occasionally cause solely deep infarcts because the superficial territory has good collateral flow; these infarcts are called *striatocapsular* because they involve the internal capsule and the adjacent basal ganglia, which are supplied by lenticulostriate branches of the MCA.[1,5,40] Tiny emboli may cause small deep or superficial infarcts.

MRI is more sensitive for the detection of brain infarcts than is CT and is also superior in detecting hemorrhagic infarction by imaging hemosiderin. Hemorrhagic infarction has long been considered characteristic of embolism, especially when the artery leading to the infarct is patent.[41] The mechanism of hemorrhagic infarction is reperfusion of ischemic zones, which occurs with spontaneous passage of the embolus, after iatrogenic opening of an occluded artery (e.g., endarterectomy, fibrinolytic treatment), or after restoration of the circulation after a period of systemic hypoperfusion. Hemorrhage occurs into proximal reperfused regions of brain infarcts.[1,5,42] At times, it is also possible to image the acute embolus on CT.[1,43]

In unselected series of stroke patients, transthoracic echocardiography (TTE) (see Chap. 13) has been variably useful in detecting sources.[1,44,45] TTE is useful in patients with known cardiac disease to clarify potential embolic sources and heart function,[5] young patients without stroke risk factors, and stroke patients who do not have lacunar infarction or ultrasound evidence of intrinsic atherostenosis of a major extracranial and intracranial artery. TEE (see Chap. 13) provides much better visualization of the aorta, atria, cardiac valves, and septal regions. Reports of TEE suggest that the diagnostic yield is 2 to 10 times that of TTE.[46,47] Aortic plaques, atrial septal aneurysms, and atrial septal defects also are much better seen with TEE (Fig. 89-3). The use of an echo-enhancing agent such as agitated saline helps detect intracardiac shunts.

Echocardiography has definite limitations. Particles as small as 2 mm can block major brain arteries but are beyond the imaging resolution of current echocardiographic technology. Also, thromboembolism is a dynamic process. When a clot forms in the heart and embolizes, there may be no residual evidence until it re-forms.[1,26] Cardiac thrombi are imaged differently on sequential echocardiograms;[1,48] even large thrombi seen on one echocardiogram can disappear later.[48]

Embolic signals are now detected by monitoring with TCD.[1,49] Embolic particles passing under TCD probes produce transient, short-duration, high-intensity signals referred to as high-intensity transient signals (HITS). Examples of HITS are show in Figs. 89-4 and 89-5. TCD monitoring of patients with atrial fibrillation,[50] cardiac surgery,[51] prosthetic valves, left ventricular assist devices, carotid artery disease, and carotid endarterectomy have shown a relatively high frequency of embolic signals. In the future, monitoring of emboli with TCD will become an important diagnostic modality to guide treatment.

PREVENTION AND TREATMENT

Early studies showed that warfarin is effective in preventing brain embolism in patients with rheumatic mitral stenosis and atrial fibrillation (AF). Previously, the intensity of anticoagulation was higher than that currently used, and brain hemorrhages and other bleeding complications were common. Trials have now shown that low-dose warfarin [International Normalized Ratio (INR) 2.0 to 3.0] is also effective in preventing brain emboli in patients with nonrheumatic AF.

In the Copenhagen Atrial Fibrillation Aspirin Anticoagulation (AFASAK) study, 1007 patients (median age, 74.2 years) with chronic, nonrheumatic AF were assigned to warfarin (INR 2.8 to 4.2), aspirin (75 mg/day), or placebo.[52] The study was halted prematurely when an analysis of effectiveness reached a predetermined level of significance in favor of warfarin treatment. The principal outcome was the composite of ischemic or hemorrhagic stroke, transient ischemic attack (TIA), and systemic embolism. The observed reduction for warfarin compared to placebo was 64 percent, an absolute risk reduction of 3.5 percent per year. An analysis by intention to treat, which excluded TIA and minor stroke, indicated a risk reduction of about 50 percent ($p < .05$) and an absolute reduction of about 1.5 percent per year.

The Stroke Prevention in Atrial Fibrillation (SPAF) study investigators evaluated warfarin and aspirin in patients with nonrheumatic AF.[53] The study evaluated two groups of patients on the basis of their eligibility for warfarin. In the first group, 627 patients who were judged eligible for warfarin were randomized to open-label warfarin (INR, 2.8 to 4.5; prothrombin time, 1.3 to 1.8 times control) or were double-blinded to either aspirin (325 mg daily, enteric-coated) or matching placebo. In the second group, 703 patients ineligible for warfarin were randomized (double-blind) to aspirin (325 mg daily, enteric-coated) or placebo. The principal outcome, a composite of ischemic stroke and systemic embolism, was decreased significantly during a mean follow-up of 1.3 years. The outcome of disabling ischemic stroke or vascular death was reduced by warfarin by 54 percent ($p = .11$), an absolute reduction of 2.6 percent per year. Aspirin also decreased the principal outcome in both study

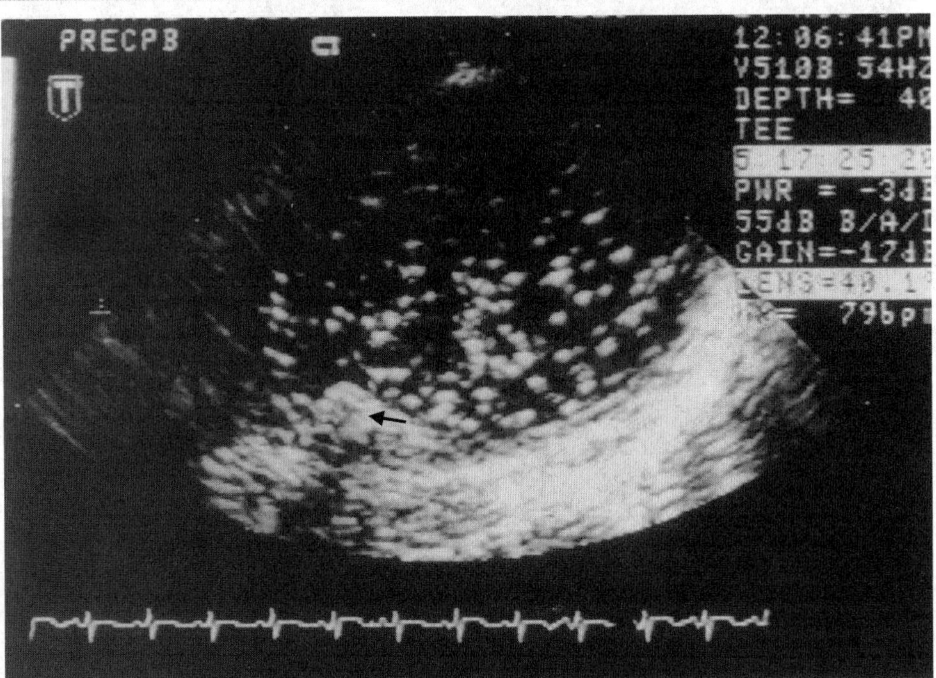

FIGURE 89-3 TEE recording during cardiac surgery from the aorta at the level of the origin of the left subclavian artery. A mobile plaque is seen protruding into the aortic lumen (small black arrow). This recording was taken after the release of aortic clamps and shows a "shower" of emboli within the aortic lumen beyond the area where the aorta was previously clamped. Submitted by Dr. Denise Barbut. (From Caplan LR. *Stroke: A Clinical Approach*, 3d ed. Boston: Butterworth-Heinemann; 2000, with permission.)

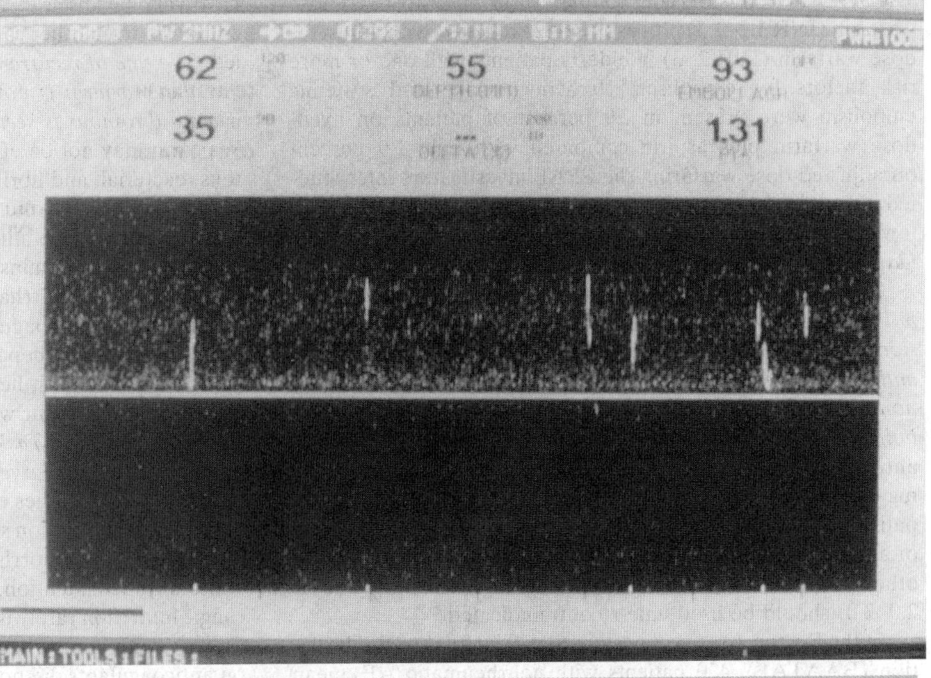

FIGURE 89-4 TCD recording from the MCA during steady-state cardiac bypass surgery at a time when the aorta was being manipulated. The white streaks represent microemboli. Submitted by Dr. Denise Barbut. (From Caplan LR. *Stroke: A Clinical Approach*, 3d ed. Boston: Butterworth-Heinemann; 2000, with permission.)

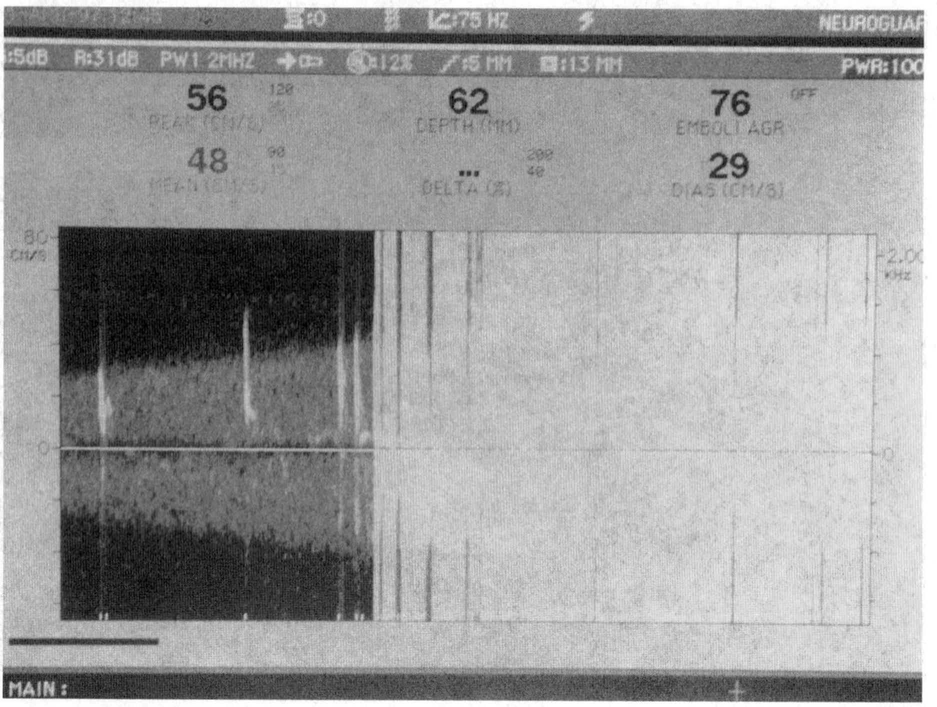

FIGURE 89-5 TCD recording from the MCA during cardiac bypass surgery. A few distinct emboli (white streaks in the left side of the figure) are followed by a massive shower of emboli ("whiteout") at the time of the release of aortic clamps. Submitted by Dr. Denise Barbut. (From Caplan LR. *Stroke: A Clinical Approach*, 3d ed. Boston: Butterworth-Heinemann; 2000, with permission.)

groups. The risk reduction was 42 percent (p = .02), and the absolute reduction was 2.7 percent per year. The outcome of disabling stroke or death was reduced 22 percent by aspirin (p = .33), an absolute reduction of about 1 percent per year. The SPAF investigators later compared low-intensity fixed-dose warfarin (INR 1.2–1.5) plus aspirin (325 mg/day) with adjusted-dose warfarin (INR 2–3) in elderly patients with one or more risk factors for embolism.[54] Ischemic stroke and systemic embolism were present in 7.9 percent of patients on fixed-dose warfarin plus aspirin compared with only 1.9 percent on adjusted-dose warfarin. The SPAF investigators later studied the effectiveness of 325 mg of aspirin in patients with low risk and found that the rate of ischemic stroke was low (2 percent per year).[55]

The SPAF study identified three risk factors for thromboembolism—recent congestive heart failure, a history of hypertension, and previous thromboembolism[56,57]*—and suggested that anticoagulation with warfarin is not indicated in patients with none of the three risk factors who are at low risk for thromboembolism (2.5 percent per year).* In such patients the dangers of anticoagulant therapy may outweigh its benefits. Aspirin (325 mg daily) probably constitutes reasonable and safe therapy for patients with lone, nonrheumatic AF who are under 60 years of age and have none of the three identified risk factors.[56–58] In other patients with AF, long-term oral warfarin therapy (INR 2.0–3.0) should be used unless contraindicated.[55,58]

In the Boston Area Anticoagulation Trial for Atrial Fibrillation (BAATAF), 420 patients with nonrheumatic AF, mean age 68 years, were randomized unblinded to warfarin (target prothrombin time ratio, 1.2 to 1.5 × control, INR 1.5 to 2.7) or to a control group whose members were allowed to take aspirin.[59] The principal outcome was ischemic stroke or systemic embolism, and the mean follow-up was 2.2 years. The incidence of stroke was reduced 86 percent in the warfarin group compared with control (p = .002), equivalent to an absolute risk reduction of 2.6 percent per year. There was no demonstrable benefit of aspirin, but the study was not designed to test aspirin.

The European Atrial Fibrillation Trial (EAFT) study group addressed the question of the optimal level of anticoagulation by reviewing the results of its own trial.[60] *No treatment effect was found with anticoagulation responses below INRs of 2.0.* The rate of thromboembolic events was lowest at INRs from 2 to 3.9; most major hemorrhages occurred at INRs of 5.0 and above. The EAFT group recommended a target of 3.0 with a range of 2 to 5.0.[60] Fixed-dose warfarin with a target of INR 1.3 to 1.5 was not as effective as standard adjusted-dose warfarin at an average INR of 2.4 even when aspirin 325 mg/day was added to the low fixed-dose warfarin in another study.

Warfarin is about 50 percent more effective than aspirin in preventing stroke in patients with atrial fibrillation who do not have valvular disease. The effectiveness of anticoagulation on embolism from other cardiac conditions has not been well studied. *The rate of recurrence of stroke in patients with MVP is so low that warfarin is not recommended for prophylaxis except when a thrombus is seen on echocardiography* (see Chap. 58). Warfarin may not be effective in preventing calcific, myxomatous, bacterial, and fibrin-platelet emboli and has been posited to worsen cholesterol crystal embolization.[61]

The timing of the initiation of warfarin anticoagulation after embolic stroke remains controversial. Embolic brain infarcts often become hemorrhagic, and serious brain hemorrhage has occurred after anticoagulation.[62–65] Large infarcts, hypertension, large bolus doses of heparin, and excessive anticoagulation have been associated with hemorrhage. Because most hemorrhagic transformations occur within 48 h, the *recommendations of the Cerebral Embolism Task Force were to avoid early anticoagulation in patients with large infarcts or hemorrhagic transformation on repeat CT.*[66] Studies of patients with cerebral and cerebellar hemorrhagic infarction show that in the vast majority, the cause is embolic, that hemorrhagic infarction occurs equally with and without anticoagulation, and that the development of hemorrhagic infarction rarely is accompanied by clinical worsening.[67,68] Patients with hemorrhagic transformation who were continued on anticoagulants did not worsen. The risk of reembolism must be balanced against the small but definite risk of important bleeding. *If the patient has a large brain infarct, heparin should be delayed and bolus heparin infusions should be avoided. If the risk of reembolism is high, immediate heparinization is advisable, whereas if the risk seems low, it is prudent to delay anticoagulants for at least 48 h.* A recent study showed that *patients with atrial fibrillation with embolic strokes who were treated with well-controlled heparin anticoagulation soon after a stroke onset fared better than did patients who were treated later.*[68,69]

Paradoxical Embolism

While once considered rare, emboli entering the systemic circulation through right-to-left shunting of blood are now often recognized with the use of newer diagnostic technologies. By far the most common potential intracardiac shunt is a residual patent foramen ovale (PFO). The high frequency of PFOs in the normal adult population has made it difficult to be certain in an individual stroke patient with a PFO whether paradoxical embolism through the PFO was the cause of the stroke or whether the PFO was merely an incidental finding. Autopsy series have shown that about 30 percent of adults have a probe-patent foramen ovale at necropsy.[70] Hagen and associates studied 956 patients with clinically and pathologically normal hearts and found a PFO in 27.3 percent.[70] The frequency of PFOs declined with age: 34.3 percent during the first three decades of life, 25.4 percent during the fourth through eighth decades, and 20.2 percent during the ninth and tenth decades. The average diameter of PFOs was 4.9 mm, and the size tended to increase with age.[70] Echocardiographic studies have shown that PFOs are more common in patients with an undetermined cause of stroke than in those in whom another etiology has been defined.[71,72]

A review of series of patients with paradoxical embolism[73] through a PFO and the author's experience allow the derivation of five criteria that, when four or more are met, establish with a high degree of certainty the presence of a paradoxical embolism.[1] The findings are (1) *a situation that promotes thrombosis of leg or pelvic veins*, e.g., long sitting in one position or recent surgery, (2) *increased coagulability*, e.g., the use of oral contraceptives, the presence of Leiden factor with resistance to activated protein C, dehydration, (3) *the sudden onset of stroke during sexual intercourse, straining at stool, or another activity that includes a Valsalva maneuver* or promotes right-to-left shunting of blood, (4) *a pulmonary embolism* within a short time before or after the neurologic ischemic event, and (5) *the absence of other putative causes of stroke after thorough evaluation.*

Brain Hypoperfusion Resulting from Cardiac Pump Failure

After cardiopulmonary resuscitation (CPR), the heart often recovers in individuals in whom the brain has been irreversibly harmed by ischemic-anoxic damage.[74] Cardiologists must be familiar with the pathology, signs, and prognosis of brain dysfunction after periods of circulatory failure.

Different brain regions have selective vulnerability to hypoxic-ischemic damage. The regions that are most remote and at the edges of a major vascular supply are more liable to injury. These zones usually have been referred to as "border zones" or "watersheds."

The cerebral cortex is most vulnerable to injury. Damage may be diffuse or "laminar," involving layers of the cortex. The hippocampus is one of the most vulnerable areas.[75,76] In the brain, the border zone regions are between the anterior cerebral artery (ACA) and the MCA and between the MCA and the PCA. Damage is usually most severe in the posterior parieto-temporooccipital region and in the frontal areas most remote from the heart, which thus are called *distal fields*. A similar border zone exists in the cerebellum between the cerebellar arteries and in the brainstem between the medial and lateral penetrating arteries. The basal ganglia and thalamus are most involved if hypoxia is severe but some circulation is preserved. This situation applies most to hanging, strangulation, drowning, and carbon monoxide exposure.[77] Cerebellar neurons, especially Purkinje's cells, also may be selectively injured.

When circulatory arrest is complete and abrupt, brainstem nuclei are especially vulnerable to necrosis, especially in young humans and experimental animals.[78] When hypoxia and ischemia are especially severe, the spinal cord also may be damaged.[79] When cortical damage is very severe and protracted, cytotoxic edema causes massive brain swelling, with cessation of blood flow and brain death.

CLINICAL FINDINGS

Very severe damage leads to mortal injury to the cortex and brainstem, irreversible coma, and brain death. When initially examined, such patients have no brainstem reflexes (pupillary, corneal, and oculovestibular and oculocephalic reflexes) and no response to stimuli except perhaps a decerebration response. These findings do not improve, and respiratory control is absent or lost.

When cerebral cortical damage is very severe but brainstem ischemic changes are reversible, brainstem reflexes are preserved but there is no meaningful response to the environment. Automatic facial movements such as blinking, tongue protrusion, and yawning usually persist. The eyes may rest slightly up and move from side to side. When this state does not improve, it is referred to as the *persistent vegetative state*[74,75,80] or "wakefulness without awareness." Laminar cortical necrosis causes seizures. These seizures are often multifocal myoclonic twitches or jerks of the facial and limb muscles that are difficult to control with anticonvulsants; oversedation should be avoided.

With severe border-zone injury, there is weakness of the arms and proximal lower extremities with preservation of face, leg, and foot movement (the "man in a barrel" syndrome). With less severe ischemia, the symptoms and signs are predominantly visual. Patients describe difficulty seeing and cannot integrate the features of large objects or scenes despite a retained ability to see small objects in some parts of their visual fields. Reading is impossible. There are features of Balint's syndrome,[74] including asimultagnosia (seeing things piecemeal or sequentially), optic ataxia (poor eye-hand coordination), and optic apraxia (difficulty in directing gaze). Apathy and inertia are also common and are due to damage to the frontal lobe. Amnesia is also very common. These patients cannot form new memories and have patchy, retrograde amnesia for events during and before hospitalization. This Korsakoff-type syndrome is due to hippocampal damage and may not be fully reversible. Amnesia may be accompanied by visual abnormalities, apathy, and confusion or may be isolated.

PROGNOSIS

Shortly after resuscitation or arrest, patients with less severe cerebral injuries show some reactivity to the environment. Eye opening and restless limb movements develop. The eyes may fixate on objects. Noise, a flashlight, or a gentle pinch arouses patients to avoid or react to stimuli. Soon these patients awaken fully and may begin to speak. Cognitive and behavioral abnormalities may be detected after the patient awakens, depending on the degree of injury.

Prognostic signs and variables have been extensively studied.[74,81,82] The initial neurologic findings and their course are helpful in predicting the outcome. Among patients who have meaningful responses to pain at 1 h, almost all survivors have preserved intellectual function. Patients who do not respond to pain by 24 h either die or remain in a vegetative state. Being comatose predicts a poor prognosis.[82] *Thus, two simple observations—the presence or absence of coma and the response to pain—predict the neurologic outcome very early.*[82]

In a study in Seattle of out-of-hospital cardiac arrests, patients who did not awaken died on average 3.5 days after arrest.[83] Of 459 patients, 183 never awakened (39 percent). Among those who did awaken, 91 (32 percent) had persistent neurologic deficits.[84] Prognosis could be made by analyzing pupillary light reflexes, eye movements, and motor responses.[84] Bystander initiation of CPR was not significantly related to awakening,[84] in contrast to another study that found that outcome was better if CPR was started by bystanders before the emergency team arrived.[85] Patients awake on admission were included in one study[85] but excluded in the other.[84] After in-hospital CPR, pneumonia, hypotension, renal failure, cancer, and a housebound state before hospitalization were significantly related to death in the hospital (see Chap. 34).[86]

DIAGNOSTIC TESTING

Neurologic imaging and other tests have proved to be relatively unhelpful, in contrast to a neurologic examination.[74] CT is used to exclude other causes of coma, such as brain hemorrhage. Electroencephalography (EEG) is helpful in studying cortical activity in unresponsive patients and assessing brain death. Similarly, the absence of responses to visual and somatosensory stimuli is a poor prognostic sign. TCD may be helpful in the evaluation of brain death.[87]

TREATMENT

Other than maintaining adequate circulation and oxygenation, treatment has not been helpful in improving outcome. Increased blood sugar correlates with a poor outcome,[88] and experimental animals subjected to circulatory arrest do worse if they have been fed glucose before the arrest. Blood calcium and the presence of free radicals and excitatory neurotoxins have all been postulated to affect neuronal cell death.[89] A multifaceted approach to therapy has been most successful.[90]

Neurologic Effects of Cardiac Drugs and Cardiac Encephalopathy

Drugs given to patients with cardiac disease often have neurologic side effects[91] (see Chap. 81). Digitalis can cause visual hallucinations, yellow vision, and general confusion.[92] Digitalis levels need not be elevated excessively; the symptoms disappear with cessation of the drug. Quinidine can cause confusion with delirium, seizures and coma, vertigo, tinnitus, and visual blurring.[93] Chronic cognitive and behavioral changes and "quinidine dementia" are less well known.[93] Similar toxicity has been seen with lithium. Patients may become acutely comatose while being treated with intravenous lidocaine. This effect has been associated with the accidental administration of very large doses; more common CNS effects of less extreme toxicity include sedation, irritability, and twitching. The twitching may progress to seizures accompanied by respiratory depression. Amiodarone often causes ataxia, weakness, tremors, paresthesias, visual symptoms, and a parkinsonian-like syndrome and occasionally causes delirium.[91]

Patients with congestive heart failure often develop an encephalopathy characterized by decreased alertness, sleepiness, a decrease in all intellectual functions, asterixis, and variability of alertness and cognitive functions from minute to minute and hour to hour.[91] These patients may not have pulmonary, liver, or renal failure or electrolyte abnormalities. This cardiac encephalopathy is probably multifactoral. Posited explanations include decreased brain perfusion resulting from low cardiac output and high central venous pressure, intracranial fluid effusion similar in etiology to pericardial and pleural effusions and ascites, and side effects of cardiac and other drugs.[91]

NEUROLOGIC AND CEREBROVASCULAR COMPLICATIONS OF CARDIAC SURGERY

The frequency of abnormalities of intellectual function and behavior after cardiac surgery is quite high.[94] Fortunately, most changes are reversible with time. The reported incidence of neurologic complications after cardiac surgery varies widely from 7 to 61 percent for transient complications and from 1.6 to 23 percent for permanent complications.[95,96]

Prospectively, transient complications have been noted in 61 percent of patients.[97] In one series, 16.8 percent of patients had stroke or encephalopathy after coronary artery bypass surgery (CABS); the encephalopathies usually cleared, and only 2 percent of these patients had severe strokes.[98]

Atherothrombotic Hemodynamically Mediated Brain Infarcts

A major concern has been that the hemodynamic and circulatory stress of heart surgery will lead to underperfusion of areas supplied by already stenosed or occluded arteries, leading to brain infarcts. This concern underlies neck auscultation for bruits, ultrasound carotid artery testing, and cerebral angiography before CABS. However, hemodynamically induced infarction related to preexisting atherosclerotic occlusive cervicocranial arterial disease is a rare complication of heart surgery. Embolism arising from cardiac and aortic sources is much more common and a much greater concern.[94] *Patients with carotid bruits have a very low rate of stroke after elective surgery.*[99] *In a retrospective study of CABS patients with known carotid disease, ipsilateral strokes occurred in 1.1 percent of arteries with 50 to 90 percent stenosis, 6.2 percent of arteries with >90 percent stenosis, and only 2 percent of vessels with carotid occlusion.*[100,101] Stroke rates vary greatly in those undergoing combined as opposed to staged procedures.[102] Definitive management of combined cerebral and coronary artery disease awaits the outcome of clinical trials. Intracranial flow and velocity do not show significant changes in patients with high-grade carotid stenosis during CABS.[103]

Most studies have relied on clinical localization of focal deficits and inference about their mechanisms. A neuroradiology study reviewed neuroimaging results from 30 patients with acute strokes in relation to CABS.[104] Only one had evidence of a hemodynamic atherostenotic mechanism. Thromboembolic infarction often occurs in the days after surgery, when cessation of anticoagulation and the activation of coagulation factors promote hypercoagulability.

In some patients, hypercoagulability related to surgery can precipitate occlusive thrombosis in atherostenotic arteries, and the newly formed thrombus can lead to intraarterial embolism. *Cardiac, aortic, and intraarterial embolism accounts for the vast majority of cardiac surgery–related focal neurologic deficits.*

Brain Embolism

A strong argument against a hemodynamic cause of many strokes is their timing. Strokes occur more frequently *after* recovery from the anesthetic. If the mechanism of stroke were hemodynamic, the major circulatory stress would be intraoperative and patients would awaken with the deficit. In two studies in which the authors recorded the timing of CABS-related strokes, only 16 percent[105] and 17 percent,[106] respectively, of patients had deficits noted immediately postoperatively. The distribution of infarcts and their multiplicity on neuroimaging scans were most consistent with embolism. Embolic infarcts may involve either the anterior or the posterior circulation.[94,98,104,105] In a series of postoperative posterior circulation strokes, the majority were embolic and followed cardiac surgery.[106]

Emboli may arise from preexisting cardiac abnormalities such as hypofunctioning ventricles and dilated atria and from aortic atheromas or postoperative arrhythmias.[94] *Mounting evidence links operative and postoperative embolism to aortic ulcerative atherosclerotic lesions. Cross-clamping of the ascending aorta and aortotomy liberate cholesterol or calcific plaque debris.*[94,107] Figure 89-1 shows the aorta of a patient who died having never awakened after CABS. Figure 89-2 shows cholesterol crystals and other debris trapped within a filter placed in the aorta at the time of unclamping.

In a series in which embolic signals were monitored during CABS surgery, 34 percent of those signals were detected as the aortic cross-clamps were removed, and another 24 percent as aortic partial occlusion clamps were removed.[107] The number of microemboli detected correlates with abnormalities of cognitive function studied after surgery.[94,108] Figure 89-3 shows microemboli within the aorta shown by TEE after the release of aortic clamps. Figures 89-4 and 89-5 show TCD recordings during manipulation of the aorta and after the release of aortic clamps.

Necropsy examination of patients dying after cardiac surgery have shown severe bilateral, predominantly border-zone infarcts.[109] The small arteries of the brain and other viscera (heart, kidney, spleen, pancreas) may be packed with birefringent cholesterol crystal emboli.[109] TEE makes it possible to detect protruding ulcerative plaques in the aorta preoperatively and intraoperatively.[94,110] Intraaortic atherosclerotic debris identified by TEE has been found to be associated with embolic events.[110] Intraoperative B-mode ultrasonography with the probe placed on the aorta also has been used to detect severe aortic atherosclerotic plaques.[111] Ultrasonic imaging showed aortic atheromas in 58 percent of patients, whereas visual examination and palpation detected plaques in only 24 percent.[111] *Atherosclerosis of the ascending aorta is a very important risk factor for post-CABS stroke.*[94] *In patients who are scheduled to undergo elective cardiac surgery, consideration should be given to having TEEs performed before surgery to evaluate cardiac lesions and thrombi, cardiac function, and aortic atheromas.*

Encephalopathy

Gilman described a diffuse CNS disorder after open heart surgery—characterized by altered levels of consciousness and activity and confusion[112]—that is now referred to as *encephalopathy*. Clinical and imaging studies usually do not show important focal neurologic signs or large focal infarcts. The incidence of encephalopathy varies.[96] In one series, 57 of 1669 (3.4 percent) CABS patients had postoperative changes in mental state, including delirium and encephalopathy.[113] In the Cleveland Clinic prospective series, 11.6 percent were "encephalopathic" on the fourth postoperative day.[98]

Encephalopathy has multiple causes. Embolization of particulate matter was considered the leading cause, and this led to technical improvements, including the introduction of membrane rather than bubble oxygenators and on-line filtration.[96] These technical advances have led to a decrease in the risk of macroemboli (>25 mm) as a cause, but they do not provide protection against microemboli of air, fat, or particles.[96]

Necropsy studies of patients who died after cardiopulmonary bypass or angiography have awakened interest in this subject.[96,114] Focal, small capillary and arteriolar dilatations (SCADs) were commonly found in the brain.[114] About one-half of SCADs show birefringent crystalline material within the dilated capillaries. SCADs could, at least in part, explain the decreased cerebral blood flow found during cardiopulmonary bypass. SCADs are iatrogenically generated microemboli, but their origin is unknown. Their morphology is most consistent with air or fat.

Other causes of encephalopathy are common. Hypoxic-ischemic insults caused by hypotension and hypoperfusion do occur. *Drugs are a very common cause of encephalopathy in the postoperative period. Particularly important are haloperidol, narcotics, and sedatives.* Morphine sometimes is used heavily intraoperatively, and opiate withdrawal with restlessness and hyperactivity can result. Agitation and restlessness are often early signs of organic encephalopathy and may lead to the administration of haloperidol, barbiturates, phenothiazines, or benzodiazepines for calming and sedation. When these drugs wear off and the patient begins to awaken, agitation may occur and more sedatives may be given. Haloperidol causes rigidity, restlessness, agitation, hallucinations, and confusion. In experimental animals, haloperidol delays recovery from strokes by months, and its use is not advised.[115] Phenothiazines and sedatives are also problematic; *in general, the use of sedatives and narcotics should be minimized and the doses should be tapered as soon as possible.*

Intracranial Hemorrhage after Cardiac Surgery

Intracerebral or subarachnoid hemorrhages after cardiac surgery have been reported occasionally, most commonly in children who had repair of congenital heart disease[116] or after cardiac transplantation.[117] The postulated mechanism involves an abrupt increase in brain blood flow with rupture of small intracranial arteries that are not prepared for the new load. Usually, there is a prolonged period when cardiac output is low, and this output is increased suddenly by the surgery. Abrupt increases in brain blood flow and pressure in other situations also have been associated with intracerebral hemorrhage.[118]

Peripheral Nerve Complications

Brachial plexus and peripheral nerve lesions frequently develop after cardiac surgery and can be confused with CNS complications.[119] In one series, new peripheral nervous system deficits occurred in 13 percent of patients.[119] The most common deficit is a unilateral brachial plexopathy characterized by shoulder pain and usually weakness and numbness in one hand. It probably is caused by the positioning of the arm during surgery, with traction on the lower trunk of the brachial plexus. Ulnar, peroneal, and saphenous nerve injuries also are common and also are related to positioning. Diaphragmatic and vocal cord paralyses probably are related to local effects of cardiac surgery on the recurrent laryngeal and phrenic nerves.

CARDIAC EFFECTS OF BRAIN LESIONS

Information is beginning to emerge on cardiac muscle changes (myocytolysis), arrhythmias, pulmonary edema, ECG changes, and sudden death resulting from brain disease and sudden emotional stresses.[120]

Cardiac Lesions

The two lesions found most commonly in the hearts of patients dying with acute CNS lesions are patchy regions of myocardial necrosis and subendocardial hemorrhage. The abnormalities range from eosinophilic staining of cells with preserved striations to transformation of myocardial cells into dense eosinophilic contraction bands. These changes have been referred to as *myocytolysis*.[120] Subendocardial petechiae and frank hemorrhages also are noted. These lesions were described in the 1950s but were considered rare.[121,122] One study found a very high incidence of myocardial abnormalities in patients dying of brain lesions that increase intracranial pressure rapidly.[123] Stress-related release of catecholamines and possibly corticosteroids may be responsible, at least in part, for the cardiac lesions found in patients with CNS lesions.[120,124–127]

Electrocardiographic and Enzyme Changes

In stroke patients, especially those with subarachnoid hemorrhage, electrocardiograms (ECGs) may show a prolonged QT interval; giant, wide, roller-coaster inverted T waves; and U waves.[128] These changes often are called *cerebral T waves*. Patients with stroke who have continuous ECG monitoring have a high incidence of T-wave and ST-segment changes, various arrhythmias, and cardiac enzyme abnormalities. ECG changes may include a prolonged QT interval, depressed ST segments, flat or inverted T waves, and U waves.[120,128–130] Less often, tall, peaked T waves and elevated ST segments are noted (see Chap. 11).

Cardiac and skeletal muscle enzymes, including the MB isoenzyme of creatine kinase (MB-CK), are often abnormal in stroke patients.[131–133] During the 4 to 7 days after a stroke, there is usually a slow rise and later a fall in serum MB-CK levels, a pattern quite different from that found in acute myocardial infarction (see Chap. 42); the temporal pattern of cardiac isoenzyme release is more compatible with smoldering low-grade necrosis, such as patchy, focal myocytolysis.[121] The ST-segment and T-wave abnormalities and cardiac arrhythmias correlate significantly with raised levels of MB-CK in stroke patients.[121]

Arrhythmias

Various cardiac arrhythmias have been found in stroke patients, most frequently sinus bradycardia and tachycardia and premature ventricular contractions.[120,129,130] Some arrhythmias are manifestations of primary cardiac problems, but others are undoubtedly secondary to the brain lesions. The incidence of sinus tachycardia and bradycardia is maximal on the first day after intracerebral hemorrhage.[134] Ventricular bigeminy, atrioventricular dissociation and block, ventricular tachycardia, atrial fibrillation, and bundle branch blocks are found less often.[134] All arrhythmias are more common in patients who have primary brainstem lesions or brainstem compression.

Pulmonary Edema

Acute pulmonary edema may complicate strokes, especially subarachnoid hemorrhage (SAH) and posterior circulation ischemia and hemorrhage.[121] Pulmonary edema has been found in 70 percent of patients with fatal SAH and correlates with the severity and suddenness of the development of raised intracranial pressure.[135]

Centrally mediated sympathetic discharges such as those caused by increased intracranial pressure produce intense systemic vasoconstriction.[136] Blood shifts from the high-resistance systemic circulation to the lower-resistance pulmonary circulation. Increased pulmonary capillary pressure leads to pulmonary hypertension and rupture of pulmonary vessels, with lung hemorrhage. The pulmonary edema fluid has a high protein content and can develop despite normal cardiac function.[121,136]

Sudden Death

Sudden death associated with stressful situations, including so-called voodoo death, must involve CNS mechanisms.[127,137,138] Ventricular fibrillation, the presumed mechanism of sudden death, can be elicited reliably by stimulation of cardiac sympathetic nerves in both normal and ischemic hearts.[139] Ischemia reduces the threshold for ventricular fibrillation.[121,140] Stress must cause CNS stimulation that triggers autonomic activation.[127] Sudden vagotonic stimulation can cause bradycardia and cardiac standstill. The effects of vagal stimulation on the development of ventricular arrhythmias are uncertain.[139] Patients with lateral medullary and lateral pontine infarcts that affect reticular formation structures die unexpectedly; these patients have a high incidence of various types of autonomic dysregulation, such as labile blood pressure, syncope, tachycardia, and flushing, as well as a failure of automatic respiration.

COEXISTENT VASCULAR DISEASES AFFECTING BOTH HEART AND BRAIN

Atherosclerosis

The most common and important vascular disease that affects both the brain and the heart is atherosclerosis. The most common cause of death in stroke patients is coronary artery disease,[141] and extra- and intracranial arterial atherosclerosis[142] is common in patients with coronary artery disease.

PATHOLOGY AND PREDOMINANT SITES OF DISEASE

In white men, the predominant atherosclerotic lesions involve the origins of the internal carotid artery (ICA) and the VA origins in the neck.[5,143] Fatty streaks and flat plaques first affect the posterior wall of the common carotid artery (CCA) opposite the flow divider between the ICA and the external carotid artery (ECA), a region of low shear stress.[144] Atherosclerotic plaques at this site do not differ from plaques in the aorta or coronary arteries (see Chap. 36). At first, plaques expand gradually and encroach on the lumen of the ICA and sometimes the CCA (Fig. 89-6). Atheromatous plaques often develop concurrently at the VA origin or spread from the parent subclavian artery to involve the VA origin.[145] When plaques reach a critical size, they affect the turbulence, flow, and motion of the arteries, causing complications to develop within the plaques. Cracking, ulcerations, and mural thrombi develop, and the overlying endothelium is damaged with the development of occlusive thrombi.[146] Fresh thrombi that are loosely adherent to vascular walls rapidly propagate and embolize. Because the ICA has no nuchal branches, a clot often propagates cranially, usually extending as far as the first branch of the ophthalmic artery, which arises from the intracranial siphon portion of the ICA. In the VA, collateral channels from the ECA and the thyrocervical trunk usually provide collateral channels that reconstitute the VA in the neck and limit the propagation of thrombi. During 2 to 3 weeks after the development of an occlusive thrombus, a clot gradually organizes and is much less likely to propagate or embolize. The reduction in cranial blood flow caused by severe stenosis or occlusion of the ICA or VA stimulates the development of collateral circulation that usually becomes adequate.

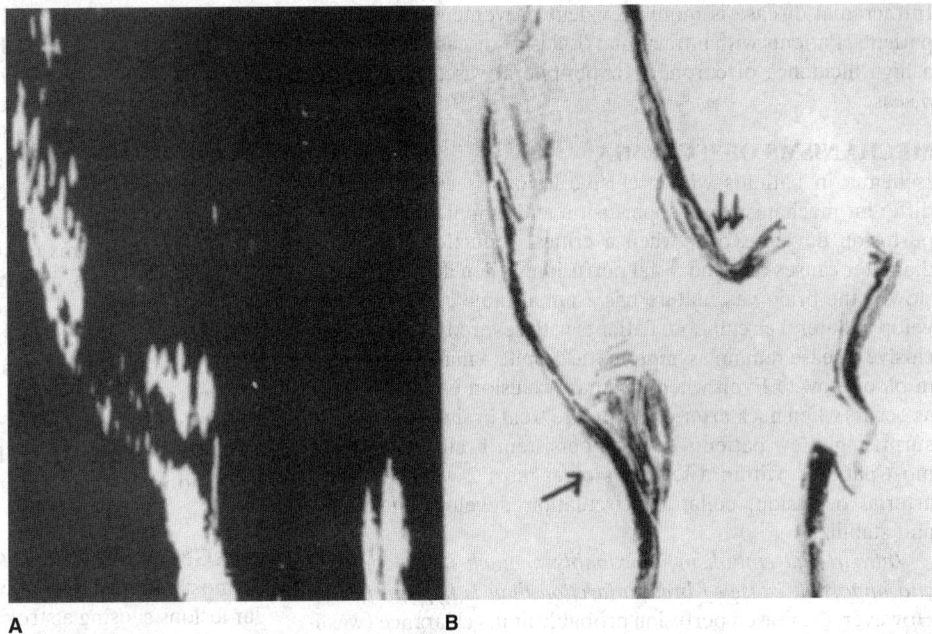

FIGURE 89-6 *A.* B-mode ultrasonic image showing plaque at internal carotid artery origin. *B.* A carotid specimen. The plaque (single arrow) is opposite the flow divider between the internal and external carotid arteries (two arrows). [From Hennerici M, Steinke W. Abbildende Ultraschallverfahren (B-scan) in duplex system. In: *Durchblutungsstorungen des Gehirns—Neue Diagnostischen Möglichkeiten*. Gutersloh: Bertelsmann; 1987, with permission.]

Figure 89-7 shows diagrammatically the sites of predilection for the development of atherosclerosis in the cervicocranial circulation. Note the concentration of these sites at branch points and flow dividers. There are important race and sex differences in the distribution of cerebral atherosclerosis.[147–149] White men usually develop lesions of the ICA and VA origins. Patients with ICA-origin disease have a high frequency of hypercholesterolemia, coronary artery disease, and peripheral vascular occlusive disease. With the exception of the basilar artery (BA) and the ICA siphon, intracranial occlusive disease develops only after extracranial disease is well established in this group. Blacks and individuals of Chinese, Japanese, and Thai ancestry have a much higher incidence of intracranial occlusive disease and a rather low frequency of extracranial disease.[147,149,150]

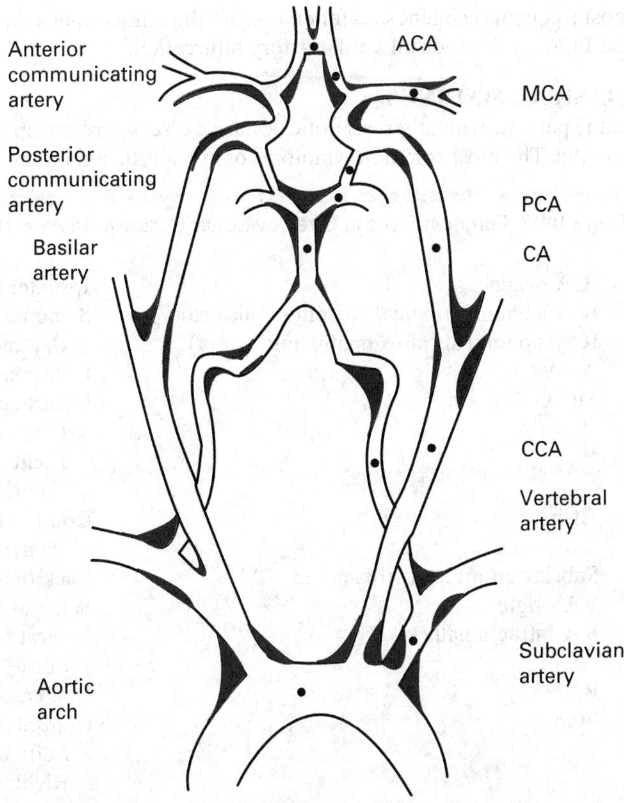

FIGURE 89-7 Sites of predilection for atherosclerotic narrowing. Dark areas represent plaques. (From Caplan LR. *Stroke: A Clinical Approach*, 3d ed. Boston: Butterworth-Heinemann; 2000, with permission.)

Intracranial disease is more prevalent in women and diabetic patients. Patients with intracranial occlusive disease do not have a high incidence of coronary or peripheral vascular occlusive disease.

MECHANISMS OF ISCHEMIA

Ischemia in patients with occlusive lesions is caused by two different mechanisms: hypoperfusion and embolism.[5,151] Hypoperfusion develops only when a critical reduction in luminal diameter causes reduced distal perfusion. When flow is reduced slowly, the brain vasculature has a remarkable capacity to develop collateral circulation. Patients with severe ICA-origin occlusive disease remain asymptomatic despite a marked decrease in blood flow.[152] Even when vascular occlusion is abrupt—e.g., as occurs when neck arteries are tied to treat brain aneurysms—surprisingly few patients develop persistent brain ischemia. In most patients, within a few days or at most 2 weeks after an arterial occlusion, collateral circulation develops maximally and stabilizes.

Intraarterial embolism is probably a much more common and important cause of brain infarction than is hypoperfusion. However, decreased perfusion probably limits clearance (washout) of emboli.[151] In patients with anterior circulation infarcts, angiography shows a very high frequency of intraarterial intracranial emboli distal to an ICA thrombosis.[153] These emboli most often involve the MCA and its branches. If angiography is repeated or performed later than 48 h after a stroke, MCA occlusion is usually not present.[5,6] Intraarterial emboli often fragment and move distally. Intraarterial embolism is also very common in the posterior circulation, where the most common donor sites are the VA origin and the intracranial VA and the most frequent recipient sites for emboli are the intracranial VA, the PCA, and the distal basilar artery bifurcation.[154]

CLINICAL FINDINGS

Many patients with atherosclerotic occlusive disease are asymptomatic. The most common symptoms of hypoperfusion or embolism are headache, TIAs, and neurologic signs related to brain infarction. Headaches are due to vascular distention or brain swelling secondary to infarction. Unaccustomed headaches often precede strokes.[5,155] TIAs are caused by hypoperfusion or intraarterial emboli. Frequent, very brief stereotyped spells precipitated by postural changes suggest a hemodynamic mechanism. In contrast, emboli cause longer, less frequent attacks.[156] In many patients with clinical TIAs—i.e., TIAs with no lasting symptoms or signs—neuroimaging tests show brain infarcts.[157] Strokes may have various temporal features, such as being maximal at outset, fluctuating, stepwise, or gradually progressive. The pattern is related to the adequacy of collateral circulation and the propagation and embolization of thrombi.

Neurologic symptoms and signs depend on the region of brain that is ischemic. Table 89-2 outlines the most common clinical patterns resulting from occlusions of the major extracranial and intracranial arteries.[5,143]

DIAGNOSTIC TESTING

In most patients, the nature and severity of the brain and vascular lesions causing a stroke can be defined. CT and MRI should localize brain lesions, distinguish between infarcts and hemorrhages, and determine the location, extent, and size of the processes. CT or MRI is usually the first test in patients with suspected stroke because the information allows clinicians to exclude nonvascular disease such as tumor or abscess, differentiate hemorrhage from ischemia and show subdural hematomas, identify the vascular territory involved, and define the extent of brain already damaged.

The vascular territory involved should be inferred by the nature of the neurologic symptoms and signs and the location of brain lesions on CT or MRI. Echocardiography, especially TEE, has dramatically improved the ability to detect potential cardiac sources of emboli (see Chap. 13).

Ultrasound techniques can be used to screen for obstructive lesions in the major extracranial and intracranial arteries in both

TABLE 89-2 Common Signs in Cerebrovascular Occlusive Disease at Various Sites

Site	Signs
ICA origin	Ipsilateral transient monocular blindness; MCA and ACA signs
ICA siphon (proximal to ophthalmic artery)	Same as ICA origin
ICA siphon (distal to ophthalmic artery)	MCA and ACA signs
ACA	Contralateral weakness of the lower limb and shoulder shrug
MCA	Contralateral motor, sensory, and visual loss Left: Aphasia Right: Neglect of left space, lack of awareness of deficit, apathy, impersistence
AChA	Contralateral motor, sensory, and visual loss, usually without cognitive changes
Subclavian artery (proximal to VA)	Lack of arm stamina, cool hand, transient dizziness, veering, diplopia
VA origin	Same as subclavian, but no ipsilateral arm or hand findings
VA intracranially	Lateral medullary syndrome; staggering and veering (cerebellar infarction)
BA	Bilateral motor weakness; ophthalmoplegia and diplopia
PCA	Contralateral hemianopia and hemisensory loss Left: alexia with agraphia Right: neglect of left visual space

ABBREVIATIONS: ICA = internal carotid artery; ACA = anterior cerebral artery; MCA = middle cerebral artery; AChA = anterior choroidal artery; VA = vertebral artery; BA = basilar artery; PCA = posterior cerebral artery.

anterior (carotid) and posterior (vertebrobasilar) circulation arteries. For extracranial use, the two most important are *B-mode scans* and *Doppler spectra*, both pulsed and continuous-wave (CW) Doppler. The anatomy of the carotid bifurcation (the CCA, proximal ICA, and ECA) and the proximal VAs can be imaged by high-frequency, 5- to 10-MHz B-mode ultrasound systems, which provide images of the vessels in real time both longitudinally and in cross section (Fig. 89-8). Plaque calcifications and clots are often difficult to image. Pulsed Doppler registers frequency shifts from moving columns of blood. Doppler analysis can show the direction and velocity of blood flow. Multigated Doppler and B-mode scanning are now used together in so-called duplex systems.[5,158] The duplex system is probably more than 90 percent effective in separating arteries that are normal or minimally narrowed from those which have moderate disease (30 to 70 percent narrowing) and those with severe narrowing (>70 percent stenosis). B-mode scanning sometimes suggests the presence of ulceration or hemorrhage in plaques that show heterogeneous images.[158] CW Doppler uses a movable probe to measure flow velocities along the carotid and vertebral arteries; the technique is less time-consuming and expensive than the duplex system and in expert hands is very accurate in detecting high-grade stenosis.[159] Ultrasound techniques cannot reliably separate complete occlusion from very high degrees of stenosis. Color-flow and power Doppler can show turbulence and altered flow dynamics.

TCD ultrasound is used to analyze the presence of intracranial arterial stenoses and provide information about the intracranial effects of extracranial occlusive lesions. The technique takes advantage of the soft spots in the temporal bones and natural foramina (the orbit and the foramen magnum) that provide windows for ultrasound recording. The depth and angle of the probe recording can be varied, allowing the recording of velocities and sound spectra from all the major intracranial arteries.[5,87,160] Major obstructive lesions are shown reliably by both extracranial ultrasound and TCD. Continuous recording of intracranial arteries with TCD is a very sensitive and accurate method of detecting emboli passing under the probes.[94,107,161] Examples of microembolic signals are shown in Figs. 89-4 and 89-5.

Magnetic resonance angiography (MRA) (see Chap. 18) provides an additional method of imaging both the extracranial and intracranial arteries for areas of stenosis and occlusion.[5,150,162] CT angiography (CTA), using a spiral (helical) CT machine and dye injected intravenously, also can image the major large craniocervical arteries.[163] Standard catheter angiography is warranted when ultrasound and CTA or MRA have not sufficiently defined the vascular lesion and treatment is clinically feasible.[5,150]

TREATMENT

For rational treatment, the following should be known: the location, nature, and severity of the occlusive lesion; the location, extent, and reversibility of the brain lesion; and the blood constituents and coagulability.[5,164] Treatment should *not* be guided solely by the temporal pattern of the symptoms, such as TIA, progressing stroke, or so-called completed stroke.[5,164] These time courses do not predict the cause and mechanism of ischemia, do not indicate whether an infarct is present, and do not identify patients who will have further or recurrent ischemia.

Physicians should first decide whether any specific therapy is indicated. Very severe neurologic deficits, serious intercurrent illnesses (dementia, cancer, etc.), and psychosocioeconomic considerations may make patients unsuitable for specific treatments. If treatment is feasible, the next questions to be considered are what brain tissue is at risk for further ischemia and what the benefit/risk ratio of specific treatments may be. To determine the tissue at risk, clinicians consider the cause and the deficit. For example, a man with a slight hemiplegia caused

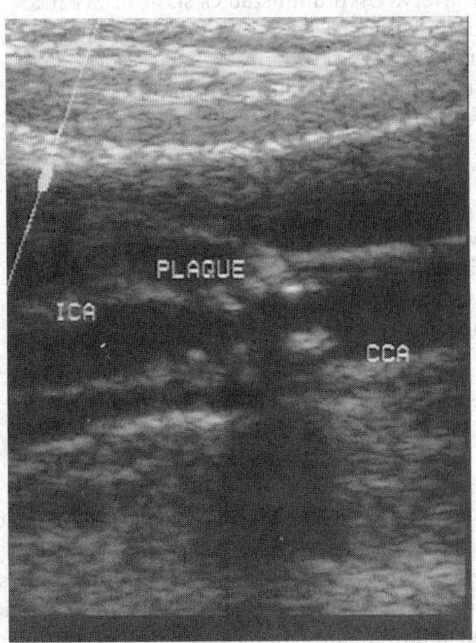

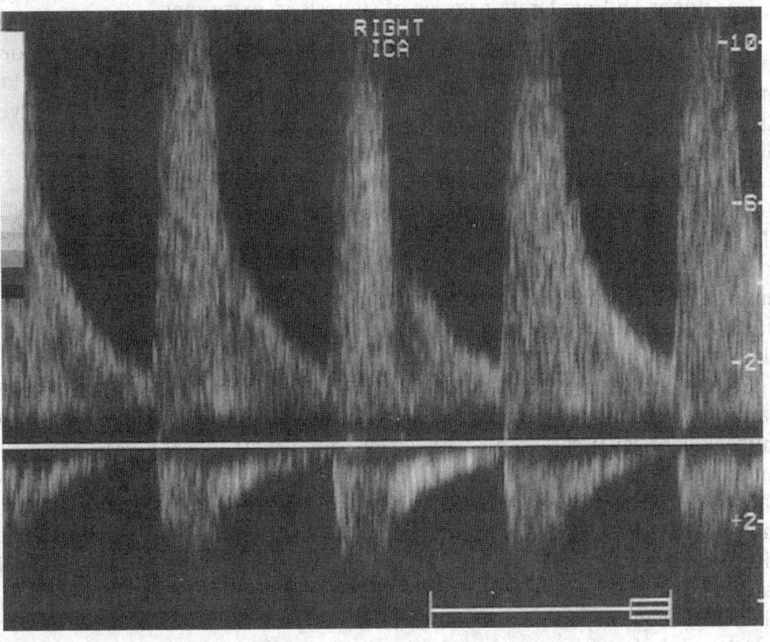

FIGURE 89-8 Duplex scan of carotid artery plaque. *A*. B-mode ultrasonic image showing plaque protruding into internal carotid artery (ICA) lumen. *B*. Doppler spectra at level of plaque showing high voltage related to stenosis.

by a small lacunar infarct in the anterior limb of the internal capsule may have infarcted the entire tissue supplied by an occluded small artery. In that case, treatment consists of controlling hypertension, the cause of the microvasculopathy. If, however, that patient has a small cortical infarct in the precentral gyrus resulting from ICA disease, the rest of the ICA territory is at risk for further ischemia and aggressive treatment is warranted. Suppose a patient has a moderate-size MCA infarct. If the patient is a Chinese woman with intrinsic atherosclerotic disease of that MCA, she may have little tissue at risk for further ischemia. No aggressive treatment should be given. If that woman's infarct is due to cardiogenic embolism, the whole remainder of the brain will be at risk for further damage from another embolus. Newer MRI techniques—diffusion-weighted and perfusion MRI—along with MRA, can show, even very soon after the symptoms begin, brain that is already infarcted and brain tissue that is underperfused but not yet infarcted.[5,163,165,166]

Patients who have little tissue at risk are not candidates for specific therapy. If there is considerable residual at-risk tissue, the guidelines for the use of anticoagulants and antiplatelet agents given in Table 89-3 are used to direct treatment, which depends on the location and severity of the causative vascular lesions. Carotid endarterectomy (CEN) has been shown to be effective in symptomatic patients with severe ICA stenosis (>70 percent).[167–170]

The Asymptomatic Carotid Artery Study (ACAS) suggested that carotid endarterectomy is slightly better than medical therapy in asymptomatic patients with severe carotid stenosis when the operation is executed by surgeons who have a record of very low surgical morbidity and mortality.[171] For CEN to be effective, the operative mortality and morbidity must not be greater than 2 to 4 percent.[167–171] Surgery is also feasible on the extracranial vertebral artery in selected patients with an intraarterial embolism from that site or with intractable posterior circulation hemodynamic ischemia, a rare occurrence.[172]

For minor and moderate degrees of stenosis in extra- and intracranial arteries, agents that alter platelet aggregation and adhesion are recommended. The most likely mechanism of ischemia in these patients is "white clot"—platelet fibrin emboli. Aspirin,[173,174] ticlopidine,[175,176] clopidogrel,[177] and a tablet containing 25 mg aspirin and 200 mg of modified-release dipyridamole given two times a day[178] have all proved effective in randomized trials that contained large numbers in patients with TIAs and minor strokes. Many nonsteroidal anti-inflammatory drugs have antiplatelet effects, as do the omega-3 fish oils containing eicosapentanoic acid. Clopidogrel is as effective as ticlopidine and has fewer serious hematologic complications[177] (see Chap. 44).

For patients with severe stenosis of large intracranial arteries, warfarin is recommended if there are no contraindications. The anticoagulant level should be kept at an INR of 2.0 to 3.0. Anticoagulation should be continued for at least 2 months. The state of the intracranial arteries can be monitored by using TCD and/or MRA or CTA.[163] The same regimen is used for patients with severe extracranial stenosis who are not operative candidates or refuse surgery. For patients with complete occlusions when first seen, heparin and then warfarin are prescribed for 2 to 3 months.[5]

Thrombolytic drugs, especially recombinant tissue-type plasminogen activator (rt-PA) and streptokinase, have been given intravenously and intraarterially in patients with acute brain ischemia. In a study in which the arterial lesions were not defined, intravenous therapy with rt-PA given within 90 min and 3 h of ischemia onset, in the aggregate provided a statistically significant benefit.[179] Unfortunately, in this and other studies, about 6 to 12 percent of patients treated with thrombolytic agents developed important intracranial bleeding. Uncontrolled studies have shown that patients with distal intracranial arterial embolic occlusions do well with intravenous thrombolytic therapy.[180–182] Patients with ICA occlusions in the neck and intracranially rarely reperfuse after intravenous thrombolytic therapy, especially if collateral circulation is poor. Intraarterially admin-

TABLE 89-3 Suggested Use of Anticoagulants and Platelet Antiaggregants

HEPARIN (STANDARD DOSE)

Short term, 2–4 weeks. Usually given by intravenous infusion, keeping APTT between 60 and 100 s (1.5–2 × control APTT).

1. Immediate therapy for definite cardiac-origin cerebral embolism (large cerebral infarct, hypertension, bacterial endocarditis, or sepsis would delay or contraindicate this use).
2. Patients with severe stenosis or occlusion of the ICA origin, ICA siphon, MCA, vertebral artery, or basilar artery with less than a large clinical deficit. Subsequent treatment could consist of warfarin or surgery.

HEPARIN (SUBCUTANEOUS MINIDOSE)

For prophylaxis of deep vein occlusion in patients immobilized by stroke (unless contraindicated) (see Chap. 60).

WARFARIN

Usually overlapped with heparin; keeping prothrombin time around INR of 2.0–3.0 (approximately 1.3–1.5 × control).

1. Long term (>3 months)
   a. Patients with cardiogenic cerebral embolization and rheumatic heart disease, atrial fibrillation with large atria or prior cerebral embolism, prosthetic valves, and some hypercoagulable states.
   b. Patients with severe stenosis of the ICA origin, ICA siphon, MCA stem, vertebral artery, and basilar artery. Used until studies show artery has been occluded for at least 3 weeks.
2. Short term (3–6 weeks)
   a. Patients with recent occlusion of the ICA, MCA, vertebral, or basilar arteries.

PLATELET ANTIAGGREGANTS (ASPIRIN, TICLOPIDINE, CLOPIDOGREL)

1. Patients with plaque disease of the extracranial and intracranial arteries without severe stenosis.
2. Patients with polycythemia or thrombocytosis and related ischemic attacks.

ABBREVIATIONS: APTT = activated partial thromboplastin time; ICA = internal carotid artery; MCA =55 middle cerebral artery; INR = International Normalized Ratio.

istered prourokinase thrombolysis also has been proved to be very effective in opening blocked intracranial arteries within the anterior circulation.[183] Patients with in situ thrombosis superimposed on preexisting severe atherostenosis do less well than do patients with embolism. The dose, timing, mode of delivery, and target group for therapy remain unsettled. The author believes that vascular imaging should precede the administration of thrombolytic agents. Brain and vascular imaging can give physicians guidance in selecting who should receive thrombolytics and by what route.[184]

Because all patients with atherosclerosis are at risk of developing more lesions, control of risk factors is very important and should be begun in the hospital. Risk factors include smoking, hyperlipidemia, obesity, inactivity, and hypertension (see Chap. 38). Blood pressure should not be lowered excessively during the acute ischemic period, as this may decrease flow in collateral arteries. Blood pressure control can be instituted 3 to 4 weeks after the stroke. Rehabilitation also must begin early.

Management of Coexisting Coronary and Cerebrovascular Disease

Many patients have both coronary and cerebrovascular occlusive disease. In candidates for both CABS and CEN, controversy surrounds which surgery should be done first or whether both procedures should be done together under the same anesthetic. *In general, the most symptomatic system should be operated on first.* Thus, if a patient has severe coronary disease with active cardiac ischemia but asymptomatic severe extracranial occlusive disease, he or she should have a CABS procedure, and CEN can be considered later.[5] By contrast, if a patient has active cerebrovascular symptoms (recent TIAs or a nondisabling stroke within the last 3 months) and minor or stable coronary symptoms, a CEN will be in order without a CABS. If the patient has active coronary and cerebrovascular symptoms, the CEN and CABS should be performed together.[185–187] The reasons for this view are as follows: (1) The morbidity and mortality of the two procedures done together are considerably higher than those of either alone. The stroke risk is especially high.[187] (2) Patients with asymptomatic bruits and even severe stenosis have a very low rate of stroke resulting from hemodynamic changes during CABS or other surgery. Most operative and postoperative strokes are cardioembolic. (3) With good medical care, the risk of myocardial infarction during CEN in patients with stable coronary disease is relatively low (see Chap. 91).

In patients considered for cardiac surgery who have symptoms of brain ischemia, it is important to define the extent of cerebrovascular disease preoperatively by noninvasive means (ultrasound and/or MRA) as well as to define cardiac and coronary artery anatomy and function. Staged surgical procedures sometimes are warranted. In some patients with excessive surgical risks, anticoagulation represents an alternative treatment. Clearly, optimal medical therapy should be instituted preoperatively and continued after surgery.

Systemic Arterial Hypertension

High blood pressure, both acute and chronic, damages deep, penetrating small intracranial arteries; accelerates the development of atherosclerosis in the extracranial and large intracranial arteries; and results in ischemic syndromes of lacunar infarction,[5,188,189] diffuse ischemic changes in white matter and basal gray matter structures (Binswanger's disease[5,190]), and intracerebral hemorrhage. Hypertension is also common in patients with aneurysmal SAH and may contribute to enlargement and rupture of aneurysms.

Hypertension especially damages the deep arteries that penetrate perpendicularly from the major intracranial arteries (Fig. 89-9) (see Chap. 51). Serial sections of these arteries in patients with hypertension show characteristic abnormalities consisting of focal microaneurysmal enlargements and small hemorrhagic extravasations through the arterial walls. Subintimal foam cells may obliterate the lumen, and pink-staining amorphous fibrinoid material is found within the walls of thickened arteries. In places, the vessels often are replaced by whorls, tangles, and wisps of connective tissue that completely obliterate the usual vascular layers, causing segmental arterial disorganization as a consequence of *lipohyalinosis* and *fibrinoid degeneration*.[5,191] Microaneurysms are common in patients with hypertensive intracerebral hemorrhages and in hypertensive older patients.[192–194]

The two major patterns of brain ischemia in patients with hypertension are *discrete lacunar infarcts* and a more *diffuse patchy white and gray matter degeneration with gliosis*. Both are caused by sclerotic changes in deep intracerebral arteries and arterioles. The term *lacunae* (hole) refers to a small, deep infarct caused by lipohyalinosis of the penetrating artery that feeds the ischemic brain tissue.[191] Other vascular pathologic processes, such as microdissections and tiny emboli, occasionally also cause lacunes.[191] Some patients are normotensive and have miniature atherosclerotic lesions (so-called microatheromas) at the orifices of the branches or within the parent arteries blocking or extending into the branches.[5,188] Amyloid angiopathy also can cause small, deep infarcts in normotensive and hypertensive patients. Single lacunes cause discrete clinical syndromes.[5,195,196] The most common syndromes are pure motor hemiparesis,[197] pure sensory stroke,[198] ataxic hemiparesis,[199] and the dysarthria–clumsy hand syndrome[200] (see Chap. 51).

Since the advent of CT and MRI, it has become widely

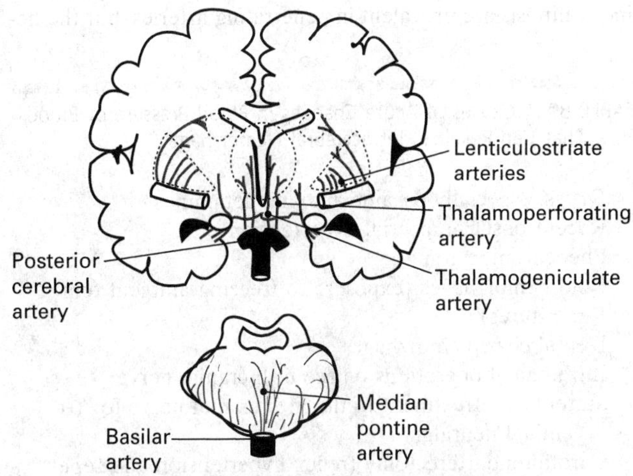

FIGURE 89-9 Deep penetrating arteries prone to the development of lipohyalinosis and microaneurysms (dark blue). Occlusion of these arteries causes lacunar infarcts, and their rupture causes intracerebral hemorrhage. (From Caplan LR. *Stroke: A Clinical Approach*, 3d ed. Boston: Butterworth-Heinemann; 2000, with permission.)

appreciated that hypertensive patients with lacunes often have more diffuse changes in the white matter of the brain that are referred to as *leuko-araiosis*.[190,201] The clinical picture consists of acute strokes; subacute progression of neurologic signs; dementia, especially the frontal lobe apathetic type; slow shuffling gait disorder; and parkinsonian, pyramidal, and pseudobulbar signs.[190,202,203] The clinical signs and gross pathology are identical to those partially described by Otto Binswanger in 1894 and 1895 and by his students Alzheimer and Nissl.[202] The deep arteries are thickened and hyalinized and show lipohyalinosis and sometimes amyloid angiopathy in regions of white matter atrophy and gliosis. Invariably, lacunar infarcts also are found. The pathogenesis most likely is related to diffuse vascular narrowing in deep arteries and altered microvascular flow and perfusion. Some studies suggest altered hemorrheology and increased blood viscosity, and some patients have had polycythemia.[190] The diagnosis is made on the basis of the clinical findings, the CT and MRI abnormalities, and the absence of cortical infarcts, larger artery occlusive disease, or cardioembolic sources.

HYPERTENSIVE INTRACEREBRAL HEMORRHAGE

Intracerebral hemorrhage (ICH) accounts for about 10 percent of all strokes.[5,6] Head trauma, vascular malformations, bleeding diatheses, drugs (especially amphetamines and cocaine), amyloid angiopathy, and intracranial aneurysms account for some cases.[192,204] Traditionally, spontaneous ICH usually has been equated with hypertensive hemorrhage. Many of these patients, however, have no history of hypertension and no associated changes of hypertensive vasculopathy at necropsy.[118,192,205,206] Acute elevations of blood pressure and/or blood flow to the brain (Table 89-4) can cause ICH through the sudden increase in blood pressure, causing breakage of capillaries and arterioles.[118,192]

Hypertensive ICH issues from the deep penetrating arteries, and so the locations parallel the distribution of those arteries. Hematomas develop in the same sites as lacunes; the most common locations are the putamen/internal capsule (30 to 40 percent), caudate nucleus (8 percent), lobar white matter (20 percent), thalamus (15 percent), pons (10 percent), and cerebellum (10 percent).[192] In fatal hematomas, microaneurysms and lipohyalinosis are prevalent in penetrating arteries, but the hematomas obscure findings in the middle of the lesions.[207] Along the outside, circumferentially, fibrin globules represent rupture sites.[207] Arterioles or capillaries rupture in the center of the lesion, suddenly increasing local tissue pressure and leading to pressure on adjacent capillaries, which then rupture. As the hematoma gradually grows on its periphery (Fig. 89-10), local tissue pressure and finally intracranial pressure increase until the hematoma is contained. Alternatively, the pressure is decompressed by the lesion emptying into the ventricular system or into the subarachnoid space on the brain surface.[5]

TABLE 89-4 Causes of Acute Changes in Blood Pressure or Blood Flow That Can Result in Intracerebral Hemorrhage

- Drugs, especially cocaine and amphetamines
- Recent onset of arterial hypertension
- Pheochromocytoma
- Cold hemorrhages (exposure to freezing ambient temperatures)
- Dental chair hemorrhages
- Intracranial operations on the fifth cranial nerve
- Stereotactic treatment of the fifth cranial nerve for trigeminal neuralgia
- Carotid endarterectomy (reflex hypertension and reperfusion)
- Cardiac transplantation, especially in children
- Surgical repair of congenital heart disease in children
- Migraine

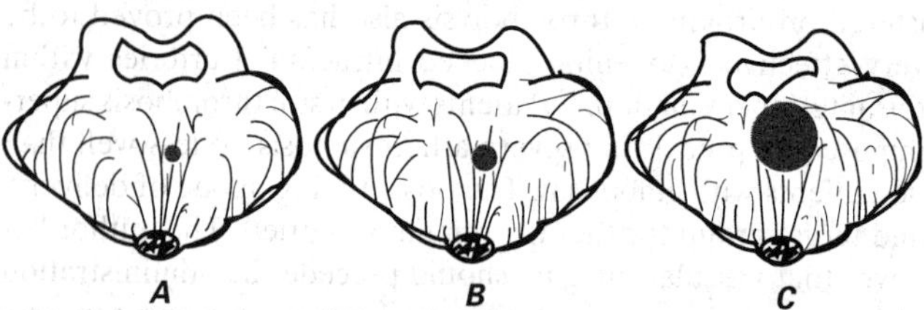

FIGURE 89-10 Gradual evolution of a hypertensive pontine intracerebral hematoma. *A*. The earliest leakage of blood from a paramedian penetrating artery. *B* and *C*. The hematoma has grown. (From Caplan LR. *Stroke: A Clinical Approach*, 3d ed. Boston: Butterworth-Heinemann; 2000, with permission.)

Clinical Findings Patients with ICH most often have a gradual evolution of neurologic signs; symptoms do not begin abruptly, as they do in SAH.[192] The first neurologic signs are related to the bleeding site; e.g., left putaminal hematoma patients may first notice right arm weakness or numbness, whereas cerebellar hematoma patients stagger and feel off balance. As the hematoma grows, the focal signs worsen. When and if the hematoma increases sufficiently in size to increase intracranial pressure, headache, vomiting, and decreased levels of alertness develop.[192] In the presence of small, restricted hemorrhages, headache is absent and the patient remains alert. The course and findings mimic so-called progressing ischemic stroke. Headache is absent or not a very prominent symptom in more than half of patients with ICH. Loss of consciousness is also not invariable but is a bad prognostic sign when present. Clinical localization of the hematoma rests on an analysis of pupillary responses, eye movements, and the presence and distribution of motor signs.

Diagnosis CT accurately shows the location, size, shape, and extent of hematomas. Also shown is the presence of ventricular and surface drainage, surrounding edema, and pressure shifts in surrounding tissues. MRI in a patient with an acute hematoma is more difficult to interpret, but old hematomas are more readily shown by imaging hemosiderin-containing cavities. Susceptibility-weighted images acquired on echo-planar machines can show even very acute intracerebral hemorrhages.[208] MRI is superior to CT in imaging arteriovenous malformations and cavernous angiomas. Lumbar puncture seldom is warranted. An atypical location, an absence of hypertension, and abnormal vascular echoes on MRI are indications for angiography.

Prognosis and Treatment Coma, increased intracranial pressure, and large hematoma size (>3 cm in one dimension on CT) all indicate a poor prognosis.[192,209] Ordinarily, severe systemic hypertension should be reduced, but not excessively. The hematoma causes increased intracranial pressure, and the spinal fluid pressure and the pressure in the dural sinuses increase pari passu. Patients with ICH can die from raised intracranial pressure. To perfuse the brain and maintain an arteriovenous pressure gradient, the systemic arterial pressure must rise. Overzealous reduction of systemic blood pressure can cause clinical deterioration. The patient's state of alertness and neurologic signs should be monitored carefully, together with the blood pressure.

Recent hematomas in the cerebral lobes, cerebellum, and right putamen sometimes are drained surgically without leaving a major deficit, at times by using stereotactic equipment with CT guidance. The indications for drainage are increased intracranial pressure and the presence of lesions that require removal (tumor, arteriovenous malformation, aneurysm).[192] When hematomas resolve, they leave a cavity, disconnecting but not destroying the overlying cortex.

Small hematomas usually resolve well without specific therapy except blood pressure control, whereas massive hematomas usually kill or maim patients before they can be treated. Medium-size hematomas (2 to 4 cm), which increase intracranial pressure and cause worsening signs or decreased consciousness while patients are under observation, are indications for drainage if they are favorably located.

Subarachnoid Hemorrhage

SAH is not caused directly by hypertension in most cases, although an abrupt increase in blood pressure (e.g., resulting from cocaine or amphetamines) sometimes can lead to SAH, as can a bleeding diathesis, trauma, and amyloid angiopathy. *The most common lesions causing SAH are abnormal vessels such as aneurysms and vascular malformations on or near the surface of the brain.* SAH involves bleeding directly into the subarachnoid space with rapid dissemination into the cerebrospinal fluid (CSF) pathways. Usually blood is released suddenly under systemic arterial pressure, causing an abrupt rise in intracranial pressure and producing headache, vomiting, and interruption of conscious behavior and memory, at least temporarily.[5,210] In some patients, the jet and spread of blood cause neck ache, backache, or sciatica instead of headache. These patients usually are agitated and restless or sleepy and have a stiff neck.

The most common cause of SAH is leakage from a berry aneurysm. Often there has been a past history of a "warning leak," that is, a sudden-onset headache unusual for the patient that lasts days and usually prevents normal daily activities.[210,211] Aneurysms most often are located at bifurcations of major intracranial arteries. The most common sites are the ICA–posterior communicating artery junction, the ACA–anterior communicating artery junction, and the MCA bifurcation. CT often can suggest the site of rupture if blood is pooled locally near a typical site.[212] Large aneurysms are occasionally visible on contrast-enhanced CT or MRI. CTA and MRA are useful tests for screening for aneurysms.[163] Lumbar puncture is very important in the diagnosis of SAH.[213] The absence of blood in the CSF effectively excludes the diagnosis of SAH if the fluid is examined within 24 h of the onset of the headache, although bleeds that are very small in volume or older than 72 h can be missed. The CSF pressure, the presence of xanthochromia, and quantification of the hemoglobin and bilirubin content of the CSF by spectrophotometry can help establish and date the bleeding and document increased intracranial pressure.[213]

The two most important complications of aneurysmal SAH are rebleeding and brain ischemia caused by vasoconstriction (so-called vasospasm). Once an aneurysm has ruptured, either a tiny cap of platelets and fibrin seals the point of rupture or continued bleeding leads to death. Lysis of the fibrin cap initiates rebleeding. Surgical clipping of the aneurysmal sac or obliteration of the aneurysm by endovascular use of balloons or other devices should be attempted before rebleeding occurs.

Vasoconstriction of arteries is thought to be due to blood or blood products that bathe the adventitia of arteries.[214–217] In the presence of a large accumulation of blood, there is a much higher incidence of arterial vasoconstriction and resultant brain ischemia and infarction. Delayed ischemia also can develop after surgery, as manipulation of vessels can precipitate or potentiate vasoconstriction. The clinical findings in patients with vasoconstriction confirmed by angiography are often those of diffuse brain swelling, such as headache, decreased alertness, and confusion. When vasoconstriction is focal or multifocal, the clinical findings are those of focal ischemia, such as hemiparesis, aphasia, and hemianopia. Vasoconstriction usually has its onset 3 to 5 days after a hemorrhage. The peak time for constriction is days 5 to 9; vasoconstriction usually improves after the second week unless rebleeding occurs.[218]

Vasoconstriction is detected by angiography in 30 to 70 percent of patients with SAH, depending on the timing of the study.[218,219] Severe vasoconstriction is manifested by a lumen size of <0.5 mm, delayed anterograde flow, and evidence of collateral filling distal to the vasoconstricted vessel. TCD is effective in monitoring for the presence of vasoconstriction, which increases blood flow velocities.[220] Single-photon emission computed tomography (SPECT) also can show regions of poor perfusion and document the presence of delayed ischemia.[221]

Many treatments have been tried to prevent or treat vasoconstriction after SAH.[217] These treatments include removal of blood by lumbar puncture and at the time of early surgery, pharmacologic agents such as calcium channel blockers to minimize contraction of the arterial wall, and hypervolemia to prevent ischemia by maintaining perfusion. At present, the most popular approaches are early surgery, nimodipine (a calcium channel blocker), and hypervolemic therapy, especially after aneurysmal clipping. Hypovolemia is common after SAH, as is hyponatremia. Hypervolemia does not reverse the vasoconstriction but helps maintain brain perfusion.

Coagulopathies

Hypercoagulability and bleeding caused by decreased coagulability affect most body organs, including the brain and heart. An increased tendency toward clotting can be caused by abnormalities of the formed blood elements or serologic factors.[222–224] Increased numbers of red blood cells and platelets and qualitative abnormalities such as sickle cell disease can cause intravascular clotting, especially in the presence of dehydration and reduced plasma volume. Excessive platelet activation, or so-called sticky platelets, also can explain increased coagulability but has proved hard to measure reliably in vitro.[225] The level of beta-thromboglobulin is a good marker for platelet activation (see Chap. 44). Serologic abnormalities may be congenital or acquired. Decreased amounts of natural anticoagulants (antithrombin III, protein C, and protein S), resistance to activated protein C, and prothrombin gene mutations can cause hypercoagulability.[222–224,226] These proteins may be decreased in patients with hypoproteinemia, especially that resulting from the nephrotic syndrome and urinary protein loss. Fibrinogen levels and the levels of various coagulation factors, such as factors VIII and XI, also may be high in patients with a prothrombotic state (see Chap. 44). In many of these patients—e.g., those on high-dose estrogen birth control pills, pregnant women, and patients with cancer—serologic and standard coagulation tests (in vitro) do not clarify the mechanism of the excessive clotting in vivo. Stroke patients may have serologic evidence of platelet activation and increased fibrin formation but decreased natural fibrinolytic and anticoagulant activity.[223,226]

Recently, measurement of various serum antiphospholipid antibodies has elicited considerable interest. The substances that usually are measured are the so-called lupus anticoagulant[227–229] and anticardiolipin antibodies. Increased activity of antiphospholipid antibodies (APLAs) is found in patients with systemic lupus erythematosus, acquired immunodeficiency syndrome (AIDS), giant-cell arteritis, and Sneddon's syndrome[229–232] (livedo reticularis and strokes) as well as in association with the use of some drugs (e.g., phenytoin, phenothiazines, procainamide, hydralazine, and quinidine). When the APLAs are not associated with other conditions and the patient has clinical evidence of excess clotting, the disorder is considered primary and is referred to as the *primary APLA syndrome*.[232–235] Patients with APLAs have an increased incidence of spontaneous abortions, venous occlusive disease of the legs and pulmonary embolism, brain infarcts (often multiple), thrombocytopenia, and false-positive syphilis serologic tests. Older patients with APLAs often also have important risk factors for stroke.[232–235]

Patients with systemic illnesses often have an elevated erythrocyte sedimentation rate, and strokes and pulmonary emboli often follow and complicate myocardial infarction (see Chap. 42). Customarily, such brain infarcts have been attributed to cardiogenic embolism, but some undoubtedly are related to thromboses precipitated by increased levels of acute-phase reactant coagulation proteins. Cancer, especially mucinous adenocarcinoma, has been associated with multiple vascular occlusions, large and tiny brain infarcts, and venous and arterial occlusions.[236]

Deficient coagulability can lead to serious intracranial bleeding. The hemorrhage can be into the brain (ICH), the CSF (SAH), or the subdural and epidural compartments. Thrombocytopenia, hemophilia, and leukemia are conditions that commonly lead to intracranial hemorrhage. The most common iatrogenic cause of bleeding is anticoagulation with heparin or warfarin.[192,237] Brain hemorrhage also has been described after fibrinolytic treatment of patients with coronary artery disease[238] and after rt-PA infusion to treat cerebrovascular occlusive disease[179–184] (see Chaps. 42 and 44).

Anticoagulant-related ICH, a catastrophic complication with high morbidity and mortality, is relatively rare considering the frequency of anticoagulant use. Anticoagulant-related hemorrhages develop more insidiously and evolve more slowly and more often than do other causes of ICH.[237] Many are erroneously attributed to brain ischemia, especially when anticoagulants have been prescribed to treat TIAs. Any patient taking anticoagulants who develops CNS symptoms should be considered to have anticoagulant-related ICH until CT or MRI excludes that diagnosis. The hematoma grows slowly and insidiously increases intracranial pressure. Many patients require surgical drainage of their hematomas to ensure survival. Anticoagulants should be stopped immediately, and their effect reversed by fresh frozen plasma or vitamin K. It is probably safe to resume anticoagulation with heparin 7 days to 2 weeks after the ICH if indicated, e.g., for prophylaxis in patients with artificial heart valves.[239] In patients treated with fibrinolytic agents, hemorrhages are most often lobar or cerebellar and may be multiple. ICH is more common when there is a past stroke, when heparin or other agents that affect coagulation are given with or after fibrinolytic agents, and when there is a hemostatic defect secondary to treatment.[239]

Arterial Dissections

Aortic dissections involving the innominate or carotid arteries (see Chap. 88) are a well-known cause of stroke and other manifestations of brain ischemia. Less well known are the syndromes produced by dissections of the extracranial and intracranial arteries, which are especially likely to occur in young, active individuals without risk factors for atherosclerosis or stroke but after trauma or chiropractic or other neck manipulations. They also are associated with fibromuscular dysplasia, Marfan's syndrome, pseudoxanthoma elasticum, and migraine.

Dissections start with a tear in the media and spread longitudinally (Fig. 89-11), often disrupting adventitial fibers or even rupturing through the adventitia to produce an extravascular hematoma and a false aneurysm or pseudoaneurysm within muscle and connective tissue. Intracranially, such a rupture can produce SAH. Other dissections cause arterial obstruction and secondary thrombosis of the narrowed vascular lumen. Most cerebrovascular dissections occur in the extracranial vessels, particularly the pharyngeal portion of the ICA and the nuchal vertebral arteries.[5,240–243]

Extracranial dissections produce sharp pain and throbbing headache; brain and retinal ischemic episodes, which may occur in rapid-fire attacks ("carotid allegro"[243]); and pressure on adjacent structures, especially cranial nerves X through XII, which exit at the skull base. Strokes, usually from embolization of

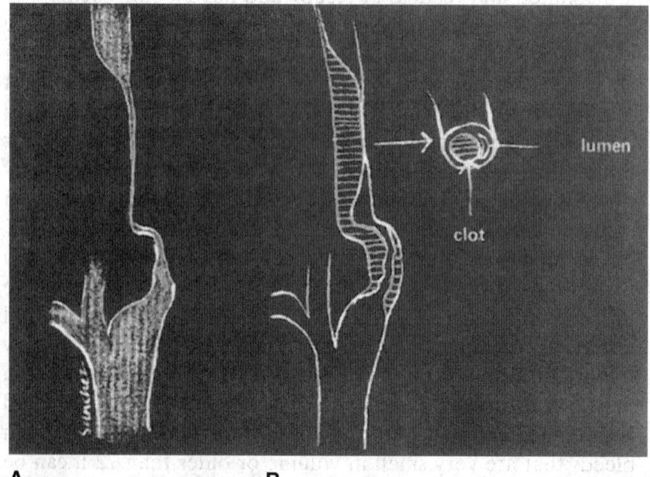

FIGURE 89-11 Diagrams of a carotid artery dissection. *A*. The lumen encroached on by the intramural clot. *B*. The dissection (cross-hatched). (From Caplan LR. *Stroke: A Clinical Approach*, 3d ed. Boston: Butterworth-Heinemann; 2000, with permission.)

clots, are common but may have a benign course. Intracranial dissections have a worse prognosis, often with vascular rupture and SAH. The diagnosis is confirmed by angiography, CT, or MRI. Ultrasound studies can be helpful in suggesting the diagnosis of dissection in the neck.[244]

Treatment consists of the use of heparin acutely, followed by warfarin. In patients in whom the dissected artery is initially occluded and remains occluded, warfarin can be stopped after 6 to 12 weeks. The author continues warfarin in other patients until there no longer is severe luminal narrowing, monitoring the dissected arteries by using noninvasive techniques (ultrasound, CTA, or MRA). Intracranial dissections with SAH have been treated surgically.[241,245]

References

1. Caplan LR. Brain embolism. In: Caplan LR, Hurst JW, Chimowitz MI. *Clinical Neurocardiology*. New York: Marcel Dekker, 1999; 35–185.
2. Aring C, Merritt H. Differential diagnosis between cerebral hemorrhage and cerebral thrombosis. *Arch Intern Med* 1935; 56: 435–456.
3. Whisnant J, Fitzgibbons J, Kurland L, Sayre GP. Natural history of stroke in Rochester, Minnesota, 1945–1954. *Stroke* 1971; 2:11–22.
4. Matsumoto N, Whisnant J, Kurland L, Okazaki H. Natural history of stroke in Rochester, Minnesota, 1955–1969. *Stroke* 1973; 4:2–29.
5. Caplan LR. *Stroke: A Clinical Approach*, 3d ed. Boston: Butterworth-Heinemann; 2000.
6. Mohr J, Caplan LR, Melski J, et al. The Harvard Cooperative Stroke registry: A prospective study. *Neurology* 1978; 28:754–762.
7. Foulkes MA, Wolf PA, Price TR, et al. The Stroke Data Bank: Design, methods, and baseline characteristics. *Stroke* 1988; 19: 547–554.
8. Kunitz S, Gross C, Heyman A, et al. The Pilot Stroke Data Bank: Definition, design and data. *Stroke* 1984; 15:740–746.
9. Bogousslavsky J, Cachin C, Regli F, et al. Cardiac sources of embolism and cerebral infarction—clinical consequences and vascular concomitants: The Lausanne Stroke Registry. *Neurology* 1991; 41:855–859.
10. Kittner SJ, Sharkness CM, Sloan M, et al. Infarcts with a cardiac source of embolism in the NINDS Stroke Data Bank: Neurologic examination. *Neurology* 1992; 42:299–302.
11. Sandok BA, Giuliani ER. Cerebral ischemic events in patients with mitral valve prolapse. *Stroke* 1982; 13:448–450.
12. Lauzier S, Barnett HJM. Cerebral ischemia with mitral valve prolapse and mitral annulus calcification. In: Furlan AJ, ed. *The Heart and Stroke*. London: Springer-Verlag; 1987:63.
13. Pomerance A, Davies MJ. Strokes: A complication of mitral leaflet prolapse. *Lancet* 1977; 2:1186.
14. Hanson MR, Conomy JP, Hodgman JR. Brain events associated with mitral valve prolapse. *Stroke* 1980; 11:499–506.
15. Jones HR, Naggar CZ, Selyan MP, et al. Mitral valve prolapse and cerebral ischemic events: A comparison between a neurology population with stroke and a cardiology population with mitral valve prolapse observed for 5 years. *Stroke* 1982; 13:451–453.
16. Pomerance A. Pathological and clinical study of calcification in the mitral valve ring. *J Clin Pathol* 1970; 23:354–361.
17. Stein JH, Soble JS. Thrombus associated with mitral valve calcification. *Stroke* 1995; 26:1697–1699.
18. DeBono DP, Warlow CP. Mitral-annulus calcification and cerebral or retinal ischemia. *Lancet* 1979; 2:383–385.
19. Benjamin EJ, Plehn JF, D'Agostino RB, et al. Mitral annular calcification and the risk of stroke in an elderly cohort. *N Engl J Med* 1992; 327:374–379.
20. Sacco RL, Ellenberg JH, Mohr JP, et al. Infarcts of undetermined cause: The NINCDS Stroke Data Bank. *Ann Neurol* 1989; 25: 382–390.
21. Galve E, Candell-Riera J, Pigrau C, et al. Prevalence, morphology, types and evaluation of cardiac valvular disease in systemic lupus erythematosus. *N Engl J Med* 1988; 319:817–823.
22. Barbut D, Borer JS, Wallerson D, et al. Anticardiolipin antibody and stroke: Possible relation of valvular heart disease and embolic events. *Cardiology* 1991; 79:99–109.
23. Cohen A, Tzourio C, Chauvel C, et al. Mitral valve strands and the risk of ischemic stroke in elderly patients. *Stroke* 1997; 28: 1574–1578.
24. Caplan LR. Mitral valve strands: What are they and what is their relation to stroke? *Neurol Network Comment* 1998; 2:11–14.
25. Kanter MC, Hart RG. Neurologic complications of infective endocarditis. *Neurology* 1991; 41:1015–1020.
26. Caplan LR. Of birds and nests and brain emboli. *Rev Neurol (Paris)* 1991; 147:265–273.
27. Amarenco P, Duyckaerts C, Tzourio C, et al. The prevalence of ulcerated plaques in the aortic arch in patients with stroke. *N Engl J Med* 1992; 326:221–225.
28. Weinberger J, Azhar S, Danisi F, et al. A new noninvasive technique for imaging atherosclerotic plaque in the aortic arch of stroke patients by transcutaneous real-time B-mode ultrasonography. *Stroke* 1998; 29:673–676.
29. The French Study of Aortic Plaques in Stroke Group. Atherosclerotic disease of the aortic arch as a risk factor for recurrent ischemic stroke. *N Engl J Med* 1996; 334:1216–1221.
30. Gacs G, Merel MD, Bodosi M. Balloon catheter as a model of cerebral emboli in humans. *Stroke* 1982; 13:39–42.
31. Fisher CM. Left hemiplegia and motor impersistence. *J Nerv Ment Dis* 1956; 123:201–218.
32. Caplan LR, Kelly M, Kase CS, et al. Infarcts of the inferior division of the right middle cerebral artery: Mirror image of Wernicke's aphasia. *Neurology* 1986; 36:1015–1020.
33. Caplan LR. Posterior cerebral artery. In: Bogousslavsky J, Caplan LR, eds. *Stroke Syndromes*. New York: Cambridge University Press; 1995:290.
34. Yammamoto Y, Georgiadis AL, Chang H-M, et al. Posterior cerebral artery territory infarcts in the New England Medical Center Posterior Circulation Registry. *Arch Neurol* 1999; 56: 824–832.
35. Mehler MF. The rostral basilar artery syndrome: Diagnosis, etiology, prognosis. *Neurology* 1989; 39:9–16.
36. Amarenco P. The spectrum of cerebellar infarctions. *Neurology* 1991; 41:973–979.
37. Fieschi C, Argentino C, Lenzi GL, et al. Clinical and instrumental evaluation of patients with ischemic stroke within the first six hours. *J Neurol Sci* 1989; 91:311–322.
38. Kushner MJ, Zanotte EM, Bastianiello S, et al. Transcranial Doppler in acute hemispheric brain infarction. *Neurology* 1991; 41:109–113.
39. Ringlestein EB, Koschorke S, Holling A, et al. Computed tomographic patterns of proven embolic brain infarcts. *Ann Neurol* 1989; 26:759–765.
40. Bladin PF, Berkovic SF. Striatocapsular infarction. *Neurology* 1984; 34:1423–1430.
41. Fisher CM, Adams RD. Observations on brain embolism. *J Neuropathol Exp Neurol* 1951; 10:92–94.
42. Fisher CM, Adams RD. Observations on brain embolism with special reference to hemorrhagic infarction. In: Furlan AJ, ed. *The Heart and Stroke*. London: Springer-Verlag; 1987:17.
43. Tomsick T, Brott T, Barsan W, et al. Thrombus localization with emergency cerebral computed tomography. *Stroke* 1990; 21:180.

44. Bergeron GA, Shah PM. Echocardiography unwarranted in patients with cerebral ischemic events. *N Engl J Med* 1981; 304:489.
45. Greenland P, Knopman D, Mikell F, et al. Echocardiography in diagnostic assessment of stroke. *Ann Intern Med* 1981; 95:51–54.
46. Tegeler CH, Downes TR. Cardiac imaging in stroke. *Stroke* 1991; 22:1206–1211.
47. Cohen A, Chauvel C. Transesophageal echocardiography in the management of transient ischemic attack and ischemic stroke. *Cerebrovasc Dis* 1996; 6(suppl 1):15–25.
48. DeWitt LD, Pessin MS, Pandian NG, et al. Benign disappearance of ventricular thrombus after embolic stroke: A case report. *Stroke* 1988; 19:393–396.
49. Markus HS, Harrison MJ. Microembolic signal detection using ultrasound. *Stroke* 1995; 26:1517–1519.
50. Tong DC, Bolger A, Albers GW. Incidence of transcranial Doppler-detected cerebral microemboli in patients referred for echocardiography. *Stroke* 1994; 25:2138–2141.
51. Barbut D, Hinton RB, Szatrowski TP, et al. Cerebral emboli detected during bypass surgery are associated with clamp removal. *Stroke* 1994; 25:2398–2402.
52. Petersen P, Boysen G, Godtfredsen J, et al. Placebo-controlled, randomized trial of warfarin and aspirin for prevention of thromboembolic complications in chronic atrial fibrillation: The Copenhagen AFASAK Study. *Lancet* 1989; 1:175–179.
53. Stroke Prevention in Atrial Fibrillation Investigators. The stroke prevention in atrial fibrillation trial: Final results. *Circulation* 1991; 84:527–539.
54. Stroke Prevention in Atrial Fibrillation Investigators. Adjusted-dose warfarin versus low-intensity fixed-dose warfarin plus aspirin for high-risk patients with atrial fibrillation: Stroke Prevention in Atrial Fibrillation III randomized clinical trial. *Lancet* 1996: 348:633–638.
55. Stroke Prevention in Atrial Fibrillation Investigators. Prospective identification of patients with nonvalvular atrial fibrillation at low risk during treatment with aspirin: Stroke prevention in Atrial Fibrillation III Study. *Circulation* 1997; 96(suppl):I-28 (Abstract).
56. The Stroke Prevention in Atrial Fibrillation Investigators. Predictors of thromboembolism in atrial fibrillation: I. Clinical features of patients at risk. *Ann Intern Med* 1992; 116:1–5.
57. The Stroke Prevention in Atrial Fibrillation Investigators. Predictors of thromboembolism in atrial fibrillation: II. Echocardiographic features of patients at risk. *Ann Intern Med* 1992; 116: 6–12.
58. Pritchett ELC. Management of atrial fibrillation. *N Engl J Med* 1992; 326:1264–1271.
59. The Boston Area Anticoagulation Trial for Atrial Fibrillation Investigators. The effect of low-dose warfarin on the risk of stroke in patients with nonrheumatic atrial fibrillation. *N Engl J Med* 1990; 323:1505–1511.
60. European Atrial Fibrillation Trial Study Group. Optimal oral anticoagulation therapy in patients with nonrheumatic atrial fibrillation and recent cerebral ischemia. *N Engl J Med* 1995; 333: 5–10.
61. Moldveen-Geronimus M, Merriam JC. Cholesterol embolization: From pathologic curiosity to clinical entity. *Circulation* 1967; 35: 946–953.
62. Shields RW Jr, Laureno R, Lachman T, et al. Anticoagulant-related hemorrhage in acute cerebral embolism. *Stroke* 1984; 15: 426–437.
63. Cerebral Embolism Study Group. Immediate anticoagulation of embolic stroke: A randomized trial. *Stroke* 1983; 13:668–676.
64. Toni D, Fiorelli M, Bastianello S, et al. Hemorrhagic transformation of brain infarct. *Neurology* 1996; 46:341–345.
65. Cerebral Embolism Task Force. Cardiogenic brain embolism: The second report of the Cerebral Embolism Task Force. *Arch Neurol* 1989; 46:727–743.
66. Pessin MS, Estol CJ, Lafranchise F, et al. Safety of anticoagulation after hemorrhagic infarction. *Neurology* 1993; 43:1298–1303.
67. Chaves CJ, Pessin MS, Caplan LR, et al. Cerebellar hemorrhagic infarction. *Neurology* 1996; 46:346–349.
68. Chamorro A, Vila N, Ascaso C, Blanc R. Heparin in acute stroke with atrial fibrillation: Clinical relevance of very early treatment. *Arch Neurol* 1999; 56:1098–1102.
69. Caplan LR. When should heparin be given to patients with atrial fibrillation-related brain infarcts? *Arch Neurol* 1999; 56:1059–1060.
70. Hagen PT, Scholz DG, Edwards WD. Incidence and size of patent foramen ovale during the first 10 decades of life: An autopsy study of 965 normal hearts. *Mayo Clin Proc* 1984; 59:17–20.
71. Lechat PH, Mas JL, Lascault G, et al. Prevalence of patent foramen ovale in patients with stroke. *N Engl J Med* 1988; 318:1148–1152.
72. Petty GW, Khanderia BK, Chu C-P, et al. Patent foramen ovale in patients with cerebral infarction: A transesophageal echocardiographic study. *Arch Neurol* 1997; 54:819–822.
73. Gautier JC, Durr A, Koussa S, et al. Paradoxical cerebral embolism with a patent foramen ovale: A report of 29 patients. *Cerebrovasc Dis* 1991; 1:193–202.
74. Caplan LR. Cardiac arrest and other hypoxic-ischemic insults. In: Caplan LR, Hurst JW, Chimowitz MI, eds. *Clinical Neurocardiology*. New York: Marcel Dekker, 1999; 1–34.
75. Dougherty JH, Rawlinson DG, Levy DE, et al. Hypoxic-ischemic brain injury and the vegetative state: Clinical and neuropathologic correlation. *Neurology* 1981; 31:991–997.
76. Cummings JL, Tomiyasu U, Read S, et al. Amnesia with hippocampal lesions after cardiopulmonary arrest. *Neurology* 1984; 34: 679–681.
77. Dooling E, Richardson EP. Delayed encephalopathy after strangling. *Arch Neurol* 1976; 33:196–199.
78. Gilles F. Hypotensive brainstem necrosis. *Arch Pathol* 1969; 88: 32–41.
79. Caronna JJ, Finkelstein S. Neurological syndromes after cardiac arrest. *Stroke* 1978; 9:517–520.
80. Levy DE, Knill-Jones RP, Plum F. The vegetative state and its prognosis following non-traumatic coma. *Ann NY Acad Sci* 1978; 315:293–306.
81. Willoughby J, Leach B. Relation of neurological findings after cardiac arrest to outcome. *Br Med J* 1974; 3:437–439.
82. Levy D, Carrona JJ, Singer BH, et al. Predicting outcome from hypoxic-ischemic coma. *JAMA* 1985; 253:1420–1426.
83. Longstreth WT, Inui TS, Cobb LA, et al. Neurologic recovery after out-of-hospital cardiac arrest. *Ann Intern Med* 1983; 38: 588–592.
84. Longstreth WT, Diehr P, Inui TS. Prediction of awakening after out-of-hospital cardiac arrest. *N Engl J Med* 1983; 308:1378–1382.
85. Thompson RG, Hallstrom AP, Cobb LA. Bystander-initiated cardiopulmonary resuscitation in the management of ventricular fibrillation. *Ann Intern Med* 1979; 90:737–740.
86. Bedell SE, Delbanco TG, Cook EF, Epstein FH. Survival after cardiopulmonary resuscitation in the hospital. *N Engl J Med* 1983; 309:569–576.
87. Caplan LR, Brass LM, DeWitt LD, et al. Transcranial Doppler ultrasound: Present status. *Neurology* 1990; 40:696–700.
88. Longstreth WT, Inui TS. High blood glucose level on hospital admission and poor neurological recovery after cardiac arrest. *Ann Neurol* 1984; 15:59–63.
89. Collins RC, Dobkin BH, Choi DW. Selective vulnerability of the brain: New insights into the pathophysiology of stroke. *Ann Intern Med* 1989; 110:992–1000.
90. Giswold S, Safar P, Rao G, et al. Multifaceted therapy after global brain ischemia in monkeys. *Stroke* 1984; 15:803–812.
91. Caplan LR. Encephalopathies and neurological effects of drugs used in cardiac patients. In: Caplan LR, Hurst JW, Chimowitz

MI, eds. *Clinical Neurocardiology*. New York: Marcel Dekker; 1999:186.
92. Closson RG. Visual hallucinations as the earliest symptom of digoxin intoxication. *Arch Neurol* 1983; 40:386.
93. Gilbert GJ. Quinidine dementia. *JAMA* 1977; 237:2093–2094.
94. Barbut D, Caplan LR. Brain complications of cardiac surgery. *Curr Probl Cardiol* 1997; 22:455–476.
95. Slogoff S, Girgis KZ, Keats AS. Etiologic factors in neuropsychiatric complications associated with cardiopulmonary bypass. *Anesth Analg* 1982; 61:903–911.
96. Gilman S. Neurological complications of open heart surgery. *Ann Neurol* 1990; 28:475–476.
97. Shaw PJ, Bates D, Cartlidge NEF, et al. Early neurological complications of coronary artery bypass surgery. *Br Med J* 1985; 291: 1384–1387.
98. Breuer AC, Furlan AJ, Hanson MR, et al. Central nervous system complications of coronary artery bypass graft surgery: Prospective analysis of 421 patients. *Stroke* 1983; 14:682–687.
99. Ropper AH, Wechsler LR, Wilson LS. Carotid bruit and the risk of stroke in elective surgery. *N Engl J Med* 1982; 307:1388–1390.
100. Furlan AJ, Craciun AR. Risk of stroke during coronary artery bypass graft surgery in patients with internal carotid artery disease documented by angiography. *Stroke* 1985; 16:797–799.
101. Sila C. Neuroimaging of cerebral infarction associated with coronary revascularization. *AJNR* 1991; 12:817–818.
102. Hertzer NR, Loop FD, Beven EG, et al. Surgical staging for simultaneous coronary and carotid disease: A study including prospective randomization. *Vasc Surg* 1989; 9:455–463.
103. VonReutern G-M, Hetzel A, Birnbaum D, et al. Transcranial Doppler ultrasound during cardiopulmonary bypass in patients with internal carotid artery disease documented by angiography. *Stroke* 1988; 19:674–680.
104. Hise JH, Nippu ML, Schnitker JC. Stroke associated with coronary artery bypass surgery. *AJNR* 1991; 12:811–814.
105. Wijdicks EFM, Jack CR. Coronary artery bypass grafting-associated stroke. *J Neuroimag* 1996; 6:20–22.
106. Tettenborn B, Caplan LR, Sloan MA, et al. Postoperative brainstem cerebellar infarcts. *Neurology* 1993; 43:471–477.
107. Barbut D, Hinton RB, Szatrowski TP, et al. Cerebral emboli detected during bypass surgery are associated with clamp removal. *Stroke* 1994; 25:2398–2402.
108. Pugsley W, Paschalis C, Treasure T, et al. The impact of microemboli during cardiopulmonary bypass on neuropsychological functioning. *Stroke* 1994; 25:1393–1399.
109. Price DL, Harris J. Cholesterol emboli in cerebral arteries are a complication of retrograde aortic perfusion during cardiac surgery. *Neurology* 1970; 20:1207–1214.
110. Karalis DG, Chandrasekaran K, Victor MF, et al. Recognition and embolic potential of intraaortic atherosclerotic debris. *J Am Coll Cardiol* 1991; 17:73–78.
111. Marshall JNG, Barzilai B, Kouchoukos N, Saffitz J. Intraoperative ultrasonic imaging of the ascending aorta. *Ann Thorac Surg* 1989; 48:339–344.
112. Gilman S. Cerebral disorders after open-heart operations. *N Engl J Med* 1965; 272:489–498.
113. Coffey CE, Massey EW, Roberts KB, et al. Natural history of cerebral complications of coronary artery bypass graft surgery. *Neurology* 1983; 33:1416–1421.
114. Moody DM, Bell MA, Challa VR, et al. Brain microemboli during cardiac surgery or aortography. *Ann Neurol* 1990; 28:477–486.
115. Feeney DM, Gonzalez A, Law WA. Amphetamine, haloperidol and experience interact to affect the rate of recovery after motor cortex injury. *Science* 1982; 217:855–857.
116. Humphreys RP, Hoffman JH, Mustard WT, Trusler GA. Cerebral hemorrhage following heart surgery. *J Neurosurg* 1975; 43: 671–675.
117. Sila CA. Spectrum of neurologic events following cardiac transplantation. *Stroke* 1989; 20:1586–1589.
118. Caplan LR. Intracerebral hemorrhage revisited. *Neurology* 1988; 38:624–627.
119. Lederman RJ, Breuer AC, Hanson MR, et al. Peripheral nervous system complications of coronary artery bypass graft surgery. *Ann Neurol* 1982; 12:297–301.
120. Caplan LR, Hurst JW. Cardiac and cardiovascular findings in patients with nervous system disease—strokes. In: Caplan LR, Hurst JW, Chimowitz MI, eds. *Clinical Neurocardiology*. New York: Marcel Dekker; 1999:303.
121. Norris JW, Hachinski V. Cardiac dysfunction following stroke. In: Furlan AJ, ed. *The Heart and Stroke*. London: Springer-Verlag; 1987:171.
122. Smith RP, Tomlinson BE. Subendocardial hemorrhages associated with intracranial lesions. *J Pathol Bacteriol* 1954; 68:327–334.
123. Kolin A, Norris JW. Myocardial damage from acute cerebral lesions. *Stroke* 1984; 15:990–993.
124. Samuels MA. Electrocardiographic manifestations of neurologic disease. *Semin Neurol* 1984; 4:453–459.
125. Myers MG, Norris JW, Hachinski V, Sole MJ. Plasma norepinephrine in stroke. *Stroke* 1981; 12:200–204.
126. Marion DW, Segal R, Thompson ME. Subarachnoid hemorrhage and the heart. *Rev Neurosurg* 1986; 18:101–106.
127. Samuels M. "Voodoo" death revisited: The modern lessons of neurocardiology. *Neurologist* 1997; 3:293–304.
128. Burch GE, Myers R, Abildskov JA. A new electrocardiographic pattern observed in cerebrovascular accidents. *Circulation* 1954; 9:719–723.
129. Dimant J, Grob D. Electrocardiographic changes and myocardial damage in patients with acute cerebrovascular accidents. *Stroke* 1977; 8:448–455.
130. Rolak LA, Rokey R. Electrocardiographic features: In: Rolak LA, Rokey R, eds. *Coronary and Cerebral Vascular Disease*. Mt. Kisco, NY: Futura; 1990:139–197.
131. Fabinyi G, Hunt D, McKinley L. Myocardial creatine kinase isoenzyme in serum after subarachnoid hemorrhage. *J Neurol Neurosurg Psychiatry* 1977; 40:818–820.
132. Neil-Dwyer G, Cruickshank J, Stratton C. Beta-blockers, plasma total creatine kinase and creatine kinase myocardial isoenzyme, and the prognosis of subarachnoid hemorrhage. *Surg Neurol* 1986; 25:163–168.
133. Myers MG, Norris JW, Hachinsky VC, et al. Cardiac sequelae of acute strokes. *Stroke* 1982; 13:838–842.
134. Stober T, Sen S, Anstatt T, Bette L. Correlation of cardiac arrhythmias with brainstem compression in patients with intracerebral hemorrhage. *Stroke* 1988; 19:688–692.
135. Wier BK. Pulmonary edema following fatal aneurysmal rupture. *J Neurosurg* 1978; 49:502–507.
136. Theodore J, Robin ED. Pathogenesis of neurogenic pulmonary edema. *Lancet* 1975; 2:749–751.
137. Engel GL. Psychologic factors in instantaneous cardiac death. *N Engl J Med* 1976; 294:664–665.
138. Lown B, Temte JV, Reich P, et al. Basis for recurring ventricular fibrillation in the absence of coronary heart disease and its management. *N Engl J Med* 1976; 294:623–629.
139. Talman WT. Cardiovascular regulation and lesions of the central nervous system. *Ann Neurol* 1985; 18:1–12.
140. Schwartz PJ, Stone HL, Brown AM. Effects of unilateral stellate ganglion blockage on the arrhythmias associated with coronary occlusion. *Am Heart J* 1976; 92:589–599.
141. Adams H, Kassell N, Mazuz H. The patients with transient ischemic attacks: Is this the time for a new therapeutic approach? *Stroke* 1984; 15:371–375.
142. Hennerici M, Aulich A, Sandmann W, Freund HJ. Incidence of asymptomatic extracranial arterial disease. *Stroke* 1981; 12: 750–758.

143. Caplan LR. Cerebrovascular disease: Large artery occlusive disease. In: Appel S, ed. *Current Neurology*, vol 87. Chicago: Year Book; 1988:179–226.
144. Zarins CK, Giddins DP, Bharadvaj BK, et al. Carotid bifurcation atherosclerosis. *Circ Res* 1983; 53:502–514.
145. Hutchinson EC, Yates DO. The cervical portion of the vertebral artery: A clinicopathologic study. *Brain* 1956; 79:319–331.
146. Fisher CM, Ojemann RG. A clinico-pathologic study of carotid endarterectomy plaques. *Rev Neurol (Paris)* 1986; 142:573–589.
147. Caplan LR, Gorelick PB, Hier DB. Race, sex, and occlusive vascular disease: A review. *Stroke* 1986; 17:648–655.
148. Gorelick PB, Caplan LR, Hier DB, et al. Racial differences in the distribution of posterior circulation occlusive disease. *Stroke* 1985; 16:785–790.
149. Feldmann E, Daneault N, Kwan E, et al. Chinese-white differences in the distribution of occlusive cerebrovascular disease. *Neurology* 1990; 40:1541–1545.
150. Caplan LR, Wolpert SM. Angiography in patients with occlusive cerebrovascular disease: Views of a stroke neurologist and neuroradiologist. *AJNR* 1991; 12:593–601.
151. Caplan LR, Hennerici M. Impaired clearance of emboli is an important link between hypoperfusion, embolism, and ischemic stroke. *Arch Neurol* 1998; 55:1475–1482.
152. Chambers BR, Norris JW. Outcome in patients with asymptomatic neck bruits. *N Engl J Med* 1986; 315:860–865.
153. Ringelstein EB, Zeumer H, Angelou D. The pathogenesis of strokes from internal carotid artery occlusion: Diagnostic and therapeutical implications. *Stroke* 1983; 14:867–875.
154. Caplan LR, Tettenborn B. Vertebrobasilar occlusive disease: Review of selected aspects. 2: Posterior circulation embolism. *Cerebrovasc Dis* 1992; 2:320–326.
155. Gorelick PB, Hier DB, Caplan LR, Langenberg P. Headache in acute cerebrovascular disease. *Neurology* 1986; 36:1445–1450.
156. Pessin MS, Hinton RC, Davis KR, et al. Mechanism of acute carotid stroke. *Ann Neurol* 1979; 6:245–252.
157. Caplan LR. Significance of unexpected (silent) brain infarcts. In: Caplan LR, Shifrin EG, Nicolaides AN, Moore WS, eds. *Cerebrovascular Ischaemia: Investigation and Management*. London: Med-Orion; 1996:423–433.
158. O'Donnell TF, Erdoes L, Mackey WC, et al. Correlation of B-mode ultrasound imaging and arteriography with pathologic findings at carotid endarterectomy. *Arch Surg* 1985; 120:443–449.
159. Zwiebel WJ, Zagzebski JA, Crummy AB, Hirscher M. Correlation of peak Doppler frequency with lumen narrowing in carotid stenosis. *Stroke* 1982; 13:386–391.
160. Hennerici M, Rautenberg W, Sitzer G, Schwartz A. Transcranial Doppler ultrasound for the assessment of intracranial arterial flow velocity: I. Examination technique and normal values. *Surg Neurol* 1986; 315:860–865.
161. Spencer MP, Thomas GI, Nicholls SC, et al. Detection of middle cerebral artery emboli during carotid endarterectomy using transcranial Doppler ultrasonography. *Stroke* 1990; 21:415–423.
162. Edelman RR, Mattle HP, Atkinson DJ, Hoogewoud HM. MR angiography. *AJR* 1990; 154:937–946.
163. Caplan LR, DeWitt LD, Breen JC. Neuroimaging in patients with cerebrovascular disease In: Greenberg J, ed. *Neuroimaging: A Companion to Adams and Victor's Principles of Neurology*. New York: McGraw-Hill; 1999:493–520.
164. Caplan LR. Treatment of cerebral ischemia: Where are we headed? *Stroke* 1984; 15:571–574.
165. Warach S, Gaa J, Siewert B, et al. Acute human stroke studied by whole brain echo planar diffusion-weighted magnetic resonance imaging. *Ann Neurol* 1995; 37:231–241.
166. Sorensen AG, Buonanno F, Gonzalez RG, et al. Hyperacute stroke: Evaluation with combined multisection diffusion-weighted and hemodynamically weighted echo-planar MR imaging. *Radiology* 1996; 199:391–401.
167. North American Symptomatic Carotid Endarterectomy Trial (NASCET) Collaborators. Beneficial effect of carotid endarterectomy in symptomatic patients with high-grade carotid stenosis. *N Engl J Med* 1991; 325:445–453.
168. Barnett HJM, Taylor DW, Eliasziw M, et al for the North American Symptomatic Carotid Endarterectomy Trial Collaborators. Benefit of carotid endarterectomy in patients with symptomatic moderate or severe stenosis. *N Engl J Med* 1998; 339:1415–1425.
169. European Carotid Surgery Trialist's Collaborative Group. MRC European Carotid Surgery Trial: Interim results for symptomatic patients with severe (70–99 percent) or with mild (0–29 percent) carotid stenosis. *Lancet* 1991; 1:1235–1243.
170. European Carotid Surgery Trialist's Collaborative Group. Randomised trial of endarterectomy for recently symptomatic carotid stenosis: Final results of the MRC European Carotid Surgery Trial (ECST). *Lancet* 1998; 351:1379–1387.
171. Executive Committee for the Asymptomatic Carotid Atherosclerosis Study. Endarterectomy for asymptomatic carotid artery stenosis. *JAMA* 1995; 273:1421–1428.
172. Berguer R, Caplan LR, eds. *Vertebrobasilar Arterial Disease*. St Louis: Quality Medical Publishers; 1991:201–261.
173. Fields WS, Lemak NA, Frankowski RF, Hardy RJ. Controlled trial of aspirin in cerebral ischemia. *Stroke* 1977; 8:301–314.
174. Antiplatelet Trialists' Collaboration. Collaborative overview of randomised trials of antiplatelet therapy. 1: Prevention of death, myocardial infarction, and stroke by prolonged antiplatelet therapy in various categories of patients. *Br Med J* 1994; 308:81–106.
175. Hass WK, Easton JD, Adams HP, et al. A randomized trial comparing ticlopidine hydrochloride with aspirin for the prevention of stroke in high risk patients. *N Engl J Med* 1989; 321:501–507.
176. Warlow CP. Ticlopidine, a new antithrombotic drug: But is it better than aspirin for long term use? *J Neurol Neurosurg Psychiatry* 1990; 53:185–187.
177. CAPRIE Steering Committee. A randomised, blinded, trial of clopidogrel versus aspirin in patients at risk of ischaemic events. *Lancet* 1996; 348:1329–1339.
178. Diener HC, Cunha L, Forbes C, et al. European Stroke Prevention Study: 2. Dipyridamole and acetylsalicylic acid in the secondary prevention of stroke. *J Neurol Sci* 1996; 143:1–13.
179. The National Institute of Neurological Disorders and Stroke rt-PA Study Group. Tissue plasminogen activator for acute ischemic stroke. *N Engl J Med* 1995; 333:1581–1587.
180. del Zoppo GJ, Poeck K, Pessin MS, et al. Recombinant tissue plasminogen activator in acute thrombotic and embolic stroke. *Ann Neurol* 1992; 32:78–86.
181. Wolpert SM, Bruckmann H, Greenlee R, et al. Neuroradiologic evaluation of patients with acute stroke treated with recombinant tissue plasminogen activator. *AJNR* 1993; 14:3–13.
182. Pessin MS, del Zoppo GJ, Furlan AJ. Thrombolytic treatment in acute stroke: Review and update of selected topics. In: Moskowitz MA, Caplan LR, eds. *Cerebrovascular Diseases: Nineteenth Princeton Stroke Conference*. Boston: Butterworth-Heinemann; 1995:409–418.
183. Furlan A, Higashida R, Wechsler L, et al. A randomized trial of intra-arterial prourokinase for acute ischemic stroke of less than 6 hours duration due to middle cerebral artery occlusion. *JAMA* 1999; 282:2003–2011.
184. Caplan LR, Mohr JP, Kistler JP, et al. Should thrombolytic therapy be the first-line treatment for acute ischemic stroke? Thrombolysis—Not a panacea for ischemic stroke. *N Engl J Med* 1997; 337:1309–1310.
185. Pettigrew LC. Surgical considerations. In: Rolak L, Rokey R,

eds. *Coronary and Cerebral Vascular Disease*. Mt Kisco, NY: Futura; 1990:349–377.
186. Hertzer NR, Loop FD, Beven EG. Management of coexistent carotid and coronary artery disease: A surgical viewpoint. In: Furlan A, ed. *The Heart and Stroke*. London: Springer-Verlag; 1987:305–318.
187. Easton JD, Hart RG. Asymptomatic carotid artery disease in patients undergoing open heart surgery: A neurologic viewpoint. In: Furlan A, ed. *The Heart and Stroke*. London: Springer-Verlag; 1987:319–327.
188. Caplan LR. Intracranial branch atheromatous disease. *Neurology* 1989; 39:1246–1250.
189. Caplan LR. Lacunar infarction: A neglected concept. *Geriatrics* 1976; 31:71–75.
190. Caplan LR. Binswanger's disease revisited. *Neurology* 1995; 45: 626–633.
191. Fisher CM. The arterial lesions underlying lacunes. *Acta Neuropathol* 1969; 12:1–15.
192. Kase CS, Caplan LR. *Intracerebral Hemorrhage*. Boston: Butterworth-Heinemann; 1994.
193. Rosenblum WI. Miliary aneurysms and "fibrinoid" degeneration of cerebral blood vessels. *Hum Pathol* 1977; 8:133–139.
194. Fisher CM. Pathological observations in hypertensive cerebral hemorrhage. *J Neuropathol Exp Neurol* 1971; 30:536–550.
195. Mohr JP. Lacunes. *Stroke* 1982; 13:3–11.
196. Fisher CM. Lacunar strokes and infarcts: A review. *Neurology* 1982; 32:871–876.
197. Fisher CM. Pure motor hemiplegia of vascular origin. *Arch Neurol* 1965; 13:30–44.
198. Fisher CM. Pure sensory stroke and allied conditions. *Stroke* 1982; 13:434–447.
199. Fisher CW. Ataxic hemiparesis. *Arch Neurol* 1978; 35:126–128.
200. Fisher CM. A lacunar stroke, the dysarthric-clumsy hand syndrome. *Neurology* 1967; 17:614–617.
201. Hachinski VC, Potter P, Merskey H. Leuko-araiosis. *Arch Neurol* 1987; 44:21–23.
202. Caplan LR, Schoene W. Subcortical arteriosclerotic encephalopathy (Binswanger disease): Clinical features. *Neurology* 1978; 28: 1206–1219.
203. Babikian V, Ropper AH. Binswanger's disease: A review. *Stroke* 1987; 18:2–12.
204. Kase CS. Intracerebral hemorrhage: Non-hypertensive causes. *Stroke* 1986; 17:590–594.
205. Bahemuka M. Primary intracerebral hemorrhage and heart weight: A clinicopathological case-control review of 218 patients. *Stroke* 1987; 18:531–536.
206. Brott T, Thalinger K, Hertzberg V. Hypertension as a risk factor for spontaneous intracerebral hemorrhage. *Stroke* 1986; 17:1078–1083.
207. Fisher CM. Pathological observations in hypertensive cerebral hemorrhages. *J Neuropathol Exp Neurol* 1971; 30:536–550.
208. Linfante I, Linas RH, Caplan LR, Warach S. MRI features of intracerebral hemorrhage within 2 hours from symptoms onset. *Stroke* 1999; 30:2263–2267.
209. Tuhrim S, Dambrosia JM, Price TR, et al. Prediction of intracerebral hemorrhage survival. *Ann Neurol* 1988; 24:258–263.
210. Adams HP, Jergenson DD, Kassell NF, Sahs AL. Pitfalls in the recognition of subarachnoid hemorrhage. *JAMA* 1980; 244: 794–796.
211. Ostergaard JR. Warning leaks in subarachnoid hemorrhage. *Br Med J* 1990; 301:190–191.
212. Weisberg L. Computed tomography in aneurysmal subarachnoid hemorrhage. *Neurology* 1979; 29:802–808.
213. Caplan LR, Flamm ES, Mohr JP, et al. Lumbar puncture and stroke. *Stroke* 1987; 18:540A–544A.
214. Heros R, Zervas NT, Varsos V. Cerebral vasospasm after subarachnoid hemorrhage: An update. *Ann Neurol* 1983; 14:599–608.
215. Kassell N, Sasaki T, Colohan A, Nazar G. Cerebral vasospasm following aneurysmal subarachnoid hemorrhage. *Stroke* 1985; 16: 562–572.
216. MacDonald RL, Weir BK. A review of hemoglobin and the pathogenesis of cerebral vasospasm. *Stroke* 1991; 22:971–982.
217. Wilkins RH. Attempts at prevention or treatment of intracranial arterial spasm: An update. *Neurosurgery* 1986; 18:808–825.
218. Weir B, Grace M, Hansen J, Rothberg C. Time course of vasospasm in man. *J Neurosurg* 1978; 48:173–178.
219. Kwak R, Niizuma H, Ohi T, Suzuki J. Angiographic study of cerebral vasospasm following rupture of intracranial aneurysms: I. Time of the appearance. *Surg Neurol* 1979; 11:257–262.
220. Sloan MA, Haley EC, Kassell NF, et al. Sensitivity and specificity of transcranial Doppler ultrasonography in the diagnosis of vasospasm following subarachnoid hemorrhage. *Neurology* 1989; 39: 1514–1518.
221. Davis S, Andrews J, Lichtenstein M, et al. A single-photon emission computed tomography study of hypoperfusion after subarachnoid hemorrhage. *Stroke* 1990; 21:252–259.
222. Hart RG, Kanter MC. Hematologic disorders and ischemic stroke: A selective review. *Stroke* 1990; 20:1111–1121.
223. Coull BM, Goodnight SH. Current concepts of cerebrovascular disease and stroke: Antiphospholipid antibodies, prothrombotic states and stroke. *Stroke* 1990; 21:1370–1374.
224. Feinberg WM, Bruck DC, Ring ME. Hemostatic markers in acute stroke. *Stroke* 1989; 20:592–597.
225. Wu K, Hoak J. Increased platelet aggregation in patients with transient ischemic attacks. *Stroke* 1975; 6:521–524.
226. Feinberg WM. Coagulation. In: Caplan LR, ed. *Brain Ischemia: Basic Concepts and Clinical Relevance*. London: Springer-Verlag; 1995:85–96.
227. Hart R, Miller V, Coull B, Bril V. Cerebral infarction associated with lupus anticoagulants: Preliminary report. *Stroke* 1984; 15: 114–118.
228. Levine SR, Welch KMA. The spectrum of neurologic disease associated with antiphospholipid antibodies, lupus anticoagulants, and anticardiolipin antibodies. *Arch Neurol* 1987; 44: 876–883.
229. Kushner M, Simonian N. Lupus anticoagulant, anticardiolipin antibodies and cerebral ischemia. *Stroke* 1989; 20:225–229.
230. Levine SR, Langer SL, Albers JW, Welch KMA. Sneddon's syndrome: An antiphospholipid antibody syndrome. *Neurology* 1988; 38:798–800.
231. Rebollo M, Vol JF, Garijil F, et al. Livedo reticularis and cerebrovascular lesions (Sneddon's syndrome): Clinical, radiologic, and pathologic features in eight cases. *Brain* 1983; 106:965–979.
232. Antiphospholipid Antibodies in Stroke Study Group (APASS). Clinical and laboratory findings in patients with antiphospholipid antibodies and cerebral ischemia. *Stroke* 1990; 21:1268–1273.
233. DeWitt LD, Caplan LR. Antiphospholipid antibodies and stroke. *AJNR* 1991; 12:454–456.
234. Asherson RA. A "primary antiphospholipid syndrome"? (editorial). *J Rheumatol* 1988; 15:1742–1746.
235. Coull BM, Boudette DN, Goodnight SH, et al. Multiple cerebral infarction and dementia associated with anticardiolipin antibodies. *Stroke* 1987; 18:1107–1112.
236. Amico L, Caplan LR, Thomas C. Cerebrovascular complications of mucinous cancers. *Neurology* 1989; 39:522–526.
237. Kase C, Robinson R, Stein R, et al. Anticoagulant-related intracerebral hemorrhage. *Neurology* 1985; 35:943–948.
238. Bovill EG, Terrin ML, Stump DC, et al. Hemorrhagic events during therapy with recombinant tissue-type plasminogen activator, heparin, and aspirin for acute myocardial infarction. *Ann Intern Med* 1991; 115:256–265.
239. Babikian V, Kase C, Pessin M, et al. Resumption of anticoagulation after intracranial bleeding in patients with prosthetic valves. *Stroke* 1988; 19:407–408.

240. Hart RG, Easton JD. Dissections of cervical and cerebral arteries. *Neurol Clin North Am* 1983; 1:255–282.
241. Anson J, Crowell RM. Cervicocranial arterial dissection. *Neurosurgery* 1991; 29:89–96.
242. Mokri B, Houser W, Sandok B, Piepgras D. Spontaneous dissections of the vertebral arteries. *Neurology* 1988; 38:880–885.
243. Ojemann RG, Fisher CM, Rich JC. Spontaneous dissecting aneurysms of the internal carotid artery. *Stroke* 1972; 3:434–440.
244. Hennerici M, Steinke W, Rautenberg W. High-resistance Doppler flow pattern in extracranial carotid dissection. *Arch Neurol* 1989; 46:670–672.
245. Berger MS, Wilson CB. Intracranial dissecting aneurysms of the posterior circulation. *J Neurosurg* 1984; 61:882–894.

CHAPTER 90

DIAGNOSIS AND MANAGEMENT OF DISEASES OF THE PERIPHERAL ARTERIES AND VEINS

Paul W. Wennberg / Thom W. Rooke

INTRODUCTION

Peripheral vascular disease (PVD) is common in the adult population.[1,2] Arterial disease, which affects 10 to 15 percent of the adult population in developed countries, is seen commonly in cardiology practices, but venous and lymphatic disease must not be ignored. The natural history of each disease, regardless of the underlying etiology, may include ischemia, pain, swelling, and ultimately ulceration. Despite its high prevalence, few individuals receive formal PVD training in internal medicine or cardiology training programs. Despite or because of this, cardiologists often are consulted on patients with peripheral atherosclerosis, deep vein thrombosis, peripheral vasculitis, and many other PVDs. Fortunately, the history and physical examination often make the diagnosis relatively straightforward. Well-defined invasive and noninvasive testing methods are available that can provide confirmation, quantification, and in some instances clarification of the diagnosis.

This chapter provides an introduction to PVD. History, physical examination, and noninvasive laboratory testing are emphasized, followed by brief discussions of specific disease entities commonly seen in cardiovascular practice. Aortic disease, cerebrovascular diseases, vascular surgery, and percutaneous interventions are discussed elsewhere (Chaps. 56, 89, 91, and 93).

ASSESSMENT OF ARTERIAL DISEASE

History

General information, including the age, gender, associated medical problems (including prior trauma, vascular and orthopedic procedures, and past or current medication use), and risk factors for atherosclerosis, should be obtained. Symptoms, including onset, progression, and aggravating or alleviating factors, should be clarified. Claudication, ischemic rest pain, and skin ulceration are the usual presenting complaints of occlusive arterial disease. The description of symptoms may be quite different from patient to patient.

Claudication

Claudication ("limping") is a stereotypical, reproducible distress in single or multiple muscle groups of the lower extremity brought on in a predictable manner by sustained exercise and relieved by rest. The distress may be described as numbness, weakness, giving way, aching, cramping, or pain. It may change in character and/or location as the causative lesion or lesions progress. Claudication occurs at a predictable distance or time, but when the workload is increased by a rapid pace, a burden, or walking uphill or over rough terrain, the distance or time shortens. When the distance to claudication abruptly decreases, one must consider thrombosis in situ or an embolic event. Claudication often worsens after a period of inactivity such as hospitalization but usually returns to baseline with reconditioning.

Claudication occurs in muscle groups rather than joints. Relief with rest is independent of position and is timely, usually within 5 to 10 min. When these criteria are not met, musculoskeletal or neurologic disorders should be suspected. While lifestyle limitation and changes in quality of life should be an integral part of the history, quantitation of disease severity by history alone is unreliable. Variability in pace, workload, and estimates of distance all are based on the patient's perception. Standardized treadmill testing utilizing ankle/brachial indexes at rest and after the completion of an exercise protocol confirms the diagnosis, determines the severity, and documents claudication distance for future follow-up.

Variants of Claudication

There are many causes of claudication, but four specific variants merit mention here (Table 90-1). In the first, a classic claudication history is obtained, but on examination, the pulses are normal and no bruits are noted. After exercise, the pedal pulses disappear, the feet become pale, proximal bruits are noted, and the ankle/brachial indexes drop. The symptoms and findings normalize within minutes of rest. Initially, this was thought to be *vasospastic claudication*,[3] but arteriography has shown occlusive disease in proximal vessels, usually of atherosclerotic origin,[4] that is subcritical at rest. During exercise, blood is shunted into collateral arterial muscular beds, depriving downstream arteries of flow. Popliteal entrapment or adventitial cystic disease of the popliteal artery also can cause this syndrome.[5]

A second variant is *pseudoclaudication*, which may be of neurogenic or muscular origin. A patient with neurogenic claudication will describe exercise-induced distress with a dysesthetic quality that clears slowly or requires a specific posture for relief, usually with the hips in flexion. Clumsiness may develop as walking progresses. Symptoms occur with prolonged standing or in fixed positions such as being seated or lying. A history of back injury should be sought. Compression of the distal spinal cord by hypertrophic bone, disk protrusion, or tumor may be the cause.[6] Arterial and neurogenic disease may coexist. In this situation, the dominant lesion can be identified by observing symptoms and measuring the arterial indexes after exercise.[7]

Muscular distress induced by exercise is common in patients with amyotrophic lateral sclerosis, muscular dystrophy, McArdle's syndrome, and other myopathies. The muscular deficits are apparent on examination. Exercise testing clarifies the status of the arterial system.

Venous claudication is described as a congestive, often "bursting" distress of the thighs and calves induced by standing, running, and sometimes walking. Relief with rest is slow and is accelerated notably when the patient reclines and elevates the legs. This type occurs with significant iliocaval obstruction. Signs of venous hypertension of the legs and lower abdomen often are noted and should be apparent during the examination.

TABLE 90-1 Differential Diagnosis of Claudication

Atherosclerosis obliterans
Arteritis (Takayasu's, giant cell)
Embolic disease/acute arterial occlusion
Degenerative joint disease (hip, back, knee)
Spinal stenosis
Myopathy
Thromboangiitis obliterans
Popliteal entrapment
Venous claudication/varicosities
Baker's cyst
Deconditioning
Aortic dissection
Aortic coarctation
Retroperitoneal fibrosis

Ischemic Distress

With severe perfusion deficits, patients can experience persistent distress of two types: rest pain and ischemic neuropathy. Rest pain is constant and agonizing in quality and is confined to the affected digits, foot, or hand and less commonly the entire limb. It may localize to sites of infarction, ulceration, or infection. Small, localized areas of ischemic pain can occur with vasculitis, microembolization, or thrombosis but more often are caused by trauma to an area with poor perfusion as a result of chronic occlusive disease. It is important to inquire about new shoes, recent trimming of callus or nails, and other potential sources of trauma. Rest pain is noted commonly at night and is relieved by dependency, i.e., hanging the limb off the bed or sleeping in a chair, or, paradoxically, with walking. Pain later becomes constant, interrupting sleep, suppressing appetite, inducing weight loss, and requiring large doses of analgesics. The area is sensitive to touch by clothing and bedding. Depression is often present. Eventually, muscular atrophy and contractures at the ankle, knee, or hip may result as the limb is passively or actively protected and held immobile.

Ischemic neuropathy is a constant distress described as aching, throbbing, burning, pulling, or tearing. It is diffuse and often affects the entire lower leg or forearm. Shifting or lancinating pain often is experienced. Exacerbation of pain may occur spontaneously, often accompanied by diffuse cyanosis and coolness of the skin.

ARTERIAL EXAMINATION

The aorta and the radial, ulnar, subclavian, carotid, femoral, popliteal, posterior tibial, and dorsalis pedis arteries are accessible to palpation, although the dorsalis pedis artery may be congenitally absent. The temporal and occipital arteries are also accessible and should be palpated when temporal arteritis is suspected. Pulses are graded on a scale of 0 to 5; 0 being absence, 4 normal, and 5 aneurysmal. When a pulse is not present, a Doppler examination should be performed to establish whether the pulse is absent, obscured by overlying tissue or edema, or simply below the level of detection by palpation. Typically, when the arterial pressure is below 60 mmHg or an ankle brachial index (ABI) is below 0.6, pedal pulses are not palpable.

Auscultation of the femoral, iliac, aortic, carotid, and subclavian areas should be performed routinely.

The abdominal aorta is best examined with the patient supine on a firm surface, with the knees flexed and the arms at the side. Examination begins with the gentle pressure of eight fingers spread across the epigastrium in an effort to appreciate diffuse pulsation. Two or three fingers of each hand gradually are brought deeper on either side of the aorta until its pulsation and dimensions are defined. Alternatively, the fingers may occupy one side, and the thumbs the opposite side. It is helpful to coach the patient to breathe and relax, penetrating deeper with each expiration and warning that modest discomfort may be felt.

The popliteal artery is more difficult to examine, especially when musculoskeletal structures are prominent or relaxation is poor. It is best approached with the patient supine with the knee relaxed and "cradled" into the fingers. The pulse sometimes may be located by palpating distally between the heads of the gastrocnemius muscle. Popliteal examination routinely should include both of these sites as well as the adductor muscle mass distal to the adductor. Aneurysms can occur at any of these three locations (Fig. 90-1).

The radial pulse is quite accessible, but the ulnar artery is subject to variation and frequently is obscured by tendons. It is a particularly important vessel because of the relatively high incidence of trauma to this artery as it crosses the wrist. Deep and superficial palmar arches connect these two arteries into an arcade that supplies the digits. The *Allen test* ascertains arch patency. This test depends on the integrity of the radial, ulnar, and palmar arch arteries. It is performed by occluding the radial and ulnar artery with firm digital pressure and having the patient exsanguinate the hand by making a fist. The hand is relaxed and partially opened when the radial or ulnar artery is released. It is imperative that the wrist be relaxed to avoid false-positive results caused by ligamentous compression.[8] The procedure then is repeated for the other artery. If the noncompressed artery is patent, flushing of the entire hand will occur within 3 s after release. Delayed refilling is diagnostic of occlusive disease in the noncompressed vessel. Digital or microcirculatory deficits are suggested if refilling is slow or absent in isolated digits.[9]

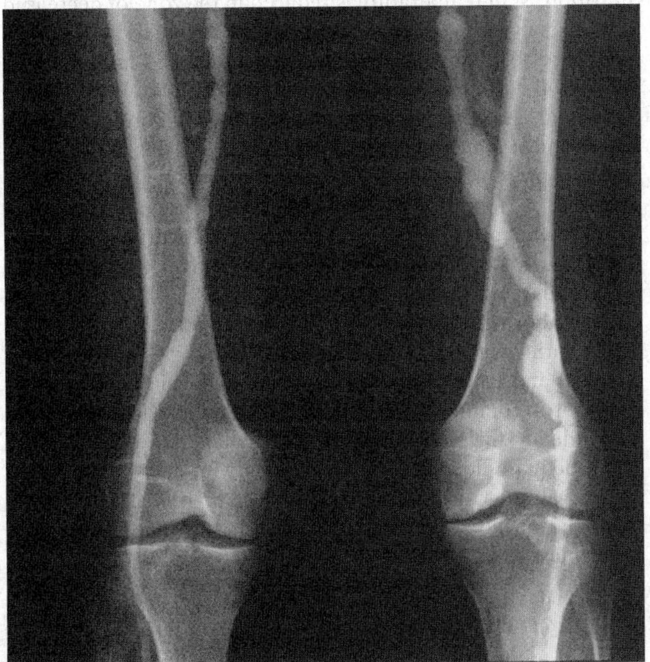

FIGURE 90-1 Popliteal artery aneurysms located at multiple levels on the left, starting at the adductor hiatus. Diffuse arteriomegaly is present on the left.

Aneurysms

Arterial aneurysms are a major cause of death and disability. Early detection allows definitive repair. The three most common aneurysms are accessible to examination, including 40 to 60 percent of abdominal aortic aneurysms and almost all popliteal and femoral aneurysms.[10–13] It should be noted that aneurysms tend to occur concurrently at multiple sites. Therefore, when a popliteal aneurysm is found, a careful search for iliac, femoral, and aortic aneurysms should be performed. The size and pulsatility of paired arteries are normally of similar magnitude. Ectasia is suspected when a pulse is larger or more forceful than expected. *Aneurysm* is defined as a focal enlargement one and one half or more times larger than the usual diameter of the artery. Arteriomegaly is present when the artery is widened, usually over a long distance, but is not yet aneurysmal (Fig. 90-1). The diagnosis is suspected when a palpable, often visible pulsation is transmitted to the fingers on each side of an enlarged vessel. Tortuosity of the carotids, abdominal aorta, and subclavian arteries can mimic an aneurysm. Ultrasound or angiographic studies may be needed to clarify the diagnosis when the examination is unclear.

Many abdominal aortic aneurysms are detected by palpation. They present as a pulsating mass below the xiphoid and above the umbilicus, often filling the epigastrium. Most aneurysms are centered to the left of the midline, but tortuosity occasionally may result in lateralization, commonly to the right. Slight discomfort is usual during examination, but significant tenderness suggests an inflammatory aneurysm, recent expansion, or a contained rupture. When the mass extends below the umbilicus, it may represent either extension into the iliac arteries or a large, overlapping aortic aneurysm. Isolated iliac aneurysms usually are hidden in the pelvis, and less than a fifth can be detected by abdominal examination or digital examination of the rectum or pelvis. Most are found incidentally on an imaging study or after the onset of symptoms.[14] Femoral aneurysms often are first noted by the patient. Popliteal lesions are easily overlooked unless the popliteal space is examined routinely at all three sites described above. Femoral and popliteal aneurysms often are first detected after acute thrombosis, distal micro- or macroembolization, or edema from perianeurysm venous compression or thrombosis.[12,13]

Most thoracic and thoracoabdominal aneurysms are diagnosed incidentally on imaging procedures but may present with pain, cough, dysphagia, hemoptysis, or dysphonia. Physical signs are late manifestations of thoracic aneurysms and may include aortic valve incompetence, unilateral or bilateral jugular venous distention, and pulsatility in the upper intercostal spaces of the precordium. Carotid and axillosubclavian aneurysms are easily diagnosed by palpation, and some present with local pain, thrombosis, or distal embolic complications.[15,16] Visceral aneurysms are rarely large enough to be palpated; 3 to 5 percent present as rupture, and the majority are found incidentally at surgery or during imaging.[17,18]

Bruits

Bruits extending into diastole suggest a high-grade stenosis. However, bruits may disappear when a critical narrowing is reached. A continuous bruit throughout systole and diastole is pathognomonic of an underlying arteriovenous fistula. Bruits may be found at an acquired fistula of paired arteries and veins (Fig. 90-2); over multiple congenital fistulas of the liver, lung, soft tissue, or skull; and over areas of tumor necrosis or prior biopsies. A supraclavicular bruit that disappears with shoulder hyperabduction may be found in young patients.[19] Finally, an epigastric bruit may represent compression of the celiac artery rather than visceral or renal artery stenosis, especially in the young, if asymptomatic, or in the absence of other vascular disease.[20]

Extensions of the Arterial Examination

The value of the Allen test in establishing patency of the radial, ulnar, and digital arteries was discussed above. Pedal perfusion traditionally has been tested by timing elevation pallor and venous refilling (Table 90-2). With the patient supine, both feet are elevated to 60° for 1 min. If no pallor is seen, perfusion is judged to be normal. The appearance of pallor within 15 s suggests poor healing capacity, and pallor without elevation is indicative of severe ischemia. The patient then sits upright, and refilling of the pedal veins is timed. Normal filling occurs in less than 15 s, filling between 30 and 45 s suggests slow healing, and values beyond 60 s confirm severe ischemia. Venous incompetence invalidates venous filling times, and the test is not practical in the presence of significant edema or obesity. Several maneuvers are used to screen for arterial, venous, and neurogenic compression syndromes of the thoracic outlet. Because these tests are frequently abnormal in the normal population and because of the complexity of the syndromes, the reader is referred to detailed reviews.[21,22]

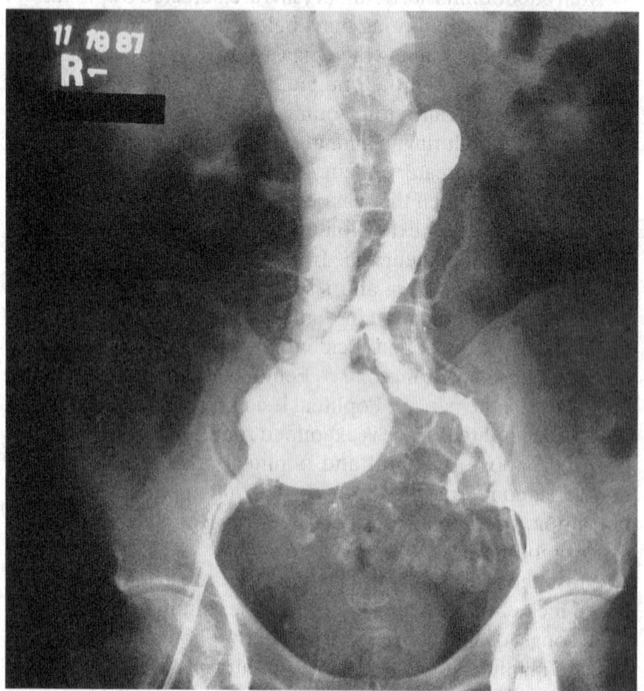

FIGURE 90-2 An aortogram in a 72-year-old who presented with worsening dyspnea over several months and a continuous bruit over the right lower quadrant. A right iliac aneurysm has ruptured, creating a fistula into the right iliac vein. Immediate contrast accumulation is seen in the inferior vena cava. After repair, the patient's symptoms from high-output cardiac failure resolved.

TABLE 90-2 Elevation Pallor and Venous Refilling

ELEVATION PALLOR[a]	
Grade	Pallor Onset
Normal	None
I	>60 s
II	<60 s
III	<30 s
IV	Without elevation
VENOUS REFILLING[b]	
Severity	Venous Refill
Normal	<15 s
Moderate	20–30 s
Severe	>40 s

[a]Feet held passively at 60° while supine.
[b]Upon sitting after elevation.

The Skin

Occlusive arterial disease can alter skin temperature, color, and nutrition. Skin temperature is reduced in the zone of decreased perfusion caused by acute or chronic occlusive disease. Differences are best felt with the dorsum of the fingers, and comparisons to the contralateral or proximal limb should be made. Profound coolness suggests severe ischemia. Chronically cool hands and feet reflect the basic vasomotor tone of some patients, not the presence of poor circulation. Limbs with neurologic damage, immobility, or reflex sympathetic dystrophy are often cool. Edema can accompany these states, obscuring pulses and therefore mimicking arterial disease. Ankle/brachial indexes differentiate occlusive disease from these vasomotor changes (see "Laboratory Assessment: Arterial Disease," below). Skin color varies with blood flow and therefore with temperature, activity, and emotional stimuli. A red or purplish color of the forefoot is common with chronic ischemia and increases with dependency; this is due to chronic arteriolar dilation in response to inadequate flow. Pallor can be seen with acute ischemia or on elevation with chronic ischemia. Skin that is chronically deprived of blood becomes thin, translucent, and shiny. Nails may thicken, and calluses may develop.

LABORATORY ASSESSMENT: ARTERIAL DISEASE

Testing usually is performed to document the severity of disease. However, confirmation or clarification of the diagnosis, monitoring of disease progression, and assessment of outcome after intervention are all appropriate indications for vascular testing. Vascular tests generally are classified as invasive (such as angiography) or noninvasive. This section focuses on noninvasive testing. Noninvasive testing of the arterial system is divided into three broad categories, depending on the type of information generated.

Anatomic Studies

Imaging techniques, including two-dimensional ultrasound, magnetic resonance imaging, computed tomography, and angiography, provide anatomic information. The presence or absence of aneurysms, dissections, stenoses, or occlusions is determined readily by these tests (Chaps. 13, 16, 17, and 18).

Hemodynamic Studies

These techniques provide information about the hemodynamic significance of a vascular lesion. These tests measure a pressure drop or an increase in flow velocity across a lesion, providing information about the hemodynamic impact of the stenosis.

Functional Studies

The information obtained by anatomic or hemodynamic testing may be insufficient to explain the symptoms or degree of impairment described by the patient. In this case, a functional vascular test can be helpful. Functional studies often involve some form of "stress testing." For example, treadmill testing is the most commonly used test to assess claudication.

CONTINUOUS-WAVE DOPPLER

The most widely used continuous-wave (CW) Doppler devices are simple hand-held units that can be purchased for a few hundred dollars and are easily carried in a coat pocket. The Doppler detects blood motion and may be used alone as a means of screening for vascular disease,[23,24] or it may be an integral part of other tests, such as segmental pressure determination (described below).

In a normal artery, the waveform is triphasic. During cardiac systole, there is forward flow in the arteries. During early diastole, the flow reverses direction (because of the elastic recoil of the peripheral arteries). Finally, during middle to late diastole, there is a return of forward flow as arterial blood runs off through the distal vessels.[25] The normal triphasic signal becomes altered by a hemodynamically significant stenosis. If the degree of stenosis is minimal, subtle changes such as dampening of the signal and/or loss of the mid-diastolic forward flow component may be noted distal to the lesion, resulting in a biphasic signal. As the severity of the stenosis worsens, the signal eventually becomes monophasic as only systolic flow is present and then is absent with occlusion. The location of a stenosis may be estimated by assessing the Doppler signal at multiple sites along the limb. CW Doppler is inexpensive and may be performed at the bedside as an extension of the vascular examination. It requires training and practice for effective use, and the information obtained may be limited by the fact that this is a "blind" technique. Duplicated vessels, anatomic variations, and obesity may reduce its accuracy.

SEGMENTAL PRESSURES AND EXERCISE TESTING

Segmental pressures are measured by placing inflatable cuffs around the limb at multiple levels and sequentially inflating and deflating them to determine the arterial pressure at each site.[25] Pneumatic cuffs typically are placed around the thigh, calf, ankle, upper or lower arm, or digits. A CW Doppler (see above) is positioned over the artery at a site distal to the pressure cuff or cuffs and is used to determine the systolic pressure at which arterial flow resumes as the cuff is deflated. The limb pressures typically are divided by a reference arterial pressure (the brachial artery systolic pressure) to create an index. The most commonly reported segmental pressure is the ABI. Severity of disease is determined by the ABI (Table 90-3).

Segmental pressures provide a simple, reproducible, inexpensive, and accurate method of determining whether arterial obstruction is present, the severity of the obstruction, and the approximate location of the obstruction or obstructions. The stress or exercise ABI identifies arterial lesions that are too minor to produce pressure changes at rest. The subject is placed on a treadmill and ambulated according to a standardized protocol. Protocols may be "fixed" (for example, 2 miles/h at a 12 percent incline for a maximum of 5 min) or utilize "graded" exercise similar to that used in cardiac exercise studies.[26] Elements of the lower extremity study (i.e., ABIs or CW Doppler analysis) are performed before and after exercise. Exercise studies can be used to identify parameters such as the minimum walking distance that will produce claudication, the walking distance at which a patient normally would stop, and the maximum walking distance.

The major disadvantage of segmental pressure measurement is that it cannot be used in patients whose blood vessels are noncompressible or poorly compressible because of calcification of the arterial wall.[27] This occurs most commonly in diabetic patients. When vessels are stiff, the cuff cannot produce sufficient pressure to obliterate blood flow and the arterial pressure cannot be determined. Even when the large vessels of the limb are noncompressible, however, the digital vessels in the toes and fingers often remain uncalcified and can be used to estimate pressure if an appropriate cuff is available. Many groups utilize the great toe index in such situations.

TABLE 90-3 The Ankle/Brachial Index

	Preexercise	Postexercise	Claudication	Walking Time, min
Normal	>0.95	>0.95	None	5
Minimal	>0.95	<0.95	None	5
Mild	>0.80	>0.50	Present late	5
Moderate	<0.80	<0.50	Present, limiting	<5
Severe	<0.50	<0.15	Early, limiting	<3

ABI is the systolic blood pressure of the higher arm/systolic blood pressure at the ankle measured in the supine position. Postexercise values are after 5 min at a 10 percent grade at 2 mph (the authors' laboratory protocol; other protocols may be used). Speed may be varied if needed.

PULSE VOLUME RECORDING

Pulse volume recording (PVR) is used to assess the arterial pulsatility of the limb.[28] A pneumatic pressure cuff is placed around the limb at a given level. The cuff is filled with air to a low pressure (typically 40 to 60 mmHg) and is connected by a flexible hose to a pressure transducer. The blood ejected from the left ventricle during cardiac systole causes a transient distention of the limb, which in turn produces a transient rise in cuff pressure. The cyclic changes in cuff pressure with each heartbeat provide an index of arterial "pulsatility." Measurements typically are made at multiple levels along the limb (as is done with segmental pressures), and the tracings are analyzed to determine whether there is a particular level at which the waveform changes shape or pulse dampening occurs.[29] When an altered pulse volume waveform is present, it can be inferred that there is a hemodynamically signficant lesion proximal to the site of the cuff.

TRANSCUTANEOUS OXIMETRY

Transcutaneous oxygen (Tcp_{O_2}) measurement is used to evaluate skin blood flow.[30] Oxygen-sensing electrodes are attached to the skin by means of adhesive rings that create an airtight seal. The seal ensures that the only oxygen that reaches the electrode has diffused from the skin. The surface temperature of the electrode is maintained at a relatively high temperature (43 to 45°C) so that the small vessels underlying the electrode are maximally dilated. Cutaneous blood flow is determined in part by the patency of the proximal arteries.[31] The amount of oxygen that diffuses out of the skin depends on numerous factors, including the arterial partial pressure of oxygen, the cutaneous blood flow, and the rate of oxygen consumption by the skin. When cutaneous blood flow is high (relative to the metabolic rate of the skin), Tcp_{O_2} may approach arterial O_2. In contrast, when cutaneous blood flow is low, Tcp_{O_2} is reduced. Tcp_{O_2} is not so much a measurement of skin blood flow as a measurement of the adequacy of cutaneous oxygen delivery. Transcutaneous oximetry has been shown to be useful in a number of situations, including evaluation of critical ischemia. It may be difficult to determine the functional severity of arterial occlusive disease solely on the basis of historical or clinical findings even when basic noninvasive testing is available. This difficulty is especially relevant when the clinician is attempting to determine whether limb revascularization is required for pain relief, ulcer healing, or limb salvage. Tcp_{O_2} can be used to predict whether the cutaneous perfusion is adequate for healing at a given amputation site (Table 90-4). Values above 40 mmHg are typically sufficient for healing, while those below 20 mmHg are not likely to heal.[32]

Certain disease states may affect the small vessels or microcirculation without involving larger arteries. When this occurs, techniques such as CW Doppler, segmental pressures, and PVR will not detect a significant abnormality. In contrast, Tcp_{O_2} measurements usually demonstrate the inadequacy of circulation when it is due to small vessel occlusive disease. Tcp_{O_2} determination is often valuable in the assessment of patients with diabetes (when noncompressible or poorly compressible vessels are present) and/or small vessel disease.[33] Although Tcp_{O_2} measurement is an accurate way to assess the severity of cutaneous ischemia, it has several limitations. These limitations include its inability to localize the occlusive disease to a particular segment or vessel and the fact that each laboratory must standardize and validate the technique before the results can be relied on for diagnostic and therapeutic decisions.[34,35]

TABLE 90-4 Interpretation of Tcp_{O_2} Values

	Rest	Elevation
Normal	45	<10
Mild	40–45	<10
Moderate	20–39	<10
Severe	20–39 or <20	>10 any
Critical	0	

Tcp_{O_2} values in mmHg at rest and after 30° elevation. A fall greater than 10 mmHg with elevation increases the degree of severity by one grade. Values less than 20 have poor potential for healing; values of 20–30 have a variable potential for healing.

Imaging Techniques

Imaging modalities such as two-dimensional (2D) real-time ultrasound, computed tomography (CT), and magnetic resonance imaging (MRI) are described in greater detail elsewhere (see Chaps. 13, 17, and 18). They increasingly are being used in place of angiography, especially for the evaluation of aneurysm, dissection, and arterial rupture. New acquisition and processing techniques are enabling CT and MR angiography (MRA) to replace conventional angiography as a means of identifying arterial stenoses and occlusions. Indeed, in diabetic patients and others at high risk of renal damage from contrast, MRA should be strongly considered if it is available and has sufficient resolution to plan surgical intervention. Continued technological advances in these noninvasive modalities may allow CT and MRI to compete with conventional angiography in all but a few selected circumstances.

ARTERIAL DISEASES OF THE LOWER EXTREMITY

Arterial Occlusive Disease

Arteriosclerosis obliterans (ASO) is the most common cause of lower extremity ischemic syndromes in western societies regardless of age.[36] The presentation varies greatly with the time course of progression, the presence and extent of collateral vessels, comorbidities, and activity of the patient. If the patient is active, intermittent claudication is the usual presenting complaint; if inactive, rest pain, ulceration, dependent rubor with edema secondary to compensatory dependency, or gangrene may be the presenting complaint.

In general, symptoms occur distal to the level of stenosis. Superficial femoral disease causes claudication of the entire calf. Both thigh and calf symptoms occur with common femoral and external iliac lesions, hip and buttock claudication alone suggests an internal iliac stenosis, and foot and calf claudication suggests popliteal or infrapopliteal disease. Impotence suggests aortoiliac disease.

PREVALENCE AND NATURAL HISTORY

There is a relatively high prevalence of ASO that increases with age.[1,36,37] The Framingham Study estimated the annual incidence of symptomatic disease at 0.3 percent and 0.1 percent for men and women, respectively.[38,39] The prevalence of intermittent claudication increases with age: 1.8 percent under age 60, 3.7 percent age 60 to 70, and just over 5 percent at age 70 and above. Risk factors for ASO reflect those for coronary disease.[40] Diabetes increases the risk of ASO threefold (higher if asymptomatic ASO is included).[41] In a hypertensive elderly population, the incidence of ASO as defined by an ABI <0.90 was slightly higher than 25 percent. The risk of death, usually from a cardiovascular event, increases dramatically as the ABI decreases.[42,43] The 5-year mortality of an ABI less than 0.85 is 10 percent; if ABI is less than 0.40, it approaches 50 percent.

The rate of progression of symptoms or the need for revascularization is slow.[44] Symptoms that have worsened at 5 years occur in approximately 20 percent of these patients.[45] The requirement for revascularization because of imminent tissue or limb loss or rest pain approaches 5 percent per year. Amputation rates are similarly low, around 1 percent per year. However, up to 15 percent of those who continue smoking undergo amputation within 5 years. Diabetic patients have an amputation rate of 25 percent over 9 years.[46-49]

TREATMENT

Aggressive *risk factor modification* should be the cornerstone of therapy in all patients. The slow rate of progression and the high incidence of vascular comorbidities indicate an optimum role for modifying the underlying atherosclerotic process. Smoking cessation is a must. Control of diabetes should be emphasized since the risk for amputation is increased in this population, although the benefit has not been documented in large arteries. Lipid lowering has a beneficial role in patients with ASO.[50,51] The goals are similar to those for patients with coronary artery disease.[52] Hypertension control should be optimized (see Chap. 51).

A *walking program* should be initiated in all patients. Bicycling and other forms of exercise used for cardiovascular conditioning unfortunately do not provide the same benefit that walking provides. The effectiveness of a structured walking program has been well demonstrated.[53-55] Twenty to 30 min 4 to 5 days per week improves exercise capacity and increases total and absolute walking distance from 50 to 300 percent. The mechanism of this improvement is not clear, but increased collateral formation or recruitment, muscle training, improved oxygen uptake, and improved mechanics of walking are all plausible.[56] Diligent foot care and protection must be emphasized, particularly in diabetic patients and those with severe reductions in ABI or Tcp_{O_2} values. Footwear must be supportive and protective, and nail care should be performed regularly by professionals.

Medical therapy for peripheral artery disease has been slow to develop. Pentoxyfilline has proved effective in some patients with ASO,[57] but stomach irritation limits its use in others. Recently, cilostazol has been approved for use for patients with claudication. It is effective in increasing walking distance, but the effect is lost when the drug is stopped. Several other medications are currently in development. Direct vasodilators have proved ineffective, although verapamil increased walking distance in one study.[58] Beta blockade has long been believed to be contraindicated for patients with ASO, but two studies have refuted this idea.[54,59] In light of the beneficial effects of beta blockade in patients with coronary artery disease, these agents should not be withheld from patients with peripheral ASO.

Revascularization should be considered in patients with rest pain, impending tissue loss, or significant limitation of lifestyle. Surgical revascularization has been available for years. Large vessel bypass surgery with synthetic graft material is well established and durable. More recently, in situ distal bypass utilizing reversed or intact saphenous vein has shown promising long-term patency. Percutaneous balloon angioplasty with or without stent placement is often useful for lesions of the proximal renal and iliac arteries. There is decreasing long-term effectiveness at more distal vessels because of the reduction in both artery size and flow rates. However, for patients at high risk for limb loss (deemed poor surgical candidates or technically unfeasible for revascularization), it is reasonable to consider angioplasty for limb salvage.

Acute Arterial Occlusion

PRESENTATION

Acute arterial occlusion presents as a clinical pentad of pain, pallor, paresthesia, paralysis, and pulselessness. The limb also may be cold. Some or all of these findings may be present. The limb is at risk if flow is not restored quickly. Distal changes caused by microembolisation also may be seen. There are two exceptions to the usual presentation of acute arterial occlusion. The first is branch vessel occlusion in the setting of acute aortic dissection. Variability may be present on examination. The pulse deficit and the area affected may migrate, causing discrepancies between examiners as the dissection progresses. The second is ergot toxicity, which usually is diagnosed only after a direct question about its use is asked.[60]

ETIOLOGY

The etiology of acute arterial occlusions is classified into three groups: trauma and dissection, thrombosis in situ, and embolism. Attention to arterial integrity is of prime importance in dealing with injuries caused by penetration (including medical interventions), crush or fracture, and deceleration injuries. In situ thrombosis occurs with both occlusive and aneurysmal disease. Any of the lesions listed in Table 90-1, aneurysms, clotting disorders, but predominantly atherosclerosis with its multiple manifestations and risk factors can be the substrate of thrombosis.

A small percentage of acute emboli come from proximal occlusive or aneurysmal arterial lesions, but the majority originate from the heart. Both the left ventricle and the left atrium may harbor a thrombus.[61] Emboli tend to be multiple and recurrent and to distribute randomly, mostly to the legs but with a significant incidence of cerebral, renal, visceral, and arm events.[62] Venous thrombi from the right side of the heart or limbs can pass across cardiac septal defects or patent foramina ovali and cause arterial events.[63]

MANAGEMENT

Immediate measures are needed to protect the limb and restore blood flow. Heparin is given to prevent clot propagation and treat the embolic source or sources.[64,65] Angiography is required to plan repair when there is preexisting occlusive or aneurysmal disease or when the etiology is uncertain. Many surgeons perform balloon embolectomy without angiography when an embolic source is certain and the vessel was previously normal. Ideally, all acute occlusions warrant repair, although the urgency is governed by the degree of ischemia. Severe ischemia is suggested by pallor at rest, profound coolness, tender or hard muscles, and loss of motor and sensory function. When severe ischemia is present, repair must occur within hours to salvage the limb. Additional time may be taken to address ancillary problems in patients with lesser degrees of ischemia, and sometimes no repair is elected when the occlusion has a minimal impact on the patient's lifestyle. If acute cardiac events create prohibitive risks for surgery, the heart may be stabilized over a few hours before embolectomy or revascularization is performed under local anesthesia.[66,67] When indicated, lysis of acute occlusion can be effective.[68–70]

PREVENTION

Acute arterial occlusion is often preventable, and conditions known to cause occlusion warrant treatment. Aneurysms, adventitial cystic disease, popliteal entrapment syndromes, and atrial myxoma are treated surgically. Treatable medical disorders include vasculitis, hematologic disorders, and thyrotoxicosis. Atrial or ventricular thrombi, atrial fibrillation, acute myocardial infarction, congestive failure, severe cardiomyopathy, and prosthetic valves all warrant chronic antithrombotic therapy to prevent thrombus formation.

Unusual Causes

Leg claudication and ischemia result from numerous disorders (Table 90-1). Many are suggested by the history (acute arterial occlusion, aortic dissection, temporal and Takayasu's arteritis, radiation therapy, ergot use, and competitive cycling), some by physical findings (coarctation, pseudoxanthoma elasticum, occluded aneurysms), and others only through imaging.

THROMBOANGIITIS OBLITERANS

Thromboangiitis obliterans (TAO), or Buerger's disease, is the most common of these disorders.[21,71–73] Buerger first described this inflammatory vasculopathy with a characteristic, highly cellular intraluminal thrombus that affects small and medium-size arteries and veins. TAO always is associated with tobacco use and may be an autoimmune response to it. TAO is seen predominantly in males in the second through fifth decades, although the incidence in women is rising. Clinically, TAO differs from atherosclerosis in that concurrent involvement of the upper extremity is common. The initial involvement is in digital, pedal, and hand vessels; progression to the calf, thigh, and forearm is brisk and occurs over a few months or years. One-third of these patients report Raynaud's phenomenon. Recurrent episodes of superficial phlebitis of the calves or forearms are seen frequently. Biopsy of acute lesions, particularly accessible veins, is diagnostic, and angiographic features are characteristic. Rare manifestations include coronary, cerebral, or visceral artery lesions. Progressive tissue loss is inevitable until tobacco exposure is stopped. Stability or improvement is variable but is possible only after all exposure to tobacco ceases.[74] Surgical sympathectomy and intravenous prostacyclin analogs can accelerate healing of ischemic lesions,[75] but amputation of damaged digits and limbs often is required.

POPLITEAL ENTRAPMENT SYNDROME

Popliteal entrapment syndrome occurs when the popliteal artery is trapped by the medial gastrocnemius or various muscular and ligamentous bands during passive dorsiflexion or active plantar flexion. The entrapment may cause claudication and (later) occlusion. It usually is seen in relatively young, healthy individuals and typically occurs with significant exertion. Surgical repair is the treatment of choice.[76] Although uncommon, entrapment syndromes can be seen at other sites.

ADVENTITIAL CYSTIC DISEASE

Adventitial cystic disease is a slowly enlarging growth in the popliteal (or occasionally common femoral) artery that is analogous in structure and content to a ganglion or mucoid cyst. It may cause claudication and subsequent occlusion. Surgical repair is the treatment of choice.[77]

TAKAYASU'S AND GIANT CELL ARTERITIS

Takayasu's arteritis and giant-cell (temporal) arteritis (GCA) are similar in pathologic process but affect different age groups. In general, Takayasu's arteritis involves arteries below the neck, and GCA involves arteries above the neck. However, involvement of the aorta and great vessels, subclavian and axillary arteries, renal and iliofemoral, profunda femoral, and superficial femoral arteries has been described with each one. Disease is usually bilateral and results in claudication that progresses briskly over a few months. Ischemia is rare. Both have characteristic clinical and laboratory findings, including an elevated sedimentation rate and typical arteriographic features. These diseases are unique among arteriopathies in that acute stenotic lesions significantly improve with steroid therapy. Adjunctive cytotoxic drugs are also useful.[78–80]

ERGOT

Ergot compounds can induce Raynaud's phenomenon, claudication, acute ischemia, and tissue infarction. These problems usually are seen in those using ergot to treat migraine headaches. Intravenous nitroprusside infusion may help acute ischemia.[60] The incidence of ergot toxicity is decreasing as alternatives for migraine treatment become available, but it should be considered in patients with ischemia and few, if any, risk factors.

FIBROMUSCULAR DYSPLASIA

Fibromuscular dysplasia has been described in almost all arteries. It usually affects women in the middle years. Renal artery disease is the most common, but carotid, mesenteric, and both upper and lower extremity diseases may be seen.

Aneurysmal Disease

Abdominal aneurysms are found in 15 percent of men over age 65 screened by ultrasound,[81] and a familial tendency for aneurysms in both males and females has been identified.[82] Effective repair of aneurysms has been available for several decades. An appreciation of three general characteristics of aneurysms allows a logical approach to management. First, aneurysms caused by degenerative etiologies progressively enlarge over years. Second, aneurysms caused by infectious or traumatic etiologies expand over days to months. Third, aneurysms tend to be multiple. Five to 10 percent of patients with an aortic aneurysm and 50 percent or more with peripheral aneurysms will have aneurysms elsewhere.[83,84] Rupture is the primary worry with thoracic, abdominal, iliac, and visceral artery aneurysms, whereas thrombosis and embolism are typical of carotid and peripheral aneurysms. Aneurysms may cause dysfunction of adjacent structures by compression or fistula formation with those structures (Fig. 90-2). Ascending thoracic aorta aneurysms may contribute to aortic valve regurgitation or dissection, particularly when caused by cystic medial necrosis or congenital defects of the arterial wall.

These patients should be screened for aneurysmal disease during examination. Further imaging should be considered if an aneurysm is found elsewhere or in the setting of unexplained occlusion of a distal artery, microembolic syndromes, limb edema (possibly caused by aneurysm compression), fistula, and any continuous bruit. Aneurysms should be sought in the setting of diseases known to cause them, including syphilis, heritable disorders of collagen, several of the vasculitides, and atherosclerosis. Hypertension, smoking, and age predispose to aneurysm formation.

Microcirculatory Disorders

There are many etiologies that produce microcirculatory disease (Table 90-5). Digital and microcirculatory ischemia may present as focal digital cyanosis, petechiae, splinter hemorrhages, ulcer, infarction, or gangrene and may be accompanied by livedo reticularis and Raynaud's phenomenon. Skin findings may be single or multiple and are usually acute. Most initial lesions heal spontaneously with little or no tissue loss. Recurrences are common and can result in loss of digits or large areas of skin (Fig. 90-3). Most etiologies are diagnosed by clinical features and selective tests. Vasculitic syndromes respond to steroids and/or cytotoxic agents. Anticoagulants are given for associated circulating anticoagulant or antiphospholipid syndromes.[85] Myeloproliferative disease and dysproteinemias are treated with chemotherapy, sometimes enhanced by plasmapheresis. Clotting syndromes are controlled with anticoagulants. Culture-sensitive antibiotics are essential for treating endocarditis, and infected prosthetic valves usually must be removed. Digital ischemia with advanced malignancy is rare and may be idiopathic or associated with coagulopathy, dysproteinemia, or marantic endocarditis.

TABLE 90-5 Etiology of Microcirculatory Disease

- Embolism
  - Arteriosclerosis obliterans
  - Anticoagulation
  - Trauma, instrumentation
  - Surgery
- Vasculitis
- Endocarditis
- Ergot toxicity
- Cold injury
- Malignancy
- Hepatitis
- Hematologic
  - Polycythemia vera
  - Thrombocytosis
  - Dysproteinemia
  - Cryoglobulinemia
  - Cold agglutinins
  - Circulating anticoagulants
- Antiphospholipid antibodies
- Thrombotic cytopenic purpura
- Heparin-induced thrombocytopenia

Microembolism

Microembolism usually originates from an ulcerative plaque or aneurysm and only rarely from the heart. Solitary lesions showering atheroemboli are readily treated surgically.[86] When lesions are found at several levels, surgical choices are more difficult. Suprarenal sources can cause progressive azotemia or intestinal ischemia and require a formidable repair.[87] Thromboulcerative disease of the entire aorta can shower emboli randomly to the brain, viscera, kidneys, skin, and muscle. Anemia, leukocytosis, azotemia, an elevated sedimentation rate, and abnormal urinary sediment usually are noted. This syndrome of diffuse microembolization often requires biopsy for differentiation from vasculitis.[88] Microembolic events may be spontaneous or can be precipitated by surgery, instrumentation, or anticoagulant therapy.[87] Antiplatelet agents may prevent recurrences when surgery is not feasible; however, efficacy is poorly documented.[89]

Vasospastic Disorders

The color and warmth of the acral parts vary considerably from person to person in a normal population, reflecting individual vasomotor tone. Livedo reticularis, acrocyanosis, and Raynaud's phenomenon are distinctive clinical syndromes manifested by abnormal color and temperature changes of the skin. These syndromes are induced or intensified as a result of stimuli from cold, emotion, or drugs. They cause spasm in digital arteries, arterioles, and perhaps venules. These disorders are usually benign, lifelong primary processes, but all three syndromes can have important secondary causes. Careful clinical examination and selective testing usually will confirm the specific etiology and define the prognosis and the direction of therapy.

LIVEDO RETICULARIS

Livedo reticularis is characterized by a persistent, symmetric, bluish lacy pattern on the extremities and sometimes the trunk that is variable in extent and intensity. It is most apparent after stimulation by cold or emotion and fades with warmth and exercise. It is first seen in childhood or at puberty and is more common in women and fair-skinned individuals. It is so common in its milder form that it often is overlooked or considered a variant of normal skin. It has been postulated that spasm of the cutaneous arterioles (with secondary dilation of the capillaries and venules) causes slow flow, increased oxygen uptake, and reduced oxyhemoglobin, producing color change. Primary livedo reticularis often is seen with acrocyanosis and primary Raynaud's disease. Treatment is rarely needed.

Secondary livedo reticularis is patchy, focal, or asymmetric in distribution and relatively late in onset; it may be complicated by local infarction or ulceration. The lesions may be elevated or tender when caused by vasculitis. Therapy is directed at the

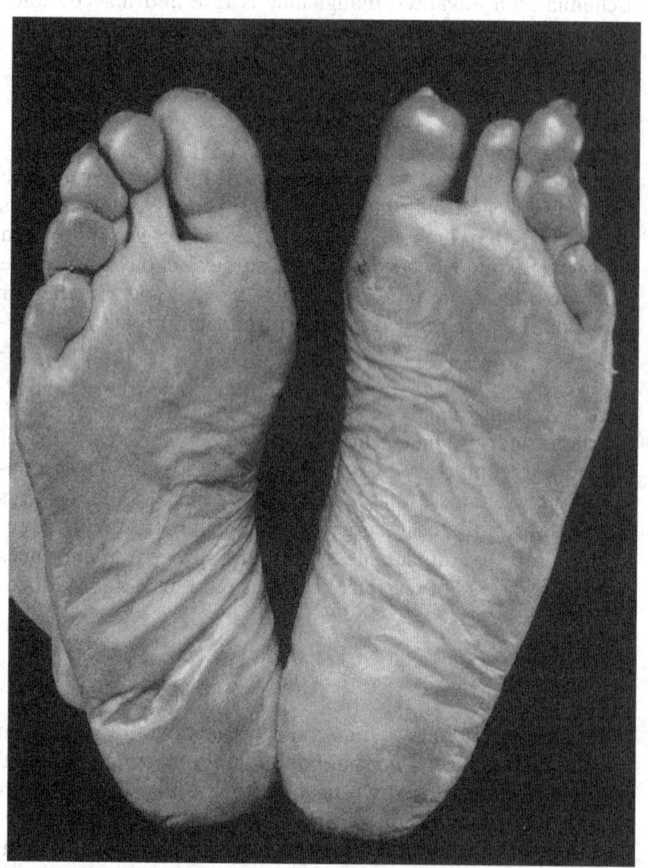

A

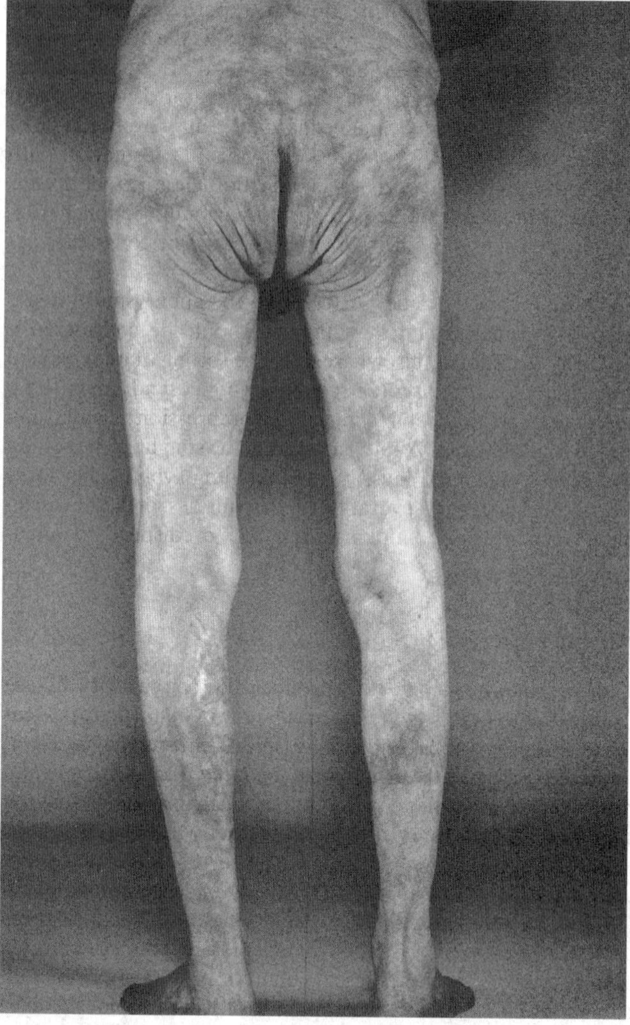

B

FIGURE 90-3 Two photographs of skin changes caused by microemboli. *A.* Cyanotic toe pads and livedo reticularis over the plantar aspect of both feet. *B.* Extensive livido reticularis in the same patient. A previously unknown 7-cm aortic aneurysm was found and repaired.

underlying cause (Table 90-6). Vasodilators and sympathectomy are of unpredictable, anecdotal value for healing painful ulcers. Hemosiderin deposition can occur in secondary and, on occasion, primary livedo reticularis. Erythema ab igne can be confused with livedo reticularis. This is a focal, well-defined lesion with broader bands of fixed red color, often with a hemosiderin stain. It is a reaction to chronic, local heat exposure such as a heating pad or fireplace.

TABLE 90-6 Etiologies of Livido Reticularis

Environmental (cold)	Reflex sympathetic dystrophy
Atheroembolism (cholesterol)	Myeloproliferative diseases
Connective tissue disease	Vasculitis
Cutaneous vasculitis	Thrombocytosis
Amantidine HCl	

ACROCYANOSIS

Acrocyanosis is a benign, persistent cyanotic discoloration and coolness of the hands (or fingers or sometimes the feet) that is seen more commonly in women. Cold and emotion intensify, whereas warmth and exercise ameliorate, the findings. Mild local edema is not uncommon and is not bothersome; associated hyperhidrosis may require treatment. Acrocyanosis is painless and does not ulcerate, but it is a bothersome cosmetic problem for some. Calcium entry blockers or alpha$_1$ antagonists often reduce the symptoms. A modest degree of acrocyanosis sometimes is seen in limbs immobilized by neurogenic deficits. Rarely, beta-blockade will induce the syndrome.

RAYNAUD'S PHENOMENON

Raynaud's phenomenon is diagnosed from history alone. It is difficult to demonstrate even with ice immersion, as generalized cooling usually is needed to bring out the findings. The syndrome is defined as episodes of blue or white color changes of the digits, often followed by reactive hyperemia during recov-

TABLE 90-7 Raynaud's Phenomenon: Secondary Causes

Collagen vascular disease	Medications
Scleroderma	Beta blockers
Mixed connective tissue disease	Ergotamine
	Methysergide
Rheumatoid arthritis	Vinblastine, bleomycin
Myositis	Estrogens
Sjögren's syndrome	Imipramine
Necrotizing vasculitis	Microcirculatory diseases
Hematologic disorders	Beurger's disease
Neurogenic	Hypothenar hammer syndrome
Thoracic outlet irritation	
Carpal tunnel syndrome	Environmental
Neuropathy	Cold injury
Myxedema	Vibration syndrome
Acromegaly	Vinyl chloride disease
Pulmonary hypertension	

ery. It is induced by cold or emotional stimuli. Many patients describe the white phase (some describe blue changing to white, and a few blue only), but most note the subsequent hyperemia. A dead, numb feeling (but rarely pain) accompanies the ischemic phase, and a dysesthetic, throbbing, or painful sensation is common during recovery. Fingers are involved more often than are toes, initially the distal digits and later the entire digit but rarely the palm. The thumbs often are spared. Recovery time is 3 to 10 min but can exceed 1 h in advanced cases, usually of secondary origin. Allen and Brown[90] defined primary Raynaud's as episodes of bilateral color changes induced by cold or emotion without evidence of ischemia or other disease for 2 years. Later development of secondary disease was noted in 2 to 5 percent of patients.[91–93] A prospective study confirmed that patients without laboratory evidence of digital occlusive, clotting, or serologic abnormalities have a benign course, with only 2 percent showing secondary causes in the subsequent decade.[94]

The causes of secondary Raynaud's phenomenon are diverse (Table 90-7). Most can be defined by history and examination, knowledge of their natural behavior, vascular laboratory measurements of digital obstruction, and clotting or serologic tests. Arteriography (from the arch through the digits) is reserved for unusual problems or for planning surgery when needed. Trophic skin changes and ischemic lesions usually reflect occlusive etiologies, while a unilateral Raynaud's suggests a secondary process.[93,95]

Most patients with primary Raynaud's phenomenon require no therapy and quickly learn to keep not only the hands but the whole body warm. Treatment of secondary forms is directed at the underlying cause when feasible. Calcium channel blockers and non-beta-adrenergic blocking sympatholytics, alone or in combination, can suppress the episodes in some patients, but drugs and sympathectomy have little impact on ischemic complications. These complications are best treated with local debridement and control of infection and pain.

UPPER EXTREMITY ARTERIAL DISEASE

Upper extremity arterial occlusive disease is less common but more varied in etiology than disease of the lower extremity. Associated vasospastic and microcirculatory disorders are more common. The origin of the brachiocephalic artery, the axillosubclavian area, and the arteries of the hand account for the majority of stenotic lesions. Problems arising in the muscular portion of the arm are less common. Causes include embolic occlusion, trauma, vasculitis, fibromuscular dysplasia, and infections. Arterial testing of the upper extremity should be performed to document the level and severity of disease, especially when lesions are progressive or symptomatic or when tissue loss is occurring or is imminent. Noninvasive testing should survey the entire limb, including the digits. Angiography should include the aortic arch and extend through the hand, with vasodilation of the digital arteries to differentiate "fixed" occlusions from vasospasm.

Chronic atherosclerotic occlusive disease is seen predominantly at the origin of the innominate or, more commonly, the left subclavian artery. Claudication is uncommon or modest because arm use is more intermittent and because the upper extremity has excellent collateral circulation. Radiologic or ultrasound evidence of flow reversal or "steal" from the vertebral artery is not uncommon, but any neurologic symptoms most often are explained by associated carotid disease rather than the subclavian lesion.[96] Acute macroemboli to the arm come predominantly from the heart and only occasionally from proximal aneurysmal or stenotic lesions. Most acute occlusions in situ reflect direct or iatrogenic trauma, thrombosis in or from an aneurysm, or a clotting disorder.

Acute or chronic microcirculatory disease of the hands may be due to numerous mechanisms (Table 90-5). Connective tissue diseases, hematologic disorders, and occupational trauma may result in microvascular disease. Raynaud's phenomenon (see above) can accompany any acute or chronic occlusive process. It also may reflect direct neural irritation at the thoracic outlet or represent a response to medications or the environment. Women who present with Raynaud's phenomenon, digital ulceration, and telangectasias over the facies should be fully evaluated for connective tissue disease, particularly scleroderma or a variant of scleroderma. In such cases, peripheral alpha blockers or calcium channel inhibitors may prove effective.[97]

Aneurysmal disease of the upper extremity is rare. When it is present, the usual location is the proximal brachiocephalic or axillosubclavian arteries. Atherosclerosis, trauma, and thoracic outlet syndrome are the most common etiologies. Thrombosis, distal micro- or macroemboli, and a painful mass are the expected presentations. Rupture is rare unless there is infection.[98]

Several specific entities should be remembered. TAO may present initially with Raynaud's phenomenon or hand ischemia. If it presents late, digital necrosis may be present. It is usually bilateral and may be associated with lower extremity involvement of ischemia, claudication, or superficial thrombophlebitis.[99] Takayasu's syndrome nearly always presents with upper extremity claudication or ischemia. Additionally, 10 percent of patients with temporal arteritis have disease of the great vessels or the proximal arm arteries. Limiting arm claudication progresses rapidly in these patients over just a few months. The process can be halted or improved with steroid therapy.[79,80]

Thoracic Outlet Syndrome

Thoracic outlet syndrome usually results from an osseous lesion (commonly a cervical rib) that causes an aneurysm or stenosis of the subclavian artery. Symptoms may be variable. This reflects the anatomy in that the artery, vein, and nervous bundle all pass through a small, dynamic space. The usual mechanism of damage is the clavicle and a cervical rib (or the first rib) impinging on the subclavian artery like a scissors. This predisposes to thrombosis and Raynaud's phenomenon (Fig. 90-4). Venous and neurogenic complaints may be present. The patient is usually young and active with progressive and frequently puzzling complaints of arm fatigue, swelling, or paresthesia.

The presence of positive thoracic outlet maneuvers does not make the diagnosis of thoracic outlet syndrome. Imaging for the presence of a functional stenosis with duplex ultrasound, the vascular laboratory, or arteriography can be used to document the presence of a functional hemodynamic change. Clinical correlation is required for the diagnosis. Resection of a cervical rib or first rib frequently is required.[100] However, improvement of symptoms is variable, particularly if they are neurogenic in origin.

Hammer Hand Syndrome

Hammer hand syndrome results from trauma to the hypothenar area caused by using the hand as a hammer or by repetitive force on levers or other devices. These activities may produce occlusion or aneurysm formation of the ulnar artery, usually at the level of the hammate bone. Digital ischemia and Raynaud's phenomenon of one or more digits can result from emboli. Improvement follows if the trauma is stopped, but continued problems require surgical treatment.[101] Vibratory tools such as chain saws, grinders, and jackhammers can induce hand dysesthesias and Raynaud's phenomenon when used for several years. Symptoms initially occur during use and later become chronic. Ischemia is a rare and late occurrence.[102]

CLINICAL ASSESSMENT: VENOUS DISEASE

Disease of the venous system is a rapidly changing area of vascular medicine. Anticoagulation therapy is undergoing refinements, surgical management of deep venous obstruction and incompetence is evolving, and new imaging techniques are enhancing diagnosis.[103,104]

Varicose Veins

Varicosities of the superficial veins begin with the incompetence of one or more valves. When proximal valves fail, the column of blood supported by the distal valves increases. As more valves become incompetent, the vein dilates and becomes tortuous. *Primary varicosities* are often a familial trait; their symptoms are exacerbated by prolonged standing, obesity, and pregnancy. *Secondary varicosities* may reflect underlying perforator and deep venous obstruction and/or incompetence, which shifts venous return to the superficial veins. Common secondary causes of varicosities include extrinsic venous compression, prior deep vein thrombosis, congenital lesions, arteriovenous fistulas, and right-sided heart disease. Edema and venous stasis changes rarely are caused by primary varicosities and usually signal the presence of an underlying secondary process. The history, examination, and (when necessary) laboratory evaluation of the deep venous system usually allow the physician to differentiate primary from secondary varicosities.

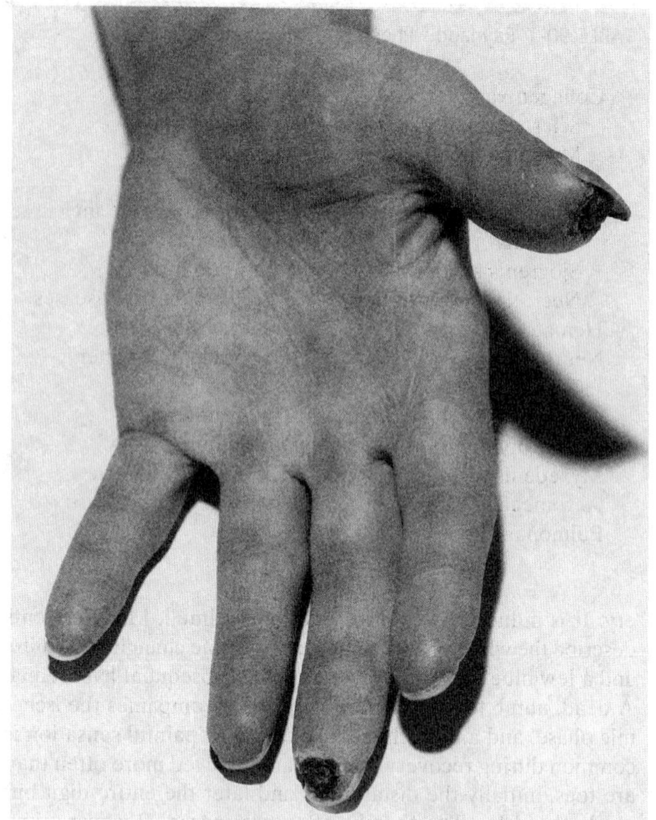

A

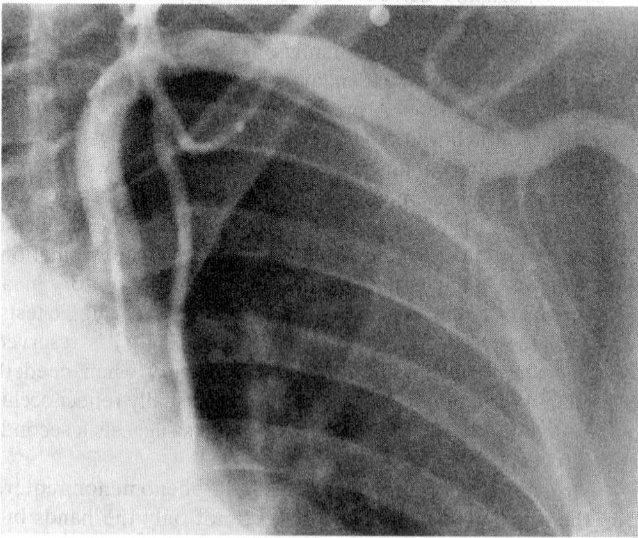

B

FIGURE 90-4 *A.* Photograph of a 24-year-old male who presented with left hand rest pain and ischemic ulcers of digits 1 and 3. He worked as a painter, during which time he experienced arm claudication. Raynaud's phenomenon was present for about 9 months. Thoracic outlet maneuvers were positive bilaterally. *B.* Selective angiography of the left subclavian artery reveals a poststenotic aneurysm with faint shadowing suggestive of thrombus. Cervical ribs were present and were resected.

Varicose veins may ache or burn with standing or prolonged sitting (especially with the legs in a dependent position). Enlargement usually occurs over time, and superficial thrombophlebitis may occur. Rarely, veins may bleed; this bleeding is often brisk despite the venous source because venous pressure is elevated when the limb is dependent. Control of bleeding therefore must include pressure and limb elevation. Both symptoms and progression can be ameliorated by the use of graduated compression hose of 20 to 30 mmHg or more. Ablation of the vein should be considered if complications or discomfort interferes with occupation or lifestyle. Sclerotherapy is effective for certain varicosities and cutaneous "spiders." Surgical removal is indicated for longer segments of proximal varicosities, especially if perforator or saphenofemoral incompetence is present.

Superficial Thrombophlebitis

The presence of a warm, tender, erythematous, and indurated linear lesion in the anatomic course of a superficial vein suggests superficial thrombophlebitis. Ultrasound can differentiate thrombophlebitis from lymphangitic streaks, erythema nodosum, and other lesions. Thrombophlebitis often occurs in a varix or at sites of indwelling catheters or needles. Active infection may be associated with needle use or with the use of illicit street drugs. In such cases, appropriate antibiotics should be used. Infected or suppurative thrombophlebitis often requires surgical removal for the infection to clear. Lesions occurring in a previously normal vein, whether single or migratory, can be idiopathic but may be associated with malignancy, thromboangiitis obliterans, or vasculitis. The lesions of the latter two conditions may be nodular rather than linear and require diagnostic biopsy.[105] An age-appropriate evaluation for underlying diseases that can predispose to clotting should be performed. Superficial thrombophlebitis is usually self-limited, but recovery can be accelerated by rest, topical warmth, and anti-inflammatory agents. Systemic anticoagulation is appropriate for lesions that progress despite conservative care and those located where the lesser or greater saphenous veins enter the deep system.[106]

Deep Vein Thrombosis

The morbidity and mortality of deep vein thrombosis (DVT) remain high. Risk factors for DVT and pulmonary embolism have been well defined in several studies (Table 90-8).[107] The manifestations of DVT are a prominent superficial venous pattern, edema, muscle turgidity, and discomfort. However, these findings may be absent or subtle. For this reason, objective testing to confirm and define the extent of DVT should be obtained whenever it is suspected. Definitive testing also establishes the need for anticoagulation and provides the means to assess clot propagation. A confirmed diagnosis facilitates treatment choices when anticoagulation is relatively or absolutely contraindicated. If the diagnosis is disproved, the cost of treatment and the risks of hemorrhage, heparin-induced thrombocytopenia, and warfarin necrosis are avoided.[108,109]

A wide spectrum of diseases can mimic DVT (Table 90-9). They are diagnosed by their clinical findings and confirmed by appropriate testing (see "Laboratory Assessment: Venous Disease," below) Less than half of patients considered to have DVT have the diagnosis confirmed when tested objectively.[110–112]

Treatment with heparin acutely and warfarin for 12 to 16 weeks is highly effective in preventing clot propagation and pulmonary embolism (see Chap. 53). The recent literature suggests treatment for a minimum of 6 to 12 months in patients with spontaneous DVT.[113] Heparin-induced thrombocytopenia

TABLE 90-8 Risk Factors for Deep Vein Thrombosis

Age	Prior superficial vein thrombosis
Immobility	Hospitalization
Recent surgery	Malignancy
Progesterone therapy	Trauma
Residency in care facility	
Prior deep vein thrombosis	

TABLE 90-9 Etiology of Edema

	One Limb	Multiple Limbs
Decreased Outflow	Deep vein thrombosis	Proximal DVT (IVC)
	Deep vein insufficiency	Bilateral DVT
	Lymphedema	Lymphedema
	Superficial varicosities	Central venous compression
	Extrinsic compression	Pregnancy
	Baker's cyst	Pelvic mass
	May-Thurner syndrome	Obesity
	Pelvic mass	Dependency/immobility
	Factitial	Renal failure
	Arterial aneurysms	Congestive heart failure
		Pulmonary hypertension
Increased Inflow	AV malformations	Pregnancy
	Klippel-Trenaunay syndrome	Drug-induced
	Orthopedic	Cushing's syndrome
	Fracture	
	Osteomyelitis	
	Charcot joint	
	Gastrocnemius or popliteal muscle rupture	
Other	Low oncotic pressure	
	Anemia	
	Hypoalbuminemia	
	Lipedema	
	Hypothyroidism	

is detected by monitoring platelets at 2- to 3-day intervals, and warfarin necrosis is avoided by overlapping heparin with warfarin for 4 to 5 days.[108,109] Low-molecular-weight heparin (adjusted for weight) has shown promise in treating uncomplicated DVT while coumadin is taking effect.[114–116] The risk of major hemorrhage from anticoagulation is 1 to 2 percent when control is strict and attention is paid to drugs that alter warfarin's effect.[117] The international normalized ratio (INR) should be followed to ensure consistency between laboratories.

Thrombus isolated to the calf is less dangerous than thrombus in the thigh, but upward of 20 percent of such thrombi can extend proximally and 10 percent embolize. Laboratory surveillance of the lesion is required if anticoagulants are not used.[118] Caval occlusive procedures (primarily percutaneously placed filters) are used when anticoagulants are contraindicated or have failed to prevent a large pulmonary embolism. If a caval filter is placed and the contraindication to anticoagulation resolves, long-term anticoagulation should be considered since the filter itself may be thrombogenic. Thrombolytic therapy[119] that is given early accelerates recovery and may reduce the incidence or severity of postphlebitic syndrome. However, well-defined indications for thrombolytic therapy in DVT have not been established. Long-term use of compression stockings to the knee (or above, if tolerated) drastically reduces the incidence of postphlebitic syndrome, venous stasis changes, and venous ulceration.[120]

PHLEGMASIA CERULEA DOLENS

Phlegmasia cerulea dolens is a rare complication of DVT that is characterized by rapid and massive edema, severe pain, and cyanosis. This most commonly occurs in the setting of extensive iliofemoral thrombosis. A third of these patients die of pulmonary embolism, and half develop distal gangrene. It is seen most commonly with advanced malignancy or severe infections but can follow surgery, fractures, and other common precipitants of thrombosis.[121] Urgent treatment, including placement of a caval filter, heparinization, and sometimes debulking of the clot by thrombectomy or thrombolysis, is essential to minimize loss of life or limb.

There are numerous causes of limb pain and swelling that clinically mimic acute DVT. Objective testing may be indicated in many cases. D-dimer,[122] duplex ultrasound, or venography will confirm acute thrombosis in about one-third of suspicious episodes.[123] Patients who have *chronic deep venous insufficiency* are most likely to be symptomatic from other conditions. These patients may have acute episodes of pain and swelling that mimic new thrombosis, especially if they are not compliant in using elastic support hose or if the limb is stressed by prolonged dependency, travel, hot weather, or increased sodium intake.

Prophylactic anticoagulation is warranted in patients with prior venous thromboembolism or known clotting disorders who are traumatized or undergo medical or surgical illness with prolonged bed rest.[104,105,124] If anticoagulation must be interrupted for a surgical procedure, baseline duplex ultrasound and postoperative surveillance ultrasound (on or about day 2) may be obtained. With this approach, new clot can be detected even when old clot is present or symptoms are masked by analgesia. When thromboembolic events occur without a recognized risk factor for venous stasis or injury, a search for venous compression, inherited or acquired clotting abnormalities, or systemic disease is appropriate. Even when the results are negative, such screening is valuable in planning the duration of therapy and establishing the prognosis.

CENTRAL VENOUS THROMBOSIS

Occlusion of the superior vena cava (SVC) or inferior vena cava (IVC) may be an acute thrombotic event or may occur gradually from extrinsic compression or extension of distal thrombosis. The acute syndromes produce massive regional swelling and discomfort. Venous collaterals are prominent in chronic occlusion. The presence of superficial collateral veins in IVC syndrome is best appreciated with the patient upright. Malignancy is the cause of over 80 percent of SVC obstructions and about half of IVC obstructions. Relatively benign causes of the SVC syndrome include indwelling catheters (common) and fibrosing mediastinitis (rarely).[125] Inferior vena caval clots often extend from leg thrombosis. Both syndromes may be the initial manifestation of a primary clotting abnormality. Thrombolytic therapy may clear thrombosis if given early, and bypass surgery is effective and durable in selected instances of either syndrome.[126]

THROMBOSIS IN OTHER VEINS

Acute and chronic hepatic vein thrombosis presents with varying degrees of hepatic failure and ascites. Clotting disorders, tumors, and congenital venous anomalies are the most common causes.[127] Acute axillosubclavian thrombosis often is attributed to unusual effort or positioning. There is often evidence of thoracic outlet obstruction. Compression by tumor or aneurysm, indwelling catheters, and clotting defects are other causes. Thrombolytic therapy can be effective when given early and should be followed by anticoagulation. Some patients with local lesions can be further improved by balloon dilatation or surgery.[128]

Chronic Venous Insufficiency

Chronic deep venous incompetence or obstruction (causing venous hypertension in the upright position) may produce chronic venous insufficiency. This is characterized by leg edema, venous dilation, and intradermal deposition of proteins and hemosiderin. Cutaneous changes of fibrosis, lichenification, cellulitis, and ulceration may follow. Edema of the foot (with sparing of the toes) differentiates edema of chronic venous insufficiency from lymphedema. Symptoms include heavy congested limbs, venous claudication, pruritus, and skin ulceration that is often painless. Prior deep venous thrombosis, chronic right-sided heart disease, and an arteriovenous fistula also may produce this syndrome. Increased ambulatory pressure can be confirmed by direct measurement or plethysmography. Both incompetence and obstruction can be documented by bidirectional Doppler, ultrasound, duplex ultrasound, or venography.[129] Once ulceration has occurred, successful management is staged. Reduction of the edema must occur first, followed by healing of the ulcer and finally lifelong control of venous hypertension utilizing rigid or elastic support at 30 to 40 mmHg of compression (or more if required). Repair or replacement of incompetent proximal valves and bypass of iliocaval obstruction are promising in only a very select subset of these patients. The initial durability of these operations is encouraging.[130,131]

LABORATORY ASSESSMENT: VENOUS DISEASE

As with arterial testing, the indications for peripheral venous testing include objective documentation and diagnosis of venous disease, assessment of severity, and monitoring of progression or regression. Venous tests may be invasive (such as venography) or noninvasive, and the information they provide may be anatomic, hemodynamic, or functional.

Anatomic Studies

Duplex ultrasound, CT, MRI/MRA, and venography are the anatomic methods available for evaluation of the venous system. Venography is considered the "gold standard" for the determination of DVT. Venous duplex ultrasound is the most commonly used method, although it has the potential advantage of differentiating acute thrombus from old thrombus on the basis of the presence or absence of distention (common with acute clot) and increased echogenicity (common with chronic clot). It is less sensitive than venography above the groin and below the knee.

Physiologic Studies

CONTINUOUS-WAVE DOPPLER

Continuous-wave Doppler detects the movement of blood. CW Doppler provides qualitative (but not quantitative) information about the presence of hemodynamically significant reflux or obstruction. When the limb is interrogated at multiple levels, localization of the abnormality may be estimated (specificity 88 percent, sensitivity 85 percent).[132] However, this is a poor technique for evaluating partially obstructing thrombus or calf DVT. Although it is relatively sensitive for detecting areas of hemodynamically significant valvular incompetence, it cannot determine the functional significance of venous incompetence. In contrast to the triphasic arterial signal, the venous signal is much more complex. The components of venous flow evaluated by CW Doppler include the following.

Spontaneity When the Doppler is placed over a large vein, a spontaneous venous flow signal should be heard. Minor repositioning should be all that is necessary to obtain a detectable flow signal in most veins. If more extraordinary measures are needed, such as elevating, compressing, or another manipulation of the limb, this suggests an abnormality in venous flow.

Phasicity Venous return varies with the respiratory cycle. Above the diaphragm, there is an increase in venous return during inspiration. Below the diaphragm, venous return decreases during inspiration because increased intraabdominal pressure during inspiration opposes venous return. A loss of phasicity with respiration suggests venous obstruction.

Augmentation If a Doppler is placed over a vein in the proximal limb (for example, the femoral vein) and a distal portion of the limb (for example, the calf) is compressed, there should be an increase in venous return. This phenomenon, which is called augmentation, occurs only if the vein is patent between the site of compression and the site of Doppler interrogation.

Competency If a normal limb is compressed proximally (for example, over the thigh) or if a Valsalva maneuver is performed, the Doppler flow signal obtained distally (for example, over the popliteal vein) should cease temporarily as flow is stopped by the closure of venous valves. If the valves are incompetent, a retrograde flow signal will be noted.

Pulsatility Unlike arterial flow, venous flow is not necessarily pulsatile. When significant pulsatility is noted, one must consider the possibility of tricuspid regurgitation, right-sided heart failure, pulmonary hypertension, volume overload, an arteriovenous fistula, or other causes of increased venous pressure with pulsatility.

Venous Plethysmography

Many plethysmographic techniques have been developed to measure the changes in limb volume that occur when venous return is enhanced or impeded. The most popular techniques are strain gauge plethysmography, air plethysmography, and impedance plethysmography. A fourth modality, photoplethysmography,[133] is not truly a plethysmographic technique but instead estimates the amount of blood in the limb by reflecting infrared light off red blood cells flowing through the cutaneous vasculature.

PLETHYSMOGRAPHY FOR VENOUS INCOMPETENCE

Venous incompetence can be diagnosed and quantified by using plethysmography.[134,135] The patient is placed in an upright position (sitting or standing), and an air cuff or strain gauge is positioned around the lower portion of the limb. Once a steady volume measurement is obtained, the patient is tipped back and the legs are elevated to drain them of blood. The plethysmographic reading falls as blood drains from the veins and the limb becomes smaller. Once the blood has been emptied, the patient is returned to the upright position and the veins refill. If the valves are competent, refilling must occur in an antegrade fashion through the arteries and capillaries. In normal individuals, this may take a minute or more. If there is venous incompetence, the veins refill quickly and the leg volume returns to baseline more rapidly than normal. The next question is whether the incompetence is superficial or deep. If the incompetence is primarily superficial, placing tourniquets around the leg and/or directly compressing the incompetent superficial vein with a finger will normalize the refilling time.

EXERCISE VENOUS PLETHYSMOGRAPHY

This approach is used to assess the function of the "muscle pump" that normally compresses the veins and ejects blood out of the limb whenever muscular contraction occurs.[134,135] As was described above, the plethysmograph is placed around the lower limb or ankle while the patient is upright (sitting or standing). Once a stable baseline volume measurement is achieved, the patient exercises the leg by a series of toe or heel raises or deep knee bends. If a treadmill is available, the patient may walk. In patients with normal venous pump function, the leg volume decreases during exercise. At the end of exercise, the volume returns to baseline as the veins refill. Legs with impaired venous pump function (caused by venous obstruction, valvular incompetence, or primary pump failure) do not decrease their plethysmographic volume normally during exercise.

OUTFLOW PLETHYSMOGRAPHY

Plethysmographic techniques also can be used to evaluate limbs for the venous obstruction seen with acute or chronic DVT. Impedance plethysmography (IPG) is the best studied and most widely employed technique.[136–138] Unlike "anatomic" tests such as venography and ultrasound scanning (i.e., tests that directly image the thrombus), functional tests such as IPG identify the presence of venous thrombi by detecting the hemodynamic abnormalities they produce. Because IPG relies on indirect evidence of venous obstruction, it may be subject to more false positives and negatives than are imaging tests. Nevertheless, the ease of performance, low cost, and reasonable overall accuracy of IPG continue to make it a useful screening tool in appropriate settings.

The basic principles that underlie IPG are simple. A high-frequency, low-intensity electrical current that is too weak to be felt by the subject is passed between two electrodes that encircle the lower limb. Between the electrodes are two other electrodes across which voltage measurements are made. The voltage difference between the "measuring" electrodes is dependent on the electrical impedance of the underlying limb. Electrical impedance is dependent on the volume of blood (or other fluid) within the limb. The rate of change in limb volume is dependent on the rate of flow, which is reflected in the rate of change in electrical impedance.

To test for the presence of DVT, the patient lies supine with the legs slightly flexed and elevated. A pneumatic compression cuff is placed around the thigh and inflated to a pressure above venous pressure but below arterial pressure (typically 40 to 50 mmHg), producing venous occlusion. As blood becomes trapped beyond the cuff, the volume of the lower leg increases and the electrical impedance and voltage change. After an inflation period of 1 to 2 min, the cuff is deflated rapidly and venous flow resumes. As blood drains from the limb, the volume and voltage change rapidly. Values for the increase in leg volume produced by cuff inflation and the decrease in leg volume 3 s after cuff deflation are plotted on a standard diagram, and the presence or absence of obstruction consistent with DVT is determined.

CLINICAL APPLICATION

The accuracy of IPG as a means of detecting proximal DVT has been studied extensively, with generally impressive results. One analysis that compared IPG with venography in 2561 limbs demonstrated a sensitivity of 93 percent, a specificity of 94 percent, and an overall accuracy of 94 percent.[132] False positives occur when conditions other than acute DVT cause and mimic venous obstruction. The most common examples include elevated venous pressure from congestive heart failure, extrinsic vein compression, and "old" nonrecanalized venous thrombi. In contrast, false-negative tests usually are due to below-the-knee thrombi or nonoccluding proximal thrombi. As one would predict, the accuracy of IPG is variable and depends on the subgroup of patients being studied. Although there is ample documentation that the test is useful when applied to symptomatic patients, concern has been raised about its reliability as a tool for screening high-risk, asymptomatic patients. Other pitfalls of testing include unsuitable body habitus (such as morbid obesity or severe limb edema) and inability on the part of the patient to cooperate during the examination. Despite these caveats, IPG offers considerable prognostic information about the likelihood of a subsequent pulmonary embolism in patients suspected of having DVT. In one report involving short-term follow-up on 1074 patients with bilaterally negative IPG, there were no fatal pulmonary emboli and only a 1 percent incidence of clinical suspicion for nonfatal pulmonary emboli.[139] Other plethysmographic techniques have demonstrated similar results. IPG is best suited for use with cooperative, anatomically suitable patients in whom there is either a clinical suspicion of acute proximal DVT or a need to demonstrate that a patient is not at high risk for pulmonary embolism.

LYMPHEDEMA

The lymphatic vessels contain valves that are similar to those in veins but even more fragile. Trauma to a lymph vessel may easily damage these valves. There are multiple lymphatic vessels or channels (deep and superficial) in each limb. In contrast to the venous system, the superficial lymphatic vessels carry the large majority of flow. These systems coalesce at the inguinal lymph nodes and continue as the iliac and paraaortic lymphatic channels, which finally empty into the thoracic duct at the left subclavian vein.

Etiology

Lymphedema is the collection of lymphatic fluid in the dermal and subcutaneous tissues and may be primary or secondary. *Primary* lymphedema may be present at birth as an isolated occurrence or as part of a congenital familial syndrome. Onset of lymphedema in the teens or early twenties is called *lymphedema praecox* (Fig. 90-5) and is seen more often in females (usually at menarche). Rarely, primary lymphedema with onset in later years is called *lymphedema tarda*. This is a diagnosis of exclusion since a secondary cause is much more likely in this age group.

Secondary lymphedema is much more common than primary. Trauma, recurrent infection, obstruction by mass, infiltrative processes, or direct damage to the lymphatic system by radiation can cause lymphatic vessel destruction. Lymphedema of an upper extremity may occur after a radical or modified radical mastectomy. Recurrent cellulitis is common in patients with lymphedema. Streptococcus, which can enter the skin through a crack in the toe webs caused by trychophytosis, further inflames and damages the lymphatic channels and the connecting lymph nodes. Repeated infection damages and eventually obliterates the vessel; preventing these infections is therefore a cornerstone of treatment.

Diagnosis

History and physical examination allow the diagnosis in the majority of cases.[140] Unlike edema and lipedema, lymphedema involves the toes. The skin is thickened and takes on a consistency termed *peau d'orange* (literally, "an orange peel"). Dependent edema also spares the toes since footwear does not allow the swelling to occur. Lipedema, which is caused by excess fatty deposits that usually are increased at the time of menarche,

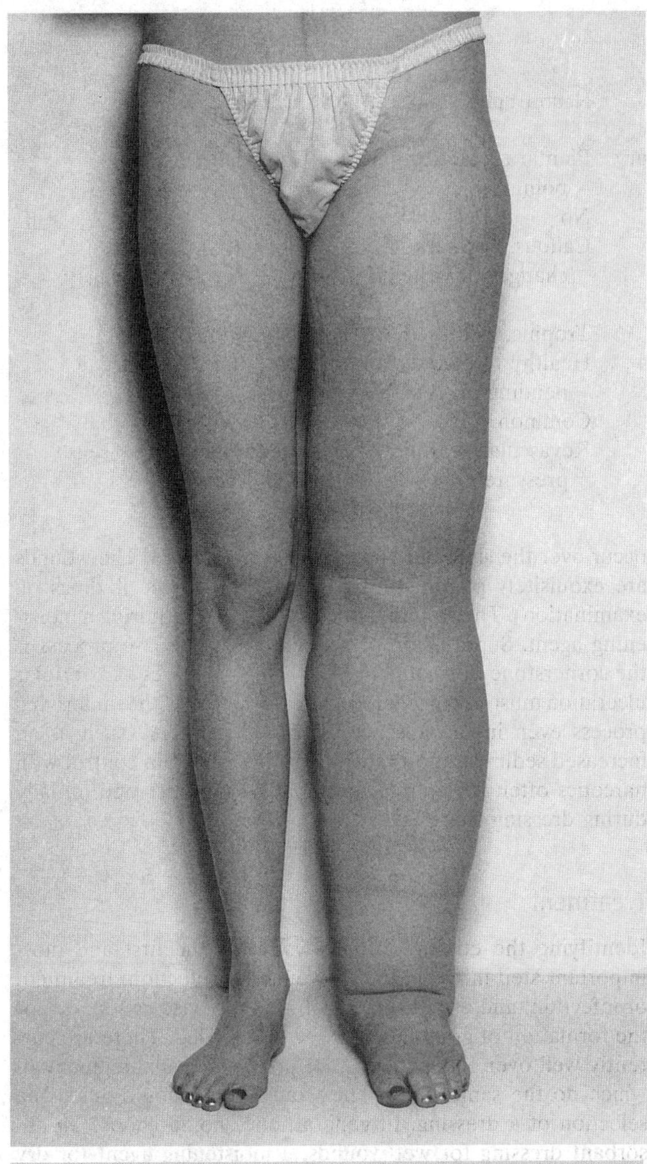

FIGURE 90-5 Photograph of a young woman with lymphedema praecox. Note the asymmetry and note that the toes are affected. The leg was reduced with elevation and compression.

is more difficult to differentiate. These fatty deposits may be asymmetric and may run in families. In lipedema, the toes are spared and there is often a ridge or fold overhanging the ankle. Lipedema and lymphedema may coexist. Laboratory testing may help differentiate the two.

Testing

Lymphangiography and lymphoscintigraphy are the two techniques currently available for direct imaging of the lymphatic system. Lymphangiography is more difficult to perform and carries a risk of lymphangitis. However, anatomic features are obtained and differentiation between primary (absence of lymphatic structures) and secondary (obstruction at a level by a mass, an injury, or lymph node hypertrophy caused by lymphoma) lymphedema often can be determined. The lymphoscintogram is based on the uptake and movement of ^{99}Tc-labeled antimony trisulfide colloid after injection between the web spaces of digits. It is easier to perform this lymphangiography and has a significantly lower risk of lymphangitis. While it has good ability to differentiate lymphedema from other causes of edema, it cannot reliably distinguish primary from secondary lymphedema.

Treatment

The mainstay of treatment for lymphedema is compression. First the leg must be reduced in size by elevation, mechanical pumping, or manual massage. Wrapping of the distal-to-proximal portion of the affected limb or limbs is required whenever the patient is up and also should be encouraged when the patient is supine. Once the leg volume has decreased, a compression garment of 40 to 50 mmHg should be worn daily and replaced two to four times per year as needed. Early and aggressive treatment of cellulitis and fungal infections helps prevent worsening.

ULCERATION

Lower and upper extremity ulceration of vascular etiology is common. However, nonvascular etiologies are also common and must be kept in mind when a properly treated ulcer does not respond to therapy. Dermatologic, oncologic, hematologic, infectious, and factitious causes must be considered in such circumstances. Ulceration caused by a vascular etiology can be classified into four categories: arterial, arteriolar, venous, and neurotrophic (Table 90-10). Multifactorial ulcerations are common, particularly in diabetic patients and immunosuppressed persons. It is beyond the scope of this section to detail the diagnosis and treatment of each, but general principals will be discussed.

Arterial Ulcers

Arterial ulcers generally are located on the distal portion of the lower extremities but may occur anywhere. A traumatic event or surgical procedure such as vein harvesting or toenail trimming often initiates the ulcer. A dense black eschar can form over a dry base. Findings of arterial insufficiency are common. The wound may be tender, and infection can occur. Healing is often problematic until oxygen delivery is increased. In such cases, revascularization is indicated. If this is not possible, external compression devices may be successful, although they are not widely available.

Venous Ulcers

Venous ulcers are relatively painless. They typically develop above the malleoli, usually after years of deep venous insufficiency. Skin changes include thickening, hemosiderin deposits, and edema. The ulcer base is wet and frequently has secondary infection. Varicose veins may cause local venous ulcers after trauma. The natural history is an enlarging ulcer that appears deep because of associated edema. Treatment requires compression and elevation. The edema must be driven out of the leg to create an environment for granulation. Compression with elastic wraps (and foam pads over the ulcer sites to provide

TABLE 90-10 Recognition of Ulcers of Vascular Etiology

Type	Venous	Arterial	Neurotrophic	Arteriolar
Location	Above medial and lateral malleoli	Shins, toes, sites of injury	Plantar surface, pressure points	Shin, calf
Pain	No, unless infected	Yes	No	Exquisite
Skin	Stasis pigmentation Thickening with lipodermatosclerosis	Shiny, pale decreased hair; may see livido	Callous, normal to changes of ischemia	Normal or "satellite" ulcers in various stages
Edges	Clean	Smooth	Trophic, calloused	Serpiginous
Base	Wet, weeping, healthy granulation	Dry, pale with eschar	Healthy to pale depending on ASO	Dry, punched-out, pale, thin eschar
Cellulitis	Common	Often	Common	No
Treatment	Compression	Revascularize	Revascularize, relieve pressure	Treat underlying disease and pain

added compression) is the treatment method of choice. If there is infection, a short course of antibiotics may be required.

Neurotrophic Ulcers

Neurotrophic ulceration is seen in all adult medical specialties. Diabetes, peripheral neuropathies, spinal cord injuries, and other causes of decreased sensation may be present. External pressure by a shoe, a brace, or a foreign body embedded in the foot may start the ulcer. The wound edges develop callus that can mask undermining. The edges must be probed bluntly to determine the extent or presence of fistula tracts. Infection is common, particularly when the decreased sensation masks the pain that infection normally causes. *Osteomyelitis* is frequently present, especially when the ulcer has been present for months and has been treated with short courses of oral antibiotics. Treatment includes relief of the pressure and debridement of the callus. Infection must be treated aggressively, and the presence of osteomyelitis must be excluded. In diabetic patients, arterial occlusive disease also may be present. Revascularization, bony debridement, or amputation often is required to prevent sepsis or achieve healing.

Arteriolar Ulcers

Arteriolar ulcers are caused by occlusion of dermal arterioles that vertically penetrate the dermal layer. This anatomy leads to the characteristic "cookie cutter" appearance and serpiginous edge seen in these ulcers. Islands or satellites of ulcers often occur over the shin, but any area can be affected. The wounds are exquisitely painful (out of proportion to the findings on examination). The wound base is usually dry, requiring a moistening agent. Suppression of the underlying disease process is the cornerstone of treatment (Table 90-11). Flares of arteriolar ulceration must be considered an exacerbation of the underlying process even in the absence of "usual markers" such as an increased sedimentation rate and antibodies. Pain control with narcotics often is required during acute episodes and initially during dressing changes.

TABLE 90-11 Etiologies of Arteriolar Ulcers

- Connective tissue diseases
  - Rheumatoid arthritis
  - Scleroderma
  - Mixed connective tissue diseases
  - Lupus erythematosus
- Vasculitis
- Malignancy
- Myeloproliferative disorders
- Inflammatory bowel disease

Treatment

Identifying the etiology of the wound is the first and most important step in treatment. In general, protection, treatment of infection, and establishment of an ulcer base conducive for the formation of granulation tissue are needed. There are currently well over 1000 wound care products available, many of which do the same thing. The wound base should guide the selection of a dressing. In general, one should choose an absorbant dressing for wet wounds, a moistening agent for dry wounds, and an antibiotic agent for infected wounds. Moisture-neutral dressings are also available. Debridement using wet-to-dry gauze or nonstick products to prevent irritation often is required. Blunt or sharp manual debridement also may be necessary.

References

1. Stoffers H, Rinkens P, Kester A, et al. The prevalence of asymptomatic and unrecognized peripheral arterial occlusive disease. *Int J Epidemiol* 1996; 25:282.
2. Elhadd T, Jung R, Newton R, et al. Incidence of asymptomatic peripheral arterial occlusive disease in diabetic patients attending a hospital clinic. *Adv Exp Med Biol* 1997; 428:45.
3. Leary W, Allen E. Intermittent claudication as a result of arterial spasm induced by walking. *Am Heart J* 1941; 22:719–725.
4. DeWesse J. Pedal pulses disappearing with exercise. *N Engl J Med* 1960; 262:1214.
5. Barnett A, Dugdale L, Ferguson I. Disappearing pulse syndrome due to myxomatous degeneration of the popliteal artery. *Med J Aus* 1966; 2:355.
6. Kavanaugh G, Svein H, Holman C, Johnson R. "Pseudoclaudica-

tion" syndrome produced by compression of the cauda equina. *JAMA* 1968; 206:2477.
7. Goodreau J, Creasy J, Flanigan D, et al. Rational approach to the differentiation of vascular and neurogenic claudication. *Surgery* 1978; 84:749.
8. Kamienski R, Barnes R. Critique of the Allen test for continuity of the palmar arch assessment by Doppler ultrasound. *Surg Gynecol Obstet* 1976; 142:861.
9. Allen E. Thromboangiitis obliterans: Methods of diagnosis of chronic occlusive arterial lesions distal to the wrist with illustrative cases. *Am J Med Sci* 1929; 178:237.
10. Lederle F, Walker J, Reinke D. Selective screening for abdominal aortic aneurysms with physical examination and ultrasound. *Arch Intern Med* 1988; 148:1753.
11. Littooy F, Stefan G, Greisler H, et al. Use of sequential B-mode ultrasonography to manage abdominal aortic aneurysms. *Arch Surg* 1989; 124:419.
12. Wychulis A, Spittell JJ, Wallace R. Popliteal aneurysms. *Surgery* 1970; 68:942.
13. Pappas C, James J, Bernatz P, Schirger A. Femoral aneurysms: Review of surgical management. *JAMA* 1964; 190:489.
14. McCready R, Pairolero P, Gilmore J, et al. Isolated iliac artery aneurysms. *Surgery* 1983; 94:688.
15. Zwolak R, Whitehouse W, Knake J, et al. Atherosclerotic extracranial carotid artery aneurysms. *J Vasc Surg* 1985; 1:415.
16. Pairolero P, Walls J, Payne W, et al. Subclavian-axillary artery aneurysms. *Surgery* 1981; 90:757.
17. Stanley J, Thompson N, Fry W. Splanchnic artery aneurysms. *Arch Surg* 1970; 101:689.
18. Trastek V, Pairolero P, Joyce J, et al. Splenic artery aneurysms. *Surgery* 1982; 91:649.
19. Perloff J. *Physical Examination of the Heart and Circulation*. Philadelphia: Saunders; 1982.
20. McLaughlin M, Colapinto R, Hobbs B. Abdominal bruits: Clinical and angiographic correlation. *JAMA* 1975; 232:1238.
21. Beven E. Thoracic outlet syndromes. In: Young JR, Graor RA, Olin JW, et al, eds. *Peripheral Vascular Diseases*. St. Louis: Mosby–Year Book; 1991:497.
22. Stoney R, Cheng S. Neurogenic thoracic outlet syndrome. In: Rutherford RB, ed. *Vascular Surgery*, 4th ed. Philadelphia: Saunders; 1995:976.
23. Strandness DJ, McCutcheon E, Rushmer R. Application of transcutaneous Doppler flowmeter in evaluation of occlusive arterial disease. *Surg Gynecol Obstet* 1966; 122:1039.
24. Strandness DJ, Schultz R, Sumner D, Rushmer R. Ultrasound flow detection: A useful technic in the evaluation of peripheral vascular disease. *Am J Surg* 1967; 113:311.
25. Johnston K. Processing continuous wave Doppler signals and analysis of peripheral arterial waveform. In: Bernstein EF, ed. *Vascular Diagnosis Problems and Solutions*, 4th ed. St. Louis: Mosby; 1993:149.
26. Regensteiner J. Exercise rehabilitation for patients with peripheral arterial disease. *Exerc Sport Sci Rev* 1995; 23:1.
27. Hobbs J, Yao J. A limitation of the Doppler ultrasound method of measuring ankle systolic pressure. *Vasa* 1974; 3:160.
28. Darling R, Raines J. Quantitative segmental pulse volume recorder: A clinical tool. *Surgery* 1973; 72:873.
29. Symes J, Graham A, Mousseau M. Doppler waveform analysis versus segmental pressure and pulse-volume recording: Assessment of occlusive disease in the lower extremity. *Can J Surg* 1984; 27:345.
30. Rooke T. The use of transcutaneous oximetry in the noninvasive vascular laboratory. *Int Angiol* 1992; 11:36.
31. Rooke T, Hollier L, Osmundson P. The influence of sympathetic nerves on transcutaneous oxygen tension in normal and ischemic lower extremities. *Angiology* 1987; 38:400.
32. Bacharach J, Rooke T, Osmundson P, et al. Predictive value of transcutaneous oxygen pressure and amputation success by use of supine and elevation measurements. *J Vasc Surg* 1992; 15:558.
33. Rooke T, Osmundson P. The influence of age, sex, smoking, and diabetes on lower limb transcutaneous oxygen tension in patients with arterial occlusive disease. *Arch Intern Med* 1990; 150:129.
34. Rooke T, Osmundson P. Variability and reproducibility of transcutaneous oxygen tension measurements in the assessment of peripheral vascular disease. *Angiology* 1989; 40:695.
35. Rooke T, Heser J, Hallett J, et al. Hemodynamic changes following the surgical revascularization of lower limbs in patients with arterial occlusive disease: A comparison of six methods. *J Vasc Technol* 1993; 17:27.
36. Criqui M, Denenberg J, Langer R, et al. The epidemiology of peripheral arterial disease: Importance of identifying the population at risk. *Vasc Med* 1997; 2:221.
37. Stoffers H, Rinkens P, Kester A, et al. The prevalence of asymptomatic and unrecognized peripheral arterial occlusive disease. *Int J Epidemiol* 1996; 2:282.
38. Kannel W, McGee D. Update on some epidemiologic features of intermittent claudication: The Framingham Study. *J Am Geriatr Soc* 1985; 33:13.
39. Brand F, Kannel W, Evans J, et al. Glucose intolerance, physical signs of peripheral arterial disease, and risk of cardiovascular events: The Framingham Study. *Am Heart J* 1998; 136:919.
40. Hooi J, Stoffers H, Kester A, et al. Risk factors and cardiovascular diseases associated with asymptomatic peripheral arterial occlusive disease: The Limburg PAOD Study: Peripheral Arterial Occlusive Disease. *Scand J Prim Health Care* 1998; 16:177.
41. Brand F, Abbott R, Kannel W. Diabetes, intermittent claudication, and risk of cardiovascular disease: The Framingham Study. *Diabetes* 1989; 38:504.
42. Criqui M, Deneberg J. The generalized nature of atherosclerosis: How peripheral arterial disease may predict adverse events from coronary artery disease. *Vasc Med* 1998; 3:241.
43. McKenna M, Wolfson S, Kuller L. The ratio of ankle and arm blood pressure as an independent risk factor of mortality. *Athero* 1991; 87:119.
44. McDaniel M, Cronenwett J. Basic data related to the natural history of intermittent claudication. *Ann Vasc Surg* 1989; 3:273.
45. Boyd A. The natural course of arteriosclerosis of the lower extremities. *Proc R Soc Med* 1962; 55:591.
46. Juergens J, Barker N, Hines EJ: Arteriosclerosis obliterans: Review of 520 cases with special reference to pathogenic and prognostic factors. *Circulation* 1960; 21:188.
47. Schadt D, Hines AJ, Juergens J, et al. Chronic atherosclerotic occlusion of the femoral artery. *JAMA* 1961; 175:937.
48. Moss SEM, Klein RM. The 14-year incidence of lower extremity amputation in a diabetic population: The Wisconsin Epidemiologic Study of Diabetic Retinopathy. *Diabetes Care* 1999; 22:951.
49. Adler A, Boyko E, Ahroni J, et al. Lower extremity amputation in diabetes: The independent effects of peripheral vascular disease. *Diabetes Care* 1999; 22:1029.
50. Hamalainen H, Ronnemaa T, Halonen J, et al. Factors predicting lower extremity amputations in patients with type 1 or type 2 diabetes mellitus: A population-based 7-year follow-up study. *J Intern Med* 1999; 246:97.
51. Migdalis I, Dimakopoulos N, Kourti A, et al. The prevalence of peripheral vascular disease in type 2 diabetic patients with and without proteinuria. *Int Angiol* 1994; 13:229.
52. Barndt R, Blankenhorn D, Crawford D, et al. Regression and progression of early femoral atherosclerosis in treated hyperlipoproteinemic patients. *Ann Intern Med* 1977; 86:139.
53. Hiatt W. Benefit of exercise conditioning for patients with peripheral arterial disease. *Circulation* 1990; 81:602.
54. Hiatt W, Stoll S, Nies A. Effect of beta-adrenergic blockers in the peripheral circulation in patients with peripheral arterial disease. *Circulation* 1985; 72:1226.

55. Lundgren F, Dahlloff A, Lundholm K, et al. Intermittent claudication—surgical reconstruction or physical training? A prospective randomized trial of treatment efficiency. *Ann Surg* 1989; 209:346.
56. Dahloff A, Bjorntorp P, Holm J, et al. Metabolic activity of skeletal muscle in patients with peripheral arterial insufficiency: Effect of physical training. *Eur J Clin Invest* 1974; 4:9.
57. Hood S, Moher D, Barber G. Management of intermittent claudication with pentoxyfilline: Meta-analysis of randomized controlled trials. *Can Med Assoc J* 1996; 155:1053.
58. Bagger J, Helligose P, Randsbaek F, et al. Effect of verapamil in intermittent claudication: A randomized, double-blind, placebo-controlled, cross-over study after individual dose response assessment. *Circulation* 1997; 95:422.
59. Radack K, Wyderski R: β-Adrenergic blocker therapy does not worsen intermittent claudication in subjects with peripheral arterial disease: A meta-analysis of randomized controlled trials. *Arch Intern Med* 1991; 151:1769.
60. Shepherd R. Ergotism. In: White RA, Hollier LH, eds. *Vascular Surgery: Basic Science and Clinical Correlations.* Philadelphia: Lippincott; 1994:177.
61. Hight D, Tilney N, Couch N. Changing clinical trends in patients with peripheral arterial emboli. *Surgery* 1976; 79:171.
62. Darling R, Austen W, Linton R. Arterial embolism. *Surg Gynecol Obstet* 1967; 124:106.
63. Meister S, Grossman W, Dexter L, Dalen J. Paradoxical embolism: Diagnosis during life. *Am J Med* 1972; 53:292.
64. Holm J, Schersten T. Anticoagulant treatment during and after embolectomy. *Acta Chir Scand* 1972; 138:683.
65. Green R, DeWeese J, Rob C. Arterial embolectomy before and after the Fogarty catheter. *Surgery* 1975; 77:24.
66. Fogarty T, Cranley J, Krause R, et al. A method for extraction of arterial emboli and thrombi. *Surg Gynecol Obstet* 1963; 116:241.
67. Thompson J, Weston A, Aigler L, et al. Arterial embolectomy after acute myocardial infarction: A study of 31 patients. *Ann Surg* 1970; 171:979.
68. McNamara T, Fischer J. Thrombolysis of peripheral arterial and graft occlusions: Improved results using high-dose urokinase. *AJR* 1985; 144:769.
69. Ouriel K, Veith F, Sasahara A. Thrombolysis or peripheral arterial surgery: Phase I results. *J Vasc Surg* 1996; 23:64.
70. Ouriel K, Vieth F, Sasahara A. Thrombolysis of Peripheral Arterial Surgery (TOPAS) investigators. A comparison of recombinant urokinase with vascular surgery as initial treatment for acute arterial occlusion of the legs. *N Engl J Med* 1998; 338:1105.
71. Lie J. The rise and fall and resurgence of thromboangiitis obliterans (Buerger's disease). *Acta Pathol Jpn* 1989; 39:153.
72. Mills J, Taylor LJ, Porter J. Buerger's disease in the modern era. *Am J Surg* 1987; 154:123.
73. Olin J, Young J, Graor R, et al. The changing clinical spectrum of thromboangiitis obliterans (Buerger's disease). *Circulation* 1990; 82:3.
74. Shigematsu H, Shigematsu K. Factors affecting the long-term outcome of Buerger's disease (thromboangiitis obliterans). *Int Angiol* 1999; 18:58.
75. Fiessinger J, Schafter M. Trial of iloprost versus aspirin treatment for critical limb ischaemia of thromboangiitis obliterans. *Lancet* 1990; 335:555.
76. Collins P, McDonald P, Lim R. Popliteal artery entrapment: An evolving syndrome. *J Vasc Surg* 1989; 10:484.
77. Ishikawa K. Cystic adventitial disease of the popliteal artery and of other stem vessels in the extremities. *Jpn J Surg* 1987; 17:221.
78. Klein R, Hunder G, Stanson A, et al. Large artery involvement in giant cell (temporal) arteritis. *Ann Intern Med* 1975; 83:806.
79. Hall S, Barr W, Lie J, et al. Takayasu arteritis: A study of 32 North American patients. *Medicine (Baltimore)* 1985; 64:89.
80. Kerr G, Hallahan C, Giordano J, et al. Takayasu arteritis. *Ann Intern Med* 1994; 120:919.
81. Bergqvist D, Bengtsson J, Sternby N. Associated atherosclerotic manifestations. In: Greenhalgh RM, Mannick JA, eds. *The Cause and Management of Aneurysms*, vol 47. London: Saunders; 1990:47.
82. Johansen K, Koepsell T. Familial tendency for abdominal aortic aneurysms. *JAMA* 1986; 256:1934.
83. Dent T, Lindenauer M, Ernst C, et al. Multiple arteriosclerotic aneurysms. *Arch Surg* 1972; 105:338.
84. Joyce J, Fairbairn JI, Kincaid O, et al. Aneurysms of the thoracic aorta: A clinical study with special reference to prognosis. *Circulation* 1964; 29:176.
85. Gastineau D, Kazmier F, Nichols W, et al. Lupus anticoagulant: An analysis of the clinical and laboratory features of 219 cases. *Am J Hematol* 1985; 19:265.
86. Karmody A, Powers S, Monaco V, et al. "Blue toe" syndrome: An indication for limb salvage surgery. *Arch Surg* 1976; 111:1263.
87. Hollier L, Kazmier F, Ochsner J, et al. "Shaggy" aorta syndrome with atheromatous embolization to visceral vessels. *Ann Vasc Surg* 1991; 5:439.
88. Richards A, Eliot R, Kanjuh V, et al. Cholesterol embolism: A multiple-system disease masquerading as polyarteritis nodosa. *Am J Cardiol* 1965; 15:696.
89. Kaufman J, Shah D, Leather R. Atheroembolism and microembolic syndromes (blue toe syndrome and disseminated atheroembolism). In: Rutherford RB, ed. *Vascular Surgery*, 4th ed. Philadelphia: Saunders; 1995:669.
90. Allen E, Brown G. Raynaud's disease: A critical review of minimal requisites for diagnosis. *Am J Med Sci* 1932; 183:187.
91. DeTakats G, Fowler E. Raynaud's phenomenon. *JAMA* 1962; 179:99.
92. Priollet P, Vayssairat M, Housset E. How to classify Raynaud's phenomenon: Long-term follow-up study of 73 cases. *Am J Med* 1987; 87:494.
93. Gifford RJ, Hines EJ. Raynaud's disease among women and girls. *Circulation* 1957; 16:1012.
94. Landry G, Edwards J, McLafferty R, et al. Long-term outcome of Raynaud's syndrome in a prospectively analyzed patient cohort. *J Vasc Surg* 1996; 23:76.
95. Coffman J. *Raynaud's Phenomenon.* New York: Oxford University Press; 1989.
96. Walker P, Paley D, Harris K. What determines the symptoms associated with subclavian artery occlusive disease? *J Vasc Surg* 1985; 2:154.
97. Rose N, Leskovsek N. Scleroderma: Immunopathogenesis and treatment. *Immunol Today* 1998; 19:499.
98. Bower T, Pairolero P, Hallet JJ, et al. Brachiocephalic aneurysms: The case for early recognition and repair. *Ann Vasc Surg* 1991; 5:125.
99. Hirai M, Shionaya S. Arterial obstruction of the upper limb in Buerger's disease: Its incidence and primary lesion. *Br J Surg* 1979; 66:124.
100. Kieffer E, Ruotolo C. Arterial complications of thoracic outlet compression. In: Rutherford RB, ed. *Vascular Surgery*, 4th ed. Philadelphia: Saunders; 1995:992.
101. Conn JJ, Bergan J, Bell J. Hypothenar hammer syndrome: Post-traumatic digital ischemia. *Surgery* 1970; 68:1122.
102. *Vibration Syndrome: Current Intelligence Bulletin 38.* Washington, DC: National Institute of Occupational Safety and Health; 1982.
103. Hirsh J, Hull R. *Venous Thromboembolism: Natural History, Diagnosis and Management.* Boca Raton, FL: CRC Press; 1987.
104. LeClerc J. *Venous Thromboembolic Disorders.* Philadelphia: Lea & Febiger; 1991.
105. Zimran A, Shilo S, Herskro C. Chronic cutaneous polyarteritis

nodosa simulating recurrent thrombophlebitis. *Isr J Med Sci* 1985; 21:154.

106. Plate G, Eklof B, Jensen R, et al. Deep venous thrombosis, pulmonary embolism, and acute surgery in thrombophlebitis of the long saphenous vein. *Acta Chir Scand* 1985; 151:242.
107. O'Fallon W, Heit J, Mohr D, et al. Predictors of recurrence after deep vein thrombosis and pulmonary embolism: A population-based cohort study. *Blood* 1998; 10:560a.
108. Ansell J, Deykin D. Heparin-induced thrombocytopenia and recurrent thromboembolism. *Am J Hematol* 1980; 8:325.
109. Colp M, Minifee P, Wolma F. Coumadin necrosis: A review of the literature. *Surgery* 1988; 103:271.
110. Haeger K. Problems of acute deep vein thrombosis: The interpretation of signs and symptoms. *Angiology* 1969; 20:219.
111. Barnes R, Wu K, Hoak J. Fallibility of the clinical diagnosis of venous thrombosis. *JAMA* 1975; 234:605.
112. Ouriel K, Whitehouse WJ, Zarins C. Combined use of Doppler ultrasound and phlebography in suspected deep venous thrombosis. *Surg Gynecol Obstet* 1984; 159:242.
113. Kearon C, Gent M, Hirsh J, et al. A comparison of three months of anticoagulation with extended anticoagulation for a first episode of idiopathic venous thrombosis. *N Engl J Med* 1999; 340:901.
114. Litin S, Heit J, Mees K. Use of low-molecular-weight heparin in the treatment of venous thromboembolic disease: Answers to frequently asked questions. *Mayo Clin Proc* 1998; 73:545.
115. Lensing A, Prins M, Davidson B, et al. Treatment of deep venous thrombosis with low-molecular-weight heparins. *Arch Intern Med* 1995; 155:601.
116. Green D, Hirsh J, Heit J, et al. Low molecular weight heparin: A critical analysis of clinical trials. *Pharmacol Rev* 1994; 46:89.
117. Robitaille P, LeClerc J, Brave G. Treatment of venous thromboembolism. In: LeClerc J, ed. *Venous Thromboembolic Disorders*. Philadelphia: Lea & Febiger; 1991:267.
118. Kakkar V, Howe C, Nicholaides A, et al. Deep vein thrombosis of the leg: Is there a higher risk group? *Am J Surg* 1970; 120:527.
119. Comerota A. Venous thromboembolism. In: Rutherford RB, ed. *Vascular Surgery*, 4th ed. Philadelphia: Saunders; 1995:1995.
120. Prandoni P, Lensing A, Cogo A, et al. The long-term clinical course of acute deep venous thrombosis. *Ann Intern Med* 1996; 125:1.
121. Brockman S, Vasko J. Phlegmasia cerulea dolens. *Surg Gynecol Obstet* 1965; 121:1347.
122. Heit J, Minor T, Andrews J, et al. Determinates of plasma D-dimer sensitivity for acute pulmonary embolism as defined by pulmonary angiography. *Arch Pathol Lab Med* 1999; 123:235.
123. LeClerc J, Jay R, Hull R. Recurrent leg symptoms following deep vein thrombosis: A diagnostic challenge. *Arch Intern Med* 1985; 145:1867.
124. Hyers T, Hull R, Weg J. Antithrombosis therapy for venous thromboembolic disease. *Chest* 1989; 95:S375.
125. Parish B, Marschke RJ, Dines D, et al. Etiologic considerations in superior vena cava syndromes. *Mayo Clin Proc* 1981; 56:407.
126. Lockridge S, Kibbe W, Doty D. Obstruction of the superior vena cava. *Surgery* 1979; 85:14.
127. Lillimoe K, Cameron J. The Budd-Chiari syndrome. In: Rutherford RB, ed. *Vascular Surgery*, 4th ed. Philadelphia: Saunders; 1995:1195.
128. Machleder H. Evaluation of a new treatment strategy for Paget-Schroetter syndrome: Spontaneous thrombosis of the axillary-subclavian vein. *J Vasc Surg* 1993; 17:305.
129. Nicholaides A, Christopoulos D, Vasdekis S. Progress in the investigation of chronic venous insufficiency. *Ann Vasc Surg* 1989; 3:278.
130. Kistner R, Ferris E. Technique of surgical reconstruction of femoral vein valve. In: Bergan JJ, Yao JST, eds. *Operative Techniques of Vascular Surgery*. New York: Grune & Stratton; 1980:291.
131. Lalka S. Management of chronic obstructive venous disease of the lower extremity. In: Rutherford RB, ed. *Vascular Surgery*, 4th ed. Philadelphia: Saunders; 1995:1862.
132. Wheeler H, Anderson FJ. Use of noninvasive tests as the basis for treatment of deep vein thrombosis. In: Rutherford RB, ed. *Vascular Diagnosis*, 4th ed. St. Louis: Mosby; 1993:862.
133. Abramowitz H, Queral L, Flinn W, et al. The use of photoplethysmography in the assessment of venous insufficiency: A comparison to venous pressure measurements. *Surgery* 1979; 86:434.
134. Katz M, Comerota A, Kerr R. Air plethysmography (APG): A new technique to evaluate patients with chronic venous insufficiency. *J Vasc Technol* 1991; 15:23.
135. Rooke T, Heser JL, Osmonson PJ. Exercise strain-gauge venous plethysmography: Evaluation of a "new" device for assessing lower limb venous incompetence. *Angiology* 1987; 43:219.
136. Brown J, Ward P, Wilkinson A, et al. Impedance plethysmography: A screening procedure to detect deep vein thrombosis. *J Bone Joint Surg* 1987; 69:264.
137. Huisman M, Buller H, TenCate J, et al. Serial impedance plethysmography for suspected deep venous thrombosis in outpatients: The Amsterdam General Practitioner Study. *N Engl J Med* 1986; 314:823.
138. Patterson R, Fowl R, Keller J, et al. The limitations of impedance plethysmography in the diagnosis of acute deep venous thrombosis. *J Vasc Surg* 1989; 9:725.
139. Wheeler H, Anderson FJ, Cardullo P, et al. Suspected deep vein thrombosis: Management by impedance plethysmography. *Arch Surg* 1982; 117:1296.
140. Campisi C. Lymphoedema: Modern diagnostic and therapeutic aspects. *Int Angiol* 1999; 18:14.

C H A P T E R 91

SURGICAL TREATMENT OF PERIPHERAL VASCULAR DISEASE

Thomas F. Dodson / Robert B. Smith III

The emergence of managed care and the advent of minimally invasive procedures have wrought an evolutionary upheaval in the field of vascular surgery, and the pace of change has accelerated, with new technology and new discoveries carrying the field into the twenty-first century. In a recent editorial, a leading medical journal[1] looked back over the most important medical developments of the past 1000 years, and the advances the editors chose to highlight were not surprising. The discovery of cells and their structures, the development of anesthesia, the elucidation of the role of microbes in disease, the development of body imaging, and the discovery of antimicrobial agents were cited, along with several others.

Vascular surgery is a relatively new entrant in the field of medicine and surgery. Its modern origins date back only about 50 years, with the first femoral-to-popliteal bypass being done in 1948 and the first abdominal aortic aneurysm being repaired in 1951.[2] The past 50 years have brought remarkable progress to this young discipline. New technologies currently being evaluated include minimally invasive surgery,[3] gene therapy,[4] the role of computers and the internet,[5-7] tissue engineering,[8] and telemedicine,[9,10] to mention just a few.

This chapter is divided into three sections: (1) carotid endarterectomy, (2) upper and lower extremity revascularization, and (3) upper and lower extremity venous thrombosis. While vascular surgery remains only a "palliative" therapy for people with atherosclerotic and venous disease, "curative" therapies no doubt await insightful and determined investigators. The scalpel will clearly yield to the gene in the days to come.[11]

CAROTID ENDARTERECTOMY

Stroke continues to be the third leading cause of death in the United States, outranked only by heart disease and cancer. There are nearly 500,000 cases of stroke each year in this country, with approximately one-third of patients dying as a result.[12] However, there has been a decline over the past four decades in both the incidence of stroke and the mortality resulting from it. In the past several years, however, evidence has suggested that this long decline in stroke mortality and morbidity may have plateaued in the Minneapolis-St. Paul area.[12] Ironically, recent data from the Mayo Clinic in Rochester, Minnesota, noted that, in the period 1985 to 1989, there was a continuance of an earlier "leveling off" of incidence rates and a suggestion that stroke rates have actually increased over the past 10 years.[13,14] While it has been suggested that "environmental factors" influence the risk of stroke, certainly, better control of hypertension, a gradual reduction in the percentage of individuals who smoke cigarettes, an increased awareness of the benefits of a physically active lifestyle, greater attention to cholesterol reduction and dietary modification, and greater use of anticoagulants in patients with atrial fibrillation have probably all contributed to the decline in stroke deaths in the United States.

In terms of who should undergo operation for carotid artery disease, we are finally on relatively firm ground. There have been six prospective randomized trials published on this topic since 1991, five of which have shown a benefit for surgery in preventing cerebral ischemia.[15-20] Data continue to come from these randomized prospective studies, and Barnett and colleagues recently reported that, based on a further review of the North American Symptomatic Carotid Endarterectomy Trial (NASCET) data, carotid endarterectomy in symptomatic patients with 50 to 69 percent stenosis produced only a "moderate" reduction in the risk of further stroke.[21] An analysis of this information noted an absolute risk reduction of 10.1 percent at 5 years for those symptomatic patients with carotid stenoses of 50 to 69 percent but also noted no benefit for patients with symptomatic stenoses of less than 50 percent. The authors further suggested that decision making regarding these patients with a moderate degree of stenosis could be aided by a full evaluation of underlying risk factors, but that their analysis did not justify a "large" increase in the rate of carotid endarterectomy. As pointed out in an editorial commenting on Barnett's paper, the accumulation of scientific data about carotid endarterectomy is "virtually unmatched in clinical surgical research,"[22] and internists and surgeons alike have embraced this information: the number of carotid endarterectomies performed in 1996—130,000—doubled the number performed in 1991.[23]

TABLE 91-1 Treatment Plan for Patients with Carotid Disease

Category of Patient	Treatment
Patients with Symptomatic Carotid Stenoses	
>80% stenosis of internal carotid artery	CEA indicated
50–79% stenosis of carotid artery but with vascular laboratory data suggesting closer to 79%	CEA probably indicated; assess risk factors
50–79% stenosis of carotid artery but with vascular laboratory data suggesting closer to 50%	CEA may be indicated; assess risk factors
<50% stenosis of carotid artery	Trial of medical therapy
Patients with Asymptomatic Carotid Stenoses	
>80% stenosis of carotid artery	CEA indicated
50–79% stenosis of carotid artery but with vascular laboratory data suggesting closer to 79%	CEA may be indicated; assess risk factors
50–79% stenosis of carotid artery but with vascular laboratory data suggesting closer to 50%	CEA not indicated
<50% stenosis of carotid artery	CEA not indicated

ABBREVIATION: CEA = carotid endarterectomy.

Our current decision making process for patients with carotid disease is outlined in Table 91-1.

With respect to preoperative imaging of patients with carotid disease, the "gold standard," cerebral arteriography, is being utilized less in an effort to reduce both the risk and the cost of the overall procedure. As noted in the previous edition of this text, the Asymptomatic Carotid Atherosclerosis Study (ACAS) and the NASCET study had 1.2 percent and 0.7 percent morbidity rates, respectively from cerebral angiography. A recent evaluation of "silent embolism" after cerebral angiography by Bendszus and colleagues from Germany raised this issue anew. By using sophisticated techniques [diffusion-weighted magnetic resonance imaging (MRI)] both before and after angiography, they were able to demonstrate 42 "bright lesions" in 23 patients (of 100 patients total) after 23 procedures.[24] It is interesting to note that no new neurologic deficits were observed in any of these patients, and the authors suggested that these changes were silent because they were located in "noneloquent brain areas." The frequency of the lesions was correlated with the amount of contrast medium, the amount of time used for fluoroscopy, the number of vessels that proved difficult to probe, and the number of catheters used.

Over the last several years, a number of papers have addressed the issue of carotid endarterectomy without angiography.[25–28] The consensus of opinion is that, with a dedicated vascular laboratory, the great majority of patients (perhaps as many as 90 percent) can be safely evaluated with an ultrasound only. Indications suggesting the need for arteriography include: (1) uncertainty about the accuracy or reliability of the vascular laboratory; (2) uncertainty about possible complete occlusion of the internal carotid artery in a patient with ongoing localizing symptoms; (3) concern about proximal or intrathoracic disease; (4) patients with "technically difficult" studies due to variant arterial anatomy; and (5) patients with symptoms and an indeterminate study.[27]

The great majority of our patients have their carotid endarterectomies done under local anesthesia with light sedation given by the anesthesiologist.[29] Others have utilized cervical block anesthesia with similarly good results.[30,31] We feel that these techniques are safer than a general anesthetic and provide moment-to-moment assessment of the patient's neurologic condition, avoiding the necessity of concern at the end of the case as the patient awakens from general anesthetic. We also shunt the patient routinely (Fig. 91-1), realizing, however, that approximately 80 percent of patients can undergo operation safely without the use of a shunt.

One change that we have made in recent years in our technique of carotid endarterectomy is an increased tendency to patch the carotid after endarterectomy. In years past, our indications for use of the patch were (1) female gender and (2) recurrent stenoses and the necessity for reoperation. Two papers that have been influential in this regard are the work of Moore and colleagues reporting on results of the ACAS study,[32] and the work of AbuRahma and colleagues reporting on a randomized prospective trial of primary closure versus patching.[33] In the former study, the authors were able

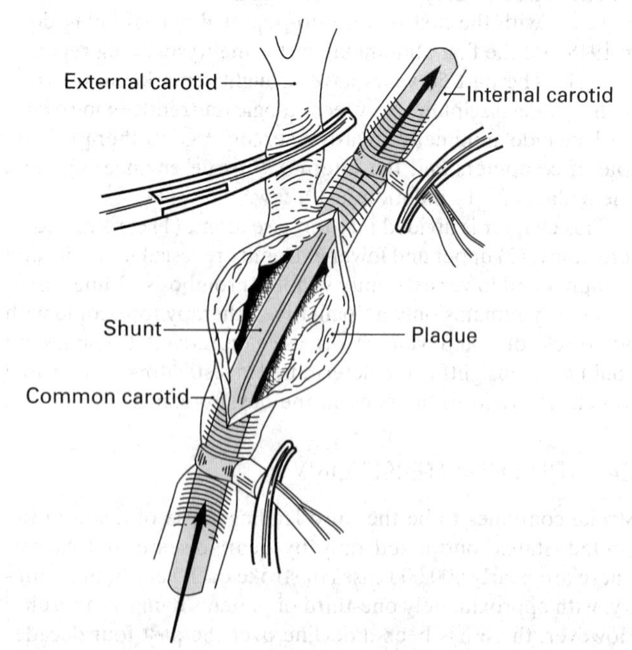

FIGURE 91-1 Indwelling shunt in place to preserve internal carotid flow during the endarterectomy.

to show an overall incidence of recurrent carotid stenosis of 4.5 percent in patients who underwent patch angioplasty, compared with an incidence of 16.9 percent in patients undergoing primary arterial repair. The second report, from West Virginia University, looked at 74 patients undergoing bilateral carotid endarterectomies with primary closure on one side and patch angioplasty on the other. Not only did patch angioplasty have a lower incidence of recurrent stenosis (1 versus 22 percent), but the total internal carotid occlusion rate was lower as well (0 versus 8 percent with primary closure). Addition of a patch adds only a few minutes to the operation, with no increase in perioperative morbidity or mortality rates.

A carotid endarterectomy performed under local anesthesia with intraoperative sedation imposes a low degree of surgical stress on the patient, with only a rare need for blood transfusion. The risk of operation rises with increases in the patient's symptoms: the asymptomatic patient has the lowest risk, about 1 percent perioperative morbidity and mortality rates; the patient with transient ischemic attacks has a perioperative risk of about 3 percent, with a doubling of the yearly stroke risk from 1 percent (in the asymptomatic patient) to 2 percent; the patient who has had a completed stroke has a perioperative risk of about 5 percent, with a yearly stroke risk of 4 percent.[34] For the past several years, we have adopted a clinical pathway for patients undergoing carotid endarterectomy that utilizes the postanesthesia care unit (PACU) for several hours after operation, with subsequent transfer to the vascular surgery ward rather than to the intensive care unit (ICU). Only patients with complications, with coexistent carotid and coronary disease awaiting cardiac surgery, or with instability are admitted to the ICU. While the majority of our patients are discharged on the second postoperative day, other groups have demonstrated the safety and cost reductions possible with discharge within 24 h of operation.[35,36]

The treatment of carotid artery disease represents a benchmark for many other common vascular problems. Large randomized studies were performed to answer difficult questions. The economic milieu made a search for more cost-effective and efficient care a necessity, and we have responded by diminishing invasive preoperative testing and markedly shortening hospital stay, both of which were accomplished without sacrifice of quality of care.[37] Other questions remain to be answered in a similar fashion.

In discussing the "best evidence-based surgical procedure for the prevention of occlusive stroke,"[38] it is important to note that all the questions about carotid disease are not settled, and certainly they never will be. The use of balloon angioplasty for the treatment of vascular stenoses has been a mainstay in the armamentarium of cardiologists and interventional radiologists since Gruentzig's work nearly three decades ago. It is no wonder that lesions in the carotid territory have beckoned to those physicians with catheter-based skills. Surgical investigators, in many cases vascular surgeons worried both about the potential for harm to their patients and about the potential loss of revenue, have expressed concern,[39] have embraced the new technology,[40] or have worked to compare the two competing methods of treatment of carotid disease.[41] One of a series of articles from the University of Alabama in Birmingham by Jordan and his colleagues on this topic showed that percutaneous transluminal angioplasty—in a retrospective review—carried a "significantly higher" neurologic risk than did carotid endarterectomy performed under regional anesthesia. In another study appearing at about the same time,[42] Naylor and colleagues reported on a prospective randomized trial of CEA versus carotid angioplasty in which the trial was stopped because of an increased number of complications in the angioplasty arm. Reporting on only 17 patients, they suspended the trial when 5 of the 7 patients who had carotid angioplasty had a stroke. None of the 10 patients who had carotid endarterectomy had complications.

To address concerns about the potential increased risk of embolic events during percutaneous angioplasty and stenting, some investigators have been evaluating filter devices that could be positioned downstream from the carotid stenosis prior to angioplasty and stenting. One such device was reported on by Ohki and colleagues recently,[43] and their data indicated that 88 percent of the particles liberated during the procedure were captured by their device. This experiment utilized carotid bifurcation plaques obtained from patients after carotid endarterectomy and subjected them to a perfusion circuit with continuous flow through the plaque. Human trials were suggested as the next step.

A statement on this important topic was issued by an American Heart Association Science Advisory group in 1998.[44] They concluded that carotid angioplasty and carotid stenting should, "with rare and infrequent exception," be undertaken only as part of a prospective, randomized trial. In that regard, after a great deal of debate, study, and discussion, our vascular center has decided to enter the Carotid Revascularization Endarterectomy versus Stent Trial (CREST) study.[45] For further discussion of this subject, please see Chap. 92.

UPPER AND LOWER EXTREMITY REVASCULARIZATION

Upper Extremity Revascularization

Chronic arterial insufficiency of the upper extremity is most often due to occlusive disease of the aortic arch branches near their origin, either the subclavian artery or the brachiocephalic trunk. Symptoms may either be limited to ischemic manifestations of the arm and hand or may include posterior circulation insufficiency of the brain due to subclavian steal syndrome. Selection of patients for surgical intervention is extremely important in this group of disorders, since many patients have few or no symptoms and should not be subjected to an operative procedure simply for the correction of an anatomic or radiologic finding.[46,47] Individuals who are significantly limited by arm claudication or those who have symptomatic subclavian steal syndrome should be thoroughly evaluated by vascular examination and complete angiography. Since the patterns of occlusive lesions are extremely variable, any surgical procedure must be carefully planned. Generally, extrathoracic bypass procedures are preferred if a normal donor artery is available; otherwise, a transthoracic procedure may be required to originate a prosthetic bypass from the aortic arch itself. A recent large series of patients with symptomatic atherosclerotic occlusive disease of the innominate artery was presented by Azakie and colleagues, from the University of California at San Francisco.[48] They operated upon 94 patients between 1960 and 1997, performing innominate endarterectomies in 72 patients and bypass grafting in 22 patients. Although there were three perioperative deaths and four strokes (three of which resolved), their long-term results were very good, with freedom from recurrence requiring operation of 99 percent at 5 years and an actuarial survival rate of 85 percent at 5 years. If an extrathoracic bypass is feasible, the operation imposes a low degree of surgical stress, and there is little likelihood of a need for blood transfusions. General anesthesia is preferred, but selected operations for poor-risk patients can be performed with local anesthesia if necessary.

Atheromatous occlusive disease of the subclavian artery is the most common lesion involving the proximal branches of the aortic arch. Extrathoracic revascularization of this vessel can be achieved by one of several techniques, depending on the pattern of obstruction and the relationship of the artery in question to a patent donor vessel. When the ipsilateral common carotid artery is patent and has minimal or no disease, it is frequently chosen as the site of arterial inflow. Perler and colleagues performed carotid-subclavian bypasses or transposition procedures on 31 individuals for a variety of conditions between 1979 and 1989. They achieved relief of symptoms in 30 patients (97 percent), with a symptom-free survival rate of 89 percent at 1 year and 84 percent at 2 years.[49]

Vein grafts are often utilized to improve flow to the upper arm or forearm. Since the demonstration of this technique in 1965 by Garrett, et al.,[50] others have published series of bypass grafts for upper limb ischemia.[51,52] In the largest such series, comprising 74 patients who underwent 95 separate operations over a 15-year period, there were no operative deaths and only a single major amputation. The survival rate was 86 percent at 5 years, with an overall patency rate of 61 percent at that time. Vein grafts were superior at all sites to prostheses.[53] A third alternative (after transthoracic or transsternal operations and extraanatomic bypasses) to improve perfusion to the upper extremity is the utilization of endovascular techniques for aortic arch lesions. A multidisciplinary approach utilizing endovascular techniques for treatment of lesions of the subclavian, innominate, and common carotid arteries was presented by the group from the Cleveland Clinic.[54] In a series of 83 patients, initial technical success was achieved in 82 of 87 procedures (94 percent), but complications occurred in 18 of 87 procedures (20.7 percent), and the 30-day mortality rate for the entire group was 4.8 percent (4 of 83 patients). The investigators acknowledged that there is "no reliable way, short of angiography, to assess anatomic patency" of the vessels that were angioplastied and stented. They also concluded that the results, particularly when complete occlusions were included in the patients being considered for intervention, "seem to favor" surgical treatment.

A more optimistic report, but involving fewer patients, was submitted recently by the cardiology group from the Lahey Clinic. They reported on 18 patients with symptomatic aortic arch vessel stenosis or occlusion.[55] This group of patients represented all patients referred to their practice over a period of 4 years, and all were treated with percutaneous techniques utilizing Palmaz stents. Primary patency was 100 percent with *no* major complications, and, at a mean follow-up of 17 months, all patients were asymptomatic, again, with, 100 percent primary patency (determined by noninvasive studies). The authors concluded by stating that percutaneous stenting should become the "preferred" therapy for the treatment of aortic arch atherosclerotic disease.

Lower Extremity Revascularization

Just as patients with asymptomatic carotid bruits have a higher risk of a cardiac ischemic event than of a stroke,[56] patients with peripheral vascular disease have an increased risk of death from cardiovascular causes. In a study of 565 men and women who were evaluated for the presence of large-vessel peripheral arterial disease (abnormal segment-to-arm blood pressure ratios or abnormal flow velocities), 67 subjects with peripheral arterial disease were identified. During a follow-up of 10 years, 21 of the 34 men (61.8 percent) and 11 of the 33 women (33.3 percent) died. In patients without evidence of arterial disease, the death rates were 16.9 percent for the men and 11.6 percent for the women.[57] The same conclusion was found by Vogt and colleagues, who demonstrated that patients with a diminished ankle-arm blood pressure index of 0.9 or less had a crude overall mortality rate about fivefold greater than that of patients with a higher value of this index.[58] Unfortunately, utilization of the ankle-brachial index (ABI) to follow the progression of lower extremity atherosclerotic disease has been found to be unreliable. In a study of 193 extremities in 114 patients with a mean follow-up of 3.3 years,[59] Porter and colleagues from Portland, Oregon, found that the ABI had a sensitivity of only 41 percent in determining the progression of disease. While the ABI was stated to be "poor" at identifying a *worsening* of vascular disease, it remains an important and easily performed screening test.

Patients with Claudication

A conservative approach to patients with claudication is generally appropriate. This conservatism is based on the fact that the outcome of local disease in the leg is relatively benign, while the outcome for the individual patient is increasingly malignant. A recent article by a TransAtlantic Inter-Society study group[60] noted that, of 100 patients presenting to a physician with claudication, 75 patients would have stability or improvement in the leg over 5 years. Of the 25 whose condition would deteriorate over this period of time, only 5 patients would require an intervention, and only 2 would require amputation. With respect to "systemic outcome," the outlook is not so sanguine. Thirty of the patients will die within 5 years, and 5 to 10 of the individuals will have a nonfatal cardiovascular event within this period of time. The majority of the deaths will be due, of course, to cardiac events.

Given that the symptom of claudication is such an ominous predictor of widespread vascular disease, risk-factor modification is the first step in the treatment of such patients. Of the four factors that are involved in patients with claudication—smoking, diabetes, dyslipidemia, and hypertension—*tobacco use is the single most important factor.*[61] In fact, patients who continue to smoke have double (60 percent) the 5-year mortality rate of patients who are able to stop smoking. Likewise, tight control of diabetes, utilization of statin agents to treat hyperlipidemia, and treatment of hypertension are all directed toward reducing further atherosclerosis, particularly in the cerebral and coronary beds.

After control of risk factors, an exercise program is the next step in the effective treatment of the claudicant. In an interesting study carried out by both the Department of Surgery and the Department of Psychiatry and Behavioral Medicine at Brown

University,[62] Patterson and colleagues found that both patients who exercised at home and those who exercised under supervision improved after a 12-week period of time. The degree of improvement was more marked in those patients who were supervised (280 percent increase) than in those who exercised at home (170 percent increase). Depending upon the degree of limitation imposed by the claudication, either type of program may be of benefit.

The next concern in the treatment of patients with claudication is the consideration of pharmacologic therapy. Pentoxifylline (Trental) was the first drug approved for treatment of claudication in the United States, but we have largely discontinued using this agent because of its cost as well as its limited clinical benefit. A relatively new drug, cilostazol (Pletal) has now been approved for use in patients with claudication, and it seems to have real potential. In a multicenter, randomized, double-blind placebo controlled trial conducted by Money and colleagues, it was found that cilostazol "significantly increased" absolute claudication distance at all measured time points.[63] Because cilostazol is a phosphodiesterase inhibitor, it should not, however, be administered in patients with congestive heart failure (see also Chap. 90).

The final issue in the evaluation of patients with claudication is that of potential intervention with an operative or endovascular approach to the underlying atherosclerotic lesion. This has been and remains a controversial topic, perhaps even more so in light of the increasing interest in catheter-based therapies. Two recent papers have addressed the topic of operative intervention. The first, from Charleston, West Virginia,[64] was an interesting study that compared patients with bilateral claudication who had saphenous vein grafts placed on one side and polytetrafluoroethylene (PTFE) grafts on the other. These were really "ideal" patients, since they were required to have two- to three-vessel runoff before entry into the study. There were no operative deaths or perioperative amputations for either procedure, and both grafts were found to have "comparable" patencies with identical limb salvage (98 percent) at 72 months. The second paper, from Shah and colleagues at Albany,[65] evaluated 409 infrainguinal reconstructions for claudication and was designed to answer the rhetorical question, "Is it worth the risk?" In this large series, they had only one limb lost due to embolization and no operative deaths. Their conclusions, even acknowledging that 18 percent of their interventions required second procedures, were that infrainguinal bypass grafting procedures were "valid treatment options" in selected patients with claudication. Contradicting what we stated earlier about the poor long-term survival in patients with claudication, they had a 93 percent cumulative patient survival rate at 4 years, compared with a 65 percent cumulative patient survival rate when operative intervention was required for limb salvage.

Percutaneous transluminal angioplasty (PTA) in patients with claudication was addressed by Whyman and colleagues in a randomized controlled trial.[66] Sixty-two patients with short femoral artery stenoses or occlusions and iliac stenoses were randomized to either PTA plus medical therapy or to medical therapy alone. At 2 years of follow-up, the PTA group and the control group "did not differ significantly" in the four categories analyzed. They concluded by stating that the addition of angioplasty to conventional medical treatment "does not confer a measurable benefit in the patient's perceived or measured walking ability after 2 years." They also acknowledged that a large randomized trial would be needed in order to settle the issue of which, if any, patients might benefit from angioplasty.

A recent paper by Golledge and colleagues, from London, looked directly at the outcomes of femoropopliteal angioplasty in 43 patients with intermittent claudication, 4 with rest pain, and 27 patients with tissue loss.[67] Although "technical success" was achieved in 67 patients (91 percent), failure of the procedure occurred in the remaining 7 patients. With respect to the 43 patients with claudication, 9 of the 43 patients with intermittent claudication still had symptoms at 1 year. Seven other patients with claudication required another intervention. In 27 of the 43 patients (63 percent), the claudication had resolved. Considering all patients, symptomatic improvement was found in only 51 percent of patients 1 year from the time of angioplasty, although approximately two-thirds of patients with intermittent claudication were symptom free at 12 months. The authors suggested that a longer period of follow-up would be required to assess durability of the angioplasty procedure.

TABLE 91-2 Outcome after Lower Extremity Revascularization

Author	Study Size	Study Methods	Results
Nicoloff et al. 1998[71]	112 patients	112 consecutive patients who underwent bypass surgery for limb salvage	7 deaths (6%); 75 patients (67%) ambulatory and 30 (27%) nonambulatory at last follow-up; ideal results felt to be "infrequent"
Pomposelli et al. 1998[69]	262 patients	262 patients, 80 years old or older, who had 299 lower extremity bypass operations; limb salvage was the indication in 96%	Limb salvage rate at 5 years 92%; patient survival 44%; patients with poor levels of ambulatory status preoperatively more likely to end up nonambulatory or to require nursing home care
Seabrook et al. 1999[70]	70 patients	70 patients who had successful in situ saphenous vein bypasses for limb-threatening ischemia	37 of 69 patients (53%) reporting no problems with revascularized limb; a significant proportion requiring the assistance of a cane, walker, or wheelchair for mobility

Patients with Rest Pain

Ischemic rest pain is frequently an intolerable symptom and implies potential loss of the foot or limb. Whereas patients with claudication are generally managed in a conservative or nonoperative manner, patients with rest pain or a nonhealing lesion are evaluated for a potential operation, frequently as outpatients in the increasingly cost-conscious environment. The question of amputation versus revascularization for rest pain or a nonhealing lesion arises, especially in the elderly.

In the previous edition of this text, we stated that about 95 percent of patients with rest pain should have an attempt at revascularization, while the remaining 5 percent, for reasons of their moribund condition, little chance of functional recovery, or irretrievable limb ischemia, should undergo amputation. We still feel that this is the correct approach, but our outlook on this aggressive approach has been colored by information gained from a number of centers in this country. The data are summarized in Table 91-2.[68–70] Basically, all the studies suggest that operation for limb salvage is a major operative intervention, and that many of these patients have "functional disabilities" that mandate continued close observation and care. One of the authors stated that "it is abundantly clear that limb-threatening ischemia is a manifestation of atherosclerosis that occurs in patients who are approaching the end of life, at a time when functional status is frequently declining rapidly and interval survival is short."[71] In an attempt to better delineate who might benefit from lower extremity bypass procedures, Kalman and colleagues, from Toronto, looked at 358 consecutive in-situ distal leg bypass procedures from 1986 to 1995.[72] They asserted that four significant variables were associated with a late lower survival rate: male gender, diabetes, chronic renal insufficiency, and a history of cerebrovascular disease. When all four variables were present, the predicted 5-year survival rate was reduced to 2 percent. The paper concluded that these variables *were* predictive of lower late survival rates and that they might be used in the decision for either revascularization or amputation.

As noted earlier, we are in a period of transition in terms of the imaging of carotid artery disease, and approaches to imaging of the vasculature of the extremities are also evolving. We continue to order arteriograms to assess the vasculature of the arms and legs, but magnetic resonance angiography (MRA) with contrast agent enhancement may ultimately supplant contrast arteriography (Fig. 91-2).[73,74] MRA has also been utilized in graft surveillance, with an accuracy of 95 percent when combined with color-flow duplex imaging.[75] We currently utilize MRA to identify runoff vessels in patients who are otherwise candidates for revascularization but in whom contrast angiography has been of poor quality or has failed to demonstrate patent runoff vessels. The utility of MRA in this setting has been confirmed by investigators who noted a limb-salvage rate of 78 percent in patients with angiographically occult runoff vessels that were detectable by MRA.[76]

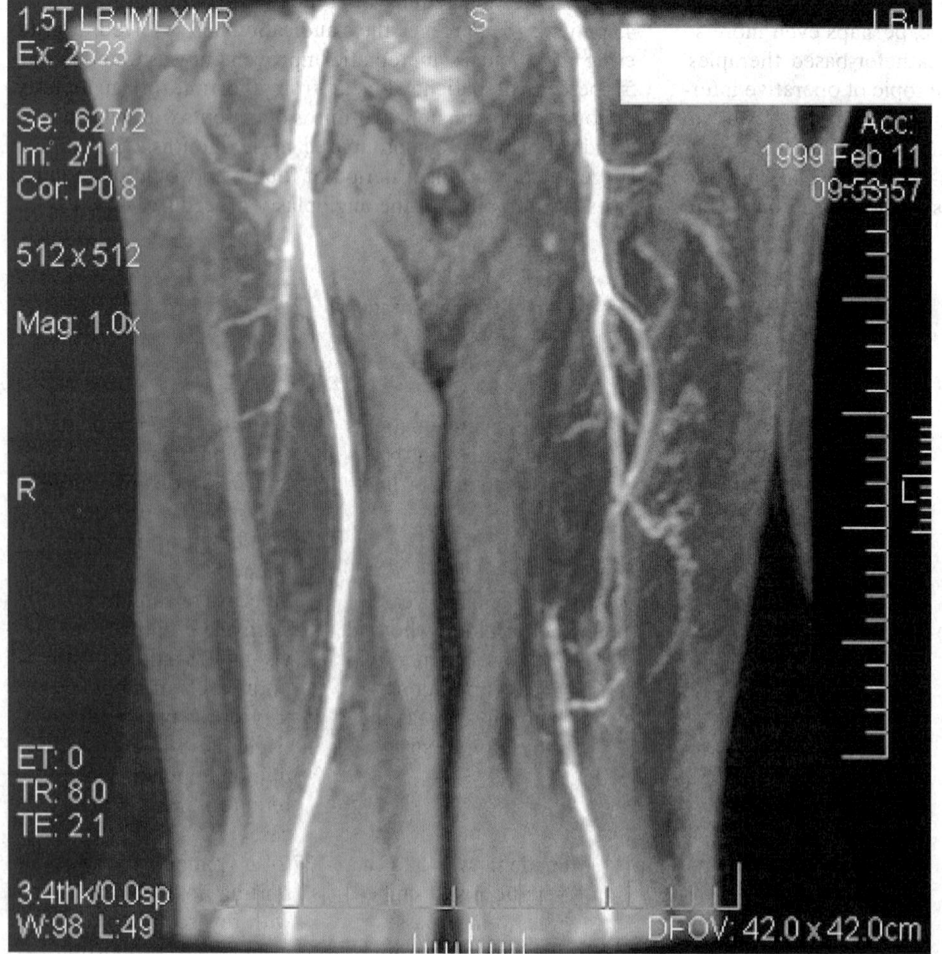

FIGURE 91-2 Magnetic resonance angiogram with gadolinium enhancement, showing left superficial femoral artery (SFA) occlusion in a patient with rest pain.

Although we prefer to utilize the greater saphenous vein as a conduit in almost all infrainguinal bypasses, there are a number of alternatives. In situations where there is inadequate autogenous material available for bypass, utilization of PTFE below the knee, in one recent series, yielded a 2-year patency of 52 percent with a limb-salvage rate of 62 percent.[77] While most investigators acknowledge the relatively poor long-term results with PTFE bypasses to infrapopliteal arteries, some authors still recommend its utilization in the above-knee position.[78,79]

Other options include the use of arm and lesser saphenous vein grafts[80]; composite sequential bypass utilizing vein sewn to PTFE[81]; use of an anastomotic vein patch, as popularized by Taylor and colleagues[82]; umbilical vein grafts[83];

distal venous arterialization,[84] and cryopreserved vein allografts.[85,86] With respect to the latter, Carpenter and colleagues have documented a primary graft patency at 1 year of 13 percent and a limb-salvage rate of 42 percent. In his more recent paper, he endeavored to define the immune response to allograft bypass and concluded that the allografts are immunogenic and prompt a T cell–mediated response. He suggested that it may be possible to modify the factor of rejection by the use of immunosuppressive medication. In a recent report by Castier, he and his colleagues, from Clichy, France, used cryopreserved *arterial* allografts in 32 patients with limb-threatening ischemia between 1993 and 1997.[87] While arterial dilatation occurred in two patent grafts (requiring replacement), the overall primary patency was 57 percent at 12 months and 39 percent at 18 months. This work remains investigational.

In the largest series on long-term results of in-situ saphenous vein bypass grafts, Shah et al. documented a cumulative secondary patency rate of 91 and 81 percent at 1 and 5 years, respectively, and a limb-salvage rate of 97 and 95 percent at 1 and 5 years, respectively.[88] These results continue to set the standard for infrainguinal reconstruction performed today. It has also been shown in a prospective, randomized, multicenter study that a comparison of in-situ (Fig. 91-3) and reversed saphenous vein bypasses revealed "no significant differences" in overall patency rates.[89] The authors concluded that surgeons should therefore be adept at both procedures. We are increasingly utilizing "vein mapping" to help locate acceptable venous conduits preoperatively; these veins include the accessory ipsilateral greater saphenous vein, the contralateral greater saphenous vein, the lesser saphenous vein, and arm veins. Again, Shah et al. have shown that utilization of "spliced" excised vein segments will yield a primary patency rate of 72 percent at 1 year and 45 percent at 4 years.[90] At present, there seem to be few fundamental impediments to the ability of vascular surgeons to operate on distal extremity vasculature. Intensive surveillance, involving utilization of duplex scanning of vein grafts at 1 month, 3 months, 6 months, and every 6 months thereafter, seems to aid in detecting graft-threatening lesions, although it also adds to cost.[91]

We have also learned, since the publication of the last edition of this text, that the addition of anticoagulation to patients in a high-risk setting after infrainguinal bypass grafting may be beneficial in promoting graft patency. In a randomized prospective trial carried out by Sarac and colleagues, from the University of Florida, the authors were able to show that, while perioperative therapy with heparin increased the wound hematoma rate, long-term anticoagulation with warfarin improved both the patency rate and the limb-salvage rate in patients at high risk for graft thrombosis.[92] A recent meta-analysis confirmed this finding and also suggested that platelet inhibitors reduced the risk of graft occlusion after infrainguinal bypass surgery.[93]

Angioplasty of the femoral, popliteal, and even tibioperoneal vessels has been recommended by some investigators.[94–99] Randomized controlled trials are needed to determine the efficacy of these approaches.[100] Endovascular techniques such as stent placement[101] and percutaneous femoropopliteal graft placement[102,103] are also being evaluated in patients with femoral and popliteal artery disease. Cost-effective analyses of femoropopliteal revascularization procedures are now available, and more are to follow.[104,105]

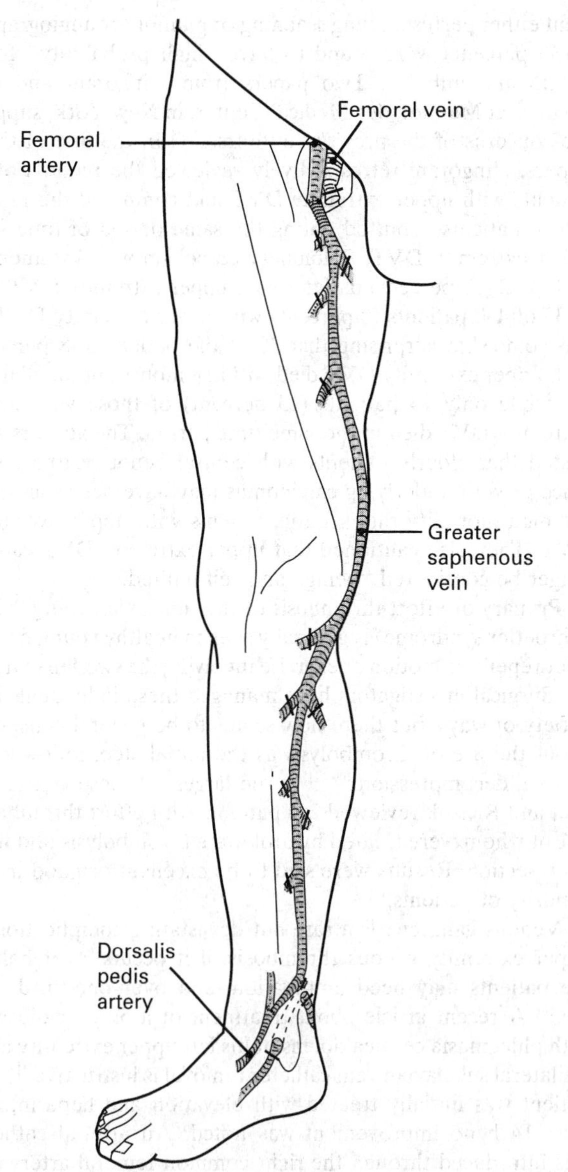

FIGURE 91-3 In-situ bypass from femoral artery to dorsalis pedis artery.

UPPER AND LOWER EXTREMITY VENOUS THROMBOSIS

Upper Extremity Venous Thrombosis

Deep venous thrombosis (DVT) of the upper extremity was thought in the past to be a rare event and to have a relatively benign outcome. However, recent information from both the United States and other countries challenges these assumptions. In a report from Padua, Italy, Prandoni and colleagues evaluated 58 patients suspected of having upper extremity DVT in the years 1990 to 1994.[106] Their evaluations revealed that 27 of the 58 patients (47 percent) had thrombosis and that central venous catheters, "thrombophilic states," and previous lower extremity thromboses were all associated with the development of upper extremity thrombosis. Of the 22 patients who underwent either perfusion lung scanning or pulmonary angiography, 8 (36 percent) were found to have "high probability" for a pulmonary embolus. Two papers from Hingorani and colleagues, at Maimonides Medical Center, in New York, support the concerns of the previous authors.[107,108] In the first of these papers, Hingorani retrospectively reviewed the records of 52 patients with upper extremity DVT and compared the results to 430 patients admitted during the same period of time with lower extremity DVT. Pulmonary embolism was documented in 9 of 52 (17 percent) patients with upper extremity DVT and in 33 of 430 patients (8 percent) with lower extremity DVT. It was somewhat surprising that 25 of the patients (48 percent) with upper extremity DVT died within 6 months of the diagnosis, while only 14 patients (13 percent) of those with lower extremity DVT died in the same time period. The authors suggested that elderly patients with central venous catheters in place or with underlying carcinomas may have been factors in the high mortality rate seen in patients with upper extremity DVT. They also cautioned that upper extremity DVT can no longer be considered "benign and self-limited."

Primary or effort thrombosis of the subclavian vein (Paget-Schroetter syndrome) is generally seen in healthy young people after repetitive motion or exercise involving the swollen extremity. Surgical investigators have managed these individuals in a variety of ways, but there now seems to be general consensus about the use of thrombolysis as the initial step, followed by surgical decompression.[109–111] In the largest of these series, Urchel and Razzuk reviewed 264 patients with effort thrombosis, 211 of whom were treated by urokinase thrombolysis and first-rib resection. Results were said to be excellent or good in the majority of patients.[111]

Venous gangrene is a rare but devastating complication of upper extremity venous thrombosis; if it occurs, over half of the patients may need amputation, and over one-third may die.[112] A recent article about treatment of a 57-year-old man with phlegmasia cerulea dolens of his left upper extremity after ipsilateral subclavian vein catheter removal is instructive.[113] The patient was initially treated with elevation and heparin, and after 14 h no improvement was noted. An arterial catheter was introduced through the right common femoral artery and positioned in the left brachial artery, and an infusion of urokinase was started. After 12 h the extremity was improved, and within 4 days the extremity appeared normal. While urokinase is not currently available, this case does illustrate the potential limb-saving ability of this and other thrombolytic agents.

Patients who develop upper extremity DVT and have contraindications to or unsuccessful use of anticoagulation have been a significant source of concern. A recent paper by Spence and associates, from Cleveland,[114] showed that superior vena cava filters can be successfully placed without undue difficulty, and, in their series of 41 patients, using four different types of filters, they had no complications and no clinical evidence of pulmonary embolism or superior vena cava syndrome.

Lower Extremity Venous Thrombosis

DVT (see also Chap. 90) of the lower extremities is an insidious and potentially lethal problem in hospitalized patients. It has been estimated that there are approximately 600,000 cases of venous thromboembolism in the United States each year.[115] Risk factors have been detailed in multiple publications and include age above 40, past history of DVT, general anesthesia, operations, pregnancy, malignant disease, hypercoagulable states, and trauma.[115] With respect to patients with cancer, an important nationwide study of patients with DVT was undertaken in Denmark to look at the potential association of primary venous thrombosis and the subsequent diagnosis of cancer.[116] Although they found the expected "strong associations" with cancers of the pancreas, ovary, liver, and brain, they concluded that an "aggressive search" for a hidden malignancy in a patient with a primary DVT was not cost effective and was therefore not indicated. Hypercoagulable states (Fig. 91-4) have received renewed attention in recent years.[115–121] A relatively new addition to abnormalities in coagulation occurred with the discovery of factor V Leiden, and this abnormality has been found in about one-fifth of patients with venous thrombosis. In an attempt to look at the risk of recurrent venous thrombosis in patients who carried the mutation, Simioni and colleagues searched for factor V Leiden in 251 unselected patients who had had a first episode of symptomatic DVT diagnosed by venography.[122] They found the mutation in 41 of the patients (16.3 percent), and, after a follow-up of 8 years, approximately 40 percent of patients had had recurrent venous thrombosis, compared to an incidence of recurrence of 18 percent in patients who did not have this mutation.

In a more recent attempt to clarify the risk of recurrent DVT in patients with and without genetic mutations, De Stefano and colleagues looked at a retrospective cohort of 624 patients who had had a first episode of DVT.[123] They looked at patients who were heterozygous carriers of factor V Leiden, patients who were heterozygous for both factor V Leiden and a prothrombin mutation, and patients who had neither mutation. In contradistinction to the previous study, they found that the risk of recurrent DVT was similar among carriers of factor V Leiden and patients without the mutation. Carriers of both factor V Leiden

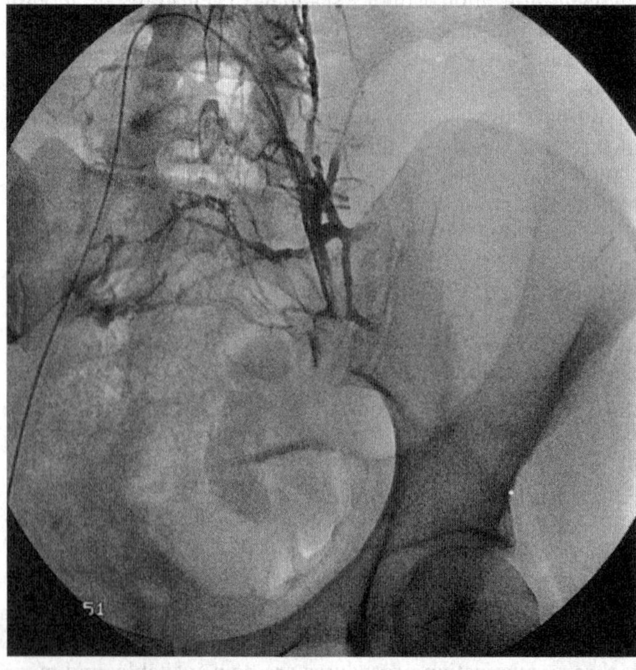

FIGURE 91-4 Venogram in a 31-year-old woman with a swollen leg, hypercoagulable state, and left iliac vein occlusion.

and the prothrombin mutation were, however, at an increased risk of recurrent DVT, and they recommended consideration of lifelong anticoagulation. Studies have documented DVT in 58 percent of trauma patients,[124] 11 percent of patients undergoing lower extremity amputation,[125] and 33 percent of patients in a medical ICU.[126] An excellent overview of the multifactoral nature of venous thrombosis was recently provided by Rosendaal, from Leiden University Medical Center, in the Netherlands.[127]

Patients with DVT are effectively treated by heparin given either by continuous intravenous infusion or by subcutaneous injection. The past decade has brought a number of changes in the therapeutic approach to patients with clot in major lower extremity veins: a 5-day course of heparin has been shown to be as effective as a 10-day course[128]; 6 months of oral anticoagulant therapy has been shown to have a lower recurrence rate than the same dose given for 6 weeks[129]; and low-molecular-weight heparin has been found effective in treating patients at home with proximal DVT.[130,131] Low-molecular-weight heparin has also been shown to be efficacious in reducing the risk of venous thromboembolism in patients with acute medical illnesses,[132] and in a recent head-to-head comparison between enoxaparin and coumadin, enoxaparin-treated patients had a lower recurrence rate of symptomatic venous thromboembolism as well as a lower incidence of bleeding.[133] A review of low-molecular-weight heparins and a look at "new" antithrombotic agents have been provided by Hirsh and colleagues, from Hamilton, Ontario.[134,135]

In recent years, there has been some enthusiasm for lytic therapy in patients with DVT. The reasoning has been that lytic therapy could lyse the clot, restore normalcy to the leg and, more importantly perhaps, to the valves of the affected leg, thereby reducing the long-term sequelae of DVT, primarily the postphlebitic syndrome, which manifests as edema, hyperpigmentation, and ulceration and occurs in up to one-third of patients (Fig. 91-5).[136] The obvious issue is weighing the risks of lytic therapy against the chronic problems of the postphlebitic syndrome. In an attempt to assemble data from a large number of patients who have undergone thrombolytic therapy for lower

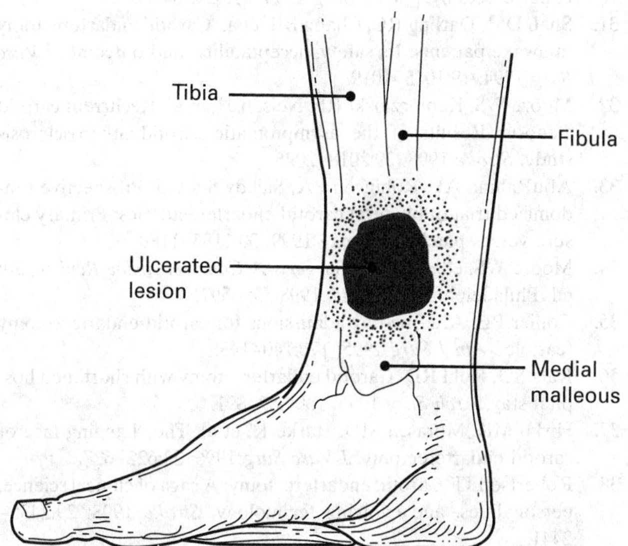

FIGURE 91-5 Venous stasis ulceration of the lower extremity after an episode of deep venous thrombosis.

extremity DVT, Mewissen and colleagues formed a venous registry and collected data from 63 centers.[137] After 312 urokinase infusions in 303 limbs of 287 patients, they found that complete lysis was achieved in 96 infusions (31 percent) and that "major" bleeding complications, most often at the puncture site, occurred in 54 patients (11 percent). Six of the patients (1 percent) developed pulmonary emboli, and there were two deaths, one from an intracranial hemorrhage and one from a pulmonary embolus. While the authors concluded that catheter-directed therapy is "safe and effective," there is currently little unanimity of opinion on this topic.

This issue was also addressed by O'Meara et al., who used decision analysis after estimating the probabilities of various adverse outcomes of treatment and found that all 36 patients interviewed were unwilling to accept an increased risk of death from lytic therapy in order to avoid the postphlebitic syndrome. In other words, in this study, all the patients selected heparin when presented with the data.[138] A recent report describing a spontaneous spinal epidural hematoma with subsequent paraplegia in an 18-year-old female after heparin and urokinase therapy for DVT lends credence to their decision.[139]

The two ends of the spectrum in patients with DVT are represented by patients with clot in their calf veins or clot in the superficial veins of the leg and patients with near total venous occlusion. While patients with clot in their calf veins and patients with clot in the superficial veins are often viewed as having benign problems, data collected over the past decade have suggested that this may be a false assumption. In one study conducted at the beginning of the last decade, investigators showed that 24 (32 percent) of 75 patients with lower extremity calf vein thrombi had propagation of their thrombi, and 11 of those 24 (46 percent) had propagation into the popliteal or larger veins of the thigh.[140] Three recent papers that looked at patients with superficial thrombophlebitis documented a high incidence of hypercoagulability in such patients,[141] extension into the common femoral vein in 9 percent of cases with pulmonary emboli in 10 percent of that group,[142] and an unexpectedly high incidence of pulmonary emboli (33 percent) in 7 of 21 patients with superficial thrombophlebitis studied by perfusion lung scanning.[143] Observations such as these would suggest that calf vein thrombi and superficial thrombi are not benign problems.

Patients with extensive clot in the lower extremities may go on to phlegmasia cerulea dolens or acute iliofemoral venous thrombosis. This condition, which is characterized by near total venous occlusion, may lead to total venous occlusion and venous gangrene. Venous thrombectomy for this condition has received renewed enthusiasm in the surgical literature,[144,145] but lytic therapy[146,147] and nonoperative therapy[148] also have their proponents.

While heparin and warfarin sodium are excellent therapy for the majority of patients with DVT, not all patients can tolerate the complications of these agents. Such patients include individuals with recent trauma, active bleeding, or hemolysis; those with complications of heparin therapy; and those with inferior vena caval clot or iliofemoral venous thrombosis.

For these patients, the treatment of choice is often the placement of a vena cava filter. In a review of their 20-year experience, Greenfield and colleagues noted a caval patency rate of 96 percent, with a rate of recurrent emboli of 4 percent.[149] There was no procedural mortality rate, and the morbidity rate was minimal. In an attempt to answer some of the questions surrounding the use of vena cava filters, Decousus and colleagues randomly assigned 400 patients with proximal DVT who were at risk for pulmonary emboli to receive a vena cava filter (200 patients) or no filter (200 patients), and, in a second aspect of the study, patients were also assigned to receive low-molecular-weight heparin or unfractionated heparin.[150] While the patients who received vena cava filters had a lower incidence of pulmonary emboli by day 12 (1.1 percent versus 4.8 percent for those who did not receive filters), there was an increased incidence of recurrent DVT in the patients receiving filters. There were no significant differences in mortality rates or other outcomes. Low-molecular-weight heparin produced a better outcome in terms of the incidence of symptomatic or asymptomatic pulmonary embolism at day 12 and also for recurrent venous thrombosis, but the results were not statistically significant. In a follow-up editorial on this subject, Haire suggested that only "well-designed comparative trials" could give us the necessary information on which to base our clinical decisions about the proper use of vena cava filters.[151]

References

1. Editors. Looking back on the millennium in medicine. *N Engl J Med* 2000; 342:42–49.
2. Friedman S. *A History of Vascular Surgery*. New York: Futura; 1989.
3. Rattner DW. Future directions in innovative minimally invasive surgery. *Lancet* 1999; 353(suppl I):12–15.
4. Hollingsworth SJ, Barker SGE. Gene therapy: Into the future of surgery. *Lancet* 1999; 353(suppl I):19–20.
5. Schneider JR, Lindsay TF. The internet and vascular surgery: A brief description of the internet, the world wide web, and some of the vascular surgical resources available. *Vasc Surg* 1997; 31:605–613.
6. Soot LC, Moneta GL, Edwards JM. Vascular surgery and the internet: A poor source of patient-oriented information. *J Vasc Surg* 1999; 30:84–91.
7. Veldenz HC, Dennis JW. The internet and education in surgery. *Am Surgeon* 1998; 64:877–880.
8. Kaihara S, Vacanti JP. Tissue engineering: Toward new solutions for transplantation and reconstructive surgery. *Arch Surg* 1999; 134:1184–1188.
9. Deaton DH, Balch D, Kesler C, et al. Telemedicine and endovascular aortic grafting. *Am J Surg* 1999; 177:75–77.
10. Wirthlin DJ, Buradagunta S, Edwards RA, et al. Telemedicine in vascular surgery: Feasibility of digital imaging for remote management of wounds. *J Vasc Surg* 1998; 27:1089–1100.
11. Isner JM, Baumgartner I, Rauh G, et al. Treatment of thromboangiitis obliterans (Buerger's disease) by intramuscular gene transfer of vascular endothelial growth factor: Preliminary clinical results. *J Vasc Surg* 1998; 28:964–975.
12. Bronner LL, Kanter DS, Manson JE. Primary prevention of stroke. *N Engl J Med* 1995; 333:1392–1400.
13. Brown RD, Whisnant JP, Sicks JD, et al. Stroke incidence, prevalence, and survival: Secular trends in Rochester, Minnesota, through 1989. *Stroke* 1996; 27:373–380.
14. Bonita R, Beaglehole R. The enigma of the decline in stroke deaths in the United States: The search for an explanation. *Stroke* 1996; 27:370–372.
15. The CASANOVA Study Group. Carotid surgery versus medical therapy in asymptomatic carotid stenosis. *Stroke* 1991; 22:1229–1235.
16. Hobson RW II, Weiss DG, Fields WS, et al. Efficacy of carotid endarterectomy for asymptomatic carotid stenosis. *N Engl J Med* 1993; 328:221–279.
17. Executive Committee for the Asymptomatic Carotid Atherosclerosis Study. Endarterectomy for asymptomatic carotid artery stenosis. *JAMA* 1995; 273:1421–1428.
18. Mayberg MR, Wilson SE, Yatsu F, et al. Carotid endarterectomy and prevention of cerebral ischemia in symptomatic carotid stenosis. *JAMA* 1991; 266:3289–3294.
19. European Carotid Surgery Trialists' Collaborative Group. MRC European carotid surgery trial: Interim results for symptomatic patients with severe (70–99%) or with mild (0–29%) carotid stenosis. *Lancet* 1991; 337:1235–1243.
20. North American Symptomatic Carotid Endarterectomy Trial Collaborators. Beneficial effect of carotid endarterectomy in symptomatic patients with high-grade carotid stenosis. *N Engl J Med* 1991; 325:445–453.
21. Barnett HJM, Taylor DW, Eliasziw M, et al. Benefit of carotid endarterectomy in patients with symptomatic moderate or severe stenosis. *N Engl J Med* 1998; 339:1415–1425.
22. Chassin MR. Appropriate use of carotid endarterectomy. *N Engl J Med* 1998; 339:1468–1471.
23. Barnett HJM, Taylor DW, Eliasziw M, et al. Benefit of carotid endarterectomy in patients with symptomatic moderate or severe stenosis. *N Engl J Med* 1998; 339:1415–1425.
24. Bendszus M, Koltzenburg MY, Burger R, et al. Silent embolism in diagnostic cerebral angiography and neurointerventional procedures: A prospective study. *Lancet* 1999; 354:1594–1597.
25. Zwolak RM. Carotid endarterectomy without angiography: Are we ready? *Vasc Surg* 1997; 31:1–9.
26. Elmore JR, Franklin DP, Thomas DD, et al. Carotid Endarterectomy: The mandate for high quality duplex. *Ann Vasc Surg* 1998; 12:156–162.
27. Collier PE. Changing trends in the use of preoperative carotid arteriography: The community experience. *Cardiovasc Surg* 1998; 6:485–489.
28. Ballotta E, Da Giau G, Abbruzzese E, et al. Carotid endarterectomy without angiography: Can clinical evaluation and duplex ultrasonographic scanning alone replace traditional arteriography for carotid surgery workup? *Surg* 1999; 126:20–27.
29. Chaikof EL Dodson TF, Thomas BL, et al. Four steps to local anesthesia for endarterectomy of the carotid artery. *Surg Gynecol Obstet* 1993; 177:308–310.
30. Allen BT, Anderson CB, Rubin VG, et al. The influence of anesthetic technique on perioperative complications after carotid endarterectomy. *J Vasc Surg* 1994; 19:834–843.
31. Shah DM, Darling RC, Chang BB, et al. Carotid endarterectomy in awake patients: Its safety, acceptability, and outcome. *J Vasc Surg* 1994; 19:1015–1019.
32. Moore WS, Kempczinski RF, Nelson JJ, et al. Recurrent carotid stenosis: Results of the asymptomatic carotid atherosclerosis study. *Stroke* 1998; 29:2018–2025.
33. AbuRahma AF, Robinson PA, Saiedy S, et al. Prospective randomized trial of bilateral carotid endarterectomies: Primary closure versus patching. *Stroke* 1999; 30:1185–1189.
34. Moore WS, ed. *Vascular Surgery: A Comprehensive Review*, 5th ed. Philadelphia: Saunders; 1998:555–597.
35. Collier PE. Are one-day admissions for carotid endarterectomy feasible? *Am J Surg* 1995; 170:140–143.
36. Katz SG, Kohl RD. Carotid endarterectomy with shortened hospital stay. *Arch Surg* 1995; 130:887–891.
37. Hirko MK, Morasch MD, Burke K. et al. The changing face of carotid endarterectomy. *J Vasc Surg* 1996; 23:622–627.
38. Robertson JT. Carotid endarterectomy: A saga of clinical science, personalities, and evolving technology. *Stroke* 1998; 29:2435–2441.
39. Beebe HG. The carotid angioplasty premise. *Vasc Surg* 1996; 30:269–273.
40. Criado FJ, Wellons E, Clark NS, et al. Evolving indication for

and early results of carotid artery stenting. *Am J Surg* 1997; 174:111–114.
41. Jordan WD Jr, Voellinger DC, Fisher WS, et al. A comparison of carotid angioplasty with stenting versus endarterectomy with regional anesthesia. *J Vasc Surg* 1998; 28:397–403.
42. Naylor AR, Bolia A, Abbott RJ, et al. Randomized study of carotid angioplasty and stenting versus carotid endarterectomy: A stopped trial. *J Vasc Surg* 1998; 28:326–334.
43. Ohki T, Roubin GS, Veith FJ, et al. Efficacy of a filter device in the prevention of embolic events during carotid angioplasty and stenting: An ex vivo analysis. *J Vasc Surg* 1999; 30:1034–1044.
44. Bettmann MA, Katzen BT, Whisnant J, et al. Carotid stenting and angioplasty: A statement for health care professionals from the Councils on Cardiovascular Radiology, Stroke, Cardiothoracic and Vascular Surgery, Epidemiology and Prevention, and Clinical Cardiology, American Heart Association. *Stroke* 1998; 29:336–338.
45. Hobson RW II, Brott T, Ferguson R, et al. CREST: Carotid revascularization endarterectomy versus stent trial. *Cardiovasc Surg* 1997; 5:457–458.
46. Fields WS, Lemak NA. Joint study of extracranial arterial occlusion. *JAMA* 1972; 222:1139–1143.
47. Hafner CD. Subclavian steal syndrome. *Arch Surg* 1976; 111:1074–1080.
48. Azakie A, McElhinney DB, Higashima R, et al. Innominate artery reconstruction: Over 3 decades of experience. *Ann Surg* 1998; 228:402–410.
49. Perler BA, Williams GM. Carotid-subclavian bypass: A decade of experience. *J Vasc Surg* 1990; 12:716–723.
50. Garrett ED, Morris GC, Howell JF, et al. Revascularization of upper extremity with autogenous vein bypass graft. *Arch Surg* 1965; 91:751–757.
51. McCarthy WJ, Flinn WR, Yao JST, et al. Result of bypass grafting for upper limb ischemia. *J Vasc Surg* 1986; 3:741–746.
52. Katz SG, Kohl RD. Direct revascularization for the treatment of forearm and hand ischemia. *Am J Surg* 1993; 165:313–316.
53. Mesh CL, McCarthy WJ, Pearce WH, et al. Upper extremity bypass grafting: A 15-year experience. *Arch Surg* 1993; 128: 795–802.
54. Sullivan TM, Gray BH, Bacharach M, et al. Angioplasty and primary stenting of the subclavian, innominate, and common carotid arteries in 83 patients. *J Vasc Surg* 1998; 28:1059–1065.
55. Hadjipetrou P, Cox S, Piemonte T, et al. Percutaneous revascularization of atherosclerotic obstruction of aortic arch vessels. *J Am Coll Cardiol* 1999; 33:1238–1245.
56. Chambers BR, Norris JW. Outcome in patients with asymptomatic neck bruits. *N Engl J Med* 1986; 9:860–865.
57. Criqui MH, Langer RD, Fronek A, et al. Mortality over a period of 10 years in patients with peripheral arterial disease. *N Engl J Med* 1992; 326:381–386.
58. Vogt MT, Cauley JA, Newman AB, et al. Decreased ankle/arm blood pressure index and mortality in elderly women. *JAMA* 1993; 270:465–469.
59. McLafferty RB, Moneta GL, Taylor LM. et al. Ability of ankle-brachial index to detect lower-extremity atherosclerotic disease progression. *Arch Surg* 1997; 132:836–841.
60. TransAtlantic Inter-Society Consensus. Management of peripheral arterial disease. *J Vasc Surg* 2000; 31:S1–S34.
61. Hiatt WR, ed. Morbidity of PAD: Medical approaches to claudication, in Hirsch AT, ed: An office-based approach to the diagnosis and treatment of peripheral arterial disease: IV. *Excerpta Medi,* 1999; 6–15.
62. Patterson RB, Pinto B, Marcus B, et al. Value of a supervised exercise program for the therapy of arterial claudication. *J Vasc Surg* 1997; 25:312–319.
63. Money SR, Heard JA, Isaacsohn JL, et al. Effect of cilostazol on walking distances in patients with intermittent claudication caused by peripheral vascular disease. *J Vasc Surg* 1998; 27:267–275.
64. AbuRahma AF, Robinson PA, Holt SM. Prospective controlled study of polytetrafluoroethylene versus saphenous vein in claudicant patients with bilateral above knee femoropopliteal bypasses. *Surg* 1999; 126:594–602.
65. Byrne J, Darling RC III, Chang BB, et al. Infrainguinal arterial reconstruction for claudication: Is it worth the risk? An analysis of 409 procedures. *J Vasc Surg* 1999; 29:259–269.
66. Whyman MR, Fowkes FGR, Kerracher EMG, et al. Is intermittent claudication improved by percutaneous transluminal angioplasty? A randomized controlled trial. *J Vasc Surg* 1997; 26:551–557.
67. Golledge J, Ferguson K, Ellis M, et al. Outcome of femoropopliteal angioplasty. *Ann Surg* 1999; 229:146–153.
68. Nicoloff AD, Taylor LM, McLafferty RB, et al. Patient recovery after infrainguinal bypass grafting for limb salvage. *J Vasc Surg* 1998; 27:256–266.
69. Pomposelli FB Jr, Arora S, Gibbons GW, et al. Lower extremity arterial reconstruction in the very elderly: Successful outcome preserves not only the limb but also residential status and ambulatory function. *J Vasc Surg* 1998; 28:215–225.
70. Seabrook GR, Cambria RA, Freischlag JA, et al. Health-related quality of life and functional outcome following arterial reconstruction for limb salvage. *Cardiovasc Surg* 1999; 7:279–286.
71. Nicoloff AD, Taylor LM, McLafferty RB, et al. Patient recovery after infrainguinal bypass grafting for limb salvage. *J Vasc Surg* 1998; 27:261.
72. Kalman PG, Johnston KW. Predictors of long-term patient survival after in situ vein leg bypass. *J Vasc Surg* 1997; 25:899–904.
73. Link J, Steffens JC, Brossmann J, et al. Iliofemoral arterial occlusive disease: Contrast-enhanced MR angiography for preinterventional evaluation and follow-up after stent placement. *Radiology* 1999; 212:371–377.
74. Sueyoshi E, Sakamoto U, Matsuoka Y, et al. Aortoiliac and lower extremity arteries: Comparison of three-dimensional dynamic contrast-enhanced subtraction MR angiography and conventional angiography. *Radiology* 1999; 210:683–688.
75. Turnipseed WD, Sproat IA. A preliminary experience with use of magnetic resonance angiography in assessment of failing lower extremity bypass grafts. *Surgery* 1992; 112:664–669.
76. Carpenter JP, Golden MA, Barker CF, et al. The fate of bypass grafts to angiographically occult runoff vessels detected by magnetic resonance angiography. *J Vasc Surg* 1996; 23:483–489.
77. Eagleton MJ, Ouriel K, Shortell C, et al. Femoral-infrapopliteal bypass with prosthetic grafts. *Surgery* 1999; 126:759–765.
78. Prendiville EJ, Yeager AN, O'Donnell TF, et al. Long-term results with the above-knee popliteal expanded polytetrafluoroethylene graft. *J Vasc Surg* 1990; 11:517–524.
79. O'Riordain DS, Buckley DJ, O'Donnell JA. Polytetrafluoroethylene in above-knee arterial bypass surgery for critical ischemia. *Am J Surg* 1992; 164:129–131.
80. Calligaro KD, Syrek JR, Dougherty MJ, et al. Use of arm and lesser saphenous vein compared with prosthetic grafts for infrapopliteal arterial bypass: Are they worth the effort. *J Vasc Surg* 1997; 26:919–927.
81. Oppat WF, Pearce WH, McMillan WD, et al. Natural history of composite sequential bypass: Ten years' experience. *Arch Surg* 1999; 134:754–758.
82. Taylor RS, Loh A, McFarland RJ, et al. Improved technique for polytetrafluoroethylene bypass grafting: Long-term results using anastomotic vein patches. *Br J Surg* 1992; 79:348–354.
83. Dardik H, Miller N, Dardik A, et al. A decade of experience with the glutaraldehyde-tanned human umbilical cord vein graft for revascularization of the lower limb. *J Vasc Surg* 1988; 7:336–346.
84. Taylor RS, Belli A, Jacob S. Distal venous arterialisation for

salvage of critically ischaemic inoperable limbs. *Lancet* 1999; 354:1962–1965.

85. Carpenter JP, Tomaszewski JE. Immunosuppression for human saphenous vein allograft bypass surgery: A prospective randomized trial. *J Vasc Surg* 1997; 26:32–42.
86. Carpenter JP, Tomaszewski JE. Human saphenous vein allograft bypass grafts: Immune response. *J Vasc Surg* 1998; 27:492–499.
87. Castier Y, Leseche G, Palombi T, et al. Early experience with cryopreserved arterial allografts in below-knee revascularization for limb salvage. *Am J Surg* 1999; 177:197–202.
88. Shah DM, Darling RC, Chang BB, et al. Long-term results of in situ saphenous vein bypass: Analysis of 2058 cases. *Ann Surg* 1995; 222:438–448.
89. Wengerter K, Veith FJ, Gupta SK, et al. Prospective randomized multicenter comparison of in situ and reversed vein infrapopliteal bypasses. *J Vasc Surg* 1991; 13:189–199.
90. Chang BB, Darling RC, Bock DEM, et al. The use of spliced vein bypasses for infrainguinal arterial reconstruction. *J Vasc Surg* 1995; 21:403–412.
91. Bergamini TM, George SM, Massey HT, et al. Intensive surveillance of femoropopliteal-tibial autogenous vein bypasses improves long-term graft patency and limb salvage. *Ann Surg* 1995; 221:507–516.
92. Sarac TP, Huber TS, Back MR, et al. Warfarin improves the outcome of infrainguinal vein bypass grafting at high risk for failure. *J Vasc Surg* 1998; 28:446–457.
93. Tangelder MJD, Lawson JA, Algra A, et al. Systematic review of randomized controlled trials of aspirin and oral anticoagulants in the prevention of graft occlusion and ischemic events after infrainguinal bypass surgery. *J Vasc Surg* 1999; 30:701–709.
94. Polak J. Femoropopliteal angioplasty with US guidance: An example of a niche market. *Radiology* 1996; 199:317–318.
95. Bakal CW, Cynamon J, Sprayregen S. Infrapopliteal percutaneous transluminal angioplasty: What we know. *Radiology* 1996; 200:36–43.
96. Fraser SCA, Al-Kutoubi MA, Wolfe JHN. Percutaneous transluminal angioplasty of the infrapopliteal vessels: The evidence. *Radiology* 1996; 200:33–36.
97. Kalman PG, Johnston KW, Sniderman KW. Indications and results of balloon angioplasty for arterial occlusive lesions. *World J Surg* 1996; 20:630–634.
98. Treiman GS, Treiman RL, Ichikawa L, et al. Should percutaneous transluminal angioplasty be recommended for treatment of infrageniculate popliteal artery or tibioperoneal trunk stenosis? *J Vasc Surg* 1995; 22:457–463.
99. Stanley B, Teague B, Raptis S, et al. Efficacy of balloon angioplasty of the superficial femoral artery and popliteal artery in the relief of leg ischemia. *J Vasc Surg* 1996; 23:679–685.
100. Bradbury AW, Ruckle CV. Angioplasty for lower-limb ischemia: Time for randomized controlled trials. *Lancet* 1996; 347:277–278.
101. White GH, Liew SC, Waugh RC, et al. Early outcome and intermediate follow-up of vascular stents in the femoral and popliteal arteries without long-term anticoagulation. *J Vasc Surg* 1995; 21:270–281.
102. Cragg AH, Dake MD. Percutaneous femoropopliteal graft placement. *Radiology* 1993; 187:643–648.
103. Shapiro MJ, Levin DC. Percutaneous femoropopliteal graft placement: Is this the next step? *Radiology* 1993; 187:618–619.
104. Hunink MGM, Cullen KA, Donaldson MC. Hospital costs of revascularization procedures for femoropopliteal arterial disease. *J Vasc Surg* 1994; 19:632–641.
105. Hunink MGM, Wong JB, Donaldson MC, et al. Revascularization for femoropopliteal disease: A decision and cost-effectiveness analysis. *JAMA* 1995; 274:165–171.
106. Prandoni P, Polistena P, Bernardi E, et al. Upper-extremity deep vein thrombosis. *Arch Intern Med* 1997; 157:57–62.
107. Hingorani A, Ascher E, Hanson J, et al. Upper extremity versus lower extremity deep venous thrombosis. *Am J Surg* 1997; 174:214–217.
108. Hingorani A, Ascher E, Lorenson E, et al. Upper extremity deep venous thrombosis and its impact on morbidity and mortality rates in a hospital-based population. *J Vasc Surg* 1997; 26:853–860.
109. Azakie A, McElhinney DB, Thompson RW, et al. Surgical management of subclavian-vein effort thrombosis as a result of thoracic outlet compression. *J Vasc Surg* 1998; 28:777–786.
110. Lee MC, Grassi CJ, Belkin M, et al. Early operative intervention after thrombolytic therapy for primary subclavian vein thrombosis: An effective treatment approach. *J Vasc Surg* 1998; 27:1101–1108.
111. Urschel HC, Razzuk MA. Neurovascular compression in the thoracic outlet: Changing management over 50 years. *Ann Surg* 1998; 228:609–617.
112. Smith BM, Shield GW, Riddell DH, et al. Venous gangrene of the upper extremity. *Ann Surg* 1985; 201:511–519.
113. Gagne PJ, Martinez JM. Treatment of upper-extremity phlegmasia cerulea dolens with intra-arterial thrombolysis. *Vasc Surg* 1999; 33:633–639.
114. Spence LD, Gironta MG, Malde HM, et al. Acute upper extremity deep venous thrombosis: Safety and effectiveness of superior vena caval filters. *Radiology* 1999; 53–58.
115. Weinmann EE, Salzman EW. Deep-vein thrombosis. *N Engl J Med* 1994; 331:1630–1641.
116. Sorensen HT, Mellemkjaer L, Steffensen FH, et al. The risk of a diagnosis of cancer after primary deep venous thrombosis or pulmonary embolism. *N Engl J Med* 1998; 338:1169–1173.
117. Svensson PJ, Dahlback B. Resistance to activated protein C as a basis for venous thrombosis. *N Engl J Med* 1994; 330:517–522.
118. Ridker PM, Hennekens CH, Lindpaintner K, et al. Mutation in the gene coding for coagulation factor V and the risk of myocardial infarction, stroke, and venous thrombosis in apparently healthy men. *N Engl J Med* 1995; 332:912–917.
119. Khamashta MA, Cuadrado MJ, Mujic F, et al. The management of thrombosis in the antiphospholipid-antibody syndrome. *N Engl J Med* 1995; 332:993–997.
120. Mandel H, Brenner B, Berant M, et al. Coexistence of hereditary homocystinuria and factor V Leiden: Effect on thrombosis. *N Engl J Med* 1996; 334:763–768.
121. Den Heijer M, Koster T, Blom HJ, et al. Hyperhomocysteinemia as a risk factor for deep-vein thrombosis. *N Engl J Med* 1996; 334:759–762.
122. Simioni P, Prandoni P, Lensing AWA, et al. The risk of recurrent venous thromboembolism in patients with an $Arg^{506} \rightarrow$Gln mutation in the gene for factor V (factor V Leiden). *N Engl J Med* 1997; 336:399–403.
123. De Stefano V, Martinelli I, Mannucci PM, et al. The risk of recurrent deep venous thrombosis among heterozygous carriers of both factor V Leiden and the G20210A prothrombin mutation. *N Engl J Med* 1999; 341:801–806.
124. Geerts WH, Code KI, Jay RM, et al. A prospective study of venous thromboembolism after major trauma. *N Engl J Med* 1994; 331:1601–1606.
125. Yeager RA, Moneta GL, Edwards JM, et al. Deep vein thrombosis associated with lower extremity amputation. *J Vasc Surg* 1995; 22:612–615.
126. Hirsch DR, Ingenito EP, Goldhaber SZ. Prevalence of deep venous thrombosis among patients in medical intensive care. *JAMA* 1995; 274:335–337.
127. Rosendaal FR. Venous thrombosis: A multicausal disease. *Lancet* 1993; 353:1167–1173.
128. Hull RD, Raskob GE, Rosenblood D, et al. Heparin for 5 days as compared with 10 days in the initial treatment of proximal venous thrombosis. *N Engl J Med* 1990; 332:1260–1264.
129. Schulman S, Rhedin AS, Lindmarker P, et al. A comparison of

six weeks with six months of oral anticoagulant therapy after a first episode of venous thromboembolism. *N Engl J Med* 1995;332:1661–1665.
130. Levine M, Gent M, Hirsh J, et al. A comparison of low-molecular-weight heparin administered primarily at home with unfractionated heparin administered in the hospital for proximal deep-vein thrombosis. *N Engl J Med* 1996; 334:677–681.
131. Koopman MMW, Prandoni P, Piovella F, et al. Treatment of venous thrombosis with intravenous unfractionated heparin administered in the hospital as compared with subcutaneous low-molecular-weight heparin administered at home. *N Engl J Med* 1996; 334:682–687.
132. Samama MM, Cohen AT, Darmon J, et al. A comparison of enoxaparin with placebo for the prevention of venous thromboembolism in acutely ill medical patients. *N Engl J Med* 1999; 341:793–800.
133. Gonzalez-Fajardo JA, Arreba E, Castrodeza J, et al. Venographic comparison of subcutaneous low-molecular weight heparin with oral anticoagulant therapy in the long-term treatment of deep venous thrombosis. *J Vasc Surg* 1999; 30:283–292.
134. Wood AJJ. Low-molecular-weight heparins. *N Engl J Med* 1997; 337:688–698.
135. Hirsh J, Weitz JI. New antithrombotic agents. *Lancet* 1999; 353:1431–1436.
136. Prandoni P, Lensing AWA, Cogo A, et al. The long–term clinical course of acute deep venous thrombosis. *Ann Intern Med* 1996; 125:1–7.
137. Mewissen MW, Seabrook GR, Meissner MH, et al. Catheter-directed thrombolysis for lower extremity deep venous thrombosis: Report of a national multicenter registry. *Radiology* 1999; 211:39–49.
138. O'Meara JJ, McNutt RA, Evans AT, et al. A decision analysis of streptokinase plus heparin as compared with heparin alone for deep-vein thrombosis. *N Engl J Med* 1994; 330:1864–1869.
139. Krieger NR, Mehigan JT. Spontaneous spinal epidural hematoma after combined urokinase and heparin thrombolytic therapy for deep venous thrombosis. *Vasc Surg* 1996; 30:67–70.
140. Lohr JM, Kerr TM, Lutter KS, et al. Lower extremity calf thrombosis: To treat or not to treat? *J Vasc Surg* 1999; 14:618–623.
141. Hanson JN, Ascher E, DePippo P, et al. Saphenous vein thrombophlebitis (SVT): A deceptively benign disease. *J Vasc Surg* 1998; 27:677–680.
142. Blumberg RM, Barton E, Gelfand ML, et al. Occult deep venous thrombosis complicating superficial thrombophlebitis. *J Vasc Surg* 1998; 27:338–343.
143. Verlato F, Zucchetta P, Prandoni P, et al. An unexpectedly high rate of pulmonary embolism in patients with superficial thrombophlebitis of the thigh. *J Vasc Surg* 1999; 30:1113–1115.
144. Juhan CM, Alimi YS, Barthelmey PJ, et al. Late results of iliofemoral venous thrombectomy. *J Vasc Surg* 1997; 25:417–422.
145. Juhan C, Alimi Y, de Mauro P, et al. Surgical venous thrombectomy. *Cardiovasc Surg* 1999; 7:586–590.
146. Elliot MS, Immelman EJ, Jeffrey P, et al. The role of thrombolytic therapy in the management of phlegmasia caerulea dolens. *Br J Surg* 1979; 66:422–424.
147. Hood DB, Weaver FA, Modrall JG, et al. Advances in the treatment of phlegmasia cerulea dolens. *Am J Surg* 1993; 166:206–210.
148. Patel KR, Paidas CN. Phlegmasia cerulea dolens: The role of nonoperative therapy. *Cardiovasc Surg* 1993; 1:518–523.
149. Greenfield LJ, Proctor MC. Twenty-year clinical experience with the Greenfield Filter. *Cardiovasc Surg* 1995; 3:199–205.
150. Decousus H, Leizorovicz A, Parent F, et al. A clinical trial of vena caval filters in the prevention of pulmonary embolism in patients with proximal deep-vein thrombosis. *N Engl J Med* 1998; 338:409–415.
151. Haire WD. Vena caval filters for the prevention of pulmonary embolism. *N Engl J Med* 1998; 338:463–464.

CHAPTER 92

NONSURGICAL INTERVENTIONS FOR CAROTID DISEASE

Samir R. Kapadia / Sanjay S. Yadav

INTRODUCTION

Stroke remains a major public health problem, and carotid artery atherosclerotic disease causes a substantial portion of all strokes. Cardiologists are frequently involved in the care of patients with carotid stenosis because many of them have either occult or symptomatic coronary artery disease. Compared to endarterectomy, carotid stenting is a less invasive procedure that provides an attractive treatment alternative for some patients, particularly those with severe cardiac comorbidities. The feasibility and safety of carotid stenting procedure as a treatment for severe carotid stenosis has improved with technological advances. This chapter outlines salient features of atherosclerotic carotid artery disease and the current status of nonsurgical treatment.

EPIDEMIOLOGY

Prevalence

Stroke killed approximately 160,000 people in 1996, accounting for approximately 1 of every 14.5 deaths in the United States.[1] Stroke ranks as the third leading cause of death, behind heart disease and cancer. More importantly, stroke is a leading cause of serious long-term disability. According to the data from the Health Care Financing Administration (HCFA), in 1995 $3.7 billion was paid to Medicare beneficiaries for stroke. The total economic burden is estimated to be $20 billion every year due to health care costs and lost productivity. Each year about 600,000 people suffer a new or recurrent stroke. About 500,000 of these are first attacks, and 100,000 are recurrent attacks. This incidence of stroke in the United States may be underestimated because of incomplete inclusion of minority populations.[2]

Atheroembolic events leading to ischemic stroke account for almost 85 percent of the acute strokes and almost two-thirds of these can be attributed to a large-vessel stenosis.[3–5] Depending upon the population studied, intracranial occlusive disease is present in 5 to 15 percent of the patients with acute ischemic strokes, whereas extracranial carotid artery disease is present in 30 to 40 percent. Although the association between carotid artery disease and neurologic sequelae dates back to ancient Greece, C. Miller Fisher was the first to clearly suggest a causal relation between extracranial carotid atherosclerosis and stroke in the modern era.[6,7]

Risk Factors

Presence and severity of carotid atherosclerosis correlates with the presence and severity of coronary atherosclerosis and peripheral vascular disease.[8–13] The risk factors for coronary atherosclerosis are also associated with carotid atherosclerosis.[14–17] The incidence of severe carotid disease increases with age in men and women. One-half of men over 75 years are found to have some carotid atherosclerosis by ultrasonography, but greater than 50 percent stenosis is present only in 5 percent.[18,19] There may be substantial racial differences in the severity and distribution of carotid atherosclerosis. Caucasian patients have predominantly extracranial carotid artery atherosclerosis, whereas African-Americans, Japanese, and Chinese have predominantly intracranial vascular lesions.[20,21] Smoking is the most important risk factor for prediction of carotid atherosclerotic disease, followed by hypertension, diabetes, male gender, and elevated systolic blood pressure.[22] Association of hypercholesterolemia with stroke has been clouded by the fact that many epidemiologic studies failed to separate ischemic and hemorrhagic strokes for analysis. Therefore, hypercholesterolemia did not always pan out to be a risk factor for "stroke."[23] Multiple studies have, however, associated increased total cholesterol, increased low-density lipoprotein cholesterol, increased triglycerides, and decreased high-density lipoprotein cholesterol with carotid atherosclerosis.[17,24–26] In patients with coronary disease, even low levels of high-density lipoprotein cholesterol without elevated levels of low-density lipoprotein or total cholesterol have been associated with carotid disease.[27] Meta-analyses with clinical trials of HMG-CoA inhibitors have further added support to the association between hypercholesterolemia and ischemic stroke.[28–30]

Natural History

The risk of stroke in asymptomatic patients with ultrasound-proven carotid atherosclerosis has been studied in observational trials. These studies have demonstrated that the % stenosis, progression of atherosclerosis between examination intervals and presence or absence of ulceration affects the outcome.[31,32] The annual risk of stroke for stenosis that is <75 percent is <1 percent, but this risk increases to 2 to 5 percent with stenosis >75 percent.[33–36] The evidence of silent brain infarction or embolization may also increase the risk for future symptomatic strokes.[37] Patients who continue to remain asymptomatic in the first year of observation have significantly lower risk of subsequent stroke than are those who are symptomatic. The majority of patients who develop stroke during the observation of an asymptomatic lesion have no warning symptoms.[31,33,35,38–42]

In symptomatic patients, the risk of subsequent neurologic events is much higher than in those asymptomatic. The risk of stroke in patients with transient ischemic attacks (TIAs) from severe carotid stenosis is approximately 10 percent within the first year, with a cumulative stroke risk of approximately 30 to 35 percent at the end of 5 years. Presence of hemispheric TIAs, recent TIA, increasing frequency of TIA, or high-grade stenosis identifies the high-risk patient population.[43]

ANATOMY

In approximately 70 percent of patients, the great vessels originate from the aortic arch with three separate ostia for the innominate, left common carotid, and left subclavian arteries. The most common anomaly is origin of the left common carotid artery from the innominate artery, which is seen in approximately 20 percent of patients—the so-called bovine arch. The common carotid artery divides into the internal and external carotid arteries at the C4–C5 intervertebral space. The internal carotid artery is posterior and lateral to the external carotid artery and ascends without branching until it enters the subarachnoid space, where it gives rise to the ophthalmic artery before dividing into the anterior and middle cerebral arteries. The carotid artery can be divided into the cervical, petrous, precavernous, cavernous, paraclenoid, and supraclenoid segments from its origin to the terminal bifurcation. The diameter of the carotid sinus is approximately 7 mm, and the diameter of the distal internal carotid at the level of the siphon is approximately 4 mm.[44] Pressure on the carotid sinus stimulates mechanoreceptors in the media and adventitia that are responsible for the carotid sinus reflex leading to bradycardia and hypotension.

The brain has an extensive collateral circulation. The most significant collaterals are provided by the circle of Willis, which consists of the anterior communicating artery uniting the right and left anterior cerebral arteries and posterior communicating arteries uniting the middle cerebral and posterior cerebral arteries. A symmetrical and normal circle of Willis is present in less than one-third of individuals.[45]

MORPHOLOGY OF DISEASE

As in other arterial beds, there is a predilection for lesions at branch points and bends. The most common site of cerebrovascular atherosclerotic disease is the carotid bifurcation affecting the outer wall of the carotid sinus and extending into the distal common carotid artery.

It was thought that atherosclerotic plaques become highly vascularized with time, and these vessels rupture, either spontaneously or as a result of trauma.[46] Plaque hemorrhage may lead to immediate obstruction of the artery but this mechanism is not as frequent as previously thought.[47] More commonly, ulceration and subsequent luminal thrombosis followed by embolism leads to symptoms.[48] Ulcers are noted much more commonly in surgical specimens than at angiography, being present in up to one-third of the plaques removed at endarterectomy.[49] In the North American Symptomatic Carotid Endarterectomy Trial (NASCET), plaque ulceration more than doubled the risk for stroke.[50] Using conventional cut-film angiography, the ulcer size can be defined by multiplying the length and width of the ulcer in millimeters. The presence of a large (>40 mm) ulcer independent of associated carotid stenosis identifies a group of patients who are at risk of stroke at the rate of 7.5 percent per year.[31,32]

Several investigators have proposed the use of noninvasive diagnostic imaging techniques, such as B-mode ultrasonography, to characterize plaque composition and to identify the high-risk, unstable carotid lesion.[51–53] An attempt has been made to characterize plaque according to the relative contribution of echogenic (high-intensity) and echolucent (low-intensity) material using the classification by Gray-Weale et al.[54] Another method is to subjectively classify the plaques as either homogeneous or heterogeneous.[55] However, these distinctions are neither reliable nor reproducible.[56] Reproducible grading of ultrasound images is not consistently achievable among experienced observers, and within-observer agreement may vary with time. Helical computed tomography has been used for studying detailed plaque morphology and composition, and studies are being performed to correlate plaque anatomy with clinical outcome.[57]

Magnetic resonance imaging is the first noninvasive imaging technique that allows reliable discrimination of lipid cores, fibrous caps, calcifications, normal media, and adventitia in human atheromatous plaques in vivo. This technique also characterizes intraplaque hemorrhage and acute thrombosis. Further investigations of plaque progression, stabilization, and rupture in human atherosclerosis are currently being conducted.[58,59]

CLINICAL PRESENTATION

Transient ischemic attack is the initial symptom of carotid stenosis in the majority of the patients with symptomatic carotid disease. If no therapy is instituted, 30 to 40 percent of these patients subsequently develop stroke. The diagnosis of TIA is based on careful history taking. By definition, symptoms resolve within 24 h of onset. The symptoms of vertebrobasilar insufficiency have to be differentiated from those of carotid artery related TIAs. The motor and sensory changes from carotid disease usually involve the contralateral face and body, whereas posterior circulation events often have bilateral or crossed deficits. Dysphasia, dysarthria, contralateral visual field loss, and amaurosis fugax are manifestations of carotid disease. Vertebrobasilar insufficiency can present with ataxia, dysarthria, diplopia, or bilateral visual field loss. Hemicranial headache can occur with TIA from carotid stenosis and occipital headaches are seen with vertebrobasilar insufficiency.

DIAGNOSIS

Ultrasonography

The standard method of studying carotid arteries is with duplex ultrasonography, which is a combination of Doppler ultrasonography and B-mode imaging with a single instrument and transducer. This allows for visualization of the vessel along with the angle of ultrasound interrogation, leading to more accurate calculations of blood flow velocity. When performed by trained sonographers using a standard protocol and with ongoing quality assurance, this method can approach 90 percent sensitivity and specificity for identification of important carotid stenosis.[60–62]

Ultrasonography of the carotid artery, particularly the intimal–medial thickness (IMT), has been used as a surrogate end point in many trials examining risk factor modification, and the severity of IMT has been found to correlate well with the degree of coronary artery disease.[11,16] Moreover, the plaque morphology and progression of disease in carotid atherosclerotic lesions have correlation with the behavior of coronary atherosclerosis lesions.[9,13,63]

Magnetic Resonance Angiography

Magnetic resonance angiography (MRA) is useful in the study of carotid bifurcation, as anatomically this is a relatively motionless, sizable, and superficial structure. The newer MRA techniques allow reliable imaging of the carotid arteries from the origin of the aortic arch to the intracranial branches.

Several MRA techniques have been proposed to assess carotid bifurcation, including 2D and 3D time-of-flight (TOF) MRA and first-pass gadolinium-enhanced MRA. Several blinded-reader studies have been published comparing MRA with conventional angiography. The results based mostly on 2D TOF MRA indicate high sensitivity (>90 percent) and high negative predictive value (>90 percent) for detecting narrowing of >70 percent by NASCET criteria. The specificity of MRA is approximately 70 percent due to artifacts from tortuous vessels, turbulence of blood flow, and other technical reasons. Combining 2D TOF with single-slab 3D TOF technique through stenotic segments may yield better sensitivity and specificity.[64–67] MRA generally overestimates the degree of stenosis and is particularly poor at distinguishing between subtotal and total occlusions. However, the combination of ultrasound and MRA may raise sensitivity and specificity to a significantly high level, reducing the need for diagnostic angiography.

Angiography

Angiography is the gold standard for diagnosis of carotid stenosis. It allows accurate measurement of luminal stenosis of the entire vessel from its origin to the intracranial branches. The plaque morphology, lesion length, and reference diameter of the vessel can be accurately determined by angiography. In patients with symptomatic carotid disease, angiography identifies intracranial stenosis in a significant number of patients.[68] It is an invasive procedure with some risk of complications such as embolization and dissection, which are rare, however.[69] Currently, angiography is used in patients where noninvasive tests give uncertain results or when percutaneous therapy is considered.

NONSURGICAL MANAGEMENT

Pharmacologic Management

Antiplatelet, anticoagulant, and antihyperlipidemic agents are the potential modes of therapy in carotid stenosis. Although there are multiple studies of these agents in therapy of stroke, few have focused on the management of carotid artery disease. In the following paragraphs the available data are briefly reviewed.

ANTIPLATELET AGENTS

A number of trials have studied the role of various antiplatelet agents or their combinations in the management of stroke. Most of these studies did not specifically investigate the patients with carotid stenosis, or did they carefully exclude patients with cardioembolic stroke. The Antiplatelet Trialists' Collaboration performed a meta-analysis of 164 randomized trials of antiplatelet drugs including over 100,000 patients to analyze the effectiveness of different antiplatelet therapies in prevention of vascular events.[70] Among primary prevention recipients there was approximately a 30 percent reduction in nonfatal myocardial infarction, but there was no reduction in the incidence of stroke. In the group with a prior stroke or TIA ($n = 7850$), the incidence of subsequent ischemic nonhemorrhagic stroke was reduced from 12.2 percent in patients receiving a placebo to 9.7 percent with antiplatelet therapy ($p < 0.01$). Interestingly, there was no difference in effectiveness between different aspirin dosages or combination regimens.

Newer antiplatelet agents, the thienopyridine derivatives ticlopidine and clopidogrel, have gained widespread use in management of cardiovascular disease. The efficacy of these agents in preventing cardiovascular events has been compared to aspirin in randomized trials. In the Ticlopidine Aspirin Stroke Study, 3069 patients with noncardiogenic TIAs or minor strokes were randomized to ticlopidine or aspirin (650 mg twice a day). There was a trend in favor of ticlopidine for preventing nonfatal stroke or death at 3 years (17 versus 19 percent; $p = 0.048$).[71] The incidence of serious adverse side effects with ticlopidine, including neutropenia and thrombotic thrombocytopenic purpura, decreases the clinical usefulness of this drug.

Clopidogrel appears to have an effectiveness similar to ticlopidine with a better side effect profile and convenient pharmacokinetics. Clopidogrel was assessed in the Clopidogrel versus Aspirin in Patients at Risk of Ischemic Events trial. This trial randomized 19,185 patients with various forms of cardiovascular disease including recent ischemic stroke to clopidogrel or aspirin.[72] The combined incidence of ischemic stroke, myocardial infarction, and vascular death at approximately 2 years favored clopidogrel (5.3 versus 5.8 percent; $p = 0.043$), although the absolute reduction in events was small (0.27 percent per year). In this study, a total of 6431 patients were randomized after an ischemic stroke from atherothrombosis (59 percent) or lacunar infarction (40 percent). The outcome of the patients receiving clopidogrel was similar to that receiving aspirin (9.7 versus 10.6 percent). Therefore, clopidogrel has at least equal efficacy compared to aspirin in preventing vascular events. Whether clopidogrel plus aspirin offers an advantage over either agent alone has not been addressed.

The best data regarding outcomes of patients with significant carotid artery stenosis treated with antiplatelet therapy are derived from the medical intervention arms of the carotid endarterectomy randomized trials.[33,73–79] In the Asymptomatic Carotid Atherosclerosis Study (ACAS), 834 patients with >60 percent stenosis were randomized to 325 mg of aspirin daily plus risk factor modification.[80] The annual risk for ipsilateral stroke or any perioperative stroke or death in patients treated with aspirin alone was extremely low, only 2.2 percent per year. Moreover, aspirin is important in these patients due to their high cardiovascular risk as highlighted in the Mayo Asymptomatic Carotid Endarterectomy Study.[77] This study did not require and even discouraged the use of aspirin or any other antiplatelet drug in the surgical cohort. After randomizing only 71 patients, the trial was prematurely terminated due to an excessive rate of myocardial infarctions in the surgical group (carotid endarterectomy 22 versus aspirin 0 percent; $p = 0.0037$). Limited data exist regarding antiplatelet treatment compared to placebo in patients with documented asymptomatic carotid artery stenosis. The impact of aspirin in preventing ipsilateral TIAs or strokes from a 50 percent carotid artery stenosis in initially asymptomatic patients was analyzed from the medical arm of the VA Cooperative Study on Asymptomatic Carotid Stenosis.[81] In the original study, 233 patients were initially randomized to aspirin, but 37 (16 percent) did not actually take any aspirin because of intolerance or noncompliance. At about 4-year follow-up, incidence of ipsilateral TIA or stroke was 37.8 percent in patients not receiving aspirin compared to only 17.4 percent in the group taking aspirin ($p = 0.005$).

In symptomatic patients, however, antiplatelet drugs appear less effective for preventing recurrent stroke. In the NASCET, 331 patients with symptomatic 70 to 99 percent carotid artery stenosis were randomized to 1300 mg aspirin daily or lower doses if the high dose was not well tolerated.[74] Despite high compliance (94 percent) with aspirin therapy, 26 percent of these patients suffered an ipsilateral stroke at 2 years of follow-up. In the European Carotid Surgery Trial (ECST), the annual risk for a major ipsilateral stroke with severe symptomatic carotid stenosis was more than 5 percent.[78]

ANTICOAGULANTS

The role of anticoagulation in patients with known carotid disease has not been adequately studied. In a meta-analysis of 16 randomized studies of anticoagulant therapy after cerebral or retinal ischemia or infarction, anticoagulant therapy was shown to be ineffective in management of these patients.[82] The Stroke Prevention in Reversible Ischemia Trial study randomized 1243 patients with prior TIA or minor stroke of noncardiac origin to aspirin 30 mg daily or anticoagulant drugs with a target International Normalized Ratio (INR) of 3.0 to 4.5.[83] The combined primary end point of vascular death, stroke, myocardial infarction, or major bleeding complication was more than twice as common in the anticoagulant group ($p < 0.05$) because of excess bleeding events. The available data do not support the use of anticoagulant therapy in the management of carotid artery disease.[44]

ANTIHYPERLIPIDEMIC AGENTS

Although earlier studies using clofibrate failed to show reduction in stroke rate,[84,85] meta-analyses from HMG-CoA reductase inhibitors (statins) have conclusively shown the efficacy of antihyperlipidemic therapy in stroke reduction.[28–30] The effect of statins on atherosclerotic plaque has been carefully studied in patients with documented carotid atherosclerosis. These trials have meticulously assessed the effects of statins on the rate of change in carotid IMT using serial ultrasound measurements. In almost every study plaque regression was observed, although the magnitude of the change was small.[86–88]

Although the primary end points of these small and other larger studies were coronary events and mortality, 3 meta-analyses [28–30] focused on the effects on stroke of cholesterol reduction by statins. The first was an overview of 16 trials, which included about 29,000 patients treated and followed-up for an average of 3.3 years.[29] The average reductions in total and low-density lipoprotein-cholesterol were large, 22 and 30 percent, respectively. Patients assigned to statins had a 29 percent reduction in risk of stroke and a 22 percent reduction in risk of total mortality. There was no evidence of any increased risk in noncardiovascular mortality or cancer. Another similar analysis by Blauw et al. from 20,438 patients concluded that approximately 4 strokes could be prevented per 1000 patients treated with statins.[30] Bucher et al. have gone further and reviewed all randomized controlled trials of any cholesterol-lowering therapy that provided data on nonfatal and fatal strokes.[28] Twenty-eight trials were included in this meta-analysis, with over 49,000 and 56,000 in the intervention and control groups, respectively. The statins had a 24 percent reduction in risk of nonfatal and fatal stroke. By contrast, the risk ratios with fibrates, resins, and dietary modification had no effect on the incidence of stroke.[28] With this quite compelling evidence, patients with hypercholesterolemia and moderate-to-high risk of coronary or cerebrovascular events should be offered intensive lipid-lowering treatment with statins.

Percutaneous Intervention

Percutaneous transcatheter techniques have been used extensively in various vascular distributions. Although carotid angioplasty had been first attempted as early as in 1977, the enthusiasm for this procedure has been limited by the fear of cerebral embolism.[89] There has been a rapid growth and invigorated interest in this procedure due to the technological advances in endovascular procedures. Percutaneous intervention of the carotid arteries, when performed safely, has many advantages over surgical treatment. The potential risks of general anesthesia and the local surgical complications of endarterectomy, such as neck hematoma, infection, cervical strain, and cranial nerve damage can be completely eliminated. Furthermore, this treatment approach is particularly appealing for patients with coexistent coronary, myocardial, or valvular heart disease.

BALLOON ANGIOPLASTY

Carotid angioplasty is of historical interest only as it has been almost completely replaced by stenting, which is a safer and more dependable procedure. Angioplasty was first reported by Mathias in 1977[90] and, in 1980, both Kerber et al.[91] and Mullan et al.[92] published case reports of successful carotid angioplasty during carotid endarterectomy. Since then, multiple case reports and observational series of angioplasty of the brachiocephalic vessels have been published, but these reports lack detailed outcome assessment and are of only historical value.[93–100] Procedural success ranged from 79 to 98 percent. Strokes occurred in 4 to 6 percent of patients, with no reported deaths during follow-up.

CAROTID STENTING

In 1994, Marks et al.[101] and Mathias[102] published the first reports of stent use in patients with high cervical carotid artery dissection and stenosis. Since then, several observational series reporting promising results of carotid stenting as a treatment option for carotid stenosis have been published.

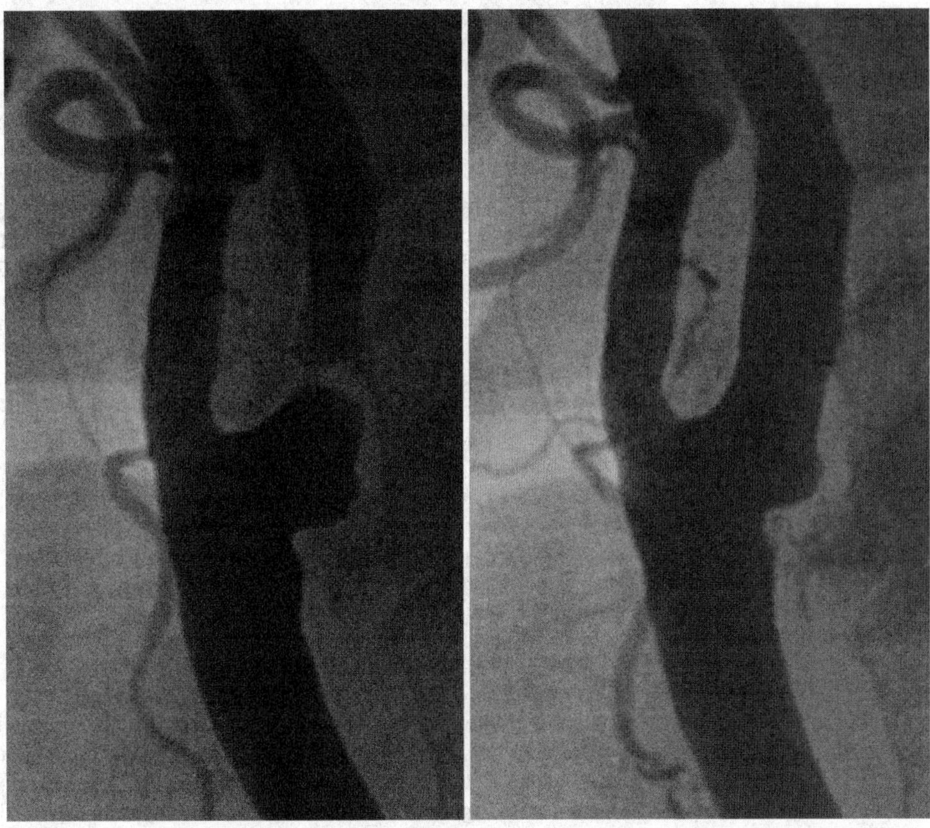

FIGURE 92-1 *A.* Severe stenosis of internal carotid artery. *B, C.* Angiogram after placement of the self-expanding SMART stent (Cordis).

Procedure Slightly different techniques of carotid stenting with similar basic principles have been reported. The goal is to access the carotid arteries with minimal manipulation of catheters, cross the lesion with least possible trauma, gently predilate the lesion, place a self-expandable stent to cover the lesion, and gently postdilate the stent to achieve an acceptable lumen. A technique utilizing a telescoping apparatus with a long sheath is popular in the United States. Various self-expandable stents are being investigated for this specific use (Fig. 92-1).[104–111] Safety and efficacy of adjuvant pharmacologic therapy for platelet inhibition is also being actively studied.

Bradycardia and hypotension are not uncommon during carotid artery stenting procedures but are typically transient. Management of more prolonged hemodynamic alterations may involve temporary transvenous pacing and/or vasoactive medications.[103] In patients with severe left ventricular systolic dysfunction or valvular heart diseases, intraprocedural hemodynamic monitoring with a pulmonary artery catheter is helpful.

Outcome Several reports of carotid stenting have been published.[104–110] Wholey and Eles reviewed carotid artery stenting data from major interventional centers in Europe, South America, and North America[111] (Table 92-1). The data were collected from surveys of the operators from various centers and also from the review of published case series. The survey included questions on patient characteristics, procedural techniques, and the results of carotid stenting. This series reported on a total of 3129 carotid artery stent placement procedures as of October 1998, 46 percent of which were performed at "high-volume" carotid stent centers in Europe and North America. One-third (37 percent) of the patients were asymptomatic. Technical success, defined as less than 30 percent residual stenosis covering a region no longer than the original lesion without any alteration of intracranial arterial anatomy, was achieved in 98.8 percent of patients. Various different stents were used depending on availability and operator preference. Stent deformation as detected by x-rays was seen in 28 instances (2 percent of all Palmaz stents), exclusively occurring with the balloon expandable Palmaz stent (Cordis, Johnson and Johnson Interventional Systems; Warren, NJ). Procedural and 30-day events were recorded. There were 74 (2.4 percent) reported TIAs. Minor strokes were defined as a new neurologic event that resulted in slight functional impairment that either completely resolved within 7 days or caused an increase in the National Institutes of Health (NIH) stroke scale of less than 4. Minor stroke rates ranged from 0 to 7 percent in different centers with a total event rate of 78 (2.49 percent). Major stroke was defined as a new neurologic deficit that persisted after 7 days and increased the NIH stroke scale by 4 or more. Major strokes were reported in 43 patients with an event rate of 1.4 percent (range 0–8 percent). Procedure-related mortality at 30 days occurred in 30 (0.96 percent) patients. Postprocedure neurologic sequelae occurred in 14 (0.79 percent) cases. Ultrasound studies were performed at 1 and 6 months poststent placement at all high-

TABLE 92-1 Results of Carotid Stenting

Study	Lesions (n)	Technical Success	30-Day Outcome Stroke	MI	Death	Mean Follow-up	Stroke After 30 Days	Restenosis
Diethrich et al.[110]	117	116 (99.1%)	10 (8.3%)	0 (0.0%)	1 (0.9%)	7.6 Months	2 (1.7%)	2 (1.7%)
Henry et al.[106]	174	173 (99.4%)	5 (2.9%)	0 (0.0%)	0 (0%)	12.7 Months	0 (0.0%)	4 (2.3%)
Laborde et al.[107]	87	87 (100%)	4 (5.3%)	0 (0.0%)	1 (1.1%)	8.7 Months	1 (1.1%)	2 (5.2%)
Wholey et al.[109]	114	108 (95%)	4 (3.5%)	1 (0.9%)	2 (1.9%)	6 Months	0 (0.0%)	1 (1.0%)
Shawl et al.[105]	96	96 (100%)	3 (3.1%)	0 (0.0%)	0 (0.0%)	8 Months	0 (0.0%)	1 (1.4%)
Yadav et al.[108]	126	126 (100%)	8 (6.3%)	0 (0.0%)	1 (0.8%)	6 Months	0 (0.0%)	4 (4.9%)
Global Experience[111]	3129	3091 (98.8%)	121 (3.9%)	—	61 (2.0%)	6 Months	14 (0.79%)	68 (2.3%)

MI = myocardial infarction.

volume centers. Restenosis defined as diameter stenosis of >50 percent was approximately 2.5 percent.

The series reported by Yadav et al., Diethrich et al., and Wholey et al. have provided the most rigorous detail of carotid stenting techniques, procedural success, and patient outcomes.[108–110] Yadav et al.[108] published their initial experience of carotid stenting in 107 consecutive patients. All procedures were successful. Patients had independent neurologic examinations before and after the procedure. Periprocedural complications included 1 stent thrombosis, 6 minor strokes, and 1 major stroke. Clinical follow-up at 30 days showed 1 additional minor stroke, 1 major stroke, 1 myocardial infarction, and 1 death not due to cerebrovascular disease. The incidence of combined end point of all strokes and death was 7.9 percent with 1.6 percent ipsilateral major stroke and death. A total of 81 (76 percent) patients underwent angiography or ultrasound evaluation 6 months after stenting. Four (4.9 percent) of these 81 patients had asymptomatic restenosis. Five asymptomatic patients had repeat intervention, with angioplasty for restenosis in 2, angioplasty for stent deformation in another 2, and endarterectomy for restenosis in 1. On 6-month follow-up, there were no strokes or deaths from cerebrovascular disease. The University of Alabama group extended their experience to 146 procedures with similar results.[112] It is important to recognize that these results were obtained in a high-risk cohort and represent the initial learning curve for carotid stenting. Of the patients treated with stenting in this series, 77 percent would have been ineligible for carotid endarterectomy on the basis of the ACAS and NASCET exclusion criteria.[74,80] The other major carotid stent series have included patients with a similar high-risk profile.

Diethrich and colleagues[110] reported their experience in 110 patients with severe carotid stenosis. Stenting was successful in 99 percent of patients. There were 7 (6.4 percent) strokes (2 major, 5 minor), 5 (4.5 percent) TIAs, and 2 asymptomatic stent occlusions in the first 30 days after the procedure. Overall, 89 percent (98) of patients had successful procedures and were free from death, surgical intervention, stroke, or stent occlusion at 30 days. During a mean of 7.6 months of follow-up, no additional neurologic events were reported.

Wholey et al. reported 114 lesions in 108 consecutive patients (58 men, mean age 70.1 years) with ≥70 percent carotid stenosis treated with percutaneous stent implantation.[111] Of these, 44 percent were asymptomatic. Stents were successfully placed in 108 (95 percent) lesions. Of the 6 technical failures, 5 were access related and 1 was due to seizures during balloon dilation. Two major (1.8 percent) and 2 minor (1.8 percent) strokes occurred, all in symptomatic patients, 1 of whom died. There were 5 (4.4 percent) TIAs and 2 (1.8 percent) brief seizure episodes during dilation. The total stroke or death rate was 5.3 percent. In the mean 6-month follow-up, there was 1 restenosis (1.0 percent) from a stent compression, which was successfully dilated. There were no neurologic sequelae, cranial palsies, or cases of stent or vessel thrombosis on follow-up.

Henry et al. reported their experience of 174 stenting procedures in 163 patients.[106] This series differs from the others as a cerebral emboli protection device was used in a small subset (n = 32, 18 percent). The majority (65 percent, 106 patients) of the patients were asymptomatic. Immediate technical success was achieved in all but 1 (99.4 percent) patient. Eight (4.6 percent) neurologic complications occurred in the periprocedural period: 3 TIA, 2 minor strokes, and 3 major strokes. Two major complications developed despite cerebral protection. Over a mean follow-up of 1 year, no ipsilateral neurologic complications were seen. Palmaz stent compression was seen in 1 patient and 4 (2.5 percent) patients were identified with restenosis.

Due to relatively small sample size and infrequent events in each series, independent predictors for procedural strokes have not been well studied. Like surgical trials, symptom status appears to correlate with the frequency of adverse neurologic outcomes after carotid stenting. This was seen in the series reported by Yadav et al., where 8 (11 percent) ipsilateral neurologic deficits or deaths were encountered after 74 procedures for symptomatic carotid stenosis and only 2 (4 percent) after 52 procedures in asymptomatic patients.[108] Similarly, Wholey et al. observed a higher stroke rate in symptomatic patients[109] than in asymptomatic patients. In a multivariate analysis of 271 carotid procedures in 231 patients, however, Mathur et al. found advanced age and long or multiple stenoses to be the independent predictors of procedural stroke.[113]

Restenosis, a long-term complication after carotid stenting, is fortunately rare. In the major carotid stent series, 33 (5 percent) of 655 carotid artery procedures were complicated by restenosis when systematically studied with either angiography or ultrasound follow-up evaluations. Stent deformation occurred in 10 (1.5 percent) patients, all occurring with the Palmaz stent. Even though only 4 (0.6 percent) cases of restenosis or stent deformation were symptomatic, 16 (24.4 percent) underwent treatment with repeat dilatation, repeat stenting, endarterectomy, or bypass grafting. As balloon-expandable stents are replaced by self-expanding stents, stent deformation has become clinically irrelevant.

The field of carotid stenting is rapidly evolving with the advent of pharmacologic and technological advances. Availability of better, tailor-made instruments, emboli protection devices, and advanced pharmacologic adjuvant therapies will make carotid stenting a more attractive procedure.

Emboli Protection Devices The major cause of stroke during carotid endarterectomy and percutaneous carotid intervention is the procedural embolization of plaque debris along with platelet and thrombin aggregates into the cerebral circulation. Transcranial Doppler monitoring, a noninvasive method to detect echogenic microemboli, has demonstrated frequent embolization during carotid endarterectomy and stenting.[114–117] Although data are limited, there appears to be a correlation between the number of emboli and neurologic outcome after endarterectomy.[116,117] Consequently, various mechanical and pharmacologic approaches to prevent distal embolization are currently under investigation to improve the safety of carotid stenting.

Various mechanical devices to prevent embolization are under investigation.[118–120] Henry et al. reported their experience in 58 carotid artery stent procedures using a prototype cerebral protection device and compared the results to 212 other patients treated without the emboli protection device.[120] This cerebral protection catheter is a low-profile, balloon-tipped device designed to block cerebral emboli when positioned in the internal carotid artery distal to the target lesion. Conceptually, the protection balloon occludes the run-off circulation to the brain, trapping any particles dislodged following balloon angioplasty or stent delivery so that they can subsequently be extracted via aspiration into the guiding catheter. In this series, there was 1 immediate neurologic complication (0.5 percent) compared to 11 (5.2 percent) in the group treated without the device. Feasibility of transient carotid occlusion without consequences and potential endothelial injury and embolization from the occlusion balloon itself, however, are important concerns that need further evaluation. An alternative mechanical embolization device that allows continued perfusion while capturing emboli has been developed (Figs. 92-2 and 92-3). This filter-type device has been tested in carotid, coronary, and peripheral interventions and should be available in the near future for rigorous randomized trials.[118]

Adjuvant Pharmacologic Therapy Pharmacologic protection against embolization is based on randomized clinical trials utilizing platelet glycoprotein IIb/IIIa inhibitors during coronary interventions. Various Gp IIb/IIIa inhibitors, especially abciximab, have been shown to be effective in reducing the ischemic complications of death, myocardial infarction, or urgent repeat revascularization after percutaneous coronary interventional procedures.[121–123]

The coronary experience has been extended to selected patients in 22 carotid stent procedures involving visible thrombus, total occlusion, or acute stroke. The preliminary data from these high-risk patients suggested relatively high bleeding complications with 2 (9 percent) central nervous system bleeding, one hemorrhagic transformation of a previously ischemic stroke and one other subarachnoid hemorrhage from a ruptured aneurysm.[124] Periprocedural glycoprotein IIb/IIIa receptor inhibition may be safer and more effective when used in a routine prophylactic manner. This approach is being currently evaluated.[124a] Other potential therapies including low molecular weight heparin or direct thrombin inhibitors have not been studied in carotid stenting procedures. Only preliminary information on the efficacy and safety of clopidogrel therapy has been available.[125]

ENDARTERECTOMY VERSUS NONSURGICAL THERAPY

Randomized trials have compared surgical therapy with medical management in symptomatic and asymptomatic carotid stenosis; however, there is no randomized trial comparing surgical therapy with contemporary carotid stenting procedure. Preliminary results from one randomized trial comparing surgery to carotid angioplasty have been reported.[73] A brief summary of these comparative trials is provided here.

Surgery versus Medical Therapy

SYMPTOMATIC DISEASE

Three pivotal studies in patients with symptomatic carotid disease have been completed and have documented improved outcomes with endarterectomy in patients with symptomatic severe carotid stenosis.

The ECST was a multicenter, randomized trial in which patients with nondisabling stroke, TIA, or retinal infarction within the preceding 6 months were randomly assigned to carotid endarterectomy or medical therapy.[78] The rate of perioperative stroke, defined as a stroke within 30 days of carotid endarterectomy or death was 7.0 percent irrespective of the stenosis severity. Patients with severe stenosis (>70 percent) assigned to surgical intervention had significant reduction in surgical death or any stroke at 3-year follow-up (12.3 versus 21.9 percent; $p < 0.01$).[76] The risk of surgical death or ipsilateral stroke by 3 years was 10.3 percent in patients assigned surgical intervention compared with 16.8 percent in patients assigned medical therapy. Patients with mild and moderate stenosis did not have an observed benefit with surgery.

The NASCET enrolled patients with 30 to 99 percent carotid artery stenosis who had experienced TIAs or nondisabling stroke within 4 months of randomization.[74] This study was undertaken in surgical centers with a documented <6 percent stroke or death rate within 30 days of carotid endarterectomy

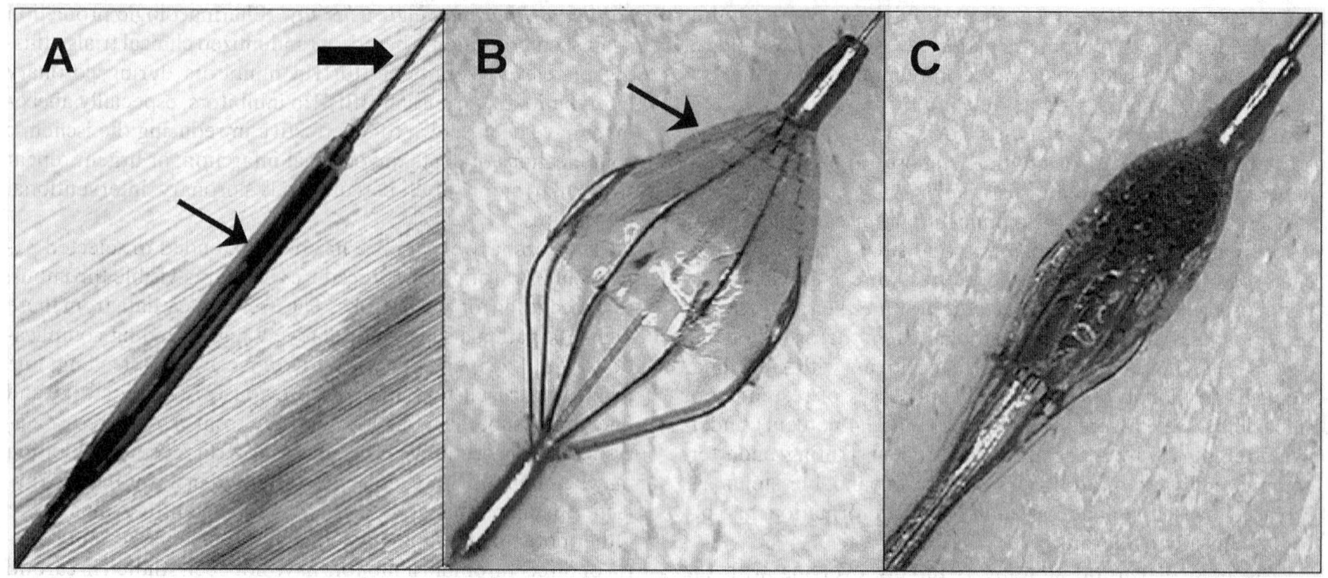

FIGURE 92-2 *A.* An emboli protection device (Angioguard, Cordis) in closed state. The bold arrow represents 0.014 in. wire that leads the device (4 French) shown by the smaller arrow. *B.* Open device with a filter with 100 μM pore size. *C.* Closed filter with captured embolic debris.

in 50 consecutive procedures performed within the preceding 24 months. Patients were stratified according to the degree of carotid stenosis (30–69 percent or 70–99 percent).

The study results from 662 patients with 70 to 99 percent stenosis were published initially.[74] The primary end point was the occurrence of nonfatal or fatal ipsilateral stroke. All patients were examined by neurologists 1, 3, 6, 9, and 12 months after entry and then every 4 months. Stroke or death occurred in 3.8 percent of patients within 30 days of surgery. The life-table estimate of the risk for ipsilateral stroke by 24-month follow-up was 9 percent in the patients treated with carotid endarterectomy compared to 26 percent in the patients treated medically (absolute risk reduction 17 percent; $p < 0.001$). The risk for any stroke (12.6 versus 27.6 percent; $p < 0.001$) and the risk for major stroke or death (8.0 versus 18.1 percent; $p < 0.01$) were also significantly reduced in patients treated with carotid endarterectomy. Review of survival curves for the occurrence of ipsilateral stroke, any stroke, any stroke or death, and other subgroups showed that the early hazard associated with surgery dissipated by 3 to 4 months and that there was persistent benefit with surgery during long-term follow-up. Subgroup analysis by the extent of carotid artery stenosis show the greatest benefit in absolute reduction of ipsilateral stroke during long-term follow-up in patients with more severe carotid disease (26 percent in the 90–99 percent group; 18 percent in the 80–89 percent group; and 12 percent in the 70–79 percent group).

A total of 2267 patients with <70 percent stenosis were also randomized to medical therapy or endarterectomy in the NASCET trial.[75] Post hoc analyses divided patients into groups with 50 to 69 percent stenosis and those with <50 percent stenosis. In patients with 50 to 69 percent stenosis, a 6.5 percent reduction in the primary end point of any ipsilateral stroke was observed by 5-year follow-up (15.7 versus 22.2 percent; $p = 0.045$). In the group with <50 percent stenosis, a nonsignificant absolute reduction of 3.8 percent was observed (14.9 versus 18.7 percent; $p = 0.16$). The risk for any stroke or death was significantly reduced in the surgical group at 5-year follow-up for patients with 50 to 69 percent stenosis (33.2 versus

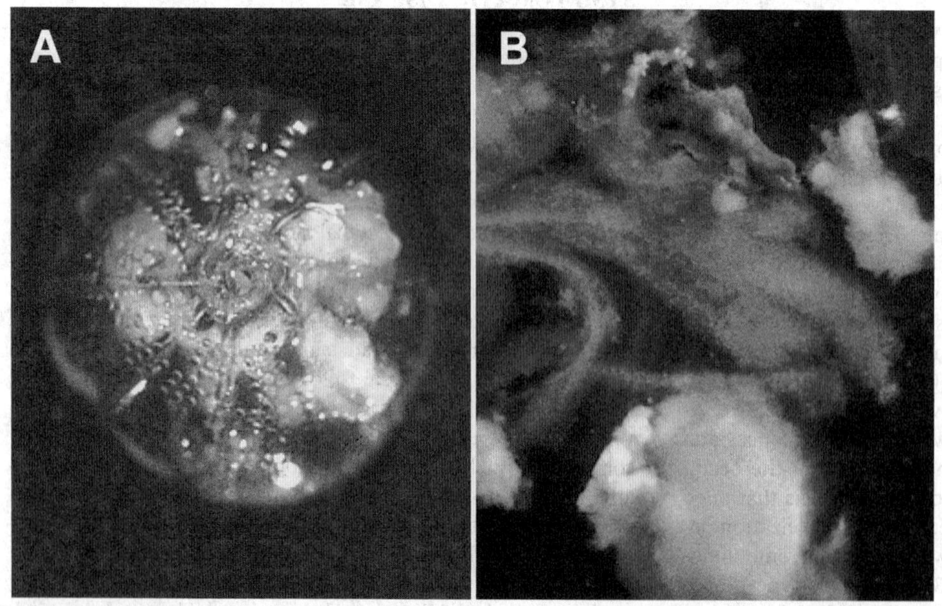

FIGURE 92-3 *A.* Filter with atheromatous embolic debris. *B.* Magnified view of typical atheromatous embolic particles retrieved during intervention.

43.3 percent; $p = 0.005$), but no reduction was observed with surgery in patients with <50 percent stenosis (36.2 versus 37 percent; $p = 0.97$).

The Veterans Affairs Cooperative Studies Program Trialist Group randomly assigned 189 men from a total of 5000 screened patients to medical therapy or endarterectomy.[79] All patients had >50 percent stenosis of the internal carotid artery ipsilateral to the presenting symptoms. Patients with TIA, transient monocular blindness, or recent small, completed strokes within last 4 months were enrolled. At a mean follow-up of 11.9 months, a significant reduction in stroke or crescendo TIAs in patients assigned to carotid endarterectomy compared with patients assigned to medical treatment was observed (7.7 versus 19.4 percent; absolute risk reduction, 11.7 percent; $p = 0.011$). The benefit of surgery was more profound in patients with internal carotid artery stenosis >70 percent (absolute risk reduction, 17.7 percent; $p = .004$). Perioperative complications (stroke or death) within 30 days of randomization occurred in 6 of 91 (6.6 percent) patients with endarterectomy (3 strokes and 3 deaths).

ASYMPTOMATIC DISEASE

The efficacy of carotid endarterectomy for patients with asymptomatic carotid artery disease is less well defined. The ACAS trial enrolled 1659 patients between 1983 and 1993 with asymptomatic carotid stenosis of ≥60 percent.[80] There was an impressively low perioperative stroke or death rate of 2.3 percent and the median follow-up of 2.7 years. The aggregate risk over 5 years for ipsilateral stroke and any perioperative stroke or death was estimated to be 5.1 percent for surgical patients and 11.0 percent for patients treated medically with aggregate risk reduction of 53 percent ($p = 0.004$). The low surgical complication rate was due in part to stringent selection criteria for participating centers, which required <3 percent incidence of stroke in the preceding 50 consecutive operations in asymptomatic patients.[126] The low rate of perioperative complications leads to the questioning of the broader application of the results to other surgical centers that may not be able to reproduce such low complication rates.[127]

The Veteran Affairs Asymptomatic Carotid Stenosis study tested endarterectomy versus aspirin treatment strategies in a randomized multicenter trial.[33] A total of 444 patients with asymptomatic carotid stenosis of ≥50 percent were randomly assigned to optimal medical treatment including antiplatelet medication (aspirin) plus carotid endarterectomy ($n = 211$) or optimal medical treatment alone ($n = 233$). Mean follow-up was approximately 4 years. The combined incidence of ipsilateral neurologic events was 8.0 percent in the surgical group and 20.6 percent in the medical group ($p = 0.001$). The incidence of ipsilateral stroke alone was high in the surgical group (4.7 percent), but was higher (9.4 percent) in the medically managed group. These differences did not reach statistical significance, however.

Operation Versus Aspirin (CASANOVA) trial randomized asymptomatic patients with 50 to 90 percent stenosis.[73] Altogether, 334 carotid endarterectomies were performed. Patients undergoing unilateral or bilateral surgery ($n = 206$) were compared with a medically treated group ($n = 160$) having either unilateral stenosis with no surgery or bilateral stenosis and surgery on the more affected side. Statistical analysis found no significant difference in the number of neurologic deficits and deaths between the two groups. However, this trial is difficult to interpret because of an almost 50 percent crossover rate from the medical to the surgical arm and the exclusion of patients with stenosis >90 percent. Another trial of patients with asymptomatic carotid artery disease is ongoing.[128]

Surgery versus Percutaneous Intervention

One randomized trial, CAVATAS, which compared surgery to percutaneous intervention, has been reported.[129] This study evaluated the safety and efficacy of percutaneous angioplasty versus endarterectomy of the carotid artery. Symptomatic patients with 70 percent stenosis were randomly assigned to angioplasty or surgery, or (if the patient was unsuitable for surgery) to angioplasty or best medical treatment. Preliminary data indicate that 253 patients were randomized to carotid endarterectomy and 251 to carotid angioplasty (of whom 25 percent received stents). A major periprocedural complication was observed in 6.3 percent of patients in both groups (M. Brown, personal communication).[44] CAVATAS-2, with a larger sample size, should provide more insights into the role of percutaneous carotid intervention.

Two important trials comparing carotid artery stenting with endarterectomy have been planned. The Carotid Revascularization Endarterectomy versus Stent Trial will randomize patients who are at low surgical risk to stenting or surgery. The primary end points for this trial are (1) any stroke, myocardial infarction, or death within 30 days, and (2) ipsilateral stroke after 30 days. This trial is planning to recruit 2500 patients, as event rate is likely to be low. A clinical events committee will adjudicate all events. The secondary end points for this study include comparisons of 30-day morbidity and mortality, long-term morbidity and mortality, restenosis rates, quality of life, and cost effectiveness for the two treatment alternatives. Multivariate analysis to identify subgroups of patients at differential risk for the two procedures will be performed.

The Stenting and Angioplasty with Protection in Patients at High Risk for Endarterectomy Trial will randomize patients at high surgical risk to carotid endarterectomy or carotid artery stenting. The high-risk patient population is defined as patients with severe cardiac comorbidities (unstable angina, valvular heart disease, or severe congestive heart failure), previous neck radiation, previous radical neck dissections, restenosis after endarterectomy, or presence of contralateral occlusion. Both de novo and restenotic lesions will be treated in symptomatic (>70 percent stenosis) or asymptomatic (>80 percent stenosis) patients. A total of 720 patients at 24 sites will be enrolled, and a parallel stent and surgical registries will be maintained for the nonrandomized patients. The primary end point is a 30-day composite of any stroke, death, or myocardial infarction. The secondary end point is 1-year ipsilateral stroke and death rate. This trial will utilize the Cordis nitinol carotid stent and Cordis Angioguard, an emboli protection device.

SUMMARY

Stroke is the leading cause of long-term serious disability in the United States, a substantial portion of which is caused by atherosclerotic carotid artery disease. The conventional risk factors for coronary atherosclerosis are also responsible for carotid atherosclerosis. Carotid stenosis is encountered in medical practice in either a symptomatic or asymptomatic state. In symptomatic patients, medical management with antiplatelet agents does not provide adequate protection against stroke. Carotid endarterectomy can help to reduce risk of subsequent stroke. Asymptomatic patients with severe carotid stenosis can benefit from surgical intervention if endarterectomy can be performed at a low operative risk.

Percutaneous carotid stenting using self-expanding stents is becoming popular for the treatment of carotid stenosis. Although this initial experience has been reported from the high-risk patient population, the results are encouraging with acceptable periprocedural stroke rates. Moreover, emboli protection devices, modern adjuvant pharmacotherapy, and modern self-expanding stents were not utilized in these studies. With rapidly expanding technology and advances in the interventional pharmacology, improvement in clinical outcome is likely. At this stage, randomized trials to compare endarterectomy with carotid stenting are warranted and are currently underway. Cautious optimism is necessary until the optimal equipment, emboli protection devices, and adjuvant pharmacotherapies are fully investigated. Until then, carotid stenting should be restricted to high-risk candidates for carotid endarterectomy including patients with severe cardiac comorbidities, previous neck surgeries or radiation or other technical contraindications for surgery.

References

1. American Heart Association. Heart and Stroke Statistical Update. *Dallas: American Heart Association.* 1999.
2. Oddone EZ, Horner RD, Sloane R, et al. Race, presenting signs and symptoms, use of carotid artery imaging, and appropriateness of carotid endarterectomy. *Stroke* 1999; 30:1350–1356.
3. Fields WS, Maslenikov V, Meyer JS, et al. Joint study of extracranial arterial occlusion. V. Progress report of prognosis following surgery or nonsurgical treatment for transient cerebral ischemic attacks and cervical carotid artery lesions. *JAMA* 1970; 211:1993–2003.
4. Hass WK, Fields WS, North RR, et al. Joint study of extracranial arterial occlusion. II. Arteriography, techniques, sites, and complications. *JAMA* 1968; 203:961–968.
5. Bamford J, Dennis M, Sandercock P, et al. The frequency, causes and timing of death within 30 days of a first stroke: The Oxfordshire Community Stroke Project. *J Neurol Neurosurg Psych* 1990; 53:824–829.
6. Fisher C. Occlusion of the carotid arteries. *Arch Neurol Psychol* 1954; 72:187–204.
7. Fisher C. Occlusion of internal carotid artery. *Arch Neurol Psychol* 1951; 65:364–377.
8. von Kemp K, van den Brande P, Peterson T, et al. Screening for concomitant diseases in peripheral vascular patients. Results of a systematic approach. *Intern Angiol* 1997; 16:114–122.
9. Saito D, Shiraki T, Oka T, et al. Morphologic correlation between atherosclerotic lesions of the carotid and coronary arteries in patients with angina pectoris. *Japan Circ J* 1999; 63:522–526.
10. Hulthe J, Wikstrand J, Emanuelsson H, et al. Atherosclerotic changes in the carotid artery bulb as measured by B-mode ultrasound are associated with the extent of coronary atherosclerosis. *Stroke* 1997; 28:1189–1194.
11. Crouse JR III, Craven TE, Hagaman AP, et al. Association of coronary disease with segment-specific intimal-medial thickening of the extracranial carotid artery. *Circulation* 1995; 92:1141–1147.
12. Wofford JL, Kahl FR, Howard GR, et al. Relation of extent of extracranial carotid artery atherosclerosis as measured by B-mode ultrasound to the extent of coronary atherosclerosis. *Arterioscler Thromb* 1991; 11:1786–1794.
13. O'Leary DH, Polak JF, Kronmal RA, et al. Carotid-artery intima and media thickness as a risk factor for myocardial infarction and stroke in older adults. Cardiovascular Health Study Collaborative Research Group. *N Engl J Med* 1999; 340:14–22.
14. Crouse JR, Toole JF, McKinney WM, et al. Risk factors for extracranial carotid artery atherosclerosis. *Stroke* 1987; 18: 990–996.
15. Howard G, Wagenknecht LE, Burke GL, et al. Cigarette smoking and progression of atherosclerosis: The Atherosclerosis Risk in Communities (ARIC) Study. *JAMA* 1998; 279:119–124.
16. Kallikazaros I, Tsioufis C, Sideris S, et al. Carotid artery disease as a marker for the presence of severe coronary artery disease in patients evaluated for chest pain. *Stroke* 1999; 30:1002–1007.
17. Salonen JT, Seppanen K, Rauramaa R, et al. Risk factors for carotid atherosclerosis: The Kuopio Ischaemic Heart Disease Risk Factor Study. *Ann Med* 1989; 21:227–229.
18. Colgan MP, Strode GR, Sommer JD, et al. Prevalence of asymptomatic carotid disease: Results of duplex scanning in 348 unselected volunteers. *J Vasc Surg* 1988; 8:674–678.
19. Josse MO, Touboul PJ, Mas JL, et al. Prevalence of asymptomatic internal carotid artery stenosis. *Neuroepidemiol* 1987; 6:150–152.
20. Heyman A, Fields WS, Keating RD. Joint study of extracranial arterial occlusion. VI. Racial differences in hospitalized patients with ischemic stroke. *JAMA* 1972; 222:285–289.
21. Leung SY, Ng TH, Yuen ST, et al. Pattern of cerebral atherosclerosis in Hong Kong Chinese: Severity in intracranial and extracranial vessels. *Stroke* 1993; 24:779–786.
22. Whisnant JP, Homer D, Ingall TJ, et al. Duration of cigarette smoking is the strongest predictor of severe extracranial carotid artery atherosclerosis. *Stroke* 1990; 21:707–714.
23. Cholesterol, diastolic blood pressure, and stroke: 13,000 strokes in 450,000 people in 45 prospective cohorts. Prospective studies collaboration. *Lancet* 1995; 346:1647–1653.
24. Salonen R, Seppanen K, Rauramaa R, et al. Prevalence of carotid atherosclerosis and serum cholesterol levels in eastern Finland. *Arteriosclerosis* 1988; 8:788–792.
25. Bonithon-Kopp C, Touboul PJ, Berr C, et al. Factors of carotid arterial enlargement in a population aged 59 to 71 years: The EVA study. *Stroke* 1996; 27:654–660.
26. Bonithon-Kopp C, Scarabin PY, Taquet A, et al. Risk factors for early carotid atherosclerosis in middle-aged French women. *Arterioscler Thromb* 1991; 11:966–972.
27. Wilt TJ, Rubins HB, Robins SJ, et al. Carotid atherosclerosis in men with low levels of HDL cholesterol. *Stroke* 1997; 28:1919–1925.
28. Bucher HC, Griffith LE, Guyatt GH. Effect of HMGcoA reductase inhibitors on stroke. A meta-analysis of randomized, controlled trials. *Ann Intern Med* 1998; 128:89–95.
29. Hebert PR, Gaziano JM, Chan KS, et al. Cholesterol lowering with statin drugs, risk of stroke, and total mortality. An overview of randomized trials. *JAMA* 1997; 278:313–321.
30. Blauw GJ, Lagaay AM, Smelt AH, et al. Stroke, statins, and cholesterol. A meta-analysis of randomized, placebo-controlled, double-blind trials with HMG-CoA reductase inhibitors. *Stroke* 1997; 28:946–950.
31. Hennerici M, Hulsbomer HB, Hefter H, et al. Natural history of asymptomatic extracranial arterial disease. Results of a long-term prospective study. *Brain* 1987; 110:777–791.
32. Autret A, Pourcelot L, Saudeau D, et al. Stroke risk in patients with carotid stenosis. *Lancet* 1987; 1:888–890.
33. Hobson RWD, Weiss DG, Fields WS, et al. Efficacy of carotid endarterectomy for asymptomatic carotid stenosis. The Veterans Affairs Cooperative Study Group. *N Engl J Med* 1993; 328: 221–227.

34. Hertzer NR, Flanagan RA Jr, Beven EG, et al. Surgical versus nonoperative treatment of symptomatic carotid stenosis: 211 patients documented by intravenous angiography. *Ann Surg* 1986; 204:154–162.
35. Hertzer NR, Flanagan RA Jr, Beven EG, et al. Surgical versus nonoperative treatment of asymptomatic carotid stenosis: 290 patients documented by intravenous angiography. *Ann Surg* 1986; 204:163–171.
36. Mansour MA, Littooy FN, Watson WC, et al. Outcome of moderate carotid artery stenosis in patients who are asymptomatic. *J Vasc Surg* 1999; 29:217–225; (discussion) 225–227.
37. Meissner I, Wiebers DO, Whisnant JP, et al. The natural history of asymptomatic carotid artery occlusive lesions. *JAMA* 1987; 258:2704–2707.
38. Chambers BR, Norris JW. Outcome in patients with asymptomatic neck bruits. *N Engl J Med* 1986; 315:860–865.
39. Chambers BR, Norris JW. The case against surgery for asymptomatic carotid stenosis. *Stroke* 1984; 15:964–967.
40. Olin JW, Fonseca C, Childs MB, et al. The natural history of asymptomatic moderate internal carotid artery stenosis by duplex ultrasound. *Vasc Med* 1998; 3:101–108.
41. Roederer GO, Langlois YE, Jager KA, et al. The natural history of carotid arterial disease in asymptomatic patients with cervical bruits. *Stroke* 1984; 15:605–613.
42. Roederer GO, Langlois YE, Lusiani L, et al. Natural history of carotid artery disease on the side contralateral to endarterectomy. *J Vasc Surg* 1984; 1:62–72.
43. Dennis M, Bamford J, Sandercock P, et al. Prognosis of transient ischemic attacks in the Oxfordshire Community Stroke Project. *Stroke* 1990; 21:848–853.
44. Mendelsohn FO, Mahaffey KW, Yadav JS. Management of atherosclerotic carotid disease: Medical, surgical and interventional aspects. In: Topol EJ, ed. *Textbook of Cardiovascular Medicine,* vol 2. NJ: Lippincott Williams & Wilkins Healthcare; 1999:1.
45. Riggs HE, Rupp C. Variation in form of the circle of Willis. The relation of variation to collateral circulation: Anatomic analysis. *Arch Neurol* 1963; 8:24–30.
46. Lusby RJ, Ferrell LD, Ehrenfeld WK, et al. Carotid plaque hemorrhage. Its role in production of cerebral ischemia. *Arch Surg* 1982; 117:1479–1488.
47. Lennihan L, Kupsky WJ, Mohr JP, et al. Lack of association between carotid plaque hematoma and ischemic cerebral symptoms. *Stroke* 1987; 18:879–881.
48. Sitzer M, Muller W, Siebler M, et al. Plaque ulceration and lumen thrombus are the main sources of cerebral microemboli in high-grade internal carotid artery stenosis. *Stroke* 1995; 26:1231–1233.
49. Imparato AM, Riles TS, Gorstein F. The carotid bifurcation plaque: Pathologic findings associated with cerebral ischemia. *Stroke* 1979; 10:238–245.
50. Eliasziw M, Streifler JY, Fox AJ, et al. Significance of plaque ulceration in symptomatic patients with high-grade carotid stenosis. North American Symptomatic Carotid Endarterectomy Trial. *Stroke* 1994; 25:304–308.
51. Reilly LM, Lusby RJ, Hughes L, et al. Carotid plaque histology using real-time ultrasonography. Clinical and therapeutic implications. *Am J Surg* 1983; 146:188–193.
52. O'Donnell TF Jr, Erdoes L, Mackey WC, et al. Correlation of B-mode ultrasound imaging and arteriography with pathologic findings at carotid endarterectomy. *Arch Surg* 1985; 120:443–449.
53. Geroulakos G, Ramaswami G, Nicolaides A, et al. Characterization of symptomatic and asymptomatic carotid plaques using high-resolution real-time ultrasonography. *Br J Surg* 1993; 80:1274–1277.
54. Gray-Weale AC, Graham JC, Burnett JR, et al. Carotid artery atheroma: Comparison of preoperative B-mode ultrasound appearance with carotid endarterectomy specimen pathology. *J Cardiovasc Surg (Torino)* 1988; 29:676–681.
55. Leahy AL, McCollum PT, Feeley TM, et al. Duplex ultrasonography and selection of patients for carotid endarterectomy: Plaque morphology or luminal narrowing? *J Vasc Surg* 1988; 8:558–562.
56. Arnold JA, Modaresi KB, Thomas N, et al. Carotid plaque characterization by duplex scanning: Observer error may undermine current clinical trials. *Stroke* 1999; 30:61–65.
57. Estes JM, Quist WC, Lo Gerfo FW, et al. Noninvasive characterization of plaque morphology using helical computed tomography. *J Cardiovasc Surg (Torino)* 1998; 39:527–534.
58. Toussaint JF, LaMuraglia GM, Southern JF, et al. Magnetic resonance images lipid, fibrous, calcified, hemorrhagic, and thrombotic components of human atherosclerosis in vivo. *Circulation* 1996; 94:932–938.
59. Shinnar M, Fallon JT, Wehrli S, et al. The diagnostic accuracy of ex vivo MRI for human atherosclerotic plaque characterization. *Arterioscler Thromb Vasc Biol* 1999; 19:2756–2761.
60. Beebe HG, Salles-Cunha SX, Scissons RP, et al. Carotid arterial ultrasound scan imaging: A direct approach to stenosis measurement. *J Vasc Surg* 1999; 29:838–844.
61. Alexandrov AV, Vital D, Brodie DS, et al. Grading carotid stenosis with ultrasound. An interlaboratory comparison. *Stroke* 1997; 28:1208–1210.
62. Alexandrov AV, Brodie DS, McLean A, et al. Correlation of peak systolic velocity and angiographic measurement of carotid stenosis revisited. *Stroke* 1997; 28:339–342.
63. Salonen JT, Salonen R. Ultrasound B-mode imaging in observational studies of atherosclerotic progression. *Circulation* 1993; 87:II56–II65.
64. Anderson CM, Saloner D, Lee RE, et al. Assessment of carotid artery stenosis by MR angiography: Comparison with x-ray angiography and color-coded Doppler ultrasound. *AJNR Am J Neuroradiol* 1992; 13:989–1003; (discussion) 1005–1008.
65. Mittl RL Jr, Broderick M, Carpenter JP, et al. Blinded-reader comparison of magnetic resonance angiography and duplex ultrasonography for carotid artery bifurcation stenosis. *Stroke* 1994; 25:4–10.
66. Pan XM, Anderson CM, Reilly LM, et al. Magnetic resonance angiography of the carotid artery combining two- and three-dimensional acquisitions. *J Vasc Surg* 1992; 16:609–615; (discussion) 615–618.
67. Pan XM, Saloner D, Reilly LM, et al. Assessment of carotid artery stenosis by ultrasonography, conventional angiography, and magnetic resonance angiography: Correlation with ex vivo measurement of plaque stenosis. *J Vasc Surg* 1995; 21:82–88; (discussion) 88–89.
68. Kappelle LJ, Eliasziw M, Fox AJ, et al. Importance of intracranial atherosclerotic disease in patients with symptomatic stenosis of the internal carotid artery. The North American Symptomatic Carotid Endarterectomy Trial. *Stroke* 1999; 30:282–286.
69. Wholey MH. Do the benefits of angiography outweigh the risks in the treatment of patients with carotid artery occlusive disease? (editorial). *Cardiovasc Intervent Radiol* 1999; 22:183–184.
70. Collaborative overview of randomised trials of antiplatelet therapy—I: Prevention of death, myocardial infarction, and stroke by prolonged antiplatelet therapy in various categories of patients. Antiplatelet Trialists' Collaboration (published erratum appears in *Br Med J* 1994; 308(6943):1540). *Br Med J* 1994; 308:81–106.
71. Bellavance A. Efficacy of ticlopidine and aspirin for prevention of reversible cerebrovascular ischemic events. The Ticlopidine Aspirin Stroke Study. *Stroke* 1993; 24:1452–1457.
72. CAPRIE Steering Committee. A randomised, blinded trial of clopidogrel versus aspirin in patients at risk of ischaemic events (CAPRIE). *Lancet* 1996; 348:1329–1339.

73. The CASANOVA Study Group. Carotid surgery versus medical therapy in asymptomatic carotid stenosis. *Stroke* 1991; 22:1229–1235.
74. North American Symptomatic Carotid Endarterectomy Trial Collaborators. Beneficial effect of carotid endarterectomy in symptomatic patients with high-grade carotid stenosis. *N Engl J Med* 1991; 325:445–453.
75. Barnett HJ, Taylor DW, Eliasziw M, et al. Benefit of carotid endarterectomy in patients with symptomatic moderate or severe stenosis. North American Symptomatic Carotid Endarterectomy Trial Collaborators. *N Engl J Med* 1998; 339:1415–1425.
76. European Carotid Surgery Trialists' Collaborative Group. MRC European Carotid Surgery Trial: Interim results for symptomatic patients with severe (70–99%) or with mild (0–29%) carotid stenosis. *Lancet* 1991; 337:1235–1243.
77. Mayo Asymptomatic Carotid Endarterectomy Study Group. Results of a randomized controlled trial of carotid endarterectomy for asymptomatic carotid stenosis. *Mayo Clin Proc* 1992; 67:513–518.
78. European Carotid Surgery Trialists' Collaborative Group. Randomised trial of endarterectomy for recently symptomatic carotid stenosis: Final results of the MRC European Carotid Surgery Trial (ECST). *Lancet* 1998; 351:1379–1387.
79. Mayberg MR, Wilson SE, Yatsu F, et al. Carotid endarterectomy and prevention of cerebral ischemia in symptomatic carotid stenosis. Veterans Affairs Cooperative Studies Program 309 Trialist Group. *JAMA* 1991; 266:3289–3294.
80. Executive Committee for the Asymptomatic Carotid Atherosclerosis Study. Endarterectomy for asymptomatic carotid artery stenosis. *JAMA* 1995; 273:1421–1428.
81. Hobson RWD, Krupski WC, Weiss DG. Influence of aspirin in the management of asymptomatic carotid artery stenosis. VA Cooperative Study Group on Asymptomatic Carotid Stenosis. *J Vasc Surg* 1993; 17:257–263; (discussion) 263–265.
82. Jonas S. Anticoagulant therapy in cerebrovascular disease: Review and meta-analysis (published erratum appears in *Stroke* 1989; 20(4):562). *Stroke* 1988; 19:1043–1048.
83. The Stroke Prevention in Reversible Ischemia Trial (SPIRIT) Study Group. A randomized trial of anticoagulants versus aspirin after cerebral ischemia of presumed arterial origin. *Ann Neurol* 1997; 42:857–865.
84. Acheson J, Hutchinson EC. Controlled trial of clofibrate in cerebral vascular disease. *Atherosclerosis* 1972; 15:177–183.
85. The treatment of cerebrovascular disease with clofibrate. Final report of the Veterans Administration Cooperative Study of Atherosclerosis, Neurology Section. *Stroke* 1973; 4:684–693.
86. Crouse JR III, Byington RP, Bond MG, et al. Pravastatin, lipids, and atherosclerosis in the carotid arteries (PLAC-II) (published erratum appears in *Am J Cardiol* 1995; 75(12):862). *Am J Cardiol* 1995; 75:455–459.
87. Furberg CD, Adams HP Jr, Applegate WB, et al. Effect of lovastatin on early carotid atherosclerosis and cardiovascular events. Asymptomatic Carotid Artery Progression Study (ACAPS) Research Group. *Circulation* 1994; 90:1679–1687.
88. MacMahon S, Sharpe N, Gamble G, et al. Effects of lowering average of below-average cholesterol levels on the progression of carotid atherosclerosis: Results of the LIPID Atherosclerosis Substudy. LIPID Trial Research Group (published erratum appears in *Circulation* 1996; 97(24):2479). *Circulation* 1998; 97:1784–1790.
89. Beebe HG, Archie JP, Baker WH, et al. Concern about safety of carotid angioplasty (editorial). *Stroke* 1996; 27:197–198.
90. Mathias K. A new catheter system for percutaneous transluminal angioplasty (PTA) of carotid artery stenoses. *Fortschr Med* 1977; 95:1007–1011.
91. Kerber CW, Cromwell LD, Loehden OL. Catheter dilatation of proximal carotid stenosis during distal bifurcation endarterectomy. *Am J Neuroradiol* 1980; 1:348–349.
92. Mullan S, Duda EE, Patronas NJ. Some examples of balloon technology in neurosurgery. *J Neurosurg* 1980; 52:321–329.
93. Brown MM, Butler P, Gibbs J, et al. Feasibility of percutaneous transluminal angioplasty for carotid artery stenosis. *J Neurol Neurosurg Psych* 1990; 53:238–243.
94. Kachel R, Basche S, Heerklotz I, et al. Percutaneous transluminal angioplasty (PTA) of supra-aortic arteries especially the internal carotid artery. *Neuroradiology* 1991; 33:191–194.
95. Tsai FY, Matovich V, Hieshima G, et al. Percutaneous transluminal angioplasty of the carotid artery. *Am J Neuroradiol* 1986; 7:349–358.
96. Higashida RT, Tsai FY, Halbach VV, et al. Cerebral percutaneous transluminal angioplasty. *Heart Dis Stroke* 1993; 2:497–502.
97. Bergeron P, Chambran P, Hartung O, et al. Cervical carotid artery stenosis: Which technique, balloon angioplasty or surgery? *J Cardiovasc Surg (Torino)* 1996; 37:73–75.
98. Kachel R. Results of balloon angioplasty in the carotid arteries. *J Endovasc Surg* 1996; 3:22–30.
99. Gil-Peralta A, Mayol A, Marcos JR, et al. Percutaneous transluminal angioplasty of the symptomatic atherosclerotic carotid arteries: Results, complications, and follow-up. *Stroke* 1996; 27:2271–2273.
100. Motarjeme A, Keifer JW, Zuska AJ. Percutaneous transluminal angioplasty of the brachiocephalic arteries. *Am J Roentgenol* 1982; 138:457–462.
101. Marks MP, Dake MD, Steinberg GK, et al. Stent placement for arterial and venous cerebrovascular disease: Preliminary experience. *Radiology* 1994; 191:441–446.
102. Mathias K. Stent placement in arteriosclerotic disease of the internal carotid artery. In: Adam A, Dondelinger RF, Mueller PR, eds. *Textbook of Metallic Stents.* Oxford: Isis Medical Media; 1997:189.
103. Mendelsohn FO, Weissman NJ, Lederman RJ, et al. Acute hemodynamic changes during carotid artery stenting. *Am J Cardiol* 1998; 82:1077–1081.
104. Theron JG, Payelle GG, Coskun O, et al. Carotid artery stenosis: Treatment with protected balloon angioplasty and stent placement. *Radiology* 1996; 201:627–636.
105. Shawl FA, Efstratiou A, Lapetina FL, et al. Stent supported carotid angioplasty (SSCA) in patients with symptomatic coronary artery disease: Acute and long term results. *J Am Coll Cardiol* 1998; 31(suppl):454A.
106. Henry M, Amor M, Masson I, et al. Angioplasty and stenting of the extracranial carotid arteries. *J Endovasc Surg* 1998; 5:293–304.
107. Laborde JC, Fajadet J, Cassagneau B, et al. Carotid stenting in patients at risk for surgery: Immediate and long-term results. *J Am Coll Cardiol* 1998; 31(suppl):63A.
108. Yadav JS, Roubin GS, Iyer S, et al. Elective stenting of the extracranial carotid arteries. *Circulation* 1997; 95:376–381.
109. Wholey MH, Jarmolowski CR, Eles G, et al. Endovascular stents for carotid artery occlusive disease. *J Endovasc Surg* 1997; 4:326–338.
110. Diethrich EB, Ndiaye M, Reid DB. Stenting in the carotid artery: Initial experience in 110 patients. *J Endovasc Surg* 1996; 3:42–62.
111. Wholey MH, Eles G. Cervical carotid artery stent placement. *Semin Interv Cardiol* 1998; 3:105–115.
112. Roubin GS, Yadav S, Iyer SS, et al. Carotid stent-supported angioplasty: A neurovascular intervention to prevent stroke. *Am J Cardiol* 1996; 78:8–12.
113. Mathur A, Roubin GS, Iyer SS, et al. Predictors of stroke complicating carotid artery stenting. *Circulation* 1998; 97:1239–1245.
114. McCleary AJ, Nelson M, Dearden NM, et al. Cerebral haemodynamics and embolization during carotid angioplasty in high-risk patients. *Br J Surg* 1998; 85:771–774.

115. Markus HS, Clifton A, Buckenham T, et al. Carotid angioplasty. Detection of embolic signals during and after the procedure. *Stroke* 1994; 25:2403–2406.
116. Gaunt ME, Martin PJ, Smith JL, et al. Clinical relevance of intraoperative embolization detected by transcranial Doppler ultrasonography during carotid endarterectomy: A prospective study of 100 patients. *Br J Surg* 1994; 81:1435–1439.
117. Ackerstaff RG, Jansen C, Moll FL, et al. The significance of microemboli detection by means of transcranial Doppler ultrasonography monitoring in carotid endarterectomy. *J Vasc Surg* 1995; 21:963–969.
118. Yadav JS, Grube E, Rowold S, et al. Detection and characterization of emboli during coronary intervention. *Circulation* 1999; 100:I780.
119. Whitlow PL, Lylyk P, Parodi P. Protected carotid stenting: Preliminary results of a multicenter trial. *Circulation* 1999; 100:I436.
120. Henry M, Amor M, Henry I, et al. Carotid angioplasty and stenting with a new cerebral protection device: The percusurge guardwire device. *Circulation* 1999; 100:I674.
121. The EPISTENT Investigators. Randomised placebo-controlled and balloon-angioplasty-controlled trial to assess safety of coronary stenting with use of platelet glycoprotein-IIb/IIIa blockade. Evaluation of platelet IIb/IIIa inhibitor for stenting. *Lancet* 1998; 352:87–92.
122. The EPILOG Investigators. Platelet glycoprotein IIb/IIIa receptor blockade and low-dose heparin during percutaneous coronary revascularization. *N Engl J Med* 1997; 336:1689–1696.
123. Tcheng JE. Glycoprotein IIb/IIIa receptor inhibitors: Putting the EPIC, IMPACT II, RESTORE, and EPILOG trials into perspective. *Am J Cardiol* 1996; 78:35–40.
124. Chastain HDI, Mt Wong P, Mathur A, et al. Does abciximab reduce complications of cerebral vascular stenting in high risk lesions? *Circulation* 1997; 96:I283.
124a. Kapadia SR, Bajzer CT, Ziada KM, et al. Initial experience of glycoprotein IIb/IIIa inhibition with abciximab during carotid stenting: A safe adjunctive therapy. *J Am Coll Cardiol* 2000; 35:86A.
125. Bajzer CT, Kapadia SR, Yadav JS. Clopidogrel use in carotid artery stenting. *Am J Cardiol* 1999; Sept 22 (abstr 15):7P.
126. Moore WS, Vescera CL, Robertson JT, et al. Selection process for surgeons in the Asymptomatic Carotid Atherosclerosis Study. *Stroke* 1991; 22:1353–1357.
127. Moore WS, Young B, Baker WH, et al. Surgical results: A justification of the surgeon selection process for the ACAS trial. The ACAS Investigators. *J Vasc Surg* 1996; 23:323–328.
128. Halliday AW, Thomas D, Mansfield A. The Asymptomatic Carotid Surgery Trial (ACST). Rationale and design. Steering Committee. *Eur J Vasc Surg* 1994; 8:703–710.
129. Sivaguru A, Venables GS, Beard JD, et al. European carotid angioplasty trial. *J Endovasc Surg* 1996; 3:16–20.

CHAPTER 93

ADVANCES IN THE MINIMALLY INVASIVE TREATMENT OF PERIPHERAL VASCULAR DISEASE

Michael L. Marin / Larry H. Hollier / Michael Poon / Valentin Fuster

INTRODUCTION

The treatment of peripheral vascular disease (PVD) is actively changing, largely as a result of an enhanced understanding of the natural history of clinically significant disease and advances in new therapeutic technologies. The recognition that the individual symptoms of PVD are frequently only a part of the broader problem of diffuse atherosclerosis continues to refocus management of patients with peripheral occlusive disease and arterial aneurysms toward more conservative therapies and the use of less invasive technology.

The use of minimally invasive approaches to PVD has exploded in the past 10 years, following similar advances in the treatment of coronary artery disease. The potential advantages to patients and in turn to the health care system are being realized in the form of reduced morbidity, shorter lengths of stay in the hospital, and a reduction in the total cost of care.

However, these advances must not proceed without clearly defined treatment benefits and acceptable long-term therapeutic durability. This chapter reviews current advances in the least invasive therapies for the treatment of occlusive and aneurysmal disease of peripheral arteries and explores the value and limitations of these approaches.

PERIPHERAL ARTERY OCCLUSIVE DISEASES

Occlusive disease of peripheral arteries includes atherosclerosis within all vessels except the intracerebral and coronary vasculature. Minimally invasive or endovascular therapy has been attempted in almost all these vascular beds; however, the success of these procedures varies. Therapeutic approaches have included atherosclerotic plaque ablation (atherectomy), thrombolytic therapy, balloon angioplasty, intravascular stents, and stented grafts.[1]

Occlusive Disease of Aortic Arch Vessels

The advantages of treating symptomatic occlusive lesions of branch vessels of the aortic arch with catheter-based techniques can be quite dramatic, with the restoration of normal circulation without the need for intrathoracic surgery. The proximal innominate, carotid, and subclavian arteries may be accessed readily through a transfemoral catheter-based approach.[2] Luminal restoration may be achieved by using several endovascular modalities, including ballon angioplasty with or without intravascular stent placement, which appears to provide the most favorable results (Fig. 93-1 and Table 93-1). Along with the potential for primary lesion restenosis, distal arterial dissections, vessel rupture, and embolization to the cerebral circulation are complications that fortunately are uncommon after endovascular treatment of occlusive lesions of proximal arch vessels.[3,4]

Internal carotid bifurcation occlusive disease is a more common lesion that has become an important and controversial area for treatment with minimally invasive endoluminal techniques (Fig. 93-2).[5] The excellent results achieved with conventional surgical procedures to correct these extracavitary lesions and a distinct tendency of these lesions to be friable and embolize with catheter manipulations have created significant concern about the future of this approach to stroke prevention.[6] However, good results have been achieved at several centers with internal carotid artery stenting, and the potential for distal em-

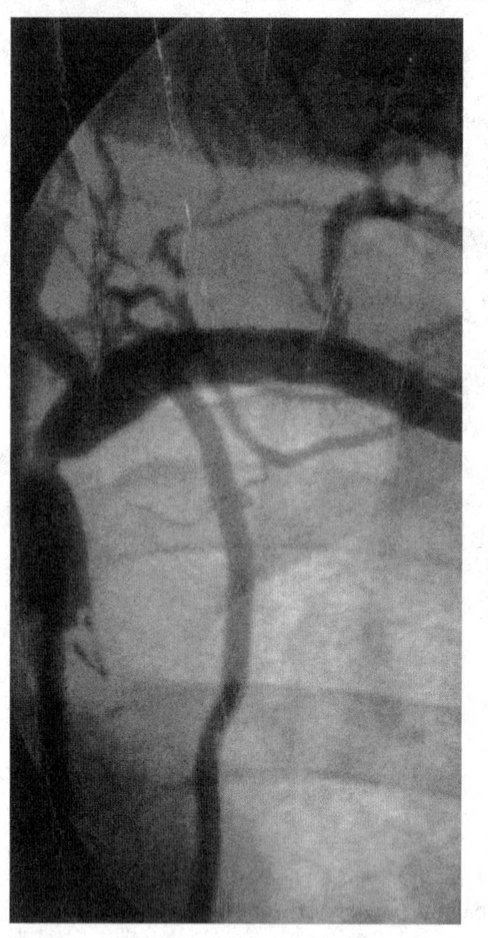

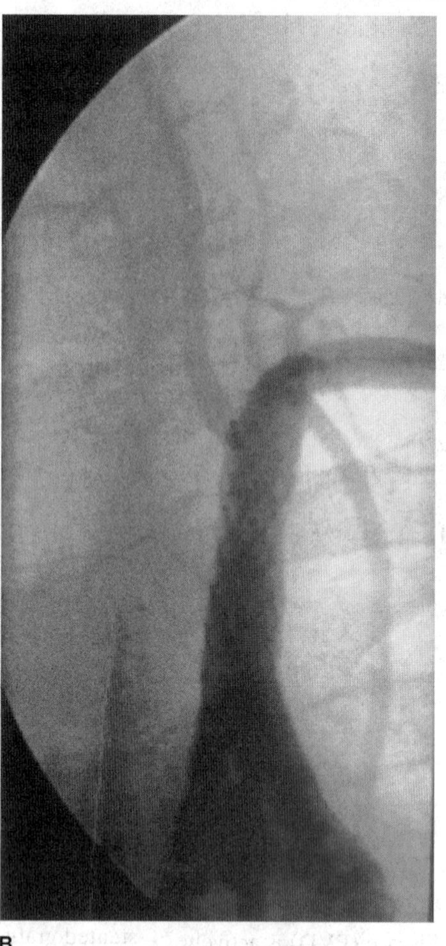

FIGURE 93-1 *A*. Aortic arch angiogram of a 63-year-old woman with left upper extremity claudication. *B*. After angioplasty with a 6-mm balloon, a residual intralesion stenosis and a vessel wall dissection prompted placement of a Palmaz balloon-expandable stent.

bolization "protection devices" to prevent thromboembolic complications may further expand the use of these procedures.[5]

Occlusive Disease of the Visceral Segment

Treatment of occlusive disease of the celiac, superior mesenteric and renal arteries can be accomplished successfully with full resolution of the underlying hemodynamically significant lesions and clinical improvement. Chronic intestinal ischemia secondary to celiac, superior, or inferior mesenteric artery occlusion and/or stenosis can have profound clinical results in select patients.[7,8] Both proximal and distal superior mesenteric artery lesions have been treated with isolated balloon angioplasty and more recently with the insertion of intravascular stents (Fig. 93-3 and Table 93-2). Despite sporadic reports of successful treatment of chronic mesenteric ischemia with endovascular treatments, comparative studies with standard surgical revascularization have not been performed.

The endoluminal treatment of renal artery stenosis has received considerable attention, particularly as improved stent technology has become available (Fig. 93-4). Early work with balloon dilatation of renal artery stenoses was limited by vessel dissections and early restenosis after treatment. This was especially true for ostial renal lesions, which probably are primarily of aortic atherosclerotic plaque origin. Recently, several careful prospective studies have demonstrated the technical effectiveness of renal stenting; however, questions remain about whether endovascular intervention for renal artery stenoses will positively affect the control of hypertension or the prevention of renal failure[9–13] (Table 93-3). Several ongoing trials may soon shed additional light on this area.[14]

Occlusive Disease of the Iliac, Femoral, Popliteal, and Tibial Arteries

Occlusive disease of the lower extremities represents a significant health problem, limiting function (ambulation) and creating significant risks for limb loss. Endovascular therapy of the iliac vessels, particularly the common iliac artery, has evolved to become standard treatment for this clinically significant problem.[15–19] Percutaneous transluminal angioplasty (PTA) with the use of supplemental stents can provide full relief of clinically

TABLE 93-1 Subclavian Artery Intervention

Type of Study	Reference	No. Vessels	Type of Lesion	Angioplasty (A) versus Stenting (S)	Technical Success, %	Follow-up, Months
Retrospective	2	43	Stenosis	A	84	15
Retrospective	3	55	Stenosis, arteritis	A	92.8	43
Retrospective	4	36	Stenosis	A	94	—

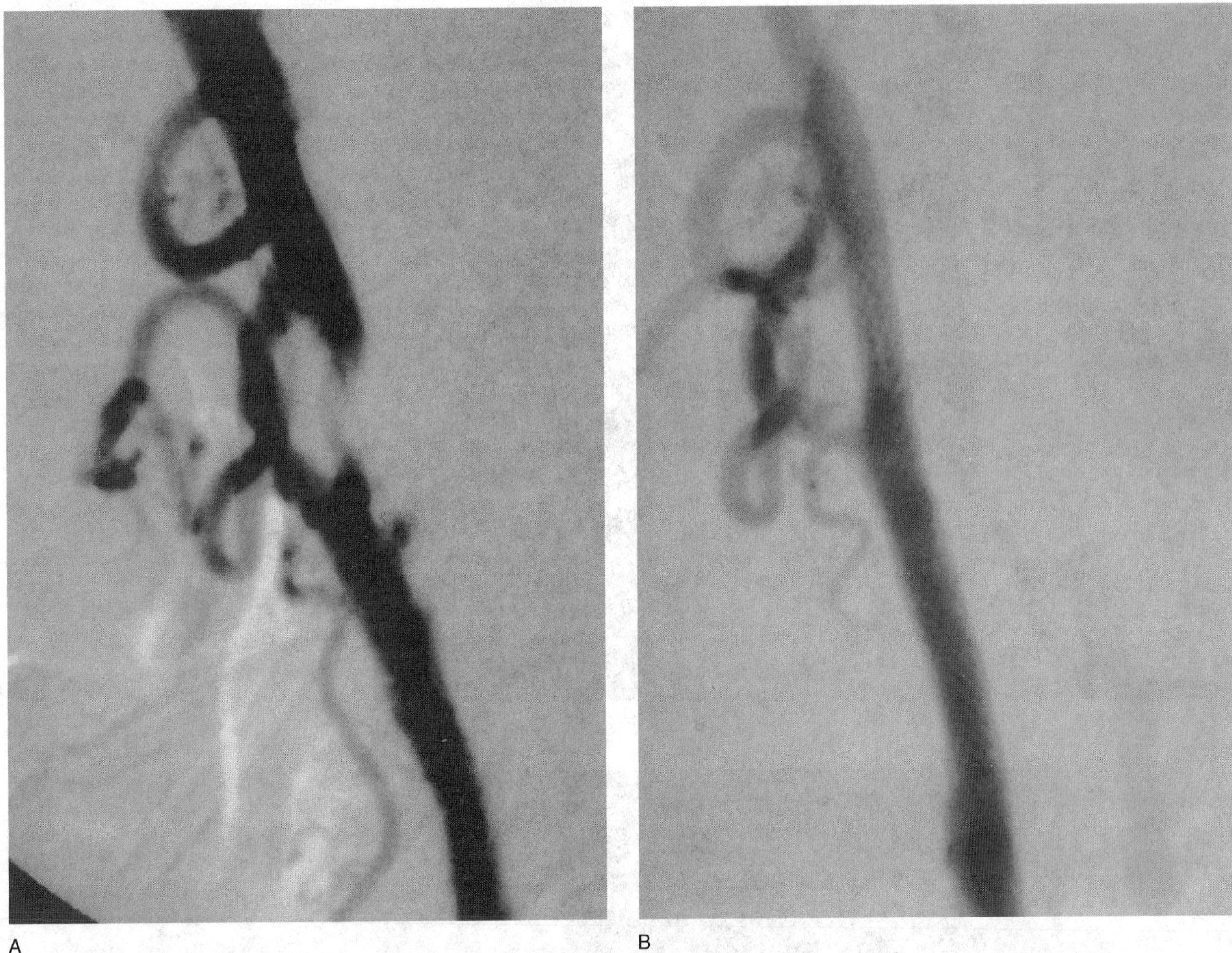

FIGURE 93-2 *A.* Carotid angiogram of an asymptomatic, high-grade left internal carotid artery stenosis. *B.* The lesion is corrected after treatment with balloon angioplasty and the implantation of a Wallstent.

important common iliac artery stenoses with good patency and relief of symptoms (Fig. 93-5 and Table 93-4).

The same results have not been fully achieved within the femoropopliteal segment of the vasculature. These regions tend to contain diffuse occlusive disease, and intervention in one isolated area of the superficial femoral or popliteal arteries often does not provide sufficient pressure gradient resolution to achieve symptomatic relief. When isolated focal lesions are present, angioplasty and occasionally stent implantation may give acceptable results (Fig. 93-6 and Table 93-5).[20–23] However, immediate successful endovascular treatment of the superficial femoral and popliteal arteries has commonly resulted in lesion restenosis or occlusion with the return of ischemic symptoms.

Some data suggest efficacy of PTA in select patients with tibial artery occlusive disease under the premise that limb salvage may be achieved, with even short-term restoration of the pedal circulation achieving the clearance of sepsis and the healing of wounds.[24–26] In select circumstances, extremities will remain healed and free from ischemic ulcers despite failure at the site of intervention (Table 93-6).

TABLE 93-2 Mesenteric Artery Intervention

Type of Study	Reference	No. Vessels	Type of Lesion	Angioplasty (A) versus Stenting (S)	Technical Success, %	Follow-up, Months
Retrospective	8	41	Stenosis	A	88	27
Retrospective	9	20	Stenosis	A	83	25

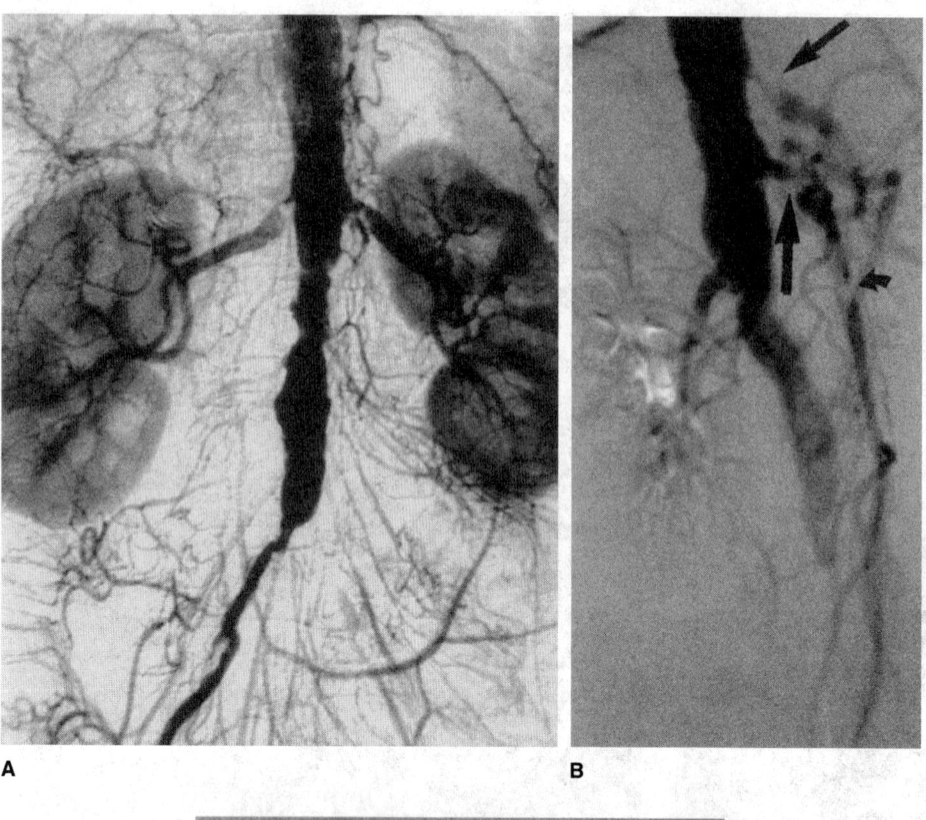

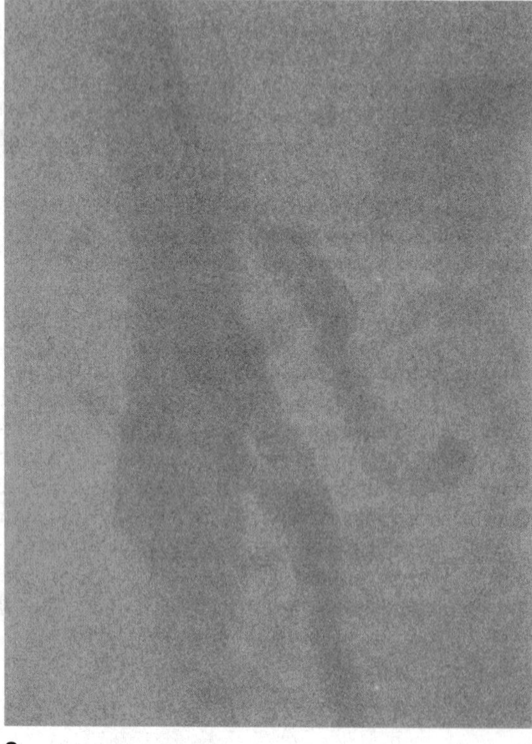

FIGURE 93-3 *A.* Mesenteric angiogram in a 69-year-old woman with a 40-lb weight loss over 16 months and severe postprandial abdominal pain. *B.* Proximal (*arrow*) and midsuperior mesenteric artery (*small arrow*) and celiac artery (*arrow*) stenoses are corrected by balloon angioplasty and Palmaz stent placement. *C.* Full resolution of abdominal symptoms and reestablishment of normal weight parameters accompanied recovery over a 4-month period after treatment.

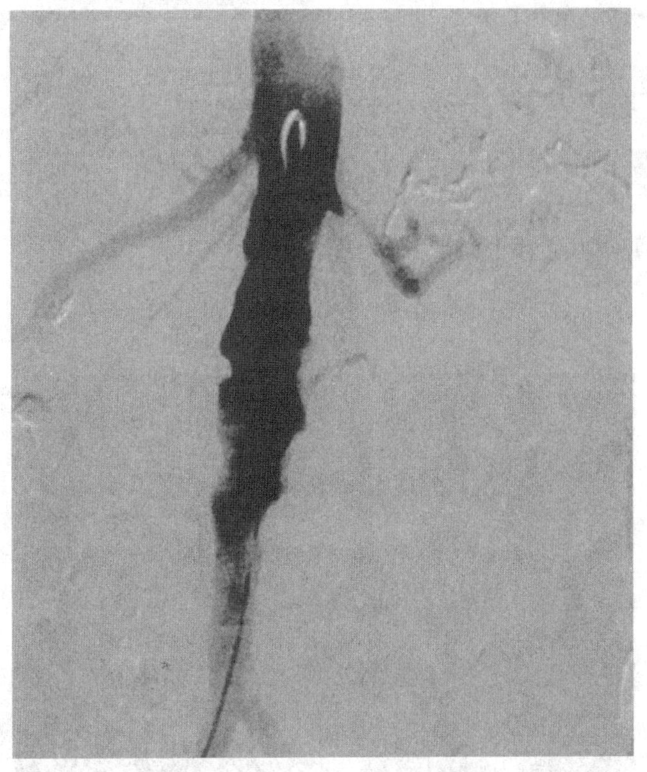
A

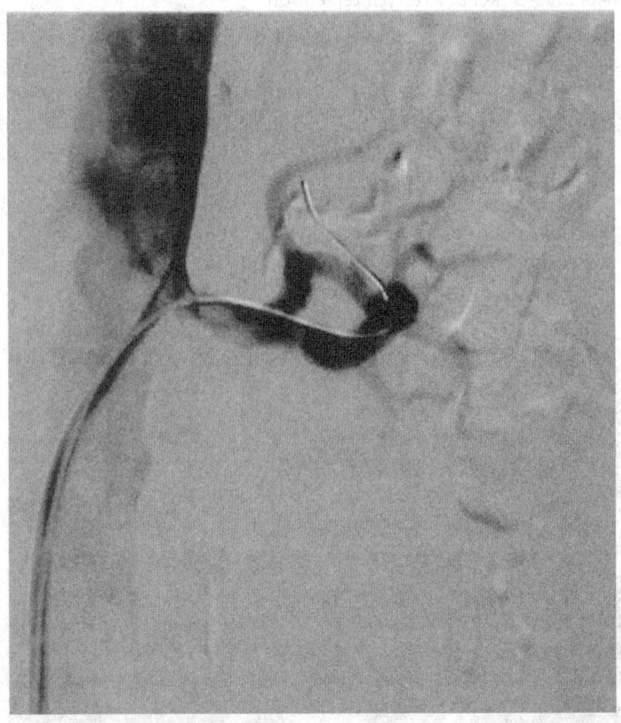
B

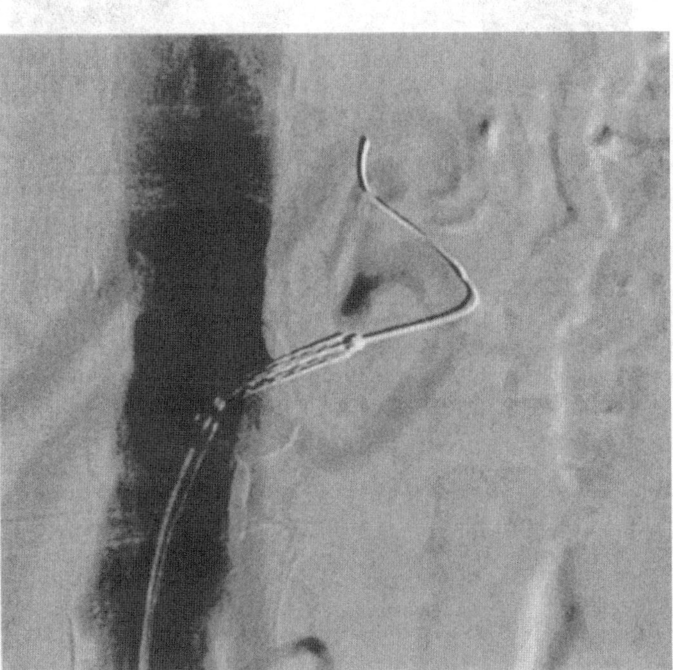
C

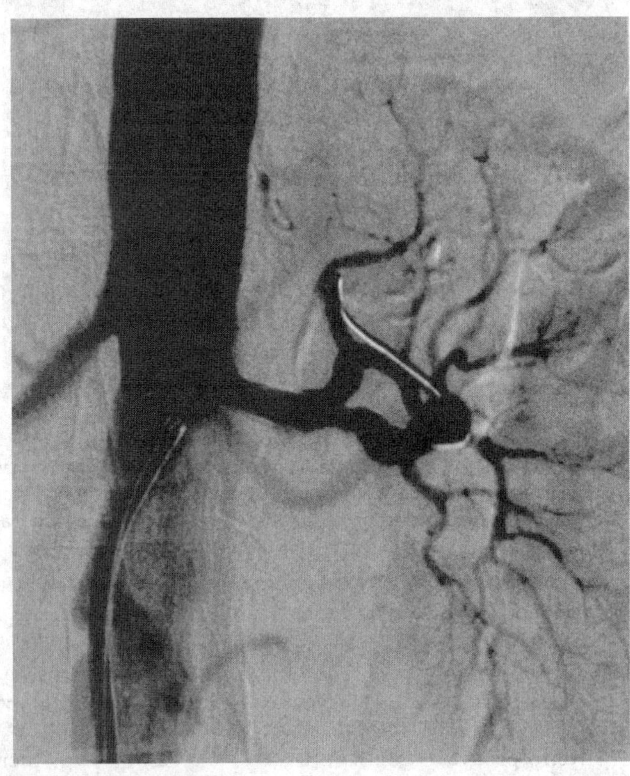
D

FIGURE 93-4 *A*. Aortogram demonstrating an isolated left renal artery stenosis in a 71-year-old woman with poorly controlled hypertension and normal renal function. *B*. Balloon angioplasty produced local dissection with residual stenosis. *C* and *D*. After implantation of an AVE stent in accordance with the SOAR trial protocol, full resolution of the hemodynamically significant lesion was achieved. The patient continues to require two medications to control her hypertension. (From Becquemin JP, Cavillon A, Haiduc F. Surgical transluminal femoropopliteal angioplasty: Multivariate analysis outcome. *J Vasc Surg* 1994; 19:495–502. Reproduced with permission from the publisher and authors.)

TABLE 93-3 Renal Artery Intervention

Type of Study	Reference	No. Vessels	Type of Lesion	Angioplasty (A) versus Stenting (S)	Technical Success, %	Follow-up, Months
Multicenter trial	10	120	Stenosis	A and S	98	8
Randomized trial	11	43	Stenosis	A and S	88	12
Retrospective	12	591	Stenosis, fibromuscular dysplasia	A	92	—
Retrospective	13	163	Stenosis	A and S	100	48
Prospective	14	74	Stenosis	A and S	100	27

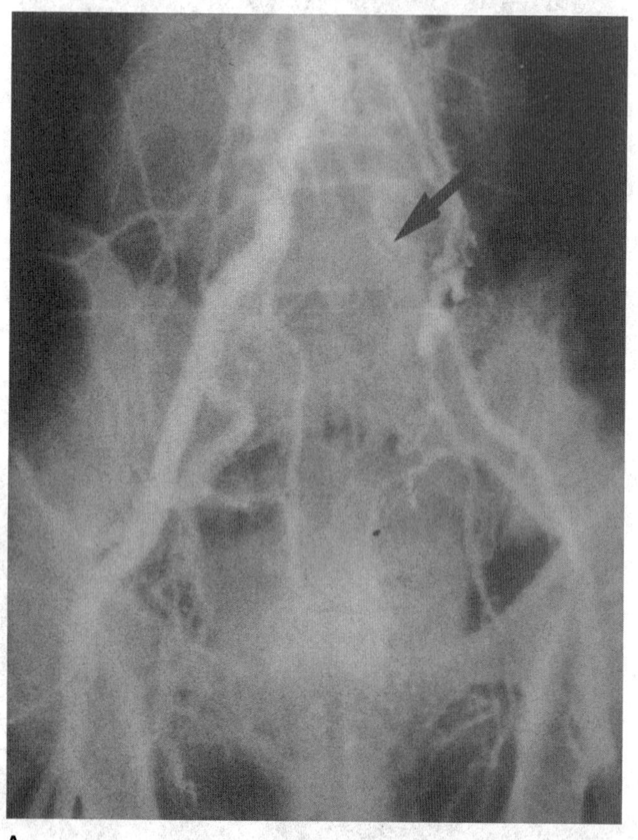

A

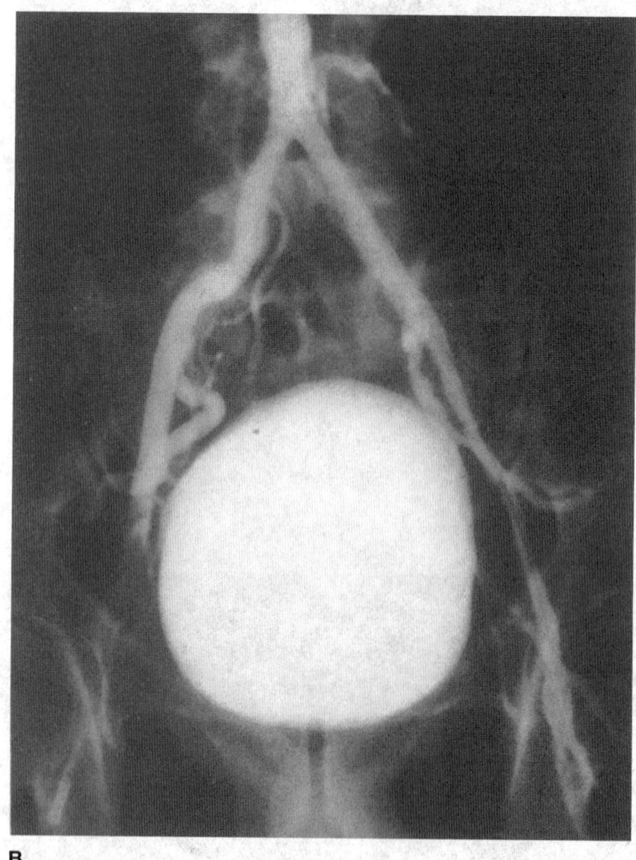

B

FIGURE 93-5 *A.* Aortogram with pelvic runoff views of a 61-year-old man with left thigh and buttock claudication and common iliac artery occlusion (*arrow*). *B.* After recannalization of the totally occluded left common iliac artery (*arrow*), normal flow was reestablished to the left leg with percutaneous balloon angioplasty and the placement of an iliac stent.

TABLE 93-4 Iliac Artery Intervention

Type of Study	Reference	No. Patients	Type of Lesion	Stent versus Angioplasty	Patency, %	Follow-up, Months
Retrospective	16	235	Stenosis/occlusive	NS*	75.4	60
Randomized trial	17	279	Stenosis/claudication	NS	78	24
Meta-analysis	18	2416†	Stenosis/claudication	NS	53	48
Multicenter trial	19	140	Stenosis/occlusive	Wallstent	71	24
Retrospective	20	238	Stenosis/occlusive	Palmaz	86	48

*NS = no significance.

†2416 patients from 14 different studies.

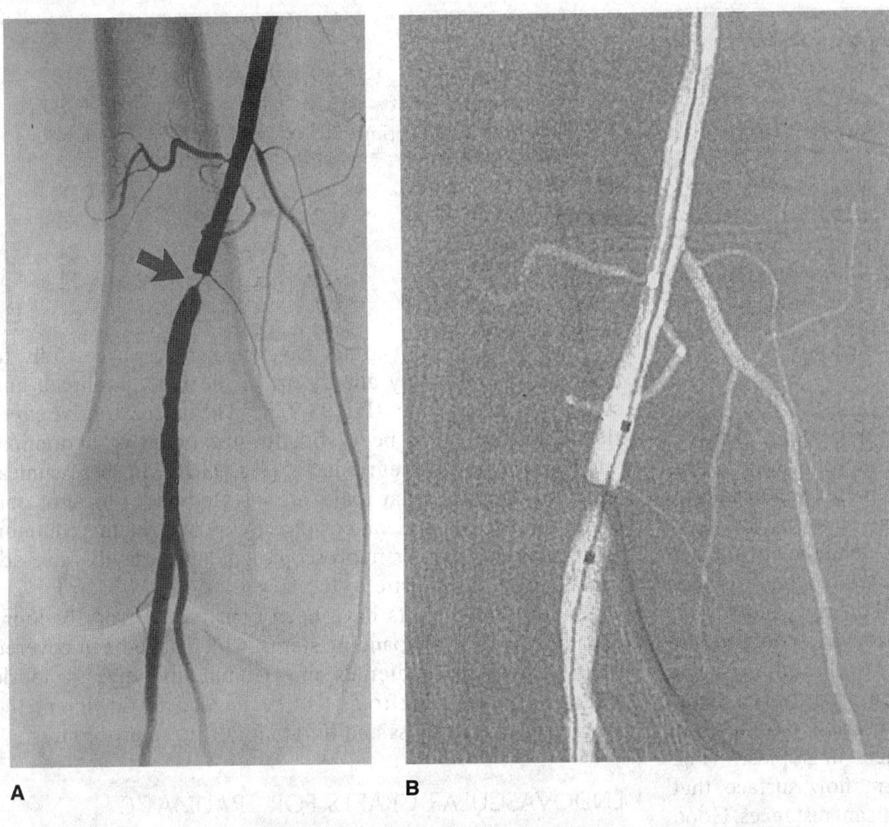

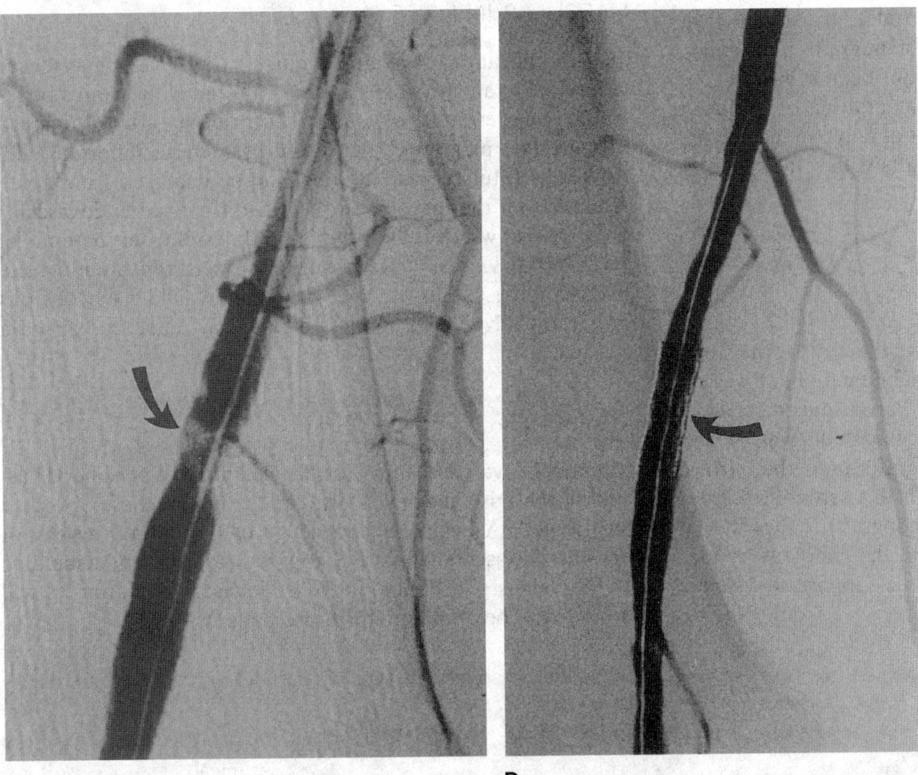

FIGURE 93-6 *A.* Angiogram of a high-grade right superficial femoral artery stenosis (*arrow*) in a 79-year-old insulin-dependent diabetic man with a right great toe infection. *B.* The isolated distal superficial femoral artery stenosis (~99%) was crossed with a balloon and dilated. *C.* Local dissection (*arrow*) and poor flow resulted. *D.* A Palmaz stent (*arrow*) repaired the dissection, with resulting good distal flow. The toe infection fully resolved; however, instent restenosis was demonstrated by ultrasonography at 6 months.

TABLE 93-5 Femoropopliteal Artery Intervention

Type of Study	Reference	No. Patients	Type of Lesion	Angioplasty (A) versus Stenting (S)	Patency, %	Follow-up, Months
Retrospective	21	96	Stenosis/occlusive	A	49	18
Retrospective	22	106	Stenosis/claudication	A	42	36
Multivariate	23	103	Stenosis	A	51	24
Retrospective	24	254	Stenosis/occlusive	A	35	72

Endovascular Stent Grafts for the Treatment of Occlusive Disease

The limitations of endoluminal therapy for treating occlusive disease occur when lesions are diffuse or multifocal, including extensive regions of the vasculature. In these circumstances, endovascular interventions are commonly not successful in achieving a durable repair. In an effort to blend the advantages of durable conventional bypass surgery employing vascular grafts with the unique traits of endoluminal therapy, endovascular stent grafts were developed.[27,28] These devices combine the unique properties of prosthetic grafts and metallic intravascular stents into a catheter-based system. When used for the treatment of occlusive disease, an endograft is inserted to completely reline a diseased vessel after long-segment angioplasty (Fig. 93-7). The endograft provides a uniform flow surface that may be extended endoluminally over significant distances. Good results have been achieved in the aortoiliac circulation (Fig. 93-8).[30] However, long-term patency of stent grafts in the superficial femoral or popliteal arteries has not been achieved.[30]

The different devices used for stent grafting of occlusive disease all employ varying combinations of polyester or polytetrafluoroethylene (PTFE) prosthetic grafts with self-expanding or balloon-expandable metallic stents.

ANEURYSMAL DISEASE OF THE AORTA AND PERIPHERAL ARTERIES

Clinical application of minimally invasive therapy for the treatment of aneurysmal disease of the aorta and peripheral vessels began in 1990 with the seminal work of Parodi and associates.[31] Expansion of the potential of intravascular stents was accomplished by the fixation of prosthetic grafts onto the surface of the metallic stent support system. In this setting, the stent functions to fix or "anastomose" the "endograft" to the internal surface of the vessel wall. By doing this, the endograft relines the vessel, assuming responsibility for the support of systemic blood pressure.

Endovascular stent grafts have been used successfully to treat peripheral artery aneurysms in the iliac, popliteal, and subclavian distributions (Fig. 93-9).[32–34] The most extensive experience, however, has been with the treatment of abdominal and thoracic aortic aneurysms[35–38] (Fig. 93-10). In these clinical situations, endovascular grafts are inserted under local or epidural anesthesia by means of direct exposure of the common femoral artery. Under fluoroscopic guidance, devices are advanced over a guidewire to the target lesion.

Endovascular grafts have been constructed from balloon-expandable or self-expanding stents, which have been covered by prosthetic graft materials, most commonly polyester fabric (Fig. 93-11). Ongoing trials will be needed to document the long-term effectiveness and durability of these procedures.

ENDOVASCULAR GRAFTS FOR TRAUMATIC VASCULAR INJURIES

The complication of a direct injury to an artery may occur secondary to an iatrogenic cause or, alternatively, from a penetrating missile or knife wound. The resulting arterial damage may produce an arterial pseudoaneurysm or an abnormal arteriovenous fistula. These injuries may be managed from a site remote from the injury with the insertion of an endovascular graft device, which relines the injured vessel from the luminal surface (Fig. 93-12).[39,40] Repairing the vessels from a remote site and avoiding surgery in the traumatized field have obvious important advantages for immediate and possible long-term success.

SUMMARY

Minimally invasive therapy for the treatment of peripheral vascular disease is changing the way patients with these disorders are treated. A complete knowledge of the natural history of peripheral vascular disease along with a clear understanding of the values and limitations of endovascular treatments will provide the best therapy for those patients.

TABLE 93-6 Tibial Artery Intervention

Type of Study	Reference	No. Vessels	Type of Lesion	Angioplasty (A) versus Stenting (S)	Technical Success, %	Follow-up, Months
Retrospective	25	417	Stenosis/occlusive	A	86	—
Retrospective	26	40	Stenosis	A	59	24
Retrospective	27	25	Stenosis	A	20	36

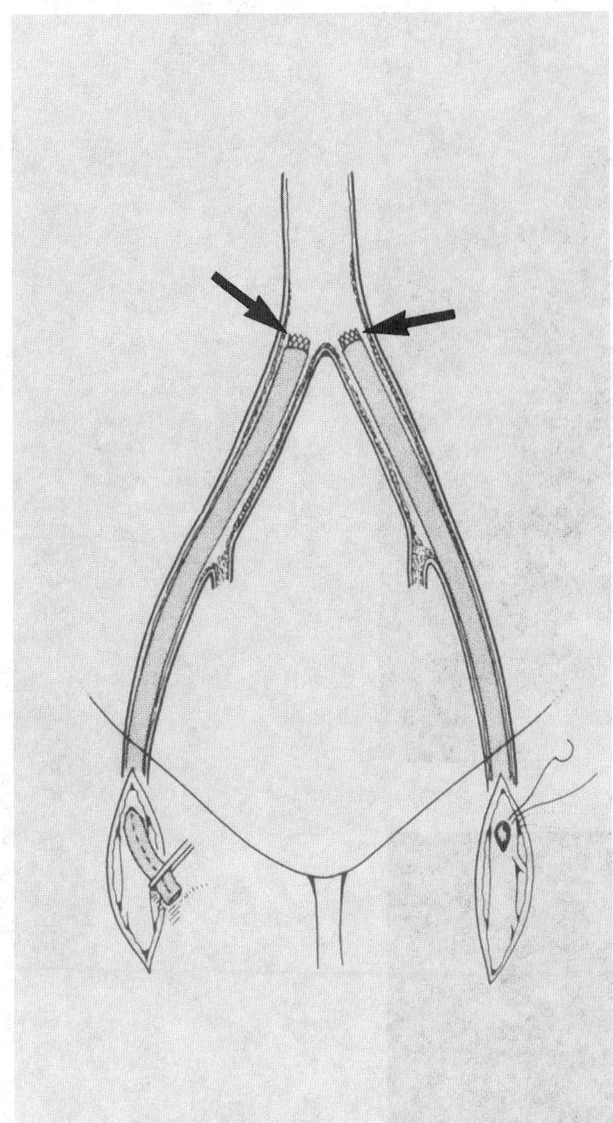

FIGURE 93-7 Artist's drawing of the technique for endovascular stent grafting of long-segment iliac artery occlusive disease. The diseased segment is recanalized with a hydrophilic guidewire. The entire diseased segment is dilated with a balloon angioplasty catheter. An endovascular stent graft is inserted to reline the diseased segment. The endograft is fixed ("anastomosed") to the proximal inflow artery with a metallic stent (*arrows*).

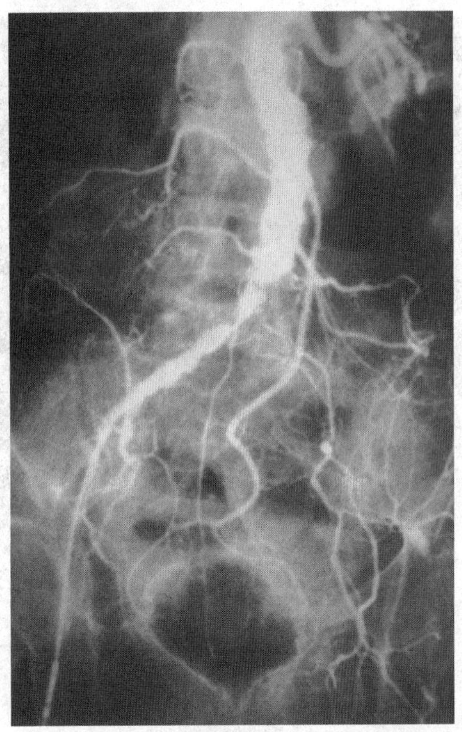

A

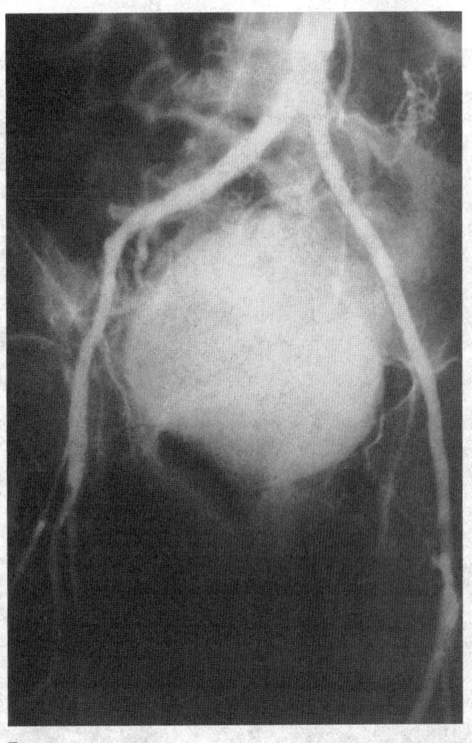

B

FIGURE 93-8 *A.* Aortogram from an 83-year-old diabetic man with limb-threatening ischemia of the left leg. Total left iliac occlusion is seen. *B.* Endovascular iliac stent graft insertion reestablished the circulation to the left leg. The right iliac stenoses were treated by balloon angioplasty.

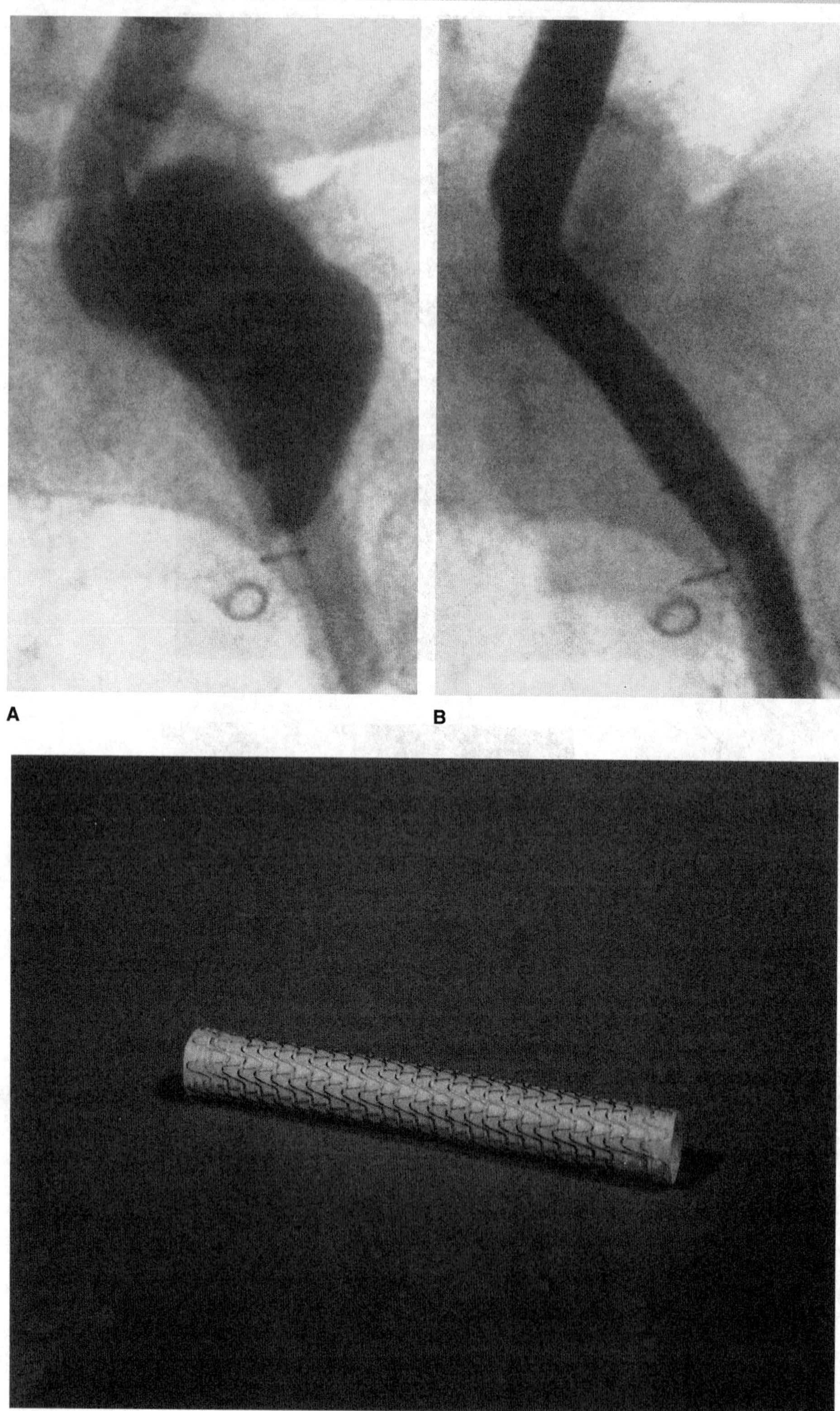

FIGURE 93-9 *A*. Angiogram of a 76-year-old man with an asymptomatic left common iliac artery aneurysm. *B*. After insertion of an endovascular stent graft, the aneurysm is fully excluded from the circulation. *C*. An example of an iliac endograft constructed from nitinol and ePTFE.

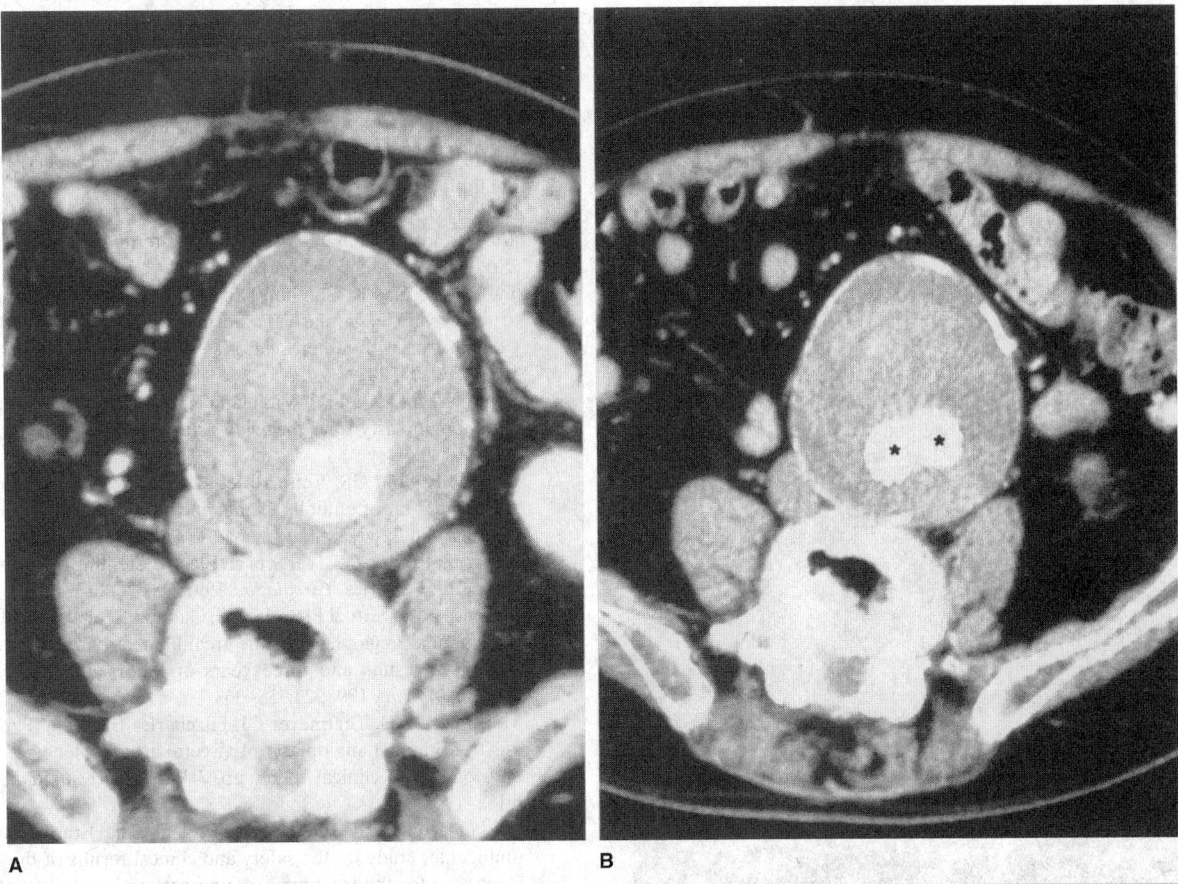

FIGURE 93-10 *A.* Computed tomography scan of a 73-year-old man demonstrated a 7-cm infrarenal abdominal aortic aneurysm. *B.* After insertion of an endovascular bifurcated stent graft, the aortic aneurysm is excluded. The two limbs of the graft are denoted with an asterisk.

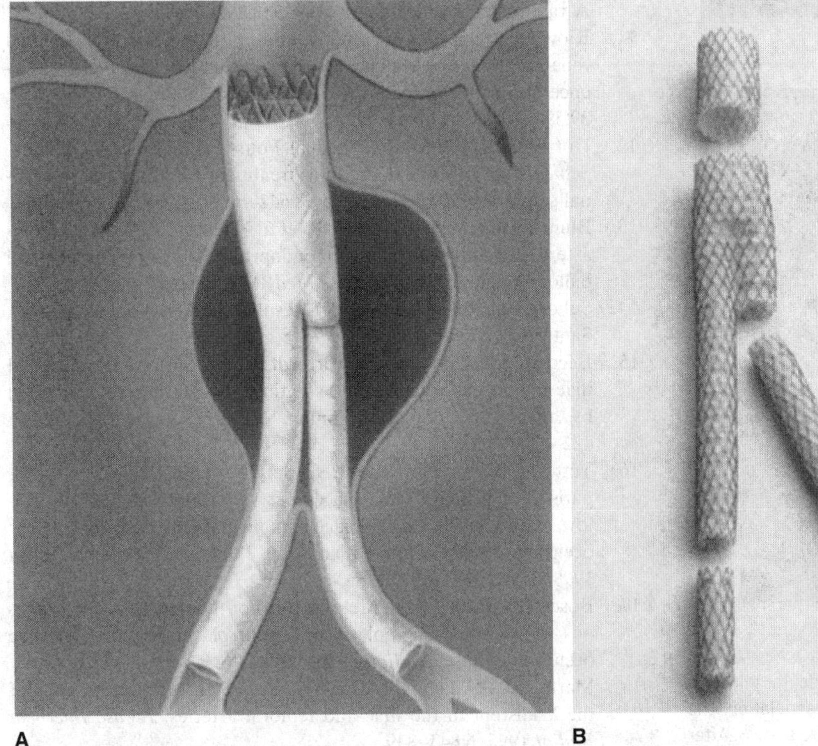

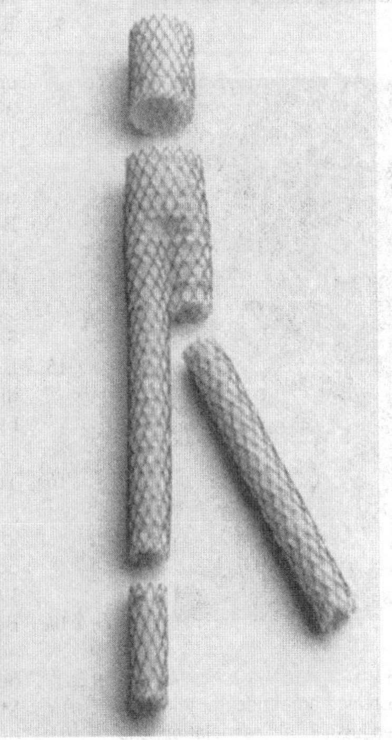

FIGURE 93-11 *A.* Photograph demonstrating the endovascular bifurcated graft technique for the treatment of abdominal aortic aneurysms. *B.* AneuRx bifurcated graft. This device combines polyester vascular graft material with a nitinol stent. Several modular pieces may be inserted to complete the reconstruction.

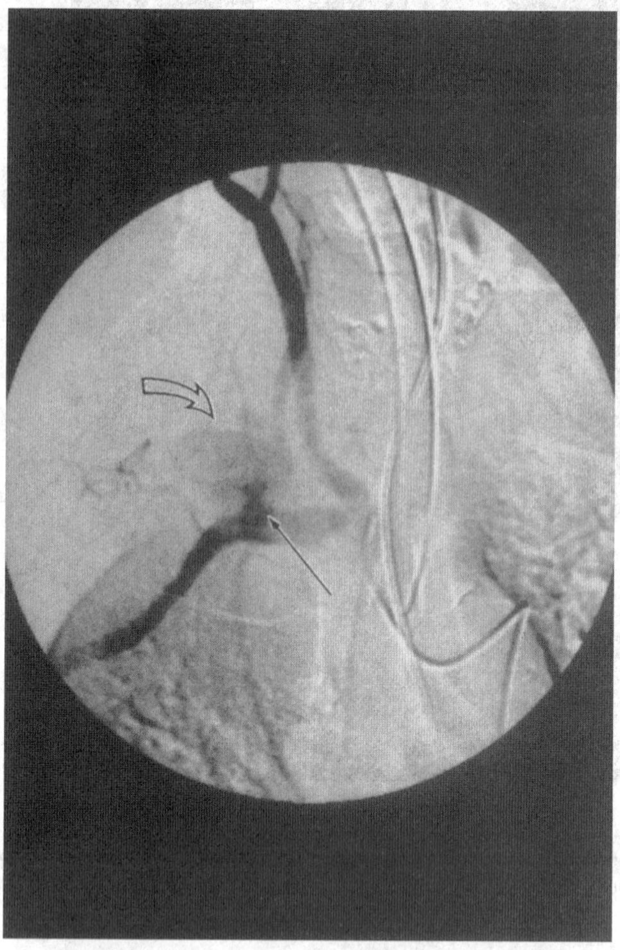

A

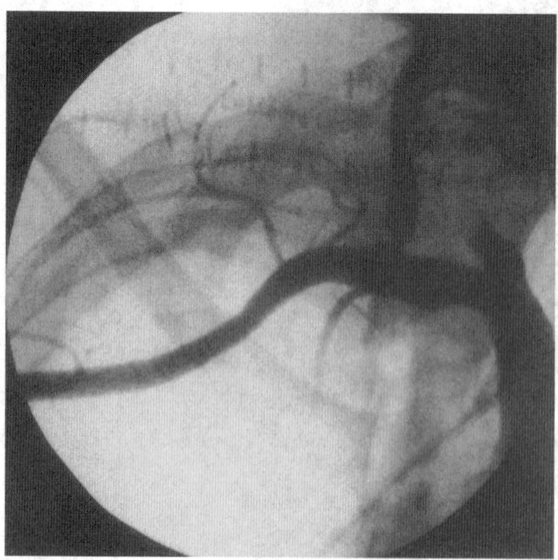

B

FIGURE 93-12 *A.* An 87-year-old woman sustained an accidental injury to the right subclavian artery during an attempted jugular vein cannulation. The site of injury (*arrow*) and the pseudoaneurysm (*open arrow*) are seen. *B.* After the insertion of a covered stent graft, the vessel injury is repaired.

References

1. Marin ML, Veith FJ. Endovascular surgery. In: Kerstein MD, White JV, eds. *Alternatives to Open Vascular Surgery*. Philadelphia: Lippincott; 1995:352.
2. Korner M, Baumgartner I, Do DD, et al. PTA of the subclavian artery and innominate arteries: Long-term results. *Vasa* 1999; 28:117–122.
3. Tyagi S, Verma PK, Gambhir DS, et al. Early and long-term results of subclavian angioplasty in aortoarteritis (Takayasu disease): Comparison with atherosclerosis. *Cardiovasc Intervent Radiol* 1998; 21:219–224.
4. Bogey WM, Demasi RJ, Vithalana R, et al. Percutaneous transluminal angioplasty for subclavian artery stenosis. *Am Surg* 1994; 60:103–106.
5. Ohki T, Roubin GS, Veith FJ, et al. Efficacy of a filter device in the prevention of embolic events during carotid angioplasty and stenting: An ex-vivo analysis. *J Vasc Surg* 1999; 30:1034–1044.
6. Yadar JS, Roubin GS, Iyer S, et al. Elective stenting of the extracranial carotid arteries. *Circulation* 1997; 95:376–381.
7. Maspes F, Mazzetti di Pietralata G, Gandini R, et al. Percutaneous transluminal angioplasty in the treatment of chronic mesenteric ischemia: Results and three years of follow-up in 23 patients. *Abdom Imaging* 1998; 23:358–363.
8. Matsumoto AH, Tegtmeyer CJ, Fitzcharles EK, et al. Percutaneous transluminal angioplasty of visceral arterial stenoses: Results and long-term, clinical follow-up. *J Vasc Intervent Radiol* 1995; 6:165–174.
9. Bakker J, Goffette PP, Henry M, et al. The Erasme study: A multicenter study on the safety and clinical results of the Palmaz stent used for the treatment of atherosclerotic ostial renal artery stenosis. *Cardiovasc Intervent Radiol* 1999; 22:468–474.
10. Van de Veb PJ, Kaatee R, Beutler JJ, et al. Arterial stenting and balloon angioplasty in ostial atherosclerotic renovascular disease: A randomized trial. *Lancet* 1999; 353:282–286.
11. Klow NE, Paulsen D, Vatne K, et al. Percutaneous transluminal renal artery angioplasty using coaxial technique: Ten years experience from 591 procedures in 419 patients. *Acta Radiol* 1998; 39:594–603.
12. Dorros G, Jaff M, Mathiak L, et al. Four year follow-up of Palmaz-Schatz stent revascularization as treatment for atherosclerotic renal stenosis. *Circulation* 1998; 98:642–647.
13. Blum U, Krumme B, Flugel P, et al. Treatment of ostial renal-artery stenoses with vascular endoprostheses after unsuccessful balloon angioplasty. *N Engl J Med* 1997; 336:459–465.
14. Suboptimal Renal Angioplasty Results (SOAR) Trial. AVE Inc., Santa Rosa, CA.
15. Becquemin JP, Allaire E, Qvarfordt P, et al. Surgical transluminal iliac angioplasty with selective stenting: Long-term results assessed by means of duplex scanning. *J Vasc Surg* 1999; 29(3): 422–429.
16. Tetteroo E, Van der Graaf Y, Bosch JL, et al. Randomized comparison of primary stent placement vs. primary angioplasty followed by selective stent placement in patients with iliac-artery occlusive disease: Dutch Iliac Stent Trial Study Group. *Lancet* 1998; 351:1153–1159.
17. Bosch JL, Hunink MG. Meta-analysis of the results of percutaneous transluminal angioplasty and stent placement for aortoiliac occlusive disease. *Radiology* 1997; 204:96–97.
18. Martin EC, Katzen BT, Benenati JF, et al. Multicenter trial of the Wallstent in the iliac and femoral arteries. *J Vasc Intervent Radiol* 1995; 6:843–849.
19. Henry M, Amor M, Ethevenot G, et al. Palmaz stent placement in iliac and femoropopliteal arteries: Primary and secondary patency in 310 patients with 2–4 year follow-up. *Radiology* 1995; 197:167–174.

20. O'Donohoe MK, Sultan S, Colgan MP, et al. Outcome of the first 100 femoropopliteal angioplasties performed in the operating theatre. *Eur J Vasc Endovasc Surg* 1999; 17:66–71.
21. Matsi PJ, Manninen HI. Impact of different patency criteria on long-term results of femoropopliteal angioplasty: Analysis of 106 consecutive patients with claudication. *J Vasc Intervent Radiol* 1995; 6:159–163.
22. Becquemin JP, Cavillon A, Haiduc F. Surgical transluminal femoropopliteal angioplasty: Multivariate analysis outcome. *J Vasc Surg* 1994; 19:495–502.
23. Johnston KW. Femoral and popliteal arteries: Reanalysis of results of balloon angioplasty. *Radiology* 1992; 183:767–771.
24. Dorros G, Jaff MR, Murphy KJ, et al. The acute outcome of tibioperoneal vessel angioplasty in 417 cases with claudication and critical limb ischemia. *Cathet Cardiovasc Diagn* 1998; 45:251–256.
25. Varty K, Bolia A, Naylor AR, et al. Infrapopliteal percutaneous transluminal angioplasty: A safe and successful procedure. *Eur J Vasc Endovasc Surg* 1995; 9:341–345.
26. Treiman GS, Treiman RL, Ichikawa L, et al. Should percutaneous transluminal angioplasty be recommended for the treatment of infrageniculate popliteal artery or tibioperoneal trunk stenosis? *J Vasc Surg* 1995; 22:457–463.
27. Marin ML, Veith FJ, Panetta TF, et al. Transfemoral stented graft treatment of occlusive arterial disease for limb salvage: A preliminary report. *Circulation* 1993; 88(4):1.
28. Cragg AH, Dake MD. Percutaneous femoropopliteal grafting: Report of a new technique (abstract). *J Vasc Intervent Radiol* 1993; 4:64.
29. Marin ML, Veith FJ, Sanchez LS, et al. Endovascular repair of aorto-iliac occlusive disease. *World J Surg* 1996; 20:679–686.
30. Cragg AH, Dake MD. Percutaneous femoropopliteal graft placement. *Radiology* 1993; 187:643–648.
31. Parodi JC, Palmaz JC, Barone HD. Transfemoral intraluminal graft implantation for abdominal aortic aneurysms. *Ann Vasc Surg* 1991; 5:491–499.
32. Marin ML, Veith FJ, Panetta TF, et al. Transfemoral endoluminal stented graft repair of a popliteal artery aneurysm. *Am J Surg* 1994; 19:754–757.
33. Marin ML, Veith FJ, Lyon RT, et al. Transfemoral endovascular repair of iliac artery aneurysms. *Am J Surg* 1995; 170:179–182.
34. Parsons RE, Marin ML, Veith FJ, et al. Midterm results of endovascular stented grafts for the treatment of isolated iliac artery aneurysms. *J Vasc Surg* 1999; 30:915–921.
35. Blum U, Voshage G, Lanmer J, et al. Endoluminal stent grafts for infrarenal abdominal aortic aneurysms. *N Engl J Med* 1997; 336:13–20.
36. Marin ML, Veith FJ, Cynamon J, et al. Initial experience with transluminally placed endovascular grafts for the treatment of complex vascular lesions. *Ann Surg* 1999; 222:449–469.
37. Dake MD, Miller DC, Semba CP, et al. Transluminal placement of endovascular stent grafts for the treatment of descending thoracic aortic aneurysms. *N Engl J Med* 1994; 331:1729–1734.
38. Temudom T, D'Ayala M, Marin ML, et al. Endovascular grafts in the treatment of thoracic aortic aneurysms and pseudoaneurysms. *Ann Vasc Surg*, 2000; 14:230–238.
39. Marin ML, Veith FJ, Panetta TF, et al. Percutaneous transfemoral insertion of a stented graft to repair a traumatic femoral arteriovenous fistula. *J Vasc Surg* 1993; 18:299–302.
40. Marin ML, Veith FJ, Panetta TF, et al. Transluminally placed endovascular stented graft repair for arterial trauma. *J Vasc Surg* 1994; 20:466–473.

PART SIXTEEN

COST-EFFECTIVE STRATEGIES, INSURANCE, AND LEGAL PROBLEMS

CHAPTER 94

COST-EFFECTIVE STRATEGIES IN CARDIOLOGY

William S. Weintraub / Harlan Krumholz

A SOCIETAL PERSPECTIVE

How do society and individuals decide to allocate resources or spend money? In capitalist societies, the invisible hand of the market guides resource use, and in principle, regulators, generally governmental agencies, ensure a "level playing field" and prevent various forms of abuse but otherwise try to stay out of the way. Free markets are guided by a principle called *willingness to pay,* which economists define as that price, governed by supply and demand, which consumers are willing to pay for a service.[1] Services in society that are deemed a "right," such as education, are not governed by free markets, since society may view that all people have a right to such services, independent of their ability to pay. Medicine is largely, although not entirely, in the class of a "right," more like education than a good governed by willingness to pay such as automobiles. When a service is not priced by willingness to pay, naturally there will be concern over how to fairly price or value it and how much of it to buy. The *value* of a service can be defined as its fair cost. The concern for value in medicine is a major societal issue. We can define *value* in health care as good care at a fair price. Whether society is achieving value in health care is a major issue all over the world.

Health care expenditures in the United States have risen dramatically in the last half of the twentieth century. Between 1960 and 1997, federal health care expenditures rose from $2.9 billion to $367 billion, and total national expenditures rose from $28.65 billion to $1.09 trillion[2] (Fig. 94-1). This represents an increase in percentage of gross national product over this period from 5.1 to 13.5 percent. This unprecedented and unparalleled increase in expense for one sector of the American economy is placing American medicine in considerable peril. The Health Care Financing Agency (HCFA) expects expenditures to double in the next 10 years, reaching 16.2 percent of the gross domestic product. The Hospital Insurance (HI) program, or Medicare Part A, pays for hospital, home health, skilled nursing, and hospice care for the aged and disabled, insuring about 39 million people in 1998. The HI program, financed primarily by

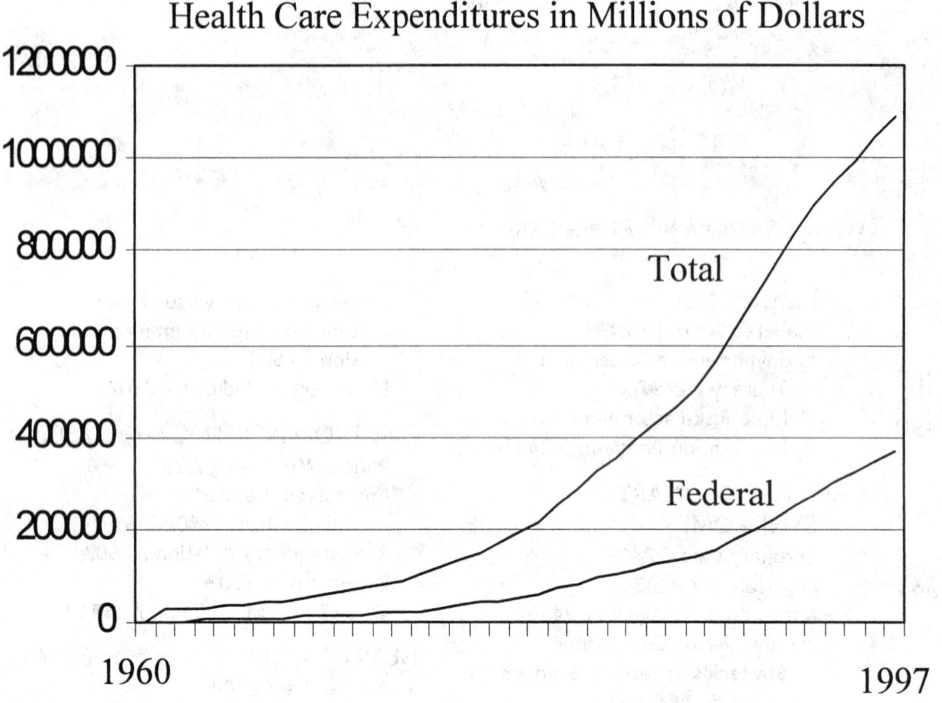

FIGURE 94-1 Increasing costs of medical services over time.

payroll taxes, mainly pays benefits for current beneficiaries, with leftover income held in a trust fund invested in U.S. Treasury securities.

A board of trustees, created by Congress, oversees annual reports on the financial status of the HI trust fund. As of 1999, income exceeds expenditures and is expected to do so for 8 more years, and by drawing down on the trust fund, benefits could continue for several years. However, given current assumptions, the HI trust fund will be depleted in 2015. In addition, there will be relatively fewer people paying and more people consuming HI resources as the population ages. It is expected that there will be 3.6 workers per HI beneficiary when the baby boom generation begins to reach age 65 in 2010, declining to 2.3 by 2030 as the last of the baby boomers reaches age 65. Current public policy has not adequately addressed how to manage the future financial status of Medicare in the United States.

Cardiovascular disease consumes substantial societal resources in economically advantaged countries and thus is responsible for a considerable part of the projected economic challenges in the future. In the United States alone, the American Heart Association estimates that the cost of cardiovascular disease in 1999 will total $286.5 billion[3] (Table 94-1). Of this total, $178.2 billion will be related to direct consumption of medical resources, and an additional $108.3 billion will be related to lost productivity due to early death and disability. Costs related to coronary artery disease (CAD) lead the other categories at $99.8 billion, but this is just a little over a third of the total. Given its magnitude, there is a strong societal interest that the $178.2 billion in direct costs is spent wisely and that the $108.3 billion in lost productivity is minimized. The field of health care economics has developed to address these societal issues.

BACKGROUND ON ECONOMIC ANALYSES

In an environment of limited resources, different societal needs compete for resources. If resources were not limited, then medical care could be provided based on clinical outcome alone, no matter how small the benefit. In such a world of inexhaustible resources, it would be reasonable to provide a treatment that benefited only 1 of every million or 10 million or 100 million individuals screened or treated. Since this is no longer and perhaps never was entirely the case, new forms of diagnostic testing and therapies, as well as existing ones, have to be justified on both an effectiveness and an economic basis. The problems of assessment of costs and comparison with outcome are especially relevant and complicated when expensive forms of therapy are used commonly and have multiple complex and interrelating indices of their effectiveness. Within medicine, these issues are perhaps most relevant to cardiovascular care because of the vast array of diagnostic and therapeutic strategies, as well as the high cost and the diversity of outcome measures.

Frequently, costs are compared between competing forms of therapeutic or diagnostic strategies. This comparison can involve performing a simulation in which costs and outcome are estimated from the literature, nonrandomized comparisons, and randomized trials. Even within randomized trials, an economic analysis can range from a simulation to a very detailed component of the trial with extensive primary data collection. For any of these designs, the simplest type of economic study is a comparison of costs, or a cost-minimization study. Such a study is useful when it is reasonable to assume that two treatment or diagnostic arms offer similar outcomes to one another.

There are three related forms of economic analyses that can be used to study relative efficacies and relative costs: cost-effectiveness, cost-utility, and cost-benefit. *Cost-effectiveness analysis measures the cost per unit of effectiveness.*[4] This form of analysis assumes that there is one overall measure of effectiveness, often survival. This method breaks down when there are multiple measures of effectiveness. For instance, one form of therapy may increase the risk of death but offer improved symptomatic status. This may, in principle, be addressed through *cost-utility analysis, in which all measures of effectiveness are incorporated into one measure called utility.*[4] Utility, however, is a very difficult parameter to measure, as will be discussed below. A third and somewhat less popular form of analysis is *cost-benefit analysis, in which measures of both cost and effectiveness are reduced to a single measure, generally dollars (or other currency).*[4] While cost-benefit analysis has not been popular in medicine due to the inherent difficulty of expressing

TABLE 94-1 Estimated Direct and Indirect Costs of Cardiovascular Diseases and Stroke, United States, 1999

	Heart Disease†	Coronary Heart Disease	Stroke	Hypertensive Disease	Congestive Heart Failure	Total Cardiovascular Disease*
DIRECT COSTS						
Hospital/nursing home	$76.4	$40.7	$24.2	$7.1	$15.0	$124.3
Physicians/other professionals	13.8	7.7	2.2	7.7	1.4	26.8
Drugs	6.6	3.2	0.3	8.1	1.0	16.0
Home health/other medical durables	5.0	1.5	2.8	1.5	2.1	11.1
Total expenditures*	$101.8	$53.1	$29.5	$24.5	$19.6	$178.2
INDIRECT COSTS						
Lost productivity/morbidity	16.5	6.9	5.4	5.0	NA	26.5
Lost productivity/mortality	64.8	39.8	10.4	3.8	1.4	81.8
Grand total*	$183.1	$99.8	$45.3	$33.3	$21.0	$286.5

*Totals may not add up due to rounding and overlap.
†This category includes coronary heart disease, congestive heart failure, and part of hypertensive disease as well as other "heart" diseases.
SOURCE: Direct costs were extrapolated from estimates for 1997 by Thomas A. Hodgson, chief economist and acting director, Division of Health and Utilization Analysis, OAEHP, CDC/NCHS. Estimates of indirect costs were made by Thomas J. Thom, statistician in the division of Epidemiology and Clinical Applications, NHLBI.

clinical outcome in monetary terms, it is, at least in theory, the most generalizable of these methods.

We can begin to understand the approach of cost-effectiveness analysis by considering two competing therapies (or tests), A and B, to treat (or diagnose) the same condition, as considered in Fig. 94-2. In the upper left-hand corner in panel 1, therapy A is more effective and less expensive than therapy B. In this setting, A is said to dominate B. Similarly in panel 4, A is less effective and more expensive than B. In this setting, B would dominate A. Commonly, however, the more effective therapy or test is also more expensive. Thus in panel 2, A is more effective but also more expensive. Similarly, in panel 3, B is more effective but also more expensive. In such a common

1: Therapy A vs B More Effective, Less Expensive	2: Therapy A vs B More Effective, More Expensive
3: Therapy A vs B Less Effective, Less Expensive	4: Therapy A vs B Less Effective, More Expensive

FIGURE 94-2 Decision matrix.

clinical situation, where a form of therapy or a test is both more effective and more expensive than a competing therapy or test, cost-effectiveness analysis can help society decide whether to allocate resources to the more effective service.

The perspective in these analyses can have an important impact on their structure and outcome. An analysis from a hospital's perspective may not include the long-term consequences of a particular clinical strategy, whereas this issue may be most important to the patient and the payer. Also, different stakeholders place different values on the outcomes and costs of medical care. For instance, physicians and patients traditionally have been more concerned about effectiveness, whereas employers and insurance companies have been more concerned about costs.

The perspective of all the various stakeholders may be viewed in aggregate as "society." To be most useful in serving societal goals, cost and cost-effectiveness analyses should be performed from a societal perspective. From a societal perspective, an economic analysis should attempt to measure all the costs and measures of outcome associated with a particular treatment. These costs should include those incurred by the patient, the costs of medical resources that could have been used for other patients, and any loss of income that the patient sustained because of poor health. Outcome should include events, quality of life, and survival. By looking at the sum of all these costs in relation to outcome, a policymaker could decide, for example, whether the public good benefited more by allocating limited health care resources to a lipid screening program or to coronary revascularization.

While it is possible, in theory, to line up the cost-effectiveness of multiple procedures into what are called *league tables,* limitations in data quality and variability in study design limit the wide applicability of such efforts.[5] An effort to create league tables was attempted in Oregon, with cost-effectiveness used to guide whether a form of therapy or a test would be funded.

This experiment was criticized and finally abandoned because of the limited amount and quality of data available, as well as concern over whether the approach was appropriate.[6] Far more common are cost-effectiveness analyses that compare two alternative treatments for a single medical condition, e.g., percutaneous transluminal angioplasty (PTCA) and coronary artery bypass grafting (CABG) for symptomatic angina. Such analyses examine the incremental cost-effectiveness of CABG compared with PTCA. In addition to focusing on a single clinical condition, the analyses most commonly limit the measured costs to direct and some portion of indirect medical costs. The purpose of these analyses is not to dictate a decision but to inform the decision-making process.

DETERMINING COSTS

Taxonomy for Costs

When considering a procedure or form of therapy, it is common to ask what it costs. An economic perspective on cost is more theoretical.[7] Economists are more concerned with how society chooses to allocate limited resources rather than with what something costs per se. Cost may be used to sum resource use when a procedure or test uses resources of several types and to permit comparison of costs between services. To accomplish the end of summarizing resource use to arrive at cost, accounting methods are used. Cost accounting has a particular taxonomy, as shown in Table 94-2.

Costs must be considered from one of several possible perspectives.[8] Thus, for a hospital, the cost is the expenses to provide a service. For payers, the cost is what the providers charge, plus their administrative expenses. In principle, cost studies often seek to determine societal costs, which should be used in cost-effectiveness analyses to gain the widest perspective. However, societal costs are never directly measurable, and thus combinations of cost proxies from one or several stakeholders, where measurable, often are used as estimates.

Costs are classified as direct or indirect.[9] Definitions of indirect costs may lead to uncertainty categorizing a particular cost. Theoretically, *direct costs* are those incurred by a stakeholder for a therapy or test, and *indirect costs* are those incurred by other societal groups. Generally, direct costs relate to the provision of medical care, whereas indirect costs are other societal costs.

TABLE 94-2 Summary of Taxonomy for Costs

- Cost perspective
  - Provider, i.e., hospital or professional
  - Payer, i.e., insurance carrier
  - Patient
- Cost category
  - Direct costs
  - Indirect costs
- Accounting method
  - Top-down
  - Bottom-up
- Costs per service
  - Average cost
  - Marginal (incremental) cost

Medical costs for a procedure such as coronary surgery can be divided into three components: in-hospital direct costs, follow-up direct costs, and indirect costs. In-patient costs comprise hospital costs (e.g., room, laboratory testing, pharmacy, etc.) and physician professional billings. Follow-up direct costs include physician office visits, outpatient testing, medications, home health providers, and additional hospitalizations. Indirect costs reflect lost patient or business opportunity or productivity costs and may be referred to as *productivity costs*.[10]

A final way of thinking about costs is that direct costs are realistically linked to a particular service, whereas indirect costs are not. This type of indirect cost is also called *overhead*.[11]

The appropriate length of time over which to measure costs depends on the procedures being studied and outcomes being measured. Thus the cost of angioplasty could be considered to be the costs of the initial hospitalization and over the first 6 months when restenosis commonly would occur. Alternatively, the cost of angioplasty could be considered the initial hospitalization alone, and the costs during the initial 6 months could be considered follow-up or induced costs, which are those generated beyond the specific time of service delivery.[12] Induced costs also could be a savings. For instance, there may be savings for stents relative to balloon angioplasty in follow-up due to less additional revascularization.

Typically, in the United States, hospital costs are used as a proxy for societal costs. What a hospital charges for a service is not its cost.[13] Measuring hospital cost is difficult and has been approached using what is called either *top-down* or *bottom-up accounting*.[14] Top-down costing involves dividing all the money spent on a hospitalization or procedure by the number of episodes of care of the particular type performed. A payer perspective would be the amount the payer pays the provider for the service. In contrast, a bottom-up approach involves individually costing all resources used for a service, i.e., supplies, equipment depreciation and facilities, salaries, etc. All methods involve a set of assumptions and limitations. When considering the cost of a specific procedure using top-down costing, it must be assumed that costs in the department in which the procedure is provided can be separated from costs in other departments. For instance, it is not clear that the cardiac catheterization laboratory costs can be clearly separated from hospital maintenance costs. There also may be variability within a department. Therefore, using identical methods to calculate the costs of angioplasty and diagnostic catheterization may not be appropriate if angioplasty consumes more resources in a period of time, such as technician time. Bottom-up methods also are limited by the ability to account for all resources consumed and to appropriately apply costs.

Another issue in measuring hospital costs is average versus marginal or incremental cost.[15] Average cost is calculated by dividing all costs for a therapy or test by the number of that particular type. In contrast, the marginal cost is the cost of the next similar procedure. Average costs include all resources used, including overhead, whose costs would not be decreased if not used. Marginal costing accepts fixed costs as a given and focuses only on variable costs or those additional resources consumed by each additional patient. Variable costs are separated analytically from fixed costs by establishing the perspective and time frame as fixed. For instance, facilities' cost is commonly considered fixed, but how should marginal personnel costs be assigned? If coronary surgery decreases as angioplasty becomes more common, do the operating room nurses remain on staff in the operating room, or will they be assigned to other duties? Because of these difficulties, most cost and cost-effectiveness studies use average costs.

Cost Measurement

Commonly used at nonfederal hospitals in the United States, there is a particularly detailed approach to top-down costing that is based on the UB92 summary of charges.[16] The UB92 is a uniform billing statement used by all third-party carriers. Charges are available for, but not limited to, such services as the surgical suite, cardiac catheterization laboratory, intensive care unit, postoperative or postprocedural floor care, respiratory therapy, supplies, electrocardiogram (ECG), telemetry, social services, etc. While hospitals will set their charges to maximize insurance reimbursements, the relationship between costs and charges, in the form global specific cost-to-charge ratios, must be developed using American Hospital Association guidelines and then filed annually with HCFA in the form of a hospital cost report, which is in the public domain.

An alternative approach is to use bottom-up cost accounting and assign cost weights to each type of resource used.[17] The sum of resources times their cost weights yields total cost. However, the methods are sufficiently laborious that they are rarely used.

Another approach is to use a payer perspective.[18] In the United States, Medicare diagnosis-related group (DRG) reimbursement rates could be used to define cost. Similar methods are available in other countries. The use of DRGs to assign cost does not account for variation in cost within that DRG and may not even reflect average resource use. While it is an excellent measure of cost from the point of view of governmental agencies, it probably does not represent as meaningful a proxy for societal cost as do provider level hospital costs.

Assessing professional medical costs is challenging. It is not sufficient to consider physicians' fees alone, since other professionals provide services.[19,20] The goal must be to capture all the professional services for a procedure. For coronary surgery, this may include such fees as the surgeon and assistants; the consultant cardiologist; and anesthesia, radiology, clinical pathology, professional components of any other testing, and any other consultants or ancillary services.[21] There is no cost-to-charge ratio, analogous to the situation for the hospital, available for physician fees to convert their charges to costs.

In the United States, there has been an effort to rationalize physician payments by developing a set of scales for services.[22] This system, the resource-based relative value scale (RBRVS), was developed over time to try to assess the relative time, physical, and cognitive efforts associated with physician services.[22] Each service is assigned a number called the relative value unit (RVU). If the profile of physician services for a procedure or hospitalization is known, then RVUs for each service may be used to develop a proxy for the physician costs. The total RVUs may be converted to a dollar figure by a conversion factor. HCFA, the federal agency that administers Medicare and Medicaid, has a standard conversion factor. The appeal of the RBRVS is that it is a relative weighting system that assigns unique weights for physician work and practice costs for each physician service by Current Procedural Terminology (CPT) code. As a result, after assigning a conversion factor, standardized estimates of the costs can be calculated and used as a gauge of physician costs. While there are still some problems with this approach, especially for the practice cost values in the RBRVS, it holds considerable promise and overcomes some of the major drawbacks of physician charge data.

Determining the costs of outpatient services presents different challenges in determining patient services use, including direct and indirect medical costs. Direct costs include physician office visits, medications, procedures and testing, rehabilitation, nursing home stays, and home health services, as well as patient out-of-pocket expenses, including travel. Assessment of these costs is difficult and complicated by insurance, since patients cannot be expected to reliably respond to how much they paid out of pocket for services and how much the insurance company paid for services. Unless there is access to a comprehensive insurance claims database, the most reasonable approach is to have patients identify the services they have received. Costs can then be attributed to the individual services and medications. Office visits and other medical services costs may be similarly estimated. Professional services can be estimated using the Medicare fee schedule, as discussed earlier. Medication costs can be estimated from compiled prices by sampling pharmacies or using published wholesale pharmaceutical prices. Using these cost estimates, a partial simulation of postdischarge direct costs may be determined.

Indirect productivity costs include missed time from work by the patient or family members. Follow-up indirect costs probably are the most difficult to determine and often are excluded as immeasurable. In any case, it is not possible to directly measure all the indirect costs. For instance, if an executive in a company has coronary surgery and is out of work for 6 weeks, there may or may not be loss of pay, but the effect on the business cannot be determined readily. Indirect costs, if measured at all, often are confined to family loss of income, and the numbers must be examined with both interest and skepticism.

Over a long time horizon, inflation must be considered. Costs must be inflated or deflated by multiplying by a constant to convert from any one year to another, based on the medical inflation rate.[23] Future costs also should be discounted to reflect the opportunity costs of current dollars, or future costs should be expressed at their present value.[24] For instance, if a policymaker were given the alternative of spending $1000 now or $1000 in 5 years to treat a given condition and obtain the same outcome, the decision would always be the latter. Costs generally are discounted at a rate of 3 percent per year.[24]

Variation in Cost

Variation in cost for a service arises from either differences in the type of measurement, as discussed earlier, or differences in resource use. Table 94-3 presents a framework for considering variation in medical costs, according to quality of care, patient, and geographic levels. These levels do not separate clearly, providing a somewhat confusing picture of the sources of variation.

TABLE 94-3 Sources of Variation in Cost

Quality of care
1. Process: Access, appropriateness, management
2. Structure: Facilities, supplies, staffing
3. Outcome: Iatrogenic complications, patients' health status

Patient level
1. Demographic: Age, sex, race
2. Disease severity: Extent of left ventricular dysfunction or severity of coronary atherosclerosis
3. Comorbidity: Cardiac or noncardiac
4. Outcome: Noniatrogenic complications, patients' health status

Geographic and non-medical economic factors
1. Facilities
2. Supplies
3. Labor

Quality of care is often broken down into the subunits of process, structure, and outcome.[25] These components of quality also may be viewed as reflecting variation in cost. For process measures of access and appropriateness, the effect on cost may be less on the individual service and more at the societal level for provision of that service. Thus, if access to coronary surgery is inadequate, the initial cost to society of coronary surgery may fall as fewer surgeries are performed, but costs may rise due to induced costs or productivity costs of failing to perform necessary surgery. However, if access to adequate diabetes care is inadequate, there may be an increase in the cost to society of inadequately treated diabetes. Similarly, if inappropriate angioplasty is being performed, then the societal cost will rise, even if the individual service is little affected. Management, on the other hand, will affect the individual service. Accordingly, if a service is handled efficiently with care maps to decrease unnecessary resource use of an overall service, such as excessive blood drawing after coronary surgery and an organized and early discharge, then costs can be decreased. Variation in management will cause variation in cost; thus, if there is variation of use of major services, such as cardiac catheterization after hospitalization for unstable angina, then costs will vary accordingly. While it may be appropriate to either perform or not perform a catheterization, the choice will affect cost. Clearly, management and appropriateness issues overlap.

Structure is related to cost. Facilities and supplies vary considerably in cost even within a single geographic location. Staffing also may vary in intensity, with some institutions having more patients being cared for by a nurse than others. Outcome also may vary with quality of care. Complications may be iatrogenic and relate to quality of care and generally increase the cost of a service. Similarly, a patient's health status may vary with quality, which will affect induced productivity costs. Thus, if there is variation in relief from angina after revascularization due to variation in quality of care, then there may be variation in ability to return to work.

Patient-level factors, such as age, gender, and race, may affect cost as much as, or perhaps more than, quality of care. Age may be thought of as similar to comorbidity, potentially raising cost. Disease severity or acuteness, however measured, also may affect costs. Thus it may cost more to perform coronary surgery or coronary angioplasty on patients with a recent acute myocardial infarction (MI) than without one.[26–28] Similarly, comorbidity may increase costs. *However, complications generally have a greater effect on costs than comorbidity or severity.*[26–28] Complications and health status outcomes related to patient-level factors do not separate cleanly from complications and heath status outcomes related to quality of care.

Finally, variation in cost may be influenced by geographic and nonmedical economic factors such as land and construction costs, cost of living, and personnel availability.[29] Also, there may be variation in cost that is independent of both quality and geography. Thus buying cooperatives of hospitals may be able to purchase supplies at greater discounts than single providers may.

Thus variation in cost of service is complicated and limits the ability to explain it. Correlates of cost variability often are studied using multivariate regression techniques.[26] While elegant, these models have significant limitations. First, studies from one or similar institutions may not be generalizable. Second, the correlates cannot always be neatly categorized, since a procedural complication may be at either the patient or provider level. Next, comorbidity, disease severity, and provider-level factors may themselves induce complications. Thus models should be developed in which patient and provider factors are correlated with outcome variables and where cost is correlated with preservice and pre- and postservice variables. Finally, cost often is not normally distributed. The distribution can be normalized to some extent by using its logarithm. However, correlating variables with the logarithm of cost is not as informative as correlating variables with cost itself.

Thus determining the specific cost of any service is difficult and, therefore, limits generalizing estimate costs outside the bounds of a particular study. In the same sense that effect sizes are considered subject to confidence intervals, cost estimates must be recognized as "estimates." This limitation also applies to using cost measurements in cost-effectiveness analyses and in constructing league tables in which several cost-effectiveness analyses are compared.

COMPARING COSTS WITH OUTCOME

Determining therapeutic or diagnostic costs independently of patient outcome is not particularly helpful for clinical decision making or setting policy. Measuring costs without considering outcomes would preclude judgments about the value of allocating resources in the health care system. The most extreme cost-minimization approach would be to stop offering medical services. However, the goal of the health care system is to maximize patient outcomes within the resource constraints. Consequently, costs and outcomes need to be considered. While it is possible to relate cost to any measure of outcome, the most generalizable approach in medicine is cost-utility analysis based on patient preference.[30]

Determination of Patient Utility and Quality-Adjusted Life Years

In the treatment of coronary artery disease, it is unusual for one measurement of outcome to be of sufficient clinical importance that all other outcome measures may be ignored in clinical decision making. While death overwhelms other outcome measures in importance, it is relatively infrequent over short periods of time for most conditions. Consequently, it is also important to consider other outcomes such as MI, unstable angina, revascularization procedures, measures of quality of life, and return to work and weigh them together. In trials comparing percutaneous coronary intervention with coronary surgery, there was no difference in mortality.[31–36] While surgery relieved angina somewhat better[31–36] at higher cost,[33,36–40] it was a disadvantage to the patient to have to undergo the surgery in the first place. Without some method to integrate various measures of outcome, it may be difficult to make an informed choice. In principle, this task may be accomplished through the determination of patient utility.

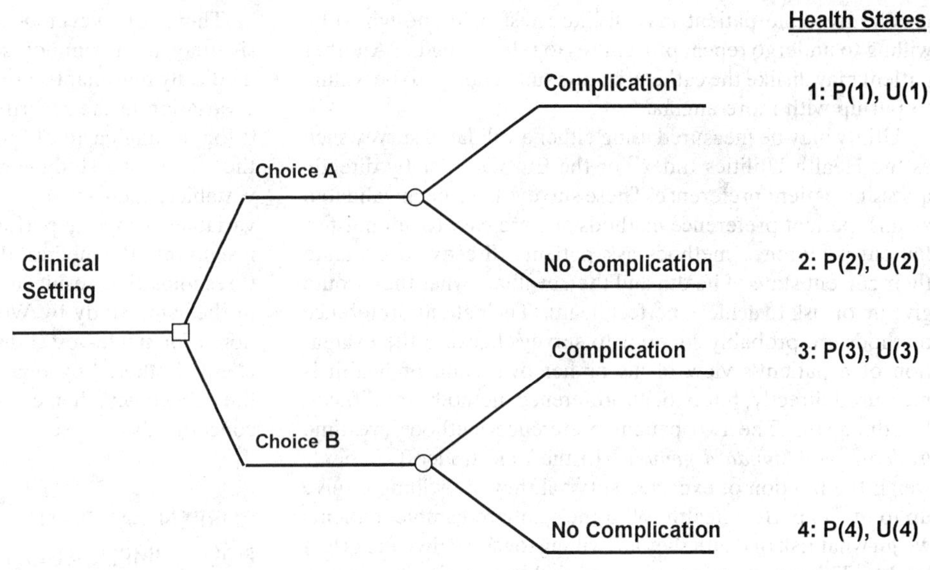

FIGURE 94-3 Idealized decision tree for a decision on diagnostic strategy or therapeutic choice.

The utility of a therapy or test is the sum of benefits, both positive and negative, that accrues to a patient over time as a result of the procedure.[41] It is, in principle, all-encompassing. We may consider the assessment of utility beginning with a decision tree (Fig. 94-3). A decision tree takes a patient at a specific point and then considers, in principal, all possible events up to some point in the future. In this model, branch points or nodes with squares represent choices and nodes with circles represent chance events. In the simplified model shown, a single choice is made, and for each choice, there are two possible outcomes. Each outcome is called a *health state*. Each health state has a utility and a probability of occurrence. The utility of choice A in Fig. 94-3 is the sum of the utility of health state 1 times its probability plus the utility of health state 2 times its probability. If choices were this easy, then the ability to determine utility of diagnostic or therapeutic strategies would be simple. However, decision trees are almost never this simple. The decision trees for diagnostic tests tend to be much more complicated than for therapeutics because a test can lead to additional tests or to a range of therapeutic alternatives. For any one treatment, there may be multiple possible health states, and the paucity of literature may make it difficult to determine the probability of different ones, much less the utility associated with each.

Utility changes over time. We may compare the utility after coronary angioplasty if a patient either does or does not suffer restenosis in Fig. 94-4. After successful angioplasty, the patient feels well and utility rises, but then the patient may suffer restenosis and utility falls. After successful redilation, utility rises again. After angioplasty not complicated by restenosis, utility gradually rises. Ultimately, the patients get to the same point, but the patient who has the episode of restenosis suffers a period of decreased utility. Utility measurement should involve patient

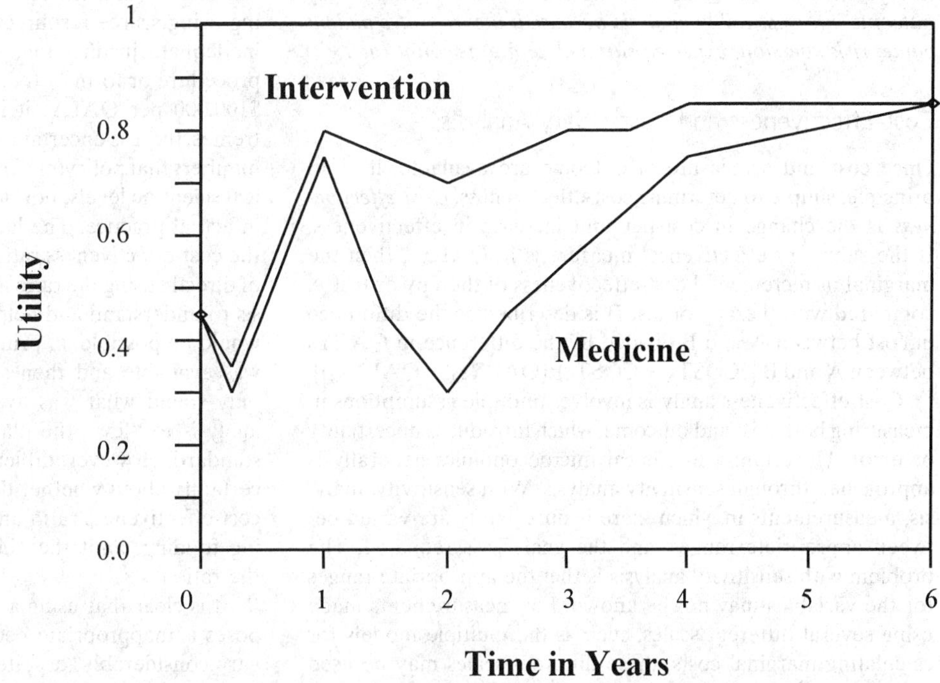

FIGURE 94-4 Theoretical time course of utility after coronary angioplasty in a patient who does not suffer restenosis (*top line*) and a patient who does suffer restenosis (*bottom line*).

preference. One patient may dislike chest pain enough to be willing to undergo repeat procedures to relieve angina. Another patient may dislike the catheterization suite enough to be willing to put up with more angina.

Utility may be measured using either a validated survey such as the Health Utilities Index[42] or the EuroQol[43] or by directly assessing patient preference. These surveys have been validated against patient preference methods and are easy to administer. Patient preference methods ask patients directly to evaluate their current state of health and then evaluate what they would give up or risk to achieve perfect health. The patient preference methods are probably superior to surveys because the evaluation of a patient's view of his or her own state of health is measured directly, but patient preference methods are difficult to administer. The two patient preference methods are time *tradeoff*[4] and *standard gamble.*[4] In the time tradeoff, patients weigh the fraction of expected survival they are willing to give up to live in perfect health. With the standard gamble, patients weigh what risk of death they are willing to take to live in perfect health. The standard gamble is probably superior because it includes the element of risk.[4]

Utility alone does not provide a final summary measure of outcome because it does not include life expectancy. This summary measure can be determined using quality-adjusted life years (QALYs), which are calculated by combining utility and survival.[44] Median or mean survival must be estimated from either the data set under consideration or from the literature. Survival, as with cost presented earlier, generally is discounted, which means that patients value a year of survival at the present time more than a year of survival in the future. The "true" discount rate for survival is unknown. Values in the literature for the discount rate have varied from 2 to 10 percent, with 3 percent being the most popular.[24] Thus, with a discount rate of 3 percent, next year's survival is 3 percent less important than this year's survival. *QALYs is the best summary measure of outcome in a cost-utility analysis because it incorporates patient value, risk aversion, expected survival, and a discount rate.*

Cost-Effectiveness and Cost-Utility Analysis

Once cost and a measure of outcome are available, it is, in principle, simple to determine cost-effectiveness. *Cost-effectiveness* is the change in cost per unit increase in effectiveness. If the summary effectiveness measure is in QALYs, then the marginal or incremental cost-effectiveness of therapy or test A compared with therapy or test B is described as the difference in cost between A and B divided by the difference in QALYs between A and B $[(\mathrm{COST}_A - \mathrm{COST}_B)/(\mathrm{QALYs}_A - \mathrm{QALYs}_B)]$.

Cost-effectiveness analysis involves multiple assumptions in measuring both cost and outcome, which introduces uncertainty or error. Uncertainty in clinical microeconomics generally is approached through sensitivity analysis. With sensitivity analysis, measurements in which there is uncertainty are varied between appropriate ranges, and the analysis is repeated. The problem with sensitivity analysis is that the appropriate ranges for the variables may not be known. For measurements made using several different scales, such as the multiple models for calculating marginal costs, these different scales may be used to perform the sensitivity analysis. For measurements that are continuous, such as professional charges, one standard deviation may be appropriate.

There is, however, no absolute standard for sensitivity analysis other than common sense and an intuitive feel for what is medically reasonable. For instance, Weinstein and Stason[45] used a variation in the severity of angina to decrease QALYs from 0 for no angina to 50 percent for severe disabling angina. If the results of a study vary significantly with changes in certain variables, then the outcome is said to be sensitive for those variables. Properly performed, sensitivity analyses should give insight into the medical decision-making process by identifying thresholds that result in changes in the process. For instance, in the same study by Weinstein and Stason,[45] a threshold was noted for single-vessel disease such that if a patient were sufficiently bothered by angina to be willing to give up 8 percent of life expectancy, then coronary surgery was indicated, excluding concerns about cost.

CURRENT AND FUTURE TRENDS AND POLICY IMPLICATIONS

Cost-effectiveness analysis in clinical medicine offers a powerful approach that may be used to help guide clinical decision making as well as for policy. To date, most cost-effectiveness analyses have been simulations. The formidable difficulties in determining cost and utility have limited the use of these tools in medical care. As the methods and science of cost-effectiveness analyses improve, these analyses should be integrated increasingly into clinical trials and applied routinely to observational databases. With the current changes in health care, accountability and cost are increasingly important, and we can expect to see more studies using these methods and greater incorporation of cost-effectiveness analysis into the medical care delivery system.

The cost-effectiveness ratio, expressed in dollars per QALY, can be used, at least in principle, to affect societal choice regarding using scarce resources. A number that is often used, with inadequate justification, is that below $50,000 per QALY, a procedure or form of therapy is cost-effective, whereas at over $100,000 per QALY, it is too expensive. Between these extremes, there is uncertainty. However, these are relatively rough numbers that policymakers may use and do not represent empirical scientific levels, nor do they reflect thresholds for decisions in actual practice. The lack of an empirical standard to which the cost-effectiveness ratio may be compared reveals the limits of directly using the ratio as opposed to cost-effectiveness analysis to understand and help inform the policymaking process. It would be possible, in principle, to figure out how much money was available and then set the limit on cost-effectiveness to only spend what was available, thus using cost-effectiveness analysis to "level the playing field" and providing a uniform standard. However, difficulties in measurement, as well as uncertainty about whether the appropriateness of using the single cost-effectiveness ratio uniformly for all major policy concerning funding, limit the ability of policymakers to directly use the ratio.

It is clear that using a single number for policymaking purposes is inappropriate because cost-effectiveness methods can vary considerably, despite recent efforts to create standards,[46] leading to different numbers. In addition, the cost-effectiveness ratio may not reflect the difference perspective of small changes made for many people with an inexpensive form of therapy versus a big change for the few for expensive therapy. Finally, cost-effectiveness analysis does not adequately reflect the variability of patient populations. Policy planners, representing society, may choose to lower the threshold for a form of therapy for the young compared with the elderly, even though the impact of age is already included in the calculation of the ratio. Thus cost-effectiveness is not designed to be used for policymaking purposes in the absence of other information but rather should help guide both clinical decision making and public policy. All this being said, the cost-effectiveness of most well established medical therapies compares well with the cost-effectiveness of other health choices, such as airbags in cars, asbestos abatement, or toxic waste control.[46]

COST-EFFECTIVENESS IN PREVENTION, DIAGNOSIS, AND THERAPY

Hyperlipidemia

Until recently, estimates of the cost-effectiveness of lipid lowering were based on decision-analytic models,[2,3,47–50] with data coming from epidemiologic studies, such as Framingham.[51] The models incorporated assumptions concerning the relationship of lipid lowering to subsequent prevention of cardiovascular events. The models also had to make assumptions concerning resource use. More recently, there have been a series of randomized trials that have shown the benefit of lipid lowering and also have included cost-effectiveness analyses (see also Chap. 38).

Education concerning lipid lowering will be inexpensive for each patient but may be quite expensive in the aggregate. A population-wide program was studied by Tosteson et al.[48] using a decision-analytic approach. A population-wide program with a cost of $4.95 per person per year and cholesterol-lowering effects on average of 2 percent reduction would prolong life at an estimated cost of only $3200 per year of life saved.

A cautionary note also was sounded by Goldman et al.[49] Using a decision-analytic model in high-risk patients, therapy with HMG-CoA reductase inhibitor was shown to dominate no therapy. However, in lower-risk populations, therapy has became much less cost-effective and is perhaps not warranted in younger patients with isolated elevation of serum lipids.

Recently, a series of clinical trials in the United States and Europe has established and more clearly defined the benefit of lipid lowering. In the Scandinavian Simvastatin Survival Study (4S),[52] 4444 men and women with a prior MI or episode of unstable angina and with total serum cholesterol between 213 and 309 mg/dL (5.5 and 8.0 mmol/L) were randomized to a low-cholesterol diet and to either placebo or simvastatin. At 5.4 years of mean follow-up, active therapy was associated with reduced all-cause mortality (30 percent; 11.5 versus 8.2 percent), reduced cardiac mortality (42 percent; 8.5 versus 5.0 percent), reduced major coronary events (34 percent; 22.6 versus 15.9 percent), and reduced cardiovascular accidents/transient ischemic attacks (37 percent; 4.3 versus 2.7 percent). Coronary revascularization procedures were reduced by 32 percent (411 versus 278), and cardiac hospitalizations were reduced by 26 percent (acute MI, 37 percent, 630 versus 395; angina, 22 percent, 401 versus 312; stroke/transient ischemic attack, 27 percent, 110 versus 80). A cost-effectiveness analysis was developed from the 4S resource clinical and resource use data, with costs attributed to these resources.[53,54] In 4S, estimated direct medical costs ranged from approximately $4000 to $30,000 per year of life gained, with therapy most cost-effective in older men with the highest baseline cholesterol and least cost-effective in younger women with the lowest baseline cholesterol. When indirect costs were included in the analyses, the estimated cost per year of life gained decreased further, with estimated net savings in the youngest patients and a cost of approximately $13,000 per year of life gained in elderly women with baseline cholesterol of 213 mg/dL.

In the West of Scotland Coronary Prevention Study (WOSCOPS), 6595 Scottish men aged 45 to 64 with moderate hypercholesterolemia [mean cholesterol 272 mg/dL (7 mmol/L) and low-density lipoprotein cholesterol >155 mg/dL (4 mmol/L)] and no history or evidence of MI were randomized to placebo or 40 mg/day pravastatin, with a mean follow-up of 4.9 years.[55] Active therapy reduced all-cause mortality by 22 percent from 4.1 to 3.2 percent, reduced cardiac mortality rates (28 percent; 1.7 versus 1.2 percent), and reduced major coronary events (31 percent; 7.9 versus 5.5 percent). No statistical difference was found in stroke (1.6 percent in placebo and pravastatin groups; 51 versus 46). Coronary revascularization procedures were reduced by 37 percent (2.5 versus 1.7 percent). Data on cardiac hospitalizations are not available. A cost-effectiveness analysis was constructed, based on the outcomes data and resource use. Cost per year of life gained (discounted at 3 to 6 percent annually) was estimated as $25,000 to $40,000, depending on risk group and model assumptions.[56]

Using data from the Pravastatin Limitation of Atherosclerosis in the Coronary Arteries[57] (PLAC I) study and the Pravastatin, Lipids, and Atherosclerosis in the Carotids (PLAC II) study and survival estimates 10 years after MI from Framingham, the Markov decision-analytic model was used to estimate the cost-effectiveness of lipid lowering in secondary prevention. Depending on specific patient risk, cost per life-year saved varied from $7124 to $12,665.

In high-risk groups, such as those with elevated low-density lipoprotein (LDL) cholesterol noted after acute MI, therapy with statins is clearly cost-effective. However, there remains considerable uncertainty as to the cost-effectiveness of therapy in lower-risk populations. Several populations, including the elderly and young groups without a prior event and moderate elevations of lipids, cannot be well assessed from present data. Furthermore, there have been no trials with lipid lowering that included patient preference or any attempt to construct QALYs.

Smoking Cessation

Cigarette smoking remains a potent and prevalent risk factor for premature death and disability. In the United States, approximately one-quarter of the men and one-fifth of the women are current cigarette smokers.[58] These 50 million individuals who annually purchase 24 billion packages of cigarettes[59] have a markedly elevated risk of cancer, pulmonary disease, and vascular disease.[60] As a result, it is estimated that about 400,000 premature deaths occur in the United States each year as a result of cigarette smoking (see also Chap. 38).

The direct medical costs attributed to cigarette smoking are substantial. The Centers for Disease Control and Prevention (CDC) conservatively estimate that medical care expenditures attributable to cigarette smoking in 1993 were $50.0 billion.

These costs included $26.9 billion for hospital expenditures, $15.5 billion for physician expenditures, $4.9 billion for nursing home expenditures, $1.8 billion for prescription drugs, and $900 million for home health services. For each pack of cigarettes sold, more than $2 was spent on medical care attributable to smoking. Of note, for each pack sold, about 90 cents of public funds was spent on medical care attributable to smoking. These estimates do not include the full range of harms caused by smoking, such as injuries from smoking-related fires or complications from premature births.

Cigarette smoking also accounts for important indirect costs such as days lost from work or disability days. Smokers reportedly are absent from work about 7 more days per year than nonsmokers. This loss in productivity associated with the health consequences of smoking is estimated to cost $47 billion.[61]

The benefit of smoking cessation is most likely to be achieved in the short term. These short-term benefits are not inconsequential. Lightwood and Glantz[62] specifically examined the short-term economic benefits of smoking cessation as a result of the rapid decline in the risk of acute MI and stroke. They estimated that a 7-year program that produced a 1 percent annual reduction in smoking prevalence would reduce the number of acute MI hospitalizations by 63,840 and the number of stroke hospitalizations by 34,261. The resulting savings would be $3.2 billion, with the prevention of about 13,000 deaths.

If all smokers quit, however, society would not realize a long-term economic benefit. Costs attributed to smoking would diminish gradually, and in the short-run, costs would be lower. However, over time, the higher survival rate as a result of smoking cessation will lead to a larger number of older individuals who will incur health care costs. As a result, the elimination of smoking would, in the long run, produce a net increase in health care costs. These increased costs would be associated with added years of life and healthier years. *Consequently, we can understand successful smoking-cessation strategies as potentially cost-effective but probably not cost saving in the long run.*

Several studies have examined the cost-effectiveness of interventions to assist smokers to quit.[63,64] These studies have overwhelmingly found effective smoking-cessation programs to be cost-effective relative to other medical interventions. Cromwell et al.[65] evaluated the cost-effectiveness of the clinical recommendations in the Agency for Health Care Policy and Research Clinical Practice Guideline on Smoking Cessation. The guideline included 15 recommended smoking-cessation interventions. The cost per smoker who successfully quit among the counseling interventions that did not include pharmacotherapy ranged from $2186 for group intensive counseling to $7922 for minimal counseling. The cost per QALY ranged from $1108 for group intensive counseling to $4015 for minimal counseling. The addition of pharmacotherapy increased the cost of the intervention but also the effectiveness. With transdermal nicotine as an adjunct therapy, the cost per QALY ranged from $1171 for group intensive counseling to $2405 for minimal counseling. With nicotine gum, it ranged from $1822 for group intensive counseling to $4542 for minimal counseling. These estimates are based on patients presenting to a primary care clinic.

Smoking-cessation programs may be even more cost-effective relative to other interventions for patients with cardiovascular disease because of their high risk of future events. Krumholz et al.[66] evaluated the cost-effectiveness of a nurse-based educational intervention for patients who had survived an acute MI. The cost-effectiveness of the program was estimated to be $220 per year of life saved. The value of these types of programs was illuminated in the sensitivity analysis. A smoking-cessation program after acute MI would remain less than $20,000 per year of life saved even if the program only produced 3 additional ex-smokers for every 1000 (baseline assumption 26 per 100) enrolled or if the program cost as much as $8840 per smoker (baseline assumption $100). Similar favorable estimates of the value of these interventions would be expected in other high-risk groups with cardiovascular disease.

Exercise

There is strikingly little information on exercise to prevent coronary artery disease. Nevertheless, the cost-effectiveness of exercise was investigated using a decision-analytic model by Jones and Eaton.[67] These investigators constructed hypothetical cohorts of sedentary men and women aged 35 to 74 years. Assuming a relative risk of 1.9 for heart disease associated with sedentary behavior, $5.6 billion would be saved annually if 10 percent of adults began a regular walking program. Alternatively, $4.3 billion could be saved if the entire sedentary population began walking regularly, accounting for costs in individuals who dislike exercising. Using the baseline assumptions, walking was found to be economically beneficial for men aged 35 to 64 years and women aged 55 to 64 years. The threshold of relative risk at which economic benefit is found for walking overall was estimated at 1.7, and for those who walk voluntarily, most adults would benefit even at a relative risk of just 1.15.

Diabetes Control

Diabetes is a common and important risk factor for cardiovascular disease. Glycemic control is related to the risk of subsequent complications.[68] As a consequence, the HbA1c level is considered an indicator of the quality of care for an organization, with recommendations for the level to be less than 7 percent.[69] Nevertheless, many diabetics do not reach this level of glycemic control (see also Chaps. 38 and Chap. 78).[70]

In economic terms, glycemic control is also important. The level of glycemic control of adult diabetics is associated with medical care expenditures. An observational study of adults with diabetes enrolled in a large health maintenance organization reported that medical care charges were strongly related to HbA1c levels.[71] An increase of 1 percent in the HbA1c level was associated with a 7 percent increase in charges. Because these patients tend to require many medical services, the impact on health care expenditures can be substantial. For example, among the patients with hypertension and heart disease, in addition to diabetes, a difference in the HbA1c level of from 9 to 10 percent was associated with a difference in costs of more than $4000 over 3 years—even after adjustment for age, sex, and other chronic conditions.

Interventions that improve glycemic control can result in fewer microvascular complications.[71,72] The resources required to produce this benefit are substantial because the interventions may include closer monitoring, increased patient education, frequent telephone contact, more clinical visits, and higher drug costs.

For type I diabetes, the Diabetes Control and Complications Trial (DCCT) may best demonstrate the benefit of these interventions.[72] This trial showed that an intensive treatment regimen decreased the risk of development or progression of retinopathy, nephropathy, and neuropathy by 50 to 75 percent. An economic analysis of the DCCT revealed that the intensive intervention was more expensive than conventional therapy by about $30,000 over the lifetime of each patient.[73] However, considering what is achieved by this investment, the cost-effectiveness of this intervention has been calculated to be $28,661 per year of life saved. With adjustments for quality of life, the intensive intervention costs $19,987 per QALY.

For type II diabetes, the United Kingdom Prospective Diabetes Study (UKPDS), the largest and longest study of this topic, demonstrated that improved blood glucose control reduces the risk of developing retinopathy and nephropathy and possibly reduces neuropathy.[74] This study and others modeled the economic impact of interventions to improve glycemic control for type II diabetes.[75] The intensive treatment doubled the cost of medical care for these patients, which was partially offset by a reduction in the number of complications. The cost-effectiveness of an intensive program was calculated to be $16,002 per QALY.

Antihypertensive Screening and Therapy

Hypertension is a risk factor for stroke, ischemic heart disease, heart failure, and end-stage renal disease (see also Chaps. 38 and Chap. 51). The Sixth Report of the Joint National Committee details our current knowledge about prevention, detection, evaluation, and treatment of hypertension.[76] The screening and treatment of hypertension in the United States, based on 1995 dollars, was estimated to cost $23.7 billion, including $6.7 billion in indirect costs for lost wages and lowered productivity.[77] The costs of the complications of hypertension would be considerably higher. The reduction in vascular events provided by screening and treating hypertension partially offsets their cost, producing a favorable cost-effectiveness ratio.

Investigators from Stanford demonstrated the value of screening in an article that was published about a decade ago.[78] The results suggest that screening is economically attractive in men and women of all ages. The ratios compared favorably with other common interventions in medicine. Men and older adults have more favorable ratios because they are more likely to have high blood pressure. In 1990 dollars, screening has a cost-effectiveness ratio of $8374 per QALY for men age 60. Screening for hypertension had the least favorable cost-effectiveness ratio, with $44,412 per QALY for 20-year-old women. In the sensitivity analysis, the ratio became less favorable as the benefit of the therapy decreased and as the cost of the medication increased.

Other investigators have examined the cost-effectiveness of treatment once a patient with hypertension is identified. A classic study in this area used a computer simulation, the CHD Policy Model, to estimate the cost-effectiveness of various antihypertensive treatments.[79] The antihypertensive and cholesterol effects of each of the medications were derived from a meta-analysis of trials that evaluated the efficacy of these agents. The CHD Policy Model, based on estimates derived from the Framingham Heart Study, calculated the effects of these changes in blood pressure and cholesterol on the incidence of coronary heart disease. They focused specifically on various antihypertensive medications in persons aged 35 through 64 years with a diastolic blood pressure of 95 mmHg or greater and no known coronary heart disease. In 1987 dollars and compared with no treatment, the cost per year of life saved was estimated to be $10,900 for propranolol, $16,400 for hydrochlorothiazide, $61,900 for prazosin hydrochloride, and $72,100 for captopril. Studies of older patients also have found that the treatment of hypertension is economically attractive.[80]

Since the publication of this study, the options for treatment have expanded. The abundance of antihypertensive strategies presents a challenge to these studies in selecting a comparison group. A strategy that is only more expensive than a competing treatment without evidence of incremental benefit will always be dominated in the analysis. The incremental advantage of many of our current treatments for hypertension over the inexpensive option of using low-dose hydrochlorothiazide is speculative and has led some observers to speculate that substantial resources are being squandered in the treatment of this condition.[81] The Sixth Joint National Committee report does recommend diuretics or beta blockers as first-line agents for managing essential hypertension. A recent economic analysis of the Joint National Committee guidelines concurred that a diuretic or beta blocker is much less expensive to achieve and maintain blood pressure control compared with a calcium-channel blocker or angiotensin-converting enzyme (ACE) inhibitor.[82]

Multiple-Risk-Factor and Community Intervention Programs

The Stanford Coronary Risk Intervention Project (SCRIP) tested the hypothesis that intensive multiple-risk-factor reduction would reduce progression of atherosclerosis in the coronary arteries of men and women compared with subjects randomly assigned to usual care.[83] Patients in the risk-reduction arm were provided individualized programs of a low-fat and low-cholesterol diet, exercise, weight loss, smoking cessation, and lipid-lowering medications. Intensive risk reduction resulted in improvements in various risk factors, including serum lipids, weight, exercise capacity, and diet, compared with relatively small changes with usual care. The risk-reduction group showed a rate of narrowing of diseased coronary artery segments 47 percent less than usual care group. There were 25 hospitalizations in the risk-reduction group for cardiac events compared with 44 with usual care. Based on data from the SCRIP program, Superko[84] estimated that when the cost savings of the reduced number of events is balanced against the cost of treatment, the prevention program would cost on average $1500 per patient per year, with a range of costing $2273 to a cost savings of $901 per patient per year.

DeBusk et al.[85] evaluated a physician-directed, nurse-managed, home-based case-management system for coronary risk-factor modification in a randomized trial during the first year after acute MI. In the hospital, specially trained nurses initiated interventions for smoking cessation, exercise training, and diet and drug therapy for hyperlipidemia. Intervention after discharge was conducted primarily by telephone and mail. In the special intervention, there was greater smoking cessation and lipid lowering as well as improved exercise performance compared with usual care. Superko[84] estimated the cost of the program at $550 per year. While a true cost-effectiveness analysis is not available, this type of program may be more attractive than other, more resource-intensive approaches.

There have been multiple studies of primary prevention programs. The 10-year results of the North Karelia project showed a 28 percent decrease in smoking, 3 percent decrease in serum cholesterol, and 3 percent decrease for systolic blood pressure.[86] In the Pawtucket Heart Health Program, citizens of all ages participated in multilevel education, screening, and counseling programs.[87] Projected cardiovascular disease rates were 16 percent lower during the education program but lessened to 8 percent after education. The Pawtucket investigators concluded that greater risk-factor control would require a sustained community effort along with state and national efforts. Modest effects of a community intervention also were noted in the Stanford Five-City Project, with the investigators concluding that better design for intervention was needed.[88] Similarly disappointing results were noted in the Minnesota Heart Health Program.[89] In a pooled analysis of the three American programs, trends were estimated for cigarette smoking, blood pressure, total cholesterol, body mass index, and coronary heart disease mortality risk for women and men, with estimates of intervention effect in the expected direction in 9 of 12 comparisons; however, none was statistically significant.[90] Kottke et al.[91] conducted a simulation based on clinical trial data, which suggested that only a population approach can prevent the majority of deaths from cardiovascular disease. However, the implementation of such programs to date has not been entirely satisfactory, and it is difficult to draw any conclusions concerning cost-effectiveness. Well-designed programs with control or resources and adequate data to conduct cost-effectiveness studies would appear to still be needed.

ACUTE CORONARY SYNDROMES

Coronary Care

Patients with an acute MI often suffer life-threatening complications that require rapid, high-level intervention. Consequently, the standard of care is to admit patients with an acute MI to a coronary care unit. Admission to these units is costly, and relatively few patients benefit from the units' advanced capabilities. The value of this triage for specific groups of patients can be illuminated through an economic analysis (see also Chap. 42).

To address this issue, Tosteson et al.[92] made use of clinical and resource use data from 12,139 emergency department patients who presented with acute chest pain. They compared a coronary care unit with admission to an intermediate care facility with central electrocardiographic monitoring and personnel to detect and treat in-hospital complications. Information on the effectiveness of coronary care units is sparse, particularly in this setting of alternatives with some of the same capabilities. Based on data from the Multicenter Chest Pain Study, the authors estimated that mortality for patients with an acute MI would be 15 percent higher for admission to an intermediate care unit compared with a coronary care unit.[93] Using this assumption, the value of admission to a coronary care unit varied depending on the age of the patient and the initial probability of an acute MI. In 1992 dollars, for patients who were 55 to 64 years old and had a 1 percent probability of MI, admission to a coronary care unit had a cost-effectiveness ratio of $1.4 million per year of life saved, whereas the same aged patients with a 99 percent probability of an MI had a cost-effectiveness ratio of $15,000 per year of life saved. The cost-effectiveness ratio was less than $75,000 per year of life saved if the probability of MI exceeded 20 percent. The cost-effectiveness of coronary care units was less favorable for younger patients because of their higher underlying risk of a life-threatening complication.

Reperfusion

With the advent of information about the efficacy of thrombolytic therapy for the treatment of patients with suspected acute MI, interest turned to the economic value of this intervention. Since the two largest and earliest trials of thrombolytic therapy used streptokinase, the early economic evaluations focused on this agent.[94–98]

A cost-effectiveness analysis published in 1992 examined the use of streptokinase compared with no treatment.[94] The investigators focused on the treatment of elderly patients with suspected acute MI, a group for which there is less enthusiasm about using thrombolytic therapy. Based on data available from GISSI-1 and ISIS-2, the relative benefit of thrombolytic therapy was assumed to be lower in elderly patients and the risk of thrombolytic therapy was assumed to be higher, but the absolute risk of an acute MI was much higher compared with younger patients. The smaller relative reduction in the higher risk associated with MI offset the higher risk of complications. Thus the decision analysis suggested that thrombolytic therapy was economically attractive over a broad range of assumptions about the risks and benefits. After considering the costs of the treatment, complications, and long-term health care of survivors, the authors estimated that the cost-effectiveness ratio of streptokinase compared with conventional medical therapy was $21,200 per year of life saved for an 80-year-old patient. The authors calculated similar estimates for younger patients. Several studies have found similar results. One analysis has even suggested that thrombolytic therapy could be cost saving because of its impact on reducing rehospitalization[98] (see also Chap. 42).

With the emergence of tissue-type plasminogen activator (tPA) as a more expensive and more effective alternative to streptokinase, studies addressed whether the incremental benefit was large enough to justify the incremental cost. The GUSTO trial investigators performed a substudy to address this issue specifically.[99] The investigators collected detailed information about resource consumption in a subgroup of the GUSTO subjects. They found that both treatment groups were similar in their use of resources in the year after enrollment. The treatment groups had a mean length of hospital stay of 8 days, including an average of 3.5 days in the intensive care unit. During the initial hospitalization, the treatment groups had a similar rate of CABG (13 percent) and PCTA (31 percent). Overall, the 1-year health costs, excluding the difference in the cost of the thrombolytic agent, were $24,990 per patient treated with tPA and $24,575 per patient treated with streptokinase. The major difference in the cost of the therapies was the cost of the drugs: $2750 for tPA and $320 for streptokinase. The primary analysis assumed no increase in costs for the tPA group after the first year. Based on the GUSTO results and an estimate of the patients' life expectancy, the additional life expectancy per patient treated with tPA was estimated to be 0.14 years.

Based on these estimates, the authors concluded that the cost-effectiveness ratio of using tPA instead of streptokinase was $32,678 per year of life saved. This ratio varied considerably based on the infarction site and the age of the patient. In general, the younger and lower-risk patients had higher cost-effectiveness ratios. For example, the cost-effectiveness ratio for tPA in a patient aged 40 years or younger with an inferior MI was $203,071 per year of life saved compared with $13,410 per year of life saved for a person aged 75 years or older with an anterior MI. An analysis conducted independent of the GUSTO trial reached similar conclusions.[100] Comparisons with other new agents await strong evidence of their superiority to tPA.

Mechanical approaches to reperfusion have been employed with increasing frequency. The clinical or economic advantage of primary angioplasty remains controversial.[101–103] Several studies have suggested a substantial advantage of primary angioplasty.[104–106] Economic analyses based on early studies suggested that primary angioplasty is associated with a reduction in mortality without increasing cost.[107,108] Other recent clinical studies of actual practice, however, have provided less impressive results associated with the use of primary angioplasty,[103,109] making estimates of the effectiveness more difficult.

A fundamental problem in this area is that the field is moving rapidly. Changes in costs and techniques require rapid access to recent data in order to develop relevant economic models. For example, stents, initially considered to be contraindicated in acute MI because of concerns that they would incite thrombus formation, are becoming the standard for primary mechanical reperfusion therapy. As evidence of the efficacy of stents accumulates, there will be a need to examine their economic impact compared with balloon angioplasty and thrombolytic therapy. Also, as more rapid discharge protocols evolve for patients who receive reperfusion therapy, the balance of costs and effectiveness may shift.[110]

Antithrombotic Agents

Aspirin reduces mortality and morbidity for patients with acute coronary syndromes. As a result of the marked benefit and the minimal cost of the therapy, no formal economic analysis of aspirin for the treatment of acute coronary syndromes has been published in the mainstream journals. The ISIS-2 trial found that aspirin avoided 25 deaths for every 1000 patients with suspected acute MI.[111] In addition, the 1 month of aspirin therapy in ISIS-2 was associated with halving the risk of stroke or reinfarction. Aspirin avoided about 10 reinfarctions and 3 strokes for every 1000 patients treated. The avoidance of complications would likely translate into cost savings, leading aspirin to be considered a "strongly dominant" therapy.

Heparin for the treatment of acute MI also has not been formally evaluated in an economic analysis because it has not been shown to provide a strong benefit for acute MI in the aspirin era.[112] In addition, while aspirin plus heparin is the standard of care for patients hospitalized with unstable angina, a metaanalysis of the unstable angina studies found only borderline significant results in favor of heparin.[113] Given the uncertainty about its effectiveness, heparin would only be a favored therapy if there were evidence that heparin reduces cost. No studies have revealed an economic advantage to heparin therapy in this setting.

New agents are emerging with increasing frequency. For example, low-molecular-weight heparin is emerging as an effective therapy for unstable angina.[114] The greater cost and benefit of this new treatment make it ideal for economic analyses. Mark et al.[115] performed an economic analysis for a subset of patients enrolled in the Efficacy and Safety of Subcutaneous Enoxaparin in Non-Q-Wave Coronary Events Study Group (ESSENCE).[115] Patients treated with enoxaparin had lower resource use during the initial hospitalization, and this benefit persisted at 30 days, with a cumulative cost savings associated with enoxaparin of $1172 ($p$ = 0.04). The investigators concluded that enoxaparin both improves important clinical outcomes and saves money relative to therapy with standard unfractionated heparin, making it a strongly dominant therapy.

The use of a monoclonal antibody fragment against the platelet receptor glycoprotein IIb/beta IIIa inhibitors is growing. Treatment of high-risk patients undergoing coronary revascularization reduces the short-term risk of death, MI, or coronary revascularization.[116] An economic analysis of the EPIC trial found that the use of this therapy for high-risk patients was associated with a cost savings of $622 per patient during the initial hospitalization from reduced acute ischemic events.[117] During the 6-month follow-up, the therapy decreased repeat hospitalization rates by 23 percent (p = 0.004) and repeat revascularization by 22 percent (p = 0.04), producing a mean $1270 savings per patient (exclusive of drug cost) (p = 0.018). If the cost of the drug were less than $1270, then the strategy would be effective and cost saving.

The Randomized Efficacy Study of Tirofiban for Outcomes and Restenosis (RESTORE) trial found that in patients undergoing coronary angioplasty for acute coronary syndromes, tirofiban protects against early adverse cardiac events related to abrupt closure.[118] A subsequent economic analysis reported that the use of tirofiban (including drug costs) was not associated with an increase in health care costs.[119]

Neither of these studies directly examined the use of this agent in patients with acute ischemic syndromes. Future studies (with economic substudies), such as the TACTICS (Treat Angina with Aggrastat and Determine Cost of Therapy with Invasive or Conservative Therapy)–TIMI 18 trial will address this issue.[120]

Invasive versus Conservative Strategies in Non-ST-Segment Elevation Acute Coronary Syndromes

The relative value of an invasive strategy with early catheterization and possible revascularization compared with a conservative strategy with exercise testing in patients with unstable angina or non-ST-segment elevation acute MI has been studied in several clinical trials with equivocal results to date.[121–123] None of these trials included an economic component. An invasive versus a conservative strategy for non-ST-segment acute coronary syndromes is currently being studied in the TACTICS–TIMI 18 trial. It will be the first trial in this area with a formal cost and cost-effectiveness analysis built into the structure of the trial.[120,124]

Beta-Blocker Therapy

Beta-blocker therapy has been shown to reduce mortality following an acute MI.[125] Goldman et al.[126] conducted the most widely cited economic analysis of the costs and effectiveness of beta-blocker therapy. Using data from the literature, they estimated that beta-blocker therapy produced a relative reduction in mortality of 25 percent in years 1 to 3 after an MI and a 7 percent reduction for years 4 to 6. They evaluated the cost-effectiveness of the therapy under the assumption that the benefit did not persist after year 6. Costs were calculated using 1987 dollars. The investigators stratified potential patients by their estimated mortality into low, medium, and high risk: 1.5, 7.5, and 13 percent, respectively, in the first year. The cost-effectiveness ratio was strongly associated with the underlying risk of the patient. For a 45 year-old man with low risk, the cost-effectiveness ratio was $23,457, with medium risk it was $5890, and with high risk it was $3623.

ACE Inhibition

Several large randomized trials have demonstrated a reduction in acute MI for patients with left ventricular dysfunction after an acute MI who are treated with an ACE inhibitor.[127] Tsevat et al.[128] examined the cost-effectiveness of this intervention using resource use, survival, and health-related quality of life information from the Survival and Ventricular Enlargement (SAVE) trial, a randomized trial of captopril for survivors of an anterior MI with an ejection fraction of 40 percent or less. The investigators conservatively estimated that the benefit of captopril did not persist beyond 4 years. The trial found that captopril improved survival at 3.5 years by about 20 percent. Costs were calculated in 1991 dollars. The cost-effectiveness ranged from $60,800 per QALY for 50-year-old patients to $3600 for 80-year-old patients. McMurray et al.[129] also found that ACE inhibitors are an economically attractive intervention after MI.

Rehabilitation

In a decision-analytic model, Ades et al.[130] studied the cost-effectiveness of cardiac rehabilitation to coordinate exercise training and secondary prevention after acute MI. The cost-effectiveness of cardiac rehabilitation, in dollars per year of life saved, was calculated by combining published results of randomized trials of cardiac rehabilitation on mortality rates, epidemiologic studies of long-term survival in the overall postinfarction population, and studies of patient charges for rehabilitation services and averted medical expenses for hospitalizations after rehabilitation. Cardiac rehabilitation participants had an incremental life expectancy of 0.202 years. In 1988, the average cost of rehabilitation and exercise testing was $1485, partially offset by averted cardiac rehospitalizations of $850 per patient. A cost-effectiveness value of $2130 per year of life saved was determined for the late 1980s, projected to a value of $4950 per year of life saved in 1995. A sensitivity analysis was conducted to support these findings.

REVASCULARIZATION

Societal Burden

Revascularization, either by CABG or PTCA, represents an expensive form of therapy for the treatment of angina pectoris and, in some patients, the prolongation of life. The societal burden is substantial with over 367,000 CABG and over 482,000 PTCA procedures performed in 1996.[3] These numbers represent a 227 percent increase in CABG since 1979 and a 213 percent increase in PTCA since 1987. Given the difficulties in estimating cost, all cost figures across multiple institutions and health care systems must be considered "best guess" estimates. Nonetheless, the American Heart Association estimates the average cost of coronary surgery at $44,820 and of percutaneous coronary intervention of $20,370 in 1995. These costs may be too low if estimation of in-hospital costs is too high or too low or if induced and productivity costs are not accounted for adequately. If these numbers are accurate, the cost of coronary surgery is approximately $16 billion and angioplasty $10 billion.

Variation in Costs

The variation in costs of revascularization has been investigated in a number of studies. Within institutions, only a fraction of the variation in costs of coronary surgery or coronary angioplasty can be accounted for by either patient-level or procedural-level factors.[23,26–28,131] Complications predict variation to a greater extent. A study from Emory University, for instance, found that the hospital component of the cost of coronary surgery in 1990 dollars was $16,776 if there were no complications, $17,794 with one complication, $23,624 with three complications, and $50,609 with five or more complications.[26] In a study from Duke University, the surgeon was found to be responsible for much of the variability in cost of coronary surgery.[28] Data from the Cleveland Clinic, Emory University, and others have shown that complications also account for more of the variability in cost of angioplasty than preprocedural or procedural data.[26–28] The need for emergent bypass surgery has been shown to be a strong determinant of hospital costs after coronary angioplasty.[27,131] However, the ability to account for variation in cost is best described when length of stay is added to the models.[23,26,131]

Length of stay represents a summary variable that may include multiple unmeasured or unidentified variables and, when studied in models with other variables, may confound or obscure the effect of clinical variables on cost. This problem is apparent within single institutions. Considering broader groups of institutions in different geographic regions will result in even greater variation. Medicare data suggest that hospital-level variables account for some of the variability in hospital costs of coronary surgery, whereas geographic and other provider factors also account for additional variability in the angioplasty costs.[29,132] However, the ability to account for variation in cost across multiple institutions is modest.[132]

The evaluation of cost as well as cost-effectiveness of these procedures is complicated by technological improvements and changes in the delivery of health care. In addition, care maps and other efforts to improve efficiency have dramatically decreased the incidence of complications, shortened length of stay, and cut costs.[131,132] Just as these improvements may not be reflected in published clinical trials concerning outcomes, the available cost-effectiveness analyses also will not entirely reflect either technologic improvements nor increased efficiency in health care delivery.

Coronary surgery has improved in recent years with greater use of arterial grafts, improved anesthesia and cardioplegia, and the introduction of less invasive coronary surgery. In this regard, outcome and costs in 1996 dollars in 12,266 patients undergoing coronary bypass surgery between 1988 and 1996 at Emory University were evaluated.[23] The patients became sicker, especially with more hypertension, diabetes, prior MIs, and a decrease in ejection fraction over the period. Mortality tended to decrease from 4.7 to 2.7 percent ($p = 0.07$). After accounting for increasing indices of severity of disease over the period, there was a significant decrease in mortality (odds ratio 0.90 per year; $p = 0.0001$). The Q-wave MI rate fell from 4.1 to 1.3 percent ($p < 0.0001$). Mean hospital cost decreased from $22,689 to $15,987, and postoperative length of stay decreased from 9.2 to 5.9 days. After accounting for other variables, cost decreased by $1118 per year and length of stay by 0.55 days per year.

PTCA also has improved with technological improvements, especially coronary stents. Stent procedures have improved with better deployment and less need for full anticoagulation. Thus, in the era of stents plus ticlopidine or clopidogrel, stents do not add as much to the cost of intervention as during the era of full anticoagulation. In this regard, Peterson et al.[133] showed that the in-hospital cost of balloon angioplasty in 109 patients studied between 1995 and 1996 was $10,219. In 64 patients from 1993 to 1995, the cost of PTCA with stenting plus warfarin was $15,793, and in 217 patients undergoing PTCA with stenting plus ticlopidine the cost was $13,065. Improvements in PTCA services between 1990 and 1997 in 1997 dollars were investigated in 17,399 patients undergoing PTCA at Emory University.[131] Mortality changed little from 0.63 to 0.88 percent ($p = 0.84$). The Q-wave MI rate fell from 0.68 to 0.24 percent ($p = 0.036$). Emergent coronary surgery fell from 3.50 to 1.56 percent ($p < 0.0001$). Mean hospital cost decreased from $9816 to $7442 ($p < 0.0001$), and the length of stay after the procedure decreased from 2.81 to 2.00 days ($p < 0.0001$).

Some technologic improvements have been specifically subjected to economic analyses. The use of stents was compared with balloon angioplasty in the STRESS trial.[134] In this relatively early evaluation of stents, there was less additional revascularization and less restenosis with stents but no difference in survival. Costs were higher with stents, due to the prolonged hospitalization and full anticoagulation. Stents ultimately may dominate balloon angioplasty, since hospital stay is now likely to be similar, as stent costs decline while additional procedures continue to be avoided. In both the EPIC and RESTORE trials, the costs of PTCA with and without glycoprotein IIb/IIIa antagonists during balloon angioplasty in the setting of unstable angina or non-Q-wave MI was studied.[135,136] In both studies, there was improved outcome with glycoprotein IIb/IIIa blockade, with little or no increase in costs. A formal cost-effectiveness analysis of glycoprotein IIb/IIIa blockade for balloon angioplasty has been published in preliminary form.[137] Finally, a purely theoretical paper has suggested that a therapy costing in the range of $1000 that decreases restenosis after coronary angioplasty by 50 percent could offer a cost-effectiveness ratio of $16,000 per QALY.[138]

Coronary Surgery versus Medicine

Coronary surgery has been compared with medicine in three major clinical trials conducted in the 1970s and early 1980s (see Chap. 48). None of these trials incorporated cost assessment or cost-effectiveness analyses in their designs. However, the cost-effectiveness of coronary surgery was studied in a relatively early, although detailed decision-analytic study by Weinstein and Stason.[45] Costs included those of surgery, medical management of angina, and treatment of future MIs. CABG was shown to increase unadjusted life expectancy by 0.6 year in patients with two-vessel disease and 6.9 years in patients with left main coronary disease. With one-vessel disease, a gain in quality-adjusted life expectancy may be noted, due to less angina after surgery. For patients with severe angina, the cost-effectiveness of CABG ranged from $3800 per QALY gained in left main disease to $30,000 in one-vessel disease.

Coronary Surgery versus Percutaneous Coronary Intervention

The cost-effectiveness of CABG versus PTCA was first assessed using a decision-analytic model by Wong et al.[139] 8 years after the Weinstein and Stason article.[45] This article was published after PTCA was more established but before the era of stents and before results of randomized trials comparing PTCA with CABG. The model predicted that patients treated with PTCA would have more additional revascularization procedures than patients treated with CABG but that cost would be similar in the long term. In patients with angiographically suitable two-vessel disease, PTCA was found to be a reasonable alternative to CABG. Even in patients with three-vessel disease, bypass surgery was only slightly better than angioplasty.

CABG versus PTCA as an initial revascularization strategy has been compared in a series of six randomized trials from the late 1980s and early 1990s.[31–36] These trials showed little difference in death or MI except in the subgroup with treated diabetes, for which several trials showed a benefit to coronary surgery.[32,140] However, there generally was less angina and less need for additional revascularization procedures after coronary surgery. Cost analyses were performed in the EAST and BARI trials in the United States, ERACI in Argentina, RITA in the United Kingdom, and GABI in Germany.[36–40]

In the EAST trial, Weintraub et al.[37] examined the in-hospital and 3-year costs of patients randomized to revascularization with coronary surgery or coronary angioplasty. While the in-hospital costs of surgery were higher than those of angioplasty, there was little difference in 3-year costs. This was due to the need for additional procedures in many of the angioplasty patients.

BARI[32] was a multicenter trial with 1829 patients and included prospective information on economic costs and quality of life in 934. The initial cost of angioplasty was $21,113 and coronary surgery was $32,247 ($p < 0.001$). However, by 5 years, the costs were much closer, $56,225 for angioplasty and $58,889 for surgery ($p = 0.047$). The costs were surprisingly and disturbingly high in both treatment arms, and there was considerable overlap. The BARI trial showed that CABG dominated PTCA for treated diabetics with three-vessel disease.

Two European randomized trials of PTCA and CABG have included economic end points: the RITA trial[36,38] of 1011 patients and the GABI trial[33] of 358 patients. In the GABI trial, the initial procedural costs were $16,562 for CABG and $5000 for PTCA. After 1 year, the authors found that there was little increase in cumulative costs in the CABG group, whereas the cumulative costs for the PTCA group were $11,250.[33] Similar results were found in the RITA trial, where initially there were much higher costs in the CABG group, but by 2 years the cumulative costs in the PTCA group were 80 percent of those for the CABG group.[38] Cost at 3 years in the ERACI trial also was higher in the CABG group than in the PTCA group but had narrowed from in-hospital costs.[40]

Other than for treated diabetics in the BARI trial, there are inadequate data to perform a cost-effectiveness analysis comparing PTCA with CABG from any of the trials to date because the difference in symptomatic status makes it necessary to include utility assessment. This is essential because if there is no difference in survival, and life years alone were the measure of outcome, then the decision could be made on the basis of cost alone. There are three more contemporary trials comparing PTCA with CABG. There is ARTS in Europe and Israel and ERACI II in Argentina. Preliminary data from ERACI II suggest that PTCA with stenting may dominate CABG, but this is a small trial with only preliminary data in late 1999.[141] There is an ongoing trial in the United Kingdom, continental Europe, and Canada, SoS, which is comparing contemporary coronary intervention with stents with coronary bypass surgery. SoS will incorporate a formal cost-effectiveness analysis with utility assessment (see also Chap. 45).

PTCA versus Medicine

The cost-effectiveness of PTCA compared with medicine also was assessed as part of the now somewhat historical paper by Wong et al.[139] referred to earlier concerning the comparison of PTCA with CABG. This study suggested that in patients with severe angina or documented ischemia, angioplasty was cost-effective for single-vessel disease. PTCA has been compared with medicine in three randomized trials, ACME,[142] AVERT,[143] and RITA II.[144] All showed less angina with PTCA. AVERT and RITA II found more cardiovascular events with angioplasty. However, these trials have been small, underpowered to examine hard end points, and have largely included low-risk patients. None included a formal cost or cost-effectiveness analysis. In the ongoing COURAGE trial, a larger cohort of 3260 higher-risk patients, all treated with the best available medical therapy, are being randomized to PTCA with medicine versus medicine alone. COURAGE includes a formal cost-effectiveness analysis with utility assessment by direct patient preference.

ELECTROPHYSIOLOGY

Patient Monitoring

Monitoring involves multiple areas, including Holter monitoring, cardiac event recording, and monitoring in the hospital. Event recorders were compared with a 48-h monitor in a randomized trial by Kinlay et al.[145] using a randomized crossover trial design in 43 patients with palpitations. Event monitors were twice as likely to provide a diagnostic rhythm strip ECG during symptoms as the 48-h monitor. Event monitors dominated continuous monitors with cost savings.

Implantable Cardiac Defibrillators

Implantable cardiac defibrillators (ICDs) have become widely used to prevent sudden cardiac death in patients at high risk (see also Chap. 31). The cost-effectiveness of this therapy has been investigated with decision-analytic models as well as within the context of randomized trials. Kupersmith et al.[146] investigated the cost-effectiveness of ICD implantation using a decision-analytic model. These investigators based their model on a patient population of 218 well-characterized patients for whom the time of first appropriate discharge was determined.[147] All patients underwent electrophysiologic testing. The authors assumed that the time of first appropriate shock would have been the time of death without the ICD, which was compared with observed mortality. Costs were based on the Medicare fee schedule. Cost-effectiveness was \$31,100 per year of life saved. At an ejection fraction of less than 25 percent and greater than or equal to 25 percent, cost-effectiveness was \$44,000 and \$27,200 per year of life saved. Endocardial ICDs became popular at the time of this study and decreased the cost-effectiveness ratio to \$25,700 per year of life saved.

Owens et al.[148] also developed a decision-analytic model, but with a different construction and a somewhat different question. Specifically, ICDs were compared with amiodarone in patients at high or intermediate risk using a highly detailed model with event rates from the literature and costs estimated from published cost rates in California.[149] In high-risk patients, if an ICD reduces total mortality by 20 percent, the marginal cost-effectiveness of an ICD relative to amiodarone was \$74,400 per QALY saved. If an ICD reduces mortality by 40 percent, the cost-effectiveness of ICD use was \$37,300 per QALY saved, with the results sensitive to assumptions about quality of life. Decision-analytic models were noted by Larsen et al.[149] and Kupermann et al.[150] In these studies, the cost-effectiveness of treatment with an ICD was better than that noted by Owens et al.[148] at \$30,500[150] and \$47,700[149] per life year saved, adjusted to 1995 dollars. However, the study by Owens et al.[148] considered the more superior antiarrhythmic agent amiodarone.

In a small, randomized trial conducted by Wever et al.,[151] 60 consecutive postinfarct survivors of sudden cardiac death were randomly assigned either ICD as first choice or antiarrhythmic drugs and guided by electrophysiologic testing. Fifteen patients died, 4 in the early ICD group and 11 in the electrophysiologic testing-guided strategy group ($p = 0.07$). The cost-effectiveness of ICD compared with drug therapy was \$11,315 per life year saved by early ICD implantation. If quality-of-life measures are taken into account, the cost-effectiveness of early ICD implantation was even more favorable.

Cost-effectiveness of ICD compared with conventional therapy from the MADIT trial was reported by Mushlin et al.,[152] based on 181 patients randomized in the United States. Hospital costs were estimated from the UB92 formulation of the hospital bill and converted to costs using hospital-specific cost-to-charge ratios. Corresponding physician costs were based on a national study of Medicare claims that calculated the ratio of physician to hospital costs for each DRG.[153] Additional professional costs were calculated from payment rates in the Medicare RBRVS. MADIT included epicardial implants in the beginning of the trial and endocardial implants later on. The discounted survival was 3.46 years for the ICD group and 2.66 years for the conventional therapy group to 4 years of follow-up and was associated with an incremental cost-effectiveness ratio of \$27,000 (95 percent confidence interval, \$200 to \$68,200) per life year saved. The results probably would have been more favorable if all patients were treated with endocardial implants. These results probably offer the strongest argument for the cost-effectiveness of ICDs.

Radiofrequency Ablation

Radiofrequency ablation (RFA) can be curative of supraventricular arrhythmias and offers the potential for dominating older forms of therapy (see also Chap. 28). This was studied in a small group of patients by Kalbfleisch et al.[154] The authors determined charges for radiofrequency catheter modification of the atrioventricular (AV) node in 15 patients with symptomatic AV node reentrant tachycardia despite pharmacologic therapy and compared these charges with the estimated health care charges by the same patients before the catheter procedure was performed. The duration and frequency of symptoms were 16 ± 9 years and 4.5 ± 6 episodes per month, respectively. Fourteen of the 15 patients required only one procedure for diagnosis and cure of AV node reentrant tachycardia, and 1 patient required two sessions; all underwent electrophysiologic study before discharge from the hospital to confirm the short-term efficacy of the procedure. The mean duration of the hospital stay was 3 ± 1.5 days, with a charge per patient in 1991 dollars of $15,893 ± $3338, including hospital and physician components. All patients had a successful outcome and required no additional antiarrhythmic therapy. The estimated cost of health care utilization for these 15 patients before cure of AV node reentrant tachycardia was $7651 per patient per year. While small in scale, and with less than optimal costing methods, this study reflects dominance of RFA. A similar costing study from Australia of RFA compared with continued medical therapy also showed dominance of the procedure.[155] RFA in 20 patients was compared with surgical treatment in 20 patients and medical therapy in 12 patients in the nonrandomized comparison. RFA dominated medical therapy. Surgical therapy was slightly more efficacious, but at much higher cost.[156]

A more sophisticated decision-analytic model was created by Hogenhuis et al.[157] In four groups of patients with Wolff-Parkinson-White syndrome, those with (1) prior cardiac arrest, (2) paroxysmal supraventricular tachycardia or atrial fibrillation (PSVT/AF) with hemodynamic compromise, (3) PSVT/AF without hemodynamic compromise, and (4) no symptoms, the authors developed a cost-effectiveness analysis examining five clinical management strategies: (1) observation, (2) observation until a cardiac arrest dictates the need for therapy, (3) initial drug therapy guided by noninvasive monitoring, (4) initial RFA, and (5) initial surgical ablation. A model was developed that included the risks of cardiac arrest, PSVT/AF, drug side effects, procedure-related complications and mortality, the efficacy of drugs and RFA, and cost. RFA was assumed to have an overall efficacy of 92 percent in preventing cardiac arrest and arrhythmias. The model predicted that RFA would yield life expectancy greater than or equal to other strategies. In cardiac arrest survivors and patients who have had PSVT/AF with hemodynamic compromise, the model suggested that RFA would prolong survival at a lower cost. For patients with PSVT/AF without hemodynamic compromise, the marginal cost-effectiveness of attempted RFA ranged from $6600 for 20-year-olds to $19,000 for 60-year-olds per QALY gained. However, for asymptomatic patients, RFA costs ranged from $174,000 for 20-year-olds to $540,000 for 60-year-olds per QALY gained.

Pacemakers

There is a paucity of cost-effectiveness data concerning pacemakers. This may be so because in the classic indication of heart block they are so clearly life-saving that even if they do not dominate no therapy, there can be little doubt about their cost-effectiveness (see also Chap. 31). Some effort has gone into resource utilization issues. Stamato et al.[158] performed a cost-minimization study in which they showed that charges and probably costs will be lower with implantation in a catheterization laboratory as opposed to the operating room. The cost-effectiveness of dual-chamber DDD pacing compared with single-chamber VVI pacing was studied using a decision-analytic model by Sutton and Bourgeois.[159]

Over a 10-year period, a computer model calculated the incidence and prevalence of atrial fibrillation, stroke, permanent disability, heart failure, and mortality in six patient categories: sick sinus syndrome paced VVI, sick sinus syndrome and atrioventricular block upgraded to DDD, sick sinus syndrome paced DDD from the outset, atrioventricular block paced VVI and those upgraded to DDD, and atrioventricular block paced initially DDD. Survival and functional capacity were improved with DDD pacing both for sick sinus syndrome and for atrioventricular block. DDD pacing also was less expensive in the long term, with health care costs in follow-up being a number of times more expensive than the pacemaker. In appropriate patients, DDD pacing dominates VVI pacing. Other efforts have gone into establishing guidelines to ensure the appropriate use of pacemakers.[160–163]

Care of Atrial Fibrillation

The major risk of atrial fibrillation is embolic stroke. The cost-effectiveness of anticoagulation was considered using a decision-analytic model by Gage et al.[164] The authors obtained the probabilities of adverse outcomes from trials involving anticoagulation for nonvalvular atrial fibrillation. They noted a 22 percent reduction in ischemic stroke with aspirin therapy from a metaanalysis[165] and a 68 percent reduction with warfarin therapy from the atrial fibrillation investigators' collaborative analysis of five clinical trials.[166] The authors obtained utility estimates by interviewing 74 patients with atrial fibrillation, using the time tradeoff method for three degrees of severity of stroke and for daily therapy with aspirin or warfarin. Costs were estimated, based on the literature. For patients at medium risk of stroke (i.e., patients with atrial fibrillation and one additional stroke risk factor, including a history of stroke, transient ischemic attack, hypertension, diabetes, or heart disease), the cost-effectiveness of warfarin therapy as compared with aspirin therapy was $8000 (range, $200 to $30,000) per QALY. Both warfarin and aspirin dominated no therapy. For patients at low risk of stroke (i.e., isolated atrial fibrillation), quality-adjusted life expectancy was 6.70 years with warfarin therapy, 6.69 years with aspirin therapy, and 6.51 years with no therapy. The marginal cost-effectiveness of warfarin over aspirin was $370,000 per QALY saved in the base case. If the annual rate of stroke were 0.5 percent higher in low-risk patients, warfarin treatment would cost $66,000 per QALY. Aspirin dominated no therapy.

In a decision-analytic model from Sweden, Gustafsson et al.[167] found that anticoagulation dominated no therapy, and in a decision-analytic model from the United Kingdom, Lightowlers and McGuire[168] found anticoagulation to be cost-effective and dominate no therapy in higher-risk patients.

Recent efforts have focused on strategies for managing cardioversion, antiarrhythmic therapy, and anticoagulation. Eckman et al.[169] constructed a decision-analytic model considering the base case of a 65-year-old man with nonvalvular atrial fibrillation. Cardioversion followed by a combination of amiodarone and warfarin was the most effective strategy, yielding a gain of 2.3 QALYs compared with no therapy. The marginal cost-effectiveness ratio of cardioversion followed by aspirin with amiodarone was $33,800 per QALY and without amiodarone was $10,800 per QALY. Cardioversion followed by amiodarone and warfarin had a marginal cost-effectiveness ratio of $92,400 per QALY compared with amiodarone and aspirin.

Catherwood[170] constructed a similar decision-analytic model considering multiple strategies involving cardioversion followed by aspirin, amiodarone, and warfarin. Strategies involving cardioversion dominated no cardioversion. For patients at high risk of stroke (5.3 percent per year), cardioversion alone followed by repeated cardioversion plus amiodarone therapy on relapse was cost-effective at $9300 per QALY compared with cardioversion alone followed by warfarin therapy on relapse. This strategy also was preferred for moderate-risk patients (3.6 percent per year), but with a higher cost-effectiveness ratio of $18,900 per QALY. In the lowest-risk patients (1.6 percent per year), cardioversion alone followed by aspirin therapy on relapse was preferred.

Another issue concerning the care of patients with atrial fibrillation is the role of transesophageal echocardiography in avoiding prolonged anticoagulation prior to cardioversion. This was investigated using a decision-analytic model by Seto et al.[171] The authors studied the cost-effectiveness of three strategies: (1) conventional therapy with transthoracic echocardiography and warfarin therapy for 1 month before cardioversion, (2) initial transthoracic echo followed by transesophageal echo and early cardioversion if no thrombus was detected, and (3) initial transesophageal echo with early cardioversion if no thrombus is detected. With strategies 2 and 3, if a thrombus was seen, a follow-up transesophageal echo was performed. If no thrombus was seen, cardioversion was performed. All strategies used anticoagulation before and extending for 1 month after cardioversion. Life expectancy, utilities, event probabilities, and cost were ascertained from the literature. Strategy 3 (cost, $2774; QALYS, 8.49) dominated strategy 2 (cost, $3106; QALYs, 8.48) and conventional therapy (cost, $3070; QALYs, 8.48). The study demonstrated that transesophageal echo-guided cardioversion dominated conventional therapy if the risk of stroke after transesophageal echo negative for atrial thrombus is slightly less than that after conventional therapy. However, the issue of the best way to facilitate cardioversion to minimize periprocedural stroke is not yet certain.

HEART FAILURE

Perspective

Heart failure is a major medical problem in economically advantaged countries. In the United States, the approximate prevalence of congestive heart failure is 4.6 million, with an incidence of 400,000 new cases a year and approximately 870,000 hospitalizations a year. Furthermore, hospitalizations for heart failure have increased by 130.8 percent between 1979 and 1996.[3] In 1995, the Health Care Financing Agency paid $3.4 billion to Medicare beneficiaries for heart failure, and it is the single most common cause of hospitalizations over the age of 65.[2] The American Heart Association estimates the total annual direct and indirect care costs of heart failure at $21 billion dollars.[3]

Heart failure differs from other areas of consideration in this chapter because it is a disease process rather than a single form of therapy or service. Thus the economics of heart failure and cost-effectiveness strategies must approach it as a process and then consider breaking the process down. Heart failure must be considered a process in which patients have a baseline health state, with associated baseline continuing costs for medication and office visits as well as productivity costs. The patient may then decompensate, resulting in a hospitalization, presumably with a somewhat worse health state and associated costs. Efforts will then be made to return the patient to his or her baseline health state and maintain him or her there. Finally, patients may be considered for transplantation to try to reverse or partially reverse heart failure, also with associated cost (see also Chaps. 21 and Chap. 22).

Digoxin

Despite over 200 years of experience, the role of digoxin in the treatment of congestive heart failure remains uncertain. In the absence of adequate clinical data, the cost-effectiveness data similarly will be limited. Nonetheless, Ward et al.[172] developed a decision-analytic model concerning digoxin withdrawal in patients with stable heart failure. The clinical sequelae of digoxin withdrawal came from the Prospective Randomized Study of Ventricular Failure and Efficacy of Digoxin (PROVED) and Randomized Assessment of Digoxin and Inhibitors of Angiotensin-Converting Enzyme (RADIANCE) trials.[173,174] Costs were estimated from hospital and Medicare data. Outcomes included treatment failures, digoxin toxicity, and health care costs. Continuation of digoxin therapy in patients with heart failure nationally would avoid 185,000 office visits, 27,000 emergency visits, and 137,000 hospital admissions for heart failure, but with 12,500 cases of digoxin toxicity. The net annual savings would be $406 million (90 percent confidence interval, $106 to $822 million). Sensitivity analysis showed that digoxin is cost saving if the incidence of digoxin toxicity is 33 percent or less. Thus digoxin therapy was found to dominate withdrawal of digoxin in stable heart failure.

In a large randomized trial study, the effect of digoxin on mortality and hospitalization in patients with heart failure and left ventricular ejection fractions of 0.45 or less were randomly assigned to digoxin (3397 patients) or placebo (3403 patients) in addition to diuretics and ACE inhibitors.[175] While there was no effect on mortality, there were 26.8 percent hospitalizations in the digoxin groups versus 34.7 percent in the placebo group ($p < 0.001$). Although no formal cost-effectiveness analysis is available, Mark estimated that the digoxin therapy is at least cost neutral and probably cost saving.[176]

ACE Inhibition

The efficacy of ACE inhibition in preserving left ventricular size and in prolonging survival in patients with heart failure has been established in a series of clinical trials. In a meta-analysis of 32 trials totaling 7105 patients, the mortality rate in patients randomized to ACE inhibitor was 15.8 percent compared with 21.9 percent for placebo (odds ratio, 0.77; 95 percent confidence interval, 0.67 to 0.88).[177] None of these trials included prospective economic evaluations. However, there have been several decision-analytic analyses based on these trials.

Tsevat et al.[128] studied the effectiveness of ACE inhibition after MI, and the results are reviewed in that section. Glick et al.[178,179] developed a decision-analytic model based on the SOLVD trial. SOLVD was an 83-center trial in which 2569 patients with symptomatic heart failure and ejection fractions of 35 percent or less received either the ACE inhibitor enalapril or placebo. At 41.4 months of follow-up, enalapril decreased mortality and hospitalization by 16 and 26 percent, respectively. Costs were estimated based on HCFA reimbursement rates in 1992 dollars. For patients with heart failure, enalapril dominates placebo in the short term and is highly economically attractive in the long term. Enalapril saved approximately $717 per patient over the period of the SOLVD treatment trial. When trial data were projected over a patient's lifetime, therapy with enalapril produced a cost utility ratio of $115 per QALY. As pointed out by Boyko et al.,[180] there is variation in the cost of ACE inhibitors, and as these agents become less expensive, their cost-effectiveness ratio may become even more attractive.

Somewhat more general in the treatment of heart failure is the Paul et al.[181] decision-analytic model based on the SOLVD and VheFt I and II trials. These trials considered the strategies of (1) standard therapy (digoxin and diuretics) with no vasodilator agents, (2) hydralazine hydrochloride-isosorbide dinitrate combination, and (3) ACE inhibition with enalapril. Using data from three major randomized, controlled trials to estimate treatment efficacy, mortality rates, and hospitalization rates, the cost was $5600 per year of life gained with hydralazine–isosorbide dinitrate compared with standard therapy. Compared with the hydralazine–isosorbide dinitrate combination therapy, the incremental cost-effectiveness ratio for enalapril therapy was $9700 per year of life saved.

The cost-effectiveness of ACE inhibition also has been studied in Europe using decision-analytic techniques. In mild heart failure, Kleber[182] found ACE inhibition to be cost-effective but not cost saving. However, in the Netherlands, van Hout et al.[183] found ACE inhibition to dominate not using ACE. Similarly, in a study from the United Kingdom based on SOLVD, Hart et al.[184] found that ACE therapy potentially could dominate not using ACE therapy.

Beta Blockade

Recently, beta blockade, especially with carvedilol, has been added to the therapeutic armamentarium for heart failure. There have been four randomized trials in 1094 patients with New York Heart Association class II to IV symptoms and left ventricular ejection fraction of 0.35 or less.[185] The series of trials was terminated early, based on a finding of a 65 percent mortality reduction in patients receiving carvedilol (95 percent confidence interval, 39 to 82 percent). Delea, et al.[186] constructed a decision-analytic model estimating life expectancy and health care costs for patients with heart failure receiving carvedilol plus conventional therapy (digoxin, diuretics, and ACE inhibitors) or conventional therapy alone. Benefit estimates were based on the carvedilol trial results, assuming either "limited benefits" persisting for 6 months, the average duration of follow-up in the clinical trials, or "extended benefits" persisting for 6 months and then declining gradually over 3 years. For conventional therapy alone, estimated life expectancy was 6.67 years, and for carvedilol it was 6.98 and 7.62 years, assuming limited and extended benefits, respectively. Expected lifetime costs of heart failure–related care were estimated at $28,756 for conventional therapy and $36,420 and $38,867 for carvedilol, assuming limited and extended benefits, respectively. Cost per life year saved for carvedilol was $29,477 and $12,799 under limited and extended benefits assumptions, respectively. Thus the cost-effectiveness of cardvedilol remains in a reasonable range but is not as attractive as ACE inhibition.

Disease Management Strategies

Heart failure is particularly well suited to developing strategies, such as the development of heart failure clinics, to improve management. Evaluating treatment strategies is difficult because (1) it is difficult to construct randomized trials logistically, (2) there may be contamination in which the management strategy is used to some extent in the control arm, (3) there may be differences between programs that are inherent in different medical centers that make collaboration for multisite efforts difficult, and (4) different health care systems may vary substantially. These variations also may limit generalizability. The difficulties in mounting trials to evaluate outcome of management strategies is a similar limitation for randomized trials. Nonetheless, several small efforts have been made.

Rich et al.[187] conducted a randomized trial using a nurse-directed, multidisciplinary intervention on readmission rate within 90 days of hospital discharge, quality of life, and costs for elderly patients admitted to the hospital with heart failure. The intervention was comprised of educating the patient and family, diet, early discharge planning, reviewing medications, and intensive follow-up. Survival for 90 days without readmission was achieved in 91 of the 142 patients in the treatment group versus 75 of the 140 patients with conventional care ($p = 0.09$). There were 53 readmissions in the treatment group versus 94 in the control group (risk ratio, 0.56; $p = 0.02$). The number of readmissions for heart failure was reduced by 56.2 percent in the treatment group (54 versus 24 in the control group; $p = 0.04$). In the control group, 23 patients (16.4 percent) had more than one readmission versus 9 (6.3 percent) in the treatment group (risk ratio, 0.39; $p = 0.01$). In a subgroup of 126 patients, quality-of-life scores at 90 days improved more from baseline in the treatment group ($p = 0.001$). Because of the reduction in hospital admissions, the total cost of care was $460 less per patient in 1994 dollars in the treatment group, confirming strong dominance for the management strategy.

Weinberger et al.[188] studied 1396 patients hospitalized with chronic diseases, half of whom had congestive heart failure, who were randomized to intensive medical management versus usual care. There were more repeat hospitalizations in the specialized care group. This seemingly contradictory finding[188] reveals that disease management is not easily subjected to scientific scrutiny.

West et al.[189] and Kornowski et al.[190] studied a disease management strategy based on outpatient care rather than focusing on patients being discharged. In a study in Israel, Kornowski et al.[190] analyzed outcome of 42 patients aged 78 ± 8 years with New York Heart Association congestive heart failure class III or IV who were examined at home weekly by local internists and a trained paramedical team. The year before, entry to the home-care program was compared with the first year of home surveillance. Functional status (ability to perform daily activities on a 1 to 4 scale) improved from 1.4 ± 0.9 to 2.3 ± 0.7 ($p < 0.001$). The total hospitalization rate fell from 3.2 ± 1.5 to 1.2 ± 1.6 hospitalizations per year and length of stay from 26 ± 14 to 6 ± 7 days per year ($p < 0.001$ for both). Cardiovascular admissions fell from 2.9 ± 1.5 to 0.8 ± 1.1 hospitalizations per year and stay from 23 ± 13 to 4 ± 4 days per year ($p < 0.001$). This study showed improved outcome but at an uncertain tradeoff in resource use between increased home visits and decreased hospitalizations for the intervention.

West et al.[189] used a strategy of physician-led but nurse-managed, home-based heart failure management not involving home visits. Nurses directed the implementation of guidelines for pharmacologic and dietary therapy by frequent telephone contact of 51 patients with heart failure for 138 ± 44 days. Compared with the period before enrollment, sodium intake fell by 38 percent ($p = 0.0001$), vasodilator doses increased ($p = 0.01$), and functional status and exercise capacity improved significantly ($p = 0.01$). Compared with the 6 months before enrollment, general medical and cardiology visits declined by 23 and 31 percent, respectively (both $p < 0.03$), and emergency room visits for heart failure and for all causes declined 67 and 53 percent, respectively (both $p < 0.001$). Compared with 1 year before enrollment, hospitalization rates for heart failure and for all causes declined 87 and 74 percent ($p = 0.001$). Thus this strategy improved clinical outcome for heart failure while reducing resource use, again suggesting strong dominance.

Rich[191] and Philbin[192] have both reviewed disease management programs. Between 1983 to 1998, 16 studies, 10 observational and 6 randomized trials, of multidisciplinary heart failure disease management programs were published in the English language literature. All studies reported reduced hospitalization, and several studies reported improved quality of life, functional capacity, patient satisfaction, and compliance. All studies that included a cost analysis found the disease management programs to be cost-effective. Rich[191] suggested that current data are limited by generalizability to the more heterogeneous population of patients with heart failure, and the feasibility of translating specific disease management programs into diverse practice environments, and how to individualize the programs for each patient. While the impact of heart failure disease management programs on survival is also unknown, these programs appear to be cost-effective at reducing morbidity and improving quality of life in selected patients with heart failure.

Heart Transplantation

Heart transplantation remains sufficiently infrequent, with just 2290 in the United States in 1997, that its overall impact on cost from a public health standpoint is small (see also Chap. 22). The American Heart Association estimates the average cost of transplants at $253,200, with an annual follow-up cost of $21,200.[3] Cardiac transplantation has not been subjected to rigorous cost-effectiveness analysis, perhaps because of inadequate natural history data with which to compare transplant patients. Although cardiac transplantation is certainly expensive, these patients generally would have a life expectancy of a few weeks to months in the absence of the transplant. In a somewhat preliminary, and now dated study, Evans[193] showed that overall cost-effectiveness of heart transplant was estimated at $44,300 per year of life saved.

DIAGNOSIS

Establishing the cost-effectiveness of diagnostic testing is considerably more difficult than it is for therapeutics because diagnostics by themselves rarely affect outcome. Rather, diagnostics generally lead to a range of choices of therapeutic options with the potential for very different outcomes. Thus decision-analytic models with diagnostics tend to be more complicated than with therapeutics, and consequently, the uncertainty is much greater. Randomized trials with diagnostics are also quite unusual. Thus such cost-effectiveness analyses as exist are essentially all decision-analytic simulations.

Testing for CAD

Garber and Solomon[194] evaluated the cost-effectiveness of noninvasive and direct coronary angiography in the diagnosis of CAD. The tests evaluated included treadmill exercise ECG, planar thallium imaging, single-photon-emission computed tomography, stress echocardiography, and positron-emission tomography, all followed by coronary angiography, if positive, and finally, direct coronary angiography. Survival was based on the medically or surgically treated patients in the CASS study. How survival after angioplasty was calculated is not clear. Based on a metaanalysis of trials comparing angioplasty with medicine, surgery was assumed to have 1.6 times the ability of angioplasty to relieve symptoms. Sensitivities and specificities of testing were developed from a metaanalysis of the literature. Positron-emission tomography (PET) was the most sensitive noninvasive test and exercise testing the least sensitive. Single-photon emission computed tomography (SPECT) was nearly as sensitive as and somewhat less specific than PET (specificity, 0.77 for SPECT and 0.82 for PET). Stress echocardiography is more specific than PET (0.88 compared with 0.82) but less sensitive (0.76 compared with 0.91). There were no published data on the sensitivity of PET for detecting severe (left main and three-vessel) coronary disease, but planar thallium imaging, SPECT, and echocardiography are highly sensitive for detecting severe disease. These figures are based on studies that included small numbers of patients. Exercise testing is not as sensitive (see also Chap. 40).

Little difference in life expectancy was noted with the various strategies, but somewhat more variation to QALYs because the calculation of QALYS gives credit to strategies that improve symptoms rapidly. Nonetheless, the differences amounted to a couple of weeks over approximately 12 years in men and 14 years in women. Costing was based on Medicare payments.

Single-photon emission computed tomography (SPECT) had higher QALYs at higher cost than stress echocardiography with a marginal cost-effectiveness ratio of $64,000 in 65-year-old men to nearly $150,000 in 45-year-old women. Positron emission tomography (PET) generally produced slightly better outcomes than SPECT but at much greater cost. While immediate angiography dominated PET in every group, immediate angiography was more expensive than SPECT with a margin from about $80,000 in 65-year-old men to nearly $200,000 in 45-year-old women.

Strategies in which patients are neither tested nor treated initially are not no-cost strategies, since patients may experience an MI and undergo medical or surgical treatment in the future.

Thus the cost-effectiveness of stress echocardiography compared with no testing ranges from $31,000 per QALY in 65-year-old men to $98,000 per QALY in 45-year-old women.

At a different prevalence of disease, the ranking of tests changes somewhat. For 55-year-old men with a 75 percent pretest risk for disease, initial angiography becomes more attractive (it will be chosen whenever a cost-effectiveness ratio of $45,000 is acceptable), and stress echocardiography remains preferable to exercise testing (with a cost-effectiveness ratio of $22,000 per QALY. At a 25 percent prevalence of disease, echocardiography seems to be the most attractive test under most circumstances; single-photon-emission computed tomography (SPECT) would be chosen over echocardiography only if a cost-effectiveness ratio of $110,000 is considered acceptable, and immediate angiography would be chosen over SPECT only at a cost-effectiveness ratio of $355,000. Thus stress echocardiography remains a cost-effective strategy at a wide range of prevalence of disease, whereas immediate angiography is a cost-effective choice when the pretest probability of disease is high.

Somewhat similar analyses have been offered by Kim et al.[195] and Kuntz et al.[196] The study by Kim et al.[195] specifically studied women. In a 55-year-old woman with definite angina, direct angiography was found to be appropriate, with a marginal cost-effectiveness of $17,000 per QALY. This figure rises as the probability of angina falls, and in the midrange of probabilities, echocardiography was felt to be preferable. In the study by Kuntz et al.,[196] the incremental cost-effectiveness of direct coronary angiography compared with exercise echocardiography was $36,400 per QALY in a 55-year-old man. For 55-year-old men with atypical angina, exercise echocardiography compared with exercise electrocardiography at a cost of $41,900 per QALY. If exercise echocardiography was not available, exercise single-photon-emission computed tomography (SPECT) cost $54,800 per QALY saved compared with exercise electrocardiography. For a 55-year-old man with nonspecific chest pain, the cost-effectiveness of exercise electrocardiography compared with no testing was $57,700 per QALY.

These studies can be criticized easily for making multiple assumptions. However, the end result is quite reasonable. *In patients with chest pain in the intermediate range of probabilities, a test that includes myocardial imaging, either echocardiography or single-photon-emission computed tomography (SPECT), is appropriate, with echo more appropriate in the lower probability range and SPECT in the higher probability range.* Immediate angiography is appropriate as the probability of disease rises. In lower-risk populations, a treadmill exercise test is probably appropriate, and ultimately, in very low-risk populations, in the single digits of pretest probability, reassurance and watchful waiting would be the strategy of choice.

Triage after MI

The proper evaluation of patients after acute MI in terms of assessment of residual ischemia has remained uncertain. The alternatives are to do nothing and follow patients clinically, to obtain an exercise ECG, to obtain an exercise ECG along with an imaging test, or to perform cardiac catheterization. There are no adequate randomized trials in this area and certainly none that include a cost-effectiveness analysis.

Thus this area has been explored exclusively with decision-analytic models. Dittis et al.[197] developed a model with the options of exercise ECG, exercise thallium scintigraphy, and coronary angiography, followed by CABG surgery for patients with left main coronary disease only or patients with left main disease, three-vessel disease, or single- or double-vessel disease and a significant amount of myocardium in jeopardy. Proceeding directly to angiography for risk stratification was the most effective approach, lowering expected mortality from 8 percent to approximately 3 percent. However, the marginal costs for this strategy were high. The most cost-effective approach was to screen patients initially with exercise ECG.

The approach of using the exercise ECG as a screen after MI was studied by Kuntz et al.,[198] who developed a decision-analytic model for representative patient subgroups based on relevant clinical characteristics. The model estimates QALYs and direct lifetime costs for two strategies: coronary angiography and treatment guided by its results versus initial medical therapy without angiography. Decision-tree chance-node probabilities were estimated from pooled data of randomized clinical trials, and additional relevant literature costs were estimated with the use of the Medicare Part A database; quality-of-life adjustments were derived from a survey of 1051 patients who had had a recent acute MI. The incremental cost-effectiveness ratios for coronary angiography and treatment guided by its result, compared with initial medical therapy without angiography, varied from $17,000 to over $1 million per QALY gained. Patient subgroups with severe postinfarction angina or a strongly positive exercise tolerance test typically had cost-effectiveness ratios of less than $50,000 per QALY gained. In addition, most patient subgroups with a prior MI had cost-effectiveness ratios of less than $50,000 per QALY of life gained, even with a negative exercise test result.

CONCLUSIONS

Health care economics offer a powerful set of tools for establishing cost and overall measures of outcome and relating cost to outcome. These tools have been used increasingly in cardiovascular medicine for the purposes of gaining greater insight to facilitate improved patient management but also to help guide public policy. These tools have been applied widely now in cardiovascular medicine, with peer-reviewed literature on cost and often cost-effectiveness analysis, in most areas of cardiovascular medicine. However, the methods of measurement and analysis have varied widely, limiting the ability to compare studies and thus generalize the findings. A recent effort in the United States[24] should provide a guide to investigators performing cost-effectiveness analyses to perform them in a more standard manner. The quality of data available in many areas probably poses a greater problem. Over time, however, the quality of data and of scholarship should increase, making economic studies ever more meaningful and relevant to the practice of medicine.

ACKNOWLEDGMENT

We thank Lesley Wood for her careful editorial review.

References

1. Allenet B, Sailly J-C. Willingness of pay as a measure of benefit in health. *J D'Econ Med* 1999; 17:301–326.

2. *http://www.hcfa.gov.*
3. *1999 Heart and Stroke Statistical Update.* Dallas: American Heart Association; 1998.
4. Drummond MF, Stoddart GL, Torrance GW. *Methods for the Economic Evaluation of Health Care Programmes.* Oxford, England: Oxford University Press; 1990:74–167.
5. Kupersmith J, Holmes-Rovner M, Hogan A, et al. Cost-effectiveness analysis in heart disease: II. Preventive therapies. *Prog Cardiovasc Dis* 1995; 37:243–271.
6. Borna S, Sundaram S. An approach to allocating limited health resources. *J Health Soc Behav* 1999; 11:85–94.
7. Schlander M. Rational resource allocation in the health care system: I. Why rationing may become inevitable. *Med Welt* 1999; 50:36–41.
8. Weintraub WS, Warner CD, Mauldin PD, et al. Economic winners and losers after introduction of an effective new therapy depend on the type of payment system. *Am J Managed Care* 1997; 3:743–749.
9. Weintraub WS. Microeconomic methods in cardiovascular care. In: Talley JD, Mauldin PD, Becker ER, eds. *Cost-Effective Diagnosis and Treatment of Coronary Artery Disease.* Baltimore: Wiliams & Wilkins; 1999:17–29.
10. Rothermich EA, Pathak DS. Productivity-cost controversies in cost-effectiveness analysis: Review and research agenda. *Clin Ther* 1999; 21:255–267.
11. Evans DB. Principles involved in costing. *Med J Aust* 1990; 153:S10–S12.
12. Hlatky MA. Analysis of costs associated with CABG and PTCA. *Ann Thorac Surg* 1996; 61:S30–S32.
13. Finkler SA. The distinction between costs and charges. *Ann Intern Med* 1982; 96:102–109.
14. Finkler SA, Ward DM. *Essentials of Cost Accounting for Health Care Organizations*, 2d ed. Rockville, MD: Aspen Publications; 1999:11–43.
15. Hlatky MA, Lipscomb J, Nelson C, et al. Resource use and cost of initial coronary revascularization: coronary angioplasty versus coronary bypass surgery. *Circulation* 1990; 82(suppl IV):IV-208–IV-213.
16. Weintraub WS, Mauldin PD, Talley JD, et al. Determinants of hospital costs in acute myocardial infarction. *Am J Managed Care* 1996; 2:977–986.
17. Lefebvre C, Van Der Perre T. Activity based costing. *Acta Hospital* 1994; 34:5–16.
18. Coulam RF, Gaumer GL. Medicare's prospective payment system: A critical appraisal. *Health Care Financ Rev* 1991; 13:45–77.
19. Becker ER, Mauldin PD, Weintraub WS. CABG and PTCA physician practice profiles using the resource-based relative value scale (RBRVS): Better methods for explaining the variation. *Clin Res* 1994; 42:225A.
20. Becker ER, Mauldin PD, Bernadino ME. Using physician work RVUs to profile surgical packages: methods and results for kidney transplant surgery. *Best Pract Benchmark Healthcare* 1996; 3:140–146.
21. Becker ER, Mauldin PD, Culler SD, et al. Applying the resource-based relative-value scale to the Emory Angioplasty versus Surgery Trial. *Am J Cardiol* 2000; 85:685–691.
22. Hsiao WC, Braun P, Yntema D, et al. Estimating physicians' work for a resource-based relative value scale. *N Engl J Med* 1998; 319:835–841.
23. Weintraub WS, Craver JM, Jones EL, et al. Improving cost and outcome of coronary surgery. *Circulation* 1998; 98:23–28.
24. Gold MR, Siegel JE, Russell LB, et al. *Cost-Effectiveness in Health and Medicine.* New York: Oxford University Press; 1996.
25. Quality of Care and Outcomes Research in CVD and Stroke Working Groups. Measuring and improving quality of care: A report from the American Heart Association/American College of Cardiology First Scientific Forum on Assessment of Healthcare Quality in Cardiovascular Disease and Stroke. *Circulation* 2000; 101:1483–1493.
26. Mauldin PD, Weintraub WS, Becker E. Predicting hospital charges and costs for coronary surgery from pre-operative and post-operative variables. *Am J Cardiol* 1994; 74:772–775.
27. Ellis SG, Miller DP, Brown KJ, et al. In-hospital costs of percutaneous coronary revascularization: Critical determinants and implications. *Circulation* 1995; 92:741–747.
28. Mark DB, Gardner LH, Nelson CL, et al. Long-term costs of therapy for CAD: A prospective comparison of coronary angioplasty, coronary bypass surgery and medical therapy in 2258 patients. *Circulation* 1993; 88(2):I-480.
29. Topol EJ, Ellis SG, Cosgrove DM, et al. Analysis of coronary angioplasty practice in the United States with an insurance-claims database. *Circulation* 1993; 87:1489–1497.
30. Harris RA. Nease RF Jr. The importance of patient preferences for comorbidities in cost-effectiveness analyses. *J Health Econ* 1997; 16:113–119.
31. King SB III, Lembo NJ, Weintraub WS, for the EAST Investigators. A randomized trial comparing coronary angioplasty with coronary bypass surgery. *N Engl J Med* 1994; 331:1044–1050.
32. The BARI Investigators. Comparison of coronary bypass surgery with angioplasty in patients with multivessel disease. *N Engl J Med* 1996; 335:217–225.
33. Hamm CW, Reimers J, Ischinger T, et al. A randomized study of coronary angioplasty compared with bypass surgery in patients with symptomatic multivessel coronary artery disease. *N Engl J Med* 1994; 331:1037–1043.
34. CABRI Trial Participants. First-year results of CABRI (Coronary Angioplasty versus Bypass Revascularization Investigation). *Lancet* 1995; 346:1179–1184.
35. Rodriguez A, Boullon F, Perez-Balino N, et al. Argentine randomized trial of percutaneous transluminal coronary angioplasty versus coronary artery bypass surgery in multivessel disease (ERACI): In-hospital results and 1-year follow-up. *J Am Coll Cardiol* 1993; 22:1060–1067.
36. The RITA Investigators. Coronary angioplasty versus coronary artery bypass surgery: the Randomized Intervention Treatment of Angina (RITA) trial. *Lancet* 1993; 341:573–580.
37. Weintraub WS, Mauldin PD, Becker E, et al. A comparison of the costs of and quality of life after coronary angioplasty or coronary surgery for multivessel coronary artery disease: Results from the Emory Angioplasty versus Surgery Trial (EAST). *Circulation* 1995; 92:2831–2840.
38. Hlatky MA, Rogers WJ, Johnstone I, et al. Medical care costs and quality of life after randomization to coronary angioplasty or coronary bypass surgery. *N Engl J Med* 1997; 336:92–99.
39. Sculpher MJ, Seed P, Henderson RA, et al. Health service costs of coronary angioplasty and coronary artery bypass surgery: The Randomized Intervention Treatment of Angina (RITA) trial. *Lancet* 1994; 344:927–930.
40. Rodriguez A, Mele E, Peyregne E, et al. Three-year follow-up of the Argentine Randomized Trial of Percutaneous Transluminal Coronary Angioplasty versus Coronary Artery Bypass Surgery in Multivessel Disease (ERACI). *J Am Coll Cardiol* 1996; 27:1178–1184.
41. Alchian A. The meaning of utility measurement. *Am Econ Rev* 1953; 143:26–50.
42. Feeny DH, Torrance GW, Furlong WJ. Health utilities index. In: Spilker B, ed. *Quality of Life and Pharmacoeconomics in Clinical Trials.* Philadelphia: Lippincott-Raven; 1996:239–252.
43. Cook TA, O'Regan M, Galland RB. Quality of life following percutaneous transluminal angioplasty for claudication. *Eur J Vasc Endovasc Surg* 1996; 11:191–194.
44. Loomes G, McKenzie L. The use of QALYs in health care decision making. *Soc Sci Med* 1989; 28:299–308.

45. Weinstein MC, Stason WB. Cost effectiveness of coronary artery bypass surgery. *Circulation* 1982; 66(suppl III):56–65.
46. Tengs TO, Adams ME, Pliskin JS, et al. Five-hundred life-saving interventions and their cost-effectiveness. *Risk Anal* 1995; 15:369–390.
47. Schulman KA, Kinosian B, Jacobson TA, et al. Reducing high blood cholesterol level with drugs: Cost-effectiveness of pharmacologic management. *JAMA* 1990; 264:3025–3033.
48. Tosteson AN, Weinstein MC, Hunink MG, et al. Cost-effectiveness of populationwide educational approaches to reduce serum cholesterol levels. *Circulation* 1997; 95:24–30.
49. Goldman L, Weinstein MC, Goldman PA, et al. Cost-effectiveness of HMG-CoA reductase inhibition for primary and secondary prevention of coronary heart disease. *JAMA* 1991; 265:1145–1151.
50. Garber AM, Browner WS, Hulley SB. Cholesterol screening in asymptomatic adults, revisited. *Ann Intern Med* 1996; 124: 518–531.
51. Abbott RD, McGee D, Kannel WB, et al. The probability of developing certain cardiovascular disease in eight years at specified values of some characteristics. In: Kannel WB, Wolf PA, Garrison RJ, eds. *The Framingham Study: An Epidemiological Investigation of Cardiovascular Disease* (publication no. NIH 87:2284). Bethesda: US Department of Health, Education & Welfare; 1987:sec 37.
52. Randomized trial of cholesterol lowering in 4444 patients with coronary heart disease: The Scandinavian Simvastatin Survival Study. *Lancet* 1994; 344:1383–1389.
53. Pedersen TR, Kjekshus J, Berg K, et al. Cholesterol lowering and the use of healthcare resources: Results of the Scandinavian Simvastatin Survival Study. *Circulation* 1996; 93:1796–1802.
54. Johannesson M, Jonsson B, Kjekshus J, et al. Cost effectiveness of simvastatin treatment to lower cholesterol levels in patients with coronary heart disease. *N Engl J Med* 1997; 336:332–336.
55. Shepherd J, Cobbe SM, Ford I, et al. Prevention of coronary heart disease with pravastatin in men with hypercholesterolemia. *N Engl J Med* 1995; 333:1301–1307.
56. Caro J, Klittich W, McGwire A, et al. The West of Scotland Coronary Prevention Study: Economic benefit analysis of primary prevention with pravastatin. *Br Med J* 1997; 315:1577–1582.
57. Ashraf T, Hay JW, Pitt B, et al. Cost-effectiveness of pravastatin in secondary prevention of coronary artery disease. *Am J Cardiol* 1996; 78:409–414.
58. State-specific prevalence among adults of current cigarette smoking and smokeless tobacco use and per capita tax-paid sales of cigarettes—United States, 1997. *MMWR* 1998; 47:922–926.
59. US Department of Agriculture. *Tobacco Situation and Outlook Report* (publication no. TBS-227). Washington: US Department of Agriculture, Economic Research Service, Commodity Economics Division; June 1994.
60. US Department of Health and Human Services. *Reducing the Health Consequences of Smoking: 25 Years of Progress.* A Report of the Surgeon General (DSS Publication No. CDC89;8411). U.S. Department of Health and Human Services, Public Health Service, Centers for Disease Control, Center for Chronic Disease Prevention and Health Promotion, Office on Smoking and Health; 1989.
61. MacKenzie TD, Bartecchi CF, Schrier RW. The human costs of tobacco use. *N Engl J Med* 1994; 330:975–980.
62. Lightwood JM, Glantz SA. Short-term economic and health benefits of smoking cessation. *Circulation* 1997; 96:1089–1096.
63. Warner KE. Cost effectiveness of smoking-cessation therapies: Interpretation of the evidence—and implications for coverage. *Pharmacoeconomics* 1997; 11:538–549.
64. Meenan RT, Stevens VJ, Hornbrook MC, et al. Cost-effectiveness of a hospital-based smoking cessation intervention. *Med Care* 1998; 36:670–678.
65. Cromwell J, Bartosch WJ, Fiore MC, et al. Cost-effectiveness of the clinical practice recommendations in the AHCPR guideline for smoking cessation. *JAMA* 1997; 278:1759–1766.
66. Krumholz HM, Chen BJ, Tsevat J, et al. Cost-effectiveness of a smoking cessation program after myocardial infarction. *J Am Coll Cardiol* 1993; 22:1703–1705.
67. Jones TF, Eaton CB. Cost-benefit analysis of walking to prevent coronary heart disease. *Arch Farm Med* 1994; 3:703–710.
68. Moss SE, Klein R, Klein BEK, et al. The association of glycemia and cause-specific mortality in a diabetic population. *Arch Intern Med* 1994; 154:2473–2479.
69. American Diabetes Association. Standards of medical care for patients with diabetes mellitus. *Diabetes Care* 1997; 20(suppl 1):S5–S13.
70. Hayward RA, Manning WG, Kaplan SH, et al. Starting insulin therapy in patients with type 2 diabetes: Effectiveness, complications and resource utilization. *JAMA* 1997; 278:1663–1669.
71. Gilmer TP, O'Connor PJ, Manning W, et al. The cost to health plans of poor glycemic control. *Diabetes Care* 1997; 20:1847–1853.
72. The Diabetes Control and Complications Trial Research Group. Intensive diabetes treatment and complications in IDDM. *N Engl J Med* 1993; 329:977–986.
73. The Diabetes Control and Complications Trial Research Group. Lifetime benefits and costs of intensive therapy as practiced in the diabetes control and complications trial. *JAMA* 1996; 276: 1409–1415.
74. UK Prospective Diabetes Study Group. Intensive blood-glucose control with sulphonylureas or insulin compared with conventional treatment and risk of complications in patients with type 2 diabetes. *Lancet* 1998; 352:837–853.
75. Eastman RC, Javitt JC, Herman WH, et al. Model of complications of NIDDM: II. Analysis of the health benefits and cost-effectiveness of treating NIDDM with the goal of normoglycemia. *Diabetes Care* 1997; 20:735–744.
76. The sixth report of the joint national committee on prevention, detection, evaluation, and treatment of high blood pressure. *Arch Intern Med* 1997; 157:2413–2446.
77. Dustan HP, Roccella EJ, Garrison HH. Controlling hypertension: A research success story. *Arch Intern Med* 1996; 156:1926–1935.
78. Littenberg B, Garber AM, Sox HC Jr. Screening for hypertension. *Ann Intern Med* 1990; 112:192–202.
79. Edelson JT, Weinstein MC, Tosteson AN, et al. Long-term cost-effectiveness of various initial monotherapies for mild to moderate hypertension. *JAMA* 1990; 263:407–413.
80. Johannesson M, Dahlof B, Lindholm LH, et al. The cost-effectiveness of treating hypertension in elderly people: An analysis of the Swedish Trial in Old Patients with Hypertension (STOP Hypertension). *J Intern Med* 1993; 234:317–323.
81. Moser M. Why are physicians not prescribing diuretics more frequently in the management of hypertension? *JAMA* 1998; 279:1813–1816.
82. Ramsey SD, Neil N, Sullivan SD, et al. An economic evaluation of the JNC hypertension guidelines using data from a randomized controlled trial. Joint National Committee. *J Am Board Fam Pract* 1999; 12:105–114.
83. Haskell WL, Alderman EL, Fair JM, et al. Effects of intensive multiple risk factor reduction on coronary atherosclerosis and clinical cardiac events in men and women with coronary artery disease: The Stanford Coronary Risk Intervention Project (SCRIP). *Circulation* 1994; 89:975–990.
84. Superko HR. Sophisticated primary and secondary atherosclerosis prevention is cost effective. *Can J Cardiol* 11(suppl C): 35C–40C.
85. DeBusk RF, Miller NH, Superko HR, et al. A case-management system for coronary risk factor modification after acute myocardial infarction. *Ann Intern Med* 1994; 120:721–729.

86. Puska P, Tuomilehto J, Nissinen A, et al. Ten years of the North Karelia project. *Acta Med Scand* 1985; 701(suppl):66–71.
87. Carleton RA, Lasater TM, Assaf AR, et al. The Pawtucket Heart Health Program: Community changes in cardiovascular risk factors and projected disease risk. *Am J Public Health* 1995; 85:777–785.
88. Winkleby MA, Taylor CB, Jatulis D, et al. The long-term effects of a cardiovascular disease prevention trial: The Stanford five-city project. *Am J Public Health* 1996; 86:1773–1779.
89. Luepker RV, Rastam L, Hannan PJ, et al. Community education for cardiovascular disease prevention: Morbidity and mortality results from the Minnesota Heart Health Program. *Am J Epidemiol* 1996; 144:351–362.
90. Winkleby MA, Feldman HA, Murray DM. Joint analysis of three U.S. community intervention trials for reduction of cardiovascular disease risk. *J Clin Epidemiol* 1997; 50:645–658.
91. Kottke TE, Puska P, Salonen JT. et al. Projected effects of high-risk versus population-based prevention strategies in coronary heart disease. *Am J Epidemiol* 1985; 121:697–704.
92. Tosteson AN, Goldman L, Udvarhelyi IS, et al. Cost-effectiveness of a coronary care unit versus an intermediate care unit for emergency department patients with chest pain. *Circulation* 1996; 94:143–150.
93. Beamer AD, Lee TH, Cook EF, et al. Diagnostic implications for myocardial ischemia of the circadian variation of the onset of chest pain. *Am J Cardiol* 1987; 60:998–1002.
94. Krumholz HM, Pasternak RC, Weinstein MC, et al. Cost effectiveness of thrombolytic therapy with streptokinase in elderly patients with suspected acute myocardial infarction. *N Engl J Med* 1992; 327:7–13.
95. Laffel GL, Fineberg HV, Braunwald E. A cost-effectiveness model for coronary thrombolysis/reperfusion therapy. *J Am Coll Cardiol* 1987; 5(suppl B):79B–90B.
96. Simoons ML, Vos J, Martens LL. Cost-utility analysis of thrombolytic therapy. *Eur Heart J* 1991; 12:694–699.
97. Midgette AS, Wong JB, Beshansky JR, et al. Cost-effectiveness of streptokinase for acute myocardial infarction: A combined meta-analysis and decision analysis of the effects of infarct location and of likelihood of infarction. *Med Decis Making* 1994; 14:108–117.
98. Herve C, Castiel D, Gaillard M, et al. Cost-benefit analysis of thrombolytic therapy. *Eur Heart J* 1990; 11:1006–1010.
99. Mark DB, Hlatky MA, Califf RM, et al. Cost effectiveness of thrombolytic therapy with tissue plasminogen activator as compared with streptokinase for acute myocardial infarction. *N Engl J Med* 1995; 332:1418–1424.
100. Kalish SC, Gurwitz JH, Krumholz HM, et al. A cost-effectiveness model of thrombolytic therapy for acute myocardial infarction. *J Gen Intern Med* 1995; 10:321–330.
101. Lange RA, Hillis LD. Should thrombolysis or primary angioplasty be the treatment of choice for acute myocardial infarction? Thrombolysis—the preferred treatment. *N Engl J Med* 1996; 335:1311–1312.
102. Grines CL. Should thrombolysis or primary angioplasty be the treatment of choice for acute myocardial infarction? Primary angioplasty—the strategy of choice. *N Engl J Med* 1996; 335(17):1313–1316.
103. Berger AK, Schulman KA, Gersh BJ, et al. Primary coronary angioplasty versus thrombolysis for the management of acute myocardial infarction in elderly patients. *JAMA* 1999; 282: 341–348.
104. Grines CL, Browne KF, Marco J, et al. A comparison of immediate angioplasty with thrombolytic therapy for acute myocardial infarction. The Primary Angioplasty in Myocardial Infarction Study Group. *N Engl J Med* 1993; 328:673–679.
105. Gibbons RJ, Holmes DR, Reeder GS, et al. Immediate angioplasty compared with the administration of a thrombolytic agent followed by conservative treatment for myocardial infarction. The Mayo Coronary Care Unit and Catheterization Laboratory Groups. *N Engl J Med* 1993; 328:685–691.
106. Zijlstra F, de Boer MJ, Hoorntje JC, et al. A comparison of immediate coronary angioplasty with intravenous streptokinase in acute myocardial infarction. *N Engl J Med* 1993; 328:680–684.
107. Reeder GS, Bailey KR, Gersh BJ, et al. Cost comparison of immediate angioplasty versus thrombolysis followed by conservative therapy for acute myocardial infarction: A randomized prospective trial. Mayo Coronary Care Unit and Catheterization Laboratory Groups. *Mayo Clin Proc* 1994; 69:5–12.
108. The PAMI Trial Investigators. Analysis of the relative costs and effectiveness of primary angioplasty versus tissue-type plasminogen activator: The Primary Angioplasty in Myocardial Infarction (PAMI) trial. *J Am Coll Cardiol* 1997; 29:901–907.
109. Every NR, Parsons LS, Hlatky M, et al. A comparison of thrombolytic therapy with primary coronary angioplasty for acute myocardial infarction: Myocardial Infarction Triage and Intervention Investigators. *N Engl J Med* 1996; 335:1253–1260.
110. Grines CL, Marsalese DL, Brodie B, et al. Safety and cost-effectiveness of early discharge after primary angioplasty in low risk patients with acute myocardial infarction. PAMI-II Investigators: Primary Angioplasty in Myocardial Infarction. *J Am Coll Cardiol* 1998; 31:967–972.
111. Randomised trial of intravenous streptokinase, oral aspirin, both, or neither among 17,187 cases of suspected acute myocardial infarction: ISIS-2. ISIS-2 (Second International Study of Infarct Survival) Collaborative Group. *Lancet* 1988; 2:349360.
112. Collins R, Peto R, Baigent C, et al. Aspirin, heparin, and fibrinolytic therapy in suspected acute myocardial infarction. *N Engl J Med* 1997; 336:847–860.
113. Oler A, Whooley MA, Oler J, et al. Adding heparin to aspirin reduces the incidence of myocardial infarction and death in patients with unstable angina. *JAMA* 1996; 276:811–815.
114. Cohen M, Demers C, Gurfinkel EP, et al. A comparison of low-molecular-weight heparin with unfractionated heparin for unstable coronary artery disease: Efficacy and Safety of Subcutaneous Enoxaparin in Non-Q-Wave Coronary Events Study Group (ESSENCE). *N Engl J Med* 1997; 337:447–452.
115. Mark DB, Cowper PA, Berkowitz SD, et al. Economic assessment of low-molecular-weight heparin (enoxaparin) versus unfractionated heparin in acute coronary syndrome patients: Results from the ESSENCE randomized trial. Efficacy and Safety of Subcutaneous Enoxaparin in Non-Q wave Coronary Events (unstable angina or non-Q-wave myocardial infarction). *Circulation* 1998; 97:1702–1707.
116. Topol EJ, Califf RM, Weisman HF, et al. Randomised trial of coronary intervention with antibody against platelet IIb/IIIa integrin for reduction of clinical restenosis: Results at six months. The EPIC Investigators. *Lancet* 1994; 343:881–886.
117. Mark DB, Talley JD, Topol EJ, et al. Economic assessment of platelet glycoprotein IIb/IIIa inhibition for prevention of ischemic complications of high-risk coronary angioplasty. The EPIC Investigators. *Circulation* 1996; 94:629–635.
118. Topol EJ, Ferguson JF, Weisman HF, et al. Long-term protection from myocardial ischemic events in a randomized trial of brief integrin beta-3 blockade with percutaneous coronary intervention. *JAMA* 1997; 278:479–484.
119. Weintraub WS, Culler S, Boccuzzi SJ, et al. Economic impact of GPIIB/IIIA blockade after high-risk angioplasty: Results from the RESTORE trial. Randomized Efficacy Study of Tirofiban for Outcomes and Restenosis. *J Am Coll Cardiol* 1999; 34:1061–1066.
120. Weintraub WS, Culler SD, Kosinski A, et al. Economics, health-related quality of life, and cost-effectiveness methods for the TACTICS (Treat Angina with Aggrastat [tirofiban] and Determine Cost of Therapy with Invasive or Conservative Strategy): TIMI 18 trial. *Am J Cardiol* 1999; 83:317–322.

121. Braunwald E, McCabe CH, Cannon CP, et al. Effects of tissue plasminogen activator and a comparison of early invasive and conservative strategies in unstable angina and non-Q-wave myocardial infarction: Results of the TIMI IIIB trial. *Circulation* 1994; 89:1545–1556.
122. Boden WE, O'Rourke RA, Crawford MH, et al. Outcomes in patients with acute non-Q-wave myocardial infarction randomly assigned to an invasive as compared with a conservative management strategy. *N Engl J Med* 1998; 338:1785–1792.
123. Ragmin F, Wallentin L, Swahn E, et al. Invasive compared with non-invasive treatment in unstable coronary-artery disease: FRISC II prospective randomised multicentre study. *Lancet* 1999; 354:708–715.
124. Cannon CP, Weintraub WS, Demopoulos LA, et al. Invasive versus Conservative Strategies in Unstable Angina and Non-Q Wave Myocardial Infarction Following Treatment with Tirofiban: Rationale and study design of the International TACTICS-TIMI 18 trial. *Am J Cardiol* 1998; 82:731–736.
125. Yusuf S, Peto R, Lewis J, et al. Beta blockade during and after myocardial infarction: An overview of the randomized trials. *Prog Cardiovasc Dis* 1985; 27:335–371.
126. Goldman L, Sia ST, Cook EF, et al. Costs and effectiveness of routine therapy with long-term beta-adrenergic antagonists after acute myocardial infarction. *N Engl J Med* 1988; 319:152–157.
127. Brown NJ, Vaughan DE. Angiotensin-converting enzyme inhibitors. *Circulation* 1998; 97:1411–1420.
128. Tsevat J, Duke D, Goldman L, et al. Cost-effectiveness of captopril therapy after myocardial infarction. *J Am Coll Cardiol* 1995; 26:914–919.
129. McMurray JJ, McGuire A, Davie AP, et al. Cost-effectiveness of different ACE inhibitor treatment scenarios post-myocardial infarction. *Eur Heart J* 1997; 18:1411–1415.
130. Ades PA. Pashkow FJ. Nestor JR. Cost-effectiveness of cardiac rehabilitation after myocardial infarction. *J Cardpulm Rehabil* 1997; 17:222–231.
131. Weintraub WS, Ghazzal ZMB, Douglas JS Jr, et al. Trends in outcome and costs of coronary intervention in the 1990s. *Circulation* 1997; 96:I-456.
132. Cowper PA, DeLong ER, Peterson ED, et al. Geographic variation in resource use for coronary artery bypass surgery. IHD Port Investigators. *Med Care* 1997; 35:320–333.
133. Peterson ED, Cowper PA, Zidar JP, et al. In-hospital costs of coronary stenting (with or without Coumadin) compared to angioplasty. *Circulation* 1996; 94:1891A.
134. Cohen DJ, Krumholz HM, Sukin CA, et al. In-hospital and one-year economic outcomes after coronary stenting or balloon angioplasty: Results from a randomized clinical trial. *Circulation* 1995; 92:2480–2487.
135. Mark DB, Talley JD, Topol EJ, et al. Economic assessment of platelet glycoprotein IIb/IIIa inhibition for prevention of ischemic complications of high-risk coronary angioplasty: EPIC Investigators. *Circulation* 1996; 94:629–635.
136. Weintraub WS, Culler S, Boccuzzi SJ, et al. Economic impact of GPIIB/IIIA blockade after high-risk angioplasty: Results from the RESTORE trial. *J Am Coll Cardiol* 1999; 34:1061–1066.
137. Weintraub WS, Boccuzzi SJ, Shen Y, et al. Targeting patients for thrombus inhibition after angioplasty: Clinical and economic implications. *J Am Coll Cardiol* 1997; 29:500A.
138. Weintraub WS. Evaluating the cost of therapy for restenosis: Considerations for brachytherapy. *Int J Radiat Oncol Biol Phys* 1996; 36:949–958.
139. Wong JB, Sonnenberg FA, Salem DN, et al. Myocardial revascularization for chronic stable angina: Analysis of the role of percutaneous transluminal coronary angioplasty based on data available in 1989. *Ann Intern Med* 1990; 113:852–871.
140. Detre KM, Guo P, Holubkov R, et al. Coronary revascularization in diabetic patients: A comparison of the randomized and observational components of the bypass angioplasty revascularization investigation (BARI). *Circulation* 1999; 99:633–640.
141. Rodriguez A, Palacios IF, Navia J, et al. Argentine Randomized Study: Coronary angioplasty with stenting versus coronary artery bypass surgery in patients with multiple vessel disease (ERACI II): 30-day and long-term follow-up results. *Circulation* 1999; 100:I-234.
142. Parisi AF, Folland ED, Hartigan P, on behalf of the Veterans Affairs ACME Investigators. Comparison of angioplasty with medical therapy in the treatment of single-vessel coronary artery disease. *N Engl J Med* 1992; 326:10–16.
143. Pitt B, Waters D, Brown WV, et al. Aggressive lipid-lowering therapy compared with angioplasty in stable coronary artery disease. *N Engl J Med* 1999; 341:70–76.
144. Chamberlain DH, Fox KAA, Henderson RA, et al. Coronary angioplasty versus medical therapy for angina: The second randomised intervention treatment of angina (RITA-2) trial. *Lancet* 1997; 350:461–468.
145. Kinlay S, Leitch JW, Neil A, et al. Cardiac event recorders yield more diagnoses and are more cost-effective than 48-hour Holter monitoring in patients with palpitations: A controlled clinical trial. *Ann Intern Med* 1996; 124(1 pt 1):16–20.
146. Kupersmith J, Hogan A, Guerrero P, et al. Evaluating and improving the cost-effectiveness of the implantable cardioverter-defibrillator. *Am Heart J* 1995; 130(3 pt 1):507–515.
147. Levine JH, Mellits ED, Baumgardner RA, et al. Predictors of first discharge and subsequent survival in patients with automatic implantable cardioverter defibrillators. *Circulation* 1991; 84: 558–566.
148. Owens DK, Sanders GD, Harris RA, et al. Cost-effectiveness of implantable cardioverter defibrillators relative to amiodarone for prevention of sudden cardiac death. *Ann Intern Med* 1997; 126: 1–12.
149. Larsen GC, Manolis AS, Sonnenberg FA, et al. Cost-effectiveness of the implantable cardioverter-defibrillator: Effect of improved battery life and comparison with amiodarone therapy. *J Am Coll Cardiol* 1992; 19:1323–1334.
150. Kuppermann M, Luce BR, McGovern B, et al. An analysis of the cost effectiveness of the implantable defibrillator. *Circulation* 1990; 81:91–100.
151. Wever EF, Hauer RN, Schrijvers G, et al. Cost-effectiveness of implantable defibrillator as first-choice therapy versus electrophysiologically guided, tiered strategy in postinfarct sudden death survivors. *Circulation* 1996; 93:489–496.
152. Mushlin AI, Hall WJ, Zwanziger J, et al. The cost-effectiveness of automatic implantable cardiac defibrillators: Results from MADIT. Multicenter Automatic Defibrillator Implantation Trial. *Circulation* 1998; 97:2129–2135.
153. Mitchell JB, Surge RT, Lee AJ, et al. *Per Case Prospective Payment for Episodes of Hospital Care* (final report prepared for the Health Care Financing Administration under contract no 500-92-0020). Waltham, MA: Health Economics Research; 1995.
154. Kalbfleisch SJ, Calkins H, Langberg JJ, et al. Comparison of the cost of radiofrequency catheter modification of the atrioventricular node and medical therapy for drug-refractory atrioventricular node reentrant tachycardia. *J Am Coll Cardiol* 1992; 19:1583–1587.
155. Kertes PJ, Kalman JM, Tonkin AM. Cost effectiveness of radiofrequency catheter ablation in the treatment of symptomatic supraventricular tachyarrhythmias. *Aust NZ J Med* 1993; 23: 433–436.
156. Weerasooriya HR, Murdock CJ, Harris AH, et al. The cost-effectiveness of treatment of supraventricular arrhythmias related to an accessory atrioventricular pathway: Comparison of catheter ablation, surgical division and medical treatment. *Aust NZ J Med* 1994; 24:161–167.
157. Hogenhuis W, Stevens SK, Wang P, et al. Cost-effectiveness of

radiofrequency ablation compared with other strategies in Wolff-Parkinson-White syndrome. *Circulation* 1993; 88(suppl II):II-437–II-446.

158. Stamato NJ, O'Toole MF, Enger EL. Permanent pacemaker implantation in the cardiac catheterization laboratory versus the operating room: An analysis of hospital charges and complications. *Pacing Clin Electrophysiol* 1992; 15:2236–2239.
159. Sutton R, Bourgeois I. Cost benefit analysis of single and dual chamber pacing for sick sinus syndrome and atrioventricular block: An economic sensitivity analysis of the literature. *Eur Heart J* 1996; 17:574–582.
160. Falk RH. Impact of prospective peer review on pacemaker implantation rates in Massachusetts. *J Am Coll Cardiol* 1990; 15:1087–1092.
161. Parsonnet V. Role of peer review of pacemaker implantations. *J Am Coll Cardiol* 1990; 15:1093–1094.
162. Dreifus LS, Fisch C, Griffin JC, et al. Guidelines for implantation of cardiac pacemakers and antiarrhythmia devices. *Circulation* 1991; 84:455–467.
163. Ray SG, Griffith MJ, Jamieson S, et al. Impact of the recommendations of the British Pacing and Electrophysiology Group on pacemaker prescription and on the immediate costs of pacing in the Northern Region. *Br Heart J* 1992; 68:531–534.
164. Gage BF, Cardinalli AB, Albers GW, et al. Cost-effectiveness of warfarin and aspirin for prophylaxis of stroke in patients with nonvalvular atrial fibrillation. *JAMA* 1995; 274:1839–1845.
165. Barnett HJM, Eliasziw M, Meldrum HE. Drugs and surgery in the prevention of ischemic stroke. *N Engl J Med* 1995; 332:238–248.
166. Laupacis A, Boysen G, Connolly S, et al. Risk factors for stroke and efficacy of antithrombotic therapy in atrial fibrillation: Analysis of pooled data from five randomized controlled trials. *Arch Intern Med* 1994; 154:1449–1457.
167. Gustafsson C, Asplund K, Britton M, et al. Cost-effectiveness of primary stroke prevention in atrial fibrillation: Swedish national perspective. *Br Med J* 1992; 305:1457–1460.
168. Lightowlers S, McGuire A. Cost-effectiveness of anticoagulation in nonrheumatic atrial fibrillation in the primary prevention of ischemic stroke. *Stroke* 1998; 29:1827–1832.
169. Eckman MH, Falk RH, Pauker SG. Cost-effectiveness of therapies for patients with nonvalvular atrial fibrillation. *Arch Intern Med* 1998; 158:1669–1677.
170. Catherwood E, Fitzpatrick WD, Greenberg ML, et al. Cost-effectiveness of cardioversion and antiarrhythmic therapy in nonvalvular atrial fibrillation. *Ann Intern Med* 1999; 130:625–636.
171. Seto TB, Taira DA, Tsevat J, et al. Cost-effectiveness of transesophageal echocardiographic-guided cardioversion: A decision analytic model for patients admitted to the hospital with atrial fibrillation. *J Am Coll Cardiol* 1997; 29:122–130.
172. Ward RE, Gheorghiade M, Young JB, et al. Economic outcomes of withdrawal of digoxin therapy in adult patients with stable congestive heart failure. *J Am Coll Cardiol* 1995; 26:93–101.
173. Uretsky BF, Young JB, Shahidi FE, et al. Randomized study assessing the effect of digoxin withdrawal in patients with mild to moderate chronic congestive heart failure: Results of the PROVED trial. *J Am Coll Cardiol* 1993; 22:955–962.
174. Packer M, Gheorghiade M, Young JB, et al. Withdrawal of digoxin from patients with chronic heart failure treated with angiotensin-converting-enzyme inhibitors. *N Engl J Med* 1993; 329:1–7.
175. Garg R, Gorlin R, Smith T, et al. The effect of digoxin on mortality and morbidity in patients with heart failure. *N Engl J Med* 1997; 336:525–533.
176. Mark, DB. Medical economics in cardiovascular medicine. In: Topol EJ, ed. *Cardiovascular Medicine*. Philadelphia: Lippincott-Williams & Wilkins; 1997:1193.
177. Garg R, Yusuf S, for the Collaborative Group on ACE Inhibitor Trials. Overview of randomized trials of angiotensin-converting-enzyme inhibitors on mortality and morbidity in patients with heart failure. *JAMA* 1995; 273:1450–1456.
178. The SOLVD Investigators. Effect of enalapril on survival in patients with reduced left ventricular ejection fractions and congestive heart failure. *N Engl J Med* 1991; 325:293–302.
179. Glick H, Cook J, Kinosian B, et al. Costs and effects of enalapril therapy in patients with symptomatic heart failure: An economic analysis of the Studies of Left Ventricular Dysfunction (SOLVD) treatment trial. *J Cardiac Failure* 1995; 1:371–379.
180. Boyko WL Jr, Glick HA, Schulman KA. Economics and cost-effectiveness in evaluating the value of cardiovascular therapies. ACE inhibitors in the management of congestive heart failure: Comparative economic data. *Am Heart J* 1999; 137:S115–S119.
181. Paul SD, Kuntz KM, Eagle KA, et al. Costs and effectiveness of angiotensin converting enzyme inhibition in patients with congestive heart failure. *Arch Intern Med* 1994; 154:1143–1149.
182. Kleber FX. Socioeconomic aspects of ACE inhibition in the secondary prevention in cardiovascular disease. *Am J Hypertens* 1994; 7:112S–116S.
183. Van Hout BA, Wielink G, Bonsel GJ, et al. Effects of ACE inhibitors on heart failure in the Netherlands: A pharmacoeconomic model. *Pharmacoeconomics* 1993; 3:387–397.
184. Hart W, Rhodes G, McMurray J. The cost effectiveness of enalapril in the treatment of chronic heart failure. *Br J Med Econ* 1993; 6:91–98.
185. Packer M, Bristol MR, Cohn JN, et al. The effect of carvedilol on morbidity and mortality in patients with chronic heart failure. *N Engl J Med* 1996; 334:1349–1355.
186. Delea TE, Vera-Llonch M, Richner RE, et al. Cost effectiveness of carvedilol for heart failure. *Am J Cardiol* 1999; 83:890–896.
187. Rich MW, Beckham V, Wittenberg C, et al. A multidisciplinary intervention to prevent the readmission of elderly patients with congestive heart failure. *N Engl J Med* 1995; 333:1190.
188. Weinberger M, Oddone EZ, Henderson WG. Does increased access to primary care reduce hospital readmissions? Veterans Affairs Cooperative Study Group on Primary Care and Hospital Readmission. *N Engl J Med* 1996; 334:1441–1447.
189. West JA, Miller NH, Parker KM, et al. A comprehensive management system for heart failure improves clinical outcomes and reduces medical resource utilization. *Am J Cardiol* 1997; 79: 58–63.
190. Kornowski R, Zeeli D, Averbuch M, et al. Intensive home-care surveillance prevents hospitalization and improves morbidity rates among elderly patients with severe congestive heart failure. *Am Heart J* 1995; 129:762–766.
191. Rich MW. Heart failure disease management: A critical review. *J Cardiac Failure* 1999; 5:64–75.
192. Philbin EF. Comprehensive multidisciplinary programs for the management of patients with congestive heart failure. *J Gen Intern Med* 1999; 14:130–135.
193. Evans RW. Cost-effectiveness analysis of transplantation. *Surg Clin North Am* 1986; 66:603–616.
194. Garber AM, Solomon NA. Cost-effectiveness of alternative test strategies for the diagnosis of coronary artery disease. *Ann Intern Med* 1999; 130:719–728.
195. Kim C, Kwok YS, Saha S, et al. Diagnosis of suspected coronary artery disease in women: A cost-effectiveness analysis. *Am Heart J* 1999; 137:1019–1027.
196. Kuntz KM, Fleischmann KE, Hunink MG, et al. Cost-effectiveness of diagnostic strategies for patients with chest pain. *Ann Intern Med* 1999; 130:709–718.
197. Dittus RS, Roberts SD, Adolph RJ. Cost-effectiveness analysis of patient management alternatives after uncomplicated myocardial infarction: A model. *JAMA* 1987; 10:869–878.
198. Kuntz KM, Tsevat J, Goldman L, et al. Cost-effectiveness of routine coronary angiography after acute myocardial infarction. *Circulation* 1996; 94:957–965.

CHAPTER 95

INSURANCE ISSUES IN PATIENTS WITH HEART DISEASE

Michael B. Clark / William T. Friedewald

INSURANCE MEDICINE AND CARDIOLOGY

The purpose of insurance is to provide for financial relief in the event of significant economic loss. Insurance usually takes the form of a contract—a legal agreement between insurer and insured—specifying those losses that are to be covered and the insurance benefit agreed upon. Under specific conditions, including definable losses that occur by chance within large populations at risk, the laws of probability can be applied, using actuarial methods to predict the total amount of loss for a group of individuals over some defined period of time.[1] For life and health insurance, an evaluation process described as *insurance underwriting* serves to identify the potential risk of loss for each individual. When a premium proportional to that risk is assessed, the result is an insurance system that allows for economic risk to be spread over large groups of people, with contributions from each insured proportional to the risk assumed by the insurer for that individual.

These concepts of insurance and insurance underwriting are not new; insurance for commercial ventures existed in some form by the Middle Ages, and life insurance had appeared by the seventeenth century. Private medical insurance, usually for catastrophic illnesses, was available in the 1800s.[2] Within the past 100 years, there has been an explosion in the amount of life and health insurance available and in the diversity of insurance products. This includes group employee-sponsored health and life insurance, insurance options offered by health maintenance and managed care organizations, and government-sponsored health insurance plans for indigent, disabled, and elderly populations. Within the medical community, the impact of this changing insurance climate has been enormous.[3,4] Nevertheless, as medical care providers and as consultants, cardiologists continue to play an important role in insurance underwriting evaluation.

MEDICAL UNDERWRITING FOR LIFE INSURANCE

Medical Risk Assessment

As a first step in the risk assessment process for an insurance applicant with a cardiac impairment, the patient's physician submits medical information to the insurance company in the form of the Attending Physician Statement (APS). This may include an outline of recent medical history and will often contain office and hospital records for review. Clinical problems identified in the APS are analyzed for severity of disease, extent of clinical evaluation, and thoroughness of clinical follow-up to provide data for risk assessment.

After the development of any additional information provided by authorized query to one of the national insurance company data-base exchanges, the next step in the medical underwriting evaluation involves, in most cases, the insurance medical examination. Comprehensive history taking and physical examination are routine in these examinations. Noninvasive cardiac testing may also be required by the insurance company, particularly if large amounts of insurance are requested or if additional information is required to permit a proper assessment of cardiac risk. A cardiology consultant may serve as a member of the medical underwriting team itself at this stage, reviewing all of the cardiac information obtained as part of the evaluation, including electrocardiograms and stress test tracings.

To complete the risk assessment process, each medical condition identified during the medical underwriting evaluation must be correlated with long-term survival data relevant to that disease process. From these data, a mortality ratio is derived (observed deaths in a population of individuals affected by the condition divided by the expected deaths for a comparable standard population).[5,6] This quantitative prognostic index serves as a standard, which is useful for comparing mortality projections among the various medical conditions. In general, the higher the mortality ratio calculated for a particular impairment, the greater the mortality and, thus, the greater the relative risk assumed by the company to provide insurance for individuals affected by that impairment. The mortality ratios calculated for various medical conditions are integrated into a table of risk classes or "ratings"; applicants within a rating class are grouped together to be assessed similar insurance premiums. The relationship of risk class to premium is complex and often varies by company and by insurance product, but the final result is coverage for financial loss, with the contribution to the total insurance pool proportional to the medical risk assumed by the insurance company. This equitable arrangement has the additional benefit of making insurance coverage possible for many people with cardiac disease who would otherwise be uninsurable.[7,8]

Published data relevant to mortality assessment derive from several sources. Excellent long-term follow-up data are available for insured populations based on medical conditions, demographic characteristics, and personal habits identified at the time of original insurance application (Table 95-1). Results are usually expressed as mortality ratios to address directly the prognostic, as opposed to diagnostic, significance of examination and laboratory abnormalities, such as "heart murmur on exam" or "low serum albumin." This information, while particularly relevant to insurance underwriting, may not be directly comparable to standard mortality data derived from the general population, as the insured population data more precisely relate to large groups of *selected* individuals (those people willing and able to purchase life insurance). A further limitation of such data is that they typically involve follow-up intervals as long as 20 to 30 years. Significant medical advances, as well as changes in demographics or personal lifestyles that occur during the period of study, may significantly limit the applicability of the information developed.

Long-term clinical and epidemiologic studies published in the medical literature are also useful for mortality assessment and are generally readily available for most medical impairments. In such studies, the survival data as reported can be extrapolated to provide actuarial information useful to the calculation of mortality risk. A common shortcoming in such clinical studies, however, is the single reporting of the observed mortality for the population recruited into the study without sufficient information to allow one to extrapolate the findings to the larger population from which they were selected.[9] This actuarial problem for many of the studies reported in the clinical literature was recently identified in a review[10] of a reported study of survivors of asymptomatic myocardial infarction.[11] "Good long-term prognosis" was the conclusion of the clinical investigation, which followed 48 patients with a mean age of 36 years for approximately 6 years; the observed mortality in this population was 10 percent for the entire period. However, reference to the U.S. Standard Life Tables (1979–1981) reveals a much lower expected mortality (approximately 1.46 percent) at this age for the same length of follow-up. The estimated mortality ratio of 685 percent (10 percent/1.46 percent × 100) represents a high substandard risk level for life insurance purposes, even though it may represent good clinical results in young patients with severe cardiac disease.

CORONARY HEART DISEASE: ANGINA PECTORIS AND MYOCARDIAL INFARCTION

One long-term follow-up study in the insured population[12] has shown initial and short-term mortality following the diagnosis of coronary disease to be relatively high (estimated at up to 1150 percent of standard mortality depending on the presenting manifestations of disease) and quite variable for clinical subpopulations. This initial period of unstable risk is followed by a plateau phase during which the mortality rate (found to be close to 390 percent of standard) is relatively stable and thus more predictable. Other studies in insured individuals have confirmed this pattern,[13,14] which has led to the common practice of postponing consideration for life insurance for periods of up to 1 year following the initial presentation of coronary heart disease (CHD). Over the next several years, the excess *short-term* mortality demonstrated for this disease is reflected in a series of short-term extra premium charges. Upon reaching the more predictable plateau phase, a permanent, somewhat substandard rating is usually applied to correspond to the more stable but still greater than expected mortality rate seen in individuals with CHD.

To facilitate appropriate risk assessment, special attention is directed to the presence of known CHD risk factors, such as high blood pressure, diabetes mellitus, hyperlipidemia, smoking history, and obesity. In addition, a strong family history of cardiovascular disease has been confirmed in studies in insured as well as in

TABLE 95-1 Mortality Ratios in Cardiac Impairments: Selected Data

Medical Finding or Condition	Age Interval, Years	Number of Patients	Mortality Ratio, Percent
ECG findings in males	40–64	21,415	
Axis deviation (symptomatic)			225
Axis deviation (asymptomatic)			139
ST depression (symptomatic)			420
ST depression (asymptomatic)			220
Heart murmurs	50–59	21,295	
Apical systolic (not transmitted to neck; presumed functional)			114
Apical systolic (transmitted)			178
Basal systolic			276
Acute myocardial infarction	30–59	1,608	145
Coronary bypass reoperation	50–59	1,608	145

SOURCE: Adapted from Refs. 14, 33, 36, and 37.

other broader-based epidemiologic populations to be an independent risk factor for coronary heart disease, with mortality ratios in insureds of 189 and 121 percent for men and women, respectively.[14]

Long-term prognosis in patients with CHD may be influenced by intercurrent clinical interventions, such as the use of thrombolytic drugs or the performance of coronary angioplasty and coronary bypass surgery.[36,37] Commonly, life insurance consideration for patients having undergone these procedures is initially postponed to allow for review of the clinical course soon after the intervention. Underwriting risk assessment after this initial period is quite similar to that for the coronary syndromes, as described above, with particular consideration given to the status of left ventricular function before and after intervention, the number and extent of coronary artery lesions seen on coronary angiography, and the results of electrocardiographic, echocardiographic, and radionuclide stress testing. In addition, the presence or absence of coronary artery risk factors, in particular smoking, will influence the level of the final medical rating. The frequency and thoroughness of follow-up care may also influence the medical underwriter in otherwise borderline cases.

Mortality risk assessment is considerably more difficult when only limited information is available. For example, the record from the patient's physician may include, in its assessment of an individual presenting with chest pain, a simple statement such as "possible angina, trial of nitroglycerin initiated" with no further cardiac testing indicated at the time of insurance review. For purposes of risk assessment, this information would commonly be rated as "definite angina" until further clinical follow-up or noninvasive cardiac testing results were made available. Exercise electrocardiograms are, in general, routinely required for applicants requesting large amounts of insurance, although some insurance companies have recently discontinued this requirement. Even for such companies, however, these tests continue to be ordered when indicated by the presence of strong risk factors for CHD or by suggestive clinical presentations documented in the attending physician's medical summary forwarded to the insurance company. An abnormal stress test will, in most cases, result in a recommendation for a less than standard insurance rating. These judgments can be revised, however, based on supplementary evidence provided by the applicant's personal physician, including the results of stress testing with cardiac imaging or the findings on coronary angiography.

HIGH BLOOD PRESSURE

Since 1925, the life insurance industry has published several major comprehensive studies demonstrating increased mortality among insured populations with high blood pressure.[15–17] All of these show a direct, nearly linear relation between systolic and diastolic blood pressure and mortality. The 1979 Blood Pressure Study[17] dealt in the main with the mortality experience between 1954 and 1972 of 4,350,000 men and women aged 15 to 60. An estimated 530,000 of these men and women had borderline or definite high blood pressure, obviously an unusually large population of people with this diagnosis. During this study's follow-up phase, the first effective (and later routinely) used treatment for high blood pressure was introduced in the United States, and thus the 1979 study, unlike previous studies, was influenced by the increasing use of antihypertensive medication. Mortality ratios for mildly or moderately hypertensive individuals were approximately 20 percent lower than for those with more severe elevations of blood pressure. In a subgroup of applicants who were taking antihypertensive medication at the time of entry and whose blood pressure was well controlled, mortality was closer to normal (mortality ratio in males under 50 years of age at the time of insurance review, 175 percent; in males over 50 years old, 95 percent). More recently, the Multiple Medical Impairment Study underscored the necessity for adequate blood pressure control. Identification of elevated blood pressure as part of the insurance risk assessment examination was found to impact negatively on the mortality experience of most of the other medical impairments studied.[18] It follows, then, that consideration of less than standard or declined insurance applications would generally apply only to patients with untreated hypertension, for noncompliance with prescribed medical regimens, or with hypertension complicated by end-organ damage (ventricular hypertrophy or cerebrovascular or renal disease). Although such developments are often identified in the clinical record, at times additional testing is performed by the insurance company and may include electrocardiography and qualitative urinary protein measurement. On rare occasions, echocardiography may be ordered to assess the degree of cardiac impairment as a result of long-standing hypertension where other clues are ambiguous or contradictory.

VALVULAR HEART DISEASE

The Medical Impairment Study of 1983 provided long-term survival data in the insured population with heart murmurs.[14] Information extracted from that study has been used to provide mortality projections in people with valvular heart disease (Table 95-1). Advances in cardiac diagnostic technology since publication of that study, particularly the development of echocardiographic and Doppler imaging systems, have allowed better definition of valvular pathology. With these and other advances in medical and surgical intervention, it has become more difficult to accumulate data concerning the natural history of unoperated cardiac valvular impairments.[19,20]

Mitral Valve Prolapse

This is, at present, the most common valve condition reported to insurance companies. Although most such patients are offered standard insurance rates, a small subset of patients with frequent chest pain, cardiac arrhythmias, and significant mitral regurgitation may be rated below standard.[21]

Congenital Valvular Heart Disease

Most companies postpone consideration of life insurance for an infant with known or suspected congenital heart disease until the child reaches 1 or 2 years of age. Even then, the history must include a definitively proven diagnosis as well as successful repair of all surgically correctable lesions before the applicant can be considered for life insurance. After successful restoration of normal cardiac hemodynamics, most applicants with congenital defects—including those with atrial and ventricular septal defects, corrected pulmonic stenosis, patent ductus, or coarctation of the aorta (once blood pressure has returned to normal)—can be considered as standard risks.[22] Uninsurable applicants would include most cases of transposition of the great vessels, Ebstein's anomaly, anomalous venous return, and Eisenmenger's syndrome.

Congenital bicuspid aortic valve remains a difficult clinical and underwriting problem.[8] Estimation of prognosis in this impairment when applicants present in the second and third decades of life is often problematic. In the absence of associated echocardiographic evidence of left ventricular enlargement, most companies are willing to assess this risk as only mildly substandard. Left ventricular dilatation or hypertrophy seen on echocardiography, or the presence by Doppler analysis of any significant degree of aortic stenosis or regurgitation, will usually require a more substantial rating assessment.

Acquired Valvular Heart Disease

To perform risk assessment in applicants known to have acquired valvular disease, the underwriter will usually first consider the clinical and electrocardiographic findings on the insurance examination. The degree of cardiac enlargement and severity of left ventricular dysfunction will also be considered and will commonly be outlined in the APS. The medical underwriter will also give consideration to the attendant risk of anticipated surgical valve repair or replacement as well as to the risk of lifelong anticoagulation following such surgery. Applicants with valvular disease who show evidence of marked cardiomegaly, especially with prior history or physical examination findings consistent with left-sided or right-sided heart failure, cannot usually be offered life insurance. Other significant complications, such as new-onset atrial fibrillation or systemic embolization, will usually result in a postponement for up to 1 year prior to reconsideration. In most other cases, life insurance can be offered, albeit at rates significantly below standard.[8,20,23] Early follow-up studies of patients undergoing surgical procedures that preserve the native cardiac valve have demonstrated an improvement in perioperative and short-term postoperative survival.[21] As more complete long-term data in patients undergoing these procedures become available, further liberalization of risk penalties may be possible.

OTHER CARDIAC DISEASES OR ABNORMAL LABORATORY FINDINGS

Cardiomyopathy

Insurance risk assessment of the applicant with cardiomyopathy is based on the initial clinical presentation of the patient and the subsequent clinical and physiologic evaluation. Life insurance cannot usually be offered to those diagnosed with dilated (congestive) cardiomyopathy or amyloid heart disease. Systemic diseases with cardiac involvement, such as scleroderma and sarcoidosis, are most often assessed on the basis of overall disease activity and response to therapy. Insurance, however, may be available to many in this latter group of patients, albeit at rates below standard.[8]

Evaluation of the asymptomatic individual with a strong family history of inheritable heart disease or in whom a heart murmur has been discovered may at times produce findings consistent with the obstructive or nonobstructive cardiomyopathies. Complete information concerning the natural history of these impairments is not yet available, particularly in the mild, asymptomatic cases.[24] In the past, many clinical reports were of severe and fatal outcomes, leading many insurance companies to decline or rate highly any applicant with an established diagnosis of hypertrophic cardiomyopathy.[8] More recent experience in defining mortality outcomes in hypertrophic cardiomyopathy has been much more favorable[25,26] and may allow for more favorable mortality risk assessment in the future.[27]

Arrhythmias

Most insurance companies will consider applicants who give a history of paroxysmal or chronic atrial arrhythmias in the context of the presence and severity of coexisting cardiac disease. One series in an insured population with paroxysmal atrial tachycardia noted mortality rates quite similar to those of the standard population; the mortality ratio for this condition was estimated to be 73 percent.[14] This can be contrasted with mortality ratios of 700 percent or greater in the presence of atrial fibrillation.[28] In the apparently asymptomatic young individual with new-onset atrial arrhythmias, particular attention is paid to social history and habits such as smoking or excessive alcohol use. In the middle-aged or older applicant, the possibility of asymptomatic coronary heart disease must also be assessed.

Ventricular arrhythmias have remained a difficult risk-assessment problem. In many cases, isolated ventricular ectopy can be rated in the context of the underlying cardiac impairment, such as coronary artery or valvular heart disease. Particular attention is directed during the review of the medical record to the results of clinical cardiac evaluation, including stress testing and noninvasive analysis of cardiac function.[29] Survivors of sudden death will, in most cases, be declined—a situation that may change as long-term data on the benefits of automatic implantable defibrillator (AID) become available. This change would probably apply to those patients in whom AID implantation has been performed as prophylaxis in the setting of high clinical risk for sudden death[30] (see also Chap. 33).

Heart Transplantation

Heart transplantation techniques and immunosuppressive strategies have continued to evolve and have been associated with significant improvement in 5- to 10-year survival (see also Chap. 22). Most insurance companies would continue to decline such patients, however, until additional long-term survival data became available.

Insurance Laboratory Evaluation Abnormalities

Life insurance underwriting protocols generally include a clinical laboratory panel with a full lipid profile and a resting electrocardiogram. Depending on the age of the applicant and the amount of life insurance requested, additional testing, including stress testing and echocardiography, may be required. In most cases, abnormalities revealed during this laboratory evaluation are fully consistent with the clinical history as reported in the APS. In a minority of applicants, however, medical history is scanty or medical records are unavailable. In such patients, medical underwriting risk assessment is then based primarily on the findings from the insurance physical and laboratory examination. Studies in insured as well as in general populations provide the necessary mortality projections for underwriting risk assessment using these parameters (Table 95-1). The Medical Impairment Study (1983), for example, confirmed the benign prognosis of incidental bradycardia found on insurance examination, with mortality ratios of 73 to 80 percent reported.[14] On the other hand, a relative mortality of 250 percent was found for the finding of tachycardia.[14] Additional information is available to perform risk assessment for findings such as overweight and underweight,[12,31] low serum albumin,[32] and an abnormal electrocardiogram.[33,34]

HEALTH AND DISABILITY INSURANCE

Health insurance continues to evolve in terms of overall cost, quality, and availability within the current environment of health care reform. Further, the delivery of health care under managed care plans by both governmental and employer insurance plans has begun to redefine many aspects of the traditional patient–doctor, doctor–doctor, and doctor–insurer relationships.[3,4]

Within this environment, cardiologists remain vitally important, functioning both as clinical consultants to primary care providers as well as professional consultants to managed care organizations and indemnity insurance plans. This latter role deserves special emphasis. Cardiologists will often be called upon to provide the expertise essential to the determination of the medical necessity and appropriateness of care for health insurance case management and claim review. Assessment of new technology in its evolution from experimental procedure to accepted standard of care is a particularly important responsibility of the insurance consultant in the managed care environment.[35]

The role of the physician in disability determination is more complex, often requiring legal interpretation of disability based on the results of medical data available. The expertise of medical specialists—including physiatrists, physical and occupational therapists, and social workers—may be required for complete evaluation and recommendations. In general, thorough analysis coupled with appropriate goal-directed therapy often allows for return to work in a supportive environment accommodated to individual needs.

For practical purposes, the patient with known heart disease of any kind is going to have difficulty in obtaining standard individual health or disability insurance. As in patients with high blood pressure, however, effective subclassification of patients and effective new therapies may allow insurance to become available to more and more patients who were considered unacceptable insurance risks in the past.

ACKNOWLEDGMENTS

We gratefully acknowledge the work of Dr. M. Irene Ferrer and Dr. Joseph A. Wilber in previous editions of this textbook, from which we drew for this current chapter.

References

1. Morton GA. *Principles of Life and Health Insurance.* Atlanta: Life Office Management Association; 1984.
2. Brackenridge RDC, Brown AE. A historical survey of the development of life assurance. In: Brackenridge RDC, Elder WJ, eds. *Medical Selection of Life Risks,* 3rd ed. New York: Stockton Press; 1992:3–17.
3. Billi JE, Wise CG, Bills EA, Mitchell RL. Potential effects of managed care on specialty practice at a university medical center. *N Engl J Med* 1995; 333:979–983.
4. Weisbuch JB, Roberts NK. Without the denominator, where is the quality improvement paradigm in the nation's health care reform? *J Ins Med* 1995; 27:12–14.
5. Pokorski RJ. Mortality methodology and analysis seminar test. *J Ins Med* 1995; 20:20–45.
6. Seltzer F. Choosing a standard for adjusted mortality rates. *Stat Bull* 1996; 77:13–19.
7. Cumming GR, Croxson R. Cardiovascular disorders: Part I. Coronary heart disease. In: Brackenridge RDC, Elder WJ, eds. *Medical Selection of Life Risks,* 3rd ed. New York: Stockton Press; 1992:251–323.
8. Croxson RS. Cardiovascular disorders: Part II. Other cardiovascular disorders. In: Brackenridge RDC, Elder WJ, eds. *Medical Selection of Life Risks,* 3rd ed. New York: Stockton Press; 1992:324–431.
9. Singer RB. Pitfalls of inferring annual mortality from inspection of published survival curves. *J Ins Med* 1994; 26:333–338.
10. Iacovino JR. A "quick hit" method to assess insurance mortality from a clinical article. *J Ins Med* 1994; 26:317–318.
11. Negus BH. Coronary anatomy and prognosis of young, asymptomatic survivors of myocardial infarction. *Am J Med* 1994; 96:354–358.
12. Clarke RD. Mortality of impaired lives 1964–73 (abstr). *J Inst Act* 1979; 100 (part 1). In: Lew EA, Gajewski J, eds. *Medical Risks: Trends in Mortality by Age and Time Elapsed.* New York: Praeger; 1990:7–120.
13. Jarvis HJ. Development of the diabetic, coronary, and blood pressure pools (abstr). *Cooperation internationale pour les assurances des risques aggraves,* 1986. In: Lew EA, Gajewski J, eds. *Medical Risks: Trends in Mortality by Age and Time Elapsed.* New York: Praeger; 1990:7–122.
14. Medical Impairment Study 1983 (abstr) I. Boston: Society of Actuaries and Association of Life Insurance Medical Directors of America, 1986. In: Lew EA, Gajewski J, eds. *Medical Risks: Trends in Mortality by Age and Time Elapsed.* New York: Praeger; 1990:6–78.
15. *Build and Blood Pressure Study 1959.* Chicago: Society of Actuaries; 1959.
16. *Mortality Investigation of Declined Lives in Japan.* Tokyo: The Life Insurance Association of Japan; 1979.
17. *Blood Pressure Study 1979.* Boston: Society of Actuaries and Association of Life Insurance Medical Directors of America; 1980.
18. *Multiple Medical Impairment Study.* Westwood, MA: Center for Medico-Actuarial Statistics of MIB, Inc.; 1998.
19. Borer JS, Kligfield P. Aortic regurgitation: Making management decisions. *ACC Curr J Rev* 1995; 4:30–32.
20. MacKenzie BR. Long-term mortality and complications of Bjork-Shiley spherical-disc valves—A life table analysis. *J Ins Med* 1992; 24:128–132.
21. Jeresaty RM. Mitral valve prolapse: An update. In: Arnold CB, ed. *Transactions of The American Academy of Insurance Medicine: One Hundred and First Annual Meeting.* Tampa, FL: Klay Printing; 1993:24–33.
22. Singer RB, Gajewski J. Cardiovascular diseases I. In: Lew EA, Gajewski J, eds. *Medical Risks: Trends in Mortality by Age and Time Elapsed, 1.* New York: Praeger; 1990:6-30–6-38.
23. Cumming GR. Survival after valve replacement. In: Arnold CB, ed. *Transactions of The America Academy of Insurance Medicine: One Hundred and First Annual Meeting.* Tampa, FL: Klay Printing; 1993:40–55.

24. Elliott PM, Saumarez RC, McKenna WJ. Recent clinical advances in hypertrophic cardiomyopathy. *Heart Failure* 1995; 11:15–25.
25. Cannan CR, Reeder GS, Bailey KR, et al. Natural history of hypertrophic cardiomyopathy: A population-based study, 1976 through 1990. *Circulation* 1995; 92:2488–2495.
26. Ten Cate FJ. Prognosis of hypertrophic cardiomyopathy. *J Ins Med* 1996; 28:42–45.
27. Iacovino JR. The nonmortality of hypertrophic cardiomyopathy in an unselected, community diagnosed and treated population. *J Ins Med* 1996; 28:51–54.
28. Gajewski J, Singer RB. Mortality in an insured population with atrial fibrillation. *JAMA* 1981; 245:1540–1544.
29. Chait L. Electrocardiography. In: Brackenridge RDC, Elder WJ, eds. *Medical Selection of Life Risks,* 3rd ed. New York: Stockton Press; 1992:433–472.
30. Gorlin R. Cost-effectiveness of ICD therapy for ventricular arrhythmias. *Prim Cardiol* 1995; 21:32–38.
31. *Build Study 1979.* Boston: Society of Actuaries and Association of Life Insurance Medical Directors of America; 1980.
32. Segel L. Serum albumin: "Phoenix" of the blood profile. *On the Risk* 1995; 11:81–83.
33. Rose G, Baxter PJ, Reid DD, McCartney P. Prevalence and prognosis of electrocardiographic findings in middle-aged men (abstr). *Br Heart J* 1978; 40:636–643. In: Lew EA, Gajewski J, eds. *Medical Risks: Trends in Mortality by Age and Time Elapsed.* New York: Praeger; 1990.
34. Ferrer MI. A survey of 19,734 electrocardiograms obtained in insurance applicants. *J Ins Med* 1985; 16:6–13.
35. Privette M, ed. Court overrules HCFA 1986 investigational devices payment policy. *Cardiology* 1996; 25:4.
36. Singer RB. Comparative mortality by sex and age in residents of Rochester, Minnesota, with acute myocardial infarction during 1960–1979 (sudden deaths included). *J Ins Med* 1995–1996; 27:235–240.
37. Hutchinson R. Additional follow-up of patients with coronary bypass reoperation at Cleveland Clinic. *J Ins Med* 1994; 26: 324–328.

CHAPTER 96

CARDIAC EVALUATIONS FOR LEGAL PURPOSES

Elliot L. Sagall* / Ira S. Nash

INTRODUCTION

This chapter describes for the physician the scope of the legal areas where issues concerning heart disorder are key elements of the litigation. The following topics will be discussed: (a) the essential components of a medicolegal cardiac evaluation; (b) the legal and medical concepts, definitions, and criteria for determinations of diagnosis and the time of occurrence of specific cardiac lesions, causality, disability, medical malpractice, prognosis, life expectancy, and other medicolegal assessments; and (c) the formulation of a report of the physician's findings and opinions that will be meaningful and helpful to the legal forum assigned to resolve the disputed medical problems of the case in hand.

The socioeconomic ramifications of heart disease have long been a source of vexing legal as well as medical problems with no easy resolution as yet forthcoming. Nationwide, claims instituted by heart patients and/or their beneficiaries alleging heart disorder, disability, and cardiac death as a workplace or accidental injury or as due to the negligent action of a health care provider are burgeoning in number and scope. The existence of a heart disorder may also be the key issue in the legal determination of an individual's physical capacity to participate as a defendant or witness in a legal proceeding, to drive a motor vehicle, to pilot an airplane, to engage in "substantial" gainful activity, to write a legally valid will or contract, to enable an insurer to recover some of the moneys paid to a worker as compensation for a work-related injury, or to invalidate a life insurance policy. It may be the basis for suit by a disabled employee against the employer for illegal job discrimination.

The rapidly expanding interrelationships of heart disorders and the law necessarily will involve physicians who examine and treat cardiac patients more and more frequently in one or combinations of several roles, as follows: (a) as a factual witness called upon to present the history personally received and the findings of physical and other examinations performed and treatment rendered; (b) as an expert witness called by one side or the other in a legal dispute to present opinions on the issues under consideration; (c) as an impartial witness called by the presiding judicial arbiter for opinion testimony; or (d) as a defendant in a suit for medical malpractice.

The question of a cardiac patient's eligibility for certain statutory or common law benefits is basically a legal rather than a medical issue. Accordingly, the ultimate determination is assigned to a court, jury, administrative agency, commissioner, referee, or some other duly appointed person or persons referred to as a *fact finder.* The legal resolution of disputed issues of a medical nature, however, almost invariably necessitates consideration of expert medical opinion testimony. Crucial areas such as diagnosis, extent, degree, and causation of disability, the existence and time frame of "conscious" pain and suffering, the necessity and reasonableness of past and projected medical and surgical treatment, the charges rendered, the role of preexisting conditions, losses of bodily functions, scarring and disfigurement, reduction of life expectancy, prognosis, whether an "end result" has been reached, and the many other items that determine damages to be awarded to the victim of a cardiac injury or benefits available under covering workers' compensation or other legislative acts, and the causal relationship of each to the alleged injury, generally require medical substantiation or refutation.

LEGAL ACTIONS REQUIRING CARDIAC MEDICAL EVALUATIONS

The spectrum of legal actions where medical evaluations relating to cardiology become key issues is vast, varied, and limited only by the ingenuity and imagination of the claimants' attorneys.[1-3] The most common areas include the following:

1. Claims brought under various state workers' compensation statutes and similar federal legislation (e.g., the Federal Longshoremen's and Harbor Workers' Compensation Act and the Federal Employees' Compensation Act), where cardiac disorder disability, treatment, or death is alleged

* This chapter is dedicated to the memory of Dr. Elliot L. Sagall.

a consequence of a work-related heart "injury" or an "occupational disease."

2. Tort claims under common law seeking damages for alleged cardiac "injury" due to negligence on the part of another person or persons, including suits for medical malpractice.
3. Claims against insurers, including the Social Security Disability Insurance program, for pensions, covered medical expenses, losses of income, or accidental death benefits resulting from heart disease.
4. Questions as to the fitness of a person with a heart disorder to return to a specific job, to drive a motor vehicle, to operate machinery or other equipment, to pilot an airplane, to participate in a legal proceeding, to serve a prison sentence, or to prepare a will.
5. Claims instituted by insurers alleging preexistent heart disease as a basis for qualifying under "second injury funds" for reimbursement of workers' compensation benefits, the voiding of an insurance contract by reason of the applicant's fraudulent concealment of a preexisting heart disorder, or the nonpayment of special benefits provided in the insurance contract for death or injury due to an accident because of the contribution of a preexistent cardiac disorder.
6. Claims under the Americans with Disabilities Act.

Of these, the most commonly encountered are claims that a cardiac disorder is a workplace injury covered by the applicable workers' compensation statute.

Although individual state and federal workers' compensation acts differ somewhat in requirements for eligibility and benefits provided to injured workers and their dependents,[4] the fundamental social principle common to all compensation statutes is that the financial costs of work-related injuries should be assumed to a large extent by the employer as an expense of production and not by the injured worker or by public funds. Without exception, all compensation acts embrace the basic concept that the right to compensation for work-incurred injury is provided to the injured employee without regard to fault or to demonstrable negligence of the employer. Legal defenses available under common law to employers to avoid or to mitigate liability such as assumption of the risk of the job by the employee's acceptance of the employment or contributory negligence by the employee or fellow employees are specifically excluded from workers' compensation. In turn, the benefits potentially accruing to an injured employee are generally limited to a portion of the lost wages plus allowances for dependents and reasonable and necessary medical expenses. Items such as pain and suffering and loss of consortium, which may play a large role in the determination of an award to an injured person in actions for tort (negligence) under common law, are excluded. In workers' compensation, legal liability attaches to the employer (or insurance carrier) for the consequences of an injury, including heart disorder, disability, or death,[1,4–8] demonstrated to have occurred during "the course of" and to have arisen "out of" employment—a formula that has aptly been characterized as "deceptively simple and litigiously prolific."

Under some compensation statutes, the basic formula of compensable injury has been modified by specific legislative restrictive definitions that require that the alleged work injury be suffered "by accident" or be due to "unusual stress" or to "stress greater than normal nonwork life" or to have been contributed "substantially" to by the work. In most jurisdictions, an identified time and place of injury must be demonstrated for coverage to apply. And in one compensation act (Wyoming's), further restriction has been placed for legal acceptance of an alleged work-related cardiac injury in that no more than 4 h must elapse between the claimed time of injury and the first clinical manifestations of same.[9]

The imposition of these restrictions indicates a legislative attempt to distinguish alleged work-related heart injuries from those that occur as a result of the natural progression of the underlying disease—an effort not often successful. Along these lines, one state (Nevada) even went so far as to exclude "coronary thrombosis, coronary occlusion, or any other ailment or disorder of the heart, and any death or disability ensuing therefrom" as an injury by accident arising out of and in the course of employment, except under certain circumstances for firefighters, police officers, prison guards, and several other favored categories of public employees.[10]

In many states the concept of "accidental disability"* for purposes of workers' compensation or retirement has been extended for certain named occupational groups, particularly uniformed police and firefighters, by legislative inclusion in the covering statutes of a presumption of job causation for disabling heart disease or hypertension. Although theoretically rebuttable, such presumptions, from a practical viewpoint, generally cannot be overcome, particularly if the worker has no clear risk factors for heart disease. The result is that applicants under these laws (commonly referred to as "Heart Laws") often need only establish the existence of a disabling heart disorder or hypertension and not the causal connection to the employment, although in some jurisdictions, (e.g., Massachusetts) the existence of significant nonemployment risk factors such as tobacco abuse may overcome the presumption of job-related causation. The Massachusetts statute 11 is a typical example:

> Notwithstanding the provisions of any general or special law to the contrary . . . any condition of impairment of health caused by hypertension and heart disease resulting in total or partial disability or death to a uniformed member of a paid fire department or permanent member of a police department . . . shall, if he successfully passed a physical examination on entry into such service which examination failed to reveal any evidence of such condition, be presumed to have been suffered in line of duty, unless the contrary be shown by competent evidence.[11]

The first step in the process of determining eligibility of an applicant for the benefits provided under this statute usually is an examination by a medical panel appointed for the purpose of determining the existence of heart disease or hypertension, the resulting job disability, and job causation. The medical

* Accidental disability retirement applies to a permanent work incapacity as a result of a work-related injury or a hazard experienced in the performance of job duties. Ordinary disability retirement applies to permanent work incapacity due to sickness or injury that is not job-related. Since the financial benefits of an accidental disability retirement generally are significantly greater than those of an ordinary disability retirement in that the awards usually are free from federal and state income tax, applicants for disability understandably seek the greater "take-home" pay of an "accidental disability."

panel's findings, however, are only advisory and are not binding on the designated retirement board. Since the etiology of most forms of heart disease and hypertension is not currently known, the medical panel, most often, cannot provide "competent evidence" to offset the legislative presumption of job causation embodied in the covering statute. An accidental disability can then be awarded if the medical panel has found the existence of a disabling cardiac or hypertensive condition. The applicant's task under many of these statutes is further eased by the definition of *job disability* as an incapability of the applicant to perform the full range or "all" of the duties, including response to emergency situations inherent in the course of police or firefighting activities. The legal dependents of retirees under the Heart Law do not automatically receive death benefits. They usually have the burden of establishing by medical evidence that the death was causally related to the condition for which retirement was awarded. Thus, a statement on a death certificate that the immediate cause of death was "cardiac arrest" is not sufficient to establish legal causation, since cardiac arrest is frequently only a terminal event, not necessarily related to a condition of preexistent heart disease or hypertension. However, medical opinion that the death was hastened to some degree (even by as short a period as seconds to minutes) by reason of reduced cardiac reserve related to the underlying heart disorder may be sufficient to satisfy the legal issue of causality.

Particularly important in adjudication of claims for cardiac injury, disability, or death under workers' compensation and in actions in tort for injury due to negligence is the universal legal acceptance of the common law precept that prior infirmity is no bar to benefits even though the injured person would not have suffered injury, as is the case in most cardiac claims, had there not been underlying heart disease. Legally, the injured person may be entitled to benefits if it can be shown that the employment or an act of negligence in some way aggravated a preexisting condition to lead to injury, disability, or death sooner than would otherwise have been expected during the natural history of the underlying disorder. Under many state compensation acts, the burden of proving job causation generally assigned to the claimant is eliminated when the worker is found deceased or otherwise medically unable to testify at the place of employment. By the statutory adoption of presumption of work relationship in such situations, the burden of disproving causation is placed upon the employer. Under the Federal Longshoremen's and Harbor Workers' Compensation Act, a set of presumptions effectively requires that the employer establish noncausation to the job for almost all medical conditions that may render an employee permanently or partially disabled from work.[12]

Under actions in tort in common law, recovery of "damages" may be obtained when the plaintiff or those claiming through the plaintiff can show that the disorder and its consequences arose from or were aggravated by the negligent activity of another (commonly referred to as a *tortfeasor*). Unlike the doctrine of workers' compensation, liability in actions of tort is predicated on fault. To be awarded "damages," the injured party must show (1) that the defendant owed the plaintiff a duty, i.e., the duty to adhere to an accepted standard of medical care and the duty to refrain from negligence; (2) that the defendant's conduct breached that duty; (3) that the plaintiff suffered injuries or "harms"; (4) that the defendant's negligent conduct was the proximate cause of the damage (harms) allegedly suffered by the plaintiff; and (5) that the victim's own negligence did not contribute to his or her harms (the *doctrine of contributory negligence*). Again, susceptibility to injury by reason of preexisting infirmity does not bar recovery.

Actions in tort alleging cardiac injury most commonly arise from motor vehicle accidents where it is claimed that a myocardial contusion, an acute coronary artery occlusion, an acute myocardial infarction, a cardiac death, or some other acute cardiac episode resulted from, or was hastened by, physical trauma or the psychological consequences of the accident. Most difficult in both medical determinations and legal handling are those situations where it is alleged that a preexisting condition of stable angina pectoris has been aggravated, as evidenced by a change in a preexisting symptom complex, but with no objective evidence to support the claimed aggravation. Another commonly encountered vexing medicolegal problem is whether a fatal cardiac episode was "the result of" or "the cause of" an accident—a determination also of importance when insurance contracts provide double indemnity or other specified benefits for "accidental" death or injury. Other frequently encountered actions in tort involving cardiac patients are those in which it is alleged that heart problems have stemmed from trauma or stress subsequent to negligent conduct, such as from falling objects, slipping, and other accidentally induced falls; from exposure to food poisonings; from toxic fumes; from menacing animals; and from long-term psychological "stress." In addition, the Americans with Disabilities Act, initially phased in on July 26, 1992, promises new areas of litigation by prohibiting employment discrimination against an employee "who meets the skill, experience, education and other job-related requirements of a position held or desired, and who, with or without reasonable accommodation, can perform the essential functions of a job."[13]

Medical malpractice suits fall within the province of actions in tort and are subject to the same legal considerations affecting all claims for "damages" due to "negligence." In malpractice cases, as with other actions in tort, the aggrieved patient or those acting for the plaintiff have the burden of demonstrating (1) that the defendant breached a standard of care owed, and (2) that this breach caused the plaintiff "harm." In evidentiary proof, the plaintiff must define by expert medical opinion the standard of care alleged to have been breached. The plaintiff must further establish the existence of alleged "harms" or "damage" and also must then show, again by expert medical opinion, that the alleged deviation from the acceptable standard of care was the cause of the claimed "damages." Finally, in many jurisdictions it must further be demonstrated that the plaintiff's conduct did not negligently contribute to the claimed harms. Unless all these criteria are satisfied, a directed verdict for the defendant may be ordered by the judge.

In some legal actions, the known existence of a prior cardiac disorder is of importance in the assessment of financial awards. Under the Second Injury Funds of the Federal Longshoremen's and Harbor Workers' Compensation Act and of many state workers' compensation acts, some financial relief is afforded the employer or insurer for disability payments to an injured worker if it can be demonstrated that the work incapacity following an accepted or assigned work injury was made substantially greater than would otherwise have been the case because of a known preexistent medical condition or that death would not have occurred without the preexisting physical impairment.

In other instances, the demonstration of a heart disorder may be of key importance in a legal decision as to whether a worker can return to a prior job that an employer claims involves physical or psychological stress potentially harmful to a person with known heart disease or where the operation of machinery by a person subject to sudden incapacity, as from an acute cardiac dysrhythmia, would endanger others; whether a person should be rejected from driving a motor vehicle, particularly one used in public transportation, or from piloting an airplane; whether a heart patient can participate in a court trial as a defendant or witness or serve a prison term, write a valid will, or be forced to pay alimony or other financial assessment; whether certain items claimed as income-tax–deductible medical expenses are medically justified as treatment; whether an insurance contract can be voided because of the applicant's fraudulent concealment of a known cardiac disorder in the original application for the policy; and in other situations where the question of preexistent heart disorder may be of importance for legal and insurance determinations of eligibility for "accidental death" benefits.

A large area of litigation involving heart disorder concerns the many applicants for disability benefits under the Social Security Disability Insurance Program, public welfare programs, the Veterans Administration service- and non-service-related pensions, and privately purchased disability, accident, and health insurance contracts. In most of these situations, the legal issue to be decided is the work capacity of the individual, as defined in the covering statute or insurance contract, based on a demonstrated medical condition, not the question of causation. Miscellaneous legal actions that may require expert medical opinions on heart disorders and their consequences include determination of the existence and extent of "conscious pain and suffering" as an element of tort "damages," losses of bodily functions under certain workers' compensation statutes, reduction of life and/or work-year expectancy due to a cardiac disorder or worsening thereof, projected reasonable medical expenses of future treatment in a cardiac patient, relation of coronary artery bypass grafting or other treatments to a compensable myocardial infarction, prognosis, projected life span, and other medicolegal issues.

THE CARDIOLOGIST IN THE COURTROOM

It is in the role of an expert witness that cardiologists most often find themselves involved with the legal profession. Any duly licensed physician, however, whether a general practitioner or a specialist, is considered legally qualified to present opinion testimony when the medical issues in hand are not a matter of common knowledge. The appropriateness of a particular physician's competency to testify as an expert, however, can be raised by either side of the dispute and put before the court for its evaluation on the basis of the physician's training, experience, and demonstrated bias. Once a physician has been accepted as an expert witness, the weight to be attached to the medical conclusions presented is determined by a legally appointed fact-finding body. Since the current state of scientific knowledge in cardiology often does not provide clear-cut answers to many of the courtroom medical questions, there is often a difference between the conclusions reached by the expert witnesses called by the two sides in a case. In such instances, the legal fact finder can adopt the opinion believed most likely to conform to the facts and reach a decision on that basis. In some legal actions the fact finder may elect to call on an outside court-appointed physician for an "impartial" opinion. Thus, almost every legal decision in medical matters has to be supported by the testimony of a physician "expert witness." It is imperative, therefore, that legal decisions should be in accord with the main current of medical thinking and the testimony of the "experts" should be within the boundaries of presently acceptable scientific beliefs and concepts.

The physician who testifies as an expert witness need not have personally examined the claimant or even have any personal knowledge of the claimant's medical condition prior to or following an alleged incident. The medical expert may reach conclusions solely from a review of the medical records and other factual data that have been admitted into evidence. Alternatively, the expert may be presented by either counsel with a hypothetical question that contains a set of facts to be utilized for the conclusions reached and the opinions expressed. The law, however, does require that those facts put forth in hypothetical questions be supported by the evidence presented in the case. Thus, the fact finder cannot adopt the opinion expressed by an expert in answer to a hypothetical question unless the evidence on hand is sufficient to establish the truth of the supposition. When the factual evidence is conflicting, as is frequently the case, it is within the province of the fact finder to determine which evidence is to be believed and adopted as "factual."

The hypothetical question posed to a medical expert in courtroom proceedings need not include all the evidence previously presented in the case. It may be limited to a partisan recital of that evidence most favorable to the proponent's side. The adversary party, in cross-examination of the expert, however, can propose a counterhypothetical recital of alleged facts to provide data omitted or now added to the original question. The medical expert can then be asked whether the newly assumed facts alter the opinions previously expressed. In this manner, both parties in the legal dispute have full opportunity to pose to medical experts respective versions of what they believe is factual. Again, however, the ultimate determination of medical issues for legal purposes rests with the duly appointed fact finder, not with the medical experts.

Generally, it is not sufficient for an expert witness to present conclusions alone without supporting reasoning. The basis on which the opinion rendered rests also may be subject to attack in cross-examination so that the testimony presented can be weighed by the fact finder. In formulating an opinion, the medical expert must appreciate the degree of certainty required in reaching medical conclusions in a legal forum. The legal system recognizes the current inability of medical science to answer definitively and with absolute certainty many of the medical questions raised in individual cases. Yet the legal body responsible for final legal resolution must answer as best it can all the issues raised at the time of trial. Legal proof cannot be equated with scientific proof. In civil cases, decisions are based primarily upon standards such as a preponderance of the evidence and clear and convincing evidence. In criminal matters, the requirements are more stringent, usually beyond a reasonable doubt. The law generally requires that answers to medical questions be expressed in terms of reasonable medical certainty or probability rather than mere possibility. In essence, this means that the conclusions reached by an expert are believed to be more likely than not true even though the level of certainty would not be acceptable to a body of scientists. In accord with this legal philosophy, reasonable medical certainty generally means reasonable legal certainty—a far less exacting criterion of proof than that required for medical scientific certainty.

In cases involving cardiac claims, as in most civil cases, the burden of proof generally is placed on the claimant, who must show by a preponderance of supporting evidence, including expert opinion when necessary, that the allegations are true. For example, in a claim alleging a cardiac disorder and its consequences as a workplace injury, the claimant must provide the fact finder with sufficient supporting medical expert testimony attesting not only to the existence of a cardiac disorder but also to its causal relationship to some element of the employment. A claimant's burden of proof generally is not met when a medical expert merely acknowledges the possibility of the truth of the allegations rather than asserting their probability. Phraseology frequently employed by physicians in medical reports and testimony such as *may, could,* or *might have* serves no useful purpose in the courtroom. Additionally, the burden of proof is not met, nor is it sustained, when the medical supportive conclusions are shown to be based on speculation, rather than on reasonable medical certainty, or when the medical expert admits that acceptance and denial of the allegations are equal possibilities that cannot be differentiated.

As pointed out earlier in this chapter, under many workers' compensation acts, when a worker is found dead or unable to testify at the place of employment, the burden of disproving causation by the job is placed on the employer. The Federal Longshoremen's and Harbor Workers' Compensation Act even goes a step further by stating, "In any proceeding for the enforcement of a claim for compensation under this Act it shall be presumed, in the absence of substantial evidence to the contrary. . . . That the claim comes within the provisions of this Act. . . ."[12] In actions for medical malpractice the burden of proof of lack of causation by negligence may be shifted to the defendant health care provider when the doctrines of *res ipsa loquitur* ("the thing speaks for itself") and the *captain of the ship,* i.e., the operating room surgeon, become applicable. When expert medical opinions presented by the respective litigants contradict or conflict, the fact finder must choose between them. The choice is subject to reversal on appeal to a higher court only when contrary to the weight of the evidence or the result of an error in legal procedure. Since the legal fact finder often lacks an adequate scientific background, legal decisions may appear contrary to medical thinking.

THE MEDICOLEGAL CARDIAC EVALUATION

Medical examinations and evaluations performed specifically for legal and insurance reasons necessarily emphasize aspects of the medical situation not customarily addressed by physicians, since the primary purpose of such evaluations is the answering of legal questions and not the providing of medical care.

The scope of potential medicolegal questions where heart disorder is germane to the litigation is too broad to be reviewed completely here. Certain inquiries, however, are fundamental to most claims alleging cardiac injury, dysfunction, or death. These are (1) the cardiac diagnosis accepted legally as established in a given claimant; (2) the time of onset of each specific cardiac lesion; (3) the causal relation, if any, between the factor or factors under legal examination and the cardiac disorder found; (4) the medical determination of the impairment based on the claimant's overall cardiovascular status; and (5) the medical considerations in allegations of professional negligence. Additionally, in some legal actions arising under workers' compensation and some insurance policies, questions as to the role of preexisting disease or infirmity in contributing to the covered impairment or death may be of paramount importance in determining eligibility for benefits as well as the amount of benefits to be paid by the employer or insurer.

Defining the Cardiac Diagnosis

From the medical viewpoint, the diagnosis is the foundation on which the treatment of the patient is constructed. From the legal viewpoint, the diagnosis is the foundation upon which many decisions and rulings concerning issues of causation, eligibility for disability and retirement pensions, awards for damages, and many other matters arising in the litigation on hand are made. Although the diagnosis has to be made by a physician based upon medical data, legally it is considered only one of the various factual determinations in the case. The diagnosis reached by a physician after the gathering, reviewing, and studying of the medical data is, in essence, merely an opinion based on the individual examiner's specialized training, study, experience, and interpretation of the medical findings. As such, it is open to question both medically and legally as to reasonableness, accuracy, and completeness. Since different examiners may make different diagnoses, opinions expressed in court are subject to interrogation by counsel during cross-examination. The cardiac diagnosis should be established in each instance as fully as possible in terms of (1) an etiologic diagnosis that describes the underlying disease processes; (2) an anatomic diagnosis that describes the specific structural abnormalities (lesions) found in the cardiovascular examination; and (3) a physiologic diagnosis that describes the resulting disturbances of cardiovascular action and function. These should be delineated in generally accepted terminology, such as recommended by the Criteria Committee of the New York Heart Association in that committee's publication, "Nomenclature and Criteria for Diagnosis of the Heart and Great Vessels."[14] Because of varying connotations and implications, nonspecific terms, such as heart attack, coronary, mild or massive heart attack, and heart disease, without adequate qualification as to specific meaning, should not be employed in the cardiac evaluator's written report or testimony. Similarly, umbrella terms, such as *unstable angina, preinfarction angina, acute coronary deficiency,* and *acute coronary insufficiency,* should be avoided unless they are precisely defined.

The etiologic diagnosis should be reached after consideration of both the structural and functional disturbances found. If two or more etiologic bases for a person's heart disorder are present, each should be listed. Legally, the identification of the etiologic basis of a cardiac disorder or disorders becomes important in a causality assessment where worsening of a preexistent cardiac condition is claimed as a "personal injury" (and must be differentiated from the expected natural progression) and in legal actions where an estimation of life expectancy is of importance in determining awards for "damages" or in settlement proceedings.

The anatomic diagnosis comprises that component of the total cardiac diagnosis that describes the specific structural lesions present in the heart and great vessels. A complete description of the anatomic alterations often constitutes an important aspect of the legal determinations of a cardiac "personal injury" and of disability. Thus, for example, there may be considerable differences in the benefits or awards available legally for the sustaining of an episode of prolonged ischemic cardiac pain when diagnosed as an intermediate coronary syndrome with no documented new myocardial damage or when diagnosed as acute myocardial necrosis with resulting permanent new or added heart damage.

Anatomic lesions of the heart and great vessels frequently can be delineated clinically on the basis of the history, the findings of physical examination, and the results of specialized cardiac diagnostic studies. Certain anatomic lesions, e.g., a coronary artery thrombotic occlusion, however, cannot be diagnosed with reasonable certainty unless established by coronary angiography or other reliable objective means. Thus, diagnoses of *coronary thrombosis* and *microscopic myocardial necrosis,* terms not infrequently encountered in cardiac medicolegal reports and expert testimony, should usually be reserved for the radiologist or pathologist. When more than one anatomic abnormality is found, each should be included in the final diagnosis.

The physiologic diagnosis specifies the alterations in cardiovascular dynamics and function that have resulted from the cardiac pathology. The physiologic diagnosis may include a description of the cardiac rhythm; disturbances in cardiac impulse conduction; disturbances in supravalvular, valvular, or subvalvular function; malfunctions of prostheses, homografts, and cardiac pacemakers; disturbances in myocardial pump action; disturbances in intravascular pressures; abnormal communications (shunts) in the heart or great vessels; and the anginal syndromes. A cardiac diagnosis presented in the courtroom should be supported, wherever possible, by objective measures of cardiac structure and function, where indicated and within limitations of practicality and risk. A diagnosis based solely on a claimant's history, although in many cases the only diagnostic tool available to the medical expert, is not on secure grounds and, accordingly, is subject to strong attack on cross-examination. Many symptoms common to cardiac disorders, such as chest pain, shortness of breath on exertion, palpitations, and fatigue, are not pathognomonic for heart disorder. Symptoms alone are difficult to evaluate, since they may be exaggerated for self-serving purposes. Symptoms, per se, also defy quantifying. In contrast, the severity of symptoms in cardiac patients often does not correlate with the degree and severity of the found impairment of heart structure and function, and some cardiac disorders may result in no, minimal, or nonspecific symptoms.

The physician performing a cardiac evaluation for legal purposes must determine whether the patient-claimant had heart disease prior to the alleged potentially harmful exposure under legal consideration and, if so, whether there was a change in the preexistent cardiac status after the exposure. If a change is found, the physician must then define its nature and extent and whether it is permanent or temporary. It is also important to distinguish between a demonstrated structural change in a preexisting heart disorder and an alleged hastening of an expected consequence.

Diagnoses, as with other medical opinions, presented to a legal forum must be established in terms of reasonable medical certainty. Possible, potential, or suspected heart disorder has no place in the courtroom or in other legal determinations.

Timing the Onset of Cardiac Lesions

Determining the time of onset of specific cardiac pathology is an essential part of many cardiac medicolegal evaluations. It is often the crux of causation or of eligibility for the benefits of an insurance contract. Because of the variability of clinical presentations, individual differences in response to and manifestations of illness, and the frequent initial "silent" development of many cardiac pathologies, it may be impossible to time the onset of cardiac conditions within the precise framework sought by the law. Yet, the time of onset of cardiac lesions and dysfunction must be defined by the cardiac examiner as best as it can be with reasonable medical certainty and probability.

Determining the time of onset of a myocardial infarction may be difficult because of variable clinical presentations. The classic textbook presentation of sudden crushing anterior chest pain associated with profuse diaphoresis, dyspnea, and weakness is a generally acceptable index of the occurrence at that time of significant discrete acute myocardial tissue necrosis, although the possibility that some degree of myocardial necrosis has occurred previously (silently or with atypical manifestations) cannot be excluded. In some patients, an acute myocardial infarction, although evident at a later date on an electrocardiogram or at postmortem examination, is clinically silent. In other patients, the clinical picture is one of waxing and waning ischemic symptoms or signs over the course of 1 or more days with or without a bout of classic, prolonged chest discomfort. In patients with previous angina pectoris, an acute myocardial infarction may be manifested by an anginal attack of greater severity and duration or of radiation and location different from that previously experienced.

Unless otherwise determinable, the time of onset of a cardiac arrhythmia generally is accepted as the time of occurrence of identifying symptoms such as palpitations or a sudden collapse, as with a cardiac arrest due to ventricular tachycardia or fibrillation. The time of onset of coronary atherosclerotic, valvular, hypertensive, and most other heart disorders generally cannot be determined medically with any greater accuracy other than that the underlying etiologic condition must have been present for some time (usually only measurable in months or years) prior to the initial clinical manifestations. The occurrence of sudden collapse, acute pulmonary edema, cardiogenic shock, or severe pain provides an index of the time of rupture of an aortic aneurysm of a cardiac valve, papillary muscle, or of chordae tendineae, or infarcted myocardium. However, the commencement of the pathophysiologic processes underlying such rupture cannot be pinpointed with accuracy because of subtle or absent manifestations for a variable period of time preceding the catastrophic event.

Assessment of Causality

The determination of causation is vital to legal actions in which a heart disorder or its consequences is claimed as a compensable "work injury," as an injury due to "negligence," or as an "accident" under an insurance contract in which benefits are specifically provided for injury, disability, or death due to an "accident" rather than "illness." In general, legal claims of cardiac injury or sudden cardiac death generally allege as *a* or *the* cause of (1) an isolated, specifically identified incident, event, accident, trauma, or exposure; (2) a complication of medical or surgical treatment or other alleged so-called triggers[5,6] or (as in a malpractice action) a negligent treatment or negligent failure to institute indicated treatment; (3) a set of repetitive, cumulative factors[7] that, although subliminal individually, have combined in additive effect to produce cardiovascular harm (e.g., repeated subthreshold inhalation of carbon monoxide); (4) a long-term "overall" job or situational physical or psychological "stress"; or (5) a combination of one or more of the preceding.[6,7] In such actions, the claimant must first establish the existence of a cardiac disorder that can be accepted as an "injury" and then establish a causal connection between such injury and the alleged harmful consequences (disability, medical and surgical treatment and diagnostic expenses, pain and suffering, death, and other items of "harms") for which benefits are claimed. The claimant usually has the further burden of disproving any contributions to the alleged harms from intervening causes or from personal negligence if such charges are raised by the defendant.

In disputed issues involving causality questions in medical disorders, the legal fact finder must rely on the evidence put forth by the respective litigants, particularly expert medical opinion testimony. Physicians presenting such testimony in cause-and-effect assessments must appreciate the different weights assigned by the legal profession to the various elements that comprise a legal causality determination from those assigned by the medical profession to a pure medical assessment of causality (see Table 96-1). Causation often means one thing to a physician and quite another to an attorney, judge, or administrative hearing official. On occasions, medical opinion testimony based on traditional medical concepts of causality differs dramatically from answers based primarily on legal concepts utilized by a fact finder in reaching courtroom decisions.

TABLE 96-1 Medical Versus Legal Emphasis in Causality Assessment

Medical Emphasis	Legal Emphasis
The etiologic bases of a disease or disorder	The proximate ("triggering") cause of an injury, disability, or death
The causes of disease	A cause of injury, disability, or death
The producing cause of the entire disorder	An aggravation of a preexisting condition
The key role of preexisting disease	"The victim is taken as found," not as a normal, healthy person, but subject to whatever existing medical disorders were present at the time of exposure
The end result was inevitable because of the expected progression of the preexisting disease	A determination of whether the end result was hastened, not the time amount of hastening
The degree of aggravation was small in the light of the entire clinical picture	The crux is aggravation, not degree
The alleged causative element(s) not unique or unusual	The key element is the causative element(s), not the characteristics
The multiplicity of causes and their interrelationships	The key is the causative element(s) under legal scrutiny, independent of other coexisting or interrelating causes
Scientific proof of causation required	Establishment of causation generally is defined in terms of reasonable medical certainty, i.e., probable vs. possible, more likely than not, a 50.1% chance of relationship
Equally consistent theories of causation acceptable in differential diagnosis and choice of therapies	Equally consistent theories of causation do not satisfy standards for legal proof
The ultimate answer to causations can be deferred, pending new scientific advances	The issue of causation must be decided legally when presented
In assessment of damages (harms), there should be an apportionment of the role of each causative element	Generally, a total responsibility is assigned for the end result, if such is deemed due to a legally indicated exposure

SOURCE: Adapted from Sagall and Reed,[3] Sagall,[18] and Danner and Sagall.[19]

There are many differences between the medical and legal approaches to solving causality problems.[15–20] The physician, for example, in viewing a patient's medical problems, instinctively searches for the basic cause or causes underlying the overall disorder, whereas legal and judiciary professionals generally limit their concern to the one or more items under legal scrutiny as an "injury," independent of other causes. The physician generally defines cause as the production of a new condition or a new pathology or dysfunction, whereas the law in its definition accepts the aggravation of an underlying disorder by the worsening, hastening, or acceleration of its progression. The law thus includes in its framework of causation not only the production of a de novo condition but also the "triggering" or "proximate precipitation" of a new stage of pathology or of a new dysfunction in an underlying disorder and the worsening of an ongoing pathologic process. Physicians are reluctant to assign causal responsibility when the degree of aggravation of a preexisting condition is small in relation to the extent of the underlying abnormality or when the degree of hastening of an inevitable end result is minor. The law, in comparison, emphasizes the fact of hastening or aggravation, not the quantitative aspects. The crux of legal causation thus is the occurrence of an aggravation of an underlying disorder, not the degree to which it was aggravated, or the hastening of an end result, not the extent to which it was hastened.

Physicians are usually impressed that the alleged injury would not have occurred in the absence of a preexisting disorder that rendered the patient susceptible to harm from the alleged exposure. Legal fact finders, however, see it as immaterial that the event in question would not have caused injurious consequences had the victim been in good or average health. In all personal injury legal actions, the victim is "taken as he is found." Preexisting infirmity does not bar legal recovery, nor is it an acceptable excuse to relieve a defendant from legal responsibility or to mitigate the damages to be assessed. An illustration is the case of the proverbial "straw that broke the camel's back." To the physician, the proverb emphasizes the obvious predisposition to break down because of existing overload. The physician thus assigns the cause of the camel's collapse to the prior strain on his back, not to the added straw. The law, in comparison, asserts that although loaded to the breaking point, the back had held up without breaking. Accordingly, the added straw must be viewed as the cause of the collapse and the person who placed the straw on that loaded back as legally responsible for the consequences. Most often, the assignment of legal liability in such situations is made without attempt to apportion a percentage of harm between the triggering straw and the preexisting load. Unfortunately, the many current deficiencies in medical knowledge concerning the etiology and pathogenesis of most cardiac disorders and the limitations of presently available cardiac diagnostic testing procedures often prevent defining precisely the complete cardiac diagnosis, the nature and extent of the underlying pathology, the pathophysiologic mechanisms that have led to the end result, the sequence in which pathologic lesions have developed, the time of onset of certain lesions, and the answers to the many medical questions that may be of key importance in the legal matter on hand. The medical determination of causation is further made difficult because the very nature of most cardiac disorders categorized legally as personal injuries does not, in contrast to lesions such as burns or lacerations, present clinical or pathologic features pathognomonic of trauma or of an external cause. Thus, the question of whether some identified external element or stress played a contributory or precipitating role in their development or whether the disorder found stemmed from the natural, expected progression of an underlying cardiac disease unrelated to and unaffected by the item under legal scrutiny quite frequently is not amenable to clear-cut answers.

Similarly, differences in the provisions of the individual state and territorial workers' compensation acts under which most cardiac claims arise, differences in legal philosophy among the many persons assigned fact-finding roles in disputed litigation, subtle differences in claims that are seemingly identical, and the often diametrically opposed medical conclusions presented in a given case by equally competent medical experts preclude the formulation of legal standards of causality that can be applied uniformly to cover all instances. Accordingly, each case must be decided, both medically and legally, on its own set of facts and medical testimony. Certain precepts, however, should govern medical assessments of causality in cardiac claims. For an alleged causal connection to be accepted in a cardiac case as probable or with reasonable medical certainty, the following criteria should be satisfied:

- The cardiac diagnosis should be delineated completely and established, as far as reasonably possible, by objective means, and those portions of the cardiac condition under consideration as potential "injuries" specified.
- The alleged causative element presented for legal consideration should be one that is currently recognized medically and scientifically as capable, under appropriate circumstances, of producing the heart disorder or injury found.
- Conversely, the cardiac condition or dysfunction diagnosed must be one generally recognized medically as a possible result of the alleged harmful exposure.
- The time interval elapsing between the alleged noxious exposure and the medically manifest evidence of heart damage or dysfunction must be consistent with currently accepted scientific concepts of pathogenesis.
- The proposed cause-and-effect relation, although not always fully explainable in terms of present-day scientific knowledge, must still be consistent with current scientific concepts.

As an aid to medical assessment of causality in coronary artery heart disease and its ischemic sequelae, the reader is referred to the "Report of the American Heart Association's Committee on Stress, Strain, and Heart Disease."[20] Although originally published in 1977, the conclusions of this committee, supported by more recent studies,[21–32] are currently valid with only minor modification, have not been supplanted by any other formal set of medical causality guidelines, and are generally accepted by the medical profession. The conclusions currently pertinent to a medical assessment of causality in cardiac claims are subsequently summarized:

- Long-term repetitive physical effort, such as is inherent in many occupations, cannot currently be regarded medically as a causative element in the development of atherosclerotic coronary heart disease. Such activity, if playing any role in this disease process, is believed beneficial by preventing or slowing the rate of atherosclerotic progression.[20]
- Long-term repeated physical effort of work and/or nonwork activities in persons with underlying heart disease theoretically may hasten the development of congestive heart failure by reason of the additional workload imposed upon an already weakened heart. It is not possible within the present state of medical knowledge, however, to determine in any given heart patient when congestive heart failure would have occurred as the result of the expected natural progression of the underlying cardiac disorder in the absence of such exertional efforts; hence in these situations a causative or aggravating role to such stress most often cannot be assigned with "reasonable medical certainty."[20]
- Continued, psychological emotional stress and job demands to which an individual may have been subjected over a protracted period of time, though commonly accepted by the public and many physicians, have not been established scientifically as a causative or worsening agent in the genesis or acceleration of atherosclerotic disease,[20–36] although the possibility of some contribution cannot be excluded in individual cases.
- A single, isolated, identified physical or emotional stress in individuals rendered susceptible by reason of preexistent heart disease, is capable of eliciting adverse cardiac responses that, in turn, can "trigger" or hasten certain cardiac lesions and dysfunctions such as an attack of angina pectoris, a myocardial infarction, a sudden cardiac dysrhythmia, sudden

cardiac death, rupture of a diseased cardiac structure, coronary artery vasospasm, and flash pulmonary edema.[20-32]

- The shorter the time interval between the exposure of an individual to a potentially noxious stimulus and the appearance of clinical or pathologic evidence of new heart disease or dysfunction, the more likely there is a causal relation between the two. Conversely, the farther apart in time, the less likely is a cause-and-effect relation.[20]
- The exposure of a person with underlying heart disease to a stimulus potentially capable of eliciting harmful cardiovascular responses does not necessarily mean that such will be elicited, even when the exposure would be advised against medically because of the possibility of ensuing harm.[20]

The elements most often accepted by workers' compensation adjudicators in cardiac cases as work-related competent-producing causes of injury, disability, or death are identified incidents of physical work effort (usual, unusual, or of a degree greater than accustomed nonwork exertion, depending on the covering compensation act requirements); adverse work environments, (e.g., excessive heat or cold); and acute psychological trauma such as a heated argument or a sudden fright; an accidental electric shock; a severe nonpenetrating blow or other mechanical injury to the chest; and adverse cardiac reactions to medical, surgical, corrective, and rehabilitative therapy of an industrial injury not originally involving the cardiovascular system.

Nationwide, burgeoning claims under workers' compensation alleging illnesses such as coronary heart disease, hypertension, stroke, gastrointestinal disorders, and neuropsychiatric states as initiated or worsened by overall job-related "stress" are straining the workers' compensation system.[36] Frequently cited as "harmful" to the cardiovascular system are adverse mental reactions stemming from harassment by superiors, frustration from dealing with the public, tension created by imposed deadlines and quotas, boredom or excessive responsibility in job duties, threats of job termination or changes, insufficient vacations and time off, changing work shifts, long work hours, and ongoing business financial problems. In the cardiac "stress" cases that have reached state supreme court levels on appeals, the decisions have been mixed and have not established uniform case law precedents. For example, note the following cases:

- In New Hampshire, medical opinion that the continuing "stress" of a failing business over a 2-year period did not cause the fatal myocardial infarction suffered by the owner on a Sunday morning at home was upheld and compensation to his widow denied.[37]
- In contrast, a Rhode Island trial commissioner's denial of compensation to the widow of a newspaper sports editor who suffered a fatal cerebral hemorrhage at home was reversed. The court concluded that medical testimony that the deceased was suffering from high blood pressure of the type that would rise whenever he was under stress plus evidence that the decedent attended a professional football game earlier in the day of his death that placed him "under pressure" to meet a reporting deadline were sufficient to support the claim that his death that night was due to a cerebral hemorrhage resulting from aggravation of his preexisting hypertension.[38]
- In Colorado, the denial of compensation by the Industrial Commission to the widow of a fire department lieutenant with preexisting mitral valve prolapse and hypertension who died at home on the tenth day of a vacation absence from work was vacated. As grounds for the reversal and for an award of compensation, the court concluded that uncontroverted testimony from the fire chief, coworkers, and widow that the decedent had suffered a great deal of cumulative tension and frustration relating to his being overlooked in favor of junior firefighters for promotion and to his differing from superiors in department training and communication policies qualified this "stress" as an injury or occupational disease arising out of and in the course of employment. On this basis, the court remanded the claim to the referee to make specific findings whether the job-related stress was the proximate cause of the death. The decedent's doctor testified that the likely cause of death was an irregular heart rhythm that, when combined with a preexisting mitral valve prolapse and job-related stress, resulted in a fatal arrhythmia. The doctor further testified that the imminence of the decedent's return to work may have exacerbated his stress level, and was a contributory cause of his death.[39]
- In Connecticut, the court affirmed a commissioner's decision that unjust criticism of a bank employee on a number of occasions by superiors so aggravated her condition of obstructive coronary disease as to lead to a continued work disability from angina pectoris. This despite the presence of multiple coronary atherosclerosis risk factors including extensive cigarette smoking, obesity, and a positive family history of premature coronary disease.[40]

Major risk factors for coronary heart disease, such as cigarette smoking, elevated blood cholesterol, diabetes mellitus, hypertension, and positive family history of coronary disease, are often put forth by defense counsels as mitigating elements arguing against the claim's validity in questions of causality in coronary heart disease. Conversely, in a New Hampshire Supreme Court decision, the absence of identified risk factors in a firefighter with catheter-documented coronary atherosclerotic disease was deemed to support the *prima facie* presumption in the state's Workers' Compensation Act that heart disease in firefighters is occupationally related.[41]

In evaluating the role of risk factors in cardiac claims, it should be recognized that risk factors are of importance primarily in epidemiologic studies applicable to groups, not to an individual. For any given person, the presence or absence of medical background risk factors does not necessarily indicate the premature development of this condition. Thus, although statistically related to the presence of coronary heart disease, generally accepted risk factors for coronary atherosclerosis cannot be viewed medically as legally causative elements in the production of the disease.

Not all cardiac claims require legal causality determinations. For example, in claims instituted under the Social Security Disability Insurance Program, the primary issue is whether the applicant is unable to engage in substantial gainful employment as defined in the covering statute, not the medical or legal relationship of the disability to a particular causative element. Similarly, eligibility for benefits in most privately acquired insurance contracts is based on the fact of disability, generally independent of cause.

Evaluation of Disability

Evaluation of disability for legal and insurance purposes is a complex process necessarily involving more than one professional discipline. The evaluation generally requires interrelating the fields of medicine, law, insurance, judiciary, vocational counseling, and rehabilitation. As a minimum, a cardiac disability evaluation is twofold: first, a medical assessment must be made both in terms of what the patient cannot do and what the patient should not do by reason of the cardiac disorder and, second, there must be a legal translation of the medically determined impairment into the specific definition of disability in the applicable statute or insurance contract. The latter often involves questions concerning disability being total versus partial, permanent, house-confining, and other qualifying or restrictive adjectives that may affect benefits. As with most medicolegal evaluations, contested claims for disability benefits are decided by legal or administrative fact finders, with the physician's role limited to providing the fact finder with medical data and opinion testimony that can be utilized in reaching a conclusion. As a minimum, the physician examining a patient-claimant for disability evaluation purposes should attempt to determine the following issues:

- The full cardiac diagnosis, including etiology when known, and all anatomic and functional derangements found, together with the supporting clinical evidence.
- The clinical manifestations of the disorder revealed by the medical examination, including all subjective complaints and, more important, all objective confirmatory findings that support the presence of a heart disease or disorder medically recognized as capable of producing the symptoms alleged as the basis for disability.
- The impairment in the patient's physical activities and mental capacity in terms of limitations of walking, stair climbing, standing, sitting, reaching, lifting, bending, pushing, pulling, gripping, running, work hours, work pace, ability to concentrate, and capacity to work under conditions of tension, heat, cold, etc.
- The restrictions of nonwork and work activities medically imposed to prevent an aggravation of the underlying heart disorder or to prevent further heart damage, such as advice to post-myocardial infarction patients not to subject themselves to sudden bursts of strenuous physical effort. In those instances where the law requires that causation be apportioned between the parties (e.g., work-related versus non-work-related disabilities), the physician may be asked to furnish an opinion as to the causation of each of the impairments found. For example, in claims based on myocardial infarction, the physician may be asked what aspects of the impairments found are related to the underlying coronary atherosclerotic disease for which there may not be legal liability and what are related to the myocardial infarction itself for which there may exist legal responsibility.

In those situations where a patient-claimant has impairments coexisting from cardiac as well as noncardiac disorders, the physician may be asked to separate the impairments due to each disorder and, in assessing the overall combined impairments, whether noncardiac impairments magnify those attributable to the heart disorder. Where workers' compensation acts provide second injury funds, the examining or treating physician may be asked whether the disability from a cardiac injury in an employee with a known physical impairment from a congenital or acquired heart condition was made substantially greater by the combined effects of such impairment and subsequent personal injury.

In reaching the conclusions expressed in the medical assessment of disability, all currently available objective means of diagnosis and measurement of cardiac function should be used within practical limits of risk to the patient, cost of the testing, and value of the information to be obtained. Wherever feasible, medical evaluations of disability should be based on objective findings to obviate depending only on subjective complaints, which are often unreliable because they are self-serving. Medical assessments of cardiac impairment are significantly hampered by the following items:

1. Reliance on subjective complaints.
2. Individual variations in symptoms, motivation, adjustment, and return-to-work desires among persons with similar cardiac abnormalities.
3. Limitations of currently available means for quantitative measurement of cardiac functional reserves.
4. Frequent discrepancy between objective findings and subjective complaints.
5. Difficulties in transferring the results of objective test measurements, such as those of exercise stress testing, into the variable environment of the workplace or other real-life settings.
6. Susceptibility of most cardiac impairments to sudden change so that an impairment assessment or disability evaluation at a given date may be invalid for a later time.

The definition of disability from cardiovascular and/or other conditions for adults to qualify for benefits under the Social Security Insurance program requires an "inability to engage in any substantial gainful employment by reason of any medically determinable physical or mental impairment which can be expected to result in death or has lasted or is expected to last for a continuous period of not less than 12 months." The listing of impairment for each major body system, the applicable medical criteria, and the key concepts of medical evaluations are outlined and defined in the agency's handbook, *Disability Evaluation under Social Security,* [42] and on its web site on the Internet. [43]

In workers' compensation, for both cardiac and noncardiac conditions, administrators in more and more states have turned to the American Medical Association's *Guides to the Evaluation of Permanent Impairment*[44] for determinations of qualifying disability, as well as for rating the impairment in terms of percentage degree of functional loss that may qualify the injured worker for additional benefits in addition to lost wages. The New York Heart Association's[14] grading system of cardiac functional capacity provides an easily understood, readily applicable guide to the medical description of cardiovascular impairment:

Class I. Patients with cardiac disease, but without resulting limitation of physical activity. Ordinary physical activity does not cause undue fatigue, palpitation, dyspnea, or anginal pain.

Class II. Patients with cardiac disease resulting in slight limitations of physical activity. They are comfortable at rest. Ordinary physical activity results in fatigue, palpitation, dyspnea, or anginal pain.

Class III. Patients with marked limitation of physical activity.

They are comfortable at rest. Less than ordinary physical activity causes fatigue, palpitation, dyspnea, or anginal pain.

Class IV. Patients with cardiac disease resulting in inability to carry on any physical activity without discomfort. Symptoms of heart failure or of the anginal syndrome may be present even at rest. If any physical activity is undertaken, discomfort is increased.

For further discussion of medical evaluations and legal definitions of disability under a variety of situations plus extensive legal and medical references to disability assessments the reader is referred to the *Disability Handbook* of Balsam and Zabin[45] and its updated supplements.[46] The legal aspects of commonly sought medical assessments of physical impairment by third-party physicians and the legal relationship of the third-party physician and the person being examined are discussed by Rothstein.[47]

As with causality assessments, medical and legal assessments of disability may vary considerably because of the difference in emphasis necessarily placed by each profession on individual aspects of the impairment in the disability rating process. Although a physician might consider a patient not disabled and, therefore, employable, the fact finder may declare the same person disabled from work activity under the terms of the applicable law or insurance contract. Here the physician must appreciate that in reaching the legal decision as to work capacity, the fact finder frequently has to include nonmedical elements such as age, sex, educational background, motivation, and prior work training and experience. Additionally, the fact finder's decision may be influenced by the availability of certain types of employment in the local or national labor market, the problems imposed by transportation to and from work sites, language or other communication problems, and other factors that, as a practical matter, so restrict a given person's opportunity for gainful employment as to make that individual practically disabled from gainful employment although medically cleared for work.

It is also important to recognize that because of differing statutory and contractual definitions, a person declared disabled and awarded benefits under one disability program may not be deemed eligible for benefits under another program. Thus, an award for disability by one agency or insurer does not, by itself, bind another agency or insurer. Each insurance contract or other disability benefit program or statute must be considered individually and separately for each claim raised, although the claim in each instance is based on the same medical disorders and impairments.

Prognosis and Life Expectancy Assessments

When considering a lump sum settlement of a disputed cardiac claim or when setting up a dollar reserve to cover future benefits, defendant attorneys and insurers often ask their cardiology expert for an opinion as to a claimant's future course, anticipated future treatment, and/or life expectancy. Estimates of the number of years a claimant with heart disease can reasonably be expected to live not only are utilized legally to establish economic and other losses in the consideration of awards for "damages" in tort cases of cardiac injury, but also may be significant in limiting potential "damages" by reason of the heart condition's expected reduction of life span in cases where the legal liability is for a noncardiac injury.[48] Prognostic and life expectancy determinations realistically have to be based to a large extent upon statistical considerations and parameters in reported series involving large numbers of patients. While statistical conclusions do not necessarilly apply to a given individual patient, a medical assessment of a cardiac patient's expected need for and extent of future treatment and of life expectancy, formulated after thorough medical examination and based on valid scientific guidelines, can be relatively accurate within certain ranges and, of practical usefulness to the legal resolution of cardiac claims of persons with heart disease.

Determination of Malpractice

The risk of a physician being sued for professional negligence is an inescapable fact of today's professional life. Choosing cardiology as a specialty increases this risk[49] because of a variety of reasons, particularly (1) the ever-present threat of sudden, unpredicted death due to the nature of heart diseases; (2) the inherent hazards and complications of invasive procedures and cardiac surgery; (3) the often-encountered lack of clear-cut diagnostic evidence or an atypical clinical presentation in the early stages of an acute myocardial infarction; (4) the unavoidable mortality and morbidity associated with heroic medical and surgical treatment of desperately ill patients in the end stages of heart disease; and (5) the many problems involved in obtaining informed consent for procedures beyond the understanding of most lay persons, particularly when frightened by the threats of a cardiac illness.

In medical malpractice cases, those instituting the claim have the legal burden of demonstrating by factual and opinion evidence (1) that the defendant doctor or other health care provider owed a duty to the plaintiff as is legally and morally implied in the physician-patient relationship; (2) that the defendant violated that duty by breaching the standard of care; (3) that the patient suffered injury or harm; (4) that the physician or other health care provider's negligence was the proximate cause of that harm; and (5) in some jurisdictions, that the patient's conduct did not negligently contribute to the alleged harm (the doctrine of contributory negligence). Unless all these elements are established in the courtroom by the plaintiff, the legal action will fail.

The evidentiary proof required of the plaintiff in establishing the bases of his or her action generally necessitates that expert medical opinion be provided that (1) defines the standard of care due the plaintiff by the defendants; (2) establishes the breach or failure to conform to that standard of care; (3) defines the injuries or "harms" claimed; and (4) causally relates the harms found to the claimed negligent action or failure to act on the part of the defendants. Should a patient suffer harm during the course of medical diagnosis and treatment, the physician and/or other health care providers may be liable, separately or additionally, to two other legal actions. The first constitutes charges that the patient was not given sufficient information by the responsible professional persons to allow a legally valid "informed" consent to be made to a medically prescribed diagnostic test or treatment that resulted in injury. Therefore, performance of the procedure or treatment was legally an "assault," subject to evidentiary requirements less stringent than those required in actions in tort as well as protected by a different statute of limitations. The second possible legal action is one based on alleged breach of contract should a particular result or cure allegedly promised not be achieved. In both of these actions, supportive expert medical opinions may not be necessary to substantiate the claim, since the legal issue in dispute often hinges on the factual determination of whether the defendant physician did or did not say what the patient alleges and not a separate demonstration of professional negligence.

Medical evaluation of a malpractice claim requires a careful review of all the claimant's medical records with particular attention, first, to whether the defendant's professional actions were in accord with generally accepted and proper standards of professional conduct and, second, to whether the alleged "harms" were causally related to the defendant's professional actions or failure to act.

As discussed in detail in Chap. 97, clinical practice guidelines are intended to help improve medical practice by providing clear and well-documented statements regarding appropriate medical services for particular medical conditions. Such guidelines can therefore, at least in theory, act as objective references for the standard of care in medical malpractice suits. Indeed, one of the factors that has promoted the development of practice guidelines has been the belief that physicians could model their practices on the guideline recommendations and avoid the tendency to practice "defensive medicine"—a pattern of excessive diagnostic testing and interventions designed to avoid legal liability.[50] The actual impact of practice guidelines on medical malpractice has been more complex.

First, practice guidelines have not uniformly been accepted as admissible evidence by the courts.[50] In some cases, courts have held that the guidelines are "hearsay" and could not be admitted into evidence unless the experts who developed them testified directly and were subject to cross-examination. In other cases, the courts have allowed the use of guidelines at trial, but have not automatically granted them status as a valid statement of the standard of practice. Most observers now believe that guidelines will be routinely admissible into evidence and granted appropriate weight as long as there is expert testimony offered to attest to the guideline's validity and authority.[51]

It is also the case that guidelines may be used as both a "sword" and "shield"[52] in particular cases of malpractice. That is, physicians may be sued for their failure to meet published guidelines, even as many had hoped that guidelines would protect physicians from frivolous suits. The most extensive examination of this issue[53] found that in a review of 259 cases of medical malpractice, clinical practice guidelines were cited in 17. Of those, guidelines were used to build a case against the physician (inculpatory) in 12 cases and to provide a defense for the physician (exculpatory) in 4 cases. The authors acknowledge that their study was biased, in that the presence of exculpatory guidelines may have prevented plaintiffs from pursuing a malpractice claim. Nevertheless, a survey of malpractice attorneys reported in the same paper found that guidelines were more than twice as likely to be used as inculpatory rather than exculpatory once a suit was filed.[53]

In a medical evaluation of alleged professional negligence, the fact that a patient suffered injurious effects during or after a prescribed treatment or procedure does not by itself raise a legal presumption of negligence as a causative factor. A physician is not legally responsible for a poor patient outcome unless it is proved that it followed from lack of professional care and diligence ordinarily possessed by others in the profession.

THE MEDICOLEGAL CARDIAC EXAMINATION

The techniques employed in medicolegal cardiac examinations are essentially the same as in medical examinations performed for treatment purposes. Generally, the basic components of history taking, physical examination, resting electrocardiogram, and chest roentgenogram plus review and study of the available medical records suffice. In claims where the patient-claimant is not available for examination, the evaluation may have to be made entirely on the basis of medical records. Rarely do the legal questions require the employment of more advanced diagnostic testing. In such cases, the recommending physician must keep in mind the information it can be expected to provide, the limitations of results, the pitfalls in interpretation, the availability and cost of the procedure, and the inherent risks and hazards to the patient. All must be weighed carefully against the legal need for the information to be obtained.

When cardiac disorders have legal consequences, the content of the medical history ultimately accepted by the legal arbiter frequently makes or breaks the action instituted by the plaintiff-claimant. For example, in many workers' compensation cases there is often no dispute concerning insurance coverage and the presence of a disabling cardiac disorder for which benefits might be available under the law; rather, the key issue is whether a work-connected factor played a role in precipitating, triggering, hastening, aggravating, or otherwise "causing" the disorder. The crucial element in such causality assessments frequently is the medical history ultimately accepted by the fact finder as depicting the sequence of events and circumstances surrounding the occurrence of cardiac symptoms. In those situations where it is alleged or where it can be anticipated that it will later be alleged that the patient's heart disorder arose in some part out of employment, thereby entitling the person to workers' compensation benefits for disability, the examining physician should inquire about and include in the written history the sequence of events preceding and leading to the onset of symptoms for which the patient sought medical attention. Inquiry should also be made as to the specific work activities engaged in before, during, and after an alleged cardiac incident; whether these were customary and usual for the employee; and whether there were associated environmental conditions that could have intensified the potential physiologic demands. Similarly, in situations where mechanical trauma is alleged to be a cause of heart injury, as in tort cases involving motor vehicle accidents, inquiry should be directed to the exact type of mechanical forces involved, particularly the point or points of bodily contact; the effect on the patient's body; the development and objective evidence of trauma such as cuts, external bleeding, and ecchymoses; and the precise time and sequence of occurrence of symptoms and signs consistent with cardiac injury. The list of potential questions that may be pertinent in the medicolegal history thus is virtually endless. In each case, therefore, the examiner's questioning must be tailored to provide the information needed to reach a reasonable medical conclusion for the facts on hand. Hospital records generally contain more than one written history. Significant historic facts, often of key legal significance, may be found in the admitting histories and progress notes of attending physicians, interns, residents, nurses, and medical students and in reports of consultants and occupational and physical therapists as well as in less obvious places, such as in requests for x-rays, laboratory determinations, and various diagnostic tests and reports. Accordingly, the physician asked to make a medical evaluation for legal purposes should request the complete hospital records rather than only the discharge summary.

Because the medical history is derived by an interview between a physician and a patient and simultaneously or later transposed into a written record, it is subject to many limitations of content, distortion, and error that may affect its legal value. Many of these limitations stem from a failure of the interviewer to ask pertinent questions, a failure of the interviewed patient to understand the questions asked or to respond appropriately, a bias of the interviewer, and self-serving motives of the patient. Typically, histories contained in hospital records are devoid of those items that later are of key importance in legal resolution of the claim. This is quite common in the history recorded at the time the patient is first seen with an actual or suspected acute myocardial infarction. In such situations, brevity in history taking is essential because of the urgent need to establish a diagnosis and institute lifesaving therapy rapidly. Characteristically, such histories make no mention of details relevant to causation that are crucial in later legal actions. In many instances, the attending physician, not aware of the potential legal actions that may stem from the patient's cardiac disorder, fails to record the detailed history necessary to resolve the legal aspects of the patient's illness, making it necessary to obtain a detailed history at a later date when the patient has become less reliable because of elements of financial or other gain associated with the institution of a claim for benefits.

THE MEDICOLEGAL REPORT

The report prepared by the physician of the cardiac evaluation is an important document with far-reaching practical consequences.[54] For the attorney or insurer to whom it is addressed, the report forms the basis for determining the pretrial acceptance or denial of the claim, the consideration of settlement negotiations, the pretrial preparation, and the courtroom presentation of the medical aspects of the case. For the physician, the time put forth in compiling a comprehensive medical report of the examination findings, summary of medical records, and conclusions drawn therefrom will later provide a useful refresher of the pertinent medical findings and the bases for the conclusions reached should the matter come to trial at some later date. Carelessly composed, poorly prepared, or obviously biased medical reports frequently prove damaging and embarrassing to the physician called upon to testify at trial.

The composition of a medical report for legal and insurance purposes differs from that of the usual medical report in that it often requires inclusion of information not directly related to the treatment of a patient but essential for answering the various medical questions posed by the impending litigation. In most situations, the medicolegal report of a cardiac examination and findings is best presented in narrative form. As a minimum such a report should cover the following topics, preferably in the order listed:

- A recounting of the history personally related to the examining physician by the patient-claimant or outlined in the medical records reviewed, with particular emphasis on the sequence of events leading to the seeking of medical attention. In a workers' compensation claim, adequate facts must be recorded in the medical history as to the overall job duties and requirements, including consideration of possible noxious occupational exposures and psychological "stress." There should also be detailed recounting of the work activity before, during, and after an alleged cardiac event. In an automobile accident or other situation where trauma is alleged as a cause of a cardiac "injury," there should be a description of the mechanical aspects of the contact or psychological sequelae. The significant past medical history should be detailed, with particular reference to recognized background medical risk factors favoring premature development of atherosclerotic coronary heart disease and the existence of prior heart disorder or of other conditions that might affect the patient's susceptibility to cardiac injury and/or current medical status.
- A chronologic listing, with summary of the contents deemed important, of the various hospital and medical reports and other data reviewed by the physician and utilized in the formulation of the opinions reached. If death has occurred, the pertinent findings of autopsy should be included.
- A detailing of the physical examination findings with description of all the abnormalities detected as well as the important negatives.
- The results of the various diagnostic studies performed or utilized by the examining physician in reaching conclusions of the evaluation.
- A statement of the complete cardiac diagnosis with substantiating reasons.
- The examiner's opinion concerning each of the various medicolegal questions posed in the individual case with substantiating reasons that support the conclusions expressed.

The medicolegal report should conclude with the physician's signature in black ink for photocopy purposes and a certification—a simple maneuver that in many cases suffices for the report to be accepted into evidence without need for the personal appearance of the author to verify its authenticity. The following is an example that has been successfully employed:

> CERTIFICATION: I hereby swear that I am a physician duly licensed in the state of __________ and further state that this written report of __________ pages dated __________ represents my report concerning __________ and is signed under the pains and penalties of perjury pursuant to the laws of this state, as cited in Chapter ______, Section ______.
> Signed ____________________
> Board-certified in Internal Medicine and Cardiovascular Diseases

Finally, it is imperative that the physician submitting a medicolegal report recognize that the report, in most cases, will be made available to opposing counsel in sufficient time for detailed close study and conference with his or her medical expert in preparation for a potential intensive cross-examination.

References

1. McNiece HF. *Heart Disease and the Law*. Englewood Cliffs, NJ: Prentice-Hall; 1961.
2. Sagall EL, Reed BC. *The Heart and the Law—A Practical Guide to Medicolegal Cardiology*. New York: Macmillan; 1968.

3. Sagall EL, Reed BC. *The Law and Clinical Medicine*. Philadelphia: Lippincott; 1970.
4. "Analysis of Workers' Compensation Laws," prepared and published annually by the Chamber of Commerce of the United States, 1615 H Street, NW, Washington, DC 20062; 1999.
5. Sagall EL. Heart disease, workmen's compensation and the practicing physician. *N Engl J Med* 1961; 264:699–705.
6. Sagall EL. Compensable heart disease. *Trial* 1969; 5:29–31.
7. LaDou J, Mulryan LE, McCarthy KJ. Cumulative injury or disease claims: An attempt to define employers' liability for workers' compensation. *Am J Law Med* 1980; 6:1–28.
8. Sullivan RT. Heart injuries under workers' compensation: Medical and legal considerations. *Suffolk Univ Law Rev* 1980; 14:1365–1401.
9. Wyo Stat §27-12-603(b) (1977).
10. (a) Nev Rev Stat Ann, Title 53, Ch 616.110 (1985). (b) Nev Rev Stat Ann, Title 53, Ch 617.457 (1973).
11. Mass. Gen. Laws Ch 32 §94 (1956).
12. Longshoremen's and Harbor Workers' Compensation Act, Amendments of 1972, Sec. 20.
13. The Americans with Disabilities Act 42 U.S.C. 12101, et seq.
14. Criteria Committee of the New York Heart Association. *Nomenclature and Criteria for Diagnosis of Diseases of the Heart and Great Vessels*, 9th ed. Boston: Little, Brown; 1994.
15. Small B. Gaffing at a thing called cause: Medico-legal conflicts in the concept of causation. *Texas Law Rev* 1953; 31:630–659.
16. Sagall EL. Heart disease and the law—medico-legal considerations of causality. *Tenn Law Rev* 1963; 30:517–535.
17. Sagall EL, Reed BC. The legal assessment of causality. *Med Sci* 1967; 18(July):51–54.
18. Sagall EL. Causality assessment—Medical vs. legal. *Trial* 1969; 5(June/July):59–60.
19. Danner D, Sagall EL. Medicolegal causation: A source of professional misunderstanding. *Am J Law Med* 1977; 3:303–308.
20. American Heart Association. Report of the Committee on Stress, Strain, and Heart Disease. *Circulation* 1977; 55:825A–835A.
21. Muller JE, Toffler GH, Stone PH. Circadian variation and triggers of onset of acute cardiovascular disease. *Circulation* 1989; 79:733–743.
22. Brodsky MA, Allen BJ. Stress, cardiac arrhythmias, and sudden cardiac death. *Pract Cardiol* 1989; 15:49A–55A.
23. Muller JE, Toffler GH, eds. A symposium: Triggering and circadian variation of acute cardiovascular disease. *Am J Cardiol* 1990; 66:1G–70G.
24. Johnson RJ. Sudden death during exercise. A cruel turn of events. *Postgrad Med* 1992; 92:195–206.
25. Mittleman MA, Maclure M, Toffler GH, et al. Triggering of acute myocardial infarction by heavy physical exertion. Protection against triggering by regular exertion. *N Engl J Med* 1993; 329:1677–1690.
26. Muller JE, Abela GS, Nesto RW, Toffler GH. Triggers, acute risk factors and vulnerable plaques: The lexicon of a new frontier. *J Am Coll Cardiol* 1994; 23:809–813.
27. Taylor CB. Anger, angina, and ischemia. *J Myocard Ischem* 1994; 6:11–17.
28. Gottdiener JS, Krantz DS, Howell RH, et al. Induction of silent myocardial ischemia with mental stress testing: Relation to triggers of ischemia during daily life activities and to ischemic functional severity. *J Am Coll Cardiol* 1994; 24:1645–1651.
29. Maron BJ, Poliac LC, Kaplan JA, Myeller FO. Blunt impact to the chest leading to sudden death from cardiac arrest during sports activities. *N Engl J Med* 1995; 333:337–342.
30. Mittleman MA, Maclure M, Sherwood JB, et al. Triggering of acute myocardial onset by episodes of anger. *Circulation* 1995; 92:1720–1725.
31. Gabbay FH, Krantz DS, Kop WJ, et al. Triggers of myocardial ischemia during daily life in patients with coronary artery disease: Physical and mental activities, anger and smoking. *J Am Coll Cardiol* 1996; 27:585–592.
32. Krantz DS, Kop WJ, Gabbay FH, et al. Circadian variation of ambulatory myocardial ischemia. Triggering by daily activities and evidence of an endogenous circadian component. *Circulation* 1996; 93:1364–1371.
33. Sagall EL, Reed BC. Heart disorder due to emotional stress: Medical and legal aspects. *Med Counterpoint* 1969; 1(April): 15–43.
34. *Proceedings of the Conference on Stress, Strain, Heart Disease and the Law*, Boston, Jan. 26–28, 1978. US Government Printing Office, Publication 790-281-412/107, 1979.
35. *Stress in the Workplace: Costs, Liability and Prevention*. Rockville, MD: The Bureau of National Affairs; 1987.
36. Hlatky MA, Lam LC, Lee KL, et al. Job strain and the prevalence and outcome of coronary artery disease. *Circulation* 1995; 92:327–333.
37. *New Hampshire Supply Company, Inc. et al. v. Edith Steinberg et al.* 121 N.H. 506, 433 A.2d 1247 (1981).
38. *Helen F. Mulcahey v. New England Newspapers, Inc.* 488 A.2d 681 (R.I. 1985).
39. *City of Boulder v. Barbara E. Streeb et al.* 706 P.2d 786 (Colo. 1985).
40. *Rosalie McDonough v. Connecticut Bank and Trust Company et al.* 204 Conn. 104 527 A.2d 664 (1987).
41. *Cunningham v. City of Manchester Fire Department*. 129 N.H. 232.
42. *Disability Evaluation under Social Security*. DHEW Publication No. 05-10089, Washington, DC, US Government Printing Office, February 1986.
43. http://www.ohsu.edu/disability/adult.html.
44. Committee on Rating of Mental and Physical Impairment, American Medical Association. *Guides to the Evaluation of Permanent Impairment*, 4th ed. Chicago: American Medical Association; 1993.
45. Balsam A, Zabin AP. *Disability Handbook*. Colorado Springs: Shepard's/McGraw-Hill; 1990.
46. Balsam A, Zabin AP. *Disability Handbook. 1995 cumulative supplement*. Current through December, 1994. Colorado Springs: Shepard's/McGraw-Hill; 1995.
47. Rothstein MA. Legal issues in the medical assessment of physical impairment by third-party physicians. *J Leg Med* 1984; 5:503–548.
48. Sagall EL. Life expectancy determination. *Trial* 1969; 5(Aug/Sep):59–62.
49. Sagall EL, Lucas I, eds. *Malpractice Hazards in Cardiology* (proceedings, symposium, Boston, May 12, 1971). Boston: Massachusetts Heart Association; 1973.
50. Eagle KA, Lee TH, Brennan TA, et al. Task force 2: Guideline implementation. *J Am Coll Cardiol* 1997; 29:1141–1147.
51. Jacobson PD. Legal and policy considerations in using clinical practice guidelines. *Am J Cardiol* 1997; 80:74H–79H.
52. Pelly JE, Newby L, Tito F, et al. Clinical practice guidelines before the law: Sword or shield? *Med J Aust* 1998; 169:330–333.
53. Hyams AL, Brandenburg JA, Lipsitz SR, et al. Practice guidelines and malpractice litigation: A two-way street. *Ann Intern Med* 1995; 122:450–455.
54. Sagall EL. Physician's medical report. *Trial* 1972; 8(Jan/Feb):59–62.

C H A P T E R 97

PRACTICE GUIDELINES IN CARDIOVASCULAR CARE

Ira S. Nash

INTRODUCTION

The delivery of medical care in the United States is an enormous enterprise which now accounts for approximately 14 percent of the entire economic activity of the nation and for which about $1 trillion changes hands each year.[1] The rapid growth of medical expenditures throughout the 1970s and 1980s—and, in particular, the burden of those expenditures borne by businesses through their provision of employee health insurance benefits—fostered an intense and unprecedented scrutiny of the practice of medicine. This scrutiny, which has continued to grow, is actually just a single component of a broader transformation in the delivery of medical care, which has been termed the "industrialization" of medicine. Kleinke describes this as a movement to "rationalize health care delivery, measure the costs and benefits of treatments, and compare the outcomes of different providers."[2] He goes on to say that "the compulsion to identify, measure and emulate 'best practices' is the essence of true industrialization." Others have referred to this being nothing less than a "revolution" in medical care.[3]

Physicians, long accustomed to the autonomous, small-scale practice of medicine, are understandably often bewildered by this transformation and are, as a rule, unschooled in the techniques required to understand and lead it.[4] This chapter deals with one of the new tools—clinical practice guidelines—which have the potential to keep physicians in the forefront of medicine's transformation and simultaneously to facilitate the transformation itself.

We first address the context in which practice guidelines have achieved their current prominence. Next, the nature of guidelines is presented, including the criteria by which the value of particular guidelines may be judged and how specific guidelines are and ought to be developed. Following the general discussion of guidelines, we present the key provisions of the most important practice guidelines in cardiovascular medicine. Finally, the success of practice guidelines in improving cardiovascular medicine is examined.

QUALITY OF CARE

Practice Variation

One of the most striking aspects of the delivery of medical care in the United States is its enormous inhomogeneity.[5-7] Much of the evidence of this practice variation comes from the examination of treatments for cardiovascular illnesses. Substantial differences in the way cardiology is practiced—what diagnostic tests are performed, what interventions are undertaken, how specific diseases or syndromes are approached—have been well documented across an array of patient and provider characteristics. African Americans are offered coronary angiography and revascularization less frequently than whites with similar disease severity.[8,9] Rates of rehospitalization after acute infarction differ markedly among different cities, in the absence of clinical differences among the populations.[10] Following a myocardial infarction, one is much more likely to undergo catheterization in Texas than New York,[11] or in the South compared with New England.[12] As the cost, complexity, and potential benefit of medical care (and cardiac care in particular) have grown, so too has the importance of addressing this variation. Which of the different approaches to care is "right"? Which leads to the greatest benefit for patients? Could similar benefits be achieved at a lower cost? How could one tell? Addressing these and related questions is the essence of evaluating the quality of medical care. Evaluating the quality of care is a necessary prerequisite for improving it.

Defining Quality

Many different definitions of quality have been proposed. Leaders in the field have suggested that this multiplicity of definitions may make sense, given the complexity of medical care and the wide range of specific, local goals associated with assessing its quality.[13] The Institute of Medicine put forth a definition of the quality of medical care which has been widely adopted: "the degree to which health services for individuals and populations increase the likelihood of desired health outcomes and are consistent with current professional knowledge."[14] Simply put, good medical practice is necessarily based on sound medical knowledge, and if done right, benefits patients. Note that even under the best of circumstances, quality medical care improves the *likelihood* of good outcomes but cannot guarantee them. A patient with cardiogenic shock on the basis of an extensive myocardial infarction is at high risk of dying even with the best medical care. Likewise, many patients will recover without incident after an infarction even if they do not receive effective therapies such as thrombolysis or postinfarction beta blockade. It is therefore inappropriate to examine only patient outcomes (such as mortality following an infarction) to judge the quality of care they received.

Measuring Quality: Structure, Process, and Outcome

A more complete assessment of the quality of care depends on considering three fundamental components of medical practice, which, taken together, paint a more complete picture: the structure, process, and outcome of care.[15] The structure of care is a characterization of the environment in which care is delivered. The process of care encompasses the myriad steps in the actual delivery of services, and the outcome of care is some result of interest to patients or providers. Consider, as an example, the assessment of the quality of care provided by a cardiac catheterization laboratory.

The structure of care provided by the lab includes the physical attributes of the facility, such as the modernity of the fluoroscopic equipment and the sophistication of the patient hemodynamic monitor. Perhaps less obviously, it also encompasses the staffing levels of the laboratory (e.g., nurse/patient ratios, nurse/technologist ratios), the level of training of the personnel (e.g., advanced cardiac life support certification, or "cross-training" of nursing and technical staff), and the maintenance of the equipment (e.g., the frequency of radiation safety inspections and film processor calibration). The structure of the laboratory also extends beyond its own physical boundaries. Is the laboratory a free-standing facility? Is it in a community hospital, where it may be used for general vascular radiology as well as coronary angiography? Is there a cardiac surgical program at the same institution?

The process of care addresses what providers do and how they do it. For the catheterization laboratory, this runs the gamut from how patients are scheduled for their procedure (indeed, how they are identified as candidates for a procedure) through the steps that are taken to prepare them for the catheterization (including patient education and the solicitation of informed consent) and all the details of the procedure and postprocedure care. Clearly, this includes an enormous number of potential points of quality assessment. How are patients prepared for the catheterization? Do cardiology trainees perform part (or all) of the procedure under supervision? How are patients monitored after their procedure? Are there dedicated personnel who remove the arterial introducing sheaths? How much heparin is used? How long are patients required to stay in bed? The list goes on.

Finally, an assessment of the quality of the laboratory may rightfully include an examination of the outcomes of the patients who were treated. This may include traditional outcomes such as complications and mortality, but can also be construed more broadly to include "patient-centered outcomes" such as patients' satisfaction with the care they received[16,17] or the functional capacity of patients who have undergone percutaneous interventions.[18]

Quality Assessment and Improvement

With the dimensions of quality more broadly drawn, the assessment and improvement of care can be specified more precisely with reference to the definition of quality offered by the Institute of Medicine. This assessment may then, in turn, form the basis for quality improvement or for comparisons among providers. Some component of the structure, process, or outcome of a particular aspect of medical care must be selected, defined, and measured. In order for the quality assessment to be meaningful (and, ultimately useful as a vehicle for improving care), certain criteria must be met.[19,20]

First, the focus of the assessment must be something under the control of the providers of care. There may be particular health outcomes which are of interest to patients and providers; but if they remain outside the ability of medical care to influence them, then measuring them would neither inform a judgment about the quality of care delivered nor form the basis for improving it. For example, the frequency with which patients with hypertrophic cardiomyopathy experience potentially life-threatening arrhythmias is of great interest to affected patients and their physicians. Yet tracking such events in a given population says little about the quality of medical care they received, since there are no therapies currently available that can reliably influence the outcome.

A measurable outcome of care must therefore be linked with a controllable structure or process of care. The mortality associated with coronary artery bypass graft (CABG) surgery is arguably the most intensively tracked outcome in all of medicine and has drawn the attention of a large number of investigators[21–24] as well as government agencies.[25,26] One critical factor in making this outcome a useful quality measure is that it can be influenced by changing the environment and processes of care.[27] Mortality following CABG depends, in part, on how well patients are treated. Tracking outcomes can therefore stimulate examination of, and changes in, the way care is delivered which can then result in improved outcomes.[28]

A measurable process of care can also be the focus of quality assessment and improvement activities as long as it is closely linked to an important health outcome. The National Cooperative Cardiovascular Project (CCP), sponsored by the Health Care Finance Administration (HCFA), is an excellent example of a large-scale quality assessment and improvement project predicated on this principle.[29] Drawing on a large body of randomized controlled clinical trials of therapies for patients with acute myocardial infarction, investigators developed a series of quality indicators. These indicators were measures of specific processes of care; that is, they specified which patients received which therapy. Based on the evidence from clinical trials, the investigators also specified which patients *should* get which therapy. They determined in this way the percentage of candidates for a given therapy who actually received it. Since the clinical trials established, for example, the connection between early aspirin administration and improved survival,[30] measuring the extent to which patients actually did receive aspirin serves as a measure of the quality of the care delivered. In situations such as this, where process and outcome are so well linked by clinical evidence, measuring some specific step in the delivery of care instead of the final outcome offers several important advantages. First, it provides an important efficiency. Since every patient treated for a particular condition such as myocardial infarction is exposed to a system of care but only a small percentage of patients (regardless of the care they receive) is likely to experience a particular outcome such as death, many more patients must be studied if the quality of care they receive is to be judged solely on the outcomes they experience.

Mant and Hicks[31] estimated the relative numbers of patients required to detect differences in the quality of care provided to patients with acute myocardial infarction based on process versus outcome measures. After applying estimates of the efficacy of a variety of medical therapies for myocardial infarction derived from randomized trials, they constructed a model for calculating the sample size needed to detect a given difference in mortality between two hospitals treating populations with the same risk of dying. For example, detecting a reduction in mortality from 30 percent (the assumed baseline mortality in the absence of any effective therapies) to 25 percent (achievable with the adoption of 31 percent of effective interventions) with a power of 80 percent and a significance level of 5 percent, would require the examination of records from nearly 1300 patients with myocardial infarction. To detect the difference in frequency of use of effective therapeutic interventions that could lead to a reduction in mortality of the same magnitude (the process instead of the outcome of care), they derived a minimum sample size of only 27 patients. Clearly, tremendous economy of effort could be achieved by focusing on process instead of outcome.

In addition, if only the outcomes of care are tracked, then any efforts directed at improving outcomes must still ultimately identify and improve those aspects of the delivery of care which drive the outcome. So, for example, if hospitals tracked only infarction mortality without measuring the extent to which their patients receive aspirin, then the discovery of high mortality rates would necessarily lead to an investigation of care, including critical steps such as the use of aspirin. Following aspirin utilization directly focuses attention where it must eventually be paid.[32]

Another criterion that any useful quality measure must fulfill rests on the fact that resources devoted to assessing one aspect of care are necessarily unavailable for a similar examination of some other aspect of care.[33] Maximizing the impact of quality assessment and improvement activities therefore requires prioritization in favor of high-cost, prevalent conditions. One of the most important reasons why cardiovascular medicine has come under so much scrutiny is the large economic impact of cardiovascular disease and its treatment.[34]

Finally, a range of practical issues must be considered in choosing a useful measure of the structure, process, or outcome of care. The collection of necessary data must be feasible within the constraints of time and resources. Quality measures must also be reliable (measurable in a consistent way over time), valid (a true measure of what one hopes to measure), and sensitive to change over time and differences among systems of care.

Ultimately, regardless of which type of quality measure is selected, its interpretation often rests on comparing local findings or practices against an objective standard. Such standards serve to link the desired health outcomes, which are the centerpiece of the definition of quality, with the elements of care that providers can control. They specify the setting and conditions or particular processes of care which, if adhered to, maximize the likelihood of good patient outcomes. These compilations of standards are clinical practice guidelines.

CLINICAL PRACTICE GUIDELINES

Definition

In 1989, a new federal agency, The Agency for Health Care Policy and Research (AHCPR) was created with the charge to "enhance the quality, appropriateness, and effectiveness of health care services, through the establishment of a broad base of scientific research and through the promotion of improvements in clinical practice and in the organization, financing and delivery of health care services."[35] Specifically included in the legislation was the charge that the agency put forth "clinically relevant guidelines that may be used by physicians, educators, and health care practitioners to assist in determining how diseases, disorders, and other health conditions can most effectively and appropriately be prevented, diagnosed, treated and managed clinically."[36] In order to assist the newly formed agency in fulfilling its mandate, the Institute of Medicine convened an advisory committee, which issued its report in 1990.[37] That report defined practice guidelines as "systematically developed statements to assist practitioner and patient decisions about appropriate health care for specific clinical circumstances."[38] The intended utility of practice guidelines was expressed in a follow-up report by the Institute of Medicine in 1992[39]: "Scientific evidence and clinical judgement can be systematically combined to produce clinically valid, operational recommendations for appropriate care that can and will be used to persuade clinicians, patients, and others to change their practices in ways that lead to better health outcomes and lower health care costs." While the report acknowledged the existence of substantial barriers to the realization of this ideal, it remains a concise statement of the potential utility of practice guidelines.

Other Aids to Clinical Practice

As the perceived need to improve the quality of care has grown, so too has the range of tools available to practitioners. Many of these share some characteristics of practice guidelines. Unfortunately, there is no universal agreement about the names used to describe them, which has led to some confusion. *Medical review criteria* are "systematically developed statements that can be used to assess the appropriateness of specific health care decisions, services, and outcomes."[40] These are generally derived from clinical practice guidelines and allow for their application in assessing and improving care. They may be "restatements of specific guideline recommendations into forms suitable for . . . review of clinical practice."[41] For example, the AHCPR guideline for the management of congestive heart failure states that patients with a reduced ejection fraction (EF) should be treated with an angiotensin converting enzyme (ACE) inhibitor.[42] The medical review criterion derived from that recommendation states that "patients with EF ≤35 percent should be receiving an ACE inhibitor at appropriate doses unless hyperkalemic, documented intolerance, patient hypotensive."[41] The standards by which care was judged in the CCP were also medical review criteria.

Another quality improvement tool closely related to practice guidelines is a *critical pathway.* A critical pathway may also be referred to as a critical path, a clinical pathway, a clinical plan, a care map, or a care plan[43] (although others have drawn distinctions among these[44]). These are usually locally developed, highly detailed accounts of how the process of care should unfold for a focused episode of care. They typically deal with the direction and coordination of inpatient services for a particular diagnosis or procedure. For instance, a CABG critical pathway may specify what each of several different providers of care should do during each day of a patient's stay. This would include items such as nursing instruction in the use of incentive spirometry on postoperative day 1, the removal of chest tubes by the surgeon on day 3, climbing stairs with the physical therapist on day 5, and so on. Developing explicit statements of this sort forces groups of providers to examine their practices and achieve local consensus about how care should be delivered, and the final products serve as real-time references to those caring for patients.

For critical pathways, clinical practice guidelines or other statements regarding the quality of medical care to achieve their intended effect, the tools themselves must be of high quality, and they must be used in an effective way.

Guideline Attributes

Several observers have suggested lists of attributes which good practice guidelines should have. The Institute of Medicine report lists eight important qualities[45] (Table 97-1). *Validity* implies that the guidelines, if adopted, will actually lead to the anticipated improvements in health outcomes and/or cost of care. *Reliability or reproducibility* is achieved if another group of guideline developers would create equivalent guidelines, if they relied on the same evidence, and if the guidelines are "interpreted and applied consistently by practitioners."[45] Good

TABLE 97-1 Desirable Attributes of Clinical Practice Guidelines Identified by the Institute of Medicine

Validity	Clarity
Reliability	Multidisciplinary development
Clinical applicability	Scheduled review
Flexibility	Documentation

SOURCE: From Field and Lohr,[45] with permission.

guidelines should also have clear *clinical applicability,* so that they pertain to a broad, well-defined, and explicitly stated population. Guidelines must also allow for some *flexibility* of medical practice and acknowledge the appropriate role of clinical judgment and possible exceptions to broad dictates. *Clarity* of recommendations is another important attribute and should be promoted through the use of precise definitions of terms, unambiguous recommendations, and a variety of presentation techniques. Ideally, guidelines should be developed through *a multidisciplinary process,* which elicits the input of a broad range of stakeholders in the field. Given the rapid pace of medical research and the attendant changes in clinical practice over time, good guidelines should include a provision for *scheduled revision* or an "expiration date." Finally, the institute report suggests that good guidelines should be *well documented,* so that users will know the "procedures followed in developing guidelines, the participants involved, the evidence used, the assumptions and rationales accepted, and the analytic methods employed."[45]

The Evidence-Based Medicine Working Group has put forth its own criteria for judging the quality of practice guidelines. They posed a series of questions, the affirmative answers to which indicate a good guideline[46]:

- Were all important options and outcomes clearly specified?
- Was an explicit and sensible process used to identify, select, and combine evidence?
- Was an explicit and sensible process used to consider the relative value of different outcomes?
- Is the guideline likely to account for important recent developments?
- Has the guideline been subject to peer review and testing?
- Are practical, clinically important recommendations made?
- How strong are the recommendations?

They conclude: "A good guideline, based on solid scientific evidence and an explicit process for judging the value of alternative practices, allows you to review, at one sitting, links between multiple options and outcomes."[47]

Weingarten endorsed this same series of questions to assess the quality of practice guidelines,[48] but Selker offered a slightly different set of criteria.[49] He proposed that guidelines must have the following attributes to warrant adoption:

- Face validity: they must appear "reasonable and appropriate to relevant experts in the field."
- Content validity: they must be based on sound medical evidence.
- Clinical practicality: they must balance specificity with flexibility.
- Consensus validity: they must reflect the achievement of consensus by affected parties.
- Demonstrated safety and effectiveness: they should be tested and proved useful in clinical trials.
- Transportability: they must be useful across a range of practice settings.
- Timeliness: they should be up to date, reflecting current medical knowledge.

Achieving each of these goals is a challenging task for guideline developers, as the promulgators of the standards have themselves acknowledged. It is also not a trivial process even to determine whether these quality criteria are met.

That is why The American Medical Association (AMA), which compiles a list of practice guidelines,[50] has included guidelines based on how they were developed rather than on their content.

How Do Guidelines Measure Up?

There are now a huge number of practice guidelines put forth by a large number of organizations and dealing with a broad array of clinical issues. The AMA directory lists nearly 2000 guidelines by roughly 80 organizations dealing with issues from allergy testing to wound care.[50] The National Guideline Clearinghouse, a collaborative effort of the AHCPR, the AMA, and the American Association of Health Plans, has more restrictive criteria for inclusion than the AMA directory and still lists over 550 practice guidelines on its web site.[51] With such a large number of guidelines in the published literature, a number of investigators have attempted to assess how well they fulfill the criteria discussed above.

Shaneyfelt and colleagues explicitly judged a total of 279 clinical practice guidelines published between 1985 and 1997.[52] They first devised an evaluation tool that consisted of 25 specific standards that guidelines should ideally fulfill. These criteria were separated into standards of development and format, standards of evidence identification and summary, and standards on the formulation of recommendations. No attempt was made to prioritize the standards, and the authors acknowledge that it is extremely unlikely that any guideline would fulfill all of them. Nevertheless, they reported that the guidelines met a mean of only 43.1 percent of the quality standards and concluded that most guidelines "do not adhere well to established methodologic standards," especially in regard to how the underlying medical evidence is gathered and critically combined.[52] Cook and Giacomini, in an accompanying editorial, commented that the findings revealed "the diversity of guideline methodologies . . . and [are a] call for greater transparency of guideline reporting and more rigorous peer review."[53] Parmley, in a critique[54] of an abbreviated version[55] of the AHCPR guidelines for congestive heart failure,[42] made similar observations regarding the importance (and practical difficulty) of peer review of clinical practice guidelines. In order to create guidelines of the highest quality, their development should follow an organized process.

Guideline Development

Although some of the desirable attributes of guidelines discussed previously—such as multidisciplinary input—speak to how guidelines should be developed, some groups have approached the process of guideline development more explicitly. Task Force 1 of the 28th Bethesda Conference of the American College of Cardiology detailed eight phases of successful clinical practice guideline development.[56] Within each of these phases, they outlined specific tasks to be accomplished (Table 97-2).

Perhaps no other step in guideline development is as critical as systematically evaluating the strength of the evidence upon which recommendations are based. Unless, as is rarely the case, all of the available evidence supports a particular clinical approach, guideline developers must weigh one bit of evidence against another. Even in the less problematic circumstance of general concordance of the available data, the quality of the data may have important implications for the confidence the guideline drafters have in one or more of their recommendations.

Some research findings (or other pieces of evidence) reported in the medical literature are more reliable than others. That is, some reported findings are likely to be a true effect, while others may be only an artifact of a study design flaw or a statistical quirk. There is a generally accepted hierarchy of study design, based on the premise that the systematic minimization of potential bias improves the reliability of research results.[57] The most reliable research results come from randomized controlled trials (RCTs),[58] and among RCTs, those that re-

TABLE 97-2 Phases of Guideline Development and Associated Tasks Identified by the 28th Bethesda Conference

Phase 1. Administrative oversight
- Task 1. Identify specific goals
- Task 2. Prioritize possible guideline topics
- Task 3. Review the literature to define task, costs, and time line

Phase 2. Select expert panel
- Task 1. Members must bring expertise, diversity, enthusiasm, and commitment
- Task 2. Convene panel electronically (videoconference, e-mail) to begin plans
- Task 3. Confirm outline, map patient care algorithm

Phase 3. Literature search and evidence review
- Task 1. Computerized literature search
- Task 2. Match literature to guideline outline, rate evidence
- Task 3. Create evidence tables for each topic
- Task 4. Base wording of recommendations on strength of relevant evidence

Phase 4. Consensus process
- Task 1. Converge on recommendations by an explicit process

Phase 5. Computerize guideline documents in format for clinical use
- Task 1. Link recommendations with related evidence
- Task 2. Create preformatted documents to capture data and facilitate care
- Task 3. Create database to store information regarding guideline compliance

Phase 6. Test and revise guideline
- Task 1. Expert panel tests computerized guideline in actual patient care
- Task 2. Final revision of guidelines based on testing

Phase 7. Disseminate guideline
- Task 1. Publish printed version, disseminate computerized version
- Task 2. Encourage local customization

Phase 8. Revise and refine guideline
- Task 1. Maintain ongoing literature review
- Task 2. Refine management strategies based on patient outcomes associated with guideline use

SOURCE: From Jones et al.,[56] with permission.

cruited larger cohorts of patients are generally more reliable than smaller studies.[57] In descending order of reliability (ascending vulnerability to bias), the remaining sources of data are cohort studies, case-control studies, case series and registries, and case reports and expert opinion.[57] The AHCPR guideline developers have divided the different levels of available evidence into three classes. A-level evidence is derived from RCTs (both large and small), meta-analyses of RCTs, well-conducted cohort studies, and metanalyses of well-conducted cohort studies. B-level evidence is drawn from studies with other kinds of designs. C-level evidence is based on expert opinion only.[57] Other guideline developers have adopted a similar method of ranking the evidence upon which their recommendations rest.[59]

Although evidence of consistently high quality may form the basis for strong guideline recommendations, it must be noted that there are legitimate circumstances where this concordance is violated. If several large RCTs provide conflicting conclusions, then the quality of the available evidence may be high but the recommendation necessarily weak. On the other hand, if there is such universal agreement that a particular element of care is so essential that no RCT is ever likely to be done (e.g., the necessity of examining a patient[56]), then a strong recommendation may be appropriate in the absence of rigorous evidence. Guideline developers have therefore developed separate systems for indicating the strength of their recommendations.

A very good system for classifying recommendations is used by the Joint Task Force on Practice Guidelines of the American College of Cardiology (ACC) and the American Heart Association (AHA). They use the classification scheme in Table 97-3 to summarize the indications for a particular treatment or therapy. This classification has been slightly modified in some of the joint ACC/AHA guidelines. For example, in the guideline for the treatment of myocardial infarction,[59] class I indications are those which are "beneficial, useful, and effective." In the guidelines on assessing cardiac risk in patients undergoing noncardiac surgery,[60] class I indications are defined as those where the treatment is "of benefit." The preoperative evaluation guidelines also do not distinguish between classes IIa and IIb. The myocardial infarction guidelines have a more forceful description of class III indications than the preoperative evaluation guidelines, stating that the procedure or treatment "may be harmful," while the other guidelines state that class III procedures and treatments are just "not necessary." Despite these minor variations, the broad classes remain uniform in basic meaning across all of the ACC/AHA guidelines.

TABLE 97-3 American College of Cardiology/American Heart Association Classification of Guideline Recommendations

Class I: Conditions for which there is evidence and/or general agreement that a given procedure or treatment is of benefit

Class II: Conditions for which there is conflicting evidence and/or a divergence of opinion about the usefulness or efficacy of a procedure or treatment

- Class IIa: weight of evidence in favor or usefulness or efficacy
- Class IIb: usefulness or efficacy is less well established

Class III: Conditions for which there is evidence and/or general agreement that the procedure/treatment is not useful/effective and in some cases may be harmful

Guideline Implementation

Clinical practice guidelines are a tool for improving patient care. Much of that potential can be realized only by changing physician behavior, since physicians are ultimately responsible for directing care. Even a well-crafted guideline, then, will not benefit patients unless and until it actually changes how doctors act under particular circumstances.

Multiple studies have demonstrated that just making information available to physicians is generally insufficient to change their practice.[61] Successful implementation of clinical practice guidelines must therefore go beyond making the guidelines themselves accessible through publication in the medical literature or by electronic means. The extent to which cardiovascular clinical practice guidelines have been successful in improving care is reviewed later in this chapter. Here, we review some of the barriers to guideline implementation and the strategies for overcoming them.

Perhaps the greatest barrier to guideline implementation is the complexity of the health care delivery system itself. Medical care is provided in a broad range of settings, from private physicians' offices to large academic medical centers and by a host of practitioners with different levels of interest and expertise in particular clinical conditions. Given the financial pressure present in many medical delivery systems, guideline implementation may well be seen as another burden or expense rather than as an aid to clinical practice. Even if guideline adoption is seen as desirable, limitations of physician time and practice resources may hinder efforts to move forward. Where physician time and practice resources do not constrain efforts at guideline adoption, the complexity and diversity of clinical encounters still make routine application of uniform standards of practice difficult. The inadequacy of many clinical information systems, which under ideal circumstances could identify patients who meet guideline criteria and remind providers of current recommendation, is another important institutional barrier to successful guideline implementation.[62]

Skepticism among clinicians about the value of guidelines is also a significant barrier to their implementation. This skepticism, in turn, may be a result of a general mistrust of "cookbook"[54] approaches to clinical practice, a rejection of national (in favor of local) standards of practice,[63] concerns regarding malpractice liability,[64] or differences in physician training and experience.[65] Certainly, deficiencies in the guidelines themselves—including conflicting recommendations among different guidelines addressing the same conditions, lack of clarity of recommendations, or any other failure of the guidelines to achieve the high standards discussed previously—contribute to physician skepticism and decrease the likelihood of successful guideline implementation.[66]

Just as the barriers to guideline implementation are diverse, there is no single proven strategy for successful guideline adoption. For guideline developers, close attention to the principles of rigorous data synthesis and the straightforward presentation of well-documented recommendations is essential. Explicit discussion of potential conflicts with other guidelines and the reasons for different recommendations should be included. Guideline writers should include clear statements regarding the limitations of their own guidelines with respect to the patients or conditions to which they apply. Guideline developers should also recognize that guidelines are not "self-implementing."[67]

Those who are charged with implementing practice guidelines must be prepared to address the barriers discussed above. Clear demonstration of the value of guideline adoption, through the feedback of local data demonstrating improvements in patient outcomes, is often part of a successful strategy. Simultaneous development of the infrastructure to support clinical practice guidelines, including modifying the incentives of clinicians and investing in clinical information systems, is also helpful.

CARDIOVASCULAR CLINICAL PRACTICE GUIDELINES

Finding Practice Guidelines

Clinical practice guidelines in cardiovascular medicine have been developed by many different organizations on a wide array of topics. New guidelines are constantly being produced in order to cover new subjects and to incorporate new data about previously addressed conditions. Just keeping track of the guidelines themselves has become challenging for clinicians and policymakers. Fortunately, there are several ways to find relevant guidelines.

Most clinical practice guidelines are published in peer-reviewed medical journals. Often, the journals are the official publication of the same parent organization that produced the guideline. So, for example, the guidelines compiled by the American College of Physicians/American Society of Internal Medicine are published in the *Annals of Internal Medicine;* those of the American College of Chest Physicians appear in *Chest,* and the guidelines of the joint efforts of the ACC/AHA are published in both the *Journal of the American College of Cardiology* and *Circulation.* Guidelines by lesser-known groups are also generally published in mainstream journals. Even government agencies, which have their own publishing capabilities, often seek to have part or all of their guidelines published in journals as well. As a consequence, a computer search of the MEDLINE database of peer-reviewed journals can produce a list of many of the sought guidelines. This process is far from perfect, however, in part because of the wide variety of key terms used to index published guidelines.

The National Library of Medicine periodically publishes the results of its own electronic searches of the medical literature as part of its series *Current Bibliographies in Medicine.* One such search for practice guidelines, prepared in 1992, utilized a total of 39 search terms to obtain a comprehensive list.[68] Such a search strategy is not only daunting for even the most facile users of computerized medical database search engines but also inevitably yields a large number of references of minimal relevance, which must then be manually culled from the bibliography in a rather laborious fashion.

Guidelines have been compiled by other parties as well. The American Medical Association annually publishes its *Clinical Practice Guideline Directory.*[50] Although the guidelines themselves are not included in the directory, there are listings of guidelines by subject and sponsoring organization as well as sections on guidelines in development, contact information for all the sponsoring groups, bibliographic references for published guidelines, and a listing of withdrawn (obsolete or superseded) guidelines.

The electronic compendium of guidelines maintained by the National Guideline Clearinghouse[51] is very useful. This searchable web site allows the user to specify the subject and/or sponsor of guidelines. The interface is user-friendly, and the list generated by the search contains links to the specified guideline. So, for example, if one specifies *cardiovascular disease,* a total of 55 listed guidelines is presented, along with suggested search terms ("*heart disease,* "*vascular disease,* etc., and the number of guidelines fitting those search criteria). The links allow a user to go directly from the list to a brief summary of the guideline prepared by the National Guideline Clearinghouse as well as to the full text of a particular guideline, often at the web site of the sponsoring organization.

Categorizing Cardiovascular Clinical Practice Guidelines

The large number of cardiovascular clinical practice guidelines, as well as their detail and rapid evolution, makes it impossible to present a comprehensive discussion of all of their provisions here. For example, the 1996 ACC/AHA guidelines for the management of patients with acute myocardial infarction[59] are 100 pages long and cover every aspect of myocardial infarction care, from the prophylactic use of antiarrhythmic agents to the indications for temporary transvenous pacing. An even more focused guideline, such as the physician monograph from the National Cholesterol Education Program (NCEP) on cholesterol management in patients with established coronary heart disease,[69] is over 25 pages long and contains information and detailed recommendations about dietary management as well as dosing information about specific lipid-lowering medications.

Instead of trying to present all cardiovascular guidelines, the most prominent guidelines are presented here and several of their key findings and recommendations are discussed. These guidelines generally follow the criteria previously outlined. The guidelines are divided into five broad categories, which are discussed in turn. The first group are those dealing with the assessment and treatment of risk factors for cardiovascular disease. The second group includes the guidelines for screening asymptomatic populations for the presence of specific cardiovascular diseases. Next, we review the guidelines that pertain to the diagnosis and treatment of established cardiovascular conditions. The fourth group of guidelines speaks to the application of various technologies for diagnosis and treatment. The final group covers specific interventions and/or treatments.

Assessment and Treatment of Risk Factors for Cardiovascular Disease

Because cardiovascular and, in particular, coronary disease may present in sudden and catastrophic fashion, attention has long been paid to identifying those factors that may predict the development of overt disease. More recently, the accumulation of compelling data demonstrating the efficacy of risk-factor interventions in improving clinical outcomes[70,71] has reinforced the value of risk-factor modification. In addition, the identification of previously unrecognized risk factors continues[72,73] to focus attention on the prevention of cardiovascular illness.

HYPERTENSION

The most comprehensive and definitive guideline on hypertension is the Sixth Report of the Joint National Committee on Prevention, Detection, Evaluation and Treatment of High Blood Pressure, commonly referred to as JNC VI.[74] The JNC report is divided into four sections. The first provides introductory information, including data on the prevalence of hypertension and its clinical consequences. It also includes a discussion of the workings of the JNC, such as the methodology they used to evaluate the quality and reliability of available scientific evidence for each of their recommendations. The second section addresses blood pressure measurement and the clinical evaluation of hypertensive patients. Section 3 covers the prevention and treatment of high blood pressure, and the final section deals with special populations and situations.

Section 1 of JNC VI concludes that:

- "Hypertension awareness, treatment, and control rates have increased during the last 3 decades."[74]
- Age-adjusted mortality rates for stroke and coronary heart disease (CHD) declined during the same period of time.
- End-stage renal disease and congestive heart failure (important consequences of uncontrolled hypertension) are increasing.
- RCTs are the best source of information, but they have some limitations.
- Prevention and treatment of hypertension and target-organ damage should remain public health priorities.

Section 2 defines normal and elevated blood pressure (Table 97-4). It also proposes that blood pressure be evaluated as part of a more comprehensive cardiovascular risk assessment, so that a patient with other risk factors would have his blood pressure controlled more vigorously than someone without other risk factors (Table 97-5). Similarly, hypertensive damage to another organ system should trigger more intensive antihypertensive efforts (Table 97-6). This approach, of recommending intensified treatment of a particular risk factor—in this case, hypertension—based on both the degree to which that risk factor is present and the presence of other risk factors or overt cardiovascular disease, is a general model of most guidelines for risk-factor modification. It implicitly recognizes that risk factors do not operate independently of one another[75] and that a particular patient's overall cardiovascular risk reflects the integration of many different factors.[76,77]

Section 3 details the myriad treatment options open to clinicians for the control of hypertension. The major conclusions are as follows:

- Lifestyle modification can lower blood pressure and prevent cardiovascular disease.
- Diuretics and beta blockers should be chosen as initial therapy in the absence of specific indications for other agents.

Details are also provided concerning the treatment of hypertensive emergencies and strategies that may be employed to improve patient compliance with antihypertensive regimens.

TABLE 97-4 Blood Pressure Classification from JNC VI[a]

Category	Systolic Blood Pressure, mmHg		Diastolic Blood Pressure, mmHg
Optimal	<120	and	<80
Normal	<130	and	<85
High normal	130–139	or	85–89
Stage 1 hypertension	140–159	or	90–99
Stage 2 hypertension	160–179	or	100–109
Stage 3 hypertension	≥180	or	≥110

[a]When systolic and diastolic pressures fall into different categories, the patient is assigned on the basis of the higher of the two categories. Elevated readings should be based on the average of two or more readings, taken at each of two more visits after initial screening.

SOURCE: From JNC VI,[74] with permission.

TABLE 97-5 Cardiovascular Risk Stratification in Patients with Hypertension

Major risk factors
- Smoking
- Dyslipidemia
- Diabetes mellitus
- Age >60 years
- Sex (men and postmenopausal women)
- Family history of cardiovascular disease (women <65 years or men <55 years)

Target organ damage/clinical cardiovascular disease
- Heart diseases
  - Left ventricular hypertrophy
  - Angina or prior myocardial infarction
  - Prior coronary revascularization
  - Heart failure
- Stroke or transient ischemic attack
- Nephropathy
- Peripheral arterial disease
- Retinopathy

SOURCE: From JNC VI,[74] with permission.

HYPERLIPIDEMIA

There are several important guidelines that address the assessment and management of hyperlipidemia as a risk factor for cardiovascular disease. The oldest, and still most influential from a national policy perspective, is the second report of the adult treatment panel of the NCEP.[78] The NCEP subsequently published a physician monograph (and accompanying patient education materials) addressing cholesterol management in patients with established coronary heart disease.[69] The American College of Physicians issued a clinical guideline on screening asymptomatic adults for the presence of hyperlipidemia in

1996,[79] which proved to be quite controversial.[80,81] Finally, the AHA has issued several related scientific statements regarding cholesterol assessment and management as a primary preventive measure for individuals without CHD[82] or as a secondary measure for those who do have CHD.[83,84] The AHA guidelines are in close agreement with those of the NCEP, and the key recommendations of the latter are presented.

As with the hypertension guidelines discussed previously, the NCEP recommends a comprehensive assessment of overall cardiovascular risk as the basis for clinical decision making. The risk factors to be assessed are shown in Table 97-7 and are slightly different from the risk factors listed in Table 97-5, though the broad overlap between the two lists is apparent. Note that a high level of high-density lipoprotein (HDL) cholesterol is considered a "negative risk factor." That is, an individual with an HDL cholesterol above 60 mg/dL may be treated as if he or she had one fewer other risk factors.

The key treatment recommendations of the NCEP are summarized in Table 97-8. Note that treatment is to be based on the level of low-density lipoprotein (LDL) cholesterol rather than on the total cholesterol. For patients at greatest risk for future morbid events—those with established CHD—the goal of treatment is the achievement of an LDL cholesterol of ≤100 mg/dL through a combination of dietary and drug therapy. For those without established CHD but with two or more risk factors (Table 97-7), the LDL goal is <130 mg/dL. For individuals at low risk, the LDL goal is <160 mg/dL. Differential thresholds for the initiation of drug and dietary therapy are recommended. This approach is echoed in the AHA statements.

The dietary therapy recommended by the NCEP is summarized by the Step I and Step II Diets.[78] The Step I Diet, recommended by the AHA for the general population, is characterized by a total dietary fat intake of <30 percent of total calories, with <10 percent of total calories derived from saturated fat. Dietary cholesterol should be limited to <300 mg per day. The Step II Diet calls for a reduction in total calories derived from saturated fat to <8 percent and a reduction in dietary cholesterol to <200 mg per day.

The NCEP guidelines were issued prior to the availability of clinical trials evidence demonstrating the efficacy of HMG-CoA reductase inhibitors (statins) in reducing mortality and morbidity from CHD.[70] These data were the basis for the recommendations in the AHA statements that statin drugs are the first choice for lowering LDL cholesterol in those individuals identified as candidates for drug treatment provided that they have no specific contraindications to the medications and their tryglyceride levels are below 400 mg/dL.[84]

TABLE 97-6 Risk Stratification and Treatment of High Blood Pressure

	Risk Group		
Blood Pressure Stage	A	B	C
High-normal	Lifestyle modification	Lifestyle modification	Drug therapy[a]
1	Lifestyle modification (up to 12 months)	Lifestyle modification (up to 6 months)[b]	Drug therapy
2	Drug therapy	Drug therapy	Drug therapy

Risk group A: No risk factors; no target-organ damage or clinical cadiovascular disease.
Risk group B: At least one risk factor not including diabetes mellitus; no target-organ damage or clinical cardiovascular disease.
Risk group C: Target-organ damage or clinical cardiovascular disease and/or diabetes mellitus, with or without other risk factors.
[a]Consider drug therapy as initial therapy if multiple risk factors present.
[b]For those with heart failure, renal insufficiency, or diabete mellitus.
SOURCE: From JNC VI,[74] with permission.

DIABETES MELLITUS

The assessment and management of this complex disease is beyond the scope of this chapter. However, insofar as diabetes is a major risk factor for the development of cardiovascular disease, the recommendations of the AHA for diabetes management as a means of both primary[82] and secondary[84] prevention of CHD are quite simple. Both documents call for "appropriate hypoglycemic therapy to achieve near normal fasting plasma glucose as indicated by HbA1c" and "treatment of other risk factors" in accord with other guidelines.

Addressing a related issue, the ACC and the American Diabetes Association have issued a joint statement of recommendations for diagnosing CHD in patients with diabetes.[85]

CIGARETTE SMOKING

The link between cigarette smoking and cardiovascular disease is firmly established. Smoking cessation is therefore an important component of risk-factor modification for the prevention of cardiovascular disease. The definitive guideline on smoking cessation was produced by the AHCPR.[86] This provides extensive background information and a careful review of the efficacy of available methods of promoting smoking cessation. A much more concise document, in the form of a science advisory from

TABLE 97-7 Non-LDL-Cholesterol Risk Factors for CHD Identified by the National Cholesterol Education Program

Positive risk factors
- Age: male ≥45 years; female ≥55 (or premature menopause without hormone replacement)
- Family history: premature (<55 years in men, <65 years in women) CHD in first-order relative
- Current cigarette smoking
- Hypertension: blood pressure ≥140/90 or use of antihypertensive medication
- Low HDL cholesterol: <35 mg/dL
- Diabetes mellitus

Negative risk factor
- High HDL cholesterol: ≥60 mg/dL

SOURCE: From the Expert Panel on Detection, Evaluation, and Treatment of High Blood Cholesterol in Adults,[78] with permission.

TABLE 97-8 Treatment Recommendations of the National Cholesterol Education Program

Patient Category	LDL Level at Which to Initiate Treatment mg/dL		
	Dietary Treatment	Drug Treatment	LDL Goal, mg/dL
No CHD and fewer than two risk factors	≥160	≥190	<160
No CHD and two or more risk factors	≥130	≥160	<130
Established CHD	>100	≥130[a]	≤100

[a]Drug therapy should be considered if the LDL cholesterol is between 100 and 129 mg/dL.

SOURCE: From the Expert Panel on Detection, Evaluation, and Treatment of High Blood Cholesterol in Adults,[78] with permission.

the AHA,[87] is a useful reference for most physicians. Although science advisories are not labeled as "practice guidelines" by the AHA, they fulfill the definition of a practice guideline offered earlier in this chapter and so are considered here. The AHA advisory recommends the following smoking cessation steps:

- Every smoker should be counseled to quit on every physician office visit; maintenance should be discussed with all ex-smokers.
- Every patient should be asked about tobacco use.
- Clinicians should receive training in smoking cessation counseling.
- Office systems to facilitate cessation programs should be established.

The "minimal intervention" to promote smoking cessation should include the following elements:

- Asking about smoking
- Recommending cessation
- Helping those who want to quit through the provision of educational materials, referral to specialists, or other community resources
- Scheduling a quit date
- Arranging for follow-up

Although the authors acknowledge the barriers to successful smoking cessation, they review a large body of evidence supporting the efficacy of the recommended interventions.

OBESITY

Obesity is defined by the National Heart Lung and Blood Institute of the National Institutes of Health (NIH) as a body mass index—BMI = [weight (kg)/height (m)^2]—of 30 kg/m^2 or more; overweight is defined as a BMI of 25 to 29.9 kg/m^2.[88] Although traditionally considered to increase the risk of CHD only through its influence on other risk factors such as hypertension, hyperlipidemia, and diabetes, obesity is now recognized as a risk factor for CHD in its own right.[89] In addition to the NIH guidelines, the American Association of Clinical Endocrinologists (AACE) and the American College of Endocrinology (ACE) have jointly issued a position statement on obesity.[90] The NIH guidelines are summarized here. The principal recommendations are:

- The use of the BMI as a tool to assess overweight and obesity
- Comprehensive assessment of other cardiovascular risk factors
- The establishment of clear goals for weight loss, with an initial goal of a 10 percent reduction in body weight, followed by additional weight loss as needed and an ongoing weight maintenance program
- Weight loss should be achieved primarily through the reduction of dietary calories
- Physical activity should be part of a comprehensive weight reduction program
- Drug therapy with FDA-approved agents should be considered for those individuals with a BMI ≥30
- Weight loss surgery should be considered for individuals with severe obesity, defined as a BMI >40, or a BMI >35 in the presence of other significant comorbidities

PHYSICAL INACTIVITY

As is the case with obesity, physical inactivity is an independent risk factor for coronary artery disease.[91] Two important guidelines have formulated recommendations for increasing the general level of physical activity among the general population. The Consensus Statement of the NIH, while not presented as a formal guideline, reports as its intent "to advance understanding of the . . . issue in question and to be useful to health professionals and the public"[92] and so fulfills the definition of a generic guideline. The Statement on Exercise of the AHA[91] is a conceptually similar document.

The NIH document states that "All Americans should engage in regular physical activity at a level appropriate to their capacity, needs and interest. Children and adults alike should set a goal of accumulating at least 30 minutes of moderate-intensity physical activity on most, and preferably, all days of the week."[92]

The AHA recommendations are very similar: ". . . dynamic exercise of the large muscles for extended periods of time (30–60 minutes, three to six times weekly) is recommended. This may include short periods of moderate intensity . . . that total 30 minutes on most days."[91]

Screening for Cardiovascular Diseases

There are few nationally recognized clinical practice guidelines that primarily address the issue of screening for cardiovascular disease in the asymptomatic population. The use of specific technologies that are sometimes used as screening tools is discussed later in this chapter. This section addresses the recommendations for screening per se. All of the guidelines in this section are part of the *Guide to Clinical Preventive Services,* a comprehensive document dealing with the detection and prevention of a broad range of conditions, which was developed by the U.S. Preventive Services Task Force.[93]

CORONARY ARTERY DISEASE

Screening for coronary disease among asymptomatic individuals was not recommended. The guideline states:

> There is insufficient evidence to recommend for or against screening middle-aged and older men and women for asymptomatic coronary artery disease. . . . Recommendations against routine screening can be made on other grounds for individuals who are not at high risk of developing clinical heart disease. Routine screening is not recommended as part of the periodic health visit or preparticipation sports examination for children, adolescents, or young adults.[93]

The guideline left open the question of the utility of screening individuals at high risk, stating that such screening would be justified if the results would influence treatment. The task force also found that screening individuals in certain occupations (e.g., airline pilots) may be justified on public health grounds.

CAROTID ARTERY STENOSIS

The U.S. Preventive Services Task Force recommendations regarding screening for asymptomatic carotid artery stenosis are very similar to those regarding screening for coronary artery disease.[94] The guidelines state that there is insufficient evidence to recommend for or against general screening, whether by ultrasound or other techniques. Rather, they recommend discussing the potential value of screening with patients who may be at high risk. Even that recommendation is qualified, in that it applies only if high-quality vascular surgery (defined as surgical mortality and morbidity from carotid endarterectomy of less than 3 percent) is available.

ABDOMINAL AORTIC ANEURYSM

Screening for abdominal aortic aneurysm is the third and final cardiovascular condition addressed by the screening guidelines of the U.S. Preventive Services Task Force.[95] Here again, they report that there is insufficient evidence to recommend for or against routine screening. While stating that there is no evidence, even in high-risk populations, that screening leads to lower morbidity and mortality, the guidelines concede that clinicians may wish to screen selected high-risk patients because of the significant prevalence of the disease and the efficacy of surgical repair. Screening is recommended only for patients who are candidates for abdominal surgery, regardless of their risk.

Established Cardiovascular Conditions

There are five broad cardiovascular conditions for which well-formulated clinical practice guidelines have been written. These are atrial fibrillation, chronic stable angina, heart failure, myocardial infarction, and valvular heart disease. The AHCPR also issued clinical practice guidelines for unstable angina,[96] but these were published in 1994, and the approach to unstable angina has progressed very rapidly since that time. As a result, those guidelines are not included here.

ATRIAL FIBRILLATION

The best guidelines available for the approach to patients with atrial fibrillation are those that were prepared by a committee sponsored by the AHA.[97] Although the document produced was not formally labeled a practice guideline, it contains specific evidence-based recommendations intended to guide clinical practice.

The guideline establishes three therapeutic goals for each patient with atrial fibrillation: rate control, maintenance of sinus rhythm, and the prevention of thromboembolism. The first goal should be achieved for all patients, whereas the approach to the other two requires a careful weighing of individualized risks and benefits. The recommendations for achieving each of these goals are presented below.

Rate Control Control of the ventricular response to atrial fibrillation avoids a tachycardia-induced myopathy and reduces patients' symptoms.[97] It can be achieved by pharmacologic or nonpharmacologic means. The guidelines recommend the intravenous use of verapamil, diltiazem, or a beta blocker for acute rate control and the same drugs in oral formulations for chronic use. They state that digoxin is less effective and should be considered a front-line agent only in patients who also have congestive heart failure and also that some patients will require combination therapy. Nonpharmacologic rate control can be achieved with catheter ablation or modification of the AV node.

Maintanence of Sinus Rhythm Sinus rhythm preserves atrioventricular synchrony, maintains cardiac output, and reduces symptoms associated with an irregular rhythm. Restoration of sinus rhythm may also reduce the risk of future thromoboembolic events. Despite these important goals, there are few data to guide rational clinical decision making regarding overall strategies of cardioversion and antiarrhythmic drug therapy. The document states that the "selection of an antiarrhythmic agent should be individualized and will depend in part on renal and hepatic function, concomitant illnesses and drugs, and cardiovascular function."[97]

Preventing Thromboembolism The guidelines recommend identifying patients with atrial fibrillation who are at high risk for stroke based on the presence of one or more "high-risk variables." These are age >65 years, hypertension, prior stroke or transient ischemic attack (TIA), diabetes, or recent heart failure. Individuals at high risk should be treated with warfarin titrated to an International Normalized Ratio (INR) of 2.0 to 3.0. Low-risk patients may be treated with 325 mg of aspirin daily. For all individuals who are undergoing elective cardioversion by electrical or pharmacologic means, anticoagulants should be administered for at least 3 weeks prior and 4 weeks after.

CHRONIC STABLE ANGINA

Definitive guidelines for the management of patients with chronic stable angina were recently published.[98] These are particularly valuable because they represent the collaborative effort not just of the ACC and the AHA but also of the American College of Physicians—American Society of Internal Medicine (ACP-ASIM).

The guidelines clearly specify a rational, evidence-based approach to the patient with angina, beginning with establishing the diagnosis. A useful classification of chest pain is presented to aid the clinician in determining the risk of ischemic heart disease. Chest pain should be considered (definite) angina if it:

1. Is substernal in location, with a characteristic quality and duration
2. Is provoked by exertion or emotional stress
3. Is relieved by rest or nitroglycerin

Chest pain that fulfills two of the preceding criteria is considered probable or atypical angina and chest pain that meets one or fewer of the criteria is considered noncardiac chest pain, not angina.

The assessment of patients presenting with chest pain is outlined in a flow diagram (Fig. 97-1). The key elements of the assessment algorithm are the risk stratification of the patient on clinical grounds; the exclusion of other, related conditions such as unstable angina or acute myocardial infarction; and the evaluation of possible precipitating factors, such as anemia and hyperthyroidism. Those patients who, after such an assessment, are thought to have a high probability of coronary artery disease are then candidates for the treatment algorithms specifying the approach to stress testing and angiography (Fig. 97-2) and treatment (Fig. 97-3).

The guidelines recommend (class I) cardiac catheterization and coronary angiography for a particular subset of patients with chronic stable angina. They include patients with

- Disabling chronic stable angina (Canadian Cardiovascular Society classes III and IV) despite medical therapy
- High-risk criteria on noninvasive testing regardless of anginal severity
- Angina who have survived sudden cardiac death or have serious ventricular arrhythmias
- Angina and symptoms and signs of congestive heart failure
- Clinical characteristics that indicate a high likelihood of severe coronary artery disease

Pharmacologic treatment of patients with angina (Fig. 97-3) should be directed at reducing symptoms as well as lowering the risk of future ischemic events. The key elements of the treatment include:

- Aspirin unless specifically contraindicated
- Beta blockers unless specifically contraindicated
- Calcium antagonists and/or long-acting nitrates when beta blockers are contraindicated, fail to control symptoms, or are associated with intolerable side effects
- Sublingual nitroglycerin or nitroglycerin spray for the immediate relief of angina
- Lipid-lowering therapy for appropriate patients (see guidelines for hyperlipidemia, above)

In addition to the medications specified above, the guidelines urge a comprehensive treatment plan according to the following mnemonic:

A. Aspirin and antianginals
B. Beta blockers and blood pressure control
C. Cigarette smoking cessation and cholesterol reduction
D. Diet and diabetes control
E. Education and exercise

Intensive efforts at risk factor identification and modification are considered essential elements of the treatment of all patients with chronic angina, and the spe-

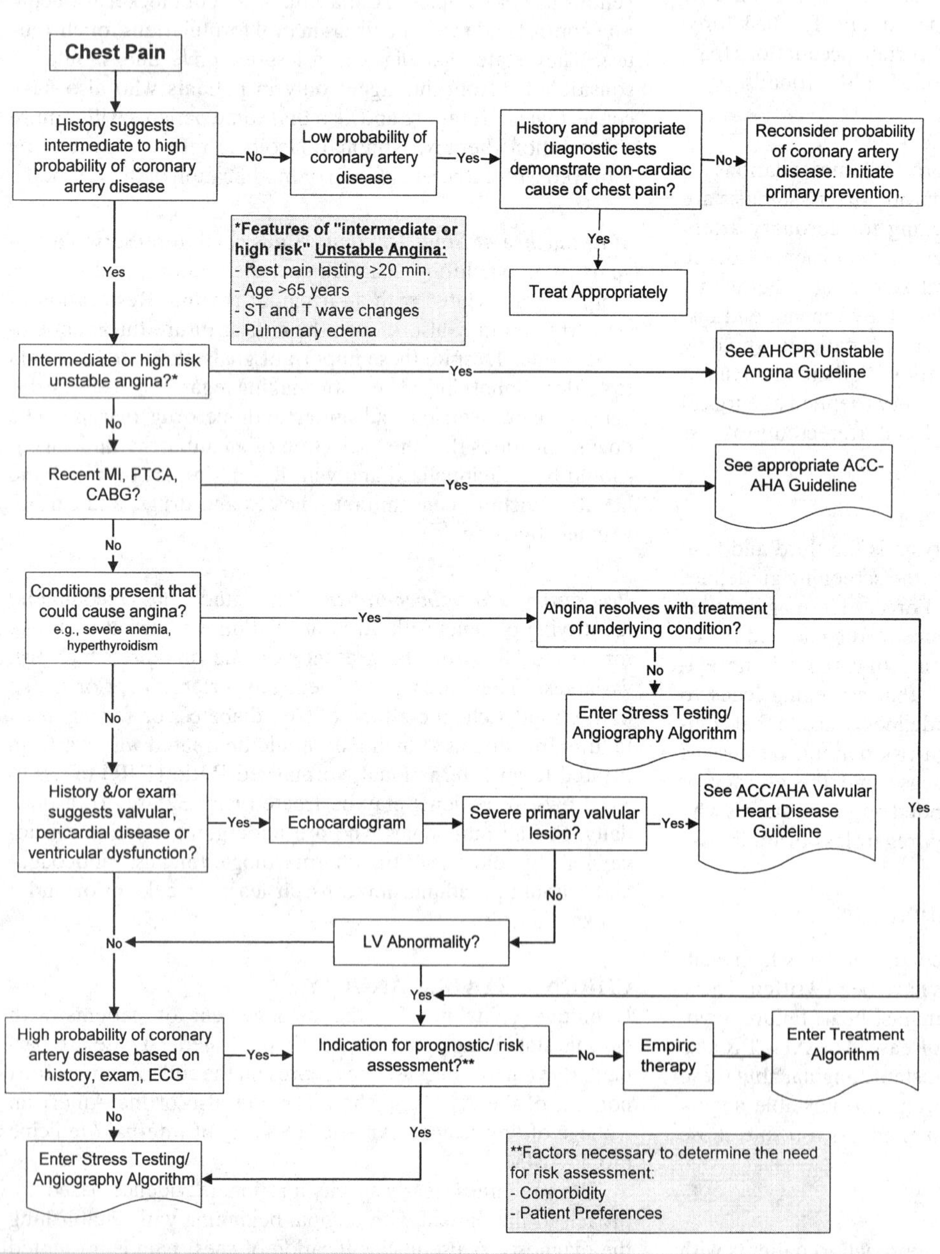

FIGURE 97-1 Algorithm for the clinical assessment of patients with chest pain. (From Gibbons et al.,[98] with permission.)

cific recommendations follow the guidelines for risk factor modification discussed earlier in this chapter.

HEART FAILURE

Two major guidelines exist to help the clinician in the care of patients with congestive heart failure and/or depressed left ventricular function. The AHCPR published its guidelines in 1994.[42] The ACC and AHA published their joint guidelines in 1995.[99] Both documents address the role of diagnostic testing in heart failure and make recommendations about appropriate pharmacologic therapy.

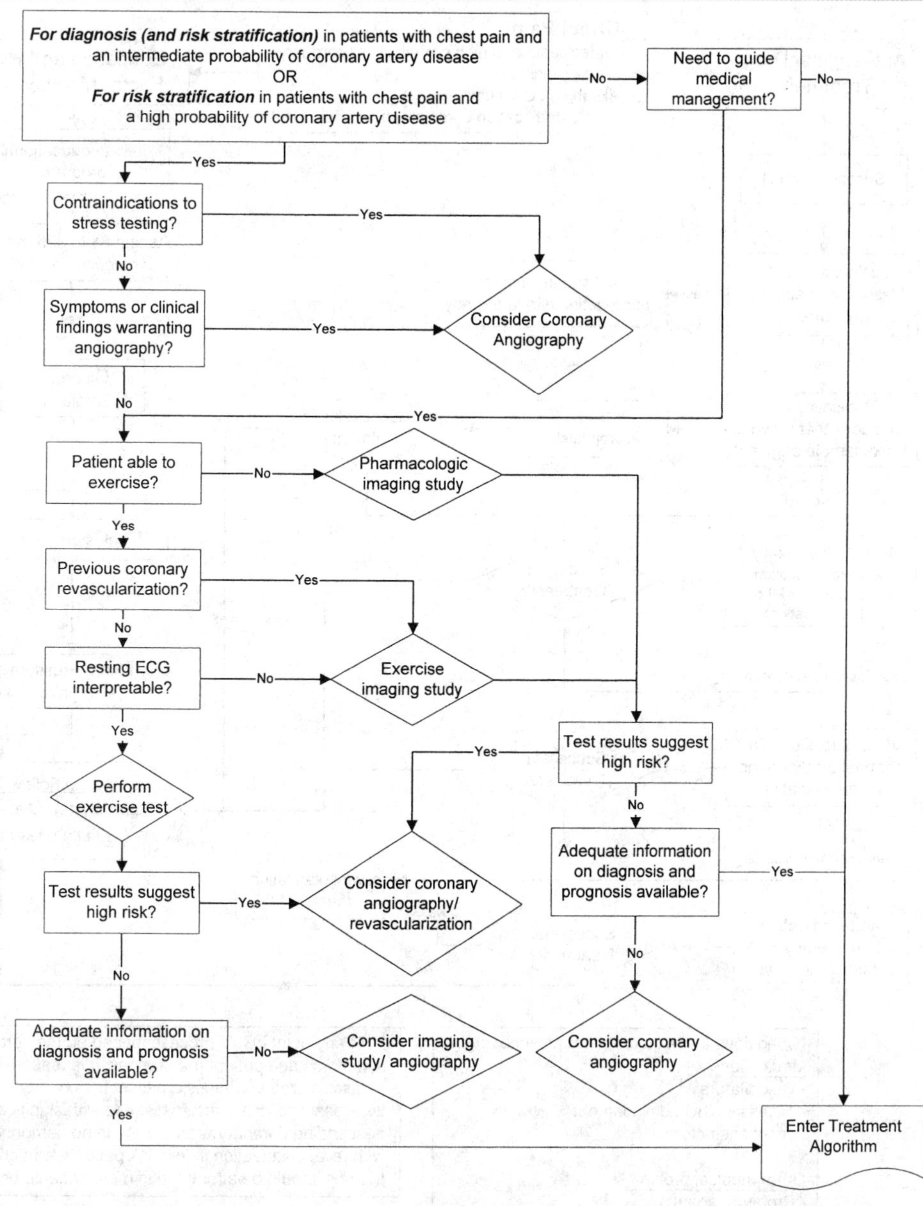

FIGURE 97-2 Algorithm for the use of stress testing and angiography in patients with angina. (From Gibbons et al.,[98] with permission.)

Diagnostic Testing For patients with chronic or stabilized heart failure, the ACC/AHA guidelines identify the following elements of the diagnostic workup as class I:

- Complete blood count and urinalysis
- Blood serum: electrolytes, blood urea nitrogen, creatinine, glucose, phosphorus, magnesium, calcium, and albumin levels
- Thyroid-stimulating hormone levels
- Chest radiograph and electrocardiogram
- Transthoracic echocardiogram
- Noninvasive stress testing to detect ischemia in patients who would be candidates for revascularization
- Coronary arteriography in patients with a previous infarction who would be candidates for revascularization
- Cardiac catheterization and coronary arteriography in patients with angina, those with large areas of ischemia on noninvasive testing and those at risk for CHD who are undergoing surgical correction of noncoronary cardiac lesions

The AHCPR guidelines are generally consistent with these recommendations. Among the diagnostic tests and procedures that are not *routinely* recommended by either guidelines (although allowances are made for exceptions) are:

- Endomyocardial biopsy
- Multiple echocardiograms or radionuclide ventriculograms as a means of routine follow-up
- Holter monitoring or signal-averaged electrocardiography

Pharmacologic Treatment The two major guidelines are also very similar in their recommendations regarding drug treatment for heart failure. The class I recommendations of the ACC/AHA are:

- Angiotensin converting enzyme (ACE) inhibitors for all patients with reduced left ventricular ejection fraction unless contraindicated
- Hydralazine and isosorbide dinitrate in patients who cannot take ACE inhibitors
- Digoxin in patients with heart failure due to systolic dysfunction not adequately responsive to ACE inhibitors and diuretic drugs
- Digoxin in patients with atrial fibrillation and rapid ventricular rates
- Diuretic drugs for patients with fluid overload

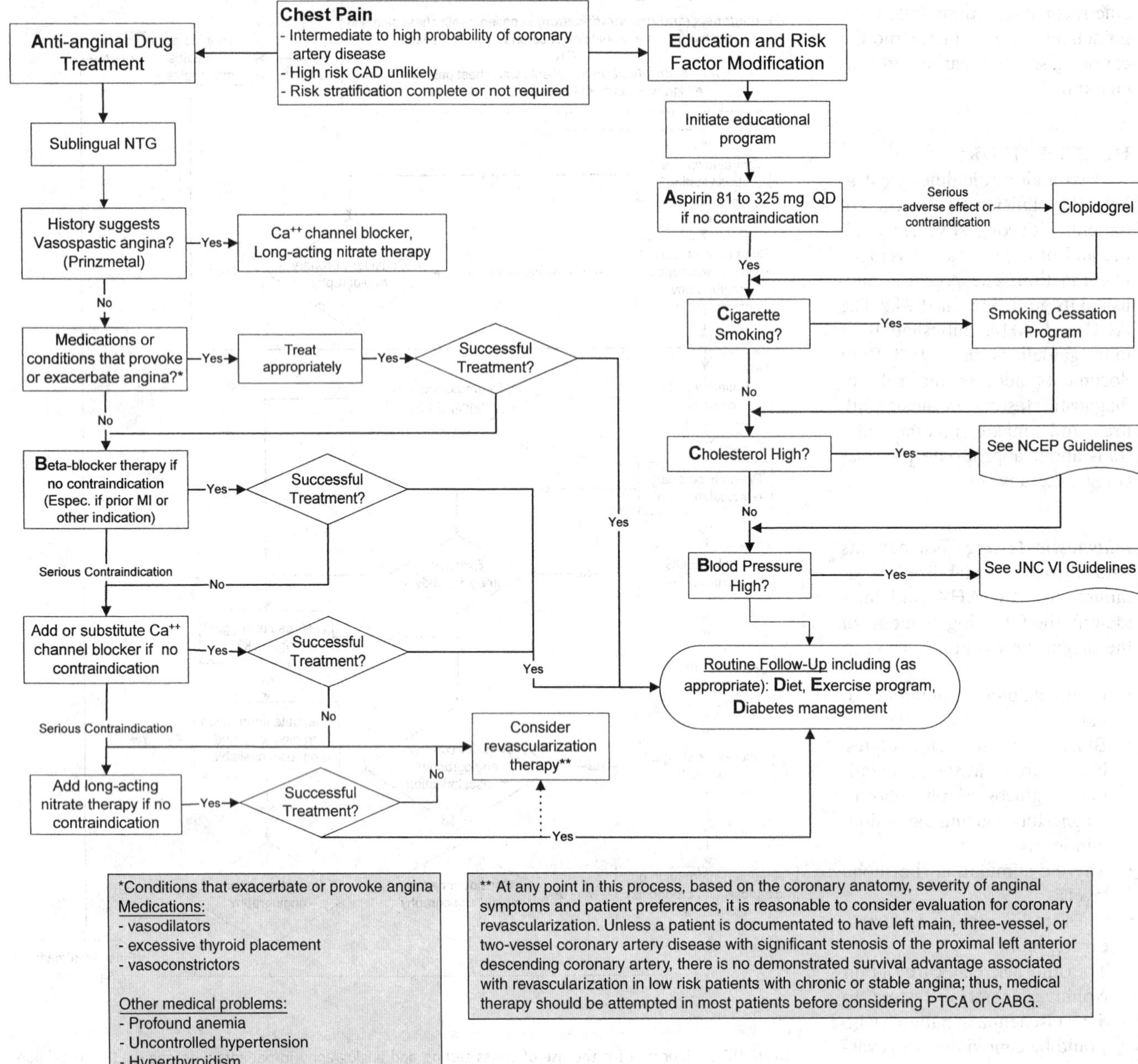

FIGURE 97-3 Algorithm for the treatment of chronic stable angina. (From Gibbons et al.,[98] with permission.)

- Anticoagulation in patients with atrial fibrillation or a previous history of systemic or pulmonary embolism
- Beta blockers for high risk patients after an acute myocardial infarction

Note that the routine use of beta blockers was not recommended in these guidelines. Newer evidence in support of the use of these agents is reviewed in Chap. 21. Among the treatments that are not recommended by the ACC/AHA (class III) are:

- Drugs with positive inotropic effect in the absence of systolic dysfunction
- Treatment of asymptomatic arrhythmias

The AHCPR guidelines also indicate that routine anticoagulation of heart failure patients is not indicated.

MYOCARDIAL INFARCTION

The ACC/AHA guidelines for the care of acute myocardial infarction are the most definitive and up to date. These were originally published in 1990,[100] revised in 1996,[59] and updated again in 1999.[101] The most important class I recommendations from the 1999 guideline update are presented.

With regard to prehospital and initial emergency department management, the following are class I recommendations:

- Availability of 911 emergency access
- Availability of emergency medical services with the capability of defibrillating patients in the field
- Emergency department standards to assure clinical evaluation of patients at risk for myocardial infarction (MI) within 10 min of hospital arrival and thrombolysis (if indicated) within 30 min
- Oxygen for all patients with pulmonary congestion or demonstrated arterial desaturation
- Aspirin for all patients without clear contraindication
- Intravenous nitroglycerin for the first 24 to 48 h in patients with CHF, large anterior infarcts, persistent ischemia, or hypertension

Strategies for early coronary revascularization are also highlighted. Pharmacologic thrombolysis and direct coronary angioplasty are considered alternative therapies, based on locally available resources and expertise. Class I indications for thrombolysis include:

- ST elevation >0.1 mV in two or more contiguous leads, time to therapy 12 h or less, and age less than 75 years
- Bundle branch block that obscures ST analysis and clinical history suggestive of acute infarction

Class I indications for primary angioplasty are:

- As an alternative to thrombolysis in patients who meet the same electrocardiographic criteria, in whom the procedure can be performed within 90 min (time to balloon inflation) of presentation, by operators who perform ≥75 procedures per year in centers that perform ≥200 procedures per year and have cardiac surgical programs
- In patients who are within 36 h of infarction and develop cardiogenic shock and in whom revascularization can be accomplished within 18 h of the development of shock

The class I indications for emergent or urgent coronary artery bypass graft surgery are:

- Failed angioplasty with persistent pain or hemodynamic instability, given suitable coronary anatomy
- Persistent or refractory ischemia in patients who are not suitable candidates for percutaneous intervention
- Coincident CABG at the time of surgical repair of postinfarction ventricular septal defect (VSD) or mitral regurgitation

Key pharmacologic therapy (class I) for patients with acute infarction, beyond the use of thrombolytics are:

- Heparin in all patients undergoing percutaneous or surgical revascularization
- Early (intravenous) beta blockers for patients without contraindications who can be treated within 12 h, or who have continuing or recurrent ischemia or tachyarrhythmias
- ACE inhibitors within 24 h in patients with anterior infarctions, clinical heart failure, or demonstrated left ventricular systolic dysfunction (ejection fraction <40 percent)

Of note, there are no class I indications for calcium channel blockers or magnesium, so that these agents should not be considered part of the routine management of MI patients. Secondary prevention—the long-term, postdischarge management of MI patients—is also addressed by the guidelines. The critical class I indications for secondary prevention include:

- Management of lipids, through the initiation of the Step II Diet in all patients, and the use of lipid-lowering agents in patients with an LDL cholesterol of >125 mg/dL
- Long-term use of beta blockers in all but low-risk patients
- Long-term use of aspirin in all patients
- Long-term anticoagulation in patients unable to take aspirin and in those with atrial fibrillation or left ventricular thrombus

The guidelines also address the indications for coronary angiography and revascularization in patients who did not undergo primary angioplasty. Such a strategy is not recommended as a routine procedure after successful thrombolysis but is indicated in the presence of:

- Spontaneous or easily provoked ischemia early after infarction
- Hemodynamic instability
- A planned repair of a mechanical complication of infarction (VSD, mitral regurgitation)

VALVULAR HEART DISEASE

There are few areas of clinical decision making in cardiology as complex as the assessment and management of patients with valvular heart disease. The reader is referred to Chaps. 55 through 58 for a comprehensive discussion of the approach to particular valvular lesions, since the complexity of their management precludes a complete discussion here. This section briefly presents some of the key elements of the ACC/AHA guideline pertaining to valvular heart disease.[102]

Class I indications for the assessment of patients with known or suspected valvular heart disease include the following:

- Echocardiography for diastolic, continuous, holosystolic, or loud systolic murmurs, or in patients with murmurs and signs or symptoms of heart failure, ischemia or endocarditis
- Catheterization prior to valve replacement surgery

Specific indications for the use of percutaneous balloon valvotomy for aortic stenosis and mitral stenosis are presented. There are no class I indications for balloon aortic valvotomy, and it should not be considered a satisfactory alternative to surgery for aortic valve replacement. Mitral valvotomy is indicated (class I) in symptomatic patients with a mitral valve area of <1.5 cm^2 and valvular morphology favorable to balloon valvotomy as long as there is no atrial thrombus present and no significant mitral regurgitation.

The guidelines present useful flow diagrams to aid the clinician in dealing with particularly challenging circumstances, such as determining the appropriate timing for valve repair or replacement in patients with chronic mitral regurgitation (Fig. 97-4) and chronic aortic regurgitation (Fig. 97-5).

The use of anticoagulants in patients with prosthetic heart valves is also discussed. Class I indications for the use of warfarin include:

- All patients for the first 3 months following valve replacement surgery (INR 2.5 to 3.5)
- Mechanical aortic or mitral prosthesis

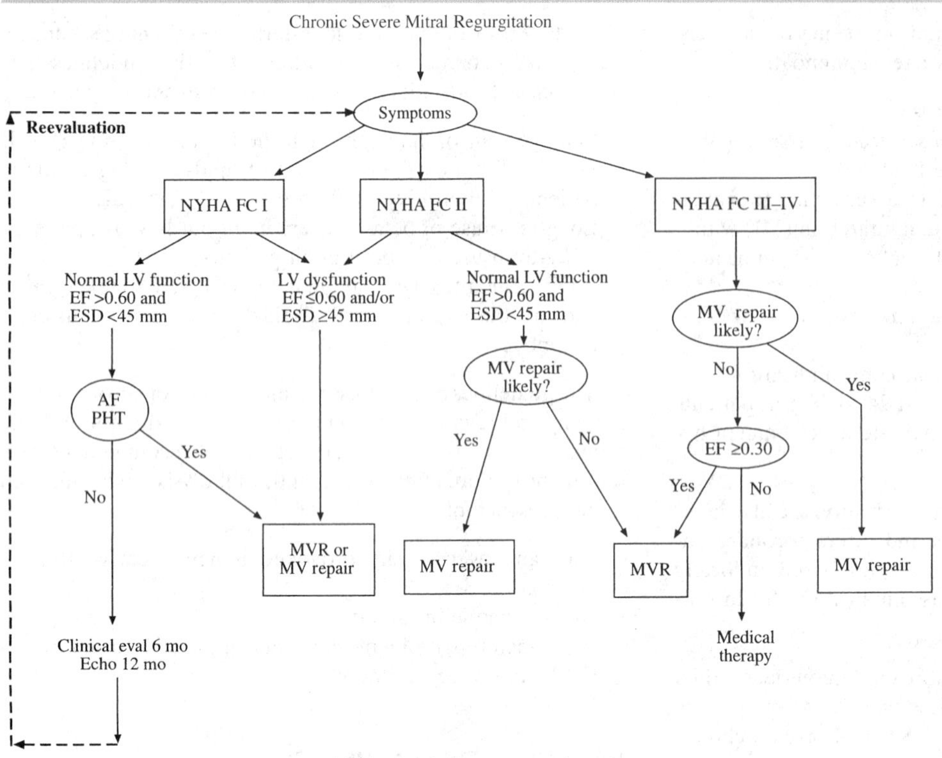

FIGURE 97-4 Algorithm for the management of patients with chronic severe mitral regurgitation. AF, atrial fibrillation; EF, ejection fraction; ESD, end-systolic diameter; FC, functional class; MV, mitral valve; NYHA, New York Heart Association; PHT, pulmonary hypertension. (From Bonow et al.,[102] with permission.)

- Bioprosthetic aortic or mitral valve in the presence of atrial fibrillation, left ventricular dysfunction, previous thromboembolism, or hypercoagulable state

Use of Cardiovascular Technology

Cardiovascular medicine is extremely technology-intensive and is becoming more so with the continuous development of new and highly sophisticated techniques for patient assessment and treatment. This section presents the highlights of clinical practice guidelines that have been developed to aid physicians in the rational use of this technology. There are national guidelines on exercise testing, echocardiography, coronary angiography, and electrophysiologic testing. We also present recommendations for risk-stratifying patients with known or suspected cardiac disease prior to noncardiac surgery, since this risk assessment often depends on the use of the other technologies discussed.

EXERCISE TESTING

The most authoritative practice guidelines for exercise testing are a product of the ACC/AHA Task Force on Practice Guidelines.[103] Those guidelines describe the following class I indications:

- As a diagnostic tool in patients with an intermediate pretest probability of coronary artery disease (CAD) and an electrocardiogram with less than 1 mm of resting ST-segment depression
- As a means of risk assessment in patients with known or suspected CAD
- Before discharge following myocardial infarction, for prognosis, assessment of medical therapy, or activity prescription
- Evaluation of exercise capacity in patients with heart failure
- Demonstration of ischemia prior to planned coronary revascularization or reassessment of symptoms following revascularization
- Identification of appropriate programmable parameters for patients with rate-adaptive pacemakers

The ACC/AHA Task Force has also produced guidelines for the use of radionuclide imaging in both with and without exercise testing,[104] as has the Society of Nuclear Medicine.[105]

ECHOCARDIOGRAPHY

There is considerable overlap between the previously discussed ACC/AHA guideline on valvular heart disease[102] and the ACC/AHA guideline devoted specifically to the use of echocardiography.[106] Once again, key class I indications for the use of echocardiography are presented:

- Evaluation of heart murmurs in symptomatic patients or in patients whose murmur has a moderate probability of reflecting structural heart disease
- Assessment of hemodynamic severity of known valvular lesions
- Evaluation of the patient with known or suspected endocarditis in order to assess the degree of hemodynamic compromise or to detect and characterize vegetations
- Evaluation of patients with known valvular lesions (or prosthetic valves) who have a change in functional status
- Evaluation of left ventricular function in ischemic heart disease, heart failure, or symptoms suggestive of either
- Evaluation of suspected pericardial disease, including trauma, constriction, pericarditis, or pericardial tamponade
- Evaluation of possible cardiac masses
- Evaluation of possible aortic dissection, aneurysm, or rupture (may be best accomplished via transesophageal techniques)
- Evaluation of pulmonary hypertension and/or suspected pulmonary embolism
- Search for a cardiac source of systemic or cerebral embolism
- Evaluation of possible underlying structural heart disease in patients with arrhythmias or syncope

Additional class I indications are listed for the evaluation of critically ill or hemodynamically unstable patients as well as patients with congenital heart disease.

CORONARY ANGIOGRAPHY

Cardiac catheterization is performed more than a million times per year in the United States, and the frequency of its use continues to grow.[107] The ACC/AHA guidelines on coronary angiography[107] seek to provide a framework for the appropriate use of this technique. The class I indications for coronary angiography include:

- Canadian Cardiovascular Society class III or IV angina despite medical therapy
- High-risk criteria on noninvasive testing, including depressed left ventricular function, a large stress-induced (especially anterior) perfusion defect, or a strongly positive treadmill exercise test
- Resuscitation following an episode of sudden cardiac death
- Unstable angina (in high- or intermediate-risk patients) that has not fully responded to medical therapy
- Recurrent symptoms within 9 months of prior percutaneous coronary intervention
- As an alternative to thrombolytic therapy for acute MI (if done with an intent to perform percutaneous transluminal coronary angioplasty)
- Spontaneous or easily provoked ischemia in the immediate postinfarction period or as a precursor to the surgical repair of a mechanical complication of acute infarction
- Hemodynamic instability in the peri- or immediate postinfarction period
- Prior to valve surgery or balloon valvotomy in patients with ischemic symptoms or at high risk for CAD
- Prior to surgical correction of congenital heart disease in patients at high risk for CAD on the basis of symptoms, risk factors, or particular congenital lesions
- Heart failure due to systolic dysfunction with noninvasive evidence of underlying CAD

The preceding list is not exhaustive, either in its presentation of indications considered by the guidelines or in terms of other settings when coronary angiography may be appropriate. As the guidelines themselves state: "This report is not intended to provide strict indications and contraindications for coronary angiography because, in the individual patient, multiple other considerations may be relevant, including the family setting, occupational needs, and individual lifestyle preferences."[107]

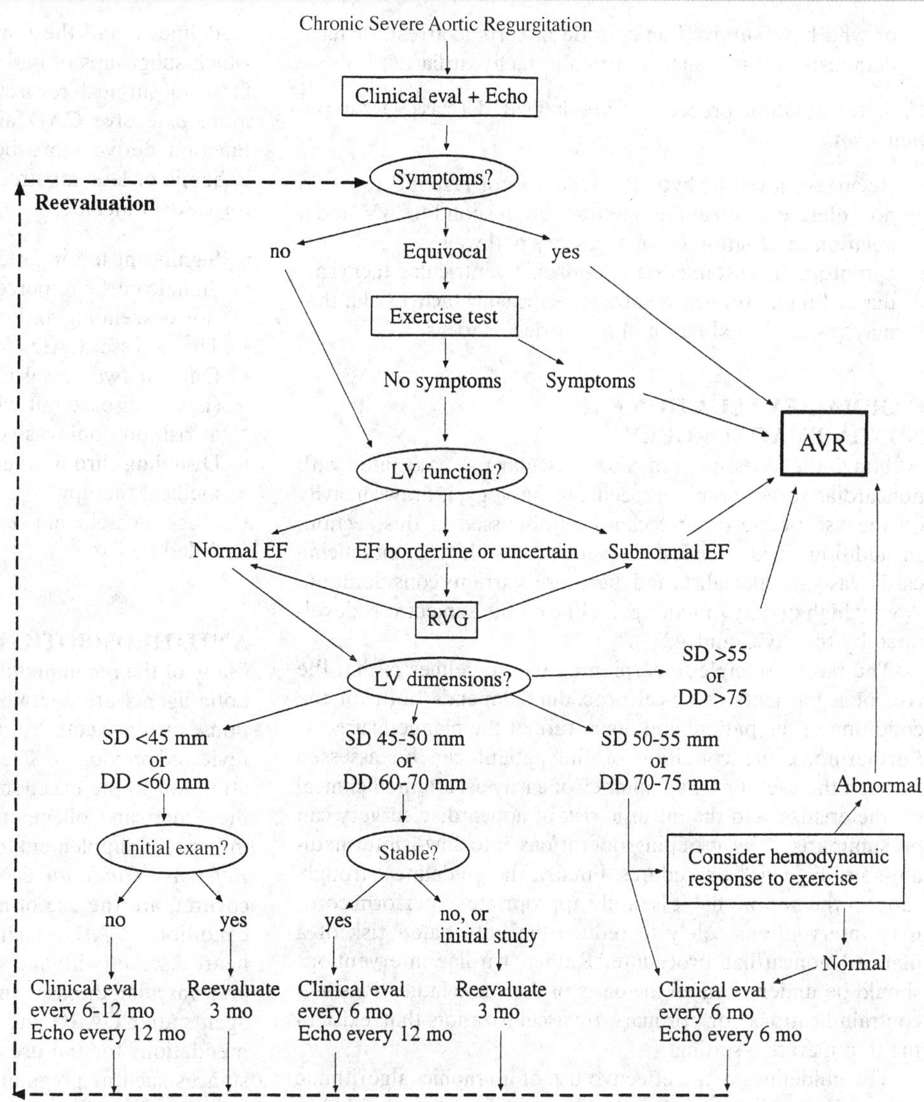

FIGURE 97-5 Algorithm for the management of patients with chronic severe aortic regurgitation. DD, end-diastolic dimension; RVG, radionuclide ventriculography; SD, end-systolic dimension. (From Bonow et al.,[102] with permission.)

ELECTROPHYSIOLOGIC TESTING

The North American Society of Pacing and Electrophysiology, the American College of Cardiology, and the AHA collaborated to produce guidelines for invasive electrophysiologic testing and catheter ablation procedures, which were published in 1995.[108] Class I indications for electrophysiologic testing identified by the guidelines include patients with

- Sinus node dysfunction as the suspected cause of symptoms
- Second- or third-degree AV block who remain symptomatic following pacemaker insertion and in whom another arrhythmia is suspected as the cause of symptoms
- Narrow QRS complex tachycardias who do not respond to or do not tolerate medical therapy
- The Wolff-Parkinson-White syndrome who have survived an episode of cardiac arrest, have unexplained syncope, or are candidates for ablation of an accessory pathway
- Suspected structural heart disease with unexplained syncope,

or who have survived an episode of cardiac arrest, or have demonstrated sustained ventricular tachycardia

Catheter ablation procedures are indicated (class I) for patients with

- Recurrent atrial arrhythmias who do not respond to or do not tolerate medical therapy but may respond to AV nodal ablation or ablation of an accessory pathway
- Symptomatic sustained monomorphic ventricular tachycardia or bundle branch reentrant ventricular tachycardia that may respond to ablation of a ventricular focus

CARDIAC EVALUATION FOR NONCARDIAC SURGERY

Although the assessment of cardiovascular risk associated with noncardiac surgery is not a specific technology, it draws heavily on the use of the other techniques discussed in this section. In addition, it is a major clinical responsibility of practicing cardiovascular specialists and therefore warrants consideration. A very high quality practice guideline on the subject was developed by the ACC and AHA.[60]

The basic principle underpinning the guidelines is that the risk of a particular surgical procedure depends both on the condition of the patient and the nature of the planned surgery. Furthermore, the condition of the patient can be assessed through the use of a small number of easily ascertained clinical characteristics, and the intrinsic risk of noncardiac surgery can be summarized by grouping operations into low-, intermediate-, and high-risk procedures. Finally, the guidelines strongly support the notion that it is rarely appropriate to perform coronary interventions solely to reduce the anticipated risk of a planned noncardiac procedure. Rather, cardiac interventions should be undertaken on the basis of the same indications and contraindications for coronary revascularization that exist in the nonoperative setting.

The guidelines make effective use of a graphic, algorithmic approach to risk assessment that has also been reproduced in pocket form as a quick reference. The principal algorithm is reproduced as Fig. 97-6. High-risk surgical procedures include emergent major operations, aortic and major vascular procedures, and those anticipated to involve large shifts of fluids or prolonged time under anesthesia. Intermediate-risk procedures include carotid endarterectomy as well as orthopedic and prostate operations. Low-risk surgeries include cataract extractions, breast procedures, and endoscopies.

Specific Interventions and Treatments

The range of specific cardiovascular interventions and therapies for which specific guidelines exist is broad. The following four areas were chosen to illustrate this range: CABG, the use of antithrombotic therapies, the implantation of cardiac pacemakers and antiarrhythmia devices, and the use of cardiac rehabilitation programs.

CORONARY ARTERY BYPASS GRAFT SURGERY

As the ACC/AHA guidelines on the subject state, "CABG surgery is among the most common operations performed in the world and accounts for more resources expended in cardiovascular medicine than any other single procedure."[109] The guidelines detail the randomized trial evidence that identifies which subgroups of patients with CAD derive the most benefit from surgical revascularization. In general, patients with more extensive CAD and depressed left ventricular systolic function derive more benefit than similar patients with less ischemia or less impaired ventricles. Specific class I indications for CABG include:

- Significant left main coronary artery stenosis
- Significant (≥70 percent) stenosis of the proximal left anterior descending and proximal left circumflex arteries
- Three-vessel CAD
- One- or two-vessel CAD without left anterior descending (LAD) disease but with a large area of viable myocardium at risk on noninvasive testing
- Disabling chronic angina or ongoing unstable angina despite medical therapy
- Ongoing ischemia or hemodynamic instability following a failed PTCA

ANTITHROMBOTIC THERAPY

Many of the recommendations regarding the use of antithrombotic agents are contained in guidelines for particular conditions, such as acute MI and atrial fibrillation, which have been reviewed previously. They are mentioned here primarily to draw attention to the excellent compilation of recommendations by the American College of Chest Physicians. These were detailed in a special supplement to *Chest*[110] and summarized in the *Quick Reference Guide for Clinicians* in 1999.[111] Among the subjects covered are the use of antithrombotic agents in the following conditions: CAD, ischemic stroke, atrial fibrillation, valvular heart disease (with and without prosthetic valves), and peripheral vascular disease. In addition, the role of antithrombotic agents after CABG and PTCA is reviewed, along with recommendations for the use of these agents under special circumstances such as pregnancy, and the management of excessive anticoagulation.

PACEMAKERS AND ANTIARRHYTHMIC DEVICES

The guidelines for the use of these devices come from the ACC and the AHA.[112] Class I indications for the implantation of a permanent pacemaker generally depend on the presence of a bradycardic rhythm and an established connection between the rhythm and symptoms. These include:

- Third-degree AV block associated with:
  - —Symptomatic bradycardia, or the need for drugs (for other conditions) that induce symptomatic bradycardia
  - —Periods of asystole ≥3 s or an escape rate <40 beats per minute (even in the absence of symptoms)
  - —Postoperative AV block not expected to resolve
  - —Neuromuscular disorders with associated AV block
- Second-degree AV block with associated symptomatic bradycardia
- Intermittent third-degree AV block or type II second-degree AV block with chronic bifascicular or trifascicular block
- Persistent and symptomatic second- and third-degree AV block following MI
- Transient second- or third-degree infranodal AV block with associated bundle branch block

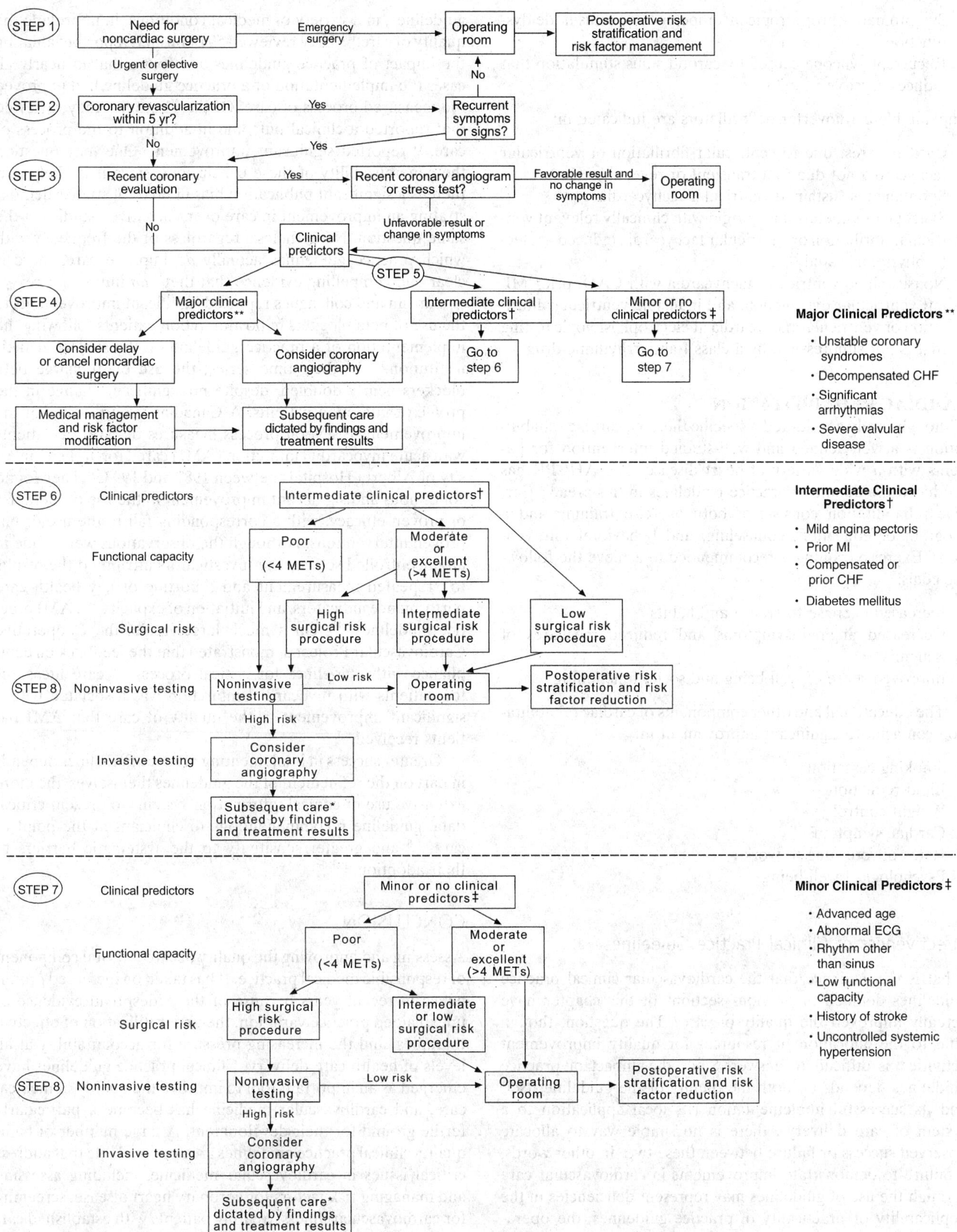

FIGURE 97-6 Algorithm for the preoperative assessment of cardiac risk. (From Eagle et al.,[60] with permission.)

- Symptomatic chronotropic incompetence or sinus node dysfunction
- Recurrent syncope caused by carotid sinus stimulation that induces asystole of >3 s

Implantable cardioverter defibrillators are indicated in:

- Cardiac arrest due to ventricular fibrillation or ventricular tachycardia not due to a transient or reversible cause
- Spontaneous sustained ventricular tachycardia
- Syncope of undetermined origin with clinically relevant ventricular fibrillation or ventricular tachycardia induced at electrophysiologic study
- Nonsustained ventricular tachycardia with CAD, prior MI, left ventricular dysfunction, and inducible ventricular fibrillation or ventricular tachycardia at electrophysiologic testing that is not suppressible by a class I antiarrhythmic drug

CARDIAC REHABILITATION

Although rarely considered a specific therapy, cardiac rehabilitation is a well-defined and well-studied intervention for patients with a wide variety of heart disease. The AHCPR has produced the definitive practice guidelines in this area.[113] Cardiac rehabilitation consists of both exercise training and a program of education, counseling, and behavioral interventions. Exercise training is recommended to achieve the following goals:

- Increased exercise tolerance and habits
- Decreased anginal symptoms and reduced measures of ischemia
- Improved sense of well-being and social functioning

The educational and other components of cardiac rehabilitation can achieve significant improvement in:

- Smoking cessation
- Lipid reduction
- Weight control
- Cardiac symptoms
- Rates of returning to work
- Psychological well-being

Effectiveness of Clinical Practice Guidelines

What is the evidence that the cardiovascular clinical practice guidelines detailed in previous sections of this chapter have actually improved the quality of care? The question, though vital to the allocation of resources for quality improvement activities, is difficult to answer. Since the impact of practice guidelines depends on both the quality of the guideline itself and its successful implementation (its local application to a system of care delivery), there is no simple way to allocate observed success or failure between these two. In other words, a failure to demonstrate improvements in cardiovascular care through the use of guidelines may represent deficiencies in the applicability or practicality of practice guidelines, the operational failure of implementing them locally, or some combination of both. In addition, it is challenging to perform randomized trials of guideline use. Fortunately, there are data to suggest that guidelines can improve care. Grimshaw and Russell compiled the most rigorous assessment of the success of practice guidelines, in a variety of medical conditions, in improving the quality of care.[114] They reviewed 59 published reports evaluating the impact of practice guidelines and found that in nearly all cases the implementation of a practice guideline had improved the measured process of care. Of the 11 studies they reviewed that reported a clinical outcome in addition to the process of care, 9 reported significant improvement. One may question the generalizability of these conclusions, since it is likely that there is a significant publication bias in favor of studies demonstrating an improvement in care over "negative" studies of the same question. Nevertheless, regardless of the frequency with which practice guidelines actually *do* improve care, there is clear and compelling evidence that they *can* improve care.

Sarasin and colleagues reported significant improvements in the use of beta blockers in postinfarction patients following the implementation of a practice guideline on the subject at their institution.[115] In their time series, the use of discharge beta blockers nearly doubled, despite no significant change in the profile of infarction patients. A Canadian group looked at the improvement in several process measures of care for patients with acute myocardial infarction (AMI) cared for at the University of Alberta Hospitals between 1987 and 1993.[116] They found continuous and significant improvement in the use of therapies of proven efficacy, with a corresponding fall in the use of unproven interventions. Although the observations were made in an uncontrolled setting, the investigators attributed the results to "repeated measurement and reporting of key health care performance indicators, and initiation of explicit . . . AMI practice guidelines."[116] On a much larger scale, the Cooperative Cardiovascular Project demonstrated that the feedback on compliance with guidelines for critical process of care measures for patients with myocardial infarction was associated with a significant improvement in the quality of care that AMI patients received.[117]

Greater success in implementing practice guidelines depends in part on the refinement of the guidelines themselves, the more extensive use of clinical information systems to present critical data, guideline recommendations to clinicians at the point of care, [118] and greater sensitivity to the systematic barriers to their adoption.[119,120]

CONCLUSION

Assessing and improving the quality of care is a vital component of responsible medical practice. It has taken on increased prominence in recent years because of the widespread evidence of unexplained practice variation, the underutilization of effective therapies, and the increasing pressure for accountability at all levels of health care delivery. Clinical practice guidelines have emerged as an important tool to improve the quality of medical care, and cardiovascular medicine has become a particularly fertile ground for their development. A large number of high-quality clinical practice guidelines are now available that address critical issues in cardiovascular medicine, including assessing and managing risk factors for coronary heart disease, screening for cardiovascular illness, treating patients with established cardiovascular illness, and applying technology and therapies appropriately. When they are based on dependable, rigorous evidence, written in clear language, and implemented with sensitivity to the myriad local issues that can thwart their success, clinical practice guidelines can help improve patient care.

References

1. Health Care Financing Administration, 1999. ⟨http://www.hcfa.gov/stats/nhe-oact⟩
2. Kleinke JD. Medicine's industrial revolution. *Wall Street Journal,* August 21, 1995, p A7.
3. Relman AS. Assessment and accountability: The third revolution in medical care. *N Engl J Med* 1988; 319:1220–1222.
4. Berwick DM, Nolan TW. Physicians as leaders in improving health care: A new series in Annals of Internal Medicine. *Ann Intern Med* 1998; 128:289–292.
5. Wennberg JE, Gittelsohn AM. Small area variations in health care delivery. *Science* 1973; 321:1168–1173.
6. Chassin MR, Kosecoff J, Park RE, et al. Variations in the use of medical and surgical services by the Medicare population. *N Engl J Med* 1986; 314:285–290.
7. Gornick ME, Eggers PW, Reilly TW, et al. Effects of race and income on mortality and use of services among Medicare beneficiaries. *N Engl J Med* 1996; 335:791–799.
8. Ayanian JZ, Udvarhelyi S, Gatsonis CA, et al. Racial differences in the use of revascularization procedures after coronary angiography. *JAMA* 1993; 269:2642–2646.
9. Peterson ED, Wright SM, Daley J, et al. Racial variation in cardiac procedure use and survival following acute myocardial infarction in the Department of Veteran Affairs. *JAMA* 1994; 271:1175–1180.
10. Fisher ES, Wennberg JE, Stukel TA, et al. Hospital readmission rates for cohorts of Medicare beneficiaries in Boston and New Haven. *N Engl J Med* 1994; 331:989–995.
11. Guadagnoli E, Hauptman PJ, Ayanian JZ, et al. Variation in the use of cardiac procedures after acute myocardial infarction. *N Engl J Med* 1995; 333:573–578.
12. Pilote L, Califf RM, Sapp S, et al. Regional variation across the United States in the management of acute myocardial infarction. *N Engl J Med* 1995; 333:565–572.
13. Blumenthal D. Quality of care—What is it? *N Engl J Med* 1996; 335:891–894.
14. Institute of Medicine. *Medicare: A Strategy for Quality Assurance.* Washington, DC: National Academy Press; 1990.
15. Donabedian A. *Explorations in Quality Assessment and Monitoring: Vol 1. The Definition of Quality and Approaches to Its Assessment.* Ann Arbor, MI: Health Administration Press; 1980.
16. Nash IS. Improving outcomes of percutaneous coronary intervention. *Am Heart J* 1999; 137:979–982.
17. Cleary P, Edgman-Levitan S. Health care quality: Incorporating consumer perspectives. *JAMA* 1997; 278:1608–1612.
18. Nash IS, Curtis LH, Rubin H. Predictors of patient reported physical and mental health six months after percutaneous coronary revascularization. *Am Heart J* 1999; 138:422–429.
19. Hammermeister KE, Shroyer AL, Sethi GK, Grover FL. Why it is important to demonstrate linkages between outcomes of care and processes and structures of care. *Med Care* 1995; 33(10 suppl):OS5–OS16.
20. Siu A. personal communication.
21. Williams SV, Nash DB, Goldfarb. Differences in mortality from coronary bypass graft surgery at five teaching hospitals. *JAMA* 1991; 266:810–815.
22. O'Connor GT, Plume SK, Olmstead EM, et al. Multivariate prediction of in-hospital mortality associated with coronary artery bypass graft surgery: Northern New England Cardiovascular Disease Study Group. *Circulation* 1992; 85:2110–2118.
23. Luft HS, Romano PS. Chance, continuity, and change in hospital mortality rates: Coronary artery bypass graft patients in California hospitals, 1983–1989. *JAMA* 1993; 270:331–337.
24. Hannan EL, Kilburn H, Bernard H, et al. Coronary artery bypass surgery: The relationship between in-hospital mortality rate and surgical volume after controlling for clinical risk factors. *Med Care* 1991; 29:1094–1107.
25. New York State Department of Health. *Coronary Artery Bypass Surgery in New York State, 1994–1996.* Albany, NY: New York State Department of Health; 1998.
26. Pennsylvania Health Care Cost Containment Council. *Pennsylvania's Guide to Coronary Artery Bypass Graft Surgery 1994–1995.* Harrisburg, PA: Pennsylvania Health Care Cost Containment Council; 1998.
27. Kasper JF, Plume SK, O'Connor GT. A methodology for QI in the coronary artery bypass grafting procedure involving comparative process analysis. *QRB Quality Rev Bull* 1992; 18(4):129–133.
28. Dziuban SW, McIlduff JB, Miller SJ, Dal Col RH. How a New York cardiac surgery program uses outcomes data. *Ann Thorac Surg* 1994; 58:1871–1876.
29. Ellerbeck EF, Jencks SF, Radford MJ, et al. Quality of care for Medicare patients with acute myocardial infarction. *JAMA* 1995; 273:1509–1514.
30. ISIS-2 (Second International Study of Infarct Survival) Collaborative Group. Randomised trial of intravenous streptokinase, oral aspirin, both, or neither among 17,187 cases of suspected acute myocardial infarction: ISIS-2. *Lancet* 1988; 2:349–360.
31. Mant J, Hicks N. Detecting differences in quality of care: The sensitivity of measures of process and outcome in treating acute myocardial infarction. *Br Med J* 1995; 311:793–796.
32. Saketkhou BB, Conte FJ, Noris M, et al. Emergency department use of aspirin in patients with possible acute myocardial infarction. *Ann Intern Med* 1997; 127:126–129.
33. Casalino LP. The unintended consequences of measuring quality on the quality of medical care. *N Engl J Med* 1999; 341:1147–1150.
34. Topol EJ, Califf RM. Scorecard cardiovascular medicine: Its impact and future directions. *Ann Intern Med* 1994; 120:65–70.
35. Public Law 101-239, the Omnibus Budget Reconciliation Act of 1989, section 901.
36. Public Law 101-239, the Omnibus Budget Reconciliation Act of 1989, section 912.
37. Field MJ, Lohr KN, eds. *Clinical Practice Guidelines: Directions for a New Program.* Washington, DC: National Academy Press; 1990.
38. Field MJ, Lohr KN, eds. *Clinical Practice Guidelines: Directions for a New Program.* Washington, DC: National Academy Press; 1990:8.
39. Field MJ, Lohr KN, *Guidelines for Clinical Practice: From Development to Use.* Washington, DC: National Academy Press; 1992:4.
40. Field MJ, Lohr KN, eds. *Clinical Practice Guidelines: Directions for a New Program.* Washington, DC: National Academy Press; 1990:50.
41. Hadorn DC, Baker DW, Kamberg CJ, Brook RH. Phase II of the AHCPR-sponsored heart failure guideline: Translating practice recommendations into review criteria. *Jt Comm J Qual Improv* 1996; 22:265–276.
42. Konstam MA, Dracup K, Baker DW, et al. *Heart Failure: Evaluation and Care of Patients with Left Ventricular Systolic Dysfunction. Clinical Practice Guideline No. 11.* Rockville, MD: US Department of Health and Human Services, Agency for Health Care Policy and Research; 1994.
43. Pearson SD, Goulart-Fisher D, Lee TH. Critical pathways as a strategy for improving care: Problems and potential. *Ann Intern Med* 1995; 123:941–948.
44. Ritchie JL, Forrester JS, Jones RH, et al. 28th Bethesda conference: Practice guidelines and the quality of care. *J Am Coll Cardiol* 1997; 29:1125–1179.
45. Field MJ, Lohr KN, eds. *Clinical Practice Guidelines: Directions for a New Program.* Washington, DC: National Academy Press; 1990:59.
46. Hayward RSA, Wilson MC, Tunis SR, et al. User's guide to the medical literature: VIII. How to use clinical practice guide-

lines. A: Are the recommendations valid? *JAMA* 1995; 274: 570–574.

47. Wilson MC, Hayward RAS, Tunis SR, et al. User's guide to the medical literature: VIII. How to use clinical practice guidelines. B: What are the recommendations and will they help you in caring for your patients? *JAMA* 1999; 274:1630–1632.
48. Weingarten S. Using practice guidelines compendiums to provide better preventive care. *Ann Intern Med* 1999; 130:454–458.
49. Selker HP. Criteria for adoption of medical practice guidelines. *Am J Cardiol* 1993; 71:339–341.
50. American Medical Association. *Clinical Practice Guidelines Directory 1999*. Chicago: American Medical Association; 1999.
51. http://www.guidelines.gov/index.asp
52. Shaneyfelt TM, Mayo-Smith MF, Rothwangle J. Are guidelines following guidelines? The methodological quality of clinical practice guidelines in the peer-reviewed medical literature. *JAMA* 1999; 281:1900–1905.
53. Cook D, Giacomini M. The trials and tribulations of clinical practice guidelines. *JAMA* 1999; 281:1950–1951.
54. Parmley WW. Clinical practice guidelines: Does the cookbook have enough recipes? *JAMA* 1994; 272:1374–1375.
55. Baker DW, Konstam MA, Bottorff M, Pitt B. Management of heart failure, I: Pharmacologic treatment. *JAMA* 1994; 272: 1361–1366.
56. Jones RH, Ritchie JL, Fleming BB, et al. Task Force 1: Clinical practice guideline development, dissemination and computerization. *J Am Coll Cardiol* 1997; 29:1133–1141.
57. Hadorn DC, Baker D, Hodges JS, et al. Rating the quality of evidence for clinical practice guidelines. *J Clin Epidemiol* 1996; 49:749–754.
58. U.S. Preventive Services Task Force. *Guide to Clinical Preventive Services*. Baltimore, MD: Williams & Wilkins; 1989.
59. Ryan TJ, Anderson JL, Antman EM, et al. ACC/AHA guidelines for the management of patients with acute myocardial infarction: A report of the American College of Cardiology/American Heart Association Task Force on Practice Guidelines (Committee on Management of Acute Myocardial Infarction). *J Am Coll Cardiol* 1996; 28:1328–1428.
60. Eagle KA, Brundage BH, Chiatman BR, et al. ACC/AHA guidelines for perioperative cardiovascular evaluation for noncardiac surgery: A report of the American College of Cardiology/American Heart Association Task Force on Practice Guidelines (Committee on Perioperative Cardiovascular Evaluation for Noncardiac Surgery). *J Am Coll Cardiol* 1996; 27:910–948.
61. Lee TH, Pearson SD, Johnson PA, et al. Failure of information as an intervention to modify clinical management: A time-series trial in patients with acute chest pain. *Ann Intern Med* 1995; 122:434–437.
62. Field MJ, Lohr KN, eds. *Clinical Practice Guidelines: Directions for a New Program*. Washington, DC: National Academy Press; 1990:12.
63. Grimshaw JM, Russell IT. Achieving health gain through clinical guidelines: II. Ensuring guidelines change medical practice. *Quality Health Care* 1994; 3:45–51.
64. Pelly JE, Newby L, Tito F, et al. Clinical practice guidelines before the law: Sword or shield? *Med J Aust* 1998; 169:330–333.
65. Chodoff P, Crowley K. Clinical practice guidelines: Roadblocks to their acceptance and implementation. *J Outcomes Mgt* 1995; 2(2):5–10.
66. Grol R, Dalhuijsen J, Thomas S, et al. Attributes of clinical guidelines that influence use of guidelines in general practice: Observational study. *Br Med J* 1998; 317:858–861.
67. Field MJ, Lohr KN, eds. *Clinical Practice Guidelines: Directions for a New Program*. Washington, DC: National Academy Press; 1990:78.
68. Scannell KM, Miller N, Glock M. *Current Biographies in Medicine 92-14: Practice Guidelines*. Washington, DC: National Library of Medicine; 1992.
69. National Cholesterol Education Program. *Cholesterol Lowering in the Patient with Coronary Heart Disease: Physician Monograph*. National Institutes of Health Publication 97-3794. Bethesda, MD: National Institutes of Health; 1997.
70. Scandinavian Simvastatin Survival Study Group. Randomised trial of cholesterol lowering in 4444 patients with coronary heart disease: The Scandinavian Simvastatin Survival Study (4S). *Lancet* 1994; 344:1001–1009.
71. Sacks FM, Pfeffer MA, Moye LA, et al. The effect of pravastatin on coronary events after myocardial infarction in patients with average cholesterol levels. *N Engl J Med* 1996; 335:1001–1009.
72. Ridker PM. Are associations between infection and coronary disease causal or due to confounding? *Am J Med* 1999; 106:376–377.
73. Bostom AG, Selhub J. Homocysteine and arteriosclerosis: Subclinical and clinical disease associations. *Circulation* 1999; 99:2361–2363.
74. Joint National Committee on Prevention, Detection, Evaluation and Treatment of High Blood Pressure. The sixth report of the Joint National Committee on Prevention, Detection, Evaluation and Treatment of High Blood Pressure. *Arch Intern Med* 1997; 157:2413–2446.
75. Pasternak RC, Grundy SM, Levy D, et al. Spectrum of risk factors for coronary heart disease. *J Am Coll Cardiol* 1996; 27:978–990.
76. Swan HJC, Gersh BJ, Grayboys TB, et al. Evaluation and management of risk factors for the individual patient (case management). *J Am Coll Cardiol* 1996; 27:1030–1039.
77. Grundy SM, Paternak R, Greenland P, et al. Assessment of cardiovascular risk by use of multiple-risk-factor assessment equations: A statement for healthcare professionals from the American Heart Association and the American College of Cardiology. *Circulation* 1999; 100:1481–1492.
78. Expert Panel on Detection, Evaluation, and Treatment of High Blood Cholesterol in Adults. Summary of the second report of the National Cholesterol Education Program (NCEP) Expert Panel on Detection, Evaluation, and Treatment of High Blood Cholesterol in Adults (Adult Treatment Panel II). *JAMA* 1993; 269:3015–3023.
79. Garber AM, Browner WS, Hulley SB. Clinical guideline, part 2: Cholesterol screening in asymptomatic adults, revisited. *Ann Intern Med* 1996; 124:518–531.
80. Task Force on Risk Reduction, American Heart Association. Cholesterol screening in asymptomatic adults: No cause to change. *Circulation* 1996; 93:1067–1068.
81. Garber AM, Browner WS. Cholesterol screening guidelines: Consensus, evidence, and common sense. *Circulation* 1997; 95:1642–1645.
82. Consensus Panel Statement. Guide to primary prevention of cardiovascular diseases. *Circulation* 1997; 95:2330.
83. Grundy SM, Balady GJ, Criqui MH, et al. When to start cholesterol-lowering therapy in patients with coronary heart disease: A statement for healthcare professionals from the American Heart Association Task Force on Risk Reduction. *Circulation* 1997; 95:1683–1685.
84. Consensus Panel Statement. Preventing heart attack and death in patients with coronary disease. *Circulation* 1995; 92:2–4.
85. Summary report from the Consensus Development Conference on Diagnosis of Coronary Heart Disease in People with Diabetes. (http://www.acc.org)
86. Fiore MC, Bailey WC, Cohen SJ, et al. *Smoking Cessation: Clinical Practice Guideline No 18*. Rockville, MD: U.S. Department of Health and Human Services, Public Health Service, Agency for Health Care Policy and Research; 1996.
87. Ockene IS, Houston-Miller, N. Cigarette smoking, cardiovascular disease, and stroke: A statement for healthcare professionals

from the American Heart Association. *Circulation* 1997; 96:3243–3247.

88. *Obesity Education Initiative: Clinical Guidelines on the Identification, Evaluation, and Treatment of Overweight and Obesity in Adults.* Bethesda, MD: National Institutes of Health, National Heart, Lung, and Blood Institute; 1998.
89. Eckel RH, for the Nutrition Committee. Obesity and heart disease: A statement for healthcare professionals from the Nutrition Committee, American Heart Association. *Circulation* 1997; 96:3248–3250.
90. AACE/ACE Obesity Task Force. AACE/ACE position statement on the prevention, diagnosis, and treatment of obesity. *Endocrinol Pract* 1997; 3:162–208.
91. Fletcher GF, Balady G, Blair SN, et al. Statement on exercise: Benefits and recommendations for physical activity programs for all Americans: A statement for health professionals by the Committee on Exercise and Cardiac Rehabilitation of the Council on Clinical Cardiology, American Heart Association. *Circulation* 1996; 94:857–862.
92. *Physical Activity and Cardiovascular Health: National Institutes of Health Consensus Statement.* Bethesda, MD: National Institutes of Health; 1995; 13(3):1–33.
93. *Guide to Clinical Preventive Services,* 2d ed. Baltimore, MD: Williams & Wilkins; 1996:3–14.
94. *Guide to Clinical Preventive Services,* 2d ed. Baltimore, MD: Williams & Wilkins; 1996:53–61.
95. *Guide to Clinical Preventive Services,* 2d ed. Baltimore, MD: Williams & Wilkins; 1996:67–72.
96. Braunwald E, Mark DB, Jones RH, et al. *Unstable Angina: Diagnosis and Management. Clinical Practice Guideline No. 10.* AHCPR Publication no. 94-0602. Rockville, MD: Agency for Health Care Policy and Research and the National Heart, Lung, and Blood Institute, Public Health Service, U.S. Department of Health and Human Services; March 1994.
97. Prystowsky EN, Benson DW, Fuster V, et al. Management of patients with atrial fibrillation: A statement for healthcare professionals from the Subcommittee on Electrocardiography and Electrophysiology, American Heart Association. *Circulation* 1996; 93:1262–1277.
98. Gibbons RJ, Chatterjee K, Daley J, et al. ACC/AHA/ACP-ISM guidelines for the management of patients with chronic stable angina: A report of the American College of Cardiology/American Heart Association Task Force on Practice Guidelines (Committee on Management of Patients with Chronic Stable Angina). *Circulation* 1999; 99:2829–2848.
99. Ritchie JL, Cheitlin MD, Eagle KA, et al. Guidelines for the evaluation and management of heart failure: A report of the American College of Cardiology/American Heart Association Task Force on Practice Guidelines (Committee on Evaluation and Management of Heart Failure). *J Am Coll Cardiol* 1995; 26:1376–1398.
100. Gunnar RM, Bourdillon PDV, Dixon DW, et al. Guidelines for the early management of patients with acute myocardial infarction: A report of the American College of Cardiology/American Heart Association Task Force on Assessment of Diagnostic and Therapeutic Cardiovascular Procedures (Subcommittee to Develop Guidelines for the Early Management of Patients with Acute Myocardial Infarction). *J Am Coll Cardiol* 1990; 16:249–292.
101. Ryan TJ, Antman EM, Brooks NH, et al. 1999 update: ACC/AHA guidelines for the management of patients with acute myocardial infarction: Executive summary and recommendations: A report of the American College of Cardiology/American Heart Association Task Force on Practice Guidelines (Committee on Management of Acute Myocardial Infarction). *Circulation* 1999; 100:1016–1030.
102. Bonow RO, Carabello B, deLeon AC Jr, et al. ACC/AHA guidelines for the management of patients with valvular heart disease: A report of the American College of Cardiology/American Heart Association Task Force on Practice Guidelines (Committee on Management of Patients with Valvular Heart Disease). *J Am Coll Cardiol* 1998; 32:1486–1588.
103. Gibbons RJ, Balady GJ, Beasley JW, et al. ACC/AHA guidelines for exercise testing: A report of the American College of Cardiology/American Heart Association Task Force on Practice Guidelines (Committee on Exercise Testing). *J Am Coll Cardiol* 1997; 30:260–311.
104. Ritchie JL, Bateman TM, Bonow RO, et al. ACC/AHA guidelines for clinical use of cardiac radionuclide imaging: A report of the American College of Cardiology/American Heart Association Task Force on Practice Guidelines (Committee on Radionuclide Imaging). *J Am Coll Cardiol* 1995; 25:521–547.
105. Strauss HW, Miller DD, Wittry MD, et al. *Procedure Guideline for Myocardial Perfusion Imaging.* Reston, VA: Society of Nuclear Medicine; 1999.
106. Cheitlan MD, Alpert JS. ACC/AHA guidelines for the clinical application of echocardiography: A report of the American College of Cardiology/American Heart Association Task Force on Practice Guidelines (Committee on Clinical Application of Echocardiography). *Circulation* 1997; 95:1686–1744.
107. Scanlon PJ, Faxon DP, Audet AM, et al. ACC/AHA guidelines for coronary angiography: A report of the American College of Cardiology/American Heart Association Task Force on Practice Guidelines (Committee on Coronary Angiography), developed in collaboration with the Society for Cardiac Angiography and Interventions. *J Am Coll Cardiol* 1999; 33:1756–1816.
108. Zipes DP, DiMarco JP, Gillette PC, et al. ACC/AHA guidelines for clinical intracardiac electrophysiological and catheter ablation procedures: A report of the American College of Cardiology/American Heart Association Task Force on Practice Guidelines (Committee on Clinical Intracardiac Electrophysiologic and Catheter Ablation Procedures), developed in collaboration with the North American Society of Pacing and Electrophysiology. *Circulation* 1995; 92:673–691.
109. Eagle KA, Guyton RA, Davidoff R, et al. ACC/AHA guidelines for coronary artery bypass graft surgery: A report of the American College of Cardiology/American Heart Association Task Force on Practice Guidelines (Committee to Revise the 1991 Guidelines for Coronary Artery Bypass Graft Surgery). *J Am Coll Cardiol* 1999; 34:1262–1347.
110. American College of Chest Physicians. *Fifth ACCP Consensus Conference on Antithrombotic Therapy. Chest* 1998; 144 (suppl):439S–769S.
111. Dalen JE, Hirsh J, for the American College of Chest Physicians. *Fifth ACCP Consensus Conference on Antithrombotic Therapy (1998): Summary Recommendations.* Northbrook, IL: American College of Chest Physicians; 1999.
112. Gregoratos G, Cheitlin MD, Conill A, et al. ACC/AHA guidelines for implantation of cardiac pacemakers and antiarrhythmia devices: A report of the American College of Cardiology/American Heart Association Task Force on Practice Guidelines (Committee on Pacemaker Implementation). *J Am Coll Cardiol* 1998; 31:1175–1209.
113. USDHHS. *Cardiac Rehabilitation: Clinical Practice Guideline No. 16.* Rockville, MD: U.S. Department of Health and Human Services, Agency for Health Care Policy and Research, 1995.
114. Grimshaw JM, Russell IT, Effect of clinical guidelines on medical practice: A systematic review of rigorous evaluations. *Lancet* 1993; 342:1317–1322.
115. Sarasin FP, Maschiangelo ML, Schaller MD, et al. Successful implementation of guidelines for encouraging the use of beta blockers in patients after acute myocardial infarction. *Am J Med* 1999; 106:499–505.

116. Montague T, Taylor L, Martin S, et al. Can practice patterns and outcomes be successfully altered? Examples from cardiovascular medicine. *Can J Cardiol* 1995; 11:487–492.
117. Marciniak TA, Ellerbeck EF, Radford MJ, et al. Improving the quality of care for Medicare patients with acute myocardial infarction: Results from the Cooperative Cardiovascular Project. *JAMA* 1998; 279:1351–1357.
118. Tierney WM, Overhage JM, Takesue BY, et al. Computerizing guidelines to improve care and patient outcomes: The example of heart failure. *JAMA* 1995; 2:316–322.
119. Cabana MD, Rand CS, Powe NR, et al. Why don't physicians follow clinical practice guidelines? A framework for improvement. *JAMA* 1999; 282:1458–1465.
120. James PA, Cowan TM, Graham RP. Patient-centered clinical decisions and their impact on physician adherence to clinical guidelines. *J Fam Pract* 1998; 46:311–318.

CHAPTER 98

BEHAVIORAL MEDICINE IN THE TREATMENT OF HEART DISEASE

Thomas G. Pickering / Karina Davidson / William Gerin

In an assessment of the causes of death in the United States in 1993, McGinnis and Foege[1] estimated that approximately 50 percent of deaths (the majority of which were due to heart disease) were attributable to behavioral or lifestyle factors, including tobacco use, poor diet, physical inactivity, and alcohol consumption. Although genetic factors undoubtedly contribute to individual susceptibility to these factors, a prime ingredient is individual behavior. The costs of treating heart disease are escalating at an alarming rate because of the widespread use of sophisticated and increasingly expensive treatments such as coronary artery stents and gene therapy. Most efforts to contain the rise in health care costs have focused on limiting supply (a largely unfulfilled promise of managed care) and imposing some sort of rationing. However, in 1993, Fries and associates[2] pointed out that restricting demand could achieve the same objective. They identified six factors, including four that are relevant to this chapter:

1. Much disease is preventable.
2. Risky behavior costs money. Lifetime medical costs, which averaged $225,000 per person, are clearly related to health behavior habits; for example, those costs are approximately one-third higher in smokers than in nonsmokers.
3. Self-management can result in savings. Several studies have shown that providing medical consumers with information about and guidelines for self-management can lower the use of medical services 10 percent or more.
4. Health behavior promotion at work has reduced medical costs. This has been documented in numerous studies.

This chapter focuses on the major behavioral and psychological factors that influence the course of heart disease and discusses how they can be treated. The behavioral factors are smoking, obesity, and physical inactivity, and the psychological factors are hostility, depression, and anxiety.

A dramatic example of the effects of environmental and psychosocial factors on cardiovascular disease is provided by a recent analysis of changing mortality rates in Russia.[3] Over a 4-year period after the breakup of the Soviet Union, life expectancy declined 5 years, most of which could be attributed to increased mortality in men age 25 to 64 resulting from accidents and cardiovascular disease. Factors that might have contributed to those changes include economic instability, stress, depression, and increased intake of alcohol and tobacco. An equally dramatic example of the influence of lifestyle factors comes from the Honolulu Heart Program, in which it was found that retired men who walked less than 1 mile a day were nearly twice as likely to die over a 12-year period than were men who walked more than 2 miles daily.[4]

Psychosocial factors can influence the course of chronic disease by two main pathways: by inducing behavioral or lifestyle patterns, such as smoking, that are injurious and through a direct effect of social and environmental factors such as socioeconomic status and stress on the disease process. Individual characteristics interact with both pathways, influencing how people choose their lifestyles and how they react to stress. An example of the multiplicity of pathways linking psychosocial factors and disease is provided by hostility, a personality characteristic that has been shown to be a risk factor for coronary heart disease. It has been hypothesized that hostile persons show an exaggerated cardiovascular reactivity to stress, which contributes to the development of atherosclerosis or may trigger an acute event (see below). Hostile persons are also more likely to smoke and less likely to quit.[5]

Although it is widely accepted that behavioral and lifestyle factors may play an important role in the development of coronary heart disease, most practicing cardiologists are not involved in the primary prevention of disease as much as they are in the treatment of existent disease. One factor that is not widely appreciated is how important lifestyle and psychological factors can be in influencing the progression of established coronary heart disease. For example, a study at the Mayo Clinic evaluated a cohort of 381 patients referred to a cardiac rehabilitation unit after hospitalization for an acute coronary event [unstable angina, myocardial infarction (MI), bypass surgery, or angioplasty]. In addition to the traditional risk factors, patients were evaluated for psychological distress (a term that includes depression and vital exhaustion). Over a 6-month follow-up period, it was found that persons high in psychological distress were three times more likely to be hospitalized for recurrent coronary events [i.e., an odds ratio (OR) of 3.05]; other less powerful predictive factors included no previous bypass procedure (OR = 2.73), diabetes (OR = 2.65), and ejection fraction <40 percent (OR = 1.98). Interestingly, smoking and the use of beta blockers did not predict relapse. A second example comes from a study of patients undergoing coronary angioplasty, after which new cardiac events occur in 20 to 30 percent of patients within 1 year. The study found that after controlling for standard risk factors, men who scored high on anger had a threefold increase in the rate of recurrent events compared with men with lower scores.[6]

BASIC PRINCIPLES OF BEHAVIORAL MEDICINE

It has long been recognized that knowledge alone does not provide sufficient motivation to change behavior.[7] A fundamental problem is that intervention studies commonly produce improvements in the behavior being manipulated that last a few weeks or months, but by 1 year there is almost always a relapse. An example is the Trials of Hypertension Prevention, in which patients were asked to reduce their weight or salt intake (Fig. 98-1).

Some of the basic principles that may be employed to obtain sustained behavioral change can be illustrated by the example of dietary intervention, but the same principles apply to modalities such as smoking cessation and exercise.

TABLE 98-1 Stages of Change

1. Precontemplation. Patient is not yet thinking about changing behavior
2. Contemplation. Patient is considering but is not yet ready to engage in behavior change
3. Preparation. Patient intends to take action in the next month
4. Action. Patient begins actual process of behavior change
5. Maintenance. Patient develops strategies to prevent relapse

As with other types of behavioral intervention, many studies of dietary intervention have reported disappointing or at best modest lipid-lowering results even when trained dietitians and knowledgeable health professionals were involved in the intervention process.[8–10] One reason for these disappointing results is suggested by recent behavioral studies that indicate that the method used to deliver dietary interventions may be less than optimal. Earlier intervention studies typically applied a didactic, informative approach with little attention paid to what now are recognized as important differences in learning styles or levels of motivation to change behavior.[11] More recent behavioral models identify psychosocial factors that influence food choices and delineate the process of motivating changes in behavior.[12] Several behavioral models have evolved, and these models are potentially additive. The social learning theory model incorporates behavior modification methods that include cognitive, interpersonal, and environmental influences on behavior.[13] The basic components of this approach include self-monitoring and analysis of behavior; self-management, including stimulus control of external cues; the replacement of less desirable (i.e., high-fat foods) behaviors with more desirable behaviors; and the reinforcement of desirable behaviors.[7] Strongly related is the construct of "self-efficacy,"[14] which refers to a person's degree of confidence that she or he has the ability to gain control over specific behaviors, such as eating and dieting. Increased self-efficacy has been found to be a critical element in motivation to engage in healthy behaviors.[14]

Over the last decade, research on the stages of change model has yielded valuable insights regarding how, why, and when persons will change behavior.[15] This model suggests that behavior change is achieved through a series of stages: precontemplation, contemplation, preparation, action, and maintenance[16] (Table 98-1).

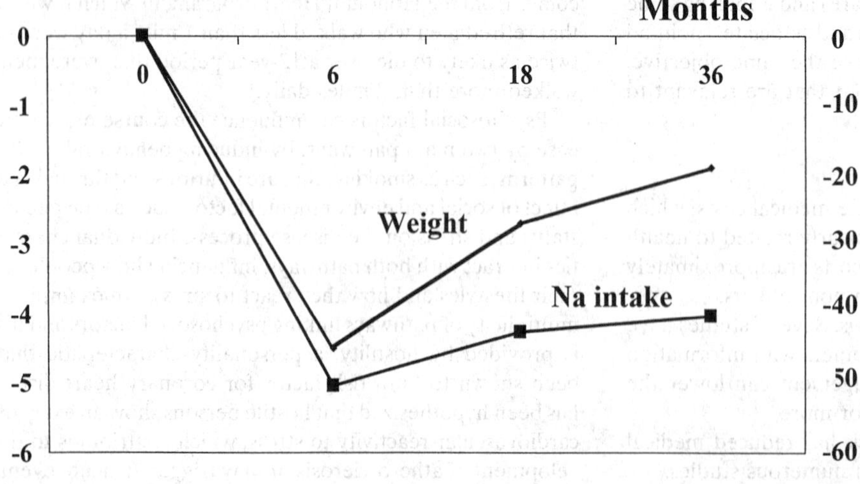

FIGURE 98-1 The trials of hypertension prevention.

Since most dietary intervention studies have applied approaches suitable for the action stage, it is not surprising that adherence has been disappointing. It is likely that many participants were overwhelmed, uncommitted, or simply not ready to adopt the recommended eating pattern.

Barriers to Behavioral Intervention and the Role of Collaborative Management of Patients with Heart Disease

A basic issue in the treatment of behavioral and lifestyle factors is the concept of collaborative management. Heart disease is usually chronic, and its successful management requires active collaboration between the patient and the health care providers. There is a large gap between the care that is prescribed and what is actually achieved. A classic example is control of hypertension, in which despite the availability of numerous powerful medications, blood pressure is adequately controlled in fewer than one-third of patients.[17] Some of the barriers to the more successful implementation of recommended lifestyle and other changes are summarized in Table 98-2. These barriers can be categorized as relating to the patient, the physician, or the health care system.

Patients often lack the knowledge and motivation to make behavior changes, and the training of cardiologists rarely includes behavior and behavioral intervention. Physicians generally have a low opinion of the effectiveness of behavioral interventions and little incentive to implement them, let alone the time. Because neither patients nor physicians have pressured the health care system to recognize the importance of making these changes, behavioral interventions rarely are reimbursed.

Despite these limitations, health care providers can and should use behavioral techniques to improve self-care in patients with chronic illnesses such as heart disease. These techniques include contracting with the patient to reach specific goals, evaluating the patient's readiness for self-care, breaking self-care tasks into small manageable steps, providing personalized feedback to the patient, self-monitoring of health-related behaviors, enlisting social support, and checking the patient's commitment to key tasks. One of the first steps is to define problems clearly. Physicians usually are concerned with items such as poor compliance and unhealthy behavior, while patients are more concerned with symptoms and emotional distress. Few physicians ask patients to identify the biggest problems they face in managing illness.

In light of the lack of training in behavioral techniques and the severe time limitations of cardiologists, the solution to this dilemma ideally should be a team approach. Behavioral interventions tend to require relatively large amounts of time, but a lot can be achieved by persons whose training and time is less costly than those of the physician. These persons include nurses, psychologists, dietitians, and social workers.

At the end of this chapter specific strategies are discussed that can be used easily by the physician to help patients make the necessary changes in their behavior.

TABLE 98-2 Barriers to Implementation of Behavioral Changes

Barriers
Patient
Lack of knowledge
Lack of motivation
Low self-efficacy (confidence in the ability to effect changes)
Unreadiness to commit to behavior change
Lack of access to care
Social and cultural factors
Physician
Time constraints
Problem-based focus
Perceived ineffectiveness of interventions
Lack of behavioral skills
Lack of incentives
Health care system
Focus on acute care
Failure to provide team approach
Failure to provide reimbursement
Lack of policies and standards

SMOKING CESSATION

Smoking kills more than 400,000 Americans every year, and more than half of these deaths are due to cardiovascular disease and stroke. Smoking has been recognized for many years as one of the "big three" risk factors for cardiovascular disease (the others being hypertension and hyperlipidemia) and is responsible for about 30 percent of cardiovascular morbidity and mortality.[18] Smoking more than doubles the incidence of coronary artery disease and increases mortality 70 percent.[19] The economic cost of tobacco smoking has been estimated to be over $50 billion a year. The risks associated with smoking are almost completely reversible after quitting,[20,21] and smoking cessation has been shown to be one of the most cost-effective interventions in the field of medicine.[22] However, smoking cessation programs rarely are reimbursed by health insurance programs.

AHCPR Guidelines

The science and effectiveness of smoking cessation programs have been reviewed extensively by the Agency for Health Care Policy (AHCPR), which issued its guidelines in 1996.[18] The guidelines stress that health care clinics such as cardiology practices are ideal settings for the promotion of smoking cessation treatments. More than 70 percent of smokers report that they see a physician at least once a year.[23] The guidelines emphasize that a variety of effective strategies can be adopted, some very simple and others more complex. The recommended steps are summarized below.

- Clearly, step 1 is to identify smokers. Although this seems obvious, data show that only about 50 percent of smokers report ever having been asked by a physician if they smoked.[24]
- Step 2 is advising a smoker to quit, an intervention that takes 3 min at most. Although this may seem trivial, an analysis of several studies has shown that the quit rate will increase from 7.9 percent to 10.2 percent, an increment that may seem insubstantial except that each smoker who quits will add up to 15 years to his or her life expectancy.[18] Moreover, this

number will increase with each succeeding examination in which the physician advises the patient to quit.

- Step 3 is the assessment of a smoker's willingness to quit. The mnemonic STOP is advocated: *s*upport from the physician in the quit attempt; *t*ry, acknowledging that the patient is making a commitment to try, not necessarily to quit; *o*ptions, reviewing the various treatment options open to the patient; and *p*icking a quit day.
- Step 4 deals with a smoker who is unwilling to attempt to quit. This involves promoting the patient's readiness to quit, and emphasizes the four Rs: personal *r*elevance to the patient's medical and social situation, the *r*isks associated with smoking, the *r*ewards of quitting, and the *r*epetition of a stop-smoking message. A good way to assess a patient's readiness to quit is to use the stages of change model described above.[25] The important message here is that all smokers should be given advice about smoking, but the advice should differ according to the patient's stage of change.
- Step 5 deals with the strategy that is chosen for a patient who is willing to quit. A general rule is that "more is better," or that the quit rate is proportional to the amount of effort that is put into it. The options, which are not mutually exclusive, include counseling, which has two basic components: providing social support and boosting skills in problem solving. Other components include the use of nicotine replacement therapy, which can be delivered in a variety of ways, including gum, skin patches, and nasal sprays. A number of clinical trials have shown that the nicotine patches can double quit rates.[26] Finally, the use of the antidepressant drug bupropion (Zyban) has been found to be very effective. A study published after the AHCPR guidelines were published found that bupropion approximately doubled the quit rate[27] and that the best results were obtained with a combination of counseling, nicotine patches, and bupropion treatment.

Nicotine Gum and Patch

Since 1995, nicotine gum (Nicorette) and nicotine skin patches (Nicoderm, Nicotrol) have been approved as over-the-counter drugs. The gum is available in 2- or 4-mg doses, and it is recommended that one to two pieces be chewed per hour. The lower dose is for persons who smoke fewer than 25 cigarettes daily, and the higher dose is for those who smoke more. The regular dose is used for 6 weeks, followed by 6 weeks of tapering.

The Nicotrol patch label instructs patients to use the patch for 16 h a day for 6 weeks, with no tapering period. The Nicoderm CQ patch is used for 16 h a day at a high dose (21 mg/day) for 6 weeks, followed by 14 mg/day for 2 weeks and then 7 mg/day for 2 weeks. Both the gum and the patch have been subjected to several placebo-controlled clinical trials that have shown that the use of either one leads to an approximate doubling of the quit rate.[28]

Nicotine Nasal Spray and Inhaler

The spray is available as a prescription drug (Nicotrol nasal spray) that is designed to deliver the nicotine more rapidly than does the gum or patch. It is administered once or twice per hour for up to 3 months. Its use doubles the quit rate; side effects include sore throat and rhinitis, both of which are usually transient.[28] Another prescription formulation is the Nicotrol inhaler, which has pharmacokinetics similar to those of the nicotine gum. Its effectiveness is comparable to that of the other nicotine replacement therapies.[28]

Bupropion

Bupropion originally was developed as an antidepressant, for which it is not very effective. As an antismoking adjuvant, it is available in a long-acting form as Zyban, which has been found to lead to a doubling of the quit rate. The recommended dose is 300 mg/day, which is started 1 week before the quit date and continued for 7 to 12 weeks. It has been found to work equally well whether or not the smoker is depressed, suggesting that its antidepressant activity is not its primary mode of action.[29] Side effects include dry mouth and insomnia.

Reimbursement Issues

One of the reasons why so little attention is given to smoking cessation programs is that those programs rarely are reimbursed by insurance companies. A survey of managed care companies found that only 9 percent reimbursed physicians for implementing the AHCPR recommendations fully, while another 39 percent reimbursed partially and 53 percent did not reimburse at all.[30] Approximately half the companies surveyed were not aware of the existence of the guidelines. Whereas 54 percent of managed care organizations (MCOs) offered some self-help materials for smokers, only 17.6 percent provided reimbursement for bupropion use.

The almost total lack of reimbursement for smoking cessation programs stands in stark contrast to the reimbursement for the treatment of the other two major risk factors for heart disease: hypertension and hyperlipidemia. Smoking cessation has been labeled "the gold standard of health care cost-effectiveness"[22] and is dramatically more cost-effective in terms of life-years saved (LYS) than is treatment for hypertension or hyperlipidemia with medications (Table 98-3).

One commonly given reason why smoking cessation is not reimbursed more often is that the benefits are delayed for about 5 to 10 years, which may be longer than the life span of many

TABLE 98-3 Cost-effectiveness of Treatment of the Big Three Cardiovascular Risk Factors

Intervention	Cost per Life-Year Saved, $
Smoking cessation[a]	
Brief advice from doctor	1000–3000
High intensity	6000–15,000
Treatment of hypertension[b]	11,000–72,000
Treatment of hyperlipidemia[c]	9000–297,000

SOURCE: [a]From Warner.[22] [b]From Edelson JT, Weinstein MC, Tosteson AN, et al. Long-term cost-effectiveness of various initial monotherapies for mild to moderate hypertension [see comments]. *JAMA* 1990; 266:407. [c]From Hay JW, Wittels EH, Gotto AMJ. An economic evaluation of lovastatin for cholesterol lowering and coronary artery disease reduction [see comments]. *Am J Cardiol* 1991; 67:789.

MCOs; hence, no net cost savings for the MCO will result from the program. However, this is a double standard: Coronary bypass surgery and angioplasty are reimbursed routinely, and no one ever questions whether they reduce health care costs for an MCO, which clearly they do not.

In light of these numbers, why do so few physicians pay attention to smoking cessation? There are several reasons: First, physicians are not trained in behavioral techniques such as counseling even though this is an activity to which they devote substantial time. They believe that their patients already know that smoking is harmful and that counseling is unlikely to have a significant effect. Second, the fact that it is not reimbursed automatically gives counseling a low priority. Thus, it has been established that brief (3 mins or so) counseling from a physician can double the spontaneous quit rate of smokers, which is about 2.5 percent per year. If a physician counsels 100 patients per year, 95 percent will continue to smoke, a dispiritingly large number for the physician. However, of the 2.5 smokers who quit as a result of physician counseling—in addition to the other 2.5 smokers who will quit spontaneously—one ex-smoker will avoid a premature smoking-related death and another will gain up to 15 years of life expectancy. The cost of this benefit will have been 3 h and 20 min of the physician's time.

DIETARY INTERVENTIONS

Dietary factors have a substantial impact on the development of cardiovascular disease (CVD). Many studies show that saturated fat and lipid intake is associated with rates of CVD-related death and all-cause mortality.[31,32] On the basis of epidemiologic and observational studies in men, women, African-Americans, and elderly persons as well as postmortem angiographic studies in young persons, the National Institutes of Health and the European Atherosclerosis Society have concluded that the level of serum lipids is a causal factor in coronary artery disease.[32–34]

Low-density lipoprotein cholesterol (LDL-C) and other components of the lipid profile are affected by dietary interventions.[35] This has led to strong recommendations by the National Cholesterol Education Program that dietary counseling should form the basis of lipid-regulating regimens for both the prevention and the clinical management of CVD.[36] Reductions in lipid levels are readily achievable through careful adherence to dietary changes.

Compared with pharmacologic intervention, dietary intervention has produced less net reduction in total cholesterol (TC) and LDL-C levels in randomized trials.[37] However, two secondary intervention trials—one with medication (Scandinavian Simvastatin Survival Study) and one with a Mediterranean, alpha-linolenic-rich diet (Lyon Diet Heart Study)—reported remarkably similar reductions in cardiac deaths over 5 years.[8–10,38]

Comprehensive reviews of dietary intervention studies[11,32,39] lead to the conclusion that aggressive treatment with a diet low in total and saturated fat produces lowered serum lipid levels and positive angiographic changes as well as potentially helping improve angina and other non-lipid-related symptoms. However, achieving and maintaining dietary adherence on a long-term basis remains a major challenge.

On the basis of the cumulative scientific evidence from epidemiologic and controlled clinical trials, the National Cholesterol Education Program (NCEP) advocated diet as the cornerstone of treatment in its reports of the Adult Treatment Panel as well as in its Population Based Panel and Pediatric Panel reports.[36,40] In 1989, both NCEP and the American Heart Association (AHA) announced populationwide recommendations for step I and step II diets as primary strategies for the prevention and treatment of high blood lipids.[36,41]

The last two decades have seen improvement in some aspects of the U.S. diet and corresponding declines in blood lipid levels.[11,39] Although the vast majority of U.S. adults still eat more than the recommended 30 percent of total calories as fat, the country as a whole has had a major downward shift in total fat intake.

Obesity and weight are increasing at epidemic rates, however, especially among young women and children.[34] This is due to other factors, such as levels of inactivity, and other aspects of the diet such as energy sources. For example, a potential contributor is the low intake of total dietary fiber. The AHA recommends 25 to 30 g of dietary fiber a day from whole grains, vegetables, and fruits. Because the population eats on average less than half the recommended daily minimum of five servings of fruits and vegetables, the intake of more energy-dense but nutrient-poor foods is the likely consequence.[34] It has been estimated that 52 million Americans are candidates for diet therapy to reduce high blood lipids; however, according to several surveys, fewer than 10 percent have been prescribed such diets.[42,43]

Other Nutrients, Antioxidants, and Homocysteine

Other nutrients have been explored in regard to their impact on blood lipids. The antioxidant vitamins E and C and beta-carotene delay and reduce the oxidation of LDL-C in vitro and may be especially important among smokers.[44–47] Observational studies in female nurses and male health professionals have reported favorable reductions in coronary heart disease (CHD) risk among those who take vitamin E supplements, but no intervention trials have been completed.[46] The use of vitamin E supplements was associated with a 35 percent reduction in CHD after adjustment for other risk factors, multiple vitamins, beta-carotene, and vitamin C.[45,46] Conversely, iron has been suggested to serve as a prooxidant in the arterial wall, potentially contributing to LDL-C oxidation, endothelial injury, and myocardial injury.[48] Studies on iron and the risk of CHD have been inconclusive.

Elevated levels of homocysteine damage endothelial cells and promote arterial occlusion.[49] Homocysteine is produced by the demethylation of methionine, an amino acid found mainly in animal protein foods. This conversion is dependent on folic acid, with vitamins B_6- and B_{12}-dependent enzymes playing a role as well. If these factors are reduced or inactivated, elevations in homocysteine can result. Diets rich in dark green and yellow fruits and vegetables and whole grains that provide an optimal amount of 400 mg/day of folate are adequate to produce serum folate levels of 15 μmol/L.

OBESITY

Independent of the qualitative objectives of dietary adherence, obesity directly and indirectly plays a major causal role in CHD and stroke.[50] It contributes to dyslipidemia, diabetes, and hypertension, and its strong association with reduced physical activity further exacerbates cardiovascular disease.[51–53] The national prevalence of obesity is currently estimated at 30 percent among adults and children.[54,55]

Excess body weight has been causally linked with deleterious changes in the lipoprotein profile.[51] Several studies have documented the fact that lipoprotein abnormalities are induced with weight gain and reversed with weight loss.[56,57] Particularly in obese children, even small degrees of weight loss can result in dramatic normalization of the lipid profile.[57]

In summary, the research strongly suggests that a diet reduced in total and saturated fat, lipids, trans-fatty acids, homocysteine, sodium, and excess calories and increased in dietary fiber (especially soluble fiber), antioxidants, folate, vitamin B_6, and n-3 fatty acids will lower cardiovascular risk for most persons. The resulting diet is rich in fruits and vegetables, whole grains and cereals, low-fat and skim dairy products, and fish, lean meats, and/or soy protein foods. Foods should be cooked without added saturated fat or cooked in a small amount of liquid vegetable oil, preferably olive oil, canola oil, or another monounsaturated nonhydrogenated liquid oil. Egg yolks should be limited to fewer than two per week.

Prevention and Treatment of Obesity

A recent National Institutes of Health (NIH) conference on voluntary methods for weight loss and control concluded that most existing adult obesity interventions are ineffective, with one-third to two-thirds of the lost weight being regained in 1 year and almost all the weight being regained within 5 years.[55] Training and calorie restrictions and the use of packaged diet food are not effective in the long term. The greatest success in treating the obese adult has occurred with combined dietary fat restriction, behavioral skill development, and regular exercise.[58,59] Other effective strategies include family-oriented interventions and booster sessions.[60] Pharmacologic appetite suppressants and gene therapy may offer promising options in the future for some patients, but inevitably diet and energy balance must be addressed.

Practical Steps toward Achieving Dietary Adherence

In a review of 30 studies reporting changes in fat intake, Barnard and coworkers[61] summarized the factors that were commonly associated with increased adherence. Those factors include the following:

- Stricter limits on fat intake. The lower the limit, the closer the average level of adherence.
- Frequent monitoring. At least monthly monitoring is recommended.
- Vegetarian diets. The use of a vegetarian diet more often achieved recommended fat intake than did nonvegetarian approaches.
- Initial residential components. These components provide intensive training, monitoring, provision of food, and group support in the short term, resulting in better adherence to self-selected diets in the long term. However, these components may be impractical in many cases.
- Family involvement. Involvement by family members results in improved adherence.
- Group support. This is not mandatory but can be helpful.
- Providing food. Entire meals are not required, but some provision of acceptable products is important.
- Symptomatic patients. These patients appear to be more motivated to comply with dietary regimens; healthy, high-risk patients appear to be less motivated.

Relevant sources of total and saturated fat and lipids should be identified before one attempts to prescribe a new dietary pattern for any patient. Two large-scale controlled clinical trials reported that meats, fats and oils, dairy foods, and baked goods contributed more total and saturated fat to the diets of adults than did any other food groups.[62,63] Fortunately, there are now many acceptable alternatives to these high-fat foods. Substitution of lower-fat or fat-free versions for high-fat foods (e.g., skim milk for whole milk, fat-free salad dressing for full-fat salad dressing) and the addition of more servings of fruits, vegetables, and grains to compensate for fewer servings of high-fat meats, dairy products, and baked goods are essential components. The food industry has responded aggressively to the request for lower-fat and no-fat products. The greater challenge lies in achieving the desired shift to a higher intake of foods with complex carbohydrates.

Changing Dietary Behavior One Patient at a Time

On the basis of these behavioral principles and the accumulated knowledge about diet and risk reduction, Van Horn and Kavey[34] have made the following suggestions, which can help promote successful dietary adherence:

- Start with dietary assessment and then individualize the dietary intervention. Assessing baseline intake is the only way to identify the foods that are contributing the most saturated fat and lipids to a patient's diet. In adults, this is often meats, fats, and sweets. In children, it is often whole-milk dairy products. In children who consume the recommended four servings of dairy foods per day, it may be possible to achieve adherence to the step I diet (≤10% saturated fat acids) by switching to skim milk and low-fat dairy products at school and at home.
- Provide clear, identifiable goals for each person. For example, current food labels make it possible to establish a fixed "fat gram goal" rather than following the less precise recommendations to get less than 30 percent of calories from total fat. This provides each person with an objective target he or she can self-monitor. Similarly, establishing the goal number of servings of fruits, vegetables, and grains can further help an individual achieve increased fiber, folate, and antioxidant intake.
- Assess the current state of change and determine the person's level of confidence (self-efficacy) in achieving a self-determined adherence goal. Reassess the person's status at each subsequent visit.
- Encourage self-monitoring through the use of food records and/or other simplified fat and fiber goal-counting records. Also, encourage the use of nonfood self-rewards when goals are met.
- Promote the benefit of adopting other health-oriented behaviors, including exercise, relaxation techniques, and stress reduction.
- Prevent relapse through ongoing follow-up, reassessment, and the establishment of new goals as needed.

- Patients who are referred to registered dietitians or other trained nutrition counselors may require relatively few follow-up sessions. Comprehensive feedback on dietary adherence can be provided to the referring physician by these other health professionals for consideration in determining future treatment plans.

EXERCISE

Physical inactivity is widely recognized as a major risk factor for cardiovascular disease, and numerous studies have shown that even mild exercise can reduce the probability of morbid events and even improve longevity. Only 22 percent of adults engage in 30 min or more of light to moderate exercise five or more times a week, the recommended amount for cardiovascular benefit.[64] Despite the fact that patients with cardiac disease are seen regularly by both cardiologists and primary care physicians, most physicians do not counsel their patients about physical activity.[65,66] One of the goals of the national Health Promotion Objectives for the year 2000 is to increase to at least 50 percent the number of primary care physicians who assess and advise their patients about exercise.

Two studies have investigated the efficacy of exercise counseling by physicians. Both used the stages of change model described above. One study, the Physician-based Assessment and Counseling for Exercise (PACE),[67] gave patients a brief questionnaire in the waiting room to assess their readiness for change: precontemplation, not intending to exercise; contemplation, willing to consider becoming more active; and active, already exercising. Physicians were given a manual describing the intervention and spent about 5 min describing it to the patients. There was also a 10-min follow-up call from a health educator. This simple intervention resulted in an approximate doubling in the number of minutes of walking per week in the intervention group (an average increase of 37 min) without any significant change in the controls. However, the participants in this study were followed for only 6 weeks. A second trial, Physically Active for Life (PAL),[68] used a similar design and demonstrated a marginally significant positive effect at 6 weeks, but the effect disappeared when assessed at 8 months. One reason for the more disappointing results in PAL might have been that the participants were older (average age, 65).

Whereas it is often recommended that exercise should occur in bouts of 30 min or so, there is evidence that shorter bouts can be equally effective in improving cardiovascular fitness. One study[69] compared the effects of a single 30-min bout, three 10-min bouts, and bouts of 5 min or more totaling 30 min and found that all three produced roughly the same degree of improvement in blood pressure and body fat.

As with any form of behavioral intervention, a number of methods help improve adherence to exercise regimens. The first is to educate and motivate patients about the benefits of exercise (moving them from precontemplation to contemplation). The second is to set reasonable goals that can be increased gradually over time. It may be helpful for the patient and the interventionist to agree on a "behavioral contract" with a date set for achieving a particular goal. Self-monitoring is also helpful (keeping a log of daily activities, for example), and feedback and reinforcement should be provided regularly to the participant. It is also important to identify barriers that may hinder progress and find ways to overcome them. For example, if a patient has no easy means of getting to a gym, a home exercise program can be recommended.

PSYCHOSOCIAL RISK FACTORS

Stress, depression, anger and hostility, the type A behavior pattern, and anxiety have been proposed as possible cardiovascular disease risk factors. Unfortunately, the supporting or contradictory evidence for each construct is often considered interchangeable in the evaluation of its role in the development and manifestation of cardiovascular disease. Each construct, however, is theoretically and operationally distinct from the others, and the empirical support for each one as a cardiovascular disease risk factor varies. Further, recent technology and animal experiments suggest that some of these psychosocial factors contribute to the pathogenesis of cardiovascular disease whereas others do not.[70]

Stress

Stress is listed as one of the major factors causing heart disease when patients and lay persons are asked and is listed more frequently than high blood pressure and high lipids by those persons.[71] However, the investigation of stress as a cardiovascular disease risk factor has been vexed by definitional difficulties. Stress to the layperson typically encompasses, among other issues, work and family stress, social isolation, and the occurrence of recent acute and chronic life events. Work stress, which is defined as having low control over the way in which work is done but high work demands, has been implicated as a reliable and consistent predictor of the progression of hypertension,[72] carotid atherosclerosis,[73] and cardiac events and death.[74–76] Other theorists have argued that work stress is better assessed as low job control, and this index of work stress also has been found to predict future cardiac events.[77] Family stress rarely has been studied in regard to its relation to cardiovascular disease recurrence and mortality. However, it has been hypothesized that women with dual roles—both family and work stress—would have increased cardiovascular disease incidence, but in fact these women seem to have lower cardiovascular disease risk.[78]

Social isolation (few friends, family members, or close others) and perceived lack of social support consistently have been found to predict acute MI and cardiac death. As has been noted by Rozanski and colleagues,[70] the relative risks in the most recent 15 studies indicate a threefold mortality risk for cardiovascular disease patients who are socially isolated and/or perceive poor social support.

Acute mental stress such as the sudden loss of a loved one or an earthquake consistently has been shown to provoke silent myocardial ischemia and predict increased cardiovascular disease incidence and death in epidemiologic studies.[79]

Depression

Depressive symptoms and depressive disorders predict cardiac recurrence and mortality with a relative risk ranging from 2.6 to 7.8 in cardiac patients.[80–83] These risk ratios remain when all other known predictors of MI recurrence are controlled for, and depressive symptoms predict MI recurrence in a gradient fashion. Thus, there is considerable evidence that a cardiac patient who is depressed is at substantially higher risk for a future event. As is reviewed in Chap. 79, many studies have examined the mechanisms that may underlie this relationship as well as some interventions that may reduce this excess risk.

Anxiety

There have been fewer investigations of the relation of anxiety to cardiac disease and recurrence.[81,82,84,85] Most studies of anxiety disorders have examined the increased occurrence of cardiovascular disease mortality in psychiatric patients known to have some type of anxiety disorder,[86–88] although some small studies have found a relation between anxiety and sudden cardiac death in cardiovascular disease patients.[70] However, anxiety symptoms were not associated with MI recurrence in these studies. Rozanski and associates, among others,[70,89,90] have hypothesized that anxiety disorders and the associated symptoms may cause an alteration in cardiac autonomic tone through impaired vagal control, reduced heart rate variability, or both to cause an increased risk of sudden cardiac death in cardiac patients. A further discussion of the role of anxiety and related disorders can be found in Chap. 79.

Type A Behavior Pattern

Friedman and Rosenman[91] first proposed that a constellation of competitive, hostile, time-pressured behaviors constitutes a personality trait ("type A") that predisposes patients to cardiovascular disease. Although the Western Collaborative Group study found a twofold risk for cardiovascular disease and a fivefold MI recurrence risk in those in the type A-B categorization, several later studies failed to find that difference.[92] Many theorists have suggested that hostility, or the tendency to view others with suspicion and skepticism, may be the toxic component of the type A behavioral pattern and that this component should be evaluated independently for its prediction of increased risk in cardiac patients. Four small studies of cardiovascular disease patients found that the presence of a high level of hostility is associated with more rapid progression of atherosclerosis, more ischemia, a faster rate of restenosis after angioplasty, and a higher probability of recurrent MI.[6,93–96]

Psychosocial Interventions

In light of the emphasis cardiovascular disease patients place on stress and psychosocial factors as contributors to their disease and some of the recent evidence suggesting that psychosocial factors predict cardiovascular disease recurrence and death, offering psychosocial interventions for cardiovascular disease patients seems reasonable. However, there are many different types of interventions that are aimed at different psychosocial factors and different outcomes.

Linden and associates[97] conducted a meta-analysis of 23 controlled psychosocial intervention studies. All the patients were receiving standard medical and surgical care, and most additionally were receiving standard cardiac rehabilitation interventions. For follow-up periods of less than 2 years, there was a 41 percent reduction in mortality and a 46 percent reduction in MI recurrence as a result of psychosocial interventions. There were also significant and clinically meaningful reductions in measures of psychosocial distress such as depression and anxiety and in cardiovascular risk factors such as blood pressure and lipid levels. Only three randomized trials reported results for more than 2 years of follow-up, and in none of them did the effects of psychosocial intervention on mortality or MI recurrence remain significant.

Two large studies of psychosocial interventions merit special comment. In 1989, Frasure-Smith and coinvestigators reported favorable survival results for post-MI patients (n = 229) who received a home- and telephone-based stress-monitoring nursing intervention. As a result of this outcome, a larger randomized trial of a similar intervention was conducted (n = 1376). In this trial, there was no overall survival impact of the program, and in elderly women, there was increased cardiac and all-cause mortality.[98] In the second study, Jones and West[99] conducted a randomized controlled psychological intervention trial in 2328 post-MI patients and also found no difference in cardiac event recurrence and mortality at 12 months of follow-up. Two important features of these studies may explain their negative results. First, neither one actually achieved the objective of significantly reducing stress when this is operationalized as decreased scores on standardized depression and anxiety scales. Second, neither study screened patients to determine whether they in fact exhibited any symptoms of stress or of the psychological factor that was targeted by the intervention. Frasure-Smith[100] conducted a reanalysis of her original nursing intervention and reported that only patients who reported distress during hospitalization benefited from the psychosocial intervention; this is consistent with the author's speculation that those not at risk for psychosocial difficulties will not benefit from a psychosocial intervention. However, firm conclusions about the efficacy of psychosocial interventions in cardiac patients awaits larger randomized trials that target those at risk. A trial of this sort has recently been funded by NIH, to examine the efficacy of cognitive-behavioral interventions on cardiac, psychosocial, and cardiovascular disease risk factor outcomes in lonely and/or depressed post-MI patients.

Clinical Implications

Because of the dearth of large, randomly assigned psychosocial interventions, there is not yet sufficient evidence to recommend or caution against psychosocial interventions for altering cardiac outcomes in patients with CHD. There is, however, ample evidence that improvement in psychosocial functioning can be obtained through the use of standardized, empirically supported therapy protocols administered by mental health professionals to patients who are at psychosocial risk. Improving the quality of life and decreasing the psychological distress of cardiac patients also may have other benefits. First, many of the mechanisms proposed to account for the association between psychosocial factors and cardiovascular disease are behavioral. Thus, decreasing depressive symptoms is hypothesized to decrease smoking rates, increase engagement in physical activity, and improve dietary habits.[101] Second, decreasing psychosocial distress is thought to increase patient compliance with physicians' recommendations, but testing these behavioral mechanisms, as well as the pathophysiologic mechanisms addressed elsewhere, awaits larger, controlled trials.

Cardiologists should be aware of psychosocial risk factors present in their patients. Asking about social support and recent symptoms of depression will identify patients at increased risk of event recurrence or death. Referring such patients to mental health specialists for further diagnostic and intervention investigations may improve patients' quality of life and their behavioral risk factor profile, if not their cardiac outcome.

Cost Implications

Thorough cost-effectiveness and cost-offset analyses are being conducted in some of the recent psychosocial trials. For example, the average cost of adding a behavioral intervention to the treatment of a cardiac patient in one study was $790.[102] The longest and most comprehensive psychosocial intervention (for reducing type A behavior), the Recurrent Coronary Care Project in California, showed MI recurrence decreases for the intervention patients, but treatment required an average of 58 hours per patient. This amount of therapy, when delivered in a group format, as occurred in this trial, would cost on average $1200 per patient.

COMPLIANCE: THE KEY TO SUCCESSFUL INTERVENTIONS

The evidence for the intervention strategies reviewed in this chapter points to the inescapable conclusion that changing lifestyle habits can significantly reduce the risk for cardiovascular disease. No matter how efficacious the intervention strategy is, however, it is doomed to failure unless the patient complies with the requirements of the intervention. Nonadherence crosses treatment regimens, age and gender groups, and socioeconomic strata and, moreover, varies across the treatment course.[1,2] Thus, persons are asked to change their diets, eat less, exercise more, quit smoking, reduce the amount of stress they experience, and change the ways in which they express anger. These changes are difficult. Knowledge of the risks is clearly insufficient to produce changes; most persons know by now that smoking is bad for them, that their diet could be improved, and so on. These behaviors, however, are reinforcing in their own right. Smoking is pleasurable, as is the avoidance of nicotine withdrawal; high-fat foods taste good; and exercise is time-consuming and may be boring and even painful for many persons. Coping with stress and anger means having to examine one's life in ways that may be unpleasant and even traumatic. Thus, poor health habits that may have been reinforced over the course of a lifetime are very resistant to change. Clearly, it is vitally important to begin establishing healthy behavior habits early in life; however, parents and teachers may provide poor models for these behaviors, having been enculturated in a time during which such concerns were virtually nonexistent.

Much of the adherence problem occurs early in treatment. It has been estimated that 50 percent of persons discontinue participation in cardiac rehabilitation programs within the first year.[3] The smoking cessation literature reports a 79 percent relapse rate in the first 6 months.[4] Not only are early adherence problems likely, early adherence rates are predictive of longer-term adherence.[5–7]

The primary care physician and the cardiologist can play a major role in helping persons alter poor health habits and establish healthy behaviors. A physician is regarded by many patients as a source of authority and can have a large impact on behavior change.[103] In addition, a physician can refer patients to other health professionals, such as nutrition and exercise counselors and stress- and anger-reduction therapists. This often does not occur, however, for a number of reasons. First, while most physicians are undoubtedly aware of the importance of healthy behaviors, they may be convinced that patients will not engage in them or may not know how to suggest such changes or to whom to refer these patients. Second, given the current reimbursement climate, many physicians have only a very few minutes to spend with each patient.

The fact is that a great deal is now known about how to maximize the likelihood that patients will adhere to health behavior regimens. One review provides a great amount of detail concerning these regimens[104]; a brief summary is provided below that briefly describes strategies that have been demonstrated to be successful in improving compliance to cardiovascular disease behavioral intervention strategies.

- Signed agreements. A written contract is drawn up between the patient and the physician or other health professional in which a specific set of behaviors to be followed by the patient is agreed on. These behaviors should be as specific as possible (e.g., number of calories per day, number of servings of fruits and vegetables per day, number of minutes of cardiovascular-strengthening exercise, number of hours of stress-reduction therapy). Behavioral logs should be maintained by the patient.
- Behavioral skill training. Patients can attend classes that teach healthy cooking, proper stretching techniques before and after exercise, and how to respond to an anger-provoking situation. Patients may want to engage in healthy behaviors, but without the skills, they tend to fall back on old behaviors.
- Self-monitoring. Many patients are truly unaware of the extent to which they engage in certain unhealthy behaviors. It is useful to have them monitor the number of cigarettes they smoke, their daily intake of fat (current packaging requirements make this relatively easy), and so on. The first step in changing behavior is to establish a baseline so that the patient can see improvement.
- Self-efficacy enhancement. Patients' confidence in their ability to engage in a particular behavior, such as eating in more healthy ways or exercising with a specified frequency, has been shown to be an important factor in their motivation to engage in these behaviors. Self-monitoring (discussed above) provides a baseline level and can document improvement. Even small changes will increase a patient's self-efficacy for a given behavior, so that he or she is motivated to continue. This will produce additional positive change, which then enhances self-efficacy even more, and so on. The physician or other health professional can focus on such improvement as a means of further enhancing the patient's self-efficacy for behavior change.
- Telephone and/or mail contact. Such reminders have been shown to have a positive effect on compliance.
- Spouse and/or social support. A great deal of research has shown that others in the patient's social environment can have a dramatic impact on compliance. When a physician discusses behavior change with the patient, it is helpful for such a support person to be present as well. If an exercise and/or diet regimen is agreed on, possibly using a contract, as was described above, having a support person participate will significantly enhance the likelihood that the patient will

stay with the program. Having an immediate other, such as a spouse, continue in her or his own unhealthy behavior patterns, conversely, such as continuing to smoke or to express anger in an abusive or unhealthy manner, will hinder the possibility for change on the part of the patient.

- Stages of change. Earlier in this chapter, it was noted that different persons may be in different stages of readiness to change behavior.[16] Thus, one patient may be ready only to begin discussing the need to stop smoking, while another may be ready to begin the actual quitting. Research shows that it is helpful to tailor advice to the patient's current stage of readiness. The techniques described above are clearly additive; more than one may be combined usefully to help the patient comply. It is also clear that in trying, many patients will fail. However, it is worth noting that a patient cannot quit smoking until she or he first *tries* to quit, and so efforts to produce this behavior are a good investment of the physician's time.
- The authors strongly recommend that primary care physicians develop a network of health care professionals who can support their efforts and to whom patients can be referred for help with specific intervention strategies.
- Physicians are a long way from eliminating the need for medication and surgical intervention for cardiovascular disease. However, the situation is better than it was only a relatively short time ago. If physicians advocate such strategies, prescribe them, discuss them with patients, and refer patients to other health professionals, a substantial proportion of the need for more traditional interventions can be eliminated.

CONCLUSIONS

The potential applications of behavioral techniques in cardiology are enormous and largely unrealized. In principle, they can help prevent the onset of disease, treat it once it is established, and be used in conjunction with virtually any other kind of treatment. In practice, few cardiologists have the time or interest to pay much attention to them despite the demonstrated efficacy of many programs. Future success depends on better education of physicians, the incorporation of a team approach, and recognition of the value of behavioral interventions by third-party payers.

References

1. McGinnis JM, Foege WH. Actual causes of death in the United States. *JAMA* 1993; 270:2207.
2. Fries JF, Koop CE, Beadle CE, et al. Reducing health care costs by reducing the need and demand for medical services: The Health Project Consortium. *N Engl J Med* 1993; 329:321.
3. Notzon FC, Komarov YM, Ermakov SP, et al. Causes of declining life expectancy in Russia. *JAMA* 1998; 279:793.
4. Hakim AA, Petrovitch H, Burchfiel CM, et al. Effects of walking on mortality among nonsmoking retired men. *N Engl J Med* 1998; 338:94.
5. Lipkus IM, Barefoot JC, Williams RB, et al. Personality measures as predictors of smoking initiation and cessation in the UNC Alumni Heart Study. *Health Psychol* 1994; 13:149.
6. De Leon CFM, Kop WJ, de Swart HB, et al. Psychosocial characteristics and recurrent events after percutaneous transluminal coronary angioplasty. *Am J Cardiol* 1996; 77:252.
7. Glanz K. Nutrition education for risk factor reduction and patient education: A review. *Prev Med* 1999; 14:721.
8. De Lorgeril M, Renaud S, Mamelle N, et al. Mediterranean alpha-linolenic acid-rich diet in secondary prevention of coronary heart disease. *Lancet* 1994; 343:1454.
9. Randomized trial of cholesterol lowering in 4,444 patients with coronary heart disease: Scandinavian Simvastatin Survival Study (4S). *Lancet* 1994; 344:1383.
10. Walden CE, Retzlaff BM, Buck BL, et al. Lipoprotein lipid response to the National Cholesterol Education Program Step II diet by hypercholesterolic and combined hyperlipidemic women and men. *Arterioscler Thromb Vasc Biol* 1997; 17:375.
11. Buefel RR. Assessment of the U.S diet in national nutrition surveys: National collaborative efforts and NHANES. *Am J Clin Nutr* 1994; 59(suppl):1645.
12. Glanz K, Eriksen MP. Individual and community models for dietary behavior change. *J Nutr Educ* 1993; 25:80.
13. Bandura A. *Social Foundations of Thought and Action: A Social Cognitive Theory*. Englewood Cliffs, NJ: Prentice-Hall; 1986.
14. Bandura A. *Self-Efficacy: The Exercise of Control*. New York: Freeman; 1997.
15. Prochaska JO, DiClemente CC. Transtheoretical therapy: Toward a more integrative model of change. *Psycho Ther Res Pract* 1982; 19:276.
16. Prochaska JO, DiClemente CC, Norcross JC. In search of how people change: Applications to addictive behaviors. *Am Psychol* 1992; 47:1102.
17. The sixth report of the Joint National Committee on prevention, detection, evaluation, and treatment of high blood pressure. *Arch Intern Med* 1997; 157:2413.
18. Fiore MC, Jorenby DE, Baker TB. Smoking cessation: Principles and practice based upon the AHCPR Guideline, 1996: Agency for Health Care Policy and Research. *Ann Behav Med* 1997; 19:213.
19. Weintraub WS, Klein LW, Seelaus PA, et al. Importance of total life consumption of cigarettes as a risk factor for coronary artery disease. *Am J Cardiol* 1985; 55:669.
20. Rosenberg L, Kaufman DW, Helmrich SP, et al. The risk of myocardial infarction after quitting smoking in men under 55 years of age. *N Engl J Med* 1985; 313:1511.
21. Gordon T, Kannel WB, McGee D, et al. Death and coronary attacks in men after giving up cigarette smoking: A report from the Framingham study. *Lancet* 1974; 2:1345.
22. Warner KE. Smoking out the incentives for tobacco control in managed care settings. *Tob Control* 1998; 7(suppl):S50.
23. Tomar SL, Husten CG, Manley MW. Do dentists and physicians advise tobacco users to quit? *J Am Dent Assoc* 1996; 127:259.
24. Anda RF, Remington PL, Sienko DG, et al. Are physicians advising smokers to quit? The patient's perspective. *JAMA* 1987; 257:1916.
25. Prochaska JO, Di Clemente CC, Velicer WF, et al. Standardized, individualized, interactive, and personalized self-help programs for smoking cessation. *Health Psychol* 1993; 12:399.
26. Silagy C, Mant D, Fowler G, et al. Meta-analysis on efficacy of nicotine replacement therapies in smoking cessation. *Lancet* 1994; 343:139.
27. Jorenby DE, Leischow SJ, Nides MA, et al. A controlled trial of sustained-release bupropion, a nicotine patch, or both for smoking cessation. *N Engl J Med* 1999; 340:685.
28. Hughes JR, Goldstein MG, Hurt RD, et al. Recent advances in the pharmacotherapy of smoking. *JAMA* 1999; 281:72.
29. Hayford KE, Patten CA, Rummans TA, et al. Efficacy of bupropion for smoking cessation in smokers with a former history of major depression or alcoholism. *Br J Psychiatry* 1999; 174:173.
30. McPhillips-Tangum C. Results from the first annual survey on addressing tobacco in managed care. *Tob Control* 1998; 7(suppl): S11.
31. Keys A. *Seven Countries: A Multivariate Analysis of Death and*

Coronary Heart Disease. Cambridge, MA: Harvard University Press; 1980.
32. Levine G, Keaney J, Vita J. Cholesterol reduction in cardiovascular disease. *N Engl J Med* 1995; 332:512.
33. Lipid Research Clinics Program. The Lipid Research Clinics Coronary Primary Prevention Trial results: I. Reduction in incidence of coronary heart disease. *JAMA* 1984; 251:351.
34. Van Horn L, Kavey RE. Diet and cardiovascular disease prevention: What works? *Ann Behav Med* 1997; 19:197–212.
35. Greenland P, Hayman L. Making cardiovascular disease prevention a reality. *Ann Behav Med* 1997; 19:193.
36. National Cholesterol Education Program: *Report of the Expert Panel on Population Strategies for Blood Cholesterol Reduction*. DHHS Publication No. (NIH) 90-30-46. Bethesda, MD: U.S. Department of Health and Human Services, Public Health Service, National Institutes of Health, National Heart, Lung and Blood Institute; 1990.
37. Holme I. An analysis of randomized trials evaluating the effect of cholesterol reduction on total mortality and coronary heart disease incidence. *Circulation* 1990; 82:1916.
38. Renaud S, de Lorgeril M, Delaye J, et al. Cretan Mediterranean diet for prevention of coronary heart disease. *Am J Clin Nutr* 1995; 61(suppl):1360S.
39. *Nationwide Food Consumption Survey, Continuing Survey of Food Intake by Individuals: Women 19–50 Years and Children 1–5 Years, 4 Days*. Washington, DC: U.S. Department of Agriculture, Human Nutrition Information Service; 1996.
40. Expert Panel on Detection Evaluation and Treatment of High Blood Cholesterol in Adults. Summary of the Second Report of the National Cholesterol Education Program (NCEP) Expert Panel on Detection, Evaluation, and Treatment of High Blood Cholesterol in Adults (Adult Treatment Panel II). *JAMA* 1993; 269:3015.
41. LaRosa JC, Hunninghake D, Bush D, et al. The cholesterol facts: A summary of the evidence relating dietary facts, serum cholesterol, and coronary heart disease: A joint statement by the American Heart Association and the National Heart, Lung, and Blood Institute. *Circulation* 1990; 81:1721.
42. Sempos C, Cleeman J, Carroll M, et al. Prevalence of high blood cholesterol among U.S. adults. *JAMA* 1993; 269:3009.
43. Schucker B, Wittes JT, Santanello NC, et al. Change in cholesterol awareness and action: Results from national physician and public surveys. *Arch Intern Med* 1991; 151:666.
44. Stone NJ. Diet, blood cholesterol levels, and coronary heart disease. *Coron Artery Dis* 1993; 4:871.
45. Princen HM, Van Poppel G, Vogelezang C, et al. Supplementation with vitamin E but not beta-carotene in vivo protects low density lipoprotein from lipid peroxidation in vitro: Effect of cigarette smoking. *Arterioscler Thromb* 1992; 12:554.
46. Stamler MJ, Hennekens CH, Manson JE, et al. Vitamin E consumption and the risk of coronary disease in women. *N Engl J Med* 1993; 328:1444.
47. Steinberg D, Parthasarathy S, Carew TE, et al. Beyond cholesterol: Modifications of low-density lipoprotein that increase its atherogenicity. *N Engl J Med* 1989; 320:915.
48. Hoffman RM, Garewal IIS. Antioxidants and the prevention of coronary heart disease. *Arch Intern Med* 1995; 155:241.
49. Boushey CJ, Beresford SAA, Omenn GS, et al. A quantitative assessment of plasma homocysteine as a risk factor for vascular disease: Probable benefits of increasing folic acid intakes. *JAMA* 1995; 274:1049.
50. Hubert HB, Feinleib M, McNamara PM, et al. Obesity as an independent risk factor for cardiovascular disease: A 26-year follow-up of participants in the Framingham Heart Study. *Circulation* 1983; 67:968.
51. Denke MA, Sempos CT, Grundy SM. Excess body weight: An underrecognized contributor to high blood cholesterol levels. *Arch Intern Med* 1993; 153:1093.
52. Medalie JH, Papier CM, Goldbourt U, et al. Major factors in the development of diabetes mellitus in 10,000 men. *Arch Intern Med* 1975; 135:811.
53. Tobian L. Hypertension and obesity. *N Engl J Med* 1978; 298:46.
54. McCarron D. Calcium metabolism in hypertension. *Keio J Med* 1995; 44:105.
55. Health implications of obesity: National Institutes of Health Consensus Development Conference Statement. *Ann Inter Med* 1985; 103:1073.
56. Wood PD, Stefanick ML, Williams PT, et al. The effects on plasma lipoprotein of a prudent weight-reducing diet, with or without exercise, in overweight men and women. *N Engl J Med* 1988; 319:1173.
57. Becque MD, Katch VL, Rocchini AP, et al. Coronary risk incidence of obese adolescents: Reduction by exercise plus diet intervention. *Pediatrics* 1988; 81:605.
58. O'Leary KD, Wilson GT. *Behavior Therapy: Application and Outcome*. Englewood Cliffs, NJ: Prentice-Hall; 1975.
59. Brownell KD, Heckerman C, Westlake R. The behavior control: A descriptive analysis of a large scale program. *J Clin Psychol* 1979; 35:864.
60. Garner D, Wooley S. Confronting the failure of behavior and dietary treatments for obesity. *Clin Psychol Rev* 1991; 11:729.
61. Barnard N, Akhtar A, Nicholson A. Factors that facilitate compliance to lower fat intake. *Arch Fam Med* 1995; 4:153.
62. Tinker L, Burrows E, Henry H, et al. The Women's Health Initiative: Overview of the nutrition components. In: Krummel D, Kris-Etherton P, eds. *Nutrition in Women's Health*. Garthersberg, MD: Aspen; 1996:510.
63. Dolecek TA, Milas NC, Van Horn LV, et al. A long-term nutrition intervention experience: Lipid responses and dietary adherence patterns in the Multiple Risk Factor Intervention Trial (MRFIT). *J Am Diet Assoc* 1986; 86:752.
64. U.S. Department of Health and Human Services. *Healthy People 2000: National Health Promotion and Disease Prevention Objectives*. DHHS Publication No. (PHS) 91-50212. Washington, DC: U.S. Department of Health and Human Services; 1990.
65. Wells KB, Lewis CE, Leake B, et al. The practices of general and subspecialty internists in counseling about smoking and exercise. *Am J Public Health* 1986; 76:1009.
66. Orleans CT, George LK, Houpt JL, et al. Health promotion in primary care: A survey of U.S. family practitioners. *Prev Med* 1985; 14:636.
67. Calfas KJ, Long BJ, Sallis JF, et al. A controlled trial of physician counseling to promote the adoption of physical activity. *Prev Med* 1996; 25:225.
68. Goldstein MG, Pinto BM, Lynn H, et al. Physician-based physical activity counseling for middle-aged and older adults: A randomized trial. *Ann Behav Med* 1999; 21:40.
69. Coleman KJ, Raynor HR, Mueller DM, et al. Providing sedentary adults with choices for meeting their walking goals. *Prev Med* 1999; 28:510.
70. Rozanski A, Blumenthal JA, Kaplan J. Impact of psychological factors on the pathogenesis of cardiovascular disease and implications for therapy. *Circulation* 1999; 99:2192.
71. Kirkland SA, MacLean DR, Langille DB, et al. Knowledge and awareness of risk factors for cardiovascular disease among Canadians 55 to 74 years of age: Results from the Canadian Heart Health Surveys, 1986–1992. *Can Med Assoc J* 1999; 161(suppl 8):S10.
72. Schnall PL, Schwartz JE, Landsbergis PA, et al. A longitudinal study of job strain and ambulatory blood pressure: Results from a three year follow up. *Psychosom Med* 1999; 60:697.
73. Lynch J, Krause N, Kaplan GA, et al. Work place demands,

economic reward, and progression of carotid atherosclerosis. *Circulation* 1997; 96:302.

74. Karasek RA, Baker D, Marxer F, et al. Job decision latitude, job demands, and cardiovascular disease: A prospective study of Swedish men. *Am J Public Health* 1981; 75:694.
75. Karasek RA, Theorell T, Schwartz JE, et al. Job characteristics in relation to the prevalence of myocardial infarction in the U.S. Health Examination Survey (HESS) and the Health and Nutrition Examination Survey (HAINES). *Am J Public Health* 1988; 78:910.
76. Theorell T, Tsutsumi A, Hallqist J, et al. Decision latitude, job strain, and myocardial infarction: A study of working men in Stockholm. *Am J Public Health* 1998; 88:382.
77. Johnson JV, Stewart W, Hall EM, et al. Long-term psychosocial work environment and cardiovascular mortality among Swedish men. *Am J Public Health* 1996; 86:324.
78. Gove WR. Gender differences in mental and physical illness: The effects of fixed roles and nurturant roles. *Soc Sci Med* 1984; 19(2):77.
79. Gabbay FH, Krantz DS, Kop WJ, et al. Triggers of myocardial ischemia during daily life in patients with coronary artery disease: Physical and mental activities, anger and smoking. *J Am Coll Cardiol* 1996; 27:585.
80. Frasure-Smith N, Lesperance F, Juneau M, et al. Gender, depression, and one-year prognosis after myocardial infarction. *Psychosom Med* 1999; 61:26.
81. Denollet J, Brutsaert DL. Personality, disease severity, and the risk of long-term cardiac events in patients with a decreased ejection fraction after myocardial infarction. *Circulation* 1998; 97:167.
82. Hermann C, Brand-Driehorst S, Kaminsky B, et al. Diagnosis groups and depressed mood as predictors of 22-month mortality in medical patients. *Psychosom Med* 1998; 60:570.
83. Frasure-Smith N, Lesperance F, Talajic M. Depression and 18-month prognosis after myocardial infarction. *Circulation* 1995; 91:999.
84. Frasure-Smith N, Lesperance F, Talajic M. The impact of negative emotions on prognosis following myocardial infarction: Is it more than depression? *Health Psychol* 1995; 14:388.
85. Moser DK, Dracup K. Is anxiety early after myocardial infarction associated with subsequent ischemic and arrhythmic events? *Psychosom Med* 1996; 58:395.
86. Haines AP, Imeson JD, Meade TW. Phobic anxiety and ischemic heart disease. *Br Med J* 1987; 295:297.
87. Kawachi I, Colditz GA, Ascherio A, et al. Prospective study of phobic anxiety and risk of coronary heart disease in men. *Circulation* 1994; 89:1992.
88. Kawachi I, Sparrow D, Vokonas PS, et al. Symptoms of anxiety and risk of coronary heart disease: The Normative Aging Study. *Circulation* 1994; 90:2225.
89. Kawachi I, Sparrow D, Vokonas PS, et al. Decreased heart rate variability in men with phobic anxiety (data from the Normative Aging Study). *Am J Cardiol* 1995; 75:882.
90. Watkins LL, Grossman P, Krishnan R, et al. Anxiety and vagal control of heart risk. *Psychosom Med* 1998; 60:498.
91. Friedman M, Rosenman RH. Association of specific overt behavior pattern with blood and cardiovascular findings: Blood cholesterol level, blood clotting time, incidence of arcus senilis, and clinical coronary artery disease. *JAMA* 1959; 169:1286.
92. Miller TQ, Turner CW, Tindale RS, et al. Reasons for the trend toward null findings in research on Type A behavior. *Psychol Bull* 1991; 110:469.
93. Koskenvuo M, Kaprio J, Rose RJ, et al. Hostility as a risk factor for mortality and ischemic heart disease in men. *Psychosom Med* 1988; 50:330.
94. Hecker MHL, Chesney MA, Blacks GW, et al. Coronary-prone behaviors in the Western Collaborative Group Study. *Psychosom Med* 1988; 50:153.
95. Dembroski TM, MacDougall JM, Costa PT, et al. Components of hostility as predictors of sudden death and myocardial infarction in the Multiple Risk Factor Intervention Trial. *Psychosom Med* 1989; 51:514.
96. Lau J, Antman EM, Jimenez-Silva J, et al. Cumulative meta-analysis of therapeutic trials for myocardial infarction. *N Engl J Med* 1992; 327:248.
97. Linden W, Stossel C, Maurice J. Psychosocial interventions for patients with coronary artery disease: A meta-analysis. *Arch Intern Med* 1996; 156:745.
98. Frasure-Smith N, Lesperance F, Prince RH, et al. Randomized trial of home-based psychosocial nursing intervention for patients recovering from myocardial infarction. *Lancet* 1997; 350:473.
99. Jones DA, West RR. Psychological rehabilitation after myocardial infarction: Multicentre randomized controlled trial. *Br Med J* 1996; 313:1517.
100. Frasure-Smith N. In-hospital symptoms of psychological stress as predictors of long-term outcome after acute myocardial infarction in men. *Am J Cardiol* 1991; 67:121.
101. Davidson K, Jonas B, Dixon K, et al. Do depression symptoms predict early hypertension incidence in young adults from the CARDIA study? *Arch Intern Med* 2000; 160:1495.
102. Oldridge N, Furlong W, Feeny D, et al. Economic evaluation of cardiac rehabilitation soon after acute myocardial infarction. *Am J Cardiol* 1993; 72:154.
103. Caggiula A, Watson J, Kuller L, et al. Cholesterol-lowering intervention program: Effect of the Step I diet in community office practices. *Arch Intern Med* 1996; 156:1205.
104. Ammerman A, Caggiula A, Elmer PJ, et al. Putting medical practice guidelines into practice: The cholesterol model. *Am J Prev Med* 1994; 10:209.

INDEX

NOTE: Boldface numbers indicate the start of the main discussion of the topic; numbers followed by an *f* or a *t* refer to figures and tables, respectively.

C

D

F

H

J

K

M

O

Q

R

U

ISBN 0-07-135693-2

90000

9 780071 356930

FUSTER/HURST'S THE HEART
SET

ISBN 0-07-135696-7

90000

9 780071 356961

FUSTER/HURST'S THE HEART
VOL. 2

Part 7

SYSTEMIC ARTERIAL HYPERTENSION

Part 8

PULMONARY HYPERTENSION AND PULMONARY DISEASE

Part 9

VALVULAR HEART DISEASE

Part 10

CONGENITAL HEART DISEASE

Part 11

CARDIOMYOPATHY AND SPECIFIC HEART MUSCLE DISEASES

Part 12

PERICARDIAL DISEASES AND ENDOCARDITIS